Neurology
of the Newborn

Joseph J. Volpe

Bronson Crothers Distinguished Professor of Neurology
Harvard Medical School
Neurologist-in-Chief Emeritus
Children's Hospital
Boston, Massachusetts

Neurology
of the Newborn

FIFTH EDITION

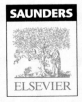

SAUNDERS

ELSEVIER

SAUNDERS
ELSEVIER

1600 John F. Kennedy Boulevard
Suite 1800
Philadelphia, PA 19103-2899

NEUROLOGY OF THE NEWBORN, FIFTH EDITION   ISBN: 978-1-4160-3995-2
Copyright © 2008, 2001 by Saunders, an imprint of Elsevier Inc.

Notice

Knowledge and best practice in this field are constantly changing. As new research and
experience broaden our knowledge, changes in practice, treatment, and drug therapy may
become necessary or appropriate. Readers are advised to check the most current information
provided (i) on procedures featured or (ii) by the manufacturer of each product to be
administered, to verify the recommended dose or formula, the method and duration of
administration, and contraindications. It is the responsibility of practitioners, relying on their
own experience and knowledge of the patient, to make diagnoses, to determine dosages and
the best treatment for each individual patient, and to take all appropriate safety precautions. To
the fullest extent of the law, neither the Publisher nor the Author assumes any liability for any
injury and/or damage to persons or property arising out of or related to any use of the material
contained in this book.

The Publisher

Library of Congress Cataloging-in-Publication Data

Volpe, Joseph J.
    Neurology of the newborn/Joseph J. Volpe. – 5th ed.
        p.; cm.
    Includes bibliographical references and index.
    ISBN 978-1-4160-3995-2
    1. Newborn infants–Diseases. 2. Pediatric neurology. I. Title.
    [DNLM: 1. Nervous System Diseases. 2. Infant, Newborn, Diseases. 3. Infant, Newborn.
WS 340 V899n 2008]

RJ290.V64 2008
618.92'01–dc22

2007044207

Acquisitions Editor: Judy Fletcher
Publishing Services Manager: Frank Polizzano
Project Manager: Lee Ann Draud
Design Direction: Ellen Zanolle
Cover design: Ellen Zanolle

Printed in the United States of America

Last digit is the print number: 9 8 7 6 5 4 3 2 1

To my wife,
Sara,
for her love and understanding,
without which this book would not be possible

Preface to the Fifth Edition

The nearly 30 years since publication of the first edition of this book have been a period of extraordinary development in the discipline of the neurology of the newborn. In 1981, at the time of publication of the first edition, there was a sense of a new frontier to be pioneered. Currently articles on neonatal neurology are abundant in the major journals in pediatrics, child neurology, and related disciplines. Current-day annual meetings of scientific societies of pediatrics and child neurology are dominated by research and clinical presentations on the neurology of the newborn. Thus, the field now has matured fully into a discipline in its own right.

The fifth edition of this book has been completely updated and extensively revised. All of the changes have been incorporated into an organization that is identical to that of the previous editions. Thus, the four initial chapters establish the foundation of the remainder of the book. These four chapters deal with the development of the nervous system, the disorders caused by anomalous development, the clinical neurological examination, and the specialized techniques in the neurological evaluation. The fifth chapter, concerning neonatal seizures, serves as an effective bridge between the initial chapters and the later, disease-focused chapters, because neonatal seizure is a key manifestation of many of the neurological disorders dealt with later in the book. The next 19 chapters focus on the neurological disorders, with a strong clinical emphasis. However, as in the past, the lessons learned from basic and clinical research are brought to the bedside in the discussions of the diseases.

This book is intended for a broad audience, that is, from the most highly specialized neonatal physicians to those with a more general perspective. I have attempted to generate a systematic, readable, and comprehensive synthesis of the neurology of the newborn that will be of value to all individuals who care for the infant, both in the critical neonatal period and later. The clinical discussions are buttressed by information generated from the most recent diagnostic methodologies, by the results of promising new therapies, and by insights gained from basic research in such relevant disciplines as neuroscience, genetics, and developmental biology. Attempting to do all this has been stimulating and challenging, and I apologize if I have oversimplified in some areas and displayed my ignorance in others. After five editions I hope that these two problems are few.

Previous readers will recognize that I place great value on the liberal use of tables to synthesize major points throughout the book. This edition contains approximately 550 tables. Many of these are new, many replace earlier tables, and many of the original tables contain new information. As with tables, I value greatly the illustrative power of figures, in the form of flow diagrams, experimental findings, clinical and pathological specimens, and all types of brain imaging. This edition contains approximately 665 figures, many of which are new. Moreover, many of the original figures have been replaced with better examples of the relevant findings.

The extraordinary progress in the study of the neurology of the newborn is reflected in part by the explosion of new literature in the relevant disciplines. This edition contains approximately 12,500 references, nearly 3000 more than in the previous edition. The enormous increase in the relevant literature between the last and current edition is a tangible reflection of the intense interest in this extraordinarily important field. Every chapter contains many new citations as part of the updating of the entire book.

I have been extremely fortunate to have the help of many very talented and dedicated people in the preparation of this book. As she did for the previous two editions, Irene Miller performed the simply incredible task of typing and retyping the entire book: text, tables, legends, and references. She manipulated and renumbered the 12,500 references with aplomb; to this day, I don't understand how she did it so efficiently and without losing her mind. Janine Zieg prepared many new flow diagrams and schematics and updated many others with great skill and patience, particularly because I revised them incessantly. Sarah Andiman ably assisted in this endeavor. My young colleague, Dr. Omar Khwaja, spent many hours at the computer helping a computer-naïve author with illustrations; he contributed important images and helped restore the value of some originals. Finally, as in previous editions, I acknowledge the support and patience at Elsevier of Judy Fletcher, with whom I have worked for almost 20 years since the third edition and who supervised the overall project. Ellen Zanolle designed the fetching cover and successfully convinced a stodgy author that covers should be eye-catching. Lee Ann Draud superbly led the production efforts. Not only was her Elsevier group so tolerant of my obsessive pursuit of perfection, but they allowed me to add new references until the very end of 2007.

Joseph J. Volpe, MD

Preface to the First Edition

The neurology of the newborn is a topic of major importance because of the preeminence of neurological disorders in neonatology today. The advent of modern perinatal medicine, accompanied by striking improvements in obstetrical and neonatal care, has changed the spectrum of neonatal disease drastically. Many previously dreaded disorders such as respiratory disease have been controlled to a major degree. At the same time, certain beneficial results of improved care, for example, markedly decreased mortality rates for premature infants, have been accompanied by neurological disorders that would not have had time to evolve in past years.

This major importance of neonatal neurological disease has stimulated efforts by workers in many disciplines to recognize, understand, treat, and ultimately prevent such disease. This book is an attempt to bring together the knowledge gained from these efforts and to present my current understanding of the neurology of the newborn. Because of the diversity of knowledge that I have attempted to bring to bear upon the problems discussed in this book, I may have oversimplified in certain areas and displayed my own ignorance in others. Nevertheless, I have written the material in the hope that it will be of value to all health professionals involved in the care and follow-up of the newborn infant with neurological disease.

The prime focus of the discussions of neonatal neurological disease throughout this book is the clinical evaluation of the infant, that is, what we can learn from observation of the setting and mode of presentation of the disease and the disturbances of neurological function apparent on careful examination. The theme that recurs most often is that careful clinical assessment, in the traditional sense, is the prerequisite and the essential foundation for understanding the neurological disorders of the newborn. The infant does not advertise his or her neurological disorder with the drama that older children and adults exhibit, but with patience and diligence we can discover a treasure of important clinical clues when we elicit a complete history and perform a careful physical examination. It is this quality of discovery with simple techniques that has made the neurology of the newborn so stimulating for me, and I hope that this book can lead the reader to similar discoveries.

With accomplishment of the essential first step of definition of the clinical problem, we can turn in a rational way to the increasingly sophisticated means of studying the infant's deranged neural structure and function. Although my emphasis is, first, on the simplest and least invasive techniques for providing us with the necessary information, we are in an era when sophisticated and informative procedures such as imaging the brain itself can be done in a safe and effective way.

The final process in our understanding the infant with a neurological disorder requires an awareness of a burgeoning corpus of information derived from studies in human and experimental pathology, physiology, biochemistry, and related fields. Of necessity, often we must extrapolate to our newborn patient data obtained from animals. Such extrapolation must always be made cautiously, and yet we cannot ignore the many lessons learned from the laboratory that have proved invaluable in our understanding of neonatal neurological disease. In this book, on the one hand, I attempt to synthesize in a comprehensible manner relevant material from a diversity of disciplines and, on the other hand, try very hard not to oversimplify what are clearly very complex issues.

I believe that the neurology of the newborn has come of age and, indeed, should be viewed as a discipline in its own right. I hope that in some way this book will contribute to establishing that status. My most fervent hope is that this discipline excites the interests and efforts of others concerned with the neonatal patient and that, through concerted actions, the greatest possible benefits accrue to the infant with neurological disease.

Acknowledgments

It is with pleasure and eagerness that I acknowledge with gratitude the help of so many over the years. I am grateful to Dr. Raymond Adams, who introduced me to neurology and neuropathology and provided a model of scholarship in medicine that I have since striven to achieve; to Dr. C. Miller Fisher, who taught me the inestimable value of looking carefully at the patient and never denying observations that did not fit preconceived notions; and to Dr. E. P. Richardson, Jr., who taught me neuropathology and provided a framework for study on which I remain dependent.

I owe enormous gratitude to Dr. Philip Dodge, who stimulated me to study pediatric neurology and, after my training, guided me to the neurology of the newborn. To this day he has been a continual source of support and inspiration.

I gratefully acknowledge the help and contributions of many investigators with an interest in the newborn. Their work is included on many of the pages of this book, and although acknowledgment is made in those places, I take this particular opportunity to thank them again for their generosity. Many other physicians involved in the care of newborns have shared their unusual and interesting cases with me; I thank them for their stimulation and education. Many faculty, fellows, and house officers at St. Louis Children's Hospital and Boston Children's Hospital have helped me immeasurably in the study of neonatal patients. My collaborators in clinical and basic research, especially Drs. Hannah Kinney, Paul Rosenberg, Frances Jensen, and Timothy Vartanian, have been wonderful partners in our pursuit of discovery and creativity in the study of the newborn brain. Finally, my colleagues in neonatal neurology at Boston Children's Hospital, Drs. Adre du Plessis, Janet Soul, and Omar Khwaja, have been a constant source of stimulation. I am grateful for all of these contributions.

Joseph J. Volpe, MD

CONTENTS

HUMAN BRAIN DEVELOPMENT

Neural Tube Formation and Prosencephalic Development

An understanding of the development of the nervous system is essential for an understanding of neonatal neurology. An obvious reason for this contention is the wide variety of disturbances of neural development that are flagrantly apparent in the neonatal period. In addition, all the insults that affect the fetus and newborn, and that are the subject matter of most of this book, exert their characteristic effects in part because the brain is developing in many distinctive ways and at a very rapid rate. As I discuss further in Chapter 2, a strong likelihood exists that many of these common insults exert deleterious and far-reaching effects on certain aspects of neural development—effects that until now have escaped detection by available techniques.

In Chapters 1 and 2, I emphasize the aspect of normal development that has been deranged, the structural characteristics of the abnormality, and the neurological consequences. It is least profitable to attempt to characterize exhaustively all the presumed *causes* of these abnormalities of the developmental program. Although a few examples of environmental agents that insult the developing human nervous system at specific time periods and produce a defect are recognized, few of these agents leave an identifying stamp. This obtains particularly because, in the first two trimesters of gestation, the developing brain is not capable of generating the glial and other reactions to injury that serve as useful clues to environmental insults that occur at later time periods. The occasional example of a virus, chemical, drug, or other environmental agent that has been shown to produce a disorder of brain development is mentioned only in passing. However, I emphasize genetic considerations whenever possible because of their importance in parental counseling. Therefore, the organizational framework is the chronology of normal development of the human nervous system. A brief review of the major developmental events that occur most prominently during each time period is presented, followed by a discussion of the disorders that result when such development is deranged.

This chapter is devoted to the first two major processes involved in human brain development: formation of the neural tube and the subsequent formation of the prosencephalon. These early processes are discussed separately from later events because, together, the early processes result in the essential form of the central nervous system (CNS) and can be considered the neural components of *embryogenesis*. The later

developmental events, relating largely to the intrinsic structure of the CNS, can be considered the neural components of *fetal* development.

MAJOR DEVELOPMENTAL EVENTS AND PEAK TIMES OF OCCURRENCE

The major developmental events and their peak times of occurrence are shown in Table 1-1. The time periods are those during which the *most rapid progression* of the developmental event occurs. Although some overlap exists among these time periods, it is valid and convenient to consider the overall maturational process in terms of a sequence of individual events.

Termination Period

In a discussion of the timing of the disorders, the time periods shown in Table 1-1 are obviously of major importance. Nonetheless, it is necessary to recognize that an aberration of a developmental event need not be caused by an insult impinging *at the time of the event*. Thus, a given malformation may not have its onset after the developmental event is completed, but the developmental program may be injured *at any time before* the event is under way. The concept of a *termination period* (i.e., the time in the development of an organ after which a specific malformation cannot occur by any teratogenic mechanism) was enunciated by Warkany.[1] Thus, in the discussion of timing of malformations, I state that the onset of a given defect could occur *no later than* a given time.

PRIMARY NEURULATION AND CAUDAL NEURAL TUBE FORMATION (SECONDARY NEURULATION)

Normal Development

Neurulation refers to the inductive events that occur on the dorsal aspect of the embryo and result in the formation of the brain and spinal cord. These events can be divided into those related to the formation of brain and spinal cord exclusive of those segments caudal to the lumbar region (i.e., *primary neurulation*) and those related to the later formation of the lower sacral segments of the spinal cord (i.e., *caudal neural tube formation* or *secondary neurulation*). Primary neurulation and secondary neurulation are discussed separately.

TABLE 1-1	Major Events in Human Brain Development and Peak Times of Occurrence
Major Developmental Event	**Peak Time Of Occurrence**
Primary neurulation	3–4 weeks of gestation
Prosencephalic development	2–3 months of gestation
Neuronal proliferation	3–4 months of gestation
Neuronal migration	3–5 months of gestation
Organization	5 months of gestation to years postnatally
Myelination	Birth to years postnatally

Primary Neurulation

Primary neurulation refers to formation of the neural tube, exclusive of the most caudal aspects (see later). The time period involved is the third and fourth weeks of gestation (Table 1-2). The nervous system begins on the dorsal aspect of the embryo as a plate of tissue differentiating in the middle of the ectoderm (Fig. 1-1). The underlying notochord and chordal mesoderm induce formation of the neural plate, which is formed at approximately 18 days of gestation.[2,3] Under the continuing inductive influence of the chordal mesoderm, the lateral margins of the neural plate invaginate and close dorsally to form the neural tube. During this closure, the neural crest cells are formed, and these cells give rise to dorsal root ganglia, sensory ganglia of the cranial nerves, autonomic ganglia, Schwann cells, and cells of the pia and arachnoid (as well as melanocytes, cells of the adrenal medulla, and certain skeletal elements of the head and face). The neural tube gives rise to the CNS. The first fusion of neural folds occurs in the region of the lower medulla at approximately 22 days. Closure generally proceeds rostrally and caudally, although it is not a simple, zipper-like process.[4-9] The anterior end of the neural tube closes at approximately 24 days, and the posterior end closes at approximately 26 days. This posterior site of closure is at approximately the upper sacral level, and the most caudal cord segments are formed by a different developmental process occurring later (i.e., canalization and retrogressive differentiation, as discussed later).[10-12] Interaction of the neural tube with the surrounding mesoderm gives rise to the dura and axial skeleton (i.e., the skull and the vertebrae).

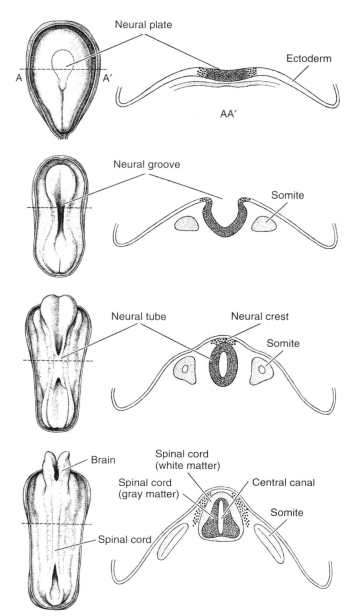

Figure 1-1 **Primary neurulation.** Schematic depiction of the developing embryo: external view (*left*) and corresponding cross-sectional view (*right*) at about the middle of the future spinal cord. Note the formation of the neural plate, neural tube, and neural crest cells. (*From Cowan WM: The development of the brain*, Sci Am *241:113-133, 1979.*)

TABLE 1-2	Primary Neurulation
Peak Time Period	
3–4 weeks of gestation	
Major Events	
Notochord, chordal mesoderm → neural plate → neural tube, neural crest cells	
Neural tube → brain and spinal cord → dura, axial skeleton (cranium, vertebrae), dermal covering	
Neural crest → dorsal root ganglia, sensory ganglia of cranial nerves, autonomic ganglia, and so forth	

The deformations of the developing neural plate required to form the neural folds, and subsequently the neural tube, depend on a variety of cellular and molecular mechanisms.[7-9,12-34] The most important cellular mechanisms involve the function of the cytoskeletal network of microtubules and microfilaments. Under the influence of vertically oriented microtubules, cells of the developing neural plate elongate, and their basal portions widen. Under the influence of microfilaments oriented parallel to the apical surface, the apical portions of the cells constrict. These deformations produce the stresses that lead to formation of the neural folds and then the neural tube.

TABLE 1-3	Caudal Neural Tube Formation (Secondary Neurulation)
Peak Time Period	
Canalization: 4–7 weeks of gestation	
Retrogressive differentiation: 7 weeks of gestation to after birth	
Major Events	
Canalization: undifferentiated cells (caudal cell mass) → vacuoles → coalescence → contact central canal of rostral neural tube	
Retrogressive differentiation: regression of caudal cell mass → ventriculus terminalis, filum terminale	

TABLE 1-4	Disorders of Primary Neurulation: Neural Tube Defects
Order of Decreasing Severity	
Craniorachischisis totalis	
Anencephaly	
Myeloschisis	
Encephalocele	
Myelomeningocele, Chiari type II malformation	

Concerning molecular mechanisms, a particular role of surface glycoproteins, particularly cell adhesion molecules, involves cell-cell recognition and adhesive interactions with extracellular matrix (i.e., to cause adhesion of the opposing lips of the neural folds). Other critical molecular events include action of the products of certain regional patterning genes (especially bone morphogenetic proteins and sonic hedgehog), homeobox genes, surface receptors, and transcription factors. The relative importance of these molecular characteristics is currently under intensive study.

Caudal Neural Tube Formation (Secondary Neurulation)

Formation of the caudal neural tube (i.e., the lower sacral and coccygeal segments) occurs by the sequential processes of canalization and retrogressive differentiation. These events, sometimes called *secondary neurulation*, occur later than those of primary neurulation and result in development of the remainder of the neural tube (Table 1-3). At approximately 28 to 32 days, an aggregate of undifferentiated cells at the caudal end of the neural tube (caudal cell mass) begins to develop small vacuoles. These vacuoles coalesce, enlarge, and make contact with the central canal of the portion of the neural tube previously formed by primary neurulation.[2] Not infrequently, accessory lumens remain and may be important in the genesis of certain anomalies of neural tube formation (see later). The process of canalization continues until approximately 7 weeks, when retrogressive differentiation begins. During this phase, from 7 weeks to sometime after birth, regression of much of the caudal cell mass occurs. Remaining structures are the ventriculus terminalis, primarily located in the conus medullaris, and the filum terminale.

Disorders

Disturbances of the inductive events involved in primary neurulation result in various errors of neural tube closure, which are accompanied by alterations of axial skeleton as well as of overlying meningovascular and dermal coverings. The resulting disorders are considered next, in order of decreasing severity (Table 1-4). Disorders of caudal neural tube formation (i.e., occult dysraphic states) are discussed in the final section.

Craniorachischisis Totalis

Anatomical Abnormality. In craniorachischisis, essentially total failure of neurulation occurs. A neural plate–like structure is present throughout, and no overlying axial skeleton or dermal covering exists (Fig. 1-2).[35,36]

Timing and Clinical Aspects. Onset of craniorachischisis totalis is estimated to be no later than 20 to 22 days of gestation.[2] Because most such cases are aborted spontaneously in early pregnancy, and only a few have survived to early fetal stages, the incidence is unknown.

Anencephaly

Anatomical Abnormality. The essential defect of anencephaly is failure of *anterior* neural tube closure. Thus, in the most severe cases, the abnormality extends from the level of the lamina terminalis, the site of final closure at the most rostral portion of the neural tube, to the foramen magnum, the approximate site of onset of anterior neural tube closure.[2,36] When the defect in the skull extends through the level of the foramen magnum, the abnormality is termed *holoacrania* or *holoanencephaly*. If the defect does not extend to the foramen magnum, the appropriate term is *merocrania* or *meroanencephaly*. The most common variety of anencephaly is involvement of the forebrain and variable amounts of upper brain stem. The exposed neural tissue is represented by a hemorrhagic, fibrotic, degenerated mass of neurons and glia with little definable structure. The frontal bones above the supraciliary ridge, the parietal bones, and the squamous part of the occipital bone are usually absent. This anomaly of the skull imparts a remarkable, froglike appearance to the patient when viewed face on (Fig. 1-3).

Timing and Clinical Aspects. Onset of anencephaly is estimated to be no later than 24 days of gestation.[2] Polyhydramnios is a frequent feature.[37] Approximately 75% of the infants are stillborn, and the remainder die in the neonatal period (see later). The disorder is not rare, and epidemiological studies reveal striking variations in prevalence as a function of geographical location, sex, ethnic group, race, season of the year, maternal age, social class, and history of affected siblings.[36,38-42] Anencephaly is relatively more common in whites than in blacks, in the Irish than in most other ethnic groups, in girls than in boys (especially in preterm infants), and in infants of particularly young or particularly old mothers.[36,39,43] The risk increases with decreasing social class and with the history of

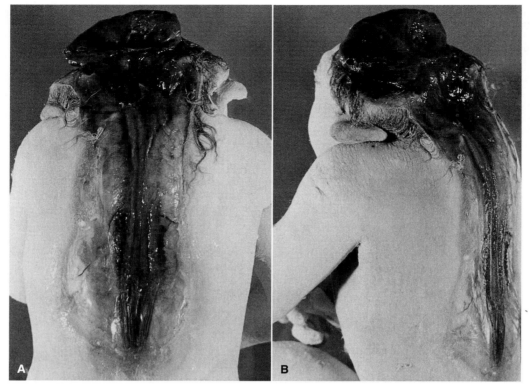

Figure 1-2   Craniorachischisis. Dorsal (**A**) and dorsolateral (**B**) views of a human fetus. *(Courtesy of Dr. Ronald Lemire.)*

affected siblings in the family. Since the late 1970s, the incidence of anencephaly, like that of myelomeningocele (see later), has been declining. Rates of occurrence of anencephaly decreased from approximately 0.4 to 0.5 per 1000 live births in 1970 to approximately 0.2 per 1000 live births in 1989.[40,44] In the United States this decline has been more apparent in Hispanic and non-Hispanic white infants than in black infants,[40,45-47] and this finding is of potential relevance to pathogenesis. Both genetic and environmental influences appear to operate in the genesis of anencephaly (see the later discussion of myelomeningocele). This defect is identified readily prenatally by cranial ultrasonography in the second trimester of gestation (Fig. 1-4).[48]

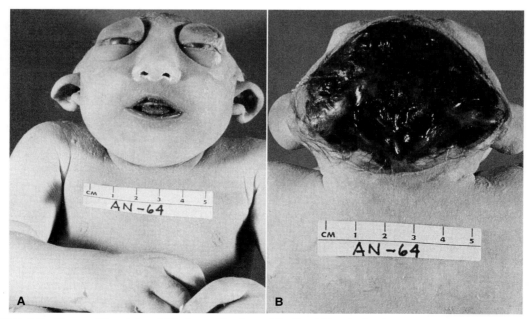

Figure 1-3   Anencephaly. Face-on (**A**) and dorsal (**B**) views. *(Courtesy of Dr. Ronald Lemire.)*

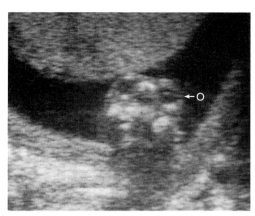

Figure 1-4 Ultrasonogram of anencephaly at 17 weeks of gestation. Note the symmetrical absence of normal structures superior to the orbits (O). *(From Goldstein RB, Filly RA: Prenatal diagnosis of anencephaly: Spectrum of sonographic appearances and distinction from the amniotic band syndrome,* AJR Am J Roentgenol *151:547-550, 1988.)*

TABLE 1-6 Survival in Anencephaly
No Intensive Care (n = 181)*
40% alive at 24 hours
15% alive at 48 hours
2% alive at 7 days
None alive at 14 days
Intensive Care (n = 6)[†]
Birth to 7 days: 5/6 alive at 7 days
After extubation: death at 8 days (2/5), 16 days (1/5), 3 weeks (1/5), and 2 months (1/5)

*Data from Baird PA, Sadovnick AD: Survival in infants with anencephaly, *Clin Pediatr* 23:268-271, 1984.
[†] Data from Peabody JL, Emery JR, Ashwal S: Experience with anencephalic infants as prospective organ donors, *N Engl J Med* 321:344-350, 1989.

Systematic prenatal detection and elective termination of pregnancy of all infants with anencephaly resulted in no anencephalic births over a 2-year period in one large university hospital in the eastern United States.[46]

Renewed investigation of the neurological function and survival of anencephalic infants was provoked by interest in the 1990s in the use of organs of such infants for transplantation.[49-53] Because lack of function of the entire brain, including the brain stem, is obligatory for the diagnosis of brain death in the United States, the finding of persistent clinical signs of brain stem function of anencephalic infants supported by neonatal intensive care in the first week of life is of major importance (Table 1-5).[54-56] Moreover, with such neonatal intensive care, including intubation, most infants survived for at least 7 days after extubation (Table 1-6).[54] This survival with intensive care is strikingly different from the situation with no intensive care, in which no more than 2% of liveborn anencephalic infants survive to 7 days (see Table 1-6).[39,57,58] The persistence of brain stem function and of viability is consistent with the not uncommon finding at neuropathological study of a rudimentary brain stem.[36,39]

Myeloschisis

Anatomical Abnormality. The essential defect of myeloschisis is failure of *posterior neural tube closure.*

TABLE 1-5 Brain Stem Function in Anencephaly	
Clinical Feature	**Number (Total n = 12)**
Reactive pupils	3
Spontaneous eye movements	4
Oculocephalic responses	6
Corneal reflex	6
Auditory response	5
Suck, root, and gag responses	7
Spontaneous respiration	12

Adapted from data in Peabody JL, Emery JR, Ashwal S: Experience with anencephalic infants as prospective organ donors, *N Engl J Med* 321:344-350, 1989.

A neural plate–like structure involves large portions of the spinal cord and manifests as a flat, raw, velvety structure with no overlying vertebrae or dermal covering.

Timing and Clinical Aspects. Onset of myeloschisis is no later than 24 days of gestation.[2] Most infants with myeloschisis are stillborn and merge with the category of more restricted defect of neural tube closure (i.e., myelomeningocele). Myeloschisis is often associated with anomalous formation of the base of skull and upper cervical region that results in retroflexion of the head on the cervical spine.[59,60] This constellation is termed *iniencephaly.*

Encephalocele

Anatomical Abnormality. Encephalocele may be envisioned as a *restricted disorder of neurulation* involving *anterior neural tube closure.* This concept, however, must be understood with the awareness that the precise pathogenesis of this disorder remains unknown. The lesion occurs in the occipital region in 70% to 80% of cases (Fig. 1-5).[61-65] A less common site is the frontal region, where the encephalocele may protrude into the nasal cavity. Cases of frontal lesions are relatively more common in Southeast Asia than in Western Europe or North America.[66-68] Least common lesion sites are the temporal and parietal regions.[69] In the typical occipital encephalocele, the protruding brain is usually derived from the occipital lobe and may be accompanied by dysraphic disturbances involving cerebellum and superior mesencephalon. The neural tissue in an encephalocele usually connects to the underlying CNS through a narrow neck of tissue. The protruding mass, most often occipital lobe, is represented usually by a closed neural tube with cerebral cortex, exhibiting a normal gyral pattern, and subcortical white matter. As many as 50% of cases are complicated by hydrocephalus.[70] Encephaloceles located in the low occipital (below the inion) or high cervical regions and combined with deformities of lower brain stem and of base of skull and upper cervical vertebrae characteristic of the Chiari type II malformation (associated with myelomeningocele [see later]) comprise the Chiari type III malformation.[71] This type of encephalocele contains

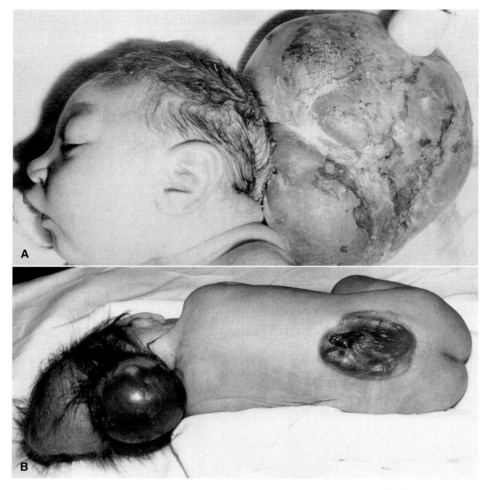

Figure 1-5 Encephalocele. A, Newborn with a large occipital encephalocele. **B,** Newborn with both an occipital encephalocele and a thoracolumbar myelomeningocele. *(Courtesy of Dr. Marvin Fishman.)*

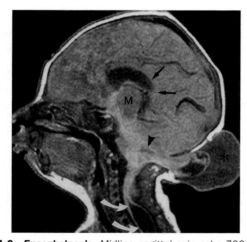

Figure 1-6 Encephalocele. Midline sagittal spin echo 700/20 magnetic resonance imaging scan demonstrates a low occipital encephalocele containing cerebellar tissue. The cystic portions (*asterisk*) within the herniated cerebellum are of uncertain origin. The posterior aspect of the corpus callosum (*straight black arrows*) is not clear and is probably dysgenetic. The third ventricle is not seen, but the massa intermedia (M) is very prominent. The tectum is deformed and is not readily identified. The fourth ventricle (*arrowhead*) is deformed and displaced posteriorly. A syrinx (*curved white arrows*) is present in the middle to lower cervical spinal cord. *(From Castillo M, Quencer RM, Dominguez R: Chiari III malformation: Imaging features,* AJNR Am J Neuroradiol 13:107-113, 1992.)

cerebellum in virtually all cases and occipital lobes in approximately one half of cases (Fig. 1-6).[71] Partial or complete agenesis of the corpus callosum occurs in two thirds of cases. Anomalies of venous drainage (aberrant sinuses and deep veins) occur in about one half of patients and must be considered in surgical approaches to these lesions.[71]

Timing and Clinical Aspects. Onset of the most severe lesions is probably no later than the approximate time of anterior neural tube closure (26 days) or shortly thereafter. Later times of onset are likely for the lesions that involve primarily or only the overlying meninges or skull.[36] (Approximately 10% to 20% of the occipital lesions contain no neural elements and thus are appropriately referred to as *meningoceles*.) Infants with encephaloceles not uncommonly exhibit associated malformations.[64,72] A frequent CNS anomaly is subependymal nodular heterotopia.[73] The most commonly recognized syndromes associated with encephalocele are Meckel syndrome (characterized by occipital encephalocele, microcephaly, microphthalmia, cleft lip and palate, polydactyly, polycystic kidneys, ambiguous genitalia, other deformities[66]) and Walker-Warburg syndrome (see Chapters 2 and 19). These disorders, as well as several other less common syndromes associated with encephalocele, are inherited in an autosomal recessive manner.[64,72,74] Maternal hyperthermia

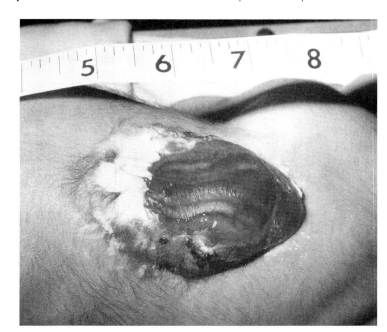

Figure 1-7   Newborn with a large thoracolumbar myelomeningocele. The white material is vernix. Note the neural plate–like structure in the middle of the lesion. *(Courtesy of Dr. Marvin Fishman.)*

between 20 and 28 days of gestation has been associated with an increased incidence of occipital encephalocele,[72] as well as with other neural tube defects (see later). Diagnosis by intrauterine ultrasonography in the second trimester has been well documented.[75-79] Diagnosis before fetal viability has been followed by elective termination; later diagnosis may allow delivery by cesarean section.

Neurosurgical intervention is indicated in most patients.[62,64] Exceptions include those with massive lesions and marked microcephaly. Surgery is necessary in the neonatal period for ulcerated lesions that are leaking cerebrospinal fluid (CSF). An operation can be deferred if adequate skin covering is present. Preoperative evaluation has been facilitated by the use of computed tomography (CT) and, especially, magnetic resonance imaging (MRI) scans.[71,80,81] Outcome is difficult to determine precisely because of variability in selection for surgical treatment. In a combined surgical series of 40 infants,[62,63] 15 infants (38%) died, many of whose complications can be managed more effectively now in neurosurgical facilities. Of the 25 survivors, 14 (56%) were of normal intelligence, although often with motor deficits, and 11 (44%) exhibited both impaired intellect and motor deficits. Outcome is more favorable for infants with anterior encephaloceles than those with posterior encephaloceles. Thus, in one series of 34 cases, mortality was 45% for infants with posterior defects and 0% for those with anterior defects. Normal outcome occurred in 14% of the total group with posterior defects and in 42% of those with anterior defects.[64]

Myelomeningocele

Anatomical Abnormality. The essential defect in myelomeningocele is *restricted failure of posterior neural tube closure.* Approximately 80% of lesions occur in the lumbar (thoracolumbar, lumbar, lumbosacral) area, presumably because this is the last area of the neural tube to close.[62] The neural lesion is represented by a neural plate or abortive neural tube–like structure in which the ventral half of the cord is relatively less affected than the dorsal. Most of the lesions are associated with dorsal displacement of the neural tissue, such that a sac is created on the back (Fig. 1-7). This dorsal protrusion is associated with an enlarged subarachnoid space ventral to the cord. The axial skeleton is uniformly deficient, and an incomplete although variable dermal covering is present. The defects of the spinal column were studied in detail by Barson[82] and consist of a lack of fusion or an absence of the vertebral arches, resulting in bilateral broadening of the vertebrae, lateral displacement of pedicles, and a widened spinal canal. The caudal extent of the vertebral changes is usually considerably greater than the extent of the neural lesion.

Timing. Onset of myelomeningocele is probably no later than 26 days of gestation.[2] This period in the fourth week of gestation is the time for normal neural tube closure. Studies of *early human embryos with dysraphic states* support this conclusion by providing histological evidence for dysraphism at *developmental stages before completion of neural tube closure.*[83]

Clinical Aspects. Myelomeningocele and its variants are the most important examples of faulty neurulation, because affected infants usually survive. As with anencephaly, earlier studies showed the highest incidences in certain areas of Ireland, Great Britain, northern Netherlands, and northern China.[41,42] A large variation in incidences in the United States is apparent, ranging in earlier studies from 0.6 per 1000 live births in Memphis, Tennessee, to 2.5 per 1000 in Providence, Rhode Island.[40,84] Over approximately the last 2 to 3 decades, the incidence has declined in Great Britain, the United States, and several other countries, even before the advent of folic acid supplementation

TABLE 1-7   **Correlations Among Motor, Sensory, and Sphincter Function, Reflexes, and Segmental Innervation**

Major Segmental Innervation*	Motor Function	Cutaneous Sensation	Sphincter Function	Reflex
L1–L2	Hip flexion	Groin (L1) Anterior, upper thigh (L2)	—	—
L3–L4	Hip adduction Knee extension	Anterior, lower thigh and knee (L3) Medial leg (L4)	—	Knee jerk
L5–S1	Knee flexion Ankle dorsiflexion Ankle plantar flexion	Lateral leg and medial foot (L5) Sole of foot (S1)	—	Ankle jerk
S1–S4	Toe flexion	Posterior leg and thigh (S2) Middle of buttock (S3) Medial buttock (S4)	Bladder and rectal function	Anal wink

*Segmental innervation for motor and sensory functions overlaps considerably; correlations shown are approximate.

(see later).[40-42,44,85-95] In the United States, overall incidences of myelomeningocele were 0.5 to 0.6 per 1000 live births in 1970 and 0.2 to 0.4 per 1000 live births in 1989.[40] In California, the incidence per 1000 live births in 1994 was 0.47 in non-Hispanic whites, 0.42 in Hispanics, 0.33 in African Americans, and 0.20 in Asians.[41,42]

The major clinical features relate primarily to the nature of the primary lesion, the associated neurological features, and hydrocephalus. Approximately 80% of myelomeningoceles seen at birth occur in the lumbar, thoracolumbar, or lumbosacral regions (see Fig. 1-7). Neural tissue of most lesions appears platelike.

Neurological Features. The disturbances of neurological function, of course, depend on the level of the lesion. Particular attention should be paid to examination of motor, sensory, and sphincter function. Moreover, in the first days of life, motor function subserved by segments caudal to the level of the lesion is common, but then it generally disappears after the first postnatal week.[96] Table 1-7 lists some of the important correlations among motor, sensory, and sphincter function, reflexes, and segmental innervation. Assessment of the functional level of the lesion allows reasonable estimates of potential future capacities. Thus, most patients with lesions below S1 ultimately are able to walk unaided, whereas those with lesions above L2 usually are wheelchair dependent for at least a major portion of their activities.[97-102] Approximately one half of patients with intermediate lesions are ambulatory (L4, L5) or primarily ambulatory (L3) with braces or other specialized devices and crutches. Considerable variability exists between subsequent ambulatory status and apparent neurological segmental level, especially in patients with midlumbar lesions.[100,103,104] Good strength of iliopsoas (hip flexion) and of quadriceps (knee extension) muscles is an especially important predictor of ambulatory potential rather than wheelchair dependence.[103,104] Deterioration to a lower level of ambulatory function than that expected from segmental level occurs over years, and this tendency is worse in the absence of careful management. In addition, patients with lesions as high as thoracolumbar levels, at least as young children, can use standing braces or other specialized devices to be upright and can be taught to "swivel walk."[98,105] Indeed, continuing improvements in ambulatory aids and their use are constantly increasing the chances for ambulation in children with higher lesions (see "Results of Therapy").

Segmental level also is an important determinant of the likelihood of development of scoliosis. Most patients with lesions above L2 ultimately exhibit significant scoliosis, whereas this complication is unusual in patients with lesions below S1.

Hydrocephalus. Several clinical features are helpful in evaluating the possibility of hydrocephalus. First, on examination, *the status of the anterior fontanelle and the cranial sutures* should be noted. A full anterior fontanelle and split cranial sutures are helpful signs for the diagnosis of increased intracranial pressure, if the meningomyelocele is not leaking CSF. In the latter case, the CSF leak at the site of the primary lesion serves as decompression, and the signs may be absent. *Evaluation of the head size* provides useful information. If the head circumference is more than the 90th percentile, approximately a 95% chance exists that appreciable ventricular enlargement is present.[106] If the head circumference is less than the 90th percentile, an approximately 65% chance of hydrocephalus still exists.[106] The *site of the lesion* is also helpful in predicting the presence or imminent development of hydrocephalus. With occipital, cervical, thoracic, or sacral lesions, the incidence of hydrocephalus is approximately 60%; with thoracolumbar, lumbar, or lumbosacral lesions, the incidence of hydrocephalus is approximately 85% to 90%.[106-108]

Signs of increased intracranial pressure are not prerequisites for the diagnosis of hydrocephalus in the newborn and, indeed, are observed in only approximately 15% of newborns with myelomeningocele.[109] Serial ultrasound scans are important because progressive ventricular dilation, without rapid head growth or signs of increased intracranial pressure, occurs in infants with myelomeningocele,[109,110] in a manner analogous to the development of hydrocephalus after

TABLE 1-8 Hydrocephalus and Myelomeningocele

Temporal Features
Most rapid progression occurring in first postnatal month
Dilation of ventricles before rapid head growth or before
signs of increased intracranial pressure or both

Etiological Features
Chiari type II hindbrain malformation with obstruction of
fourth ventricular outflow or flow of cerebrospinal fluid
through posterior fossa
Associated aqueductal stenosis

Importance
Major cause of neurological morbidity, especially if
complicated by infection
Effective control correlated with ultimate neurological
function

intraventricular hemorrhage (see Chapter 11). The most common time for hydrocephalus with myelomeningocele to be accompanied by overt clinical signs is 2 to 3 weeks after birth; more than 80% of infants who have hydrocephalus with myelomeningocele and who do not undergo shunting procedures exhibit such clinical signs by 6 weeks of age (Table 1-8).[108,109]

Chiari Type II Malformation. The *Chiari type II malformation* is central for causation of both clinical deficits related to brain stem dysfunction, a serious complication in a minority of patients with myelomeningocele, and hydrocephalus, a serious complication in most patients with myelomeningocele (see earlier). Nearly every case of thoracolumbar, lumbar, and lumbosacral myelomeningocele is accompanied by the Chiari type II malformation. The major features of this lesion include (1) inferior displacement of the medulla and the fourth ventricle into the upper cervical canal, (2) inferior displacement of the lower cerebellum through the foramen magnum into the upper cervical region, (3) elongation and thinning of the upper medulla and lower pons and persistence of the embryonic flexure of these structures,

and (4) a variety of bony defects of the foramen magnum, occiput, and upper cervical vertebrae.

Hydrocephalus associated with the Chiari type II malformation probably results primarily from one or both of two basic causes (see Table 1-8). The first is the hindbrain malformation that blocks either the fourth ventricular CSF outflow or the CSF flow through the posterior fossa. The second is aqueductal stenosis, which may be associated with the Chiari type II malformation in approximately 40% to 75% of the cases.[109,111,112] Aqueductal atresia is present in an additional 10%. Studies of human embryos and fetuses with myelomeningocele support the concept that the Chiari type II hindbrain malformation is a primary defect and not a result of hydrocephalus.[82] Moreover, studies of a mutant mouse with defective neurulation ("Splotch") provide insight into the mechanism by which myelomeningocele may lead to the Chiari type II malformation.[18] Thus, in this model it is clear that the Chiari type II malformation results because of growth of hindbrain in a posterior fossa that is too small. The abnormally small posterior fossa is caused by a lack of the normal distention of the developing ventricular system, including the fourth ventricle; the lack of distention occurs largely because of the open neural tube defect. Hydrocephalus then results from the Chiari type II malformation, as described earlier. Additionally supportive of this formulation is the demonstration that closure of the myelomeningocele in the second trimester of fetal life, before the most rapid growth of the cerebellum, results in upward displacement of the inferiorly herniated cerebellar vermis, expansion of the posterior fossa, improvement in CSF flow, and reduced need for ventriculoperitoneal shunting for hydrocephalus (see later) (Fig. 1-8).[113,114]

Clinical features directly referable to the hindbrain anomaly of the Chiari type II malformation (i.e., not to hydrocephalus) are probably more common than is recognized. In one carefully studied series of 200 infants, one third exhibited feeding disturbances

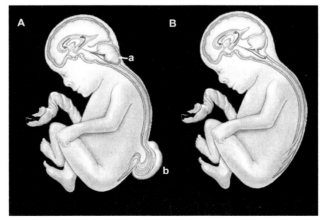

Figure 1-8 **Pathogenetic formulation for the Chiari type II malformation and the effect of treatment.** See text for details. In **A**, Chiari malformation (a) and the open myelomeningocele (b) are shown. The negative pressure generated from drainage of cerebrospinal fluid from the open myelomeningocele (b) results in the inferior displacement of the cerebellum (a) and thereby the Chiari type II malformation. **B**, After fetal closure, positive back pressure reduces the cerebellar hernia and expands the posterior fossa. *(From Sutton LN, Adzick NS, Bilaniuk LT, Johnson MP, et al: Improvement in hindbrain herniation demonstrated by serial fetal magnetic resonance imaging following fetal surgery for myelomeningocele, JAMA 282:1826-1831, 1999.)*

TABLE 1-9	Relation of Brain Stem Dysfunction to Mortality in Myelomeningocele		
Clinical Features		**Number**	**Mortality**
Stridor		10	0
Stridor and apnea		4	25%
Stridor, apnea, cyanotic spells, and dysphagia		5	60%
Total		19	21%

Adapted from Charney EB, Rorke LB, Sutton LN, Schut L: Management of Chiari II complications in infants with myelomeningocele, *J Pediatr* 111:364-371, 1987.

TABLE 1-10	Brain Stem Malformations in Myelomeningocele	
Total with Brain Stem Malformation		76%
Defective myelination		44%
Hypoplasia of cranial nerve nuclei		20%
Hypoplasia or aplasia of olives		20%
Hypoplasia or aplasia of basal pontine nuclei		16%
Hypoplasia of tegmentum		4%

Adapted from Gilbert JN, Jones KL, Rorke LB, Chernoff GF, et al: Central nervous system anomalies associated with meningomyelocele, hydrocephalus, and the Arnold-Chiari malformation: Reappraisal of theories regarding the pathogenesis of posterior neural tube closure defects, *Neurosurgery* 18:559-564, 1986.

(associated with reflux and aspiration), laryngeal stridor, or apneic episodes (or all three).[115] In one third of these affected infants, death was "directly or indirectly attributed to these problems." Indeed, in this and similar series, at least one half of the deaths of infants with myelomeningocele can be attributed to the hindbrain anomaly (despite treatment of the back lesion and hydrocephalus).[18,115-118] In a cumulative series of 142 infants, the median age at onset of symptoms referable to brain stem compromise was 3.2 months.[117] The clinical syndromes of brain stem dysfunction and their relation to mortality are presented in Table 1-9.[117,119,120] The 19 affected infants represented 13% of those with myelomeningocele. The principal clinical abnormalities in this and related studies reflect lower brain stem dysfunction and include vocal cord paralysis with stridor, abnormalities of ventilation of both obstructive and central types (especially during sleep), cyanotic spells, and dysphagia.[118,119,121-128] The full constellation of stridor, apnea, cyanotic spells, and dysphagia is associated with a high mortality (see Table 1-9). Such sensitive assessments of brain stem function as brain stem auditory-evoked responses, polysomnography, pneumographic ventilatory studies, and somatosensory-evoked responses yield abnormal results in infants with myelomeningocele in approximately 60% of cases and are the neurophysiological analogues of the clinical deficits.[118,129-133] The clinical abnormalities of brain stem function have three primary causes. First, they relate in part to the brain stem malformations, which involve cranial nerve and other nuclei, and are present in most cases at autopsy (Table 1-10).[112] Second, compression and traction of the anomalous caudal brain stem by hydrocephalus and increased intracranial pressure may play a role, especially in the vagal nerve disturbance that results in the vocal cord paralysis and stridor. Third, ischemic and hemorrhagic necrosis of brain stem is often present and may result from the disturbed arterial architecture of the caudally displaced vertebrobasilar circulation.[119]

Other Anomalies of the Central Nervous System. Other anomalies of the CNS have been described with myelomeningocele and the Chiari type II malformation. Perhaps most important of these are abnormalities of cerebral cortical development. In earlier studies, the pathological finding of microgyria was described in 55% to 95% of cases.[134,135] Whether this finding reflected a true cortical dysgenesis was not clear, but its presence was of major potential importance because of a relationship with the intellectual deficits that occur in a minority of these patients. Moreover, the occurrence of seizures in approximately 20% to 25% of children with myelomeningocele may be accounted for in part by such cortical dysgenesis.[136-138] This issue was clarified considerably by a careful neuropathological study of 25 cases of myelomeningocele (Table 1-11). Fully 92% of the brains showed evidence of cerebral cortical dysplasia, and 40% had overt polymicrogyria.[112] Thus, impaired neuronal migration was a common feature.

Other anomalous features, such as cranial lacunae, hypoplasia of the falx and tentorium, low placement of the tentorium, anomalies of the septum pellucidum, anterior and inferior "pointing" of the frontal horns, thickened interthalamic connections, and widened foramen magnum, are of uncertain clinical significance. However, they are visualized readily to varying degrees with CT, MRI, and cranial ultrasonography.[66,139-141] Anomalies in position of cerebellum are observable in utero by ultrasonography or MRI.[142,143] Cerebellar dysplasia, including heterotopias, is definable neuropathologically in 72% of cases.[112]

Management. Management of the patient with myelomeningocele, or of any patient with a neural tube defect, should begin with the following question: How could this have been prevented? Indeed, *prevention* must be considered the primary goal for the future. Major advances have been made in this direction (see later).

TABLE 1-11	Cerebral Cortical Malformations in Myelomeningocele	
Total with Cerebral Cortex Dysplasia		92%
Neuronal heterotopias		44%
Polymicrogyria (with disordered lamination)		40%
Disordered lamination only		24%
Microgyria, normal lamination		12%
Profound migrational disturbances		24%

Adapted from Gilbert JN, Jones KL, Rorke LB, Chernoff GF, et al: Central nervous system anomalies associated with meningomyelocele, hydrocephalus, and the Arnold-Chiari malformation: Reappraisal of theories regarding the pathogenesis of posterior neural tube closure defects, *Neurosurgery* 18:559-564, 1986.

TABLE 1-12	Incidence of Ventriculoperitoneal Shunt Placement after Fetal Surgery
Upper Level of Lesion	**Shunt Placement No. (%)**
T10–T12	5/5 (100%)
L1–L3	33/43 (77%)
L4–L5	19/52 (37%)
S1	6/16 (37%)
Total group	63/116 (54%)*

*Historical controls, 85% to 90%.
Data from Bruner JP, Tulipan N, Reed G, Davis GH, et al: Intrauterine repair of spina bifida: Preoperative predictors of shunt-dependent hydrocephalus, *Am J Obstet Gynecol* 190:1305-1312, 2004.

The first issue that must be faced in a newborn with myelomeningocele is whether the newborn should receive anything more than conservative, supportive care (e.g., tender nursing care and oral feedings). A decision for no surgical intervention must be made with a clear understanding of the prognosis of the lesion (see "Results of Therapy"). If an infant is to receive more than supportive therapy, the major consideration must be the management of the myelomeningocele and the complicating hydrocephalus. Most neurosurgeons in the United States operate on the back lesion and the associated hydrocephalus in nearly every newborn with myelomeningocele.[117,144,145] Although the therapies are best discussed by the appropriate surgical specialists, a brief review is necessary here.

Myelomeningocele. The first issue to be addressed in the management of the myelomeningocele is the possibility of *antenatal therapy*. Experimental and clinical data raise the possibility that exposure of the open neural tube to amniotic fluid and to the intrauterine pressure and mechanical stresses associated with labor and delivery can injure the spinal cord and worsen the neurological outcome.[7,146-150] Indeed, because of experimental evidence that prolonged exposure of the dysplastic spinal cord to the intrauterine environment before labor may accentuate the neurological deficits, and that covering the lesion may prevent this deterioration, *human fetal surgery* in the 20th to 30th weeks of gestation has been performed.[113,114,151-155] Although an endoscopic approach was used in initial studies, currently a hysterotomy is performed, and the lesion is covered with dura and skin. In one study of 42 infants treated in utero at 20 to 26 weeks of gestation and followed postnatally, 24 (57%) with thoracic or lumbar level defects had lower extremity function better than predicted from the anatomical level of the lesion.[114] Particularly striking has been the apparent decrease in need for postnatal shunt placement for hydrocephalus (Table 1-12).[114,155] Thus, overall, 54% of 116 infants treated in utero at a mean gestational age of 25 weeks required postnatal shunt placement, compared with approximately 85% to 90% of historical control infants not treated in utero. Notably, reversal of the hindbrain herniation of the Chiari type II malformation was a consistent finding[114] and may underlie the decrease in need for shunt placement. This beneficial effect of intrauterine repair on the hindbrain herniation was predicted by experiments in fetal lambs.[156] The promising findings with intrauterine surgery has led to a large randomized clinical trial in the United States.

Consistent with the possibility of mechanical injury during labor, the results of a retrospective review of 160 carefully studied cases of myelomeningocele suggest that *delivery by cesarean section* before the onset of labor may result in better subsequent motor function than vaginal delivery or delivery by cesarean section after a period of labor (Table 1-13).[157] Overall, infants delivered by cesarean section before the onset of labor had a mean level of paralysis 3.3 segments below the anatomical level of the spinal lesion, compared with 1.1 and 0.9 for infants delivered vaginally or delivered by cesarean section after the onset of labor, respectively. This variance is large enough to make the difference between the child's being ambulatory or wheelchair bound. Thus, scheduled delivery by cesarean section before the onset of labor should be considered for the fetus with meningomyelocele, particularly if prenatal ultrasonography and karyotyping rule out the presence of severe hydrocephalus, chromosomal abnormality, or multiple systemic anomalies.

The prevalent notion is that *early closure of the back lesion* (within the first 24 to 72 hours) is optimal. The rationale for this approach has been the prevention of infection and the loss of motor function that may occur after the first days of life (see earlier). The prevention of infection is supported by several studies.[115,158,159] A study of 110 infants suggests that closure of the back

TABLE 1-13	Level of Motor Paralysis at 2 Years of Age as a Function of Exposure to Labor and Type of Delivery			
		FUNCTIONAL LEVEL OF PARALYSIS (%)		
Labor/Delivery	**Mean Anatomical Level***	**Sacral or No Paralysis**	**L4 or L5**	**T12–L3**
No labor: cesarean section	L1.1	45	34	21
Labor: cesarean section	L1.0	20	29	51
Labor: vaginal delivery	L2.5[†]	14	55	31
All exposed to labor		16	47	37

*Based on radiographs of the spine.
[†]$P < .001$ compared with both cesarean section groups; by chance, the newborns in the vaginal delivery group had a significantly more favorable (i.e., lower) anatomical level.
Data from Luthy DA, Wardinsky T, Shurtleff DB, Hollenbach KA, et al: Cesarean section before the onset of labor and subsequent motor function in infants with meningomyelocele diagnosed antenatally, *N Engl J Med* 324:662-666, 1991; total number, 160.

lesion is not indicated so urgently. In infants whose lesions were closed in the first 48 hours, the incidence of ventriculitis was 10% (5/52) versus 12% (4/32) when lesions were closed in 3 to 7 days and 8% (1/12) when lesions were closed after 7 days.[160] Moreover, lower extremity paralysis was neither worsened by delay of surgery nor improved by surgical treatment within 48 hours. On balance, it would appear most prudent to close the back as promptly as possible (within the first 24 to 72 hours) but not to feel compelled to proceed so rapidly as to interfere with rational decision making.

In addition, value for the use of prophylactic antibiotics from the first 24 hours of life to the time of surgery is suggested by the results of two studies.[160,161] In the later and larger study, ventriculitis developed in only 1 of 73 infants (1%) receiving broad-spectrum antibiotic prophylactic therapy, compared with 5 of 27 (19%) who did not receive antibiotics.[161]

Details of the operative repair of myelomeningocele are discussed in other sources.[145,162,163] Techniques to minimize the risk of subsequent development of tethered cord are important.

Hydrocephalus. The management of the commonly associated hydrocephalus depends, first, on identification of the condition in the affected child. The findings of rapid head growth, bulging anterior fontanelle, and split cranial sutures are obvious, and an ultrasound scan can define the severity and the pattern of the ventricular dilation. More difficult is identification of low-grade hydrocephalus, often with no clinical signs, with CSF pressure in the normal range and with ventricles that are moderately dilated but not necessarily increasing disproportionately in size. Often such patients are considered to have "arrested" hydrocephalus. Later observations of similar patients have demonstrated a discrepancy in performance versus verbal intelligence quotient (IQ) scores, with the latter higher than the former. This discrepancy is considered consistent with a hydrocephalic state, which benefits from placement of a shunt.[164,165] Improvements in performance scores and decreases in ventricular size have been described in studies of such patients.[164] These data suggest that earlier use of shunt placement improves the cognitive outcome of infants with myelomeningocele (see next section). Value for nonsurgical therapy (e.g., isosorbide) to alleviate the need for shunt placement, suggested by earlier studies,[166,167] was not demonstrated in a later study.[168] This therapy, however, may delay the need for shunt placement; such temporization is useful for the infant too small or too sick to undergo a shunt procedure.

When a shunt is considered appropriate in the first weeks of life, a ventriculoperitoneal system is used.[115,116,169] Although controlled data are not available, in several studies of apparently comparable series of patients, intelligence appeared to be better preserved if ventriculoperitoneal shunts were performed more liberally.[170,171] Such an apparent benefit for the early treatment of hydrocephalus is supported by data suggesting that the degree of ventriculomegaly identified in utero or the size of the cerebral mantle in the first week of life correlates significantly with subsequent intelligence if the hydrocephalus is treated.[172,173] This conclusion must be interpreted with the awareness that the incidence of shunt complications varies depending on the clinical circumstances and that shunt complications have a major deleterious effect on intellectual outcome.[106,174,175]

The dominant deleterious shunt complication is *infection.* In a study of 167 infants with myelomeningocele, the mean IQ of infants with shunt placement for hydrocephalus complicated by infection was 73; with shunt placement for hydrocephalus and no infection, the mean IQ was 95.[176] The mean IQ in infants with myelomeningocele but no hydrocephalus was 102. The similarity of IQ in infants with and without hydrocephalus suggests that the hydrocephalus per se, if adequately treated and not complicated by infection, does not have a major deleterious effect on intellectual outcome.

Brain Stem Dysfunction Associated with the Chiari Type II Malformation. Management of the clinical abnormalities of brain stem dysfunction (see Table 1-9) associated with the Chiari II malformation is difficult. Infants with stridor and obstructive apnea generally respond effectively to improved control of hydrocephalus; any additional benefit for cervical decompression is less clear.[119,121] However, infants with severe symptoms, especially cyanotic episodes related to expiratory apnea of central origin, do not respond effectively to current modes of therapy.[119,121] With progression of the condition, mortality rates in such infants exceed 50%. In a study of 17 infants who had brain stem signs in the first month of life (swallowing difficulty, 71%; stridor, 59%; apneic spells, 29%; weak cry, 18%; aspiration, 12%), and in whom functioning shunts were in place, decompressive upper cervical laminectomy resulted in complete resolution of signs in 15 (2 infants died).[127] Postoperative morbidity was least when surgery was carried out within weeks rather than months after clinical presentation.

Orthopedic and Urinary Tract Complications. Of major subsequent importance to outcome of the infant with myelomeningocele are the incidence and severity of orthopedic and urinary tract complications. The latter are the major causes of death after the first year of life. The management of these groups of complications is a major problem after the newborn period and is best discussed in another context.[177-182] However, *urodynamic evaluation in the newborn* with myelomeningocele is of major predictive value concerning the risk of subsequent decompensation of the urinary tract.[182,183] Indeed, in a study of 36 infants, 13 of 16 who had subsequent deterioration of the urinary tract had incoordination of the detrusor-external urethral sphincter in the newborn period. This incoordination was followed by such deterioration in 72% of the newborns. Thus, addition of a urodynamic evaluation in the newborn provides critical information about the urinary tract and helps to determine the optimal type and frequency of follow-up management. Subsequent therapies, such as anticholinergic medication and clean, intermittent

TABLE 1-14	Outcome of Myelomeningocele as a Function of Therapeutic Approach*
"Conservative" Therapy: 1950s Mortality: 85%–90% by 10 years Survivors: 70% ambulatory; mean IQ, 89	
"Aggressive" Therapy (Unselected Early Closure of Primary Lesion and Treatment of Hydrocephalus): 1960s Mortality: 40%–50% by 16 years Survivors: 45% ambulatory; mean IQ, 77	
"Selective" Therapy (Selected Early Closure of Primary Lesion and Treatment of Hydrocephalus): Early 1970s Mortality: 55% (most were selected for no early closure) Survivors: 80% ambulatory; 85% IQ >75	
"Aggressive-Selective" Therapy: Late 1970s to Present Mortality: 14% by 3 to 7 years Survivors: 74% ambulatory; 73% IQ >80	

*See text for references.
IQ, intelligence quotient.

catheterization, have resulted in continence for as many as 85% of patients.[18,100,115,177-179,182] Notably, orthopedic and urinary tract difficulties are very important determinants of patient and family perceptions of quality of life in adolescence.[184]

Results of Therapy. *Conservative therapy* (i.e., no early surgery), the standard of care in the 1950s, provides an approximate measure of the natural history of the disorder (Table 1-14).[185] Approximately 50% of patients managed conservatively were dead by 2 months of age, 80% by 1 year, and 85% to 90% by 10 years. Of the survivors, 70% were ambulatory (with or without aids), and their mean IQ was 89.

With the advent of early closure of the myelomeningocele and improved techniques of dealing with the hydrocephalus, *aggressive therapy*, which included unselective early operation of the primary lesion, was adopted in many medical centers in the 1960s. The results of this approach were, in some ways, disappointing (see Table 1-14).[100,185-187] Although mortality decreased markedly (40% to 50% of patients were alive at age 16 years), the quality of life suffered notably. Of the larger number of survivors, 55% were confined to wheelchairs, and most of these children were incontinent, with a mean IQ of 77.[185] Approximately 30% of survivors exhibited epilepsy.[187]

Because the policy of unselective early operation appeared to cause a larger number of severely handicapped children who required an enormous amount of medical supervision and in-hospital therapy, and whose families required a great deal of social support, Lorber[186] advocated *selective therapy*, the use of strict criteria for treatment. The criteria were designed to exclude patients who would die despite therapy or, if they survived, would be very severely handicapped. Adverse prognostic criteria were identified as follows: (1) severe paraplegia (no lower limb function other than hip flexors, adductors, and quadriceps), (2) gross enlargement of the head, (3) kyphosis, (4) associated gross congenital

anomalies, and (5) major birth injury. Shortly after the published recommendation to use such criteria, Stark and Drummond[171] reported their experience with 163 patients with myelomeningocele at a medical center (Edinburgh) that had been using criteria comparable to those recommended by Lorber for 7 years (1965 to 1971) (see Table 1-14). Approximately 50% of the Edinburgh patients were considered to have the most favorable prognosis and were selected for early closure of the back lesion and subsequent vigorous therapy. The more severely affected 50% were given only symptomatic therapy. More than 70% of the treated patients were alive at 6 years of age, whereas more than 80% of the untreated patients were dead by 3 months of age. Of treated patients, approximately 80% were ambulatory with or without aids, and 87% were free of upper urinary tract disease. The level of intelligence was higher in the selectively treated patients than in the previously reported, unselectively treated patients.[188] Thus, only 15% of patients selected for therapy exhibited an IQ of less than 75, whereas 33% of patients unselectively treated had an IQ of less than 75. The improvement in intellectual function was associated with a more liberal use of shunting procedures for hydrocephalus, a relationship noted by others.[170] In later series of children similarly selected for therapy, treated survivors exhibited a similarly better outcome than with earlier "aggressive" therapy.[189-191]

The use of selective criteria for the institution of therapy for myelomeningocele in the newborn period presented at least *two major problems*. First, some infants who could possibly have had a favorable outcome were excluded and were allowed to experience a poor outcome or to die. Second, some infants who were selected for early vigorous therapy had a poor outcome.

Perhaps in part because of the problems encountered with the use of selective criteria, as just noted, *aggressive therapy* has been favored *in the last 2 to 3 decades* in most centers in North America. Moreover, results of such therapy appear to be superior to those reported previously for selective therapy (see Table 1-14). For example, in one series of 200 consecutive, unselected infants who were treated aggressively, mortality was only 14% after 3 to 7 years of follow-up. Of the survivors, 74% were ambulatory at least a portion of the time, and 87% were continent of urination.[115] The apparent improvement in outcome relative to the earlier results of aggressive therapy relates to several factors, including improvements in diagnosis and monitoring of hydrocephalus (e.g., brain imaging), improvements in management of CSF shunts, more effective therapy of infections, and improvements in braces and other aids for ambulation.[115-117,192,193]

A largely *aggressive approach* that appears to *combine a degree of selection* (e.g., advising against early surgery for infants with major cerebral anomalies, hemorrhage, or infection; high cord lesions and "cord paralysis"; and advanced hydrocephalus) has yielded results similar to those just recorded for aggressive therapy.[116] Indeed, in a study of this "aggressive-selective" approach, fully 71% of infants were selected for early surgery because of the absence of the adverse initial findings noted. Of these infants, 79% of survivors exhibited "normal" cognitive development, and 72% were ambulatory.[116]

Conclusions. No easy answers exist to the questions of when and how to treat the newborn infant who has myelomeningocele. The widespread employment of prenatal diagnosis and termination of pregnancy, especially in the presence of associated severe cerebral or systemic anomalies, will continue to alter the spectrum of infants observed in neonatal units. The possibility of intrauterine treatment, as noted earlier, likely will have a major impact on decision making. Currently, concerning the newborn with the lesion in the absence of major irreversible parenchymal injury (e.g., complicating major hypoxic-ischemic encephalopathy or serious associated cerebral anomaly), the likelihood for intellectual impairment seems low, and aggressive therapy directed toward the back lesion and the hydrocephalus seems indicated to me. Indeed, even in the infant with major parenchymal disease, closure of the back lesion and placement of a shunt for hydrocephalus for the purposes of the infant's comfort and nursing care are reasonable. Although undue delay in onset of therapy is inappropriate, time for rational discussions with the family can be taken and should not compromise outcome. However, little enthusiasm can be marshaled for delaying decisions for management. Not only does delay lead to compromise in outcome for many patients, but it also puts the parents in an uncertain and nearly intolerable position. It is not trite to conclude that management of each patient must be determined individually. Perhaps no other problem in neonatal medicine necessitates as much perception and sensitivity on the part of primary physicians. They must be able to make as precise a prognostic formulation as possible in the context of current medical knowledge and the facilities available to them and the patient's family. Of equal importance, physicians must have the sensitivity toward the family and the patient that is needed to estimate the impact of the disease on everyone concerned.

Etiology: Genetic and Environmental Considerations. Prevention of myelomeningocele and other neural tube defects necessitates understanding of their causes. Recognized causes of such defects include (1) multifactorial inheritance, (2) single mutant genes (e.g., the autosomal recessively inherited Meckel syndrome), (3) chromosomal abnormalities (e.g., trisomies of chromosomes 2, 7, 9, 13, 14, 15, 16, 18, and 21 and duplications of chromosomes 1, 2, 3, 6, 7, 8, 9, 11, 13, 16, 20, and X), (4) certain rare syndromes of uncertain modes of transmission, (5) specific teratogens (e.g., aminopterin, thalidomide, valproic acid, carbamazepine), and (6) specific phenotypes of unknown causes (e.g., cloacal exstrophy and myelocystocele).[42,90,194-197] Of defects resulting from these causes, most cases ($\approx$80%) are encompassed within the group in which the neural tube defect is the only major congenital abnormality and inheritance is multifactorial (i.e., dependent on a genetic predisposition that is polygenic and influenced by minor additive genetic variation at several gene loci).[92,198] Environmental influences may play an important role on this substrate.

Factors establishing the combined influence of both genetic and environmental influences are summarized in Tables 1-15 and 1-16. Factors establishing the *genetic role* include (1) a preponderance in female patients, (2) ethnic differences that persist after geographical migration, (3) increased incidence with parental consanguinity, (4) increased rate of concordance in apparently monozygotic twin pairs, and (5) increased

TABLE 1-15 Factors Influencing Differences in Prevalence of Myelomeningocele		
Factor	Time Period	Prevalence
Country		
England/Wales	1996	0.32
Finland	1996	0.41
Norway	1996	0.57
Northern Netherlands	1996	0.63
Region of Country		
Northern China	1992–1993	2.92
Southern China	1992–1993	0.26
Time Period		
Eastern Ireland	1980	2.7
Eastern Ireland	1984	0.6
Ethnic/Racial (California)		
Non-Hispanic White	1990–1994	0.47
Hispanic	1990–1994	0.42
African-American	1990–1994	0.33
Asian	1990–1994	0.20
Prenatal Diagnosis and Elective Termination (England/Wales)		
Live and stillbirths	1996	0.09
Live and stillbirths and terminations	1996	0.31

Data from Mitchell LE, Adzick NS, Melchionne J, Pasquariello PS, et al: Spina bifida, *Lancet* 364:1885-1895, 2004.

TABLE 1-16	Maternal Risk Factors for Myelomeningocele	
Factor		**Relative Risk**
Previous affected pregnancy (same partner)		30
Inadequate intake of folic acid		2–8
Pregestational diabetes		2–10
Intake of valproic acid or carbamazepine		10–20
Low vitamin B_{12}		3
Obesity		1.5–3.5
Hyperthermia		2

Data from Mitchell LE, Adzick NS, Melchionne J, Pasquariello PS, et al: Spina bifida, *Lancet* 364:1885-1895, 2004.

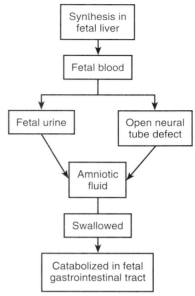

Figure 1-9 Physiology and pathophysiology of alpha-fetoprotein in utero.

incidence in siblings (as well as in second-degree and, to a lesser extent, third-degree relatives) and in children of affected patients.[41,84,90,92,194,196,198-204] The possibility of important *environmental influences* is suggested particularly by large variations in incidence as a function of geographical location and time period of study (see Table 1-15). Particularly potent data to suggest environmental influences relate to long-term trends in incidence. For example, in the northeastern United States, an epidemic period could be defined between approximately 1920 and 1949, with a peak between 1929 and 1932.[205] Since the late 1980s, a prominent steady decline in incidence has occurred in both the United States and Great Britain (see earlier).[40-42,84,88,90,91,93,95,206] The *interaction of environmental and genetic influences* has been demonstrated in experimental studies of the curly-tail mouse, in which a neural tube defect is inherited as an autosomal recessive trait.[7,207] Among *specific environmental influences*, a particularly important role for *folate deficiency* during the period of neural tube formation is suggested by experimental and clinical studies (see later). Other environmental factors, such as prenatal exposure to maternal hyperthermia, maternal diabetes mellitus, valproic acid (see Chapter 24), carbamazepine (see Chapter 24), maternal obesity, and low maternal vitamin B_{12} concentrations, also are of varying importance (see Table 1-16).[41,89,92,195,208-223]

The increased incidence of neural tube defects in siblings of index cases (see Table 1-16) has had major importance for *genetic counseling*. However, precise estimates of risks in subsequent siblings must take into account the population under study (see Table 1-15). A striking relationship between recurrence risk and the level of the myelomeningocele in the index case has been shown.[203] Thus, the risk for recurrence in a sibling was 7.8% if the index case had a lesion at T11 or above but only 0.7% if the lesion was below T11. A decline in the risk of neural tube defect as birth order increases also has been defined[111,200]; for example, in a study in Albany, New York, the risk for subsequent affected siblings (1.4%) was significantly less than for previously affected siblings (3.1%).[201]

Prenatal Diagnosis: Alpha-Fetoprotein and Ultrasonography. Prenatal suspicion of the presence of a neural tube defect is based primarily on the determination of levels of *alpha-fetoprotein in maternal serum.* This protein is the major protein component of human fetal serum and can be detected 30 days after conception. Serum levels of alpha-fetoprotein peak at approximately 10 to 13 weeks of gestation. Increased levels of alpha-fetoprotein in amniotic fluid occur with open neural tube defects; the mechanism for the elevated levels is thought to represent transudation of the protein from the membranes covering the lesion (Fig. 1-9).[224]

Until the mid-1980s, amniocentesis for detection of elevated levels of alpha-fetoprotein in amniotic fluid was the most common, albeit invasive procedure for suspicion of an open neural tube defect. Several reports in the late 1970s indicated that determination of *maternal serum alpha-fetoprotein levels* was useful for screening for neural tube defects.[225-229] The largest study involved measurements in more than 18,000 pregnant women in the United Kingdom.[225] The optimal time for measurement was shown to be 16 to 18 weeks of pregnancy. Subsequent experience in Scotland,[226] Sweden,[230] Wales,[231] and the United States[232,233] confirmed the high sensitivity of the analysis of alpha-fetoprotein in serum, and large-scale screening programs now are well established.[92,231,233,234] The diagnosis and anatomical details of the neural tube defect are then elucidated by ultrasonography and perhaps MRI.[78,79,92,231,235-239] The earliest ultrasonographic features include changes in the configuration of the posterior fossa, in addition to the lesion itself. Fetal MRI is the most valuable means to identify anatomical details (Fig. 1-10).

Primary Prevention. Prenatal diagnosis of neural tube defects and termination of pregnancy involving an affected fetus are effective methods of *secondary* prevention. However, a method of primary prevention would be more widely acceptable. Evidence now shows that folate *supplementation* around the time of conception

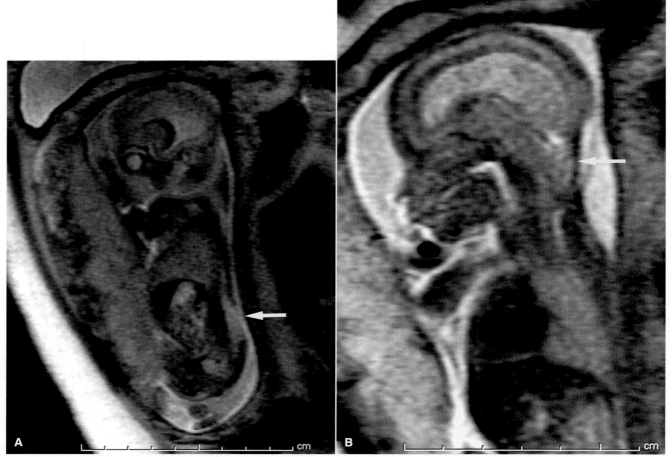

Figure 1-10 **Fetal magnetic resonance imaging at 20 weeks of gestation.** In **A**, a large thoracolumbosacral myelomeningocele (*arrow*) is apparent. In **B**, note the low-lying cerebellum (*arrow*), characteristic of a Chiari type II malformation; mild ventriculomegaly is also present. (*Courtesy of Dr. Omar Khwaja.*)

and therefore neural tube closure has a major preventive effect on the occurrence of neural tube defects.[7,41,42,92,95,206,240-281]

The effect of *multivitamin supplementation* before and during early pregnancy on recurrence of neural tube defects was first studied definitively by Smithells and colleagues,[240-243] in a recruited series of women with histories of births of one or more previously affected children. The multivitamin supplement contained "physiological" quantities of vitamins, such as folate, riboflavin, ascorbic acid, and vitamin A. The results of the study were striking. Of 454 women taking supplements, only 3 (0.7%) had recurrences, whereas of 519 women not taking supplements, 24 (4.7%) had

recurrences. Although the study was criticized for several methodological issues,[282,283] the data were promising. A subsequent study by Smithells and co-workers[248] showed a similarly striking effect. A non-controlled study in the United States on women identified largely by elevated serum alpha-fetoprotein levels, measured in a single regional laboratory, confirmed the beneficial role of folate-containing multivitamins (Table 1-17).[246] Moreover, the beneficial effect of folate was related clearly to the time during pregnancy when neural tube closure occurs.

After the aforementioned study, the British Medical Research Council completed an extremely important multicenter study.[250] Women were assigned randomly

TABLE 1-17	Effect of Folate-Containing Multivitamins on Prevalence of Neural Tube Defects			
	WEEKS 1–6		**WEEKS 7+ ONLY**	
Multivitamin	**No.**	**NTD (per 1,000)**	**No.**	**NTD (per 1,000)**
With folate	10,713	0.9	7,795	3.2
Without folate	926	3.2		

NTD, neural tube defect.
Adapted from Milunsky A, Jick H, Jick SS, Bruell CL, et al: Multivitamin/folic acid supplementation in early pregnancy reduces the prevalence of neural tube defects, *JAMA* 262:2847-2852, 1989.

TABLE 1-18	Role of Folic Acid in Prevention of Neural Tube Defects: Multicenter, Randomized, Double-Blind Clinical Trial*			
RANDOMIZATION GROUP		**OCCURRENCE OF NEURAL TUBE DEFECT**		
Folic Acid	**Other Vitamins**	**No. Affected/Total No.**		**Relative Risk: Folic Acid versus Nonfolic Acid**
+	−	1/242 } 3/483 (0.6%)		0.17
+	+	2/241 }		
−	−	10/243 } 17/477 (3.6%)		
−	+	7/234 }		

*Includes women who were not already pregnant at the time of randomization and who completed treatment period (until 12th week of pregnancy). Data from MRC Vitamin Study Research Group: Prevention of neural tube defects: Results of the Medical Research Council Vitamin Study, *Lancet* 338:131-137, 1991.

to four groups allocated to receive one of the following regimens of supplementation: folate and a multivitamin supplementation of "other vitamins," folate alone, "other vitamins" alone, or no folate or "other vitamins" (Table 1-18). The results were decisive in demonstrating the preventive effect and the specific role of folate (versus other components of the previously used multivitamin preparations). The overall reduction in neural tube defects was 83%. The findings clearly had major implications for the primary prevention of neural tube defects. On the basis of this study, the U.S. Centers for Disease Control and Prevention recommended an increase in folic acid intake by 0.4 mg/day for women from the time they plan to become pregnant through the first 3 months of pregnancy.[284] The folate was not recommended to be administered as a multivitamin preparation because of the potential danger for toxicity from excessive amounts of other vitamins in the multivitamin preparation. Because of the uncertainty of the degree of risk from the folate supplementation, the initial recommendations were directed only to women who had had a previous pregnancy complicated by a neural tube defect, as in the British study. Subsequently, two studies showed a preventive effect of periconceptional folic acid exposure on the occurrence of neural tube defects in populations of women without a prior affected child.[253,254] These observations were followed by the recommendation of the U.S. Public Health Service and the American Academy of Pediatrics that "all women capable of becoming pregnant consume 0.4 mg of folic acid daily to prevent neural tube defects."[285]

The optimal methods of folate supplementation and dose of the supplement are not totally clarified.[286,287] Public educational campaigns, albeit useful, have not been entirely successful, especially because as many as 50% of pregnancies are unplanned, and only a few of the "nonplanners" are reached by such campaigns.[287,288] In 1998, the U.S. Food and Drug Administration mandated fortification of all enriched grain products with folate. Similar programs have been instituted in many other countries and have resulted in an approximately 50% reduction in prevalence of neural tube defects.[95,206,276-278,280,289,289a] However, the British Medical Research Council study used a 4 mg (rather than 0.4 mg) daily folate dose and achieved an 83% reduction in prevalence of lesions. Thus, one expert in the field recommended a public health policy that includes "both the mandatory fortification of flour and a recommendation that all women planning a pregnancy take 5 mg of folic acid per day."[279]

The mechanism of the beneficial effect of folate is not established. One report raised the possibility that autoantibodies against folate receptors are present in as many as 75% of women who have had a pregnancy complicated by a neural tube defect.[290] The autoantibody-mediated block of cellular folate uptake by folate receptors could be bypassed by administered folate because the latter is reduced and methylated in vivo and is transported into cells by the reduced folate carrier. A related possibility is that the beneficial effect of folate could involve *the metabolism of homocysteine to methionine*, a reaction catalyzed by methionine synthase and necessitating a metabolite of folic acid (5-methyltetrahydrofolate).[7,41,269,271-273,291-294] A critical enzyme in synthesis of 5-methyltetrahydrofolate, *methylenetetrahydrofolate reductase*, is defective in 12% to 20% of cases of neural tube defects.[269,294] One biochemical result of this disturbance is an elevation of homocysteine, which has been shown to produce neural tube defects in avian embryos.[293] Another potential mechanism of a defect in homocysteine conversion to methionine is a disturbance in methylation reactions, for which methionine is crucial.[269,281] Transmethylations of DNA, proteins, and lipids have far-reaching metabolic consequences.[269,281]

Occult Dysraphic States

Anatomical Abnormality. Occult dysraphic states are characterized by overt abnormalities involving vertebral, overlying dermal structures or both and by neural lesions that are often subtle or even nonexistent (Table 1-19). These disorders are distinguished from the disorders of primary neurulation not only by their usual caudal locus but also particularly by the presence of intact skin over the lesions. Often the abnormality is so well concealed that it goes undetected for years, hence the term *occult*. A basic relation to disorders of primary neurulation is indicated by the finding that 4.1% of siblings of patients with occult dysraphic states exhibit disorders of primary neurulation, most often myelomeningocele or anencephaly.[295]

The *principal developmental abnormality* involves the separation of overlying ectoderm from the developing neural tube, a developmental event often termed

TABLE 1-19	Disorders of Caudal Neural Tube Formation: Occult Dysraphic States

Order of Time of Origin during Development

Myelocystocele
Diastematomyelia-diplomyelia
Meningocele-lipomeningocele
Lipoma, teratoma, other tumors
Dermal sinus with or without "dermoid" or "epidermoid" cyst
"Tethered cord" (without any of the above)

disjunction. Failure of this separation impairs the insertion of mesoderm between the ectoderm and neural tube and, as a consequence, results in disturbed development of vertebrae and related mesodermal tissue. Although disturbances in disjunction may occur at any level of the neuraxis, they are most common in the region of the caudal neural tube and are thus often classified, as I do here, among disorders of caudal neural tube formation.[296] The disjunctional failure results most conspicuously in ectodermal abnormalities, dermal tracts and sinuses, abnormalities of mesodermally derived tissue (e.g., vertebral defects, lipomatous masses), and caudal neural tube abnormalities.

Because caudal neural tube formation by the processes of canalization and retrogressive differentiation results in the conus medullaris and filum terminale, it is not surprising that almost invariable and unifying findings in these disorders are abnormalities of the conus and filum. The conus is usually prolonged, and the filum terminale is thickened. Moreover, these structures frequently are "tethered" or fixed at their caudal end by fibrous bands, lipoma, extension of dermal sinus, or related lesions. This fixation is thought to impair the normal mobility of the lower spinal cord, and as a consequence, movements of the trunk such as flexion and extension transmit tension through the prolonged conus to the spinal cord and cause injury.[297-299] This explanation of the neural injury complements the "traction" concept (i.e., because of its tethered caudal end, the cord sustains a traction injury caused by the differential growth of the vertebral column and the neural tissue). This concept of differential growth as the sole cause of the injury is contradicted by the finding that differential growth is slight between approximately the 26th week of gestation, when the cord is at the level of the third lumbar segment, and maturity, when the cord is at the level of the first or second lumbar segment.[82,300] Nevertheless, contributory importance for traction associated with tethering in the genesis of the injury is indicated by studies of mitochondrial oxidative metabolism of cord in vivo in affected patients by dual-wavelength reflection spectrophotometry.[301] Thus, distinct disturbances observed intraoperatively improved markedly on release of the tethered cord.

With the occult dysraphic states, as noted earlier, the neural lesion is often rather subtle, and the major overt abnormality involves mesodermally derived structures (especially the vertebrae), the overlying dermal structures, or both. Thus, vertebral defects occur in 85% to 90% of cases and consist most commonly of laminar defects over several segments; other skeletal abnormalities include a widened spinal canal and sacral deformities.[2,62,81,298,299,302-304] Approximately 80% of affected infants exhibit a dermal lesion in the lumbosacral area, consisting of abnormal collections of *hair*, cutaneous *dimples* or *tracts*, superficial cutaneous *abnormalities* (e.g., hemangioma), or a subcutaneous *mass* (see later).

Timing. The neural lesions, in approximate order of time of origin during neural development, are myelocystocele, diastematomyelia-diplomyelia, meningocele-lipomeningocele, lipoma (other tumors), dermal sinus with or without "dermoid" or "epidermoid" cyst, and "tethered cord" alone (see Table 1-19). Less common (although related) lesions include anterior dysraphic disturbances, such as neurenteric cyst and anterior meningocele, and the *caudal regression syndrome.* This latter rare disorder is characterized by dysraphic changes primarily of the sacrum and coccyx, with atrophic changes of muscles and bones of the legs; the neural anomalies range from minor fusion of spinal nerves and sensory ganglia to agenesis of the distal spinal cord.[305] Approximately 15% to 20% of patients are infants of diabetic mothers, and approximately 0.3% of infants of diabetic mothers exhibit the lesion.[306-310] (Infants of diabetic mothers also exhibit a 15- to 20-fold increased risk, relative to infants of nondiabetic mothers, of anencephaly or myelomeningocele.[310]) Because the lower genitourinary tract and anorectal structures are developing simultaneously and in close proximity to the caudal neural tube, the lesions listed in Table 1-19 are not uncommonly associated with anorectal and genitourinary abnormalities.[81] Indeed, the presence of such lesions should be considered in infants with abnormalities of caudal neural tube formation.

In *myelocystocele,* a localized cystic dilation of the central canal of the caudal neural tube is present.[2,311] The frequent association with cloacal exstrophy, omphalocele, imperforate anus, severe vertebral defects, and other malformations makes this one of the most severe malformations of the newborn period.[2] The onset of this lesion is estimated to be 28 days of gestation. In *diastematomyelia,* the spinal cord is bifid.[2,81,298,303,304,312,313] The lesion is most common in the lumbar region. In some cases, the spinal cord is separated by a bony, cartilaginous, or fibrous septum protruding from the dorsal surface of the vertebral body, whereas in other cases no septum is present (the term *diplomyelia* is sometimes used for the latter cases). Because many types of duplication of the developing caudal neural tube may occur during canalization, it is postulated that persistence of these tubes could result in diastematomyelia. The duplications may occur because of splitting of the notochord with impaired induction of both the neural tube and the vertebrae. *Meningocele* over the lower spine is rare as an isolated lesion and is not associated with hydrocephalus or neurological deficits, unlike disorders of primary neurulation.[2,303] More cases are associated with infiltration of fibrofatty tissue that is contiguous with a subcutaneous lipoma (i.e., *lipomeningocele*).[2,314,315] *Subcutaneous lipoma* with intradural extension is more common without an accompanying meningocele. Less commonly, other *tumors* may be observed.[316-319] By far the most common of these tumors is teratoma, although neuroblastoma, ganglioneuroma, hemangioblastoma, and related neoplasms, presumably originating from germinative tissue in the primitive caudal cell mass, or arteriovenous malformation, may occur. Congenital *dermal sinus* consists usually of a dimple in the lumbosacral region from which a small sinus tract proceeds inwardly and rostrally. The tract may enlarge subcutaneously into a cyst that contains predominantly dermal structures ("dermoid") or epidermal structures ("epidermoid"). Extension of the tract into the vertebral canal may cause neurological symptoms as a result of compression, tethering, or infection. These lesions result from an invagination of ectoderm that is carried by the canalized neural tube as it separates from the surface.[2] With *tethered cord*, the conus is prolonged, the filum abnormal, and the caudal end of the cord fixed by fibrous bands.[2,81,298,299,303]

The relative frequency of the several occult dysraphic states differs somewhat, according to the source of the cases. Thus, in one large surgical series of 73 patients, dermal sinus with or without cyst accounted for approximately 35% of cases; lipoma accounted for approximately 30% of cases. Diastematomyelia and anterior meningocele were much less common.[302] Very frequent accompanying features, and sometimes the sole and predominant abnormalities, were the prolongation of the conus and a defective filum terminale. In a series of 144 cases of caudal lesions observed in a children's hospital, as in the surgical series, lipoma was similarly common (40% of cases), and diastematomyelia was similarly uncommon (4% of cases), but dermal sinus with or without cyst accounted for only 10% of cases.[316] Sacrococcygeal teratoma composed 12% and myelocystocele 8% of cases in this less selected series. In another children's hospital–based series of 104 cases, data were similar except that diastematomyelia accounted for approximately 25% of cases.[303]

Clinical Aspects. In the newborn period, the clinical features most suggestive of an occult dysraphic state are the *dermal stigmata* (Table 1-20). Thus, abnormal collections of hair, subcutaneous mass, superficial cutaneous abnormalities (e.g., hemangioma, skin tag, cutis aplasia, pigmented macule), or cutaneous dimples or tracts, should raise suspicion of a disorder of caudal neural tube formation.[298,299,303,317,320-327] The incidence of associated spinal dysraphism with various cutaneous stigmata in one large series was as follows: "hairy patch," 4 of 10; subcutaneous mass, 6 of 6; hemangioma, 2 of 11; skin tag 1 of 7; cutis aplasia, 1 of 1; "simple dimple" (midline, <5 mm, and <2.5 cm above the anus), 0 of 160; atypical dimples, 3 of

TABLE 1-20	Neonatal Clinical Features Most Suggestive of Occult Dysraphic State

Abnormal collection of hair
Subcutaneous mass
Cutaneous abnormalities (hemangioma, skin tag, cutis aplasia, pigmented macule)
Cutaneous dimples or tracts

13; and atypical dimples and other skin lesions, 5 of 7.[324] Although neurological deficits are most unusual in the newborn, motor or sensory disturbances in the legs or feet or sphincter abnormalities occasionally may be detected.

The most common clinical presentations for occult dysraphic states later in infancy include delay in development of sphincter control, delay in walking, asymmetry of legs or abnormalities of feet (e.g., pes cavus and pes equinovarus), and pain in the back or lower extremities. Recurrent meningitis is an uncommon, although dangerous, feature. Similarly, rapid neurological deterioration, although unusual, may occur (see later). In the older child or adolescent, the major clinical features are gait disturbance, abnormality of sphincter function, development of a foot deformity, and scoliosis.

Management. Management of the newborn with a skin lesion suggestive of an occult dysraphic state usually includes radiography of the spine. However, before the age of 1 year, ossification of the posterior spinal elements is insufficient to be certain that no abnormality is present. Moreover, even in older infants and children, 10% to 15% of patients with occult dysraphic states have normal spine radiographs. An important noninvasive initial evaluation is *ultrasonography*, a procedure made possible in the newborn in part because of the poor ossification of posterior spinal elements.[328,329,329a] Visualization of the spinal cord, subarachnoid space, conus medullaris, and filum terminalis and real-time ultrasonographic observation of the mobility of the cord have allowed identification of a variety of occult dysraphic states.[328,329] If both radiography and ultrasonography findings of the spine are normal, no neurological signs exist, and the only clinical finding is a simple dimple or flat hemangioma, many clinicians consider further radiological study to be unnecessary in the neonatal period and clinical follow-up appropriate. My inclination most often, however, is to perform *an MRI.*

If a skeletal abnormality or other abnormality is present on the radiographs or sonogram, or if the findings are equivocal, MRI is clearly indicated. MRI has added enormously to assessment (Fig. 1-11).[81,311,313,322,330] MRI is especially valuable for demonstrating the sagittal and coronal topography of the intravertebral and extravertebral components; only bony lesions are not as effectively visualized by MRI as by CT. Indeed, CT is especially useful in demonstrating anomalous bony structures and diastematomyelia spurs.[303,323]

Surgery is performed primarily to *prevent* development of neurological deficits.[303,312,323,325] The optimal

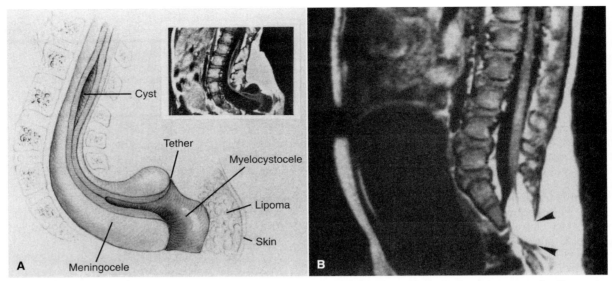

Figure 1-11 **Disorders of caudal neural tube formation. A,** Myelocystocele: artist's drawing of the meningocele surrounding the myelocystocele and related abnormalities. *Inset*: T1-weighted magnetic resonance imaging (MRI), sagittal view, showing a T12–L3 intramedullary cyst, terminal myelocystocele, meningocele, and lipoma dorsal and superior to the meningocele and myelocystocele. **B,** Lipomyelomeningocele with tethered cord. Sagittal, partial saturation (T1-weighted) MRI, 5 mm–thick section shows spinal cord to extend to level of S1 and S2. At this level, a fatty mass envelops the distal spinal cord. The fatty mass extends through a vertebral defect (*arrowheads*) into subcutaneous soft tissues that are enlarged by the lipoma. (**A,** *From Peacock WJ, Murovic JA: Magnetic resonance imaging in myelocystoceles: Report of two cases,* J Neurosurg *70:804-807, 1989.* **B,** *From Packer RJ, Zimmerman RA, Sutton LN, et al: Magnetic resonance imaging of spinal cord disease of childhood,* Pediatrics *78:251-256, 1986.*)

timing of surgery in the infant with few or even no neurological signs is controversial, but the combination of excellent preoperative imaging with MRI, microsurgical techniques, and intraoperative monitoring of cord function by evoked potentials has so decreased morbidity that treatment in the neonatal period before the onset of symptoms has been recommended.[298,331,332] Moreover, neurological deficits may develop in young infants suddenly, and these deficits may persist partially or totally despite prompt surgical treatment.[298,299,333,334] The mechanism of this sudden deterioration may represent vascular insufficiency produced by tension on a tethered cord, angulation of the cord around fibrous or related structures, or a direct effect of a tumor (e.g., lipoma) or cyst. Surgical release of the tethered cord combined with removal of the tumor or cyst will prevent such deterioration and may partially reverse deficits recently acquired.

PROSENCEPHALIC DEVELOPMENT

Normal Development

Prosencephalic development occurs by inductive interactions under the primary influence of the prechordal mesoderm. The peak time period involved is the second and third months of gestation, with the earliest prominent phases in the fifth and sixth weeks of gestation (Table 1-21).[2,335,336] The major inductive relationship of concern is between the notochord-prechordal mesoderm and the forebrain (see Table 1-21). This interaction occurs ventrally at the rostral end of the embryo; thus, the term *ventral induction* is sometimes used. The inductive interaction influences formation of much of the *face* as well as the *forebrain*, and hence severe

disorders of brain development at this time also usually result in striking facial anomalies.

Development of the prosencephalon is considered best in terms of three sequential events (i.e., *prosencephalic formation, prosencephalic cleavage,* and *midline prosencephalic development*) (see Table 1-21). *Prosencephalic formation* begins at the rostral end of the neural tube at the end of the first month and the beginning of the second month, shortly after the anterior neuropore closes. *Prosencephalic cleavage* occurs most actively in the fifth and sixth weeks of gestation and includes three basic cleavages of the prosencephalon: (1) horizontally, to form the paired optic vesicles, olfactory bulbs, and tracts; (2) transversely, to separate the telencephalon from diencephalon; and (3) sagittally, to form, from the telencephalon, the paired cerebral hemispheres, lateral ventricles, and basal ganglia (see Table 1-21). The third event, *midline prosencephalic development*, occurs from the latter half of the second month

TABLE 1-21   Prosencephalic Development
Peak Time Period 2–3 months

Major Events
Prechordal mesoderm → face and forebrain
Prosencephalic development
  Prosencephalic formation
  Prosencephalic cleavage
    Paired optic and olfactory structures
    Telencephalon → cerebral hemispheres
    Diencephalon → thalamus, hypothalamus
Midline prosencephalic development
    Corpus callosum, septum pellucidum, optic nerves
    (chiasm), hypothalamus

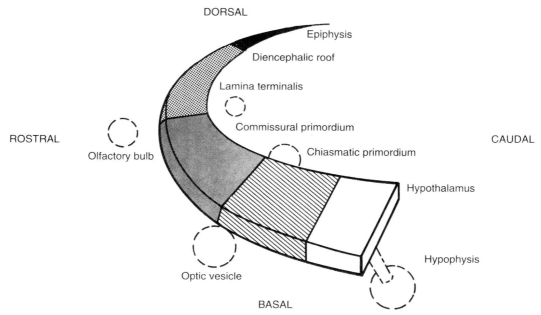

Figure 1-12 **Prosencephalic midline is represented by a series of independent but closely related segments.** Note particularly the commissural, chiasmatic, and hypothalamic primordia or plates. *(From Leech RW, Shuman RM: Holoprosencephaly and related cerebral midline anomalies: A review.* J Child Neurol *1:3-18, 1986.)*

through the third month, when three crucial thickenings or plates of tissue become apparent (Fig 1-12); from dorsally to ventrally, these are the commissural, chiasmatic, and hypothalamic plates. These structures are important in the formation, respectively, of the corpus callosum and the septum pellucidum, the optic nerve-chiasm, and the hypothalamic structures. The most prominent of these midline developments is formation of the corpus callosum, the earliest components of which appear at approximately 9 weeks; by 12 weeks, an independent corpus callosum is definable at the commissural plate. The callosum is formed by cortical axons that are attracted to the midline by specialized glial cells that express chemoattractants of the Netrin family. After crossing, these axons do not recross because of the expression of the chemorepellent protein Slit, which activates the Roundabout (Robo) receptor.[337] The first regions of the callosum to form are derived from crossing axons, so-called *pioneering axons* from the cingulate cortex, which enter the rostrum (the region inferior to the genu) and the anterior body.[337, 337a, 337b] This development is followed by formation of the genu and finally, posteriorly, the splenium. The basic structure is completed by approximately 20 weeks of gestation.[335,337-339] Subsequent thickening of this structure occurs as a result of growth of crossing fibers during organizational events (see later).

Major insights into the molecular genetic determinants of forebrain development have been gained in recent years.[337a,337b,340-352a] The genes involved are crucial for dorsoventral patterning in the developing forebrain. The most important molecular pathway in prosencephalic development is the *sonic hedgehog signaling pathway*, consisting of critical ventralizing molecules. Sonic hedgehog protein (*Shh*) is a secreted product of the prechordal mesoderm. Before secretion,

cholesterol is required for modification of *Shh* at its C-terminus (an event relevant to causes of holoprosencephaly; see later). Secreted *Shh* activates a receptor, *Patch*, which, in turn, leads to activation of several other genes (e.g., *GLI2*) and transcription factors that enter the nucleus to modify gene transcription. A second major molecular pathway, the so-called *nodal pathway*, is initiated by bone morphogenetic proteins, key dorsalizing molecules. The transcriptional regulators induced in this pathway include *TGIF, TDGFI,* and *FASTI.* Additional genes, such as *ZIC2*, also may play a role in prosencephalic formation. The clinical relevance of these insights includes the importance of performing mutation analysis of these genes in selected patients with disorders of prosencephalic development (see later).

Disorders

Disorders of prosencephalic development are considered best in terms of the three major events described earlier (i.e., prosencephalic formation from the rostral end of the neural tube, prosencephalic cleavage, and midline prosencephalic development) (Table 1-22). The spectrum of pathology varies from a profound derangement (e.g., aprosencephaly) to certain disturbances of midline prosencephalic development (e.g., isolated agenesis of the corpus callosum) that are sometimes not detected during life.

Aprosencephaly and Atelencephaly

Anatomical Abnormality. Aprosencephaly and atelencephaly are the most severe of the disorders of prosencephalic development.[353-365] In *aprosencephaly*, the entire process fails to occur, and the result is an absence of formation of both telencephalon and diencephalon, with a prosencephalic remnant located at the

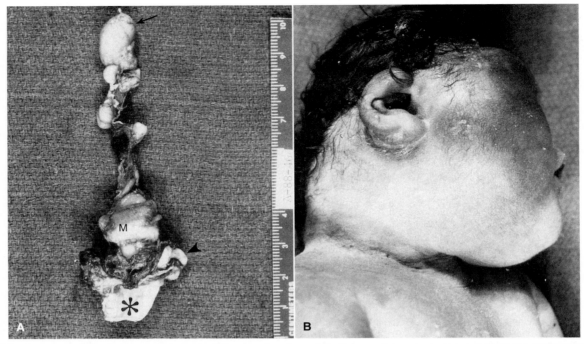

Figure 1-13   Aprosencephaly. A, Gross photograph of the dorsal surface of the intracranial contents showing near-total absence of prosence-phalon with rudimentary ball-like structures (*arrow*), cysts (the largest cyst was ruptured during fixation), malformed midbrain (M), and relatively normal-appearing lower brain stem (*medulla, asterisk*). The cerebellum is a vestigial remnant (*arrowhead*). **B,** Lateral view of the head in aprosen-cephaly. Note evidence of minimal cranial volume above the ears and supraorbital regions, as in anencephaly, but with normal hair and dermal covering. *(From Kim TS, Cho S, Dickson DW: Aprosencephaly: Review of the literature and report of a case with cerebellar hypoplasia, pigmented epithelial cyst and Rathke's cleft cyst,* Acta Neuropathol *79:424-431, 1990.)*

rostral end of a rudimentary brain stem (Fig. 1-13A). In *atelencephaly*, the anomaly is less severe in that the diencephalon is relatively preserved. When the telencephalon is absent and the diencephalon is only rudimentary, the term *atelencephalic aprosencephaly* has been used. The findings of calcific vasculopathy and calcification in the remaining neural tissue have led to the suggestion that, in some cases, these disorders may result from an encephaloclastic event shortly after neurulation. These anomalies are distinguishable from anencephaly most readily by the presence of an intact, although flattened, skull and intact scalp (Fig. 1-13B).

Timing. The disorders presumably have their origin no later than the onset of prosencephalic development at the beginning of the second month of gestation.

TABLE 1-22   Disorders of Prosencephalic Development
Prosencephalic Formation Atelencephaly/atelencephaly
Prosencephalic Cleavage Holoprosencephaly/holotelencephaly
Midline Prosencephalic Development Agenesis of corpus callosum Agenesis of septum pellucidum (with or without cerebral clefts) Septo-optic dysplasia Septo-optic–hypothalamic dysplasia

A slightly later time of origin may be operative in cases that appear to be related to a destructive process.

Clinical Aspects. Aprosencephaly-atelencephaly is characterized by a strikingly small cranium with little volume apparent above the supraorbital ridges (see Fig. 1-13B). However, as noted earlier, distinction from anencephaly is based easily on the intact skull and dermal covering. Facial anomalies (including cyclopia or absence of eyes) that bear similarities to those associated with holoprosencephaly (see later) are associated much more commonly with aprosencephaly than with atelencephaly. Similarly, anomalies of external genitalia and limbs are more common with aprosencephaly than with atelencephaly. Aprosencephaly is a lethal condition; most examples have been fetal specimens or involved patients who died in the neonatal period. Survival for approximately a year with little neurological function except breathing has been observed with atelencephaly.

Holoprosencephalies

Anatomical Abnormality. The holoprosencephalic-holotelencephalic group of disorders represents the next most severe derangements of prosencephalic development and specifically involves prosencephalic cleavage (see Table 1-22). In this category of disorders, the malformation of the forebrain may be so severe that there is marked disturbance of formation of both telencephalon and diencephalon; the term *holoprosencephaly* is most appropriate. The essential abnormality is a

Chapter 1 Neural Tube Formation and Prosencephalic Development

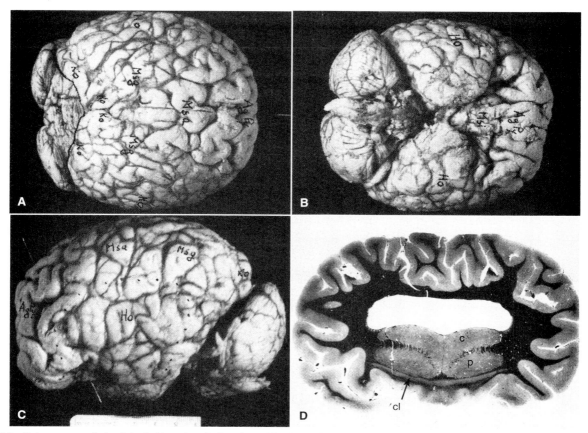

Figure 1-14 **Holoprosencephaly. A** to **D**, Note the single-sphered forebrain. **D**, Basal ganglia fused in the midline are caudate (c), putamen (p), and claustrum (cl). *(Courtesy of Dr. Paul Yakovlev.)*

failure of the horizontal, transverse, and sagittal cleavages of the prosencephalon. In the more common of the severe cases, in which the telencephalon remains as a single-sphered structure but the diencephalon is somewhat less affected, the term *holotelencephaly* may be more appropriate. In general, the term *holoprosencephaly* is used for the entire spectrum of cleavage disorders. Because the olfactory bulbs and tracts are nearly always absent in this category of disorders, the term *arrhinencephaly* has been used. Because the primary defect in these disorders is failure of prosencephalic development, and indeed the limbic structures representative of the rhinencephalon are present, the term *arrhinencephaly* is in fact a misnomer in these disorders and is best discarded.[335]

The *four major neuropathological varieties of holoprosencephaly* are distinguished principally according to the severity of the abnormality of cleavage of cerebral hemispheres and deep nuclear structures. The major neuropathological features of the most severe disturbance, appropriately characterized as *alobar holoprosencephaly*, include a single-sphered cerebral structure with a common ventricle, fusion of basal ganglia and thalamus, a membranous roof over the third ventricle that is often distended into a large cyst posteriorly, absence of the corpus callosum, as well as absence of the olfactory bulbs and tracts, and hypoplasia of the optic nerves or the presence of only a single optic nerve (Figs. 1-14 and 1-15).[2,66,81,340,346,347,351,365-378]

The cerebral cortex surrounding the single ventricle exhibits the cytoarchitecture of the hippocampus and other limbic structures, and the most striking abnormality is the essentially total failure of development of the supralimbic cortex, the hallmark of the human cerebrum (see Fig. 1-14).[335] The cortical mantle often shows heterotopias and other signs of subsequently disordered neuronal migration.[367,368,379] In *semilobar holoprosencephaly*, failure of separation of the anterior hemispheres with presence of a posterior portion of the interhemispheric fissure, less severe fusion of deep nuclear structures, and absence of the *anterior* portion of the corpus callosum (this finding is opposite of all other types of callosal hypoplasia, in which the posterior callosum is absent or deficient) are noted. In *lobar holoprosencephaly*, the cerebral hemispheres are nearly fully separated, deep nuclear structures are nearly or totally separated (by brain imaging), and the posterior callosum is well developed, although the anterior callosum may be somewhat underdeveloped. In the least severe, middle interhemispheric variant or *syntelencephaly*, only the posterior frontal and parietal regions fail to separate, and only the body of the corpus callosum is deficient. Microcephaly is present in the majority of infants with semilobar and lobar holoprosencephaly. Hydrocephalus is present in the majority of infants with alobar holoprosencephaly usually in association with the large dorsal cyst of the third ventricle, secondary

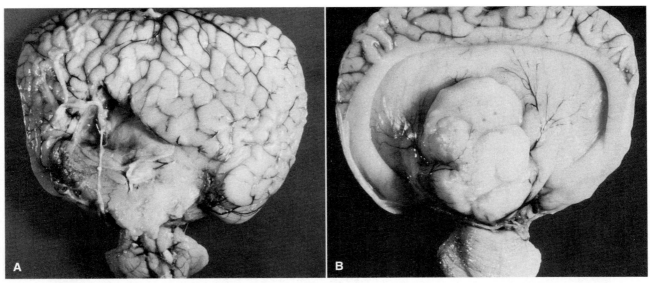

Figure 1-15 Holoprosencephaly. **A**, Dorsal view; note the single-sphered forebrain and membranous roof over the third ventricle that is distended into a posterior cyst. **B**, After removal of the cyst; note the exposed and fused thalami and basal ganglia in the midline.

to marked fusion of thalamus and impaired egress of CSF through the aqueduct.

Timing. Onset of the holoprosencephalies is no later than the fifth and sixth weeks of gestation. A particularly critical impaired event (i.e., the evagination of the cerebral hemispheres through sagittal cleavage of the prosencephalon) occurs at approximately 35 days of gestation.[2] The olfactory bulbs and tracts are not discernible until approximately 42 days of gestation, and thus the frequent absence of olfactory structures is understandable.

Clinical Aspects. The frequency of holoprosencephaly, which is distinctly less than that of the particularly common dysraphic disturbances discussed earlier, is approximately 1 in 10,000 live births.[66,351,365,371,374] The incidence is more than 60-fold greater in studies of aborted human embryos, a finding that indicates that most cases are eliminated prenatally.[371,380]

The *facial anomaly* in the most severe case is represented by a single median eye ("cyclops"), or even no eye at all, and a rudimentary nasal structure, the proboscis, often located above the midline orbit.[340,347,371,372,374,378,381] There may be no nasal structures at all. Less severe facial deformities include marked ocular hypotelorism with or without a proboscis (ethmocephalus) and ocular hypotelorism with a flat, single-nostril nose (cebocephaly [i.e., facial appearance of the *Cebus*]) (Figs. 1-16 and 1-17). Still less severe deformities include mild to moderate ocular hypotelorism (less commonly, ocular hypertelorism), a flat but double-nostril nose, and median cleft lip and palate, often with an absent philtrum and similar features with bilateral cleft lip and palate.[371,372,374] In the least affected cases, the facial deformity may be difficult to detect, or indeed there may be no facial deformity at all. The cases with the most severe facial malformations are consistently associated with severe

holoprosencephaly, but the converse is not true; alobar holoprosencephaly is unassociated with significant facial abnormality in approximately 10% of cases.[374] Abnormalities of other organ systems occur in approximately 75% of cases of holoprosencephaly and consist primarily of disturbances of cardiac, skeletal, genitourinary, and gastrointestinal development, understandable in view of the similar time periods of rapid development.[2]

The *neurological features* in the most severe cases are obvious from the neonatal period. Infants exhibit frequent apneic spells, stimulus-sensitive tonic spasms, various abnormalities of hypothalamic function (e.g., poikilothermia, diabetes insipidus, or inappropriate antidiuretic hormone secretion), and virtually total failure of neurological development.[351,365,371,372,379,382-385] Seizures occur in a large minority, and especially in infants with cytogenetic abnormalities, the most severe forms of holoprosencephaly result in death in the first year. However, prolonged survival is common with the less severe forms of holoprosencephaly. Subsequent neurological deficits relate to the nature of the neuropathological features.[351,365,376,386] The degree of failure of cerebral cleavage correlates with the cognitive deficits, hypothalamic cleavage with the endocrinopathies, and basal ganglia and thalamic cleavage with dystonia and impaired motor function. Still less severely affected children may escape clinical detection until later in infancy or childhood.[340,351,365,371,372,376-388] Ultrasound scan provides useful information in the neonatal period regarding the nature and extent of the maldevelopment (Fig. 1-18). MRI is most valuable (Fig. 1-19).

Etiology: Genetic Considerations. Causes of holoprosencephaly include chromosomal abnormalities, monogenic syndromic disorders, monogenic nonsyndromic disorders, and effects of teratogens (Table 1-23). The relative distribution of these causes varies

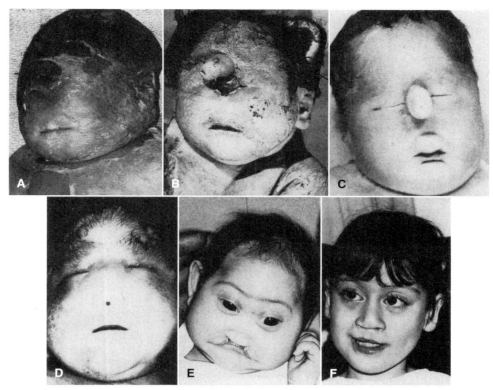

Figure 1-16   Spectrum of dysmorphic faces associated with variable degrees of holoprosencephaly. A, Cyclopia without proboscis formation. Note the single central eye. **B**, Cyclopia with proboscis. **C**, Ethmocephaly. Ocular hypotelorism with the proboscis located between the eyes. **D**, Cebocephaly. Ocular hypotelorism with a single-nostril nose. **E**, Median cleft lip, flat nose, and ocular hypotelorism. **F**, Ocular hypotelorism and surgically repaired cleft lip. *(From Cohen MM Jr: Perspectives on holoprosencephaly. I. Epidemiology, genetics, and syndromology, Teratology 40:211-235, 1989.)*

considerably with the method of case ascertainment, but the following discussion represents a general consensus of available data. Approximately 60% of cases of holo-prosencephaly are related to *chromosomal disorders*, and trisomy 13 accounts for approximately one half of these (see Table 1-23).[347,351,374] Six chromosomal regions, involving chromosomes 2,3,7,13,18, or 21, have been implicated in holoprosencephaly.[340,347,374] Holoprosencephaly is particularly characteristic of

trisomy 13.[340,347,351,371,372,374,389,390] The disorder also has been observed with 10% mosaicism of trisomy 13 and with deletion 13 and ring 13.[371,372,383,389-391] Additional chromosomal abnormalities have involved chromosome 18 in particular, as well as chromosomes 2, 3, 7, and 21.[340,347,371-374,383,389-397]

Monogenic multiple malformation syndromes account for approximately 25% of cases (see Table 1-23).[74,351,398] Particularly noteworthy is the relationship with

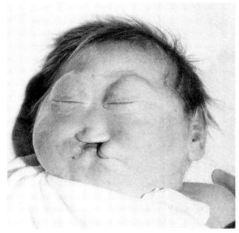

Figure 1-17   Newborn with holoprosencephaly. Note the ocular hypotelorism, flat, single-nostril nose, and severe median cleft lip and palate. *(Courtesy of Dr. Marvin Fishman.)*

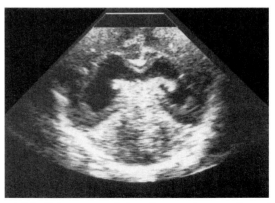

Figure 1-18   Holoprosencephaly, ultrasound scan. Coronal scan shows a single ventricle straddling fused thalami in the midline. The mushroom-shaped structures extending into the ventricle from the medial surfaces are choroid plexus. *(Courtesy of Dr. Gary D. Shackelford.)*

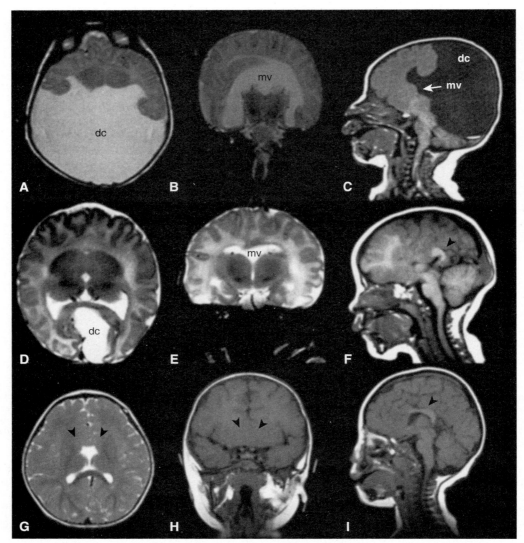

Figure 1-19 **A** to **C**, **Magnetic resonance imaging (MRI) of a newborn with alobar holoprosencephaly (HPE).** Axial T2-weighted image (**A**) demonstrates failure of separation of the two hemispheres and thalami, and a large dorsal cyst (dc). Coronal T2-weighted image (**B**) shows a continuity of gray matter in the midline without an interhemispheric fissure. The ventricular system is composed of a single midline monoventricle (mv). Sagittal T1-weighted image (**C**) shows absence of the corpus callosum and a monoventricle that communicates with the dorsal cyst. **D** to **F**, MRI of a 3-year-old patient with *semilobar* HPE. Axial T2-weighted image (**D**) shows absence of interhemispheric fissure anteriorly. The posterior hemispheres are well separated, and the posterior horns of the lateral ventricles are well formed. A dorsal cyst is present (dc). Coronal T2-weighted image (**E**) of the same patient shows a monoventricle (mv) and partial nonseparation of the thalamic nuclei. A sagittal T1-weighted image (**F**) of a different patient with semilobar HPE demonstrates absence of the genu and body of the corpus callosum, but presence of the splenium (*arrowhead*). **G** to **I**, MRI of a 16-month-old infant with *lobar* HPE. Axial T2-weighted image (**G**) shows cerebral hemispheres that are fairly well separated both anteriorly and posteriorly. The fontal horns are underdeveloped (*arrowheads*). Coronal T1-weighted image (**H**) shows failure of complete separation of the frontal lobes with continuity of gray matter in the inferior frontal regions (*arrowheads*). A sagittal T1-weighted image (**I**) demonstrates that the body and splenium of the corpus callosum are present (*arrowhead*), but the genu is not developed. *(From Hahn JS, Barkovich AJ, Stashinko EE, Kinsman SL, et al: Factor analysis of neuroanatomical and clinical characteristics of holoprosencephaly,* Brain Dev *28:413-419, 2006.)*

Smith-Lemli-Opitz syndrome, a disorder of cholesterol biosynthesis, in view of the importance of cholesterol for the sonic hedgehog signaling pathway (see earlier discussion). These syndromic disorders are inherited as autosomal recessive (Smith-Lemli-Opitz syndrome, pseudotrisomy 13, Meckel syndrome) or autosomal dominant (Pallister-Hall syndrome, velocardiofacial syndrome) traits.

Monogenic nonsyndromic disorders account for approximately 15% to 20% of cases of holoprosencephaly (see Table 1-23). The genes discussed earlier regarding prosencephalic development have been implicated.

The most common (37%) of these involve sonic hedgehog and autosomal dominant inheritance.* In the autosomal dominant cases, considerable intrafamilial variability of the phenotype can occur. Parents may exhibit such relatively inconspicuous features as hypotelorism, iris coloboma, hyposmia, single maxillary central incisor (Fig. 1-20), absent frenulum, microcephaly, or mild cognitive deficits. *Clearly, careful examination of the parents (and other family members) is essential.*

---

*See references 340,345,347,351,371,372,383,392,393,398-405.

TABLE 1-23	Etiological Background of Holoprosencephaly*

Chromosomal
Chromosome 13: trisomy 13 ring 13, deletion 13
Chromosome 18: trisomy 18, ring 18, deletion 18
Chromosomes 2,3,7,21: deletions, trisomies

Monogenic Syndromic
Smith-Lemli-Opitz
Pseudotrisomy 13
Pallister-Hall
Meckel
Velocardiofacial

Monogenic Nonsyndromic
SHH
PTCH
GLI2
TGIF
TDGF1
FAST1
Z1C2

Teratogenic Agents
Maternal diabetes
Others
Sporadic

*See text for references.

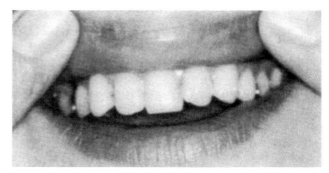

Figure 1-20 Autosomal dominant holoprosencephaly. Mother of an infant with alobar holoprosencephaly. Note the single central maxillary incisor. Computed tomography scan of mother was normal, and she had normal intelligence. *(From Hennekam RCM, Van Noort G, de la Fuente FA, Norbruis OF: Agenesis of the nasal septal cartilage: Another sign in autosomal dominant holoprosencephaly, Am J Med Genet 39:121-122, 1991.)*

Teratogenic influences can be operative although the extent of their role in origin requires further study. Holoprosencephaly occurs in as many as 1% to 2% of infants of diabetic mothers, including gestational diabetics.[351,371,372,406] Moreover, the occurrence of holoprosencephaly in lambs born to ewes that ingested a toxic plant alkaloid raises the possibility of environmental etiological factors.[407] Because this alkaloid appears to alter cholesterol metabolism, and as noted earlier, cholesterol is involved in sonic hedgehog signaling crucial for forebrain development, a pathogenetic mechanism is suggested.[345-347] Whether agents that perturb cholesterol biosynthesis (e.g., statin drugs) play an etiological role remains to be established.

Holoprosencephaly has been reported in infants with prenatal exposure to antiepileptic drugs, alcohol, retinoic acid, and cytomegalovirus infection, but the extent of the role of these factors in origin remains unclear.[351] Prenatal diagnosis of holoprosencephaly, including the more severe types of accompanying facial anomalies, can be made by ultrasonography.[408-410] Detection of chromosomal abnormalities or genetic mutations by preimplantation diagnosis has been reported.[411]

Disorders of Midline Prosencephalic Development

The principal disorders of midline prosencephalic development are considered best in terms of the normal events centered around the commissural, chiasmatic, and hypothalamic plates. The specific disorders observed according to the plate most affected are shown in Table 1-24. The abnormalities of midline prosencephalic development can be considered the least severe of the spectrum of abnormalities of prosencephalic development (Fig. 1-21). These midline disorders are discussed best in two broad categories: abnormalities of corpus callosum and of septum pellucidum.

Anatomical Abnormality. *Agenesis of the corpus callosum,* complete or partial, is a striking abnormality (Fig. 1-22).[336,337,337a,337b,412-417] The superomedial aspects of the lateral ventricles are deformed by the fibers of the cerebral hemispheres that were destined to cross in the corpus callosum and that, with agenesis, instead course longitudinally as the bundles of Probst (Fig. 1-22B). With partial agenesis, the posterior portion is nearly always affected. (A notable exception is the anterior involvement that occurs when partial agenesis is associated with the holoprosencephalies.[373]) Agenesis of the corpus callosum in *selected* series, identified by MRI scan, has been associated with other brain anomalies in most cases[337,337a,337b,412,413,417-419a]; the most commonly associated anomalies are the Chiari II malformation, cerebellar vermian hypoplasia, and disorders of neuronal migration (see Chapter 2). In three large series, approximately 25% to 45% of cases were accompanied by migrational disorder.[413,417,418]

TABLE 1-24	Disorders of Midline Prosencephalic Development	
Region Affected		**Disorder**
Commissural plate		Agenesis of corpus callosum and/or septum pellucidum
Commissural and chiasmatic plates		Septo-optic dysplasia
Commissural, chiasmatic, and hypothalamic plates		Septo-optic–hypothalamic dysplasia

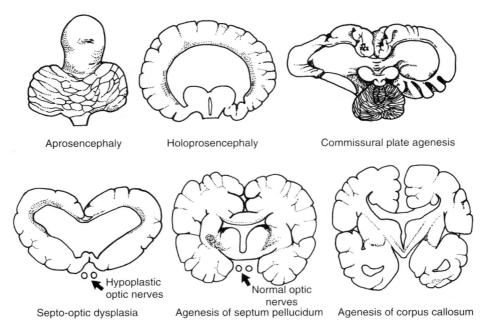

Aprosencephaly   Holoprosencephaly   Commissural plate agenesis

Hypoplastic optic nerves
Septo-optic dysplasia

Normal optic nerves
Agenesis of septum pellucidum

Agenesis of corpus callosum

Figure 1-21 **Schematic depiction of the spectrum of defects of prosencephalic development.** *(From Leech RW, Shuman RM: Holoprosencephaly and related cerebral midline anomalies: A review, J Child Neurol 1:3-18, 1986.)*

The association with disorders of neuronal migration may relate to the finding that callosal development and neuronal migration occur concurrently in human brain development.

Absence of the septum pellucidum, like agenesis of the corpus callosum, is an important clue to the presence of other, clinically more serious abnormalities of prosencephalic development or of concomitant developmental events (e.g., neuronal migration).[336,420-438] In addition, the septum pellucidum can be destroyed by concomitant hydrocephalus or by contiguous ischemic lesions (e.g., porencephaly). Thus, it is understandable that in one large MRI series of absence of the septum pellucidum, this anomaly was never seen as an isolated finding; it was associated with holoprosencephaly, agenesis of the corpus callosum, septo-optic dysplasia, schizencephaly, basilar encephalocele, hydrocephalus (as a result of aqueductal stenosis or the Chiari II malformation), and porencephaly-hydranencephaly.[412]

One prominent example of these disorders is the *syndrome of absence of septum pellucidum with schizencephaly* (often mistakenly termed *porencephaly*) (Fig. 1-23 and Table 1-25).[412,421,425-428,430,436,439]

Minor disturbances of development of the septum pellucidum (i.e., cavum septi pellucidi) have a slight association with later cognitive deficits.[423,424,431,432,440] Thus, when the two leaves of the septum pellucidum fail to fuse as the fetal brain matures, so-called *cavum septi pellucidi* results. This finding is clearly abnormal only after the neonatal period because all premature infants exhibit an ultrasonographically demonstrable cavum up to 34 weeks of gestation, and 36% of term infants still have a small (mean, 0.5 cm) cavum.[424,441] Nevertheless, a large cavum septi pellucidi (>1 cm) in a term newborn should be viewed with suspicion, although previous suggestions of a relatively high association with subsequent cognitive deficits appear to be related largely to selection bias.[440]

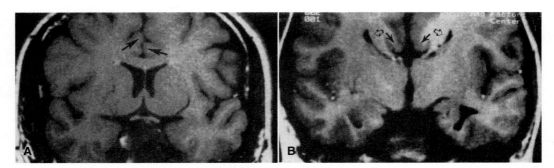

Figure 1-22 **Agenesis of the corpus callosum, coronal magnetic resonance imaging scans. A,** Normally inverted cingulate gyri (*arrows*) with normal corpus callosum. **B,** Everted cingulate gyri (*solid arrows*) with complete agenesis of corpus callosum. Inversion of the cingulate gyrus results from normal callosal formation; everted cingulate gyri are therefore a sign of callosal dysgenesis. Crescentic lateral ventricles (*open arrows*) result from the impression of medial ventricular wall by longitudinally oriented callosal bundles (i.e., Probst bundles). *(From Barkovich AJ, Norman D: Anomalies of the corpus callosum: Correlation with further anomalies of the brain, AJNR Am J Neuroradiol 9:493-501, 1988.)*

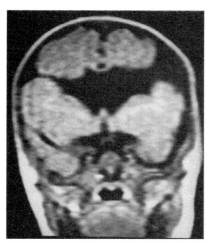

Figure 1-23 Agenesis of the septum pellucidum with schizencephaly. Coronal magnetic resonance imaging scan shows complete absence of the septum pellucidum and bilateral schizencephalic clefts in a 2-month-old infant who had neonatal seizures.

Timing. Agenesis of the corpus callosum has its origin no later than 9 to 20 weeks of gestation, peak time of development of this structure (see earlier). Because the posterior portion is the last portion to form, it is perhaps understandable that partial agenesis affects posterior components and that the relevant developmental disturbance for partial agenesis occurs later during callosal development than the disturbance for complete agenesis.

Agenesis of the septum pellucidum has its origin no later than approximately the end of the period for formation of the corpus callosum (i.e., ≈20 weeks of gestation). This structure develops during formation of the corpus callosum, in the medial inferior aspect of the commissural plate,[442] and the corpus callosum is completed first. The timing of minor abnormalities of the septum pellucidum (e.g., cavum) clearly is much later, because the rostral-caudal process of fusion of the two leaves of the septum does not commence until near the time of birth.

Clinical Aspects. *Agenesis of the corpus callosum* without other recognized abnormality of the CNS can be asymptomatic or can at least necessitate sophisticated neuropsychological tests of interhemispheric processing to detect an abnormality.[413,414,443-445] Most cases reported in hospital-based or clinic-based series are associated with other anomalies of the nervous system,[337,412-415,417,418,446,447] principally Chiari II malformation (with myelomeningocele and characteristic brain stem anomaly), cerebellar vermian hypoplasia, encephalocele (basilar type [i.e., frontonasal or sphenoid]), more severe defect of prosencephalic development (holoprosencephaly), or anomaly of neuronal migration (schizencephaly, lissencephaly, pachygyria, polymicrogyria, marked neuronal heterotopias). Not surprisingly, the neurological features of large *hospital-based* series of infants and children with agenesis (complete or partial) of the corpus callosum are not subtle. In one study (n = 63), 85% had cognitive deficits, and more than 90% had neuromotor disturbances.[418] Rarely, massive dorsal cystic expansion of the third ventricle occurs and produces hydrocephalus.[416,448,449] The associated anomalies determine the major features of the clinical syndrome. Important examples of the more than 50 syndromes associated with agenesis or hypoplasia of the corpus callosum include autosomal recessive disorders (Walker-Warburg syndrome, Fukuyama muscular dystrophy, Joubert syndrome, Andermann syndrome, Meckel syndrome), autosomal dominant disorders (familial septo-optic dysplasia, Sotos syndrome, Rubinstein-Taybi syndrome, lissencephaly type 1 [LISI], X-linked lissencephaly with ambiguous genitalia [XLAG], X-linked lissencephaly [XLIS], hydrocephalus due to stenosis of the aqueduct of Sylvius [HSAS], Aicardi syndrome [see next paragraph]), and metabolic disorders (nonketotic hyperglycinemia, pyruvate dehydrogenase complex deficiency, fumarase deficiency).

One important disorder characterized by agenesis of the corpus callosum in female infants, not discussed elsewhere in this book, is the *Aicardi syndrome*.[450-461] Agenesis of the corpus callosum, with chorioretinal lacunae and female gender, is a hallmark of the syndrome (Table 1-26). The neurological features (e.g., infantile spasms, other seizures, and cognitive deficits) are related principally to accompanying defects of neuronal migration. These consist primarily of periventricular neuronal heterotopias and polymicrogyria. At least 80% of affected infants subsequently exhibit severe mental retardation. The disorder is believed to be an X-linked dominant, male-lethal mutation, and the moderate degree of phenotypic variability appears to be related to nonrandom X-inactivation.[450]

TABLE 1-25	Syndrome of Absence of Septum Pellucidum with Schizencephaly*
Neuropathology	
Absence of septum pellucidum	
Cerebral cleft: unilateral (60%), narrow (75%), associated with primary fissures	
Heterotopias	
Gyral abnormalities	
Clinical	
Hemiparesis-quadriparesis (80%)	
Seizures (50%)	
Mental retardation (50%); normal cognition (15%)	

*See text for references. Numbers are rounded off.

TABLE 1-26	Aicardi Syndrome: Major Features
Female preponderance	
Chorioretinal lacunae	
Agenesis of corpus callosum: complete, 70%; partial, 30%	
Infantile spasms	
Cerebral cortical polymicrogyria	
Cerebral neuronal heterotopias	
Intracranial cysts (interhemispheric or in vicinity of third ventricle)	
Costovertebral defects	

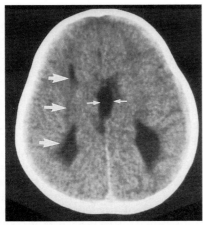

Figure 1-24 **Agenesis of the corpus callosum.** Computed tomography scan in a 14-day-old infant shows a midline, superiorly displaced third ventricle (*small arrows*) visible on this high cut between abnormally straight lateral ventricles (*large arrows*).

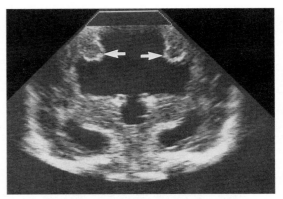

Figure 1-26 **Agenesis of the corpus callosum.** Coronal ultrasound scan shows absence of the corpus callosum and presence of Probst longitudinal callosal bundles indenting the dorsomedial aspect of the lateral ventricles (*arrows*).

Although easily identified by MRI or CT scan (see Fig. 1-22; Fig. 1-24), agenesis of the corpus callosum also is identified readily in the newborn by ultrasonography.[462,463] Characteristic features on sagittal views are elevation of the third ventricle, radial orientation of gyri (instead of the normal horizontal orientation) producing a "sunburst" appearance (Fig. 1-25), and, on coronal views, widely separated frontal horns, concave medial border, and Probst bundles (Fig. 1-26). Identification of agenesis of the corpus callosum, in my opinion, is an indication for MRI to evaluate the possibility of associated neuronal migrational disturbance.

The clinical features of *absence of septum pellucidum*, as with agenesis of the corpus callosum, depend principally on the associated disorders (see the earlier discussion of anatomical abnormality). In general, the associated disorders are detected best by MRI. Table 1-25 lists the clinical features of one of the more prominent of these disorders (i.e., absence of septum pellucidum with schizencephaly). The most crucial aspect of the neuropathology in this disorder, the schizencephalic cerebral cleft, may not be apparent

on CT scan; MRI is critical in the evaluation. One report has identified a patient with mitochondrial complex III deficiency.[433] A rare autosomal recessive form has been shown to be related to a mutation in a homeobox gene, *HESX1*, crucial for development of forebrain, eyes, and pituitary gland.[439] One series emphasized the association of craniofacial dysmorphisms, brain abnormalities (callosal agenesis, schizencephaly, heterotopias), and endocrinopathies.[438]

The clinical features of septo-optic dysplasia are most apparent after the neonatal period. In addition to optic nerve hypoplasia and associated visual deficit, disturbances of hypothalamic-pituitary function are common.[428,430,435,437,438,464] In one selected series of infants referred to an endocrine clinic, approximately 60% exhibited diabetes insipidus, 80% had multiple pituitary hormone deficiencies, 60% had genitalia anomalies resulting from hypogonadotrophic hypogonadism, and, importantly, 75% had persistent *neonatal hypoglycemia*.[435] In a large selected series of children with optic nerve hypoplasia reported from a pediatric ophthalmology clinic, although only a minority had absence of septum pellucidum, fully 72% had endocrinopathy, especially disturbances of growth hormone homeostasis.[437] Indeed, optic nerve hypoplasia and septo-optic dysplasia should be considered on

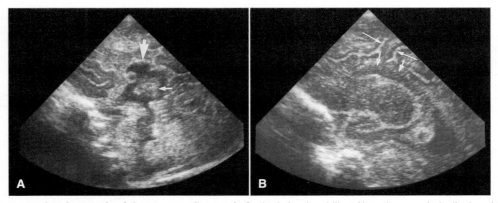

Figure 1-25 **Ultrasonography of agenesis of the corpus callosum. A,** Sagittal view in midline. Note the superiorly displaced third ventricle (*large arrow*). Massa intermedia (*small arrow*) is visible within third ventricle. **B,** Parasagittal view. Note the medial cortical sulci radiating superiorly (*long arrows*) instead of horizontally and the absence of the normally echogenic pericallosal sulcus (*short arrows*).

TABLE 1-27	Major Causes of Hydrocephalus Overt at Birth in 127 Cases	
Cause	**Percentage (%)**
Aqueductal stenosis	33
Myelomeningocele: Chiari type II malformation	28
"Communicating" hydrocephalus	22
Dandy-Walker malformation	7
Other	10

Data from Mealey J Jr, Gilmor RL, Bubb MP: The prognosis of hydrocephalus overt at birth, *J Neurosurg* 39:348-355, 1973; and McCullough DC, Balzer-Martin LA: Current prognosis in overt neonatal hydrocephalus, *J Neurosurg* 57:378-383, 1982.

a continuum of a heterogeneous group of disorders of midline development. Thus, these disorders, related to defective development of the commissural and chiasmatic plates, often also involve the hypothalamic plate. Moreover, seizure disorders and cognitive deficits, perhaps related to accompanying errors in neuronal migration, also may occur. Clearly, the clinical aspects of these several disorders of midline prosencephalic development (see Table 1-24) overlap and merge with the clinical features of migrational defects discussed in Chapter 2.

CONGENITAL HYDROCEPHALUS: FETAL AND NEONATAL

Congenital hydrocephalus refers to a state of progressive ventricular enlargement apparent from the first days of life and, by implication, with onset in utero. In the following discussion, fetal hydrocephalus and neonatal hydrocephalus are distinguished on the basis of the time of diagnosis of the hydrocephalus, and the conditions are considered separately. The information provided concerning hydrocephalus identified in utero by ultrasonography and MRI (i.e., fetal hydrocephalus) is based on review of approximately 650 previously reported cases,[76,465-488] as well as approximately 30 personal (unpublished) cases. Concerning hydrocephalus identified initially at birth or the first few days of life, information is based on approximately 370 previously reported cases,[489-494] as well as approximately 35 personal (unpublished) cases.

Discussion of congenital hydrocephalus is pertinent to this chapter because, although the cause is heterogeneous, most cases appear to be disorders in development of the brain and its CSF circulatory system. Moreover, the critical timing of the development of the CSF pathways occurs in close proximity to the events of development just discussed.

Anatomical Abnormalities

Abnormalities anywhere in the CSF pathway from formation in the choroid plexus to absorption in the arachnoidal villi can cause hydrocephalus of intrauterine onset. Indeed, the *spectrum of causes* varies somewhat, according to the selection bias of the reported

series (i.e., whether identified in utero or in the immediate postnatal period).

The major causes of *neonatal* hydrocephalus, as identified in two large series conducted in neonatal neurosurgical services, are presented in Table 1-27.[489,490] In these studies, aqueductal stenosis accounted for approximately one third of cases. Although most examples of aqueductal stenosis are nonfamilial, an X-linked variety associated with adducted thumbs and, commonly, agenesis of the corpus callosum is important to recognize because of its consistent relationship with subsequent mental retardation.[495] This disorder has been shown to be related to a mutation in the neural cell adhesion molecule, L1CAM.[495-499] Additional genetic varieties of aqueductal stenosis included autosomal recessive inheritance, with a normal phenotype, and X-linked or autosomal recessive inheritance with the VACTERL association (vertebral anomalies, anal atresia, cardiovascular anomalies, tracheoesophageal fistula, renal dysplasia, limb defects).[500] Myelomeningocele with the Chiari type II malformation, "communicating" hydrocephalus, and the Dandy-Walker malformation accounted for most of the remaining cases of neonatal hydrocephalus. Much less common is hydrocephalus as a result of intrauterine infection (e.g., toxoplasmosis and cytomegalovirus; see Chapter 20), tumor (e.g., choroid plexus papilloma; see Chapter 23), (intrauterine) intraventricular hemorrhage, and malformation of the vein of Galen (see Chapter 23).

The distribution of major causes of hydrocephalus identified in utero (i.e., *fetal* hydrocephalus) is different from the distribution reported for neonatal cases (Table 1-28).[76,465-471,473-486,488] Thus, the most common cause is holoprosencephaly (with or without myelomeningocele), a disorder with a poor outcome because of the disturbance of prosencephalic development. The other causes are generally similar to those of neonatal hydrocephalus. However, with fetal hydrocephalus, the severity of the hydrocephalus tends to be greater. Moreover, myelomeningocele associated with fetal hydrocephalus tends to be large. Overall, the incidence of serious associated brain anomalies in fetal hydrocephalus is generally approximately 60% to 70%. These anomalies have major implications with respect to outcome and management (see later).

Timing

In view of the heterogeneity of causes of congenital hydrocephalus, definition of a single time of onset of the disorder is not possible. However, the most important developmental processes in this context occur at approximately 6 to 10 weeks of gestation.[2,501,502] Specifically, at this time, three events critical for the development of the CSF pathways occur: (1) development of the secretory epithelium in the choroid plexus, (2) perforation of the roof of the fourth ventricle, and (3) formation of the subarachnoid spaces. Impairments of the last two processes bear a relationship with the genesis of the hydrocephalus associated with the Dandy-Walker malformation and communicating

TABLE 1-28	Major Causes of Fetal Hydrocephalus (n = 38)		
Cause		**Percentage (%)**	**Mean DQ/IQ**
Holoprosencephaly		45	
with myelomeningocele		27	48
without myelomeningocele		18	42
Myelomeningocele (isolated)		25	75
Dandy-Walker malformation		10	66
X-linked hydrocephalus		10	10
"Primary" hydrocephalus		10	60

DQ, development quotient; IQ, intelligence quotient.
Data from Futagi Y, Suzuki Y, Toribe Y, Morimoto K: Neurodevelopmental outcome in children with fetal hydrocephalus, *Pediatr Neurol* 27:111-116, 2002.

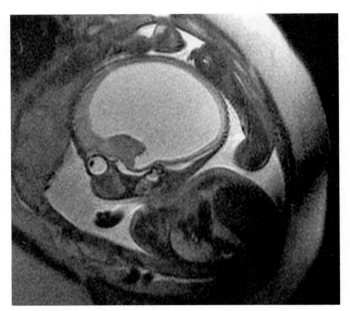

Figure 1-27   Fetal hydrocephalus at 31 weeks of gestation: intrauterine magnetic resonance imaging scan. The fetus is in the breech position. Note the marked ventriculomegaly. Other views showed aqueductal stenosis and partial agenesis of the corpus callosum. *(Courtesy of Dr. Omar Khwaja.)*

hydrocephalus. The critical timing for hydrocephalus with holoprosencephaly is during this exact period (see discussion of holoprosencephaly earlier). The key timing for development of aqueductal stenosis is probably later (i.e., between 15 and 17 weeks of gestation, the period of rapid elongation of the mesencephalon and evolution of the normal constriction of the aqueduct).[465] Similar timing may be appropriate for the hydrocephalus associated with the Chiari malformation and myelomeningocele, because aqueductal stenosis is a common cause of the disturbance in CSF dynamics (see earlier). Clearly, of course, the inflammatory processes that cause intrauterine onset of hydrocephalus (e.g., toxoplasmosis) develop still later as a consequence of the derangement in CSF flow or absorption resulting from the associated ependymitis and arachnoiditis.

Clinical Features

In *neonatal hydrocephalus*, the clinical presentation (i.e., markedly enlarged head, full anterior fontanelle, and separated cranial sutures) is similar to, although more severe than, that described for the later postnatal development of hydrocephalus with myelomeningocele (see earlier). Careful neonatal assessment should be made for signs of specific etiological types of congenital hydrocephalus, such as the flexion deformity of the thumbs characteristic of approximately 50% of cases of X-linked aqueductal stenosis,[383,493,496-499,503-505] the occipital cranial prominence of the Dandy-Walker formation, and the chorioretinitis of intrauterine infection by toxoplasmosis or cytomegalovirus. Serial assessments of neurological status, rate of head growth, signs of increased intracranial pressure, and ventricular size (by cranial ultrasonography) are of particular value in documenting the severity and rapidity of progression of the hydrocephalic process. A careful assessment of the cerebral parenchyma by MRI is valuable for detection of the size of the cerebral mantle, associated anomalies of the cerebrum (e.g., disorder of neuronal migration), evidence of parenchymal destruction (e.g., calcification, cysts), and likely sites of

disturbance of CSF dynamics (based on topographical distribution of ventricular dilation).

The widespread use of intrauterine ultrasonography has led increasingly to the diagnosis of *fetal hydrocephalus*.[75,466-474,476-486,488,506-510] Before 24 weeks of gestation, the ventricles dilate with usually no change in biparietal diameter, and not until after 32 to 34 weeks of gestation does head growth consistently increase with progression of ventricular dilation. The most prominent additional clinical features are the occurrence of major extraneural anomalies in 40% to 50% of cases of fetal hydrocephalus, major CNS anomalies in 60% to 70%, and extraneural or CNS anomalies (or both) in 80%. These anomalies have a dominant effect on outcome (see the following section). MRI is most effective for assessment of fetal hydrocephalus and associated CNS anomalies (Fig. 1-27).

Management and Outcome

Management of infants with *neonatal hydrocephalus* (i.e., hydrocephalus overt at birth) should begin, as in other infants with major neurological diseases, with the same question: How could this have been prevented? Indeed, the advent of intrauterine diagnosis by ultrasonography has raised the possibilities of delivery of the infant before marked progression of the disorder and perhaps even of intrauterine treatment (see later). When the hydrocephalus is discovered at the time of delivery, however, the decision about how to treat the infant is obviously made after birth. In earlier years, available data suggested a very unfavorable outlook for affected infants,[489] but later experience indicated a considerable improvement in prognosis with modern neurosurgery[490] and reason for a more aggressive program of intervention.

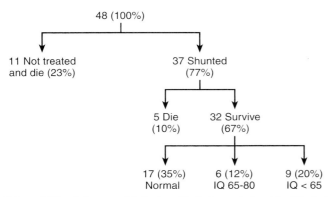

48 (100%)

11 Not treated
and die (23%)

37 Shunted
(77%)

5 Die
(10%)

32 Survive
(67%)

17 (35%)
Normal

6 (12%)
IQ 65-80

9 (20%)
IQ < 65

Figure 1-28 Outcome of infants with hydrocephalus identified at birth. Data are derived from study of 48 infants. Percentage figures in parentheses are proportions of the total group of 48. IQ, intelligence quotient. *(From McCullough DC, Balzer-Martin LA: Current prognosis in overt neonatal hydrocephalus,* J Neurosurg *57:378-383, 1982.)*

This improvement relates in large part to better neonatal intensive care and neurosurgical techniques. Of 48 infants reported by McCullough and Balzer-Martin,[490] 11 were not treated, primarily because of severe neural tube defects, and died; 37 (77%) underwent shunt placement at an average age of 11 weeks (Fig. 1-28). Of the 37 infants with shunts, 86% survived. On follow-up of these survivors, 17 (46%) were normal, 6 (16%) had an IQ between 65 and 80, and 9 (24%) had an IQ less than 65. Thus, of the total group of 48 infants, only approximately one third exhibited normal intelligence. The most decisive predictors of favorable outcome were the size of the cerebral mantle before shunt placement and the origin of the hydrocephalus. Of the four major etiological categories (see Table 1-27), the mean IQ was highest for infants with communicating hydrocephalus (score of 109) and myelomeningocele (score of 108), and lowest for infants with aqueductal stenosis (score of 71) and Dandy-Walker malformation (score of 45). The poorer outlook in the last two categories may relate to associated cerebral abnormalities, especially with the Dandy-Walker malformation, consisting primarily of cerebral neuronal migrational defects and agenesis of the corpus callosum (see the following

section on posterior fossa CSF collections).[383,491,511-513] Later data from the same institution showed a somewhat improved outcome; 43% of infants evaluated at birth with hydrocephalus were normal on follow-up.[483] The relatively favorable results in this population of infants with hydrocephalus overt at birth (see Fig. 1-28) led to the conclusion that the infant with neonatal hydrocephalus should receive a ventriculoperitoneal shunt "except in extreme instances (severe birth defects and minimal cerebral tissue)."[490] The difficulty of using even the amount of cerebral tissue as a major criterion and the remarkable ability of neonatal hydrocephalic brain to reconstitute its cerebral mantle after ventricular decompression are illustrated by the patient whose CT scans are shown in Figure 1-29. Indeed, rapid recovery from cortical visual impairment following correction of prolonged shunt malfunction (many months) in infants with congenital hydrocephalus attests to the potential plasticity of hydrocephalic brain.[514]

Rational management of *fetal ventricular dilation* necessitates understanding of the natural history.[75,466-480,482-486,488,491,506-508,510,515] In one carefully studied series of 47 infants with fetal ventriculomegaly, 54% of the original group died in utero, primarily because of elective termination provoked by the finding of serious neural or extraneural anomalies or both (Fig. 1-30).[471] Of the 22 survivors, only 2 clearly exhibited unequivocal progression of ventriculomegaly in utero; these infants were delivered vaginally and developed normally after ventriculoperitoneal shunt. Of the 19 infants who had stable ventriculomegaly, 9 exhibited signs after delivery of increased intracranial pressure and underwent placement of a ventriculoperitoneal shunt. The 3 infants in this series who had subsequent neurological deficits had associated anomalies. Indeed, *all infants with subsequent neurological deficits had anomalies.* Thus, of the surviving newborns, 64% were normal on follow-up, and none of these had anomalies. Clearly, the poorer outcome in fetal hydrocephalus compared with neonatal hydrocephalus relates to the associated anomalies. This principle is illustrated by the more recent observations summarized in Table 1-28.[486]

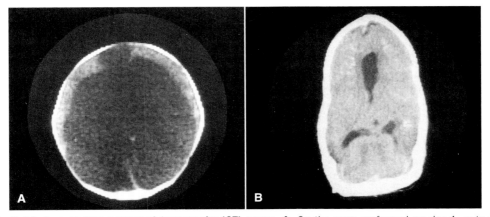

Figure 1-29 Congenital hydrocephalus: computed tomography (CT) scans. A, On the scan performed on day 1, note the essentially total absence of recognizable cerebral mantle in the occipital region and extreme attenuation of the mantle anteriorly. **B,** CT scan at 12 months (11 months after placement of ventriculoperitoneal shunt). Note the marked increase in thickness of the cerebral mantle.

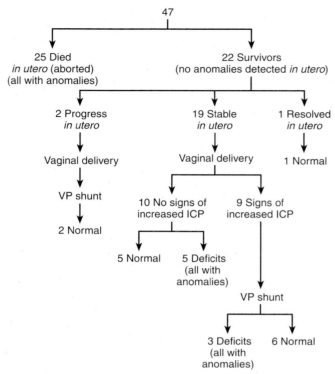

Figure 1-30 **Outcome of infants with ventriculomegaly identified in utero.** Data are derived from study of 47 fetuses. ICP, intracranial pressure; VP, ventriculoperitoneal. *(Data from Hudgins RJ, Edwards MS, Goldstein R, et al: Natural history of fetal ventriculomegaly,* Pediatrics *82:692-697, 1988).*

This discussion of fetal hydrocephalus excludes those cases that exhibit *isolated mild fetal ventriculomegaly. Ventriculomegaly* is defined as an axial diameter greater than 10 mm across the atrium of the posterior or anterior of the lateral ventricles.[510] (The normal atrial diameter is constant at a mean of 7.6 ± 0.6 mm from 14 to 38 weeks of gestation.) Fetal hydrocephalus is present at diameters greater than 15 mm; isolated fetal ventriculomegaly is the term used for diameters of 10 to 15 mm. With the latter, outcome is characterized by a risk of approximately 10% to 35% for neurological handicap, often mild and usually related to associated neural anomalies. These infants are evaluated in utero to exclude associated neural and extraneural disorders, as described later for fetal hydrocephalus.

The suggestions from studies of fetal primates that intrauterine decompression of hydrocephalus is beneficial,[112,516-518] and the demonstration that placement of a ventriculoamniotic shunt is possible in utero in the human fetus,[487,488,519,520] raised the possibility that antepartum intervention may be indicated in the fetus with hydrocephalus. Two problems with this approach are obvious. First, it is unclear that placement of a shunt in utero rather than in the neonatal period improves outcomes in the human patient. Second, it is clear from the data just described that most examples of poor outcome with fetal hydrocephalus relate to the associated severe developmental anomalies, which, of course, would not benefit from such intervention and sometimes can be difficult to identify in utero.

Indeed, review of the experience described in Figure 1-30 suggests that in only two cases did progressive fetal ventriculomegaly occur; with prompt postnatal placement of a shunt, the infants were normal on follow-up. Thus, in that series, no clear case existed of a fetus that could have had an improved outcome with intrauterine intervention.[471] Indeed, in a study of 41 fetuses treated with intrauterine shunting in the 1980s, procedure-related mortality was 10%, and outcome of survivors was not improved.[521] However, in a more recent review of 39 cases of fetal hydrocephalus treated by intrauterine shunting in Brazil, no procedure-related deaths were recorded, and 67% of infants later exhibited an IQ higher than 70.[487] Nevertheless, it is apparent that the treated fetal cases were highly selected and were not representative of the general population of fetal hydrocephalus, because *no* cases of holoprosencephaly were included, infants with chromosomal defects were excluded, and approximately 50% were uncomplicated aqueductal stenosis.[487]

A reasonable and currently accepted *obstetrical approach to the fetus with hydrocephalus* is essentially as follows.[471,488,506] First, after the diagnosis of hydrocephalus is made, thorough sonographic evaluation should be directed toward measurement of changes in ventricular size, cortical thickness, detection of any major associated anomalies (e.g., open neural tube defects and renal or cardiac anomalies), and documentation of progression. Second, amniocentesis is advisable to evaluate chromosomal abnormalities associated with hydrocephalus (e.g., trisomy 13 and trisomy 18), fetal sex (with history of X-linked aqueductal stenosis), alpha-fetoprotein levels, and cytomegalovirus or *Toxoplasma* infection (by polymerase chain reaction testing). Third, maternal serological examination should further assess the possibility of intrauterine infection, which is associated with a poor prognosis in the presence of hydrocephalus. Fourth, fetal MRI is obtained to assess the size of the cerebral mantle and the presence of neural anomalies. If the preceding evaluations do not indicate a poor prognosis, if progression of ventriculomegaly is documented, and if amniotic fluid lecithin-to-sphingomyelin ratios indicate mature fetal lungs, delivery by cesarean section is indicated. If the fetus is too immature for delivery, close sonographic follow-up of ventricular size is important; if progression of ventricular dilation is rapid, corticosteroid therapy for induction of lung maturity and cesarean section are indicated. Delivery in a center with modern neurosurgical facilities is critical (see later), although not all infants exhibit postnatal progression and require ventriculoperitoneal shunt.[485,508] Whether intrauterine shunting should be considered in selected cases, because of the possibility of injury to the cerebral mantle by progressive hydrocephalus,[522] is unresolved. This issue is under study.[488]

Conclusions

Decisions concerning management of congenital hydrocephalus differ considerably according to the time of diagnosis of the hydrocephalus. Thus, when the obstetrician is faced with the diagnosis of intrauterine hydrocephalus, the options range from elective termination of pregnancy to prompt delivery by cesarean section. In general, termination of pregnancy is a possibility only if the diagnosis is established before the time of fetal viability. The most critical obstetrical task is to determine the presence of major congenital abnormalities, commonly associated with intrauterine hydrocephalus, or of major cerebral injury as a result of intrauterine infection; both problems are clear indicators of a poor ultimate prognosis. Should these indicators be absent, prompt delivery (after induction of lung maturity if necessary) is most appropriate. A temporizing role for intrauterine ventricular decompression remains unclear. Postnatally, the therapeutic decisions are similar although perhaps less difficult. I believe that placement of a ventriculoperitoneal shunt is indicated in virtually all cases, because nursing care and comfort of even the infant with a clearly unfavorable neurological prognosis are facilitated greatly by shunt placement.

CEREBELLAR MALFORMATIONS AND POSTERIOR FOSSA CEREBROSPINAL FLUID COLLECTIONS

Cerebellar malformations are discussed best in this context because the most critical embryonic time period for development of cerebellar form and cellular structure occurs in the second and third months of gestation, as for prosencephalic development (discussed earlier). Because most cerebellar malformations manifest clinically after the neonatal period, I emphasize here principally those that are likely to be encountered in the newborn. As with other developmental events, I briefly review normal cerebellar development first and then consider the major cerebellar malformations.

Normal Development

The primordia of the cerebellar hemispheres appear in the fifth gestational week as bilateral thickenings in the lateral aspects of the dorsal surface of the rhombencephalon (i.e., the rhombic lips).[81,523] By continued growth of this region, the primitive vermis and cerebellar hemispheral anlage become apparent by 12 to 13 weeks. During the latter part of this period, two migrational events occur. Progenitor cells in the subependymal germinative zones of the rhombic lip, adjacent to the fourth ventricle, generate (1) neurons that migrate radially to form the dentate nucleus and other roof nuclei and the Purkinje cells and (2) neurons that migrate tangentially over the surface of the cerebellum to form the external granule cell layer. The latter cells later in gestation and postnatally then migrate inward through the molecular layer and Purkinje cells to form the internal granule cells of the mature cerebellum.

The *roof* of the fourth ventricle initially consists only of the choroid plexus and the anterior and posterior membranous areas. The anterior membranous area is incorporated into the choroid plexus.[81] The posterior membranous area remains and eventually cavitates to form the midline foramen of Magendie.[524] A disturbance in the temporal aspects of this process appears to be involved in the genesis of the Dandy-Walker malformation (see later).

Disorders

Cerebellar malformations, considered in this context of developmental events of the second and third months of gestation, are diverse and extensive.[81,523-525] In Table 1-29 I provide a list of those most commonly encountered in the newborn period and divide them, perhaps simplistically, into those that affect primarily the vermis or primarily the hemispheres (with or without accompanying vermian involvement). In the following section, I discuss the vermian disorders in varying detail. Those disorders involving the hemispheres (see Table 1-29) either manifest clinically after the neonatal period (e.g., most familial varieties[526-538]) or are discussed elsewhere in this book (e.g., prematurity [see Chapter 8], lissencephalies [see Chapter 2], congenital muscular dystrophies [see Chapter 19], metabolic disorders [see Chapters 15 and 16], and cytomegalovirus infection [see Chapter 20]).

TABLE 1-29 **Cerebellar Malformations and Posterior Fossa Cerebrospinal Fluid Collections**
Cerebellar Malformations
Primarily Involving Vermis
Dandy-Walker malformation
Joubert syndrome: "molar tooth" malformations
Rhombencephalosynapsis
Primarily Involving Cerebellar Hemispheres (with or without Vermis)
Prematurity (especially with associated cerebral white matter injury)
Familial
Lissencephalies with cerebellar hypoplasia (*REELIN* and some cases of *LIS1* and *XLIS*)
Congenital muscular dystrophies (Fukuyama, Walker-Warburg, muscle-eye-brain)
Metabolic disorders (especially peroxisomal and mitochondrial disorders; glutaric acidemia, type 2; congenital disorder of glycosylation, type 1)
Congenital cytomegalovirus infection
Posterior Fossa Fluid Collections
Enlarged fourth ventricle
Enlarged cisterna magna (secondary to developmental cerebellar hypoplasia or to cerebellar atrophy)
Arachnoidal cyst

Posterior fossa CSF collections also are discussed here because some of the most prominent of these include cerebellar malformations (e.g., Dandy-Walker malformation). Additionally, some of these fluid collections may suggest a cerebellar malformation.

Dandy-Walker Malformation

Anatomical abnormality. *Dandy-Walker malformation* accounts for approximately 5% to 10% of congenital hydrocephalus cases and consists of three major abnormalities: (1) complete or partial agenesis of the cerebellar vermis, (2) cystic dilation of the fourth ventricle, and (3) enlargement of the posterior fossa with a resulting high position of the tentorium (and torcular and lateral sinus) (Table 1-30).[18,81,359,421,523,539-552] Hydrocephalus, an additional important feature, usually appears in overt form after the neonatal period (see later). Associated abnormalities of the CNS occur in as many as 70% of cases, with the clinically most important examples being agenesis of the corpus callosum and a variety of defects of neuronal migration (see Table 1-30). The fundamental hindbrain abnormality relates to defective formation of the cerebellar vermis and the roof of the fourth ventricle. During development of the fourth ventricular roof, the foramen of Magendie usually opens before the foramina of Luschka. The disturbance in Dandy-Walker malformation appears to be primarily a delay or total failure of cavitation of the posterior membranous area of the developing roof of the fourth ventricle (see "Normal Development" earlier) to form the foramen of Magendie, thus allowing a buildup of CSF and development of the cystic dilation of the fourth ventricle. Despite the subsequent opening of the foramina of Luschka (usually patent in Dandy-Walker malformation), cystic dilation of the fourth ventricle persists, and CSF flow is impaired. Thus, in this context, the Dandy-Walker malformation can be viewed as a localized defect in differentiation of the roof of the newly closed neural tube in the region of the hindbrain.

Timing. The timing of the development of the Dandy-Walker malformation is not entirely clear. However, the major time period of foramina development is the second and third months of gestation (i.e., the peak time period of midline prosencephalic development, as discussed earlier).[2,81,359] This time period also overlaps that of neuronal migration (see Chapter 2). Thus, agenesis of the corpus callosum and defects of neuronal migration are not unexpected as important accompaniments to the Dandy-Walker malformation (see Table 1-30).

Clinical aspects. The clinical spectrum of the Dandy-Walker malformation is difficult to define decisively from published writings because the disorder often is a component of another disorder. For example, in one series (n = 50) of fetal cases, karyotype (when available) was abnormal in 46%.[552] Moreover, the Dandy-Walker malformation is a feature of many syndromes, including Rubinstein-Taybi, Meckel-Gruber, Coffin-Siris, Ellis-van Creveld, and Smith-Lemli-Optiz syndromes,

TABLE 1-30	Dandy-Walker Malformation: Neuropathology
Primary	
Enlargement of posterior fossa (elevated tentorium)	
Cystic dilation of fourth ventricle	
Agenesis of cerebellar vermis	
Hydrocephalus	
Associated	
Agenesis of the corpus callosum (20%–30%)	
Cerebral neuronal heterotopias ($\approx$15%)	
Cerebral gyral abnormalities ($\approx$10%)	
Aqueductal stenosis ($\approx$5%–10%)	
Abnormalities of inferior olivary and/or dentate nuclei ($\approx$20%)	
Occipital encephalocele (10%–15%)	
Syringomyelia ($\approx$5%–10%)	
One or more of the above (50%–70%)	
Systemic anomalies (especially cardiac) (30%–40%)	

among others, many of which are autosomal recessive traits. Nevertheless, certain clinical aspects are consistent.[18,359,421,539-546,549-551]

The *dominant clinical feature* in early infancy is the occurrence of hydrocephalus, with a striking occipital prominence to the cranium and a large cystic dilation of the fourth ventricle, enlarging the posterior fossa (Fig. 1-31). However, pronounced hydrocephalus is present in only a minority of cases in the neonatal period. Nevertheless, because of widespread prenatal and neonatal ultrasonography, more cases now are identified in utero and in the neonatal period, despite the absence of a rapidly enlarging head and overt signs of increased intracranial pressure. By 3 months of age, approximately 75% of patients exhibit hydrocephalus, and ultimately 90% or more have hydrocephalus. Indeed, in some cases of Dandy-Walker malformation, hydrocephalus may not develop until adulthood.

Other important clinical features include the accompanying anomalies of CNS and extraneural structures. The data shown in Table 1-30 are derived from a combination of reports, based both on brain imaging in vivo and on postmortem examination. In general, the incidences of associated CNS anomalies in purely autopsy series are approximately twice those shown in Table 1-30. Systemic anomalies are present in approximately 30% to 40% of cases and include serious cardiac and urinary tract defects.

Outcome is related to the severity both of the malformation and of the associated anomalies, as well as the degree of hydrocephalus (see Table 1-28).[18,359,421,523,539-546,549] The severity of these features, in turn, is reflected in the usual time of diagnosis as shown in Table 1-31. For cases identified in utero or in the neonatal period, outcome has been generally unfavorable: nearly 40% die, and 75% of survivors exhibit cognitive deficits. *However, the most fundamental determinants of outcome are the associated neural and extraneural anomalies, and if these can be excluded by imaging studies, outcome is markedly better.*

Management is complicated by the presence of the cystic dilation of the fourth ventricle and by the generalized ventriculomegaly.[541-545] Direct unroofing of

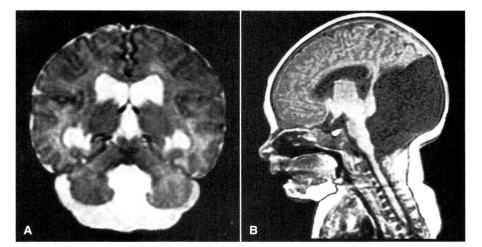

Figure 1-31 Dandy-Walker malformation. Magnetic resonance imaging (MRI) scans from a 5-day-old infant. **A**, Coronal T2-weighted scan shows agenesis of the cerebellar vermis with an enlarged fourth ventricle expanding into a posterior fossa cyst. The corpus callosum is hypoplastic. The lateral and third ventricles are enlarged, consistent with hydrocephalus. **B**, Sagittal T1-weighted MRI scan shows absence of the cerebellar vermis, a dilated fourth ventricle, and an enlarged posterior fossa.

the fourth ventricular cyst in general is not effective.[543] Shunting of only the fourth ventricle theoretically would be effective if the aqueduct were freely patent. Unfortunately, in Dandy-Walker malformation, the aqueduct functionally does not allow adequate flow of CSF, and thus the preferred approach is to shunt both the cyst and the lateral ventricle at the same time, and then connect the two catheters by a Y-connector to the peritoneal catheter.[543,545] Some neurosurgeons prefer to place a ventriculoperitoneal shunt first and later add a shunt of the posterior fossa cyst if the former shunt is not effective.[544]

Joubert Syndrome–Related Disorders and the "Molar Tooth" Malformation

Joubert syndrome classically has referred to the autosomal recessively inherited constellation of marked cerebellar vermis hypoplasia, hypotonia, ataxia, cognitive impairment, abnormal eye movements, and breathing (Table 1-32).[523,525,553-563] The *anatomical features* include a small, dysplastic vermis, dysplasias and heterotopias of the roof nuclei, absence of decussation of the superior cerebellar peduncles (and the pyramidal and pontine tracts), multiple brain stem nuclear abnormalities, and thinning of the pontomesencephalic junction.[81] The resulting neuroradiological hallmark of this cerebellar midbrain-hindbrain malformation, especially on axial MRI images, is a triangular ("bat-wing" shaped) fourth ventricle, the small cerebellar vermis, and large, straight (uncrossed) cerebellar peduncles, the "molar tooth" malformation (Fig. 1-32).[81] In

recent years, genetic studies have defined at least five genetic loci, and clinical studies have shown eight overlapping related phenotypes. As a consequence, the term, *Joubert syndrome–related disorders* has been used.[562,563]

The *clinical features* in the neonatal period most commonly include hyperpnea intermixed with apnea, hypotonia, and an unusual craniofacial appearance (prominent forehead, high rounded eyebrows, epicanthal folds, upturned nose, and an open mouth)

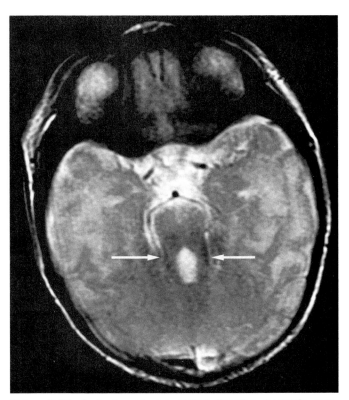

Figure 1-32 Joubert syndrome–related disorder: magnetic resonance imaging scan. The infant was 21 days old and had clinical features as described in the text. Note the prominent, straight superior cerebellar peduncles (*arrows*) and triangular fourth ventricle (i.e., the "molar tooth" malformation). (*Courtesy of Dr. Omar Khwaja.*)

TABLE 1-31	Dandy-Walker Malformation: Outcome*	
Time of Diagnosis	**Mortality (%)**[†]	**Subnormal Intelligence (% of Survivors)**
Prenatal or newborn	38	75
After newborn period	10	25

*See text for references.
[†]Often related to systemic anomalies.

TABLE 1-32	Usual Clinical Presentation of Major Posterior Fossa Cerebrospinal Fluid Collections in Infancy
Disorder	**Clinical Presentation**
Enlarged Fourth Ventricle	
Dandy-Walker malformation	Hydrocephalus
Joubert syndrome: familial vermian agenesis	Episodic hyperpnea, abnormal eye movements
Trapped fourth ventricle	Enlarging fourth ventricle with signs of brain stem dysfunction or of increased intracranial pressure after intraventricular hemorrhage or meningitis; hydrocephalus
Enlarged Cisterna Magna	Asymptomatic; hypotonia, tremor; nonprogressive macrocephaly
Arachnoidal Cyst	Posterior fossa mass, hydrocephalus

(see Table 1-32).[523,525,555,559-563] The respiratory disturbance usually improves spontaneously over the ensuing weeks and months. Nystagmus ("jerky" eye movements) may be apparent in the neonatal period and may be replaced months later by the more characteristic oculomotor apraxia. Ataxia and cognitive deficits are apparent later. In one large series (n = 29), 40% of patients attended regular school, albeit with prominent speech difficulties, and 60% had more overt cognitive disability.[559] Other features may include retinal dystrophy, coloboma, renal abnormalities, and hepatic fibrosis.

At least five *gene loci* have been identified with Joubert syndrome–related disorders: *JBTS1* (chromosome 9), *JBTS2* (chromosome 11), *JBTS3* (chromosome 6), *JBTS4* (chromosome 2), and *JBTS5* (chromosome 12).[562] The best studied thus far is *JBTS3*, which is characterized clinically by the features noted earlier as well as by cerebral abnormalities (e.g., polymicrogyria, corpus callosum abnormalities, and seizures).[562,563] The gene involved is *AHI1*, encoding the Jouberin protein, a presumed signalling molecule expressed in embryonic hindbrain and forebrain.[558,563] The developmental defect involves cerebral, brain stem, and cerebellar development, perhaps at the levels of patterning, migration, and axon pathfinding.

Rhombencephalosynapsis

Rhombencephalosynapsis, a rare disorder, is characterized by agenesis or hypoplasia of the vermis, fusion of the cerebellar hemispheres, and fusion of the dentate nuclei and cerebellar peduncles (see Table 1-29).[81,525,564-568] Clinical features appear after the neonatal period, but I discuss the disorder here because diagnosis by fetal MRI now is the most common means of initial recognition of the disorder. Fetal MRI usually has been obtained because the screening ultrasound scan showed ventriculomegaly.

The *anatomical features* are identified best postnatally by MRI. The vermian agenesis and dorsal fusion of the cerebellar hemispheres are striking (Fig. 1-33). Because of fusion of the dentate nuclei, the posterior fourth ventricle looks pointed and is sometimes referred to as having a "keyhole" appearance. Ventriculomegaly is present in 80% of reported cases, and absence of the septum pellucidum and abnormalities of the corpus callosum are observed in 60% to 70%. A relation of the abnormality to disturbed midline

development of the forebrain is supported by the latter findings, as well as by the frequent accompaniment of fused thalami.

Clinical findings later in infancy and childhood have ranged from mild truncal ataxia and normal cognitive abilities to severe cerebellar deficits, cerebral palsy, and mental retardation. Progressive ventricular dilation has resulted in shunt placement in approximately 30% of cases.

Posterior Fossa Cerebrospinal Fluid Collections

Prominent posterior fossa CSF collections are best considered in three major categories: enlargement of the fourth ventricle, enlargement of the cisterna magna (mega cisterna magna), and arachnoidal cyst (see Table 1-32). Enlarged fourth ventricle is a feature especially of developmental disorders of vermian development (particularly Dandy-Walker malformation and Joubert syndrome), as discussed earlier. Only trapped fourth

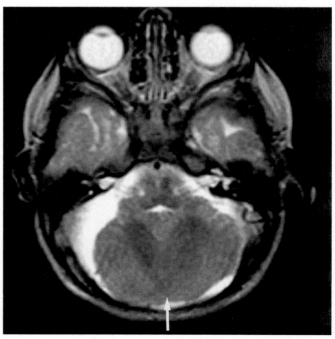

Figure 1-33 Rhombencephalosynapsis in a newborn: magnetic resonance imaging scan. Note the fused cerebellar hemispheres (*arrow*) and the lack of recognizable vermis characteristic of this lesion. *(Courtesy of Dr. Omar Khwaja.)*

ventricle is considered here. The usual clinical presentations of these three major categories of posterior fossa CSF collections are shown in Table 1-32.

Trapped fourth ventricle results when both the aqueduct and the outflow of the fourth ventricle are obstructed by an inflammatory process, provoked by blood or bacterial meningitis. This striking syndrome is usually accompanied by hydrocephalus and rapidly increasing fourth ventricular size, with brain stem compression and a neurological syndrome with prominent brain stem dysfunction. Shunting of the fourth ventricle and lateral ventricles is usually indicated.

Enlargement of the cisterna magna is the second major category of posterior fossa CSF collections and is separable from Dandy-Walker malformation because cystic dilation of the fourth ventricle does not exist, the cerebellar vermis is present, and the posterior fossa is not enlarged. An enlarged cisterna magna may result from developmental disturbance of the cerebellar hemispheres (see earlier) (see Table 1-29). These abnormalities are readily identified by the nature of the cerebellar hemispheral abnormality. Large cisterna magna may be an apparently isolated abnormality with apparently normal cerebellar hemispheres and as such may be a marker for other developmental disturbances of brain, because in one large hospital-based series, developmental and neurological abnormalities were observed in 62% of such cases.[569] Enlarged cisterna magna is also a common feature of benign infantile macrocephaly (see Chapter 3).

Arachnoidal cyst is the third major category of prominent posterior fossa CSF collections (see Table 1-32). Such cysts do not communicate with the fourth ventricle or with the subarachnoid space in the posterior fossa. They rarely manifest in the neonatal period; the usual clinical presentation is later in infancy and childhood either as a posterior fossa mass, simulating a tumor, or as a cause of hydrocephalus because of obstruction of CSF flow in the posterior fossa or at the outflow of the fourth ventricle. Some of these cysts may enlarge later, perhaps because they represent failure of the normal involution of Blake's pouch, the transient developmental evagination of the anterior membranous area of the fourth ventricular roof that, accordingly, appears to contain CSF-secreting choroid plexus.[547]

REFERENCES

1. Warkany J: *Congenital Malformations*, Chicago: 1971, Mosby.
2. Lemire RJ, Loeser JD, Leech RW, Alvord EC Jr: *Normal and Abnormal Development of the Human Nervous System*, Hagerstown, MD: 1975, Harper & Row.
3. Monsoro-Burq AH, Bontoux M, Vincent C, Ledouarin NM: The developmental relationships of the neural tube and the notochord: Short and long term effects of the notochord on the dorsal spinal cord, *Mech Dev* 53:157-170, 1995.
4. Geelan JA, Langman J: Closure of the neural tube in the cephalic region of the mouse embryo, *Anat Rec* 189:625-640, 1977.
5. Seller MJ: Sex, neural tube defects, and multisite closure of the human neural tube, *Am J Med Genet* 58:332-336, 1995.
6. Golden JA, Chernoff GF: Multiple sites of anterior neural tube closure in humans: Evidence from anterior neural tube defects (anencephaly), *Pediatrics* 95:506-510, 1995.
7. Manning S, Madsen J, Jennings R: Pathophysiology, prevention and potential treatment of neural tube defects, *Ment Retard Dev Disabil Res Rev* 6:6-14, 2000.
8. Copp AJ, Greene ND, Murdoch JN: Disheveled: Linking convergent extension with neural tube closure, *Trends Neurosci* 28:453-456, 2003.
9. Detrait ER, George TM, Etchevers HC, Gilbert JR, et al: Human neural tube defects: Developmental biology, epidemiology, and genetics, *Neurotoxicol Teratol* 27:515-524, 2005.
10. Copp AJ, Brook FA: Does lumbosacral spina bifida arise by failure of neural folding or by defective canalisation? *J Med Genet* 26:160-1666, 1989.
11. Copp AJ, Brook FA, Estibeiro AS, Shum W, et al: *The Embryonic Development of Mammalian Neural Tube Defects: Progress in Neurobiology*, London: 1990, Pergamon Press.
12. Harding BN, Copp AJ: Malformations. In Graham DI, Lantos PL, editors: *Greenfield's Neuropathology*, 7, London: 2002, Arnold Publishers.
13. Jacobson M: *Developmental Neurobiology*, New York: 1991, Plenum Press.
14. Karfunkel P: The mechanisms of neural tube formation, *Int Rev Cytol* 38:245-271, 1974.
15. Nagele RG, Bush KT, Kosciuk MC, Hunter ET, et al: Intrinsic and extrinsic factors collaborate to generate driving forces for neural tube formation in the chick: A study using morphometry and computerized three-dimensional reconstruction, *Dev Brain Res* 50:101-111, 1989.
16. Morriss-Kay GM, Crutch B: Culture of rat embryos with beta-D-xyloside: Evidence of a role for proteoglycans in neurulation, *J Anat* 134:491-506, 1982.
17. Hay ED: Extracellular matrix, *J Cell Biol* 91:S205-S223, 1981.
18. McLone DG, Suwa J, Collings JA: Neurulation: Biochemical and morphological studies on primary and secondary neural tube defects. In Marlin AE, editor: *Concepts in Pediatric Neurosurgery*, Basel: 1983, Karger.
19. van Straaten HW, Hekking JW, Beursgens JP, Terwindt-Rouwenhorst E, et al: Effect of the notochord on proliferation and differentiation in the neural tube of the chick embryo, *Development* 107:793-803, 1989.
20. Copp AJ, Bernfield M: Accumulation of basement membrane-associated hyaluronate is reduced in the posterior neuropore region of mutant (curly tail) mouse embryos developing spinal neural tube defects, *Dev Biol* 130:583-590, 1988.
21. Copp AJ, Bernfield M: Glycosaminoglycans vary in accumulation along the neuraxis during spinal neurulation in the mouse embryo, *Dev Biol* 130:573-582, 1988.
22. Bernfield M, Sanderson RD: Syndecan, a developmentally regulated cell surface proteoglycan that binds extracellular matrix and growth factors, *Philos Trans R Soc Lond [Biol]* 327:171-186, 1990.
23. Chen WH, Morrisskay GM, Copp AJ: Genesis and prevention of spinal neural tube defects in the curly tail mutant mouse: Involvement of retinoic acid and its nuclear receptors RAR-beta and RAR-gamma, *Development* 121:681-691, 1995.
24. Hol FA, Geurds MPA, Chatkupt S, Shugart YY, et al: PAX genes and human neural tube defects: An amino acid substitution in PAX1 in a patient with spina bifida, *J Med Genet* 33:655-660, 1996.
25. Zhang J, Hagopian-Donaldson S, Serbedzija G, Elsemore J, et al: Neural tube, skeletal and body wall defects in mice lacking transcription factor AP-2, *Nature* 381:238-241, 1996.
26. Schorle H, Mejer P, Buchert M, Jaenisch R, et al: Transcription factor AP-2 essential for cranial closure and craniofacial development, *Nature* 381:235-238, 1996.
27. Huang LS, Voyiazakis E, Markenson DF, Sokol KA, et al: apo B gene knockout in mice results in embryonic lethality in homozygotes and neural tube defects, male infertility, and reduced HDL cholesterol ester and apo A-I transport rates in heterozygotes, *J Clin Invest* 96:2152-2161, 1995.
28. Milunsky A: Congenital defects, folic-acid, and homoeobox genes, *Lancet* 348:419-420, 1996.
29. Smith JL, Schoenwolf GC: Neurulation: Coming to closure, *Trends Neurosci* 20:510-517, 1997.
30. Jungbluth S, Koentges G, Lumsden A: Coordination of early neural tube development by BDNF/trkB, *Development* 124:1877-1885, 1997.
31. Andaloro VJ, Monaghan DT, Rosenquist TH: Dextromethorphan and other N-methyl-D-aspartate receptor antagonists are teratogenic in the avian embryo model, *Pediatr Res* 43:1-7, 1998.
32. Sadler TW: Mechanisms of neural tube closure and defects, *Ment Retard Dev Disabil Res Rev* 4:247-253, 1998.
33. LeDouarin NM, Halpern ME: Discussion point. Origin and specification of the neural tube floor plate: Insights from the chick and zebrafish, *Curr Opin Neurobiol* 10:23-30, 2000.
34. Boyles AL, Hammock P, Speer MC: Candidate gene analysis in human neural tube defects, *Am J Med Genet C Semin Med Genet* 135C:9-23, 2005.
35. Larroche J-C: Malformations of the nervous system. In Adams JH, Corsellis JAN, Duchen LW, editors: *Greenfield's Neuropathology*, New York: 1984, Wiley & Sons.
36. Lemire RJ, Siebert JR: Anencephaly: Its spectrum and relationship to neural tube defects, *J Craniofac Genet Dev Biol* 10:163-174, 1990.
37. Book JA, Rayner S: A clinical and genetical study of anencephaly, *Am J Hum Genet* 2:61-84, 1950.
38. Nakano KK: Anencephaly: A review, *Dev Med Child Neurol* 15:383-400, 1973.

39. Melnick M, Myrianthopoulos NC: Studies in neural tube defects. II. Pathologic findings in a prospectively collected series of anencephalics, *Am J Med Genet* 26:797-810, 1987.

40. Yen IH, Khoury MJ, Erickson JD, James LM, et al: The changing epidemiology of neural tube defects: United States, 1968-1989, *Am J Dis Child* 146:857-861, 1992.

41. Mitchell LE, Adzick NS, Melchionne J, Pasquariello PS, et al: Spina bifida, *Lancet* 364:1885-1895, 2004.

42. Mitchell LE: Epidemiology of neural tube defects, *Am J Med Genet C Semin Med Genet* 135C:88-94, 2005.

43. Fedrick J: Anencephalus: Variation with maternal age, parity, social class and region in England, Scotland and Wales, *Ann Hum Genet* 34:31-38, 1970.

44. Roberts HE, Moore CA, Cragan JD, Fernhoff PM, et al: Impact of prenatal diagnosis on the birth prevalence of neural tube defects: Atlanta, 1990-1991, *Pediatrics* 96:880-883, 1995.

45. Snyder RD, Fakadej AF, Riggs JE: Anencephaly in the United States, 1968-1987: The declining incidence among white infants, *J Child Neurol* 6:304-305, 1991.

46. Limb CJ, Holmes LB: Anencephaly: Changes in prenatal detection and birth status, 1972 through, 1990, *Am J Obstet Gynecol* 170:1333-1338, 1994.

47. Williams LJ, Rasmussen SA, Flores A, Kirby RS, et al: Decline in the prevalence of spina bifida and anencephaly by race/ethnicity: 1995-2002, *Pediatrics* 116:580-586, 2005.

48. Goldstein RB, Filly RA: Prenatal diagnosis of anencephaly: Spectrum of sonographic appearances and distinction from the amniotic band syndrome, AJR, *Am J Roentgenol* 151:547-550, 1988.

49. Arras JD, Shinnar S: Anencephalic newborns as organ donors: A critique, *JAMA* 259:2284-2285, 1988.

50. Shewmon DA, Capron AM, Peacock WJ, Schulman BL: The use of anencephalic infants as organ sources: A critique, *JAMA* 261:1773-1781, 1989.

51. Medearis DN Jr, Holmes LB: On the use of anencephalic infants as organ donors, *N Engl J Med* 321:391-393, 1989.

52. Kohrman AF, Clayton EW, Frader JE, Grodin MA, et al: Infants with anencephaly as organ sources: Ethical considerations, *Pediatrics* 89:1116-1119, 1992.

53. Council on Ethical, and Judicial Affairs: The use of anencephalic neonates as organ donors, *JAMA* 273:1614-1618, 1995.

54. Peabody JL, Emery JR, Ashwal S: Experience with anencephalic infants as prospective organ donors, *N Engl J Med* 321:344-350, 1989.

55. Ashwal S, Schneider S, Tomasi G, Peabody JL: Neurological findings and brain death determination in twelve liveborn anencephalic infants, *Ann Neurol* 26:437-438, 1989.

56. Ashwal S, Peabody JL, Schneider S, Tomasi LG, et al: Anencephaly: Clinical determination of brain death and neuropathologic studies, *Pediatr Neurol* 6:233-239, 1990.

57. Baird PA, Sadovnick AD: Survival in infants with anencephaly, *Clin Pediatr* 23:268-271, 1984.

58. Baird PA, Sadovnick AD: Survival in liveborn infants with anencephaly [letter], *Am J Med Genet* 28:1019-1020, 1987.

59. Gartman JJ, Melin TE, Lawrence WT, Powers SK: Deformity correction and long-term survival in an infant with iniencephaly: Case report, *J Neurosurg* 75:126-130, 1991.

60. Erdincler P, Kaynar MY, Canbaz B, Kocer N, et al: Iniencephaly: Neuroradiological and surgical features. Case report and review of the literature, *J Neurosurg* 89:317-320, 1998.

61. Ingraham FD, Scott HW: Arnold-Chiari malformation, *N Engl J Med* 229:108, 1943.

62. Matson D: *Neurosurgery of Infancy and Childhood*, Springfield, IL: 1969, Charles C Thomas.

63. Mealey J Jr, Dzenitis AJ, Hockey AA: The prognosis of encephaloceles, *J Neurosurg* 32:209-218, 1970.

64. Brown MS, Sheridan-Pereira M: Outlook for the child with a cephalocele, *Pediatrics* 90:914-919, 1992.

65. Rowland CA, Correa A, Cragan JD, Alverson CJ: Are encephaloceles neural tube defects? *Pediatrics* 118:916-923, 2006.

66. Friede RL: *Developmental Neuropathology*, 2nd, New York: 1989, Springer-Verlag.

67. Rapport RL 2d, Dunn RC Jr, Alhady F: Anterior encephalocele, *J Neurosurg* 54:213-219, 1981.

68. Richards CGM: Frontoethmoidal meningoencephalocele: A common and severe congenital abnormality in Southeast Asia, *Arch Dis Child* 67:717-719, 1992.

69. Curnes JT, Oakes WJ: Parietal cephaloceles: Radiographic and magnetic resonance imaging evaluation, *Pediatr Neurosci* 14:71-76, 1988.

70. von Brandensky G, Klick A: Encephalocele und hydrocephalus, *Z Kinderchir* 7:583, 1969.

71. Castillo M, Quencer RM, Dominguez R: Chiari III malformations: Imaging features, AJNR, *Am J Neuroradiol* 13:107-113, 1992.

72. Cohen MM Jr, Lemire RJ: Syndromes with cephaloceles, *Teratology* 25:161-172, 1982.

73. Roelens FA, Barth PG, Van Der Harten JJ: Subependymal nodular heterotopia in patients with encephalocele, *Eur J Paediatr Neurol* 3:59-63, 1999.

74. Jones KL: *Smith's Recognizable Patterns of Human Malformation*, 6th ed, Philadelphia: 2006, Elsevier Saunders.

75. Chervenak FA, Isaacson G, Mahoney MJ, Tortora M, et al: The obstetric significance of holoprosencephaly, *Obstet Gynecol* 63:115-121, 1984.

76. Chervenak FA, Berkowitz RL, Tortora M, Hobbins JC: The management of fetal hydrocephalus, *Am J Obstet Gynecol* 151:933-942, 1985.

77. Chatterjee MS, Bondoc B, Adhate A: Prenatal diagnosis of occipital encephalocele, *Am J Obstet Gynecol* 153:646-647, 1985.

78. Nadel AS, Green JK, Holmes LB, Frigoletto FD Jr, et al: Absence of need for amniocentesis in patients with elevated levels of maternal serum alpha-fetoprotein and normal ultrasonographic examinations, *N Engl J Med* 323:557-561, 1990.

79. Hansen AR, Madsen JR: Antenatal neurosurgical counseling: Approach to the unborn patient, *Pediatr Clin North Am* 51:491-505, 2004.

80. Byrd SE, Harwood-Nash DC, Fitz CR, Rogovitz DM: Computed tomography in the evaluation of encephaloceles in infants and children, *J Comput Assist Tomogr* 2:81-87, 1978.

81. Barkovich AJ: *Pediatric Neuroimaging*, 4th ed, Philadelphia: 2005, Lippincott Williams & Wilkins.

82. Barson AJ: Spina bifida: The significance of the level and extent of the defect to the morphogenesis, *Dev Med Child Neurol* 12:129-144, 1970.

83. Osaka K, Tanimura T, Hirayama A, Matsumoto S: Myelomeningocele before birth, *J Neurosurg* 49:711-724, 1978.

84. Myrianthopoulos NC, Melnick M: Studies in neural tube defects. I. Epidemiologic and etiologic aspects, *Am J Med Genet* 26:783-796, 1987.

85. Windham GC, Edmonds LD: Current trends in the incidence of neural tube defects, *Pediatrics* 70:333-337, 1982.

86. Stein SC, Feldman JG, Friedlander M, Klein RJ: Is myelomeningocele a disappearing disease? *Pediatrics* 69:511-514, 1982.

87. Adams MM, Greenberg F, Khoury MJ, Marks JS, et al: Trends in clinical characteristics of infants with spina bifida: Atlanta, 1972-1979, *Am J Dis Child* 139:514-517, 1985.

88. Leech RW, Payne GG Jr: Neural tube defects: Epidemiology, *J Child Neurol* 6:286-287, 1991.

89. Bound JP, Francis BJ, Harvey PW: Neural tube defects, maternal cohorts, and age: A pointer to aetiology, *Arch Dis Child* 66:1223-1226, 1991.

90. Lemire RJ: Neural tube defects, *JAMA* 259:558-562, 1988.

91. Stone DH: The declining prevalence of anencephalus and spina bifida: Its nature, causes and implications, *Dev Med Child Neurol* 29:541-546, 1987.

92. Seller MJ: Risks in spina bifida, *Dev Med Child Neurol* 36:1025-1041, 1994.

93. Murphy M, Seagroatt V, Hey K, O'Donnell M, et al: Neural tube defects, 1974-94: Down but not out, *Arch Dis Child* 75:F133-F134, 1996.

94. Olney R, Mulinare J: Epidemiology of neural tube defects, *Ment Retard Dev Disabil Res Rev* 4:241-246, 1998.

95. Gucciardi E, Pietrusiak MA, Reynolds DL, Rouleau J: Incidence of neural tube defects in Ontario, 1986-1999, *CMAJ* 167:237-240, 2002.

96. Sival DA, van Weerden TW, Vles JS, Timmer A, et al: Neonatal loss of motor function in human spina bifida aperta, *Pediatrics* 114:427-434, 2004.

97. McLaughlin JF, Shurtleff DB: Management of the newborn with myelodysplasia, *Clin Pediatr* 18:463-476, 1979.

98. Liptak GS, Shurtleff DB, Bloss JW, Baltus-Hebert E, et al: Mobility aids for children with high-level myelomeningocele: Parapodium versus wheelchair, *Dev Med Child Neurol* 34:787-796, 1992.

99. Coniglio SJ, Anderson SM, Ferguson JEI: Functional motor outcome in children with myelomeningocele: Correlation with anatomic level on prenatal ultrasound, *Dev Med Child Neurol* 38:675-680, 1996.

100. Hunt GM, Poulton A: Open spina bifida: A complete cohort reviewed, 25 years after closure, *Dev Med Child Neurol* 37:19-29, 1995.

101. Williams EN, Broughton NS, Menelaus MB: Age-related walking in children with spina bifida, *Dev Med Child Neurol* 41:446-449, 1999.

102. Verhoef M, Barf HA, Post MW, van Asbeck FW, et al: Functional independence among young adults with spina bifida, in relation to hydrocephalus and level of lesion, *Dev Med Child Neurol* 48:114-119, 2006.

103. McDonald CM, Jaffe KM, Mosca VS, Shurtleff DB: Ambulatory outcome of children with myelomeningocele: Effect of lower-extremity muscle strength, *Dev Med Child Neurol* 33:482-490, 1991.

104. McDonald CM, Jaffe KM, Shurtleff DB, Menelaus MB: Modifications to the traditional description of neurosegmental innervation in myelomeningocele, *Dev Med Child Neurol* 33:473-481, 1991.

105. Liptak GS, Masiulis BS: Letter, *Pediatrics* 74:165, 1984.

106. Lorber J: Systematic ventriculographic studies in infants born with meningomyelocele and encephalocele, *Arch Dis Child* 36:381, 1961.

107. Meyer-Heim AD, Klein A, Boltshauser E: Cervical myelomeningocele—follow-up of five patients, *Eur J Paediatr Neurol* 7:407-412, 2003.

108. Rintoul NE, Sutton LN, Hubbard AM, Cohen BA, et al: A new look at myelomeningoceles: Functional level, vertebral level, shunting, and the implications for fetal intervention, *Pediatrics* 109:409-413, 2002.

109. Stein SC, Schut L: Hydrocephalus in myelomeningocele, *Childs Brain* 4:413-419, 1979.

110. Bell WO, Sumner TE, Volberg FM: The significance of ventriculomegaly in the newborn with myelodysplasia, *Childs Nerv Syst* 3:239-241, 1987.

111. Peach B: Arnold-Chiari malformation: Anatomic features of 20 cases, *Arch Neurol* 12:613-621, 1965.

112. Gilbert JN, Jones KL, Rorke LB, Chernoff GF, et al: Central nervous system anomalies associated with meningomyelocele, hydrocephalus, and the Arnold-Chiari malformation: Reappraisal of theories regarding the pathogenesis of posterior neural tube closure defects, *Neurosurgery* 18:559-564, 1986.

113. Sutton LN, Adzick NS, Bilaniuk LT, Johnson MP, et al: Improvement in hindbrain herniation demonstrated by serial fetal magnetic resonance imaging following fetal surgery for myelomeningocele, *JAMA* 282:1826-1831, 1999.

114. Johnson MP, Sutton LN, Rintoul N, Crombleholme TM, et al: Fetal myelomeningocele repair: Short-term clinical outcomes, *Am J Obstet Gynecol* 189:482-487, 2003.

115. McLone DG, Dias L, Kaplan WE, Sommers MW: Concepts in the management of spina bifida. In Marlin AE, editor: *Concepts in Pediatric Neurosurgery*, Basel: 1985, Karger.

116. McLaughlin JF, Shurtleff DB, Lamers JY, Stuntz JT, et al: Influence of prognosis on decisions regarding the care of newborns with myelodysplasia, *N Engl J Med* 312:1589-1594, 1985.

117. Worley G, Schuster JM, Oakes WJ: Survival at, 5 years of a cohort of newborn infants with myelomeningocele, *Dev Med Child Neurol* 38:816-822, 1996.

118. Kirk VG, Morielli A, Brouillette RT: Sleep-disordered breathing in patients with myelomeningocele: The missed diagnosis, *Dev Med Child Neurol* 41:40-43, 1999.

119. Charney EB, Rorke LB, Sutton LN, Schut L: Management of Chiari II complications in infants with myelomeningocele, *J Pediatr* 111:364-371, 1987.

120. Dahl M, Ahlsten G, Carlson H, Ronne-Engström E, et al: Neurological dysfunction above cele level in children with spina bifida cystica: A prospective study to three years, *Dev Med Child Neurol* 37:30-40, 1995.

121. Cochrane DD, Adderley R, White CP, Norman M, et al: Apnea in patients with myelomeningocele, *Pediatr Neurosurg* 16:232-239, 1990.

122. Davidson Ward SL, Jacobs RA, Gates EP, Hart LD, et al: Abnormal ventilatory patterns during sleep in infants with myelomeningocele, *J Pediatr* 109:631-634, 1986.

123. Hesz N, Wolraich M: Vocal-cord paralysis and brainstem dysfunction in children with spina bifida, *Dev Med Child Neurol* 27:528-531, 1985.

124. Hays RM, Jordan RA, McLaughlin JF, Nickel RE, et al: Central ventilatory dysfunction in myelodysplasia: An independent determinant of survival, *Dev Med Child Neurol* 31:366-370, 1989.

125. Swaminathan S, Paton JY, Davidson Ward SL, Jacobs RA, et al: Abnormal control of ventilation in adolescents with myelodysplasia, *J Pediatr* 115:898-903, 1989.

126. Oren J, Kelly DH, Todres ID, Shannon DC: Respiratory complications in patients with myelodysplasia and Arnold-Chiari malformation, *Am J Dis Child* 140:221-224, 1986.

127. Vandertop WP, Asai A, Hoffman HJ, Drake JM, et al: Surgical decompression for symptomatic Chiari II malformation in neonates with myelomeningocele, *J Neurosurg* 77:541-544, 1992.

128. Putnam PE, Orenstein SR, Pang D, Pollack IF, et al: Cricopharyngeal dysfunction associated with Chiari malformations, *Pediatrics* 89:871-876, 1992.

129. Barnet AB, Weiss IP, Shaer C: Evoked potentials in infant brainstem syndrome associated with Arnold-Chiari malformation, *Dev Med Child Neurol* 35:42-48, 1993.

130. Worley G, Erwin CW, Schuster JM, Park Y, et al: BAEPs in infants with myelomeningocele and later development of Chiari II malformation-related brainstem dysfunction, *Dev Med Child Neurol* 36:707-715, 1994.

131. Petersen MC, Wolraich M, Sherbondy A, Wagener J: Abnormalities in control of ventilation in newborn infants with myelomeningocele, *J Pediatr* 126:1011-1015, 1995.

132. Taylor MJ, Boor R, Keenan NK, Rutka JT, et al: Brainstem auditory and visual evoked potentials in infants with myelomeningocele, *Brain Dev* 18:99-104, 1996.

133. Waters KA, Forbes P, Morielli A, Hum C, et al: Sleep-disordered breathing in children with myelomeningocele, *J Pediatr* 132:672-681, 1998.

134. Peach B: Arnold-Chiari malformation: Morphogenesis, *Arch Neurol* 12:527, 1965.

135. Ingraham FD, Swan H, Hamlin H: *Spina Bifida and Cranium Bifidum*, Cambridge, MA: 1944, Harvard University Press.

136. Bartoshesky LE, Haller J, Scott RM, Wojick C: Seizures in children with meningomyelocele, *Am J Dis Child* 139:400-402, 1985.

137. Noetzel MJ, Blake JN: Prognosis for seizure control and remission in children with myelomeningocele, *Dev Med Child Neurol* 33:803-810, 1991.

138. Talwar D, Baldwin M, Horbatt CI: Epilepsy in children with meningomyelocele, *Pediatr Neurol* 13:29-32, 1995.

139. Naidich TP: Cranial CT signs of the Chiari II malformation, *J Neuroradiol* 8:207-227, 1981.

140. Naidich TP, McLone DG, Fulling KH: The Chiari II malformation. IV. The hindbrain deformity, *Neuroradiology* 25:179-197, 1983.

141. Klucznik RP, Wolpert SM, Anderson MJ: Congenital and developmental abnormalities of the brain. In Patterson AS, editor: *MRI in Pediatric Neuroradiology*, St. Louis: 1992, Mosby.

142. Benacerraf BR, Stryker J, Frigoletto FD Jr: Abnormal US appearance of the cerebellum (banana sign): Indirect sign of spina bifida, *Radiology* 171:151-153, 1989.

143. Babcook CJ, Goldstein RB, Barth RA, Damato NM, et al: Prevalence of ventriculomegaly in association with myelomeningocele: Correlation with gestational age and severity of posterior fossa deformity, *Radiology* 190:703-707, 1994.

144. Marlin AE: The initial treatment of the child with myelomeningocele: A practice survey of the American Society for Pediatric Neurosurgery (ASPN). In Marlin AE, editor: *Concepts in Pediatric Neurosurgery*, Basel: 1990, Karger.

145. Kaufman BA: Neural tube defects, *Pediatr Clin North Am* 51:389-419, 2004.

146. Heffez DS, Aryanpur J, Hutchins GM, Freeman JM: The paralysis associated with myelomeningocele: Clinical and experimental data implicating a preventable spinal cord injury, *Neurosurgery* 26:987-992, 1990.

147. Heffez DS, Aryanpur J, Rotellini N, Hutchins GM, et al: Intrauterine repair of experimental surgically created dysraphism, *Neurosurgery* 32:1005-1010, 1993.

148. Epstein F, Marlin A, Hochwald G, Ransohoff J: Myelomeningocele: A progressive intra-uterine disease, *Dev Med Child Neurol* 18:12-15, 1976.

149. Korenromp MJ, van Gool JD, Bruinese HW, Kriek R: Early fetal leg movements in myelomeningocele [letter], *Lancet* 1:917-918, 1986.

150. Meuli M, Meulisimmen C, Hutchins GM, Yingling CD, et al: In utero surgery rescues neurological function at birth in sheep with spina bifida, *Nat Med* 1:342-347, 1995.

151. Liechty KW, Adzick NS: Prospects for fetal therapy of neural tube defects, *Ment Retard Dev Disabil Res Rev* 4:291-295, 1998.

152. Bruner JP, Richards WO, Tulipan NB, Arney TL: Endoscopic coverage of fetal myelomeningocele in utero, *Am J Obstet Gynecol* 180:153-158, 1999.

153. Bruner JP, Tulipan N, Paschall RL, Boehm FH, et al: Fetal surgery for myelomeningocele and the incidence of shunt-dependent hydrocephalus, *JAMA* 282:1819-1825, 1999.

154. Simpson JL: Fetal surgery for myelomeningocele, *JAMA* 282:1873-1874, 1999.

155. Bruner JP, Tulipan N, Reed G, Davis GH, et al: Intrauterine repair of spina bifida: Preoperative predictors of shunt-dependent hydrocephalus, *Am J Obstet Gynecol* 190:1305-1312, 2004.

156. Paek BW, Farmer DL, Wilkinson CC, Albanese CT, et al: Hindbrain herniation develops in surgically created myelomeningocele but is absent after repair in fetal lambs, *Am J Obstet Gynecol* 183:1119-1123, 2000.

157. Luthy DA, Wardinsky T, Shurtleff DB, Hollenbach KA, et al: Cesarean section before the onset of labor and subsequent motor function in infants with meningomyelocele diagnosed antenatally, *N Engl J Med* 324:662-666, 1991.

158. Sharrard WJW, Zachary RB, Lorber J, Bruce AM: A controlled trial of immediate and delayed closure of spina bifida cystica, *Arch Dis Child* 38:18, 1963.

159. Raine PA, Young DG: Bacterial colonisation and infection in lesions of the central nervous system, *Dev Med Child Neurol Suppl* 35:111-116, 1975.

160. Charney EB, Weller SC, Sutton LN, Bruce DA, et al: Management of the newborn with myelomeningocele: Time for a decision-making process, *Pediatrics* 75:58-64, 1985.

161. Charney EB, Melchionni JB, Antonucci DL: Ventriculitis in newborns with myelomeningocele, *Am J Dis Child* 145:287-290, 1991.

162. McCullough DC, Johnson DL: Myelomeningocele repair: Technical considerations and complications. In Marlin AE, editor: *Concepts in Pediatric Neurosurgery*, Basel: 1988, Karger.

163. Teichgraeber JF, Riley WB, Parks DH: Primary skin closure in large myelomeningoceles, *Pediatr Neurosci* 15:18-22, 1989.

164. Hammock MK, Milhorat TH, Baron IS: Normal pressure hydrocephalus in patients with myelomeningocele, *Dev Med Child Neurol Suppl* 37:55-68, 1976.

165. Badell Ribera A, Shulman K, Paddock N: The relationship of non-progressive hydrocephalus to intellectual functioning in children with spina bifida cystica, *Pediatrics* 37:787-793, 1966.

166. Lorber J: Isosorbide in the medical treatment of infantile hydrocephalus, *J Neurosurg* 39:702-711, 1973.

167. Lorber J, Salfield S, Lonton T: Isosorbide in the management of infantile hydrocephalus, *Dev Med Child Neurol* 25:502-511, 1983.

168. Liptak GS, Gellerstedt ME, Klionsky N: Isosorbide in the medical management of hydrocephalus in children with myelodysplasia, *Dev Med Child Neurol* 34:150-154, 1992.

169. Stark GD, Drummond MB, Poneprasert S, Robarts FH: Primary ventriculo-peritoneal shunts in treatment of hydrocephalus associated with myelomeningocele, *Arch Dis Child* 49:112-117, 1974.

170. Naglo AS, Hellstrom B: Results of treatment in myelomeningocele, *Acta Paediatr Scand* 65:565-569, 1976.

171. Stark GD, Drummond M: Results of selective early operation in myelomeningocele, *Arch Dis Child* 48:676-683, 1973.

172. Hunt GM, Holmes AE: Factors relating to intelligence in treated cases of spina bifida cystica, *Am J Dis Child* 130:823-827, 1976.

173. Coniglio SJ, Anderson SM, Ferguson JE: Developmental outcomes of children with myelomeningocele: Prenatal predictors, *Am J Obstet Gynecol* 177:319-326, 1997.

174. Laurence KM: A case of unilateral megalencephaly, *Dev Med Child Neurol* 6:585-590, 1964.

175. Storrs BB: Ventricular size and intelligence in myelodysplastic children. In Marlin AE, editor: *Concepts in Pediatric Neurosurgery*, Basel: 1988, S. Karger.

176. McLone DG, Czyzewski D, Raimondi AJ, Sommers RC: Central nervous system infections as a limiting factor in the intelligence of children with myelomeningocele, *Pediatrics* 70:338, 1982.

177. Liptak GS, Bloss JW, Briskin H, Campbell JE, et al: The management of children with spinal dysraphism, *J Child Neurol* 3:3-20, 1988.

178. Uehling DT, Smith J, Meyer J, Bruskewitz R: Impact of an intermittent catheterization program on children with myelomeningocele, *Pediatrics* 76:892-895, 1985.

179. Lie HR, Lagergren J, Rasmussen F, Lagerkvist B, et al: Bowel and bladder control of children with myelomeningocele: A Nordic study, *Dev Med Child Neurol* 33:1053-1061, 1991.

180. Sherk HH, Uppal GS, Lane G, Melchionni J: Treatment versus nontreatment of hip dislocations in ambulatory patients with myelomeningocele, *Dev Med Child Neurol* 33:491-494, 1991.

181. Swank M, Dias L: Myelomeningocele: A review of the orthopaedic aspects of 206 patients treated from birth with no selection criteria, *Dev Med Child Neurol* 34:1047-1052, 1992.

182. Kasabian NG, Bauer SB, Dyro FM, Colodny AH, et al: The prophylactic value of clean intermittent catheterization and anticholinergic medication in newborns and infants with myelodysplasia at risk of developing urinary tract deterioration, *Am J Dis Child* 146:840-843, 1992.

183. Bauer SB, Hallett M, Khoshbin S, Lebowitz RL, et al: Predictive value of urodynamic evaluation in newborns with myelodysplasia, *JAMA* 252:650-652, 1984.

184. Bier JA, Prince A, Tremont M, Msall M: Medical, functional, and social determinants of health-related quality of life in individuals with myelomeningocele, *Dev Med Child Neurol* 47:609-612, 2005.

185. Laurence KM: Effect of early surgery for spina bifida cystica on survival and quality of life, *Lancet* 1:301-304, 1974.

186. Lorber J: Spina bifida cystica: Results of treatment of 270 consecutive cases with criteria for selection for the future, *Arch Dis Child* 47:854-873, 1972.

187. Hunt GM: Open spina bifida: Outcome for a complete cohort treated unselectively and followed into adulthood, *Dev Med Child Neurol* 32:108-118, 1990.

188. Lorber J: Results of treatment of myelomeningocele: An analysis of 524 unselected cases, with special reference to possible selection for treatment, *Dev Med Child Neurol* 13:279-303, 1971.

189. Tew B, Evans R, Thomas M, Ford J: The results of a selective surgical policy on the cognitive abilities of children with spina bifida, *Dev Med Child Neurol* 27:606-614, 1985.

190. Evans RC, Tew B, Thomas MD, Ford J: Selective surgical management of neural tube malformations, *Arch Dis Child* 60:415-419, 1985.

191. Hagelsteen JH, Lagergren J, Lie HR, Rasmussen F, et al: Disability in children with myelomeningocele: A Nordic study, *Acta Paediatr Scand* 78:721-727, 1989.

192. Shurtleff DB: Letter, *Pediatrics* 74:164, 1984.

193. Steinbok P, Irvine B, Cochrane DD, Irwin BJ: Long-term outcome and complications of children born with meningomyelocele, *Childs Nerv Syst* 8:92-96, 1992.

194. Holmes LB, Driscoll SG, Atkins L: Etiologic heterogeneity of neural-tube defects, *N Engl J Med* 294:365-369, 1976.

195. Martínez-Frías M-L: Valproic acid and spina bifida [letter], *Lancet* 338:196-197, 1991.

196. Hall JG, Solehdin F: Genetics of neural tube defects, *Ment Retard Dev Disabil Res Rev* 4:269-281, 1998.

197. Lynch SA: Syndromes associated with neural tube defects, *Am J Med Genet C Semin Med Genet* 9999:1-8, 2005.

198. Carter CO: Clues to the aetiology of neural tube malformations, *Dev Med Child Neurol* 16:3-15, 1974.

199. Carter CO, Evans K: Children of adult survivors with spina bifida cystica, *Lancet* 2:924-926, 1973.

200. Lorber J: The family history of spina bifida cystica, *Pediatrics* 35:598, 1965.

201. Janerich DT, Piper J: Shifting genetic patterns in anencephaly and spina bifida, *J Med Genet* 51:101, 1978.

202. Toriello HV, Higgins JV: Occurrence of neural tube defects among first-, second-, and third-degree relatives of probands: Results of a United States study, *Am J Med Genet* 15:601-606, 1983.

203. Hall JG, Friedman JM, Kenna BA, Popkin J, et al: Clinical, genetic, and epidemiological factors in neural tube defects, *Am J Hum Genet* 43:827-837, 1988.

204. Chatkupt S, Skurnick JH, Jaggi M, Mitruka K, et al: Study of genetics, epidemiology, and vitamin usage in familial spina bifida in the United States in the, 1990s, *Neurology* 44:65-70, 1994.

205. MacMahon B, Yen S: Unrecognised epidemic of anencephaly and spina bifida, *Lancet* 1:31-33, 1971.

206. Stevenson RE, Allen WP, Pai GS, Best R, et al: Decline in prevalence of neural tube defects in a high-risk region of the United States, *Pediatrics* 106:677-683, 2000.

207. Seller MJ, Adinolfi M: The curly-tail mouse: An experimental model for human neural tube defects, *Life Sci* 29:1607-1615, 1981.

208. Layde PM, Edmonds LD, Erickson JD: Maternal fever and neural tube defects, *Teratology* 21:105-108, 1980.

209. Shiota K: Neural tube defects and maternal hyperthermia in early pregnancy: Epidemiology in a human embryo population, *Am J Med Genet* 12:281-288, 1982.

210. Zimmerman AW: Hyperzincemia in anencephaly and spina bifida: A clue to the pathogenesis of neural tube defects? *Neurology* 34:443-450, 1984.

211. Rosa FW: Spina bifida in infants of women treated with carbamazepine during pregnancy, *N Engl J Med* 324:674-677, 1991.

212. Ehlers K, Sturje H, Merker H-J, Nau H: Valproic acid-induced spina bifida: A mouse model, *Teratology* 45:145-154, 1992.

213. Smith MS, Edwards MJ, Upfold JB: The effects of hyperthermia on the fetus, *Dev Med Child Neurol* 28:806-809, 1986.

214. Smith MS, Upfold JB, Edwards MJ, Shiota K, et al: The induction of neural tube defects by maternal hyperthermia: A comparison of the guinea-pig and human, *Neuropathol Appl Neurobiol* 18:71-80, 1992.

215. Warkany J: Teratogen update: Hyperthermia, *Teratology* 33:365-371, 1986.

216. Sandford MK, Kissling GE, Joubert PE: Neural tube defect etiology: New evidence concerning maternal hyperthermia, health and diet, *Dev Med Child Neurol* 34:661-675, 1992.

217. Ray JG, Blom HJ: Vitamin B_{12} insufficiency and the risk of fetal neural tube defects, *Q J Med* 96:289-295, 2003.

218. Greene MF: Diabetic embryopathy, 2001: Moving beyond the "diabetic milieu," *Teratology* 63:116-118, 2001.

219. Hernandez-Diaz S, Werler MM, Walker AM, Mitchell AA: Neural tube defects in relation to use of folic acid antagonists during pregnancy, *Am J Epidemiol* 153:961-968, 2001.

220. Matalon S, Schechtman S, Goldzweig G, Ornoy A: The teratogenic effect of carbamazepine: A meta-analysis of, 1255 exposures, *Reprod Toxicol* 16:9-17, 2002.

221. Watkins ML, Rasmussen SA, Honein MA, Botto LD, et al: Maternal obesity and risk for birth defects, *Pediatrics* 111:1152-1158, 2003.

222. Milunsky A, Ulcickas M, Rothman KJ, Willett W, et al: Maternal heat exposure and neural tube defects, *JAMA* 268:882-885, 1992.

223. Shaw GM, Todoroff K, Velie EM, Lammer EJ: Maternal illness, including fever and medication use as risk factors for neural tube defects, *Teratology* 57:1-7, 1998.

224. Brock DJ: Mechanisms by which amniotic-fluid alpha-fetoprotein may be increased in fetal abnormalities, *Lancet* 2:345-346, 1976.

225. Wald NJ, Cuckle H, Brock JH, Peto R, et al: Maternal serum-alpha-fetoprotein measurement in antenatal screening for anencephaly and spina bifida in early pregnancy: Report of U.K. collaborative study on alpha-fetoprotein in relation to neural-tube defects, *Lancet* 1:1323-1332, 1977.

226. Ferguson-Smith MA, Rawlinson HA, May HM, Tait HA, et al: Avoidance of anencephalic and spina bifida births by maternal serum-alpha fetoprotein screening, *Lancet* 1:1330-1333, 1978.

227. Macri JN, Haddow JE, Weiss RR: Screening for neural tube defects in the United States: A summary of the Scarborough Conference, *Am J Obstet Gynecol* 133:119-125, 1979.

228. Milunsky A, Alpert E, Neff RK, Frigoletto FD Jr: Prenatal diagnosis of neural tube defects. IV. Maternal serum alpha-fetoprotein screening, *Obstet Gynecol* 55:60-66, 1980.

229. Haddow JE, Macri JN: Prenatal screening for neural tube defects, *JAMA* 242:515-516, 1979.

230. Schnittger A, Kjessler B: Alpha-fetoprotein screening in obstetric practice, *Acta Obstet Gynecol Scand Suppl* 119:1-47, 1984.

231. Roberts CJ, Evans KT, Hibbard BM, Laurence KM, et al: Diagnostic effectiveness of ultrasound in detection of neural tube defect: The South Wales experience of 2509 scans (1977-1982) in high-risk mothers, *Lancet* 2:1068-1069, 1983.

232. Macri JN, Weiss RR: Prenatal serum alpha-fetoprotein screening for neural tube defects, *Obstet Gynecol* 59:633-639, 1982.

233. Main DM, Mennuti MT: Neural tube defects: Issues in prenatal diagnosis and counselling, *Obstet Gynecol* 67:1-16, 1986.

234. Persson PH, Kullander S, Gennser G, Grennert L, et al: Screening for fetal malformations using ultrasound and measurements of alpha-fetoprotein in maternal serum, *Br Med J (Clin Res Ed)* 286:747-749, 1983.

235. Hood VD, Robinson HP: Diagnosis of closed neural tube defects by ultrasound in second trimester of pregnancy, *Br Med J* 2:931, 1978.

236. Hobbins JC, Grannum PA, Berkowitz RL, Silverman R, et al: Ultrasound in the diagnosis of congenital anomalies, *Am J Obstet Gynecol* 134:331-345, 1979.

237. Harwood SJ, Pinsker MC: Detection of fetal anencephaly using real-time ultrasound, *South Med J* 72:223-225, 1979.
238. Morrow RJ, McNay MB, Whittle MJ: Ultrasound detection of neural tube defects in patients with elevated maternal serum alpha-fetoprotein, *Obstet Gynecol* 78:1055-1057, 1991.
239. Penso C, Redline RW, Benacarrl BR: A sonographic sign which predicts which fetuses with hydrocephalus have an associated neural tube defect, *Ultrasound Med* 6:307-311, 1986.
240. Smithells RW, Sheppard S, Schorah CJ, Seller MJ, et al: Possible prevention of neural-tube defects by periconceptional vitamin supplementation, *Lancet* 1:339-340, 1980.
241. Smithells RW, Sheppard S, Schorah CJ, Seller MJ, et al: Apparent prevention of neural tube defects by periconceptional vitamin supplementation, *Arch Dis Child* 56:911-918, 1981.
242. Smithells RW: Neural tube defects: Prevention by vitamin supplements, *Pediatrics* 69:498-499, 1982.
243. Smithells RW, Nevin NC, Seller MJ, Sheppard S, et al: Further experience of vitamin supplementation for prevention of neural tube defect recurrences, *Lancet* 1:1027-1031, 1983.
244. Laurence KM, James N, Miller MH, Tennant GB, et al: Double-blind randomised controlled trial of folate treatment before conception to prevent recurrence of neural-tube defects, *Br Med J (Clin Res Ed)* 282:1509-1511, 1981.
245. Laurence KM: Neural tube defects: A two-pronged approach to primary prevention, *Pediatrics* 70:648-650, 1982.
246. Milunsky A, Jick H, Jick SS, Bruell CL, et al: Multivitamin/folic acid supplementation in early pregnancy reduces the prevalence of neural tube defects, *JAMA* 262:2847-2852, 1989.
247. Mulinare J, Cordero JF, Erickson JD, Berry RJ: Periconceptional use of multivitamins and the occurrence of neural tube defects, *JAMA* 260:3141-3145, 1988.
248. Smithells RW, Sheppard S, Wild J, Schorah CJ: Prevention of neural tube defect recurrences in Yorkshire: Final report [letter], *Lancet* 2:498-499, 1989.
249. Laurence KM: Folic acid to prevent neural tube defects [letter], *Lancet* 338:379-380, 1991.
250. MRC Vitamin Study Research Group: Prevention of neural tube defects: Results of the Medical Research Council Vitamin Study, *Lancet* 338:131-137, 1991.
251. Holmes-Siedle M, Lindenbaum RH, Galliard A: Recurrence of neural tube defect in a group of at-risk women: A 10 year study of Pregnavite Forte F, *J Med Genet* 29:134-135, 1992.
252. Oakley GP: Folic acid preventable spina bifida and anencephaly, *JAMA* 269:1292-1293, 1993.
253. Werler MM, Shapiro S, Mitchell AA: Periconceptional folic acid exposure and risk of occurrent neural tube defects, *JAMA* 269:1257-1261, 1993.
254. Czeizel AE, Dudas I: Prevention of the, 1st occurrence of neural-tube defects by periconceptional vitamin supplementation, *N Engl J Med* 327:1832-1835, 1992.
255. Holmes-Siedle M, Dennis J, Lindenbaum RH, Galliard A: Long term effects of periconceptional multivitamin supplements for prevention of neural tube defects: A 7-year to, 10-year follow up, *Arch Dis Child* 67:1436-1441, 1992.
256. Holmes LB: Prevention of neural tube defects, *J Pediatr* 120:918-919, 1992.
257. Bendich A: Folic acid and neural tube defects: Introduction to part II, *Life Sci* 1200:108-111, 1993.
258. Wald N: Folic acid and the prevention of neural tube defects, *Life Sci* 1200:112-129, 1993.
259. Mulinare J: Epidemiologic association of multivitamin supplementation and occurrence of neural tube defects, *Life Sci* 1200:130-136, 1993.
260. Mills JL: Effects of recent research on recommendation for periconceptional folate supplement use, *Life Sci* 1200:137-145, 1993.
261. Bower C, Stanley FJ, Nicol DJ: Maternal folate status and the risk for neural tube defects: The role of dietary folate, *Life Sci* 1200:146-155, 1993.
262. Schorah CJ, Habibzadeh N, Wild J, Smithells RW: Possible abnormalities of folate and vitamin B12 metabolism associated with neural tube defects, *Ann NY Acad Sci* 678:81-91, 1995.
263. Shaw GM, Schaffer D, Velie EM, Morland K, et al: Periconceptional vitamin use, dietary folate, and the occurrence of neural tube defects, *Epidemiology* 6:219-226, 1995.
264. Oakley GP, Erickson JD, Adams MJ: Urgent need to increase folic acid consumption, *JAMA* 274:1717-1718, 1995.
265. Gordon N: Folate metabolism and neural tube defects, *Brain Dev* 17:307-311, 1995.
266. Crandall BF, Corson VL, Goldberg JD, Knight G, et al: Folic acid and pregnancy, *Am J Med Genet* 55:134-135, 1995.
267. Khoury MJ, Shaw GM, Moore CA, Lammer EJ, et al: Does periconceptional multivitamin use reduce the risk of neural tube defects associated with other birth defects? Data from two population-based case-control studies, *Am J Med Genet* 61:30-36, 1996.
268. Daly S, Mills JL, Molloy AM, Conley M, et al: Minimum effective dose of folic acid for food fortification to prevent neural-tube defects, *Lancet* 350:1666-1669, 1997.
269. Eskes TKAB: Neural tube defects, vitamins and homocysteine, *Eur J Pediatr* 157:S139-S141, 1998.
270. Watkins ML: Efficacy of folic acid prophylaxis for the prevention of neural tube defects, *Ment Retard Dev Disabil Res Rev* 4:282-290, 1998.
271. Copp AJ, Fleming A, Greene NDE: Embryonic mechanisms underlying the prevention of neural tube defects by vitamins, *Ment Retard Dev Disabil Res Rev* 4:264-268, 1998.
272. Barber RC, Lammer EJ, Shaw GM, Greer KA, et al: The role of folate transport and metabolism in neural tube defect risk, *Mol Genet Metabol* 66:1-9, 1999.
273. Finnell RH, Greer KA, Barber RC, Piedrahita JA: Neural tube and craniofacial defects with special emphasis on folate pathway genes, *Crit Rev Oral Biol Med* 9:38-53, 1998.
274. Honein MA, Paulozzi LJ, Mathews TJ, Erickson JD, et al: Impact of folic acid fortification of the US food supply on the occurrence of neural tube defects, *JAMA* 285:2981-2986, 2001.
275. Mills JL, England L: Food fortification to prevent neural tube defects: Is it working? *JAMA* 285:3022-3023, 2001.
276. Van Dyke DC, Berg MJ: Folic acid and prevention of birth defects, *Dev Med Child Neurol* 44:426-429, 2002.
277. Ray JG, Meier C, Vermeulen MJ, Boss S, et al: Association of neural tube defects and folic acid food fortification in Canada, *Lancet* 360:2047-2048, 2002.
278. Mills JL, Signore C: Neural tube defect rates before and after food fortification with folic acid, *Birth Defects Res A Clin Mol Teratol* 70:844-845, 2004.
279. Wald NJ: Folic acid and the prevention of neural-tube defects, *N Engl J Med* 350:101-103, 2004.
280. Lopez-Camelo JS, Orioli DM, Dutra MDG, NazerHerrera J, et al: Reduction of birth prevalence rates of neural tube defects after folic acid fortification in Chile, *Am J Med Genet A* 135:120-125, 2005.
281. Blom HJ, Shaw GM, den Heijer M, Finnell RH: Neural tube defects and folate: Case far from closed, *Nat Rev Neurosci* 7:724-731, 2006.
282. Elwood JM: Can vitamins prevent neural tube defects? *CMAJ* 129:1088-1092, 1983.
283. Wald NJ, Polani PE: Neural-tube defects and vitamins: The need for a randomized clinical trial, *Br J Obstet Gynaecol* 91:516-523, 1984.
284. Rush D, Rosenberg IH: Folate supplements and neural tube defects, *Nutr Rev* 50:25-26, 1992.
285. American Academy of Pediatrics Committee on Genetics: Folic acid for the prevention of neural tube defects, *Pediatrics* 104:325-327, 1999.
286. Rader JI, Schneeman BO: Prevalence of neural tube defects, folate status, and folate fortification of enriched cereal-grain products in the United States, *Pediatrics* 117:1394-1399, 2006.
287. Brent RL, Oakley GP Jr: The folate debate, *Pediatrics* 117:1418-1419, 2006.
288. Brent RL, Oakley GP, Mattison DR: The unnecessary epidemic of folic acid–preventable spina bifida and anencephaly, *Pediatrics* 106:825-827, 2000.
289. Klusmann A, Heinrich B, Stopler H, Gartner J, et al: A decreasing rate of neural tube defects following the recommendations for periconceptional folic acid supplementation, *Acta Paediatr* 94:1538-1542, 2005.
289a. De Wals P, Tairou F, Van Allen MI, Uh SH, et al: Reduction in neural-tube defects after folic acid fortification in Canada, *N Engl J Med* 357:135-142, 2007.
290. Rothenberg SP, daCosta MP, Sequeira JM, Cracco J, et al: Autoantibodies against folate receptors in women with a pregnancy complicated by a neural-tube defect, *N Engl J Med* 350:134-142, 2004.
291. Steegers-Theunissen RP, Boers GH, Blom HJ, Nijhuis JG, et al: Neural tube defects and elevated homocysteine levels in amniotic fluid, *Am J Obstet Gynecol* 172:1436-1441, 1995.
292. van der Put NMJ, van den Heuvel LP, Steegers-Theunissen RPM, Trijbels FJM, et al: Decreased methylene tetrahydrofolate reductase activity due to the 677C - ->T mutation in families with spina bifida offspring, *J Mol Med* 74:691-694, 1996.
293. Rosenquist TH, Ratashak SA, Selhub J: Homocysteine induces congenital defects of the heart and neural tube: Effect of folic acid, *Proc Natl Acad Sci U S A* 93:15227-15232, 1997.
294. Christensen B, Arbour L, Tran P, Leclerc D, et al: Genetic polymorphisms in methylenetetrahydrofolate reductase and methionine synthase, folate levels in red blood cells, and risk of neural tube defects, *Am J Med Genet* 84:151-157, 1999.
295. Carter CO, Evans KA, Till K: Spinal dysraphism: Genetic relation to neural tube malformations, *J Med Genet* 13:343-350, 1976.
296. Harding BN, Surtees R: Metabolic and neurodegenerative diseases of childhood. In Graham DI, Lantos PL, editors: *Greenfield's Neuropathology, 7*, London: 2002, Arnold Publishers.
297. Grant DN: Spinal dysraphism, *Postgrad Med J* 48:493-495, 1972.
298. McLone DG, La Marca F: The tethered spinal cord: Diagnosis, significance, and management, *Semin Pediatr Neurol* 4:192-208, 1997.

299. Cornette L, Verpoorten C, Lagae L, Plets C, et al: Closed spinal dysraphism: A review on diagnosis and treatment in infancy, *Eur J Paediatr Neurol* 2:179-185, 1998.

300. Sahin F, Selcuki M, Ecin N, Zenciroglu A, et al: Level of conus medullaris in term and preterm neonates, *Arch Dis Child* 77:F67-F69, 1997.

301. Yamada S, Zinke DE, Sanders D: Pathophysiology of "tethered cord syndrome," *J Neurosurg* 54:494-503, 1981.

302. Anderson FM: Occult spinal dysraphism: A series of 73 cases, *Pediatrics* 55:826-835, 1975.

303. Scatliff JH, Kendall BE, Kingsley DP, Britton J, et al: Closed spinal dysraphism: Analysis of clinical, radiological, and surgical findings in 104 consecutive patients, *AJNR Am J Neuroradiol* 10:269-277, 1989.

304. Pang D: Split cord malformation. I. A unified theory of embryogenesis for double spinal cord malformations, *Neurosurgery* 31:451-480, 1992.

305. Towfighi J, Housman C: Spinal cord abnormalities in caudal regression syndrome, *Acta Neuropathol* 81:458-466, 1991.

306. Kitzmiller JL, Cloherty JP, Younger MD, Tabatabaii A, et al: Diabetic pregnancy and perinatal morbidity, *Am J Obstet Gynecol* 131:560-580, 1978.

307. Assemany SR, Muzzo S, Gardner LI: Syndrome of phocomelic diabetic embryopathy (caudal dysplasia), *Am J Dis Child* 123:489-491, 1972.

308. Rusnak SL, Driscoll SG: Congenital spinal anomalies in infants of diabetic mothers, *Pediatrics* 35:989, 1965.

309. Mills JL: Malformations in infants of diabetic mothers, *Teratology* 25:385-394, 1982.

310. Becerra JE, Khoury MJ, Cordero JF, Erickson JD: Diabetes mellitus during pregnancy and the risks for specific birth defects: A population-based case-control study, *Pediatrics* 85:1-9, 1990.

311. Peacock WJ, Murovic JA: Magnetic resonance imaging in myelocystoceles: Report of two cases, *J Neurosurg* 70:804-807, 1989.

312. Gower DJ, Del Curling O, Kelly DLJ, Alexander EJ: Diastematomyelia: A 40-year experience, *Pediatr Neurosci* 14:90-96, 1988.

313. Harwood-Nash DC, McHugh K: Diastematomyelia in 172 children: The impact of modern neuroradiology, *Pediatr Neurosurg* 16:247-251, 1990.

314. Seeds JW, Jones FD: Lipomyelomeningocele: Prenatal diagnosis and management, *Obstet Gynecol* 67:S34-S37, 1986.

315. Seeds JW, Powers SK: Early prenatal diagnosis of familial lipomyelomeningocele, *Obstet Gynecol* 72:469-471, 1988.

316. Lemire RJ, Beckwith JB: Pathogenesis of congenital tumors and malformations of the sacrococcygeal region, *Teratology* 25:201-213, 1982.

317. Baraitser P, Shieff C: Cutaneomeningo-spinal angiomatosis: The syndrome of Cobb. A case report, *Neuropediatrics* 21:160-161, 1990.

318. Michaud LJ, Jaffe KM, Benjamin DR, Stuntz JT, et al: Hemangioblastoma of the conus medullaris associated with cutaneous hemangioma, *Pediatr Neurol* 4:309-312, 1988.

319. Langer JC, Harrison MR, Schmidt KG, Silverman NH, et al: Fetal hydrops and death from sacrococcygeal teratoma: Rationale for fetal surgery, *Am J Obstet Gynecol* 160:1145-1150, 1989.

320. Higginbottom MC, Jones KL, James HE, Bruce DA, et al: Aplasia cutis congenita: A cutaneous marker of occult spinal dysraphism, *J Pediatr* 96:687-689, 1980.

321. Hall DE, Udvarhelyi GB, Altman J: Lumbosacral skin lesions as markers of occult spinal dysraphism, *JAMA* 246:2606-2608, 1981.

322. Albright AL, Gartner JC, Wiener ES: Lumbar cutaneous hemangiomas as indicators of tethered spinal cords, *Pediatrics* 83:977-980, 1989.

323. Pang DL, Hoffman HJ, Rekate HL: Split cord malformation. II. Clinical syndrome, *Neurosurgery* 31:481-500, 1992.

324. Kriss VM, Desai NS: Occult spinal dysraphism in neonates: Assessment of high-risk cutaneous stigmata on sonography, *AJR Am J Roentgenol* 171:1687-1692, 1998.

325. Ackerman LL, Menezes AH: Spinal congenital dermal sinuses: A 30-year experience, *Pediatrics* 112:641-647, 2003.

326. Tubbs RS, Wellons JC, 3rd, Iskandar BJ, Oakes WJ: Isolated flat capillary midline lumbosacral hemangiomas as indicators of occult spinal dysraphism, *J Neurosurg* 100:86-89, 2004.

327. Piatt JH Jr: Skin hemangiomas and occult dysraphism, *J Neurosurg* 100:81-82; discussion 82, 2004.

328. Scheible W, James HE, Leopold GR, Hilton SV: Occult spinal dysraphism in infants: Screening with high-resolution real-time ultrasound, *Radiology* 146:743-746, 1983.

329. Naidich TP, Fernbach SK, McLone DG, Shkolnik A: John Caffey Award. Sonography of the caudal spine and back: Congenital anomalies in children, *AJR Am J Roentgenol* 142:1229-1242, 1984.

329a. Lowe LH, Johanek AJ, Moore CW: Sonography of the neonatal spine: Part 2, spinal disorders, *AJR Am J Roentgenol* 188:739-744, 2007.

330. Packer RJ, Zimmerman RA, Sutton LN, Bilaniuk LT, et al: Magnetic resonance imaging of spinal cord disease of childhood, *Pediatrics* 78:251-256, 1986.

331. Naidich TP, McLone DG, Mutluer S: A new understanding of dorsal dysraphism with lipoma (lipomyeloschisis): Radiologic evaluation and surgical correction, *AJR Am J Roentgenol* 140:1065-1078, 1983.

332. Hoffman HJ, Taecholarn C, Hendrick EB, Humphreys RP: Management of lipomyelomeningoceles: Experience at the Hospital for Sick Children, Toronto, *J Neurosurg* 62:1-8, 1985.

333. Dubowitz V, Lorber J, Zachary RB: Lipoma of the cauda equina, *Arch Dis Child* 40:207, 1965.

334. Pasternak JF, Volpe JJ: Lumbosacral lipoma with acute deterioration during infancy, *Pediatrics* 66:125-128, 1980.

335. Yakovlev PI: Pathoarchitectonic studies of cerebral malformations. I. Arrhinencephalies (holotelencephalies), *J Neuropathol Exp Neurol* 18:22, 1959.

336. Leech RW, Shuman RM: Holoprosencephaly and related midline cerebral anomalies: A review, *J Child Neurol* 1:3-18, 1986.

337. Richards LJ, Plachez C, Ren T: Mechanisms regulating the development of the corpus callosum and its agenesis in mouse and human, *Clin Genet* 66:276-289, 2004.

337a. Paul LK, Brown WS, Adolphs R, Tyszka JM, et al: Agenesis of the corpus callosum: Genetic, developmental and functional aspects of connectivity, *Nat Rev Neurosci* 8:287-299, 2007.

337b. Ren T, Anderson A, Shen WB, Huang H, et al: Imaging, anatomical, and molecular analysis of callosal formation in the developing human fetal brain, *Anat Rec A Discov Mol Cell Evol Biol* 288:191-204, 2006.

338. Kier EL, Truwit CL: The normal and abnormal genu of the corpus callosum: An evolutionary, embryologic, anatomic, and MR analysis, *AJNR Am J Neuroradiol* 17:1631-1641, 1996.

339. Kier EL, Truwit CL: The lamina rostralis: Modification of concepts concerning the anatomy, embryology, and MR appearance of the rostrum of the corpus callosum, *AJNR Am J Neuroradiol* 18:715-722, 1997.

340. Muenke M: Holoprosencephaly as a genetic model for normal craniofacial, development, *Dev Biol* 5:294-301, 1994.

341. Rubenstein JLR, Shimamura K, Martinez S, Puelles L: Regionalization of the prosencephalic neural plate, *Annu Rev Neurosci* 21:445-477, 1998.

342. Chiang C, Litingtung Y, Lee E, Young KE, et al: Cyclopia and defective axial patterning in mice lacking sonic hedgehog gene function, *Nature* 383:407-413, 1996.

343. Belloni E, Muenke M, Roessler E, Traverso G, et al: Identification of sonic hedgehog as a candidate gene responsible for holoprosencephaly, *Nature* 14:353-356, 1996.

344. Roessler E, Belloni E, Gaudenz K, Jay P, et al: Mutations in sonic hedgehog gene cause holoprosencephaly, *Nat Genet* 14:357-360, 1996.

345. Rubenstein JLR, Beachy PA: Patterning of the embryonic forebrain, *Curr Opin in Neurobiol* 8:18-26, 1998.

346. Golden JA: Holoprosencephaly: A defect in brain patterning, *J Neuropathol Exp Neurol* 57:991-999, 1998.

347. Muenke M, Cohen MM: Genetic approaches to understanding brain development: Holoprosencephaly as a model, *Ment Retard Dev Disabl Res Rev* 6:15-21, 2000.

348. Nanni L, Croen LA, Lammer EJ, Muenke M: Holoprosencephaly: Molecular study of a California population, *Am J Med Genet* 90:315-319, 2000.

349. Sarnat HB, Flores-Sarnat L: Neuropathologic research strategies in holoprosencephaly, *J Child Neurol* 16:918-931, 2001.

350. Rallu M, Corbin JG, Fishell G: Parsing the prosencephalon, *Nature Rev Neurosci* 3:943-951, 2002.

351. Hahn JS, Plawner LL: Evaluation and management of children with holoprosencephaly, *Pediatr Neurol* 31:79-88, 2004.

352. Sarnat HB: CNS malformations: Gene locations of known human mutations, *Eur J Paediatr Neurol* 9:427-431, 2005.

352a. El-Jaick KB, Powers SE, Bartholin L, Myers KR, et al: Functional analysis of mutations in TGIF associated with holoprosencephaly, *Mol Genet Metab* 90:97-111, 2007.

353. Garcia CA, Duncan C: Atelencephalic microcephaly, *Dev Med Child Neurol* 19:227-232, 1977.

354. Iivanainen M, Haltia M, Lydecken K: Atelencephaly, *Dev Med Child Neurol* 19:663-668, 1977.

355. Kim TS, Cho S, Dickson DW: Aprosencephaly: Review of the literature and report of a case with cerebellar hypoplasia, pigmented epithelial cyst and Rathke's cleft cyst, *Acta Neuropathol* 79:424-431, 1990.

356. Adkins WN, Kaveggia EG: Sporadic case of apparent aprosencephaly, *Am J Med Genet* 3:311-314, 1979.

357. Lurie IW, Nedzed MK, Lazjuk GI, Kirillova IA, et al: The XK-aprosencephaly syndrome [letter], *Am J Med Genet* 7:231-234, 1980.

358. Lurie IW, Nedzved MK, Lazjuk GI, Kirillova IA, et al: Aprosencephaly-atelencephaly and the aprosencephaly (XK) syndrome, *Am J Med Genet* 3:301-309, 1979.

359. Martin RA, Carey JG: A view and case report of aprosencephaly and the XK aprosencephaly syndrome, *Am J Med Genet* 11:369-371, 1982.

360. Siebert JR, Warkany J, Lemire RJ: Atelencephalic microcephaly in a 21-week human fetus, *Teratology* 34:9-19, 1986.

361. Siebert JR, Kokich VG, Warkany J, Lemire RJ: Atelencephalic microcephaly: Craniofacial anatomy and morphologic comparisons with holoprosencephaly and anencephaly, *Teratology* 36:279-285, 1987.

362. Harris CP, Townsend JJ, Norman MG, White VA, et al: Atelencephalic aprosencephaly, *J Child Neurol* 9:412-416, 1994.

363. Ippel PF, BreslauSiderius EJ, Hack WWM, vanderBlij HF, et al: Atelencephalic microcephaly: A case report and review of the literature, *Eur J Pediatr* 157:493-497, 1998.

364. Kakita A, Hayashi S, Arakawa M, Takahashi H: Aprosencephaly: Histopathological features of the rudimentary forebrain and retina, *Acta Neuropathol* 102:110-116, 2001.
365. Hahn JS, Barkovich AJ, Stashinko EE, Kinsman SL, et al: Factor analysis of neuroanatomical and clinical characteristics of holoprosencephaly, *Brain Dev* 28:413-419, 2006.
366. Kobori JA, Herrick MK, Urich H: Arhinencephaly: The spectrum of associated malformations, *Brain* 110:237-260, 1987.
367. Mizuguchi M, Morimatsu Y: Histopathological study of alobar holoprosencephaly. 2. Marginal glioneural heterotopia and other gliomesenchymal abnormalities, *Acta Neuropathol* 78:183-188, 1989.
368. Mizuguchi M, Morimatsu Y: Histopathological study of alobar holoprosencephaly. 1. Abnormal laminar architecture of the telencephalic cortex, *Acta Neuropathol* 78:176-182, 1989.
369. Souza JP, Siebert JR, Beckwith JB: An anatomic comparison of cebocephaly and ethmocephaly, *Teratology* 42:347-357, 1990.
370. Rössing R, Friede RL: Holoprosencephaly with retroprosencephalic extracerebral cyst, *Dev Med Child Neurol* 34:177-181, 1992.
371. Cohen MM Jr: Perspectives on holoprosencephaly. I. Epidemiology, genetics, and syndromology, *Teratology* 40:211-235, 1989.
372. Cohen MM Jr: Perspectives on holoprosencephaly. III. Spectra, distinctions, continuities, and discontinuities, *Am J Med Genet* 34:271-288, 1989.
373. Oba H, Barkovich AJ: Holoprosencephaly: An analysis of callosal formation and its relation to development of the interhemispheric fissure, *AJNR Am J Neuroradiol* 16:453-460, 1995.
374. Olsen CL, Hughes JP, Youngblood LG, Sharpe Stimac M: Epidemiology of holoprosencephaly and phenotypic characteristics of affected children: New York State, 1984-1989, *Am J Med Genet* 73:217-226, 1997.
375. Simon EM, Hevner R, Pinter JD, Clegg NJ, et al: Assessment of the deep gray nuclei in holoprosencephaly, *AJNR Am J Neuroradiol* 21:1955-1961, 2000.
376. Plawner LL, Delgado MR, Miller VS, Levey EB, et al: Neuroanatomy of holoprosencephaly as predictor of function: Beyond the face predicting the brain, *Neurology* 59:1058-1066, 2002.
377. Lewis AJ, Simon EM, Barkovich AJ, Clegg NJ, et al: Middle interhemispheric variant of holoprosencephaly: A distinct cliniconeuroradiologic subtype, *Neurology* 59:1860-1865, 2002.
378. Yamada S, Uwabe C, Fujii S, Shiota K: Phenotypic variability in human embryonic holoprosencephaly in the Kyoto collection, *Birth Defects Res A Clin Mol Teratol* 70:495-508, 2004.
379. Takahashi S, Miyamoto A, Saino T, Inyaku F: Alobar holoprosencephaly with diabetes insipidus and neuronal migration disorder, *Pediatr Neurol* 13:175-177, 1995.
380. Matsunaga E, Shiota K: Holoprosencephaly in human embryos: Epidemiologic studies of 150 cases, *Teratology* 16:261-272, 1977.
381. DeMyer W, Zeman W, Palmer CG: The face predicts the brain: Diagnostic significance of median facial anomalies for holoprosencephaly (arrhinencephaly), *Pediatrics* 34:256-263, 1964.
382. Smith DW, Patau K, Therman E, et al: The D-1 trisomy syndrome, *J Pediatr* 62:326-341, 1963.
383. Warkany J, Lemire RJ, Cohen MM Jr: *Mental Retardation and Congenital Malformations of the Central Nervous System*, Chicago: 1981, Year Book.
384. Hasegawa Y, Hasegawa T, Yokoyama T, Kotoh S, et al: Holoprosencephaly associated with diabetes insipidus and syndrome of inappropriate secretion of antidiuretic hormone, *J Pediatr* 117:756-758, 1990.
385. Louis ED, Lynch T, Cargan AL, Fahn S: Generalized chorea in an infant with semilobar holoprosencephaly, *Pediatr Neurol* 13:355-357, 1995.
386. Roesler CP, Paterson SJ, Flax J, Hahn JS, et al: Links between abnormal brain structure and cognition in holoprosencephaly, *Pediatr Neurol* 35:387-394, 2006.
387. Shanks DE, Wilson WG: Lobar holoprosencephaly presenting as spastic diplegia, *Dev Med Child Neurol* 30:383-386, 1988.
388. Biancheri R, Rossi A, Tortori-Donati P, Stringara S, et al: Middle interhemispheric variant of holoprosencephaly: A very mild clinical case, *Neurology* 63:2194-2196, 2004.
389. Holmes LB, Driscoll S, Atkins L: Genetic heterogeneity of cebocephaly, *J Med Genet* 11:35-40, 1974.
390. Münke M: Clinical, cytogenetic, and molecular approaches to the genetic heterogeneity of holoprosencephaly, *Am J Med Genet* 34:237-245, 1989.
391. Lorch V, Fojaco R, Bauer CR: Cebocephalus associated with trisomy 13-15 mosaicism, *Arch Neurol* 35:163-165, 1978.
392. Uchida IA, McRae KN, Wang HC, Ray M: Familial short arm deficiency of chromosome 18 concomitant with arrhinencephaly and alopecia congenita, *Am J Hum Genet* 17:410, 1965.
393. Emberger JM, Marty-Double C, Pincemin D, Caderas de Kerleau J: [Holoprosencephaly by triploidy 69 XXX in a 5 month old fetus], *Ann Genet* 19:191-193, 1976.
394. Spinner NB, Eunpu DL, Austria JR, Mamunes P: Holoprosencephaly in a newborn girl with 46,XX,i(18q), *Am J Med Genet* 39:11-12, 1991.
395. Hamada H, Arinami T, Koresawa M, Kubo T, et al: A case of trisomy 21 with holoprosencephaly: The fifth case, *Jinrui Idengaku Zasshi* 36:159-163, 1991.
396. Estabrooks LL, Rao KW, Donahue RP, Aylsworth AS: Holoprosencephaly in an infant with a minute deletion of chromosome 21(q22.3), *Am J Med Genet* 36:306-309, 1990.
397. Helmuth RA, Weaver DD, Wills ER: Holoprosencephaly, ear abnormalities, congenital heart defect, and microphallus in a patient with 11q-mosaicism, *Am J Med Genet* 32:178-181, 1989.
398. Lazaro L, Dubourg C, Pasquier L, LeDuff F, et al: Phenotypic and molecular variability of the holoprosencephalic spectrum, *Am J Med Genet A* 129:21-24, 2004.
399. Pfitzer P, Muntefering H: Cyclopism as a hereditary malformation, *Nature* 217:1071-1072, 1968.
400. Berry SA, Pierpont ME, Gorlin RJ: Single central incisor in familial holoprosencephaly, *J Pediatr* 104:877-880, 1984.
401. Hennekam RC, Van Noort G, de la Fuente FA, Norbruis OF: Agenesis of the nasal septal cartilage: Another sign in autosomal dominant holoprosencephaly [letter], *Am J Med Genet* 39:121-122, 1991.
402. Ardinger HH, Bartley JA: Microcephaly in familial holoprosencephaly, *J Craniofac Genet Dev Biol* 8:53-61, 1988.
403. Kato M, Nanba E, Akaboshi S, Shiihara T, et al: Sonic hedgehog signal peptide mutation in a patient with holoprosencephaly, *Ann Neurol* 47:514-516, 2000.
404. Marini M, Cusano R, DeBiasio P, Caroli F, et al: Previously undescribed nonsense mutation in SHH caused autosomal dominant holoprosencephaly with wide intrafamilial variability, *Am J Med Genet A* 117:112-115, 2003.
405. Hehr U, Gross C, Diebold U, Wahl D, et al: Wide phenotypic variability in families with holoprosencephaly and a sonic hedgehog mutation, *Eur J Pediatr* 163:347-352, 2004.
406. Barr M Jr, Hanson JW, Currey K, Sharp S, et al: Holoprosencephaly in infants of diabetic mothers, *J Pediatr* 102:565-568, 1983.
407. Binns W, James LF, Shupe JL, Thacker EJ: Cyclopian-type malformation in lambs, *Arch Environ Health* 5:106, 1962.
408. Chervenak FA, Isaacson G, Hobbins JC, Chitkara U, et al: Diagnosis and management of fetal holoprosencephaly, *Obstet Gynecol* 66:322-326, 1985.
409. McGahan JP, Nyberg DA, Mack LA: Sonography of facial features of alobar and semilobar holoprosencephaly, *AJR Am J Roentgenol* 154:143-148, 1990.
410. Nyberg DA, Mack LA, Bronstein A, Hirsch J, et al: Holoprosencephaly: Prenatal sonographic diagnosis, *AJR Am J Roentgenol* 149:1051-1058, 1987.
411. Verlinsky Y, Rechitsky S, Verlinsky O, Ozen S, et al: Preimplantation diagnosis for sonic hedgehog mutation causing familial holoprosencephaly, *N Engl J Med* 348:1449-1454, 2003.
412. Barkovich AJ, Norman D: Absence of the septum pellucidum: A useful sign in the diagnosis of congenital brain malformations, *AJNR Am J Neuroradiol* 9:1107-1114, 1988.
413. Utsunomiya H, Ogasawara T, Hayashi T, Hashimoto T, et al: Dysgenesis of the corpus callosum and associated telencephalic anomalies: MRI, *Neuroradiology* 39:302-310, 1997.
414. Taylor M, David AS: Agenesis of the corpus callosum: A United Kingdom series of 56 cases, *J Neurol Neurosurg Psychiatry* 64:131-134, 1998.
415. Nissenkorn A, Michelson M, Ben-Zeev B, Lerman-Sagie T: Inborn errors of metabolism: A cause of abnormal brain development, *Neurology* 56:1265-1272, 2001.
416. Barkovich AJ, Simon EM, Walsh CA: Callosal agenesis with cyst: A better understanding and new classification, *Neurology* 56:220-227, 2001.
417. Sztriha L: Spectrum of corpus callosum agenesis, *Pediatr Neurol* 32:94-101, 2005.
418. Bedeschi MF, Bonaglia MC, Grasso R, Pellegri A, et al: Agenesis of the corpus callosum: Clinical and genetic study in 63 young patients, *Pediatr Neurol* 34:186-193, 2006.
419. Hetts SW, Sherr EH, Chao S, Gobuty S, et al: Anomalies of the corpus callosum: An MR analysis of the phenotypic spectrum of associated malformations, *AJR Am J Roentgenol* 187:1343-1348, 2006.
419a. Fratelli N, Papageorghiou AT, Prefumo F, Bakalis S, et al: Outcome of prenatally diagnosed agenesis of the corpus callosum, *Prenat Diagn* 27:512-517, 2007.
420. Hale BR, Rice P: Septo-optic dysplasia: Clinical and embryological aspects, *Dev Med Child Neurol* 16:812-817, 1974.
421. Barkovich AJ, Kjos BO, Norman D, Edwards MS: Revised classification of posterior fossa cysts and cystlike malformations based on the results of multiplanar MR imaging, *AJNR Am J Neuroradiol* 10:977-988, 1989.
422. Barkovich AJ, Fram EK, Norman D: Septo-optic dysplasia: MR imaging, *Radiology* 171:189-192, 1989.
423. Breeding LM, Bodensteiner JB, Cowan L, Higgins WL: The cavum septi pellucidi: A magnetic resonance imaging study of prevalence and clinical associations in a pediatric population, *J Neuroimaging* 1:115-118, 1991.
424. Bodensteiner JB, Schaefer GB: Wide cavum septum pellucidum: A marker of disturbed brain development, *Pediatr Neurol* 6:391-394, 1990.
425. Aicardi J, Goutières F: The syndrome of absence of the septum pellucidum with porencephalies and other developmental defects, *Neuropediatrics* 12:319-329, 1981.
426. Shimozawa N, Ohno K, Takashima S, Takakura H, et al: The syndrome of the absence of a septum pellucidum with porencephaly, *Brain Dev* 8:632-636, 1986.

427. Menezes L, Aicardi J, Goutières F: Absence of the septum pellucidum with porencephalia: A neuroradiologic syndrome with variable clinical expression, *Arch Neurol* 45:542-545, 1988.
428. Kuriyama M, Shigematsu Y, Konishi K, Konishi Y, et al: Septo-optic dysplasia with infantile spasms, *Pediatr Neurol* 4:62-65, 1988.
429. Leech RW, Shuman RM: Midline telencephalic dysgenesis: Report of three cases, *J Child Neurol* 1:224-232, 1986.
430. Ouvrier R, Billson F: Optic nerve hypoplasia: A review, *J Child Neurol* 1:181-188, 1986.
431. Schaefer GB, Bodensteiner JB, Thompson JN: Subtle anomalies of the septum pellucidum and neurodevelopmental deficits, *Dev Med Child Neurol* 36:554-559, 1994.
432. Bodensteiner JB, Schaefer GB, Craft JM: Cavum septi pellucidi and cavum vergae in normal and developmentally delayed populations, *J Child Neurol* 13:120-121, 1998.
433. Schuelke M, Krude H, Finckh B, Mayatepek E, et al: Septo-optic dysplasia associated with a new mitochondrial cytochrome b mutation, *Ann Neurol* 51:388-392, 2002.
434. Miller SP, Shevell MI, Patenaude Y, Poulin C, et al: Septo-optic dysplasia plus: A spectrum of malformations of cortical development, *Neurology* 54:1701-1703, 2000.
435. Traggiai C, Stanhope R: Endocrinopathies associated with midline cerebral and cranial malformations, *J Pediatr* 140:252-255, 2002.
436. Stevens CA, Dobyns WB: Septo-optic dysplasia and amniotic bands: Further evidence for a vascular pathogenesis, *Am J Med Genet A* 125:12-16, 2004.
437. Ahmad T, Garcia-Filion P, Borchert M, Kaufman F, et al: Endocrinological and auxological abnormalities in young children with optic nerve hypoplasia: A prospective study, *J Pediatr* 148:78-84, 2006.
438. Polizzi A, Pavone P, Iannetti P, Manfre L, et al: Septo-optic dysplasia complex: A heterogeneous malformation syndrome, *Pediatr Neurol* 34:66-71, 2006.
439. Dattani MT, Martinez-Barbera JP, Thomas PQ, Brickman JM, et al: Molecular genetics of septo-optic dysplasia, *Horm Res* 53:26-33, 2000.
440. Pauling KJ, Bodensteiner JB, Hogg JP, Schaefer GB: Does selection bias determine the prevalence of the cavum septi pellucidi? *Pediatr Neurol* 19:195-198, 1998.
441. Mott SH, Bodensteiner JB, Allan WC: The cavum septi pellucidi in term and preterm newborn infants, *J Child Neurol* 7:35-38, 1992.
442. Barkovich AJ, Norman D: Anomalies of the corpus callosum: Correlation with further anomalies of the brain, *AJNR Am J Neuroradiol* 9:493-501, 1988.
443. Sanders RJ: Sentence comprehension following agenesis of the corpus callosum, *Brain Lang* 37:59-72, 1989.
444. Koeda T, Takeshita K: Tactile naming disorder of the left hand in two cases with corpus callosum agenesis, *Dev Med Child Neurol* 35:65-69, 1993.
445. Friefeld S, MacGregor DL, Chuang S, Saint-Cyr J: Comparative study of inter- and intrahemispheric somatosensory functions in children with partial and complete agenesis of the corpus callosum, *Dev Med Child Neurol* 42:831-838, 2000.
446. Bodensteiner JB, Breen L, Schwartz TL, Schaefer GB: Hypoplastic corpus callosum in ocular albinism: Indication of a global disturbance of neuronal migration, *J Child Neurol* 5:341-343, 1990.
447. Hartmann H, Uyanik G, Gross C, Hehr U, et al: Agenesis of the corpus callosum, abnormal genitalia and intractable epilepsy due to a novel familial mutation in the Aristaless-related homeobox gene, *Neuropediatrics* 35:157-160, 2004.
448. Young JN, Oakes WJ, Hatten HP: Dorsal third ventricular cyst: An entity distinct from holoprosencephaly, *J Neurosurg* 77:556-561, 1992.
449. Griebel ML, Williams JP, Russell SS, Spence GT, et al: Clinical and developmental findings in children with giant interhemispheric cysts and dysgenesis of the corpus callosum, *Pediatr Neurol* 13:119-124, 1995.
450. Neidich JA, Nussbaum RL, Packer RJ, Emanuel BS, et al: Heterogeneity of clinical severity and molecular lesions in Aicardi syndrome, *J Pediatr* 116:911-917, 1990.
451. Nielsen KB, Anvret M, Flodmark O, Furuskog P, et al: Aicardi syndrome: Early neuroradiological manifestations and results of DNA studies in one patient, *Am J Med Genet* 38:65-68, 1991.
452. Donnenfeld AE, Packer RJ, Zackai EH, Chee CM, et al: Clinical, cytogenetic, and pedigree findings in 18 cases of Aicardi syndrome, *Am J Med Genet* 32:461-467, 1989.
453. Molina JA, Mateos F, Merino M, Epifanio JL, et al: Aicardi syndrome in two sisters, *J Pediatr* 115:282-283, 1989.
454. Roland EH, Flodmark O, Hill A: Neurosonographic features of Aicardi's syndrome, *J Child Neurol* 4:307-310, 1989.
455. Hamano S, Yagishita S, Kawakami M, Ito F, et al: Aicardi syndrome: Postmortem findings, *Pediatr Neurol* 5:259-261, 1989.
456. Tagawa T, Mimaki T, Ono J, Tanaka J, et al: Aicardi syndrome associated with an embryonal carcinoma, *Pediatr Neurol* 5:45-47, 1989.
457. Bertoni JM, von Loh S, Allen RJ: The Aicardi syndrome: Report of 4 cases and review of the literature, *Ann Neurol* 5:475-482, 1979.
458. Menezes AV, MacGregor DL, Buncic JR: Aicardi syndrome: Natural history and possible predictors of severity, *Pediatr Neurol* 11:313-318, 1994.
459. Rosser TL, Acosta MT, Packer RJ: Aicardi syndrome: Spectrum of disease and long-term prognosis in 77 females, *Pediatr Neurol* 27:343-346, 2002.
460. Aicardi J: Aicardi syndrome, *Brain Dev* 27:164-171, 2005.
461. Palmer L, Zetterlund B, Hard AL, Steneryd K, et al: Aicardi syndrome: Presentation at onset in Swedish children born in 1975-2002, *Neuropediatrics* 37:154-158, 2006.
462. Atlas SW, Shkolnik A, Naidich TP: Sonographic recognition of agenesis of the corpus callosum, *AJR Am J Roentgenol* 145:167-173, 1985.
463. Fawer C-L, Calame A, Anderegg A, Deonna T, et al: Agenesis of the corpus callosum: Real-time ultrasonographic diagnosis and autopsy findings, *Helv Paediatr Acta* 40:371-380, 1985.
464. Hellstrom A, Wiklund LM, Svensson E, Stromland K, et al: Midline brain lesions in children with hormone insufficiency indicate early prenatal damage, *Acta Paediatr* 87:528-536, 1998.
465. Friedman JM, Santos-Ramos R: Natural history of X-linked aqueductal stenosis in the second and third trimesters of pregnancy, *Am J Obstet Gynecol* 150:104-106, 1984.
466. Cochrane DD, Myles ST: Management of intrauterine hydrocephalus, *J Neurosurg* 57:590-596, 1982.
467. Chervenak FA, Berkowitz RL, Romero R, Tortora M, et al: The diagnosis of fetal hydrocephalus, *Am J Obstet Gynecol* 147:703-716, 1983.
468. Cochrane DD, Myles ST, Nimrod C, Still DK, et al: Intrauterine hydrocephalus and ventriculomegaly: Associated anomalies and fetal outcome, *Can J Neurol Sci* 12:51-59, 1985.
469. Bromley B, Frigoletto FD Jr, Benacerraf BR: Mild fetal lateral cerebral ventriculomegaly: Clinical course and outcome, *Am J Obstet Gynecol* 164:863-867, 1991.
470. Amato M, Hüppi P, Durig P, Kaiser G, et al: Fetal ventriculomegaly due to isolated brain malformations, *Neuropediatrics* 21:130-132, 1990.
471. Hudgins RJ, Edwards MS, Goldstein R, Callen PW, et al: Natural history of fetal ventriculomegaly, *Pediatrics* 82:692-697, 1988.
472. Pober BR, Greene MF, Holmes LB: Complexities of intraventricular abnormalities, *J Pediatr* 108:545-551, 1986.
473. Renier D, Sainte-Rose C, Pierre-Kahn A, Hirsch JF: Prognostic des hydrocéphalies anténatales, *Presse Med* 18:168-172, 1989.
474. Pretorius DH, Davis K, Manco-Johnson ML, Manchester D, et al: Clinical course of fetal hydrocephalus: 40 cases, *AJR Am J Roentgenol* 144:827-831, 1985.
475. Serlo W, Kirkinen P, Jouppila P, Herva R: Prognostic signs in fetal hydrocephalus, *Childs Nerv Syst* 2:93-97, 1986.
476. Nyberg DA, Mack LA, Hirsch J, Pagon RO, et al: Fetal hydrocephalus: Sonographic detection and clinical significance of associated anomalies, *Radiology* 163:187-191, 1987.
477. Renier D, Sainte-Rose C, Pierre-Kahn A, Hirsch JF: Prenatal hydrocephalus: Outcome and prognosis, *Childs Nerv Syst* 4:213-222, 1988.
478. Drugan A, Krause B, Canady A, Zador IE, et al: The natural history of prenatally diagnosed cerebral ventriculomegaly, *JAMA* 261:1785-1788, 1989.
479. Stirling HF, Hendry M, Brown JK: Prenatal intracranial haemorrhage, *Dev Med Child Neurol* 31:807-811, 1989.
480. Benacerraf BR: Fetal hydrocephalus: Diagnosis and significance [editorial], *Radiology* 169:858-859, 1988.
481. Hanigan WC, Gibson J, Kleopoulos NJ, Cusack T, et al: Medical imaging of fetal ventriculomegaly, *J Neurosurg* 64:575-580, 1986.
482. Leidig E, Dannecker G, Pfeiffer KH, Salinas R, et al: Intrauterine development of posthaemorrhagic hydrocephalus, *Eur J Pediatr* 147:26-29, 1988.
483. Rosseau GL, McCullough DC, Joseph AL: Current prognosis in fetal ventriculomegaly, *J Neurosurg* 77:551-555, 1992.
484. Levitsky DB, Mack LA, Nyberg DA, Shurtleff DB, et al: Fetal aqueductal stenosis diagnosed sonographically: How grave is the prognosis? *AJR Am J Roentgenol* 164:725-730, 1995.
485. Kirkinen P, Serlo W, Jouppila P, Ryynanen M, et al: Long-term outcome of fetal hydrocephaly, *J Child Neurol* 11:189-192, 1996.
486. Futagi Y, Suzuki Y, Toribe Y, Morimoto K: Neurodevelopmental outcome in children with fetal hydrocephalus, *Pediatr Neurol* 27:111-116, 2002.
487. Cavalheiro S, Moron AF, Zymberg ST, Dastoli P: Fetal hydrocephalus-prenatal treatment, *Childs Nerv Syst* 19:561-573, 2003.
488. Davis GH: Fetal hydrocephalus, *Clin Perinatol* 30:531-539, 2003.
489. Mealey J Jr, Gilmor RL, Bubb MP: The prognosis of hydrocephalus overt at birth, *J Neurosurg* 39:348-355, 1973.
490. McCullough DC, Balzer-Martin LA: Current prognosis in overt neonatal hydrocephalus, *J Neurosurg* 57:378-383, 1982.
491. Hanigan WC, Morgan A, Shaaban A, Bradle P: Surgical treatment and long-term neurodevelopmental outcome for infants with idiopathic aqueductal stenosis, *Childs Nerv Syst* 7:386-390, 1991.
492. Fernell E, Uvebrant P, von Wendt L: Overt hydrocephalus at birth: Origin and outcome, *Childs Nerv Syst* 3:350-353, 1987.
493. Halliday J, Chow CW, Wallace D, Danks DM: X linked hydrocephalus: A survey of a 20 year period in Victoria, Australia, *J Med Genet* 23:23-31, 1986.

494. Fernell E, Hagberg B, Hagberg G, von Wendt L: Epidemiology of infantile hydrocephalus in Sweden. II. Origin in infants born at term, *Acta Paediatr Scand* 76:411-417, 1987.

495. Wong EV, Kenwrick S, Willems P, Lemmon V: Mutations in the cell adhesion molecule LI cause mental retardation, *Trends Neurosci* 18:168-172, 1995.

496. Schrander Stumpel C, Howeler C, Jones M, Sommer A, et al: Spectrum of X-linked hydrocephalus (HSAS), MASA syndrome, and complicated spastic paraplegia (SPG1): Clinical review with six additional families, *Am J Med Genet* 57:107-116, 1995.

497. Yamasaki M, Thompson P, Lemmon V: CRASH Syndrome: Mutations in L1CAM correlate with severity of the disease, *Neuropediatrics* 28:175-178, 1997.

498. Takahashi S, Makita Y, Okamoto N, Miyamoto A, et al: L1CAM mutation in a Japanese family with X-linked hydrocephalus: A study for genetic counseling, *Brain Dev* 19:559-562, 1997.

499. Sztriha L, Vos YJ, Verlind E, Johansen J, et al: X-linked hydrocephalus: A novel missense mutation in the L1CAM gene, *Pediatr Neurol* 27:293-296, 2002.

500. Haverkamp F, Wolfle J, Aretz M, Kramer A, et al: Congenital hydrocephalus internus and aqueduct stenosis: Aetiology and implications for genetic counselling, *Eur J Pediatr* 158:474-478, 1999.

501. McComb JG: Cerebrospinal fluid physiology of the developing fetus, *AJNR Am J Neuroradiol* 13:595-599, 1992.

502. Catala M: Carbonic anhydrase activity during development of the choroid plexus in the human fetus, *Childs Nerv Syst* 13:364-368, 1997.

503. Holtzman RN, Garcia L, Koenigsberger R: Hydrocephalus and congenital clasped thumbs: A case report with electromyographic evaluation, *Dev Med Child Neurol* 18:521-524, 1976.

504. Willems PJ, Vits L, Raeymaekers P, Beuten J, et al: Further localization of X-linked hydrocephalus in the chromosomal region-xq28, *Am J Hum Genet* 51:307-315, 1992.

505. Serville F, Lyonnet S, Pelet A, Reynaud M, et al: X-linked hydrocephalus-clinical heterogeneity at a single gene locus, *Eur J Pediatr* 151:515-518, 1992.

506. Vintzileos AM, Ingardia CJ, Nochimson DJ: Congenital hydrocephalus: A review and protocol for perinatal management, *Obstet Gynecol* 62:539-549, 1983.

507. Birnholz J: Fetal neurology. In Sanders RC, Hill M, editors: *Ultrasound Annual*, New York: 1984, Raven Press.

508. Glick PL, Harrison MR, Nakayama DK, Edwards MS, et al: Management of ventriculomegaly in the fetus, *J Pediatr* 105:97-105, 1984.

509. Zlotogora J, Sagi M, Cohen T: Familial hydrocephalus of prenatal onset, *Am J Med Genet* 49:202-204, 1994.

510. Wyldes M, Watkinson M: Isolated mild fetal ventriculomegaly, *Arch Dis Child Fetal Neonatal Ed* 89:F9-13, 2004.

511. Hart MN, Malamud N, Ellis WG: The Dandy-Walker syndrome: A clinicopathological study based on 28 cases, *Neurology* 22:771-780, 1972.

512. Tal Y, Freigang B, Dunn HG, Durity FA, et al: Dandy-Walker syndrome: Analysis of 21 cases, *Dev Med Child Neurol* 22:189-201, 1980.

513. Hirsch JF, Pierre-Kahn A, Renier D, Sainte Rose C, et al: The Dandy-Walker malformation: A review of 40 cases, *J Neurosurg* 61:515-522, 1984.

514. Connolly MB, Jan JE, Cochrane DD: Rapid recovery from cortical visual impairment following correction of prolonged shunt malfunction in congenital hydrocephalus, *Arch Neurol* 48:956-957, 1991.

515. Den Hollander NS, Vinkesteijn A, Schmitz-van Splunder P, Catsman-Berrevoets CE, et al: Prenatally diagnosed fetal ventriculomegaly: Prognosis and outcome, *Prenat Diagn* 18:557-566, 1998.

516. Michejda M, Hodgen GD: In utero diagnosis and treatment of non-human primate fetal skeletal anomalies. I. Hydrocephalus, *JAMA* 246:1093-1097, 1981.

517. Michejda M, Patronas N, DiChiro G, Hodgen GD: Fetal hydrocephalus. II. Amelioration of fetal porencephaly by in utero therapy in nonhuman primates, *JAMA* 251:2548-2552, 1984.

518. Michejda M, Queenan JT, McCullough D: Present status of intrauterine treatment of hydrocephalus and its future, *Am J Obstet Gynecol* 155:873-882, 1986.

519. Clewell WH, Johnson ML, Meier PR, Newkirk JB, et al: A surgical approach to the treatment of fetal hydrocephalus, *N Engl J Med* 306:1320-1325, 1982.

520. Bannister CM: Fetal neurosurgery: A new challenge on the horizon, *Dev Med Child Neurol* 26:827-830, 1984.

521. Manning FA, Harrison MR, Rodeck C: Catheter shunts for fetal hydronephrosis and hydrocephalus: Report of the International Fetal Surgery Registry, *N Engl J Med*, 3151986.

522. Oi SZ, Yamada H, Kimura M, Ehara K, et al: Factors affecting prognosis of intrauterine hydrocephalus diagnosed in the third trimester, *Neurol Med Chir* 30:456-461, 1990.

523. ten-Donkelaar HJ, Lammens M, Wesseling P, Thijssen HOM, et al: Development and developmental disorders of the human cerebellum, *J Neurol* 250:1025-1036, 2003.

524. Patel S, Barkovich AJ: Analysis and classification of cerebellar malformations, *AJNR Am J Neuroradiol* 23:1074-1087, 2002.

525. Boltshauser E: Cerebellum-small brain but large confusion: A review of selected cerebellar malformations and disruptions, *Am J Med Genet A* 126:376-385, 2004.

526. Sarnat HB, Alcalá H: Human cerebellar hypoplasia: A syndrome of diverse causes, *Arch Neurol* 37:300-305, 1980.

527. Tomiwa K, Baraitser M, Wilson J: Dominantly inherited congenital cerebellar ataxia with atrophy of the vermis, *Pediatr Neurol* 3:360-362, 1987.

528. Fenichel GM, Phillips JA: Familial aplasia of the cerebellar vermis: Possible X-linked dominant inheritance, *Arch Neurol* 46:582-583, 1989.

529. Mathews KD, Afifi AK, Hanson JW: Autosomal recessive cerebellar hypoplasia, *J Child Neurol* 4:189-194, 1989.

530. Dooley JM, LaRoche GR, Tremblay F, Riding M: Autosomal recessive cerebellar hypoplasia and tapeto-retinal degeneration: A new syndrome, *Pediatr Neurol* 8:232-234, 1992.

531. Guzzetta F, Mercuri E, Bonanno S, Longo M, et al: Autosomal recessive congenital cerebellar atrophy: A clinical and neuropsychological study, *Brain Dev* 15:439-445, 1993.

532. Shevell MI, Majnemer A: Clinical features of developmental disability associated with cerebellar hypoplasia, *Pediatr Neurol* 15:224-229, 1996.

533. Gardner RJM, Coleman LT, Mitchell LA, Smith LJ, et al: Near-total absence of the cerebellum, *Neuropediatrics* 32:62-68, 2001.

534. Wassmer E, Davies P, Whitehouse WP, Green SH: Clinical spectrum associated with cerebellar hypoplasia, *Pediatr Neurol* 28:347-351, 2003.

535. Zafeiriou DI, Vargiami E, Boltshauser E: Cerebellar agenesis and diabetes insipidus, *Neuropediatrics* 35:364-367, 2004.

536. Yapici Z, Eraksoy M: Non-progressive congenital ataxia with cerebellar hypoplasia in three families, *Acta Paediatr* 94:248-253, 2005.

537. Glass HC, Boycott KM, Adams C, Barlow K, et al: Autosomal recessive cerebellar hypoplasia in the Hutterite population, *Dev Med Child Neurol* 47:691-695, 2005.

538. Boycott KM, Flavelle S, Bureau A, Glass HC, et al: Homozygous deletion of the very low density lipoprotein receptor gene causes autosomal recessive cerebellar hypoplasia with cerebral gyral simplification, *Am J Hum Genet* 77:477-483, 2005.

539. Bordarier C, Aicardi J: Dandy-Walker syndrome and agenesis of the cerebellar vermis: Diagnostic problems and genetic counselling, *Dev Med Child Neurol* 32:285-294, 1990.

540. Russ PD, Pretorius DH, Johnson MJ: Dandy-Walker syndrome: A review of fifteen cases evaluated by prenatal sonography, *Am J Obstet Gynecol* 161:401-406, 1989.

541. Maria BL, Zinreich SJ, Carson BC, Rosenbaum AE, et al: Dandy-Walker syndrome revisited, *Pediatr Neurosci* 13:45-51, 1987.

542. Golden JA, Rorke LB, Brucke DA: Dandy-Walker syndrome and associated anomalies, *Pediatr Neurosci* 13:38-44, 1987.

543. Edwards MS, Raffel C: Discussion of articles by Maria et al and Golden et al, *Pediatr Neurosci* 13:45-51, 1987.

544. Bindal AK, Storrs BB, McLone DG: Management of the Dandy-Walker syndrome, *Pediatr Neurosurg* 16:163-169, 1990.

545. Osenbach RK, Menezes AH: Diagnosis and management of the Dandy-Walker malformation: 30 years of experience, *Pediatr Neurosurg* 18:179-189, 1992.

546. Estroff JA, Scott MR, Benacerraf BR: Dandy-Walker variant-prenatal sonographic features and clinical outcome, *Radiology* 185:755-758, 1992.

547. Strand RD, Barnes PD, Poussaint TY, Estroff JA, et al: Cystic retrocerebellar malformations: Unification of the Dandy-Walker complex and the Blake's pouch cyst, *Pediatr Radiol* 23:258-260, 1994.

548. Tortori Donati P, Fondelli MP, Rossi A, Carini S: Cystic malformations of the posterior cranial fossa originating from a defect of the posterior membranous area. Mega cisterna magna and persisting Blake's pouch: Two separate entities, *Childs Nerv Syst* 12:303-308, 1996.

549. Tan E-C, Takagi T, Karasawa K: Posterior fossa cystic lesions-magnetic resonance imaging manifestations, *Brain Dev* 17:418-424, 1995.

550. Elterman RD, Bodensteiner JB, Barnard JJ: Sudden unexpected death in patients with Dandy-Walker malformation, *J Child Neurol* 10:382-384, 1995.

551. Ondo WG, Delong GR: Dandy-Walker syndrome presenting as opisthotonus: Proposed pathophysiology, *Pediatr Neurol* 14:165-168, 1996.

552. Ecker JL, Shipp TD, Bromley B, Benacerraf B: The sonographic diagnosis of Dandy-Walker and Dandy-Walker variant: Associated findings and outcomes, *Prenat Diagn* 20:328-332, 2000.

553. Joubert M, Eisenring JJ, Robb JP, Andermann F: Familial agenesis of the cerebellar vermis: A syndrome of episodic hyperpnea, abnormal eye movements, ataxia, and retardation, *Neurology* 19:813-825, 1969.

554. Steinlin M, Schmid M, Landau K, Boltshauser E: Follow-up in children with Joubert syndrome, *Neuropediatrics* 28:204-211, 1997.

555. Maria BL, Hoang KB, Tusa RJ, Mancuso AA, et al: "Joubert syndrome" revisited: Key ocular motor signs with magnetic resonance imaging correlation, *J Child Neurol* 12:423-430, 1997.

556. Sztriha L, Al-Gazali LI, Aithala GR, Nork M: Joubert's syndrome: New cases and review of clinicopathologic correlation, *Pediatr Neurol* 20:274-281, 1999.

557. Anderson JS, Gorey MTP, Pasternak JF, Trommer BL: Joubert's syndrome and prenatal hydrocephalus, *Pediatr Neurol* 20:403-405, 1999.

558. Dixon-Salazar T, Silhavy JL, Marsh SE, Louie CM, et al: Mutations in the AHI1 gene, encoding Jouberin, cause Joubert syndrome with cortical polymicrogyria, *Am J Hum Genet* 75:979-987, 2004.
559. Hodgkins PR, Harris CM, Shawkat FS, Thompson DA, et al: Joubert syndrome: Long-term follow-up, *Dev Med Child Neurol* 46:694-699, 2004.
560. Janecke AR, Muller T, Gassner I, Kreczy A, et al: Joubert-like syndrome unlinked to known candidate loci, *J Pediatr* 144:264-269, 2004.
561. Morava E, Dinopoulos A, Kroes HY, Rodenburg RJ, et al: Mitochondrial dysfunction in a patient with Joubert syndrome, *Neuropediatrics* 36:214-217, 2005.
562. Valente EM, Marsh SE, Castori M, Dixon-Salazar T, et al: Distinguishing the four genetic causes of Jouberts syndrome-related disorders, *Ann Neurol* 57:513-519, 2005.
563. Valente EM, Brancati F, Silhavy JL, Castori M, et al: AHI1 gene mutations cause specific forms of Joubert syndrome-related disorders, *Ann Neurol* 59:527-534, 2006.

564. Toelle SP, Valcinkaya C, Kocer N, Deonna T, et al: Rhombencephalosynapsis: Clinical findings and neuroimaging in 9 children, *Neuropediatrics* 33:209-214, 2002.
565. Odemis E, Cakir M, Aynaci FM: Rhombencephalosynapsis associated with cutaneous pretibial hemangioma in an infant, *J Child Neurol* 18:225-228, 2003.
566. Napolitano M, Righini A, Zirpoli S, Rustico M, et al: Prenatal magnetic resonance imaging of rhombencephalosynapsis and associated brain anomalies: Report of 3 cases, *J Comput Assist Tomogr* 28:762-765, 2004.
567. Demaerel P, Morel C, Lagae L, Wilms G: Partial rhombencephalosynapsis, *AJNR Am J Neuroradiol* 25:29-31, 2004.
568. Chemli J, Abroug M, Tlili K, Harbi A: Rhombencephalosynapsis diagnosed in childhood: Clinical and MRI findings, *Eur J Paediatr Neurol* 11:35-38, 2007.
569. Bodensteiner JB, Gay CT, Marks WA, Hamza M, et al: Macro cisterna magna: A marker for maldevelopment of the brain? *Pediatr Neurol* 4:284-286, 1988.

Chapter 2

Neuronal Proliferation, Migration, Organization, and Myelination

The awesome complexity of the human brain begins its evolution after the essential external form is established by the events described in Chapter 1. The events that follow are proliferation of the brain's total complement of neurons, migration of those neurons to specific sites throughout the central nervous system (CNS), the series of organizational events that results in the intricate circuitry characteristic of the human brain, and, finally, the ensheathment of this circuitry with the neural-specific membrane, myelin. These events span a period from the second month of gestation to adult life, including the perinatal period. Aberrations of neural development may be an important consequence of many perinatal insults; this consequence heretofore was not clearly recognized.

This chapter reviews the normal aspects of neuronal proliferation, migration, organization, and myelination. A discussion follows regarding the disorders encountered when normal development goes awry.

NEURONAL PROLIFERATION

Normal Development

Major proliferative events occur initially between 2 and 4 months of gestation, with the peak time period quantitatively in the third and fourth months (Table 2-1). All neurons and glia are derived from the ventricular and subventricular zones, present in the subependymal location at every level of the developing nervous system. This highly critical process clearly relates to the ultimate integrity of every system within the neural apparatus.

Valuable quantitative information concerning cellular proliferation is derived from studies of the deposition of brain DNA, the chemical correlate of cell number, or from direct counting by optical and stereological methods (Fig. 2-1).[1,2] Two phases can be distinguished: the first, occurring from approximately 2 to 4 months of gestation, is associated primarily with generation of *radial glia and neuronal proliferation;* the second, occurring from approximately 5 months of gestation to 1 year (or more) of life, is associated primarily with *glial multiplication* (see later discussion concerning organizational events). Similarly, some neuronal formation occurs later than 4 months of gestation, principally in the cerebral subventricular zone and the cerebellar external granule cell layer (see later). Finally, proliferation of the *vascular tree,* arterial before

venous, is particularly active during the phase of neuronal proliferation.[3-6] Initially, a leptomeningeal plexus of vessels appears; this is followed in the third month by radially oriented, primarily unbranched vessels, which in the fourth and later months develop horizontal branching (Fig. 2-2).[4,6]

The fundamental aspects of cell proliferation in the wall of the neural tube were described first on the basis of morphological observations by Sauer in 1935.[7,8] They then were delineated further by the use of radioautography with [³H]thymidine-labeled DNA by Sidman, Rakic, Berry, and others 2 to 3 decades later, still later by Caviness, Rakic, and co-workers with bromodeoxyuridine-labeled DNA,[9-20] and most recently by immunocytochemistry, computer-assisted serial electron micrographic reconstruction, and time-lapse multiphoton imaging (Fig. 2-3).[21-23b] Cells in the periphery of the *ventricular zone* were shown to replicate their DNA, migrate toward the luminal surface, and divide; the two daughter cells then were noted to migrate back to the periphery of the ventricular zone. This *to-and-fro migration,* or *interkinetic nuclear migration,* is repeated each time DNA replication and mitosis occur in the ventricular zone. In some regions of the forebrain, a *subventricular zone* of proliferating cells can be identified (see Fig. 2-3). In the monkey cerebrum, studied in detail by Rakic and co-workers and by others,[13,16,19,21-26] the ventricular zone gives birth to most neurons, and the subventricular zone is the point of origin of some later-appearing neurons (e.g., upper layers of cerebral cortex and later subplate neurons) and most glia. When cells withdraw from the mitotic cycle and cease proliferative activity, they migrate into the intermediate zone on their way to forming the cortical plate (see later discussion). The elegant work of Caviness and co-workers defined

TABLE 2-1	Neuronal Proliferation
Peak Time Period
3–4 months
Major Events
Ventricular zone and subventricular zone are the sites of proliferation.
Proliferative units are produced by symmetrical divisions of progenitor cells.
Proliferative units later enlarge by asymmetrical divisions of progenitor cells before neuronal migration.

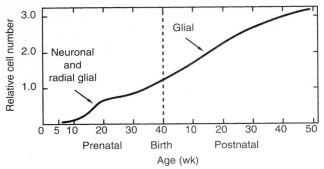

Figure 2-1 **Relative cell number in human forebrain as a function of age.** Total content of forebrain DNA is used to estimate relative cell number. Note that the curve has two phases of rapid increase in cell number. See text for details. *(Adapted from Dobbing J, Sands J: Quantitative growth and development of human brain*, Arch Dis Child *48:757–767, 1973.)*

the G_1 phase of the cell cycle as the molecular "control point" for these critical proliferative events.[20,27]

Rakic's studies of monkey cortical development led him to the conclusion that, in the earliest phases of proliferation, progenitor cells divide *symmetrically* into two additional progenitor cells, and that "proliferative units" of neuronal progenitor cells develop in this way (see later and see also Table 2-1).[16,25,26,28] This process determines the number of proliferative units in the ventricular-subventricular zones. Later, at a time comparable to the second half of the second month of gestation in the human, the number of these proliferative units becomes stable as the progenitor cells begin to divide asymmetrically (i.e., each division results in dissimilar cells, one of which is a stem cell and the other a postmitotic neuronal cell). These asymmetrical divisions determine the *size* of each proliferative unit (see Table 2-1). As the proliferative phase progresses, proportionately more postmitotic neuronal cells and fewer stem cells are produced.[19] Rakic concluded that the neurons of these proliferative units migrate together in a column to form the neuronal columns of the cerebral cortex (Fig. 2-4).[28] Other factors can become operative to determine the complete functional organization of the cerebral cortex (see later discussion of migration), but the general principle is the generation of neuronal units in the ventricular-subventricular zones with subsequent migration

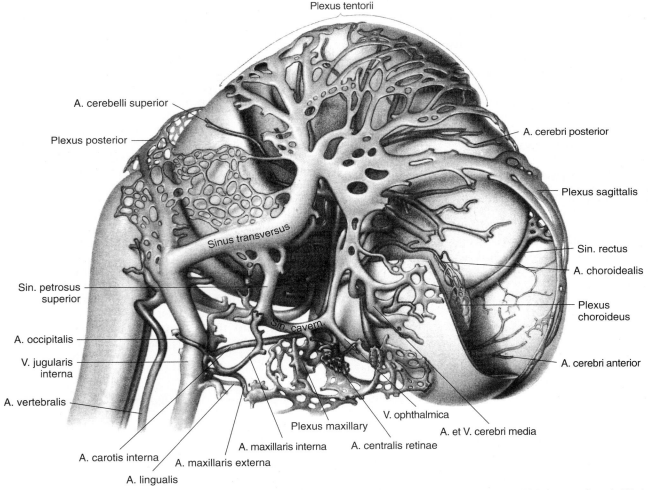

Figure 2-2 **Reconstruction of the perineural vascular territory of the brain (intracranial vasculature) of a stage 20 human embryo (≈51 days, ≈18 to 22 mm).** The dural venous sinuses, the arachnoidal arterial and venous systems, and the pial plexus that characterize the adult brain are already recognizable at this age. The wall of the cerebral cortex (cerebral vesicle) has been opened to demonstrate that, at this age, its intrinsic vascularization has not started, but that of the choroid plexus is already under way. A, artery; cavern, cavernous; sin, sinus; V, vein. *(From Streeter GL:* Contributions to Embryology, *vol. 8. Carnegie Institute of Embryology, 1918.)*

Figure 2-3   Cerebral wall during cortical plate development. Schematic drawing of the cerebral wall during development of the mammalian cortical plate (CP) to demonstrate the major zones: ventricular (V), subventricular (S), intermediate (I), and marginal (M). *(From Rakic P: Timing of major ontogenetic events in the visual cortex of the rhesus monkey. In Buchwald NA, Brazier MAB, editors:* Brain Mechanisms in Mental Retardation, *New York: 1975, Academic Press.)*

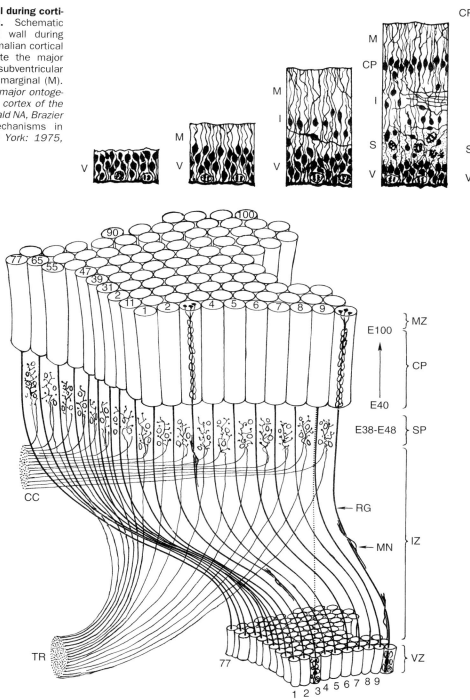

Figure 2-4   The relation between a small patch of the proliferative, ventricular zone (VZ) and its corresponding area within the cortical plate (CP) in the developing cerebrum. Although the cerebral surface in primates expands and shifts during prenatal development, ontogenetic columns (outlined by cylinders) may remain attached to the corresponding proliferative units by the grid of radial glial fibers. Neurons produced between E40 and E100 by a given proliferative unit migrate in succession along the same clonally related radial glial guides (RG) and stack up in reverse order of arrival within the same ontogenetic column. Each migrating neuron (MN) first traverses the intermediate zone (IZ) and then the subplate (SP), which contains subplate neurons and "waiting" afferents from the thalamic radiation (TR) and ipsilateral and contralateral corticocortical connections (CC). After entering the cortical plate, each neuron bypasses earlier generated neurons and settles at the interface between the CP and marginal zone (MZ). As a result, proliferative units 1 to 100 produce ontogenetic columns 1 to 100 in the same relative position to each other without a lateral mismatch (e.g., between proliferative unit 3 and ontogenetic column 9, indicated by a *dashed line*). Thus, the specification of cytoarchitectonic areas and topographic maps depends on the spatial distribution of their ancestors in the proliferative units, whereas the laminar position and phenotype of neurons within ontogenetic columns depend on the time of their origin. *(From Rakic P: Specification of cerebral cortical areas,* Science *241:170-176, 1988.)*

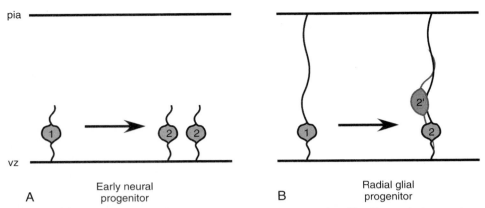

Figure 2-5 **Two types of neuronal progenitors.** In **A**, as occurs especially early in neuronal proliferation, a single neural precursor (1) gives rise to two identical precursors (2), that is, a symmetrical division. In **B**, as occurs especially later in neuronal proliferation, a radial neuronal progenitor (radial glial progenitor or radial glial cell) (1) divides asymmetrically into dissimilar cells, that is, an identical radial progenitor (2) and a postmitotic neuronal cell (2′) that migrates along the fiber of its clonally related radial progenitor to ultimately reach the cerebral cortex.

of these groups. Rakic showed that the distinguishing features of the kinetics of neuronal proliferation in primates versus species with smaller neocortices are a longer cell-cycle duration and, particularly, a more prolonged developmental period of neuronal proliferation.[19] Because of the latter, the total number of proliferative units of neuronal cells generated is much greater in the primate.

At *least two types of neuronal progenitors are present in the ventricular zone:* (1) a short neural precursor that has a ventricular endfoot and a leading process of variable length and (2) the radial glial cell that spans the entire cortical plate with contacts at both the ventricular and pial surfaces (Fig. 2-5).[23] The former progenitor previously was considered the principal neuronal precursor cell. An exciting advance in the understanding of neuronal proliferation was the identification of the *radial glial cell as another major neuronal progenitor in the ventricular zone.*[22,23,23a,23b,29-38] Previously, the major roles of this cell were considered to be, initially, a glial guide for migrating neurons and, later, a source of astrocytes (see later). However, more recent studies based on immunocytochemical and molecular techniques indicate that radial glial cells give rise to many neurons generated in the ventricular zone, particularly radially migrating excitatory projection cortical neurons. Thus, the term *radial glial cell* (which I continue to use) may ultimately be replaced by "radial glial progenitor" or "radial progenitor." When the radial glial cell functions as a neuronal progenitor, the clonally related neuron so generated then migrates along the parent radial glial fiber (see Fig. 2-5). These elegant proliferative events involving the radial glial cell as neuronal progenitor are modulated by several key signaling pathways involving the Notch receptor, the ErbB receptor (through the ligand neuregulin), and the fibroblast growth factor receptor.[28,38,39] Other critical molecular determinants include beta-catenin, a protein that functions in the decision of progenitors to proliferate or differentiate.[40] Finally, of particular importance in the regulation of radial glial production of neurons are calcium waves propagating through connexin channels of the radial

glial cell.[35] Calcium entry is critical in the regulation of the cell cycle.

Subsequent to neurogenesis, radial cells produce astrocytes and probably other glial cells (e.g., oligodendroglia).[36] Additionally, more recent data indicate that radial glial cells also give rise to cells that persist in the subventricular zone of *adult* brain as stem cells capable of producing neurons.[36] The multiple functions of radial glial cells are summarized in Table 2-2.

Disorders

Disorders of neuronal proliferation would be expected to have a major impact on CNS function. Because of difficulties in quantitating neuronal populations, however, proliferative disorders often are difficult to define by conventional neuropathological examination. Even when the disorder is so extreme that the brain is grossly undersized (i.e., micrencephaly) or oversized (i.e., macrencephaly), defining the nature and severity of the proliferative derangement is also difficult by conventional techniques. (Although theoretically there is the possibility that the disorders relate to alterations in later-occurring normal apoptotic events, I consider these to be disorders of proliferation until evidence of an apoptotic disorder is recorded.) In the following discussion, I focus on these two extremes of apparent proliferative disorders, but I emphasize that conclusions about the nature of the disorders can be made only cautiously.

Micrencephaly

Disorders apparently related to impaired neuronal proliferation are categorized under the term *primary micrencephaly*, to distinguish the disorder from micrencephalies secondary to destructive disease (Table 2-3).

TABLE 2-2	Functions of Radial Glial Cells
Progenitors for cortical neurons	
Guides of neuronal migration	
Progenitors for astrocytes and oligodendrocytes	
Neural stem cells found in subventricular zone of adult brain	

TABLE 2-3	Disorders of Neuronal Proliferation: Primary Micrencephaly*
Familial	
Autosomal recessive (micrencephaly vera)	
Autosomal dominant	
X-linked recessive	
Genetics unclear (ocular abnormalities)	
Teratogenic	
Irradiation	
Metabolic-toxic (e.g., fetal alcohol syndrome, related to cocaine, hyperphenylalaninemia)	
Infection (rubella, cytomegalovirus)	
Syndromic (Multiple Systemic Anomalies)	
Chromosomal	
Familial	
Sporadic	
Sporadic (Nonsyndromic)	

*Excluded are cases of congenital microcephaly secondary principally to destructive disease (hypoxia-ischemia, infection) developing after the conclusion of cerebral neuronal proliferation.

TABLE 2-4	Radial Microbrain
Term newborns: death, birth–30 days	
Brain weight 16–50 g (normal, 350 g)	
No evidence for destructive process	
Normal residual germinal matrix at term	
Normal cortical lamination	
Cortical neurons 30% of normal number	
Cortical neuronal columns decreased in number	
Neuronal complement of each column normal	

Data from Evrard P, de Saint-Georges P, Kadhim HJ, Gadisseux J-F: Pathology of prenatal encephalopathies. In French JH, Harel S, Casaer P, editors: *Child Neurology and Developmental Disabilities*, Baltimore: 1989, Paul H. Brookes.

proliferative events, which generates by *symmetrical* divisions of neuronal progenitors the total *number* of proliferative units, is based on the finding of a marked reduction in number of cortical neuronal columns but an apparent normal complement of the neurons per column (i.e., normal size of columns) (Fig. 2-6).[5]

The latter relates to hypoxic-ischemic, infectious, metabolic, or other destructive events, occurring usually *following completion* of cerebral neuronal proliferative events near the end of the fourth month of gestation (see Chapters 8, 9, 14, 15, 16, and 20). The primary micrencephalies that have been shown most clearly to be related to impaired neuronal proliferation include the autosomal recessively inherited disorders, often categorized as *micrencephaly vera*. Thus, in the context of this chapter, I discuss these conditions in most detail.

Micrencephaly Vera. *Micrencephaly vera* refers to a heterogeneous group of disorders that appear to have, as the common denominator, small brain size because of a derangement of proliferation (see Table 2-3). Thus, no evidence of intrauterine destructive disease or of gross derangement of other developmental events (e.g., neurulation, prosencephalic cleavage, neuronal migration) exists, and the abnormal brain size is apparent as early as the third trimester of gestation). The brain is generally well formed, although the gyrification pattern may be simplified to a variable degree. As noted earlier, the clearest examples of micrencephaly vera are the autosomal recessively inherited micrencephalies, and I use this term only for these examples of primary micrencephaly. I first discuss *radial microbrain*, an informative but rare and particularly severe type of micrencephaly vera, and then the more common varieties of micrencephaly vera.

Anatomical Abnormality: Radial Microbrain. Radial microbrain is a rare disorder of particular interest because it appears to provide the first clear example of a disturbance in number of proliferative units.[5,41] The major features of the seven cases studied carefully by Evrard and colleagues[5,41] are outlined in Table 2-4. The extremely small brain has no marked gyral abnormality, no evidence of a destructive process, and no disturbance of cortical lamination. The conclusion that the disturbance involves the early phase of

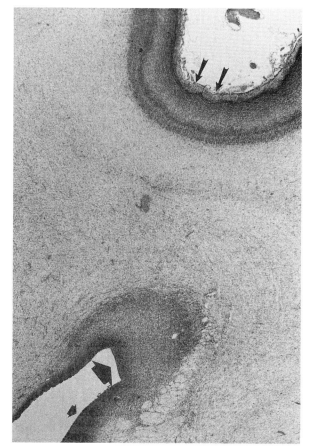

Figure 2-6 **Radial microbrain.** Brain of a full-term newborn with the pathological picture of radial microbrain described in the text. Note the normal cortical lamination *(long arrows)* and the normal residual germinative zone *(both short arrows)*. From Evrard P, de Saint-Georges P, Kadhim HJ, et al: Pathology of prenatal encephalopathies. In French JH, Harel S, Casaer P, editors: Child Neurology and Developmental Disabilities, *Baltimore: 1989, Paul H. Brookes.)*

Timing and Clinical Aspects: Radial Microbrain. The presumed timing of radial microbrain is no later than the earliest phase of proliferative events in the second month of gestation. The essential abnormality involves the symmetrical divisions of progenitors to form additional progenitors and thereby the number of proliferative units. Later proliferative events that determine the size of each column proceed normally, as evidenced not only by the normal neuronal complement of each column but also by the presence of a normal residual amount of germinal matrix at term (see Fig. 2-6).

The clinical features are not entirely clear, because this anomaly is rare. The reported cases have been full-term newborns who died in the first month of life. The distinction from anencephaly and aprosencephaly-atelencephaly is based on the presence of an intact skull and dermal covering, in contrast to anencephaly, and of a normal external appearance of cerebrum and ventricles, observable by ultrasonography, in contrast to aprosencephaly-atelencephaly. The disorder is notably familial, probably of autosomal recessive inheritance.

Anatomical Abnormality: Micrencephaly Vera. As noted earlier, the designation *micrencephaly vera* refers to a heterogeneous group of autosomal recessive disorders that appear to have, as the common denominator, small brain size because of a derangement of proliferation (see Table 2-3). In recent years, remarkable insights into the genetics and molecular bases of these disorders have been gained (see later).

The anatomical studies of Evrard and colleagues[5,41] provide insight into the fundamental disturbance in micrencephaly vera, at least in a prototypical autosomal recessive variety (Table 2-5). The brain is small (clearly more than several standard deviations below the mean) but not so strikingly as in the tiny radial microbrain. Simplification of gyral pattern exists with no other external abnormality and no evidence of a destructive process. The number of cortical neuronal columns appears normal, but the neuronal complement of each column, especially the superficial cortical layers, is decreased markedly. Additional evidence of disturbance of the later proliferative events that determine size of cortical neuronal columns is the absence of residual germinal matrix in the 26-week fetal brain studied by Evrard and colleagues (Fig. 2-7). The deficiency in neurons of the superficial cortical layers may explain the simplification of gyral pattern (see the later discussion of gyral development in migrational disorders).

Timing and Clinical Aspects: Micrencephaly Vera. The presumed timing of the micrencephaly vera group of disorders involves the period of later proliferative events by asymmetrical divisions of neuronal progenitors, that is, onset at approximately 6 weeks in the human, with later rapid progression until approximately 18 weeks (see earlier). The most severely undersized brains are expected to have the earliest onsets and the most marked deficiency of neurons in each cortical column.

The *clinical presentation* of infants with the prototypical autosomal recessive forms of micrencephaly vera is interesting in that, as newborns, most affected infants do not show striking neurological deficits or seizures. This presentation is in contrast to that of other varieties of micrencephaly, that is, intrauterine destructive disease or other developmental derangement (e.g., migrational defect). Rare autosomal recessive forms of micrencephaly with severe neuronal migrational defects (i.e., microlissencephaly) are more likely to be accompanied by neurological deficits and seizures (see the later discussion of disorders of neuronal migration).

Magnetic resonance imaging (MRI) has been invaluable in the assessment of micrencephaly vera, especially for evaluation of gyral development and the presence of associated migrational abnormalities.[42] Most commonly, gyral formation is variably simplified (Fig. 2-8), and the term *microcephaly with simplified gyri* is often used.[42-50] Simplification of the gyral pattern often is not obvious. Rare cases are associated with severe migrational disturbances, such as lissencephaly, periventricular heterotopia, or posterior fossa deficits, especially cerebellar hypoplasia.[45,47,48,51-53]

Etiology: Autosomal Recessive Micrencephaly. At least six gene loci have been identified for autosomal recessive primary micrencephaly, or micrencephaly vera. Four of the genes have been identified (Table 2-6).[46,54-59] Perhaps not unexpectedly, the genes play key roles in mitosis. *Microcephalin* is crucial for cell cycle control, chromosome condensation, and DNA repair. *CDK5RAP2* is a centrosomal protein involved in microtubular function necessary for formation of the mitotic spindle. *ASPM* also is necessary for microtubular function at the poles of the mitotic spindle, and *CENPT* similarly is involved in formation of the mitotic spindle.

Etiology: Other Disorders. The four major etiological categories for primary micrencephaly, in addition to the autosomal recessive group just discussed, are familial, teratogenic, syndromic, and sporadic (see Table 2-3). *Familial syndromes* are most critical to detect because of implications for genetic counseling. In addition to the autosomal recessive group (see earlier), these inherited varieties include autosomal dominant and X-linked recessive types, as well as familial types with ocular

---

TABLE 2-5	Micrencephaly Vera: Autosomal Recessive Type

No evidence for destructive process
No evidence for migrational defect
No apparent defect in number of cortical neuronal columns
Cortical neuronal columns with marked decrease in neurons of layers II and III
No residual germinal matrix at 26 weeks of gestation ("premature exhaustion" of matrix)

From Evrard P, de Saint-Georges P, Kadhim HJ, Gadisseux J-F: Pathology of prenatal encephalopathies. In French JH, Harel S, Casaer P, editors: *Child Neurology and Developmental Disabilities*, Baltimore: 1989, Paul H. Brookes.

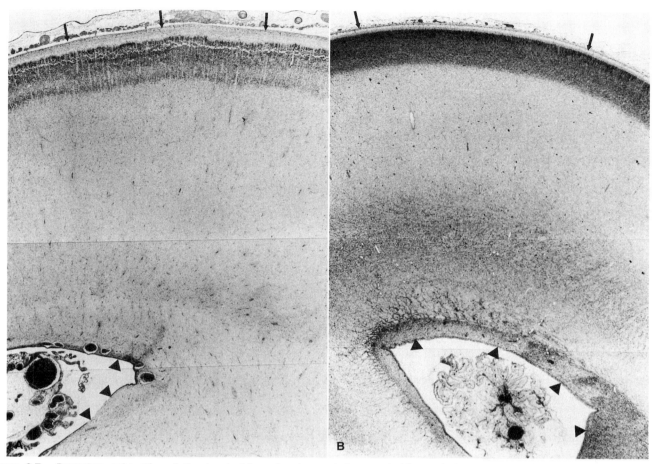

Figure 2-7   Premature exhaustion of the germinal layer in microcephaly vera. A, Microcephaly vera, human fetal forebrain, 26 weeks of gestation. B, Normal human fetal forebrain, 26 weeks, same cortical region for comparison. The germinal layer (*arrowheads*), cerebral cortex (*arrows*), and intervening cerebral white matter are visible. In microcephaly vera (A), the germinal layer is exhausted at this age, and the white matter is almost devoid of late migrating glial and neuronal cells. Cortical layers VI to IV are normal, whereas the two superficial layers are almost missing. (*From Evrard P, de Saint-Georges P, Kadhim HJ, et al: Pathology of prenatal encephalopathies. In French JH, Harel S, Casaer P, editors*: Child Neurology and Developmental Disabilities, *Baltimore: 1989, Paul H. Brookes.*)

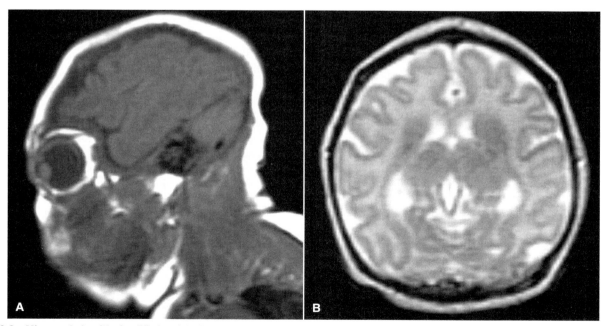

Figure 2-8   Microcephaly with simplified gyri. In **A**, the sagittal T1-weighted magnetic resonance imaging (MRI) scan shows marked microcephaly. In **B**, the axial T2-weighted MRI scan shows simplification of the gyral pattern. No other dysgenetic abnormalities are present, nor is any evidence of destructive disease manifest. *(Courtesy of Dr. Omar Khwaja.)*

TABLE 2-6   **Autosomal Recessive Primary Micrencephaly (Micrencephaly Vera): Molecular Genetics**

Locus	Gene/Protein	Function
MCPH 1	Microcephalin	Cell cycle control
MCPH 3	CDK5RAP2 (**c**yclin-**d**ependent **k**inase-5 **r**egulatory **a**ssociated **p**rotein-2)	Mitotic spindle formation
MCPH 5	ASPM (**a**bnormal **s**pindle in **m**icrocephaly)	Mitotic spindle formation
MCPH 6	CENPJ (**c**entromere-**a**ssociated **p**rotein **J**)	Mitotic spindle formation

MCPH, Autosomal recessive primary micrencephaly.

abnormalities and variable genetics.[60-74] These ocular abnormalities may include chorioretinopathy that can be confused with the chorioretinitis of intrauterine infection (see Chapter 20). One such disorder is *Cohen syndrome*, which is inherited in an autosomal recessive manner. Of the unusual cases of micrencephaly with autosomal dominant inheritance, intellect subsequently is usually either spared or only mildly defective; patients generally have no facial dysmorphism, although digital anomalies and rare syndromic varieties have been reported.[71,74] X-linked recessive inheritance of micrencephaly has been described, albeit less commonly than autosomal recessive inheritance.

The best-documented *teratogenic agent* producing micrencephaly is irradiation, such as by atomic bomb or radiation therapy for tumor or ankylosing spondylitis, particularly before 18 weeks of gestation (see Table 2-3).[75-77] The most critical period in the Nagasaki-Hiroshima experience was 8 to 15 weeks.[77] Maternal alcoholism or cocaine abuse (see Chapter 24) and maternal hyperphenylalaninemia have been associated with micrencephaly. Micrencephaly, usually with mental retardation, occurs in as many as 75% to 90% of (nonphenylketonuric) children of women with phenylketonuria; the risk for the fetus correlates with the severity of the maternal hyperphenylalaninemia.[78-88] With dietary treatment, the risk declines to as low as 8% when phenylalanine levels are controlled before conception and to 18% when control is achieved by 10 weeks of pregnancy.[89] When control is not achieved until 20 to 30 weeks, the incidence of microcephaly increases to 40%. Rarer intrauterine teratogens for micrencephaly include anticonvulsant drugs (see Chapter 24), organic mercurials, and excessive ingestion of vitamin A or vitamin A analogues (see Chapter 24).[90] Finally, among intrauterine infections that may cause micrencephaly (see Chapter 20), rubella is the best candidate for an agent that may produce micrencephaly through an impairment of proliferation rather than principally through a destructive process. Cytomegalovirus infection may also act in this way, although disturbances of neuronal migration and destructive lesions contribute to the condition. Human immunodeficiency virus characteristically produces micrencephaly (without major destructive lesions) after the neonatal period, although neonatal cases have been reported (see Chapter 20).

Syndromic cases, that is, those with multiple associated systemic anomalies, may be related to chromosomal disorders or monogenic (familial) defects, or they may occur sporadically (see Table 2-3). In one consecutive sample of congenital microcephaly, syndromic disorders accounted for only 6% of cases.[91] The nature of the proliferative disorder in this diverse group is generally not known and is not discussed further. Clinical details are available in standard sources.[73]

Sporadic nonsyndromic cases, that is, those with no related family history, identifiable teratogen, or recognizable syndrome, are the most common varieties of micrencephaly vera (see Table 2-3).[91,92] No associated systemic or other neural malformations can be identified. The nature of the proliferative disturbance is generally unknown.

Macrencephaly

Anatomical Abnormality. The designation *macrencephaly* signifies a large brain and is a feature of a heterogeneous group of disorders that have not been well defined from the neuropathological standpoint. Nevertheless, several entities clearly exist in which the brain is generally well formed but is unusually large (see Table 2-5). Genetic varieties, suggestive of a derangement in the developmental program for neuronal proliferation, have been defined (see following discussion). As with micrencephaly, however, the conclusion that we are dealing with proliferative disorders can be made only tenuously until central neuronal populations can be quantified more accurately. This discussion *excludes* other rare disorders of macrocephaly, such as enlargement of the skull (craniometaphyseal dysplasia, hemoglobinopathy), subdural hematoma or effusion (see Chapters 10, 21, 22), hydrocephalus (see Chapters 1, 11, 21), metabolic disorders (see Chapter 15), or degenerative disorders (Alexander disease, Canavan disease [see Chapter 16]).

Timing and Clinical Aspects. Although neuronal proliferation in the cerebrum is an event that occurs principally during the third and fourth months of gestation, this time period may be prolonged in disorders of excessive proliferation. Alternatively, abnormal proliferation may occur at the appropriate time during development but at an excessive rate. Additionally, a later-occurring defect of normal apoptosis or programmed cell death (see later section on organization) perhaps could lead to macrencephaly. The issues of mechanism are unresolved and await development of suitable experimental models for elucidation.

The *clinical syndrome* in the several types of macrencephaly (Table 2-7) varies from no apparent neurological deficit (e.g., autosomal dominant, isolated macrencephaly) to severe recalcitrant seizures and mental retardation (e.g., autosomal recessive, isolated

TABLE 2-7	Disorders of Neuronal Proliferation: Macrencephaly

Isolated Macrencephaly
Familial
Autosomal dominant (relation to ''benign enlargement of extracerebral spaces'' or ''external hydrocephalus'')
Autosomal recessive
Sporadic

Associated Disturbance of Growth
Achondroplasia
Beckwith syndrome
Cerebral gigantism
Fragile X syndrome (see ''Chromosomal Disorders'' below)
Marshall-Smith syndrome
Thanatophoric dysplasia
Weaver syndrome

Neurocutaneous Syndromes
Multiple hemangiomatosis
Lipomas, hemangiomas, lymphangiomas, pseudo-papilledema (Bannayan-Riley-Ruvalcaba)
Asymmetrical hypertrophy, hemangiomata, varicosities (Klippel-Trenaunay-Weber)
Asymmetrical hypertrophy, telangiectatic lesions, flame nevus of the face (cutis marmorata telangiectatica congenita)
Neurofibromatosis,* tuberous sclerosis,† Sturge-Weber syndrome†
Epidermal nevus syndrome (see ''Unilateral Macrencephaly'' below)

Chromosomal Disorders
Fragile X syndrome (relative macrencephaly)
Klinefelter syndrome

Unilateral Macrencephaly (Hemimegalencephaly)
Isolated
Syndromic: epidermal nevus syndrome, Proteus syndrome (most common)

*Neurocutaneous disorder of cellular proliferation causing macrencephaly and affecting primarily nonneuronal elements (i.e., glia).
†Neurocutaneous disorders of cellular proliferation but not usually associated with neonatal macrencephaly.

macrencephaly, or unilateral macrencephaly). In other types of the disorder, extraneural features may dominate the clinical presentation (e.g., associated growth disorders and certain neurocutaneous syndromes). Some of these individual clinical aspects are mentioned briefly in the following discussion.

Familial, Isolated Macrencephaly. Perhaps the most common variety of macrencephaly occurs in the familial setting and in the absence of any other extraneural findings. For this group, I use the term *familial, isolated macrencephaly*. Two genetic types can be recognized: autosomal dominant and autosomal recessive; the former is much more common.

In familial, isolated macrencephaly of the *autosomal dominant type*, the head is usually large at birth (>90th percentile in ≈50%) and continues to grow postnatally at a relatively rapid rate.[93,94] Neurological deficits are rarely striking, and development and ultimate level of intelligence are in the normal range in approximately 50% to 60% of cases. Mental retardation is present in only approximately 10%. The genetic component of this syndrome is overlooked frequently until the head circumference of the parents is measured. The diagnosis of fetal macrocephaly of this type was made in the 34th week of pregnancy in a woman with benign macrocephaly.[95]

Related to autosomal dominant macrencephaly is a syndrome of macrocephaly, categorized under several names: *benign enlargement of extracerebral spaces, benign subdural effusions of infancy*, and *idiopathic external hydrocephalus*.[94,96-102] The clinical features described in the previous paragraph are present, and brain imaging studies show prominent extracerebral subarachnoid spaces and a large brain (Fig. 2-9). The cisterna magna especially may be prominent. In some cases, subdural and subarachnoid fluid appears to be present; the distinction is best made by MRI scan.[96] Head growth in the first year is rapid, and infants not overtly macrocephalic at birth attain rates of head growth at the 97th percentile or slightly higher. Accelerating

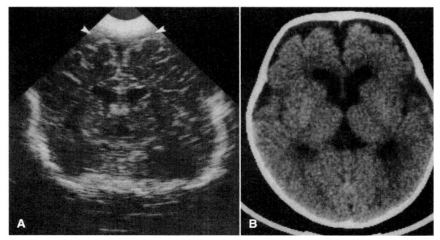

Figure 2-9 ''Benign'' macrocephaly. **A,** Coronal sonogram demonstrates mild ventricular enlargement and moderate extra-axial fluid over the convexities *(arrowheads)*. **B,** Axial computed tomography scan shows similar findings. *(From Babcock DS, Han BK, Dine MS: Sonographic findings in infants with macrocrania, AJNR Am J Neuroradiol 9:307-313, 1988.)*

head growth ceases by approximately 1 year, and over the next several years extracerebral spaces become smaller, although the brain is clearly larger than average. Because of the large brain size, if the infant is first evaluated after the second year of life, isolated macrencephaly will be observed. Because as many as 90% of these infants have a parent with a large head, the genetic features are similar to those of autosomal dominant isolated macrencephaly. The similarity of the clinical features and genetics suggests that these may represent different forms of the same fundamental disorder. Those unusual patients with isolated macrencephaly that conforms to *autosomal recessive inheritance* are more likely to exhibit definite mental retardation, epilepsy, and motor deficits.[90]

Sporadic, Isolated Macrencephaly. Isolated macrencephaly with no evidence of a familial disorder by history and after measurement of parental head circumference occurs only slightly less often than the autosomal dominant disorder described previously.[93,103,104] The clinical course is similar.

Associated Disturbance of Growth. Macrencephaly may be associated with generalized disorders of growth, such as achondroplasia, Beckwith syndrome, cerebral gigantism (Sotos syndrome), fragile X syndrome, Marshall-Smith syndrome, thanatophoric dysplasia, and Weaver syndrome (see Table 2-7).[73,93,105-108] Except in Beckwith syndrome, which is complicated by neonatal hypoglycemia, neurological features in the neonatal period are unusual. The precise neuropathological correlates for the macrencephaly in these disorders remain to be defined. The gene mutated or deleted in Sotos syndrome, *NSD1*, encodes a nuclear receptor binding protein that may be involved in proliferative events.

Neurocutaneous Syndromes. Several of the neurocutaneous disorders are associated with evidence of excessive cellular proliferation within the CNS, sometimes with overt macrencephaly, and evidence of excessive proliferation of mesodermal structures (see Table 2-7). Macrencephaly occurs most consistently in this context in the multiple hemangiomatosis syndromes.[73,109-115]

In *neurofibromatosis*, an autosomal dominant disorder, the principal proliferative abnormality involves glia, particularly astrocytes. (Thus, the onset of the proliferative disorder in this disease primarily occurs after the time period of neuronal proliferative events.) Approximately 40% of infants exhibit more than five café-au-lait spots larger than 5 mm at birth.[116-122] Approximately 40% to 50% of such infants have macrocephaly, usually after the neonatal period.[123,124] Consistent with the predominantly glial rather than neuronal involvement in the disorder, the megalencephaly relates primarily to increases in cerebral *white matter* volume, primarily in frontal and parietal areas.[125] Relative macrocephaly with generalized glial tumors has been documented by prenatal ultrasound.[126] Hemimegalencephaly with neonatal seizures and associated neuronal migrational defects also have been observed.[127,128] Of the glial tumors that are the hallmark of this disease, optic nerve glioma and plexiform neuroma of the eyelid have been observed in the newborn, albeit rarely.[117,122] The gene for this disorder, located on chromosome 17, *NF1*, has been shown to encode a protein involved in the negative regulation of a key signal transduction pathway, the Ras pathway, which transmits mitogenic signals to the nucleus.[120-122,129,130] Thus, loss of the neurofibromatosis protein, neurofibromin, leads to increased mitogenic signaling and thereby to the proliferative abnormalities characteristic of the disorder.

In *Sturge-Weber disease*, a sporadic disorder, the principal abnormality affects leptomeningeal blood vessels. Thus, the time of onset is probably coincident with that for neuronal proliferation. Data suggest that the fundamental defect in this disorder is a failure of development of superficial cortical veins that diverts blood to the developing leptomeninges, with the formation of abnormal vascular channels as a consequence.[131] Abnormalities of fibronectin in cerebral vessels may play a role in the genesis of the vascular abnormality.[132] The characteristic facial port-wine stain is described in Chapter 3; the overall incidence of clinical manifestations of Sturge-Weber disease (glaucoma or seizures) is 2% to 8% in patients with unilateral facial lesions and 24% in patients with bilateral facial lesions.[131,133,134] Identification of the newborn with intracranial involvement is difficult. Seizures and cerebral calcification (identified by computed tomography [CT]) have been noted only occasionally in newborns (Fig. 2-10).[42,135-138] Cerebral calcifications most commonly appear after 6 months of age and often considerably later.[114,131,139-141] MRI appears to be the most useful imaging study in the first year[42,114,131,134,140-143]; the principal findings are cerebral cortical and white matter changes in the region of the leptomeningeal angiomatosis, angiomatous alteration of overlying calvaria, and atypically located, congested deep cerebral veins.[114,140,142] Gadolinium-enhanced MRI is the gold standard for demonstration of the leptomeningeal vascular lesion (Fig. 2-11).[42,114,131,140-142] The choroid plexus is enlarged on the side of the leptomeningeal lesion, presumably because of the diversion of venous blood into the deep venous system, as a consequence of the lack of superficial cortical venous drainage (see earlier discussion). On single photon emission tomographic studies, decreased cortical perfusion may be observed in the region of the vascular lesion.[131,141,144,145] MRI perfusion studies also may be useful in detecting perfusion deficits.[146] Infants with Sturge-Weber syndrome who have bilateral cerebral disease have a much poorer outcome (8% with average intelligence) than those with unilateral cerebral disease (45% with average intelligence).[134,138,144,145,147,148]

In *tuberous sclerosis*, the principal proliferative abnormality affects both neurons and glia. The neuropathological and molecular aspects of these disorders indicate that tuberous sclerosis also reflects abnormal migration and differentiation (see later).[149-151] The critical neonatal cutaneous feature is a depigmented, ash

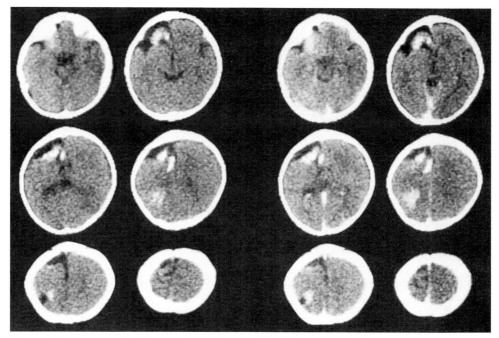

Figure 2-10 **Sturge-Weber disease, computed tomography (CT) scan.** This infant exhibited seizures on the fifth day of life. The CT scan was obtained at the age of 4 months. *Left,* Conventional CT scan. *Right,* Contrast-enhanced CT scan. Note marked atrophy and calcification in the left frontal region and, to a lesser extent, in the left parietal region. Only scant contrast enhancement is apparent. *(From Kitihara T, Maki U: A case of Sturge-Weber disease with epilepsy and intracranial calcification at the neonatal period,* Eur Neurol *17:8-12, 1978.)*

leaf–shaped macule. Seizures may occur in the neonatal period.[149,152-155] Cardiac tumors (rhabdomyomata) are characteristic and uncommonly may lead to neurological features by causing cardiac failure, arrhythmias, or cerebral emboli (personal cases). Cardiac rhabdomyomata have been identified in affected fetuses and are usually the first clue to prenatal diagnosis.[156,157] The diagnosis

of tuberous sclerosis is established in 80% to 95% of fetuses with cardiac rhabdomyomata.[158,159] The natural history of these tumors is favorable—virtually all regress at least partially.[159] Subependymal nodules, the most common cerebral lesion detected in utero, have been identified as early as 21 weeks.[160] Indeed, I consider the most useful *constellation of features for*

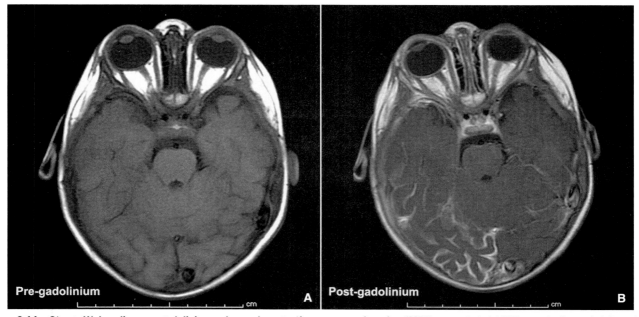

Pre-gadolinium **A** Post-gadolinium **B**

Figure 2-11 **Sturge-Weber disease, gadolinium-enhanced magnetic resonance imaging (MRI) scan. A,** Axial MRI scan before administration of gadolinium in an infant with a port-wine stain shows no definite abnormality. **B,** The scan after gadolinium enhancement shows diffuse leptomeningeal enhancement in the right occipital and temporal regions. The findings are characteristic of Sturge-Weber disease. *(Courtesy of Dr. Omar Khwaja.)*

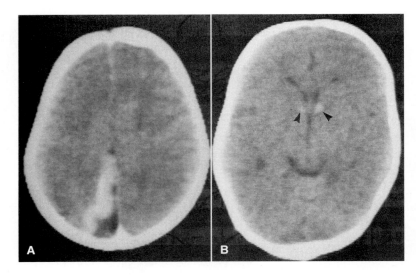

Figure 2-12 **Tuberous sclerosis, computed tomography scan.** This infant exhibited generalized seizures and depigmented macules at 4 weeks of age. Note, **A**, the striking cortical tuberous change in the left occipital region and, **B**, the small subependymal nodules *(arrowheads)* near the heads of both caudate nuclei.

the diagnosis of tuberous sclerosis in the neonatal period to consist of the depigmented macule, cardiac rhabdomyoma, subependymal nodule, and cortical tuber. In one large series, approximately 90% of newborns studied by MRI exhibited the latter two cerebral lesions.[157] Neuropathological features include both the characteristic subependymal and cerebral cortical-subcortical collections of abnormal neurons and glia (i.e., subependymal nodules and cortical tubers) and heterotopic collections of similar cells in the cerebral white matter, often arranged in radial bands.[161-166] The cells are often bizarre, large, and poorly differentiated, exhibiting features of both neurons and astrocytes. Subependymal giant cell astrocytoma has been reported in newborns with tuberous sclerosis[157,167-169] but more typically it appears in older children. Both CT scanning and ultrasonography can be useful in diagnosis (Figs. 2-12 and 2-13).[42,152,153,170,171] However, MRI has proven of particular value in the neonatal period and demonstrates the subependymal collections, the cortical tubers, and the white matter lesions especially well (Fig. 2-14).[42,157,165,166,168,172-174] Because of the unmyelinated cerebral white matter in the newborn, the cortical tubers (hypointense on T1-weighted images, hyperintense on T2-weighted images) have signal characteristics opposite those exhibited by older children with the disorder.[42,166]

The tuberous sclerosis phenotype is associated with dysfunction of genes on either chromosome 9 or chromosome 16.[130,175-177] The disorder, although autosomal dominant, is associated with a high spontaneous mutation rate. Overall, approximately 80% of cases are sporadic.[150,151] The genes, *TSC1* on chromosome 9 and *TSC2* on chromosome 16, encode the respective

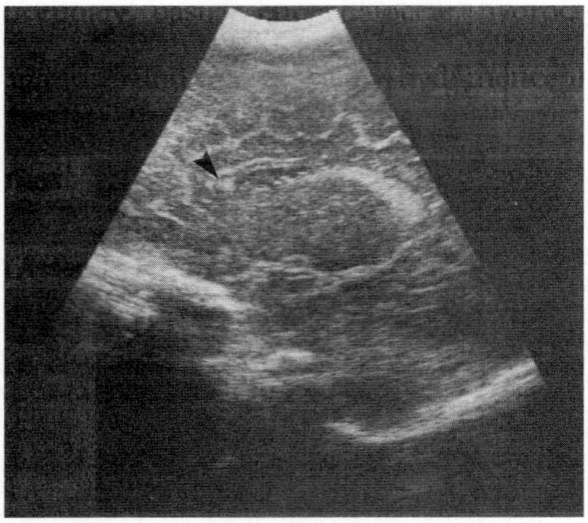

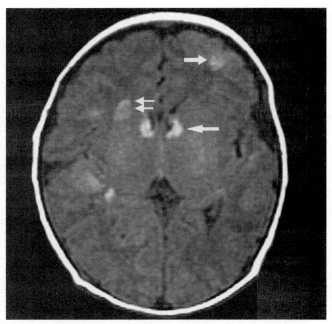

Figure 2-14 **Tuberous sclerosis, magnetic resonance imaging (MRI) scan.** This 11-day-old infant was identified in utero with a cardiac rhabdomyoma. On this axial T1-weighted MRI, note the multiple cortical tubers *(thick arrow)*, subependymal nodules *(thin arrow)*, and radial cerebral white matter lesion *(double arrow)*. *(Courtesy of Dr. Omar Khwaja.)*

Figure 2-13 **Tuberous sclerosis, ultrasound scan.** This infant exhibited depigmented macules with myoclonic seizures at 3 weeks of age. The parasagittal ultrasound scan shows an echogenic subependymal nodule *(arrowhead)* that was also seen on a computed tomography scan.

proteins, hamartin and tuberin.[150,151] Hamartin and tuberin interact to form a complex, and this complex is involved in molecular signaling critical for cell proliferation, cell growth, and cell adhesion/migration.[150,151] Disturbance of these processes underlies the proliferative abnormalities (subependymal nodules, astrocytomas, and cardiac, renal, and other tumors), the abnormalities of cell size (large, bizarre cells in nodules and tubers) and the radial white matter disturbances (apparent disturbances in radial migration and release of migrating cells from the radial glial progenitor). The *TSC2* mutations result in the most severe phenotypes and account for the majority of neonatal cases.

Chromosomal Disorders. The possibility that the fragile X syndrome may include a proliferative abnormality is raised by the finding of absolute or relative macrocephaly in approximately 40% of infants.[178,179] However, a disturbance of cerebral organizational events appears to be the dominant neural abnormality in fragile X syndrome (see later). Rarer chromosomal disorders with macrencephaly are Klinefelter syndrome and partial trisomy of chromosome 7.[90,180,181]

Unilateral Macrencephaly (Hemimegalencephaly). Unilateral macrencephaly represents, at least in part, a localized disorder of cell proliferation within the CNS. The anatomical data suggest excessive proliferation of both neurons and astrocytes, but also defects in subsequent migration of neurons and in cortical organization. In this disorder, enlargement of one hemisphere, or a portion thereof, occurs, often accompanied by abnormal cortical gyration, a disordered and unusually thick cortex, large and sometimes bizarre neurons, heterotopic neurons in subcortical white matter, and increased number and often size of astrocytes.[95,182-196]

The *clinical syndrome* in isolated and syndromic cases consistently has included severe seizures from early infancy, usually in the neonatal period, with subsequent severely disturbed neurological development.[95,193-210] The cranial asymmetry in unilateral macrencephaly may be overlooked in the newborn if the skull is not examined carefully, especially from above. CT scanning demonstrates a degree of enlargement of the hemisphere or a portion thereof that initially may be suggestive of a congenital neoplasm. MRI scanning is the best imaging method to demonstrate the neuronal heterotopias and abnormalities of cerebral cortical gyration (Fig. 2-15). Electroencephalography (EEG) in the infants with earliest onset of seizures may demonstrate a characteristic pattern of larger-amplitude triphasic complexes. Seizures are usually recalcitrant to therapy. Hemispherectomy, as early as the first months of life, has been followed by improved outcome.[195,200-202,208,211] Prognosis after hemispherectomy depends primarily on the functional status of the contralateral hemisphere. Positron emission tomographic studies of cerebral glucose utilization showed cortical hypometabolism in the contralateral hemisphere in four of eight infants, and this abnormality correlated with a poorer outcome after hemispherectomy.[211] Related

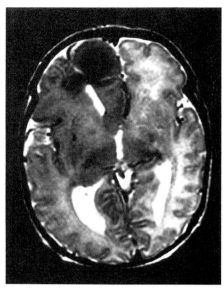

Figure 2-15 Hemimegalencephaly, magnetic resonance imaging (MRI) scan. This T2-weighted axial MRI shows an enlarged right hemisphere with right frontal pachygyria. Note also the enlarged right lateral ventricle and anomalous configuration of the right frontal horn. The left hemisphere is normal. *(From Flores-Sarnat L: Hemimegalencephaly. I. Genetic, clinical, and imaging aspects, J Child Neurol 16:373-384, 2002.)*

physiological studies showed that the nonmalformed hemisphere is secondarily impaired with persistent clinical and electrical seizures as early as the first months of life, and early hemispherectomy is beneficial.[212] Indeed, bilateral neuropathological changes, albeit with less severe changes in the contralateral hemisphere, have been described.[191]

Syndromic varieties of hemimegalencephaly are multiple but most commonly include epidermal nevus syndrome, Proteus syndrome, and hypomelanosis of Ito.[195] A relatively rare neurocutaneous disorder, *epidermal nevus syndrome*, is associated with hemimegalencephaly in approximately one half of cases.[195,205,213-215] The clinical neurological and neuropathological features are essentially similar to those just described for sporadic cases of hemimegalencephaly.[205,213,216-224] The characteristic cutaneous feature is illustrated in Figure 2-16. Many infants exhibit facial hemihypertrophy as a result of lipomatous-hamartomatous lesions of the lower half of the cheek. In *Proteus syndrome*, unilateral or generalized hypertrophy of the body; thickened, hyperpigmented skin; lipomata; lymphangiomata; and hemangiomata, macrodactyly, and a curious gyriform appearance of the plantar surface of the feet may accompany the hemimegalencephaly.

MIGRATION

Normal Development

Neuronal migration refers to the remarkable series of events whereby millions of nerve cells move from their sites of origin in the ventricular and subventricular zones to the loci within the CNS, where they will reside for life. The *peak time period* for this occurrence is

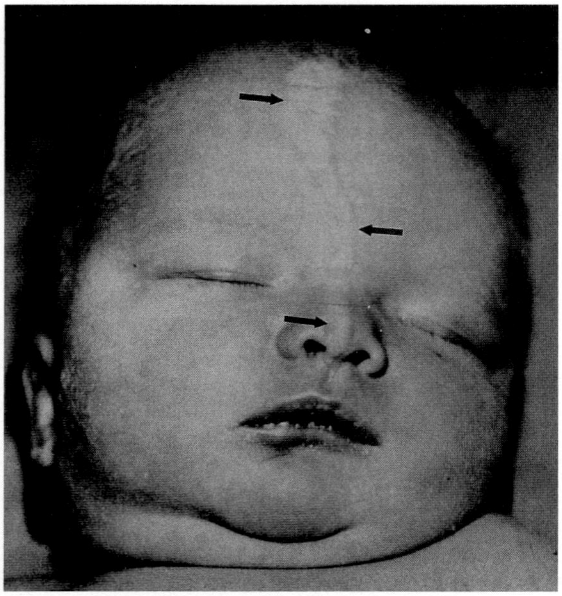

Figure 2-16 **Epidermal nevus syndrome.** This infant was 48 hours old. Note the midline linear nevus *(arrows)*. *(From Chalhub EG, Volpe JJ, Gado MH: Linear nevus sebaceous syndrome associated with porencephaly and nonfunctioning major cerebral venous sinuses, Neurology 25:857-860, 1975.)*

TABLE 2-8	**Neuronal Migration**
Peak Time Period	
3–5 months	
Major Events	
Cerebrum	
Radial migration: cerebral cortex (projection neurons), deep nuclei	
Tangential migration: cerebral cortex (interneurons)	
Cerebellum	
Radial migration: Purkinje cells, dentate nuclei	
Tangential migration: external → internal granule cells	

the third to fifth months of gestation, although neuronal migration can be detected in certain areas of the cerebrum as early as the second month and slightly after the fifth month (Table 2-8). Regulation of the timing and direction of these many simultaneous migrations must be highly ordered, but only recently has insight been gained into these control mechanisms (see later).

Two Basic Varieties of Neuronal Migration

The major features of cell migration in the primate were defined initially, particularly by the classic studies of Sidman and Rakic,[24-26,225-228] who used primarily autoradiographic, electron microscopic, and Golgi techniques. Later work used immunocytochemical and retroviral methods and the study of genetically manipulated animals to elaborate earlier observations.[23a,25,26,31,41,228-261] *Two basic varieties* of cell migration have been delineated: *radial* and *tangential* (see Table 2-8). In the *cerebrum*, radial migration of cells from their origin in the ventricular and subventricular zones is the primary mechanism for formation of the cortex and deep nuclear structures. *Radial migration* gives rise to the *projection neurons* of the cortex. These neurons emanate primarily from the *dorsal region of the subependymal germinative zones*. *Tangential migration* of neurons generated in the *ventral aspect of the subependymal germinative zones* results in the *gamma-aminobutyric acid (GABA)–expressing interneurons* of the cerebral cortex.[23a,249,250,253,254,258,259,262] These neuronal precursors migrate parallel to the surface of the cortex and proceed in one of three streams (i.e., through the subventricular zone, the intermediate zone, or the marginal zone) before terminal radial movement to arrive in the cortical plate. In the *cerebellum*, radial migration causes the genesis of Purkinje cells, the dentate nucleus, and other roof nuclei. Tangential migration of cells that originate in the germinal zones in the region of the rhombic lip and migrate over the surface of the cerebellum forms the well-known *external granular layer*. These cells then migrate radially inward to form the *internal granule cell layer* of the cerebellar cortex. Thus, during their journey from their point of origin in the ventricular zone, the granule cells exhibit both radial and tangential migration.

Migration to Cerebral Cortex

The basic pattern of cell migration for formation of the cerebral cortex is shown in Figures 2-17 and 2-18. Two basic modes of cell migration are apparent (see Fig. 2-18). The first and earlier mechanism is movement by translocation of the cell body (i.e., somal translocation) (Table 2-9).[258,263] This mode of migration probably results in the formation of the preplate (see Fig. 2-17). This layer of neurons later is split by the arrival of the cortical plate neurons into a superficial layer nearest the pial surface, which produces the Cajal-Retzius and related neurons of the marginal zone, and a deeper layer, which becomes the subplate neurons. The preplate neurons and the subsequently formed Cajal-Retzius and subplate neurons are critical for the progression of neuronal migration (see later).

The second mode of migration, leading to the formation of most of the cerebral cortex, occurs by radial migration (see Figs. 2-17 and 2-18). These cells are generated by the radial glial progenitors discussed earlier (see the discussion of proliferation). The clonally related neuron migrates along the parental radial glial fiber, which extends to the pial surface. Initially, cells are generated in the *ventricular zone*, and then they migrate relatively rapidly and synchronously through the intermediate zone in waves to the developing cortical plate. At *later stages*, as shown by Rakic[24-26,226-228] in studies of the monkey visual cortex, the neurons are generated especially in the *subventricular zone* (see Fig. 2-17). By labeling dividing cells with [³H]thymidine at various times during development and then determining where the labeled cells appear in the cortical plate, Rakic showed that cells that migrate first take the deepest positions in the cortex, whereas those migrating later take more superficial positions. By *20 to 24 weeks* of gestation, the human cerebral cortex essentially has its *full complement* of neurons.

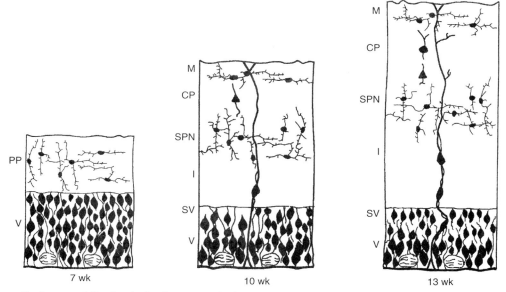

Figure 2-17   **Schematic diagram of the developing human cerebral cortex at the gestational ages indicated.** The pial surface is at the top and the ventricular surface at the bottom of each depiction of the cerebral wall. CP, cortical plate; I, intermediate zone; M, marginal zone; PP, preplate zone; SPN, subplate neurons; SV, subventricular zone; V, ventricular zone. A radial glial fiber is shown traversing the cerebral mantle in the two right schematics and is not labeled.

How do the migrating cells know how to reach where they are going? In the major process of radial migration, radial glial cells serve as the guides for migration of young neurons from their sites of origin in the ventricular and, later, subventricular zones across a distance that can be many times greater than the length of their leading processes to their ultimate position in the cortical plate (see Table 2-9; Fig. 2-19).* The elaboration of the structure of the

_____

*See references 25,26,31,41,227-231,239,245,248,249,251-253,255, 256,258-260,264-266.

radial glial fiber system has been clarified by immuno-cytochemical and ultramicroscopic studies, especially by Caviness and others.[229-231,239,255,256,258] Initially, the system is uniformly radial in alignment, and in the ventricular zone the fibers appear to separate columns of germinative cells, the proliferative units described by Rakic in the primate (see earlier). The radial glial system in the developing cerebral wall forms fascicles of fibers rather than isolated fibers. With the rapid growth of the cerebral wall, and particularly the intermediate zone, the fiber fascicles develop distinct curves with definite region-specific changes in

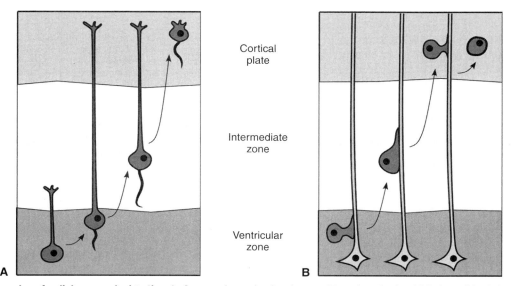

Figure 2-18   **Two modes of radial neuronal migration.** In **A**, an early mechanism is somal translocation in which the cell body is translocated from the point of origin in the ventricular zone to the cortical plate. In **B**, a later and predominant mechanism is radial migration, in which cells are generated by radial glial progenitors, and the clonally related neuron migrates along the parent radial glial fiber. Tangential migration differs from radial migration (see text).

TABLE 2-9 **Migration to Cerebral Cortex**

Initially, neurons migrate by translocation of the cell body (somal translocation). Later and predominantly, neurons migrate by following radial glial guides (i.e., the fibers of their clonally related radial progenitors).

Simultaneous with this radial migration, tangential migration parallel to the surface of the cortex (followed by radial migration to the cortex) results in the GABA-expressing interneurons of the cortex.

Proliferative units of the ventricular zone migrate through the radial glial scaffolding to become the ontogenetic neuronal columns of cerebral cortex.

Migration through subplate neurons and ''waiting'' thalamo-cortical and corticocortical afferents is likely important for later neuronal development (e.g., synaptogenesis).

Early-arriving neurons take deep positions in cortex, and later-arriving neurons take superficial positions (i.e., ''inside-out'' pattern).

GABA, gamma-aminobutyric acid.

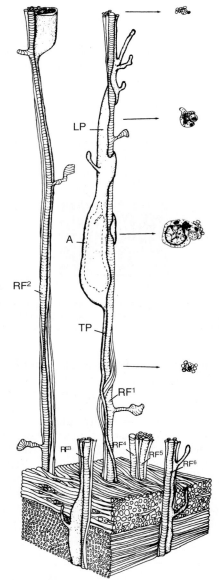

Figure 2-19 **Three-dimensional reconstruction of migrating neurons, based on electron micrographs of semiserial sections.** Note the apposition of the migrating neuron (A), with its leading process (LP) and attenuated trailing process (TP), to the guiding radial glial fiber (RF). As discussed in the text, the migrating neuron and the radial glial progenitor are clonally related. *(From Sidman RL, Rakic P: Neuronal migration, with special reference to developing human brain: A review, Brain Res 62:1-35, 1973.)*

trajectory (Fig. 2-20). Nevertheless, the dominant feature remains the migration of apparent clonally related columns of cells among the same radial glial fascicles, again likely related to the proliferative units described earlier.[237] As the migrating neurons approach the cortical plate, the radial glial fascicles begin to defasciculate, and radial fibers tend to penetrate the cortex more as single fibers.[230] This occurrence develops at the junction of the upper intermediate zone and the subplate zone, an important site for neuronal heterotopias in disorders of neuronal migration (see later).

Insights into the *key molecular determinants of neuronal migration* have been gained in recent years (Table 2-10). I present a brief discussion here of some of the best-studied molecules; further review of molecular determinants is provided later in the discussions of the molecular aspects of individual disorders of migration. Roles for molecules on preplate neurons (and the later Cajal-Retzius and subplate neurons), radial glia, and migrating neurons have been established. From *preplate neurons and the Cajal-Retzius cells of the marginal zone*, such extracellular matrix molecules as fibronectin and chondroitin and heparan sulfate proteoglycans clearly are crucial.[232,249,258,267-269] The secreted glycoprotein, reelin, lacking in the mutant mouse ''reeler'' with a neuronal migrational disorder, is an important product of the Cajal-Retzius cells.[251,253,257,258,266,270-274] Platelet-activating factor acetylhydrolase, lacking in one form of human lissencephaly (see later), suggests an important role for a molecule related to platelet-activating factor, a notion further supported by in vitro studies.[249,275-277] Neurons with GABA receptors in the preplate, Cajal-Retzius cells, and perhaps migrating neurons also now appear to be involved in migrational events.[266,278]

Important molecular determinants of migration on *radial glia* include three signaling pathways, involving erb B4 receptors, Notch receptors and brain lipid-binding protein (BLBP) (see Table 2-10).[249,251,253,279,280] The first of these are the surface ligands for neuregulin located on *migrating neurons* (see Table 2-10). An additional and well-characterized surface molecule of importance on migrating neurons is the surface

glycoprotein, astrotactin.[281,282] Doublecortin is the product of a gene on the X chromosome and is involved in double cortex (band) heterotopia in female patients and lissencephaly in male patients, important human neuronal migration disorders (see later).[252,253,257,258,283-287] This protein, expressed in migrating neurons at the growing end, is involved in an intracellular signaling pathway important for neuronal migration. Doublecortin is a microtubule-associated protein, which plays a role in microtubule polymerization and thereby may be involved in neuronal migration by mediating the cytoskeletal changes required for such movement.[252,253,258] The gene

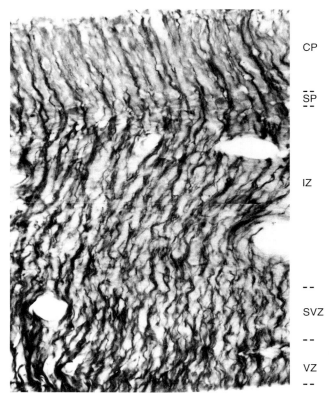

CP

SP

IZ

SVZ

VZ

Figure 2-20   Glial fiber alignment at E15 in the developing rat. The glial fibers ascend almost radially through the ventricular (VZ) and subventricular zone (SVZ). Within the intermediate zone (IZ), the fiber fascicles become arced medially to laterally. At the level of the IZ-subplate (SP) interface, they again become inflected to a radial alignment, orthogonal to the pial surface, which is maintained across the cortical strata. This coronal 6-μm plastic section was immunostained with RC2 antibody for radial glial fibers. Bar = 20 μm; CP, cortical plate. *(From Gadisseux JF, Evrard P, Misson JP, Caviness VS: Dynamic structure of the radial glial fiber system of the developing murine cerebral wall: An immunocytochemical analysis,* Dev Brain Res *50:55-67, 1989.)*

responsible for the human neuronal migration disorder, periventricular heterotopia, *filamin 1*, encodes a neuronal actin cross-linking protein that transduces ligand-receptor binding into actin reorganization, critical for locomotion of many cell types.[258,288] Involvement of neuronal calcium channels, glutamate, and *N*-methyl-D-aspartate (NMDA) receptors is supported by the work particularly of Rakic and coworkers, but also of others.[243,244,251,252,289-294] Thus, selective blockage of N-type, but not of L-and T-type, calcium channels inhibits neuronal migration. N-type calcium channels are involved primarily in release of neurotransmitters. That the neurotransmitter involved is glutamate, which acts on the NMDA receptor, is suggested by the demonstration that blockers of NMDA receptors, but not of non-NMDA receptors, inhibit neuronal migration (Fig. 2-21). Axonal release of glutamate may be the source of the glutamate that acts on the migrating neuron.

Radial glial cells have *additional functions*, aside from guidance of neuronal migration (see Table 2-2 and earlier discussion). Thus, the initial role of these cells is as neuronal progenitors. Generation of neurons is followed by the role as radial glial guides. Still later, these cells give rise to astrocytes and oligodendroglia, and the cellular progeny of the radial glial cell will then serve as a source of neural stem cells in the subventricular zone of the mature brain.

Disorders

Disorders of neuronal migration usually cause overt disturbances of neurological function with clinical deficits often apparent from the first days of life. Seizures are most often the dominant early neurological sign with the more severe migrational disturbances. The advent of MRI scanning markedly increased the ability to identify these disorders in vivo, demonstrated the relatively high prevalence of these disorders, and

TABLE 2-10 Selected Key Molecular Determinants of Neuronal Migration	
Preplate neurons (also marginal [Cajal-Retzius] zone and subplate neurons) and extracellular matrix	Fibronectin, chondroitin, and heparan sulfate Fukutin proteoglycans GABA receptors Integrins Laminin Reelin
Radial glia	erb B⁴ receptors Brain lipid binding protein (BLBP)
Migrating neurons	Notch receptors Neuregulin Astrotactin Doublecortin Platelet-activating factor acetylhydrolase (subunit 1) Filamin 1 Cyclin-dependent kinase-5 (cdk-5) Neural cell adhesion molecule (NCAM) *N*-methyl-D-aspartate (NMDA) receptors Calcium channels GABA receptors

GABA, gamma-aminobutyric acid.

TABLE 2-11	Disorders of Neuronal Migration
Order of Decreasing Severity	
Schizencephaly	
Lissencephaly: pachygyria	
Polymicrogyria	
Heterotopia	
Focal cerebrocortical dysgenesis	
Possible Concomitant Abnormalities of Corpus Callosum	

showed their broad clinical expression (see later discussion). The major disorders are listed in Table 2-11 in order of decreasing severity.

Gyral Abnormality in Migrational Disorders

The hallmark of the migrational disorders is an aberration of gyral development. Formation of the many secondary and tertiary gyri of the human brain occurs after neuronal migration has ceased (Fig. 2-22).[3,295-298]

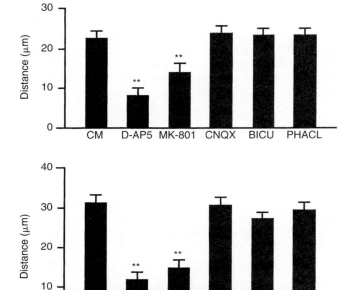

Figure 2-21 **The effect of antagonists to inotropic receptors on the migration of cerebellar granule cells.** All preparations were obtained from 10-day-old mice. Each column shows the mean length of the migration route for at least 100 labeled cells. The small bar is the standard error of the mean. Each antagonist to specific *N*-methyl-d-aspartate (NMDA) (D-AP5, MK-801), non-NMDA (CNQX), gamma-aminobutyric acid A (GABAA) (bicuculline [BICU]), or GABAB (phaclofen [PHACL]) receptors was added to the tissue culture medium in separate experiments 2 hours after staining, and preparations were maintained for an additional 2 hours (**A**) to 4 hours (**B**). The mean distance of cell displacement after the addition of 10 μm CNQX, 10 μm BICU, or 500 μm PHACL was not significantly different from values obtained in control slice preparations (CM) at each time point. However, addition of 100 μm D-AP5 or 10 μm MK-801 (NMDA antagonists) inhibited cell movement. Mean migratory distance was obtained by subtracting the mean displacement of the cell soma at 2 hours in culture from the total length of the migratory pathway. The *double asterisks* indicate statistical significance ($P < .01$). *(From Komuro H, Rakic P: Modulation of neuronal migration by NMDA receptors,* Science 260:95-97, 1993.)*

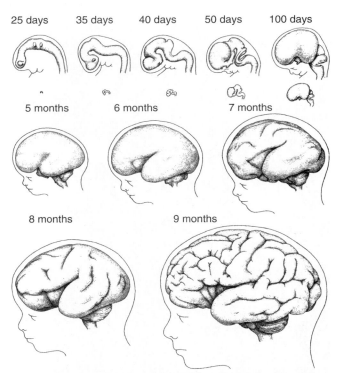

Figure 2-22 **Schematic depiction of gyral development in human brain.** Note the particularly prominent changes in the last 3 months of gestation. *(From Cowan WM: The development of the brain,* Sci Am 241:113-133, 1979.)*

The fastest increase in number of the major gyri occurs between 26 and 28 weeks of gestation.[295] Further elaboration of these gyri continues during the third trimester and shortly after birth.[295] The stimulus for gyral formation appears to be the remarkable increase in surface area of cerebral cortex that occurs during this period, particularly the difference in increase in surface area of the outer versus the inner cortical layers.[299] In the normal cortex, the surface area of the outer cortical layers is greater than the inner layers, and this discrepancy leads to compressive stresses that may lead to gyral formation. These relative increases in cortical surface area require the complement of neurons provided by migrational events. In lissencephaly, in which all cortical layers fail to receive their full complement of neurons, no gyri develop. In polymicrogyria, the surface area of outer cortical regions is much greater than that of inner cortical regions, and the result is an excess of gyri.[299] In addition, gyral development may be stimulated by the forces produced by growth of cerebral white matter axons originating in the cortex, the concept of *tension-based morphogenesis*.[300]

Corpus Callosum Defect in Migrational Disorders

In addition to gyral abnormality, a common feature of migrational disorders is hypoplasia or agenesis of the corpus callosum; occasionally, absence of the septum pellucidum also accompanies these disorders. Development of the corpus callosum (the major interhemispheric commissure) and of the septum is associated temporally and causally with the migrational events in the cerebrum (see Chapter 1). Thus, the timing of these aspects of midline prosencephalic development occurs almost coincidentally with the major neuronal migrational events for formation of cerebral cortex. Moreover, normal elaboration of cortical-cortical callosal fibers requires normal progression of neuronal migration to cerebral cortex. The frequent concurrence of hypoplasia or agenesis of the callosum with the migrational disorders discussed is therefore understandable.

Schizencephaly

Anatomical Abnormality. *Schizencephaly* is the most severe, yet restricted, of the cortical malformations (see Table 2-11).[301-309] A complete agenesis of a portion of the germinative zones and thereby the cerebral wall is believed to exist, leaving seams or clefts. The pial-ependymal seam is characteristic (Fig. 2-23). In the walls of the clefts, the cortical plate exhibits the hallmarks of migrational disturbance (e.g., a thick, microgyric cortex and large neuronal heterotopias). In bilateral lesions, schizencephaly in one hemisphere may be accompanied by polymicrogyria or focal cortical dysplasia in the other. The lips of the clefts may become widely separated, and dilation of the lateral ventricles may occur. Hydrocephalus often complicates such open-lipped lesions, especially when bilateral (see later). These open-lipped lesions, when bilateral, may be referred to incorrectly as hydranencephaly, a later destructive lesion of the cerebral hemispheres; when they are unilateral, they may be referred to incorrectly as porencephaly, a destructive lesion of one hemisphere. Indeed, it is now clear that unilateral and bilateral schizencephalies can be familial and probably account for previous reports of "familial porencephaly."[148,310-317] Gray matter (often polymicrogyric), lining the lesion and demonstrable on brain imaging, especially MRI, is the key finding indicative of schizencephaly.

The advent of MRI expanded greatly the understanding of anatomical and clinical aspects of schizencephaly. Indeed, several previous notions that were based almost exclusively on study of autopsy cases (i.e., that schizencephaly is rare, bilateral, and associated invariably with severe neurological deficits) were shown to be incorrect. Thus, in two large series, 67 cases were collected, and schizencephaly was unilateral in 63% (Table 2-12).[318] The clefts tended to be in the regions of the rolandic and sylvian fissures and involved predominantly frontal areas. Subsequent series confirmed these observations.[306]

Timing and Clinical Aspects. Onset of the developmental disturbance that leads to schizencephaly is considered to be no later than the beginning of migrational events in the cerebrum in the third month of gestation. The possibility that destructive lesions operate in the third or fourth month of gestation, perhaps injuring both the germinative zones and migrating

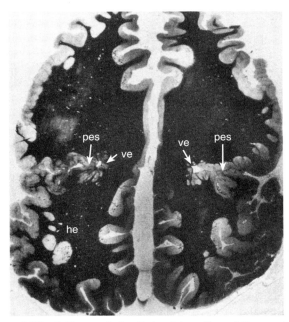

Figure 2-23 Schizencephaly. Horizontal section of the cerebrum, stained for myelin. Note the symmetrical clefts in the axis of the central fissures, pial-ependymal seams (pes), portion of lateral ventricles (ve), polymicrogyric cortex in margins of clefts, and neuronal heterotopias, especially on the left (he). *(From Yakovlev PI, Wadsworth RC: Schizencephalies: A study of the congenital clefts in the cerebral mantle. I. Clefts with fused lips, J Neuropathol Exp Neurol 5:116, 1946.)*

TABLE 2-12	Schizencephaly: Anatomical (Magnetic Resonance Imaging) and Clinical Features	
Feature	**Percentage**
Anatomical	
Unilateral	63%
Bilateral	37%
Closed clefts	42%
Open clefts	58%
Frontal	44%
Frontoparietal	30%
Parietal, temporal, or occipital	26%
Associated septo-optic dysplasia	39%
Anatomical-Clinical Correlates	
Cognitive Disturbances (Prominent)	
Bilateral	100%
Unilateral	24%
Motor Disturbances	
Bilateral	86%
Unilateral	77%
Frontal	84%
Not frontal	29%
Open lip	94%
Closed lip	22%
Seizure Disorder	
Bilateral	72%
Unilateral	60%
Hydrocephalus	
Open lip	52%
Closed lip	0%

Data from Barkovich AJ, Kjos BO: Schizencephaly: Correlation of clinical findings with MR characteristics, *AJNR Am J Neuroradiol* 13:85-94, 1992 and Packard AM, Miller VS, Delgado MR: Schizencephaly: Correlations of clinical and radiologic features, *Neurology* 48:1427-1434, 1997 and based on a cumulative series of 67 cases.

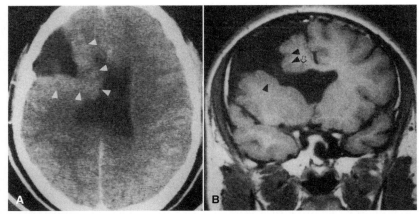

Figure 2-24 **Unilateral schizencephaly with separated lips. A,** Contrast-enhanced axial computed tomography scan shows deep infolding of the cortex in the right frontal region, apparently pressing on the right lateral ventricle *(arrowheads)*. (This cortical gray matter lining of the cleft is important in distinction from a destructive lesion, such as porencephaly.) **B,** Coronal SE 600/20 magnetic resonance imaging scan shows the infolding to be a large cleft in apparent continuity with lateral ventricle. (The pial-ependymal seam may not be demonstrable or may be disrupted.) Continuity of gray matter through the cleft is clearly shown *(arrowheads)*, as is the focus of heterotopic gray matter along the roof of the right lateral ventricle *(open arrow)*. The septum pellucidum is absent, consistent with the diagnosis of septo-optic dysplasia. *(From Barkovich AJ, Norman D: MR imaging of schizencephaly, AJNR Am J Neuroradiol 9:297-302, 1988.)*

neurons on radial glial fibers, is raised by multiple reports.[304,309,319-321] However, the demonstration, at least in certain rare familial cases, of a defect in the homeobox gene, EMX2, supports the notion that schizencephaly most often is a disorder of the developmental program.[252,315,322-324] This gene, specifically expressed in neuroblasts of the ventricular zone, is involved in the structural patterning of the developing forebrain, including neuronal migration. Nevertheless, a multifactorial origin of schizencephaly is supported by the association with fetal cytomegalovirus infection (which can cause both dysgenetic and destructive effects) and systemic abnormalities secondary to vascular disruption.[309,325]

The clinical features of schizencephaly have begun to be clarified by the study of patients identified by MRI. The lesion may be suspected because of the appearance of a focal ventricular dilation on ultrasonogram or CT scan or occasionally because of visualization of a gray matter–lined cleft on CT scan (Fig. 2-24A).[306,307,326,327] However, far more sensitive for identification of schizencephaly is MRI (Fig. 2-24B).[42,307,308,318,326,328,329] The salient feature is the lining of the cleft by cerebral cortex, often thickened by pachygyric or polymicrogyric cortex with heterotopias. The clinical spectrum is clearly broader than was previously expected. Severity relates to extent and

distribution of cerebral involvement (see Table 2-11).[306,307,318,330] In two series, prominent cognitive disturbances were present with all bilateral lesions but only 24% of unilateral lesions.[316,318] (I have seen one patient who had bilateral clefts with average intelligence.) Motor disturbances are nearly invariable with frontal and with open-lipped lesions (see Table 2-12).[306,307,316,318] Seizures may begin as late as adult life in patients with schizencephaly.[307,316,331,332] Hydrocephalus complicates approximately 50% of open-lipped lesions (see Table 2-12), although the mechanism for the impaired cerebrospinal fluid dynamics is unclear.[316] Agenesis of the septum pellucidum occurs in 70% of cases, and accompanying septo-optic dysplasia occurs in 10% to 25% (see Chapter 1).[307] Agenesis or hypoplasia of the corpus callosum occurs in 30% of cases of schizencephaly.[307]

Lissencephaly and Pachygyria

Anatomical Abnormality. In *lissencephaly* (i.e., "smooth brain"), the brain has few or no gyri.* Two basic anatomical types of lissencephaly can be distinguished (Tables 2-13 and 2-14). In *type I lissencephaly,* the cerebral wall is similar to that of an approximately

---

*See references 5,41,90,248,252,253,257,258,261,262,303,333-347.

TABLE 2-13	**Major Varieties of Type I Lissencephaly: Etiology/Genetics**			
Disorders	**Gene Locus**	**Protein**	**Function**
Isolated lissencephaly (LIS1)	17p13.3	PAFAH	Cytoskeleton (microtubules/dynein)
Miller-Dieker syndrome (LIS1)	17p13.3	PAFAH 14-3-3ε	Cytoskeleton(microtubules/dynein)
Isolated lissencephaly (XLIS)	Xq22.3	Doublecortin	Cytoskeleton (microtubules)
XLAG	Xp22	ARX	Homeobox
LCHb	7q22	Reelin	Neuron/radial glial cell interactions

ARX, an Aristaless-related homeobox transcription factor encoded by the gene *ARX;* LCHb, lissencephaly with cerebellar hypoplasia b; PAFAH, platelet-activating factor acetylhydrolase; XLAG, X-linked lissencephaly with abnormal genitalia.

TABLE 2-14   Major Varieties of Type II ("Cobblestone") Lissencephaly: Etiology/Genetics

Disorder	Gene Locus	Protein	Function
Fukuyama congenital muscular dystrophy	9q31-32	Fukutin	Glycosylation
Walker-Warburg syndrome	9q34.1	POMT1	Glycosylation
Muscle-eye-brain disease	1p34	POMGnT1	Glycosylation

POMGnT1, protein O-mannose N-acetylglucosaminyltransferase; POMT1, protein O-mannosyltransferase 1.

12-week-old fetus (Fig. 2-25A and B). The layers consist, from the pial surface, of an outermost relatively cell-poor marginal layer, a diffuse cellular layer containing primarily pyramidal and other neurons characteristic of lower layers of cortex, a zone of heterotopic neurons in columns, and an innermost band of white matter. The pathological features indicate that the diffuse cellular layer contains neurons that were destined to constitute the deep layers of cortex but were never displaced by subsequent migrations, the neurons of which constitute the heterotopic layer. In *type II lissencephaly* the appearance is quite different (Fig. 2-25C). The cortex is represented by clusters and circular arrays of neurons, with no recognizable organization or lamination, separated by glial and vascular septa. Large heterotopic collections of neurons are prominent. Notable, however, are the protrusions over the cortical surface where neurons have migrated through the pia. These protrusions cause the cortical surface to be irregular or "pebbly" in appearance.

In *pachygyria*, the features are similar to those described for lissencephaly but are less marked.* The gyri are relatively few, are unusually broad, and are associated with an abnormally thick cortical plate (Fig. 2-26, parasagittal region). The microscopic features are similar to those of lissencephaly, although the abnormalities are less marked (Fig. 2-27). Pachygyria should be considered *on a continuum with lissencephaly*, because, depending on the nature of the genetic disturbance,

*See references 5,41,252,253,257,258,261,303,339-341,343,345, 348-353.

lissencephaly syndromes may be characterized principally by pachygyria rather than by lissencephaly (see later).

Timing. The onset of lissencephaly-pachygyria is considered to be no later than the third and fourth months of gestation. This conclusion is based on the anatomical features of the lesions, as well as cases in which putative teratogenic exposures could be documented.[5,303,341,354]

Clinical Aspects: Type I Lissencephaly. The clinical aspects of lissencephaly-pachygyria are considered best in terms of those disorders characterized by type I and type II disease (see Tables 2-13 and 2-14). Thus, eight genetic disorders are recognized, five resulting in type I lissencephaly. Approximately 60% of cases of type I lissencephaly are caused by defects of the chromosome 17p13.3 gene (*LIS1*), and approximately one half of the remaining cases are caused by defects of the Xq22.3 gene *XLIS* or *DCX* (see Table 2-12). (The *XLIS* cases account for nearly all the male infants in the non-*LIS1* group.) Both lissencephaly with cerebellar hypoplasia b (reelin deficiency) and X-linked lissencephaly with abnormal genitalia (XLAG) are much less common.

The *clinical features* of the major form of type I lissencephaly (*LIS1*, isolated lissencephaly related to the chromosome 17p13.3 locus), are summarized in Table 2-15.* Despite the major brain anomaly,

*See references 248,252,253,257,258,261,262,341,344,346,355-369.

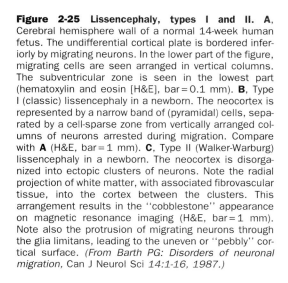
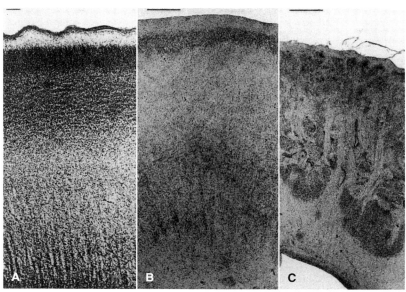

Figure 2-25 Lissencephaly, types I and II. A, Cerebral hemisphere wall of a normal 14-week human fetus. The undifferential cortical plate is bordered inferiorly by migrating neurons. In the lower part of the figure, migrating cells are seen arranged in vertical columns. The subventricular zone is seen in the lowest part (hematoxylin and eosin [H&E], bar = 0.1 mm). **B,** Type I (classic) lissencephaly in a newborn. The neocortex is represented by a narrow band of (pyramidal) cells, separated by a cell-sparse zone from vertically arranged columns of neurons arrested during migration. Compare with **A** (H&E, bar = 1 mm). **C,** Type II (Walker-Warburg) lissencephaly in a newborn. The neocortex is disorganized into ectopic clusters of neurons. Note the radial projection of white matter, with associated fibrovascular tissue, into the cortex between the clusters. This arrangement results in the "cobblestone" appearance on magnetic resonance imaging (H&E, bar = 1 mm). Note also the protrusion of migrating neurons through the glia limitans, leading to the uneven or "pebbly" cortical surface. *(From Barth PG: Disorders of neuronal migration,* Can J Neurol Sci *14:1-16, 1987.)*

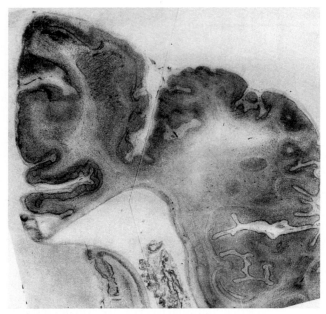

Figure 2-26 **Pachygyria and polymicrogyria.** Coronal section of the parietal lobe, parasagittal region, and lateral convexity from an infant with Zellweger cerebrohepatorenal syndrome (Nissl stain for cell bodies). Note the pachygyric cortex in the parasagittal region and the polymicrogyric cortex over the lateral convexity. *(From Volpe JJ, Adams RD: Cerebro-hepato-renal syndrome of Zellweger: An inherited disorder of neuronal migration, Acta Neuropathol [Berl] 20:175-198, 1972.)*

TABLE 2-15	Major Neurological Features of Type I Isolated Lissencephaly

Normal head size at birth → microcephaly in the first year
Hypotonia → hypertonia later in infancy
Paucity of movement, feeding disturbance
Seizures (common evolution to infantile spasms or Lennox-Gastaut syndrome in early infancy)
Electroencephalogram severely disordered with high amplitude and rapid frequency

microcephaly usually is *not* present at birth, but characteristically develops in the first year. The craniofacial appearance is generally unremarkable, except for bitemporal hollowing of the skull and a small jaw. Marked hypotonia and paucity of movement are characteristic. Spasticity does not develop until later in the first year or even after that. Neonatal seizures can occur, but characteristically seizures develop in the first 6 months as infantile spasms or as akinetic-myoclonic seizures with grossly disordered findings on the EEG (Lennox-Gastaut syndrome). The EEG is always abnormal; particularly characteristic is high-amplitude, fast activity, occurring in approximately 75% of patients with type I lissencephaly. Bursts of sharp and slow-wave complexes, interspersed with periods of voltage depression, are also common features of the EEG. Infants with primarily pachygyria rather than lissencephaly have less severe clinical deficits, including occasionally only mild subsequent impairment of

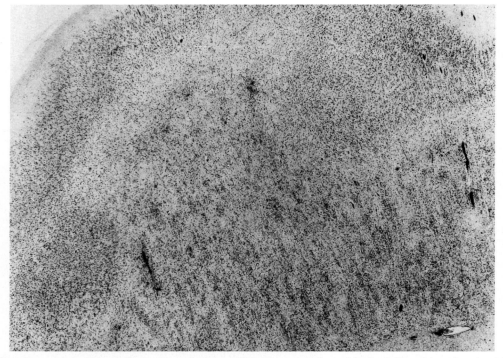

Figure 2-27 **Pachygyric cortex in the specimen shown in Figure 2-26** (Nissl stain for cell bodies). The pial surface is at the upper left-hand corner, and the subcortical white matter is at the lower right-hand corner. Note the broad layer of heterotopic neurons arranged in columns and nests, separated from the pachygyric cortex by a sparsely cellular region. The neurons of the pachygyric cortex, at higher magnification, had the characteristics of pyramidal neurons of deeper cortical layers, not displaced by subsequent migrations. *(From Volpe JJ, Adams RD: Cerebro-hepato-renal syndrome of Zellweger: An inherited disorder of neuronal migration, Acta Neuropathol [Berl]) 20:175-198, 1972.)*

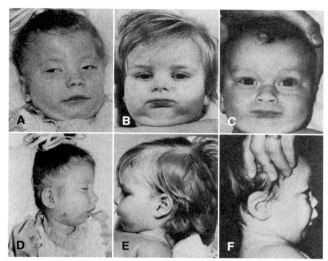

Figure 2-28   Miller-Dieker syndrome. A to **C**, Frontal and, **D** to **F**, lateral views of three infants. See text for details. *(From Dobyns WB: The neurogenetics of lissencephaly, Neurol Clin 7:89-105, 1989.)*

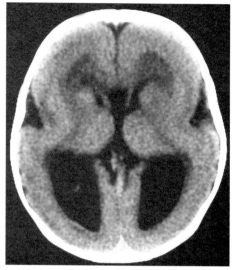

Figure 2-29   Lissencephaly, type I, computed tomography scan. Note the smooth cortical surface and colpocephaly (dilation of trigone and occipital horns of lateral ventricles). *(From Dobyns WB: The neurogenetics of lissencephaly, Neurol Clin 7:89-105, 1989.)*

intellect. In general, however, neurological outcome in *LIS1* isolated lissencephaly is characterized ultimately by mental retardation, spastic quadriparesis, and seizures.

The clinical features of the second major form of type I lissencephaly related to the chromosome 17p13.3 locus, the *Miller-Dieker syndrome*, are different from those of isolated lissencephaly because of the additional presence of craniofacial abnormalities.[73,248,257,258,261,364,370,371] Thus, in addition to the bitemporal hollowing and small jaw observed with isolated lissencephaly, patients have a characteristic facial appearance with a short nose with upturned nares, a long and protuberant upper lip with a thin vermilion border, and a relatively flattened midface (Fig. 2-28). Additional characteristic features of Miller-Dieker syndrome include cardiac malformations (20% to 25%), genital anomalies in male infants (70%), a sacral dimple (70%), deep palmar creases (65% to 70%), and clinodactyly (40% to 45%). Neurological features are similar to those described for isolated lissencephaly, although generally the disturbances are even more marked, consistent with the uniformly severe degree of the lissencephaly.

The *clinical aspects* of the *major X-linked form of type I lissencephaly* (i.e., those related to a defect in the *DCX* [or *XLIS*] gene), are similar to those described for isolated lissencephaly caused by *LIS1*. The clinical features, of course, occur in hemizygous male infants, whereas heterozygous female infants exhibit subcortical band heterotopia (see later).

The *clinical aspects* of the *rarer* form of X-linked lissencephaly (i.e., *XLAG*) are somewhat distinctive.[372-376] Particularly characteristic features include severe *neonatal* seizures (onset in >50% in the first hour of life and in utero in 20%), hypothermia, severe diarrhea, and ambiguous genitalia (micropenis, cryptorchidism). The epileptic syndrome is especially severe and relates to the particular involvement of GABAergic interneurons (see later). The lissencephaly is accompanied also

by complete agenesis of the corpus callosum. The full syndrome occurs in hemizygous male infants, although less severe phenotypes occur as a function of the severity of the genetic abnormality. Heterozygous female infants often exhibit agenesis of the corpus callosum and epilepsy.

The *clinical aspects* of *lissencephaly with cerebellar hypoplasia b*, related to a defect in *RELN*, which encodes reelin, are difficult to define decisively because of the paucity of careful clinical descriptions.[257,377-379] Perhaps most notable is the presence of microcephaly *at birth*, rather than the postnatal development of microcephaly, as in other varieties of type I lissencephaly. The term *lissencephaly with cerebellar hypoplasia b* is used to distinguish these cases from lissencephaly with cerebellar hypoplasia a. The latter are examples of type I lissencephaly secondary to either *LIS1* or *DCX* gene defects (see earlier) that may be accompanied by prominent hypoplasia of the cerebellar vermis and mild hypoplasia of the cerebellar hemispheres. By contrast, the reelin-related cases exhibit *severe* hypoplasia of the *entire* cerebellum, which also lacks folia.

The *radiological features* of type I lissencephaly may include a distinctive appearance on CT scan (Fig. 2-29). However, MRI provides superior definition of the parenchymal lesion (Figs. 2-30 and 2-31). Indeed, insight into the likely genetic lesion can be gained by evaluating the degree of lissencephaly and pachygyria, any anteroposterior gradient, agenesis of the corpus callosum, and the degree of cerebellar hypoplasia (see Fig. 2-31).[257] Thus, of *LIS1* cases, the cortex is very thick, posterior more than anterior involvement is apparent, and Miller-Dieker cases have even more severe lissencephaly than do isolated cases. *DCX* cases have anterior more than posterior involvement. *XLAG* cases have only a moderately thick cortex and prominent agenesis of the corpus callosum. Reelin cases have a moderately thick, pachygyric cortex with striking cerebellar hypoplasia. A uniform accompanying feature

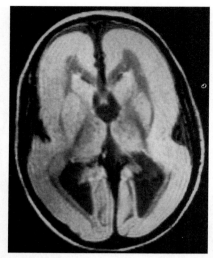

Figure 2-30 **Lissencephaly, type I, magnetic resonance imaging (MRI) scan**. Note the smooth cortical surface and colpocephaly, as described in the Figure 2-29 legend. The cerebral parenchymal features are visualized better by MRI than by computed tomography.

in all genetic types is colpocephaly (i.e., dilation of the trigone, occipital horns, and temporal horns of the lateral ventricles). The ventricular dilation of colpocephaly occurs in the trigone and occipital horns because of underdevelopment of the corpus callosum and calcarine sulci and in the temporal horns because of failure of inversion of the hippocampus.[363]

Etiology/Genetics: Type 1 Lissencephaly. The five major genetic varieties of type I lissencephaly appear to involve three different mechanisms of migrational failure (see Table 2-13). The *LIS1* cases, both isolated lissencephaly and Miller-Dieker syndrome, and the *DCX (XLIS)* cases have a defect in the pace of migration. XLAG appears to involve a defect in tangential more than radial migration. The *RELN* cases appear to be related to a defect in migrating neuron and radial glial interactions.

Isolated lissencephaly (LIS1) secondary to a deficiency in PAFAH1B1 *(LIS1)* involves a disturbance in migration because of abnormal function of the cytoskeleton.[257,258,260,262,380,381] This protein is the

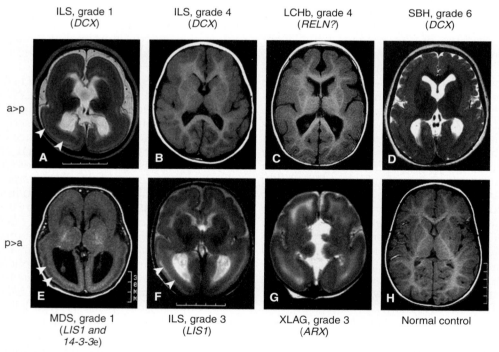

Figure 2-31 **Lissencephaly, type I, magnetic resonance imaging scans.** In contrast to a normal control (**H**), all types of lissencephaly (**A** to **G**) have absent or broad gyri and an abnormally thick cortex, except for subcortical band heterotopia (SBH), resulting from *DCX* mutation in heterozygous female infants (SBH is discussed in the text with heterotopias rather than with lissencephaly-pachygyria). The anteroposterior or rostrocaudal gradient of lissencephaly is strictly correlated with the causative gene. Specifically, mutations of *DCX* or *RELN* result in a more severe anterior than posterior (a>p) gradient (**A** to **D**), whereas mutations of *LIS1* with or without 14-3-3ε or *ARX* lead to a more severe posterior than anterior (p>a) gradient (**E** to **G**). The absolute thickness of the cortex and the presence of a cell-sparse zone also differ based on the causative gene. In patients with mutations of *DCX* (**A** and **B**) or *LIS1* (**E** and **F**), the cortex is very thick, typically 10 to 20 mm, and prominent cell-sparse zones are seen in areas of agyria (*arrowheads* in **A**, **E**, and **F**). In patients with lissencephaly with cerebellar hypoplasia group b (**C**, which resembles patients with known *RELN* mutations, although a mutation has not been demonstrated in this patient) or *ARX* (**G**) mutations, the cortex is only moderately thick, typically 5 to 10 mm, and cell-sparse zones are never seen, even in areas of agyria (**G**). In lissencephaly with cerebellar hypoplasia group b (LCHb) with or without proven *RELN* mutations, other images show an abnormal hippocampus and severe cerebellar hypoplasia (not shown). In male infants with X-linked lissencephaly with abnormal genitalia (XLAG) caused by *ARX* mutations, other images demonstrate poorly demarcated basal ganglia often with small cysts, immature white matter, and agenesis of the corpus callosum (not shown). In heterozygous female infants, mutations of *DCX* result in SBH (**D**), whereas mutations of *ARX* often result in agenesis of the corpus callosum (not shown). ILS, isolated lissencephaly; MDS, Miller-Dieker syndrome; XLAG, X-linked lissencephaly with abnormal genitalia. *(From Kato M, Dobyns WB: Lissencephaly and the molecular basis of neuronal migration,* Hum Mol Genet *12:R89-R96, 2003.)*

noncatalytic alpha subunit of the isoform Ib of platelet-activating factor acetylhydrolase. This *LIS1*-encoded protein interacts with microtubules and cytoplasmic dynein motors, crucial for both somal translocation and cell motility.

Miller-Dieker syndrome, of course, shares the PAFAH defect but because the disorder relates to a deletion, other genes are disturbed.[253,257,258,364,370,382] The protein, 14-3-3ε, appears to be the key additional defect in this more severe lissencephaly syndrome.[371] Deficiency of 14-3-3ε results in mislocalization of the *LIS1* protein and accentuates the dynein motor disturbance and thereby neuronal migration.

Isolated lissencephaly, secondary to the X-linked DCX (XLIS) gene and deficiency of *doublecortin*, appears also to be mediated at the level of the cytoskeleton.[248,257,258,283,383-385] *Doublecortin* is a microtubule-associated protein that binds to tubulin and is necessary for microtubule polymerization. Thus, as with the two *LIS1* disorders, a defect in the cytoskeleton and thereby in cell motility results.

XLAG involves a second mechanism of migration disturbance.[257,258,373,375,376] The gene involved, *ARX*, is a homeobox gene that encodes a protein critical for *tangential* migration. The result of the mutation is a marked deficiency of GABAergic interneurons, because, as noted earlier, tangential rather than radial migration is the mechanism for movement of neurons destined to be interneurons from the ventricular zone to the cortex. The severe deficiency of GABAergic neurons likely underlies the striking clinical feature of prenatal and early neonatal seizures and intractable infantile seizures (see the earlier discussion of clinical aspects).

Lissencephaly with cerebellar hypoplasia b, related to the *RELN* gene, involves a third mechanism of disturbed migration. *RELN* encodes a glycoprotein, reelin, secreted by horizontally oriented Cajal-Retzius cells in the preplate and marginal zones and is crucial for -signaling to migrating neurons on radial glial cells.[257,258,261] Reelin appears to function as a stop signal and in neuronal and radial glial cell interactions. The result of reelin deficiency is a cortex that is abnormally cellular in its most superficial zone and is inverted (i.e., early migrating pyramidal cells are the uppermost layer). Preplate-like cells accumulate in the marginal zone, a finding suggesting that the preplate has not been split by the migrating cortical neurons. Related phenomena occur in cerebellum to cause the severe cerebellar hypoplasia.

Other causes of type I lissencephaly, albeit rare, are worthy of note. A role for vascular insult during the third to fourth months of gestation has been suggested.[357,364,365,386] Moreover, lissencephalypachygyria has been documented with fetal cytomegalovirus infection (see Chapter 20) and with a variety of inborn errors of metabolism (e.g., pyruvate dehydrogenase deficiency, Zellweger syndrome, glutaric acidemia [type 2, nonketotic hyperglycinemia]; see Chapters 14, 15 and 16). Rare autosomal recessive forms with marked neonatal microcephaly and lissencephaly, the most severe form of microcephaly with simplified gyri

discussed among proliferative disorders, have been reported (see earlier).[42,345,387-389]

Recurrence risks for type 1 lissencephaly depend on the genetic type.[261] Thus, *LIS1* isolated lissencephaly, which is caused by de novo mutations, has a recurrence risk of approximately 1% (because of the theoretical risk of germline mosaicism in either parent). Miller-Dieker syndrome is related to de novo deletions in approximately 80% (recurrence risk of ≈1%), and in 20%, to inheritance of a deletion from a parent carrying a balanced chromosomal rearrangement. In the latter, recurrence risk is higher and depends on the nature of the rearrangement. With *XLIS* lissencephaly, the mother may be a carrier even if the brain MRI does not show subcortical band heterotopia.[385] Even if the mother is not a carrier, the risk of harboring germline mosaicism places a recurrence risk at about 5%. With XLAG, the carrier status of the mother should be evaluated because the phenotype in girls and women can be very mild. Thus far, the few families reported with reelin deficiency lissencephaly have exhibited autosomal recessive inheritance.

Clinical Aspects: Type II Lissencephaly. The three disorders consistently associated with type II lissencephaly are Fukuyama congenital muscular dystrophy, Walker-Warburg syndrome, and muscle-eye-brain disease (see Table 2-14).[252,253,390-403] As noted earlier, these disorders are characterized by lissencephaly in which protrusions of neurons are found over the surface of the brain and thereby render a "bumpy" or "pebbly" configuration to the cortical surface. In type II lissencephaly, the ectopic clusters of neurons within the cortex, separated by fibroglial vascular tissue that extends radially from the cerebral white matter, result in a typical MRI appearance, termed "cobblestone" lissencephaly (see later). The migrational defect is unique and is similar for the three disorders (see later). In addition to type II lissencephaly, these disorders also share congenital muscular dystrophy as a prominent clinical feature. Fukuyama congenital muscular dystrophy and muscle-eye-brain disease are discussed most appropriately with diseases of muscle (see Chapter 19). The clinical aspects of Walker-Warburg syndrome are described here.

The major *clinical features* of Walker-Warburg syndrome in many respects are different from those for the type I lissencephalic disorders (Table 2-16). Macrocephaly (84%), either apparent at birth (58%) or developing postnatally (26%), retinal malformations (100%), congenital muscular dystrophy (100%), cerebellar malformation (100%), and type II lissencephaly (100%) are characteristic.[390-393,401-403] Type II lissencephaly and the retinal, cerebellar, and muscular abnormalities are necessary for the diagnosis. The neurological features (e.g., severe seizure disorders and mental retardation) are similar to those identified for type I lissencephaly. However, the severe muscle disease, accompanied by elevated serum creatine kinase, accentuates the marked hypotonia and weakness observed with lissencephaly. Death in the first year is common.

TABLE 2-16 **Major Clinical Features of Walker-Warburg Syndrome**

Macrocephaly	84%
Present at birth	58%
Develops postnatal	26%
Type II lissencephaly	100%*
Cerebellar malformation	100%*
Ventricular dilation/hydrocephalus	95%
Retinal malformation	100%*
Anterior chamber abnormality	76%
Congenital muscular dystrophy	100%*

*Necessary for diagnosis.
Data from Dobyns WB: The neurogenetics of lissencephaly, *Neurol Clin* 7:89-105, 1989.

The *radiological features* are similar to those for type I lissencephaly in terms of the agyric brain and the concurrence of agenesis or hypoplasia of the corpus callosum or septum pellucidum. However, because of the different cerebral cortical microscopic pathological features (see earlier discussion), a slightly uneven cortex is apparent. Moreover, as noted earlier, irregular projections of the underlying white matter into the cortex lead to the term "cobblestone" lissencephaly (Fig. 2-32). The latter appearance is more clearly apparent after the neonatal period. The most characteristic distinguishing features of Walker-Warburg syndrome include the presence of cerebellar malformation and, invariably, vermian agenesis or hypoplasia, as well as complete Dandy-Walker malformation (50%) and posterior encephalocele (25% to 35%) (see Fig. 2-32; Fig. 2-33). The ventricular dilation (95%) can be

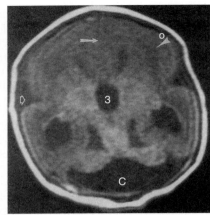

Figure 2-32 **Magnetic resonance imaging scan, type II lissencephaly in Walker-Warburg syndrome.** At the level of the third ventricle, a smooth cortical surface, open and shallow sylvian fissures *(open arrow)*, a Dandy-Walker cyst (C), and enlargement of the lateral and third (3) ventricles are demonstrated. A lack of cerebral gray-white matter interdigitation is seen (o, *arrowhead*) adjacent to a thickened cortical mantle. The "cobblestone" appearance of the cortex is faintly visible in the right frontal region and will become more apparent after the neonatal period. The anterior interhemispheric fissure is obliterated as a result of leptomeningeal thickening and proliferation *(arrow)*. The ventricular dilation and cerebellar malformation are characteristic of the syndrome (see text). *(From Rhodes RE: Walker-Warburg syndrome, AJNR Am J Neuroradiol 13:123-126, 1992.)*

distinguished from the colpocephaly of type I lissencephaly by involvement of the third and fourth ventricles and by the presence of the macrocephaly of hydrocephalus. Some of these distinguishing features are recalled by the eponymic designation for this

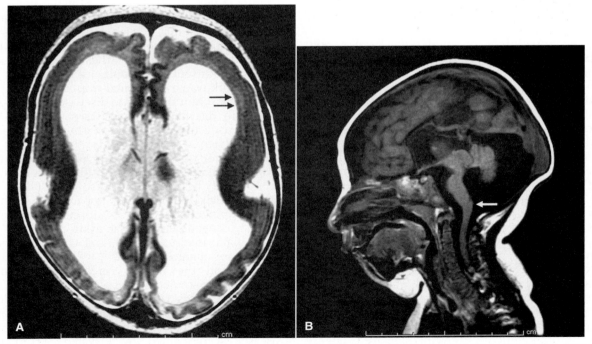

Figure 2-33 **Magnetic resonance imaging scan, type II lissencephaly, Walker-Warburg syndrome.** Note in **A** the hydrocephalus, smooth cortical surface anteriorly and pachygyric cortex posteriorly, and, barely observable, the interdigitations of white matter into the cortex with a resulting "cobblestone" appearance (arrows). In **B**, note the dysgenetic corpus callosum, cerebellar hypoplasia, and anomalous kinking of the lower brain stem *(arrow)*, all characteristic of Walker-Warburg syndrome. *(Courtesy of Dr. Omar Khwaja.)*

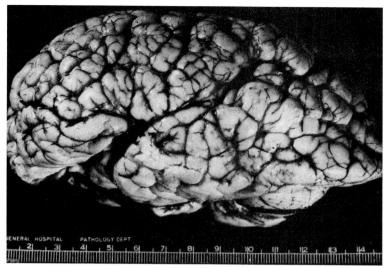

Figure 2-34 Lateral view of the cerebrum from an infant with Zellweger syndrome. Note the area of polymicrogyria, anterior to the sylvian fissure, involving the convexity of the frontal lobe. *(From Volpe JJ, Adams RD: Cerebro-hepato-renal syndrome of Zellweger: An inherited disorder of neuronal migration,* Acta Neuropathol [Berl] *20:175-198, 1972.)*

syndrome: HARD ± E, *h*ydrocephalus, *a*gyria, *r*etinal *d*ysplasia, *e*ncephalocele. I suggest an alternative, CHARM ± E, to add *c*erebellar and *m*uscle.

Etiology/Genetics: Type II Lissencephaly. The three autosomal recessive disorders that result in cobblestone lissencephaly occur because of a *failure of neurons to terminate their radial migration to the cerebral cortex.* Indeed, these neurons migrate through the glia limitans at the pial surface of the cortex and into the subarachnoid space.[258,398,399,403,404] The fundamental disturbance involves glycosylation of alpha-dystroglycan, a protein secreted particularly by astrocytes but also by neurons. Secreted alpha-dystroglycan interacts with beta-dystroglycan in the glial plasma membrane and with laminin of the extracellular matrix. The glia limitans consists of the apposed astrocytic end feet and the overlying extracellular matrix. Because the interactions of alpha-dystroglycan require correct glycosylation of the protein, failure of glycosylation is associated with gaps in the glia limitans, protrusion of neurons through these gaps, and failure of neurons to organize themselves within the cortical plate. The three mutant genes are involved in glycosylation, especially by encoding glycosyl transferases, as shown in Table 2-14. The molecular details require further delineation because the precise role of fukutin in glycosylation remains to be clarified, and only 10% to 20% of Walker-Warburg cases exhibit the protein O-mannosyl transferase defect.[399,402] In muscle, correctly glycosylated alpha-dystroglycan is required to interact with extracellular laminin and sarcolemmal betadystroglycan, which is bound to dystrophin. In the three disorders, failure of this interaction leads to degeneration of the muscle fiber and "dystrophy" (see Chapter 19).

Polymicrogyria

Anatomical Abnormality. Polymicrogyria is characterized by a great number of small plications in the cortical surface, rendering to the external aspect of the cerebrum the appearance of a wrinkled chestnut (Fig. 2-34). The multitude of small gyri are arranged in complicated festoon-like or glandular formations, appearing to result from fusion of their molecular layers (see Fig. 2-26, lateral convexity).[261,405-407]

Two basic varieties of polymicrogyria, layered and unlayered, can be distinguished from the microscopic appearance (Table 2-17 and Fig. 2-35; see Fig. 2-26).[5,41,261,303,408,409] In the *"classic," layered* variety, the cerebral cortex has four distinct layers. Thus, a relatively intact outermost molecular layer, a richly cellular second layer consisting of normal superficial cortical neurons, a cell-poor, gliotic layer in place of normal deeper cortical neurons, and a fourth layer of relatively preserved neurons arranged in columns are noted (see Fig. 2-35A). The cerebral white matter is much more abundant than in lissencephaly-pachygyria. This type of polymicrogyria often coexists in the margins of more severe ischemic destructive lesions (hydranencephaly) or in association with destructive infectious processes (e.g., toxoplasmosis or cytomegalovirus infection).[5,303,409-413] In the *nonlayered* variety of polymicrogyria, the neurons destined primarily (although not exclusively) for the outer cortical layers appear to have been impeded in their migrations. The result is a poorly laminated or nonlaminated cortex, which, after the outermost cell-poor molecular layer, consists of an ill-defined zone of larger pyramidal cells (appropriate for deeper cortex) followed by a stream of heterotopic neurons; many of these neurons are smaller pyramidal and granular cells (appropriate

TABLE 2-17 Major Varieties of Polymicrogyria
Layered: "classic" four-layered, probably postmigrational and related to destructive process
Unlayered: "nonclassic," not four-layered, migrational defect, accompanied by heterotopias and other consequences of migrational disorder

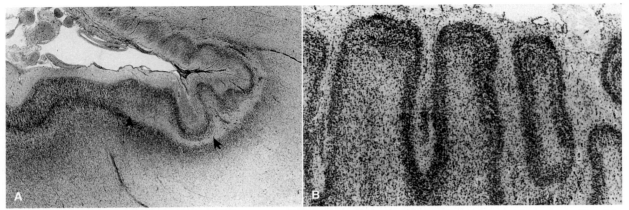

Figure 2-35   **Microgyria. A,** "Classic," layered microgyria, with transition between the microgyric and normal cortex. The aneuronal band *(arrow)* of the microgyric segment is continuous with layers III and IV of the normal cortex *(arrowhead).* Layer II of the microgyric cortex and layer II of the normal cortex are continuous (Nissl stain ×30). **B,** Unlayered microgyria in a microencephalic newborn with convulsions and general hypertonia. Note the heterotopic neurons in the subcortical white matter (hematoxylin and eosin, ×87). *(**A,** From Dias MJM, Rijckevorsel GH, Landrieu P, Lyon LG: Prenatal cytomegalovirus disease and cerebral microgyria: Evidence for perfusion failure, not disturbance of histogenesis, as the major cause of fetal cytomegalovirus encephalopathy, Neuropediatrics 15:18-24, 1984; **B,** from Barth PG: Disorders of neuronal migration, Can J Neurol Sci 14:1-16, 1987.)*

for superficial cortical layers) (see Figs. 2-26 and 2-35B). The heterotopic neurons in cerebral white matter are arranged in columns, apparently "glued" to the radial glial fibers.[5] This type of polymicrogyria is characteristic of that seen in Zellweger syndrome (see later discussion).

Timing. The two varieties of polymicrogyria appear to have differing times of onset. The nonlayered variety represents a disorder of neuronal migration, and the classic four-layered variety is a postmigrational disorder. The first type includes cases, such as patients with Zellweger syndrome (see Fig. 2-26), with concomitant migrational defects present in the cerebrum as well as in the brain stem or cerebellum. In these instances, the deepest collection of neurons appears to represent heterotopic neurons arrested during migration. Disturbance of neuronal migration as one basic cause of polymicrogyria is supported further by the occurrence of polymicrogyria in index patients and siblings of infants with Miller-Dieker lissencephaly syndrome and in the cerebral hemisphere contralateral to unilateral schizencephaly (see earlier discussion).[414] The time of onset of this nonlayered variety of polymicrogyria appears to be generally no later than the fourth to fifth months of gestation.

The second variety of polymicrogyria includes those cases with evidence of laminar neuronal necrosis in the cortex *after the apparent completion of migration.* Such examples of this postmigrational polymicrogyria include those cases associated with carbon monoxide exposure at approximately 20 to 24 weeks,[415,416] as well as with other, less well-defined intrauterine insults.[303,411,417-422] In these patients, the sparsely cellular gliotic third layer represents an area of laminar cortical necrosis, and the fourth layer is composed not of heterotopic neurons but of neurons of the deeper layers of previously formed cortex. The *postnatal* evolution of polymicrogyria and periventricular leukomalacia has been documented in a premature infant

from 31 weeks' postconceptional age, thereby documenting the postmigrational development of encephaloclastic polymicrogyria.[413] Some examples of polymicrogyria associated with cytomegalovirus infection, vascular anomalies, ischemic events, or metabolic abnormalities (mitochondrial disorders) could reside in the maldevelopmental categories, encephaloclastic categories, or both.[413,423-427] Indeed, the demonstration of lissencephaly-pachygyria in some infants with cytomegalovirus infection (see earlier discussion) documents clearly the potential for this viral infection to impair migratory events directly. A few observations suggest that some cases of polymicrogyria are caused by an encephaloclastic process *during* neuronal migration that interfered with the migrational events and produced polymicrogyria, that is, a combination of encephaloclastic and maldevelopmental varieties.[319,407,428,429] An experimental model that supports such a pathogenesis has been described.[430,431]

Clinical Aspects. The best example of a clinically well-defined, autosomal recessive disorder of neuronal migration with polymicrogyria and pachygyria is *Zellweger cerebrohepatorenal* syndrome.[5,190,432-437] The neurological syndrome in these infants is startling and is characterized by marked generalized weakness with severe hypotonia, severe recurrent seizures, and absence or marked impairment of high-level responses to visual, auditory, or somesthetic stimuli. Other features of the syndrome include a distinctive craniofacial appearance, hepatomegaly, multiple renal cortical cysts, and stippled calcification of the patellae. A disturbance of peroxisomal biogenesis is indicated by the demonstrations of absence of peroxisomes in the liver and other tissues and certain metabolic abnormalities (e.g., elevated levels of pipecolic acid and very-long-chain fatty acids and decreased levels of plasmalogens; see Chapter 16). Very-long-chain fatty acids are important constituents of plasma

TABLE 2-18 Potential Importance of Very-Long-Chain Fatty Acids in Neuronal Migration

Disease	Very-Long-Chain Fatty Acids	Plasmalogens	Neuronal Migration
Zellweger syndrome	↑	↓	Abnormal
Neonatal adrenoleukodystrophy	↑	↓	Abnormal
Bifunctional enzyme	↑	Normal	Abnormal
Rhizomelic chondrodysplasia punctata	Normal	↓	Normal

Data from Moser HW: The peroxisome: Nervous system role of a previously underrated organelle. The 1987 Robert Wartenberg lecture, *Neurology* 38:1617-1627, 1988 and Kaufmann WE, Theda C, Naidu S, et al: Neuronal migration abnormality in peroxisomal bifunctional enzyme defect, *Ann Neurol* 39:268-271, 1996.

membranes in the brain; the possibility that the accumulation of these compounds may interfere with normal membrane properties crucial for neuronal migration along radial glial fibers is suggested by the consistent relationship among generalized peroxisomal disorders between this abnormality (rather than others) and abnormal neuronal migration (Table 2-18).[438] This notion is supported further by the occurrence of polymicrogyria in an infant with deficiency of peroxisomal bifunctional enzyme, in which the impairment of peroxisomal function was confined to very-long-chain fatty acids (and bile acid intermediates).[425,439]

The clinical features of *sporadic cases* of generalized polymicrogyria are not well defined, although seizures are often recorded. In general, a broad range of clinical features has been reported, from severely impaired neurological development and intractable epilepsy to only selective disturbances of neurological function.[261] Unilateral polymicrogyria is a well-documented substrate for congenital hemiplegia.[440] Polymicrogyria may accompany other dysgenetic disorders, which have distinctive clinical features (e.g., a form of Joubert syndrome, Aicardi syndrome, Smith-Lemli-Opitz syndrome, periventricular nodular heterotopia; see Chapter 1).[261,441-443] The postnatal and postmigrational development of bilateral perisylvian polymicrogyria was documented by MRI in a premature infant with periventricular leukomalacia.[413] Focal polymicrogyria is a prominent feature of focal cerebrocortical dysgenesis, the clinical aspects of which are discussed separately later.

Growing numbers of *bilateral symmetrical polymicrogyria syndromes*, some familial, have been recognized (Table 2-19).[444-458a] The clinical features in most of these disorders occur after the neonatal period. A prominent exception is the bilateral perisylvian polymicrogyric syndromes, many of which are characterized by pseudobulbar palsy with oral-buccal-lingual deficits,

TABLE 2-19 Bilateral Symmetrical Polymicrogyria Syndromes

Topography	Genetics
Frontal	Sporadic
Frontoparietal	GPR56 (a G-protein–coupled receptor)
Perisylvian	Heterogeneous (includes Xq28 locus)
Parasagittal (Parieto-occipital)	Sporadic
Generalized	16q locus

feeding disturbances, and facial diparesis, as well as seizures from early infancy.

The *radiological diagnosis* of polymicrogyria in the *neonatal period* is often difficult, even with MRI (Fig. 2-36).[42,459] This difficulty relates in part to the lack of myelination and the less prominent gray-white matter junction in the newborn than at later ages.

Neuronal Heterotopias

Anatomical Abnormality. The least severe of the migrational disturbances, *neuronal heterotopias*, are collections of nerve cells in the periventricular region or in subcortical white matter, apparently arrested during radial migration from the subependymal germinative zones. Such collections are constant accompaniments of the more severe migrational disorders. At the other end of the spectrum, small collections of neurons in cerebral white matter are not unusual as incidental findings at autopsy.

Two major varieties of cerebral neuronal heterotopias are recognized (Table 2-20). The heterotopic collections in the periventricular (subependymal) region occur near the site of origin of neuroblasts in

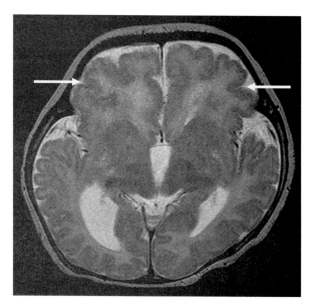

Figure 2-36 Magnetic resonance imaging (MRI) scan, polymicrogyria. This axial T2-weighted MRI scan from an infant with seizures shows bilateral symmetrical frontal polymicrogyria *(arrows)*. Note the multiple but very small sulcal indentations of the cerebral cortex. The cortical surface thus appears somewhat smooth. The distinction from lissencephaly is aided by noting that the cortex is not thick. Also notable are underopercularization of the sylvian fissure and colpocephaly (dilation of occipital horns). *(Courtesy of Dr. Omar Khwaja.)*

TABLE 2-20	Major Varieties of Cerebral Neuronal Heterotopias

Periventricular (subependymal)
Cerebral white matter
  Laminar: subcortical band or double cortex
  Nodular: focal or diffuse

the germinative ventricular and subventricular zones (Fig. 2-37). In the cerebral white matter, heterotopias may occur in a subcortical laminar distribution or as focal or diffuse nodular collections in the white matter. Those in the periventricular region are usually nodular and are termed *periventricular nodular heterotopia, periventricular heterotopia,* or *subependymal heterotopia* (see later). Those in the cerebral white matter that occur as a diffuse laminar band below the cerebral cortex are termed *band heterotopia* or *double cortex* (see later discussion).

Timing and clinical aspects. The onset of neuronal heterotopias is presumed to be no later than the last weeks of migrational events (i.e., no later than ≈20 weeks of gestation). The *clinical features* of disorders associated with cerebral neuronal heterotopias were clarified considerably by the advent of MRI scanning.[252,253,284,303,366,460-489] The clinical manifestations of nearly all cases of cerebral neuronal heterotopias begin after the neonatal period. Thus, a detailed discussion is not presented here. Periventricular heterotopia and band heterotopia (or double cortex) provide insights into mechanisms of neuronal migration and are described briefly. Focal or nodular cerebral white matter heterotopias exhibit clinical features related to the size and location of the heterotopias and are most likely to be encountered in the newborn as a feature of disorders discussed elsewhere in this book.[42,303,425,467-472,474-477,490-494] This latter diverse group is summarized in Table 2-21.

The two most common heterotopic lesions, periventricular heterotopia and band heterotopia of the double cortex syndrome, are of particular interest. (Table 2-22).[52,252,253,284,288,349,366,383,462,464,467-480,484-489,495-502] The most common genetic forms of these two lesions are X linked. An unusual autosomal recessive type of periventricular heterotopia (with microcephaly) is also recognized (see Table 2-22). In *X-linked*

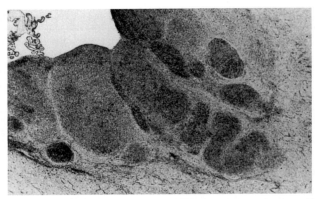

Figure 2-37 Periventricular heterotopic nodular masses. The patient is a newborn (hematoxylin and eosin, ×12.7). *(From Barth PG: Disorders of neuronal migration, Can J Neurol Sci 14:1-16, 1987.)*

periventricular heterotopia, the anatomical defect is caused by a failure of *initiation of migration.*[258] The gene involved is *filamin* which encodes filamin-1, an actin-binding protein expressed at high levels in the ventricular zone of the developing cerebrum and crucial for the initial cytoskeletal rearrangement for initiation of migration. Because of random X inactivation, neurons with the mutant gene active do not initiate migration and remain in the periventricular region, whereas neurons with the normal gene migrate normally. In the autosomal recessive variety of the disorder, related to a mutation of the *ARGEF* gene (ADP ribosylation factor, GEF-2), critical for vesicle trafficking, the mechanism for failure of some neuroblasts to initiate migration is less clear. Importantly, in this disorder, a derangement of neuronal proliferation also occurs, and severe congenital microcephaly results.

In the *double cortex syndrome,* the diffuse laminar heterotopia appears to occur because, as a consequence of random X inactivation, one population of neurons contains only the abnormal gene and thus fails to migrate fully to the cortical plate (see Table 2-22). The characteristic locus of this laminar heterotopia beneath the cerebral cortex is at the site of the critical interface of the intermediate zone and subplate neurons (Fig. 2-38). Presumably the mutated doublecortin is unable to effect the critical interaction between the migrating neurons and the subplate neurons required to penetrate this region and form the cortical plate.[248,252,253,257,258,261,285] As discussed earlier,

TABLE 2-21	Disorders Associated with Neuronal Heterotopias as the Major Manifestation of Migrational Disturbance*

Metabolic disorders: neonatal adrenoleukodystrophy, glutaric aciduria type II, nonketotic hyperglycinemia, Leigh disease, Menkes disease, GM_2-gangliosidosis, Hurler disease, Zellweger syndrome, bifunctional enzyme deficiency, carnitine palmitoyltransferase deficiency
Myotonic dystrophy
Neurocutaneous syndromes: neurofibromatosis, tuberous sclerosis, incontinentia pigmenti, Ito hypomelanosis, linear nevus sebaceus, encephalocraniocutaneous lipomatosis, Ehlers-Danlos syndrome
Multiple congenital anomaly syndromes: Smith-Lemli-Opitz, Potter, de Lange, orofacial-digital, Meckel-Gruber, Coffin-Siris
Chromosomal syndromes: trisomy 18, trisomy 13, deletion 4p, trisomy 21
Fetal toxic exposures: carbon monoxide, isotretinoic acid, ethanol, organic mercurial

*See text for references. This *excludes* disorders commonly associated with prominent gyral abnormalities (i.e., schizencephaly, lissencephaly, pachygyria, polymicrogyria). *Uncommonly*, some of the disorders listed here may also have migrational defects severe enough to have accompanying gyral abnormalities. The genetic disorders summarized in Table 2-22 are not repeated here.

TABLE 2-22 Major Genetic Syndromes with Cerebral Heterotopias*

Type of Heterotopia	Seizures	Major Cognitive Deficits	Mode of Inheritance	Manifestation in Males	Location of Gene	Gene or Gene Product
Periventricular heterotopia	Common	Uncommon	X-linked dominant	Lethal(?)*	Xq28	Filamin 1
Periventricular heterotopia (and microcephaly)	Common	Common	Autosomal recessive	As in females	20q11	*ARGEF*
Double cortex (band or laminar)	Common	Common	X-linked dominant	Lissencephaly	Xq23	Doublecortin

*Occasional male patients exhibit periventricular heterotopia.

hemizygous male infants with the doublecortin defect develop lissencephaly, and the fundamental role of doublecortin involves microtubule dynein motor function.

Focal Cerebral Cortical Dysgenesis (Dysplasia)

With the advent of MRI scanning and removal of cortical anomalies for intractable epilepsy, focal disorders of the final stages of neuronal migration to cerebral cortex have been increasingly recognized. The lesions have been described as focal cerebral cortical *dysgeneses* or *dysplasias*.[252,253,464,503-541] The *anatomical descriptions* have not varied appreciably and consist of aberrations of gyral formation (polymicrogyric or pachygyric in appearance), a cerebral cortical plate without normal lamination, and heterotopic neurons in subcortical white matter. The lesions studied most often in specimens obtained at epilepsy surgery may exhibit impaired lamination with normal appearing neurons or large, dysmorphic (misshapen) neurons. Large cells with immunocytochemical properties of neurons, glia, and multipotent neuroepithelial cells, termed *balloon cells*, may also be present. Those cases with dysmorphic large neurons, with or without the balloon cells, are

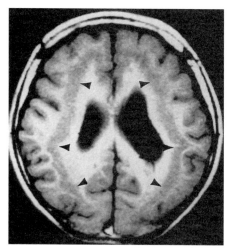

Figure 2-38 Magnetic resonance imaging (MRI) scan, band heterotopia or double cortex syndrome. This T1-weighted MRI scan shows a symmetrical band of heterotopic subcortical gray matter *(arrowheads)* underlying a cerebral cortex with a normal convolutional pattern. *(From Miura K, Watanabe K, Maeda N, et al: Magnetic resonance imaging and positron emission tomography of band heterotopia, Brain Dev 15:288-290, 1993.)*

categorized as cortical dysplasia of Taylor. Because MRI has been the basis of the anatomical diagnosis in most cases, and the finding of a "thick" cortical plate with heterotopic gray matter is the prominent feature, it has not been clear whether all the lesions are related more to focal polymicrogyria than to pachygyria. Indeed, the descriptive term *macrogyria* is sometimes used to describe the MRI appearance. Based on the cytological features, these lesions appear to represent not only disturbances of late neuronal migration but also abnormalities of proliferative and organizational events.

The *clinical syndromes* have been dominated by seizure disorders (Table 2-23) and relate in considerable part to the topography of the lesions. The seizure disorders usually begin after the neonatal period. However, in two large series, neonatal seizures occurred in approximately 35% of cases of Taylor-type focal cortical dysplasia. Notably, among the 19 patients without balloon cells, approximately 60% had neonatal onset, whereas only 15% of the 15 patients with balloon cells exhibited neonatal seizures.[538,541]

Agenesis of the Corpus Callosum, Abnormality of Septum Pellucidum, and Colpocephaly

Agenesis of the corpus callosum is a common accompaniment of the major disorders of neuronal migration, as noted in the previous discussions of the specific disorders. The reasons for the relationship are at least twofold. First, the timing of callosal formation and that of neuronal migration are nearly coincident (see discussion of midline prosencephalic development in Chapter 1). Second, the disturbance of neocortical development caused by the migrational failure is followed by a deficiency in corticocortical fibers destined for the callosum. The first of these reasons may explain the additional frequent accompaniment of neuronal migrational disorder with absence or hypoplasia of the septum pellucidum or persistently wide cavum of the septum pellucidum.

Colpocephaly, the disproportionate enlargement of trigones, occipital horns, and usually temporal horns of the lateral ventricles, also is a frequent accompaniment of neuronal migrational disorders. As discussed previously (see lissencephaly), the enlargement of the trigones and occipital horns stems from failure of development of the splenium of the corpus callosum and the calcarine fissure, and the enlargement of the temporal horns results from failure of inversion of the

TABLE 2-23   Major Clinical Syndromes Associated with Focal Cerebral Cortical Dysplasia*

Site of Dysgenesis	Clinical Syndromes
Frontal, temporal, or parietal	Complex or simple partial seizures, hemiparesis (frontal lesions)
Temporal (hippocampus)	Neonatal (subtle) seizures, later multiple seizures, mental retardation
Left frontotemporal	Developmental dyslexia
Frontal (rolandic)	Focal myoclonus, focal clonic seizures, hemiparesis
Bilateral perisylvian	Facial diplegia, dysarthria-dysphagia, generalized seizures, mental retardation
Occipital	Congenital hemianopia

*See text for references.

hippocampus, normally provoked by full neocortical development.[42,363,542] Disproportionate enlargement of the trigone and occipital horns of the lateral ventricles can be observed in any destructive disorder with particular involvement of periventricular white matter, such as periventricular leukomalacia, other encephaloclastic processes, or any developmental disorder associated with impairment of myelination (see later discussion of myelination).[543-547] Because the ventricular dilation associated with these diverse processes is also often characterized as *colpocephaly*, the term has lost distinctive meaning.

ORGANIZATION

Normal Development

Organizational events occur in a peak time period from approximately the fifth month of gestation to several years after birth. However, these complex processes may continue for many more years in human cerebrum. The major developmental features include the following: (1) establishment and differentiation of the subplate neurons; (2) attainment of proper alignment, orientation, and layering of cortical neurons; (3) elaboration of dendritic and axonal ramifications; (4) establishment of synaptic contacts; (5) cell death and selective elimination of neuronal processes and synapses; and (6) proliferation and differentiation of glia (Table 2-24). These events are of particular importance because they establish the elaborate circuitry that distinguishes the human brain, and they set the stage for the final developmental event, myelination.

Subplate Neurons

The importance of the subplate neurons in cerebral organizational events was defined by an elegant series

TABLE 2-24   Organization

Peak Time Period
5 months' gestation–years postnatal

Major Events
Subplate neurons: establishment and differentiation
Lamination: alignment, orientation, and layering of cortical plate neurons
Neurite outgrowth: dendritic and axonal ramifications
Synaptogenesis
Cell death and selective elimination of neuronal processes and of synapses
Glial proliferation and differentiation

of studies both in experimental animals and human brain.[266,548-565] Cells destined to be subplate neurons are generated in the germinative zones and migrate both radially and tangentially to the primitive marginal zone at approximately 7 weeks of gestation *before* generation and migration of neurons of the cortical plate (Fig. 2-39 and Table 2-25). Initially, these cells are part of the preplate that is split by approximately 10 weeks of gestation by the developing cortical plate into the subplate neurons below and the Cajal-Retzius neurons of the marginal zone above. (The cortical plate neurons give rise to layers II through VI of the cerebral cortex.) The subplate neurons rapidly exhibit morphological differentiation and express a variety of receptors for neurotransmitters (GABA, excitatory amino acids), neuropeptides, and growth factors (nerve growth factor, neuropeptide gamma, somatostatin, calbindin). The subplate neurons elaborate a dendritic arbor with spines, receive synaptic inputs from ascending afferents from thalamus and distant cortical sites, and extend axonal collaterals to overlying cerebral cortex and to other cortical and subcortical sites (thalamus, other cortical regions, corpus callosum).

The *functions of the subplate neurons* now appear to be particularly far-reaching (see Table 2-25).[548-556,559-561,563-565] Thus, they provide a site for synaptic contact for axons ascending from thalamus and other cortical sites, termed *waiting* thalamocortical and corticocortical afferents because their neuronal targets in the cortical plate have not yet arrived or differentiated. These afferents presumably would undergo degeneration if they did not have the subplate neurons as transient targets. Moreover, the subplate neurons have been shown to establish a functional synaptic link between these waiting afferents and their cortical targets. This link could exert a trophic influence on the cortical neuronal targets by the release of neuropeptides or excitatory amino acid neurotransmitter by the subplate axon terminals. A third function appears to be the guidance by subplate axons entering cerebral cortex of the ascending axons to their targets. Indeed, if the subplate neurons are eliminated, thalamocortical afferents destined for the overlying cortex fail to move superiorly into the cortex at the appropriate site and continue to grow aimlessly in the subcortical region. A fourth function of subplate neurons is involvement in cerebral cortical organization; for example, ocular dominance columns in visual cortex fail to develop if underlying subplate neurons are eliminated during development. Related to this role is the importance for subplate neurons in cortical synaptic development and function. A fifth

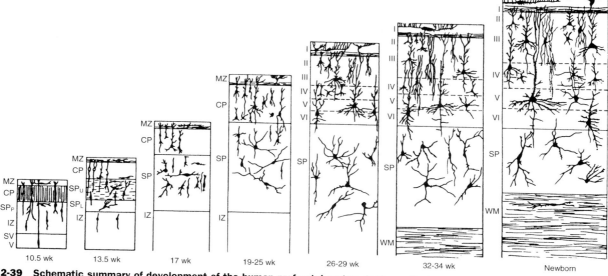

Figure 2-39 Schematic summary of development of the human prefrontal cortex. At the earliest age studied (10.5 weeks), the preplate zone has been split by the early-arriving neurons of the cortical plate into neurons of the marginal zone (MZ) above and of the subplate zone (SP) below. Note the exuberant neuronal development of the subplate zone into the third trimester of gestation. CP, cortical plate; IZ, intermediate zone; SP_L, subplate zone (lower); SP_P, subplate-preplate zone; SP_U; subplate zone (upper); SV, subventricular zone; V, ventricular zone; WM, white matter. *(From Mrzljak L, Uylings HBM, Kostovic I, et al: Prenatal development of neurons in the human prefrontal cortex. I. A qualitative Golgi study, J Comp Neurol 271:355-386, 1988.)*

function appears to be mediated by the descending axon collaterals from the subplate neurons; these collaterals appear to "pioneer" or guide the initial projections from cerebral cortex toward subcortical targets (e.g., thalamus, corpus callosum, and other cortical sites).

Concomitant studies of subplate neurons of developing *human* cerebral cortex provide a crucial link with the experimental studies (see Fig. 2-39; Fig. 2-40).[559,561-563,565-569] The subplate neuron layer in human cortex reaches a peak between approximately 24 and 32 weeks of gestation. At this peak time, the width of the subplate is approximately four times that of the cortical plate. Programmed cell death (apoptosis) of this layer appears to begin generally late in the third trimester, and approximately 90% of subplate neurons have disappeared after approximately the sixth month of postnatal life. Slightly different time courses for peak development and regression of the subplate neurons exist for somatosensory and visual cortices. Clearly, the time periods when the functions of the subplate neurons must be operative in the developing human brain correspond closely to the times of occurrence of a variety of periventricular hemorrhagic and ischemic lesions (see Chapters 9 and 11). If these lesions disrupt the subplate neurons or their axonal collaterals to subcortical or cortical sites, the functions described earlier would be impaired, and the impact on cortical neuronal development and on a variety of crucial projection systems could be enormous. *Indeed, the major portion of the striking increase in cerebral cortical volume in the last trimester of gestation consists of the extensive elaboration of the afferent fibers, previously "waiting" in contact with subplate neurons, as they enter the cerebral cortex.*[559] As noted later, this increase in cerebral cortical volume is blunted by injury to cerebral white matter in the premature infant.

Lamination and Neurite Outgrowth

Attainment of the proper alignment, orientation, and layering of cortical neurons (i.e., lamination) occur as neuronal migration ceases. These events are among

TABLE 2-25	Importance of Subplate Neurons in Development of Cerebral Cortex

Natural History

SPNs are generated and migrate beneath the pial surface as part of the preplate *before* generation and migration of neurons of the cortical plate.

Early-arriving cortical plate neurons split the preplate into the overlying marginal zone and the subplate.

SPNs rapidly exhibit morphological differentiation and transiently express a variety of receptors for neurotransmitters and growth factors.

SPNs elaborate a dendritic tree, receive synaptic inputs, and extend axonal projections to cortical and subcortical sites.

The zone of SPNs is most prominent between approximately 22 and 34 weeks of gestation.

Approximately 90% of SPNs undergo programmed cell death postnatally.

Functions

Site of synaptic contact for "waiting" thalamocortical and corticocortical afferents before formation of cortical plate

Functional link between "waiting" afferents and cortical targets

Axonal guidance into cerebral cortex for ascending afferents

Involvement in cerebral cortical organization and synaptic development

"Pioneering" axonal guidance for projections from cortex to subcortical targets

SPN, subplate neuron.

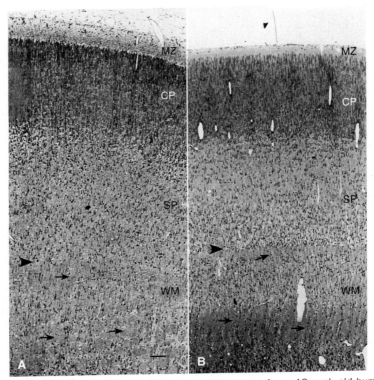

Figure 2-40 **Cytoarchitectonics of the subplate zone in the visual area.** Shown are, **A**, an 18-week old human and, **B**, a E78 monkey fetus displayed in plastic sections 1 μm thick. The subplate zone (SP) is characterized by low cell density and presence of mature neurons. The border between the subplate zone and the white matter (WM) is relatively sharp because of the presence of well-delineated fiber bundles *(arrows)* in the white matter. External limit of fibers is marked by the *arrowhead.* Note remarkable similarities between the lamination pattern and the cortical plate (CP)–subplate thickness ratio in man and monkey. The bar (=100 μm) applies to both illustrations. MZ, marginal zone. *(From Kostovic I, Rakic P: Developmental history of the transient subplate zone in the visual and somatosensory cortex of the macaque monkey and human brain,* J Comp Neurol *297:441-454, 1990.)*

the earliest in cortical organization.[5,570-572] Neurite outgrowth (i.e., the elaboration of dendritic and axonal ramifications) next becomes the dominant developmental activity in the cerebral cortex.

The most significant early studies of neurite outgrowth in human cerebral cortex were made in 1939 by Conel,[573] whose Golgi-Cox preparations of cerebral cortex from birth to 2 years of age demonstrated progressive enrichment of the dendritic and axonal plexus, with much smaller increases in size and no proportionate increases in number of individual neurons. The remarkable elaboration of dendritic branching that results can be seen in the cerebrum of a normal child, shown in Figure 2-41. The studies of Mrzljak and coworkers[566] showed similar events in frontal cortex before birth (see Fig. 2-39). Accompanying the elaboration of dendritic and axonal ramifications are the appearance of synaptic elements, the development of neurofibrils, and an increase in size of endoplasmic reticulum within the cytoplasm of cells. The biochemical correlates of these changes are increasing cerebral content of RNA and protein relative to DNA. Immunocytochemical studies document parallel expression of a variety of neurotrophins, neurotransmitters (NMDA, alpha-amino-3-hydroxy-5-methyl-4-isoxazolepropionic acid [AMPA]/kainate, GABA, and glycine receptors), surface glycoconjugates, and cytoskeletal components.[574-587] The maturational changes occur relatively rapidly in the hippocampus, whereas

they occur over a more protracted period in the supralimbic region; the latter, of course, is of great significance, because it is the locus of the major association areas. Dendritic development in the human occurs earlier in thalamus and brain stem than in cerebral cortical regions.[588,589] These findings were amplified by studies by Purpura, Huttenlocher, Marin-Padilla, Rakic, and other investigators, who used electron microscopic and immunocytochemical methods as well as Golgi techniques.[566,569,582-586,590-601]

One study of developing human brain demonstrated the strikingly active axonal development in the cerebrum over the last trimester of gestation and in the early postnatal period (Fig. 2-42).[586] Thus, immunostaining with GAP-43, a protein expressed on *growing* axons, shows exuberant expression in the cerebral white matter to approximately the subplate region at 20 weeks, to the cortical plate at 27 weeks, within the cortex at 37 weeks, and into the first year of life. This differential pattern may reflect, at 20 weeks, growth of axons from thalamus to subplate neurons, and at 27 weeks, from subplate neurons to cerebral cortex. At 37 weeks, the increase in cerebral cortical expression of GAP-43 may reflect the increase in cortical penetration of thalamic ascending fibers no longer waiting at the subplate layer, in corticocortical fibers, and in descending cortical fibers, initially pioneered by subplate axons (see earlier). These findings are consistent with more recent studies with different techniques by

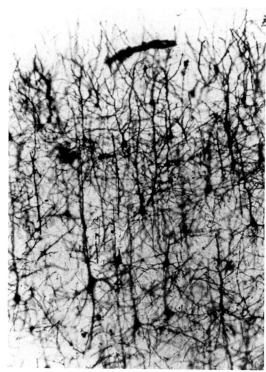

Figure 2-41   Golgi preparation (×80) of the middle frontal gyrus from a 6-year-old child without known neurological disease. Note the abundant and complex horizontal and tangential dendritic branches. *(From Buchwald NA, Brazier MAB, editors:* Brain Mechanisms in Mental Retardation, *New York: 1975, Academic Press.)*

Kostovic and co-workers.[565] Although more data are needed on these issues, it is clear that the *last trimester of human gestation is a period of rapid axonal development.*

The relationship between neurite outgrowth in cortex and development of functional capacity can be illustrated in human visual cortex during the third trimester (Fig. 2-43). Most impressive are the appearance and elaboration of basilar dendrites and the tangential spread of apical dendrites. This dendritic development is accompanied by the appearance of dendritic spines, that is, sites of synaptic contact (see the discussion of synaptic development). These anatomical expressions of differentiation are paralleled by the neurophysiological expression of maturation of the visual evoked potential (see Fig. 2-43). Such detailed relationships between dendritic structural development and specific details of neurophysiological development have been studied in depth in developing animals.[602]

The progress of dendritic differentiation depends on the establishment of afferent input and presumably synaptic activity.[294,566,574,580,581,590,603-608] In certain developing neural systems, the importance of receiving and making proper connections has been emphasized as highly critical for further organization. At least part of the influence of these connections is mediated by the functional activity generated through them (see the earlier discussion of subplate neurons).[609-612] This role of functional activity has implications for the effects of a variety of environmental stimuli on the postnatal progress of organizational development.[574,580] Neuronal activity initiates its effects on dendritic development by inducing calcium influx, both through activation of glutamate receptors, principally the NMDA receptor, but likely also GluR2-deficient AMPA receptors (see Chapter 6), and by opening of voltage-dependent calcium channels.[606,607] The calcium-mediated effects include both a direct impact on the actin and microtubular components of the cytoskeleton and on several adhesion molecules and major indirect effects by activating multiple signaling pathways that target nuclear transcription factors and thereby many genes involved in dendritic development. Studies of developing human cerebral cortex show transient exuberant expression of calcium-permeable glutamate receptors in cortical neurons during this perinatal period.[613,614]

A striking increase in cerebral cortical volume accompanies these developmental changes in cortical neurons. That this phenomenon is particularly rapid in the human infant from approximately 28 to 40 weeks after conception has been shown by quantitative MRI measurements of cortical gray matter volumes.[615] Thus, a fourfold increase in cerebral cortical gray matter volume could be documented (Fig. 2-44). The changes in cortical gyral development and cortical surface area that accompany and presumably are caused by the increase in cortical volume can be seen by MRI (Fig. 2-45).[616] Advanced diffusion-based MRI imaging known as *tractography* provides further insight into the changes in fiber tract development in the living premature infant.[617]

Synaptic Development

Synaptic formation differs appreciably among regions in the human brain. The number of dendritic spines, the sites of synaptic contacts, in the medullary reticular formation reaches a peak at 34 to 36 weeks of gestation and declines rapidly after birth (see the later discussion of disorders of organizational events).[618] In the cerebrum, synapses are observed initially on neurons of the subplate and of the marginal zone (i.e., neurons of the primitive preplate). For example, in the hippocampus, synapses in these regions are abundant as early as 15 and 16.5 weeks of gestation (Table 2-26).[619] With Golgi preparations, Purpura and co-workers[595-598,620] defined the subsequent progression of dendritic spine development in the human cortex from the fifth month of gestation (Fig. 2-46). Initially, dendrites appear as thick processes with only a few fine spicules. As development progresses, a great number and variety of dendritic spines appear. In the visual cortex, synaptogenesis is fastest between 2 and 4 months after term, a time also critical for the development of function in the visual cortex, and maximal synaptic density is attained at 8 months (Fig. 2-47).[598,620] Synapse elimination then begins, and by age 11 months, approximately 40% of synapses have been lost. In the frontal cortex, the time course of synaptic formation and of elimination differs somewhat from that in the visual cortex; maximal synaptic density is reached at approximately 15 to 24 months, and

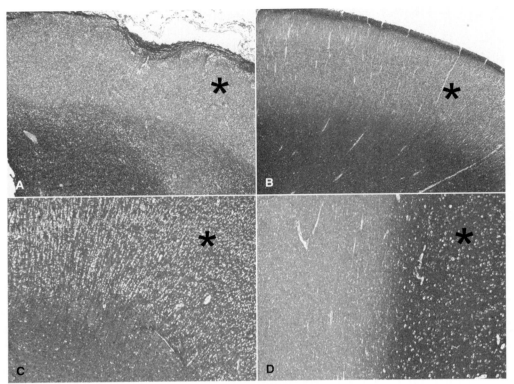

Figure 2-42 **GAP-43 expression in developing human parietal white matter and cortex.** The cortex is indicated by an asterisk. **A**, Note, at 20 postconceptional (PC) weeks, evidence for strong expression in the subcortical white matter to a region below the cortical plate, possibly the concentration of subplate neurons. **B**, At 27 PC weeks, the expression begins to enter the cerebral cortex. **C**, By 37 PC weeks, diffuse expression in cortex and decreased expression in white matter are apparent. **D**, At 144 PC weeks (i.e., ≈2 years of age), expression is prominent in cortex but not in white matter (sections (40; bars = 200 μm). See text for interpretations. *(From Haynes RL, Borenstein NS, DeSilva TM, Folkerth RD, et al: Axonal development in the cerebral white matter of the human fetus and infant,* J Comp Neurol *484:156-167, 2005.)*

synapse elimination, although reaching the same loss of 40%, is more gradual.[620,621] In the prefrontal cortex, synapse elimination extends into midadolescence.[621] Elegant studies in the monkey exhibit more uniformity in the temporal features of synaptogenesis among cortical regions, but the basic principles are formation of earliest synapses in the marginal and subplate zones, an increase in synapses in cortical plate to a peak in excess of the adult number, and a subsequent period of synaptic elimination.[622-625]

The factors that stimulate synaptic formation and development in developing brain initially include activity-independent events (i.e., molecular mechanisms involved in targeting), followed by activity-dependent events occurring after the development of receptors on target neurons and the generation of electrical activity (see the previous discussion on neurite outgrowth).[574,580,603,626-629] Many molecules and signaling pathways are involved in dendritic spine development and remodeling. The two principal themes are modulation of the following: (1) ion channels, especially calcium-permeable channels, by neurotransmitters, especially glutamate; and (2) cell surface receptors by a variety of ligands. The intracellular events lead ultimately to effects on actin-binding proteins and the actin cytoskeleton, with resulting changes in spine shape, size, and motility.[629] The importance of synaptogenesis and synapse elimination in the *plasticity* of the developing nervous system and in the potential

effect of experiential factors on developing neural function, including cognitive function, could be enormous.

Cell Death and Selective Elimination of Neuronal Processes and Synapses

Cell death and selective elimination of neuronal processes and synapses, or "regressive events" in brain development, are now recognized to be highly critical (see Table 2-24).[572,598,630-644] Results of studies in a variety of developing neuronal systems showed that after formation of neuronal collections by the "progressive" processes of proliferation and migration, *cell death* occurs.[572,634,638-645] Although variable in degree among neuronal regions, typically about half of the neurons in a given collection die before final maturation. This process of cell death is initiated and sustained by the expression of specific genes and their transcription products that actively kill the neuron.[634,638,641,643] Critical in the final phases of the sequence to cell death is the activation of a family of cysteine proteases, known as *caspases*.[643] The term *programmed cell death* has been used to emphasize that this is an active developmental process, although more commonly the term *apoptosis*, a Greek-rooted word referring to the naturally occurring seasonal loss or falling of flowers, is used to refer to this developmentally determined cell death.[572,634,638,639,641-644]

The factors that activate this death system appear to relate to competition of neurons for limited amounts of

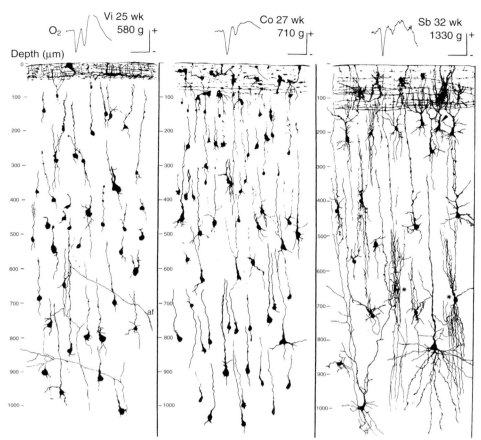

Figure 2-43 **Camera lucida composite drawings of neurons in the visual (calcarine) cortex of human infants of indicated gestational ages.** Note the appearance and elaboration of basilar dendrites and the tangential spread of apical dendrites, as well as the accompanying maturation of the visual evoked response *(top). (Courtesy of Dr. Dominick Purpura.)*

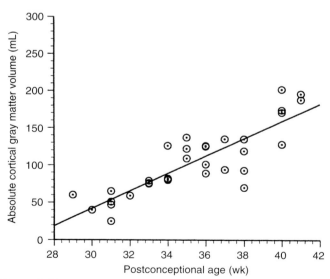

Figure 2-44 **Cerebral cortical gray matter volume as a function of postconceptional age.** Quantitative volumetric magnetic resonance imaging determinations of absolute cerebral cortical gray matter volume as a function of postconceptional age in a series (*n*=35) of preterm and full-term infants. *(From Huppi PS, Warfield S, Kikinis R, et al: Quantitative magnetic resonance imaging of brain development in premature and mature newborns,* Ann Neurol *43:224-235, 1998.)*

trophic factors, generated by the target, afferent input, or associated glia. This loss of neurons appears to serve two major functions in development: quantitative adjustments (numerical matching) of interconnecting populations of neurons and elimination of projections that are aberrant or otherwise incorrect (refinement of synaptic connections or error correction).[633,634,638,640,641,646] Failure of cell death or overactivation of this process clearly could have major deleterious implications for brain development and subsequent function.

Neural organization is refined further by a second regressive event, *selective elimination of neuronal processes and synapses.* This event primarily causes the removal of terminal axonal branches and their synapses, although even larger-scale elimination of a total pathway also occurs. Vivid demonstrations of synapse elimination are apparent in the developing brain stem and cortex of the human infant (see earlier). The determinants of selective elimination of neuronal processes and synapses are similar to those described for cell death. Activation of the NMDA type of glutamate receptor appears to be an important step in synapse elimination during development.[637] An additional crucial role of the specific region of cerebral cortex in determining the pattern of selective elimination of its terminal axons was shown by studies with cortical transplants in developing rats.[647] Thus, cortical neurons transplanted

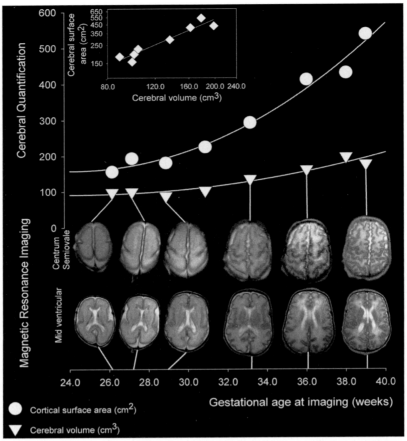

Figure 2-45 Measurements of cortical surface area and volume by advanced magnetic resonance imaging (MRI) *(upper)* and conventional MRI images of gyral development *(lower)* during the last 14 weeks of gestation. Data were derived from study of 113 preterm infants. *(From Kapellou O, Counsell SJ, Kennea NL, Dvet L, et al: Abnormal cortical development after premature birth shown by altered allometric scaling of brain growth, PLoS Med 3:e265, 2006.)*

to another region of cortex (as explants) eliminated their distal axon collaterals in the same way as did neurons of the host cortical region (into which they were transplanted), rather than in the way neurons of the donor region eliminated their distal collaterals.

The observations that cell death and elimination of neuronal processes and synapses occur during the organizational period of development have implications for the frequent demonstration that the *plasticity* of developing brain decreases as this period is completed.[630,634,638,639,648-657] It is likely that the regressive events described in this section are modified when the brain is injured and that neuronal processes and synapses destined for elimination can be retained if needed to preserve function. In addition, new projections may develop in response to injury during the

period in which the brain has the capacity to carry out organizational events. In favor of one or both of these predictions is the demonstration in both human infants and experimental models that, after neonatal cerebral lesions, ipsilateral corticospinal tract projections can be demonstrated and presumably can ameliorate the functional deficit.[652-654,658-671] The demonstration of an ipsilateral corticospinal projection until early childhood in humans suggests that retention of a normally occurring ipsilateral corticospinal tract, which otherwise is eliminated during development, is the crucial event in this form of plasticity.[654,662,672,673] The possible additional role of assumption of motor functions by ipsilateral cerebrum adjacent to the lesion is suggested by other studies.[662,665,674]

Glial Proliferation and Differentiation

Astrocytes, oligodendrocytes, and microglia are the major glial cells of the CNS. Glial proliferation and differentiation are of major importance in developing brain; glial cells clearly outnumber neurons in the CNS. In fact, in human cerebral cortex, glial cells outnumber neurons by approximately 1.25 to 1 and are almost the exclusive cell type in white matter.[675]

Astrocytic and oligodendrocytic lineage, proliferation, and differentiation have been the topics of intense

TABLE 2-26	**Synaptic Formation and Elimination in Human Cerebral Cortex**

First synapses involve the subplate neurons (e.g., 15–16-week fetal hippocampus).
Synaptogenesis in the cortical plate is most active postnatally.
Approximately 40% of synapses are eliminated subsequently.

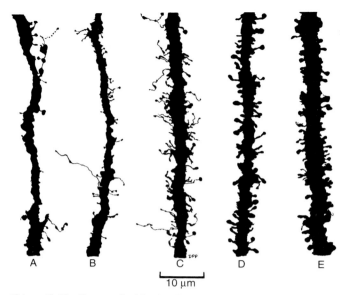

Figure 2-46 Camera lucida drawings of proximal apical dendritic segments of motor cortex pyramidal neurons during development. **A**, 18-week-old fetus; **B**, 26-week-old fetus; **C**, 33-week-old preterm infant; **D**, 6-month-old infant; **E**, 7-year-old child. The early phase of dendritic spine differentiation in proximal apical segments is associated with the development of long, thin spines and relatively few stubby and mushroom-shaped spines. The latter two types are prominent in the postnatal period and early childhood. *(Courtesy of Dr. Dominick Purpura.)*

TABLE 2-27	Glial Lineage and Differentiation in Forebrain

Astrocytes and Oligodendrocytes
Astrocytes are generated primarily *before* oligodendrocytes.
Astrocytic and oligodendroglial progenitors are principally subventricular cells and radial glia.
Proliferation of these progenitors occurs at their sites of origin and locally (during and after migration).

Microglia
Microglia originate from bone marrow-derived monocytes.
Sites of entry from the circulation include the ventricular and subventricular zones.
Migration proceeds through the cerebral white matter during middle to late gestation and then to cortex near term.

investigation in experimental systems in recent years,[237,676-711] and initial data also are emerging from studies of human brain.[577,676,700,712-725] The observations are not entirely consistent, but my best attempt at a synthesis is shown in Table 2-27. In general, astrocytes are generated primarily before oligodendrocytes. The progenitors of both astrocytes and oligodendrocytes initially are cells of the subventricular

zone and probably radial glia (see the earlier discussion of proliferation). Radial glial progenitors may give rise to a glial restricted progenitor that then generates astrocytes or oligodendrocytes. Proliferation of glia, unlike that of neurons, also may occur locally, during and after migration.

Astrocytes play a variety of complex nutritive and supportive roles in relation to neuronal homeostasis and in the reaction to metabolic and structural insults. For example, astrocytes avidly take up glutamate and convert it to glutamine by the action of the astrocyte-specific enzyme glutamine synthetase; this removal of glutamate from the extracellular space is crucial for protection against excitotoxic injury with ischemia, seizures, or hypoglycemia (see Chapters 5, 6, 8, and 12). Other functions include a wide variety of roles in inflammation, immune responses, production of trophic and neuroprotective factors (e.g., antioxidants), and tissue remodeling after injury.[572]

Oligodendroglial proliferation and differentiation are crucial for myelination and thus are discussed later in relation to that major developmental event. *Microglia* comprise the resident and immune cells of the brain and originate principally if not entirely from bone marrow–derived monocytes.[572] These cells enter the CNS (especially brain stem and spinal cord) in the first trimester, and in the cerebrum microglia become apparent in the second trimester within the marginal zone, the boundary of the cortical plate and subplate, and the ventricular-subventricular zones (see Table 2-27).[726-732a] A study of developing human cerebrum from 20 weeks of gestation made the striking observation that microglial cells during the second and third trimesters were primarily in the active (ameboid morphology) state and could be seen to migrate progressively from ventricular-subventricular zones to the cerebral white matter (20 to 35 weeks) and then to the cerebral cortex.[733] Migration may occur along white matter tracts, radially oriented vasculature, and residual radial glial cells.[729,733] Although the prevailing notion is that these cells *enter* the ventricular-subventricular zones through the circulation, whether any of these cells may *originate* in the ventricular-subventricular zones is unresolved. *The critical point is that the cerebral white matter is heavily populated with activated microglia during a period when developmental events are active and a*

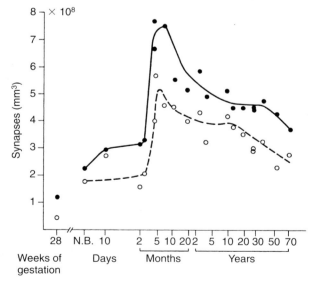

Figure 2-47 Synaptic density in layer I and layer II/III of the striate cortex. *Open circles* represent layer I; *closed circles* represent layer II/III. Note the striking increase in the first postnatal year and the subsequent decline. *(From Huttenlocher PR, de Courten C: The development of synapses in striate cortex of man, Hum Neurobiol 6:1-9, 1987.)*

variety of insults can lead to white matter injury (see Chapters 6 and 8).

Microglial cells play key roles during brain development, involving vascularization,[729] apoptosis,[644] axonal development,[586] and later myelination.[734] In addition to these key beneficial roles, these cells, when activated by such insults as hypoxia-ischemia or infection-inflammation, can release such substances as cytokines and reactive oxygen and nitrogen species, which could injure, as "innocent bystanders," differentiating oligodendrocytes of the premature infant or neurons of the term infant (see Chapter 6).

DISORDERS

The normative data just reviewed define a critical period in brain development that includes the *perinatal period*. Unfortunately, little is known about disorders of this phase of neural maturation. This ignorance is caused primarily by the inadequacy of standard neuropathological techniques to evaluate the complex circuitry and synaptic connections of human brain. Earlier, only a few studies using appropriate techniques, such as the Golgi method for staining neuronal processes, were available, and it was often not clear whether the changes observed were primary or secondary, or specific or nonspecific. Although the latter uncertainties often persist, in recent years the advent of advanced immunocytochemical methodologies, the delineation of molecular genetic defects, and the use of genetically manipulated animals provided new insights into the identity and the basis of organizational disorders. Moreover, MRI techniques (e.g., quantitative volumetric MRI, diffusion tensor MRI, and functional MRI) are clarifying these issues in the living infant (see later discussions and Chapter 4). In Table 2-28, disorders are classified according to whether deficits in organizational events appear to be the *most significant*

TABLE 2-28 **Disorders of Organization**

Primary Disturbance
Mental retardation (idiopathic), with or without seizures
Fragile X syndrome
Rett syndrome
Infantile autism
Down syndrome
Angelman syndrome
Duchenne muscular dystrophy
Other rare disorders

Potential Disturbance
Premature infants
  Periventricular leukomalacia
  Postnatal dexamethasone
  Hypothyroxinemia
  Ventilator dependence
Nutrition and breast-feeding: long-chain polyunsaturated
  fatty acids
Experiential effects
Other perinatal and postnatal insults

Associated Disturbance
Diverse (see text)

---

neuropathological lesion (primary disturbance), a likely but not entirely proven lesion (*potential disturbance*), or an *associated lesion (associated disturbance)*.

Primary Disturbance

Mental Retardation with or without Seizures. Several studies in which the Golgi technique was used showed abnormalities of development of dendritic branching and spines in children with idiopathic mental retardation with or without seizures.[594,595,735-739] The children in these studies had no anatomical evidence for destructive disease, metabolic disorder, or other developmental aberration (see Table 2-28). Huttenlocher,[594,738] using the Golgi technique and quantitative estimation of dendritic branching, initially studied 11 brains from individuals with severe mental retardation of unknown cause. In six of these brains, severe defects in the number, length, and spatial arrangement of dendritic branching and in dendritic spines, the sites of synaptic contacts, were demonstrated. The relative sparsity of horizontal and tangential dendritic branches is shown clearly in Figure 2-48. Four of the six affected children with marked dendritic abnormalities had, in addition to severe mental retardation, histories of infantile myoclonic seizures and hypsarrhythmic EEGs.[594,738,739] Moreover, Purpura[595,735] demonstrated, in a cerebral biopsy specimen of a severely retarded infant, marked abnormalities of dendritic spines, characterized principally by a marked

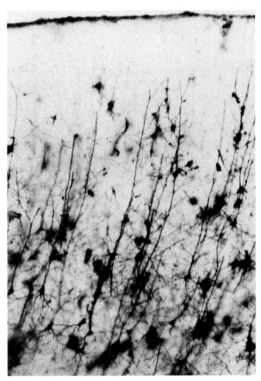

Figure 2-48 **Golgi preparation (×80) of the middle frontal gyrus from a 10-year-old child with severe mental retardation of unknown origin.** Note the relative sparsity of horizontal and tangential dendritic branches (compare with Fig. 2-41). *(From Buchwald NA, Brazier MAB, editors:* Brain Mechanisms in Mental Retardation, *New York: 1975, Academic Press.)*

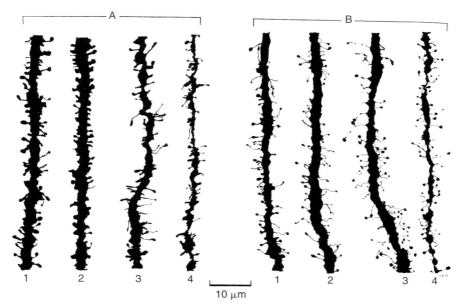

Figure 2-49 Camera lucida drawings of dendritic segments of motor cortex neurons, rapid Golgi preparations, from a normal infant and a mentally retarded infant. **A,** From a normal 6-month-old infant: 1 and 2, proximal apical dendritic segments with a predominance of stubby and mushroom-shaped spines; 3 and 4, distal apical dendritic segment and basilar dendritic segment with many more thin spines. **B,** From a 10-month-old infant with mental retardation of unknown origin: 1, 2, 3, proximal apical and, 4, basilar dendritic segments. Note the presence in the proximal segments (1, 2, 3) of many long, thin spines, comparable to the appearance of the cortex in normal preterm infants (see Fig. 2-39). *(Courtesy of Dr. Dominick Purpura.)*

reduction in short, thick-necked spines (Fig. 2-49). This finding was the only detectable defect in the biopsy specimen and after extensive clinical and laboratory studies yielded negative results.

Insight into a major mechanism in the production of such defects was provided first by the work of Purpura and co-workers.[736,737] Golgi studies of cerebral cortex from five children with mental retardation and seizures (two in one family) demonstrated striking dendritic abnormalities, the most prominent of which was the formation of distinct varicosities along the dendritic

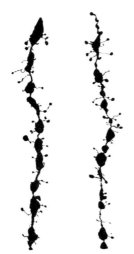

Figure 2-50 Camera lucida drawings of distal dendritic segments from an infant with mental retardation and seizures. Note the irregular varicosities of the dendritic segments. *(From Purpura DP, Bodick N, Suzuki K, et al: Microtubule disarray in cortical dendrites and neurobehavioral failure. I. Golgi and electron microscopic studies, Brain Res 281:287-297, 1982.)*

processes (Fig. 2-50). Ultrastructural studies showed an aberration of microtubules with loss of the usual parallel array of these structures. These findings indicated that a *disturbance of cytoskeletal structures,* so critical for maintenance of cell shape and for outgrowth of dendrites and axons, can cause a severe dendritic abnormality and marked neurological disturbance.[737]

More recent work has begun to delineate the molecular bases for at least some of these cases.[629] X-linked genes have been shown to be particularly important, perhaps accounting in part for the higher incidence of mental retardation in male than in female patients.[740,741] The greatest insight into X-linked mental retardation disorders involves fragile X syndrome and Rett syndrome (discussed subsequently). However, many other genes have been identified. Prominent among these are four X-linked genes found mutated in families with mental retardation that encode proteins known as Rho guanine nucleotide exchange factor 6 (ARHGEF6), oligophrenin-1, p21-activated kinase, and guanine dissociation inhibitor 1.[741,742] These proteins are involved in signaling pathways that regulate the actin cytoskeleton, so critical for neurite outgrowth, dendritic spine formation and morphology, and neurotransmitter release. This rapidly evolving field may lead to insights into potential therapies.

Rett Syndrome. Rett syndrome, a remarkable disorder observed in full form only in female patients, constitutes one of the most common causes of mental retardation in girls and women.[743,744] The disorder is characterized clinically by onset of deceleration of rate of head growth in the first months of life, loss of purposeful hand movement near the end of the first year, and development of stereotypical hand movements, autism, ataxia, microcephaly, seizures, and mental retardation before the age of 5 years.[745] The course is progressive until early childhood, when it becomes essentially static. The neuropathology consists of a small brain with an apparent disturbance of neuronal development, characterized by dendritic spine abnormalities (decreased spine density, simplified branching) and small, densely packed neurons.[746-748] Disturbed synaptogenesis has been identified.[749,750] The gene involved encodes an X-linked methyl-CpG-binding protein 2 (MeCP2) that selectively binds CpG dinucleotides and mediates transcriptional repression.[744,750-752] The specific genes apparently not repressed in Rett syndrome and causing the neuropathological features remain to be determined. Initial data indicate a critical role of MeCP2 in regulation of activity-dependent dendritic growth and synaptic maturation.[753] The disorder in its full form occurs only in female patients because of the predilection for the responsible mutations to occur in the paternal germline; thus, male children receive the paternal Y chromosome.[752] (A rare male disorder secondary to MeCP2 defects is described in Chapter 16.)

Infantile Autism. Infantile autism is a dramatic syndrome characterized by deficits in language and cognitive spheres and by behavioral abnormalities, particularly involving social interactions. Multiple causes are recognized, and indeed several of the organizational disorders delineated in this section cause pronounced autistic phenomena (e.g., fragile X syndrome, Rett syndrome). The neuropathology in infantile autism is characterized by microscopic neuronal abnormalities consistent with an organizational defect. Thus, the regions particularly affected are the frontal cerebral cortex (impaired columnar structure), limbic cortex (small neurons, increased density), cerebellum (reduced numbers of Purkinje cells), and cerebellar relay nuclei, such as the inferior olive (enlarged neurons in young patients and small neurons in adult patients).[754-757a] Additionally, evidence indicates brain overgrowth of postnatal onset that is most apparent in the first 2 years of life and is accompanied by relative macrocephaly.[758-761] The basis of the latter is unclear, although the possibility of enhanced, albeit anomalous axonal growth has been raised.[761] Overall, available data suggest a complex disturbance of principally neuronal organizational events.

Down Syndrome. Striking abnormalities of dendritic and axonal development have been described in infants with Down syndrome.[595,629,741,762-770] Significant aberrations of other aspects of brain development previously have not been consistently described in Down syndrome, and thus these well-defined organizational defects may represent the essential neuropathology of this common cause of mental retardation.

The abnormalities in Down syndrome are alterations in cortical lamination, reduced dendritic branching, diminished dendritic spines and synapses, giant spines, and abnormal spine shape.[595,741,762,764-770] Abnormalities are not apparent before 22 weeks of gestation (i.e., before the rapid progression of organizational events). In the first months of postnatal life, an excess in dendritic branching precedes the consistent decrease observed after approximately 6 months of age. This sequence of excessive initial branching followed by deficits is similar to that seen in certain animal models of impaired dendritic development. Notably, neurons of layers II and IV, which use GABA as a neurotransmitter, are deficient in number, and this disturbance would be expected to result in decreased inhibitory activity (i.e., hyperexcitability) in the cerebral cortex in Down syndrome. Two additional factors favor hyperexcitability in the cortex in Down syndrome: the specific nature of the disturbances of ion channels and the shape of dendrite spines. Together with decreased inhibitory activity, these three factors may explain the 5% to 10% incidence of seizures in these patients.[771,772] The demonstration of a defect in antioxidant capacity in Down syndrome neurons, with resulting free radical–mediated cell death, provides another important possible cause for the neuronal disturbance in Down syndrome.[773]

Fragile X Syndrome. Fragile X syndrome is the most common form of inherited mental retardation and is a disorder of male patients.[774-778a] The diagnosis was formerly based on the cytogenetic finding of a fragile site on the X chromosome, which is induced when cells are grown in medium with low folic acid and thymidine. Highly accurate direct DNA diagnostic testing is now widely available for identification of the fragile X syndrome.[777] The molecular defect involves the presence of a large amplification of a trinucleotide repeat sequence in the fragile X gene (a similar genetic amplification involves the abnormal gene in myotonic dystrophy; see Chapter 19). The neuropathology is notable for abnormal dendritic spine morphology (Fig. 2-51) by Golgi analysis of neocortical neurons.[741,776,778-780] The principal findings are an increase in long dendritic spines, fewer short spines, more immature-appearing spines, and fewer mature-appearing spines. The brain otherwise has no overt abnormalities. That the dendritic abnormality is related to the genetic defect is supported by the finding of similarly abnormal dendritic spines in fragile X gene *(FMR1)* knockout mice.[778a,781-783] Thus, these observations may indicate that the crucial morphological disturbance in this common form of mental retardation involves cortical dendritic development. The mechanism of this disturbed development appears to relate to the obligatory role played by the fragile X mental retardation protein (FMRP) in controlling cytoskeletal organization during neuronal development.[778a,784]

Angelman Syndrome. Angelman syndrome, or *happy puppet syndrome*, is identified usually after the first 6 months of life, when the prominent findings are developmental delay, ataxia, seizures, hypotonia, paroxysms of laughter, postnatally developing microbrachycephaly, and a characteristic facial appearance with macrostomia and prognathia.[785-797] The disorder is associated with a microdeletion of chromosome 15q11-13 (identifiable in ≈70% of cases), which is

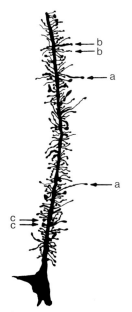

Figure 2-51 Composite camera lucida drawing of Golgi-stained, neocortical, apical dendrite in patients with fragile X syndrome. Note the long, tortuous spines with prominent terminal heads (a) and irregular dilations (b) admixed with an apparent decrease of normal short, stubby spines (c). *(From Hinton VJ, Brown WT, Wisniewski K, Rudelli RD: Analysis of neocortex in three males with the fragile X syndrome,* Am J Med Genet *41:289-294, 1991.)*

the same site as the chromosomal defect in Prader-Willi syndrome. The source of the abnormal chromosome in Angelman syndrome is the mother, and in the Prader-Willi syndrome, it is the father. The critical gene affected in Angelman syndrome appears to be *UBE3A*, the product of which functions in protein ubiquitination; the latter targets proteins for proteolysis and is crucial in brain development.[798,799] This gene is imprinted in brain; only the maternal copy normally is expressed.[799] A Golgi analysis of an affected woman showed a prominent decrease in dendritic arborization of pyramidal neurons in layers III and V and a significant decrease in the numbers of dendritic spines in apical layer III dendrites and basal layer V dendrites.[800] No other definite neuropathological abnormalities were present in the cerebrum; thus, the morphological substrate for the mental retardation and, perhaps, seizures in this disorder may involve a defect in dendritic development. A second case showed an irregular distribution of cortical neurons of layer III, but Golgi analysis was not performed.[801] More data are needed.

Duchenne Muscular Dystrophy. A consistent feature of Duchenne muscular dystrophy is mild impairment of intellect. The neuropathological substrate for this disturbance is unclear. In careful studies of more than 30 patients by conventional neuropathology,[802,803] no abnormality was recognized. However, Golgi study of cortical neurons in three patients revealed reduced length and branching of apical and basal dendrites of pyramidal neurons.[803] This observation suggests that abnormal dendritic development and arborization may underlie the intellectual abnormality in this

disease. The findings may be explainable by the demonstration that the absent protein in this disorder, dystrophin, is present normally not only in muscle but also in neurons.[804,805] Because dystrophin is associated with the cytoskeletal network, which is crucial for dendritic outgrowth, the abnormalities defined by Golgi analysis may be related directly to the absence of dystrophin in neurons. Dystrophin has been shown to be absent in neurons in Duchenne muscular dystrophy,[806] and initial data suggest that the absence of the brain isoforms of the gene are correlated with the severity of cerebral dysfunction.[807]

Other Disorders. Disorders that initial data suggest may be related to a primary disturbance of organizational events were the topic of two reports. Lyon and co-workers[808] described three infants, including two sisters, with a severe congenital encephalopathy manifested by an absent or minimal response to sensory stimuli and profound weakness and hypotonia. At autopsy, the predominant finding was a marked deficiency of cerebral axons with an associated marked decrease in size of corpus callosum and cerebral white matter. Multiple axonal swellings were present in the remaining axons. These authors postulated a primary disorder of axonal development and suggested that "the anomaly may be due to extension of the normal phenomenon of axonal elimination, related to a primary defect of the cytoskeleton." Disorders with somewhat similar findings have been reported.[809,810] More data are clearly needed.

Roessmann and co-workers described two infants with impaired motor development, with involvement of both bulbar and peripheral muscles and accompanying spasticity from the *first days of life*.[811] The most prominent finding at postmortem examination was the absence of corticospinal tract fibers below the level of the internal capsule. The possibility exists that absent or disturbed signals from the targets of these axons during development result in failure of innervation and, as a consequence, secondary axonal elimination. A similar phenomenon may underlie the absence of pyramidal tracts in X-linked aqueductal stenosis, the genetic disorder in which this finding has been recorded most consistently.[812]

Potential Disturbance

A growing body of data suggests that organizational events may be altered by a variety of common perinatal and postnatal events. Because morphological studies have been few, the possibility of an organizational disturbance currently can be regarded as potential, albeit likely.

Premature Infants. Premature infants with cerebral white matter injury (i.e., *periventricular leukomalacia*), later exhibit diminished volume of cerebral cortex, a finding made by advanced volumetric MRI and suggesting a disturbance in cerebral cortical development (see Chapter 8).[813] The cerebral cortical disturbance is also accompanied by diminished volume of thalamus and basal ganglia. The cortical disturbance does not

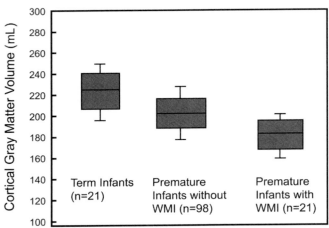

Figure 2-52 Cerebral cortical gray matter volume. Cerebral cortical gray matter volume, determined by three-dimensional volumetric magnetic resonance imaging at term age, in 21 term infants, 98 premature infants without moderate to severe white matter injury (WMI), and 21 premature infants with moderate to severe WMI (nearly exclusively noncystic WMI). See text for details. *(Redrawn from Inder TE, Warfield SK, Wang H, Huppi PS, et al: Abnormal cerebral structure is present at term in premature infants, Pediatrics 115:286-294, 2005.)*

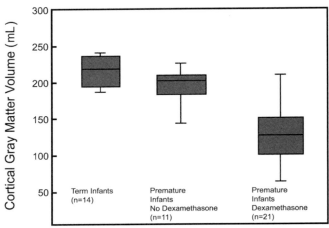

Figure 2- 53 Cerebral cortical gray matter volume. Cerebral cortical gray matter volume, determined by three-dimensional volumetric magnetic resonance imaging at term age, in 14 term infants, 11 premature infants not treated with dexamethasone, and 7 premature infants treated with dexamethasone. See text for details. *(Redrawn from Murphy BP, Inder TE, Huppi PS, Warfield S, et al: Impaired cerebral cortical gray matter growth after treatment with dexamethasone for neonatal chronic lung disease, Pediatrics 107:217-221, 2001.)*

require the relatively uncommon overtly cystic type of periventricular leukomalacia, but rather it occurs after the more common noncystic disease (Fig. 2-52) (see Chapters 8 and 9). The decreased cerebral cortical volumes have been noted by MRI volumetric studies performed as early as term equivalent,[615,814-817a] as well as later in childhood.[818-824]

The neuropathological substrate of the disturbed cerebral cortical volumetric development is unknown. Indeed, whether the volumetric changes reflect underdevelopment or atrophy after injury or a combination of dysgenetic and destructive influences remains to be elucidated. The cellular elements of concern are cerebral cortical neurons, underlying subplate neurons, descending and ascending axons in white matter, and neurons of deep nuclear structures, especially thalamus. These components constitute an interconnected interactive neuronal-axonal unit, and disturbance of one of the elements could lead to disturbance in cortical development, particularly at the levels of dendritic development and axonal ramification into the cortex, the two developmental events most responsible for the normal increase in volume of cerebral cortex over the third trimester (see earlier). The anatomical, mechanistic, and clinical issues related to this neuronal-axonal abnormality of prematurity are examined in detail in Chapters 8 and 9.

Postnatal dexamethasone treatment of preterm infants may cause a disturbance in cerebral cortical neuronal organizational events (see Table 2-28).[813] *Glucocorticoids* administered postnatally to premature infants are recognized widely to lead to a decreased incidence of bronchopulmonary dysplasia and to be associated with numerous short-term adverse systemic effects.[825,826] Still more concerning, long-term adverse neurological effects have been identified.[827-830] These observations led the American Academy of Pediatrics and the Canadian Pediatric Society to recommend that systemic dexamethasone not be used routinely for prevention or treatment of chronic lung disease and that the use of corticosteroids in general be limited to "exceptional" clinical circumstances.[827] Consistent with the neurological sequelae, a report of a small group of premature infants treated with high-dose dexamethasone showed, at term, a significant reduction in cerebral cortical gray matter volume quantitated by three-dimensional volumetric MRI (Fig. 2-53).[831] These observations, reminiscent of those just discussed in relation to premature infants with periventricular white matter injury, raise the possibility of a disturbance in cerebral cortical development. Disturbances of dendritic and axonal development have been identified in nonhuman primates treated with dexamethasone early in development.[832] Because nearly all studies of the adverse neurological effects of postnatal glucocorticoids have involved dexamethasone, a compound shown experimentally to impair neuronal development and potentially to enhance neuronal injury,[826] the possibility of less or no neurotoxicity with the administration of other glucocorticoids has been raised. Four recent reports[818,833,833a,833b] suggested that hydrocortisone could be such an agent. In one large study, 60 preterm infants were evaluated at a mean age of 8 years by quantitative MRI. Twenty-five had been treated with hydrocortisone as newborns (mean age at onset, 18 days; dose, 5 mg/kg/day for 1 week; total duration after taper, 26 days), and 35 were not treated. At 8 years of age, cerebral cortical gray matter, white matter, and hippocampal volumes did not differ between the two groups, and scores on the Wechsler Intelligence Scale for Children also were similar. In a later report, hydrocortisone therapy had no subsequent adverse effect at school age on hippocampal metabolism (assessed by proton MRI spectroscopy) or short-term memory.[833]

Why may hydrocortisone therapy not be associated with long-term neurological deficits when dexamethasone is associated with such deficits? One possible contributing factor is that hydrocortisone in brain binds preferably to the mineralocorticoid receptor, whereas dexamethasone binds preferably to the glucocorticoid receptor.[834,835] Activation of the glucocorticoid receptor leads to adverse neuronal effects.[836,837] A possible contributory deleterious role related to the excitotoxic effects of sulfites contained in the dexamethasone preparation is suggested by in vitro studies.[838] However, despite these interesting observations, the mechanisms of the neurological effects of dexamethasone in the premature newborn are likely still more complex and remain to be clarified. Although it is possible that the pharmacological doses of hydrocortisone used in the two studies showing no adverse effect[818,833] may be preferable to dexamethasone, it will require a larger experience to ensure that the former steroid regimen is completely free of any adverse effects of cerebral cortical neuronal organizational events.

Some studies suggested that the common *transient hypothyroxinemia* of premature infants is associated with subsequent cognitive disturbances and cerebral palsy.[839-847] The neonatal thyroid deficit is more severe and prolonged and the adverse outcome is more pronounced in the most preterm infants.[847] The value of neonatal therapy with thyroid hormone is unresolved. The anatomical substrate for these deficits is unknown, but abundant experimental data show that thyroid hormone is crucial for both neuronal and glial differentiation.[848-852]

The possibility that the cumulative effect of the adverse events associated with *ventilator dependence* in premature infants could play a role in a disturbance of organizational events was suggested by a careful anatomical study.[618] Thus, in this Golgi study of the medulla oblongata of ventilator-dependent infants, decreased numbers of dendritic spines, abnormally thin dendrites, and long, thin dendritic spines were documented (Fig. 2-54).[618] These abnormalities were not observed in premature infants who did not require mechanical ventilation. The potential causes of these disturbances of dendritic development were not clear.

Nutrition, Long-Chain Polyunsaturated Fatty Acids and Breast-Feeding.

The deleterious effects of infant undernutrition and the apparent beneficial effects of breast-feeding on cognitive development together suggest that nutritional factors can have an impact on organizational events (see Table 2-28).[853-866] Longer-chain polyunsaturated fatty acids, which are especially abundant in neuronal and retinal membranes, are critical for neurological and retinal development, can have beneficial effects on neurological and visual function in infants, and are present in considerable amounts in breast milk relative to at least certain formula milks.[860,867-880] Therefore, it is possible that one key determinant of these effects of breast-feeding on neuronal development is the level of such fatty acids in the infant's diet.

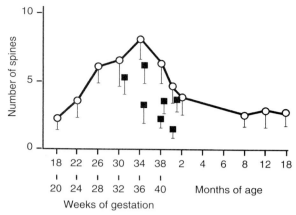

Figure 2-54 **Developmental changes of dendrite spine density.** Developmental changes of dendrite spine density (number of spines per 25 μm) in the medullary reticular formation of ventilator-dependent prematurely born infants *(black squares)* and controls *(open circles)*. *(From Takashima S, Mito T: Neuronal development in the medullary reticular formation in sudden infant death syndrome and premature infants,* Neuropediatrics *16:76-79, 1985.)*

Experiential Effects. The potential impact of *experiential* factors in regulation of cortical organization is suggested by the demonstration that variations in maternal care or related alterations in the environment in experimental animals result in an increase in synaptogenesis.[860,881,882] Particularly elegant experiments in normal and preterm monkeys showed that premature visual stimulation results in increases in size and proportions of various synapses, presumably by alterations in normal synaptic modification or elimination.[883] Visual experience of premature infants is associated with an accentuation of the development of visual evoked potentials, a finding consistent with enhancement of dendritic and axonal development and synaptogenesis (see earlier).[884] Additionally, a randomized clinical trial of an individualized developmental care program showed, at 9 months' corrected age, improved neurobehavorial function, quantitative EEG evidence of enhanced maturation, and diffusion-tensor MRI evidence of more advanced cerebral fiber tract development.[885] More data clearly are needed in these promising areas.

Other Perinatal and Postnatal Insults. Because *its time of rapid developmental progression coincides with the perinatal period,* it is most reasonable to ask whether the very frequent specific insults that affect the human brain in the perinatal period (e.g., hypoxia-ischemia, acidosis, intracranial hemorrhage, posthemorrhagic hydrocephalus, infection, and specific sensory deprivations or excesses) may exert serious consequences on these aspects of brain development. Considerable precedent for deleterious effects of *various perinatal insults* on organizational events is provided by studies with *experimental animals.*[832,881,883,886-906] Initial studies of later cortical neuronal development in "undamaged" areas adjacent to ischemic cortical injury in human infants showed dendritic aberrations that could contribute importantly to subsequent cognitive deficits and epilepsy.[907] It is a clinical truism

TABLE 2-29	Myelination
Peak Time Period	
Birth–years postnatally	
Major Events	
Oligodendroglial proliferation, migration, differentiation, and alignment → myelin sheaths	

that some children affected by one or more perinatal insults may exhibit neurological sequelae that are more severe than would be predicted from the extent of injury recognized by the usual brain imaging or neuropathological techniques. To what extent such sequelae are related to deficits in organizational development is a major topic for further research.

Associated Disturbance

In several carefully executed studies, defects in organizational events were demonstrated in such diverse disorders as congenital rubella,[908] phenylketonuria,[909] Rubinstein-Taybi syndrome,[910] trisomy 13-15,[911] trisomy 18,[912] Zellweger syndrome,[190] and maternal phenylketonuria syndrome (i.e., microcephalic child of a mother with phenylketonuria).[913] It appears unlikely that the defects represent the major or primary developmental disturbance in these disorders. In two patients with congenital rubella, heterotopic neurons (i.e., a migrational defect) and significant retardation of myelination were also noted. In patients with phenylketonuria and Rubinstein-Taybi syndrome, a similar disturbance of myelination accompanied the cytoarchitectural disturbances of cerebral cortex. The most dramatic neuropathological disturbance in trisomy 13-15 involves prosencephalic cleavage (see Chapter 1).

A common feature of trisomy 18 is periventricular heterotopias, and a consistent feature of Zellweger syndrome is major disturbance of neuronal migration (see earlier). Maternal phenylketonuria syndrome is associated most commonly with microcephaly. Nevertheless, a *contributory role* for defects in cortical organization in the genesis of the neurological deficits in these and other disorders is suggested by the studies cited.

MYELINATION

Normal Development

Myelination is characterized by the acquisition of the highly specialized myelin membrane around axons. The time period of myelination in the human is long, beginning in the second trimester of pregnancy and continuing into adult life.[572,914-917] Myelination within the CNS, particularly the forebrain, generally progresses most rapidly after birth (Table 2-29). The process of myelination begins with proliferation of oligodendroglia, which align along axons. The plasma membranes of the oligodendroglia become elaborated as the myelin membrane of the CNS.[572,701,710,915,918,919] Thus, myelination is considered best in two phases: first, oligodendroglial proliferation and differentiation, and second, myelin deposition around axons.

Oligodendroglial Development

The progression of the oligodendroglial lineage proceeds through four basic stages, beginning with the oligodendroglial progenitor and continuing successively with the preoligodendrocyte, the immature oligodendrocyte, and the mature oligodendrocyte (Fig. 2-55).[699-701,708-710,718,721,722,920] Oligodendrocytes originate from progenitors in the subventricular zone

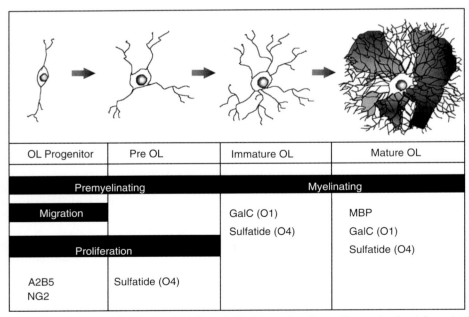

OL Progenitor	Pre OL	Immature OL	Mature OL
Premyelinating		Myelinating	
Migration		GalC (O1)	MBP
		Sulfatide (O4)	GalC (O1)
Proliferation			Sulfatide (O4)
A2B5 NG2	Sulfatide (O4)		

Figure 2-55 **Progression of the oligodendroglial lineage (OL) through the four major stages.** The predominant forms in the premature infant are the O4+O1- and O4+O1+ forms. See text for details. *(From Back SA, Volpe JJ: Cellular and molecular pathogenesis of periventricular white matter injury, Ment Retard Dev Disabil Res Rev 3:96-107, 1997.)*

and also from radial glial progenitors (see earlier). The early phase in oligodendroglial lineage arising from progenitors is a mitotically active migratory cell recognized by the monoclonal antibodies A2B5 and NG2. This cell is generated from midgestation to the early postnatal period.[699-701,718,721,722,921] As this cell migrates into the cerebral white matter, oligodendroglial differentiation proceeds to the preoligodendrocyte, a multipolar cell that retains proliferative capacity and is recognized by a monoclonal antibody to sulfatide (O4). The waves of migration of these cells may be the anatomical correlate of the periventricular bands visualized on MRI scans of the premature infant.[922,923] *The O4-positive preoligodendrocyte is the predominant oligodendroglial phase before term and accounts for 90% of the total oligodendroglial population until 28 weeks of gestation.*[721] The O4 cell differentiates into the postmitotic immature oligodendrocyte, a richly multipolar cell recognized by a monoclonal antibody to galactocerebroside (O1).[699-701,718] The proportion of O1 cells among the entire oligodendroglial population rises from 5% to 10% before 28 weeks of gestation to 30% to 40% during the premature period and to approximately 50% at term. In the third trimester of gestation, the O1 cells can be observed to develop striking linear extensions as they wrap around axons in preparation for myelination. This premyelination encasement of axons contributes to an important MRI correlate, the increase in *directionality* of water diffusion measured as relative anisotropy (Fig. 2-56).[707,924,925] This process is followed by differentiation to the mature

oligodendrocyte, a strikingly multipolar cell with membrane sheets and recognition by antibodies to myelin basic protein and proteolipid protein. This cell becomes the predominant oligodendroglial stage in the months following term and gives rise to myelination.

The molecular determinants of this process include a variety of growth factors, hormones, cytokines, surface receptors, and secreted ligands.[699-701,710,920,926-931a] These molecules include basic fibroblast growth factor, neurotrophin-3, platelet-derived growth factor, insulin-like growth factors, nerve growth factor, transferrin, iron, members of the interleukin-6 family, thyroid hormone, neuregulin, erbB receptors, semaphorins, neuropilin receptors, ephrin, Eph receptors, Nogo, and Nogo receptors.

Programmed cell death is an important feature of oligodendroglial development, as it is for neurons (see earlier). Data show that approximately 50% of oligodendroglia will undergo apoptosis during development.[695,696]

Myelination in Human Brain Regions

The most informative of the anatomical descriptions of the *progress of myelination in the human brain* are those by Yakovlev and Lecours[932] and Gilles, Kinney, and co-workers.[916,917,933] Using the Loyez method for staining myelin, Yakovlev and Lecours defined the development of myelin in 25 areas of the human nervous system (Fig. 2-57). Because approximately 7 to 10 myelin lamellae are necessary for resolution by light microscopy, it is not surprising that electron microscopic data demonstrated that the onset of myelination in various brain areas occurs several weeks or more before the onset indicated in Figure 2-57. Nevertheless, the data shown from Yakovlev and Lecours[932] provide important information. Several general points can be made on the basis of current knowledge. First, myelination begins in the peripheral nervous system, where motor roots myelinate before sensory roots. Second, shortly thereafter and before birth, myelin appears in the CNS in the brain stem and cerebellum in components of some major sensory systems (e.g., medial lemniscus for somesthetic stimuli; lateral lemniscus, trapezoid body, and brachium of the inferior colliculus for auditory stimuli) and in components of some major motor systems (e.g., corticospinal tract in the midbrain and pons and superior cerebellar peduncle). In general, however, and in contrast to the peripheral nervous system, myelination in *central sensory systems tends to precede that in central motor systems.*[932] Third, myelination within the cerebral hemispheres, particularly those regions involved in higher level associative functions and sensory discriminations (e.g., association areas, intracortical neuropil, and cerebral commissures), occurs well after birth and progresses over decades.

A study of 162 cases at a single children's hospital provided further insight into the progress of myelination from prenatal life through childhood.[572,916,917] General agreement exists between these data and those obtained by Yakovlev and Lecours[932] with a smaller sample size. The median post-term age at

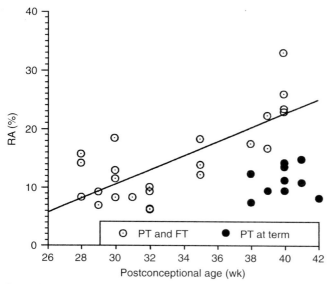

Figure 2-56 **Diffusion tensor magnetic resonance imaging determination of relative anisotropy (RA) in the cerebral white matter of normal preterm (PT) and term (FT) infants** *(open circles)* **as a function of postconceptional age.** Note the striking increase in RA, indicative of increasing directionality of diffusion, perhaps related at least in part to oligodendroglial ensheathment of axons, with maturation. The lower values of the preterm infants studied at term *(closed circles)* suggest a deleterious effect of prematurity on this process (see text for details). *(From Huppi PA, Maier SE, Peled S, et al: Microstructural development of human newborn cerebral white matter assessed in vivo by diffusion tensor magnetic resonance imaging,* Pediatr Res *44:584-590, 1998.)*

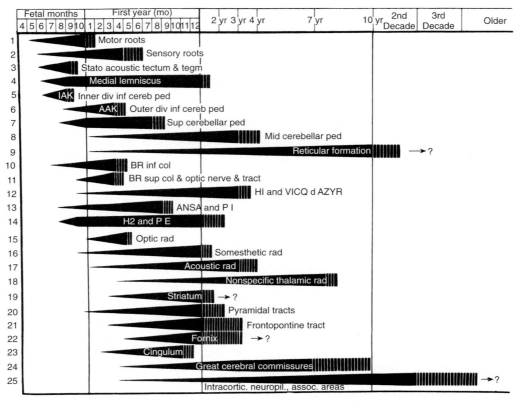

Figure 2-57   Myelogenetic cycles in the human brain. The width and length of the graphs indicate progression in the intensity of staining and the density of myelinated fibers. The vertical strips at the end of the graphs indicate the approximate age range of termination of myelination. *(Courtesy of Dr. Paul Yakovlev.)*

which mature myelin was observed in selected brain areas in this study is depicted in Table 2-30. The similarity between these data and the findings made in vivo by MRI (see Chapter 4) is striking, although MRI showed myelin somewhat earlier, especially in the preterm infant (e.g., myelin in the posterior limb of the internal capsule at 36 postconceptional weeks versus 44 weeks in the anatomical study).[934] This difference may relate to the ability of MRI to detect very early myelin wrapping. Five major general rules concerning cerebral myelination in the human can be derived from the elegant anatomical study of Kinney and co-workers: (1) proximal pathways myelinate before distal pathways, (2) sensory pathways myelinate

before motor pathways, (3) projection pathways myelinate before cerebral associative pathways, (4) central cerebral sites myelinate before cerebral poles, and (5) occipital poles myelinate before frontotemporal poles.[572,917] The latter two points are illustrated in Figure 2-58. Overall, the fastest changes in myelination occurred within the first 8 postnatal months.[917]

Disorders

Unequivocal documentation of developmental disturbances of myelin formation in the human has been hindered considerably by the inadequacy of standard neuropathological techniques in quantifying the

TABLE 2-30 Median Age When Mature Myelin Is Reached		
Brain Region	**Posterior Frontoparieto-occipital Sites**	**Anterior Frontotemporal Sites**
Internal capsule	Posterior limb, 4 weeks*	Anterior limb, 47 weeks
Sensory radiation	Optic radiation, 12 weeks	Heschl gyrus, 48 weeks
Corpus callosum	Body, 20 weeks	Rostrum, 47 weeks
	Splenium, 25 weeks	
Central white matter	Precentral gyrus, 30 weeks	Temporal lobe, 79 weeks
	Posterior frontal, 40 weeks	Temporal pole, 82 weeks
	Posterior parietal, 59 weeks	Frontal pole, 79 weeks
	Occipital pole, 47 weeks	

*Age shown is *post-term age* at which 50% of infants attain mature myelin; for postconceptional age, add 40 weeks.
Data from Brody BA, Kinney HC, Kloman AS, Gilles FH: Sequence of central nervous system myelination in human infancy. I. An autopsy study of myelination, *J Neuropathol Exp Neurol* 46:283-301, 1987.

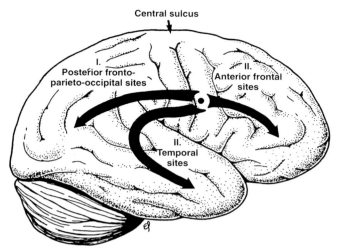

Figure 2-58   Progression of myelination. This drawing of the cerebrum depicts the progression of myelination in telencephalic sites from the central sulcus outward to the poles, with the posterior sites preceding the anterior frontotemporal sites.

degree of myelination in brain. Moreover, the most commonly used brain imaging technique in the past, CT, provides little information concerning myelination in the human infant. The advent of MRI provided considerable capability for monitoring of myelination (see Chapter 4), and MRI is invaluable in defining disturbances of human myelination (see later). Of particular importance are quantitative volumetric MRI determinations and diffusion tensor MRI studies of relative anisotropy (see later).

At least one series of cases does appear to qualify as representative of an inherited disorder of deficient myelination in the human cerebrum (see the following discussion). Moreover, the hypomyelination after cerebral white matter injury in the premature infant also is a clear example of hypomyelination. Additionally, amino acid and organic acid disturbances, hypothyroidism, and undernutrition in early infancy appear to impair brain development principally at the level of myelination. These several disorders are categorized in Table 2-31 as *primary disturbances of myelination*, that is, those in which the *most significant neuropathological*

TABLE 2-31   Disorders of Myelination
Primary Disturbance
Cerebral white matter hypoplasia
Prematurity
Periventricular leukomalacia
Other
Amino and organic acidopathies
Hypothyroidism
Postnatal undernutrition
18q–syndrome
Potential Disturbance
Perinatal/early infancy insults
Iron deficiency
Associated Disturbance
Diverse (see text)

disturbance involves myelination. Disorders in which a derangement of myelination is an *associated defect* or is a *likely but unproved lesion* are categorized as *associated* or *potential disturbances*, respectively (see Table 2-28). (Leukodystrophies and degenerative disorders caused by aberrations of myelin or glial metabolism are described in Chapter 16.)

Primary Disturbance

Cerebral white matter hypoplasia. Chattha and Richardson[935] reported the clinical and neuropathological features of 12 patients with severe intellectual impairment and spastic quadriparesis that were present from the first weeks of life but were nonprogressive. Pregnancy, labor, and delivery were essentially uneventful. Neurological deficits, particularly seizures, were apparent in the neonatal period. Subsequent neurological development was severely impaired. The unifying and outstanding neuropathological feature was a marked deficiency in cerebral white matter, most conspicuous in the centrum ovale (Fig. 2-59). Neurons were normal in appearance, and no gliosis, sign of inflammation, or other indication of a destructive process was present. An inherited developmental aberration in myelin formation was supported by the finding that the series included a set of three affected siblings, and in two other cases a family history of affected siblings was elicited. The biochemical basis of the disorder in myelin formation awaits elucidation. The use of MRI in evaluation of similar patients may lead to further delineation of this disorder. The cases are reminiscent of the murine mutants (e.g., "quaking" and "jimpy" mice) with deficient myelin formation.[936,937] Recently, an autosomal recessive disorder with hypomyelination of the central and peripheral nervous systems, as well as congenital cataract, has been defined.[937a] The central nervous system hypomyelination was principally supratentorial. Definition of the molecular genetics of this disorder will be important.

The decrease in cerebral white matter without evidence of destructive disease in the patients just described is similar to that recorded in the familial disorders of "axonal development" by Lyon and co-workers[808] and others.[809,810] In the latter cases, axonal abnormalities were identifiable, and this finding may be the crucial distinction from the cases of cerebral white matter hypoplasia.

Prematurity. Premature birth may lead to subsequent impairment of developmental events related to myelination, especially as a sequel to periventricular leukomalacia (see Chapters 8 and 9). *Periventricular leukomalacia* results in injury to cerebral white matter, characterized most commonly (80% to 90% of cases) by a diffuse abnormality consisting of astrogliosis and injury to premyelinating oligodendrocytes.[938-940] Fewer patients (10% to 20% of cases) also exhibit focal necrosis with loss of all cellular elements and with subsequent cyst formation (see Chapter 8). Either variety leads to hypomyelination documented by neuropathological study, the results of conventional brain imaging, including ultrasonography and MRI, and

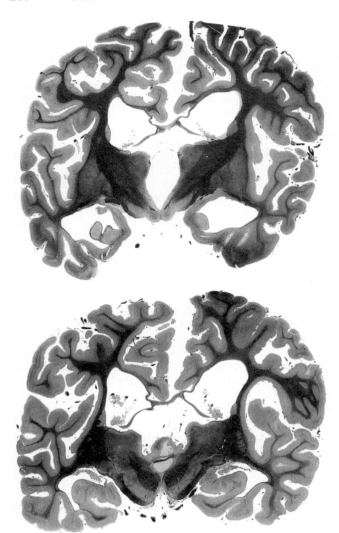

Figure 2-59 **Cerebral white matter hypoplasia.** Coronal sections of the cerebrum are stained for myelin *(black)*. Note the marked diminution in cerebral myelin, including the corpus callosum. As a consequence of the myelin disturbance, ventricular size increases. *(From Chattha AS, Richardson EP Jr: Cerebral white-matter hypoplasia,* Arch Neurol *34:137-141, 1977.)*

measurements of cerebral myelinated white matter volume, as early as term and later in childhood (see also Chapter 9).[814,817,941-953] The myelination defect relates to a presumed loss of premyelinating oligodendrocytes that therefore do not differentiate to myelin-producing mature oligodendrocytes.

Whether factors associated with prematurity, *other than* cerebral white matter injury, result in impaired myelination is unclear. Imaging studies of premature infants without signs of cystic periventricular leukomalacia demonstrate apparent disturbances in subsequent myelination.[817,818] However, as noted earlier, cystic disease accounts for the minority of cases of cerebral white matter injury, and most available studies with later MRI in the neonatal period did not use imaging methodology or timing capable of identifying the more common noncystic disease. Indeed, when careful diffusion-based MRI was used in large cohorts of premature infants, nearly 80% exhibited signs of cerebral white

matter abnormality by term equivalent (see Chapters 8 and 9 for more details). Moreover, the finding of markedly lower relative anisotropy in cerebral white matter of premature infants at term when compared with white matter of term infants further suggests a disturbance of oligodendroglial development and subsequent myelination (see Fig. 2-56) (see earlier). Thus, currently available data indicate that subsequent hypomyelination of premature infants is a sequel to diffuse injury to cerebral white matter, specifically to premyelinating oligodendrocytes.

Amino and organic acidopathies. A disturbance in myelination has been well documented in several amino acidopathies, such as maple syrup urine disease,[954] phenylketonuria,[909,955] homocystinuria,[956] and nonketotic hyperglycinemia,[956] as well as in organic acidopathies (ketotic hyperglycinemia) (see Chapters 14 and 15) (see Table 2-31).[956] The earliest change is vacuolation of myelin, which then evolves to deficient myelination. The microscopic sequence is similar to that observed in mutant mice with deficient myelin formation (see earlier). The disturbance of myelination has been documented by MRI (see Chapters 14 and 15). The mechanisms by which an amino acid disturbance leads to impaired myelination are not clear, but one explanation could be a disturbance in synthesis of myelin proteins.[957] The possibility that concomitant or preceding deficits in organizational events (e.g., elaboration of axonal ramifications, glial proliferation, or differentiation) are involved in the genesis of the myelin abnormality is raised by the organizational defects observed in phenylketonuria.[909] On balance, however, current data suggest that the primary disturbance of brain development in these patients involves myelination.

Hypothyroidism. A disturbance in myelination may be the principal neuropathological abnormality in congenital hypothyroidism (see Table 2-31). A substantial experimental literature documented impaired myelination with hypothyroidism, studied either in the intact animal or in cultured glial cells.[958-961] The report of a hypothyroid infant who was carefully studied by MRI also suggests that the principal deleterious effect of congenital hypothyroidism and the beneficial effect of therapy thereof are on the progress of myelination.[962] Moreover, data concerning the relation between timing of therapy and intellectual outcome suggest that the crucial period begins perhaps late in fetal life or in the first weeks of postnatal life.[963-967] In addition, however, the amount of thyroxine in the first 2 years is correlated with intellectual outcome, a finding further implicating the time period of myelination or oligodendroglial proliferation-differentiation or both.[968] Further data, particularly with quantitative MRI assessments of myelination, will be of interest. Finally, a disturbance of myelination is not likely to be the only important disturbance in congenital hypothyroidism, because experimental thyroid deficiency is known to impair neuronal differentiation (see earlier),[969,970] also an active process during the time period of importance in congenital hypothyroidism. Moreover, the adverse effect of maternal hypothyroxinemia during early pregnancy on neonatal neurological function raises this possibility in the human.[971] However, to my knowledge, no data are available on neuronal differentiation (e.g., Golgi analyses) in human infants dying with congenital hypothyroidism.

The earlier discussion in the section on the deleterious effects of the transient hypothyroxinemia of the premature infant on organizational events and on subsequent cognitive and motor development is relevant here. Whether a defect in myelination occurs in that context remains to be established but is plausible in view of the crucial role of thyroid hormone in oligodendroglial differentiation, as noted earlier.

Undernutrition. The effect of undernutrition in early infancy on brain development was discussed earlier in relation to disorders of organizational events. Relevant data in the context of myelination include the demonstration of a 20% to 30% reduction in cerebrosides and a 15% to 20% reduction in plasmalogens (important myelin lipids) in the cerebral white matter of malnourished infants.[972] The composition of the myelin from these infants was found to be normal, and thus decreased formation of chemically normal myelin was postulated to occur in malnutrition.[973] Results of a later study confirmed these findings.[974] The observation of Chase and Martin[975] that severe undernutrition to 4 months of age results in a permanent reduction in intelligence quotient may also be relevant in this context. Long-term follow-up studies of children undernourished in infancy generally confirm the deleterious effects on intelligence and school performance, although the roles of other factors related to deficient environmental stimulation, "social deprivation," and confounding deleterious biological factors remain to be defined clearly.[860,865,976-984] Nevertheless, the important effects of undernutrition in infancy on organizational events in the human suggest an important role for impaired neuronal differentiation or synaptogenesis as well. The developmental events particularly affected could relate principally to the timing of the insult.

Deletion 18q Syndrome. A well-recognized syndrome caused by partial deletion of the long arm of chromosome 18 (18q–) may include a primary disturbance of myelination (see Table 2-31). This disorder is characterized by postnatal microcephaly, dysmorphisms of the craniofacial region, limbs, and genitalia, and a neurological syndrome manifested by mental retardation, hypotonia, deafness, and aberrant behavior.[73] Approximately 95% of affected patients exhibit disturbances of myelination, characterized by delayed onset of myelination, low rate of the process, and diminished final levels of myelin.[985-987] The myelin disturbance, readily detected by MRI, apparently results because the deletion includes the gene for myelin basic protein.[988] Myelin basic protein is a key structural protein of mature myelin and plays a major role in myelin accretion and compaction.

Potential Disturbance

Perinatal/Early Infantile Insults. As indicated for organizational events, the time of rapid developmental progression of myelination in human cerebrum includes the neonatal period, and indeed it proceeds most rapidly during a potentially "vulnerable" or "critical" period of the first 8 months of life (see Table 2-31) (see earlier). It is reasonable to ask whether perinatal insults, such as hypoxia-ischemia, metabolic disturbances, intracranial hemorrhage, posthemorrhagic hydrocephalus, and administration of various drugs, may exert serious consequences on this specific aspect of brain development. The initial positive MRI findings in premature infants discussed earlier are relevant in this context. Considerable precedent is available from studies in animals and cultured systems.[989-998]

Iron Deficiency. Iron deficiency in infancy, a very common disorder, is associated with cognitive, motor, and behavioral deficits that may be related to impaired myelination (see Table 2-31). Iron deficiency in this context is usually related to dietary deficiency but also to breast-feeding and prematurity.[879,999,1000] Indeed, as many as 10% of infants 1 to 2 years of age in the United States and 15% of breast-fed Canadian infants exhibit iron deficiency. Because premature birth deprives the infant of the primary period of fetal iron deposition (i.e., the third trimester), the risks are still higher in these infants. Although the data are not entirely consistent, most studies show impaired motor, cognitive, and behavioral development in iron-deficient infants.[879,999-1003] Although the deleterious effects are generally modest, they may be irreversible if treatment is not prompt. Supportive of an effect on central myelination is the finding on studies of auditory and visual evoked potentials of prolonged latencies, without impairment of amplitudes.[1001,1004,1005] The maturational decline in latencies relate to acquisition of myelin, whereas changes in amplitude relate more to neuronal development (see Chapter 4). Additionally supportive of an effect on myelination is the recognition of the crucial role of iron in myelination.[710,879,999,1006] Moreover, transferrin concentrations in oligodendrocytes increase during myelination and reach a peak at the height of myelination. Finally, transferrin is involved in the regulation of the transcription of the myelin basic protein gene and has a synergistic enhancing effect on myelination with insulin-like growth factor I.[710] Because iron plays a critical role in neurotransmitter metabolism, the neural effects of iron deficiency may extend beyond an impairment of myelination.

Associated Disturbance

Defects in myelination have been recorded in congenital rubella,[908] Rubinstein-Taybi syndrome,[910] and Down syndrome.[1007] As reviewed previously, however, when careful studies of other aspects of brain development were performed, associated defects in such features as cortical organization were present. Whether the deficits in organizational events could lead to the deficit in myelination is not clear. It is likely that the advent of quantitative MRI methods will lead to elucidation of many other disorders in which impaired myelination is an associated defect.

REFERENCES

1. Dobbing J, Sands J: Quantitative growth and development of human brain, *Arch Dis Child* 48:757-767, 1973.
2. Samuelsen GB, Larsen KB, Bogdanovic N, Laursen H, et al: The changing number of cells in the human fetal forebrain and its subdivisions: A stereological analysis, *Cereb Cortex* 13:115-122, 2003.
3. Lemire RJ, Loeser JD, Leech RW, Alvord EC Jr: *Normal and Abnormal Development of the Human Nervous System*, Hagerstown, MD: 1975, Harper & Row.
4. Norman MG, O'Kusky JR: The growth and development of microvasculature in human cerebral cortex, *J Neuropathol Exp Neurol* 45:222-232, 1986.
5. Evrard P, de Saint-Georges P, Kadhim HJ, Gadisseux J-F: Pathology of prenatal encephalopathies. In French JH, Harel S, Casaer P, editors: *Child Neurology and Developmental Disabilities*, Baltimore: 1989, Paul H. Brookes.
6. Marin-Padilla M: Embryonic vascularization of the mammalian cerebral cortex. In Peters A, Jones EG, editors: *Cerebral Cortex*, New York: 1988, Plenum.
7. Sauer FC: The cellular structure of the neural tube, *J Comp Neurol* 63:13-31, 1935.
8. Sauer FC: Mitosis in the neural tube, *J Comp Neurol* 62:377, 1935.
9. Sidman RL, Miale IL, Feder N: Cell proliferation and migration in the primitive ependymal zone: An autoradiographic study of histogenesis in the nervous system, *Exp Neurol* 1:322-333, 1959.
10. Sidman RL, Angevine JB: Autoradiographic analysis of time of origin of nuclear versus cortical components of mouse telencephalon, *Anat Rec* 142:326-341, 1962.
11. Rakic P, Sidman RL: Supravital DNA synthesis in the developing human and mouse brain, *J Neuropathol Exp Neurol* 27:246-276, 1968.
12. Berry M, Rogers AW, Eayrs JF: Pattern of cell migration during cortical histogenesis, *Nature* 203:591-593, 1964.
13. Rakic P: Limits of neurogenesis in primates, *Science* 227:1054-1056, 1985.
14. Caviness VS, Takahashi T: Proliferative events in the cerebral ventricular zone, *Brain Dev* 17:159-163, 1995.
15. Takahashi T, Nowakowski RS, Caviness VS: Cell cycle parameters and patterns of nuclear movement in the neocortical proliferative zone of the fetal mouse, *J Neurosci* 13:820-833, 1993.
16. Rakic P: A small step for the cell, a giant leap for mankind: A hypothesis of neocortical expansion during evolution, *Trends Neurosci* 18:388-838, 1995.
17. Caviness VS, Takahashi T, Nowakowski RS: Numbers, time and neocortical neuronogenesis: A general developmental and evolutionary model, *Trends Neurosci* 18:379-383, 1995.
18. Takahashi T, Nowakowski RS, Caviness VS: The leaving or Q fraction of the murine cerebral proliferative epithelium: A general model of neocortical neuronogenesis, *J Neurosci* 16:6186-6196, 1996.
19. Kornack DR, Rakic P: Changes in cell-cycle kinetics during the development and evolution of primate neocortex, *Proc Natl Acad Sci U S A* 95:1242-1246, 1998.
20. Caviness VS, Takahashi T, Nowakowski RS: Neocortical malformation as consequence of nonadaptive regulation of neurogenetic sequence, *Ment Retard Dev Disabil Res Rev* 6:22-33, 2000.
21. Zecevic N, Chen YH, Filipovic R: Contributions of cortical subventricular zone to the development of the human cerebral cortex, *J Comp Neurol* 491:109-122, 2005.
22. Howard B, Chen YH, Zecevic N: Cortical progenitor cells in the developing human telencephalon, *Glia* 53:57-66, 2006.
23. Gal JS, Morozov YM, Ayoub AE, Chatterjee M, et al: Molecular and morphological heterogeneity of neural precursors in the mouse neocortical proliferative zones, *J Neurosci* 26:1045-1056, 2006.
23a. Noctor SC, Martinez-Cerdeno V, Kriegstein AR: Contribution of intermediate progenitor cells to cortical histogenesis, *Arch Neurol* 64:639-642, 2007.
23b. Mo Z, Moore AR, Filipovic R, Ogawa Y, et al: Human cortical neurons originate from radial glia and neuron-restricted progenitors, *J Neurosci* 27:4132-4145, 2007.
24. Rakic P: Timing of major ontogenetic events in the visual cortex of the rhesus monkey. In Buchwald NA, Brazier M, editors: *Brain Mechanisms in Mental Retardation*, New York: 1975, Academic Press.
25. Rakic P: Specification of cerebral cortical areas, *Science* 241:170-176, 1988.
26. Rakic P: Defects of neuronal migration and the pathogenesis of cortical malformations, *Prog Brain Res* 73:15-37, 1988.

27. Caviness VS, Goto T, Tarui T, Takahashi T, et al: Cell output, cell cycle duration and neuronal specification: A model of integrated mechanisms of the neocortical proliferative process, *Cereb Cortex* 13:592-598, 2003.
28. Rakic P: Less is more: Progenitor death and cortical size, *Nat Neurosci* 8:981-982, 2005.
29. Noctor SC, Flint AC, Weissman TA, Wong WS, et al: Dividing precursor cells of the embryonic cortical ventricular zone have morphological and molecular characteristics of radial glia, *J Neurosci* 22:3161-3173, 2002.
30. Kriegstein A, Parnavelas JG: Changing concepts of cortical development, *Cereb Cortex* 13:i-ii, 2003.
31. Weissman T, Noctor SC, Clinton BK, Honig LS, et al: Neurogenic radial glial cells in reptile, rodent and human: From mitosis to migration, *Cereb Cortex* 13:550-559, 2003.
32. Fishell G, Kriegstein AR: Neurons from radial glia: The consequences of asymmetric inheritance, *Curr Opin Neurobiol* 13:34-41, 2003.
33. Li HD, Babiarz J, Woodbury J, Kane-Goldsmith N, et al: Spatiotemporal heterogeneity of CNS radial glial cells and their transition to restricted precursors, *Dev Biol* 271:225-238, 2004.
34. Zecevic N: Specific characteristic of radial glia in the human fetal telencephalon, *Glia* 48:27-35, 2004.
35. Weissman TA, Riquelme PA, Ivic L, Flint AC, et al: Calcium waves propagate through radial glial cells and modulate proliferation in the developing neocortex, *Neuron* 43:647-661, 2004.
36. Merkle FT, Tramontin AD, Garcia-Verdugo JM, Alvarez-Buylla A: Radial glia give rise to adult neural stem cells in the subventricular zone, *Proc Natl Acad Sci U S A* 101:17528-17532, 2004.
37. Gotz M, Barde YA: Radial glial cells: Defined and major intermediates between embryonic, stem cells and CNS neurons, *Neuron* 46:369-372, 2005.
38. Ever L, Gaiano N: Radial "glial" progenitors: Neurogenesis and signaling, *Curr Opin Neurobiol* 15:29-33, 2005.
39. Lasky JL, Wu H: Notch signaling, brain development, and human disease, *Pediatr Res* 57:104R-109R, 2005.
40. Chenn A, Walsh CA: Regulation of cerebral cortical size by control of cell cycle exit in neural precursors, *Science* 297:365-369, 2002.
41. Evrard P, Miladi N, Bonnier C, Gressens P: Normal and abnormal development of the brain. In Rapin I, Segalowitz SJ, editors: *Handbook of Neuropsychology, vol. 6: Child Neuropsychology*, Amsterdam: 1992, Elsevier Science Biomedical Division.
42. Barkovich AJ: *Pediatric Neuroimaging*, 4th ed. Philadelphia: 2005, Lippincott Williams & Wilkins.
43. Barkovich AJ, Ferriero DM, Barr RM, Gressens P, et al: Microlissencephaly: A heterogeneous malformation of cortical development, *Neuropediatrics* 29:113-119, 1998.
44. Hanefeld FA: Oligogyric microcephaly, *Neuropediatrics* 30:102-103, 2001.
45. Dobyns WB, Barkovich AJ: Microcephaly with simplified gyral pattern (oligogyric microcephaly) and microlissencephaly: Reply, *Neuropediatrics* 30:104-106, 2001.
46. Dobyns WB: Primary microcephaly: New approaches for an old disorder, *Am J Med Genet* 112:315-317, 2002.
47. Klinge L, Schaper J, Wieczorek D, Voit T: Microlissencephaly in microcephalic osteodysplastic primordial dwarfism: A case report and review of the literature, *Neuropediatrics* 33:309-313, 2003.
48. Sztriha L, Dawodu A, Gururaj A, Johansen JG: Microcephaly associated with abnormal gyral pattern, *Neuropediatrics* 35:346-352, 2004.
49. Faravelli F, D'Arrigo S, Bagnasco I, Selicorni A, et al: Oligogyric microcephaly in a child with Williams syndrome, *Am J Med Genet A* 117:169-171, 2003.
50. Seeman P, Gebertova K, Paderova K, Sperling K, et al: Nijmegen breakage syndrome in, 13% of age-matched Czech children with primary microcephaly, *Pediatr Neurol* 30:195-200, 2004.
51. Kelley RI, Robinson DL, Puffenberger EG, Strauss KA, et al: Amish lethal microcephaly: A new metabolic disorder with severe congenital microcephaly and 2-ketoglutaric aciduria, *Am J Med Genet* 112:318-326, 2002.
52. Sheen VL, Ganesh VS, Topcu M, Sebire G, et al: Mutations in ARFGEF2 implicate vesicle trafficking in neural progenitor proliferation and migration in the human cerebral cortex, *Nat Genet* 36:69-76, 2004.
53. Sztriha L, Johansen JG, Al-Gazali LI: Extreme microcephaly with agyria-pachygyria, partial agenesis of the corpus callosum, and pontocerebellar dysplasia, *J Child Neurol* 20:170-172, 2005.
54. Suri M: What's new in neurogenetics? Focus on "primary microcephaly," *Eur J Pediatr Neurol* 7:389-392, 2003.
55. Xu XZ, Lee J, Stern DF: Microcephalin is a DNA damage response protein involved in regulation of CHK1 and BRCA1, *J Biol Chem* 279:34091-34094, 2004.
56. Trimborn M, Bell SM, Felix C, Rashid Y, et al: Mutations in microcephalin cause aberrant regulation of chromosome condensation, *Am J Hum Genet* 75:261-266, 2004.
57. Woods CG: Human microcephaly, *Curr Opin Neurobiol* 14:112-117, 2004.
58. Woods CG, Bond J, Enard W: Autosomal recessive primary microcephaly (MCPH): A review of clinical, molecular, and evolutionary findings, *Am J Hum Genet* 76:717-728, 2005.
59. Shen J, Eyaid W, Mochida GH, Al-Moayyad F, et al: ASPM mutations identified in patients with primary microcephaly and seizures, *J Med Genet* 42:725-729, 2005.

60. Fisch RO, Ketterling WC, Schacht LE, Letson RD: Ocular abnormalities of a child associated with familial microcephaly, *Am J Ophthalmol* 76:260-264, 1973.
61. McKusick VA, Stauffer M, Knox DL, Clark DB: Chorioretinopathy with hereditary microcephaly, *Arch Ophthalmol* 75:597-600, 1966.
62. Grizzard WS, O'Donnell JJ, Carey JC: The cerebro-oculo-facio-skeletal syndrome, *Am J Ophthalmol* 89:293-298, 1980.
63. Jarmas AL, Weaver DD, Ellis FD, Davis A: Microcephaly, microphthalmia, falciform retinal folds, and blindness: A new syndrome, *Am J Dis Child* 135:930-933, 1981.
64. Renier WO, Gabreels FJ, Jasper HH: An X-linked syndrome with microcephaly, severe mental retardation, spasticity, epilepsy and deafness, *J Ment Defic Res* 1:27-40, 1982.
65. Siber M: X-linked recessive microencephaly, microphthalmia with corneal opacities, spastic quadriplegia, hypospadias and cryptorchidism, *Clin Genet* 26:453-456, 1984.
66. Merlob P, Steier D, Reisner SH: Autosomal dominant isolated ("uncomplicated") microcephaly, *J Med Genet* 25:750-753, 1988.
67. Bawle E, Horton M: Autosomal dominant microcephaly with mental retardation, *Am J Med Genet* 33:382-384, 1989.
68. Cowie VA: Microcephaly: A review of genetic implications in its causation, *J Ment Defic Res* 31:229-233, 1987.
69. Rossi LN, Candini G, Scarlatti G, Rossi G, et al: Autosomal dominant microcephaly without mental retardation, *Am J Dis Child* 141:655-659, 1987.
70. Harbord MG, Lambert SR, Kriss A, Brett EM, et al: Autosomal recessive microcephaly, mental retardation with nonpigmentary retinopathy and a distinctive electroretinogram, *Neuropediatrics* 20:139-141, 1989.
71. Opitz JM, Holt MC: Microcephaly: General considerations and aids to nosology, *J Craniofac Genet Dev Biol* 10:175-204, 1990.
72. Manning FJ, Bruce AM, Berson EL: Electroretinograms in microcephaly with chorioretinal degeneration, *Am J Ophthalmol* 109:457-463, 1990.
73. Jones KL: *Smith's Recognizable Patterns of Human Malformation*, 6th ed. Philadelphia: 2006, Elsevier Saunders.
74. Innis JW, Asher JH, Poznanski AK, Sheldon S: Autosomal dominant microcephaly with normal intelligence, short palpebral fissures, and digital anomalies, *Am J Med Genet* 71:150-155, 1997.
75. Miller RW, Blot WJ: Small head size after in-utero exposure to atomic radiation, *Lancet* 2:784-787, 1972.
76. Schull WJ, Norton S, Jensh RP: Ionizing radiation and the developing brain, *Neurotoxicol Teratol* 12:249-260, 1990.
77. Yamazaki JN, Schull WJ: Perinatal loss and neurological abnormalities among children of the atomic bomb: Nagasaki and Hiroshima revisited, 1949 to 1989, *JAMA* 264:605-609, 1990.
78. Lenke RR, Levy HL: Maternal phenylketonuria and hyperphenylalaninemia: An international survey of the outcome of untreated and treated pregnancies, *N Engl J Med* 303:1202-1208, 1980.
79. Waisbren SE, Levy HL: Effects of untreated maternal hyperphenylalaninemia on the fetus: Further study of families identified by routine cord blood screening, *J Pediatr* 116:926-929, 1990.
80. Diamond A: Phenylalanine levels of 6–10 mg/dl may not be as benign as once thought, *Acta Paediatr* 83:89-91, 1994.
81. Levy HL, Walsbren SE, Lobbregt D, Allred E, et al: Maternal mild hyperphenylalaninaemia: An international survey of offspring outcome, *Lancet* 344:1589-1594, 1994.
82. Levy HL, Ghavami M: Maternal phenylketonuria: A metabolic teratogen, *Teratology* 53:176-184, 1996.
83. Jardim LB, Palma-Dias R, Silva LCS, Ashton-Prolla P, et al: Maternal hyperphenylalaninaemia as a cause of microcephaly and mental retardation, *Acta Paediatr* 85:943-946, 1996.
84. Hanley WB, Platt LD, Bachman RP, Buist N, et al: Undiagnosed maternal phenylketonuria: The need for prenatal selective screening or case finding, *Am J Obstet Gynecol* 180:986-994, 1999.
85. Koch R, Friedman E, Azen C, Hanley W, et al: The international collaborative study of maternal phenylketonuria status report 1998, *Ment Retard Dev Disabil Res Rev* 5:117-121, 1999.
86. Waisbren SE: Developmental and neuropsychological outcome in children born to mothers with phenylketonuria, *Ment Retard Dev Disabil Res Rev* 5:125-131, 1999.
87. Rouse B, Matalon R, Koch R, Azen C, et al: Maternal phenylketonuria syndrome: Congenital heart defects, microcephaly, and developmental outcomes, *J Pediatr* 136:57-61, 2000.
88. Platt LD, Koch R, Hanley WB, Levy HL, et al: The International Study of Pregnancy Outcome in Women with Maternal Phenylketonuria: Report of a 12-year study, *Am J Obstet Gynecol* 182:326-333, 2000.
89. Rouse B, Azen C: Effect of high maternal blood phenylalanine on offspring congenital anomalies and developmental outcome at ages 4 and 6 years: The importance of strict dietary control preconception and throughout pregnancy, *J Pediatr* 144:235-239, 2004.
90. Warkany J, Lemire RJ, Cohen MM Jr: *Mental Retardation and Congenital Malformations of the Central Nervous System*, Chicago: 1981, Year Book.
91. Vargas JE, Allred EN, Leviton A, Holmes LB: Congenital microcephaly: Phenotypic features in a consecutive sample of newborn infants, *J Pediatr* 139:210-214, 2001.
92. Krauss MJ, Morrissey AE, Winn HN, Amon E, et al: Microcephaly: An epidemiologic analysis, *Am J Obstet Gynecol* 188:1484-1489, 2003.
93. DeMeyer W: Megalencephaly in children: Clinical syndromes, genetic patterns, and differential diagnosis from other causes of megalocephaly, *Neurology* 22:634-643, 1972.
94. Laubscher B, Deonna T, Uske A, van Melle G: Primitive megalencephaly in children: Natural history, medium term prognosis with special reference to external hydrocephalus, *Eur J Pediatr* 149:502-507, 1990.
95. De Rosa MJ, Secor DL, Barsom M, Fisher RS, et al: Neuropathologic findings in surgically treated hemimegalencephaly: Immunohistochemical, morphometric, and ultrastructural study, *Acta Neuropathol (Berl)* 84:250-260, 1992.
96. de Vries LS, Smet M, Ceulemans B, Marchal G, et al: The role of high resolution ultrasound and MRI in the investigation of infants with macrocephaly, *Neuropediatrics* 21:72-75, 1990.
97. Babcock DS, Han BK, Dine MS: Sonographic findings in infants with macrocrania, *AJNR Am J Neuroradiol* 9:307-313, 1988.
98. Maytal J, Alvarez LA, Elkin CM, Shinnar S: External hydrocephalus: Radiologic spectrum and differentiation from cerebral atrophy, *AJR Am J Roentgenol* 148:1223-1230, 1987.
99. Alvarez LA, Maytal J, Shinnar S: Idiopathic external hydrocephalus: Natural history and relationship to benign familial macrocephaly, *Pediatrics* 77:901-907, 1986.
100. Hamza M, Bodensteiner JB, Noorani PA, Barnes PD: Benign extracerebral fluid collections: A cause of macrocrania in infancy, *Pediatr Neurol* 3:218-221, 1987.
101. Nickel RE, Gallenstein JS: Developmental prognosis for infants with benign enlargement of the subarachnoid spaces, *Dev Med Child Neurol* 29:181-186, 1987.
102. Wilms G, Vanderschueren G, Demaerel PH, Smet MH, et al: CT and MR in infants with pericerebral collections and macrocephaly: Benign enlargement of the subarachnoid spaces versus subdural collections, *AJNR Am J Neuroradiol* 14:855-860, 1993.
103. Pettit RE, Kilroy AW, Allen JH: Macrocephaly with head growth parallel to normal growth pattern: Neurological, developmental, and computerized tomography findings in full-term infants, *Arch Neurol* 37:518-521, 1980.
104. Sandler AD, Knudsen MW, Brown TT, Christian RM: Neurodevelopmental dysfunction among nonreferred children with idiopathic megalencephaly, *J Pediatr* 131:234-320, 1997.
105. Ott JE, Robinson A: Cerebral gigantism, *Am J Dis Child* 117:357-368, 1969.
106. Dodge PR, Holmes SJ, Sotos JF: Cerebral gigantism, *Dev Med Child Neurol* 25:248-252, 1983.
107. Kurotaki N, Imaizumi K, Harada N, Masuno M, et al: Haploinsufficiency of NSD1 causes Sotos syndrome, *Nat Genet* 30:365-366, 2002.
108. Nagai T, Matsumoto N, Kurotaki N, Harada N, et al: Sotos syndrome and haploinsufficiency of NSD1: Clinical features of intragenic mutations and submicroscopic deletions, *J Med Genet* 40:285-289, 2003.
109. Zonana J, Rimoin DL, Davis DC: Macrocephaly with multiple lipomas and hemangiomas, *J Pediatr* 89:600-603, 1976.
110. Stephan MJ, Hall BD, Smith DW, Cohen MM Jr: Macrocephaly in association with unusual cutaneous angiomatosis, *J Pediatr* 87:353-359, 1975.
111. Bannayan GA: Lipomatosis, angiomatosis, and macroencephalia, *Arch Pathol Lab Med* 92:1-5, 1971.
112. Riley HD, Smith WR: Macrocephaly, pseudopapilledema and multiple hemangiomata, *Pediatrics* 26:293-297, 1960.
113. Dvir M, Beer S, Aladjem M: Heredofamilial syndrome of mesodermal hamartomas, macrocephaly, and pseudopapilledema, *Pediatrics* 81:287-290, 1988.
114. Pont MS, Elster AD: Lesions of skin and brain: Modern imaging of the neurocutaneous syndromes, *AJR Am J Roentgenol* 158:1193-1203, 1992.
115. Lapunzina P, Gairi A, Delicado A, Mori MA, et al: Macrocephaly-cutis marmorata telangiectatica congenita: Report of six new patients and a review, *Am J Med Genet A* 130:45-51, 2004.
116. Feinman NL, Yakovac WC: Neurofibromatosis in childhood, *J Pediatr* 76:339, 1970.
117. Listernick R, Charrow J: Neurofibromatosis type, 1 in childhood, *J Pediatr* 116:845-853, 1990.
118. Korf BR: Diagnostic outcome in children with multiple cafe au lait spots, *Pediatrics* 90:924-927, 1992.
119. Fois A, Calistri L, Balestri P, Vivarelli R, et al: Relationship between cafe-au-lait spots as the only symptom and peripheral neurofibromatosis (NF1): A follow-up study, *Eur J Pediatr* 152:500-504, 1993.
120. Gutmann DH, Aylsworth A, Carey JC, Korf B, et al: The diagnostic evaluation and multidisciplinary management of neurofibromatosis 1 and neurofibromatosis 2, *JAMA* 278:51-57, 1997.
121. Feldkamp MM, Gutmann DH, Guha A: Neurofibromatosis type 1: Piecing the puzzle together, *Can J Neurol Sci* 25:181-191, 1998.
122. Ward BA, Gutmann DH: Neurofibromatosis 1: From lab bench to clinic, *Pediatr Neurol* 32:221-228, 2005.
123. North KN: Clinical aspects of neurofibromatosis 1, *Eur J Pediatr Neurol* 2:223-231, 1998.
124. North KN: Neurofibromatosis 1 in childhood, *Semin Pediatr Neurol* 5:231-241, 1998.

125. Cutting LE, Cooper KL, Koth CW, Mostofsky SH, et al: Megalencephaly in NF1. Predominantly white matter contribution and mitigation by ADHD, *Neurology* 59:1388-1394, 2002.
126. Drouin V, Marret S, Petitcolas J, Eurin D, et al: Prenatal ultrasound abnormalities in a patient with generalized neurofibromatosis type 1, *Neuropediatrics* 28:120-121, 1997.
127. Cusmai R, Curatolo P, Mangano S, Cheminal R, et al: Hemimegalencephaly and neurofibromatosis, *Neuropediatrics* 21:179-182, 1990.
128. Balestri P, Vivarelli R, Grosso S, Santori L, et al: Malformations of cortical development in neurofibromatosis typ. 1, *Neurology* 61:1799-1801, 2003.
129. Gutmann DH, Collins FS: Recent progress toward understanding the molecular biology of von Recklinghausen neurofibromatosis, *Ann Neurol* 31:555-561, 1992.
130. Gutmann DH: Recent insights into neurofibromatosis type 1. Clear genetic progress, *Arch Neurol* 55:778-780, 1998.
131. Griffiths PD: Sturge-Weber syndrome revisited: The role of neuroradiology, *Neuropediatrics* 27:284-294, 1996.
132. Comi AM, Weisz CJC, Highet BH, Skolasky RL, et al: Sturge-Weber syndrome: Altered blood vessel fibronectin expression and morphology, *J Child Neurol* 20:572-577, 2005.
133. Tallman B, Tan OT, Morelli JG, Piepenbrink J, et al: Location of port-wine stains and the likelihood of ophthalmic and/or central nervous system complications, *Pediatrics* 87:323-327, 1991.
134. Thomas-Sohl KA, Vaslow DF, Maria BL: Sturge-Weber syndrome: A review, *Pediatr Neurol* 30:303-310, 2004.
135. Nellhaus G, Haberland C, Hill BJ: Sturge-Weber disease with bilateral intracranial calcifications at birth and unusual pathologic findings, *Acta Neurol Scand* 43:314-347, 1967.
136. Kitahara T, Maki Y: A case of Sturge-Weber disease with epilepsy and intracranial calcification at the neonatal period, *Eur Neurol* 17:8-12, 1978.
137. Pascual-Castroviejo I, Diaz-Gonzalez C, Garcia-Melian RM, Gonzalez-Casado I, et al: Sturge-Weber syndrome: Study of 40 patients, *Pediatr Neurol* 9:283-288, 1993.
138. Sujansky E, Conradi S: Sturge-Weber syndrome: Age of onset of seizures and glaucoma and the prognosis for affected children, *J Child Neurol* 10:49-58, 1995.
139. Terdjman P, Aicardi J, Sainte Rose C, Brunelle F: Neuroradiological findings in Sturge-Weber syndrome (SWS) and isolated pial angiomatosis, *Neuropediatrics* 22:115-120, 1991.
140. Martí-Bonmati L, Menor F, Poyatos C, Cortina H: Diagnosis of Sturge-Weber syndrome: Comparison of the efficacy of CT and MR imaging in 14 cases, *AJR Am J Roentgenol* 158:867-871, 1992.
141. Griffiths PD, Boodram MB, Blaser S, Armstrong D, et al: (99m)Technetium HMPAO imaging in children with the Sturge-Weber syndrome: A study of nine cases with CT and MRI correlation, *Neuroradiology* 39:219-224, 1997.
142. Sperner J, Schmauser I, Bittner R, Henkes H, et al: MR-imaging findings in children with Sturge-Weber syndrome, *Neuropediatrics* 21:146-152, 1990.
143. Enjolras O, Chiron C, Diebler C, Merland JJ: New trends for an early diagnosis of the Sturge-Weber syndrome [in French], *Rev Eur Dermatol MST* 3:21-26, 1991.
144. Maria BL, Neufeld JA, Rosainz LC, Ben-David K, et al: High prevalence of bihemispheric structural and functional defects in Sturge-Weber syndrome, *J Child Neurol* 13:595-605, 1998.
145. Maria BL, Neufeld JA, Rosainz LC, Drane WE, et al: Central nervous system structure and function in Sturge-Weber syndrome: Evidence of neurologic and radiologic progression, *J Child Neurol* 13:606-618, 1998.
146. Evans AL, Widjaja E, Connolly DJ, Griffiths PD: Cerebral perfusion abnormalities in children with Sturge-Weber syndrome shown by dynamic contrast bolus magnetic resonance perfusion imaging, *Pediatrics* 117:2119-2125, 2006.
147. Bebin EM, Gomez MR: Prognosis in Sturge-Weber disease: Comparison of unihemispheric and bihemispheric involvement, *J Child Neurol* 3:181-184, 1988.
148. Berg RA, Aleck KA, Kaplan AM: Familial porencephaly, *Arch Neurol* 40:567-569, 1983.
149. Curatolo P, Verdecchia M, Bombardieri R: Tuberous sclerosis complex: A review of neurological aspects, *Eur J Pediatr Neurol* 6:15-23, 2002.
150. Narayanan V: Tuberous sclerosis complex: Genetics to pathogenesis, *Pediatr Res* 29:404-409, 2003.
151. Au KS, Williams AT, Gambello MJ, Northrup H: Molecular genetic basis of tuberous sclerosis complex: From bench to bedside, *J Child Neurol* 19:699-709, 2004.
152. Yoshimura K, Hayashi Y, Nakae Y, Nara T, et al: Brain and cardiac tumors with neonatal tuberous sclerosis [abstract], *Brain Dev* 12:358, 1990.
153. Sugita K, Itoh K, Takeuchi Y, Cho H, et al: Tuberous sclerosis: Report of two cases studied by computer-assisted cranial tomography within one week after birth, *Brain Dev* 7:438-443, 1985.
154. Lago P, Boniver C, Casara GL, Laverda AM, et al: Neonatal tuberous sclerosis presenting with intractable seizures, *Brain Dev* 16:257-259, 1994.
155. Miller SP, Tasch T, Sylvain M, Farmer J-P, et al: Tuberous sclerosis complex and neonatal seizures, *J Child Neurol* 13:619-623, 1998.

156. Bordarier C, Lellouch-Tubiana A, Robain O: Cardiac rhabdomyoma and tuberous sclerosis in three fetuses: A neuropathological study, *Brain Dev* 16:467-471, 1995.
157. Datta AN, Hahn CD, Sahin M: Clinical presentation and diagnosis of tuberous sclerosis complex in infancy, 2007, *J Child Neurol* (in press).
158. Milunsky A, Shim SH, Ito M, Jaekle RK, et al: Precise prenatal diagnosis of tuberous sclerosis by sequencing the TSC2 gene, *Prenat Diagn* 25:582-585, 2005.
159. Fesslova V, Villa L, Rizzuti T, Mastrangelo M, et al: Natural history and long-term outcome of cardiac rhabdomyomas detected prenatally, *Prenat Diagn* 24:241-248, 2004.
160. Levine D, Barnes P, Korf B, Edelman R: Tuberous sclerosis in the fetus: Second-trimester diagnosis of subependymal tubers with ultrafast MR imaging, *AJR Am J Roentgenol* 175:1067-1069, 2000.
161. Probst A, Ohnacker H: Tuberous sclerosis in a premature infant [author's transl], *Acta Neuropathol (Berl)* 40:157-161, 1977.
162. Barth PG, Stam FC, von der Harten JJ: Tuberous sclerosis and dysplasia of the corpus callosum: Case report of their combined occurrence in a newborn, *Acta Neuropathol (Berl)* 42:63-64, 1978.
163. Thibault JH, Manuelidis EE: Tuberous sclerosis in a premature infant: Report of a case and review of the literature, *Neurology* 20:139-146, 1970.
164. Seidenwurm DJ, Barkovich AJ: Understanding tuberous sclerosis, *Radiology* 183:23-24, 1992.
165. Griffiths PD, Martland TR: Tuberous sclerosis complex: The role of neuroradiology, *Neuropediatrics* 28:244-252, 1997.
166. Inoue Y, Nemoto Y, Murata R, Tashiro T, et al: CT and MR imaging of cerebral tuberous sclerosis, *Brain Dev* 20:209-221, 1998.
167. Oikawa S, Sakamoto K, Kobayashi N: A neonatal huge subependymal giant cell astrocytoma: Case report, *Neurosurgery* 35:748-750, 1994.
168. Area G, Pacheco E, Alfonso I, Duchowny MS, et al: Characteristic brain magnetic resonance imaging (MRI) findings in neonates with tuberous sclerosis complex, *J Child Neurol* 21:280-285, 2006.
169. Raju GP, Urion DK, Sahin M: Neonatal subependymal giant cell astrocytoma: New case and review of literature, *Pediatr Neurol* 36:128-131, 2007.
170. Frank LM, Chaves-Carballo E, Earley LM: Early diagnosis of tuberous sclerosis by cranial ultrasonography, *Arch Neurol* 41:1302-1303, 1984.
171. Legge M, Sauerbrei E, Macdonald A: Intracranial tuberous sclerosis in infancy, *Radiology* 153:667-668, 1984.
172. Bell DG, King BF, Hattery RR, Charboneau JW, et al: Imaging characteristics of tuberous sclerosis, *AJR Am J Roentgenol* 156:1081-1086, 1991.
173. Stricker T, Zuerrer M, Martin E, Boesch C: MRI of two infants with tuberous sclerosis, *Neuroradiology* 33:175-177, 1991.
174. Griffiths PD, Bolton P, Verity C: White matter abnormalities in tuberous sclerosis complex, *Acta Radiol* 39:482-486, 1998.
175. Kandt RS: Tuberous sclerosis: The next step, *J Child Neurol* 8:107-111, 1993.
176. Franz DN: Diagnosis and management of tuberous sclerosis complex, *Semin Pediatr Neurol* 5:253-267, 1998.
177. Crino PB, Henske EP: New developments in the neurobiology of the tuberous sclerosis complex, *Neurology* 53:1384-1390, 1999.
178. Simko A, Hornstein L, Soukup S, Bagamery N: Fragile X syndrome: Recognition in young children, *Pediatrics* 83:547-552, 1989.
179. Chudley AE, Hagerman RJ: Fragile X syndrome, *J Pediatr* 110:821-831, 1987.
180. Budka H: Megalencephaly and chromosomal anomaly, *Acta Neuropathol (Berl)* 43:263-266, 1978.
181. Drigo P, Carra S, Laverda AM, Artifoni L: Macrocephaly and chromosome disorders: A case report, *Brain Dev* 18:312-315, 1996.
182. Fitz CR, Harwood-Nash DC, Boldt DW: The radiographic features of unilateral megalencephaly, *Neuroradiology* 15:145-148, 1978.
183. Mikhael MA, Mattar AG: Malformation of the cerebral cortex with heterotopia of the gray matter, *J Comput Assist Tomogr* 2:291-296, 1978.
184. Laurence KM: The natural history of spina bifida cystica, *Arch Dis Child* 39:41, 1964.
185. Townsend JJ, Nielsen SL, Malamud N: Unilateral megalencephaly: Hamartoma or neoplasm? *Neurology* 25:448-453, 1975.
186. Bignami A, Palladini G, Zappella M: Unilateral megalencephaly with nerve cell hypertrophy: An anatomical and quantitative histochemical study, *Brain Res* 9:103-114, 1968.
187. Tjiam AT, Stefanko S, Schenk VW, de Vlieger M: Infantile spasms associated with hemihypsarrhythmia and hemimegalencephaly, *Dev Med Child Neurol* 20:779-798, 1978.
188. Manz HJ, Phillips TM, Rowden G, McCullough DC: Unilateral megalencephaly, cerebral cortical dysplasia, neuronal hypertrophy, and heterotopia: Cytomorphometric, fluorometric cytochemical, and biochemical analyses, *Acta Neuropathol (Berl)* 45:97-103, 1979.
189. Robain O, Lyon G: Familial microcephalies due to cerebral malformation: Anatomical and clinical study, *Acta Neuropathol (Berl)* 20:96-109, 1972.
190. Takashima S, Chan F, Becker LE, Houdou S, et al: Cortical cytoarchitectural and immunohistochemical studies on Zellweger syndrome, *Brain Dev* 13:158-162, 1991.
191. Jahan R, Mischel PS, Curran JG, Peacock WJ, et al: Bilateral neuropathologic changes in a child with hemimegalencephaly, *Pediatr Neurol* 17:344-349, 1997.

192. Tsuru A, Mizuguchi M, Uyemura K, Becker LE, et al: Immunohistochemical expression of cell adhesion molecule L1 in hemimegalencephaly, *Pediatr Neurol* 16:45-49, 1997.

193. Woo CLF, Chuang SH, Becker LE, Jay V, et al: Radiologic-pathologic correlation in focal cortical dysplasia and hemimegalencephaly in 18 children, *Pediatr Neurol* 25:295-303, 2001.

194. D'Agostino MD, Bastos A, Piras C, Bernasconi A, et al: Posterior quadrantic dysplasia or hemi-hemimegalencephaly: A characteristic brain malformation, *Neurology* 62:2214-2220, 2004.

195. Flores-Sarnat L: Hemimegalencephaly. I. Genetic, clinical, and imaging aspects, *J Child Neurol* 16:373-384, 2002.

196. Flores-Sarnat L, Sarnat HB, Davila-Gutierrez G, Alvarez A: Hemimegalencephaly. II. Neuropathology suggests a disorder of cellular lineage, *J Child Neurol* 18:776-785, 2003.

197. Paladin F, Chiron C, Dulac O, Plouin P, et al: Electroencephalographic aspects of hemimegalencephaly, *Dev Med Child Neurol* 31:377-383, 1989.

198. Fusco L, Vigevano F: Reversible operculum syndrome caused by progressive epilepsia partialis continua in a child with left hemimegalencephaly, *J Neurol Neurosurg Psychiatry* 54:556-558, 1991.

199. Konkol RJ, Maister BH, Wells RG, Sty JR: Hemimegalencephaly: Clinical, EEG, neuroimaging, and IMP-SPECT correlation, *Pediatr Neurol* 6:414-418, 1990.

200. Vigevano F, Di Rocco C: Effectiveness of hemispherectomy in hemimegalencephaly with intractable seizures, *Neuropediatrics* 21:222-223, 1990.

201. Vigevano F, Bertini E, Boldrini R, Bosman C, et al: Hemimegalencephaly and intractable epilepsy: Benefits of hemispherectomy, *Epilepsia* 30:833-843, 1989.

202. Appleton R, Gardner-Medwin D, Mendelow D: Hemispherectomy for intractable seizures [letter], *Dev Med Child Neurol* 33:273-274, 1991.

203. Bermejo AM, Martin VL, Arcas J, Perez HA, et al: Early infantile epileptic encephalopathy: A case associated with hemimegalencephaly, *Brain Dev* 14:425-428, 1992.

204. Tagawa T, Futagi Y, Arai H, Mushiake S, et al: Hypomelanosis of Ito associated with hemimegalencephaly: A clinicopathological study, *Pediatr Neurol* 17:180-184, 1997.

205. Bonioli EV, Bertola A, Di Stefano A, Bellini C: Sebaceous nevus syndrome: Report of two cases, *Pediatr Neurol* 17:77-79, 1997.

206. Alfonso I, Papazian O, Villalobos R, Acosta JI: Similar brain SPECT findings in subclinical and clinical seizures in two neonates with hemimegalencephaly, *Pediatr Neurol* 19:132-134, 1998.

207. Ohtsuka Y, Ohno S, Oka E: Electroclinical characteristics of hemimegalencephaly, *Pediatr Neurol* 20:390-393, 1999.

208. Battaglia D, Di Rocco C, Iuvone L, Acquafondata C, et al: Neurocognitive development and epilepsy outcome in children with surgically treated hemimegalencephaly, *Neuropediatrics* 30:307-313, 1999.

209. Mohamedbhai AG, Miyan AMH, Lacombe D: Neonatal Proteus syndrome? *Am J Med Genet* 112:228-230, 2002.

210. Antonelli A, Chiaretti A, Amendola T, Piastra M, et al: Nerve growth factor and brain-derived neurotrophic factor in human paediatric hemimegalencephaly, *Neuropediatrics* 35:39-44, 2004.

211. Rintahaka PJ, Chugani HT, Messa C, Phelps ME: Hemimegalencephaly: Evaluation with positron emission tomography, *Pediatr Neurol* 9:21-28, 1993.

212. Soufflet C, Bulteau C, Delalande T, Pinton F, et al: The nonmalformed hemisphere is secondarily impaired in young children with hemimegalencephaly: A pre- and postsurgery study with SPECT and EEG, *Epilepsia* 45:1375-1382, 2004.

213. Dobyns WB, Garg BP: Vascular abnormalities in epidermal nevus syndrome, *Neurology* 41:276-278, 1991.

214. Kwa VIH, Smitt JHS, Verbeeten BWJ, Barth PG: Epidermal nevus syndrome with isolated enlargement of one temporal lobe: A case report, *Brain Dev* 17:122-125, 1995.

215. Gurecki PJ, Holden KR, Sahn EE, Dyer DS, et al: Developmental neural abnormalities and seizures in epidermal nevus syndrome, *Dev Med Child Neurol* 38:716-723, 1996.

216. Pavone L, Curatolo P, Rizzo R, Micali G, et al: Epidermal nevus syndrome: A neurologic variant with hemimegalencephaly, gyral malformation, mental retardation, seizures, and facial hemihypertrophy, *Neurology* 41:266-271, 1991.

217. Hager BC, Dyme IZ, Guertin SR, Tyler RJ, et al: Linear nevus sebaceous syndrome: Megalencephaly and heterotopic gray matter, *Pediatr Neurol* 7:45-49, 1991.

218. Sakuta R, Aikawa H, Takashima S, Ryo S: Epidermal nevus syndrome with hemimegalencephaly: Neuropathological study, *Brain Dev* 13:260-265, 1991.

219. Sarwar M, Schafer ME: Brain malformations in linear nevus sebaceous syndrome: An MR study, *J Comput Assist Tomogr* 12:338-340, 1988.

220. Chalhub EG, Volpe JJ, Gado MH: Linear nevus sebaceous syndrome associated with porencephaly and nonfunctioning major cerebral venous sinuses, *Neurology* 25:857-860, 1975.

221. el-Shanti H, Bell WE, Waziri MH: Epidermal nevus syndrome: Subgroup with neuronal migration defects, *J Child Neurol* 7:29-34, 1992.

222. McCall S, Ramzy MI, Cure JK, Pai GS: Encephalocraniocutaneous lipomatosis and the Proteus syndrome: Distinct entities with overlapping manifestations, *Am J Med Genet* 43:662-668, 1992.

223. Kousseff BG: Hypothesis: Jadassohn nevus phakomatosis—a paracrinopathy with variable phenotype, *Am J Med Genet* 43:651-661, 1992.

224. Griffiths PD, Welch RJ, Gardner-Medwin D, Cholkar A, et al: The radiological features of hemimegalencephaly including three cases associated with Proteus syndrome, *Neuropediatrics* 25:140-144, 1994.

225. Sidman RL, Rakic P: Neuronal migration, with special reference to developing human brain: A review, *Brain Res* 62:1-35, 1973.

226. Rakic P: Cell migration and neuronal ectopias in the brain, *Birth Defects* 11:95-129, 1975.

227. Rakic P: Neuronal migration and contact guidance in the primate telencephalon, *Postgrad Med J* 54:25-40, 1978.

228. Rakic P: Principles of neural cell migration, *Experientia* 46:882-891, 1990.

229. Gadisseux JF, Evrard P, Misson JP, Caviness VS: Dynamic structure of the radial glial fiber system of the developing murine cerebral wall: An immunocytochemical analysis, *Dev Brain Res* 50:55-67, 1989.

230. Gadisseux JF, Kadhim HJ, van den Bosch de Aguilar P, Caviness VS, et al: Neuron migration within the radial glial fiber system of the developing murine cerebrum: An electron microscopic autoradiographic analysis, *Dev Brain Res* 52:39-56, 1990.

231. Misson J-P, Edwards MA, Yamamoto M, Caviness VS: Identification of radial glial cells within the developing murine central nervous system: Studies based upon a new immunohistochemical marker, *Dev Brain Res* 44:95-108, 1988.

232. Liesi P: Extracellular matrix and neuronal movement, *Experientia* 46:900-907, 1990.

233. Austin CP, Cepko CL: Cellular migration patterns in the developing mouse cerebral cortex, *Development* 110:713-732, 1990.

234. Walsh C, Cepko CL: Cell lineage and cell migration in the developing cerebral cortex, *Experientia* 46:940-947, 1990.

235. Walsh C, Cepko CL: Clonally related cortical cells show several migration patterns, *Science* 241:1342-1345, 1988.

236. Gray GE, Leber SM, Sanes JR: Migratory patterns of clonally related cells in the developing central nervous system, *Experientia* 46:929-940, 1990.

237. Luskin MB, Pearlman AL, Sanes JR: Cell lineage in the cerebral cortex of the mouse studied in vivo and in vitro with a recombinant retrovirus, *Neuron* 1:635-647, 1988.

238. Crandall JE, Misson JP, Butler D: The development of radial glia and radial dendrites during barrel formation in mouse somatosensory cortex, *Dev Brain Res* 55:87-94, 1990.

239. Gadisseux JF, Evrard PH, Misson JP, Caviness VS: Dynamic changes in the density of radial glial fibers of the developing murine cerebral wall: A quantitative immunohistological analysis, *J Comp Neurol* 321:1-9, 1992.

240. O'Rourke NA, Dailey ME, Smith SJ, Mcconnell SK: Diverse migratory pathways in the developing cerebral cortex, *Science* 258:299-302, 1992.

241. Mrzljak L, Uylings HBM, Van Eden CG, Judas M: Neuronal development in human prefrontal cortex in prenatal and postnatal stages, *Prog Brain Res* 85:185-222, 1990.

242. Zecevic N: Cellular composition of the telencephalic wall in human embryos, *Early Hum Dev* 32:131-149, 1993.

243. Komuro H, Rakic P: Selective role of N-type calcium channels in neuronal migration, *Science* 257:806-809, 1992.

244. Komuro H, Rakic P: Modulation of neuronal migration by NMDA receptors, *Science* 260:95-97, 1993.

245. Rakic P: Radial versus tangential migration of neuronal clones in the developing cerebral cortex, *Proc Natl Acad Sci U S A* 92:11323-11327, 1995.

246. Leber SM, Sanes JR: Migratory paths of neurons and glia in the embryonic chick spinal cord, *J Neurosci* 15:1236-1248, 1995.

247. O'Rourke NA, Chenn A, McConnell SK: Postmitotic neurons migrate tangentially in the cortical ventricular zone, *Development* 124:997-1005, 1997.

248. Gleeson JG, Walsh CA: New genetic insights into cerebral cortical development. In Galaburda AM, Christen Y, editors: *Normal and Abnormal Development of Cortex*, Berlin: 1997, Springer-Verlag.

249. Pearlman AL, Faust PL, Hatten ME, Brunstrom JE: New directions for neuronal migration, *Curr Opin Neurobiol* 8:45-54, 1998.

250. Komuro H, Rakic P: Distinct modes of neuronal migration in different domains of developing cerebellar cortex, *J Neurosci* 18:1478-1490, 1998.

251. Hatten ME: Central nervous system neuronal migration, *Annu Rev Neurosci* 22:511-539, 1999.

252. Walsh CA: Genetic malformations of the human cerebral cortex, *Neuron* 23:19-29, 1999.

253. Walsh CA: Genetics of neuronal migration in the cerebral cortex, *Ment Retard Dev Disabil Res Rev* 6:34-40, 2000.

254. Zecevic N, Rakic P: Development of layer I neurons in the primate cerebral cortex, *J Neurosci* 21:5607-5619, 2001.

255. Rakic P: Elusive radial glial cells: Historical and evolutionary perspective, *Glia* 43:19-32, 2003.

256. Rakic P: Developmental and evolutionary adaptations of cortical radial glia, *Cereb Cortex* 13:541-549, 2003.

257. Kato M, Dobyns WB: Lissencephaly and the molecular basis of neuronal migration, *Hum Mol Genet* 12:R89-R96, 2003.

258. Bielas S, Higginbotham H, Koizumi H, Tanaka T, et al: Cortical neuronal migration mutants suggest separate but intersecting pathways, *Annu Rev Cell Dev Biol* 20:593-618, 2004.

259. Kriegstein AR, Noctor SC: Patterns of neuronal migration in the embryonic cortex, *Trends Neurosci* 27:392-399, 2004.

260. Kanatani S, Tabata H, Nakajima K: Neuronal migration in cortical development, *J Child Neurol* 20:274-279, 2005.

261. Guerrini R, Filippi T: Neuronal migration disorders, genetics, and epileptogenesis, *J Child Neurol* 20:287-299, 2005.

262. McManus MF, Golden JA: Neuronal migration in developmental disorders, *J Child Neurol* 20:280-286, 2005.

263. Nadarajah B, Brunstrom JE, Grutzendler J, Wong ROL, et al: Two modes of radial migration in early development of the cerebral cortex, *Nat Neurosci* 4:143-150, 2001.

264. Rakic P: Mode of cell migration to the superficial layers of fetal monkey neocortex, *J Comp Neurol* 145:61-83, 1972.

265. Antanitus DS, Choi BH, Lapham LW: The demonstration of glial fibrillary acidic protein in the cerebrum of the human fetus by indirect immunofluorescence, *Brain Res* 103:613-616, 1976.

266. Marin-Padilla M: Cajal-Retzius cells in the development of the neocortex, *Trends Neurosci* 21:64-71, 1998.

267. Sheppard AM, Hamilton SK, Pearlman AL: Changes in the distribution of extracellular matrix components accompany early morphogenetic events of mammalian cortical development, *J Neurosci* 11:3928-3942, 1991.

268. Stipp CS, Litwack ED, Lander AD: Cerebroglycan: An integral membrane heparan sulfate proteoglycan that is unique to the developing nervous system and expressed specifically during neuronal differentiation, *J Cell Biol* 124:149-160, 1994.

269. Sheppard AM, Brunstrom JE, Thornton TN, Gerfen RW, et al: Neuronal production of fibronectin in the cerebral cortex during migration and layer formation is unique to specific cortical domains, *Dev Biol* 172:504-518, 1995.

270. Rakic P, Caviness VS: Cortical development: View from neurological mutants two decades later, *Neuron* 14:1101-1104, 1995.

271. D'Arcangelo G, Nakajima K, Miyata T, Ogawa M, et al: Reelin is a secreted glycoprotein recognized by the CR-50, *J Neurosci* 17:23-31, 1997.

272. Meyer G, Goffinet AM: Prenatal development of reelin-immunoreactive neurons in the human neocortex, *J Comp Neurol* 397:29-40, 1998.

273. Frotscher M, Haas CA, Forster E: Reelin controls granule cell migration in the dentate gyrus by acting on the radial glial scaffold, *Cereb Cortex* 13:634-640, 2003.

274. Tissir F, Goffinet AM: Reelin and brain development, *Nature Rev Neurosci* 4:496-505, 2003.

275. Albrecht U, AbuIssa R, Ratz B, Hattori M, et al: Platelet-activating factor acetylhydrolase expression and activity suggest a link between neuronal migration and platelet-activating factor, *Dev Biol* 180:579-593, 1996.

276. Clark GD, McNeil RS, Swann JW, Bix GJ: Platelet-activating factor produces neuronal growth cone collapse, *Neuroreport* 6:2569-2575, 1995.

277. Clark GD, Mizuguchi M, Antalffy B, Barnes J, et al: Predominant localization of the LIS family of gene products to Cajal-Retzius cells and ventricular neuroepithelium in the developing human cortex, *J Neuropathol Exp Neurol* 56:1044-1052, 1997.

278. Manent JB, Demarque M, Jorquera I, Pellegrino C, et al: A noncanonical release of GABA and glutamate modulates neuronal migration, *J Neurosci* 25:4755-4765, 2005.

279. Rio C, Rieff HI, Qi P, Corfas G: Neuregulin and erbB receptors play a critical role in neuronal migration, *Neuron* 19:39-50, 1997.

280. Anton ES, Marchionni MA, Lee KF, Rakic P: Role of GGF/neuregulin signaling in interactions between migrating neurons and radial glia in the developing cerebral cortex, *Development* 124:3501-3510, 1997.

281. Fishell G, Hatten ME: Astrotactin provides a receptor system for CNS neuronal migration, *Development* 113:755-765, 1991.

282. Zheng C, Heintz N, Hatten ME: CNS gene encoding astrotactin, which supports neuronal migration along glial fibers, *Science* 272:417-419, 1996.

283. Gleeson JG, Allen KM, Fox JW, Lamperti ED, et al: Doublecortin, a brain-specific gene mutated in human X-linked lissencephaly and double cortex syndrome, encodes a putative signaling protein, *Cell* 92:63-72, 1998.

284. Gleeson JG, Minnerath SR, Fox JW, Allen KM, et al: Characterization of mutations in the gene doublecortin in patients with double cortex syndrome, *Ann Neurol* 45:146-153, 1999.

285. Gleeson JG, Lin PT, Flanagan L, Walsh CA: Doublecortin is a microtubule-associated protein and is expressed widely by migrating neurons, *Neuron* 23:257-271, 1999.

286. Francis F, Koulakoff A, Boucher D, Chafey P, et al: Doublecortin is a developmentally regulated, microtubule-associated protein expressed in migrating and differentiating neurons, *Neuron* 23:247-256, 1999.

287. Friocourt G, Koulakoff A, Chafey P, Boucher D, et al: Doublecortin functions at the extremities of growing neuronal processes, *Cereb Cortex* 13:620-626, 2003.

288. Fox JW, Lamperti ED, Eksioglu YZ, Hong SE, et al: Mutations in filamin 1 prevent migration of cerebral cortical neurons in human periventricular heterotopia, *Neuron* 21:1315-1325, 1999.

289. Rossi DJ, Slater NT: The developmental onset of NMDA receptor-channel activity during neuronal migration, *Neuropharmacology* 32:1239-1248, 1993.

290. Rakic P, Komuro H: The role of receptor/channel activity in neuronal cell migration, *J Neurobiol* 26:299-315, 1995.

291. Hirai K, Yoshioka H, Kihara M, Hasegawa K, et al: Inhibiting neuronal migration by blocking NMDA receptors in the embryonic rat cerebral cortex: A tissue culture study, *Dev Brain Res* 114:63-67, 1999.

292. Behar TN, Scott CA, Greene CL, Wen XL, et al: Glutamate acting at NMDA receptors stimulates embryonic cortical neuronal migration, *J Neurosci* 19:4449-4461, 1999.

293. Kumada T, Komuro H: Completion of neuronal migration regulated by loss of Ca2+ transients, *Proc Natl Acad Sci U S A* 101:8479-8484, 2004.

294. Reiprich P, Kilb W, Luhmann HJ: Neonatal NMDA receptor blockade disturbs neuronal migration in rat somatosensory cortex in vivo, *Cereb Cortex* 15:349-358, 2005.

295. Chi JG, Dooling EC, Gilles FH: Gyral development of the human brain, *Ann Neurol* 1:86-93, 1977.

296. Larroche JC: *Developmental Pathology of the Neonate*, New York: 1977, Excerpta Medica.

297. Welker W: Why does cerebral cortex fissure and fold? A review of determinants of gyri and sulci. In Jones EG, Peters A, editors: *Cerebral Cortex*, New York: 1990, Plenum.

298. Ruoss K, Lovblad K, Schroth G, Moessinger AC, et al: Brain development (sulci and gyri) as assessed by early postnatal MR imaging in preterm and term newborn infants, *Neuropediatrics* 32:69-74, 2001.

299. Richman DP, Stewart RM, Hutchinson JW: Mechanical model of brain convolutional development, *Science* 189:18-24, 1975.

300. Van Essen DC: A tension-based theory of morphogenesis and compact wiring in the central nervous system, *Nature* 385:313-318, 1997.

301. Yakovlev PI, Wadsworth RC: Schizencephalies: A study of the congenital clefts in the cerebral mantle. I. Clefts with fused lips, *J Neuropathol Exp Neurol* 5:116-137, 1946.

302. Yakovlev PI, Wadsworth RC: Schizencephalies: A study of the congenital clefts in the cerebral mantle. II. Clefts with hydrocephalus and lips separated, *J Neuropathol Exp Neurol* 5:169-181, 1946.

303. Barth PG: Disorders of neuronal migration, *Can J Neurol Sci* 14:1-16, 1987.

304. Barth PG: Schizencephaly and nonlissencephalic cortical dysplasias, *AJNR Am J Neuroradiol* 13:104-106, 1992.

305. Senol U, Karaali K, Aktekin B, Yilmaz S, et al: Dizygotic twins with schizencephaly and focal cortical dysplasia, *AJNR Am J Neuroradiol* 21:1520-1521, 2000.

306. Denis D, Chateil J-F, Brun M, Brissaud O, et al: Schizencephaly: Clinical and imaging features in, 30 infantile cases, *Brain Dev* 22:475-483, 2000.

307. Granata T, Freri E, Caccia C, Setola V, et al: Schizencephaly: Clinical spectrum, epilepsy, and pathogenesis, *J Child Neurol* 20:313-318, 2005.

308. Lim CCT, Yin H, Loh NK, Chua VGE, et al: Malformations of cortical development: High-resolution MR and diffusion tensor imaging of fiber tracts at, *AJNR Am J Neuroradiol* 26:61-64, 2005.

309. Curry CJ, Lammer EJ, Nelson V, Shaw GM: Schizencephaly: Heterogeneous etiologies in a population of 4 million California births, *Am J Med Genet A* 137:181-189, 2005.

310. Robinson RO: Familial schizencephaly, *Dev Med Child Neurol* 33:1010-1012, 1991.

311. Zonana J, Adornato BT, Glass ST, Webb MJ: Familial porencephaly and congenital hemiplegia, *J Pediatr* 109:671-674, 1986.

312. Hilburger AC, Willis JK, Bouldin E, Henderson-Tilton A: Familial schizencephaly, *Brain Dev* 15:234-236, 1993.

313. Haverkamp F, Zerres K, Ostertun B, Emons D, et al: Familial schizencephaly: Further delineation of a rare disorder, *J Med Genet* 32:242-244, 1995.

314. Bonnemann GC, Meinecke P: Bilateral porencephaly, cerebellar hypoplasia and internal malformations: Two siblings representing a probably new autosomal recessive entity, *Am J Med Genet* 63:428-433, 1996.

315. Granata T, Farina L, Faiella A, Cardini R, et al: Familial schizencephaly associated with EMX2 mutation, *Neurology* 48:1403-1406, 1997.

316. Packard AM, Miller VS, Delgado MR: Schizencephaly: Correlations of clinical and radiologic features, *Neurology* 48:1427-1434, 1997.

317. Aguglia U, Gambardella A, Breedveld GJ, Oliveri RL, et al: Suggestive evidence for linkage to chromosome, 13qter for autosomal dominant type, 1 porencephaly, *Neurology* 62:1613-1615, 2004.

318. Barkovich AJ, Kjos BO: Schizencephaly: Correlation of clinical findings with MR characteristics, *AJNR Am J Neuroradiol* 13:85-94, 1992.

319. Norman MG: Bilateral encephaloclastic lesions in a 26 week gestation fetus: Effect on neuroblast migration, *Can J Neurol Sci* 7:191-194, 1980.

320. Bordarier C, Robain O, Ponsot G: Bilateral porencephalic defect in a newborn after injection of benzol during pregnancy, *Brain Dev* 13:126-129, 1991.

321. Mancini J, Lethel V, Hugonenq C, Chabrol B: Brain injuries in early foetal life: Consequences for brain development, *Dev Med Child Neurol* 43:52-55, 2001.

322. Brunelli S, Faiella A, Capra V: Germline mutations in the homeobox gene EMX2 in patients with severe schizencephaly, *Nat Genet* 12:94-96, 1996.

323. Gulisano M, Broccoli V, Pardini C, Boncinelli E: Emx1 and Emx2 show different patterns of expression during proliferation and differentiation of the developing cerebral cortex in the mouse, *Eur J Neurosci* 8:1037-1050, 1996.

324. Muzio L, Mallamaci A: Emx1, Emx2 and Pax6 in specification, regionalization and arealization of the cerebral cortex, *Cereb Cortex* 13:641-647, 2003.

325. Iannetti P, Nigro G, Spalice A, Faiella A, et al: Cytomegalovirus infection and schizencephaly: Case reports, *Ann Neurol* 43:123-127, 1998.

326. Chamberlain MC, Press GA, Bejar RF: Neonatal schizencephaly: Comparison of brain imaging, *Pediatr Neurol* 6:382-387, 1990.

327. Buckley AR, Flodmark O, Roland EH, Hill A: Neuronal migration abnormalities can still be diagnosed by computed tomography! *Pediatr Neurosci* 14:222-229, 1988.

328. Barkovich AJ, Chuang SH, Norman D: MR of neuronal migration anomalies, *AJNR Am J Neuroradiol* 8:1009-1017, 1988.

329. Barkovich AJ, Norman D: MR imaging of schizencephaly, *AJNR Am J Neuroradiol* 9:297-302, 1988.

330. Aniskiewicz AS, Frumkin NL, Brady DE, Moore JB, et al: Magnetic resonance imaging and neurobehavioral correlates in schizencephaly, *Arch Neurol* 47:911-916, 1990.

331. Yasumori K, Hasuo K, Nagata S, Masuda K, et al: Neuronal migration anomalies causing extensive ventricular indentation, *Neurosurgery* 26:504-507, 1990.

332. Leblanc R, Tampieri D, Robitaille Y, Feindel W, et al: Surgical treatment of intractable epilepsy associated with schizencephaly, *Neurosurgery* 29:421-429, 1991.

333. Miller JQ: Lissencephaly in two siblings, *Neurology* 18:841-850, 1963.

334. Norman RM: Malformations of the nervous system, birth injury, and diseases of early life. In Blackwood W, McMenemy WH, Meyer A, et al, editors: *Greenfield's Neuropathology*, Baltimore: 1967, Williams & Wilkins.

335. Dieker H, Edwards RH, Zurhein G: The lissencephaly syndrome, *Birth Defects* 5:53, 1969.

336. Garcia CA, Dunn D, Trevor R: The lissencephaly (agyria) syndrome in siblings: Computerized tomographic and neuropathologic findings, *Arch Neurol* 35:608-611, 1978.

337. Norman MG, Roberts M, Sirois J, Tremblay LJ: Lissencephaly, *Can J Neurol Sci* 3:39-46, 1976.

338. Dobyns WB, Stratton RF, Greenberg F: Syndromes with lissencephaly. I. Miller-Dieker and Norman-Roberts syndromes and isolated lissencephaly, *Am J Med Genet* 18:509-526, 1984.

339. Crome L: Pachygyria, *J Pathol Bacteriol* 71:335-352, 1956.

340. Hanaway J, Lee SI, Netsky NG: Pachygyria: Relation of findings to modern embryologic concepts, *Neurology* 18:791-799, 1968.

341. Aicardi J: The agyria-pachygyria complex: A spectrum of cortical malformations, *Brain Dev* 13:1-8, 1991.

342. Squier MV: Development of the cortical dysplasia of type-II lissencephaly, *Neuropathol Appl Neurobiol* 19:209-213, 1993.

343. Sebire G, Goutieres F, Tardieu M, Landrieu P, et al: Extensive macrogyri or no visible gyri: Distinct clinical, electroencephalographic, and genetic features according to different imaging patterns, *Neurology* 45:1105-1111, 1995.

344. Dobyns WB, Andermann E, Andermann F, Czapansky-Beilman D, et al: X-linked malformations of neuronal migration, *Neurology* 47:331-339, 1996.

345. Barkovich AJ, Kuzniecky RI, Dopbyns WB, Jackson GD, et al: A classification scheme for malformations of cortical development, *Neuropediatrics* 27:59-63, 1996.

346. Fogli A, Guerrini R, Moro F, Fernandez-Alvarez E, et al: Intracellular levels of the LIS1 protein correlate with clinical and neuroradiological findings in patients with classical lissencephaly, *Ann Neurol* 45:154-161, 1999.

347. Forman MS, Squier W, Dobyns WB, Golden JA: Genotypically defined lissencephalies show distinct pathologies, *J Neuropathol Exp Neurol* 64:847-857, 2005.

348. Ferrie CD, Jackson GD, Giannakodimos S, Panayiotopoulos CP: Posterior agyria-pachygyria with polymicrogyria: Evidence for an inherited neuronal migration disorder, *Neurology* 45:150-153, 1995.

349. Fox JW, Walsh CA: Neurogenetics '99: Periventricular heterotopia and the genetics of neuronal migration in the cerebral cortex, *J Hum Genet* 65:19-24, 1999.

350. Kato M, Takizawa N, Yamada S, Ito A, et al: Diffuse pachygria with cerebellar hypoplasia: A milder form of microlissencephaly or a new genetic syndrome, *Ann Neurol* 46:660-663, 1999.

351. Ramirez D, Lammer EJ, Johnson CB, Peterson CD: Autosomal recessive frontotemporal pachygyria, *Am J Med Genet A* 124:231-238, 2004.

352. Rossi M, Guerrini R, Dobyns WB, Andria G, et al: Characterization of brain malformations in the Baraitser-Winter syndrome and review of the literature, *Neuropediatrics* 34:287-292, 2003.

353. Kurul S, Cakmakci H, Dirik E: Agyria-pachygyria complex: MR findings and correlation with clinical features, *Pediatr Neurol* 30:16-23, 2004.

354. Choi BH, Lapham LW, Amin-Zaki L, Saleem T: Abnormal neuronal migration, deranged cerebral cortical organization, and diffuse white matter astrocytosis of human fetal brain: A major effect of methylmercury poisoning in utero, *J Neuropathol Exp Neurol* 37:719-733, 1978.

355. de Rijk-van Andel JF, Arts WF, Barth PG, Loonen MC: Diagnostic features and clinical signs of 21 patients with lissencephaly type 1, *Dev Med Child Neurol* 32:707-717, 1990.

356. Gastaut H, Pinsard N, Raybaud C, Aicardi J, et al: Lissencephaly (agyria-pachygyria): Clinical findings and serial EEG studies, *Dev Med Child Neurol* 29:167-180, 1987.

357. Hayward JC, Titelbaum DS, Clancy RR, Zimmerman RA: Lissencephaly-pachygyria associated with congenital cytomegalovirus infection, *J Child Neurol* 6:109-114, 1991.

358. Harbord MG, Boyd S, Hall-Craggs MA, Kendall B, et al: Ataxia, developmental delay and an extensive neuronal migration abnormality in 2 siblings, *Neuropediatrics* 21:218-221, 1990.

359. de Rijk-van Andel JF, Arts WF, de Weerd AW: EEG and evoked potentials in a series of 21 patients with lissencephaly type I, *Neuropediatrics* 23:4-9, 1992.

360. Ledbetter SA, Kuwano A, Dobyns WB, Ledbetter DH: Microdeletions of chromosome 17p13 as a cause of isolated lissencephaly, *Am J Hum Genet* 50:182-189, 1992.

361. Pavone L, Gullotta F, Incorpora G, Grasso S, et al: Isolated lissencephaly: Report of four patients from two unrelated families, *J Child Neurol* 5:52-59, 1990.

362. Krawinkel M, Steen HJ, Terwey B: Magnetic resonance imaging in lissencephaly, *Eur J Pediatr* 146:205-208, 1987.

363. Barkovich AJ, Koch TK, Carrol CL: The spectrum of lissencephaly: Report of ten patients analyzed by magnetic resonance imaging, *Ann Neurol* 30:139-146, 1991.

364. Dobyns WB: The neurogenetics of lissencephaly, *Neurol Clin* 7:89-105, 1989.

365. Dobyns WB, Elias ER, Newlin AC, Pagon RA, et al: Causal heterogeneity in isolated lissencephaly, *Neurology* 42:1375-1388, 1992.

366. Palmini A, Andermann F, de Grissac H, Tampieri D, et al: Stages and patterns of centrifugal arrest of diffuse neuronal migration disorders, *Dev Med Child Neurol* 35:331-339, 1993.

367. Mori K, Hashimoto T, Tayama M, Miyazaki M, et al: Serial EEG and sleep polygraphic studies on lissencephaly (agyria-pachygyria), *Brain Dev* 16:365-373, 1994.

368. Hodgkins PR, Kriss A, Boyd S, Chong K, et al: A study of EEG, electroretinogram, visual evoked potential, and eye movements in classical lissencephaly, *Dev Med Child Neurol*, 42:48-52, 2000.

369. Pilz DT, Matsumoto N, Minnerath S, Mills P, et al: LIS1 and XLIS (DCX) mutations cause most classical lissencephaly, but different patterns of malformation, *Hum Mol Genet* 7:2029-2037, 1998.

370. Dobyns WB, Curry CJR, Hoyme HE, Turlington L, et al: Clinical and molecular diagnosis of Miller-Dieker syndrome, *Am J Hum Genet* 48:584-594, 1991.

371. Toyo-oka K, Shionoya A, Gambello MJ, Cardoso C, et al: 14-3-3epsilon is important for neuronal migration by binding to NUDEL: A molecular explanation for Miller-Dieker syndrome, *Nat Genet* 34:274-285, 2003.

372. Bonneau D, Toutain A, Laquerriere A, Marret S, et al: X-linked lissencephaly with absent corpus callosum and ambiguous genitalia (XLAG): Clinical, magnetic resonance imaging, and neuropathological findings, *Ann Neurol* 51:340-349, 2002.

373. Uyanik G, Aigner L, Martin P, Cros C, et al: ARX mutations in X-linked lissencephaly with abnormal genitalia, *Neurology* 61:232-235, 2003.

374. Hahn A, Gross C, Uyanik G, Hehr U, et al: X-linked lissencephaly with abnormal genitalia associated with renal phosphate wasting, *Neuropediatrics* 35:202-205, 2004.

375. Kato M, Das S, Petras K, Kitamura K, et al: Mutations of ARX are associated with striking pleiotropy and consistent genotype-phenotype correlation, *Hum Mutat* 23:147-159, 2004.

376. Kato M, Dobyns WB: X-linked lissencephaly with abnormal genitalia as a tangential migration disorder causing intractable epilepsy: Proposal for a new term, "interneuronopathy," *J Child Neurol* 20:392-397, 2005.

377. Ross ME, Swanson K, Dobyns WB: Lissencephaly with cerebellar hypoplasia (LCH): A heterogeneous group of cortical malformations, *Neuropediatrics* 32:256-263, 2001.

378. Hong SE, Shugart YY, Huang DT, Al Shahwan S, et al: Autosomal recessive lissencephaly with cerebellar hypoplasia is associated with human RELN mutations, *Nat Genet* 26:93-96, 2000.

379. Chang BS, Duzcan F, Kim S, Cinbis M, et al: The role of RELN in lissencephaly and neuropsychiatric disease, *Am J Med Genet B Neuropsychiatr Genet* 144:58-63, 2007.

380. Koizumi H, Tanaka T, Gleeson JG: Doublecortin-like kinase functions with doublecortin to mediate fiber tract decussation and neuronal migration, *Neuron* 49:55-66, 2006.

381. Elias RC, Galera MF, Schnabel B, Briones MR, et al: Deletion of, 17p13 and LIS1 gene mutation in isolated lissencephaly sequence, *Pediatr Neurol* 35:42-46, 2006.

382. Sheen VL, Ferland RJ, Harney M, Hill RS, et al: Impaired proliferation and migration in human Miller-Dieker neural precursors, *Ann Neurol* 60:137-144, 2006.

383. Gleeson JG, Luo RF, Grant PE, Guerrini R, et al: Genetic and neuroradiological heterogeneity of double cortex syndrome, *Ann Neurol* 47:265-269, 2000.

384. LoTurco J: Doublecortin and a tale of two serines, *Neuron* 41:175-177, 2004.

385. Leventer RJ: Genotype-phenotype correlation in lissencephaly and sub-cortical band heterotopia: The key questions answered, *J Child Neurol* 20:307-312, 2005.

386. Stewart RM, Richman DP, Caviness VS: Lissencephaly and pachygyria: Architectonic and topographical analysis, *Acta Neuropathol (Berl)* 31:1, 1975.

387. Al Shawan SA, Bruyn GW, Al Deeb SM: Lissencephaly with pontocerebellar hypoplasia, *J Child Neurol* 11:241-243, 1996.

388. Kroon AA, Smit BJ, Barth PG, Hennekam RCM: Lissencephaly with extreme cerebral and cerebellar hypoplasia: A magnetic resonance imaging study, *Neuropediatrics* 27:273-276, 1996.

389. Sztriha L, Al-Gazali L, Varady E, Nork M, et al: Microlissencephaly, *Pediatr Neurol* 18:362-365, 1998.

390. Dobyns WB, Pagon RA, Armstrong D, Curry CJ, et al: Diagnostic criteria for Walker-Warburg syndrome, *Am J Med Genet* 32:195-210, 1989.

391. Rhodes RE, Hatten HP Jr, Ellington KS: Walker-Warburg syndrome, *AJNR Am J Neuroradiol* 13:123-126, 1992.

392. Miller G, Ladda RL, Towfighi J: Cerebro-ocular dysplasia—muscular dystrophy (Walker Warburg) syndrome: Findings in 20-week-old fetus, *Acta Neuropathol (Berl)* 82:234-238, 1991.

393. Bordarier C, Aicardi J, Goutieres F: Congenital hydrocephalus and eye abnormalities with severe developmental brain defects: Warburg's syndrome, *Ann Neurol* 16:60-65, 1984.

394. Aida N, Tamagawa K, Takada K, Yagishita A, et al: Brain MR in Fukuyama congenital muscular dystrophy, *AJNR Am J Neuroradiol* 17:605-613, 1996.

395. Haltia M, Leivo I, Somer H, Pihko H, et al: Muscle-eye-brain disease: A neuropathological study, *Ann Neurol* 41:173-180, 1997.

396. Santavuori P, Valanne L, Autti T, Haltia M, et al: Muscle-eye-brain disease: Clinical features, visual evoked potentials and brain imaging in 20 patients, *Eur J Pediatr Neurol* 1:41-47, 1998.

397. Kanoff RJ, Curless RG, Petito C, Siatkowski RM, et al: Walker-Warburg syndrome: Neurologic features and muscle membrane structure, *Pediatr Neurol* 18:76-80, 1998.

398. Ross ME: Neurobiology: Full circle to cobbled brain, *Nature* 418:376-377, 2002.

399. Yamamoto T, Kato V, Karita M, Kawaguchi M, et al: Expression of genes related to muscular dystrophy with lissencephaly, *Pediatr Neurol* 31:183-190, 2004.

400. Longman C, Mercuri E, Cowan F, Allsop J, et al: Antenatal and postnatal brain magnetic resonance imaging in muscle-eye-brain disease, *Arch Neurol* 61:1301-1306, 2004.

401. Vervoort VS, Holden KR, Ukadike KC, Collins JS, et al: POMGnT1 gene alterations in a family with neurological abnormalities, *Ann Neurol* 56:143-148, 2004.

402. Currier SC, Lee CK, Chang BS, Bodell AL, et al: Mutations in POMT1 are found in a minority of patients with Walker-Warburg syndrome, *Am J Med Genet A* 133:53-57, 2005.

403. Furuta A, Takashima S, Yokoo H, Rothstein JD, et al: Expression of glutamate transporter subtypes during normal human corticogenesis and type II lissencephaly, *Dev Brain Res* 155:155-164, 2005.

404. Yamamoto T, Kato Y, Kawaguchi M, Shibata N, et al: Expression and localization of fukutin, POMGnT1, and POMT1 in the central nervous system: Consideration for functions of fukutin, *Med Electron Microsc* 37:200-207, 2004.

405. Bielschowsky M, Rose M: Uber die Pathoarchitektonik der micro und pachygyren Rinde und Bezeichnungen zur Morphogenie normaler Rindengebiete, *J Psychol Neurol* 38:42, 1929.

406. Crome L: Microgyria, *J Pathol Bacteriol* 64:479-495, 1952.

407. Barkovich AJ, Rowley H, Bollen A: Correlation of prenatal events with the development of polymicrogyria, *AJNR Am J Neuroradiol* 16:822-827, 1995.

408. Billette de Villemeur T, Chiron C, Robain O: Unlayered polymicrogyria and agenesis of the corpus callosum: A relevant association? *Acta Neuropathol (Berl)* 83:265-270, 1992.

409. Dias MJM, Harmant-van Rijckevorsel G, Landrieu P, Lyon G: Prenatal cytomegalovirus disease and cerebral microgyria: Evidence for perfusion failure, not disturbance of histogenesis, as the major cause of fetal cytomegalovirus encephalopathy, *Neuropediatrics* 15:18-24, 1984.

410. Bordarier C, Robain O: Familial occurrence of prenatal encephaloclastic damage: Anatomoclinical report of, 2 cases, *Neuropediatrics* 20:103-106, 1989.

411. Bordarier C, Robain O: Microgyric and necrotic cortical lesions in twin fetuses: Original cerebral damage consecutive to twinning, *Brain Dev* 14:174-178, 1992.

412. Toti P, De Felice C, Palmeri ML, Villanova M, et al: Inflammatory pathogenesis of cortical polymicrogyria: An autopsy study, *Pediatr Res* 44:291-296, 1998.

413. Inder TE, Huppi PS, Zientara GP, Holling EE, et al: The postmigrational development of polymicrogyria documented by magnetic resonance imaging from 31 weeks postconceptional age, *Ann Neurol* 45:798-801, 1999.

414. Van Allen M, Clarren SK: A spectrum of gyral anomalies in Miller-Dieker (lissencephaly) syndrome, *J Pediatr* 102:559-564, 1983.

415. Bankl H, Jellinger K: Central nervous system injuries following fetal carbon monoxide poisoning, *Beitr Pathol Anat* 135:350-376, 1967.

416. Hallervorden J: Uber eine Kohlenoxyvergiftung im Fetalleben mit Entwicklungsstorung der Hirnrinde, *Allg Atschr Psychiatr* 124:289-297, 1949.

417. de Leon GA: Observations on cerebral and cerebellar microgyria, *Acta Neuropathol (Berl)* 20:278-287, 1972.

418. Jacob H: Die feinere Oberflachengestaltung der Hirnwindungen: Die Hirnwarzenbildung und die Mikropolygyrie, *Z Neurol Psychiatr* 170:64, 1940.

419. Richman DP, Stewart RM, Caviness VS Jr: Cerebral microgyria in a 27-week fetus: An architectonic and topographic analysis, *J Neuropathol Exp Neurol* 33:374-384, 1974.

420. du Plessis AJ, Kaufmann WE, William MD, Kupsky WJ: Intrauterine-onset myoclonic encephalopathy associated with cerebral cortical dysgenesis, *J Child Neurol* 8:164-170, 1993.

421. Guerrini R, Dubeau F, Dulac O, Barkovich AJ, et al: Bilateral parasagittal parieto-occipital polymicrogyria and epilepsy, *Ann Neurol* 41:65-73, 1997.

422. Sugama S, Kusano K: Monozygous twin with polymicrogyria and normal co-twin, *Pediatr Neurol* 11:62-63, 1994.

423. Crome L, France NE: Microgyria and cytomegalic inclusion disease in infancy, *J Clin Pathol* 12:427, 1959.

424. Kammoun F, Tanguy A, Boesplug-Tanguy O, Bensahel H, et al: Club feet with congenital perisylvian polymicrogyria possibly due to bifocal ischemic damage of the neuraxis in utero, *Am J Med Genet A* 126:191-196, 2004.

425. Nissenkorn A, Michelson M, Ben-Zeev B, Lerman-Sagie T: Inborn errors of metabolism: A cause of abnormal brain development, *Neurology* 56:1265-1272, 2001.

426. DelleUrban LAB, Righini A, Rustico M, Triulzi F, et al: Prenatal ultrasound detection of bilateral focal polymicrogyria, *Prenat Diagn* 24:808-811, 2004.

427. van Straaten HL, van Tintelen JP, Trijbels JM, van den Heuvel LP, et al: Neonatal lactic acidosis, complex I/IV deficiency, and fetal cerebral disruption, *Neuropediatrics* 36:193-199, 2005.

428. McBride MC, Kemper TL: Pathogenesis of four-layered microgyric cortex in man, *Acta Neuropathol (Berl)* 57:93-98, 1982.

429. Van Bogaert P, Donner C, David P, Rodesch F, et al: Congenital bilateral perisylvian syndrome in a monozygotic twin with intrauterine death of the co-twin, *Dev Med Child Neurol* 38:166-171, 1996.

430. Humphreys P, Rosen GD, Press DM, Sherman GF, et al: Freezing lesions of the developing rat brain: A model for cerebrocortical microgyria, *J Neuropathol Exp Neurol* 50:145-160, 1991.

431. Rosen GD, Sherman GF, Galaburda AM: Radial glia in the neocortex of adult rats: Effects of neonatal brain injury, *Dev Brain Res* 82:127-135, 1994.

432. Volpe JJ, Adams RD: Cerebro-hepato-renal syndrome of Zellweger: An inherited disorder of neuronal migration, *Acta Neuropathol (Berl)* 20:175-198, 1972.

433. Powers JM, Moser HW, Moser AB, Upshur JK, et al: Fetal cerebrohepatorenal (Zellweger) syndrome: Dysmorphic, radiologic, biochemical, and pathologic findings in four affected fetuses, *Hum Pathol* 16:610-620, 1985.

434. Kelley RI: Review: The cerebrohepatorenal syndrome of Zellweger, morphologic and metabolic aspects, *Am J Med Genet* 16:503-517, 1983.

435. Moser AE, Singh I, Brown FR III, Solish GI, et al: The cerebrohepatorenal (Zellweger) syndrome: Increased levels and impaired degradation of very-long-chain fatty acids and their use in prenatal diagnosis, *N Engl J Med* 310:1141-1146, 1984.

436. Evrard P, Caviness VS Jr, Prats-Vinas J, Lyon G: The mechanism of arrest of neuronal migration in the Zellweger malformation: An hypothesis bases upon cytoarchitectonic analysis, *Acta Neuropathol (Berl)* 41:109-117, 1978.

437. Powers JM, Tummons RC, Caviness VS Jr, Moser AB, et al: Structural and chemical alterations in the cerebral maldevelopment of fetal cerebro-hepato-renal (Zellweger) syndrome, *J Neuropathol Exp Neurol* 48:270-289, 1989.

438. Moser HW: The peroxisome: Nervous system role of a previously underrated organelle. The 1987 Robert Wartenberg lecture, *Neurology* 38:1617-1627, 1988.

439. Kaufmann WE, Theda C, Naidu S, Watkins PA, et al: Neuronal migration abnormality in peroxisomal bifunctional enzyme defect, *Ann Neurol* 39:268-271, 1996.

440. Pascual-Castroviejo I, Pascual-Pascual SI, Viano J, Martinez V, et al: Unilateral polymicrogyria: A common cause of hemiplegia of prenatal origin, *Brain Dev* 23:216-222, 2001.

441. Dixon-Salazar T, Silhavy JL, Marsh SE, Louie CM, et al: Mutations in the AHI1 gene, encoding Jouberin, cause Joubert syndrome with cortical polymicrogyria, *Am J Hum Genet* 75:979-987, 2004.

442. Aicardi J: Aicardi syndrome, *Brain Dev* 27:164-171, 2005.

443. Wieck G, Leventer RJ, Squier WM, Jansen A, et al: Periventricular nodular heterotopia with overlying polymicrogyria, *Brain* 128:2811-2821, 2005.

444. Kuznicky R, Andermann F, Guerrini R: The epileptic spectrum in the congenital bilateral perisylvian syndrome: CBPS Multicenter Collaborative Study, *Neurology* 44:379-385, 1994.

445. Sebire G, Husson B, Dusser A, Navelet Y, et al: Congenital unilateral perisylvian syndrome: Radiological basis and clinical correlations, *J Neurol Neurosurg Psychiatry* 61:52-56, 1996.

446. Gropman AL, Barkovich AJ, Vezina LG, Conry JA, et al: Pediatric congenital bilateral perisylvian syndrome: Clinical and MRI features in 12 patients, *Neuropediatrics* 28:198-203, 1997.
447. Yamamoto T, Koeda T, Maegaki Y, Tanaka C, et al: Bilateral opercular syndrome caused by perinatal difficulties, *Eur J Pediatr Neurol* 2:73-77, 1997.
448. Barkovich AJ, Hevner R, Guerrini R: Syndromes of bilateral symmetrical polymicrogyria, *AJNR Am J Neuroradiol* 20:1814-1821, 1999.
449. Guerreiro MM, Andermann E, Guerrini R, Dobyns WB, et al: Familial perisylvian polymicrogyria: A new familial syndrome of cortical maldevelopment, *Ann Neurol* 48:39-48, 2000.
450. Nevo Y, Segev Y, Gelman Y, Rieder-Grosswasser I, et al: Worster-Drought and congenital perisylvian syndromes: A continuum? *Pediatr Neurol* 24:153-155, 2001.
451. Chang BS, Piao X, Bodell A, Basel-Vanagaite L, et al: Bilateral frontoparietal polymicrogyria: Clinical and radiological features in 10 families with linkage to chromosome 16, *Ann Neurol* 53:596-606, 2003.
452. Piao X, Basel-Vanagaite L, Straussberg R, Grant PE, et al: An autosomal recessive form of bilateral frontoparietal polymicrogyria maps to chromosome 16q12.2–21, *Am J Hum Genet* 70:1028-1033, 2002.
453. Piao X, Hill RS, Bodell A, Chang BS, et al: G protein-coupled receptor-dependent development of human frontal cortex, *Science* 303:2033-2036, 2004.
454. Chang BS, Piao X, Giannini C, Cascino GD, et al: Bilateral generalized polymicrogyria (BGP): A distinct syndrome of cortical malformation, *Neurology* 62:1722-1728, 2004.
455. Suresh PA, Deepa C: Congenital suprabulbar palsy: A distinct clinical syndrome of heterogeneous aetiology, *Dev Med Child Neurol* 46:617-625, 2004.
456. Huppke P, Gartner J: Perisylvian polymicrogyria in Landau-Kleffner syndrome, *Neurology* 64:1660, 2005.
457. Luat AF, Bernardi B, Chugani HT: Congenital perisylvian syndrome: MRI and glucose PET correlations, *Pediatr Neurol* 35:21-29, 2006.
458. Piao X, Chang BS, Bodell A, Woods K, et al: Genotype-phenotype analysis of human frontoparietal polymicrogyria syndromes, *Ann Neurol* 58:680-687, 2005.
458a. Robin NH, Taylor CJ, McDonald-McGinn DM, Zackai EH, et al: Polymicrogyria and deletion 22q11.2 syndrome: Window to the etiology of a common cortical malformation, *Am J Med Genet A* 140:2416-2425, 2006.
459. Takanashi J, Barkovich AJ: The changing MR imaging appearance of polymicrogyria: A consequence of myelination, *AJNR Am J Neuroradiol* 24:788-793, 2003.
460. Tohyama J, Kato M, Koeda T, Inagaki M, et al: The "double cortex" syndrome, *Brain Dev* 15:83-84, 1993.
461. Yamaguchi E, Hayashi T, Kondoh H, Tashiro N, et al: A case of Walker-Warburg syndrome with uncommon findings, *Brain Dev* 15:61-66, 1993.
462. Hashimoto R, Seki T, Takuma Y, Suzuki N: The "double cortex" syndrome on MRI, *Brain Dev* 15:57-60, 1993.
463. Zisch R, Artmann W: MRI in the diagnosis of heterotopic gray matter: Report of three cases first discovered in adulthood, *Neuroradiology* 33:527-528, 1991.
464. Barkovich AJ, Kjos BO: Gray matter heterotopias: MR characteristics and correlation with developmental and neurologic manifestations, *Radiology* 182:493-499, 1992.
465. Kamuro K, Tenokuchi Y-I: Familial periventricular nodular heterotopia, *Brain Dev* 15:237-241, 1993.
466. Huttenlocher PR, Taravath S, Mojtahebi S: Periventricular heterotopia and epilepsy, *Neurology* 44:51-55, 1994.
467. De Volder AG, Gadisseux J-FA, Michel CJ, Maloteaux J-MV, et al: Brain glucose utilization in band heterotopia: Synaptic activity of "double cortex," *Pediatr Neurol* 11:290-294, 1994.
468. Barkovich AJ, Guerrini R, Battaglia G, Kalifa G, et al: Band heterotopia: Correlation of outcome with magnetic resonance imaging parameters, *Ann Neurol* 36:609-617, 1994.
469. Franzoni E, Bernardi B, Marchiani V, Crisanti AF, et al: Band brain heterotopia: Case report and literature review, *Neuropediatrics* 26:37-40, 1995.
470. Miura K, Watanabe K, Maeda N, Matsumoto A, et al: Magnetic resonance imaging and positron emission tomography of band heterotopia, *Brain Dev* 15:288-290, 1993.
471. Eksioglu YZ, Scheffer IE, Cardenas P, Knoll J, et al: Periventricular heterotopia: An X-linked dominant epilepsy locus causing aberrant cerebral cortical development, *Neuron* 16:77-87, 1996.
472. Dubeau F, Tampieri D, Lee N, Andermann E, et al: Periventricular and subcortical nodular heterotopia: A study of 33 patients, *Brain* 118:1273-1287, 1995.
473. Musumeci SA, Ferri R, Elia M, Scuderi C, et al: A new family with periventricular nodular heterotopia and peculiar dysmorphic features, *Arch Neurol* 54:61-64, 1997.
474. Li LM, Dubeau F, Andermann F, Fish DR, et al: Periventricular nodular heterotopia and intractable temporal lobe epilepsy: Poor outcome after temporal lobe resection, *Ann Neurol* 41:662-668, 1997.
475. Dobyns WB, Guerrini R, Czapansky-Beilman DK, Pierpont MEM, et al: Bilateral periventricular nodular heterotopia with mental retardation and syndactyly in boys: A next X-linked mental retardation syndrome, *Neurology* 49:1042-1047, 1997.
476. Ono J, Mano T, Andermann E, Harada K, et al: Band heterotopia or double cortex in a male: Bridging structures suggest abnormality of the radial glial guide system, *Neurology* 48:1701-1703, 1997.
477. Berg MJ, Schifitto G, Powers JM, Martinez-Capolino C, et al: X-linked female band heterotopia-male lissencephaly syndrome, *Neurology* 50:1143-1146, 1998.
478. Puche A, Rodriquez T, Domingo R, Casas C, et al: X-linked subcortical laminar heterotopia and lissencephaly: A new family, *Neuropediatrics* 29:276-278, 1998.
479. Preis S, Engelbrecht V, Huang Y, Steinmetz H: Focal grey matter heterotopias in monozygotic twins with developmental language disorder, *Eur J Pediatr* 157:849-852, 1998.
480. Sisodiya SM, Free SL, Thom M, Everitt AE, et al: Evidence for nodular epileptogenicity and gender differences in periventricular nodular heterotopia, *Neurology* 52:336-341, 1999.
481. Pinard J-M, Feydy A, Carlier R, Perez N, et al: Functional MRI in double cortex: Functionality of heterotopia, *Neurology* 54:1531-1533, 2000.
482. Iannetti P, Spalice A, Raucci U, Perla FM: Functional neuroradiologic investigations in band heterotopia, *Pediatr Neurol* 24:159-163, 2001.
483. Barkovich AJ, Kuzniecky RI: Gray matter heterotopia, *Neurology* 55:1603-1608, 2000.
484. Sheen VL, Dixon PH, Fox JW, Hong SE, et al: Mutations in the X-linked filamin 1 gene cause periventricular nodular heterotopia in males as well as in females, *Hum Mol Genet* 10:1775-1783, 2001.
485. Guerrini R, Mei D, Sisodiya S, Sicca F, et al: Germline and mosaic mutations of FLN1 in men with periventricular heterotopia, *Neurology* 63:51-56, 2004.
486. Sheen VL, Jansen A, Chen MH, Parrini E, et al: Filamin A mutations cause periventricular heterotopia with Ehlers-Danlos syndrome, *Neurology* 64:254-262, 2005.
487. Chang BS, Ly J, Appignani B, Bodell A, et al: Reading impairment in the neuronal migration disorder of periventricular nodular heterotopia, *Neurology* 64:799-803, 2005.
488. Battaglia G, Chiapparini L, Franceschetti S, Freri E, et al: Periventricular nodular heterotopia: Classification, epileptic history, and genesis of epileptic discharges, *Epilepsia* 47:86-97, 2006.
489. Parrini E, Ramazzotti A, Dobyns WB, Mei D, et al: Periventricular heterotopia: Phenotypic heterogeneity and correlation with Filamin A mutations, *Brain* 129:1892-1906, 2006.
490. Ishikawa A, Fukushima N, Wagatsuma Y, Soma T, et al: Magnetic resonance imaging of heterotopic gray matter, *Brain Dev* 9:60-61, 1987.
491. Esquivel EE, Pitt MC, Boyd SG: EEG findings in hypomelanosis of Ito, *Neuropediatrics* 22:216-219, 1991.
492. Palm L, Blennow G, Brun A: Infantile spasms and neuronal heterotopias. A report on six cases, *Acta Paediatr Scand* 75:855-859, 1986.
493. Palm L, Hägerstrand I, Kristoffersson U, Blennow G, et al: Nephrosis and disturbances of neuronal migration in male siblings: A new hereditary disorder, *Arch Dis Child* 61:545-548, 1986.
494. Smith AS, Weinstein MA, Quencer RM, Muroff LR, et al: Association of heterotopic gray matter with seizures: MR imaging. Work in progress, *Radiology* 168:195-198, 1988.
495. Barkovich AJ, Jackson DE Jr, Boyer RS: Band heterotopias: A newly recognized neuronal migration anomaly, *Radiology* 171:455-458, 1989.
496. Palmini A, Andermann F, Aicardi J, Dulac O, et al: Diffuse cortical dysplasia, or the "double cortex" syndrome: The clinical and epileptic spectrum in 10 patients, *Neurology* 41:1656-1662, 1991.
497. Vigevano F, Fusco L, DiCapua M, Ricci S, et al: Benign infantile familial convulsions, *Eur J Pediatr* 151:608-612, 1992.
498. DiMario FJ, Cobb RJ, Ramsby GR: Familial band heterotopias simulating tuberous sclerosis, *Neurology* 43:1424-1426, 1993.
499. Guerrini R, Dobyns WB: Bilateral periventricular nodular heterotopia with mental retardation and frontonasal malformation, *Neurology* 51:499-503, 1998.
500. Jan MM: Outcome of bilateral periventricular nodular heterotopia in monozygotic twins with megalencephaly, *Dev Med Child Neurol* 41:486-488, 1999.
501. Sheen VL, Topcu M, Berkovic SF, Yalnizoglu D, et al: Autosomal recessive form of periventricular heterotopia, *Neurology* 60:1108-10112, 2003.
502. Nagano T, Morikubo S, Sato M: Filamin A and FILIP (Filamin A–interacting protein) regulate cell polarity and motility in neocortical subventricular and intermediate zones during radial migration, *J Neurosci* 24:9648-9657, 2004.
503. Hardiman O, Burke T, Phillips J, Murphy S, et al: Microdysgenesis in resected temporal neocortex: Incidence and clinical significance in focal epilepsy, *Neurology* 38:1041-1047, 1988.
504. Kuzniecky R, Garcia JH, Faught E, Morawetz RB: Cortical dysplasia in temporal lobe epilepsy: Magnetic resonance imaging correlations, *Ann Neurol* 29:293-298, 1991.
505. Palmini A, Andermann F, Olivier A, Tampieri D, et al: Focal neuronal migration disorders and intractable partial epilepsy: Results of surgical treatment, *Ann Neurol* 30:750-757, 1991.
506. Palmini A, Andermann F, Olivier A, Tampieri D, et al: Focal neuronal migration disorders and intractable partial epilepsy: A study of 30 patients, *Ann Neurol* 30:741-749, 1991.

507. Verdú A, Ruiz-Falco ML: Eating seizures associated with focal cortical dysplasia, *Brain Dev* 13:352-354, 1991.

508. Graff-Radford NR, Bosch EP, Stears JC, Tranel D: Developmental Foix-Chavany-Marie syndrome in identical twins, *Ann Neurol* 20:632-635, 1986.

509. Becker PS: Developmental Foix-Chavany-Marie syndrome: Polymicrogyria or macrogyria? *Ann Neurol* 27:693-694, 1990.

510. Kuzniecky R, Andermann F, Tampieri D, Melanson D, et al: Bilateral central macrogyria: Epilepsy, pseudobulbar palsy, and mental retardation—a recognizable neuronal migration disorder, *Ann Neurol* 25:547-554, 1989.

511. Galaburda AM, Sherman GF, Rosen GD, Aboitiz F, et al: Developmental dyslexia: Four consecutive patients with cortical anomalies, *Ann Neurol* 18:222-233, 1985.

512. Cohen M, Campbell R, Yaghmai F: Neuropathological abnormalities in developmental dysphasia, *Ann Neurol* 25:567-570, 1989.

513. Kaufmann WE, Galaburda AM: Cerebrocortical microdysgenesis in neurologically normal subjects: A histopathologic study, *Neurology* 39:238-244, 1989.

514. Hynd GW, Semrud-Clikeman M, Lorys AR, Novey ES, et al: Brain morphology in developmental dyslexia and attention deficit disorder/hyperactivity, *Arch Neurol* 47:919-926, 1990.

515. Hynd GW, Semrud-Clikeman M: Dyslexia and brain morphology, *Psychol Bull* 106:447-482, 1989.

516. Humphreys P, Kaufmann WE, Galaburda AM: Developmental dyslexia in women: Neuropathological findings in three patients, *Ann Neurol* 28:727-738, 1990.

517. Tychsen L, Hoyt WF: Occipital lobe dysplasia: Magnetic resonance findings in two cases of isolated congenital hemianopia, *Arch Ophthalmol* 103:680-682, 1985.

518. Berry-Kravis E, Huttenlocher PR, Wollmann RL: Isolated congenital malformation of hippocampal formation as a cause of intractable neonatal seizures [abstract], *Ann Neurol* 26:485, 1989.

519. Prats JM, Garaizar C, Uterga JM, Urroz MJ: Operculum syndrome in childhood: A rare cause of persistent speech disturbance, *Dev Med Child Neurol* 34:359-366, 1992.

520. Shevell MI, Carmant L, Meagher-Villemure K: Developmental bilateral perisylvian dysplasia, *Pediatr Neurol* 8:299-302, 1992.

521. Guerrini R, Dravet C, Raybaud C, Roger J, et al: Epilepsy and focal gyral anomalies detected by MRI: Electroclinicomorphological correlations and follow-up, *Dev Med Child Neurol* 34:706-718, 1992.

522. Guerrini R, Dravet C, Raybaud C, Roger J, et al: Neurological findings and seizure outcome in children with bilateral opercular macrogyric-like changes detected by MRI, *Dev Med Child Neurol* 34:694-705, 1992.

523. Galaburda AM: Developmental dyslexia, *Rev Neurol* 149:1-3, 1993.

524. Meencke HJ, Veith G, Mcconnell RL, Andermann F, et al: Migration disturbances in epilepsy, *Epilepsy Res*:31-40, 1992.

525. Andermann F: Epilepsia partialis continua and other seizures arising from the precentral gyrus: High incidence in patients with Rasmussen syndrome and neuronal migration disorders, *Brain Dev* 14:338-339, 1992.

526. Fusco L, Bertini E, Vigevano F: Epilepsia partialis continua and neuronal migration anomalies, *Brain Dev* 14:323-328, 1992.

527. Kuzniecky R, Andermann F, Guerrini R: Congenital bilateral perisylvian syndrome: Study of, 31 patients, *Lancet* 341:608-612, 1993.

528. Ótsubo H, Hwang PA, Jay V, Becker LE, et al: Focal cortical dysplasia in children with localization-related epilepsy: EEG, MRI, and SPECT findings, *Pediatr Neurol* 9:101-107, 1993.

529. Quirk JA, Kendall B, Kingley DPE, Boyd SG, et al: EEG features of cortical dysplasia in children, *Neuropediatrics* 24:193-199, 1993.

530. Kuzniecky R, Morawetz R, Faught E, Black L: Frontal and central lobe focal dysplasia: Clinical, EEG and imaging features, *Dev Med Child Neurol* 37:159-166, 1995.

531. Barkovich AJ, Kuzniecky RI, Bollen AW, Grant PE: Focal transmantle dysplasia: A specific malformation of cortical development, *Neurology* 49:1148-1152, 1997.

532. Yoshimura K, Hamada F, Tomoda T, Wakiguchi H, et al: Focal pachypolymicrogyria in three siblings, *Pediatr Neurol* 18:435-438, 1998.

533. Barkovich AJ, Peacock W: Sublobar dysplasia: A new malformation of cortical development, *Neurology* 50:1383-1387, 1998.

534. Spreafico R, Battaglia G, Arcelli P, Andermann F, et al: Cortical dysplasia: An immunocytochemical study of three patients, *Neurology* 50:27-36, 1998.

535. Chan S, Chin SS, Nordli DR, Goodman RR, et al: Prospective magnetic resonance imaging identification of focal cortical dysplasia, including the non-balloon cell subtype, *Ann Neurol* 44:749-757, 1998.

536. Casanova MF, Buxhoeveden DP, Cohen M, Switala AE, et al: Minicolumnar pathology in dyslexia, *Ann Neurol* 52:108-110, 2002.

537. Casanova MF, Araque J, Giedd J, Rumsey JM: Reduced brain size and gyrification in the brains of dyslexic patients, *J Child Neurol* 19:275-281, 2004.

538. Mackay MT, Becker LE, Chuang SH, Otsubo H, et al: Malformations of cortical development with balloon cells: Clinical and radiologic correlates, *Neurology* 60:580-587, 2003.

539. Palmini A, Najm I, Avanzini G, Babb T, et al: Terminology and classification of the cortical dysplasias, *Neurology* 62(Suppl):S2-S8, 2004.

540. Brambati SM, Termine C, Ruffino M, Stella G, et al: Regional reductions of gray matter volume in familial dyslexia, *Neurology* 63:742-745, 2004.

541. Lawson JA, Birchansky S, Pacheco E, Jayakar P, et al: Distinct clinicopathologic subtypes of cortical dysplasia of Taylor, *Neurology* 64:55-61, 2005.

542. Baker LL, Barkovich AJ: The large temporal horn: MR analysis in developmental brain anomalies versus hydrocephalus, *AJNR Am J Neuroradiol* 13:115-122, 1992.

543. Noorani PA, Bodensteiner JB, Barnes PD: Colpocephaly: Frequency and associated findings, *J Child Neurol* 3:100-104, 1988.

544. Herskowitz J, Rosman NP, Wheeler CB: Colpocephaly: Clinical, radiologic, and pathogenetic aspects, *Neurology* 35:1594-1598, 1985.

545. Bodensteiner J, Gay CT: Colpocephaly: Pitfalls in the diagnosis of a pathologic entity utilizing neuroimaging techniques, *J Child Neurol* 5:166-168, 1990.

546. Landman J, Weitz R, Dulitzki F, Shuper A, et al: Radiological colpocephaly: A congenital malformation or the result of intrauterine and perinatal brain damage, *Brain Dev* 11:313-316, 1989.

547. Nigro MA, Wishnow R, Maher L: Colpocephaly in identical twins, *Brain Dev* 13:187-189, 1991.

548. Luskin MB, Shatz CJ: Studies of the earliest generated cells of the cat's visual cortex: Cogeneration of subplate and marginal zones, *J Neurosci* 5:1062-1075, 1985.

549. McConnell SK, Ghosh A, Shatz CJ: Subplate neurons pioneer the first axon pathway from the cerebral cortex, *Science* 245:978-982, 1989.

550. Allendoerfer KL, Shelton DL, Shooter EM, Shatz CJ: Nerve growth factor receptor immunoreactivity is transiently associated with the subplate neurons of the mammalian cerebral cortex, *Proc Natl Acad Sci U S A* 87:187-190, 1990.

551. Friauf E, McConnell SK, Shatz CJ: Functional synaptic circuits in the subplate during fetal and early postnatal development of cat visual cortex, *J Neurosci* 10:2601-2613, 1990.

552. Antonini A, Shatz CJ: Relation between putative transmitter phenotypes and connectivity of subplate neurons during cerebral cortical development, *Eur J Neurosci* 2:744-761, 1990.

553. Ghosh A, Antonini A, McConnell SK, Shatz CJ: Requirement for subplate neurons in the formation of thalamocortical connections, *Nature* 347:179-181, 1990.

554. Friauf E, Shatz CJ: Changing patterns of synaptic input to subplate and cortical plate during development of visual cortex, *J Neurophysiol* 66:2059-2071, 1991.

555. Ghosh A, Shatz CJ: Involvement of subplate neurons in the formation of ocular dominance columns, *Science* 255:1441-1443, 1992.

556. Ghosh A, Shatz CJ: A role for subplate neurons in the patterning of connections from thalamus to neocortex, *Development* 117:1031-1047, 1993.

557. Volpe JJ: Subplate neurons: Missing link in brain injury of the premature infant, *Pediatrics* 97:112-113, 1996.

558. De Azevedo LC, Hedin-Pereira C, Lent R: Callosal neurons in the cingulate cortical plate and subplate of human fetuses, *J Comp Neurol* 386:60-70, 1997.

559. Kostovic I, Judas M: Correlation between the sequential ingrowth of afferents and transient patterns of cortical lamination in preterm infants, *Anat Rec* 267:1-6, 2002.

560. Kanold PO, Kara P, Reid RC, Shatz CJ: Role of subplate neurons in functional maturation of visual cortical columns, *Science* 301:521-525, 2003.

561. Kanold PO: Transient microcircuits formed by subplate neurons and their role in functional development of thalamocortical connections, *Neuroreport* 15:2149-2153, 2004.

562. Bystron I, Molnar Z, Otellin V, Blakemore C: Tangential networks of precocious neurons and early axonal outgrowth in the embryonic human forebrain, *J Neurosci* 25:2781-2792, 2005.

563. McQuillen PS, Ferriero DM: Perinatal subplate neuron injury: Implications for cortical development and plasticity, *Brain Pathol* 15:250-260, 2005.

564. Ohshiro T, Weliky M: Subplate neurons foster inhibition, *Neuron* 51:524-526, 2006.

565. Kostovic I, Jovanov-Milosevic N: The development of cerebral connections during the first 20–45 weeks' gestation, *Semin Fetal Neonatal Med* 11:415-422, 2006.

566. Mrzljak L, Uylings H, Kostovic I, Van Eden CG: Prenatal development of neurons in the human prefrontal cortex. I. A qualitative Golgi study, *J Comp Neurol* 271:355-386, 1988.

567. Kostovic I, Lukinovic N, Judas M, Bogdanovic N, et al: Structural basis of the developmental plasticity in the human cerebral cortex: The role of the transient subplate zone, *Metab Brain Dis* 4:17-23, 1989.

568. Marin-Padilla M: Early ontogenesis of the human cerebral cortex. In Peters A, Jones EG, editors: *Cerebral Cortex*, New York: 1988, Plenum.

569. Kostovic I, Rakic P: Developmental history of the transient subplate zone in the visual and somatosensory cortex of the macaque monkey and human brain, *J Comp Neurol* 297:441-454, 1990.

570. Evrard P, Gressens P, Volpe JJ: New concepts to understand the neurological consequences of subcortical lesions in the premature brain [editorial], *Biol Neonate* 61:1-3, 1992.

571. Marin-Padilla M: Ontogenesis of the pyramidal cell of the mammalian neocortex and developmental cytoarchitectonics: A unifying theory, *J Comp Neurol* 321:233-240, 1992.

572. Kinney HC, Armstrong DL: Perinatal neuropathology. In Graham DI, Lantos PE, editors: *Greenfield's Neuropathology, 7*, London: 2002, Arnold.
573. Conel J: *The Postnatal Development of the Human Cerebral Cortex*, Cambridge, MA: 1939, Harvard University Press.
574. Johnston MV: Neurotransmitters and vulnerability of the developing brain, *Brain Dev* 17:301-306, 1995.
575. Grunnet ML: A lectin and synaptophysin study of developing brain, *Pediatr Neurol* 13:157-160, 1995.
576. Yuen EC, Howe CL, Li Y, Holtzman DM, et al: Nerve growth factor and the neurotrophic factor hypothesis, *Brain Dev* 18:362-368, 1996.
577. Aquino DA, Padin C, Perez JM, Peng D, et al: Analysis of glial fibrillary acidic protein, neurofilament protein, actin and heat shock proteins in human fetal brain during the second trimester, *Dev Brain Res* 91:1-10, 1996.
578. Ohyu J, Yamanouchi H, Takashima S: Immunohistochemical study of microtubule-associated proteins, 5 (MAP5) expression in the developing human brain, *Brain Dev* 19:541-546, 1997.
579. Sarnat HB, Nochlin D, Born DE: Neuronal nuclear antigen (NeuN): A marker of neuronal maturation in the early human fetal nervous system, *Brain Dev* 20:88-94, 1998.
580. Flint AC, Liu XL, Kriegstein AR: Nonsynaptic glycine receptor activation during early neocortical development, *Neuron* 20:43-53, 1998.
581. Bardoul M, Levallois C, Konig N: Functional AMPA/kainate receptors in human embryonic and foetal central nervous system, *J Chem Neuroanat* 14:79-85, 1998.
582. Pomeroy SL, Kim JYH: Biology and pathobiology of neuronal development, *Ment Retard Dev Disabil Res Rev* 6:41-46, 2000.
583. Hevner RF: Development of connections in the human visual system during fetal mid-gestation: A diL-tracing study, *J Neuropathol Exp Neurol* 59:385-392, 2000.
584. Honig LS, Herrmann K, Shatz CJ: Developmental changes revealed by immunohistochemical markers in human cerebral cortex, *Cereb Cortex* 6:794-806, 1996.
585. ten-Donkelaar HJ, Lammens M, Wesseling P, Hori A, et al: Development and malformations of the human pyramidal tract, *J Neurol* 251:1429-1442, 2004.
586. Haynes RL, Borenstein NS, DeSilva TM, Folkerth RD, et al: Axonal development in the cerebral white matter of the human fetus and infant, *J Comp Neurol* 484:156-167, 2005.
587. Luo L, O'Leary DD: Axon retraction and degeneration in development and disease, *Annu Rev Neurosci* 28:127-156, 2005.
588. Mojsilovic J, Zecevic N: Early development of the human thalamus: Golgi and Nissl study, *Early Hum Dev* 27:119-144, 1991.
589. Takashima S, Mito T, Becker LE: Dendritic development of motor neurons in the cervical anterior horn and hypoglossal nucleus of normal infants and victims of sudden infant death syndrome, *Neuropediatrics* 21:24-26, 1990.
590. Marin-Padilla M: Prenatal and early postnatal ontogenesis of the human motor cortex: A Golgi study. I. The sequential development of the cortical layers, *Brain Res* 23:167-183, 1970.
591. Gruner JE: The maturation of human cerebral cortex in electron microscopy study of post-mortem punctures in premature infants, *Biol Neonate* 16:243-255, 1970.
592. Molliver ME, Kostovic I, van der Loos H: The development of synapses in cerebral cortex of the human fetus, *Brain Res* 50:403-407, 1973.
593. Marin-Padilla M: Abnormal neuronal differentiation (functional maturation) in mental retardation, *Morphogenesis and Malformation of Face and Brain*, New York: 1975, Alan R. Liss.
594. Huttenlocher PR: Synaptic and dendritic development and mental defect. In Buchwald NA, Brazier MAB, editors: *Brain Mechanisms in Mental Retardation*, New York: 1975, Academic Press.
595. Purpura DP: Dendritic differentiation in human cerebral cortex: Normal and aberrant developmental patterns, *Adv Neurol* 12:91-134, 1975.
596. Paldino AM, Purpura DP: Branching patterns of hippocampal neurons of human fetus during dendritic differentiation, *Exp Neurol* 64:620-631, 1979.
597. Paldino AM, Purpura DP: Quantitative analysis of the spatial distribution of axonal and dendritic terminals of hippocampal pyramidal neurons in immature human brain, *Exp Neurol* 64:604-619, 1979.
598. Huttenlocher PR, de Courten C, Garey LJ, van der Loos H: Synaptogenesis in human visual cortex: Evidence for synapse elimination during normal development, *Neurosci Lett* 33:247-252, 1982.
599. Krmpotic-Nemanic J, Kostovic I, Kelovic Z, Nemanic D, et al: Development of the human fetal auditory cortex: Growth of afferent fibres, *Acta Anat* 116:69-73, 1983.
600. Marin-Padilla M: Structural organization of the human cerebral cortex prior to the appearance of the cortical plate, *Anat Embryol* 168:21-40, 1983.
601. Becker LE, Armstrong DL, Chan F, Wood MM: Dendritic development in human occipital cortical neurons, *Brain Res* 315:117-124, 1984.
602. Harris KM, Jensen FE, Tsao B: Three-dimensional structure of dendritic spines and synapses in rat hippocampus (CA1) at postnatal day 15 and adult ages: Implications for the maturation of synaptic physiology and long-term potentiation, *J Neurosci* 12:2685-2705, 1992.
603. Goodman CS, Shatz CJ: Developmental mechanisms that generate precise patterns of neuronal connectivity, *Cell* 72:77-98, 1993.
604. Schlaggar BL, Fox K, Oleary DM: Postsynaptic control of plasticity in developing somatosensory cortex, *Nature* 364:623-626, 1993.
605. Aizawa H, Hu SC, Bobb K, Balakrishnan K, et al: Dendrite development regulated by CREST, a calcium-regulated transcriptional activator, *Science* 303:197-202, 2004.
606. Konur S, Ghosh A: Calcium signaling and the control of dendritic development, *Neuron* 46:401-405, 2005.
607. Chen Y, Wang PY, Ghosh A: Regulation of cortical dendrite development by Rap1 signaling, *Mol Cell Neurosci* 28:215-228, 2005.
608. Chen YC, Ghosh A: Regulation of dendritic development by neuronal activity, *J Neurobiol* 64:4-10, 2005.
609. Baker RE, Ruijter JM, Bingmann D: Effect of chronic exposure to high magnesium on neuron survival in long-term neocortical explants of neonatal rats in vitro, *Int J Dev Neurosci* 9:597-606, 1991.
610. Baker RE, Ruijter JM, Bingmann D: Elevated potassium prevents neuronal death but inhibits network formation in neocortical cultures, *Int J Dev Neurosci* 9:339-345, 1991.
611. Ruijter JM, Baker RE, De Jong BM, Romijn HJ: Chronic blockade of bioelectric activity in neonatal rat cortex grown in vitro: Morphological effects, *Int J Dev Neurosci* 9:331-338, 1991.
612. Baker RE, Ruijter JM: Chronic blockade of bioelectric activity in neonatal rat neocortex in vitro: Physiological effects, *Int J Dev Neurosci* 9:321-329, 1991.
613. Talos DM, Fishman RE, Park H, Folkerth RD, et al: Developmental regulation of alpha-amino-3-hydroxy-5-methyl-4-isoxazole-propionic acid receptor subunit expression in forebrain and relationship to regional susceptibility to hypoxic/ischemic injury. I. Rodent cerebral white matter and cortex, *J Comp Neurol* 497:42-60, 2006.
614. Talos DM, Follett PL, Folkerth RD, Fishman RE, et al: Developmental regulation of alpha-amino-3-hydroxy-5-methyl-4-isoxazole-propionic acid receptor subunit expression in forebrain and relationship to regional susceptibility to hypoxic/ischemic injury. II. Human cerebral white matter and cortex, *J Comp Neurol* 497:61-77, 2006.
615. Huppi PS, Warfield S, Kikinis R, Barnes PD, et al: Quantitative magnetic resonance imaging of brain development in premature and mature newborns, *Ann Neurol* 43:224-235, 1998.
616. Kapellou O, Counsell SJ, Kennea NL, Dyet L, et al: Abnormal cortical development after premature birth shown by altered allometric scaling of brain growth, *PLoS Med* 3:e265, 2006.
617. Yoo SS, Park HJ, Soul JS, Mamata H, et al: In vivo visualization of white matter fiber tracts of preterm- and term-infant brains with diffusion tensor magnetic resonance imaging, *Invest Radiol* 40:110-115, 2005.
618. Takashima S, Mito T: Neuronal development in the medullary reticular formation in sudden infant death syndrome and premature infants, *Neuropediatrics* 16:76-79, 1985.
619. Kostovic I, Seress L, Mrzljak L, Judas M: Early onset of synapse formation in the human hippocampus: A correlation with Nissl-Golgi architectonics in, 15- and 16.5-week-old fetuses, *Neuroscience* 30:105-116, 1989.
620. Huttenlocher PR, de Courten C: The development of synapses in striate cortex of man, *Hum Neurobiol* 6:1-9, 1987.
621. Huttenlocher PR, Dabholkar AS: Regional differences in synaptogenesis in human cerebral cortex, *J Comp Neurol* 387:167-178, 1997.
622. Zecevic N, Bourgeois JP, Rakic P: Changes in synaptic density in motor cortex of rhesus monkey during fetal and postnatal life, *Dev Brain Res* 50:11-32, 1989.
623. Rakic P, Bourgeois JP, Eckenhoff MF, Zecevic N, et al: Concurrent overproduction of synapses in diverse regions of the primate cerebral cortex, *Science* 232:232-235, 1986.
624. Bourgeois J-P, Goldman-Rakic PS, Rakic P: Synaptogenesis in the prefrontal cortex of rhesus monkeys, *Cereb Cortex* 4:78-96, 1994.
625. Rakic P, Bourgeois JP, Goldmanrakic PS: Synaptic development of the cerebral cortex: Implications for learning, memory, and mental illness. In Van Pelt J, Corner MA, Uylings HBM, et al, editors: *The Self-Organizing Brain: From Growth Cones to Functional Networks*, New Haven, CT: 1994, Yale University School of Medicine.
626. Kalil RE: Synapse formation in the developing brain, *Sci Am* 261:76-79, 1989.
627. LoTurco JJ, Blanton MG, Kriegstein AR: Initial expression and endogenous activation of NMDA channels in early neocortical development, *J Neurosci* 11:792-799, 1991.
628. Patterson PH, Nawa H: Neuronal differentiation factors/cytokines and synaptic plasticity, *Neuron* 10:123-137, 1993.
629. Ethell IM, Pasquale EB: Molecular mechanisms of dendritic spine development and remodeling, *Prog Neurobiol* 75:161-205, 2005.
630. Purves D, Lichtman JW: Elimination of synapses in the developing nervous system, *Science* 210:153-157, 1980.
631. Hamburger V, Oppenheim RW: Naturally occurring neuronal death in vertebrates, *Neurosci Comment* 1:39-41, 1982.
632. Rakic P, Riley KP: Overproduction and elimination of retinal axons in the fetal rhesus monkey, *Science* 219:1441-1444, 1983.
633. Cowan WM, Fawcett JW, O'Leary DD, Stanfield BB: Regressive events in neurogenesis, *Science* 225:1258-1265, 1984.

634. Oppenheim RW: Cell death during development of the nervous system, *Annu Rev Neurosci* 14:453-501, 1991.
635. Koester SE, O'Leary DM: Functional classes of cortical projection neurons develop dendritic distinctions by class-specific sculpting of an early common pattern, *J Neurosci* 12:1382-1393, 1992.
636. Campbell G, Shatz CJ: Synapses formed by identified retinogeniculate axons during the segregation of eye input, *J Neurosci* 12:1847-1858, 1992.
637. Rabacchi S, Bailly Y, Delhayebouchaud N, Mariani J: Involvement of the N-methyl d-aspartate (NMDA) receptor in synapse elimination during cerebellar development, *Science* 256:1823-1825, 1992.
638. Ferrer I, Soriano E, Delrio JA, Alcantara S, et al: Cell death and removal in the cerebral cortex during development, *Prog Neurobiol* 39:1-43, 1992.
639. Oppenheim RW, Schwartz LM, Shatz CJ: Neuronal death, *A tradition of dying* i:1111-1115, 1992.
640. Janec E, Burke RE: Naturally occurring cell death during postnatal development of the substantia nigra pars compacta of rat. In Conn PM, editor: *Molecular and Cellular Neurosciences*, San Diego: 1993, Academic Press.
641. Allsopp T: Life and death in the nervous system, *Trends Neurosci* 16:1-4, 1993.
642. Narayanan V: Apoptosis in development and disease of the nervous system. I. Naturally occurring cell death in the developing nervous system, *Pediatr Neurol* 16:9-13, 1997.
643. Bergeron L, Yuan J: Sealing one's fate: Control of cell death in neurons, *Curr Opin Neurobiol* 8:55-63, 1998.
644. Rakic S, Zecevic N: Programmed cell death in the developing human telencephalon, *Eur J Neurosci* 12:2721-2734, 2000.
645. Driscoll M, Chalfie M: Developmental and abnormal cell death in C. elegans, *Trends Neurosci* 15:15-19, 1992.
646. Catsicas S, Thanos S, Clarke PG: Major role for neuronal death during brain development: Refinement of topographical connections, *Proc Natl Acad Sci U S A* 84:8165-8168, 1987.
647. O'Leary DD, Stanfield BB: Selective elimination of axons extended by developing cortical neurons is dependent on regional locale: Experiments utilizing fetal cortical transplants, *J Neurosci* 9:2230-2246, 1989.
648. Kolb B, Whishaw IQ: Plasticity in the neocortex: Mechanisms underlying recovery from early brain damage, *Prog Neurobiol* 32:235-276, 1989.
649. Chugani HT, Muller R-A, Chugani DC: Functional brain reorganization in children, *Brain Dev* 18:347-356, 1996.
650. Nieman G, Grodd W, Schoning M: Late remission of congenital hemiparesis: The value of MRI, *Neuropediatrics* 27:197-201, 1996.
651. Lebeer J: How much brain does a mind need? Scientific, clinical and educational implications of ecological plasticity, *Dev Med Child Neurol* 40:352-357, 1998.
652. Staudt M, Gerloff C, Grodd W, Holthausen H, et al: Reorganization in congenital hemiparesis acquired at different gestational ages, *Ann Neurol* 56:854-863, 2004.
653. Johnston MV: Clinical disorders of brain plasticity, *Brain Dev* 26:73-80, 2004.
654. Krageloh-Mann I: Imaging of early brain injury and cortical plasticity, *Exp Neurol* 190(Suppl):S84-S90, 2004.
655. Staudt M, Erb M, Braun C, Gerloff C, et al: Extensive peri-lesional connectivity in congenital hemiparesis, *Neurology* 66:771, 2006.
656. Staudt M, Braun C, Gerloff C, Erb M, et al: Developing somatosensory projections bypass periventricular brain lesions, *Neurology* 67:522-525, 2006.
657. Jacola LM, Schapiro MB, Schmithorst VJ, Byars AW, et al: Functional magnetic resonance imaging reveals atypical language organization in children following perinatal left middle cerebral artery stroke, *Neuropediatrics* 37:46-52, 2006.
658. Ono K, Shimada M, Yamano T: Reorganization of the corticospinal tract following neonatal unilateral cortical ablation in rats, *Brain Dev* 12:226-236, 1990.
659. Ono K, Yamano T, Shimada M: Formation of an ipsilateral corticospinal tract after ablation of cerebral cortex in neonatal rat, *Brain Dev* 13:348-351, 1991.
660. Barth TM, Stanfield BB: The recovery of forelimb-placing behavior in rats with neonatal unilateral cortical damage involves the remaining hemisphere, *J Neurosci* 10:3449-3459, 1990.
661. Farmer SF, Harrison LM, Ingram DA, Stephens JA: Plasticity of central motor pathways in children with hemiplegic cerebral palsy, *Neurology* 41:1505-1510, 1991.
662. Lewine JD, Astur RS, Davis LE, Knight JE, et al: Cortical organization in adulthood is modified by neonatal infarct: A case study, *Radiology* 190:93-96, 1994.
663. Maegaki Y, Yamamoto T, Takeshita K: Plasticity of central motor and sensory pathways in a case of unilateral extensive cortical dysplasia: Investigation of magnetic resonance imaging, transcranial magnetic stimulation, and short-latency somatosensory evoked potentials, *Neurology* 45:2255-2261, 1995.
664. Uematsu J, Ono K, Yamano T, Shimada M: Development of corticospinal tract fibers and their plasticity. II. Neonatal unilateral cortical damage and subsequent development of the corticospinal tract in mice, *Brain Dev* 18:173-178, 1996.
665. Muller R-A, Watswon CE, Muzik O, Chakraborty PK, et al: Motor organization after early middle cerebral artery stroke: A PET study, *Pediatr Neurol* 19:294-298, 1998.
666. Maegaki Y, Maeoka Y, Ishii S, Eda I, et al: Central motor reorganization in cerebral palsy patients with bilateral cerebral lesions, *Pediatr Res* 45:559-567, 1999.
667. Chu D, Huttenlocher PR, Levin DN, Towle VL: Reorganization of the hand somatosensory cortex following perinatal unilateral brain injury, *Neuropediatrics* 31:63-69, 2000.
668. Thickbroom GW, Byrnes ML, Archer SA, Nagarajan L, et al: Differences in sensory and motor cortical organization following brain injury early in life, *Ann Neurol* 49:320-327, 2001.
669. Briellmann RS, Abbott DF, Caflisch U, Archer JS, et al: Brain reorganization in cerebral palsy: A high-field functional MRI study, *Neuropediatrics* 33:162-165, 2002.
670. Born AP, Miranda MJ, Rostrup E, Toft PB, et al: Functional magnetic resonance imaging of the normal and abnormal visual system in early life, *Neuropediatrics* 31:24-32, 2000.
671. Kim YH, Jang SH, Han BS, Kwon YH, et al: Ipsilateral motor pathway confirmed by diffusion tensor tractography in a patient with schizencephaly, *Neuroreport* 15:1899-1902, 2004.
672. Muller K, Kass-Iliyya F, Reitz M: Ontogeny of ipsilateral corticospinal projections: A developmental study with transcranial magnetic stimulation, *Ann Neurol* 42:705-711, 1997.
673. Eyre JA, Taylor JP, Villagra F, Smith M, et al: Evidence of activity-dependent withdrawal of corticospinal projections during human development, *Neurology* 57:1543-1554, 2001.
674. Rutherford MA, Pennock JM, Cowan FM, Dubowitz LM, et al: Does the brain regenerate after perinatal infarction? *Eur J Pediatr Neurol* 1:13-17, 1997.
675. Pope A, Schoffeniels E, Franck G: Neuroglia: Quantitative aspects. In Tower DB, Hertz L, editors: *Dynamic Properties of Glial Cells*, New York: 1978, Pergamon Press.
676. Cameron RS, Rakic P: Glial cell lineage in the cerebral cortex: A review and synthesis, *Glia* 4:124-137, 1991.
677. Misson JP, Takahashi T, Caviness VS Jr: Ontogeny of radial and other astroglial cells in murine cerebral cortex, *Glia* 4:138-148, 1991.
678. Knapp PE: Studies of glial lineage and proliferation in vitro using an early marker for committed oligodendrocytes, *J Neurosci Res* 30:336-345, 1991.
679. Hardy R, Reynolds R: Proliferation and differentiation potential of rat forebrain oligodendroglial progenitors both in vitro and in vivo, *Development* 111:1061-1080, 1991.
680. Gray GE, Sanes JR: Lineage of radial glia in the chicken optic tectum, *Development* 114:271-283, 1992.
681. Raff MC, Miller RH, Noble M: A glial progenitor cell that develops in vitro into an astrocyte or an oligodendrocyte depending on culture medium, *Nature* 303:389-396, 1983.
682. Galileo DS, Gray GE, Owens GC, Majors J, et al: Neurons and glia arise from a common progenitor in chicken optic tectum: Demonstration with two retroviruses and cell type-specific antibodies, *Proc Natl Acad Sci U S A* 87:458-462, 1990.
683. Niehaus A, Stegmuller J, DiersFenger M, Trotter J: Cell-surface glycoprotein of oligodendrocyte progenitors involved in migration, *J Neurosci* 19:4948-4961, 1999.
684. Lopes-Cardozo M, Sykes JE, Van der Pal RH, van Golde LM: Development of oligodendrocytes: Studies of rat glial cells cultured in chemically-defined medium, *J Dev Physiol* 12:117-127, 1989.
685. Culican SM, Baumrind NL, Yamamoto M, Pearlman AL: Cortical radial glia: Identification in tissue culture and evidence for their transformation to astrocytes, *J Neurosci* 10:684-692, 1990.
686. Ingraham CA, McCarthy KD: Plasticity of process-bearing glial cell cultures from neonatal rat cerebral cortical tissue, *J Neurosci* 9:63-69, 1989.
687. Choi BH: Prenatal gliogenesis in the developing cerebrum of the mouse, *Glia* 1:308-316, 1988.
688. Goldman JE, Geier SS, Hirano M: Differentiation of astrocytes and oligodendrocytes from germinal matrix cells in primary culture, *J Neurosci* 6:52-60, 1986.
689. Levine SM, Goldman JE: Embryonic divergence of oligodendrocyte and astrocyte lineages in developing rat cerebrum, *J Neurosci* 8:3992-4006, 1988.
690. Hirano M, Goldman JE: Gliogenesis in rat spinal cord: Evidence for origin of astrocytes and oligodendrocytes from radial precursors, *J Neurosci Res* 21:155-167, 1988.
691. Gard AL, Pfeiffer SE: Two proliferative stages of the oligodendrocyte lineage (A2B5+O4− and O4+GalC−) under different mitogenic control, *Neuron* 5:615-625, 1990.
692. Warrington AE, Pfeiffer SE: Proliferation and differentiation of O4+ oligodendrocytes in postnatal rat cerebellum: Analysis in unfixed tissue slices using anti-glycolipid antibodies, *J Neurosci Res* 33:338-353, 1992.
693. Goldman JE: Regulation of oligodendrocyte differentiation, *Trends Neurosci* 15:359-362, 1992.
694. Gressens P, Richelme C, Kadhim HJ, Gadisseux JF, et al: The germinative zone produces the most cortical astrocytes after neuronal migration in the developing mammalian brain, *Biol Neonate* 61:4-24, 1992.

695. Barres Ba, Hart IK, Coles HSR, Burne JF, et al: Cell death in the oligodendrocyte lineage, *J Neurobiol* 23:1221-1230, 1992.
696. Barres BA, Hart IK, Cotes HSR, Burne JF, et al: Cell death and control of cell survival in the oligodendrocyte lineage, *Cell* 70:31-46, 1992.
697. Levison SW, Chuang C, Abramson BJ, Goldman JE: The migrational patterns and developmental fates of glial precursors in the rat subventricular zone are temporally regulated, *Development* 119:611-622, 1993.
698. Luskin MB, Parnavelas JG, Barfield JA: Neurons, astrocytes, and oligodendrocytes of the rat cerebral cortex originate from separate progenitor cells: An ultrastructural analysis of clonally related cells, *J Neurosci* 13:1730-1750, 1993.
699. Back SA, Volpe JJ: Cellular and molecular pathogenesis of periventricular white matter injury, *Ment Retard Dev Disabil Res Rev* 3:96-107, 1997.
700. Kinney HC, Back SA: Human oligodendroglial development: Relationship to periventricular leukomalacia, *Semin Pediatr Neurol* 5:180-189, 1998.
701. Porter B, Tennekoon G: Myelin and disorders that affect the formation and maintenance of this sheath, *Ment Retard Dev Disabil Res Rev* 6:47-58, 2000.
702. Colognato H, ffrench-Constant C: Mechanisms of glial development, *Curr Opin Neurobiol* 14:37-44, 2004.
703. Zerlin M, Milosevic A, Goldman JE: Glial progenitors of the neonatal subventricular zone differentiate asynchronously, leading to spatial dispersion of glial clones and to the persistence of immature glia in the adult mammalian CNS, *Dev Biol* 270:200-213, 2004.
704. Noble M, Proschel C, MayerProschel M: Getting a GR(I)P on oligodendrocyte development, *Dev Biol* 265:33-52, 2004.
705. Cai J, Qi YC, Hu XM, Tan M, et al: Generation of oligodendrocyte precursor cells from mouse dorsal spinal cord independent of Nkx6 regulation and Shh signaling, *Neuron* 45:41-53, 2005.
706. Marshall CAG, Novitch BG, Goldman JE: Olig2 directs astrocyte and oligodendrocyte formation in postnatal subventricular zone cells, *J Neurosci* 25:7289-7298, 2005.
707. Drobyshevsky A, Song SK, Gamkrelidze G, Wyrwicz AM, et al: Developmental changes in diffusion anisotropy coincide with immature oligodendrocyte progression and maturation of compound action potential, *J Neurosci* 25:5988-5997, 2005.
708. Yue T, Xian K, Hurlock E, Xin M, et al: A critical role for dorsal progenitors in cortical myelination, *J Neurosci* 26:1275-1280, 2006.
709. Nguyen L, Borgs L, Vandenbosch R, Mangin JM, et al: The Yin and Yang of cell cycle progression and differentiation in the oligodendroglial lineage, *Ment Retard Dev Disabil Res Rev* 12:85-96, 2006.
710. de Vellis J, Carpenter E: Development. In Siegel GJ, Albers RW, Brady ST, et al, editors: *Basic Neurochemistry: Molecular, Cellular, and Medical Aspects*, vol. 7, London: 2006, Elsevier.
711. Abematsu M, Kagawa T, Fukuda S, Inoue T, et al: Basic fibroblast growth factor endows dorsal telencephalic neural progenitors with the ability to differentiate into oligodendrocytes but not gamma-aminobutyric acidergic neurons, *J Neurosci Res* 83:731-743, 2006.
712. Roessmann U, Gambetti P: Astrocytes in the developing human brain: An immunohistochemical study, *Acta Neuropathol (Berl)*, 70:308-313, 1986.
713. Elder GA, Major EO: Early appearance of type II astrocytes in developing human fetal brain, *Brain Res* 470:146-150, 1988.
714. Mahajan RG, Mandal S, Mukherjee KL: Cathepsin D and 2′,3′-cyclic nucleotide 3′-phosphohydrolase in developing human foetal brain, *Int J Dev Neurosci* 6:117-123, 1988.
715. Aloisi F, Giampaolo A, Russo G, Peschle C, et al: Developmental appearance, antigenic profile, and proliferation of glial cells of the human embryonic spinal cord: An immunocytochemical study using dissociated cultured cells, *Glia* 5:171-181, 1992.
716. Armstrong DD: The neuropathology of the Rett syndrome, *Brain Dev* 14(Suppl):S89-S98, 1992.
717. Marin-Padilla M: Prenatal development of fibrous (white matter), protoplasmic (gray matter), and layer, 1 astrocytes in the human cerebral cortex: A Golgi study, *J Comp Neurol*, 357:554-572, 1995.
718. Rivkin MJ, Flax J, Mozel R, Osthanondh R, et al: Oligodendroglial development in human fetal cerebrum, *Ann Neurol* 38:92-101, 1995.
719. Ozawa H, Nishida A, Mito T, Takashima S: Development of ferritin-positive cells in cerebrum of human brain, *Pediatr Neurol* 10:44-48, 1994.
720. Back SA, Khan R, Gan X, Rosenberg PA, et al: A new alamar blue viability assay to rapidly quantify oligodendrocyte death, *J Neurosci Meth* 91:47-54, 1999.
721. Back SA, Luo NL, Borenstein NS, Levine JM, et al: Late oligodendrocyte progenitors coincide with the developmental window of vulnerability for human perinatal white matter injury, *J Neurosci* 21:1302-1312, 2001.
722. Back SA, Luo NL, Borenstein NS, Volpe JJ, et al: Arrested oligodendrocyte lineage progression during human cerebral white matter development: Dissociation between the timing of progenitor differentiation and myelinogenesis, *J Neuropathol Exp Neurol* 61:197-211, 2002.
723. Jakovcevski I, Zecevic N: Sequence of oligodendrocyte development in the human fetal telencephalon, *Glia* 49:480-491, 2005.
724. Rakic S, Zecevic N: Early oligodendrocyte progenitor cells in the human fetal telencephalon, *Glia* 41:117-127, 2003.

725. DeAzevedo LC, Fallet C, Moura-Neto V, Daumas-Duport C, et al: Cortical radial glial cells in human fetuses: Depth-correlated transformation into astrocytes, *J Neurobiol* 55:288-298, 2003.
726. Gould SJ, Howard S: An immunohistological study of macrophages in the human fetal brain, *Neuropathol Appl Neurobiol* 17:383-390, 1991.
727. Rezaie P, Patel K, Male DK: Microglia in the human fetal spinal cord: Patterns of distribution, morphology and phenotype, *Dev Brain Res* 115:71-81, 1999.
728. Rezaie P, Male D: Colonisation of the developing human brain and spinal cord by microglia: A review, *Microsc Res Tech* 45:359-382, 1999.
729. Rezaie P, Male D: Differentiation, ramification and distribution of microglia within the central nervous system examined, *Neuroembryology* 1:29-43, 2002.
730. Rezaie P, Bohl J, Ulfig N: Anomalous alterations affecting microglia in the central nervous system of a fetus at 12 weeks of gestation: Case report, *Acta Neuropathol (Berl)*, 107:176-180, 2004.
731. Rezaie P, Male D: Mesoglia and microglia: A historical review of the concept of mononuclear phagocytes within the central nervous system, *J Hist Neurosci* 11:325-374, 2002.
732. Rezaie P, Dean A, Male D, Ulfig N: Microglia in the cerebral wall of the human telencephalon at second trimester, *Cereb Cortex* 15:938-949, 2005.
732a. Monier A, Evrard P, Gressens P, Verney C: Distribution and differentiation of microglia in the human encephalon during the first two trimesters of gestation, *J Comp Neurol* 499:565-582, 2006.
733. Billiards SS, Haynes RL, Folkerth RD, Trachtenberg FL, et al: Development of microglia in the cerebral white matter of the human fetus and infant, *J Comp Neurol* 497:199-208, 2006.
734. Hamilton SP, Rome LH: Stimulation of in vitro myelin synthesis by microglia, *Glia* 11:326-335, 1994.
735. Purpura DP: Dendritic spine "dysgenesis" and mental retardation, *Science* 186:1126-1128, 1974.
736. Bodick N, Stevens JK, Sasaki S, Purpura DP: Microtubular disarray in cortical dendrites and neurobehavioral failure. II. Computer reconstruction of perturbed microtubular arrays, *Brain Res* 281:299-309, 1982.
737. Purpura DP, Bodick N, Suzuki K, Rapin I, et al: Microtubule disarray in cortical dendrites and neurobehavioral failure. I. Golgi and electron microscopic studies, *Brain Res* 281:287-297, 1982.
738. Huttenlocher PR: Dendritic development in neocortex of children with mental defect and infantile spasms, *Neurology* 24:203-210, 1974.
739. Huttenlocher PR: Dendritic and synaptic pathology in mental retardation, *Pediatr Neurol* 7:79-85, 1991.
740. Patterson MC, Zoghbi HY: Mental retardation: X marks the spot, *Neurology* 61:156-157, 2003.
741. Chechlacz M, Gleeson JG: Is mental retardation a defect of synapse structure and function? *Pediatr Neurol* 29:11-17, 2003.
742. Zanni G, Saillour Y, Nagara M, Billuart P, et al: Oligophrenin 1 mutations frequently cause X-linked mental retardation with cerebellar hypoplasia, *Neurology* 65:1364-1369, 2005.
743. Amir RE, Van den Veyver IB, Schultz R, Malicki DM, et al: Influence of mutation type and X chromosome inactivation on Rett syndrome phenotypes, *Ann Neurol* 47:670-679, 2000.
744. Amir RE, Van den Veyver IB, Wan M, Tran CQ, et al: Rett syndrome is caused by mutations in X-linked MECP2, encoding methyl-CpG-binding protein 2, *Nat Genet* 23:185-188, 1988.
745. Hagberg B: Clinical manifestations and stages of Rett syndrome, *Ment Retard Dev Disabil Res Rev* 8:61-65, 2002.
746. Armstrong DD: Neuropathology of Rett syndrome, *Ment Retard Dev Disabil Res Rev* 8:72-76, 2002.
747. Armstrong DD, Deguchi M, Antallfy B: Survey of MeCP2 in the Rett syndrome and the non–Rett syndrome brain, *J Child Neurol* 18:683-687, 2003.
748. Armstrong DD: Can we relate MeCP2 deficiency to the structural and chemical abnormalities in the Rett brain? *Brain Dev* 27(Supp. 1):S72-S76, 2005.
749. Fukuda T, Itoh M, Ichikawa T, Washiyama K, et al: Delayed maturation of neuronal architecture and synaptogenesis in cerebral cortex of Mecp2-deficient mice, *J Neuropathol Exp Neurol* 65:537-544, 2006.
750. Kaufmann WE, Johnston MV, Blue ME: MeCP2 expression and function during brain development: Implications for Rett syndrome's pathogenesis and clinical evolution, *Brain Dev* 27(Suppl 1):S77-S87, 2005.
751. Shahbazian MD, Zoghbi HY: Rett syndrome and MeCP2: Linking epigenetics and neuronal function, *Am J Hum Genet* 71:1259-1272, 2002.
752. Van den, Veyver IB, Zoghbi HY: Genetic basis of Rett syndrome, *Ment Retard Dev Disabil Res Rev* 8:82-86, 2002.
753. Zhou Z, Hong EJ, Cohen S, Zhao W-N, et al: Brain-specific phosphorylation of MeCP2 regulates activity-dependent Bdnf transcription, dendritic growth, and spine maturation, *Neuron* 52:255-269, 2006.
754. Belmonte MK, Allen G, Beckel-Mitchener A, Boulanger LM, et al: Autism and abnormal development of brain connectivity, *J Neuroscience* 24:9228-9231, 2004.
755. Pelphrey K, Adolphs R, Morris JP: Neuroanatomical substrates of social cognition dysfunction in autism, *Ment Retard Dev Disabil Res Rev* 10:259-271, 2004.
756. Palmen SJMC, vanEngeland H, Hof PR, Schmitz C: Neuropathological findings in autism, *Brain* 127:2572-2583, 2004.

757. Bauman ML, Kemper TL: Neuroanatomic observations of the brain in autism: A review and future directions, *Int J Dev Neurosci* 23:183-187, 2005.

757a. Minshew NJ, Williams DL: The new neurobiology of autism: Cortex, connectivity, and neuronal organization, *Arch Neurol* 64:945-950, 2007.

758. Fidler DJ, Bailey JN, Smalley SL: Macrocephaly in autism and other pervasive developmental disorders, *Dev Med Child Neurol* 42:737-740, 2000.

759. Sparks BF, Friedman SD, Shaw DW, Aylward FH, et al: Brain structural abnormalities in young children with autism spectrum disorder, *Neurology* 59:184-192, 2002.

760. Dementieva YA, Vance DD, Donnelly SL, Elston LA, et al: Accelerated head growth in early development of individuals with autism, *Pediatr Neurol* 32:102-108, 2005.

761. Courchesne E, Pierce K: Brain overgrowth in autism during a critical time in development: Implications for frontal pyramidal neuron and interneuron development and connectivity, *Int J Dev Neurosci* 23:153-170, 2005.

762. Marin-Padilla M: Structural abnormalities of the cerebral cortex in human chromosomal aberrations: A Golgi study, *Brain Res* 44:625-629, 1972.

763. Takashima S, Becker LE, Armstrong DL, Chan F: Abnormal neuronal development in the visual cortex of the human fetus and infant with Down syndrome: A quantitative and qualitative Golgi study, *Brain Res* 225:1-21, 1981.

764. Petit TL, LeBoutillier JC, Alfano DP, Becker LE: Synaptic development in the human fetus: A morphometric analysis of normal and Down's syndrome neocortex, *Exp Neurol* 83:13-23, 1984.

765. Ross MH, Galaburda AM, Kemper TL: Down syndrome: Is there a decreased population of neurons? *Neurology* 34:909-916, 1984.

766. Becker LE, Armstrong DL, Chan F: Dendritic atrophy in children with Down's syndrome, *Ann Neurol* 20:520-526, 1986.

767. Takashima S, Ieshima A, Nakamura H, Becker LE: Dendrites, dementia and the Down syndrome, *Brain Dev* 11:131-133, 1989.

768. Wisniewski KE: Down syndrome children often have brain with maturation delay, retardation of growth, and cortical dysgenesis, *Am J Med Genet Suppl* 7:274-281, 1990.

769. Becker L, Mito T, Takashima S, Onodera K: Growth and development of the brain in Down syndrome. In Epstein CJ, editor: *The Morphogenesis of Down Syndrome: Proceedings of the National Down Syndrome Society Conference on Morphogenesis and Down Syndrome, Held in New York (Progress in Clinical and Biological Research)*, New York: 1991, Wiley-Liss.

770. Vuksic M, Petanjek Z, Rasin M, Kostovic I: Perinatal growth of prefrontal layer III pyramids in Down syndrome, *Pediatr Neurol* 27:36-38, 2002.

771. Stafstrom CE, Patxot OF, Gilmore HE, Wisniewski KE: Seizures in children with Down syndrome: Etiology, characteristics and outcome, *Dev Med Child Neurol* 33:191-200, 1991.

772. Pueschel SM, Louis S, McKnight P: Seizure disorders in Down syndrome, *Arch Neurol* 48:318-320, 1991.

773. Busciglio J, Yankner BA: Apoptosis and increased generation of reactive oxygen species in Down's syndrome neurons, *Nature* 378:776-779, 1995.

774. Mandel J-L, Hagerman R, Froster U, Brown WT, et al: Fifth international workshop on the fragile X and X-linked mental retardation, *Am J Med Genet* 43:5-27, 1992.

775. Goldson E, Hagerman RJ: The fragile X syndrome, *Dev Med Child Neurol* 34:826-832, 1992.

776. Hinton VJ, Brown WT, Wisniewski K, Rudelli RD: Analysis of neocortex in three males with the fragile X syndrome, *Am J Med Genet* 41:289-294, 1991.

777. Tarleton JC, Saul RA: Molecular genetic advances in fragile X-syndrome, *J Pediatr* 122:169-185, 1993.

778. Beckel-Mitchener A, Greenough WT: Correlates across the structural, functional, and molecular phenotypes of fragile X syndrome, *Ment Retard Dev Disabil Res Rev* 10:53-59, 2004.

778a. Koukoui SD, Chaudhuri A: Neuroanatomical, molecular genetic, and behavioral correlates of fragile X syndrome, *Brain Res Brain Res Rev* 53:27-38, 2007.

779. Irwin SA, Patel B, Idupulapati M, Harris JB, et al: Abnormal dendritic spine characteristics in the temporal and visual cortices of patients with fragile-X syndrome: A quantitative examination, *Am J Med Genet* 98:161-167, 2001.

780. Hessl D, Rivera SM, Reiss AL: The neuroanatomy and neuroendocrinology of fragile X syndrome, *Ment Retard Dev Disabil Res Rev* 10:17-24, 2004.

781. Comery TA, Harris JB, Willems PJ, Oostra BA, et al: Abnormal dendritic spines in fragile X knockout mice: Maturation and pruning deficits, *Pro Natl Acad Sci* 94:5401-5404, 1997.

782. McKinney BC, Grossman AW, Elisseou NM, Greenough WT: Dendritic spine abnormalities in the occipital cortex of C57BL/6 Fmr1 knockout mice, *Am J Med Genet B Neuropsychiatr Genet* 136:98-102, 2005.

783. Galvez R, Greenough WT: Sequence of abnormal dendritic spine development in primary somatosensory cortex of a mouse model of the fragile X mental retardation syndrome, *Am J Hum Genet A* 135A:155-160, 2005.

784. Lu R, Wang HP, Liang Z, Ku L, et al: The fragile X protein controls microtubule-associated protein, 1B translation and microtubule stability in brain neuron development, *Proc Natl Acad Sci U S A* 101:15201-15206, 2004.

785. Fryburg JS, Breg WR, Lindgren V: Diagnosis of Angelman syndrome in infants, *Am J Med Genet* 38:58-64, 1991.

786. Van Lierde A, Atza MG, Giardino D, Viani F: Angelman's syndrome in the first year of life, *Dev Med Child Neurol* 32:1011-1016, 1990.

787. Yamada KA, Volpe JJ: Angelman's syndrome in infancy, *Dev Med Child Neurol* 32:1005-1011, 1990.

788. Zori RT, Hendrickson J, Woolven S, Whidden EM, et al: Angelman syndrome: Clinical profile, *J Child Neurol* 7:270-280, 1992.

789. Knoll JHM, Wagstaff J, Lalande M: Cytogenetic and molecular studies in the Prader-Willi and Angelman syndromes: An overview, *Am J Med Genet* 46:2-6, 1993.

790. Leonard CM, Williams CA, Nicholls RD, Agee OF, et al: Angelman and Prader-Willi syndrome: A magnetic resonance imaging study of differences in cerebral structure, *Am J Med Genet* 46:26-33, 1993.

791. Williams CA, Angelman H, Claytonsmith J, Driscoll DJ, et al: Angelman syndrome: Consensus for diagnostic criteria, *Am J Med Genet* 56:237-238, 1995.

792. Guerrini R, De Lorey TM, Bonanni P, Moncla A, et al: Cortical myoclonus in Angelman syndrome, *Ann Neurol* 40:39-48, 1996.

793. Viani F, Romeo A, Viri M, Mastrangelo M, et al: Seizure and EEG patterns in Angelman's syndrome, *J Child Neurol, 10* 1995..

794. Hou J-W, Wang P-J, Wang T-R: Angelman syndrome assessed by neurological and molecular cytogenetic investigations, *Pediatr Neurol* 16:17-22, 1997.

795. Minassian BA, DeLorey TM, Olsen RW, Philippart M, et al: Angelman syndrome: Correlations between epilepsy phenotypes and genotypes, *Ann Neurol* 43:485-493, 1998.

796. Dan B, Boyd SG: Angelman syndrome reviewed from a neurophysiological perspective: The UBE3A-GABRB3 hypothesis, *Neuropediatrics* 34:169-176, 2003.

797. Valente KD, Koiffmann CP, Fridman C, Varella M, et al: Epilepsy in patients with Angelman syndrome caused by deletion of the chromosome 15q11–13, *Arch Neurol* 63:122-128, 2006.

798. Kishino T, Lalanda M, Wagstaff J: UBE3A/E6-AP mutations cause Angelman syndrome, *Nat Genet* 15:70-73, 1997.

799. Rougeulle C, Glatt H, Lalande M: The Angelman syndrome candidate gene, UBE3A/E6-AP, is imprinted in brain, *Nat Genet* 17:14-15, 1997.

800. Jay V, Becker LE, Chan FW, Perry TL Sr.: Puppet-like syndrome of Angelman: A pathologic and neurochemical study, *Neurology* 41:416-422, 1991.

801. Kyriakides T, Hallam LA, Hockey A, Silberstein P, et al: Angelman's syndrome: A neuropathological study, *Acta Neuropathol (Berl)* 83:675-678, 1992.

802. Dubowitz V, Crome L: The central nervous system in Duchenne muscular dystrophy, *Brain* 92:805-808, 1969.

803. Jagadha V, Becker LE: Brain morphology in Duchenne muscular dystrophy: A Golgi study, *Pediatr Neurol* 4:87-92, 1988.

804. Lidov HGW, Byers TJ, Watkins SC, Kunkel LM: Localization of dystrophin to postsynaptic regions of central nervous system cortical neurons, *Nature* 348:725-728, 1990.

805. Lidov H, Byers TJ, Kunkel LM: The distribution of dystrophin in the murine central nervous system: An immunocytochemical study, *Neurosci* 34:167-187, 1993.

806. Kim T-W, Wu K, Black IB: Deficiency of brain synaptic dystrophin in human Duchenne muscular dystrophy, *Ann Neurol* 38:446-449, 1995.

807. Moizard MP, Billard C, Toutain A, Berret F, et al: Are Dp71 and Dp140 brain dystrophin isoforms related to cognitive impairment in Duchenne muscular dystrophy? *Am J Med Genet* 80:32-41, 1998.

808. Lyon G, Arita F, Le Galloudec E, Vallee L, et al: A disorder of axonal development, necrotizing myopathy, cardiomyopathy, and cataracts: A new familial disease, *Ann Neurol* 27:193-199, 1990.

809. Lynch BJ, Bechich MJ, Torack RM, Rust RS: Arrested maturation of cerebral neurons, axons and myelin: A new familial syndrome of newborns, *Neuropediatrics* 23:180-187, 1992.

810. Curatolo P, Cilio MR, Del Giudice E, Romano A, et al: Familial white matter hypoplasia, agenesis of the corpus callosum, mental retardation and growth deficiency: A new distinctive syndrome, *Neuropediatrics* 24:77-82, 1993.

811. Roessmann U, Horwitz SJ, Kennell JH: Congenital absence of the corticospinal fibers: Pathologic and clinical observations, *Neurology* 40:538-541, 1990.

812. Chow CW, Halliday JL, Anderson RM, Danks DM, et al: Congenital absence of pyramids and its significance in genetic diseases, *Acta Neuropathol (Berl)* 65:313-317, 1985.

813. Volpe JJ: Encephalopathy of prematurity includes neuronal abnormalities, *Pediatrics* 116:221-225, 2005.

814. Inder TE, Huppi PS, Warfield S, Kikinis R, et al: Periventricular white matter injury in the premature infant is associated with a reduction in cerebral cortical gray matter volume at term, *Ann Neurol* 46:755-760, 1999.

815. Ajayi-Obe M, Saeed N, Cowan FM, Rutherford MA, et al: Reduced development of cerebral cortex in extremely preterm infants, *Lancet* 356:1162-1163, 2000.

816. Peterson BS, Anderson AW, Ehrenkranz RA, Staib LH, et al: Regional brain volumes and their later neurodevelopmental correlates in term and preterm infants, *Pediatrics* 111:939-948, 2003.

817. Inder TE, Warfield SK, Wang H, Huppi PS, et al: Abnormal cerebral structure is present at term in premature infants, *Pediatrics* 115:286-294, 2005.
817a. Thompson DK, Warfield SK, Carlin JB, Pavlovic M, et al: Perinatal risk factors altering regional brain structure in the preterm infant, *Brain* 130:667-677, 2007.
818. Lodygensky GA, Rademaker KJ, Zimine S, Gex-Fabry M, et al: Structural and functional brain developmental after hydrocortisone treatment for neonatal chronic lung disease, *Pediatrics* 116:1-7, 2005.
819. Isaacs E, Lucas A, Chong WK, wood SJ, et al: Hippocampal volume and everyday memory in children of very low birth weight, *Pediatr Res* 47:713-720, 2000.
820. Peterson BS, Vohr B, Staib LH, Cannistraci CJ, et al: Regional brain volume abnormalities and long-term cognitive outcome in preterm infants, *JAMA* 284:1939-1947, 2000.
821. Nosarti C, Al-Asady MHS, Frangou S, Stewart AL, et al: Adolescents who were born very preterm have decreased brain volumes, *Brain* 125:1616-1623, 2002.
822. Abernethy LJ, Cooke RW, Foulder-Hughes L: Caudate and hippocampal volumes, intelligence, and motor impairment in 7-year-old children who were born preterm, *Pediatr Res* 55:884-893, 2004.
823. Reiss AL, Kesler SR, Vohr B, Duncan CC, et al: Sex differences in cerebral volumes of 8-year-olds born preterm, *J Pediatr* 145:242-249, 2004.
824. Kesler SR, Ment LR, Vohr B, Pajot SK, et al: Volumetric analysis of regional cerebral development in preterm children, *Pediatr Neurol* 31:318-325, 2004.
825. Jobe AH: Postnatal corticosteroids for preterm infants: Do what we say, not what we do, *N Engl J Med* 350:1349-1351, 2004.
826. Baud O: Postnatal steroid treatment and brain development, *Arch Dis Child* 89:96-100, 2004.
827. Committee on Fetus and Newborn: Postnatal corticosteroids to treat or prevent chronic lung disease in preterm infants, *Pediatrics* 109:330-338, 2002.
828. Yeh TF, Lin YJ, Lin HC, Huang CC, et al: Outcomes at school age after postnatal dexamethasone therapy for lung disease of prematurity, *N Engl J Med* 350:1304-1313, 2004.
829. Barrington KJ: The adverse neuro-developmental effects of postnatal steroids in the preterm infant: A systematic review of RCTs, *BMC Pediatr* 1:1, 2001.
830. Short EJ, Klein NK, Lewis BA, Fulton S, et al: Cognitive and academic consequences of bronchopulmonary dysplasia and very low birth weight: 8-year-old outcomes, *Pediatrics* 112:e359, 2003.
831. Murphy BP, Inder TE, Huppi PS, Warfield S, et al: Impaired cerebral cortical gray matter growth after treatment with dexamethasone for neonatal chronic lung disease, *Pediatrics* 107:217-221, 2001.
832. Uno H, Lohmiller L, Thieme C, Kemnitz JW, et al: Brain damage induced by prenatal exposure to dexamethasone in fetal rhesus macaques. I. Hippocampus, *Dev Brain Res* 53:157-167, 1990.
833. Rademaker KJ, Rupert M, Uiterwaal CSPM, Lieftink AF, et al: Neonatal hydrocortisone treatment related to H-1-MRS of the hippocampus and short-term memory at school age in preterm born children, *Pediatr Res* 59:309-313, 2006.
833a. Rademaker KJ, Uiterwaal CS, Groenendaal F, Venema MM, et al: Neonatal hydrocortisone treatment: Neurodevelopmental outcome and MRI at school age in preterm-born children, *J Pediatr* 150:351-357, 2007.
833b. Watterberg KL, Shaffer ML, Mishefske MJ, Leach CL, et al: Growth and neurodevelopmental outcomes after early low-dose hydrocortisone treatment in extremely low birth weight infants, *Pediatrics* 120:40-48, 2007.
834. De Kloet ER, Vreugdenhil E, Oitzl MS, Joels M: Brain corticosteroid receptor balance in health and disease, *Endocr Rev* 19:269-301, 1998.
835. Reul JM, Gesing A, Droste S, Stec IS, et al: The brain mineralocorticoid receptor: Greedy for ligand, mysterious in function, *Eur J Pharmacol* 405:235-249, 2000.
836. Almeida OF, Conde GL, Crochemore C, Demeneix BA, et al: Subtle shifts in the ratio between pro- and antiapoptotic molecules after activation of corticosteroid receptors decide neuronal fate, *FASEB J* 14:779-790, 2000.
837. Hassan AH, von Rosenstiel P, Patchev VK, Holsboer F, et al: Exacerbation of apoptosis in the dentate gyrus of the aged rat by dexamethasone and the protective role of corticosterone, *Exp Neurol* 140:43-52, 1996.
838. Baud O, Laudenbach V, Evrard P, Gressens P: Neurotoxic effects of fluorinated glucocorticoid preparation on the developing mouse brain: Role of preservatives, *Pediatr Res* 50:706-711, 2001.
839. Lucas A, Morley R, Fewtrell MS: Low triiodothyronine concentration in preterm infants and subsequent intelligence quotient (IQ) at 8 year follow up, *BMJ* 312:1132-1133, 1996.
840. Den Ouden AL, Kok JH, Verkerk PH, Brand R, et al: The relation between neonatal thyroxine levels and neurodevelopmental outcome at age 5 and 9 years in a national cohort of very preterm and/or very low birth weight infants, *Pediatr Res* 39:142-145, 1995.
841. Reuss ML, Paneth N, Pinto-Martin JA, Lorenz JM, et al: The relation of transient hypothyroxinemia in preterm infants to neurologic development at two years of age, *N Engl J Med* 334:821-827, 1996.
842. Vulsma T, Kok JH: Prematurity-associated neurologic and developmental abnormalities and neonatal thyroid function, *N Engl J Med* 334:856-857, 1996.
843. van Wassenaer AG: Effects of thyroxine supplementation on neurologic development in infants born at less than 30 weeks' gestation, *N Engl J Med* 336:21-26, 1997.
844. Reuss ML, Leviton A, Paneth N, Susser M: Thyroxine values from newborn screening of 919 infants born before 29 weeks' gestation, *Am J Public Health* 87:1693-1697, 1997.
845. Briet JM, van Wassenaer AG, Dekker FW, de Vijlder JM, et al: Neonatal thyroxine supplementation in very preterm children: Developmental outcome evaluated at early school age, *Pediatrics* 107:712-718, 2001.
846. van Wassenaer AG, Briet JM, van Baar A, Smit BJ, et al: Free thyroxine levels during the first weeks of life and neurodevelopmental outcome until the age of 5 years in very preterm infants, *Pediatrics* 109:534-539, 2002.
847. Rapaport R, Rose SR, Freemark M: Hypothyroxinemia in the preterm infant: The benefits and risks of thyroxine treatment, *J Pediatr* 139:182-188, 2001.
848. Stein SA, Adams PM, Shanklin DR, Mihailoff GA, et al: Thyroid hormone control of brain and motor development: Molecular, neuroanatomical, and behavioral studies. In Bercu BB, Shullman DI, editors: *Advances in Perinatal Thyroidology*, New York: 1991, Plenum.
849. Porterfield SP, Hendrich CE: The role of thyroid hormones in prenatal and neonatal neurological development: Current perspectives, *Endocr Rev* 14:94-106, 1993.
850. Berbel P, Auso E, Garcia-Velasco JV, Molina ML, et al: Role of thyroid hormones in the maturation and organization of the rat barrel cortex, *Neuroscience* 107:383-394, 2001.
851. Berbel P, Garcia-Velasco JW, Auso E: Influence of thyroid hormones on the development of brain cytoarchitecture and connectivity. In Morreale de Escobar G, de Vijlder JJM, Butz S, et al, editors: *The Thyroid and Brain*, Stuggart: 2003, Schattauer.
852. Cuevas E, Auso E, Telefont M, deEscobar GM, et al: Transient maternal hypothyroxinemia at onset of corticogenesis alters tangential migration of medial ganglionic eminence-derived neurons, *Eur J Neurosci* 22:541-551, 2005.
853. Cordero ME, D'Acuna E, Benveniste S, Prado R, et al: Dendritic development in neocortex of infants with early postnatal life undernutrition, *Pediatr Neurol* 9:457-464, 1993.
854. Lanting CI, Fidler V, Huisman M, Touwen B, et al: Neurological differences between 9-year-old children fed breast-milk or formula-milk as babies, *Lancet* 344:1319-1322, 1994.
855. Pollock JI: Long-term associations with infant feeding in a clinically advantaged population of babies, *Dev Med Child Neurol* 36:429-440, 1994.
856. Donma MM, Donma O: The influence of feeding patterns on head circumference among Turkish infants during the first six months of life, *Brain Dev* 19:393-397, 1997.
857. Golding J, Rogers IS, Emmett PM: Association between breast feeding, child development and behavior, *Early Hum Dev* 49(Suppl):S175-S184, 1997.
858. Gordon N: Nutrition and cognitive function, *Brain Dev* 19:165-170, 1997.
859. Richards M, Wardsworth M, Rahimi-Foroushani A, Hardy R, et al: Infant nutrition and cognitive development in the first offspring of a national UK birth cohort, *Dev Med Child Neurol* 40:163-167, 1998.
860. Gordon N: Some influences on cognition in early life: A short review of recent opinions, *Eur J Pediatr Neurol* 1:1-5, 1998.
861. Lanting CI, Patandin S, Weisglas-Kuperus N, Touwen BCL, et al: Breastfeeding and neurological outcome at 42 months, *Acta Paediatr* 87:1224-1229, 1998.
862. Vohr BR, McKinley LT: The challenge pays off: Early enchanced nutritional intake for VLBW small-for-gestation neonates improves long-term outcome, *J Pediatr* 142:459-462, 2003.
863. Hayakawa M, Okumura A, Hayakawa F, Kato Y, et al: Nutritional state and growth and functional maturation of the brain in extremely low birth weight infants, *Pediatrics* 111:991-995, 2003.
864. Latal-Hajnal B, Von Siebenthal K, Kovari H, Bucher HU, et al: Postnatal growth in VLBW infants: Significant association with neurodevelopmental outcome, *J Pediatr* 143:163-170, 2003.
865. Koscik RL, Farrell PM, Kosorok MR, Zaremba KM, et al: Cognitive function of children with cystic fibrosis: Deleterious effect of early malnutrition, *Pediatrics* 113:1549-1558, 2004.
866. Brandt I, Sticker EJ, Lentze MJ: Catch-up growth of head circumference of very low birth weight, small for gestational age preterm infants and mental development to adulthood, *J Pediatr* 142:463-468, 2003.
867. Carlson SE: Functional effects of increasing omega-3 fatty acid intake, *J Pediatr* 131:173-175, 1997.
868. Jensen CL, Prager TC, Fraley K, Chen H, et al: Effect of dietary linoleic/alpha-linolenic acid ratio on growth and visual function of term infants, *J Pediatr* 131:200-209, 1997.
869. Xiang M, Alfven G, Blennow M, Trygg M, et al: Long-chain polyunsaturated fatty acids in human milk and brain growth during early infancy, *Acta Paediatr* 89:142-147, 2000.
870. SanGiovanni JP, Parra-Cabrera S, Colditz GA, Berkey CS, et al: Meta-analysis of dietary essential fatty acids and long-chain polyunsaturated fatty acids as they relate to visual resolution acuity in healthy preterm infants, *Pediatrics* 105:1292-1298, 2000.

871. Innis SM, Gilley J, Werker J: Are human milk long-chain polyunsaturated fatty acids related to visual and neural development in breast-fed term infants? *J Pediatr* 139:532-538, 2001.

872. O'Connor DL, Hall R, Adamkin D, Auestad N, et al: Growth and development in preterm infants fed long-chain polyunsaturated fatty acids: A prospective randomized controlled trial, *Pediatrics* 108:359-371, 2001.

873. Fewtrell MS, Motley R, Abbott RA, Singhal A, et al: Double-blind, randomized trial of long-chain polyunsaturated fatty acid supplementation in formula fed to preterm infants, *Pediatrics* 110:73-82, 2002.

874. Marini A, Vegni C, Gangi S, Benedetti V, et al: Influence of different types of post-discharge feeding on somatic growth, cognitive development and their correlation in very low birthweight preterm infants, *Acta Paediatr* 92:18-33, 2003.

875. Hoffman DR, Birch EE, Castaneda YS, Fawcett SL, et al: Visual function in breast-fed term infants weaned to formula with or without long-chain polyunsaturates at 4 to 6 months: A randomized clinical trial, *J Pediatr* 142:669-677, 2003.

876. Malcolm CA, McCulloch DL, Montgomery C, Shepherd A, et al: Maternal docosahexaenoic acid supplementation during pregnancy and visual evoked potential development in term infants: A double blind, prospective, randomised trial, *Arch Dis Child Fetal Neonatal Ed* 88:F383-F390, 2003.

877. Gustafsson PA, Duchen K, Birberg U, Karlsson T: Breastfeeding, very long polyunsaturated fatty acids (PUFA) and IQ at 6 1/2 years of age, *Acta Paediatr* 93:1280-1287, 2004.

878. Bouwstra H, Dijck-Brouwer DAJ, Boehm G, Boersma ER, et al: Long-chain polyunsaturated fatty acids and neurological developmental outcome at 18 months in healthy term infants, *Acta Paediatr* 94:26-32, 2005.

879. Georgieff MK, Innis SM: Controversial nutrients that potentially affect preterm neurodevelopment: Essential fatty acids and iron, *Pediatr Res* 57:99R-103R, 2005.

880. Bouwstra H, Dijck-Brouwer J, Decsi T, Boehm G, et al: Neurologic condition of healthy term infants at 18 months: Positive association with venous umbilical DHA status and negative association with umbilical trans-fatty acids, *Pediatr Res* 60:334-339, 2006.

881. Sirevaag AM, Greenough WT: Differential rearing effects on rat visual cortex synapses. III. Neuronal and glial nuclei, boutons, dendrites, and capillaries, *Brain Res* 424:320-332, 1987.

882. Liu D, Diorio J, Day JC, Francis DD, et al: Maternal care, hippocampal synaptogenesis and cognitive development in rats, *Nat Neurosci* 3:799-806, 2000.

883. Bourgeois JP, Jastreboff PJ, Rakic P: Synaptogenesis in visual cortex of normal and preterm monkeys: Evidence for intrinsic regulation of synaptic overproduction, *Proc Natl Acad Sci U S A* 86:4297-4301, 1989.

884. Tsuneishi S, Casaer P: Effects of preterm extrauterine visual experience on the development of the human visual system: A flash VEP study, *Dev Med Child Neurol* 42:663-668, 2000.

885. Als H, Duffy FH, McAnulty GB, Rivkin MJ, et al: Early experience alters brain function and structure, *Pediatrics* 113:846-857, 2004.

886. Averill DR Jr, Moxon ER, Smith AL: Effects of Haemophilus influenzae meningitis in infant rats on neuronal growth and synaptogenesis, *Exp Neurol* 50:337-345, 1976.

887. Hicks SP, Cavanaugh MC, O'Brien ED: Effects of anoxia on the developing cerebral cortex of the rat, *Am J Pathol* 40:615-635, 1962.

888. Horn G: Thyroid deficiency and inanition: Effects of replacement therapy on development of the cerebral cortex in young albino rats, *Anat Rec* 121:63-79, 1955.

889. Oda MA, Huttenlocher PR: The effect of corticosteroids on dendritic development in the rat brain, *Yale J Biol Med* 47:155-165, 1974.

890. Schapiro S: Some physiological, biochemical, and behavioral consequences of neonatal hormone administration: Cortisol and thyroxine, *Gen Comp Endocrinol* 10:214-228, 1968.

891. West CD, Kemper TL: The effect of a low protein diet on the anatomical development of the rat brain, *Brain Res* 107:221-237, 1976.

892. Coleman PD, Riesen AH: Environmental effects on cortical dendritic fields. I. Rearing in the dark, *J Anat* 102:363-374, 1968.

893. Globus A, Scheibel AB: The effect of visual deprivation on cortical neurons: A Golgi study, *Exp Neurol* 19:331-345, 1967.

894. Valverde F: Apical dendritic spines of the visual cortex and light deprivation in the mouse, *Exp Brain Res* 3:337-352, 1967.

895. Pysh JJ, Perkins RE, Beck LS: The effect of postnatal undernutrition on the development of the mouse Purkinje cell dendritic tree, *Brain Res* 163:165-170, 1979.

896. Balazs R, Patel AJ, Hajos F: Factors affecting the biochemical maturation of the brain: Effects of hormones during early life, *Psychoneuroendocrinology* 1:25-32, 1975.

897. Bass NH, Netsky MG, Young E: Effects of neonatal malnutrition on developing cerebrum. I. Microchemical and histologic study of cellular differentiation in the rat, *Arch Neurol* 23:289-302, 1970.

898. Harris WA: Neural activity and development, *Annu Rev Physiol* 43:689-710, 1981.

899. Wiesel TN: Postnatal development of the visual cortex and the influence of environment, *Nature* 299:583-591, 1982.

900. Ferrer I, Soriano E, Marti E, Digón E, et al: Development of dendritic spines in the cerebral cortex of the micrencephalic rat following prenatal X-irradiation, *Neurosci Lett* 125:183-186, 1991.

901. Seidler FJ, Slotkin TA: Fetal cocaine exposure causes persistent noradrenergic hyperactivity in rat brain regions: Effects on neurotransmitter turnover and receptors, *J Pharmacol Exp Ther* 263:413-421, 1992.

902. Yoshioka H, Yoshida A, Ochi M, Iino S, et al: Dendritic development of cortical neurons of mice subjected to total asphyxia: A Golgi-Cox study, *Acta Neuropathol (Berl)* 70:185-189, 1986.

903. Cordero ME, Trejo M, Garcia E, Barros T, et al: Dendritic development in the neocortex of adult rats subjected to postnatal malnutrition, *Early Hum Dev* 12:309-321, 1985.

904. Greenough WT, Hwang HM, Gorman C: Evidence for active synapse formation or altered postsynaptic metabolism in visual cortex of rats reared in complex environments, *Proc Natl Acad Sci U S A* 82:4549-4552, 1985.

905. Brock JW, Prasad C: Alterations in dendritic spine density in the rat brain associated with protein malnutrition, *Dev Brain Res* 66:266-269, 1992.

906. Pascual R, Fernandez V, Ruiz S, Kuljis RO: Environmental deprivation delays the maturation of motor pyramids during the early postnatal period, *Early Hum Dev* 33:145-155, 1993.

907. Marin-Padilla M: Developmental neuropathology and impact of perinatal brain damage. III. Gray matter lesions of the neocortex, *J Neuropathol Exp Neurol* 58:407-429, 1999.

908. Kemper TL, Lecours AR, Gates MJ: Delayed maturation of the brain in congenital rubella encephalopathy, *Res Publ Assoc Res Nerv Ment Dis* 51:23, 1972.

909. Bauman ML, Kemper TL: Curtailed histoanatomic development of the brain in phenylketonuria, *J Neuropathol Exp Neurol* 30:181, 1974.

910. Pogocar S, Dyckman J, Kemper TL: Neuropathology of the Rubinstein-Taybi syndrome, *J Neuropathol Exp Neurol* 34:110, 1975.

911. Marin-Padilla M: Structural organization of the cerebral cortex (motor area) in human chromosomal aberrations: A Golgi study. I.D1 (13-15) trisomy. Patau syndrome, *Brain Res* 66:375, 1974.

912. Jay V, Chan FW, Becker LE: Dendritic arborization in the human fetus and infant with the trisomy 18 syndrome, *Dev Brain Res* 54:291-294, 1990.

913. Lacey DJ, Terplan K: Abnormal cerebral cortical neurons in a child with maternal PKU syndrome, *J Child Neurol* 2:201-204, 1987.

914. Gilles FH, Leviton A, Dooling EC: *The Developing Human Brain: Growth and Epidemiologic Neuropathology*, Boston: 1983, John Wright.

915. Bunge RP: Glial cells and the central myelin sheath, *Physiol Rev* 48:197-251, 1968.

916. Brody BA, Kinney HC, Kloman AS, Gilles FH: Sequence of central nervous system myelination in human infancy. I. An autopsy study of myelination, *J Neuropathol Exp Neurol* 46:283-301, 1987.

917. Kinney HC, Brody BA, Kloman AS, Gilles FH: Sequence of central nervous system myelination in human infancy. II. Patterns of myelination in autopsied infants, *J Neuropathol Exp Neurol* 47:217-234, 1988.

918. Del Rio-Hortega P: Tercera aportacion al conocimiento morfologico e interpretacion funcional de la oligodendroglia, *Mem Real Soc Espan Hist Nat* 14:5, 1928.

919. Quarles RH, Morell P, McFarland HF: Diseases involving myelin. In Siegel GJ, Albers RW, Brady ST, et al, editors: *Basic Neurochemistry: Molecular, Cellular, and Medical Aspects, vol. 7*, London: 2006, Elsevier.

920. Sherman DL, Brophy PJ: Mechanisms of axon ensheathment and myelin growth, *Nat Rev Neurosci* 6:683-690, 2005.

921. Kendler A, Golden JA: Progenitor cell proliferation outside the ventricular and subventricular zones during human brain development, *J Neuropathol Exp Neurol* 55:1253-1258, 1996.

922. Child A-M, Ramenghi LA, Evans DJ, Ridgeway J, et al: MR features of developing periventricular white matter in preterm infants: Evidence of glial cell migration, *AJNR Am J Neuroradiol* 19:971-976, 1998.

923. Battin MR, Maalouf EF, Counsell SJ, Herlihy AH, et al: Magnetic resonance imaging of the brain in very preterm infants: Visualization of the germinal matrix, early myelination, and cortical folding, *Pediatrics* 101:957-962, 1998.

924. Huppi PS, Maier SE, Peled S, Zientara GP, et al: Microstructural development of human newborn cerebral white matter assessed in vivo by diffusion tensor magnetic resonance imaging, *Pediatr Res* 44:584-590, 1998.

925. Kroenke CD, Bretthorst GL, Inder TE, Neil JJ: Diffusion MR imaging characteristics of the developing primate brain, *Neuroimage* 25:1205-1213, 2005.

926. Zumkeller W: The effect of insulin-like growth factors on brain myelination and their potential therapeutic application in myelination disorders, *Eur J Pediatr Neurol* 4:91-101, 1997.

927. Ahlgren SC, Wallace H, Bishop J, Neophytou C, et al: Effects of thyroid hormone on embryonic oligodendrocyte precursor cell development in vivo and in vitro, *Mol Cell Neurosci* 9:420-432, 1997.

928. Vartanian T, Fischbach G, Miller R: Failure of spinal cord oligodendrocyte development in mice lacking neuregulin, *Proc Natl Acad Sci U S A* 96:731-735, 1999.

929. Chan JR, Watkins TA, Cosgaya JM, Zhang C, et al: NGF controls axonal receptivity to myelination by Schwann cells or oligodendrocytes, *Neuron* 43:183-191, 2004.

930. Cohen RI: Visions and reflections: Exploring oligodendrocyte guidance "to boldly go where no cell has gone before," *Cell Mol Life Sci* 62:505-510, 2005.

931. Chen S, Velardez MO, Warot X, Yu ZX, et al: Neuregulin 1-erbB signaling is necessary for normal myelination and sensory function, *J Neurosci* 26:3079-3086, 2006.

931a. Zeger M, Popken G, Zhang J, Xuan S, et al: Insulin-like growth factor type 1 receptor signaling in the cells of oligodendrocyte lineage is required for normal in vivo oligodendrocyte development and myelination, *Glia* 55:400-411, 2007.

932. Yakovlev PI, Lecours AR: The myelogenetic cycles of regional maturation of the brain. In Minkowski A, editor: *Regional Development of the Brain in Early Life*, Philadelphia: 1967, FA Davis.

933. Gilles FH: Myelination in the neonatal brain, *Hum Pathol* 7:244-248, 1976.

934. Counsell SJ, Maalouf EF, Fletcher AM, Duggan PJ, et al: MR imaging assessment of myelination in the very preterm brain, *AJNR Am J Neuroradiol* 23:872-881, 2002.

935. Chattha AS, Richardson EP Jr: Cerebral white-matter hypoplasia, *Arch Neurol* 34:137-141, 1977.

936. Samorajski T, Friede RL, Reimer PR: Hypomyelination in the quaking mouse: A model for the analysis of disturbed myelin formation, *J Neuropathol Exp Neurol* 29:507-523, 1970.

937. Torii J, Adachi M, Volk BW: Histochemical and ultrastructural studies of inherited leukodystrophy in mice, *J Neuropathol Exp Neurol* 30:278-289, 1971.

937a. Biancheri R, Zara F, Bruno C, Rossi A, et al: Phenotypic characterization of hypomyelination and congenital cataract, *Ann Neurol* 62:121-127, 2007.

938. Volpe JJ: Cerebral white matter injury of the premature infant: More common than you think, *Pediatrics* 112:176-179, 2003.

939. Haynes RL, Folkerth RD, Keefe R, Sung I, et al: Nitrosative and oxidative injury to premyelinating oligodendrocytes is accompanied by microglial activation in periventricular leukomalacia in the human premature infant, *J Neuropath Exp Neurol* 62:441-450, 2003.

940. Back SA, Luo NL, Mallinson RA, O'Malley JP, et al: Selective vulnerability of preterm white matter to oxidative damage defined by F(2)-isoprostanes, *Ann Neurol* 58:108-120, 2005.

941. Cioni G, Bartalena L, Biagioni E, Boldrini A: Neuroimaging and functional outcome of neonatal leukomalacia, *Behav Brain Res* 49:7-19, 1992.

942. Fedrizzi E, Inverno M, Bruzzone MG, Botteon G, et al: MRI features of cerebral lesions and cognitive functions in preterm spastic diplegic children, *Pediatr Neurol* 15:207-212, 1996.

943. Iida K, Takashima S, Takeuchi Y, Ohno T, et al: Neuropathologic study of newborns with prenatal-onset leukomalacia, *Pediatr Neurol* 9:45-48, 1993.

944. Iida K, Takashima S, Ueda K: Immunohistochemical study of myelination and oligodendrocyte in infants with periventricular leukomalacia, *Pediatr Neurol* 13:296-304, 1995.

945. Leviton A, Gilles F: Ventriculomegaly, delayed myelination, white matter hypoplasia, and "periventricular" leukomalacia: How are they related? *Pediatr Neurol* 15:127-136, 1996.

946. Olsen P, Paakko E, Vainionpaa L, Pyhtinen J, et al: Magnetic resonance imaging of periventricular leukomalacia and its clinical correlation in children, *Ann Neurol* 41:754-761, 1997.

947. Paneth N, Rudelli R, Monte W, Rodriguez E, et al: White matter necrosis in very low birth weight infants: Neuropathologic and ultrasonographic findings in infants surviving six days or longer, *J Pediatr* 116:975-984, 1990.

948. Pellicer A, Cabanas F, Garcia-Alix A, Rodriguez JP, et al: Natural history of ventricular dilatation in preterm infants: Prognostic significance, *Pediatr Neurol* 9:108-114, 1993.

949. Rorke LB: *Pathology of Perinatal Brain Injury*, New York: 1982, Raven Press.

950. Skranes JS, Vik T, Nilsen G, Smevik O, et al: Cerebral magnetic resonance imaging and mental and motor function of very low birth weight children at six years of age, *Neuropediatrics* 28:149-154, 1997.

951. Weisglas-Kuperus N, Baerts W, Fetter W, Sauer P: Neonatal cerebral ultrasound, neonatal neurology and perinatal conditions as predictors of neurodevelopmental outcome in very low birthweight infants, *Early Hum Dev* 31:131-148, 1992.

952. Argyropoulou MI, Xydis V, Drougia A, Argyropoulou PI, et al: MRI measurements of the pons and cerebellum in children born preterm: Associations with the severity of periventricular leukomalacia and perinatal risk factors, *Neuroradiology* 45:730-734, 2003.

953. Carmody DP, Dunn SM, Boddie-Willis AS, DeMarco JK, et al: A quantitative measure of myelination development in infants, using MR images, *Neuroradiology* 46:781-786, 2004.

954. Silberman J, Dancis J, Feigin T: Neuropathological observations in maple syrup urine disease, *Arch Neurol* 5:351-363, 1961.

955. Malamud N: Neuropathology of phenylketonuria, *J Neuropathol Exp Neurol* 25:254-268, 1966.

956. Shuman RM, Leech RW, Scott CR: The neuropathology of the nonketotic and ketotic hyperglycinemias: Three cases, *Neurology* 28:139-146, 1978.

957. Prensky AL, Moser HW: Brain lipids, proteolipids, and free amino acids in maple syrup urine disease, *J Neurochem* 13:863-874, 1966.

958. Patel AJ, Hunt A, Kiss J: Neonatal thyroid deficiency has differential effects on cell specific markers for astrocytes and oligodendrocytes in the rat brain, *Neurochem Int* 15:239-248, 1989.

959. Shanker G, Amur SG, Pieringer RA: Investigations on myelinogenesis in vitro: A study of the critical period at which thyroid hormone exerts its maximum regulatory effect on the developmental expression of two myelin associated markers in cultured brain cells from embryonic mice, *Neurochem Res* 10:617-625, 1985.

960. King RA, Smith RM, Dreosti IE: Regional effects of hypothyroidism on 5'-nucleotidase and cyclic nucleotide phosphohydrolase activities in developing rat brain, *Dev Brain Res* 7:287-294, 1983.

961. Rosman NP, Malone MJ, Helfenstein M, Kraft E: The effect of thyroid deficiency on myelination of brain: A morphological and biochemical study, *Neurology* 22:99-106, 1972.

962. Alves C, Eidson M, Engle H, Sheldon J, et al: Changes in brain maturation detected by magnetic resonance imaging in congenital hypothyroidism, *J Pediatr* 115:600-603, 1989.

963. Rovet J, Ehrlich R, Sorbara D: Intellectual outcome in children with fetal hypothyroidism, *J Pediatr* 110:700-704, 1987.

964. Komianou F, Makaronis G, Lambadaridis J, Sarafidou E, et al: Psychomotor development in congenital hypothyroidism: The Greek screening programme, *Eur J Pediatr* 147:275-278, 1988.

965. Glorieux J, Dussault J, Van Vliet G: Intellectual development at age 12 years of children with congenital hypothyroidism diagnosed by neonatal screening, *J Pediatr* 121:581-584, 1992.

966. Bongers-Schokking JJ, Koot HM, Wiersma D, Verkerk PH, et al: Influence of timing and dose of thyroid hormone replacement on development in infants with congenital hypothyroidism, *J Pediatr* 136:292-297, 2000.

967. Selva KA, Harper A, Downs A, Blasco PA, et al: Neurodevelopmental outcomes in congenital hypothyroidism: Comparison of initial T4 dose and time to reach target T4 and TSH, *J Pediatr* 147:775-780, 2005.

968. Heyerdahl S, Kase BF, Lie SO: Intellectual development in children with congenital hypothyroidism in relation to recommended thyroxine treatment, *J Pediatr* 118:850-857, 1991.

969. Patel AJ, Hayashi M, Hunt A: Selective persistent reduction in choline acetyltransferase activity in basal forebrain of the rat after thyroid deficiency during early life, *Brain Res* 422:182-185, 1987.

970. Patel AJ, Hayashi M, Hunt A: Role of thyroid hormone and nerve growth factor in the development of choline acetyltransferase and other cell-specific marker enzymes in the basal forebrain of the rat, *J Neurochem* 50:803-811, 1988.

971. Kooistra L, Crawford S, van Baar AL, Brouwers EP, et al: Neonatal effects of maternal hypothyroxinemia during early pregnancy, *Pediatrics* 117:161-167, 2006.

972. Fishman MA, Prensky AL, Dodge PR: Low content of cerebral lipids in infants suffering from malnutrition, *Nature* 221:552-553, 1969.

973. Fox JH, Fishman MA, Dodge PR, Prensky AL: The effect of malnutrition on human central nervous system myelin, *Neurology* 22:1213-1216, 1972.

974. Martinez M: Myelin lipids in the developing cerebrum, cerebellum, and brain stem of normal and undernourished children, *J Neurochem* 39:1684-1692, 1982.

975. Chase HP, Martin HP: Undernutrition and child development, *N Engl J Med* 282:933-939, 1970.

976. Stoch MB, Smythe PM, Moodie AD, Bradshaw D: Psychosocial outcome and CT findings after gross undernourishment during infancy: A 20-year developmental study, *Dev Med Child Neurol* 24:419-436, 1982.

977. Galler JR, Ramsey F, Solimano G: The influence of early malnutrition on subsequent behavioral development. III. Learning disabilities as a sequel to malnutrition, *Pediatr Res* 18:309-313, 1984.

978. Rosso P: Morbidity and mortality in intrauterine growth retardation. In Senterre J, editor: *Intrauterine Growth Retardation*, New York: 1989, Raven Press.

979. Ballabriga A: Some aspects of clinical and biochemical changes related to nutrition during brain development in humans. In Evrard P, Minkowski A, editors: *Developmental Neurobiology*, New York: 1989, Raven Press.

980. Galler JR, Ramsey FC, Morley DS, Archer E, et al: The long-term effects of early kwashiorkor compared with marasmus. IV. Performance on the national high school entrance examination, *Pediatr Res* 28:235-239, 1990.

981. Rosso P: Maternal nutrition and fetal growth: Implications for subsequent mental competence, *Current Topics in Nutrition and Disease, vol. 16: Basic and Clinical Aspects of Nutrition and Brain Development*, New York: 1987, Alan R. Liss.

982. Dobbing J: Maternal nutrition in pregnancy and later achievement of offspring: A personal interpretation, *Early Hum Dev* 12:1-8, 1985.

983. Dobbing J: Infant nutrition and later achievement, *Am J Clin Nutr* 41:477-484, 1985.

984. Stein Z, Susser M: Early nutrition, fetal growth, and mental function: Observations in our species, *Current Topics in Nutrition and Disease, vol. 16: Basic and Clinical Aspects of Nutrition and Brain Development*, New York: 1987, Alan R. Liss.

985. Gay CT, Hardies LJ, Rauch RA, Lancaster JL, et al: Magnetic resonance imaging demonstrates incomplete myelination in, 18q- syndrome: Evidence for myelin basic protein haploinsufficiency, *Am J Med Genet* 74:422-431, 1997.

986. Loevner LA, Shapiro RM, Grossman RI, Overhauser J, et al: White matter changes associated with deletions of the long arm of chromosome 18 (18q- syndrome): A dysmyelinating disorder? *AJNR Am J Neuroradiol* 17:1843-1848, 1996.

987. Lancaster JL, Cody JD, Andrews T, Hardies LJ, et al: Myelination in children with partial deletions of chromosome 18q, *AJNR Am J Neuroradiol* 26:447-454, 2005.

988. Kamholz J, Spielman R, Gogolin K, Modi W, et al: The human myelin-basic-protein gene: Chromosomal localization and RFLP analysis, *Am J Hum Genet* 40:365-373, 1987.

989. Winick M: Malnutrition and brain development, *J Pediatr* 74:667-679, 1969.

990. Dobbing J: Undernutrition and the developing brain: The relevance of animal models to the human problem, *Am J Dis Child* 120:411-415, 1970.

991. Chase HP, Dorsey J, McKhann GM: The effect of malnutrition on the synthesis of a myelin lipid, *Pediatrics* 40:551-559, 1967.

992. Benton JW, Moser HW, Dodge PR, Carr S: Modification of the schedule of myelination in the rat by early nutritional deprivation, *Pediatrics* 38:801-807, 1966.

993. Wiggins RC, Fuller GN: Early postnatal starvation causes lasting brain hypomyelination, *J Neurochem* 30:1231-1237, 1978.

994. Krigman MR, Hogan EL: Undernutrition in the developing rat: Effect upon myelination, *Brain Res* 107:239-255, 1976.

995. Fuller GN, Wiggins RC: A possible effect of the methylxanthines caffeine, theophylline and aminophylline on postnatal myelination of the rat brain, *Brain Res* 213:476-480, 1981.

996. Allan WC, Volpe JJ: Reduction of cholesterol synthesis by methylxanthines in cultured glial cells, *Pediatr Res* 13:1121-1124, 1979.

997. Volpe JJ: Effects of methylxanthines on lipid synthesis in developing neural systems, *Semin Perinatol* 5:395-405, 1981.

998. Royland J, Klinkhachorn P, Konat G, Wiggins S: How much under-nourishment is required to retard brain myelin development, *Neurochem Int* 21:269-274, 1992.

999. Yager JY, Hartfield DS: Neurologic manifestations of iron deficiency in childhood, *Pediatr Neurol* 27:85-92, 2002.

1000. Gordon N: Iron deficiency and the intellect, *Brain Dev* 25:3-8, 2003.

1001. Roncagliolo M, Garrido M, Walter T, Peirano P, et al: Evidence of altered central nervous system development in infants with iron deficiency anemia at 6 mo: Delayed maturation of auditory brainstem responses, *Am J Clin Nutr* 68:683-690, 1998.

1002. Friel JK, Aziz K, Andrews WL, Harding SV, et al: A double-masked randomized control trial of iron supplementation in early infancy in healthy term breast-fed infants, *J Pediatr* 143:582-586, 2003.

1003. Lozoff B, De Andraca I, Castillo M, Smith JB, et al: Behavioral and developmental effects of preventing iron-deficiency anemia in health full-term infants, *Pediatrics* 112:846-854, 2003.

1004. Algarin C, Peirano P, Garrido M, Pizarro F, et al: Iron deficiency anemia in infancy: Long-lasting effects on auditory and visual system functioning, *Pediatr Res* 53:217-223, 2003.

1005. Sarici SU, Serdar MA, Dundaroz MR, Unay B, et al: Brainstem auditory-evoked potentials in iron-deficiency anemia, *Pediatr Neurol* 24:205-208, 2001.

1006. Connor JR, Benkovic SA: Iron regulation in the brain: Histochemical, biochemical, and molecular considerations, *Ann Neurol* 32(Suppl):S51-S61, 1992.

1007. Koo BK, Blaser S, Harwood-Nash D, Becker LE, et al: Magnetic resonance imaging evaluation of delayed myelination in Down syndrome: A case report and review of the literature, *J Child Neurol* 7:417-421, 1992.

NEUROLOGICAL
EVALUATION

Chapter 3

Neurological Examination: Normal and Abnormal Features

The neurological evaluation of the newborn comprises, as it does at other ages in pediatric medicine, the history, physical examination, and appropriate specialized studies. Relevant aspects of these three basic parts of the evaluation are illustrated in essentially every chapter of this book. Thus, enumerating all these aspects here would serve little purpose.

In this chapter, the *neonatal neurological examination* is emphasized, because an organized approach to the infant is so critical and, in fact, is the cornerstone of the neurological evaluation. My approach is organized on the framework of the neurological examination of older infants and children, but it is supplemented and modified significantly for adaptation to the newborn. Too often, an organized, systematic approach to the infant is omitted because of the morass of catheters, tubes, monitors, blindfolds, intravenous accoutrements, and the like surrounding the child. It is curiously paradoxical that these outward manifestations of our attempts to provide optimal therapy may interfere significantly with the careful clinical examination that is necessary for rational judgments regarding diagnosis, prognosis, and management. Conversely, the examiner should remember that the sick newborn, especially the premature infant, often has only tenuous control of such critical functions as respiration and cardiovascular status, and overly vigorous manipulation of the baby may have adverse consequences. The purpose of the following discussion is to describe the normal and abnormal features of the neonatal neurological examination and to illustrate the importance of these features in our understanding of neurological development and disease.

NORMAL NEUROLOGICAL EXAMINATION

In the following section, the normal features of the neonatal neurological examination are outlined (Table 3-1). Before addressing the formal neurological examination, brief discussions of determination of gestational age and evaluation of the head are necessary.

Estimation of Gestational Age

Estimation of gestational age is particularly important for several reasons. First, various aspects of the neonatal neurological evaluation change with maturation, and recognition of these changes is critical in assessing the observations. Second, certain disorders are particularly characteristic of infants who are born prematurely but

who are of average weight for gestational age, those born at term but are small for gestational age, and so forth. Third, the same insult (e.g., hypoxia-ischemia) will have a different impact on various regions of the central nervous system, in large part as a function of the gestational age of the infant.

The most helpful information for estimating gestational age is the date of the mother's last menstrual period, particularly in the smallest infants.[1,2] It is unfortunate that, too often, this information is not known precisely. Thus, various other measures have been used to estimate gestational age, including the following: anthropometric measurements, such as birth weight and head circumference; certain external characteristics; neurological evaluation; radiological study of bone maturation; certain neurophysiological parameters, especially measurement of motor nerve conduction velocity or the electroencephalogram; and cranial ultrasonographic determinations of sulcal development. All these approaches have certain merit, as well as significant limitations. Of the techniques evaluated, examination of certain external characteristics has been at least as effective as other methods.[2-4] I find four selected external characteristics to be particularly useful: the ear cartilage and its reflection in ear position, the amount of breast tissue, the characteristics of the external genitalia, and the creases of the plantar surface of the foot (Table 3-2).[3,5-10] In the first hours of life, I do not use the measurements of tone and posture for this purpose,[9,10] because in my experience these measurements are variable and are sensitive to exogenous factors, including the process of birth. However, for infants after the first hours of life, some clinicians find these evaluations useful for assessing maturation.[2,11,12] These comments are not to deny the value of recognizing the temporal characteristics of neurological maturation, as discussed in detail subsequently, but rather to emphasize that, in my experience, such characteristics are not optimal for the purposes of estimating gestational age, particularly in the immediate neonatal period.

Head: External Characteristics and Rate of Growth

External Characteristics

The external characteristics of the head to be evaluated include the size and shape (see later discussion) and the skin.

TABLE 3-1	Neonatal Neurological Examination: Basic Elements

Level of Alertness

Cranial Nerves
Olfaction (I)
Vision (II)
Optic fundi (II)
Pupils (III)
Extraocular movements (III, IV, VI)
Facial sensation and masticatory power (V)
Facial motility (VII)
Audition (VIII)
Sucking and swallowing (V, VII, IX, X, XII)
Sternocleidomastoid function (XI)
Tongue function (XII)
Taste (VII, IX)

Motor Examination
Tone and posture
Motility and power
Tendon reflexes and plantar response

Primary Neonatal Reflexes
Moro reflex
Palmar grasp
Tonic neck response

Sensory Examination

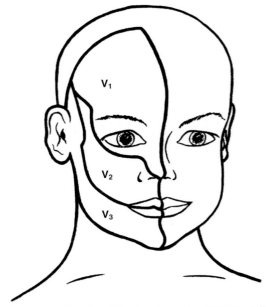

Figure 3-1 **Dermatomal distribution of the face.** Note the delineation of the three branches of the trigeminal nerve: ophthalmic (V_1), maxillary (V_2), and mandibular (V_3). (*From Enjolras O, Riche MC, Merland JJ: Facial port-wine stains and Sturge-Weber syndrome,* Pediatrics 76:48-51, 1985.)

Skin. The skin of the head should be examined carefully for the presence of dimples or tracts, subcutaneous masses (e.g., encephalocele, tumor), or cutaneous lesions, all generally discussed elsewhere in this book. In this setting, I discuss only the significance of *port-wine stains*, congenital vascular abnormalities that are present at birth and persist into adulthood. At birth, these lesions are most often pale pink, macular lesions that subsequently become dark red to purple and often nodular.[13] Port-wine stains are categorized according to their dermatomal distribution (Fig. 3-1). Their importance, apart from the significant cosmetic issue, relates principally to their association with abnormalities of choroidal vessels in the eye, which may result in glaucoma, and of meningeal and superficial cerebral vessels, which may result in cortical lesions with seizures and other neurological deficits (i.e., Sturge-Weber syndrome). The relationships between the location of the port-wine stain and the incidence of glaucoma or intracranial vascular lesion are shown in Table 3-3. In one large series, the intracranial vascular lesion of Sturge-Weber syndrome occurred in 40% to 50% of children with total involvement of V_1.[14,15] Notably, with *partial* involvement of V_1, the risk was markedly lower (1 of 17 children affected), and none of the 64 children with involvement of V_2 or V_3, or both, developed either the intracranial lesion or glaucoma.[14,15] The particular prognostic importance of involvement of V_1 was confirmed in

TABLE 3-2	External Characteristics Useful for Estimation of Gestational Age			
	GESTATIONAL AGE			
External Characteristic	**28 Weeks**	**32 Weeks**	**36 Weeks**	**40 Weeks**
Ear cartilage	Pinna soft, remains folded	Pinna slightly harder but remains folded	Pinna harder, springs back	Pinna firm, stands erect from head
Breast tissue	None	None	1–2-mm nodule	6–7-mm nodule
External genitalia: male	Testes undescended, smooth scrotum	Testes in inguinal canal, few scrotal rugae	Testes high in scrotum, more scrotal rugae	Testes descended, pendulous scrotum covered with rugae
External genitalia: female	Prominent clitoris, small, widely separated labia	Prominent clitoris, larger separated labia	Clitoris less prominent, labia majora cover labia minora	Clitoris covered by labia majora
Plantar surface	Smooth	One or two anterior creases	Two or three anterior creases	Creases cover sole

Adapted from references 3, 5, and 7 to 10.

TABLE 3-3 Relation between Location of Port-Wine Stain and Subsequent Incidence of Glaucoma or Sturge-Weber Syndrome

Location of Port-Wine Stain (Dermatomal Distribution)	Total Number	Intracranial Vascular Lesion with or without Glaucoma	Glaucoma Alone	Port-Wine Stain Only
V_1 (total) alone	4	2	1	1
V_1 (total) with other dermatomes	21	9	3	9
V_1 (partial) with or without other dermatomes	17	1	0	16
V_2 alone	29	0	0	29
V_3 alone	13	0	0	13
V_2 and V_3 (unilateral or bilateral)	22	0	0	22

Data from Enjolras O, Riche MC, Merland JJ: Facial port-wine stains and Sturge-Weber syndrome, *Pediatrics* 76:48-51, 1985.

more selected series.[16,17] The optimal timing of therapy has been the subject of debate; a large prospective study did not report treatment early in infancy and childhood to be superior to later treatment.[18-21]

Head Size and Shape. *Head circumference* is a useful measure of intracranial volume and therefore also of volume of brain and cerebrospinal fluid. Less commonly, head circumference is significantly affected by the size of extracerebral spaces, subdural and subarachnoid, or by the intracranial blood volume. Scalp edema, subcutaneous infiltration of fluid from intravenous infusion, and cephalhematoma also have obvious effects. Nevertheless, measurement of head circumference remains one of the most readily available and useful means for evaluating the status of the central nervous system in the newborn period. Longitudinal measurements in particular provide valuable information.

Head circumference is influenced by *head shape*: the more circular the head shape, the smaller the circumference needs to be to contain the same area and the same intracranial volume. Infants with relatively large occipital-frontal diameters have larger measured head circumferences than infants with relatively large biparietal diameters. This finding has important implications for evaluating the head circumference of an infant with a skull deformity such as craniosynostosis (see next paragraph). In premature infants, over the first 2 to 3 months of life, an impressive change in head shape is characterized by an increase in occipital-frontal diameter relative to biparietal diameter (Fig. 3-2). Because this alteration occurs over a matter of *weeks*, it usually does not cause major difficulties in the interpretation of head circumference, but it does need to be considered, especially in infants with unusually marked dolichocephalic change.

Craniosynostosis, defined as premature cranial suture closure, may affect one or more cranial sutures (Table 3-4).[22] Simple sagittal synostosis is most common.[22,23] The diagnosis can be suspected by the shape of the head; with synostosis of a suture, growth of the skull can occur parallel to the affected suture but not at right angles (Fig. 3-3). The "keel-shaped" head of sagittal synostosis is termed *dolichocephaly* or *scaphocephaly*, the wide head of coronal synostosis is *brachycephaly*, and the tower-shaped head of combined coronal, sagittal, and lambdoid synostosis is *acrocephaly*. A few cases of

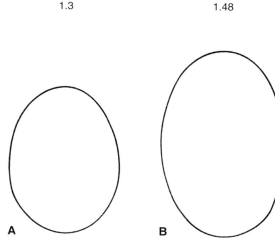
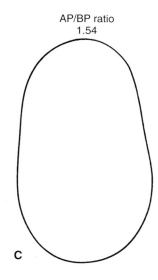

AP/BP ratio 1.3   AP/BP ratio 1.48   AP/BP ratio 1.54

Figure 3-2 Change in head shape in premature infants. Measurements of AP/BP ratio (anterior-posterior [AP] and biparietal [BP] diameters) and drawings of head shape (vertex view) of an infant, born at 28 weeks of gestation, made at, **A**, 1 week, **B**, 5 weeks, and, **C**, 11½ weeks. *(From Baum JD, Searls D: Head shape and size of pre-term low-birthweight infants,* Med Child Neurol *13:576-581, 1971.)*

A   B   C

TABLE 3-4 Distribution of Suture Involvement in Craniosynostosis

Sutures	Percentage of Cases*
Sagittal only	56
Coronal only	25
One	13
Both	12
Metopic only	4
Lambdoid only (one or both)	2
Various combinations	13

*Total of 519 patients.
Data from Matson D: *Neurosurgery of Infancy and Childhood,* Springfield, IL: 1969, Charles C Thomas.

cranial synostosis represent complex syndromes, the major features, genetics, and neurological outcome of which are summarized in Table 3-5.[24-30] The importance of early correction of synostosis for optimal cosmetic appearance and the other aspects of management are discussed in standard textbooks of neurosurgery.

Positional or deformational plagiocephaly has become a frequent clinical issue. The term *plagiocephaly* ("oblique head," from the Greek) refers to a head appearance in which the occipital region is flattened and the ipsilateral frontal area is prominent (i.e., anteriorly displaced) (Fig. 3-4). In positional or deformational plagiocephaly, caused by external molding forces, the ipsilateral ear is also displaced anteriorly, and the contralateral side of the face may appear flattened.[31,32] Torticollis may be associated and may cause a head tilt. Deformation plagiocephaly may be present at *birth*, secondary to *intrauterine* restriction to head movement as occurs with multiple gestation, abnormal uterine lie, or neck abnormality (e.g., torticollis), or it may evolve over the *first weeks to months of life*, usually secondary to *supine sleeping position* as part of the "Back to Sleep" program.[31,33] Differentiation of deformational plagiocephaly from the rare unilateral lambdoid synostosis, which can also cause occipital flattening, is usually readily made clinically. In unilateral lambdoid synostosis, the anterior displacement of the frontal area is usually less pronounced, the ear is posterior, not anterior, and is displaced inferiorly, and facial deformity is rare. Management of deformational plagiocephaly consists of parental counseling regarding head positioning with the infant supine, supervised time in the prone position, various exercises, and skull-molding helmets if necessary (see Fig. 3-4).[31,34-36]

Rate of Head Growth

Interpretation of the rate of head growth in premature infants is often difficult, in part because "normal" *postnatal* rates have been difficult to define conclusively (in contrast to normal rates of intrauterine growth, as plotted on most standard charts) and in part because commonly occurring systemic diseases and caloric deprivation in the neonatal period may interfere with brain and head growth.

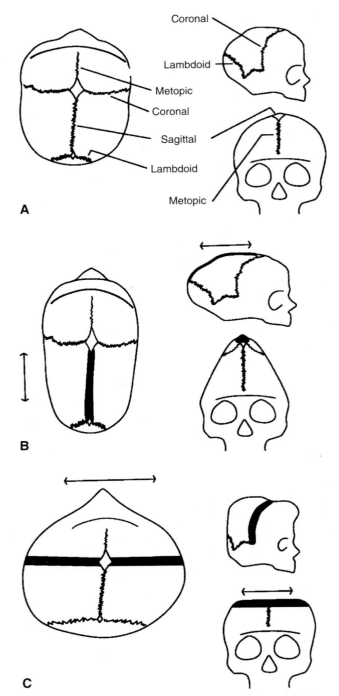

Figure 3-3 **Changes related to premature closure of cranial sutures.** Schematic diagram of, **A**, cranial sutures and changes in cranial shape with premature closure of, **B**, sagittal or, **C**, coronal sutures.

The rate of head growth in premature infants has been the subject of numerous reports.[37-50] In the *healthy premature infant*, change in the head circumference in the first days of life is minimal; indeed, a small amount of *head shrinkage* with suture overriding has been documented.[39,51] Head shrinkage reaches a peak at approximately 3 days of life, usually averages 2% to 3% of the head circumference at birth, and correlates closely with postnatal weight and urinary sodium losses. In view of these findings and the overriding of

TABLE 3-5 Craniosynostosis Syndromes

Syndrome Name	Cranium	Other Major Features	Genetics	Neurological Outcome
Crouzon	Acrocephaly (tower-shaped) with synostosis of coronal, sagittal, and lambdoid sutures	Ocular proptosis (shallow orbits) and maxillary hypoplasia	Autosomal dominant (variable expression)	Mental retardation occasional
Carpenter	Acrobrachycephaly with synostosis of coronal, sagittal, and lambdoid sutures	Lateral displacement of inner canthi, polydactyly and syndactyly of feet	Autosomal recessive	Mental retardation common
Apert	Brachycephaly with irregular synostosis, especially of coronal suture	Midfacial hypoplasia, syndactyly of fingers and toes, broad distal phalanx of thumb and big toe	Autosomal dominant (usually new mutation)	Mental retardation or borderline intelligence common
Saethre-Chotzen	Brachycephaly with synostosis of coronal suture	Prominent ear crus, maxillary hypoplasia, partial syndactyly of fingers and toes	Autosomal dominant (variable expression)	Mental retardation uncommon
Pfeiffer	Brachycephaly with synostosis of coronal and/or sagittal sutures	Hypertelorism, broad thumbs and toes, partial syndactyly of fingers and toes	Autosomal dominant	Normal intelligence usual
Antley-Bixler	Brachycephaly with multiple synostosis, especially of coronal suture	Maxillary hypoplasia, radiohumeral synostosis, choanal atresia, arthrogryposis	Autosomal recessive	Intelligence probably normal
Greig	High forehead with variable synostosis	Hypertelorism, polydactyly and syndactyly of fingers and toes	Autosomal dominant	Mild mental retardation occasional
Baller-Gerold	Synostosis of variable sutures, including metopic with trigonocephaly	Radial dysplasia with absent thumbs	Autosomal recessive	Mental retardation common
Opitz	Trigonocephaly with synostosis of metopic suture	Upward slant of palpebral fissures, epicanthal folds, narrow palate, anomalies of external ear, loose skin, variable polydactyly or syndactyly of fingers	Autosomal recessive	Mental retardation common

sutures, investigators have suggested that the head shrinkage relates to water loss from the intracranial compartment.[39]

A longitudinal study of 41 premature infants (<1500 g birth weight) with favorable neurological outcome at age 2 years, as assessed by neurological examination and Bayley Mental Developmental Scale, defined the rates of head growth shown in Table 3-6. Thus, after a period of decreasing head circumference in the first week, head growth increased by a mean of approximately 0.50 cm in the second week, 0.75 cm in the third week, and 1.0 cm per week thereafter in the neonatal period. Slower rates of head growth were observed in infants with serious systemic disorders and subsequent neurological impairment.[41] Faster rates of head growth in the first 6 weeks suggest hydrocephalus (e.g., after intraventricular hemorrhage), as detailed in Chapter 11.[38,41] "Sick" preterm infants with systemic disease often exhibit a "normal" acceleration of head growth (i.e., "catch-up" head growth) after recovery from their illness.[52] However, the smallest infants, those who weigh less than 1000 g at birth, generally do not exhibit as rapid growth as premature infants whose birth weight is greater than 2000 g and do not catch up even by 2 years of age.[45] Additionally, preterm infants born small for their gestational age often do not exhibit as rapid head growth or as effective catch-up growth as infants born average for their gestational age.[48]

The importance of duration of neonatal caloric deprivation (<85 kcal/kg/day) on head growth in the neonatal period was shown in a study of 73 preterm infants (mean gestational age, 30 ± 2 weeks) (Fig. 3-5).[53] Three phases of head growth were defined: an initial period of growth arrest or suboptimal head growth, followed by a period of catch-up growth, and terminated by a period of growth along standard curves. The duration of the period of growth arrest or suboptimal growth was directly related to the initial period of caloric deprivation and to the duration of mechanical ventilation, and the period of catch-up growth was directly related to the duration of the preceding caloric deprivation only.

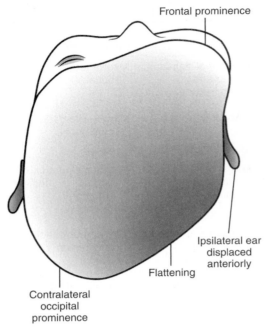

Figure 3-4 **Positional or deformational plagiocephaly.** Note the flattening of the right occiput, because the infant is placed primarily in a supine position and the infant's preferred head position is to the right. The other changes are described in the text.

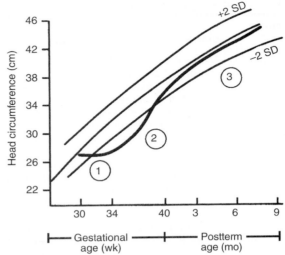

Figure 3-5 **Phases of head growth.** Phases of head growth derived from data of Georgieff and co-workers and based on study of 73 premature infants of 30±2 weeks of gestation (mean ± 2 SDs). The three phases shown are discussed in the text. *(From Georgieff MD, Hoffman JS, Pereira GR, Bernbaum J, et al: Effect of neonatal caloric deprivation on head growth and 1-year development status in preterm infants, J Pediatr 107:581-587, 1985.)*

The rate of head growth along standard curves was between the mean and 1 standard deviation (SD) below the mean for all infants except those calorically deprived the longest (4 to 6 weeks), in whom values were more than 1 SD below the mean. Indeed, such infants calorically deprived for more than 4 weeks had developmental scores lower than normal ranges at 1 year of corrected age. The deleterious effect of postnatal caloric deprivation is worse for preterm infants born small for their gestational age.[48]

Level of Alertness

The formal neonatal neurological examination should begin with assessment of the level of alertness. The *level of alertness* is perhaps the most sensitive of all neurological functions because it depends on the integrity of several levels of the central nervous system (see later). Terms used to describe this aspect of neurological function include *state*[54,55] and *vigilance*[56] (Table 3-7).

TABLE 3-6	Rates of Head Growth in Premature Infants with Favorable Neurological Outcome	
Postnatal Week	**Rate of Head Growth (cm/week)**
First	−0.60
Second	0.50
Third	0.75
After third	1.0

Data from a study of 41 premature infants (<1500 g birth weight) in Gross SJ, Oehler JM, Eckerman CO: Head growth and developmental outcome in very low-birth-weight infants, *Pediatrics* 71:70-75, 1983.

The first two states correspond to quiet and active sleep, respectively (see Chapter 4), and the next three states describe different levels of wakefulness. The level of alertness in the normal infant varies, depending particularly on time of last feeding, environmental stimuli, recent experiences (e.g., painful venipuncture), and gestational age.[57-61] Before 28 weeks of gestation, it is difficult to identify periods of wakefulness. Persistent stimulation leads to eye opening and apparent alerting for time periods measured principally in seconds. At approximately 28 weeks, however, a distinct change occurs in the level of alertness.[56] At that time, a gentle shake rouses the infant from apparent sleep and results in alerting for several minutes. Spontaneous alerting also occasionally occurs at this age. Sleep-waking cycles are difficult to observe clinically but can be shown electrophysiologically.[62] By 32 weeks, stimulation is no longer necessary; frequently, the eyes remain open, and spontaneous roving eye movements appear. Sleep-waking alternation, as defined by clinical observation, is apparent.[56] By 36 weeks, increased alertness can be observed readily, and vigorous crying appears during wakefulness. By term, the infant exhibits distinct periods of attention to visual and auditory stimuli, and it is possible to study sleep-waking patterns in detail.[58,61,63-67]

Cranial Nerves

Olfaction (I)

Olfaction, a function subserved by the first cranial nerve, is evaluated only rarely in the newborn period. In a study of 100 term and preterm infants, Sarnat observed that all normal infants of more than 32 weeks of gestation responded with sucking, arousal-withdrawal, or both, to a cotton pledget soaked with peppermint

TABLE 3-7 Major Features of Neonatal Behavioral States in Term Infants

State	Eyes Open	Respiration Regular	Gross Movements	Vocalization
1	–	+	–	–
2	–	–	±	–
3	+	+	–	–
4	+	–	+	–
5	±	–	+	+

–, absent; +, present; ±, present or absent.
Data from Prechtl HFR, O'Brien, MJ: Behavioural states of the full-term newborn: The emergence of a concept. In Stratton P, editor: *Psychobiology of the Human Newborn*, New York: 1982, John Wiley & Sons.

extract.[68] Eight of 11 infants of 29 to 32 weeks of gestation, but only one of six infants of 26 to 28 weeks of gestation also responded. Activation of orbitofrontal, olfactory cortex was detected by near-infrared spectroscopy in full-term newborns exposed to vanilla or maternal colostrum in the first weeks of life.[69]

Olfactory Discriminations. More sophisticated techniques have demonstrated *olfactory discriminations* in newborns.[70,71] Using habituation-dishabituation techniques and recordings of respiration, heart rate, and motor activity, Lipsitt and colleagues demonstrated detection and discrimination among a variety of odorants.[72-74] Mediation of discriminations at a higher level than the periphery was shown by the observation that infants, initially habituated to mixtures of odorants, exhibited dishabituation when presented with the pure components of the mixtures. A particularly interesting demonstration of olfactory discrimination in the infant involved discrimination of the odor of breast pads of the infant's mother from unused pads or those of other nursing mothers.[70,75] Infants consistently adjusted their faces and gazes toward the pads of their own mothers. Later work involving coupling of stroking with different odorants demonstrated complex associative olfactory learning in the first 48 hours of life.[70,76] That olfactory discrimination develops in utero is suggested by the demonstration of neonatal preference for the odors of amniotic fluid.[77] Finally, nutrient (breast milk or formula) odor exposure through a pacifier was shown to stimulate nonnutritive sucking during gavage feeding of premature newborns.[78]

Vision (II)

Visual responses, the afferent segment of which is subserved by the second cranial nerve, exhibit distinct changes with maturation in the neonatal period. By 26 weeks, the infant consistently blinks to light.[56,79] By 32 weeks, light provokes eye closure that persists for as long as the light is present (dazzle reflex of Peiper).[80] More sophisticated studies indicate that a series of behaviors associated with *visual fixation* can be identified by 32 weeks of gestation and can be shown to increase considerably over the next 4 weeks.[81] By 34 weeks, more than 90% of infants will track a fluffy ball of red wool.[82] At 37 weeks, the infant will turn the eyes toward a soft light.[56] By term, visual fixation and following are well developed.[83-85] For testing of visual fixation and following, I have found a most useful target to be a fluffy ball of red yarn. Opticokinetic nystagmus, elicited by a rotating drum, is present in the majority of infants at 36 weeks and is present consistently at term.[80,84,86,87]

The anatomical substrate for visual fixation and for following a moving object in the newborn may not be primarily the occipital cortex, as usually thought. Thus, two studies of newborn infants with apparent absence of occipital cortex secondary to maldevelopment (holoprosencephaly) or destructive lesion (congenital hydrocephalus, ischemic injury) suggested that these abilities are mediated at subcortical sites.[88-90] Experimental studies in subhuman primates defined such a subcortical system involving retina, optic nerves and tract, pulvinar, and superior colliculus—the so-called *collicular visual system*.[91,92] Visual abilities beyond the ability to track a moving object (i.e., visual discriminatory skills; see the following paragraphs), however, do require the geniculocalcarine cortical system.

Visual Acuity, Color, and Other Discriminations.
Elegant studies provided important information about neonatal *visual acuity*, *color perception*, *contrast sensitivity*, and *visual discrimination*.[85,93-102] Through use of the opticokinetic nystagmus response to striped patterns of varying width, investigators demonstrated that the newborn exhibits at least 20/150 vision.[103] Using a visual fixation technique, Fantz showed that the newborn attended to stripes of 1/8-inch width.[104] Visual acuity in premature infants with birth weights of 1500 to 2500 g who were studied at approximately 38 weeks of gestational age was similar to that of term infants.[99] Although studies of color perception in the newborn period often have not rigorously distinguished brightness and color, newborn infants clearly follow a colored object.[105] Color vision is demonstrable by at least as early as 2 months of age.[106,107] Contrast sensitivity increases dramatically between 4 and 9 postnatal weeks.[96]

Discrimination of a rather complex degree has been demonstrated for newborn infants.[85,94,97,98,108-114] Infants as young as 35 weeks of gestation exhibit a distinct visual preference for patterns, particularly those with a greater number of and larger details. Curved contours are favored over straight lines. Preference for novel patterns becomes apparent at 3 to 5 months.[98] Preference for patterns with facial resemblance develops between approximately 10 and 15 weeks of age,[115] and promptly thereafter discrimination occurs according to facial features.[116] The degree of contrast has a direct effect on preferences.[117] Binocular vision and appreciation of depth also appear by approximately 3 to 4 postnatal months.[94] Binocular visual acuity increases most rapidly during the same interval.[95] These higher-level visual abilities may reflect a change in the major anatomical substrate from subcortical to cortical structures.[85,92,118] Nevertheless, two studies of infants from the first days of life by functional magnetic resonance imaging (MRI) did show some evidence for activation of the visual cortex with visual stimulation; subcortical structures could not be addressed because of small anatomical size.[119,120] Infants in the first days of life also have been shown to imitate facial gestures (Fig. 3-6).[121,122] Additionally, imitation of finger movements, especially involving the left hand, has been demonstrated in healthy term infants.[123] Thus, striking changes in cortically mediated visual function occur in the first weeks and months of postnatal life. This is a period for rapid dendritic growth and synaptogenesis in visual cortex and myelination of the optic radiation (see Chapter 2).

Optic Fundi (II)

The funduscopic examination in the newborn period is facilitated considerably by the aid of a nurse and patience on the part of the examiner. The *optic disc* of the newborn lacks much of the pinkish color observed in the older infant and has a paler, gray-white appearance. This color and the less prominent vascularity of the neonatal optic disc may make distinction from optic atrophy difficult. *Retinal hemorrhages* have been observed in 20% to 40% of all newborn infants, with no association with obvious perinatal difficulties, concomitant central nervous system injury, or neurological sequelae.[80,124-126] A relationship with vaginal delivery is apparent; in one study, 38% of infants delivered vaginally exhibited retinal hemorrhages, in contrast to 3% of infants delivered by cesarean section (Table 3-8).[125] The hemorrhages generally resolve completely within 7 to 14 days. Consistent with these findings, an evaluation of eight consecutive newborns with retinal hemorrhages by MRI scan revealed no intracranial abnormalities.[127]

Pupils (III)

The pupils are sometimes difficult to evaluate in the newborn, especially the premature baby, because the eyes are often closed and resist forced opening, and the poorly pigmented iris provides poor contrast for visualizing the pupil. The size of the pupils in the premature infant is approximately 3 to 4 mm and is slightly greater in the full-term infant. Reaction to light begins to appear at approximately 30 weeks of gestation, but it is not present consistently until approximately 32 to 35 weeks.[79,128] The amplitude of the pupillary response increases markedly between 30 weeks and term (Fig. 3-7).[129] The afferent arc of this reflex leaves the optic tract before the lateral geniculate nucleus and synapses in the pretectal region of midbrain before innervating the Edinger-Westphal nucleus of the oculomotor nerve, the efferent arc of the reflex.

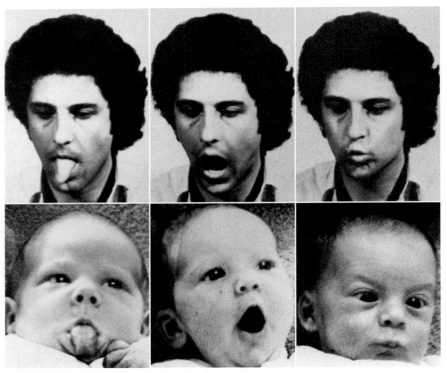

Figure 3-6 Imitation of facial gestures. Sample photographs from videotape recordings of 2- to 3-week-old infants imitating tongue protrusion, mouth opening, and lip protrusion demonstrated by an adult experimenter. *(From Meltzoff AN, Moore MK: Imitation of facial and manual gestures by human neonates, Science 198:74-78, 1977.)*

	RETINAL HEMORRHAGES	
Perinatal Factor	**No. Affected/ Total No.**	**Affected (%)**
Normal vaginal delivery	48/127	38
Abnormal vaginal delivery	22/69	32
Vaginal delivery		
Spontaneous	61/160	38
Forceps	9/36	25
Cesarean section	1/38	3

TABLE 3-8 Neonatal Retinal Hemorrhage: Influence of Perinatal Factors

Data from Besio R, Caballero C, Meerhoff E, Schwarcz R: Neonatal retinal hemorrhages and influence of perinatal factors, *Am J Ophthalmol* 87:74-76, 1979.

Extraocular Movements (III, IV, VI)

Particular attention should be paid to eye position, spontaneous eye movements, and movements elicited by the doll's eyes maneuver, vertical spin, or caloric stimulation, as well as to a variety of abnormal eye movements (see later). These oculomotor functions are subserved by cranial nerves III, IV, and VI and their interconnections within the brain stem. In most premature and some full-term infants, the eyes are slightly disconjugate at rest, with one or the other 1 to 2 mm out. (This feature is demonstrated readily by observing the light reflected off each pupil with the

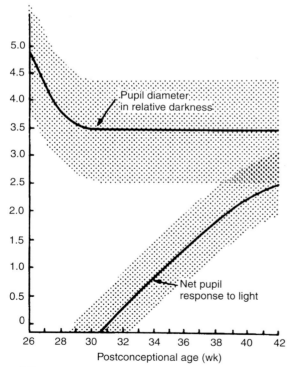

Figure 3-7 Pupil diameter in relation to light. Diameter of pupil in millimeters (mean ± SD) in term and preterm neonates in relative darkness (<10 foot-candles) and after light stimulation (600 foot-candles). *(From Isenberg SJ: Clinical application of the pupil examination in neonates, J Pediatr 118:650-652, 1991.)*

light source in the midline at approximately 2 feet from the face.)

As early as 25 weeks of gestation, full ocular movement with the *doll's eyes maneuver* can be elicited. Because interfering ocular fixation is not well developed at this stage, elicitation of lateral eye movements with the doll's eyes maneuver is much easier in the small premature infant than in the full-term infant. Another convenient means of eliciting oculovestibular responses is to spin the baby held upright; the eyes deviate in a direction opposite to the spin. Rapid maturation of this response with development of nystagmus as well as eye deviation occurs in the first 2 postnatal months.[130] Additionally, at 30 weeks of gestation, caloric stimulation with cold water leads to deviation of the eyes toward the side of the stimulated ear.[131] *Spontaneous* roving eye movements are common at approximately 32 weeks.[132] The tracking movements of the full-term and older infants at first are rather jerky and do not become smooth and gliding until approximately the third month of life.[80]

Facial Sensation and Masticatory Power (V)

Subserved by cranial nerve V (i.e., the trigeminal nerve), facial sensation is examined best with pinprick. The resulting facial grimace begins on the stimulated side of the face. If the infant has facial palsy, this response will be impaired and may be attributed mistakenly to involvement of the trigeminal nerve or nucleus. The strength of masseters and pterygoids also depends on the function of the trigeminal nerve. This strength is assessed by evaluation of sucking and by allowing the infant to bite down on the examiner's finger.

Facial Motility (VII)

The parameters of interest are the position of the face at rest, the onset of movement, and the amplitude and symmetry of spontaneous and elicited movement. Facial motility is subserved by cranial nerve VII. While the infant's face is at rest, attention should be paid to the vertical width of the palpebral fissure, the nasolabial fold, and the position of the corner of the mouth. Examination of the face should not be restricted to observation of elicited movements (e.g., crying) because the quality of *spontaneous* facial movement is of greatest importance in the assessment of cerebral lesions. Subtle lesions at all central levels are best detected by close observation of the *onset* of movement.

Audition (VIII)

The eighth cranial nerve, through its connections in the brain stem and cerebral cortex, subserves auditory function. By 28 weeks, the infant startles or blinks to a sudden, loud noise.[56] As the infant matures, more subtle responses become evident, such as cessation of motor activity, change in respiratory pattern, opening of mouth, and wide opening of eyes.[80] The relation of such responses to the development of hearing has been the subject of considerable study and controversy, but these responses likely represent the presence of at least some auditory function. Inability to elicit these responses is related usually to the failure to test in a quiet surrounding, while the baby is alert and not agitated or very hungry, and to ensure that the ear canals are free of the often copious vernix. In most cases, an infant who does not respond on the initial examination will respond when retested under more favorable conditions. More detailed evaluation of auditory function, including electrophysiological measurements (e.g., brain stem auditory evoked responses; see Chapter 4), certainly is indicated if behavioral responses are consistently absent.

Auditory Acuity, Localization, and Discriminations. More sophisticated studies have provided insight into neonatal *auditory acuity, localization,* and *discriminations.* Using the occurrence in the newborn of cardiac acceleration in relation to sound intensity, Steinschneider demonstrated a *threshold* for cardiac acceleration of approximately 40 decibels.[133] *Auditory localization* has been shown by demonstrating loss and recovery of habituation to an auditory stimulus by changing the locus of the stimulus.[134,135] *Auditory-visual coordination* in localization was shown by exposing an infant to the mother speaking before the infant through a soundproof glass screen, with her voice transmitted by a stereo system.[136,137] When the stereo system was in balance (i.e., the voice came from straight ahead), the infant was content, but when the voice appeared to come from a location different from that of the face, the infant became very upset. Maturation of connections between brain stem auditory nuclei (superior olivary nucleus, nucleus of lateral lemniscus, inferior colliculus), sensory nuclei, and facial nerve nucleus has been studied by measurement of the amplitude of the blink response to glabellar tap when the tap is preceded by an auditory tone.[138,139]

Through the use of heart rate patterns and a habituation-dishabituation model, it has been possible to demonstrate *auditory discriminations* in 3- to 5-day-old newborn infants on the basis of intensity, pitch, and rhythm. These findings are of particular interest in view of information suggesting that intensity and pitch discriminations may be mediated at subcortical levels, whereas cortical levels are required for discrimination of temporal patterns.[140] Discrimination of synthetic speech sounds according to phonemic category and of tonal sounds of different frequencies was demonstrated in newborns in the first days of life.[141-144] Discrimination of real and computer-simulated cries by newborn infants was shown by observing much restlessness and crying in infants stimulated by the real cry and considerably less such behavior in those stimulated by the computer-simulated cry.[145,146] Moreover, results of other studies indicate a preference of the newborn for human voice rather than nonhuman sounds[147] and particular preference for the mother's voice rather than another human voice.[148,149] Finally, 2- to 4-week-old infants can learn to recognize a word that their mothers repeat to them over a period of time (2 weeks) and "remember" the word for up to 2 days without intervening presentations.[150]

Studies based on optical topography or functional MRI show that newborns in the first days of life respond to normal speech with activation of the temporal regions preferentially in the left hemisphere.[151,152] These interesting observations demonstrate that the newborn brain exhibits the cortical organization to process speech and the regional specification for the left hemisphere for language. Similarly, a magnetoencephalographic study using a paradigm based on sound discrimination and important in auditory cognitive function demonstrated positive responses in newborns shortly after birth.[153]

Sucking and Swallowing (V, VII, IX, X, XII)

Sucking requires the function of cranial nerves V, VII, and XII,[80,154] swallowing requires cranial nerves IX and X, and tongue function uses cranial nerve XII. The importance of tongue function, particularly the "stripping" action of the medial tongue, was demonstrated in ultrasonographic and fiberoptic studies of neonatal feeding.[155-158] The act of feeding requires the concerted action of breathing, sucking, and swallowing.[157,159-163] Not surprisingly, the brain stem control centers for these actions, termed *pattern generators,* are closely situated.[163,164] Sucking and swallowing are coordinated sufficiently for oral feeding as early as 28 weeks.[132] This finding perhaps is not surprising because swallowing is observed in utero as early as 11 weeks of gestation.[165] The development of rooting at approximately 28 weeks is a relevant complementing feature. At this early age, however, the synchrony of breathing with sucking and swallowing is not well developed,[157] and thus oral feeding is difficult and, in fact, dangerous. By 34 weeks of gestation, however, the normal infant is able to maintain a concerted synchronous action for productive oral feeding.[161,163,166] However, maturation continues rapidly, and linkage of breathing, sucking, and swallowing is not achieved fully until 37 weeks of gestation or more.[157,163] Moreover, even in the healthy term infant, coordination of swallowing and breathing rhythms is not optimal in the first 48 hours of life.[160]

The gag reflex, subserved by cranial nerves IX and X, is an important part of the neurological evaluation in this context. A small tongue blade or a cotton-tipped swab can be used to elicit the reflex. Active contraction of the soft palate, with upward movement of the uvula and of the posterior pharyngeal muscles, should be observed.

Sternocleidomastoid Function (XI)

Function of the sternocleidomastoid muscle is mediated by cranial nerve XI. Because the function of the muscle is to flex and rotate the head to the opposite side, it is difficult to test in the newborn, especially in the premature infant. One useful maneuver with the full-term infant is to extend the head gently over the side of the bed with the child in the supine position. Passive rotation of the head reveals the configuration and bulk of the muscle, and function sometimes can be estimated if the infant attempts to flex the head.

Tongue Function (XII)

Function of tongue is mediated by cranial nerve XII. The parameters of interest are the size and symmetry of the muscle, the activity at rest, and the movement. Tongue movement is assessed best during the infant's sucking on the examiner's fingertip. The important role of the tongue in oral feeding was discussed in relation to sucking and swallowing.

Taste (VII, IX)

Taste is evaluated only rarely in the neonatal neurological examination. This function is subserved by cranial nerves VII (anterior two thirds of tongue) and IX (posterior one third of tongue). The newborn infant is very responsive to variations in taste and is capable of sharp discriminations. Lipsitt and co-workers used various parameters of sucking behavior, not only to define gustatory discriminations but also to study learning processes in the newborn.[167,168] An apparatus that allows control of the fluid to be obtained by sucking, as well as measurement of duration and frequency of sucking, has been used to demonstrate that, when presented with a sweet fluid (e.g., 15% sucrose), the infant sucks in longer bursts and with fewer rest periods than when presented with water or a salty fluid.[167-169] When sucking the sweet fluid, the heart rate increased. It was presumed from these data that the newborn infant "hedonically monitors oral stimuli and signals the pleasantness of such stimuli with the heart rate as an indicator response."[74]

Motor Examination

The major features of the motor examination to be evaluated in the neonatal period are muscle tone and the posture of limbs, motility and muscle power, and the tendon reflexes and plantar response. The postnatal age and level of alertness of the infant have an important bearing on essentially all these features. Most of the observations described next are applicable to an infant of more than 24 hours of age and in an optimal level of alertness, unless otherwise indicated.

Tone and Posture

Muscle tone is assessed best by passive manipulation of limbs with the head placed in the midline. Moreover, because tone of various muscles in part determines the posture of the limbs at rest, careful observation of posture is valuable for the proper evaluation of tone. Some investigators have devised various maneuvers of passive manipulation of limbs (e.g., approximation of heel to ear, hand to opposite ear [scarf sign], or measurement of angles of certain joints, such as the popliteal angle) to attempt to quantitate tone.[4,11,12,170] These maneuvers have not been particularly useful for me and are not discussed in detail.

Developmental Aspects. Saint-Anne Dargassies and co-workers described an approximate caudal-rostral progression in the development of tone, particularly flexor tone, with maturation.[56] At 28 weeks, resistance to passive manipulation is minimal in all limbs, but by 32 weeks, distinct flexor tone becomes apparent in the lower extremities. By 36 weeks, flexor tone is prominent in the lower extremities and is palpable in the

upper extremities. By term, passive manipulation affords appreciation of strong flexor tone in all extremities.

The posture of the infant in repose reflects these changes in tone to some extent. In my experience, these postures are apparent principally when the infant is in a slightly drowsy state. The alert infant at these various gestational ages is more active and motile, and fixed postures or so-called *preference postures* are difficult to define. This finding was well documented by Prechtl and co-workers and by others.[171-175] Nevertheless, the very quiet infant at 28 weeks often lies with minimally flexed limbs, whereas by 32 weeks one notes distinct flexion of the lower extremities at the knees and hips. By 36 weeks, flexor tone in the lower extremities results in a popliteal angle of 90%, and consistent and frequent flexion occurs at the elbows. By term, the infant assumes a flexed posture of all limbs.[56] Fisting, usually bilateral, is the predominant hand posture.[56,176] The evolution of hip (and knee) flexor tone with maturation is reflected in the developmental increase in pelvic elevation when the infant is in the prone position.[177]

Preference of Head Position. A consistent and interesting aspect of posture in newborn infants is a preference for position of the head toward the right side.[171,178-180] Prechtl and co-workers demonstrated head position toward the right side 79% of the time versus 19% toward the left and 2% toward the midline (Fig. 3-8).[171] In one study, this preference increased with gestational age,[179] whereas in another it decreased.[180] The head orientation preference may be less prominent in the first 24 hours of life.[181] This preference has not been attributable to differences in lighting, nursing practices, or other factors, but it appears to reflect a normal asymmetry of cerebral function at this age. Notably the left hemisphere, particularly the frontal region, mediates movement of the head to the right. As noted earlier, the left hemisphere appears dominant for speech perception in the newborn.

Motility and Power

The quantity, quality, and symmetry of motility and muscle power are the parameters of interest. Prechtl and co-workers[182-184] combined videotape and electrophysiological methods to describe the postnatal development of motor activity in the term infant. In the first 8 weeks, movements with a writhing quality predominate; in the period from 8 to 20 weeks, "fidgety" movements are prominent, and after the latter period, rapid large-amplitude antigravity and intentional movements ("swipes" and "swats") are prominent. In general, preterm infants exhibited similar patterns of motor development when they attained comparable postmenstrual ages, albeit with minor delays in tone and quality of movements.[175,184-186] Prechtl and others[184,187-199a] emphasized that the *quality* of *spontaneous* movements in preterm and term infants are of major importance with regard to the status of the central nervous system.

Saint-Anne Dargassies, using less sophisticated techniques, described the developmental changes in

Means and SD of head positions face to

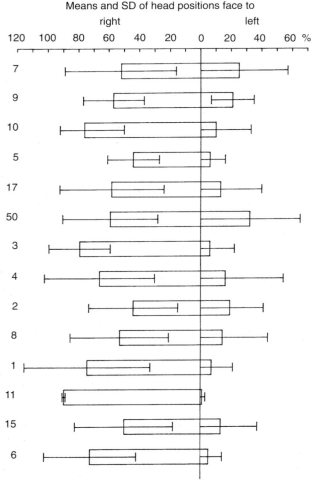

Figure 3-8 **Preference of head position.** Mean ± SD percentage of minutes from all observations in which each infant (series of 14) had face to right or left side. *(From Prechtl HF, Fargel JW, Weinmann HM, Bakker HH: Postures, motility and respiration of low-risk pre-term infants, Dev Med Child Neurol 21:3-27, 1979.)*

motility in the preterm infant.[56] At 28 weeks, movements tend to involve the entire limb or trunk and have either a slow rotational component or a fast, large-amplitude characteristic. By 32 weeks of gestation, movements are seen to be predominately flexor, especially at the hips and knees, often occurring in unison.[56] Although head turning is present, neck flexor and extensor power are negligible, as judged by complete head lag on pull to sit or when the infant is held in the sitting position. By 36 weeks, the active flexor movements of the lower extremities are stronger and often occur in an alternating rather than symmetrical fashion. Flexor movements of the upper extremities are prominent. For the first time, definite neck extensor power can be observed. When the infant is supported in the sitting position, the head is lifted off the chest and remains upright for several seconds. By term, the awake infant is particularly active if stimulated with a gentle shake. Limbs move in an alternating manner, and neck extensor power is still better. Neck flexor power becomes apparent; when the infant is pulled to a sitting position

with firm grasp of the proximal upper limbs, the head is held in the same plane as the rest of the body for several seconds.[56]

The importance of a fixed developmental program in motor development is suggested by the similarities in such development when comparing (at the same postmenstrual age) the fetus, the premature infant, and the term infant, albeit with minor exceptions.[56,63,171,175,182,184,186,191,200,201] The similarities outweigh the rather small differences.

Tendon Reflexes and Plantar Response

Tendon Reflexes. Tendon reflexes readily elicited in the term newborn are the pectoralis, biceps, brachioradialis, knee, and ankle jerks. I have considerable difficulty obtaining triceps jerks in term infants. Most of these reflexes are elicitable but less active in preterm infants. The knee jerk is often accompanied by crossed adductor responses, which should be considered normal findings in the first months of life (<10% of normal infants demonstrate crossed adductor responses after 8 months of age).[202] Useful techniques for eliciting tendon reflexes in the newborn and the frequency and intensity of the reflexes in preterm and term infants are illustrated in Figures 3-9 and 3-10.[203]

Ankle clonus of 5 to 10 beats also should be accepted as a normal finding in the newborn infant, if no other abnormal neurological signs are present and the clonus is not distinctly asymmetrical. Ankle clonus usually disappears rapidly, and the existence of more than a few beats beyond 3 months of age is abnormal.

Plantar Response. The plantar response is usually stated to be extensor in the newborn infant.[201,204] This result clearly relates to the manner in which the response is elicited. Using drag of thumbnail along the lateral aspect of the sole, Hogan and Milligan[205] observed bilateral flexion in 93 of 100 newborn infants examined. My colleagues and I[206] observed a similar result in 116 (94%) of 124 infants. In contrast, Ross and associates,[207] using drag of pin or pinstick, observed a predominance of extensor responses, with flexion in only about 5% of patients.

When evaluating the neonatal plantar response, it is necessary to consider at least four competing reflexes leading to movements of the toes. Two reflexes that result in extension are *nociceptive withdrawal* (often accompanied by triple flexion at hip, knee, and ankle) and *contact avoidance* (elicited best by stroking the dorsum of the foot, which often occurs inadvertently when holding the foot to elicit the plantar response). Two responses that lead to flexion are *plantar grasp* and *positive supporting reaction* (both elicited by pressure on the plantar aspect of the foot). Because of these competing reflexes and the relative inconsistency of responses, I consider the plantar response to be of limited value in the evaluation of the newborn infant when attempting to determine the presence of an upper motor neuron lesion.

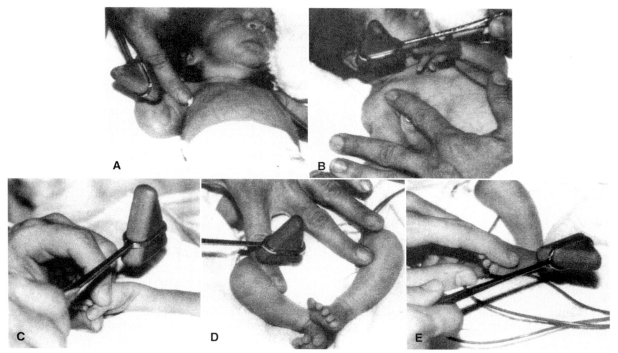

Figure 3-9   **Elicitation of deep tendon reflexes in a premature infant of 32 weeks of gestation. A** and **B**, Pectoralis major; **C**, brachioradialis; **D**, thigh adductors and crossed adductors; **E**, Achilles. *(From Kuban KC, Skouteli HN, Urion DK, Lawhon GA: Deep tendon reflexes in premature infants,* Pediatr Neurol *2:266-271, 1986.)*

Primary Neonatal Reflexes

Many primary neonatal reflexes have been described in classic writings on the neonatal examination. I find the Moro reflex, the palmar grasp, and the tonic neck response to be useful (Table 3-9). In general, I find these reflexes more valuable in assessment of disorders of lower motor neuron, nerve, and muscle than of upper motor neuron.

Moro Reflex

The *Moro reflex*, best elicited by the sudden dropping of the baby's head in relation to the trunk (the falling head should be caught by the examiner), consists of opening of the hands and extension and abduction of the upper extremities, followed by anterior flexion ("embracing") of the upper extremities and an audible cry. Hand opening is present by 28 weeks of gestation, extension and

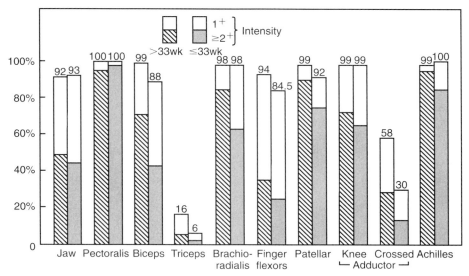

Figure 3-10   **Maturity and deep tendon reflexes.** Elicitation rate and range of intensity of deep tendon reflexes by maturity (<33 and >33 weeks of gestation). *(From Kuban KC, Skouteli HN, Urion DK, Lawhon GA: Deep tendon reflexes in premature infants,* Pediatr Neurol *2:266-271.)*

TABLE 3-9 Evolution of Moro Reflex, Palmar Grasp, and Tonic Neck Response*

Neonatal Reflex	AGE (WEEKS OF GESTATION; MONTHS POSTNATAL)		
	Onset	Well Established	Disappears
Moro reflex	28–32 weeks	37 weeks	6 months
Palmar grasp	28 weeks	32 weeks	2 months
Tonic neck response	35 weeks	1 month	6 months

*See text for details.

abduction by 32 weeks, and anterior flexion by 37 weeks.[56] Audible cry appears at 32 weeks. The Moro reflex disappears by 6 months of age in normal infants.[201,202,204]

Palmar Grasp

Palmar grasp is clearly present at 28 weeks of gestation, is strong at 32 weeks, and is strong enough and associated with enough extension of upper extremity muscles to allow the infant to be lifted from the bed at 37 weeks.[56] The palmar grasp becomes less consistent after about 2 months of age, when voluntary grasping begins to develop.

Tonic Neck Response

The *tonic neck response*, elicited by rotation of the head, consists of extension of the upper extremity on the side to which the face is rotated and flexion of the upper extremity on the side of the occiput (the lower extremities respond similarly but often not as strikingly). The term *fencing posture* is an apt description. The response appears by 35 weeks of gestation,[56] but it is most prominent about 1 month after term. It disappears by approximately 6 months of age,[202,204,208] although the changes in tone may be palpable for several additional months.[209]

Placing and Stepping

The *placing and stepping* ("walking") reactions are elicited readily by 37 weeks of gestation.[56] The former is provoked by contacting the dorsum of the foot with the edge of a table. These reflexes are commonly elicited, but their significance is not entirely clear.

Sensory Examination

Careful evaluation of sensory function is rarely part of the usual neonatal neurological examination. Most often, the imprecise description "withdrawal" is used to describe the infant's response. The premature infant of just 28 weeks of gestation discriminates touch and pain, the former resulting in alerting and slight motor activity and the latter in "withdrawal" and cry.[132] The *rooting reflex*, elicited by tactile stimulation of the perioral region, is well established by 32 weeks of gestation. By approximately 36 weeks, there is rapid turning of the head away from pinprick over the side of the face.

I routinely assess the responses of the infant to multiple (three to five) pinpricks over the medial aspect of the extremities. Responses to be observed are latency, limb movement, facial movement (i.e., grimace), vocalization (i.e., cry), and habituation. A lower-level response is extremely rapid, consists of a stereotyped response (e.g., triple flexion at hip, knee, and ankle) and is not accompanied by grimace or cry. No clear response decrement occurs with repeated trials (i.e., no habituation). A normal, higher-level response has a recognizable latency and consists usually of an apparently purposeful avoidance maneuver, usually lateral withdrawal, and grimace or cry. The response "dampens" with repeated trials; this characteristic of habituation is an important feature of the normal neonatal response.[210] In a systematic study of 130 healthy newborn infants (124 full term), my colleagues and I observed the higher-level motor response in 94%.[211]

Only since the mid-1980s has it become widely accepted that infants experience pain and that attempts to minimize pain during noxious procedures are beneficial.[212-216] Thus, infants exhibit characteristic behavioral, cardiorespiratory, hormonal, and metabolic responses to pain, retain memory of the pain for a period sufficient to modify subsequent short-term behavior, and respond beneficially to analgesic measures. Careful assessment of the quality of infant cry and of facial expressions to pain indicates appreciation of graded levels of pain.[146,212,217] Thus, the older notion that infants do not experience pain because of their "undeveloped nervous system" and therefore do not require measures to minimize pain appears finally to have been laid to rest.

ABNORMAL NEUROLOGICAL FEATURES

In the following section, the major *abnormalities* of the neonatal neurological examination are described. Whenever possible, the anatomical loci within the neuraxis that, when deranged, may cause the neurological deficits are identified. Such clinicoanatomical correlations in the newborn, in general, must be made cautiously. The organization of this discussion is identical to that used to describe the normal neonatal neurological examination.

Abnormalities of Level of Alertness

Abnormalities of the level of alertness are the most common neurological deficits observed in the neonatal period. When such abnormalities are slight, detection requires careful observation and consideration of a variety of factors, such as time of last feeding, amount of recent sleep interruptions, gestational age, and similar factors.

To ensure consistency and to avoid confusion, I use only three terms to characterize the level of alertness:

TABLE 3-10 **Levels of Alertness in the Neonatal Period**

Level of Alertness	Appearance of Infant	Arousal Response	MOTOR RESPONSES	
			Quantity	Quality
Normal	Awake	Normal	Normal	High level
Stupor				
Slight	"Sleepy"	Diminished (slight)	Diminished (slight)	High level
Moderate	Asleep	Diminished (moderate)	Diminished (moderate)	High level
Deep	Asleep	Absent	Diminished (marked)	High level
Coma	Asleep	Absent	Diminished (marked) or absent	Low level

normal, stupor, and coma (Table 3-10). These characterizations are based principally on three readily determined criteria: (1) the response to arousal maneuvers (i.e., persistent, gentle shaking, pinch, shining of a light, or ringing of a bell) and both (2) the quantity and (3) the quality of motility, both spontaneous and that elicited by pinprick of the medial extremities (see Table 3-10). Infants who are *normally alert* behave in the fashion described in the section on normal neurological findings for gestational age. Infants are considered to be *stuporous* when they have a diminished or absent arousal response and when motor responses are diminished. In slight stupor, the infant is awake but "sleepy," or "lethargic," whereas in moderate stupor, the infant appears to be asleep; in both states, an arousal response, although diminished, is present. In deep stupor, the infant not only appears to be asleep but also cannot be aroused. The distinction between deep stupor and *coma* is based primarily on the quality of the motor responses. In deep stupor, motor responses are high level (nonstereotyped, definite latency, and habituating), whereas in coma, they are low level (stereotyped, rapid onset, nonhabituating) or totally absent. Most disorders that affect the neonatal central nervous system disturb the level of alertness at some time, and longitudinal characterization of this level is the most sensitive barometer of the neurological status of the newborn infant. Use of the terminology described in Table 3-10 enables different examiners to arrive at the same conclusion about an infant's level of alertness and to do so frequently and simply.

Stupor and coma occur in older patients who have a bilateral cerebral disturbance or disturbance of the activating system of reticular gray matter present in the diencephalon (especially thalamus), midbrain, or upper pons.[218] Similar correlates may pertain to the newborn infant, but detailed clinicoanatomical correlates of stupor and coma in the newborn period are not yet available.

Abnormalities of Cranial Nerves

Olfaction

Abnormalities of olfaction, detected by the simple bedside technique in which a cotton pledget soaked with peppermint extract is used, have been demonstrated in infants with absent olfactory bulbs and tracts (i.e., disturbances of prosencephalic development, such as holoprosencephaly).[68] This simple test is also recommended for infants of diabetic mothers, because such infants carry an increased likelihood of olfactory bulb agenesis.[219] The use of olfactory stimuli by Lipsitt and others, as mentioned previously, to demonstrate function that is probably mediated at the cerebral cortical level (i.e., habituation-dishabituation) suggests the possibility that study of olfactory responses may provide a means to evaluate higher neurological function in the newborn, at least on a research basis.

Vision

Consistent failure to demonstrate visual following (or opticokinetic nystagmus with a rotating drum) in a full-term newborn is a disturbing sign. However, such failure most commonly does not relate to a *primary* disturbance in the optic nerves or tracts, but rather is usually part of a constellation of neurological abnormalities indicative of generalized or multifocal disturbance of several levels of the central nervous system. (A less common cause of apparent lack of visual responsiveness is congenital ocular motor apraxia, related usually to cerebellar vermian hypoplasia, but the characteristic head thrusting and inability to initiate saccades usually do not become apparent until head control is achieved at 2 to 3 months of age.[220]) As discussed previously (see "Normal Neurological Examination"), the earlier notion that visual following of a moving object reflected cerebral function is probably incorrect, and disturbance of such visual following suggests impairment of connections among optic nerves, tract, thalamus, and superior colliculus. Blindness is not a common finding on follow-up examination of the newborn with impaired visual following; visual following usually appears, albeit delayed, in the first weeks of life. However, if pendular, "searching" nystagmus, digital manipulation of the globe, and repetitive hand movements before the eyes appear in the first weeks or months of life, congenital blindness is likely, and the locus of the disturbance of optic pathways must be sought in the usual way.

Optic Fundi

Numerous abnormalities of the optic disc and retina may be detected in the neonatal period (Table 3-11).

Optic Disc Hypoplasia or Atrophy. Distinction of optic nerve *hypoplasia-dysplasia* and *optic atrophy* is useful. In *optic nerve hypoplasia*, the disc is quite small, one third to one half of the usual size, and occasionally is dysplastic in appearance.[221-224] Other useful findings in diagnosis are a second pigmented ring around the disc and tortuosity or abnormal origin of the vessels

TABLE 3-11	Major Abnormalities of the Optic Fundus in the Neonatal Period
Optic Disc	
Hypoplasia-dysplasia	
Atrophy	
Retina	
Retinal and preretinal hemorrhages	
Chorioretinitis	
Retinopathy of prematurity	
Retinoblastoma	

originating from the disc. The disorder is bilateral in approximately 85% of cases. This lesion accounts for approximately 25% of cases of congenital blindness,[225] it relates to a disorder during midline prosencephalic development (i.e., second and third months), and thus it may be associated with other neurological stigmata of such a disorder (see Chapter 1). Approximately 50% of affected patients subsequently exhibit other signs of cerebral abnormality (i.e., seizures and mental retardation).[222-225] The likelihood of such subsequent neurological deficits varies with the severity of hypoplasia and ranges from approximately 65% with severe bilateral hypoplasia to 40% for milder bilateral or unilateral disease. In one series of *septo-optic dysplasia* (absence of the septum pellucidum with optic hypoplasia-dysplasia), schizencephaly ("porencephaly") or agenesis of the corpus callosum was associated with 81% of patients with severe bilateral optic disease (see Chapter 1).[224] In septo-optic dysplasia, the lesion is often associated with hypothalamic-pituitary dysfunction, usually apparent after the neonatal period.[226] Neonatal hypoglycemia with seizures, however, has been reported.[222,223,227] Indeed, in one series selected from an endocrine clinic population, 75% of patients exhibited persistent neonatal hypoglycemia.[228] In approximately 50% of cases of congenital optic nerve hypoplasia with endocrine disturbance, the septum pellucidum is present on computed tomography scan. (MRI might detect hypothalamic defects in such cases.) The endocrine abnormalities are related to impairment in trophic hormone secretions (indicative of hypothalamic maldevelopment), the most common of which involves growth hormone. Impaired growth becomes apparent later in the first year or second year of life.[223,228]

In *optic atrophy*, the optic disc may be normal or nearly normal in size but is poorly vascularized and pale. (Presumably, the optic nerve has developed normally and then has been injured or affected by an ongoing metabolic or degenerative process.) Although optic atrophy in the newborn may be associated with other ocular abnormalities (e.g., glaucoma and cataracts), most cases have no such association. The origin is often attributed to injury caused by abnormalities of pregnancy, labor, or delivery, but conclusive data are lacking.

Retinal and Preretinal Hemorrhages. Retinal lesions include *retinal and preretinal hemorrhages*. The former are not of consistent clinical significance, as discussed in the earlier section on normal findings. Large preretinal hemorrhages are observed most commonly with major intracranial hemorrhage. These so-called subhyaloid hemorrhages are of ocular venous origin. Consequently, increased intracranial pressure is likely to be or to have been present.

Chorioretinitis. Chorioretinitis is observed most commonly with toxoplasmosis, cytomegalovirus, rubella, and herpes simplex infections (see Chapter 20). Chorioretinitis is nearly a constant feature of symptomatic congenital toxoplasmosis, has a predilection for the macular region, and consists of prominent necrotic lesions with striking black pigment as well as yellow scarring. In symptomatic congenital cytomegalovirus infection, retinal lesions occur in approximately 20% of affected newborns, and although the lesions bear similarities to those in toxoplasmosis, they tend to be less pigmented and more peripheral in location. The chorioretinitis of rubella is readily distinguished from that of toxoplasmosis or cytomegalovirus infection in that it consists of small areas of depigmentation and pigmentation, rendering a "salt and pepper" appearance to the retinal surface.

Retinopathy of Prematurity. The earliest vascular changes of retinopathy of prematurity are difficult to detect with certainty by direct ophthalmoscopy.[229,230] Progressive stages of the disease are more readily defined, especially by binocular indirect ophthalmoscopy. These stages include dilation and tortuosity of vessels, neovascularization, hemorrhages, intravitreous proliferation, and, finally, retinal detachment, beginning in the periphery.[230-235] A major advance in therapy has been the early use of cryotherapy (and more recently and preferably, laser therapy) to arrest progression of the disease.[234-237]

Retinoblastoma. Although only uncommonly detected in the neonatal period, retinoblastoma is important to recognize as early as possible to achieve the best possible response to therapy. The usual presenting signs are the so-called *white pupil* and *strabismus*.[229] The tumor is bilateral in about one third of cases. In approximately 10% of cases, retinoblastoma is inherited in an autosomal dominant fashion. Thus, a family history of an affected sibling should provoke a particularly thorough examination.

Pupils

The size of the pupils relates not only to the parasympathetic constrictor fibers, conveyed by the third cranial nerve, but also to sympathetic dilator fibers from the superior cervical ganglion and to systemic epinephrine from the adrenal medulla. Although afferent connections from the optic pathway may play a role in pupillary size, this part of the reflex arc is rarely the source of pupillary abnormalities in the newborn infant. Abnormal pupillary findings are of great value in clinical neurology in the localization of pathological events that occur in older infants and children. The occurrence and significance of such pupillary findings in the newborn period, however, are still not well defined.

TABLE 3-12 Major Pupillary Abnormalities and Causes in the Neonatal Period

Bilateral Increase in Size
Hypoxic-ischemic encephalopathy (reactive early, unreactive late)*
Intraventricular hemorrhage (unreactive)
Local anesthetic intoxication (unreactive)
Infantile botulism (unreactive)†

Bilateral Decrease in Size
Hypoxic-ischemic encephalopathy (reactive)

Unilateral Decrease in Size
Horner syndrome (reactive)

Unilateral Increase in Size
Convexity subdural hematoma, other unilateral mass (unreactive)
Congenital third-nerve palsy (± unreactive)
Hypoxic-ischemic encephalopathy (± unreactive)

*The most common reactivity to light is in parentheses.
†Usually midposition and unreactive.

Bilateral Increase in Pupillary Size. Bilateral increase in size of pupils that are reactive to light is seen commonly during the first hours after perinatal asphyxia in those infants who usually are not seriously affected (Table 3-12) (see Chapter 9). This finding probably relates to systemic epinephrine release in association with asphyxia.[238,239] Late in the course of serious hypoxic-ischemic encephalopathy, especially with other signs of brain stem failure, pupils may be dilated and fixed to light. A similar finding also mediated at the brain stem (midbrain) level is not unusual in massive intraventricular hemorrhage. In local anesthetic intoxication, pupils may be large and unreactive to light because of peripheral parasympatholytic effects (see Chapter 5). In infantile botulism, pupils are usually midposition in size (although they may be dilated) and unreactive to light, also secondary to peripheral synaptic effects (see Chapter 18).

Bilateral Decrease in Pupillary Size. Bilateral decrease in the size of pupils that are reactive to light (although the reaction may be difficult to detect) is seen most often once the first 12 to 24 hours after perinatal asphyxia have passed (see Table 3-12). With hypoxic-ischemic insults that have been well established for hours intrapartum, however, this miosis may be apparent earlier. The pupillary change is usually accompanied by other signs suggestive of parasympathetic discharge, such as increases in respiratory secretions and gastrointestinal motility and a relative decrease in heart rate. Whether this apparent parasympathetic predominance relates to a central autonomic disturbance or a decrease in systemic catecholamine release is unclear.

Unilateral Decrease in Pupillary Size. Unilateral decrease in size of a pupil that remains reactive to light is seen most often with Horner syndrome (see Table 3-12). In the newborn, this syndrome is almost always associated with a brachial plexus injury, which includes involvement of the eighth cervical root and first thoracic root, destined for the cervical sympathetic ganglion (see Chapter 22).

Unilateral Increase in Pupillary Size. Unilateral increase in the size of a pupil that may be sluggishly reactive or unreactive to light is very unusual in the newborn; this reflects the rarity of the uncal form of transtentorial herniation, which results in compression of the third cranial nerve and its associated parasympathetic fibers. The infrequency of the uncal syndrome is related both to the pliability of the neonatal skull and sutures and to the rarity of large *unilateral mass lesions*. In my experience, convexity subdural hematoma is the most common cause of this syndrome in the newborn infant (see Table 3-12 and Chapter 10). However, I have observed unilateral pupillary dilation secondary to transtentorial uncal herniation in neonatal bacterial meningitis.[240]

Unilateral pupillary dilation may be one feature of congenital third nerve palsy, the other features of which include weakness of medial, superior, and inferior eye movements and ptosis (see Chapter 19). The defects of extraocular movement relate to disturbed innervation of the superior, inferior, and medial rectus and inferior oblique muscles, and the ptosis relates to disturbed innervation of the levator palpebrae.

A potential cause of unilateral third nerve palsy is neonatal hypoxic-ischemic injury, documented neuropathologically as causing unilateral as well as bilateral nuclear injury in the brain stem, specifically including the third nerve nucleus (see Chapter 8). I have seen this finding in association with the brain stem neuronal injury caused by severe, abrupt, late intrapartum asphyxia (see Chapters 8 and 9).

Extraocular Movements

Abnormalities of eye position and eye movement should be sought. At least four abnormalities of eye position or eye movement may be observed in otherwise healthy term infants examined on the first 3 postnatal days.[241] Their incidence and outcome are summarized in Table 3-13 and are noted in the appropriate sections that follow.

Abnormal Eye Position. Abnormalities of eye position occur in either the horizontal plane (disconjugate) or the vertical plane (skew). Minor degrees of *disconjugate* eye position at rest or even during spontaneous and elicited movement are not unusual in apparently normal term newborns (see Table 3-13). These disappear in the newborn period. However, in small preterm infants (<1500 g), these abnormalities are more common and may persist (Table 3-14). Indeed, the incidence of *strabismus* undergoes an interesting developmental increase to a peak at 6 months of age and a nadir at 12 months, which is when approximately 15% of 155 infants in one study exhibited strabismus.[242] In another large study, strabismus was present in 10% of small preterm infants (<1501 g). On follow-up, the incidence varied from approximately 5% in infants

TABLE 3-13 Transient Abnormalities of Ocular Motility in the Term Newborn

Disorder of Ocular Motility	Percentage of Infants (N = 242)	Outcome
Disconjugate gaze (esotropia or exotropia)	9%	100% resolved in the neonatal period
Skew deviation	9%	77% resolved by 1 month; 23% later developed esotropia
Downward deviation of eyes (while awake)	2%	100% resolved by 6 months
Opsoclonus (intermittent)	3%	100% resolved by 6 months, most by 1 month

Data from Hoyt CS, Mousel DK, Weber AA: Transient supranuclear disturbances of gaze in healthy neonates, *Am J Ophthalmol* 89:708-713, 1980.

with no intraventricular hemorrhage to 16% in those with hemorrhage and to 50% in those with cystic periventricular leukomalacia.[243] In one series of preterm infants with later spastic diplegia, 90% had strabismus, and all had parieto-occipital white matter injury by MRI.[244] The high incidence of strabismus in preterm infants with white matter injury, principally located in parieto-occipital white matter, is consistent with sophisticated studies in older individuals with infantile onset of strabismus, studies suggesting that the underlying abnormality is located in parietal and occipital cortex and the connections thereof.[245]

Skew deviation of eyes (i.e., vertical disparity in eye position) is not rare in otherwise healthy term infants (see Table 3-13). Although most of these cases resolve by 1 month of age, 23% will later evolve to *esotropia*. In older patients, skew deviation is associated with lesions in the brain stem, involving either the region in or around the middle cerebellar peduncle (inferiorly displaced eye) or the medial longitudinal fasciculus (superiorly displaced eye).[246] That a similar correlation may occur in the newborn is supported by our documentation of skew deviation, with right eye down, in an infant with right intracerebellar hemorrhage and associated brain stem compression.[247] Moreover, I frequently have observed skew deviation in association with hypoxic-ischemic encephalopathy and evidence for brain stem neuronal injury, as well as with major intraventricular hemorrhage and associated brain stem dysfunction. Persistent downward deviation of eyes (*tonic downward deviation*) is a rare transient abnormality in otherwise healthy term or preterm infants

(see Table 3-13). However, the abnormality also may reflect pretectal disturbance and may thereby occur in association with paresis of upward gaze, as in hydrocephalus with a dilated third ventricle or kernicterus (see later). With the transient abnormality of the otherwise normal newborn, the doll's eyes maneuver demonstrates intact vertical gaze, thus indicating dysfunction at supranuclear levels of unknown cause. Episodic ("paroxysmal") downward deviation of eyes, lasting for several seconds, also may occur in the absence of overt neurological disease and may then resolve by 1 to 6 months of age.[248,249] Paroxysmal downward deviation also may occur later in the first year, especially in preterm infants with severe injury (periventricular leukomalacia) of posterior cerebral white matter and, perhaps, connections to the pretectal region.[250] Visual impairment is a frequent accompaniment.

Limitation of Eye Movement. Limitation of extraocular movement may occur because of isolated *nerve palsies* (see Chapter 19). Sixth nerve involvement is the most common of these palsies and causes impaired lateral eye movement with resulting medial deviation.[251,252] This nerve involvement is distinguished from esotropia (strabismus) by the doll's eyes maneuver, which fails to cause full abduction of the eye in sixth nerve palsy. Most examples of isolated sixth nerve palsy are transient; complete recovery occurs within several weeks.[251] *Duane syndrome* includes limitation of eye abduction with retraction of the globe and narrowing of the palpebral fissure on adduction of the affected eye (see Chapter 19). *Congenital fibrosis of the extraocular muscles* is a rare disorder characterized by restrictive paralysis of all extraocular muscles with essentially total ophthalmoplegia with or without ptosis (see Chapter 19).[253] *Möbius syndrome* includes defective eye abduction in approximately 80% of cases; congenital facial diplegia is the hallmark of this disorder (see later and Chapter 19).

Gaze palsies (weakness of conjugate eye movement) in the newborn are most often *horizontal* and may reflect involvement of frontal eye fields for contralateral eye movement or of gaze centers in the pons for ipsilateral eye movement. The former is more common, and both varieties occur most frequently as a feature of hypoxic-ischemic encephalopathy. These two possible anatomical loci for horizontal gaze palsies are distinguished by the doll's eyes maneuver and by caloric stimulation, which result in movement of the eyes in disturbance

TABLE 3-14 Strabismus in Survivors of Birth Weight < 1500 g*

Age of Testing	Percentage with Strabismus (n = 155)
6 weeks	18%
3 months	30%
6 months	28%*
9 months	28%
12 months	14%

*Also at 6 months, 21% of infants with strabismus had neurological abnormalities; 40% of infants with neurological abnormalities had strabismus.

Data from van Hof-Van Duin J, Evenhuis-van Leunen A, Mohn G, Baerts W, et al: Effects of very low birth weight (VLBW) on visual development during the first year after term, *Early Hum Dev* 20:255-266, 1989.

of the cerebral eye fields but not in disturbance of the pontine gaze centers. More common in the newborn period is tonic deviation of the eyes to one side as a manifestation of seizure (accompanied often by fine jerking movements of the deviated eyes) or of a postictal state. *Vertical gaze palsies* are rare in the newborn, and I have seen only defects of upward gaze with resulting downward deviation, as noted earlier. These abnormalities have occurred on the basis of presumed pretectal involvement by a massively dilated third ventricle (posthemorrhagic hydrocephalus or congenital aqueductal stenosis), major acute intraventricular hemorrhage, kernicterus, posterior fossa hemorrhage, or hypoxic-ischemic encephalopathy. Downward deviation of the eyes may be a manifestation of seizure, and the presence of fine jerking movements of the deviated eyes may help to establish this diagnosis.

Abnormal Eye Movements. Abnormal eye movements consist of the horizontal and, occasionally, the vertical jerking movements that are *seizure manifestations*, *ocular bobbing, paroxysmal downgaze or upgaze, opsoclonus, ocular flutter*, and *nystagmus. Seizures* are discussed in Chapter 5. *Ocular bobbing* is an unusual abnormality of eye movement, described originally by Fisher,[254] and is characterized by intermittent, bobbing, down and up movements of the eyes that are usually synchronous; ocular bobbing in adults is associated primarily with pontine disturbance. In the newborn, this movement can be difficult to distinguish from seizure; in my experience, ocular bobbing is primarily a rare manifestation of major intraventricular hemorrhage and severe hypoxic-ischemic encephalopathy. *Paroxysmal downgaze*, described earlier in relation to tonic downgaze, differs from ocular bobbing in its benign nature, its very brief episodic quality, and the lack of bobbing when the eyes return to the meridian. *Paroxysmal upgaze*, characterized by episodes of tonic upgaze of 15 to 30 seconds, has been documented as early as the first week of life but usually has its onset at approximately 6 months of age and is later often associated with minor cognitive deficits and ataxia.[255-257] *Opsoclonus* is a dramatic but rare abnormality of eye movement that is characterized by rapid, irregular, multidirectional conjugate jerking of the eyes. Opsoclonus can be a transient abnormality in the term newborn (see Table 3-13). In such cases, resolution usually occurs within a month, invariably by 6 months.[241,258] In older patients, opsoclonus is associated with disturbance primarily of pontine omnipause neurons. The multidirectional nature of the movements is the critical criterion for distinction from seizure. I have observed opsoclonus and *ocular flutter* (jerking similar to that of opsoclonus but confined to the horizontal plane) in infants with maple syrup urine disease, nonketotic and ketotic hyperglycinemia, and posterior fossa hemorrhage.

Nystagmus with onset at birth or the first few days of life should suggest the diagnosis of congenital nystagmus.[259-263] This disorder is characterized by rhythmic, conjugate, horizontal oscillations of both eyes. The horizontal nature of the nystagmus persists with vertical gaze, an important diagnostic point. The disorder may be familial or nonfamilial. The familial variety may be autosomal dominant, autosomal recessive, or X-linked recessive. The oscillations in an affected family member may be so reduced as to have been overlooked in the past. Visual impairment is present in the minority of patients, and static neurological deficits are present in the majority of nonfamilial (but not familial) cases with visual impairment. Because nystagmus can be observed, albeit uncommonly, in the newborn with severe visual deficit or with diencephalic or brain stem lesion (e.g., congenital tumor), a careful ophthalmological evaluation and a computed tomography or MRI scan should be obtained. Transient, idiopathic nystagmus has been described in early infancy, with mean age at disappearance at 8 months of age.[258]

Facial Sensation and Masticatory Power

Abnormality of facial sensation is rarely elicited in the newborn. I have observed several premature infants with a posterior fossa syndrome secondary to an intraventricular hemorrhage (with extension into the fourth ventricle) who had absence or impaired response to pinprick over the face bilaterally. Careful evaluation of facial sensation, not often performed in the newborn examination, may reveal more deficits than currently recognized.

Disturbance of motor function of the fifth cranial nerve is usually manifested as a defect of sucking and is rarely an isolated finding. Abnormalities of sucking and swallowing are discussed in subsequent sections.

Facial Motility

Abnormalities of facial motility should be sought when the face is at rest, at the onset of movement, during spontaneous facial movement, and during crying or grimacing. Facial weakness secondary to disturbance of the cerebrum is usually more obvious with the baby at rest or during the first movements of spontaneous facial expression and may be completely inapparent during the full movements of crying. Nuclear, cranial nerve, neuromuscular, or muscular lesions, however, are usually more obvious during elicited facial movement, such as a cry or grimace. A simple classification of the types of facial weakness that can occur in the neonatal period is provided, according to the level of the lesion in Table 3-15. Each of these specific disorders is discussed in more detail in other relevant chapters of this book.

Cerebrum. In facial weakness of cerebral origin, the upper face is spared. Other signs of cerebral deficit are usually present, such as hemiparesis, especially of an upper extremity, and seizures. The most common pathological substrate is hypoxic-ischemic encephalopathy, particularly with infarction in the distribution of the middle cerebral artery, and, less commonly, cerebral contusion. Cerebral lesions of prenatal onset (e.g., porencephaly) often have relatively less involvement of face than would be predicted on the basis of the degree of upper extremity weakness and the severity of the lesion on brain imaging. The reason for this apparent

TABLE 3-15	Major Causes of Facial Weakness in the Neonatal Period

Cerebral
Hypoxic-ischemic encephalopathy
Cerebral contusion

Nuclear
Möbius syndrome
Hypoxic-ischemic encephalopathy

Nerve
Traumatic neuropathy
Posterior fossa hematoma

Neuromuscular Junction
Myasthenia gravis
Infantile botulism

Muscle
Congenital myotonic dystrophy
Congenital muscular dystrophy
Facioscapulohumeral dystrophy
Nemaline myopathy
Myotubular myopathy
Congenital fiber type disproportion
Mitochondrial disorder: cytochrome c oxidase deficiency
Hypoplasia of depressor anguli oris muscle

facial sparing may relate to the likelihood that, during normal development of the corticobulbar system, ipsilateral terminations of each corticobulbar tract are eliminated postnatally by selective elimination of axonal processes and of synapses (see Chapter 2) but are retained when the normal contralateral input is lost. Strong support for this notion emanates from the demonstration that evaluation of older infants and children with hemiparesis revealed facial sparing when lesions occurred prenatally (82% had sparing) but not when lesions occurred beyond the neonatal period.[264] Presumably, ipsilateral terminals of the intact corticobulbar tract spared facial function, and consistent with this formulation, prenatal lesions did not show facial sparing when they were bilateral (only 8% had sparing).[264] Bilateral facial weakness of cerebral origin may be associated with weakness of sucking, swallowing, and tongue movements, as part of a congenital Foix-Chavany-Marie syndrome, secondary either to intrauterine ischemic injury or to cortical dysgenesis involving the perisylvian regions.[265]

Nucleus. Nuclear facial weakness is primarily a manifestation of Möbius syndrome and, as such, is bilateral, involves upper face and lower face (often upper more than lower), and is associated with a variety of other neurological deficits and congenital abnormalities (see Chapter 19). Difficulty with eye closure, flattened nasolabial fold, difficulty sucking, and drooling are prominent features. In view of the relative frequency of brain stem nuclear injury with perinatal asphyxia, hypoxic-ischemic encephalopathy may be associated with bilateral weakness of both the upper and lower face.

Nerve. Injury to the facial nerve is most often related to intrauterine position during labor with compression of the face against the maternal sacrum (intrauterine position is usually left occiput anterior, and thus most are left facial palsies)[266] or, less frequently, the result of forceps injury during difficult forceps extractions (see Chapter 22). Rare causes of injury to facial nerve involve compression from posterior fossa hematoma, whether intracerebellar or extraparenchymal. In nerve injuries, the upper and lower face is usually affected, and eye closure is notably poor. Because the lesion is unilateral, prominent "pulling" of the lower face toward the normal side occurs during a cry or grimace, because of the weakness of muscles on the affected side for lateral movement of the lower face. Occasionally, this pulling leads to the impression that the normal side is actually the affected side.

Neuromuscular Junction. This locus for facial weakness occurs in myasthenia gravis and infantile botulism. Bilateral facial weakness, often with ptosis, dysphagia, and generalized hypotonia, may accompany either the neonatal transient or congenital varieties of *myasthenia gravis* (see Chapter 18). Diagnosis in the newborn is made best by observation of the response to neostigmine or edrophonium. In the former, more common variety of myasthenia gravis, the mother also has the disorder. In addition to facial diplegia, the infant with *infantile botulism* exhibits unreactive pupils, dysphagia, peripheral weakness, hypotonia, and constipation.

Muscle. Generalized weakness of the face secondary to myopathic disease is associated most commonly with congenital myotonic dystrophy, congenital muscular dystrophy, facioscapulohumeral dystrophy, nemaline myopathy, myotubular myopathy, congenital fiber-type disproportion, and mitochondrial disorder (cytochrome c oxidase deficiency). These disorders often can be distinguished on clinical grounds by recognition of other features (see Chapter 19).

Restricted weakness of the face is characteristic of hypoplasia of the depressor anguli oris muscle (see Chapter 19). This disorder is characterized by an inability of the corner of the mouth to retract and be depressed. This disturbance is especially noticeable during crying. An association with cardiac and other anomalies has been defined.[267]

Audition

Definition of significant hearing loss in the newborn infant is difficult. During the clinical evaluation described in the section on normal neurological findings, it cannot be expected that minor abnormalities in auditory pathways will be detected. However, detection or at least serious suspicion of major hearing deficits usually is possible. In addition to the absence of startle and more subtle responses to sound, a sometimes valuable clue to serious hearing deficit in the alert young infant is apparent *visual hyperattentiveness* and consistent startle when the examiner approaches the child quickly from the periphery. The use of brain stem auditory evoked potentials and of evoked otoacoustic emissions is of major value (see Chapter 4). *Close follow-up and repeated examinations are important*; early diagnosis is

TABLE 3-16	Major Causes of Deafness in the Neonatal Period

Genetic
Isolated: autosomal dominant, autosomal recessive, X-linked recessive
Syndromic: associated with malformations of external ear, and ocular, skin, skeletal or systemic disease

Bilirubin and Other Toxins
Hyperbilirubinemia
Other (e.g., aminoglycosides, furosemide)

Congenital and Neonatal Infections
Congenital infections: cytomegalovirus infection, rubella, toxoplasmosis, syphilis, lymphocytic choriomeningitis
Neonatal infection: bacterial meningitis

Defects of the Head and Neck

Low Birth Weight
"Hypoxic" injury
Hyperbilirubinemia
Intracranial hemorrhage (?)
Ambient noise (?)
Additive effects (?)

Term Infant: Hypoxia-Ischemia
Perinatal asphyxia
Persistent fetal circulation

critical because language development is benefited by early corrective efforts and impaired by delay in correction (i.e., after 6 months).[268,269] Moreover, hearing loss may be *inapparent* by evoked response audiometry in the neonatal period and may appear only as a *progressive* disorder in the first 6 to 8 months of life.[270,271] Thus, the identification of the infant at risk for this subsequent hearing loss is crucial.

Serious disturbances of hearing are sometimes categorized under the popular mnemonic, the ABCDs of deafness, as follows: *A*ffected family, *B*ilirubin injury, *C*ongenital (and neonatal) infection, *D*efect of head or neck, and low birth weight ("small") (Table 3-16). Unfortunately, this mnemonic neglects the additional category of the term infant subjected to apparent hypoxic-ischemic insults, a category I have added to Table 3-16.

Genetic Deafness. Hereditary forms of deafness are common and account for approximately 50% of all cases of congenital hearing loss.[272-275] The familial genetic disorders are best categorized as those that are isolated (nonsyndromic) and those that are syndromic. In *syndromic disorders*, deficits are associated with malformations of the external ear, with eye disease (e.g., cataracts and optic atrophy), with skin disease (e.g., albinism and anhidrosis), with skeletal disease, or with other systemic disorders (e.g., thyroid disease). Many other hereditary syndromes associated with deafness manifest later in infancy and childhood. A careful family history is critical. Overall, of the genetic causes, 30% are syndromic (i.e., 15% of total congenital hearing loss), such as Pendred syndrome, Usher syndrome, Waardenburg syndrome, and brachio-oto-renal syndrome. Of these, the first two are autosomal recessive

disorders, and the latter two are autosomal dominant.[275] The remaining 70% of the genetic causes (i.e., 35% of total congenital hearing loss) are *nonsyndromic or isolated*. Autosomal dominant, autosomal recessive, X-linked recessive, and mitochondrial inheritance patterns are recognized.[275] The most common disorder involves a gene called *GJB2*, which accounts for approximately one half of the cases. The gene encodes a connexin protein involved in gap junctions and perhaps potassium influx for mechanosensory transduction in brain cells.[275]

Bilirubin and Other Toxins. Injury to cochlear nuclei secondary to marked hyperbilirubinemia is an unusual *isolated* cause of severe hearing loss (see Chapter 13).[276] Results of studies of premature infants suggest that less marked elevations of serum bilirubin level (<20 mg/dL) exert an important *additive effect* in the genesis of sensorineural hearing loss.[268,277-279] However, not all studies support this contention.[280]

The toxic effects of aminoglycosides are well known, but their contribution to serious hearing loss in the newborn period appears to be small.[273,274,276,281-283] However, agreement on this issue is not total,[284,285] and other investigators have suggested that the combination of aminoglycoside and furosemide is an important factor in neonatal hearing loss.[286] In one study of 35 newborns with sensorineural hearing loss identified by brain stem auditory evoked responses, multivariate analysis identified furosemide administration as the only significant factor.[280]

Congenital and Neonatal Infections. The classic *congenital* (*prenatal*) infection associated with deafness (i.e., rubella) is now a very uncommon cause. Congenital cytomegalovirus infection currently is the most common congenital infection that may result in serious hearing loss (see Chapter 20). However, toxoplasmosis and congenital syphilis also may cause serious hearing deficits. Lymphocytic choriomeningitis is a fifth, albeit rare prenatal infection associated with hearing loss (see Chapter 20). Bacterial meningitis is the major *neonatal* infection that may result in serious hearing deficits (see Chapter 21).

Defects of Head and Neck. Because the development of the peripheral auditory system is related intimately to the differentiation of the branchial clefts, it is understandable that auditory defects often accompany defects of head and neck. In two large series, 22% and 23% of cases of hearing impairment were related to auriculofacial anomalies.[273,274] Disturbances of the external ear and surrounding structures, some of which are hereditary (e.g., Treacher-Collins mandibulofacial dysostosis), are good examples. Other developmental defects of this type are part of a more generalized dysmorphogenesis (e.g., trisomy 13-15).

Low Birth Weight. Premature infants have a distinctly increased incidence of significant hearing loss. In an earlier series of 193 surviving preterm infants (gestational age of 28 to 36 weeks), 24 (12%) exhibited

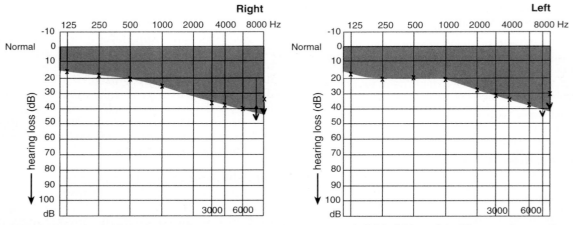

Figure 3-11 **Hearing loss in surviving preterm infants.** The abnormal audiograms of all 24 children, 8 to 10 years of age, with neurosensory hearing loss were averaged. The deficits (ordinate) were encountered particularly in the high frequencies (abscissa) and were generally symmetrical. *(From Stennert E, Schulte FJ, Vollrath M, Brunner E, et al: The etiology of neurosensory hearing defects in preterm infants,* Arch Otorhinolaryngol *221:171-182, 1978.)*

definite hearing deficits, particularly of the high-frequency, sensorineural type, on follow-up examination (Fig. 3-11).[287] Other studies indicated incidences of sensorineural hearing loss generally of approximately 5% to 10%.[277-279,283,284,286,288] More recent series suggested considerably lower incidences.[273-275]

The origin of hearing loss with prematurity is probably multifactorial. In an earlier study, a sharp relationship with recurrent "cyanotic attacks" was apparent; 11% of infants of less than 33 weeks of gestation with such attacks were found to be deaf. Later reports also supported a relationship in the premature infant between recurrent apneic spells, duration of respirator therapy, or hypoxemia and subsequent sensorineural hearing loss.[277-279,283,286] One or more of several possible bases for these relationships should be considered. The presumed basis for the relation of hearing deficits to apneic spells, duration of ventilator therapy, or hypoxemia is *hypoxic-ischemic* injury to cochlear nuclei, inferior colliculi, or both, in the brain stem (see Chapter 8). Data obtained with brain stem evoked response audiometry suggest that involvement of cochlea may also occur in hypoxic-ischemic disease (see Chapters 4 and 9). Moreover, the demonstration of neonatal *intracranial hemorrhage* involving the auditory nerve and inner ear raises the possibility that hemorrhage also plays a role.[289] A third factor, still to be defined further, is the possibility of injury to cochlear hair cells by *excessive acoustic* stimulation provided by incubator or intensive care unit noise. This notion is supported by circumstantial clinical evidence,[290,291] as well as by the observation that the cochlear hair cells of the neonatal guinea pig can be injured by noise levels attained in neonatal incubators.[290] Although it is clear that more data are needed,[276] currently a noise level of more than 45 dB is considered to be of concern in the neonatal intensive care unit.[291]

The possibility that *combined, additive effect of factors* can result in significant injury, factors that alone are not sufficient to cause injury (e.g., hypoxia, bilirubin, aminoglycosides, furosemide, and hemorrhage), must be a major topic for future research. Additive effects

of ambient noise and aminoglycosides have been described in experimental animals,[292,293] and disturbances of brain stem auditory evoked responses have been observed in premature infants treated with gentamicin.[283,294] More recent observations support the additive effects of recurrent apneic spells (and possibly prolonged respirator therapy) and hyperbilirubinemia in the premature infant.[279]

Term Infant Hypoxia-Ischemia. At least two additional groups of term infants (exclusive of those with kernicterus and congenital or neonatal infection) are at increased risk of sensorineural hearing loss: infants with perinatal asphyxia and those with persistent fetal circulation. The incidence of sensorineural hearing loss in infants with hypoxic-ischemic encephalopathy apparently secondary to *perinatal asphyxia* is variably increased. This issue is discussed in Chapter 9. The second group of infants, those with *persistent fetal circulation*, exhibited a 42% incidence of subsequent hearing loss in one series.[270] An increased risk of hearing loss after persistent fetal circulation also was observed in an earlier study.[271] In the later study of Hendricks-Munoz and Walton, two thirds of the infants with sensorineural hearing loss required hearing aids; the hearing deficits appeared after the neonatal period, in the first 6 to 8 months of life. Variables related to the hearing loss included duration of ventilation and, perhaps, use of furosemide. The former factor suggests a possible role for hypoxic-ischemic factors, but values for lowest partial pressure of arterial oxygen or arterial blood pressure did not correlate with hearing loss. However, the *duration* of hypoxemia was not addressed. More data are needed on these issues.

Sucking and Swallowing

Disturbances of sucking and of swallowing very often coexist, and even when isolated they can be difficult to distinguish. Disturbances of the gag reflex are very frequent in instances of defective swallowing, but this reflex is usually normal in instances of defective sucking alone. Specific abnormalities of sucking and

TABLE 3-17	Major Causes of Impaired Sucking and Swallowing in the Neonatal Period

Cerebral
Encephalopathies with bilateral cerebral (pyramidal) involvement: diverse causes
Extrapyramidal-adventitial movements
Congenital isolated pharyngeal dysfunction

Nuclear
Hypoxic-ischemic encephalopathy
Möbius syndrome
Werdnig-Hoffmann disease
Chiari type 2 malformation with myelomeningocele

Nerve
Traumatic facial neuropathy
Posterior fossa hematoma or tumor
Bilateral laryngeal paralysis
Familial dysautonomia (Riley-Day syndrome)

Neuromuscular Junction
Myasthenia gravis
Infantile botulism

Muscle
Congenital myotonic dystrophy
Congenital muscular dystrophy
Facioscapulohumeral dystrophy
Nemaline myopathy
Myotubular myopathy
Congenital fiber type disproportion
Mitochondrial myopathy: cytochrome c oxidase deficiency

swallowing in the newborn not uncommonly relate to a non-neurological disturbance (e.g., Pierre Robin anomalad or tracheoesophageal fistula). A framework for formulating the neurological disorders of sucking and swallowing in the newborn is presented in Table 3-17. Each of the specific disorders is discussed in more detail in other relevant chapters of this book.

Cerebrum. The most common cause of disturbances of sucking and swallowing in the newborn period is the more generalized depression of central nervous system function associated with most of the encephalopathies discussed in this text. Bilateral cerebral involvement with impaired corticobulbar function (pyramidal system) is the common denominator.

Peculiar adventitial *tongue movements* may occur as unusual findings in the newborn. I have observed tongue thrusting movements as apparent seizure manifestations, in association with serious hypoxic-ischemic injury or major intraventricular hemorrhage, and as part of the movement disorder in premature infants with severe bronchopulmonary dysplasia (see next discussion). Moreover, the feeding disturbance observed with familial dysautonomia may be accentuated by peculiar tongue rolling (see Chapter 18). The pathophysiology of these various tongue movements is unclear, but I suspect that they are mediated centrally at the level of extrapyramidal function. A well-known, albeit rare extrapyramidal disorder, *recessive guanosine triphosphate cyclohydrolase deficiency*, also is characterized by neonatal disturbances of sucking and swallowing; some cases have been responsive to treatment with L-dopa.[295]

An interesting syndrome of *congenital isolated pharyngeal dysfunction* is characterized by total paralysis of pharyngeal muscles and soft palate, with inability to swallow or gag and aspiration on attempts at feeding.[296-299] The lack of abnormality on the electromyogram suggests that this disorder is mediated centrally, above the level of the lower motor neuron. Spontaneous remission has occurred in 50% of cases within the first 6 months of life. The disorder is important to recognize because fatal aspiration has occurred in response to persistent attempts at oral feeding.

Nuclei. Involvement of the neurons of cranial nerve nuclei V, VII, XI, X, and XII, in various combinations, disturbs sucking and swallowing. The three most prominent causes of such involvement are hypoxic-ischemic injury, Möbius syndrome, and Werdnig-Hoffmann disease. Frequently, infants with the Chiari type 2 malformation and myelomeningocele have prominent impairment of lower cranial nerve function, including sucking and swallowing, as noted in Chapter 1.[300-308] The deficits presumably relate to deformation of the lower brain stem and dysfunction at the nuclear or root level.

Nerve. Involvement of the facial nerve (see previous discussion and Chapter 19) is very common, and only sucking is disturbed. In the rare case of posterior fossa hematoma or tumor, other cranial nerves can be affected, and swallowing can also be disturbed. Bilateral laryngeal paralysis may occur as an isolated abnormality of unknown cause (i.e., unassociated with Chiari type 2 malformation or other neurological defect) or in relation to birth trauma, among other possibilities (see Chapter 19). Stridor is a prominent accompanying sign. Disturbance of autonomic nerve function, as in familial dysautonomia, is a rare cause of swallowing dysfunction in the newborn (see Chapter 18).

Neuromuscular Junction. Both myasthenia gravis and infantile botulism are associated with disturbances of sucking or swallowing or both (see Chapter 18).

Muscle Involvement. Of disorders of muscle, *congenital myotonic dystrophy* is the most common cause of significant impairment of both sucking and swallowing in the newborn. Certain other myopathies can be associated with feeding disturbances, most often because of greater impairment of sucking than swallowing (see Table 3-17).

Sternocleidomastoid Function

Abnormalities of sternocleidomastoid function result in disturbed flexion and lateral rotation of the head. In the newborn, these abnormalities occur almost exclusively as a feature of *congenital torticollis*. This disorder is discussed in more detail in Chapter 19. The affected muscle is involved with a contracture that maintains the head in a slightly flexed position with slight rotation to the opposite side. This posture is most apparent when the infant is viewed from the rear.

Tongue Function

Documented abnormalities of tongue function relate primarily to defects of the neurons of the hypoglossal nucleus and of the muscle itself. The *neuronal disorders* result in atrophy and fasciculations of the tongue. The fasciculations can be detected reliably only with the tongue at rest, because all infants, especially when crying, have tremulous movements of the tongue that are virtually impossible to distinguish from fasciculations. The latter are most apparent at the periphery of the tongue at rest and, in marked examples, may give the appearance of a "bag of worms." I have observed fasciculations in newborns with Werdnig-Hoffmann disease and hypoxic-ischemic injury. Atrophy and weakness of the tongue also may occur with Möbius syndrome. A fourth disorder that may affect the nerve XII nucleus in early infancy is type II glycogen storage disease (Pompe disease), but fasciculations and weakness usually appear after the neonatal period, and *macroglossia* is common (see Chapter 18).

Involvement of *muscle of the tongue* rarely causes marked weakness. Certain infiltrations, usually resulting in macroglossia, may interfere with tongue function. These disorders include Pompe disease, generalized gangliosidosis, Beckwith syndrome, congenital hypothyroidism, angioma or hamartoma, and isolated macroglossia.

Abnormalities of the Motor Examination

Delineation of motor abnormalities in the newborn is rendered difficult by normal maturational changes in motility, tone, and character of reflexes (see previous sections). Observation of the posture and ease of passive manipulation of the limbs of infants in quiet repose must always be evaluated as functions of gestational age. Thus, a normal infant of 28 weeks of gestation may exhibit relatively little flexor or extensor tone, whereas at 32 weeks of gestation a normal infant may exhibit relatively little flexor tone in the upper extremities but considerable flexor tone in the lower extremities. Moreover, these conclusions relate to muscle *tone* and not necessarily to muscle *power*. Pathological hypertonia and hypotonia are detected readily with careful examination. The discussion that follows is based primarily on my experience with a standard clinical approach. Use of more sophisticated techniques (long-term video recordings or quantitative analyses of movement) eventually may lead to better detection of subtle deficits.[182-184,190-194,196-198,199a,309-311]

Hypertonia

Hypertonia is not as common a feature of neonatal neurological disease as is hypotonia. When present, hypertonia most often has a plastic quality, which increases with passive manipulation of the limbs and is reminiscent more of gegenhalten or of dystonia in older patients.[246] Only rarely does the increase in tone have the "clasp-knife" quality of spasticity. Neonatal hypertonia may be caused by chronic and therefore *intrauterine* injury to the corticospinal tract or

extrapyramidal system. Hypoxic-ischemic lesions are the most common cause (see Chapter 9), although markedly increased tone has been described in infants with congenital absence of the pyramidal tracts.[312] *Acute perinatal* causes of hypertonia include *meningeal inflammation,* (secondary to bacterial meningitis [see Chapter 21] or to hemorrhage [see Chapters 10 and 11]), *severe bilateral cerebral injury with brain stem release phenomena* (similar to decorticate or decerebrate posturing), *basal ganglia injury* (especially with perinatal hypoxic-ischemic insults [see Chapter 9], and *brain stem activation* (especially in infants exposed in utero to cocaine or with hyperexplexia [see Chapters 24 and 5, respectively]).

Myogenic causes of hypertonia are myotonia congenita, paramyotonia congenita, and hyperkalemic periodic paralysis (see Chapter 19). Finally, the contractures of arthrogryposis may be *mistaken* for hypertonia, and careful examination is important (see Chapter 17).

Hypotonia and Weakness

Hypotonia is the most common motor abnormality observed in neonatal neurological disorders. It is important to distinguish hypotonia from weakness, but it is unusual to observe hypotonia without at least some weakness in the newborn. Disproportionate involvement occurs, but total dissociation is rare. Hypotonia and weakness are discussed in detail in Chapters 17 to 19. Certain *patterns of weakness* are associated with the anatomical loci of disease and are reviewed briefly here.

Focal Cerebral. Focal injury to the cerebrum results in contralateral hemiparesis and a tendency of the eyes to deviate to the side of the lesion. These signs are often not striking in the newborn, but they are definite and, assuredly, detectable, contrary to what is often stated in many standard texts of neurology and neonatology. Three patterns of lateralized weakness can be defined. Hemiparesis in the term newborn most often affects the upper extremity more prominently than the lower extremity, but in the preterm newborn the opposite occurs (see Chapters 9 and 11). The upper extremity pattern of the term newborn is related usually to an arterial disturbance (primarily middle cerebral artery), with predominant involvement of the lateral cerebral convexity; the lower extremity pattern is related usually to a unilateral periventricular venous disturbance, with predominant involvement of the periventricular white matter. A third variety of focal weakness secondary to focal cerebral injury involves cortical venous infarction, which may occur in either term or preterm infants (especially with bacterial meningitis). The weakness usually involves the superior cerebral convexity and thereby causes either lower extremity monoparesis or, more likely, hemiparesis with greater involvement of lower than of upper extremity.

Parasagittal Cerebral. Parasagittal cerebral injury, as occurs after a generalized disturbance in cerebral perfusion in the term newborn, results in weakness of the proximal limbs, upper more than lower, because the lesion resides in the "watershed" region of cerebral convexities (i.e., the superomedial aspects; see Chapter 8).

Periventricular Cerebral (Bilateral). Bilateral cystic periventricular white matter injury, characteristic of the preterm infant, is secondary in largest part to disturbance of cerebral perfusion, and it results in bilateral generally symmetrical weakness of lower extremities much more than of upper extremities (see Chapter 9). Before approximately term equivalent, this pattern is very difficult to detect in the prematurely born infant. This pattern of weakness can also be observed with periventricular white matter involvement caused by hydrocephalus with dilated lateral ventricles.

Spinal Cord. Involvement of the spinal cord (e.g., spinal cord trauma) usually occurs in the cervical region and initially results in flaccid weakness of all extremities, with *sparing of the face* and the function of other cranial nerves. Involvement of sphincters is often prominent, and evolution to spasticity of the lower extremities (and upper extremities if the lesion is in the middle to upper cervical region) usually appears in weeks to months.

Lower Motor Neuron. Involvement of the lower motor neuron (e.g., Werdnig-Hoffmann disease) causes flaccid weakness of all extremities, with initial relative sparing of the face and the function of other cranial nerves. Fasciculations may be detectable, particularly in the form of "tremors" of the fingers.

Nerve Roots. Involvement of roots, as with brachial plexus injury, results in discrete and *restricted patterns of focal weakness*, according to the specific roots involved (see Chapter 22).

Peripheral Nerve. Disease of the peripheral nerves usually results in *generalized* weakness; the newborn only uncommonly exhibits the distal greater than proximal weakness characteristic of neuropathy at later ages. Peripheral nerve disease may be *focal*, such as in traumatic injury, and such restricted weakness and hypotonia reflect and suggest this possibility (see Chapter 22).

Neuromuscular Junction. Involvement of the *neuromuscular junction* (e.g., in myasthenia gravis and infantile botulism) causes generalized weakness and hypotonia. Accompanying involvement of cranial nerve function, including the face, is common (see Chapter 18).

Muscle. Disease of muscle in the newborn causes generalized weakness and hypotonia, often more prominent in proximal than in distal limbs. Certain neonatal myopathies also affect face and eye movements and swallowing (see Chapter 19).

Tendon Reflexes and Plantar Response

Abnormalities of *tendon reflexes* are frequent and important accompaniments to disturbances of the motor system in the newborn period. In general, infants with lesions *above the level of the lower motor neuron* (i.e., lesions of the cerebrum or spinal cord) exhibit preserved deep tendon reflexes but do *not* develop the characteristically hyperactive reflexes until weeks or months later (see Chapter 9). When *lower motor neuron, root*, or *nerve* is involved, deep tendon reflexes are usually *absent* or are barely detectable. Muscle power may be less affected initially; these patients may have modest muscle weakness despite absent reflexes. In disorders of the *neuromuscular junction*, the opposite often occurs, in that reflexes may be only slightly affected or unaffected, despite striking weakness. In disease of *muscle*, the decrease in deep tendon reflexes parallels the decrease in muscle power.

As indicated in the section on normal neurological findings, the *plantar response* has not been particularly helpful in my evaluation of the neonatal motor system, except in disease of lumbosacral cord or plexus. However, a distinctly asymmetrical response, in which one plantar response is extensor, should suggest disease above the level of the lower motor neuron. The most unequivocal extensor responses that I have observed in the newborn infant have accompanied spinal cord injury.

Abnormal Movements

Abnormal movements include myotonia, fasciculations, jitteriness, excessive startles, or more complex adventitial movements. Myotonia and fasciculations are motor abnormalities that have important diagnostic implications and require care for detection. Jitteriness is readily detected but is sometimes confused with other movements, such as seizure. The excessive startles of hyperexplexia are closely related (see Chapter 5). A more complex movement disorder occurs, particularly with bronchopulmonary dysplasia (see later).

Myotonia. *Myotonia* is principally observed in myotonic dystrophy and consists of sustained contraction of a muscle group, which is usually provoked by percussion. Percussion of the thenar muscles or the mentalis muscle may lead to a persistent "dimple" of the muscle that is apparent for seconds. This response is very difficult to elicit in the newborn infant (see Chapter 19).

Fasciculation. *Fasciculation*, which is spontaneous contraction of the *group* of muscle fibers that compose a motor unit, is a feature of lower motor neuron disease (e.g., Werdnig-Hoffmann disease). Fasciculations are best observed in the tongue or sometimes in the fingers (if the fingers are observed with the wrist slightly hyperextended).

Jitteriness. *Jitteriness* is a disorder of movement that is frequently observed in the newborn period; its distinction from seizure is important (see Chapter 5). The movements in jitteriness are generalized and symmetrical, have the qualities primarily of a "coarse" tremor, are exquisitely stimulus sensitive, and can be diminished effectively by gentle, passive flexion of the limbs. Frequent accompaniments are brisk deep tendon reflexes and an easily elicited Moro reflex. Jitteriness is most frequently related to insults that produce neuronal hyperirritability, such as hypoxic-ischemic encephalopathy, hypocalcemia, hypoglycemia, and drug withdrawal. However, in many infants, no definable cause exists.

Excessive Startles. Startle responses markedly excessive for the stimulation (auditory, somesthetic) that produce them is characteristic of *hyperexplexia*. As noted earlier, hypertonia is an additional feature. This disorder is discussed in Chapter 5.

Movement Disorder with Bronchopulmonary Dysplasia.

Perlman and I defined a striking movement disorder in premature infants with severe *bronchopulmonary dysplasia*.[313] The clinical features in many ways are similar to extrapyramidal movement disorders of older infants and children. Chronic hypoxemia, hypercarbia, bronchospasm, and inadequate nutrition have been present in all the patients in whom we have observed this disorder. The abnormal movements develop from approximately the third postnatal month and involve the limbs, neck, trunk, and oral-buccal-lingual structures. The limb movements are most prominent distally and consist of rapid, random, jerky movements (similar to chorea) and "restless" movements (similar to akathisia). Similar movements of the neck and face are observed; tongue movements have a "darting" quality. The oral-buccal-lingual movements are similar to the dyskinesias of elderly patients. Movements are exacerbated during episodes of respiratory failure and are attenuated during sleep. All infants have exhibited feeding disorders, largely resulting from the tongue movements. Several infants have exhibited improvement with clonazepam. The natural history has been partial or complete resolution or a static course. Neuropathological findings in the one infant studied were neuronal loss with astrocytosis in caudate, putamen, globus pallidus, and thalamus. Thus, these observations defined a previously unrecognized extrapyramidal disorder of infants with severe bronchopulmonary dysplasia; the pathogenesis may be related to chronic hypoxemia.

Abnormalities of Primary Neonatal Reflexes

Moro Reflex

The *Moro reflex* is very sensitive to the infant's level of alertness. The most common cause of a depressed or absent Moro reflex is a generalized disturbance of the central nervous system. Thus, a great variety of disorders may be responsible. An exaggerated, stereotyped, nonhabituating Moro reflex is a common neonatal feature of severe bilateral intrauterine cerebral disturbance (e.g., hydranencephaly and severe micrencephaly vera), perhaps because of release of the brain stem from inhibitory cortical influences. The most useful abnormality of the Moro reflex to elicit is distinct *asymmetry*, which is almost always a feature of root, plexus, or nerve disease. In my experience, focal

cerebral injury does not cause distinct disturbance of the Moro reflex.

Tonic Neck Reflex

As with the Moro reflex, the *tonic neck reflex* normally prominent in the 1-month-old infant may be exaggerated, stereotyped, and nonhabituating in patients with a severe fixed bilateral cerebral disturbance. When the tonic neck reflex is "obligatory" (i.e., the full response does not diminish in the normal manner if the head is maintained to the side), other focal cerebral signs such as hemiparesis are likely to be present or to evolve.

Palmar Grasp

Abnormalities of *palmar grasp* are particularly useful if asymmetrical, usually reflecting peripheral involvement (i.e., root, plexus, or nerve). As with the Moro reflex, the palmar grasp is exaggerated and nonhabituating in the presence of severe bilateral cerebral disease.[90] Marked retention of the plantar grasp beyond the first 6 months of life is more characteristic of athetoid than spastic cerebral palsy,[208] an observation suggesting an important role for the extrapyramidal motor system in the maturational disappearance of this reflex.

Abnormalities of the Sensory Examination

Abnormalities of sensation are most easily elicited and interpreted in the newborn period in peripheral lesions, especially those involving roots, and in spinal cord injury. The most illustrative of the former is the sensory deficit in infants with *brachial plexus injuries*. I have observed distinct deficits in response to pinprick in a *segmental distribution* that is usually less extensive than the deficit of motor function (see Chapter 22). Moreover, the finding of sensory deficit in the severely hypotonic infant is strongly suggestive of hypomyelinative polyneuropathy (see Chapter 18).

The major sensory abnormality in *spinal cord injury* relates to the detection of a *sensory level*, defined as the segmental level below which anesthesia or hypesthesia exists and above which normal sensation occurs. This level corresponds to the approximate segment of spinal cord primarily affected by the injury. (Only occasionally in a newborn have I been able to detect an area of *hyperesthesia* at the segment of the cord injury, as observed in older patients.) Detection of a sensory level is a particularly valuable observation, because it strongly favors the diagnosis of a spinal cord lesion.

Disturbances of sensory function that relate to *lesions of the cerebral hemispheres* are more difficult to document in the newborn period. In my experience, such lesions disturb the so-called higher-level responses described in the discussion of normal neurological findings; these responses are recognizable latency, nonstereotyped movement, accompanying grimace or cry, and habituation. This experience is consistent with the reported observation in a hydranencephalic infant with intact diencephalon but absent parietal lobes of no response decrement to pinprick on any of the administrations of the "five-trial pinprick habituation item"; in fact, the responses "tended to generalize to the whole body and

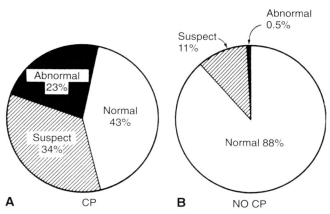

Figure 3-12 **Relation of assessment of neonatal neurological status and subsequent outcome.** Depicted are overall assessments of neurological status made in the newborn period in, **A**, infants who later exhibited cerebral palsy (CP) and, **B**, those who were free of CP. *(From Nelson KB, Ellenberg JH: Neonatal signs as predictors of cerebral palsy, Pediatrics 64:225-232, 1979.)*

increase in intensity over trials."[90] Thus, the *quality* of the response to pinprick is the critical feature in evaluating sensation with regard to cerebral lesions.

VALUE OF THE NEONATAL NEUROLOGICAL EXAMINATION

The essential value of the neurological examination in defining the locus and extent of neuropathological involvement and therefore in formulating plans of management is unequivocal in numerous examples of neurological disease. The value of performing a careful neonatal neurological examination, however, frequently is questioned on the basis of two major contentions. The first is that the usual examination permits evaluation of only function of subcortical structures,

and the second, related to the first, is that abnormal neurological findings are poor indicators of subsequent deficits of higher neurological function. I consider neither of these contentions to be supported by available data and discuss each briefly in the following sections.

Evaluation of Cerebral Function

The usual support raised for the contention that the neonatal neurological examination permits evaluation of only function of subcortical structures relates to findings of studies of hydranencephalic and anencephalic infants. Such infants often exhibit sleep-wake cycles, blink to light and sound, normal pupillary responses, and reflex extraocular movement.[90,314-316] Facial motility, limb motility, and tendon reflexes exhibit only variable impairment. However, several neurological features are conspicuously disturbed or even absent. Primary neonatal reflexes, although present, are stereotyped, elicited with very brief latencies, and not subject to habituation. Similarly, when occipital and temporal cortices are unequivocally absent, habituation to visual and auditory stimuli is absent. As noted earlier, in one well-studied case in which parietal cortex was apparently absent, habituation to pinprick was absent.[90] Moreover, contrary to the frequently stated misconception, focal cerebral lesions in the newborn result in distinct, although often subtle, focal deficits of limb movement and ocular gaze (see Chapters 9 to 11 on hypoxic-ischemic brain injury and intracranial hemorrhage). Perhaps of greatest importance is the realization that careful clinicoanatomical correlations have only recently begun to be made in neonatal neurology, especially since the advent of MRI. It is to be expected that further significant insight into the impact of cerebral injury on the neonatal neurological examination will be gained from such correlations.

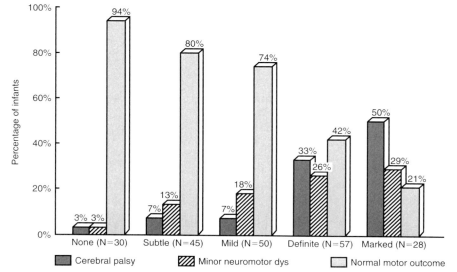

Figure 3-13 **Relationship between number and type of abnormalities observed during neonatal neurodevelopmental examination and later motor development.** Subtle abnormality, one to two minor abnormalities; mild abnormality, three to four minor abnormalities, mild neck extensor tone, or intermittent lower extremity extensor tone; definite abnormality, one major abnormality or at least five minor abnormalities; marked abnormality, at least two major abnormalities or one major and five or more minor abnormalities. *(From Allen MC, Capute AJ: Neonatal neurodevelopmental examination as a predictor of neuromotor outcome in premature infants, Pediatrics 83:498-506, 1989.)*

Role in Estimating Prognosis

The contention that the neonatal neurological examination has little predictive value for subsequent neurological abnormality is not supported by numerous studies.[12,184,199,199a,317-337] In general, the predictive power of *isolated* neurological signs in the newborn period is not great, but this fact should not detract from the very real predictive value of certain signs or combinations of signs. *Certain neonatal neurological abnormalities* were particularly valuable predictors in the large population studied as part of the Collaborative Perinatal Project of the National Institutes of Health.[317] When infants (predominately term) who subsequently developed cerebral palsy were compared with those who did not, various abnormalities of limb, neck, or trunk tone carried a 12- to 15-fold enhanced risk; diminished cry for more than 1 day carried a 21-fold enhanced risk; weak or absent sucking carried a 14-fold enhanced risk; the need for gavage or tube feedings carried a 16- to 22-fold enhanced risk; and diminished activity for more than 1 day carried a 19-fold enhanced risk. Although the actual incidence of infants exhibiting each sign who subsequently developed cerebral palsy was relatively low, usually less than 10%, the predictive power was obviously considerable and alerted the physician to neonatal neurological abnormality. Moreover, I believe that *combinations* of neurological abnormalities greatly increase predictive capacity. This belief, of course, is reasonable in that the occurrence of such combinations in the neonatal period suggests a more severe neurological disturbance. Some data support this notion.[12,184,196,199,317,318,327,331,332,334,336,337] In the aforementioned Collaborative Project, in which a combination of deficits gave the overall impression of neurological abnormality, 16% of infants later exhibited cerebral palsy. When viewed retrospectively, an overall impression of suspicious or abnormal neurological status was approximately fivefold more likely in infants who later exhibited cerebral palsy than in those who did not (Fig. 3-12).

The value of the neonatal neurological examination in estimating outcome in infants of very low birth weight also has been shown (Fig. 3-13).[326,327] A clear relationship was observed between the severity of the abnormalities at the discharge neurological examination and motor abnormalities at 1 to 5 years of age (see Fig. 3-13).[327] In the latter study, 38% of infants with any abnormality of the neonatal neurological examination at discharge developed cerebral palsy, versus 6% of infants with a normal neonatal neurological examination.[327] Of the infants who developed cerebral palsy, 80% had an abnormal neonatal neurological examination.[327] Other work has emphasized the predictive value of abnormalities of the *quality* of movements in prediction of abnormal neurological outcome.[183,184,197,198,199a]

The available data thus establish that the neonatal neurological examination is of major value, when it is carefully and thoughtfully performed. Serial examinations are especially useful. It is of critical importance to recognize, however, that *the value of the examination is greatest when it is assessed in the context of the neuropathological disorder* likely to be the cause of the neurological sign or signs. This theme of correlating clinical features with the appropriate specialized techniques for defining disorders, to reach the most meaningful diagnostic and prognostic formulations, is recurrent throughout this book.

REFERENCES

1. Sanders M, Allen M, Alexander GR, Yankowitz J, et al: Gestational age assessment in preterm neonates weighing less than 1500 grams, *Pediatrics* 88:542-546, 1991.
2. Allen MC: Assessment of gestational age and neuromaturation, *Ment Retard Dev Disabil Res Rev* 11:21-1133, 2005.
3. Finnstrom O: Studies on maturity in newborn infants. II. External characteristics, *Acta Paediatr Scand* 61:24-32, 1972.
4. Amiel-Tison C, Maillard F, Lebrun F, Breart G, et al: Neurological and physical maturation in normal growth singletons from 37 to 41 weeks' gestation, *Early Hum Dev* 54:145-156, 1999.
5. Fletcher MA: Physical assessment and classification. In Avery GB, Fletcher MA, MacDonald MG, editors: *Neonatology, Pathophysiology and Management of the Newborn*, 5th ed, Philadelphia: 1999, Lippincott Williams & Wilkins.
6. Narvey M, Fletcher MA: Physical assessment and classification. In MacDonald MG, Mullett MD, Seshia MMK, editors: *Avery's Neonatology, Pathophysiology and Management of the Newborn*, 6th ed, Philadelphia: 2005, Lippincott Williams & Wilkins.
7. Usher R, McLean F: Intrauterine growth of live-born Caucasian infants at sea level: Standards obtained from measurements in 7 dimensions of infants born between 25 and 44 weeks of gestation, *J Pediatr* 74:901-910, 1969.
8. Farr V, Kerridge DF, Mitchell RG: The value of some external characteristics in the assessment of gestational age at birth, *Dev Med Child Neurol* 8:657-660, 1966.
9. Dubowitz LM, Dubowitz V, Goldberg C: Clinical assessment of gestational age in the newborn infant, *J Pediatr* 77:1-10, 1970.
10. Ballard JL, Khoury JC, Wedig K, Wang L, et al: New Ballard score, expanded to include extremely premature infants, *J Pediatr* 119:417-423, 1991.
11. Dubowitz L, Ricciw D, Mercuri E: The Dubowitz neurological examination of the full-term newborn, *Ment Retard Dev Disabil Res Rev* 11:52-60, 2005.
12. Gosselin J, Gahagan S, Amiel-Tison C: The Amiel-Tison neurological assessment at term: Conceptual and methodological continuity in the course of follow-up, *Ment Retard Dev Disabil Res Rev* 11:34-51, 2005.
13. Tallman B, Tan OT, Morelli JG, Piepenbrink J, et al: Location of port-wine stains and the likelihood of ophthalmic and/or central nervous system complications, *Pediatrics* 87:323-327, 1991.
14. Enjolras O, Riche MC, Merland JJ: Facial port-wine stains and Sturge-Weber syndrome, *Pediatrics* 76:48-51, 1985.
15. Enjolras O, Chiron C, Diebler C, Merland JJ: New trends for an early diagnosis of the Sturge-Weber syndrome [in French], *Rev Eur Dermatol MST* 3:21-26, 1991.
16. Pascual-Castroviejo I, Diaz-Gonzalez C, Garcia-Melian RM, Gonzalez-Casado I, et al: Sturge-Weber syndrome: Study of 40 patients, *Pediatr Neurol* 9:283-288, 1993.
17. Sujansky E, Conradi S: Sturge-Weber syndrome: Age of onset of seizures and glaucoma and the prognosis for affected children, *J Child Neurol* 10:49-58, 1995.
18. Goldman MP, Fitzpatrick RE, Ruiz-Esparza J: Treatment of port-wine stains (capillary malformation) with the flashlamp-pumped pulsed dye laser, *J Pediatr* 122:71-77, 1993.
19. Strauss RP, Resnick SD: Pulsed dye laser therapy for port-wine stains in children: Psychosocial and ethical issues, *J Pediatr* 122:505-510, 1993.
20. Garden JM, Bakus AD, Paller AS: Treatment of cutaneous hemangiomas by the flashlamp-pumped pulsed dye laser: Prospective analysis, *J Pediatr* 120:555-560, 1992.
21. van der Horst CMAM, Koster PHL, de Borgie CAJM, Bossuvt PMM, et al: Effect of the timing of treatment of port-wine stains with the flash-lamp-pumped pulsed-dye laser, *N Engl J Med* 338:1028-1033, 1998.
22. Matson D: *Neurosurgery of Infancy and Childhood*, Springfield, IL: 1969, Charles C Thomas.
23. Boltshauser E, Ludwig S, Dietrich F, Landolt MA: Sagittal craniosynostosis: Cognitive development, behaviour, and quality of life in unoperated children, *Neuropediatrics* 34:293-300, 2003.
24. Jones KL: *Smith's Recognizable Patterns of Human Malformation*, 6th ed, Philadelphia: 2006, Elsevier.
25. Wiedemann HR, Grosse KR, Dibbern H: *An Atlas of Characteristic Syndromes: A Visual Aid to Diagnosis*, 2nd ed, Stuttgart: 1983, Wolfe Medical Publications.

26. Cohen MM: Proteus syndrome: Clinical evidence for somatic mosaicism and selective review, *Am J Med Genet* 47:645-652, 1993.
27. Taravath S, Tonsgard JH: Cerebral malformations in Carpenter syndrome, *Pediatr Neurol* 9:230-234, 1993.
28. Jones LJ: *Smith's Recognizable Patterns of Human Malformation*, 5th ed, Philadelphia: 1997, Saunders.
29. Wiedemann H-R, Kunze J: *Clinical Syndromes*, 3rd ed, London: 1997, Times Mirror International.
30. Jones KL: *Smith's Recognizable Patterns of Human Malformation*, 6th ed, Philadelphia: 2006, Elsevier Saunders.
31. Persing J, James H, Swanson J, Kattwinkel J: Prevention and management of positional skull deformities in infants, *Pediatrics* 112:199-202, 2003.
32. Maugans TA: The misshapen head, *Pediatrics* 110:166-167, 2002.
33. Littlefield TR, Kelly KM, Pomatto JK, Beals SP: Multiple-birth infants at higher risk for development of deformational plagiocephaly. II. Is one twin at greater risk? *Pediatrics* 109:19-25, 2002.
34. Graham JM Jr, Gomez M, Halberg A, Earl DL, et al: Management of deformational plagiocephaly: Repositioning versus orthotic therapy, *J Pediatr* 146:258-262, 2005.
35. Graham JM Jr, Kreutzman J, Earl D, Halberg A, et al: Deformational brachycephaly in supine-sleeping infants, *J Pediatr* 146:253-257, 2005.
36. Bialocerkowski A, Vladusic SL, Howell SM: Conservative interventions for positional plagiocephaly: A systematic review, *Dev Med Child Neurol* 47:563-570, 2005.
37. Sher PK, Brown SB: A longitudinal study of head growth in pre-term infants. I. Normal rates of head growth, *Dev Med Child Neurol* 17:705-710, 1975.
38. Sher PK, Brown SB: A longitudinal study of head growth in pre-term infants. II. Differentiation between "catch-up" head growth and early infantile hydrocephalus, *Dev Med Child Neurol* 17:711-718, 1975.
39. Williams J, Hirsch NJ, Corbet AJ, Rudolph AJ: Postnatal head shrinkage in small infants, *Pediatrics* 59:619-622, 1977.
40. Marks KH, Maisels MJ, Moore E, Gifford K, et al: Head growth in sick premature infants: A longitudinal study, *J Pediatr* 94:282-285, 1979.
41. Gross SJ, Eckerman CO: Normative early head growth in very low-birth-weight infants, *J Pediatr* 103:946-949, 1983.
42. Gross SJ, Oehler JM, Eckerman CO: Head growth and developmental outcome in very low-birth-weight infants, *Pediatrics* 71:70-75, 1983.
43. Casey PH, Kraemer HC, Bernbaum J, Tyson JE, et al: Growth patterns of low birth weight preterm infants: A longitudinal analysis of a large, varied sample, *J Pediatr* 117:298-307, 1990.
44. Raymond GV, Holmes LB: Head circumference standards in neonates, *J Child Neurol* 9:63-66, 1994.
45. Sheth RD, Mullett MD, Bodensteiner JB, Hobbs GR: Longitudinal head growth in developmentally normal preterm infants, *Arch Pediatr Adolesc Med* 149:1358-1361, 1995.
46. Ehrenkranz RA, Younes N, Lemons JA, Fanaroff AA, et al: Longitudinal growth of hospitalized very low birth weight infants, *Pediatrics* 104:280-289, 1999.
47. Robertson C: Catch-up growth among very-low-birth-weight preterm infants: A historical perspective, *J Pediatr* 143:145-146, 2003.
48. Brandt I, Sticker EJ, Lentze MJ: Catch-up growth of head circumference of very low birth weight, small for gestational age preterm infants and mental development to adulthood, *J Pediatr* 142:463-468, 2003.
49. Latal-Hajnal B, Von Siebenthal K, Kovari H, Bucher HU, et al: Postnatal growth in VLBW infants: Significant association with neurodevelopmental outcome, *J Pediatr* 143:163-170, 2003.
50. Lofqvist C, Engstrom E, Sigurdsson J, Hard AL, et al: Postnatal head growth deficit among premature infants parallels retinopathy of prematurity and insulin-like growth factor-1 deficit, *Pediatrics* 117:1930-1938, 2006.
51. DeSouza SW, Ross J, Milner R: Alterations in head shape of newborn infants after caesarean section or vaginal delivery, *Arch Dis Child* 51:624-627, 1976.
52. Prechtl HFR: *Continuity of Neural Functions From Prenatal to Postnatal Life*, Oxford: 1984, Spastics International Medical.
53. Georgieff MD, Hoffman JS, Pereira GR, Bernbaum J, et al: Effect of neonatal caloric deprivation on head growth and 1-year development status in preterm infants, *J Pediatr* 107:581-587, 1985.
54. Prechtl HFR, Beintema D: *The Neurological Examination of the Full Term Newborn Infant*, London: 1964, William Heinemann.
55. Brazelton TB: *Neonatal Behavioral Assessment Scale*, Philadelphia: 1973, JB Lippincott.
56. Saint-Anne Dargassies S: *Neurological Development in the Full-Term and Premature Neonate*, New York: 1977, Excerpta Medica.
57. Hall WG, Oppenheim RW: Developmental psychobiology: Prenatal, perinatal, and early postnatal aspects of behavioral development, *Annu Rev Psychol* 38:91-128, 1987.
58. McMillen IC, Kok JS, Adamson TM, Deayton JM, et al: Development of circadian sleep-wake rhythms in preterm and full-term infants, *Pediatr Res* 29:381-384, 1991.
59. Pillai M, James D: Are the behavioural states of the newborn comparable to those of the fetus? *Early Hum Dev* 22:39-49, 1990.
60. Vles JS, van Oostenbrugge R-J, Hasaart TH, Caberg H, et al: State profile in low-risk pre-term infants: A longitudinal study of 7 infants from 32-36 weeks of postmenstrual age, *Brain Dev* 14:12-17, 1992.
61. Shimada M, Segawa M, Higurashi M, Akamatsu H: Development of the sleep and wakefulness rhythm in preterm infants discharged from a neonatal care unit, *Pediatr Res* 33:159-163, 1993.
62. Scher MS, Johnson MW, Holditch-Davis D: Cyclicity of neonatal sleep behaviors at 25 to 30 weeks' postconceptional age, *Pediatr Res* 57:879-882, 2005.
63. Parmelee AH Jr, Schultz HR, Disbrow MA: Sleep patterns of the newborn, *J Pediatr* 58:241-250, 1961.
64. Parmelee AH Jr, Wenner WH, Akiyama Y, Schultz M, et al: Sleep states in premature infants, *Dev Med Child Neurol* 9:70-77, 1967.
65. Dreyfus-Brisac C: Ontogenesis of sleep in human prematures after 32 weeks of conceptional age, *Dev Psychobiol* 3:91-121, 1970.
66. Prechtl HFR, O'Brien MJ: Behavioural states of the full-term newborn: The emergence of a concept. In Stratton P, editor: *Psychobiology of the Human Newborn*, New York: 1982, John Wiley & Sons.
67. Munger DM, Bucher HU, Duc G: Sleep state changes associated with cerebral blood volume changes in healthy term newborn infants, *Early Hum Dev* 52:27-42, 1998.
68. Sarnat HB: Olfactory reflexes in the newborn infant, *J Pediatr* 92:624-626, 1978.
69. Bartocci M, Winberg J, Ruggiero C, Bergqvist LL, et al: Activation of olfactory cortex in newborn infants after odor stimulation: A functional near-infrared spectroscopy study, *Pediatr Res* 48:18-23, 2000.
70. Winberg J, Porter RH: Olfaction and human neonatal behaviour: Clinical implications, *Acta Paediatr* 87:6-10, 1998.
71. Sullivan RM, Toubas P: Clinical usefulness of maternal odor in newborns: Soothing and feeding preparatory responses, *Biol Neonate* 74:402-408, 1998.
72. Engen T, Lipsitt LP, Kaye H: Olfactory responses and adaptation in the human neonate, *J Comp Physiol Psychol* 56:73-81, 1963.
73. Engen T, Lipsitt LP: Decrement and recovery of responses to olfactory stimuli in the human neonate, *J Comp Physiol Psychol* 59:312-316, 1965.
74. Lipsitt LP: The study of sensory and learning processes of the newborn, *Clin Perinatol* 4:163-186, 1977.
75. Macfarlane A: Olfaction in the development of social preferences in the human neonate: Parent-infant interaction, *CIBA Found Symp* 33:103-117, 1975.
76. Sullivan RM, Taborsky-Barba S, Mendoza R, Itano A, et al: Olfactory classical conditioning in neonates, *Pediatrics* 87:511-518, 1991.
77. Varendi H, Christensson K, Porter RH, Winberg J: Soothing effect of amniotic fluid smell in newborn infants, *Early Hum Dev* 51:47-55, 1998.
78. Bingham PM, Abassi S, Sivieri E: A pilot study of milk odor effect on nonnutritive sucking by premature newborns, *Arch Pediatr Adolesc Med* 157:72-75, 2003.
79. Robinson J, Fielder AR: Pupillary diameter and reaction to light in preterm neonates, *Arch Dis Child* 65:35-38, 1990.
80. Peiper A: *Cerebral Function in Infancy and Childhood*, New York: 1963, Consultants Bureau.
81. Hack M, Mostow A, Miranda SB: Development of attention in preterm infants, *Pediatrics* 58:669-674, 1976.
82. Palmer PG, Dubowitz LM, Verghote M, Dubowitz V: Neurological and neurobehavioural differences between preterm infants at term and full-term newborn infants, *Neuropediatrics* 13:183-189, 1982.
83. Robinson RJ, Tizard JP: The central nervous system in the new-born, *Br Med Bull* 22:49-55, 1966.
84. Guzzetta A, Cioni G, Cowan F, Mercuri E: Visual disorders in children with brain lesions. I. Maturation of visual function in infants with neonatal brain lesions: Correlation with neuroimaging, *Eur Paediatr Neurol* 5:107-114, 2001.
85. Madan A, Good WV: Visual development in preterm infants, *Dev Med Child Neurol* 47:276-280, 2005.
86. Allen MC, Capute AJ: Assessment of early auditory and visual abilities of extremely premature infants, *Dev Med Child Neurol* 28:458-466, 1986.
87. Guzzetta A, Haataja L, Cowan F, Bassi L, et al: Neurological examination in healthy term infants aged 3-10 weeks, *Biol Neonate* 87:187-196, 2005.
88. Snyder RD, Hata SK, Brann BS, Mills RM: Subcortical visual function in the newborn, *Pediatr Neurol* 6:333-336, 1990.
89. Dubowitz LM, Mushin J, De Vries L, Arden GB: Visual function in the newborn infant: Is it cortically mediated? *Lancet* 1:1139-1141, 1986.
90. Aylward GP, Lazzara A, Meyer J: Behavioral and neurological characteristics of a hydranencephalic infant, *Dev Med Child Neurol* 20:211-217, 1978.
91. Jan JE, Wong PK, Groenveld M, Flodmark O, et al: Travel vision: "Collicular visual system"? *Pediatr Neurol* 2:359-362, 1986.
92. Cocker KD, Moseley MJ, Stirling HF, Fielder AR: Delayed visual maturation: Pupillary responses implicate subcortical and cortical visual systems, *Dev Med Child Neurol* 40:160-162, 1998.
93. Boothe RG, Dobson V, Teller DY: Postnatal development of vision in human and nonhuman primates, *Annu Rev Neurosci* 8:495-545, 1985.
94. Atkinson J: Human visual development over the first 6 months of life: A review and a hypothesis, *Hum Neurobiol* 3:61-74, 1984.
95. van Hof-Van Duin J: The development and study of visual acuity, *Dev Med Child Neurol* 31:547-552, 1989.

96. Norcia AM, Tyler CW, Hamer RD: Development of contrast sensitivity in the human infant, *Vision Res* 30:1475-1486, 1990.
97. Dobson V, Schwartz TL, Sandstrom DJ, Michel L: Binocular visual acuity of neonates: The acuity card procedure, *Dev Med Child Neurol* 29:199-206, 1987.
98. Sontheimer D: Visual information processing in infancy, *Dev Med Child Neurol* 31:787-796, 1989.
99. Hermans A, Vanhofvanduin J, Oudesluysmurphy AM: Visual acuity in low birth weight (1500-2500 g) neonates, *Early Hum Dev* 28:155-167, 1992.
100. Ipata AE, Cioni G, Boldrini A, Bottai P, et al: Visual acuity of low-risk and high-risk neonates and acuity development during the 1st-year, *Behav Brain Res* 49:107-114, 1992.
101. Van Hof-van Duin J, Heersema DJ, Groenendaal F, Baerts W, et al: Visual field and grating acuity development in low-risk preterm infants during the 1st 2 1/2 years after term, *Behav Brain Res* 49:115-122, 1992.
102. Vital-Durand F: Acuity card procedures and the linearity of grating resolution development during the 1st-year of human infants, *Behav Brain Res* 49:99-106, 1992.
103. Dayton GO Jr, Jones MH, Aiu P, Rawson RA, et al: Developmental study of coordinate movements in the human infant. I. Visual acuity in the newborn human: A study based on induced optokinetic nystagmus recorded by electrooculography, *Arch Ophthalmol* 71:865-870, 1964.
104. Fantz RL: The origin of form perception, *Sci Am* 204:66-72, 1961.
105. Chase WB: Color vision in infants, *J Exp Psychol* 20:203-207, 1937.
106. Bornstein MH, Kessen W, Weiskopf S: The categories of hue in infancy, *Science* 191:201-202, 1976.
107. Peeles DR, Teller DY: Color vision and brightness discrimination in two-month-old human infants, *Science* 189:1102-1103, 1975.
108. Fantz RL: Pattern vision in newborn infants, *Science* 140:296-299, 1963.
109. Hershenson M: Visual discrimination in the human newborn, *J Comp Physiol Psychol* 58:270-276, 1964.
110. Stechler G: Newborn attention as affected by medication during labor, *Science* 144:315-317, 1964.
111. Miranda SB: Visual abilities and pattern preferences of premature infants and full-term neonates, *J Exp Child Psychol* 10:189-205, 1970.
112. Fantz RL, Miranda SB: Newborn infant attention to form of contour, *Child Dev* 46:224-228, 1975.
113. Miranda SB, Hack M: The predictive value of neonatal visual-perceptual behaviors. In Field TM, editor: *Infants Born At Risk: Behavior and Development*, New York: 1979, SP Medical and Scientific.
114. Mirabella G, Kjaer PK, Norcia AM, Good WV, et al: Visual development in very low birth weight infants, *Pediatr Res* 60:435-439, 2006.
115. Haaf RA, Brown CJ: Infants' response to facelike patterns: Developmental changes between 10 and 15 weeks of age, *J Exp Child Psychol* 22:155-160, 1976.
116. Fagan JF III: Infant visual perception and cognition. In Brann AW Jr, Volpe JJ, editors: *Neonatal Neurological Assessment and Outcome: Seventy-seventh Ross Conference*, Columbus, OH: 1980, Ross Laboratories.
117. Farroni T, Johnson MH, Menon E, Zulian L, et al: Newborns' preference for face-relevant stimuli: Effects of contrast polarity, *Proc Natl Acad Sci U S A* 102:17245-17250, 2005.
118. Mercuri E, Atkinson J, Braddick O, Anker S, et al: The aetiology of delayed visual maturation: Short review and personal findings in relation to magnetic resonance imaging, *Eur J Paediatr Neurol* 1:31-34, 1997.
119. Born P, Leth H, Miranda MJ, Rostrup E, et al: Visual activation in infants and young children studied by functional magnetic resonance imaging, *Pediatr Res* 44:578-583, 1998.
120. Martin E, Joeri P, Loenneker T, Ekatodramis D, et al: Visual processing in infants and children studied using functional MRI, *Pediatr Res* 46:135-140, 1999.
121. Meltzoff AN, Moore MK: Imitation of facial and manual gestures by human neonates, *Science* 198:74-78, 1977.
122. Field TM, Woodson R, Greenberg R, Cohen D: Discrimination and imitation of facial expression by neonates, *Science* 218:179-181, 1982.
123. Nagy E, Compagne H, Orvos H, Pal A, et al: Index finger movement imitation by human neonates: Motivation, learning and left-hand preference, *Pediatr Res* 58:749-753, 2005.
124. Schenker JG, Gombos GM: Retinal hemorrhage in the newborn, *Obstet Gynecol* 27:521-524, 1966.
125. Besio R, Caballero C, Meerhoff E, Schwarcz R: Neonatal retinal hemorrhages and influence of perinatal factors, *Am J Ophthalmol* 87:74-76, 1979.
126. Williams MC, Knuppel RA, Obrien WF, Weiss A, et al: Obstetric correlates of neonatal retinal hemorrhage, *Obstet Gynecol* 81:688-694, 1993.
127. Smith WL, Alexander RC, Judisch GF, Sato Y, et al: Magnetic resonance imaging evaluation of neonates with retinal hemorrhages, *Pediatrics* 89:332-333, 1992.
128. Robinson RJ: Assessment of gestational age by neurologic examination, *Arch Dis Child* 41:437-443, 1966.
129. Isenberg SJ: Clinical application of the pupil examination in neonates, *J Pediatr* 118:650-652, 1991.
130. Weissman BM, DiScenna AO, Leigh RJ: Maturation of the vestibulo-ocular reflex in normal infants during the first 2 months of life, *Neurology* 39:534-538, 1989.
131. Donat JF, Donat JR, Lay KS: Changing response to caloric stimulation with gestational age in infants, *Neurology* 30:776-778, 1980.
132. Saint-Anne Dargassies S: Neurological maturation of the premature infant of 28-41 weeks' gestational age. In Falkner F, editor: *Human Development*, Philadelphia: 1966, Saunders.
133. Steinschneider A: Developmental psychophysiology. In Brackbill Y, editor: *Infancy and Early Childhood: A Handbook and Guide to Human Development*, New York: 1967, Free Press.
134. Leventhal AS, Lipsitt LP: Adaptation, pitch discrimination, and sound localization in the neonate, *Child Dev* 35:759-767, 1964.
135. Wertheimer M: Psychomotor coordination of auditory and visual space at birth, *Science* 134:18, 1961.
136. Bower TG: Development of infant behaviour, *Br Med Bull* 30:175-178, 1974.
137. Aronson E, Rosenbloom S: Space perception in early infancy: Perception within a common auditory-visual space, *Science* 172:1161-1163, 1971.
138. Anday EK, Cohen ME, Kelley NE, Hoffman HS: Reflex modification audiometry: Assessment of acoustic sensory processing in the term neonate, *Pediatr Res* 23:357-363, 1988.
139. Anday EK, Cohen ME, Hoffman HS: The blink reflex: Maturation and modification in the neonate, *Dev Med Child Neurol* 32:142-150, 1990.
140. Whitfield IC: *The Auditory Pathway*, London: 1967, Edward Arnold.
141. Eimas PD, Siqueland ER, Jusczyk P, Vigorito J: Speech perception in infants, *Science* 171:303-306, 1971.
142. Dehaene-Lambertz G, Pena M: Electrophysiological evidence for automatic phonetic processing in neonates, *Neuroreport* 12:3155-3158, 2001.
143. Cheour M, Martynova O, Naatanen R, Erkkola R, et al: Speech sounds learned by sleeping newborns, *Nature* 415:599-600, 2002.
144. Carral V, Huotilainen M, Ruusuvirta T, Fellman V, et al: A kind of auditory "primitive intelligence" already present at birth, *Eur J Neurosci* 21:3201-3204, 2005.
145. Simmer ML: Newborn's response to the cry of another infant, *Dev Psychobiol* 5:136-142, 1971.
146. Lagasse LL, Neal AR, Lester BM: Assessment of infant cry: Acoustic cry analysis and parental perception, *Ment Retard Dev Disabil Res Rev* 11:83-93, 2005.
147. Kato T, Takahashi E, Sawada K, Kobayashi N, et al: A computer analysis of infant movements synchronized with adult speech, *Pediatr Res* 17:625-628, 1983.
148. DeCasper AJ, Fifer WP: Of human bonding: Newborns prefer their mothers' voices, *Science* 208:1174-1176, 1980.
149. Ockleford EM, Vince MA, Layton C, Reader MR: Responses of neonates to parents' and others' voices, *Early Hum Dev* 18:27-36, 1988.
150. Masters JC: Developmental psychology, *Annu Rev Psychol* 32:117-128, 1981.
151. Pena M, Maki A, Kovacic D, Dehaene-Lambertz G, et al: Sounds and silence: An optical topography study of language recognition at birth, *Proc Natl Acad Sci U S A* 100:11702-11705, 2003.
152. Dehaene-Lambertz G, Dehaene S, Hertz-Pannier L: Functional neuro-imaging of speech perception in infants, *Science* 298:2013-2015, 2002.
153. Draganova R, Eswaran H, Murphy P, Huotilainen M, et al: Sound frequency change detection in fetuses and newborns: A magnetoencephalo-graphic study, *Neuroimage* 28:354-361, 2005.
154. Stevenson RD, Allaire JH: The development of normal feeding and swallowing, *Pediatr Clin North Am* 38:1439-1453, 1991.
155. Smith WL, Erenberg A, Nowak A, Franken EA Jr: Physiology of sucking in the normal term infant using real-time US, *Radiology* 156:379-381, 1985.
156. Bosma JF, Hepburn LG, Josell SD, Baker K: Ultrasound demonstration of tongue motions during suckle feeding, *Dev Med Child Neurol* 32:223-229, 1990.
157. Bu'Lock F, Woolridge MW, Baum JD: Development of co-ordination of sucking, swallowing and breathing: Ultrasound study of term and pre-term infants, *Dev Med Child Neurol* 32:669-678, 1990.
158. Eishima K: The analysis of sucking behaviour in newborn infants, *Early Hum Dev* 27:163-173, 1991.
159. Daniels H, Devlieger H, Minami T, Eggermont E, et al: Infant feeding and cardiorespiratory maturation, *Neuropediatrics* 21:9-10, 1990.
160. Bamford O, Taciak V, Gewolb IH: The relationship between rhythmic swallowing and breathing during suckle feeding in term neonates, *Pediatr Res* 31:619-624, 1992.
161. Mizuno K, Ueda A: The maturation and coordination of sucking, swallowing and respiration in preterm infants, *J Pediatr* 142:36-40, 2003.
162. Gewolb I, Bosma J, Reynolds EW, Vice FL: Integration of suck and swallow rhythms during feeding in preterm infants with and without bronchopulmonary dysplasia, *Dev Med Child Neurol* 45:344-348, 2003.
163. Rogers B, Arvedson J: Assessment of infant oral sensorimotor and swallowing function, *Ment Retard Dev Disabil Res Rev* 11:74-82, 2005.
164. Hill A, Volpe JJ: Disorders of sucking and swallowing in the newborn infant: Clinicopathological correlations. In Korobkin R, Guilleminault C, editors: *Progress in Perinatal Neurology*, Baltimore: 1981, Williams and Wilkins.
165. Miller AJ: Deglutition, *Physiol Rev* 62:129-184, 1982.
166. Casaer P, Daniels H, Devlieger H, De Cock P, et al: Feeding behaviour in preterm neonates, *Early Hum Dev* 7:331-346, 1982.

167. Lipsitt LP, Mustaine MG, Zeigler B: Effects of experience on the behavior of the young infant, *Neuropadiatrie* 8:107-133, 1977.

168. Lipsitt LP, Crook C, Booth CA: The transitional infant: Behavioral development and feeding, *Am J Clin Nutr* 41:485-496, 1985.

169. Crook CK, Lipsitt LP: Neonatal nutritive sucking: Effects of taste stimulation upon sucking rhythm and heart rate, *Child Dev* 47:518-522, 1976.

170. Amiel-Tison C: Neurological evaluation of the maturity of newborn infants, *Arch Dis Child* 43:89-93, 1968.

171. Prechtl HF, Fargel JW, Weinmann HM, Bakker HH: Postures, motility and respiration of low-risk pre-term infants, *Dev Med Child Neurol* 21:3-27, 1979.

172. Vles JS, Kingma H, Caberg H, Daniels H, et al: Posture of low-risk preterm infants between 32 and 36 weeks postmenstrual age, *Dev Med Child Neurol* 31:191-195, 1989.

173. Cioni G, Ferrari F, Prechtl HF: Posture and spontaneous motility in full-term infants, *Early Hum Dev* 18:247-262, 1989.

174. Vles JS, van Oostenbrugge R, Kingma H, Caberg H, et al: Posture during head turning in pre-term infants: A longitudinal study of 15 low-risk infants of 32-36 weeks of conceptional age, *Neuropediatrics* 20:25-29, 1989.

175. Cioni G, Prechtl HF: Preterm and early postterm motor behaviour in low-risk premature infants, *Early Hum Dev* 23:159-191, 1990.

176. Faridi MM, Rath S, Aggarwal A: Profile of fisting in term newborns, *Eur J Paediatr Neurol* 9:67-70, 2005.

177. Lacey JL, Henderson-Smart DJ, Edwards DA: A longitudinal study of early leg postures of preterm infants, *Dev Med Child Neurol* 32:151-163, 1990.

178. Turkewitz G, Gordon EW, Birch HG: Head turning in the human neonate: Spontaneous patterns, *J Genet Psychol* 107:143-158, 1965.

179. Gardner J, Lewkowicz D, Turkewitz G: Development of postural asymmetry in premature human infants, *Dev Psychobiol* 10:471-480, 1977.

180. Konishi Y, Mikawa H, Suzuki J: Asymmetrical head-turning of preterm infants: Some effects on later postural and functional lateralities, *Dev Med Child Neurol* 28:450-457, 1986.

181. Vles J, van Zutphen S, Hasaart T, Dassen W, et al: Supine and prone head orientation preference in term infants, *Brain Dev* 13:87-90, 1991.

182. Hadders-Algra M, Prechtl HFR: Developmental course of general movements in early infancy. I. Descriptive analysis of change in form, *Early Hum Dev* 28:201-213, 1992.

183. Prechtl HF: General movement assessment as a method of developmental neurology: New paradigms and their consequences, *Dev Med Child Neurol* 43:836-842, 2001.

184. Einspieler C, Prechtl HF: Prechtl's assessment of general movements: A diagnostic tool for the functional assessment of the young nervous system, *Ment Retard Dev Disabil Res Rev* 11:61-67, 2005.

185. Konishi Y, Prechtl HFR: Finger movements and fingers postures in preterm infants are not a good indicator of brain, *Early Hum Dev* 36:89-100, 1994.

186. Mercuri E, Guzzetta A, Laroche S, Ricci D, et al: Neurologic examination of preterm infants at term age: Comparison with term infants, *J Pediatr* 142:647-655, 2003.

187. Hayes MJ, Plante L, Kumar SP, Delivori-Apapadopoulos M: Spontaneous motility in premature infants: Features of behavioral activity and rhythmic organization, *Dev Psychobiol* 26:279-291, 1993.

188. Hayes MJ, Plante LS, Fielding BA, Kumar SP, et al: Functional analysis of spontaneous movements in preterm infants, *Dev Psychobiol* 27:271-287, 1994.

189. Van Der Meer AL: Keeping the arm in the limelight: Advanced visual control of arm movements in neonates, *Eur J Paediatr Neurol* 4:103-108, 1997.

190. Prechtl HFR, Einspieler C, Cioni G, Bos AF, et al: An early marker for neurological deficits after perinatal brain lesions, *Lancet* 349:1361-1363, 1997.

191. Prechtl HFR: State of the art of a new functional assessment of the young nervous system: An early predictor of cerebral palsy, *Early Hum Dev* 50:1-11, 1997.

192. Cioni G, Ferrari F, Einspieler C, Paolicelli PB, et al: Comparison between observation of spontaneous movements and neurologic examination in preterm infants, *J Pediatr* 130:704-711, 1997.

193. Cioni G, Prechtl HFR, Ferrari F, Paolicelli B, et al: Which better predicts later outcome in full-term infants: Quality of general movement or neurological examination? *Early Hum Dev* 50:71-85, 1997.

194. Bos AF, Martijn A, Okken A, Prechtl HFR: Quality of general movements in preterm infants with transient periventricular echodensities, *Acta Paediatr* 87:328-335, 1998.

195. Hadders-Algra M, Groothuis AM: Quality of general movements in infancy is related to neurological dysfunction, ADHD, and aggressive behaviour, *Dev Med Child Neurol* 41:381-391, 1999.

196. Guzzetta A, Mercuri E, Rapisardi G, Ferrari F, et al: General movements detect early signs of hemiplegia in term infants with neonatal cerebral infarction, *Neuropediatrics* 34:61-66, 2003.

197. Ferrari F, Cioni G, Einspieler C, Roversi MF, et al: Cramped synchronized general movements in preterm infants as an early marker for cerebral palsy, *Arch Pediatr Adolesc Med* 156:460-467, 2002.

198. Groen SE, de Blecourt AC, Postema K, Hadders-Algra M: General movements in early infancy predict neuromotor development at 9 to 12 years of age, *Dev Med Child Neurol* 47:731-738, 2005.

199. Paro-Panjan D, Sustersic B, Neubauer D: Comparison of two methods of neurologic assessment in infants, *Pediatr Neurol* 33:317-324, 2005.

199a. Stahlmann N, Hartel C, Knopp A, Gehring B, et al: Predictive value of neurodevelopmental assessment versus evaluation of general movements for motor outcome in preterm infants with birth weights <1500 g, *Neuropediatrics* 38:91-99, 2007.

200. Walters CE: Reliability and comparison of four types of fetal activity and of total activity, *Child Dev* 35:1249, 1964.

201. Zafeiriou DI: Primitive reflexes and postural reactions in the neurodevelopmental examination, *Pediatr Neurol* 31:1-8, 2004.

202. Paine RS, Brazelton TB, Donovan DE: Evolution of postural reflexes in normal infants and in the presence of chronic brain syndromes, *Neurology* 14:1036-1048, 1964.

203. Kuban KC, Skouteli HN, Urion DK, Lawhon GA: Deep tendon reflexes in premature infants, *Pediatr Neurol* 2:266-271, 1986.

204. Gingold MK, Jaynes ME, Bodensteiner JB, Romano JT, et al: The rise and fall of the plantar response in infancy, *J Pediatr* 135:568-570, 1998.

205. Hogan GR, Milligan JE: The plantar reflex of the newborn, *N Engl J Med* 285:502-503, 1971.

206. Rich E, Marshall R, Volpe J: Plantar reflex flexor in normal neonates [letter], *N Engl J Med* 289:1043, 1973.

207. Ross ED, Velez-Borras J, Rosman NP: The significance of the Babinski sign in the newborn: A reappraisal, *Pediatrics* 57:13-15, 1976.

208. Futagi Y, Tagawa T, Otani K: Primitive reflex profiles in infants: Differences based on categories of neurological abnormality, *Brain Dev* 14:294-298, 1992.

209. Capute AJ, Palmer FB, Shapiro BK, Wachtel RC, et al: Primitive reflex profile: A quantitation of primitive reflexes in infancy, *Dev Med Child Neurol* 26:375-383, 1984.

210. Moreau T, Birch HG, Turkewitz G: Ease of habituation to repeated auditory and somesthetic stimulation in the human newborn, *J Exp Child Psychol* 9:193-207, 1970.

211. Rich EC, Marshall RE, Volpe JJ: The normal neonatal response to pinprick, *Dev Med Child Neurol* 16:432-434, 1972.

212. Porter FL, Miller RH, Marshall RE: Neonatal pain cries: Effect of circumcision on acoustic features and perceived urgency, *Child Dev* 57:790-802, 1986.

213. Anand KJS, Hickey PR: Pain and its effects in the human neonate and fetus, *N Engl J Med* 317:1321-1329, 1987.

214. Anand KJ, Carr DB: The neuroanatomy, neurophysiology, and neurochemistry of pain, stress, and analgesia in newborns and children, *Pediatr Clin North Am* 36:795-822, 1989.

215. Porter FL, Miller JP, Cole FS, Marshall RE: A controlled clinical trial of local anesthesia for lumbar punctures in newborns, *Pediatrics* 88:663-669, 1991.

216. Schuster A, Lenard HG: Pain in newborns and prematures: Current practice and knowledge, *Brain Dev* 12:459-465, 1990.

217. Grunau RVE, Craig KD: Facial activity as a measure of neonatal pain expression. In Tyler DC, Krane EJ, editors: *Advances in Pain Research Therapy*, New York: 1990, Raven Press.

218. Plum F, Posner JB: *The Diagnosis of Stupor and Coma*, 3rd ed, Philadelphia: 1980, FA Davis.

219. Dekaban AS, Magee KR: Occurrence of neurologic abnormalities in infants of diabetic mothers, *Neurology* 8:193-200, 1958.

220. Harris CM, Hodgkins PR, Kriss A, Chong WK, et al: Familial congenital saccade initiation failure and isolated cerebellar vermis hypoplasia, *Dev Med Child Neurol* 40:775-779, 1998.

221. Walton DS, Robb RM: Optic nerve hypoplasia: A report of 20 cases, *Arch Ophthalmol* 84:572-578, 1970.

222. Margalith D, Jan JE, McCormick AQ, Tze WJ, et al: Clinical spectrum of congenital optic nerve hypoplasia: Review of 51 patients, *Dev Med Child Neurol* 26:311-322, 1984.

223. Margalith D, Tze WJ, Jan JE: Congenital optic nerve hypoplasia with hypothalamic-pituitary dysplasia: A review of 16 cases, *Am J Dis Child* 139:361-366, 1985.

224. Roberts-Harry J, Green SH, Willshaw HE: Optic nerve hypoplasia: Associations and management, *Arch Dis Child* 65:103-106, 1990.

225. Jan JE, Robinson GC, Kinnis C, MacLeod PJ: Blindness due to optic-nerve atrophy and hypoplasia in children: An epidemiological study (1944-1974), *Dev Med Child Neurol* 19:353-363, 1977.

226. Hale BR, Rice P: Septo-optic dysplasia: Clinical and embryological aspects, *Dev Med Child Neurol* 16:812-817, 1974.

227. Krause-Brucker W, Gardner DW: Optic nerve hypoplasia associated with absent septum pellucidum and hypopituitarism, *Am J Ophthalmol* 89:113-120, 1980.

228. Traggiai C, Stanhope R: Endocrinopathies associated with midline cerebral and cranial malformations, *J Pediatr* 140:252-255, 2002.

229. Friendly DS: Eye disorders in the neonate. In Avery GB, editor: *Neonatology: Pathophysiology and the Management of the Newborn*, Philadelphia: 1975, JB Lippincott.

230. Kretzer FL, Hittner HM: Retinopathy of prematurity: Clinical implications of retinal development, *Arch Dis Child* 63:1151-1167, 1988.
231. Patz A: Retrolental fibroplasia, *Surv Ophthalmol* 14:1-29, 1969.
232. Davies PA: Retinopathy of prematurity [editorial], *Dev Med Child Neurol* 32:377-378, 1990.
233. Weakley DR, Spencer R: Current concepts in retinopathy of prematurity, *Early Hum Dev* 30:121-138, 1992.
234. Phelps DL: Retinopathy of prematurity, *Pediatr Clin North Am* 40:705-714, 1993.
235. Gobel W, Richard G: Retinopathy of prematurity: Current diagnosis and management, *Eur J Pediatr* 152:286-290, 1993.
236. Phelps DL: Retinopathy of prematurity, *N Engl J Med* 326:1078-1080, 1992.
237. Javitt J, Cas RD, Chiang Y-P: Cost-effectiveness of screening and cryotherapy for threshold retinopathy of prematurity, *Pediatrics* 91:859-866, 1993.
238. Cheek DB, Malinek M, Fraillon JM: Plasma adrenalin and noradrenalin in the neonatal period, and infants with respiratory distress syndrome and placental insufficiency, *Pediatrics* 31:374-381, 1963.
239. Holden KR, Young RB, Piland JH, Hurt WG: Plasma pressors in the normal and stressed newborn infant, *Pediatrics* 49:495-503, 1972.
240. Feske SK, Carrazana EJ, Kupsky WJ, Volpe JJ: Uncal herniation secondary to bacterial meningitis in a newborn, *Pediatr Neurol* 8:142-144, 1992.
241. Hoyt CS, Mousel DK, Weber AA: Transient supranuclear disturbances of gaze in healthy neonates, *Am J Ophthalmol* 89:708-713, 1980.
242. van Hof-Van Duin J, Evenhuis-van Leunen A, Mohn G, Baerts W, et al: Effects of very low birth weight (VLBW) on visual development during the first year after term, *Early Hum Dev* 20:255-266, 1989.
243. Gibson NA, Fielder AR, Trounce JQ, Levene MI: Ophthalmic findings in infants of very low birthweight, *Dev Med Child Neurol* 32:7-13, 1990.
244. Seidl Z, Sussova J, Obenberger J, Vaneckova M, et al: Magnetic resonance imaging in diplegic form of cerebral palsy, *Brain Dev* 23:46-49, 2001.
245. Tychsen L, Lisberger SG: Maldevelopment of visual motion processing in humans who had strabismus with onset in infancy, *J Neurosci* 6:2495-2508, 1986.
246. Plum F, Posner JB: *The Diagnosis of Stupor and Coma*, Philadelphia: 1969, FA Davis.
247. Perlman JM, Nelson JS, McAlister WH, Volpe JJ: Intracerebellar hemorrhage in a premature newborn: Diagnosis by real-time ultrasound and correlation with autopsy findings, *Pediatrics* 71:159-162, 1983.
248. Kleiman MD, DiMario FJ, Leconche DA, Zaineraitis EL: Benign transient downward gaze in preterm infants, *Pediatr Neurol* 10:313-316, 1994.
249. Miller VS, Packard AM: Paroxysmal downgaze in term newborn infants, *J Child Neurol* 13:294-296, 1998.
250. Yokochi K: Paroxysmal ocular downward deviation in neurologically impaired infants, *Pediatr Neurol* 7:426-428, 1991.
251. de Grauw AJ, Rotteveel JJ, Cruysberg JR: Transient sixth cranial nerve paralysis in the newborn infant, *Neuropediatrics* 14:164-165, 1983.
252. Afifi AK, Bell WE, Menezes AH: Etiology of lateral rectus palsy in infancy and childhood, *J Child Neurol* 7:295-299, 1992.
253. Wang SM, Zwaan J, Mullaney PB, Jabak MH, et al: Congenital fibrosis of the extraocular muscles type 2, an inherited exotropic strabismus fixus, maps to distal 11q13, *Am J Hum Genet* 63:517-525, 1998.
254. Fisher CM: Ocular bobbing, *Arch Neurol* 11:543-546, 1964.
255. Hayman M, Harvey AS, Hopkins IJ, Kornberg AJ, et al: Paroxysmal tonic upgaze: A reappraisal of outcome, *Ann Neurol* 43:514-520, 1998.
256. Guerrini R, Belmonte A, Carrozzo R: Paroxysmal tonic upgaze of childhood with ataxia: A benign transient dystonia with autosomal dominant inheritance, *Brain Dev* 20:116-118, 1998.
257. Ouvrier R, Billson F: Paroxysmal tonic upgaze of childhood: A review, *Brain Dev* 27:185-188, 2005.
258. Morad Y, Benyamini OG, Avni I: Benign opsoclonus in preterm infants, *Pediatr Neurol* 31:275-278, 2004.
259. Buckley EG: The clinical approach to the pediatric patient with nystagmus, *Int Pediatr* 5:225-248, 1990.
260. Jan JE, Carruthers JD, Tillson G: Neurodevelopmental criteria in the classification of congenital motor nystagmus, *Can J Neurol Sci* 19:76-79, 1992.
261. Cibis GW, Fitzgerald KM: Electroretinography in congenital idiopathic nystagmus, *Pediatr Neurol* 9:369-371, 1993.
262. Dell'Osso LF, Weissman BM, Leigh RJ, Abel LA, et al: Hereditary congenital nystagmus and gaze-holding failure: The role of the neural integrator, *Neurology* 43:1741-1749, 1993.
263. Jan JE, Good WV, Lyons CJ, Hertle RW: Visually impaired children with sensory defect nystagmus, normal appearing fundi and normal ERGS, *Dev Med Child Neurol* 38:74-83, 1995.
264. Lenn NJ, Freinkel AJ: Facial sparing as a feature of prenatal-onset hemiparesis, *Pediatr Neurol* 5:291-295, 1989.
265. Nisipeanu P, Rieder I, Blumen S, Korczyn AD: Pure congenital Foix-Chavany-Marie syndrome, *Dev Med Child Neurol* 39:696-698, 1997.
266. Hepner WR: Some observations on facial paresis in the newborn infant: Etiology and incidence, *Pediatrics* 8:494-497, 1951.
267. Pape KE, Pickering D: Asymmetric crying facies: An index of other congenital anomalies, *J Pediatr* 81:21-30, 1972.
268. Stapells DR, Kurtzberg D: Evoked potential assessment of auditory system integrity in infants, *Clin Perinatol* 18:497-518, 1991.
269. Kennedy CR: The assessment of hearing and brainstem function. In Eyre JA, editor: *The Neurophysiological Examination of the Newborn Infant*, New York: 1992, MacKeith Press.
270. Hendricks-Munoz KD, Walton JP: Hearing loss in infants with persistent fetal circulation, *Pediatrics* 81:650-656, 1988.
271. Nield TA, Schrier S, Ramos AD, Platzker ACG, et al: Unexpected hearing loss in high-risk infants, *Pediatrics* 78:417-422, 1986.
272. Barton MD, Court SD, Waller W: Causes of severe deafness in school children in Northumberland, *BMJ* 1:1351-1355, 1962.
273. Darin N, Hanner P, Thiringer K: Changes in prevalence, aetiology, age at detection, and associated disabilities in preschool children with hearing impairment born in Goteborg, *Dev Med Child Neurol* 39:797-802, 1997.
274. Vohr BR, Carty LM, Moore PE, Letourneau K: The Rhode Island hearing assessment program: Experience with statewide hearing screening (1993-1996), *J Pediatr* 133:353-357, 1998.
275. Smith RJH, Bale JF, White KR: Sensorineural hearing loss in children, *Lancet* 365:879-890, 2005.
276. Roizen NJ: Nongenetic causes of hearing loss, *Ment Retard Dev Disabil Res Rev* 9:120-127, 2003.
277. Abramovich SJ, Gregory S, Slemick M, Stewart A: Hearing loss in very low birthweight infants treated with neonatal intensive care, *Arch Dis Child* 54:421-426, 1979.
278. Anagnostakis D, Petmezakis J, Papazissis G, Messaritakis J, et al: Hearing loss in low-birth-weight infants, *Am J Dis Child* 136:602-604, 1982.
279. Bergman I, Hirsch RP, Fria TJ, Shapiro SM, et al: Cause of hearing loss in the high-risk premature infant, *J Pediatr* 106:95-101, 1985.
280. Brown DR, Watchko JF, Sabo D: Neonatal sensorineural hearing loss associated with furosemide: A case-control study, *Dev Med Child Neurol* 33:816-823, 1991.
281. Finitzo-Hieber T, McCracken GH Jr, Brown KC: Prospective controlled evaluation of auditory function in neonates given netilmicin or amikacin, *J Pediatr* 106:129-136, 1985.
282. Colding H, Andersen EA, Prytz S, Wulffsberg H, et al: Auditory function after continuous infusion of gentamicin to high-risk newborns, *Acta Paediatr Scand* 78:840-843, 1989.
283. Ferber-Viart C, Morlet T, Maison S, Duclaux R, et al: Type of initial brainstem auditory evoked potentials (BAEP) impairment and risk factors in premature infants, *Brain Dev* 18:287-293, 1996.
284. Pettigrew AG, Edwards DA, Henderson-Smart DJ: Perinatal risk factors in preterm infants with moderate-to-profound hearing deficits, *Med J Aust* 148:174-177, 1988.
285. De Hoog M, van Zanten BA, Hop WC, Overbosch E, et al: Newborn hearing screening: Tobramycin and vancomycin are not risk factors for hearing loss, *J Pediatr* 142:41-46, 2003.
286. Salamy A, Mendelson T, Tooley WH: Developmental profiles for the brainstem auditory evoked potential, *Early Hum Dev* 6:331-339, 1982.
287. Stennert E, Schulte FJ, Vollrath M, Brunner E, et al: The etiology of neurosensory hearing defects in preterm infants, *Arch Otorhinolaryngol* 221:171-182, 1978.
288. Duara S, Suter CM, Bessard KK, Gutberlet RL: Neonatal screening with auditory brainstem responses: Results of follow-up audiometry and risk factor evaluation, *J Pediatr* 108:276-281, 1986.
289. Spector GJ, Pettit WJ, Davis G, Strauss M, et al: Fetal respiratory distress causing CNS and inner ear hemorrhage, *Laryngoscope* 88:764-784, 1978.
290. Douek E, Dodson HC, Bannister LH, Ashcroft P, et al: Effects of incubator noise on the cochlea of the newborn, *Lancet* 2:1110-1113, 1976.
291. Etzel RA, Balk SJ, Bearer CF, Miller MD, et al: Noise: A hazard for the fetus and newborn, *Pediatrics* 100:724-727, 1997.
292. Dayal VS, Kokshanian A, Mitchell DP: Combined effects of noise and kanamycin, *Ann Otol Rhinol Laryngol* 80:897-902, 1971.
293. Jauhiainen T, Kohonen A, Jauhiainen M: Combined effect of noise and neomycin on the cochlea, *Acta Otolaryngol (Stockh)* 73:387-390, 1972.
294. Cox C, Hack M, Metz D, Fanaroff A: Auditory brain stem evoked responses for screening very low birthweight infants (VLBW): Effects of gentamicin and neonatal risk factors on maturation, *Pediatr Res* 13:524-531, 1979.
295. Nardocci N, Zorzi G, Blau N, Fernandez Alvarez E, et al: Neonatal dopa-responsive extrapyramidal syndrome in twins with recessive GTPCH deficiency, *Neurology* 60:335-337, 2003.
296. Mbonda E, Claus D, Bonnier C, Evrard P, et al: Prolonged dysphagia caused by congenital pharyngeal dysfunction, *J Pediatr* 126:923-927, 1995.
297. Bellmaine SP, McCredie J, Storey B: Pharyngeal incoordination from birth to three years, with recurrent bronchopneumonia and ultimate recovery, *Aust Paediatr J* 8:137-139, 1972.
298. Ardran GM, Benson PF, Butler NR, Ellis HL, et al: Congenital dysphagia resulting from dysfunction of the pharyngeal musculature, *Dev Med Child Neurol* 7:157-166, 1965.
299. Inder TE, Volpe JJ: Recovery of congenital isolated pharyngeal dysfunction: Implications for early management, *Pediatr Neurol* 19:222-224, 1998.

300. Sieben RL, Hamida MB, Shulman K: Multiple cranial nerve deficits associated with the Arnold-Chiari malformation, *Neurology* 21:673-681, 1971.

301. Charney EB, Rorke LB, Sutton LN, Schut L: Management of Chiari II complications in infants with myelomeningocele, *J Pediatr* 111:364-371, 1987.

302. Cochrane DD, Adderley R, White CP, Norman M, et al: Apnea in patients with myelomeningocele, *Pediatr Neurosurg* 16:232-239, 1990.

303. Hesz N, Wolraich M: Vocal-cord paralysis and brainstem dysfunction in children with spina bifida, *Dev Med Child Neurol* 27:528-531, 1985.

304. Hays RM, Jordan RA, McLaughlin JF, Nickel RE, et al: Central ventilatory dysfunction in myelodysplasia: An independent determinant of survival, *Dev Med Child Neurol* 31:366-370, 1989.

305. Swaminathan S, Paton JY, Davidson Ward SL, Jacobs RA, et al: Abnormal control of ventilation in adolescents with myelodysplasia, *J Pediatr* 115:898-903, 1989.

306. Davidson Ward SL, Jacobs RA, Gates EP, Hart LD, et al: Abnormal ventilatory patterns during sleep in infants with myelomeningocele, *J Pediatr* 109:631-634, 1986.

307. Oren J, Kelly DH, Todres ID, Shannon DC: Respiratory complications in patients with myelodysplasia and Arnold-Chiari malformation, *Am J Dis Child* 140:221-224, 1986.

308. Mizuno K: Neonatal feeding performance as a predictor of neurodevelopmental outcome at 18 months, *Dev Med Child Neurol* 47:299-304, 2005.

309. Ferrari F, Cioni G, Prechtl HF: Qualitative changes of general movements in preterm infants with brain lesions, *Early Hum Dev* 23:193-231, 1990.

310. Touwen BC: Variability and stereotypy of spontaneous motility as a predictor of neurological development of preterm infants, *Dev Med Child Neurol* 32:501-508, 1990.

311. Bos A, Martijn A, van Asperen RM, Hadders-Algra M, et al: Qualitative assessment of general movements in high-risk preterm infants with chronic lung disease requiring dexamethasone therapy, *J Pediatr* 132:300-306, 1998.

312. Roessmann U, Horwitz SJ, Kennell JH: Congenital absence of the corticospinal fibers: Pathologic and clinical observations, *Neurology* 40:538-541, 1990.

313. Perlman JM, Volpe JJ: Movement disorder of premature infants with severe bronchopulmonary dysplasia: A new syndrome, *Pediatrics* 84:215-218, 1989.

314. Bates JAV: A human mid-brain preparation, *Dev Med Child Neurol* 9:780-782, 1967.

315. Hill K, Cogan D, Dodge P: Ocular signs associated with hydranencephaly, *Am J Ophthalmol* 51:267, 1961.

316. Ashwal S, Schneider S, Tomasi G, Peabody JL: Neurological findings and brain death determination in twelve liveborn anecephalic infants, *Ann Neurol* 26:437-438, 1989.

317. Nelson KB, Ellenberg JH: Neonatal signs as predictors of cerebral palsy, *Pediatrics* 64:225-232, 1979.

318. Donovan DE, Coues P, Paine RS: The prognostic implications of neurological abnormalities in the neonatal period, *Neurology* 12:910-914, 1962.

319. Del Mundo-Vallarta J, Robb JP: A follow-up study of newborn infants with perinatal complications, *Neurology* 14:413-424, 1964.

320. Prechtl HFR: Prognostic value of neurological signs in the newborn infant, *Proc R Soc Med* 58:3-22, 1965.

321. Thorn I: Cerebral symptoms in the newborn: Diagnostic and prognostic significance of symptoms of presumed cerebral origin, *Acta Paediatr Scand Suppl* 195:1-8, 1969.

322. Amiel-Tison C: Cerebral damage in full-term new-born. Aetiological factors, neonatal status and long-term follow-up, *Biol Neonat* 14:234-250, 1969.

323. Ziegler AL, Calame A, Marchand C, Passera M, et al: Cerebral distress in full-term newborns and its prognostic value: A follow-up study of 90 infants, *Helv Paediatr Acta* 31:299-317, 1976.

324. Brown JK, Purvis RJ, Forfar JO, Cockburn F: Neurological aspects of perinatal asphyxia, *Dev Med Child Neurol* 16:567-580, 1974.

325. Touwen BC, Lok-Meijer TY, Huisjes HJ, Olinga AA: The recovery rate of neurologically deviant newborns, *Early Hum Dev* 7:131-148, 1982.

326. den Ouden L, Verloove-Vanhorick SP, van Zeben-van der Aa DM, Brand R, et al: Neonatal neurological dysfunction in a cohort of very preterm and/or very low birthweight infants: Relation to other perinatal factors and outcome at 2 years, *Neuropediatrics* 21:66-71, 1990.

327. Allen MC, Capute AJ: Neonatal neurodevelopmental examination as a predictor of neuromotor outcome in premature infants, *Pediatrics* 83:498-506, 1989.

328. Geerdink JJ, Hopkins B: Qualitative changes in general movements and their prognostic value in preterm infants, *Eur J Pediatr* 152:362-367, 1993.

329. D'Eugenio DB, Slagle TA, Mettelman BB, Gross SJ: Developmental outcome of preterm infants with transient neuromotor abnormalities, *Am J Dis Child* 147:570-574, 1993.

330. de Groot L, Hoek A-M, Hopkins B, Touwen BC: Development of muscle power in preterm infants: Individual trajectories after term age, *Neuropediatrics* 24:68-73, 1993.

331. Wolf M-JB,G. Casaer P, Wolf B: Neonatal neurological examination as a predictor of neuromotor outcome at 4 months in term low-Apgar-score babies in Zimbabwe, *Early Hum Dev* 51:179-186, 1998.

332. Dubowitz L, Mercuri E, Dubowitz V: An optimality score for the neurologic examination of the term newborn, *J Pediatr* 133:406-416, 1998.

333. Majnemer A, Mazer B: Neurologic evaluation of the newborn infant: Definition and psychometric properties, *Dev Med Child Neurol* 40:708-715, 1998.

334. Mercuri E, Guzzetta A, Haataja L, Cowan F, et al: Neonatal neurological examination in infants with hypoxic ischaemic encephalopathy: Correlation with MRI findings, *Neuropediatrics* 30:83-89, 1999.

335. Amess PN, Penrice J, Wylezinska M, Lorek A, et al: Early brain proton magnetic resonance spectroscopy and neonatal neurology related to neurodevelopmental outcome at 1 year in term infants after presumed hypoxic-ischaemic brain injury, *Dev Med Child Neurol* 41:436-445, 1999.

336. Maas YGH, Mirmiran M, Hart AAM, Koppe JG, et al: Predictive value of neonatal neurological tests for developmental outcome of preterm infants, *J Pediatr* 137:100-106, 2000.

337. Als H, Butler S, Kosta S, McAnulty G: The assessment of preterm infants' behavior (APIB): Furthering the understanding and measurement of neurodevelopmental competence in preterm and full-term infants, *Ment Retard Dev Disabil Res Rev* 11:94-102, 2005.

Chapter 4

Specialized Studies in the Neurological Evaluation

In addition to the neurological examination discussed in Chapter 3, certain specialized studies are critical components of the neurological evaluation of the newborn. Most of these studies are presented in relation to relevant specific disorders throughout this book. However, certain of these specialized aspects, which are not discussed in detail elsewhere and are of definite or potential importance in the neurological evaluation, are reviewed here, including examination of the cerebrospinal fluid (CSF), certain neurophysiological studies (e.g., determination of brain stem auditory evoked responses, visual and somatosensory cortical evoked responses, and electroencephalography [EEG]), the major techniques for imaging of brain structure, certain noninvasive continuous monitoring techniques, and methods for physiological brain imaging.

CEREBROSPINAL FLUID EXAMINATION

Examination of the CSF is an important part of the evaluation of a wide variety of neurological disorders, as noted in appropriate chapters throughout this book. In this section, I focus principally on normal CSF in the newborn, particularly the newborn considered at high risk for such neurological disorders.

The principal components of the CSF examination include measurement of intracranial pressure, assessment of the color (e.g., bloody, xanthochromic) and turbidity (e.g., purulent), red blood cell (RBC) and white blood cell (WBC) counts, WBC differential count, and concentrations of protein and glucose. Other, more specialized evaluations (e.g., for microorganisms, various metabolites, and enzymes) are determined by clinical circumstances. Intracranial pressure is discussed later in this chapter in relation to noninvasive monitoring of intracranial pressure, and the other, more specialized evaluations are discussed in the relevant chapters in this book. In this section, I focus on the WBC and RBC counts and concentrations of protein and glucose.

White Blood Cell, Protein, and Glucose Concentrations

Of the several studies that address normal CSF values in the newborn,[1-12] I find the studies of Sarff and co-workers[11] and Rodriguez and co-workers[12] most informative (although all the data are generally consistent). Sarff and co-workers discussed the CSF findings in 117 high-risk infants (87 term, 30 preterm < 2500 g birth weight; 95 examined in the first week, most with clinical findings indicative of a high risk of infection, but without positive cultures for bacteria or other organisms or grossly bloody CSF) (Table 4-1). Mean values for term and preterm infants, respectively, were for WBC counts of 8 and 9 cells/mm³ (60% polymorphonuclear leukocytes), protein concentration 90 and 115 mg/dL, glucose concentrations 52 and 50 mg/dL, and ratio of CSF to blood glucose 81% and 74%. Although the ranges are wide, the values provide a useful framework for evaluation of neonatal CSF.

In a subsequent report, Rodriguez and co-workers[12] obtained more detailed data for similarly high-risk infants, but of very low birth weight (i.e., < 1500 g). When the data are expressed as a function of postconceptional age when the CSF sample was obtained, the values for the more mature infants are similar to the values obtained by Sarff and co-workers (Table 4-2). This similarity could be expected because the infants in the study by Sarff and co-workers were larger and, presumably, more mature. Notably, however, the least mature infants (26 to 28 weeks of postconceptional age) exhibited values of glucose and protein that were distinctly higher than values observed at later ages. This occurrence, as well as the finding of Sarff and co-workers that preterm infants had relatively high ratios of CSF to blood glucose (see Table 4-1), supports the notion of increased permeability of the blood-brain barrier in the small preterm infant. Moreover, increased permeability for other macromolecules (e.g., immunoglobulin G, alpha-fetoprotein) is suggested by other studies.[13-16] Although the WBC counts in the premature infants studied by Rodriguez and co-workers did not differ as a function of postconceptional age and are similar to those reported by Sarff and co-workers., the percentage of polymorphonuclear leukocytes (7%) is much lower than in the latter study. This discrepancy may be related in part to the error inherent in the study of relatively small numbers of WBCs.

These values for WBC count and protein and glucose concentrations are crucial for the evaluation of the infant with suspected bacterial meningitis or other central nervous system inflammatory processes. Although these issues are discussed in more detail later (see Chapters 20 and 21), *combinations* of abnormalities are important to recognize, and single values that are questionably abnormal are difficult to interpret conclusively.

TABLE 4-1 Cerebrospinal Fluid Findings in High-Risk Newborns		
Findings	Term	Preterm
White Blood Cell Count (cells/mm³)		
Mean ± standard deviation	8 ± 7	9 ± 6
Range	0–32	0–29
Protein Concentration (mg/dL)		
Mean	90	115
Range	20–170	65–150
Glucose Concentration (mg/dL)		
Mean	52	50
Range	34–119	24–63
Cerebrospinal Fluid/Blood Glucose (%)		
Mean	81	74
Range	24–248	55–105

Data from Sarff LD, Platt LH, McCracken GH Jr: Cerebrospinal fluid evaluation in neonates: Comparison of high-risk infants with and without meningitis, *J Pediatr* 88:473-477, 1976; based on 87 term infants and 30 low-birth-weight infants (<2500 g), 95 of whom were examined in the first week of life.

Under all circumstances, assessment of the CSF in the context of the clinical setting and the clinical features is most important.

Red Blood Cell Counts in High-Risk Newborns

Determination of "normal" values for RBC in neonatal CSF is hindered by the relatively high incidence of germinal matrix-intraventricular hemorrhage, usually clinically silent in the preterm infant (see Chapter 11) and by the likelihood that the process of birth is associated with minor amounts of subarachnoid bleeding. In the study of Sarff and co-workers,[11] the median value for RBC count was 180, with a very wide range (0 to 45,000) (Table 4-3). A similar value was obtained for premature infants in that study. In both the term and preterm infants, the most common value (mode) for RBC count was 0. However, in the report of Rodriguez and co-workers,[12] although a median value of 112 was observed, the mean was 785, and 20% of CSF samples had more than 1000 RBC/mm³ (see Table 4-3). These infants were smaller (<1500 g), but

TABLE 4-3 Red Blood Cell Counts (Cells/mm³) in Cerebrospinal Fluid of High-Risk Newborns	
SARFF AND CO-WORKERS*	
Term infants	n = 87 Median: 180 Range: 0–45,000
Preterm infants (<2500 g)	n = 30 Median: 112 Range: 0–39,000
RODRIGUEZ AND CO-WORKERS†	
Preterm infants (<1500 g)	n = 43 Mean: 785 >1000 cells/mm³ in 20% of samples

*Data from Sarff LD, Platt LH, McCracken GH Jr: Cerebrospinal fluid evaluation in neonates: Comparison of high-risk infants with and without meningitis, *J Pediatr* 88:473-477, 1976.
†Data from Rodriguez AF, Kaplan SL, Mason EO Jr: Cerebrospinal fluid values in the very low birth weight infant, *J Pediatr* 116:971-974, 1990.

ultrasonographic examinations were said to show no evidence of intracranial hemorrhage. However, exclusion of minor subarachnoid hemorrhage by cranial ultrasonography is not reliable.

The aforementioned data indicate that the finding of more than 100 RBCs/mm³ in the newborn is common and that in very-low-birth-weight infants, values greater than 1000 occur in a substantial minority in the absence of apparently clinically significant intracranial hemorrhage. Again, the importance of *combinations* of findings is important in the evaluation of the CSF for intracranial hemorrhage. Thus, the addition of xanthochromia and elevated protein concentration in CSF strongly raises the possibility of a more substantial and, clinically speaking, more important intracranial hemorrhage. This issue is discussed in more detail in Chapter 10.

NEUROPHYSIOLOGICAL STUDIES

Several specialized neurophysiological techniques have been particularly valuable in further defining the neurological maturation of the newborn. Moreover, some of these studies are commonly used in neurological diagnosis. In this section, I particularly discuss brain stem auditory evoked responses, visual evoked responses, somatosensory evoked responses, and EEG (including

TABLE 4-2 Cerebrospinal Fluid Findings in High-Risk Infants of Low Birth Weight (<1500 g)			
Postconceptional Age (Weeks)	White Blood Cell Count (cells/mm³ ± SD)	Glucose (mg/dL ± SD)	Protein (mg/dL ± SD)
26–28	6 ± 10	85 ± 39*	177 ± 60*
29–31	5 ± 4	54 ± 81	144 ± 40
32–34	4 ± 3	55 ± 21	142 ± 49
35–37	6 ± 7	56 ± 21	109 ± 53
38–40	9 ± 9	44 ± 10	117 ± 33

*Values for glucose and protein were significantly greater at 26 to 28 weeks than at subsequent postconceptional ages.
SD, standard deviation.
Data from Rodriguez AF, Kaplan SL, Mason EO Jr: Cerebrospinal fluid values in the very low birth weight infant, *J Pediatr* 116:971-974, 1990; based on 43 infants, some studied more than once, approximately 80% studied after the first week of life.

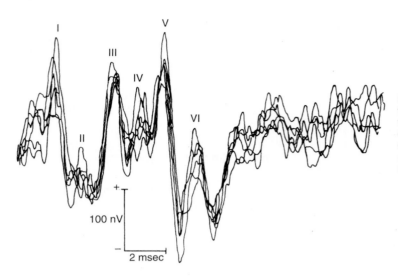

Figure 4-1 **Brainstem auditory-evoked response, major wave forms.** The responses obtained with several sequential trials were superimposed. The complete response, with the seven definable waves, is not observed in the newborn (see text for details). *(From Starr A, Amlie RN, Martin WH, Sanders S: Development of auditory function in newborn infants revealed by auditory brainstem potentials, Pediatrics 60:831-839, 1977.)*

amplitude-integrated EEG). The most widely used of these neurophysiological techniques, EEG, also is discussed regarding seizures in Chapter 5.

Brain Stem Auditory Evoked Responses

Electrophysiological investigation of the auditory system in the newborn has focused on brain stem evoked responses. However, cortical auditory evoked responses have been studied, as have visual and somatosensory evoked responses (see later sections), through computer-averaged EEG recordings obtained over the scalp after graded stimuli. Such *cortical responses* have been described in premature and full-term infants,[17-33] and these responses demonstrate that peripheral auditory stimuli are transmitted to the primary and secondary auditory cortex of the temporal lobe in the newborn period. Magnetoencephalography has been used to define the maturation of cortical evoked responses from 27 weeks of gestation to term in 18 fetuses.[34,35] This work is noteworthy for detection of a decrease in latency from 300 milliseconds at 29 weeks of gestation to 150 milliseconds at term. This novel and noninvasive technique thus not only extends insights into the maturation of auditory cortical areas during the last trimester of human gestation, but also demonstrates the applicability of magnetoencephalography to study of the fetus. Nevertheless, measurement of cortical auditory evoked potentials has been difficult to adapt to routine clinical circumstances, in part because the amplitude and latency of the observed responses vary with the infant's level of arousal and in part because of the expense of the technology (magnetoencephalography). In contrast, major attention has been paid to the earlier potentials generated from subcortical structures after auditory stimulation (i.e., the *brain stem auditory evoked response*).

Major Wave Forms and Anatomical Correlates

The brain stem auditory evoked response reflects the electrical events generated within the auditory pathways from the eighth nerve to the diencephalon and

is recorded by electrodes placed usually over the mastoid and vertex. The stimulation is usually a click or pure tone administered at a relatively rapid rate. The signal is amplified, then summed in a computer, and finally displayed by an X-Y plotter for measurements of the latency and amplitude of the various components.[23,24,36-42] To avoid movement and other artifacts, the infant is studied preferably during sleep. The complete response consists of seven components, designated consecutively by Roman numerals (Fig. 4-1).[24,36,39] Studies in animals and in adult humans indicate that the waves derive from sequential activation of the major components of the auditory pathway.[37,38,43-45] Thus, wave I represents activity of the eighth nerve, wave II the cochlear nucleus, wave III the superior olivary nucleus, wave IV the lateral lemniscus, and wave V the inferior colliculus. The precise origins of waves VI and VII remain to be established, but these waves probably are generated in the thalamus and thalamic radiations, respectively. Brain stem auditory potentials have been well defined in the newborn infant,[23,24,36,39-41,46-61] although all seven components are not observed (see later discussion).

Developmental Changes

Impressive ontogenetic changes in the brain stem auditory response have been described.[23,24,36,39,47,49,50,54,55,61-75] The most reproducible and easily definable components are waves I, III, and V; the last is sometimes fused with wave IV. Waves II, VI, and VII have generally been too variable to allow systematic study.[36] The *latencies* of the most prominent components (I, III, IV to V) decrease as a function of gestational age, with a maximal shift occurring in the weeks before 34 weeks of gestation (Fig. 4-2). Moreover, an increase in amplitude and a decrease in threshold of the response occur with increasing gestational age.

The decrease in latency of wave I with maturation indicates improvement in peripheral processing of the auditory stimulus. Whether this effect is at the level of middle ear conduction, the cochlear receptors, or the

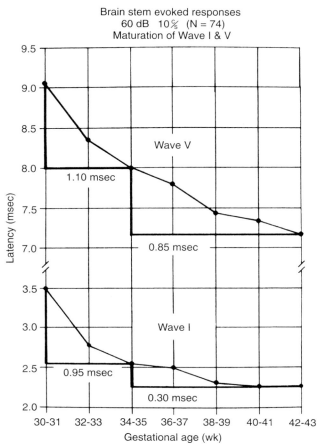

Brain stem evoked responses
60 dB 10% (N = 74)
Maturation of Wave I & V

Figure 4-2 Decrease in latencies of major waves of neonatal brain stem auditory evoked response as a function of gestational age. *(From Despland PA, Galambos R: The auditory brainstem response [ABR] is a useful diagnostic tool in the intensive care nursery, Pediatr Res 14:154-158, 1980.)*

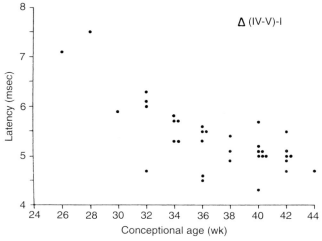

Δ (IV-V)-I

Figure 4-3 Decrease in latency of brain stem portion (i.e., time difference between waves I and IV to V) of brain stem auditory evoked response as a function of gestational age. *(From Starr A, Amlie RN, Martin WH, Sanders S: Development of auditory function in newborn infants revealed by auditory brainstem potentials, Pediatrics 60:831-839, 1977.)*

transduction of cochlear receptor potentials into eighth nerve activity (i.e., wave I) is unknown.

The time difference between wave I and the wave IV-V complex depends on transmission through the *brain stem* auditory pathway (i.e., the brain stem transmission time), and this maturational change is shown in Figure 4-3. Whether this decrease in latency relates to changes in nerve conduction velocity or synaptic efficiency is unknown. Active myelination within this brain stem system is occurring during the time period shown in Figure 4-3 (see Chapter 2); however, distinct postnatal changes in brain stem auditory evoked responses[69,70,76] appear to occur after rapid myelination has ceased.

Detection of Disorders of the Auditory Pathways

Abundant findings indicate the value of brain stem auditory evoked response studies in detecting disorders of the auditory pathways in the newborn infant.[23,24,36,39-41,53,56-61,77-104] Definition of such disorders depends on detection of responses that are abnormal in threshold sensitivity, conduction time (i.e., latency), amplitude, or conformation. In neonatal studies, deficits in threshold sensitivity and latency have been the most valuable. The general principle is

that a lesion at the periphery (middle ear, cochlea, or eighth nerve) results in a heightened threshold and a prolongation of latency of *all* the potentials, including wave I, whereas a lesion in the brain stem causes longer latencies of only those waves originating from structures distal to the lesion, with wave I spared. The essential features of these two basic abnormal patterns of brain stem auditory evoked responses observed in neonatal patients are depicted in Table 4-4.

Abnormalities of the evoked response in neonatal neurological disease are to be expected, in part because of the known neuropathological involvement of the following: the cochlear nuclei, the inferior colliculus, other brain stem nuclei, and the cochlea itself by hypoxic-ischemic insult (see Chapter 8); the cochlear nuclei, inferior colliculus and, perhaps, the cochlea or eighth nerve by hyperbilirubinemia (see Chapter 13); the eighth nerve by bacterial meningitis (see Chapter 21); the cochlea and eighth nerve by congenital viral infections (see Chapter 20); and the cochlea by intracranial hemorrhage (see Chapter 11) (Table 4-5). Indeed, brain stem evoked response audiometry has been used to describe peripheral and central disturbances in infants with congenital cytomegalovirus infection, hyperbilirubinemia, bacterial meningitis, asphyxia, persistent fetal circulation, aminoglycoside

TABLE 4-4	Two Basic Abnormal Patterns of Brain Stem Auditory Evoked Responses in Neonatal Disease	
	SITE OF DISORDER	
Response Characteristic	**Periphery**	**Brain Stem**
Threshold (wave I)	Elevated	Normal
Wave I latency	Prolonged	Normal
Wave V latency	Prolonged	Prolonged
I–V interval	Normal	Prolonged

TABLE 4-5	Probable or Proven Examples of Neonatal Neurological Disease with Abnormal Brain Stem Auditory Evoked Responses
Neurological Disorders	**Relevant Neuropathology**
Hypoxic-ischemic encephalopathy	Cochlear nuclei, inferior colliculus, cochlea
Hyperbilirubinemia	Cochlear nuclei, inferior colliculus, cochlea, eighth nerve
Bacterial meningitis	Eighth nerve
Congenital viral infection	Cochlea, eighth nerve
Intracranial hemorrhage	Cochlea

or furosemide administration, trauma to the cochlea or middle ear, and still undefined complications of low birth weight.[23,24,36,39-41,56-61,75,77,79-93,96,97,100,102,104,105,105a] The particular importance of *combinations* of these factors in the genesis of permanent deficits has been emphasized. Moreover, neonatal defects may be transient. For example, in one large study (N = 92) of term asphyxiated infants, 35% exhibited brain stem auditory evoked response deficit (increased threshold) in the first 3 days of life, but only 10% had abnormalities at 30 days.[59] Among preterm infants with birth weight less than 1500 g who were studied at term, 14% had evidence of a peripheral impairment (increased threshold), 17% a central impairment (prolonged brain stem latencies), and 4% a combined impairment, for a total of 27%.[57]

Hearing Screening

Use of the brain stem auditory evoked response as a screening device for hearing impairment in the neonate has become extremely common and is the norm in many countries.[24,39,94,98,99,102,106,107] The importance of early identification of infants with hearing impairment is based on the realization that acquisition of normal language and of social and learning skills depends on hearing.[24,39,89,98-102,106,108-114]

The most commonly recommended *screening procedure*, for preterm infants, consists of testing the infant just before hospital discharge, or at least as close to 40 weeks after conception as possible, when he or she is medically stable, and preferably in a room separate from the neonatal unit. Term infants are often tested at any point before discharge.[24,98,99,106,110,112] The initial screening procedure has consisted of conventional brain stem auditory evoked response, automated auditory evoked response, or transient evoked otoacoustic emission technique. The latter detects signals generated by cochlear outer hair cells in response to acoustic stimulation. This technique is faster and less expensive than evoked response audiometry. However, the method does not detect retrocochlear abnormalities (e.g., auditory nerve disease). Infants who fail this test are retested by auditory evoked response study, often an automated study.[106,107,112] Notably, retesting in the neonatal unit has been shown to result in reduction of failure rate by at least 80%.[114] The incidence of failure of either screening test at the time of hospital discharge is relatively high, the actual value depending on the

population studied. For low-birth-weight infants tested at term, failure rates as high as 20% to 25% are common.[24,94] Retesting infants after test failure usually is carried out after several weeks or later, often after discharge. With this approach, many infants are lost to follow-up. Because most neonates who fail the first screening procedure exhibit normal responses at the time of the retest,[24,39,49,52,53,94,98,99,106,110,114] the initial failures are likely transient, reversible disturbances, or false-positive results. For example, in one large series of more than 16,000 infants, retesting in the neonatal unit after early test failures resulted in an 80% reduction in failure rate by discharge.[114] In certain high-risk groups, the importance of later testing is emphasized by the report of hearing deficits developing in the first months of life, *after* normal results in the neonatal period.[81,82,112]

Visual Evoked Responses

Cortical Response

The *visual evoked response* refers to the electrical response, recorded usually by surface electrodes on the occipital scalp, to a standardized stimulus, the most common of which is a *light flash* of graded intensity and frequency. Flash visual evoked responses are recorded in response to red light-emitting diodes in goggles placed over the infant's eyes or in an array placed about 6 inches in front of the infant's eyes.[115-117] The fully developed response is complex, but the first two prominent waves consist of first a positive and then a negative deflection. The positive deflection is attributed to postsynaptic activation at the site of the predominant termination of visual afferents, and the negative deflection is attributed to secondary synaptic contacts in the superficial cortical layers.[118] Two features of the response are studied: the quality of the wave form and the latency between stimulus and recorded response. With flash visual evoked responses, variability in latencies can lead to difficulties in interpretation.

An alternative and generally preferable stimulus for visual evoked responses, particularly for study of visual acuity, is a shift (reversal) of a checkerboard pattern (i.e., *pattern-shift* or *pattern-reversal* visual evoked response).[37,38,115,119-121] This stimulus results in responses with less variable latencies than those obtained with a light flash stimulus. Although the technique has been used in the newborn,[37,38,115,119,120,122] including the preterm newborn,[119,120,123] experience remains limited, in part because obtaining optimal data requires that the newborn "fix" on the visual display. However, reliable data have been obtained, and this technique should prove adaptable to the newborn for wider use.

Developmental Changes

The ontogenetic changes of the visual evoked response in the human newborn have been well established.[115-117,119-121,124-136] A prolonged negative slow wave can be identified as early as 24 weeks of gestation, and this wave ultimately is replaced by the more discrete negative wave

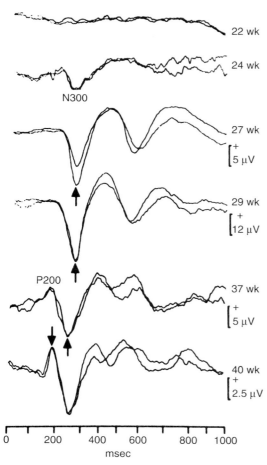

Figure 4-4 Visual evoked potentials to light-emitting diode stimulation from newborn infants, showing no recordable response at 22 weeks of postconceptional age (PCA), the emergence of N300 at 24 weeks of PCA, the late positivity following the N300 (usually ≈ 450 milliseconds), which is evident from about 27 weeks onward, and then little change until closer to term. The P200 then emerges and becomes the most prominent wave in the normal term newborn's visual evoked potential. *(From Taylor MJ: Visual evoked potentials. In Eyre JA, editor:* The Neurophysiological Examination of the Newborn Infant, *New York: 1992, MacKeith Press.)*

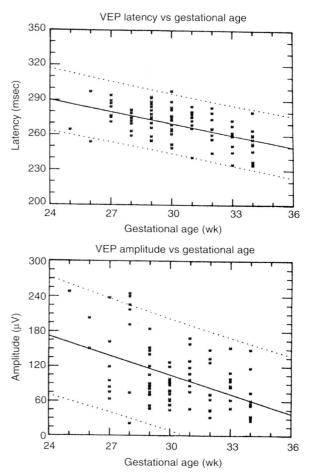

Figure 4-5 Visual evoked potential (VEP) latency and amplitude versus gestational age (ga) in weeks in 86 preterm infants. The regression line and the 95% confidence interval are indicated. (Latency = 370.7 − 3.4 × ga; amplitude = 440.4 − 11.2 × ga.) *(From Pryds O, Trojaborg W, Carlsen J, Jensen J: Determinants of visual evoked potentials in preterm infants,* Early Hum Dev *19:117-125, 1989.)*

noted earlier (Fig. 4-4). The positive wave appears between approximately 32 and 35 weeks of gestation, and by 39 weeks the visual evoked response is quite well defined. As with the components of the brain stem auditory evoked response, the latencies of both the positive and negative waves of the visual evoked response decrease in a linear fashion with increasing maturation (Fig. 4-5). This evolution in the quality and latency of the response corresponds well with the behavioral studies of visual function noted in Chapter 3. That this ontogenetic change is principally an inborn program is suggested by the finding that differences between infants born at term and healthy premature infants grown to term are small,[137] and these differences dissipate completely shortly after the time of term.[138] Although the anatomical substrate for the ontogenetic changes is undoubtedly complex, the major maturational changes correspond to the period of rapid dendritic development in the visual cortex and myelination of the optic radiations (see Chapter 2).

Detection of Disorders of the Visual Pathway

Attempts to use the neonatal visual evoked response as a measure of cerebral disturbance have been promising.[22,23,41,115,117,121,132,135,136,139-147] Premature infants with *serious hypoxemia* secondary to respiratory distress syndrome were shown to lose visual evoked responses during the insult and to regain the responses with restoration of normal blood gas levels (Fig. 4-6).[133,139] Similarly, impairment of the visual evoked response has been demonstrated in the first day after *asphyxia* in term infants, and the severity of the abnormality correlated well with poor neurological outcome.[41,135,142,147] In a study of 36 term infants who experienced "birth asphyxia" and who were studied by serial assessment of visual evoked responses, 14 of 16 infants with normal responses in the first week of life were normal on follow-up, and all 20 with abnormal responses persisting beyond the first week died or were "significantly handicapped" at 18 months of age.[147] A related observation in fetal and neonatal lambs indicates

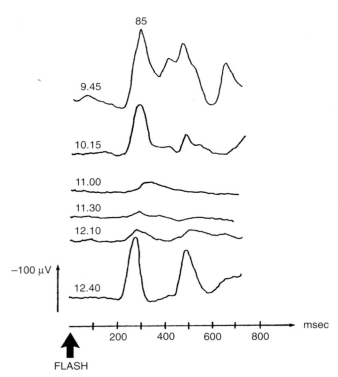

Figure 4-6 Visual evoked potentials after single flashes from a premature infant recorded at 9.45 hours after birth, at 10.15 hours after intubation and start of mechanical ventilation, at 11.00 hours during a 5-minute episode of hypoxia (partial pressure of arterial oxygen [Pao_2] = 2.9 kPa), and at 11.30, 12.10, and 12.40 hours during recovery. *(From Pryds O, Greisen G, Trojaborg W: Visual evoked potentials in preterm infants during the first hours of life,* Electroencephalogr Clin Electrophysiol *71:257-265, 1988.)*

the sensitivity of the visual evoked response to asphyxial insult.[148] Abnormalities of the visual evoked response have also been described in infants with *posthemorrhagic hydrocephalus* (see Chapter 11),[115,149,150] a finding probably reflecting the disproportionate dilation of the occipital horns of the lateral ventricles and consequent affection of the geniculocalcarine radiations. Moreover, improvement in latencies was documented immediately after ventricular tap,[150] as well as over a prolonged period after placement of ventriculoperitoneal shunt.[149] The data suggest that the determination of visual evoked responses in the neonatal period provides important information concerning cerebral function, effects of interventions, and outcome.

Somatosensory Evoked Responses

Somatosensory evoked responses have been studied most extensively in the newborn by electrical stimulation of the median nerve at the wrist or, less commonly, the posterior tibial nerve above the ankle or in the popliteal fossa and recording of the computer-averaged responses on the EEG over the contralateral parietal scalp.[41,125,151-169a] Constant primary components appear at approximately 27 weeks of age (i.e., a few weeks earlier than the comparable visual response), and the response pattern of the mature newborn appears at 37 to 38 weeks of age. As with the visual evoked response, a linear decrease in response latency

is demonstrated as a function of increasing gestational age, with the most marked decrease in the last several weeks before term (Fig. 4-7). The decrease in latencies in the somatosensory evoked response relates principally to myelination evolving in the brain stem and thalamocortical components of the somatosensory system (see Chapter 2). As with visual responses, maturation of somatosensory evoked responses does not differ significantly between term infants and healthy premature infants studied at term.

The potential clinical value of the somatosensory evoked response in the study of *disorders of the sensory*

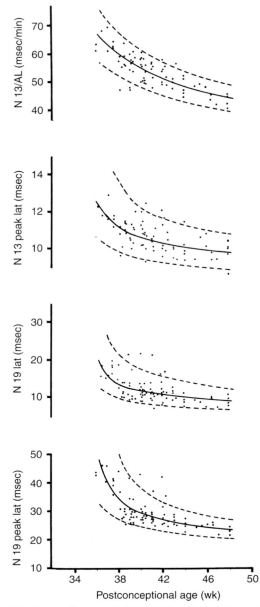

Figure 4-7 Percentile curves (P97, P50, P3) for the postconceptional age of 36 to 48 weeks estimated from the somatosensory evoked potentials of 103 normal infants. *(From Bongers-Schokking JJ, Colon EJ, Hoogland RA, Van den Brande JL, et al: Somatosensory evoked potentials in term and preterm infants in relation to postconceptional age and birth weight,* Neuropediatrics *21:32-36, 1990.)*

pathway in the newborn relates to the finding that by appropriate placement of surface electrodes closest to the presumed generator sources, the several components of this pathway can be monitored, as demonstrated in older patients.[37,38,168,169a] Thus, conduction through peripheral nerve, plexus, dorsal root, posterior column, gracile or cuneate nucleus, (contralateral) medial lemniscus, thalamus, and parietal cortex is involved. Considerable experience in adult patients indicates that evaluation of the somatosensory evoked response can provide insight into disease at various levels along this pathway. Clear application to the newborn has been demonstrated for spinal cord trauma and myelodysplasia,[170-172] as well as for a variety of cerebral abnormalities, including hypoxic-ischemic insult in the term or preterm infant, intraventricular hemorrhage and posthemorrhagic ventricular dilation in the preterm infant, hypoglycemia, and congenital hypothyroidism.[41,162-164,167-169,173-179] Because the thalamus, the thalamocortical projections, and the parietal cortex of the somatosensory system (areas interrogated by measurement of the somatosensory evoked potentials) are all involved in and are contiguous to other areas related to cognitive and motor development, persistent abnormalities in these potentials in the neonatal period may be predicted to be associated with subsequent deficits. Indeed, in a study of 63 term and preterm infants, two thirds of whom were "asphyxiated," abnormal somatosensory evoked responses in the neonatal period in 14 were associated with abnormal neurological outcome at 1 year in 11 infants; normal responses in the neonatal period occurred in 26, with normal neurological outcome in 23.[180] Prognostic value in the preterm infant is clearly less than in the term infant.[41,166]

Electroencephalogram

Normal Development

Maturation of spontaneous EEG recorded activity has been studied in considerable detail in newborn infants, often in combination with studies of sleep states.[138,169,181-214] The theme apparent from the studies of specific sensory evoked responses recurs: with increasing gestational age, impressive elaborations of measurable function occur, characterized principally by more refined organization, and whether infants are born at term or grow to term after uncomplicated premature delivery has little or no effect on these developments. The normal development of EEG patterns in the neonatal period is evaluated best in relation to sleep states. In general, active sleep is the predominant sleep state in the newborn and consists of greater than 70% of definable sleep time in the smallest premature infants and approximately 50% in term infants. In the following discussion, I review the major changes in EEG over approximately the 12 to 13 weeks before term. Development of EEG is considered best in terms of the continuity of background activity, the synchrony of this activity, and the appearance and disappearance of specific waveforms and patterns (i.e., EEG developmental landmarks) (Table 4-6).[200]

27 to 28 Weeks. Activity at this developmental stage is characteristically discontinuous, with long periods of quiescence (see Table 4-6).[200] The activity that does interrupt the quiescence occurs in generalized, rather synchronous bursts (Fig. 4-8). No distinctions between wakefulness and sleep or change in EEG to external stimulus such as loud sound (i.e., reactivity) are apparent.

29 to 30 Weeks. The discontinuity of the EEG continues at this stage, but now the activity is asynchronous (see Table 4-6; Fig. 4-9).[200] The principal developmental landmark is the appearance of *delta brushes* (i.e., delta waves of 0.3 to 1.5 Hz with superimposed fast activity in the beta range, usually 18 to 22 Hz), sometimes also called *beta-delta complexes* (Fig. 4-10).[200] These complexes appear in the central regions at this stage. In addition, temporal bursts of theta activity (4 to 6 Hz) are a second developmental landmark of this period (see Fig. 4-10). These bursts occur independently in left and right temporal areas; their sharp configuration has provoked the term *saw-tooth pattern*.

31 to 33 Weeks. At this stage, continuous activity appears during active (or rapid eye movement) sleep (see Table 4-6).[200] Moreover, although EEG is generally asynchronous, a degree of synchrony appears in active sleep. The presence of more synchrony in active sleep than in quiet sleep persists throughout the developmental period of the third trimester. The delta brushes now become more prominent in occipital and temporal areas and are apparent particularly in quiet sleep. The temporal theta bursts of earlier stages give way to temporal alpha bursts, still, however, exhibiting the sharp sawtooth pattern (Fig. 4-11).

34 to 35 Weeks. The degree of continuity in the EEG now increases further and is apparent in the awake state as well as in active sleep (see Table 4-6).[200] In concert, the degree of synchrony increases in the awake and active sleep states. Of the developmental EEG landmarks, the delta brushes now exhibit considerably higher-voltage, faster activity. The temporal theta bursts disappear during this phase. Frontal sharp wave transients (i.e., sharp waves appearing as an abrupt change from background) become apparent (Fig. 4-12) and are characteristic for their diphasic, synchronous, and generally symmetrical configuration. These normal waves should be distinguished from higher-voltage, unilateral, persistently focal, periodic, or semirhythmic sharp waves, which are abnormal and indicative of focal disease (see later discussion). At this stage, EEG becomes "reactive" to external stimuli. Most commonly, this reactivity consists of a generalized attenuation of the amount and voltage of delta activity, especially apparent in response to sound.

36 to 37 Weeks. The degree of continuity and of synchrony in the awake and active sleep states is still more

TABLE 4-6   **Developmental Aspects of Electroencephalographic Activity**

Postconceptional Age (Weeks)	CONTINUITY OF BACKGROUND ACTIVITY*			SYNCHRONY OF BACKGROUND ACTIVITY†			EEG Developmental Landmarks: Specific Waveforms and Patterns
	Awake	Quiet Sleep	Active Sleep	Awake	Quiet Sleep	Active Sleep	
27–28	–	D	D	–	++++	++++	
29–30	D	D	D	O	O	O	1. "Delta brushes" in central regions 2. Temporal theta bursts (4–6 Hz) 3. Occipital slow activity
31–33	D	D	C	+	+	++	1. "Delta brushes" in occipital-temporal regions 2. Temporal alpha bursts replace theta bursts (33 weeks) 3. Rhythmic 1.5-Hz activity in frontal leads in transitional sleep
34–35	C	D	C	+++	+	+++	1. Extremely high-voltage beta activity during "delta brushes" 2. Temporal alpha bursts disappear 3. Frontal sharp-wave transients
36–37	C	D	C	++++	++	++++	1. Central "delta brushes" disappear 2. Continuous bioccipital delta activity with superimposed 12–15-Hz activity during active sleep
38–40	C	C	C	++++	+++	++++	1. Occipital "delta brushes" decrease and disappear by 39 weeks 2. Tracé alternant pattern during quiet sleep

*C, continuous activity; D, discontinuous activity.
†O, total asynchrony; ++++, total synchrony.
EEG, electroencephalographic.
Adapted from Hrachovy RA, Mizrahi EM, Kellaway P: Electroencephalography of the newborn. In Daly DD, Pedley TA, editors: *Current Practice of Clinical Electroencephalography*, 2nd ed, New York: 1990, Raven Press.

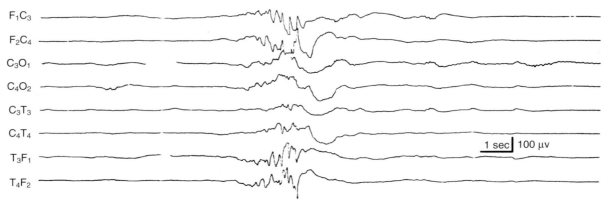

Figure 4-8   **Electroencephalogram of a male infant of 27 to 28 weeks of postconceptional age.** The bursts of generalized, bilaterally synchronous activity separated by prolonged periods of electrical quiescence are characteristic of this age. Selected sample from a 16-channel recording. *(From Hrachovy RA, Mizrahi EM, Kellaway P: Electroencephalography of the newborn. In Daly DD, Pedley TA, editors:* Current Practice of Clinical Electroencephalography, *2nd ed, New York: 1990, Raven Press.)*

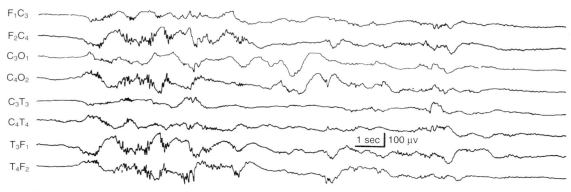

Figure 4-9 *Tracé discontinu* pattern in a male infant with a postconceptional age of 29 to 30 weeks. Selected sample from a 16-channel recording. *(From Hrachovy RA, Mizrahi EM, Kellaway P: Electroencephalography of the newborn. In Daly DD, Pedley TA, editors:* Current Practice of Clinical Electroencephalography, *2nd ed, New York: 1990, Raven Press.)*

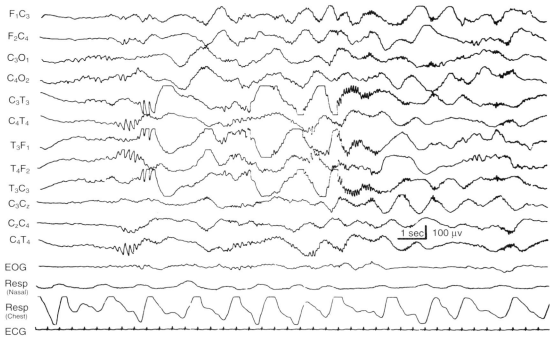

Figure 4-10 **Electroencephalogram of a female infant with a postconceptional age of 30 to 32 weeks.** *Left,* Brief bursts of 4- to 6-Hz waves of sharp configuration occurring asynchronously in the temporal regions. *Right,* Beta-delta complexes in the central and temporal regions. Selected sample from a 16-channel recording. ECG, electrocardiogram; EOG, electro-oculogram. *(From Hrachovy RA, Mizrahi EM, Kellaway P: Electroencephalography of the newborn. In Daly DD, Pedley TA, editors:* Current Practice of Clinical Electroencephalography, *2nd ed, New York: 1990, Raven Press.)*

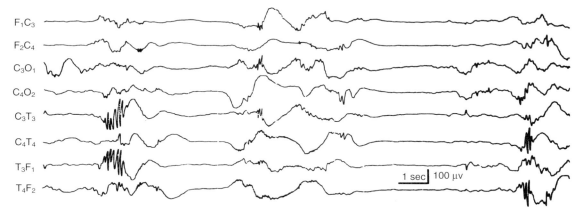

Figure 4-11 **Brief bursts of 8- to 9-Hz waves occurring bilaterally in the temporal regions in a female infant with a postconceptional age of 32 to 33 weeks.** Selected sample from a 16-channel recording. *(From Hrachovy RA, Mizrahi EM, Kellaway P: Electroencephalography of the newborn. In Daly DD, Pedley TA, editors:* Current Practice of Clinical Electroencephalography, *2nd ed, New York: 1990, Raven Press.)*

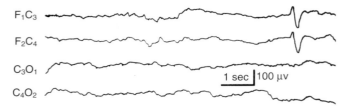

Figure 4-12 Diphasic, bilaterally synchronous and virtually symmetrical, frontal sharp waves in transitional sleep in a male infant with a postconceptional age of 36 weeks. Selected sample from a 16-channel recording. *(From Hrachovy RA, Mizrahi EM, Kellaway P: Electroencephalography of the newborn. In Daly DD, Pedley TA, editors:* Current Practice of Clinical Electroencephalography, *2nd ed, New York: 1990, Raven Press.)*

apparent (see Table 4-6).[200] At this stage, for the first time, EEG in the awake state differs from that in sleep by the presence of low-voltage activity, with a mixture of activities in the alpha, beta, theta, and delta frequency bands (Fig. 4-13). Of the developmental EEG landmarks, the delta brushes in the central region disappear. These are replaced by similar complexes in the occipital regions (i.e., bioccipital delta with superimposed 12 to 15 Hz activity, which appears during active sleep).

38 to 40 Weeks. At this stage, continuous activity now appears in quiet sleep as well as in active sleep and the awake state (see Table 4-6).[200] A considerable degree of synchrony is present in all states. The occipital delta brushes disappear, and the interesting *tracé alternant* pattern becomes apparent in quiet sleep (Fig. 4-14). This quasiperiodic tracing is characterized by periods of 3 to 15 seconds of generalized voltage attenuation, interrupted by higher-voltage, generally synchronous activity. Tracé alternant should not be confused with the more ominous burst-suppression pattern (see later discussion).

Clinical Application

The following sections focus on the application of conventional EEG in the clinical arena. The procedure requires skilled technicians and experienced interpreters of the tracing. Definitive assessment of EEG

abnormalities in the premature and term newborn requires conventional multichannel EEG. In the following discussion, I review the principal EEG abnormalities of both the premature and term newborn (Table 4-7), except for the EEG correlates of neonatal seizures (see Chapter 5).

Disordered Development. Delineation of abnormalities of EEG maturation clearly requires awareness of the normal developmental changes described in the previous section. Impairment of development level of more than 3 weeks, according to reported gestational age, is clearly abnormal.[200,215] Such disturbances are often but not necessarily associated with other EEG abnormalities, and the degree of disturbance may differ according to the state of the infant.[215-217] Abnormalities may be apparent only in quiet sleep, and thus this sleep state should be included in the EEG evaluation of the newborn.[200] Disturbed development of the EEG does not provide specific information regarding disease process and may reflect either an acute or a chronic disturbance.

Depression and Lack of Differentiation. Depression of background activity, especially of the faster frequencies, often accompanied by lack of differentiation (i.e., disappearance of the normal multiple frequencies), is common after generalized insults, especially hypoxic-ischemic insults (Fig. 4-15).[200,213,215,218,219] Other EEG abnormalities are also often present. In addition to hypoxia and ischemia, other bilateral cerebral insults may produce this EEG pattern, particularly acutely (e.g., bacterial meningitis, encephalitis, and metabolic disorders). Persistence of this EEG pattern is an unfavorable prognostic sign.

Excessively Discontinuous Activity. The development of continuous or intermittent discontinuity of EEG in the term infant is a very common feature of all neonatal encephalopathies. The most extreme of these discontinuous tracings is the *burst-suppression pattern*, which is associated with a very high likelihood of an unfavorable outcome. However, burst-suppression tracings account for the minority of excessively

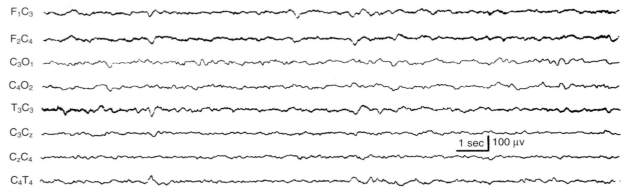

Figure 4-13 Typical awake pattern in a male term infant, characterized by a mixture of activities in the alpha, beta, theta, and delta frequency bands. Selected sample from a 16-channel recording. *(From Hrachovy RA, Mizrahi EM, Kellaway P: Electroencephalography of the newborn. In Daly DD, Pedley TA, editors:* Current Practice of Clinical Electroencephalography, *2nd ed, New York: 1990, Raven Press.)*

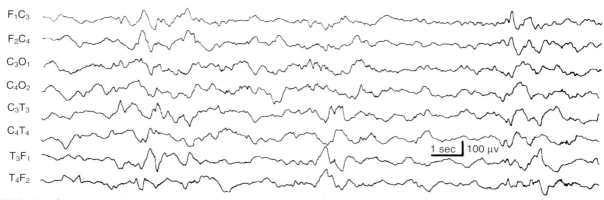

Figure 4-14 *Tracé alternant* **pattern in a male term infant.** *(From Hrachovy RA, Mizrahi EM, Kellaway P: Electroencephalography of the newborn. In Daly DD, Pedley TA, editors: Current Practice of Clinical Electroencephalography, 2nd ed, New York: 1990, Raven Press.)*

discontinuous neonatal EEGs. Recent data indicate that relatively simple analysis of the latter tracings is highly useful in predicting outcome (see later).

The *burst-suppression pattern* can be considered the most severe of the excessively discontinuous tracings just described. The EEG pattern is characterized by long periods (usually > 10 seconds) of marked depression of background activity (voltage < 5 μV), alternating with shorter periods of paroxysmal bursts, usually lasting 1 to 10 seconds and characterized by high-voltage (75 to 250 μV) theta and delta activity with intermixed spikes and waves (Fig. 4-16). This EEG pattern should be distinguished from the normal discontinuous tracing of the very immature premature infant and from the tracé alternant of quiet sleep of the infant beyond 36 weeks of gestation. Two important distinguishing features of the burst-suppression pattern are persistence of the discontinuous pattern throughout the tracing and nonreactivity (i.e., no change in the EEG with arousal attempts and painful or other stimuli). A burst-suppression pattern that is "reactive" (i.e., is altered by external stimuli) is not so uniformly associated with a poor prognosis as the nonreactive variety described here.[220-225] The poor prognosis of burst-suppression EEG is illustrated by the data depicted in Table 4-8.[226] Bacterial meningitis is the one disturbance in which I have seen a

favorable outcome, despite the finding of a burst-suppression EEG during the *acute* disease. In the group described in Table 4-8, the one infant with a favorable outcome also had acute bacterial meningitis.

Analysis of the *duration of the predominant interburst interval* (*IBI*) has proven to be a relatively simple means of *quantitation of excessively discontinuous tracings* in the term infant, and the analysis has major prognostic implications.[227] Thus, of 43 term infants (70% with hypoxic-ischemic encephalopathy) with an excessively discontinuous EEG, 10 parameters regarding the burst and IBIs were quantitated and compared with outcome. One parameter, the IBI duration that accounted for more than 50% of all IBI durations (classified into 10-second blocks), also known as *the predominant IBI duration*, predicted an unfavorable neurological outcome with high specificity (Table 4-9). Thus, IBI durations lasting longer than 30 seconds were invariably associated with an unfavorable outcome, and those with a duration of more than 20 seconds were associated with an unfavorable outcome in 92%. *Of the 43 discontinuous tracings, only 7 (16%) exhibited a burst-suppression pattern*, as defined earlier. Thus, the predominant IBI duration, *readily quantitated at the bedside*, was highly effective and, critically, applicable to the large group of excessively discontinuous tracings in term newborns with encephalopathy.

Electrocerebral Silence. Electrocerebral silence, of course, is the worst end of the continuum from depressed EEG through excessive discontinuity and burst-suppression pattern. Persistence of electrocerebral silence for 72 hours or more is indicative of cerebral death.[228,229] However, electrocerebral silence indicates cerebral cortical death and not necessarily brain stem death; if clinical evidence of persistent brain stem failure is not present, survival is possible, although in a persistent vegetative state (see Chapter 9).

Unilateral Depression of Background Activity. A marked voltage asymmetry between hemispheres of background rhythms that persists in all states is clearly different from the normal shifting asymmetries, particularly during quiet sleep (Fig. 4-17). Such persistent unilateral depressions of background activity are

---

TABLE 4-7	Major Electroencephalographic Abnormalities of the Premature and Term Newborn

Disordered development
Depression: lack of differentiation
Excessively discontinuous activity, including burst-suppression pattern
Electrocerebral silence
Unilateral depression of background activity
Periodic discharges
Multifocal sharp waves
Central positive sharp waves
Rhythmic generalized or focal alpha activity
Hypsarrhythmia

Data primarily from Hrachovy RA, Mizrahi EM, Kellaway P: Electroencephalography of the newborn. In Daly DD, Pedley TA, editors: *Current Practice of Clinical Electroencephalography*, 2nd ed, New York: 1990, Raven Press.

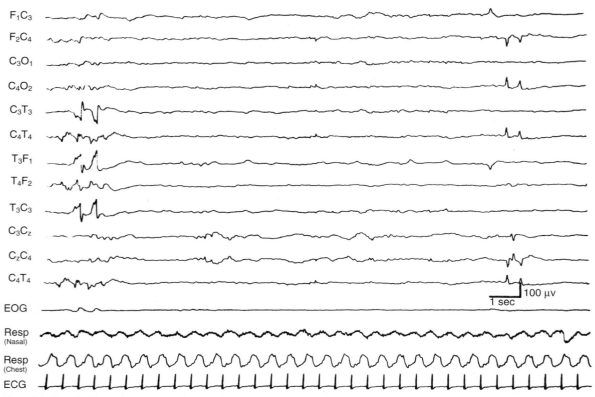

Figure 4-15 **Electroencephalogram of a male term infant who had meningitis and hypoxia at birth.** Background activity is depressed and undifferentiated, with superimposed abnormal, random sharp waves. Selected sample from a 16-channel recording. ECG, electrocardiogram; EOG, electro-oculogram. *(From Hrachovy RA, Mizrahi EM, Kellaway P: Electroencephalography of the newborn. In Daly DD, Pedley TA, editors: Current Practice of Clinical Electroencephalography, 2nd ed, New York: 1990, Raven Press.)*

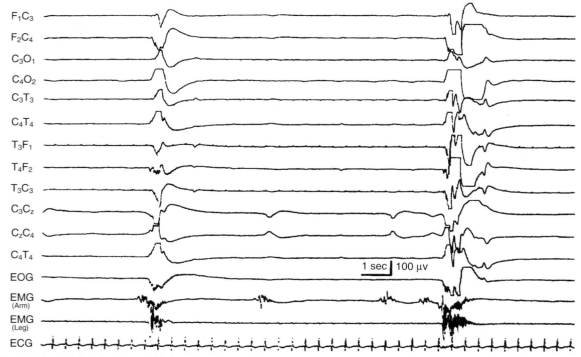

Figure 4-16 **Suppression-burst activity in a male term infant with severe neonatal hypoxia.** The bursts were associated with myoclonic jerks of the upper and lower extremities (electromyographic channels show myoclonic movement of the arm and leg). This pattern was unremitting during 90 minutes of recording and was nonreactive to intense stimuli. ECG, electrocardiogram; EMG, electromyogram; EOG, electro-oculogram. *(From Hrachovy RA, Mizrahi EM, Kellaway P: Electroencephalography of the newborn. In Daly DD, Pedley TA, editors: Current Practice of Clinical Electroencephalography, 2nd ed, New York: 1990, Raven Press.)*

TABLE 4-8 Burst-Suppression Electroencephalography in the Newborn

	Number	Percentage
Origin		
Perinatal asphyxia	12	80
Bacterial meningitis	3*	20
Central nervous system malformation	2*	13
Burst-Suppression EEG		
Onset in first week	14	93
Repeat EEG performed	8	53
Evolution to normal	4	50
Outcome		
Dead	4	27
Of 10 survivors followed		
Motor deficits	9	90
Cognitive deficits	9	90
Seizure disorder	5	50
Normal	1†	10

*One patient also experienced perinatal asphyxia.
†Infant with uncomplicated bacterial meningitis.
EEG, electroencephalography.
Data from Grigg-Damberger MM, Coker SB, Halsey CL, Anderson CL: Neonatal burst suppression: Its developmental significance, *Pediatr Neurol* 5:84-92, 1989; n = 15.

TABLE 4-9 Duration of Predominant Interburst Interval and Neurological Outcome*

Predominant Interburst Interval Duration†	Unfavorable Outcome‡
> 30 sec	10/10 (100%)
> 20 sec	12/13 (92%)
> 10 sec	24/33 (72%)

*Data from Menache CC, Bourgeois BFD, Volpe JJ: Prognostic value of neonatal discontinuous EEG, *Pediatr Neurol* 27:93-101, 2002.
†Interburst interval duration was obtained by manual measurement with classification into 10-second subintervals (1–10, 11–20, 21–30, >40 seconds); the predominant interval was defined as the interval that accounted for more than 50% of all interburst interval durations.
‡Death or moderate or severe motor and cognitive deficits were noted on follow-up.

quasiperiodic.[200,213,221,230-233] These discharges can be separated from the normal "transients" noted earlier by their higher voltage, generally longer duration, often polyphasic appearance, and persistent focality. The discharges are located more commonly in the central regions in the premature and in temporal regions in term infants (Table 4-10).[230] Neuropathological substrates are multiple in premature infants, but in the term infant the most common is infarction in the distribution of the middle cerebral artery.

Watanabe and co-workers showed the predictive value of frontal or occipital sharp waves in identification of cystic periventricular leukomalacia (Table 4-11).[233] Thus, the presence of one or both of these abnormal sharp waves was superior to the presence of positive

indicative usually of a unilateral cerebral lesion that is ischemic, hemorrhagic, or dysgenetic.

Periodic Discharges. Numerous periodic discharges may be seen in neonatal disease states. These complexes may be either strikingly periodic (Fig. 4-18) or only

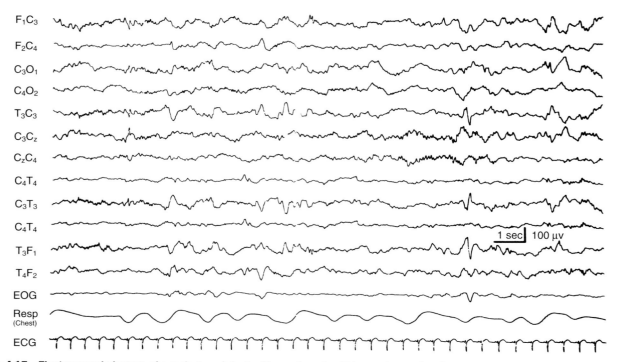

Figure 4-17 Electroencephalogram of a male term infant with a subarachnoid hemorrhage, showing suppression of background activity over the right hemisphere. Such unilateral suppressions of background activity are usually associated with an underlying structural lesion. ECG, electrocardiogram; EOG, electro-oculogram. *(From Hrachovy RA, Mizrahi EM, Kellaway P: Electroencephalography of the newborn. In Daly DD, Pedley TA, editors: Current Practice of Clinical Electroencephalography, 2nd ed, New York: 1990, Raven Press.)*

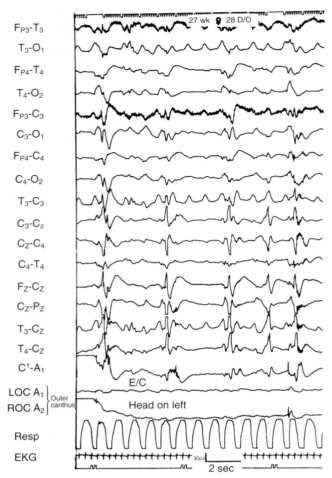

Figure 4-18 Electroencephalogram recording of a 27-week gestation, 28-day-old female infant with periodic lateralizing epileptiform discharges noted at the vertex region with a positive sharp wave morphology. This discharge was also noted with an additional electrode (C¹) referenced to the left ear. EKG, electrocardiogram; LOC, left outer canthus; ROC, right outer canthus. *(From Scher MS, Beggarly M: Clinical significance of focal periodic discharges in neonates, J Child Neurol 4:175-185, 1989.)*

rolandic sharp waves (see later) in sensitivity for identification of white matter injury.

Multifocal Sharp Waves. *Multifocal sharp waves* refer to sharp waves of high voltage and relatively long duration, occurring in multiple cerebral foci (Fig. 4-19).[200,213] These discharges tend to predominate in temporal regions and are usually accompanied by other EEG abnormalities. The types of underlying pathological features are multiple, and their specific nature determines outcome.

Central Positive Sharp Waves. These distinctive sharp waves, often termed *positive rolandic sharp waves*, are surface positive and occur either unilaterally or bilaterally in central regions (Fig. 4-20). Their particular relation to periventricular white matter injury in the premature infant has been established (see Table 4-11 and Chapter 9).[221,233-242] The apparently superior value of frontal (positive) or occipital (negative) sharp waves regarding sensitivity for white matter injury is discussed earlier (see Table 4-11).[233]

Rhythmic Generalized or Focal Alpha Frequency Activity. This rare discharge may be generalized or focal and consists of periods of rhythmic 8- to 9-Hz activity that is generally synchronous (Fig. 4-21). The activity tends to predominate in the central or temporal regions (an alpha pattern that occurs with seizure is not synchronous). This pattern has been noted with chromosomal abnormalities and inborn errors of metabolism.[200]

Hypsarrhythmia. Although the classical hypsarrhythmic EEG with infantile myoclonic spasms does not usually occur until the second month of life or later, one variety may appear in the newborn (Fig. 4-22). *Hypsarrhythmia* is characterized by periods of marked voltage attenuation, interrupted by bursts of asynchronous, high-voltage, slow activity mixed with multifocal spikes and sharp waves.[200] This pattern is differentiated from the burst-suppression pattern described earlier,

TABLE 4-10 Focal Periodic Electroencephalographic Discharges in the Newborn

	Preterm	Term
Characteristics of Discharge		
Location	Vertex-central	Temporal
Duration	<1 min	>1 min
Associated Electrographic Seizures	**35%**	**88%**
Origin		
Infarction	15%	88%
Periventricular leukomalacia	27%	0
Other structural abnormalities	27%	0
Unknown	31%	12%
Outcome		
Dead	46%	38%
Deficits	27%	50%
Normal	27%	12%

*Data from Scher MS, Beggarly M: Clinical significance of focal periodic discharges in neonates, J Child Neurol 4:175-185, 1989; n = 34 (26 preterm and 8 term).

TABLE 4-11 Frontal and Occipital Sharp Waves and Positive Rolandic or Vertex (Central) Sharp Waves in Premature Infants

Frontal or occipital sharp waves, or both, present in 100% of cases of severe PVL and in 60%–70% of cases of mild or moderate PVL

PRSs present in 65%–90% of cases of *severe* white matter lesions (i.e., PVL, periventricular hemorrhagic infarction); sensitivity lowest for the most immature infants and for mild or moderate PVL (present in 25% of cases)

PRSs generally apparent when white matter lesions are echodense but not yet cystic by ultrasonography

Lateralization or symmetry of the abnormal waves generally corresponding to lateralization or symmetry of white matter necrosis

Onset of the abnormal waves as early as 2 days, generally peaking between 5 and 14 days; *cystic* PVL noted generally 5 to 10 days later

PRS, positive rolandic sharp wave; PVL, periventricular leukomalacia.

particularly by the high voltage of the activity during the bursts; in hypsarrhythmia, voltage may reach 1000 μV, whereas in a typical burst-suppression pattern, the voltage of the bursts is usually less than 250 μV.[200]

Value of Serial Electroencephalography. The particular value of *serial* EEG in estimating outcome is pronounced.[221,224,237,243] A single EEG, particularly during the acute phase of the disease, may suggest a more ominous outcome than do subsequent EEG studies. This point is illustrated well by the data recorded in Table 4-12, based on a study of 62 infants.[237]

Amplitude-Integrated Electroencephalogram

Methodology and Rationale

Amplitude-integrated EEG (aEEG) is an increasingly used method for the continuous monitoring of cerebral electrical activity in critically ill newborns.[244] (The equipment used for application of this technique is usually termed a *cerebral function monitor*. aEEG involves a single-channel recording obtained from one pair of biparietal electrodes.[197,244-252] The EEG signal is

amplified and is then passed through a filter that attenuates activity lower than 2 Hz and higher than 15 Hz (to minimize artifacts).[244,253] The signal is processed further by amplitude and time compression before recording on a semilogarithmic scale at relatively slow speed, usually 6 cm/hour.

Among the particular values of this method are ease of application, ability to monitor continuously, *relative* ease of integration, and capacity to detect seizures, relatively severe encephalopathy, effects of drugs, and outcome. Among the disadvantages are the inability to detect hemispheric asymmetries in EEG signal, and thus certain focal lesions, and some seizures that are focal or relatively brief.

Recording

aEEG recordings are evaluated especially for background and seizure activity.[244] The major background patterns identified are termed continuous normal voltage, discontinuous normal voltage, burst suppression, continuous low voltage, and flat trace (Fig. 4-23). As described later, the last three of these are ominous tracings. Discontinuous normal voltage is considered an intermediate tracing (i.e., although most such tracings normalize within the first 24 hours, some deteriorate, and because of the latter a conventional EEG should be obtained).

Seizure activity on aEEG is characterized in general as a *rapid* rise in both the lower and upper margins of the trace (Fig. 4-24).[244] The experience of the reader is important for detection (see later).

Clinical Applications

As noted earlier, the principal clinical applications of aEEG are assessment of *term infants shortly after perinatal asphyxia* and *detection of seizures*. The value of aEEG in the former instance appears well established, whereas the role in seizure detection requires further clarification.

Assessment of Asphyxiated Term Infants. aEEG has proven very useful in assessment of the asphyxiated term newborn.[244,254-257] A particular goal has been to identify, in the first hours after birth, the likely outcome

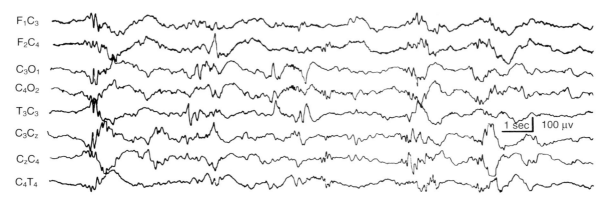

Figure 4-19 Multiple foci of abnormal, high-voltage sharp waves occurring during slow-wave sleep in a male term infant with congenital heart disease, perinatal hypoxia, and respiratory metabolic acidosis. Selected sample from a 16-channel recording. *(From Hrachovy RA, Mizrahi EM, Kellaway P: Electroencephalography of the newborn. In Daly DD, Pedley TA, editors: Current Practice of Clinical Electroencephalography, 2nd ed, New York: 1990, Raven Press.)*

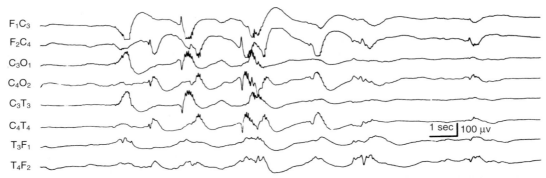

Figure 4-20 Central positive sharp waves in a male infant with an intraventricular hemorrhage; his postconceptional age is 29 to 30 weeks. Selected sample from a 16-channel recording. *(From Hrachovy RA, Mizrahi EM, Kellaway P: Electroencephalography of the newborn. In Daly DD, Pedley TA, editors: Current Practice of Clinical Electroencephalography, 2nd ed, New York: 1990, Raven Press.)*

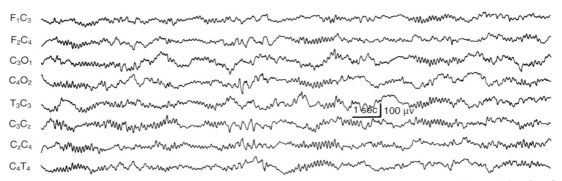

Figure 4-21 Runs of rhythmic 8- to 9-Hz activity occurring synchronously and independently in the left and right central regions in a male term infant with a chromosomal abnormality and multiple congenital anomalies. *Such alpha frequency activity may also occur in a generalized fashion.* Selected sample from a 16-channel recording. *(From Hrachovy RA, Mizrahi EM, Kellaway P: Electroencephalography of the newborn. In Daly DD, Pedley TA, editors: Current Practice of Clinical Electroencephalography, 2nd ed, New York: 1990, Raven Press.)*

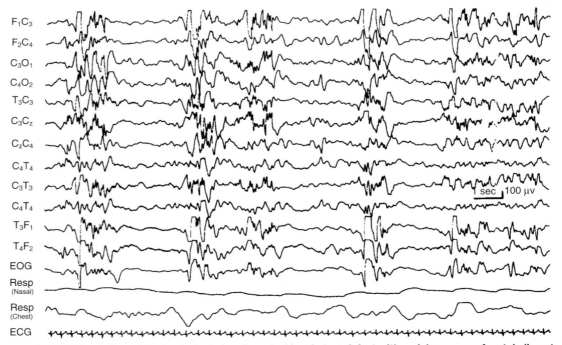

Figure 4-22 Suppression-burst variant of hypsarrhythmia in a 3-week-old male term infant with an inborn error of metabolism, type unknown. The infantile spasms in this patient were accompanied by generalized attenuation episodes in the electroencephalogram. ECG, electrocardiogram; EOG, electro-oculogram. *(From Hrachovy RA, Mizrahi EM, Kellaway P: Electroencephalography of the newborn. In Daly DD, Pedley TA, editors: Current Practice of Clinical Electroencephalography, 2nd ed, New York: 1990, Raven Press.)*

TABLE 4-12   **Serial Electroencephalograms in Preterm Infants (<1200 g) in Relation to Outcome**

EEG	OUTCOME			
	Normal	**Suspect**	**Abnormal**	**Dead**
Normal, mildly abnormal, or only one EEG moderately abnormal	76%	13%	4%	7%
Moderately abnormal (≥2 EEGs) or any markedly abnormal	6%	6%	63%	25%

EEG, electroencephalogram.
Data from Tharp BR, Scher MS, Clancy RR: Serial EEGs in normal and abnormal infants with birth weights less than 1200 grams: A prospective study with long term follow-up, *Neuropediatrics* 20:64-72, 1989; *n* = 62.

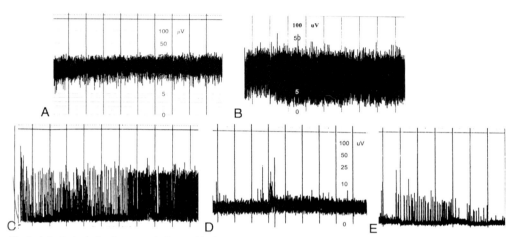

Figure 4-23   **Amplitude-integrated electroencephalographic background patterns.** Background patterns are (**A**) continuous normal voltage, (**B**) discontinuous normal voltage, (**C**) burst suppression, (**D**) continuous low voltage, and (**E**) flat trace. *(From de Vries LS, Hellstrom-Westas L: Role of cerebral function monitoring in the newborn,* Arch Dis Child Fetal Neonatal Ed *90:F201-F207, 2005.)*

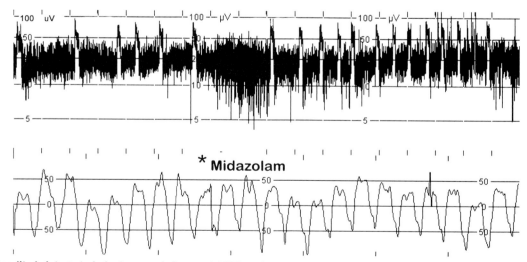

Figure 4-24   **Amplitude-integrated electroencephalogram (aEEG): seizure pattern.** Note repetitive discharges on a continuous normal voltage background pattern (*upper trace*). Simultaneous EEG (*lower trace*), displayed at the *asterisk*, shows rhythmic epileptic discharges. Midazolam was administered as shown, with no effect on repetitive discharges. *(From de Vries LS, Hellstrom-Westas L: Role of cerebral function monitoring in the newborn,* Arch Dis Child Fetal Neonatal Ed *90:F201-F207, 2005.)*

of the asphyxiated infant. The aEEG background tracings have been most useful, particularly the burst-suppression, continuous low-voltage, and flat trace patterns. In one large study, the positive predictive value for unfavorable outcome for aEEG detection of severe abnormalities at 3 hours of life was 78%, and at 6 hours, it was 86%.[258] The positive predictive value at 6 hours has been similar in other studies.[251,259] Notably, approximately 10% to 40% of infants with marked background abnormalities may normalize within 24 hours, and more than 50% of this minority group will have a favorable outcome.[255,256] Thus, monitoring the course of aEEG changes is useful, although for identification of candidates for neuroprotective therapies, such as mild hypothermia, early detection is crucial (see Chapter 9). Finally, and of additional importance, although aEEG in the first 6 hours was superior to neonatal neurological examination in identifying infants with an unfavorable short-term outcome, the *combination* of aEEG *and* the neurological examination was best, with a specificity of 94%.[254]

Detection of Seizures. The value of aEEG in detection of seizures has been assessed primarily in asphyxiated term infants.[244,252,260-262a] aEEG was not designed as a seizure monitor, although some very experienced users of the method appear skilled at seizure detection. Nevertheless, in one comparative study of aEEG and standard EEG with experienced observers, of 10 infants with ictal activity on EEG, 8 were detected by aEEG, and notably of 16 infants with interictal "multifocal epileptiform activity," only 4 were identified by aEEG.[260] Additionally, the experience of the observer is very important in aEEG detection of seizure activity. Thus, in one study involving four neonatologists with no prior experience with aEEG and trained for 3 to 5 hours in seizure detection on the aEEG tracing, only 38% of seizures were detected at the usual paper speed of 6 cm/hour.[261] Moreover, focal, low-amplitude, or brief seizures also are readily missed by aEEG.[260,261,262a]

Other Applications. aEEG has proven useful, in initial studies, for a variety of other applications. Thus, the method has been used for delineation of effects of anticonvulsant drugs (e.g., midazolam, phenobarbital),[263,264] evaluation of sleep-wake cycling in asphyxiated infants,[265] prediction of postneonatal epilepsy in asphyxiated infants,[266] definition of maturational changes in preterm infants,[267-269] and prediction of outcome in premature infants with large intraventricular hemorrhage.[270] Related methods, involving spectral analysis of the EEG and focused more on frequency than on amplitude, are in the developmental stage in the study of the premature infant.[271,272]

STRUCTURAL BRAIN IMAGING

The three major techniques for demonstrating normal and abnormal brain structure are ultrasonography, computed tomography (CT), and magnetic resonance imaging (MRI). Ultrasound scanning is the most conveniently performed of these three procedures. CT was the first of the three methods to be used clinically. MRI provides the greatest resolution and versatility, and advanced MRI techniques allow quantitation of regional volumes and fiber tracts (see later). Cranial ultrasonography and CT are long-established techniques in the study of the newborn brain and are noted only briefly here but are illustrated in most chapters of this book. I discuss MRI in more detail, including advanced MRI methods, because this modality has provided important insights into aspects of normal brain development.

Ultrasonography

Ultrasound scanning is one of several techniques that capitalize on the bone-free anterior fontanelle to provide a window into the neonatal brain.[273,274] Additionally, use of the posterior fontanelle and of the mastoid fontanelle has markedly improved the value of ultrasonography in the evaluation of posterior fossa structures. The enormous value of the technique in the study of the neonatal brain has been documented in a vast number of original papers and reviews and in several books.[274-280] The specific uses of the technique are documented throughout this book, but it is important simply to emphasize here the value of ultrasound scanning in identification of such diverse intracranial processes as the following: developmental aberrations; hypoxic-ischemic injury; subdural, germinal matrix-intraventricular, and posterior fossa hemorrhage; ventriculitis; tumors; cysts; and vascular anomalies. The basic principles of the technique and the major normal anatomical features, reviewed in previous editions of this book, are summarized in standard writings.[274,281-285]

Computed Tomography

CT scanning is an imaging technique based on the use of ionizing radiation, as in conventional radiography. Through the use of computerized image reconstruction, modern CT scanners can produce images of high resolution in only a few minutes of data acquisition. This technique is not considered in detail here, because it is now a standard radiological procedure, and its value is illustrated throughout the book. Nevertheless, in the study of the newborn, the principal disadvantages are the requirement of transport of the infant to the CT scanner and the use of ionizing radiation. Currently, CT scanning provides more definitive information than ultrasound scanning in the evaluation of most parenchymal disorders, hemorrhage or other fluid collections in the subdural and subarachnoid spaces, and most posterior fossa lesions. Except perhaps for the detection of calcification and cranial bony abnormalities, MRI provides superior resolution.

Magnetic Resonance Imaging

MRI is the most recently established conventional imaging technique in neurology. The value of this procedure in the study of the newborn brain has become increasingly clear in the past decade.[286-289] In the following discussion, I briefly review the value of MRI in defining the development of the brain. In addition to conventional MRI to provide high resolution though qualitative information, I illustrate the value of more advanced MRI techniques to provide quantitative volumetric macrostructural information and quantitative diffusion-weighted microstructural information. The basic principles of the technique, reviewed in the last edition of this book, are summarized in standard writings.[288-301]

Clinical Application

Normal Development. *Conventional MRI* is of major value in the definition of many aspects of brain development, perhaps most prominently myelination.[288,289,295,298,301-316] In general, the deposition of myelin is accompanied on T1-weighted images by an increase in signal (i.e., myelinated regions appear white) and on T2-weighted images by a decrease in signal (i.e., myelinated regions appear black). Although the choice of T1-weighted versus T2-weighted images for delineation of myelin development is not fully agreed on, emphasis on T1-weighted images in the first 6 months and on T2-weighted images after 6 months is particularly useful.[301,303,307] The progress of myelination in human brain, as defined by MRI, is depicted in Figure 4-25. The major milestones of myelination as shown by MRI are summarized in Table 4-13. The similarity between these data on myelination, defined in the living infant, and the data defined from infants at autopsy (see Chapter 2) is striking. Moreover, as with most other developmental events, myelination in healthy preterm infants is similar to that in term infants, when both groups are studied at comparable postconceptional ages.[311]

A major advance in the use of MRI for the study of normal brain development is *quantitative volumetric* MRI. Using three-dimensional imaging and tissue segmentation techniques in image processing, my colleagues and I were able to document striking changes in the growth of the brain and of major brain regions with development from 29 to 41 weeks of postconceptional age (Fig. 4-26).[317] The data show a nearly threefold increase in total brain volume, an approximately fourfold increase in cerebral cortical gray matter volume, an approximately 50% increase in unmyelinated white matter volume, and a dramatic fivefold increase in myelinated white matter volume. The increase in cortical gray matter volume occurs during the time period of rapid growth of cortical neuronal processes and exuberant influx of afferent fibers from subplate neurons and thalamus (see Chapter 2). The fastest increase in cerebral myelin occurs between 35 and 41 weeks of postconceptional age and is accompanied by prominent oligodendroglial differentiation (see Chapter 2) and the onset of cerebral myelination. Volumetric studies of children and adults who were born prematurely show decreased volumes of cerebral cortical gray matter and deep nuclear structures, especially thalamus and basal ganglia (see Chapters 2 and 9).[318-325a] Moreover, volumetric

studies as early as term equivalent have shown decreased cerebral cortical and deep nuclear volumes.[317,326-331] Additionally, the deleterious effect of postnatal dexamethasone treatment of premature infants on cerebral cortical volume has been defined by volumetric MRI analysis at term (see Chapter 2).[332,332a]

Another striking advance in the use of MRI for the study of normal brain development is the application of techniques to *quantitate water diffusion* to provide microstructural information.[333-345a,345b] Using such an advanced approach, my colleagues and I studied changes in overall water diffusion (i.e., apparent diffusion coefficient) and in preferred directionality of diffusion (i.e., relative anisotropy) in central cerebral white matter from 28 to 40 weeks of postconceptional age (Fig. 4-27).[339] The data show a striking decrease in overall water diffusion (declining apparent diffusion coefficient) (see Fig. 4-27A). At older ages, such a decline has been associated with the deposition of myelin. However, at this stage of cerebral white matter development, essentially no myelin is deposited. Insight into the likely mechanism for the decline in overall water diffusion is provided by the finding of a striking simultaneous increase in directionality of diffusion (i.e., relative anisotropy) in the same region (see Fig. 4-27B). Both the increased directionality of diffusion and the decreased overall diffusion could occur if central cerebral white matter axons were increasing in thickness and macromolecular structure or were undergoing encasement by differentiating oligodendrocytes, thereby restricting water diffusion in all directions except parallel to the fiber. Both anatomical correlates are actively evolving during this period of cerebral maturation (see Chapter 2). Both explanations could be applicable. Data in developing animals, including the subhuman primate, are consistent with these correlations.[346,347]

Still more advanced MRI techniques have provided the capability to define cortical surface area and cortical thickness. Increases in cerebral cortical surface area during the premature period are dramatic (Fig. 4-28).[348]

Disorders. The remarkable capability of MRI for delineation of a large variety of clinical disorders in newborns and young infants is illustrated throughout this book and has been reviewed by others.[288,289, 298,299,301,303,304,349] A summary of abnormalities detectable by MRI but, in my experience, readily missed by CT is provided in Table 4-14. The abnormalities include a wide variety of developmental and acquired disorders. Although MRI is clearly superior to CT in the delineation of many disorders, CT is superior to MRI in the delineation of intracranial calcification. Moreover, and perhaps most important, the use of MRI in a critically ill newborn is sometimes difficult because the infant is not easily monitored while in the bore of clinical magnets and occasionally has monitoring equipment containing ferromagnetic material. The development of nonmetallic monitoring equipment has diminished the latter difficulty, and currently even small preterm infants requiring intensive care can be imaged safely, as shown through personal experience and the work of others.[350]

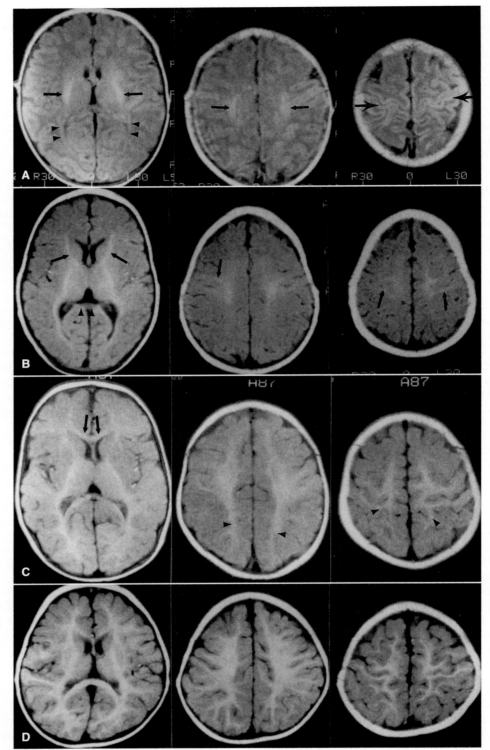

Figure 4-25 **T1-weighted magnetic resonance images of brain in healthy, A, 1-month-old, B, 4-month-old, C, 6-month-old, and, D, 8-month-old infants.** In **A**, note increased signal intensity, consistent with myelin, in posterior limb of the internal capsule (*arrows, left image*), optic radiations (*arrowheads, left image*), central corona radiata (*arrows, middle image*), and paracentral gyri (*arrows, right image*). In **B**, note the addition of increased signal in the anterior limbs of the internal capsule (*arrows, left image*) and splenium of the corpus callosum (*arrowheads, left image*), as well as intensification of the increased signal in posterior limb of the internal capsule, optic radiations, and centrum semiovale, with beginning of arborization of myelin in the paracentral regions (*arrows in middle and right images*). In **C**, note the further progression of myelination with high signal intensity not only in the splenium but also in the genu of the corpus callosum (*arrows, left image*) and increased arborization of myelin not only in paracentral regions but also in occipital areas (*arrowheads, middle and right images*). In **D**, marked progression of myelination is apparent, with nearly an adult appearance. Arborization of central white matter extends far into subcortical white matter, except in the frontal poles. *(From Barkovich AJ, Kjos BO, Jackson DE, Norman D: Normal maturation of the neonatal and infant brain: MR imaging at 1.5 T, Radiology 166:173-180, 1988.)*

TABLE 4-13	Milestones of Myelination as Shown by Magnetic Resonance Imaging*

Birth–1 Month
Dorsal midbrain
Cerebellar peduncles
Posterior limb of internal capsule
Lateral thalamus
Paracentral gyri: subcortical white matter

2–4 Months
Cerebellar white matter
Anterior limb of internal capsule
Splenium of corpus callosum
Optic radiation

4–6 Months
Genu of corpus callosum
Occipital white matter: central
Occipital white matter: peripheral (beginning)
Frontal white matter: central (beginning)

6–9 Months
Occipital white matter: peripheral
Frontal white matter: central
Frontal white matter: peripheral

*See text for references.

NONINVASIVE CONTINUOUS MONITORING TECHNIQUES

The lability of so many vital aspects of homeostasis in the newborn has made it obligatory to devise techniques for the continuous monitoring of a variety of physiological parameters. Many of these parameters have a direct bearing on the present and future integrity of the nervous system. Some of the continuous monitoring techniques (e.g., for arterial blood pressure and transcutaneous monitoring for blood gas levels) are well established and need not be discussed separately. In this section, I review three monitoring techniques that are suitable for continuous or, at least, frequent intermittent monitoring. The instrumentation for two of these techniques, measurement of intracranial pressure and cerebral blood flow (CBF) velocity, are readily available. Similarly, a third technique, near-infrared spectroscopy (NIRS), based on optical principles, has advanced rapidly through stages of research and development and has been used in clinical research.

Intracranial Pressure Monitoring

Importance of Determination

Determination of intracranial pressure is of particular importance in neonatal neurological disorders, because marked alterations of this pressure have major implications for diagnosis and management. Intracranial pressure alterations per se may lead to deleterious consequences through two basic mechanisms: *disturbances of CBF and shifts of neural structures within the cranium*. With the former consequence, cerebral perfusion pressure is related to the mean arterial blood pressure

minus the intracranial pressure. Therefore, when intracranial pressure increases, cerebral perfusion pressure decreases; if intracranial pressure increases markedly, cerebral perfusion pressure declines below the lower limit of autoregulation, and CBF may be impaired severely. Indeed, because normal arterial blood pressure in the newborn, especially the premature newborn, is relatively low, cerebral perfusion pressure already may be dangerously close to the downslope of the autoregulation curve (see Chapter 9). The other deleterious consequence of increased intracranial pressure, that is, abnormal intracranial shifts of neural structures, such as herniation of the temporal lobe through the tentorial notch or of the cerebellar tonsils through the foramen magnum, is very unusual in the newborn. The relative infrequency of temporal lobe herniation relates to the rarity of large, unilateral, supratentorial mass lesions, as well as to the relative ease of decompression of elevated pressure by the ready separation of the neonatal cranial sutures. Similarly, herniation of cerebellar tonsils through the foramen magnum requires a rapidly evolving mass in the posterior fossa, a very unusual occurrence in the newborn.

The major general causes of increased intracranial pressure in the newborn are shown in Table 4-15. These are discussed in the appropriate chapters of this book.

Anterior Fontanelle Monitors. Although lumbar puncture, placement of an epidural, subdural, or subarachnoid sensor, and ventricular puncture are well-recognized means of determining intracranial pressure, these techniques are invasive and are not readily amenable to continuous monitoring or frequent intermittent determinations in the newborn. Studies of intracranial pressure through a subarachnoid catheter in the severely asphyxiated newborn have been carried out in selected newborns (see Chapter 9).[351,352] The accessibility of the anterior fontanelle as an indicator of intracranial pressure has led to the refinement of techniques that capitalize on this anatomical peculiarity of the young infant.

Three basic devices have been applied to the anterior fontanelle to determine intracranial pressure, and the basis of the function of each is the *applanation principle*.[352-372] When the anterior fontanelle is maintained in a flat position, the pressure on each side is equal. The various devices used, their strengths and weaknesses, the manner of their application, and their validation were reviewed in previous editions of this book and have been deleted from this edition to conserve space.

Measurements of Intracranial Pressure

Normal Intracranial Pressure. Values for "normal" intracranial pressure in initial studies with anterior fontanelle monitors were difficult to determine from published data, in part because of the variability in means of application of the transducers, the sensitivity of the techniques to such factors as amount of external pressure on the sensors, and the heterogeneity of the infants studied, who usually were from intensive care facilities

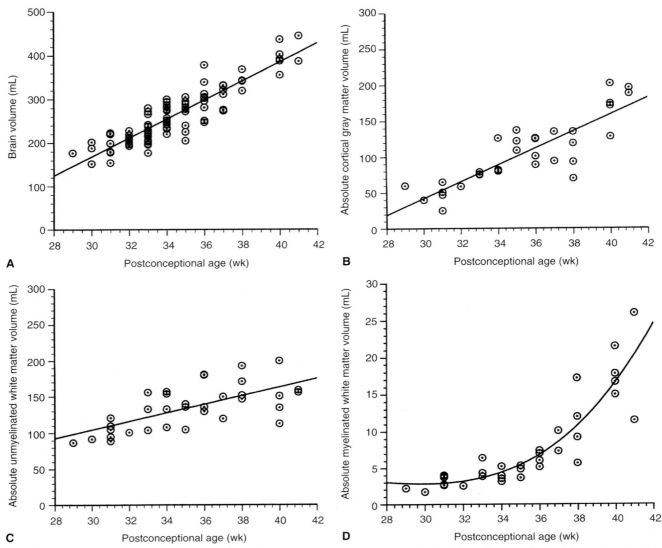

Figure 4-26 Quantitative three-dimensional volumetric magnetic resonance imaging determinations of, **A, total brain volume, B, cortical gray matter volume, C, unmyelinated white matter volume, and D, myelinated white matter volume, as a function of postconceptional age in 35 premature and full-term infants.** *(From Huppi PS, Warfield S, Kikinis R, Barnes PD, et al: Quantitative magnetic resonance imaging of brain development in premature and mature newborns, Ann Neurol 43:224-235, 1998.)*

or referral hospitals for sick infants. However, it is now apparent that these early studies overestimated the normal range of intracranial pressure in the newborn. Thus, most early studies reported that normal newborn values were 90 to 100 mm H_2O.[355,357,359,361,365] However, Welch,[373] in a study of 28 infants in the first months of life, used a simple clinical technique based on visual determination of the height of the infant's head at which the fontanelle becomes flat and obtained a mean value of 45 ± 12 mm H_2O.[373] Using a fiberoptic sensor adapted with a device that reproducibly controlled the amount of external pressure on the sensor, Walsh and Logan[364] obtained a similar value. Moreover, a study of 35 normal term infants and 25 normal preterm infants with a pneumatic-tonometric sensor obtained a value of approximately 70 mm H_2O.[362] Still later studies that employed anterior fontanelle techniques have provided values of 40 to 60 mm H_2O.[368,370,371,374] Using lumbar puncture and a sensitive pressure transducer, Kaiser and

Whitelaw[375] obtained a value of 38 ± 19 mm H_2O. Our unpublished studies in *infants not on ventilators* and free of intracranial disease, as shown by ultrasound scan, CT scan, or both, also indicate that normal intracranial pressure in the newborn is approximately 40 to 50 mm H_2O. This value is consistent with the range of approximately 30 to 70 mm H_2O obtained by lumbar puncture in newborn studies reported in 1928.[376,377]

Pathological States. Noninvasive monitoring techniques for measurement of intracranial pressure are most relevant in evaluation of infants with intraventricular hemorrhage, posthemorrhagic hydrocephalus, hypoxic-ischemic encephalopathy, bacterial meningitis, and a variety of other pathological states (see Chapters 9, 11, and 21). Examples of the striking changes defined in various states with one of the techniques (i.e., the coupled pneumatic-fiberoptic system)

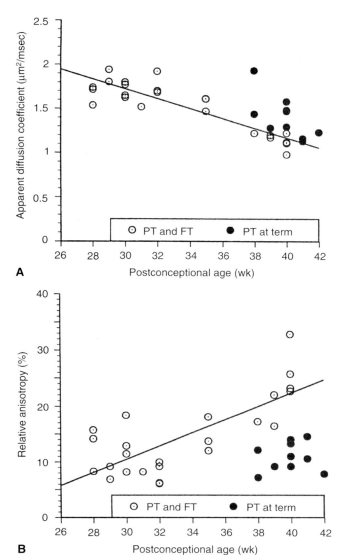

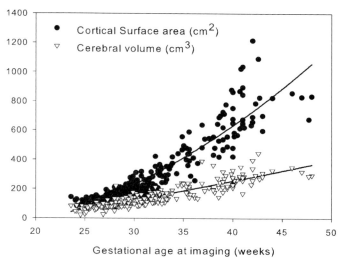

Figure 4-28 Cortical surface area and cerebral volume of preterm infants. A total of 113 preterm infants, born between 23 and 30 weeks of gestation, were studied by advanced magnetic resonance imaging (see text) to measure cortical surface area and cerebral volume over the period from birth to 48 postconceptional weeks. Note the striking increase in both surface area and volume over the last trimester and the first weeks of postnatal life. *(From Kapellou O, Counsell SJ, Kennea NL, Dyet L, et al: Abnormal cortical development after premature birth shown by altered allometric scaling of brain growth, PLoS Med 3:e265, 2006.)*

Figure 4-27 Diffusion tensor magnetic resonance imaging determinations of, A, overall water diffusion, expressed as apparent diffusion coefficient, and of, B, preferred directionality of diffusion, expressed as relative anisotropy, as a function of postconceptional age in 24 premature (PT) and full-term (FT) infants. *(From Huppi PS, Maier SE, Peled S, Zientara GP, et al: Microstructural development of human newborn cerebral white matter assessed in vivo by diffusion tensor magnetic resonance imaging, Pediatr Res 44:584-590, 1998.)*

Cerebral Blood Flow Velocity Monitoring

The anterior fontanelle of the newborn has been used to great advantage not only to image the intracranial contents by ultrasound scanning and to determine intracranial pressure by appropriate surface sensors, but also to measure the velocity of blood flow in the major cerebral arteries, especially the ascending portion of the anterior cerebral artery, by the Doppler ultrasonic

include the sharp increases in intracranial pressure documented in infants with major intracranial hemorrhage,[356] posthemorrhagic hydrocephalus,[359,368] seizures,[378] pneumothorax,[379] tracheal suctioning,[378] and head elevation.[360] Moreover, the potential value of the technique in determining the effects of certain interventions is exemplified by documentation of the immediate decreases in intracranial pressure with external ventricular drainage or lumbar puncture for treatment of posthemorrhagic hydrocephalus.[380,381] The potential importance of *serial* measurements of intracranial pressure in evaluation of presumed brain edema occurring as a consequence of hypoxic-ischemic cerebral injury is illustrated well by the work of Lupton and co-workers (see Chapter 8).[382]

TABLE 4-14	Abnormalities Detectable by Magnetic Resonance Imaging and Readily Missed by Computed Tomography

Disorders of neuronal migration
  Schizencephaly with narrow clefts
  Pachygyria
  Polymicrogyria
  Heterotopias: subependymal, subcortical
  Focal cerebral cortical dysgeneses
Partial agenesis of the corpus callosum
Disorders of myelination
Arteriovenous malformations
Focal cerebral ischemic lesions (infarcts)
  Acute: abnormality before computed tomography changes
  Chronic: demonstration of full extent of the lesion
Venous thrombosis
Parasagittal cerebral injury
Periventricular leukomalacia
Hemorrhagic lesions
  Distinction of hemorrhagic infarction from primary parenchymal hemorrhage
  Dating of hemorrhages
Virtually all lesions in posterior fossa and most lesions of spinal cord

TABLE 4-15	Increased Intracranial Pressure in the Newborn

Increased Extracerebral Volume
Blood (subdural, epidural)
CSF (communicating hydrocephalus) (subarachnoid)
Inflammatory exudate (purulent meningitis) (subarachnoid)
Effusion (subdural)

Increased Intracerebral Volume
Blood: intravascular-arterial (e.g., increased cerebral perfusion) or venous (e.g., increased central venous pressure as in pneumothorax, tracheal suctioning)
Blood: extravascular (e.g., hemorrhage)
Edema fluid: extracellular (e.g., "vasogenic," as in bacterial meningitis)
Edema fluid: intracellular (e.g., "cytotoxic," as in severe hypoxic-ischemic encephalopathy)
Mass lesion: abscess, neoplasm, vascular malformation

Increased Intraventricular Volume
Blood (e.g., intraventricular hemorrhage)
CSF (e.g., obstruction to flow at foramen of Monro, aqueduct of Sylvius, or outflow of fourth ventricle by blood, inflammatory exudate, or mass)

CSF, cerebrospinal fluid.

technique. Because the pathogenesis of a considerable proportion of the neuropathology encountered in the neonatal brain appears to relate to derangements of CBF, and because most procedures for assessing the cerebral circulation are technically difficult or invasive, or both, the Doppler ultrasonic technique has prompted considerable interest and study. In this section, I review the use of the technique to measure CBF velocity through the anterior fontanelle and by the transcranial approach, and I focus specifically on the relationship of the measurement of CBF velocity with CBF and with cerebrovascular resistance.

Basic Principles. The basic principles of the Doppler effect, the specific aspects of the available instruments, and the technique of their application were reviewed in previous editions of this book and are deleted from this edition for the purpose of conservation of space.

Quantitation of CBF velocity is based principally on calculation of either a resistance index or the area under the velocity waveforms. A typical tracing (Fig. 4-29) helps to illustrate these calculations. The *resistance index of Pourcelot*,[383,384] given by the formula RI = [S − D]/S, where RI is the resistance index and S and D are the peak systolic and end-diastolic amplitudes of flow, respectively, is useful because the index is not affected by changes in the angle of probe placement. A related index is the so-called *pulsatility index of Gosling*, given by the formula [S − D]/mean velocity. (In early neonatal studies, the resistance index often was referred to as the *pulsality index*). Changes in probe angle affect the values for S and D similarly; therefore, use of the resistance index is particularly valuable to minimize the effect of probe angle and to facilitate comparisons of serial determinations of blood flow velocity. Although the use of the resistance index is valuable for assessment

of cerebrovascular resistance, changes in the end-diastolic flow velocity are most sensitive to changes in resistance. Conversely, changes in systolic flow velocity, which also can alter the resistance index, reflect particularly pump forces, such as blood pressure and cardiac output.[385] In clinical studies concerned with patent ductus arteriosus,[386] pneumothorax,[379] hydrocephalus,[387] seizures,[378] and tracheal suctioning,[388] major changes occurred principally in diastolic flow velocity, and little or no change occurred in systolic flow velocity (see later discussion).

Whereas the resistance index can provide useful information about cerebrovascular resistance, a means for estimating changes in volemic CBF with the Doppler technique has been sought. To achieve this goal, calculation of *the area under the velocity waveform* has been used to quantitate CBF velocity tracings (see Fig. 4-29). (Most ultrasonic instruments electronically determine a mean velocity, which also reflects the area under the velocity waveforms.) Determinations of the area under the velocity waveforms (and mean velocity) have been shown in neonatal animals and in human infants to correlate with simultaneous determinations of volemic CBF (see next section). One approach includes the ultrasonic determination of vascular diameter and thereby calculation of volemic flow from the product of velocity times area (see later).[389,390]

Relation of Cerebral Blood Flow Velocity to Cerebral Blood Flow and to Cerebrovascular Resistance. The two basic determinants of CBF velocity are CBF and cerebrovascular resistance. Thus, the velocity measurement can provide information about either or both of these determinants (i.e., volemic flow and resistance). The resistance index, as described earlier, is used to evaluate cerebrovascular resistance; this index is independent of angle of insonation and is determined readily. The relationship of CBF velocity, expressed as the area under the velocity waveform (see Fig. 4-29) or its analogue, the mean velocity, with volemic CBF is given by the following equation:

$$CBF \ (cm^3/time) = CBF \ velocity \ (cm/time) \times area \ (cm^2)$$

or

$$CBF \ velocity = CBF/area$$

Area refers to the cross-sectional area of the insonated vessel. CBF velocity will increase if volemic CBF increases or if the cross-sectional area of the insonated vessel decreases. A particular relation of CBF velocity (mean or area under waveform) to volemic CBF is suggested by the demonstrations in the neonatal piglet[391] and puppy[392] of an excellent correlation between CBF velocity (quantitated as the area under the velocity waveforms) and volemic CBF measured simultaneously either by radioactive microsphere or tissue-autoradiographic techniques. A significant although less robust correlation was observed in newborn lambs.[393] Moreover, studies of human newborns show good correlations between CBF velocity (quantitated as in the animal studies) and both total CBF (measured by the

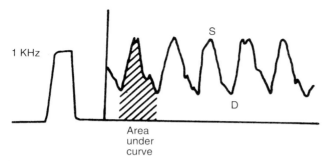

1 KHz

S

D

Area
under
curve

Figure 4-29 Cerebral blood flow velocity tracing obtained at the anterior fontanelle from the anterior cerebral artery. The deflection of the electronic internal standard is indicated to the left of the start of the tracing. S refers to peak systolic velocity, D to end diastolic velocity, and the *shaded area* to the area under one velocity waveform. The values for S and D can be used to calculate the resistance index ([S − D]/S); see text for details.

xenon-133 clearance technique)[394] and regional CBF in the distribution of the anterior cerebral artery (determined by positron emission tomography [PET]) (Table 4-16).[395] However, the *r* value for the area under the velocity waveform measurements indicated that only approximately 50% to 60% of the variance in values for CBF could be accounted for by the velocity measurements. Thus, the Doppler method was a good but not outstanding means of assessing volemic CBF.

The principal difficulty in the use of mean velocity or area under the velocity waveform to estimate changes in CBF relates to the inability to measure cross-sectional area of the insonated blood vessel. More recent developments in ultrasonic methodology may provide this ability.[389,390] The likelihood that changes in cross-sectional area do occur is shown by elegant studies in dogs, which demonstrate that large cerebral arteries account for 20% to 50% of the changes in cerebrovascular resistance that occur in response to alterations in blood pressure and blood gases.[396-399] Indeed, because in the third trimester of gestation no muscularis is present around virtually all penetrating cerebral vessels,[400] it is likely that the large extracerebral arteries (i.e., those insonated during Doppler studies and known to be invested by a muscularis[400]) are the

principal site of resistance changes, presumably by changes in their cross-sectional area. Herein lies the major difficulty for estimation of volemic CBF by Doppler. Despite this caveat, in some clinical circumstances, the technique provides useful qualitative information about cerebrovascular resistance and CBF (see later discussion).

Clinical Application

Normal Developmental Changes. Developmental changes in CBF velocity parameters have been the subject of many reports.[274,374,385,389,390,401-425] Although the data are not perfectly consistent, flow velocity generally increases in the first day of life, and resistance indices decrease. (A transient decrease in velocity and increase in resistance may occur in the first few hours after birth.) After the first postnatal day, one sees a gradual increase over the subsequent days in flow velocity (Fig. 4-30), whereas resistance indices remain more or less constant. The reasons for these changes beyond the first day are not entirely clear, but postnatal increases in blood pressure, cerebral capillary growth and recruitment, closure of the ductus arteriosus, and elevations in cerebral metabolism and blood flow (see later discussion of PET) probably play roles.

Developmental increases in volemic CBF determined by a refined Doppler method show approximately a twofold increase in flow from 32 weeks of gestation to 40 weeks.[390] The magnitude of change is similar to that obtained by PET (see later).

Changes in Cerebral Blood Flow Velocity in Neonatal Pathological States. Changes in CBF velocity have been delineated in a variety of neonatal pathological states. These findings are discussed in appropriate chapters throughout this book. In Table 4-17, I selected some of the more prominently studied states and indicated the predominant change in flow velocity (mean velocity or area under the velocity waveform) and resistance index (often termed *pulsatility index* in the literature).[274,378,379,384,386-388,391,392,394,395,407,425-460]

Clinical Value of Doppler Measurements. The previous section outlines the value of Doppler

	REGIONAL CEREBRAL BLOOD FLOW		
TABLE 4-16 Relation of Cerebral Blood Flow Velocity (CBFV) in the Anterior Cerebral Artery to Regional Cerebral Blood Flow in the Human Newborn*			
CBFV Measurement	**Frontal***	**Sylvian***	
Area under the velocity curve	0.77	0.71	$P < .001$
Resistance index	−0.67	−0.69	$P < .001$
Peak systolic flow velocity	0.21	0.17	$P > .05$
End-diastolic flow velocity	0.65	0.73	$P < .001$

*Regional CBF obtained from anterior and medial frontal cortex, in the distribution of the anterior cerebral artery, and from sylvian cortex, in the distribution of the middle cerebral artery. Values for *r* are shown. Values for left cerebral regions were used for calculations for consistency (right cerebral values did not differ significantly from left).
CBFV, cerebral blood flow velocity.
Data from Perlman JM, Herscovitch P, Corriveau S: The relationship of cerebral blood flow velocity, determined by Doppler, to regional cerebral blood flow, determined by positron emission tomography [abstract], *Pediatr Res* 19:357, 1985; *n* = 25 premature infants.

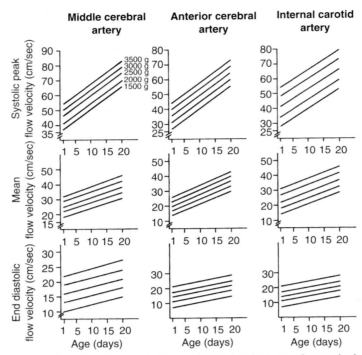

Figure 4-30 Mean reference values of cerebral blood flow velocities in middle cerebral, anterior cerebral, and internal carotid arteries from 1 to 20 days for infants of the indicated birth weights. *(From Bode H, Wais U: Age dependence of flow velocities in basal cerebral arteries,* Arch Dis Child *63:606-611, 1988.)*

measurements of CBF velocity in primarily research studies. The question of the clinical value of Doppler remains to be delineated clearly. In Table 4-18, I summarize the several situations in which I believe that Doppler measurements of CBF velocity are clinically useful. Thus, Doppler measurements are clearly useful in demonstration of cessation of CBF, whether to the entire brain (as with brain death; see next paragraph), to the distribution of a single major cerebral artery (as with cerebral infarction), or with thrombosis of a large vein or venous sinus. In addition, Doppler measurements of the resistance index are of proven value for prognostic purposes in infants with postasphyxial hypoxic-ischemic encephalopathy (see Chapter 9) and are very useful in management of posthemorrhagic hydrocephalus (see Chapter 11). Doppler, particularly color flow Doppler, is useful in identification of the

TABLE 4-17 Changes in Cerebral Blood Flow Velocity in Neonatal Pathological States*

	CEREBRAL BLOOD FLOW VELOCITY	
Pathological State	**Velocity**	**Resistance Index**
Apnea	↓	
Brain death	↓	↑
Perinatal cerebral infarction	↓↓ to 0	
Seizures	↑	↓
Marked hypercarbia	±↑	↓
Following blood transfusion for anemia	↓	↑
Polycythemia	↓	↑
"Postasphyxial" state	↓ Early, ↑ later	↓
Patent ductus arteriosus	↓	↑
Arteriovenous malformation	↑	↓
Cerebral venous thrombosis	↓↓ to 0	
Hydrocephalus	±↓	↑
Pharmacological Interventions		
Aminophylline	±↓	
Caffeine	±↓	
Doxapram	±↓	
Halothane anesthesia	↓	
Indomethacin	↓	

*See text for references.

TABLE 4-18 Clinical Value of Doppler Measurements of Cerebral Blood Flow Velocity in the Newborn*

Cessation of Cerebral Blood Flow
Brain death
Cerebrovascular occlusion (arterial or venous)

Alterations of Cerebrovascular Resistance
Hypoxic-ischemic encephalopathy
Hydrocephalus†
Arteriovenous malformation†

Ductal steal: patent ductus arteriosus†

*Does not include research applications of Doppler measurements (see text and Table 4-19 for details).
†Clinical value of Doppler measurement likely but not yet conclusively demonstrated in the newborn.

ACA   CCA

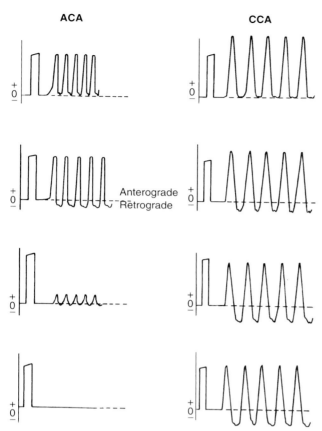

Anterograde
Retrograde

Figure 4-31 **Sequence of changes in blood flow velocity obtained from the anterior cerebral artery (ACA) and common carotid artery (CCA) with the development of brain death.** This sequence was observed over 3 to 4 days in an infant with development of brain death after hypoxic-ischemic insult. See text for details.

vascular supply and drainage of cerebral arteriovenous malformation. Finally, delineation of ductal steal, particularly retrograde flow in diastole in cerebral vessels in the presence of large patent ductus arteriosus, may prove to be of value in defining a risk for ischemic injury to brain (see Chapters 8 and 9).

Doppler Technique in the Determination of Neonatal Brain Death. McMenamin and I defined the changes in flow velocity in the anterior cerebral artery in infants who meet the clinical criteria for brain death.[427] A characteristic sequence of deterioration of the flow velocity pattern is observed (Fig. 4-31). This sequence in the cerebral circulation consists of a loss of diastolic flow, the appearance of retrograde flow during diastole, diminution of systolic flow, and the absence of detectable flow in the cerebral circulation. At the time of no detectable flow in the cerebral circulation, simultaneous study of the common carotid artery demonstrated preserved flow (presumably for the external carotid circulation; see Fig. 4-31). These findings are compatible with a progressive increase in cerebrovascular resistance and, as a consequence, a progressive decrease in cerebral perfusion secondary to diffuse cerebral necrosis. These observations indicate that the Doppler technique is a useful complement to other noninvasive methods, especially clinical assessment

and EEG, in the determination of brain death in the newborn. These initial observations were confirmed.[438,439,461] In addition, a reverberating pattern of flow with short forward flow in systole and short retrograde flow in diastole has been defined in brain-dead infants.[461] However, infants who are considered brain dead by clinical and EEG criteria may exhibit flow velocity signals in large extraparenchymal cerebral arteries, and cessation of flow velocity in cerebral arteries may occur in death of cerebrum but preservation of brain stem (and therefore capacity for survival).

Near-Infrared Spectroscopy

NIRS is an optical technique of potential value in the study of the newborn because the method is capable of providing crucial information concerning cerebral hemoglobin oxygen saturation, cerebral blood volume, CBF, cerebral oxygen delivery, cerebral venous oxygen saturation, and cerebral oxygen availability and utilization. The application of NIRS to the study of animal brain in vivo was initially shown most clearly in 1977 by Jobsis,[462] who demonstrated that absorption of near-infrared light of wave lengths between 700 to 1000 nm by soft tissue was low enough to allow spectral measurements to be made from brain when the light was directed across the cranium.

Basic Principles and Determinations

The NIRS method is based on two basic facts.[463-467] First, light in the near-infrared range can pass with relative ease through the thin skin, bone, and other tissues of the infant to allow photon transmission to occur primarily through brain. Second, by appropriate selection of near-infrared wave lengths, changes in light absorption that are characteristic of oxygenated and deoxygenated hemoglobin (Hb) and of oxidized cytochrome aa3 (i.e., cytochrome oxidase [$CytO_2$]) can be used to monitor quantitatively changes in the amounts of oxygenated hemoglobin (HbO_2) and Hb and the oxidation-reduction state of $CytO_2$, the terminal enzyme of the respiratory mitochondrial electron transport chain, which passes electrons to molecular oxygen for oxidative phosphorylation and synthesis of adenosine triphosphate (ATP) (Fig. 4-32 and Table 4-19).

NIRS instrumentation was used first in validation experiments in animals, and then in human newborns, to make *quantitative* assessment of changes in the amounts of cerebral HbO_2 and Hb, blood volume, CBF, cerebral venous oxygen saturation, and tissue oxygenation.[463,464,467-513]

The *near-infrared apparatus* (from Hamamatsu Photonics, Hamamatsu, Japan) that my colleagues and I use employs a flexible fiberoptic bundle conveying near-infrared light from laser diodes to the head. The end of the fiber bundle ("optode") is applied to the scalp in the parietal region at a site equidistant from the anterior fontanelle and the external auditory meatus. An identical bundle on the opposite side of the head (the end of which constitutes another optode) conveys transmitted light to a sensitive photomultiplier

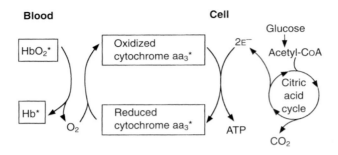

* = Measured by near infrared spectroscopy

Figure 4-32 Schematic of cerebral oxygen delivery by hemoglobin and intracellular oxygen utilization. See text for details. The *asterisk* denotes values measured by near-infrared spectroscopy. ATP, adenosine triphosphate; CoA, coenzyme A; Hb, hemoglobin; HbO₂, oxygenated hemoglobin.

TABLE 4-19 Near-Infrared Spectroscopy
Principle
By appropriate selection of near-infrared wavelengths, can detect changes in absorbance of HbO₂, Hb, and the oxidation-reduction state of cytochrome aa₃
Determinations
Continuous Measurements
Oxygen available in cerebral blood: by measuring HbO₂
Cerebral blood volume: by measuring sum of Hb and HbO₂
Cerebral perfusion: by measuring HbD (see text)
Intracellular oxygen availability or utilization: by measuring relative oxidation-reduction state of cytochrome aa₃
Serial Measurements
Cerebral blood flow: by measuring "wash-in" of HbO₂ after brief administration of oxygen
Cerebral venous oxygen saturation: by measuring the change in Hb and HbO₂ after tilting the infant head down
Cerebral function: by measuring the change in HB and HBO₂ after stimulation

Hb, deoxygenated hemoglobin; HbD, difference between oxygenated and deoxygenated hemoglobin (HbD = HbO₂ − Hb); HbO₂, oxygenated hemoglobin.

tube (Fig. 4-33). This approach generally is termed *transmission NIRS;* when placement of the optodes is such that they are not on opposite sides of the head, the term *reflectance NIRS* generally is used. There is little fundamental difference in these approaches. To prevent interference from background illumination, the head is wrapped in a light-tight bandage. A controlling computer calculates the changes in optical absorption at each wavelength and converts these into changes of HbO₂, Hb, and CytO₂.

To obtain *quantitative measurements of molar changes in HbO₂, Hb, and CytO₂ in the brain of infants,* the following calculations are important.[463] The calculation of chromophore concentrations from absorption changes makes use of the *Beer-Lambert law,* which when describing optical absorption in a highly scattering medium, may be expressed as follows:

$$\text{Absorption (OD)} = (acLB) + G$$

in which OD is optical density, a is the extinction coefficient of the chromophore (mM⁻¹/cm⁻¹), c is concentration of the chromophore (mM), L is the distance between the points where light enters and leaves the tissue (cm), B is a "pathlength factor" that takes account of the scattering of light in the tissue

(which causes the optical pathlength to be greater than L), and G is a factor related to the tissue type and measurement geometry. Assuming that L, B, and G remain constant during the study, changes in chromophore concentration can be obtained from the following expression:

$$\Delta c = \Delta OD/aLB$$

The extinction coefficients of HbO₂, Hb, and CytO₂ have been determined,[475,482] and B has been derived by several methods, all of which have given similar results. These include measurement of the time of flight of photons through tissues,[484] as well as utilization of phase-resolved spectroscopy.[482,496] In the brains of preterm infants, the value of B determined by the "time of flight" method was 4.39 (+SD 0.28).[480] Values obtained by phase-resolved spectroscopy are similar and have been shown to increase only approximately 10% by the age of 15 years.[496]

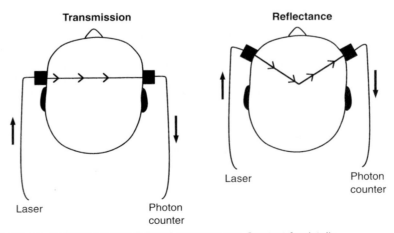

Figure 4-33 Schematic of placement of optodes in near-infrared spectroscopy. See text for details.

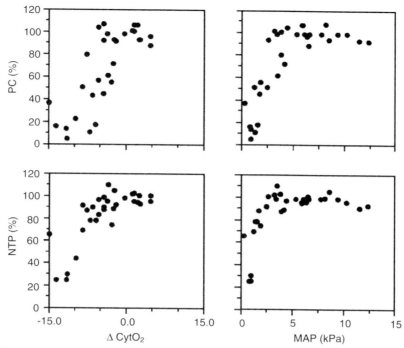

Figure 4-34 Plots obtained in neonatal piglets of phosphocreatine (PC) and nucleoside triphosphate (NTP) (primarily adenosine triphosphate [ATP]), both determined by phosphorus magnetic resonance spectroscopy, as a function of cytochrome oxidase (CytO$_2$), determined by near-infrared spectroscopy, and of mean arterial blood pressure (MAP). With the decline in MAP, PC and then NTP decrease. See text for details. *(From Tsuji M, Naruse H, Volpe JJ, Holtzman D: Reduction of cytochrome aa3 measured by near-infrared spectroscopy predicts cerebral energy loss in hypoxic piglets, Pediatr Res 37:253-259, 1995.)*

Clinical Application

Application to human infants has provided insights into the value of the NIRS in the assessment of cerebral physiology and metabolism in vivo and into potential mechanisms of brain injury in specific clinical situations. These insights are described briefly next.

Quantitative Determinations of Oxygenated Hemoglobin, Deoxygenated Hemoglobin, Cerebral Blood Volume, Cerebral Blood Flow, Cerebral Venous Oxygen Saturation, and Cytochrome Oxidase in the Newborn. A large series of studies, particularly by the research group at University College in London, initially provided major insight both into the potential value of NIRS in the study of the newborn brain and into the regulation of cerebral hemodynamics and oxygen delivery. Using the principles and background data described earlier, the British group obtained crucial quantitative data. In an initial report, Wyatt and co-workers[476] showed that cerebral HbO$_2$ decreases with a modest decrease in arterial oxygen saturation, and cerebral blood volume increases, presumably as a result of cerebral vasodilation, with an increase in arterial partial pressure of carbon dioxide (Pa$_{CO_2}$).

NIRS provides some insight into the regulation of the *oxidation-reduction state of cytochrome aa$_3$*, crucial for the assessment of oxidative metabolism, in human neonatal brain. Delpy and co-workers[477] showed that with a marked abrupt decrease in arterial oxygen saturation (from 95% to 70% in 5 minutes), a decrease in cerebral

CytO$_2$ also could be demonstrated. However, changes in CytO$_2$ in response to hypoxia are uncommon, except with marked decreases in oxygen saturation.[485] In the dog, Tamura and Chance and their co-workers[468] showed that CytO$_2$ does not begin to decrease until cerebral hemoglobin oxygen saturation decreases to approximately 10%. Using simultaneous MR spectroscopy, Chance and co-workers showed that the ratio of phosphocreatine to inorganic phosphate also did not decrease until this critical low threshold of cerebral hemoglobin oxygen saturation was reached and CytO$_2$ began to decline. Studies in neonatal piglets showed that such severe hypoxia resulted in a decline in arterial blood pressure; when the latter occurred, phosphocreatine and then ATP levels declined in parallel with CytO$_2$ levels (Fig. 4-34).[498] Similar correlations of decreases in CytO$_2$ with decreases in high-energy phosphates during postasphyxial delayed cerebral energy failure have been made.[514] These experiments showed the particular importance of cerebral *ischemia* in causing cytochrome reduction. In contrast to the relative stability of CytO$_2$ to hypoxemia, Edwards and co-workers[485] showed in the human newborn a striking relationship between *changes in Pa$_{CO_2}$ and CytO$_2$* (Fig. 4-35). In view of the potent effect of Pa$_{CO_2}$ on CBF, this observation further suggests that in the newborn, the concentration of oxidized CytO$_2$ is related closely to blood flow, a conclusion that is consistent with clinical observations that ischemia is the predominant deleterious factor in the pathogenesis of hypoxic-ischemic brain injury (see Chapters 6 and 8).

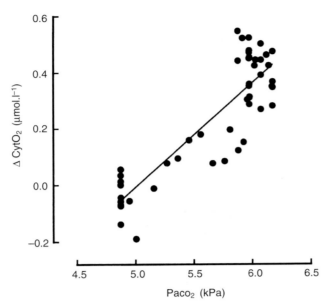

Figure 4-35 **Relationship between arterial pressure of carbon dioxide (Paco₂) and cytochrome oxidase (CytO₂) in a 1-day-old infant of 34 weeks of gestation.** Each point is an average value for a 20-second time period. *(From Edwards AD, Brown GC, Cope M, Wyatt JS, et al: Quantification of concentration changes in neonatal human cerebral oxidized cytochrome oxidase, J Appl Physiol 71:1907-1913, 1991.)*

Wyatt and co-workers[483,515] described the use of NIRS to *quantitate cerebral blood volume* and obtained a mean value in premature infants of 2.22 mL/100 g, comparing favorably with the values (2.5 mL/100 g) that my colleagues and I[515] had obtained previously by PET (see Table 4-19). Similar values were obtained by NIRS in a later study.[502] This quantitative approach was used to demonstrate an increase in cerebral blood volume to increases in Paco₂ in newborns and an increase in this reactivity of cerebral blood volume to Paco₂ with gestational age.[481] Other investigators also showed, using NIRS, that cerebral blood volume increases with increases in Paco₂ and simultaneously demonstrated by xenon-133 clearance that this increase in blood volume was associated with an increase in CBF (as expected from the vasodilation caused by increases in Paco₂).[516]

Edwards and co-workers[478] then developed a technique for *measurement of CBF*, which employs the Fick principle and the measurement by NIRS of the rate of increase in cerebral HbO₂ after an increase in arterial oxygen saturation induced by a brief inhalation of oxygen. The mean value of CBF obtained in 13 premature infants (18 mL/100g/minute) compares closely with similar values previously obtained by the techniques of xenon-133 clearance and by PET (see later and Chapter 6).[517] With the NIRS method, Wyatt and co-workers demonstrated a postnatal increase of CBF, presumably related to increased left ventricular output and decreased cerebrovascular resistance, over the first several days of life.[502] Similarly, this approach allowed the demonstration by NIRS of increasing cerebral oxygen consumption over the first weeks and months of life.[503] More recently, an increase in cerebral tissue oxygenation was shown over the same time period.[510]

Edwards and co-workers used the NIRS method for measurement of CBF to demonstrate, after injection of indomethacin to premature infants, a sharp decrease in CBF, oxygen delivery, cerebral blood volume, and reactivity of cerebral blood volume to change in Pco₂. These findings are compatible with experimental data indicating that indomethacin is a cerebral vasoconstrictor. This effect was not observed with ibuprofen.[513]

Two separate groups showed a good correlation between values of CBF obtained by NIRS and values simultaneously obtained by xenon-133 clearance.[486,494,516,518,519] The difficulties inherent with this method, dependent on the induction of an abrupt increase in HbO₂, could be overcome by the use of *indocyanine green*, a chromophore that elicits an absorption peak in the near-infrared range and is restricted to the intravascular compartment after intravenous infusion.[520-522] Studies of newborn infants have demonstrated the feasibility and potential accuracy of this technique.[521,522]

Cerebral venous oxygen saturation has been determined in the newborn by measuring the change in Hb and HbO₂ after briefly tilting the infant head-down at 15 degrees.[463,476,486,503] Cerebral venous oxygen saturation can be calculated with the assumption that the increase in cerebral blood volume consists of venous blood only. Skov and co-workers[486] showed that cerebral venous oxygen saturation is elevated in asphyxiated term infants with other indications of brain injury, consistent with the occurrence of diminished oxygen utilization after hypoxic-ischemic brain injury.

Work by our group suggests that the NIRS determination of the difference between the (arterial-weighted) HbO₂ signal and the (venous-weighted) Hb signal (i.e., HbD) correlates closely with CBF. Because HbD is obtained continuously by NIRS without manipulation of the infant, such a continuous measure of cerebral perfusion would be a major advance in the capability of NIRS. In two studies of neonatal piglets in which cerebral perfusion pressure was decreased, either by induction of hypotension[505] or by acute elevation of intracranial pressure,[523] the HbD signal changed in parallel with CBF measured simultaneously by the radioactive microsphere method (Fig. 4-36). This approach has been used to define a pressure-passive cerebral circulation in sick premature newborns[509,509a] (see Chapters 6, 8 and 9) and in infants following cardiac surgery.[524]

Value of Near-Infrared Spectroscopy in Specific Clinical Situations. Several studies documented the value of NIRS in a specific clinical situation. For example, in a study of nine preterm infants with *apnea and bradycardia*, sharp decreases in HbO₂ and in cerebral blood volume were documented. These observations suggest that both cerebral oxygen delivery and CBF were impaired.[525] This apparent impairment in CBF with apnea and bradycardia is consistent with the findings of an earlier study of similar infants by Doppler.[526] Similar but less pronounced findings have been observed during the apneic phase of *periodic breathing* in term infants.[511] In a study of *endotracheal suctioning*

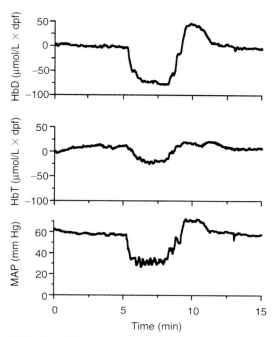

Figure 4-36 Near-infrared spectroscopic determinations in neonatal piglets during hypotension showing concordant changes between cerebral intravascular oxygenation (HbD) and mean arterial blood pressure (MAP). See text for details. HbT, total cerebral blood volume. *(From Tsuji M, du Plessis A, Taylor G, Crocker R, et al: Near infrared spectroscopy detects cerebral ischemia during hypotension in piglets, Pediatr Res 44:591-595, 1998.)*

in preterm infants, the systemic decrease in arterial hemoglobin saturation was accompanied by a decrease in cerebral hemoglobin saturation and an increase in cerebral blood volume.[527] These findings are consistent with the observations during suctioning of elevated central venous pressure and intracranial pressure in the preterm infant.[388,528] In a study of *gavage feeding* of small preterm infants, decreased cerebral blood volume and HbO_2 were documented.[512] In a study of *severely asphyxiated infants*, decreases in cerebral levels of $CytO_2$ have been demonstrated.[493] An investigation of the cerebral hemodynamic effects of *surfactant treatment* of premature infants with respiratory distress syndrome disclosed only small transient perturbations in cerebral HbO_2 concentration and in cerebral blood volume.[487] Parallel changes in the sum of HbO_2 and Hb (i.e., cerebral blood volume) and in mean arterial blood pressure during *exchange transfusion* suggested an impairment of cerebrovascular autoregulation and of changes in cerebral perfusion with this procedure.[495] With *extracorporeal membrane oxygenation*, an increase in cerebral HbO_2 and in arterial blood pressure after starting the procedure suggested the possibility of reactive hyperemia and perhaps impaired cerebrovascular autoregulation.[500] In the first 3 days of life, infants who later exhibit *severe intraventricular hemorrhage* experience fluctuations in cerebral oxygen extraction as determined by NIRS.[529] The finding is consistent with fluctuating CBF, found to be an important pathogenetic factor for such hemorrhage (see Chapter 11). With *deep hypothermic cardiac surgery with cardiopulmonary bypass* in infants, du Plessis and

co-workers[499] demonstrated a paradoxical dissociation of changes in intravascular (HbO_2) and mitochondrial ($CytO_2$) oxygenation, with a pronounced decrease in $CytO_2$ occurring during a period of rising HbO_2 (Fig. 4-37). The data suggest potentially deleterious impairments of intrinsic mitochondrial function or of delivery of intravascular oxygenation or both during the procedure. Moreover, the same group has shown a pressure-passive cerebral circulation following such surgery.[524]

Thus, it is now clear that NIRS can be applied in vivo to the human infant and can provide frequent, noninvasive, largely qualitative determinations of cerebral HbO_2 and Hb concentrations, cerebral blood volume, cerebral perfusion, oxygen delivery, cerebral venous oxygen saturation, and the oxidation state of cytochrome aa_3. The challenge for the technology is development of the capacity to provide continuous absolute values of these parameters. The currently used continuous wave instruments have not provided that capability. However, more recent work with time-resolved spectroscopy and intensity-modulated spectroscopy shows promise but will require further development.[467,530]

Utilization of NIRS for the study of *cortical activation* has been accomplished by detecting hemodynamic responses to visual, auditory, and olfactory stimulation and to pain (see Table 4-19).[531-537] The approach appears capable for detecting and generally localizing functional cortical activity in the living infant as young as 25 weeks of gestation. Initial research involved the study of the effects of visual activation in the newborn infant (Fig. 4-38).[504] Thus, with visual stimulation, an abrupt increase in cerebral blood volume, caused by an increase in both HbO_2 and Hb (findings presumably reflecting an increase in both local CBF and oxygen consumption) was documented by NIRS optodes over the occipital region. More recent studies have involved olfactory, auditory, sensorimotor, and photic stimulation, with the optodes placed on the cranium over the appropriate cortical regions.[533,534,538-540]

An extension of NIRS to accomplish more refined spatial localization includes *optical topography* and *optical tomography*. The former provides relatively rapid two-dimensional localization, valuable for functional studies, and the latter, a more detailed and slightly slower approach with multiple optodes, provides three-dimensional localization, valuable for localization of pathology.[541,542] More recent refinements of the tomographic methodology indicate a potential for functional studies as well.[543]

PHYSIOLOGICAL BRAIN IMAGING

In this section, I describe techniques that provide an image of physiological phenomena, including biochemical constituents, CBF, oxygen and glucose consumption, and neuronal activity. MR spectroscopy is crucial for biochemical information, PET for hemodynamic and metabolic insights, and functional MRI (fMRI) for neuronal activity. These methods are discussed briefly next.

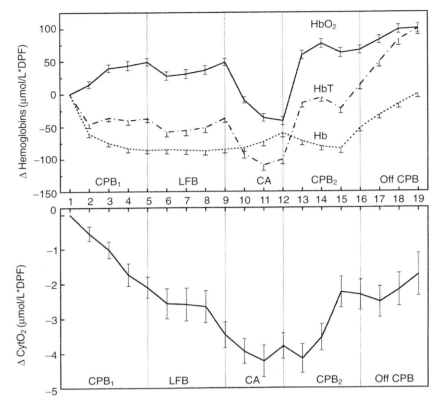

Figure 4-37   Near-infrared spectroscopic determinations of the hemoglobin (Hb) signals (*upper panel*) and of cytochrome oxidase (CytO₂) (*lower panel*) in 63 infants during deep hypothermia with core cooling cardiopulmonary bypass (**CPB₁**), low flow bypass (**LFB**), circulatory arrest (**CA**), rewarming bypass (**CPB₂**), and removal of bypass (**Off CPB**). See text for details. DPF, differential pathlength factor; HbO₂, oxygenated hemoglobin, HbT, total hemoglobin. *(From du Plessis AJ, Newburger J, Jonas RA, Hickey P, et al: Cerebral oxygen supply and utilization during infant cardiac surgery,* Ann Neurol *37:488-497, 1995.)*

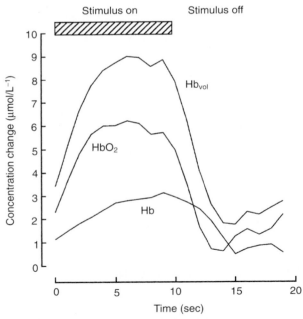

Figure 4-38   Near-infrared spectroscopic determinations of oxygenated hemoglobin (HbO₂), hemoglobin (Hb), and Hb_vol (sum of HbO₂ and Hb) over occipital cortex with visual stimulation averaged over nine cycles in the same infant. See text for details. *(From Meek JH, Firbank M, Elwell CE, Atkinson J, et al: Regional hemodynamic responses to visual stimulation in awake infants,* Pediatr Res *43:840-843, 1998.)*

Magnetic Resonance Spectroscopy

MR spectroscopy should be discussed in this context because it provides the capability for the continuous or frequent assessment of selected cerebral biochemical constituents. In the following discussion, I emphasize only the insights provided by MR spectroscopy into normal biochemical development. The clinical application of MR spectroscopy has become nearly routine and thus is cited in relevant chapters throughout the book. The basic principles of the technique, all nuclear species detectable by MR spectroscopy in vivo, and experimental studies using MR spectroscopy, were reviewed in previous editions of this book; they have been deleted from this edition for the purpose of conservation of space.

Clinical Applications

Magnetic Resonance Spectroscopic Studies in Neonatal Humans. MR spectroscopy has been applied to the study of human newborns during both normal maturation and a variety of pathological conditions.[289,306,477,544-591] The studies have addressed primarily infants who were normal or who had been asphyxiated, had sustained other ischemic injury, or had exhibited seizures; the results are described in relevant subsequent chapters. Much of the earlier work focused on phosphorus MR spectroscopy, and

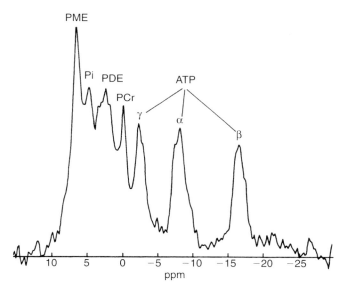

Figure 4-39 **Magnetic resonance (phosphorus-31) spectrum of normal infant.** Individual peaks are indicated. ATP, adenosine triphosphate; PCr, phosphocreatine; PDE, phosphodiesters; Pi, inorganic phosphate; PME, phosphomonoesters. *(Courtesy of Dr. Donald Younkin.)*

much of the more recent work has focused on proton MR spectroscopy.

The *phosphorus MR spectrum* of a normal infant is shown in Figure 4-39. The essential finding is the demonstration of the major phosphorus-containing constituents important for energy metabolism (the alpha, beta, and gamma forms of ATP, phosphocreatine, and inorganic phosphate[592]). In addition, peaks corresponding to phosphodiesters (largely phospholipids) and phosphomonoesters (largely ethanolamine phosphate) can be demonstrated (see later discussion). Because the concentration of hydrogen ions affects the chemical shift of inorganic phosphate but not of

phosphocreatine, the relation between the two peaks provides a measure of intracellular pH.

Normal developmental changes in phosphorus metabolites have been defined (Fig. 4-40).[556,559,579,593] A linear increase in the concentration of phosphocreatine relative to inorganic phosphorus is striking. A similar change has been noted in developing rat brain.[594] This increase in phosphocreatine reflects an increase in energy reserve that perhaps is coupled with an increase in energy demands as cerebral metabolic rate increases (see later discussion of PET). This increase in high-energy phosphates continues throughout the first 1 to 2 years of life, again in keeping with increasing cerebral metabolic rate, perhaps associated with the synaptogenesis and related aspects of cortical organizational development (see Chapter 2 and later discussion of PET).[559,579]

Accompanying the developmental change in high-energy phosphates is a decrease in phosphomonoesters and an increase in phosphodiesters (see Fig. 4-40). The phosphomonoesters consist primarily of ethanolamine phosphate, a key precursor of phospholipids of cellular membranes (including myelin), and the phosphodiesters consist primarily of the phospholipids, phosphatidylethanolamine, and phosphatidylcholine, key membrane phospholipids.[594,595] These changes appear to correlate well with the membrane proliferation associated with organizational events and with myelination (see Chapter 2).

The *proton MR spectra* of normal infants at 33 and 39 weeks of gestational age are shown in Figure 4-41. The principal peaks are the methyl protons of myoinositol, a cyclic sugar alcohol, N-acetyl–containing compounds, primarily N-acetylaspartic acid (NAA), the N-methyl protons of creatine and phosphocreatine, and the N-methyl protons of choline.[578] The methyl protons of lactate can be demonstrated when lactate is elevated. NAA is considered usually a "neuronal" marker, the

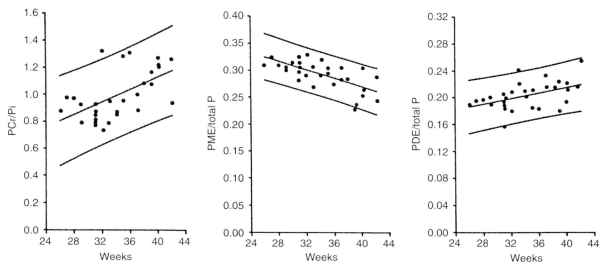

Figure 4-40 **Relationship between metabolite concentration ratios and gestational plus postnatal age in 30 infants of average weight for gestational age (AGA).** Regression lines and 95% confidence limits are shown. P, phosphorus, PCr, phosphocreatine; PDE, phosphodiesters; Pi, inorganic phosphate; PME, phosphomonoesters. *(From Azzopardi D, Wyatt JS, Hamilton PA, Cady EB, et al: Phosphorus metabolites and intracellular pH in the brains of normal and small for gestational age infants investigated by magnetic resonance, Pediatr Res 25:440-444, 1989.)*

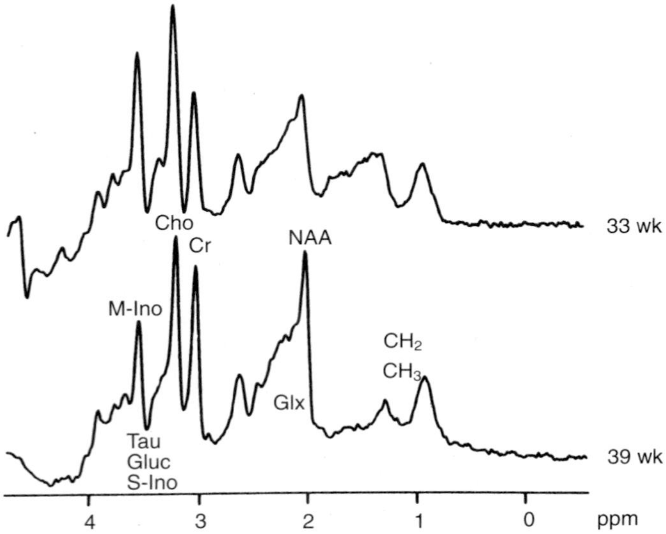

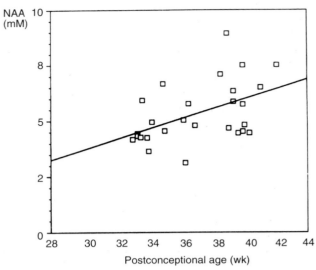

Figure 4-41 **Proton magnetic resonance spectra from the paracentral cerebral region of infants of 33 and 39 weeks of gestation.** The principal peaks are myo-inositol (M-Ino), choline (Cho), creatine (Cr), glutamate-glutamine (Glx), N-acetylaspartic acid (NAA), and methyl and methylene groups (CH_3, CH_2) of lipids and macromolecules. Note the increase in NAA with development. Glu, glucose; S-Ino, scyllo-inositol; Tau, taurine. *(From Huppi PS, Fusch C, Boesch C, Burri R, et al: Regional metabolic assessment of human brain during development by proton magnetic resonance spectroscopy in vivo and by high-performance liquid chromatography/gas chromatography in autopsy tissue, Pediatr Res 37:145-150, 1995.)*

Figure 4-42 **Proton magnetic resonance spectroscopic determinations of cerebral concentration of N-acetylaspartic acid (NAA) (squares) as a function of postconceptional age.** Note the increase in NAA with development. *(From Huppi PS, Fusch C, Boesch C, Burri R, et al: Regional metabolic assessment of human brain during development by proton magnetic resonance spectroscopy in vivo and by high-performance liquid chromatography/gas chromatography in autopsy tissue, Pediatr Res 37:145-150, 1995.)*

creatine compounds relate primarily to energy metabolism, choline-containing compounds are related primarily to membranes, and lactate accumulation occurs with anaerobic glycolysis or mitochondrial dysfunction, among other causes.[578]

Normal developmental changes in the metabolites demonstrated by proton MR spectroscopy have been defined in several studies.* The principal change is an increase in brain concentrations of NAA; the relatively low levels present in the premature infant increase approximately twofold by term (see Fig. 4-41; Fig. 4-42). Another approximately twofold increase occurs in the first year of life. The cellular origin of NAA is principally neuronal/axonal. Although studies of cells in culture indicate that the NAA concentration in immature and mature oligodendrocytes is appreciable, the levels are less than one half of those of cortical neurons.[597] Moreover, in intact tissue (e.g., transected optic nerve), 80% to 95% of the NAA is lost with axonal degeneration, despite the presence of proliferating oligodendrocyte progenitors.[598] NAA does increase in concentration in parallel with myelination, in part because of an increase of NAA in oligodendrocytes but perhaps more importantly because of axonal enlargement that accompanies myelin development.[599]

A particular value for proton MR spectroscopy in the study of infants exposed to hypoxic-ischemic insults is apparent.[289,567,573-576,578,580,587-591] In infants studied in the first days after the insult, the principal changes, discussed further in Chapter 9, consist of an increase in lactate; infants studied later ($\approx$1 week) have less

consistent abnormality of lactate but reduced NAA. The magnitude of the increases in lactate and, especially, the decreases in NAA, correlate with the severity of neurological outcome.

Positron Emission Tomography

PET has provided the capability of obtaining in vivo *regional* physiological and biochemical information about human brain in health and disease. This capability is the product of four major developments in the necessary technology, specifically, the apparatus for nuclear bombardment (i.e., the cyclotron) to produce positron-emitting isotopes, the techniques for rapid synthesis of radiopharmaceuticals necessary for biochemical and physiological studies, the mathematical models and practical algorithms to obtain the critical information from the data, and the PET instrumentation to detect the radiopharmaceuticals safely in vivo in a regional and quantitative manner.[600-604] The basic principles of PET and the methodological aspects of the most important measurements afforded by the technique were described in previous editions of this book and are deleted from this edition to conserve space.

Clinical Application

Normal Regional and Developmental Aspects. Regional aspects of *CBF* in the newborn have been defined by study principally of term infants with PET. Thus, using the $H_2{}^{15}O$ technique for determining CBF in the term newborn, my colleagues and I demonstrated highest flows in cerebral cortex and deep nuclear structures, particularly thalamus and brain stem.[605] In infants without evidence of brain injury,

---

*See references 289,306,333,564,567,570-573,578,581,582,596

TABLE 4-20	Cerebral Blood Flow Determined by Positron Emission Tomography in Premature and Term Newborns without Major Brain Injury*				
Group	Gestational Age (Weeks)	Birth Weight (g)	Age at PET Scan (Days)	Cerebral Blood Flow (mL/100 g/min)	Age at Follow-up (Months)
Premature newborns	29.8	1339	12	10.6	19
Term newborns	—	3259	17	23.1	14
Adults	—	—	—	48.4 ± 7.8	—

*Values are means derived from 10 premature and 8 term infants studied in the newborn period and found to be neurologically normal, cognitively normal, or both on follow-up.

PET, positron emission tomography.

Data from Altman DI, Powers WJ, Perlman JM, Herscovitch P, et al: Cerebral blood flow requirement for brain viability in newborn infants is lower than in adults, *Ann Neurol* 24:218-226, 1988. Mean cerebral blood flow was measured by PET with $H_2^{15}O$. The value (mean ± SD) for adults is derived from normal individuals studied by the same technique in the same laboratory; the value is from Powers WJ, Grubb RL, Darriet D, Raichle ME: Cerebral blood flow and cerebral metabolic rate of oxygen requirements for cerebral function and viability in humans, *J Cereb Blood Flow Metab* 5:600-608, 1985.

cerebral cortical flows were approximately 50% higher than flows in cerebral white matter. Higher flows in cerebral cortex versus white matter also were observed in studies of infants of approximately 36 weeks of postconceptional age by the xenon-133 clearance technique and of infants of approximately 28 weeks by single photon emission tomography.[553,606] In all studies, flows in frontal cortical regions were lower than in paracentral cortical structures. The major regional findings are similar to those obtained in neonatal animals.[607-609] Moreover, *a close coupling of CBF and cerebral metabolism is shown by similar regional differences in cerebral metabolic rates for both glucose and oxygen*.[515,604,610-616]

Developmental data for *CBF* of the human newborn have been obtained by the PET $H_2^{15}O$ technique. The observations suggest a distinct developmental change in the neonatal period (Table 4-20).[515,517,613,616,617] Thus, an approximately twofold higher mean CBF was observed in term infants versus preterm infants who did not exhibit major brain injury on follow-up (i.e., were either neurologically or cognitively normal or both on follow-up).

In addition to the apparent developmental increase in CBF over the last months of gestation, particularly noteworthy are the *low absolute values* of flow in the premature newborn. Thus, in the infants studied by PET, the mean CBF was 10.6 mL/100 g/minute (see Table 4-20). Virtually identical values were obtained by other investigators who employed the xenon-133 clearance technique after *intravenous* injection (see Chapter 6).[518,519,618-626] Values in premature newborns in the latter studies varied from approximately 10 to 20 mL/100 g/minute, with the highest values in infants who are more mature, stable, nonventilated, and beyond the first days of life.

The extent to which these absolute values for CBF obtained in human premature infants by PET and by xenon-133 clearance are indeed low is emphasized when considered in the context of ischemic thresholds in the adult. Thus, in adults studied because of cerebrovascular disease, CBF values lower than 17 to 18 mL/100 g/minute have been associated with EEG or clinical disturbance (i.e., hemiparesis).[627-632] Moreover, CBF values lower than 10 mL/100 g/minute have been observed only in infarcted tissue,[630]

and thus this level is considered a threshold of viability. Clearly, such values are compatible with normal brain structure and function in the human premature infant. In our series, three infants with mean CBF values of 4.9, 5.2, and 9.3 were subsequently normal neurologically and cognitively, and the overall outcome of premature infants with values lower than 10 mg/100 g/ minute was no different from the outcome of those with values higher than 10 mL/100 g/minute.[517] Moreover, Griesen and co-workers[621,622] showed that CBF values as low as approximately 5 mL/100 g/minute are associated with normal visual evoked responses and preserved EEG activity in premature infants.

These remarkably low values of CBF appear to be coupled to *similarly low rates of cerebral oxygen consumption*. Thus, in a study of five premature and five term infants, all values for cerebral metabolic rate for oxygen were below the threshold of viability for adult brain (i.e., 1.3 mL/100 g/minute) (Table 4-21).[613,630] Indeed, the values in the premature infants were very close to zero, particularly in cerebral white matter. Moreover, an even more prominent increase in cerebral metabolic rate for oxygen was observed between term versus preterm infants than was observed for CBF. Striking also is the low oxygen extraction fraction in both premature and term infants, and indeed in the premature infant the value was close to zero. The low oxygen extraction fraction attests further to the relative lack of interest of newborn brain in oxygen for its metabolism. Studies in a variety of animals also show striking increases in cerebral metabolic rate for oxygen with development, with the timing varying primarily with the progression of structural, biochemical, and functional parameters of brain development.[39,633-640]

The finding of very low rates of cerebral oxygen consumption thus suggests that cerebral energy requirements in the newborn, especially the premature newborn, are very low or are being met by nonoxidative metabolism of glucose, or both. Studies of developing human brain in vivo by MR spectroscopy further support the notion of low energy needs in the human infant. As discussed earlier, in their study of 30 normal preterm and term infants studied at postconceptional ages of 26 to 44 weeks, Azzopardi and co-workers[556] defined an approximately 40% increase in the ratios of phosphocreatine to inorganic

TABLE 4-21 Cerebral Metabolic Rate for Oxygen Determined by Positron Emission Tomography in Premature and Term Newborns Without Major Brain Injury

Group	Mean Birth Weight/ Gestational Age	Age at PET Scan	Mean CMRO$_2$ (mL/100 g/min)	Mean OEF	Mean CBF (mL/100 g/min)	Mean CBV (mL/100 g/min)	Age at Follow-up (Months)
Premature newborns	925 g/27 weeks	5–6 days	0.06	0.06	5.7	2.5	3–17
Term newborns	3266 g/40 weeks	6–7 days	0.80	0.21	24.7	3.6	6–12
Adults			2.87	0.37	48.4	5.1	

*Values are derived from five premature infants (with respiratory distress syndrome and small intraventricular hemorrhage) and five full-term infants (following extracorporeal membrane oxygenation for persistent fetal circulation) who were found to be neurologically normal on follow-up.

CBF, cerebral blood flow; CBV, cerebral blood volume; CMRO$_2$, cerebral metabolic rate for oxygen; OEF, oxygen extraction fraction; PET, positron emission tomography.

Data from Altman DI, Powers WJ, Perlman JM, Herscovitch P, et al: Cerebral blood flow requirement for brain viability in newborn infants is lower than in adults, *Ann Neurol* 24:218-226, 1988. CMRO$_2$ and OEF were determined by PET after inhalation of $^{15}O_2$, CBF after intravenous administration of H$_2$^{15}O, and CBV after inhalation of C^{15}O. The values for adults are derived from normal individuals studied by the same technique in the same laboratory; values are from Powers WJ, Grubb RL, Darriet D, Raichle ME: Cerebral blood flow and cerebral metabolic rate of oxygen requirements for cerebral function and viability in humans, *J Cereb Blood Flow Metab* 5:600-608, 1985.

phosphate and of phosphocreatine to ATP. These data suggest that an increase in the phosphorylation potential or energy reserve of human brain occurs during this age interval. This conclusion is supported by related studies of phosphorus metabolites of rat and guinea pig brain.[594] Finally, the possibility that lower energy demands in the late fetal and neonatal period in the human relate at least in part to lower synaptic activity is supported by electrophysiological studies. Prominent increases in the organization and the frequency of EEG activity occur in the premature infant and in the first 2 to 3 months after term (see earlier section).

In addition to low energy demands as an explanation for the low rates of cerebral oxygen consumption in the newborn, and especially the premature newborn, cerebral energy demands may be met by nonoxidative metabolism of glucose. Support for this notion originates from studies of both animals and humans. Gleason and co-workers[634] showed in the lamb that a relatively greater proportion of glucose is catabolized nonoxidatively than oxidatively in the midterm fetus relative to the situation in the adult.[634] Moreover, enzymatic studies of developing animals and human brain suggest that during early development, anaerobic glycolytic metabolism of glucose is an important pathway for glucose catabolism before oxidative glucose catabolism becomes predominant. In developing brain of the guinea pig and rat, lactate dehydrogenase activity rises dramatically before the rapid rise in activity of citrate synthase, a crucial enzyme of the tricarboxylic acid cycle, and CytO$_2$, the terminal enzyme of the electron transport chain.[641,642] Studies of human brain tissue from early prenatal life through childhood also suggest that the development of maximal oxidative metabolism of glucose may be preceded by a period of relatively prominent nonoxidative glucose catabolism.[643,644] Taken together, these data suggest that the development of the enzymatic capacity for complete aerobic utilization of glucose shows a definite correlation with the advancing development of neurological function.

The relationship of cerebral metabolism to postnatal development of human brain beyond the neonatal period was delineated by PET studies by Chugani and co-workers (Fig. 4-43).[603,604,610,645] The temporal characteristics of these later increases in cerebral metabolic rate, monitored by PET with fluorine-18–fluorodeoxyglucose, also support the link of cerebral metabolism with cortical neuronal development, particularly dendritic and axonal development, synaptogenesis, and selective elimination of neuritic processes and of synapses (see Chapter 2). Correlative studies in the developing cat support this conclusion.[646] The developmental and regional characteristics of CBF and cerebral metabolic rates for oxygen and glucose, obtained by PET and described in the preceding sections, are summarized in Table 4-22.

Pathological Studies. Regional CBF, oxygen metabolism, and glucose metabolism have been studied in preterm infants with periventricular hemorrhagic infarction and in term infants with hypoxic-ischemic encephalopathy.[604,605,611,612,614,617,647-649] The overall findings are summarized in Table 4-22, and the results are discussed in more detail in Chapters 9 and 11.

Functional Magnetic Resonance Imaging

Functional MRI (fMRI) is a method for detecting the topographic sites for neuronal activity induced by external stimulation. The approach has been used with great success in delineation of the loci of neuronal activation with a variety of cognitive and other behavioral activities. fMRI has been applied to the study of the newborn and young infant in recent years, especially in relation to visual stimulation.[650-655]

The method is based on the so-called *BOLD (blood oxygen level dependent)* response to an external stimulus. The BOLD response is related to the local ratio of deoxyhemoglobin (HbD) to oxyhemoglobin (HbO). HbD leads to a decrease in MRI signal, and HbO has no effect. In adults with an external stimulus (e.g., visual

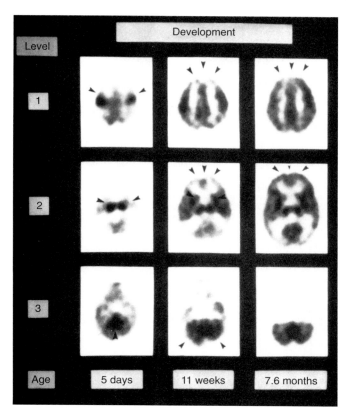

Figure 4-43   Maturation of cerebral metabolic rate for glucose, measured with fluorine-18–fluorodeoxyglucose. Note in the 5-day-old newborn the relatively high glucose metabolic rates in paracentral regions, thalamus, and brainstem-cerebellum (*arrowheads*). By 11 weeks of age, continued maturation is manifested by relatively high rates in basal ganglia and in cerebral cortical regions beyond the paracentral areas, with the prominent exception of frontal regions. By 7 to 8 months, frontal areas also exhibit relatively high glucose metabolic rates. *(From Chugani HT, Phelps ME: Maturational changes in cerebral function in infants determined by ¹⁸FDG positron emission tomography, Science 231:840-843, 1986.)*

TABLE 4-22   Principal Findings from Positron Emission Tomography Studies of Neonatal Brain*

Developmental
Regional
Initially: highest values for regional CBF and CMR-Glu in paracentral and sylvian cortex, thalamus, and brain stem
Later: increasing values in parieto-occipital and frontal cortex and in striatum
General
Initially: absolute values of mean hemispheric CBF and $CMRO_2$ below the threshold for viability in adult brain
Later: linear increase from approximately 28 weeks of gestation to term

Pathological States
Premature Infant
Periventricular hemorrhagic infarction: decrease in hemispheric CBF more extensive than predicted by conventional brain imaging (e.g., ultrasonography)
Posthemorrhagic hydrocephalus: low cerebral perfusion before CSF removal (lumbar puncture or ventricular drainage), higher after CSF removal
Term Infant
Hypoxic-ischemic encephalopathy: preponderance of pattern of decreased CBF in parasagittal cerebral regions; concomitant radionuclide brain scan or neuropathology indicates parasagittal cerebral injury; higher global CBF in the first postnatal week correlates with poorer neurological outcome.

*See text for references.
CBF, cerebral blood flow; CMR-Glu, cerebral metabolic rate for glucose; $CMRO_2$, cerebral metabolic rate for oxygen; CSF, cerebrospinal fluid.

activation), the neural activity elicited results in a marked increase in local CBF that exceeds the increase in local cerebral metabolic rate for oxygen and oxygen extraction, thereby leading to a relative increase in HbO and as a consequence a decrease in the HbD/HbO ratio. The result is an increase in MRI signal, that is, a positive BOLD response. A positive BOLD response is seen in the infant younger than 2 to 3 months, but the BOLD response in older infants is negative throughout infancy.[651-656] The negative BOLD response may result because of increased local cerebral metabolic rate for oxygen that is not met by sufficiently increased local CBF (because of immature cerebrovascular responses or because of markedly increased local cerebral metabolic rate for oxygen, caused by transiently exuberant synaptic activity) (see Chapter 2). Either response would cause an increase in the HbD/HbO ratio. *The positive BOLD response in newborns less than 2 to 3 months of age* could be the result of a local increase in CBF without a comparable increase in cerebral metabolic rate for oxygen and oxygen extraction, causing a decrease in HBD/HbO.

The limited fMRI data obtainable on newborns and very young infants have identified the *visual cortex* to be activated with *photic stimulation*.[650-652,654,656] A combined fMRI and diffusion tensor MRI study showed the fiber tract of the optic radiation leading to the activated visual cortex in a normal cerebral hemisphere and, contralateral, in an infarcted hemisphere, interruption of this tract and no activation of the cortex.[654] An fMRI study of normal 2- to 3-month-old infants demonstrated left temporal activation with speech during waking and sleeping, a finding consistent with early hemispheral specification for language.[657] Further study of other cortical functions in newborns and young infants by fMRI will be of great interest.

REFERENCES

1. Roberts MH: The spinal fluid in the newborn with especial references to intracranial hemorrhage, *JAMA* 85:500-504, 1925.
2. Waitz R: Le liquide cephalorachidien du nouveau-né, *Rev Fr Pediatr* 4:1, 1928.
3. Samson K: Die liquordiagnostik im kindesalter, *Ergeb Inn Med Kinderheilkd* 41:553, 1931.
4. Otila E: Studies on the cerebrospinal fluid in premature infants, *Acta Paediatr* 35:8-15, 1948.
5. Wyers HJG, Bakker JCW: De liquor cerebrospinalis van normale, a terme geboren neonat, *Maandschr Kindergeneeskund* 22:253-263, 1954.
6. Widell S: On the cerebrospinal fluid in normal children and in patients with acute abacterial meningoencephalitis, *Acta Paediatr Suppl* 47:1-102, 1958.
7. Naidoo BT: The cerebrospinal fluid in the healthy newborn infant, *S Afr Med J* 42:933-935, 1968.
8. Wolf H, Hoepffner L: The cerebrospinal fluid in the newborn and premature infant, *World Neurol* 2:871-877, 1961.

9. Gyllesward Å, Malmström S: The cerebrospinal fluid in immature infants, *Acta Paediatr Suppl* 51:54-62, 1962.

10. Escobedo M, Barton L, Volpe J: Cerebrospinal fluid studies in an intensive care nursery, *J Perinat Med* 3:204-210, 1975.

11. Sarff LD, Platt LH, McCracken GH Jr: Cerebrospinal fluid evaluation in neonates: Comparison of high-risk infants with and without meningitis, *J Pediatr* 88:473-477, 1976.

12. Rodriguez AF, Kaplan SL, Mason EO Jr: Cerebrospinal fluid values in the very low birth weight infant, *J Pediatr* 116:971-974, 1990.

13. Seller MJ, Adinolfi M: Levels of albumin, alpha-fetoprotein, and IgG in human fetal cerebrospinal fluid, *Arch Dis Child* 50:484-485, 1975.

14. Seller MJ, Adinolfi M: Blood-brain barrier in the human fetus [letter], *Lancet* 1:1030-1032, 1975.

15. Adinolfi M, Beck SE, Haddad SA, Seller MJ: Permeability of the blood-cerebrospinal fluid barrier to plasma proteins during foetal and perinatal life, *Nature* 259:140-141, 1976.

16. Thorley JD, Kaplan JM, Holmes RK, McCracken GH Jr, et al: Passive transfer of antibodies of maternal origin from blood to cerebrospinal fluid in infants, *Lancet* 1:651-653, 1975.

17. Akiyama Y, Schulte FJ, Schultz MA, Parmelee AH Jr: Acoustically evoked responses in premature and full term newborn infants, *Electroencephalogr Clin Neurophysiol* 26:371-380, 1969.

18. Weitzman ED, Graziani LJ: Maturation and topography of the auditory evoked response of the prematurely born infant, *Dev Psychobiol* 1:79, 1968.

19. Barnet AB, Goodwin RS: Averaged evoked electroencephalographic responses to clicks in the human newborn, *Electroencephalogr Clin Neurophysiol* 18:441, 1965.

20. Rapin I, Graziani LJ: Auditory-evoked responses in normal, brain-damaged, and deaf infants, *Neurology* 17:881-894, 1967.

21. Engel R, Young NB: Calibrated pure tone audiograms in normal neonates based on evoked electroencephalographic responses, *Neuropaediatrie* 1:149, 1969.

22. Kurtzberg D, Hilpert PL, Kreuzer JA, Vaughan HG Jr: Differential maturation of cortical auditory evoked potentials to speech sounds in normal fullterm and very low-birthweight infants, *Dev Med Child Neurol* 26:466-475, 1984.

23. Kurtzberg D, Vaughan HG Jr: Electrophysiologic assessment of auditory and visual function in the newborn, *Clin Perinatol* 12:277-299, 1985.

24. Stapells DR, Kurtzberg D: Evoked potential assessment of auditory system integrity in infants, *Clin Perinatol* 18:497-518, 1991.

25. Pasman JW, Rotteveel JJ, de Graaf R, Maassen B, et al: Detectability of auditory evoked response components in preterm infants, *Early Hum Dev* 26:129-141, 1991.

26. Rotteveel JJ, Colon EJ, deGraaf R, Notermans SLH, et al: The central auditory conduction at term date and three months after birth, *Scand Audiol* 15:75-84, 1986.

27. Rotteveel JJ, Colon EJ, Notermans LH, Stoelinga GBA, et al: The central auditory conduction at term date and three months after birth, *Scand Audiol* 15:85-95, 1986.

28. Rogers SH, Edwards DA, Henderson-Smart DJ, Pettigrew AG: Middle latency auditory evoked responses in normal term infants: A longitudinal study, *Neuropediatrics* 20:59-63, 1989.

29. Pasman JW, Rotteveel JJ, Degraaf R, Stegeman DF, et al: The effect of preterm birth on brainstem, middle latency and cortical auditory evoked responses (BMC AERs), *Early Hum Dev* 31:113-129, 1992.

30. Pasman JW, Rotteveel JJ, Maassen B, De Graaf R, et al: Diagnostic and predictive value of auditory evoked responses in preterm infants: II. Auditory evoked responses, *Pediatr Res* 42:670-677, 1997.

31. Pasman JW, Rotteveel JJ, Maassen B, Visco YM: The maturation of auditory cortical evoked responses between (preterm) birth and 14 years of age, *Eur J Paediatr Neurol* 3:79-82, 1999.

32. Fellman V, Kushnerenko E, Mikkola K, Ceponiene R, et al: Atypical auditory event-related potentials in preterm infants during the first year of life: A possible sign of cognitive dysfunction? *Pediatr Res* 56:291-297, 2004.

33. Fellman V, Huotilaninen M: Cortical auditory event-related potentials in newborn infants, *Semin Fetal Neonatal Med* 11:452-458, 2006.

34. Holst M, Eswaran H, Lowery C, Murphy P, et al: Development of auditory evoked fields in human fetuses and newborns: A longitudinal MEG study, *Clin Neurophysiol* 116:1949-1955, 2005.

35. Lowery CL, Eswaran H, Murphy P, Preissl H: Fetal magnetoencephalography, *Semin Fetal Neonatal Med* 11:430-436, 2006.

36. Starr A, Amlie RN, Martin WH, Sanders S: Development of auditory function in newborn infants revealed by auditory brainstem potentials, *Pediatrics* 60:831-839, 1977.

37. Chiappa KH, Ropper AH: Evoked potentials in clinical medicine. I, *N Engl J Med* 306:1140-1150, 1982.

38. Chiappa KH, Ropper AH: Evoked potentials in clinical medicine. II, *N Engl J Med* 306:1205-1211, 1982.

39. Kennedy CR: The assessment of hearing and brainstem function. In Eyre JA, editor: *The Neurophysiological Examination of the Newborn Infant*, New York: 1992, MacKeith Press.

40. Vohr BR, Maxon AB: Screening infants for hearing impairment, *J Pediatr* 128:710-714, 1996.

41. Majnemer A, Rosenblatt B: Evoked potentials as predictors of outcome in neonatal intensive care unit survivors: Review of literature, *Pediatr Neurol* 14:189-195, 1996.

42. Jiang ZD, Brosi DM, Wilkinson AR: Auditory neural responses to click stimuli of different rates in the brainstem of very preterm babies at term, *Pediatr Res* 51:454-459, 2002.

43. Jewett DL: Volume-conducted potentials in response to auditory stimuli as detected by averaging in the cat, *Electroencephalogr Clin Neurophysiol* 28:609-618, 1970.

44. Buchwald JS, Huang C: Far-field acoustic response: Origins in the cat, *Science* 189:382-384, 1975.

45. Starr A, Hamilton AE: Correlation between confirmed sites of neurological lesions and abnormalities of far-field auditory brainstem responses, *Electroencephalogr Clin Neurophysiol* 41:595-608, 1976.

46. Hecox K, Galambos R: Brain stem auditory evoked responses in human infants and adults, *Arch Otolaryngol* 99:30-33, 1974.

47. Schulman-Galambos C, Galambos R: Brain stem auditory-evoked responses in premature infants, *J Speech Hear Res* 18:456-465, 1975.

48. Mjoen S, Langslet A, Tangsrud SE, Sundby A: Auditory brainstem responses (ABR) in high-risk neonates, *Acta Paediatr Scand* 71:711-715, 1982.

49. Roberts JL, Davis H, Phon GL, Reichert TJ, et al: Auditory brainstem responses in preterm neonates: Maturation and follow-up, *J Pediatr* 101:257-263, 1982.

50. Salamy A, Mendelson T, Tooley WH: Developmental profiles for the brainstem auditory evoked potential, *Early Hum Dev* 6:331-339, 1982.

51. Stein L, Ozdamar O, Kraus N, Paton J: Follow-up of infants screened by auditory brainstem response in the neonatal intensive care unit, *J Pediatr* 103:447-453, 1983.

52. Shannon DA, Felix JK, Krumholz A, Goldstein PJ, et al: Hearing screening of high-risk newborns with brainstem auditory evoked potentials: A follow-up study, *Pediatrics* 73:22-26, 1984.

53. Cox LC: The current status of auditory brainstem response testing in neonatal populations, *Pediatr Res* 18:780-783, 1984.

54. Krumholz A, Felix JK, Goldstein PJ, McKenzie E: Maturation of the brainstem auditory evoked potential in premature infants, *Electroencephalogr Clin Neurophysiol* 62:124-134, 1985.

55. Jiang ZD: Maturation of the auditory brainstem in low risk preterm infants: A comparison with age-matched full term infants up to 6 years, *Early Hum Dev* 42:49-65, 1995.

56. Ferber-Viart C, Morlet T, Maison S, Duclaux R, et al: Type of initial brainstem auditory evoked potentials (BAEP) impairment and risk factors in premature infants, *Brain Dev* 18:287-293, 1996.

57. Jiang ZD, Brosi DM, Wilkinson AR: Hearing impairment in preterm very low birthweight babies detected at term by brainstem auditory evoked responses, *Acta Paediatr* 90:1411-1415, 2001.

58. Jiang ZD, Brosi DM, Wang J, Xu X, et al: Time course of brainstem pathophysiology during first month in term infants after perinatal asphyxia, revealed by MLS BAER latencies and intervals, *Pediatr Res* 54:680-687, 2003.

59. Jiang ZD, Wang J, Brosi DM, Shao XM, et al: One-third of term babies after perinatal hypoxia-ischaemia have transient hearing impairment: Dynamic change in hearing threshold during the neonatal period, *Acta Paediatr* 93:82-87, 2004.

60. Santiago-Rodriguez E, Harmony T, Bernardino M, Porras-Kattz E, et al: Auditory steady-state responses in infants with perinatal brain injury, *Pediatr Neurol* 32:236-240, 2005.

61. Wilkinson AR, Jiang A: Brainstem auditory evoked response in neonatal neurology, *Semin Fetal Neonatal Med* 11:444-451, 2006.

62. Despland PA, Galambos R: Use of the auditory brainstem responses by prematures and newborns infants, *Neuropadiatrie* 11:99-107, 1980.

63. Cox LC, Hack M, Metz DA: Brainstem-evoked response audiometry: Normative data from the preterm infant, *Audiology* 20:53, 1981.

64. Despland PA: Maturational changes in the auditory system as reflected in human brainstem evoked responses, *Dev Neurosci* 7:73-80, 1985.

65. Lasky RE, Yang E: Methods for determining auditory evoked brain-stem response thresholds in human newborns, *Electroencephalogr Clin Neurophysiol* 65:276-281, 1986.

66. Maurizi M, Almadori G, Cagini L, Molini E, et al: Auditory brainstem responses in the full-term newborn: Changes in the first 58 hours of life, *Audiology* 25:239-247, 1986.

67. Vles JSH, Casaer P, Kingma H, Swennen C, et al: A longitudinal study of brainstem auditory evoked potentials of preterm infants, *Dev Med Child Neurol* 29:577-585, 1987.

68. Collet L, Soares I, Morgon A, Salle B: Is there a difference between extra-uterine and intrauterine maturation on BAEP? *Brain Dev* 11:293-296, 1989.

69. Adelman C, Levi H, Linder N, Sohmer H: Neonatal auditory brain-stem response threshold and latency: 1 hour to 5 months, *Electroencephalogr Clin Neurophysiol* 77:77-80, 1990.

70. Lauffer H, Wenzel D: Brainstem acoustic evoked responses: Maturational aspects from cochlea to midbrain, *Neuropediatrics* 21:59-61, 1990.

71. Chiarenza GA, D'Ambrosio GM, Cazzullo G: Developmental course of brain-stem auditory evoked potentials in the first days of full term infants, *Early Hum Dev* 27:145-156, 1991.

72. Yamasaki M, Shono H, Oga M, Ito Y, et al: Changes in auditory brainstem responses of normal neonates immediately after birth, *Biol Neonate* 60:92-101, 1991.

73. Yamamoto N, Watanabe K, Sugiura J, Okada J, et al: Marked latency change of auditory brainstem response in preterm infants in the early postnatal period, *Brain Dev* 12:766-769, 1990.

74. Kohelet D, Arbel E, Goldberg M, Arlazoroff A: Brainstem auditory evoked response in newborns and infants, *J Child Neurol* 15:33-35, 2000.

75. Jiang ZD, Brosi DM, Wilkinson AR: Maximum length sequence BAER at term in low-risk babies born at 30-32 week gestation, *Brain Dev* 28:1-7, 2006.

76. Salamy A, McKean CM: Postnatal development of human brainstem potentials during the first year of life, *Electroencephalogr Clin Neurophysiol* 40:418-426, 1976.

77. Despland PA, Galambos R: The auditory brainstem response (ABR) is a useful diagnostic tool in the intensive care nursery, *Pediatr Res* 14:154-158, 1980.

78. Bergman I, Hirsch RP, Fria TJ, Shapiro SM, et al: Cause of hearing loss in the high-risk premature infant, *J Pediatr* 106:95-101, 1985.

79. Salamy A, Eldredge L, Tooley WH: Neonatal status and hearing loss in high-risk infants, *J Pediatr* 114:847-852, 2989.

80. Colding H, Andersen EA, Prytz S, Wulffsberg H, et al: Auditory function after continuous infusion of gentamicin to high-risk newborns, *Acta Paediatr Scand* 78:840-843, 1989.

81. Hendricks-Munoz KD, Walton JP: Hearing loss in infants with persistent fetal circulation, *Pediatrics* 81:650-656, 1988.

82. Nield TA, Schrier S, Ramos AD, Platzker ACG, et al: Unexpected hearing loss in high-risk infants, *Pediatrics* 78:417-422, 1986.

83. Pettigrew AG, Edwards DA, Henderson-Smart DJ: Perinatal risk factors in preterm infants with moderate-to-profound hearing deficits, *Med J Aust* 148:174-177, 1988.

84. Duara S, Suter CM, Bessard KK, Gutberlet RL: Neonatal screening with auditory brainstem responses: Results of follow-up audiometry and risk factor evaluation, *J Pediatr* 108:276-281, 1986.

85. Sohmer H, Freeman S, Gapni M, Gottein K: The depression of the auditory nerve–brain-stem evoked response in hypoxaemia: Mechanism and site of effect, *Electroencephalogr Clin Neurophysiol* 64:334-338, 1986.

86. Yasuhara A, Kinoshita Y, Hori A, Iwase S, et al: Auditory brainstem response in neonates with asphyxia and intracranial haemorrhage, *Eur J Pediatr* 145:347-350, 1986.

87. Streletz LJ, Graziani LJ, Branca PA, Desai HJ, et al: Brainstem auditory evoked potentials in fullterm and preterm newborns with hyperbilirubinemia and hypoxemia, *Neuropediatrics* 17:66-71, 1986.

88. Esbjorner E, Larsson P, Leissner P, Wranne L: The serum reserve albumin concentration for monoacetyldiaminodiphenyl sulphone and auditory evoked responses during neonatal hyperbilirubinaemia, *Acta Paediatr Scand* 80:406-412, 1991.

89. Cox C, Hack M, Aram D, Borawski E: Neonatal auditory brainstem response failure of very low birth weight infants: 8-year outcome, *Pediatr Res* 31:68-72, 1992.

90. Kitamoto I, Kukita J, Kurokawa T, Chen Y-J, et al: Transient neurologic abnormalities and BAEPs in high-risk infants, *Pediatr Neurol* 6:319-325, 1990.

91. Pettigrew AG, Edwards DA, Henderson-Smart DJ: The influence of intra-uterine growth retardation on brainstem development of preterm infants, *Dev Med Child Neurol* 27:467-472, 1985.

92. Jiang ZD, Wu YY, Zhen MS, Sun DK, et al: Development of early and late brainstem conduction time in normal and intrauterine growth retarded children, *Acta Paediatr Scand* 80:494-499, 1991.

93. Robinson RO: Familial schizencephaly, *Dev Med Child Neurol* 33:1010-1012, 1991.

94. Robinson RJ: Causes and associations of severe and persistent specific speech and language defects in children, *Dev Med Child Neurol* 33:943-962, 1991.

95. Taylor MJ, Robinson BH: Evoked potentials in children with oxidative metabolic defects leading to Leigh syndrome, *Pediatr Neurol* 8:25-29, 1992.

96. Zhang L, Jiang ZD: Development of the brainstem auditory pathway in low birthweight and perinatally asphyxiated children with neurological sequelae, *Early Hum Dev* 30:61-73, 1992.

97. Paccioretti DC, Haluschak MM, Finer NN, Robertson C, et al: Auditory brain-stem responses in neonates receiving extracorporeal membrane oxygenation, *J Pediatr* 120:464-467, 1992.

98. Mason JA, Herrmann KR: Universal infant hearing screening by automated auditory brainstem response measurement, *Pediatrics* 101:221-228, 1998.

99. Windmill IM: Universal screening of infants for hearing loss: Further justification, *J Pediatr* 133:318-319, 1998.

100. Finitzo T, Albright K, O'Neal J: The newborn with hearing loss: Detection in the nursery, *Pediatrics* 102:1452-1460, 1998.

101. Task Force on Newborn and Infant Hearing: Newborn and infant hearing loss: Detection and intervention, *Pediatrics* 103:527-530, 1999.

102. Meyer C, Witte J, Hildmann A, Hennecke K-H, et al: Neonatal screening for hearing disorders in infants at risk: Incidence, risk factors, and follow-up, *Pediatrics* 104:900-904, 1999.

103. Jiang ZD, Brosi DM, Shao XM, Wilkinson AR: Maximum length sequence brainstem auditory evoked responses in term neonates who have perinatal hypoxia-ischemia, *Pediatr Res* 48:639-645, 2000.

104. Jiang ZD, Brosi DM, Li ZH, Chen C, et al: Brainstem auditory function at term in preterm babies with and without perinatal complications, *Pediatr Res* 58:1164-1169, 2005.

105. Finitzo-Hieber T, McCracken GH Jr, Brown KC: Prospective controlled evaluation of auditory function in neonates given netilmicin or amikacin, *J Pediatr* 106:129-136, 1985.

105a. Jiang ZD, Yin R, Wilkinson AR: Brainstem auditory evoked responses in very low birth weight infants with chronic lung disease, *Eur J Paediatr Neurol* 11:153-159, 2007.

106. Vohr BR, Carty LM, Moore PE, Letourneau K: The Rhode Island hearing assessment program: Experience with statewide hearing screening (1993-1996), *J Pediatr* 133:353-357, 1998.

107. Johnson JL, White KR, Widen JE, Gravel JS, et al: A multicenter evaluation of how many infants with permanent hearing loss pass a two-stage otoacoustic emissions/automated auditory brainstem response newborn hearing screening protocol, *Pediatrics* 116:663-672, 2005.

108. Majnemer A, Rosenblatt B, Riley P: Prognostic significance of the auditory brainstem evoked response in high-risk neonates, *Dev Med Child Neurol* 30:43-52, 1988.

109. Goodman JT, Malizia KE, Durieux-Smith A, MacMurray B, et al: Bayley developmental performance at two years of age of neonates at risk for hearing loss, *Dev Med Child Neurol* 32:689-697, 1990.

110. Hayes D: State programs for universal newborn hearing screening, *Pediatr Clin North Am* 46:89-94, 1999.

111. Joint Committee on Infant Hearing: Year 2000 position statement: Principles and guidelines for early hearing detection and intervention programs, *Pediatrics* 106:798-817, 2000.

112. Hayes D: Screening methods: Current status, *Ment Retard Dev Disabil Res Rev* 9:65-72, 2003.

113. De Hoog M, van Zanten BA, Hop WC, Overbosch E, et al: Newborn hearing screening: Tobramycin and vancomycin are not risk factors for hearing loss, *J Pediatr* 142:41-46, 2003.

114. Shoup AG, Owen KE, Jackson G, Laptook A: The Parkland Memorial Hospital experience in ensuring compliance with Universal Newborn Hearing Screening follow-up, *J Pediatr* 146:66-72, 2005.

115. Taylor MJ: Visual evoked potentials. In Eyre JA, editor: *The Neurophysiological Examination of the Newborn Infant*, New York: 1992, MacKeith Press.

116. Tsuneishi S, Casaer P: Stepwise decrease in VEP latencies and the process of myelination in the human visual pathway, *Brain Dev* 19:547-551, 1997.

117. Kato T, Watanabe K: Visual evoked potential in the newborn: Does it have predictive value? *Semin Fetal Neonatal Med* 11:459-463, 2006.

118. Purpura DP, Shofer RJ, Housepian EM, Noback CR: Comparative ontogenesis of structure function relations in cerebral and cerebellar cortex. In Purpura DP, Schade JP, editors: *Progress in Brain Research*, New York: 1964, Elsevier.

119. Roy M-S, Barsoum-Homsy M, Orquin J, Benoit J: Maturation of binocular pattern visual evoked potentials in normal full-term and preterm infants from 1 to 6 months of age, *Pediatr Res* 37:140-144, 1995.

120. Kos-Pietro S, Towle VL, Cakmur R, Spire J-P: Maturation of human visual evoked potentials: 27 weeks conceptional age to 2 years, *Neuropediatrics* 28:318-323, 1997.

121. Madan A, Good WV: Visual development in preterm infants, *Dev Med Child Neurol* 47:276-280, 2005.

122. Porciatti V: Temporal and spatial properties of the pattern-reversal VEPs in infants below 2 months of age, *Hum Neurobiol* 3:97-102, 1984.

123. Harding GFA, Grose J, Wilton A, Bissenden JG: The pattern reversal VEP in short-gestation infants, *Electroencephalogr Clin Neurophysiol* 74:76-80, 1989.

124. Ellingson RJ: Cortical electrical responses to visual stimulation in the human newborn, *Electroencephalogr Clin Neurophysiol* 12:663, 1960.

125. Hrbek A, Karlberg P, Olsson T: Development of visual and somatosensory evoked responses in pre-term newborn infants, *Electroencephalogr Clin Neurophysiol* 34:225-232, 1973.

126. Graziani LJ, Korberly B: Limitations of neurologic and behavioral assessments in the newborn infant. In Gluck L, editor: *Intrauterine Asphyxia and the Developing Fetal Brain*, Chicago: 1977, Year Book.

127. Engel R, Benson RC: Estimate of conceptional age by evoked response activity, *Biol Neonat* 12:201-213, 1968.

128. Chin KC, Taylor MJ, Menzies R, Whyte H: Development of visual evoked potentials in neonates: A study using light emitting diode goggles, *Arch Dis Child* 60:1166-1168, 1985.

129. Petersen S, Pryds O, Trojaborg W: Visual evoked potentials in term light-for-gestational-age infants and infants of diabetic mothers, *Early Hum Dev* 23:85-92, 1990.

130. Apkarian P, Mirmiran M, Tijssen R: Effects of behavioural state on visual processing in neonates, *Neuropediatrics* 22:85-91, 1991.

131. Pryds O, Trojaborg W, Carlsen J, Jensen J: Determinants of visual evoked potentials in preterm infants, *Early Hum Dev* 19:117-125, 1989.

132. Häkkinen VK, Ignatius J, Koskinen M, Koivikko MJ, et al: Visual evoked potentials in high-risk infants, *Neuropediatrics* 18:70-74, 1987.

133. Pryds O, Greisen G, Trojaborg W: Visual evoked potentials in preterm infants during the first hours of life, *Electroencephalogr Clin Electrophysiol* 71:257-265, 1988.

134. Leaf AA, Green CR, Esack A, Costeloe KL, et al: Maturation of electro-retinograms and visual evoked potentials in preterm infants, *Dev Med Child Neurol* 37:814-826, 1995.

135. Mercuri E, Braddick O, Atkinson J, Cowan F, et al: Orientation-reversal and phase-reversal visual evoked potentials in full-term infants with brain lesions: A longitudinal study, *Neuropediatrics* 29:169-174, 1998.

136. Shepherd AJ, Saunders KJ, McCulloch DL, Dutton GN: Prognostic value of flash visual evoked potentials in preterm infants, *Dev Med Child Neurol* 41:9-15, 1999.

137. Engel R: Maturational changes and abnormalities in the newborn electroencephalogram, *Dev Med Child Neurol* 7:498-506, 1965.

138. Parmelee AH: Neurophysiological and behavioral organization of premature infants in the first months of life, *Biol Psychiatry* 10:501-512, 1975.

139. Graziani LJ, Katz L, Cracco Q, Cracco JB, et al: The maturation and interrelationship of EEF patterns and auditory evoked response in premature infants, *Electroencephalogr Clin Neurophysiol* 36:367-375, 1974.

140. Engel R, Fay W: Visual evoked responses at birth, verbal scores at three years, and IQ at four years, *Dev Med Child Neurol* 14:283-289, 1972.

141. Butler BV, Engel R: Mental and motor scores at 8 months in relation to neonatal photic responses, *Dev Med Child Neurol* 11:77-82, 1969.

142. Whyte HE, Taylor MJ, Menzies R, Chin KC, et al: Prognostic utility of visual evoked potentials in term asphyxiated neonates, *Pediatr Neurol* 2:220-223, 1986.

143. Placzek M, Mushin J, Dubowitz LMS: Maturation of the visual evoked response and its correlation with visual acuity in preterm infants, *Dev Med Child Neurol* 27:448-454, 1985.

144. Beverley Dw, Smith IS, Beesley P, Jones J, et al: Relationship of cranial ultrasonography, visual and auditory evoked responses with neurodevelopmental outcome, *Dev Med Child Neurol* 32:210-222, 1990.

145. Stanley OH, Fleming PJ, Morgan MH: Development of visual evoked potentials following intrauterine growth retardation, *Early Hum Dev* 27:79-91, 1991.

146. Lambert SR, Kriss A, Taylor D: Detection of isolated occipital lobe anomalies during early childhood, *Dev Med Child Neurol* 32:451-455, 1990.

147. Muttitt SC, Taylor MJ, Kobayashi JS, MacMillan L, et al: Serial visual evoked potentials and outcome in term birth asphyxia, *Pediatr Neurol* 7:86-90, 1991.

148. Woods JR Jr, Coppes V, Brooks DE, Knowles PJ, et al: Birth asphyxia. I. Measurement of visual evoked potential (VEP) in the healthy fetus and newborn lamb, *Pediatr Res* 15:1429-1432, 1981.

149. Sklar FH, Ehle AL, Clark WK: Visual evoked potentials: A noninvasive technique to monitor patients with shunted hydrocephalus, *Neurosurgery* 4:529-534, 1979.

150. McSherry JW, Walters CL, Horbar JD: Acute visual evoked potential changes in hydrocephalus, *Electroencephalogr Clin Neurophysiol* 53:331-333, 1982.

151. Desmedt JE, Manil J: Somatosensory evoked potentials of the normal human neonate in REM sleep, in slow wave sleep and in waking, *Electroencephalogr Clin Neurophysiol* 29:113-126, 1970.

152. Desmedt JE, Noel P, Debecker J, Nameche J: Maturation of afferent velocity as studied by sensory nerve potentials and by cerebral evoked potentials.In *New Developments in Electromyography and Clinical Neurophysiology*, Basel: 1973, S. Karger.

153. Cracco JB, Cracco RQ, Graziani LJ: The spinal evoked response in infants and children, *Neurology* 25:31-36, 1975.

154. Cullity P, Franks CI, Duckworth T, Brown BH: Somatosensory evoked cortical responses: Detection in normal infants, *Dev Med Child Neurol* 18:11-18, 1976.

155. Bongers-Schokking JJ, Colon EJ, Hoogland RA, Van den Brande JL, et al: Somatosensory evoked potentials in term and preterm infants in relation to postconceptional age and birth weight, *Neuropediatrics* 21:32-36, 1990.

156. Majnemer A, Rosenblatt B: Functional interhemispheric asymmetries at birth as demonstrated by somatosensory evoked potentials, *J Child Neurol* 7:408-412, 1992.

157. Pierrat V, de Vries LS, Minami T, Casaer P: Somatosensory evoked potentials and adaptation to extrauterine life: A longitudinal study, *Brain Dev* 12:376-379, 1990.

158. Laureau E, Marlot D: Somatosensory evoked potentials after median and tibial nerve stimulation in healthy newborns, *Electroencephalogr Clin Neurophysiol* 76:453-458, 1990.

159. George SR, Taylor MJ: Somatosensory evoked potentials in neonates and infants: Developmental and normative data, *Electroencephalogr Clin Neurophysiol* 80:94-102, 1991.

160. Karniski W: The late somatosensory evoked potential in premature and term infants. I. Principal component topography, *Electroencephalogr Clin Neurophysiol* 84:32-43, 1992.

161. Gibson NA, Graham M, Levene MI: Somatosensory evoked potentials and outcome in perinatal asphyxia, *Arch Dis Child* 67:393-398, 1992.

162. Cooke RWI: Somatosensory evoked potentials. In Eyre JA, editor: *The Neurophysiological Examination of the Newborn Infant*, New York: 1992, MacKeith Press.

163. de Vries LS, Eken P, Pierrat V, Daniels H, et al: Prediction of neurodevelopmental outcome in the preterm infant: Short latency cortical somatosensory evoked potentials compared with cranial ultrasound, *Arch Dis Child* 67:1177-1181, 1992.

164. White CP, Cooke RWI: Somatosensory evoked potentials following posterior tibial nerve stimulation predict later motor outcome, *Dev Med Child Neurol* 36:34-40, 1994.

165. Pierrat V, Eken P, Truffert P, Duquennoy C, et al: Somatosensory evoked potentials in preterm infants with intrauterine growth retardation, *Early Hum Dev* 44:17-25, 1996.

166. Taylor MJ, Saliba E, Laugier J: Use of evoked potentials in preterm neonates, *Arch Dis Child Fetal Neonatal Ed* 74:F70-F76, 1996.

167. Minami T, Gondo K, Nakayama H, Ueda K: Cortical somatosensory evoked potentials to posterior tibial nerve stimulation in newborn infants, *Brain Dev* 18:294-298, 1996.

168. Pihko E, Lauronen L: Somatosensory processing in healthy newborns, *Exp Neurol* 190(Suppl):S2-S7, 2004.

169. Vanhatalo S, Lauronen L: Neonatal SEP: Back to bedside with basic science, *Semin Fetal Neonatal Med* 11:464-470, 2006.

169a. Lauronen L, Nevalainen P, Wikstrom H, Parkjkonen L, et al: Immaturity of somatosensory cortical processing in human newborns, *Neuroimage* 33:195-203, 2006.

170. Abroms IF, Bresnan MJ, Zuckerman JE, Fischer EG, et al: Cervical cord injuries secondary to hyperextension of the head in breech presentations, *Obstet Gynecol* 41:369-378, 1973.

171. Duckworth T, Yamashita T, Franks CI, Brown BH: Somatosensory evoked cortical responses in children with spina bifida, *Dev Med Child Neurol* 18:19-24, 1976.

172. Reigel DH, Dallmann DE, Scarff TB, Woodford J: Intra-operative evoked potential studies of newborn infants with myelomeningocele, *Dev Med Child Neurol Suppl* 1976:42-49, 1976.

173. Majnemer A, Rosenblatt B, Riley P, Laureau E, et al: Somatosensory evoked response abnormalities in high-risk newborns, *Pediatr Neurol* 3:350-355, 1987.

174. Majnemer A, Rosenblatt B, Willis D, Lavallee J: The effect of gestational age at birth on somatosensory-evoked potentials performed at term, *J Child Neurol* 5:329-335, 1990.

175. Willis J, Duncan C, Bell R: Short-latency somatosensory evoked potentials in perinatal asphyxia, *Pediatr Neurol* 3:203-207, 1987.

176. Willis J, Duncan MC, Bell R, Pappas F, et al: Somatosensory evoked potentials predict neuromotor outcome after periventricular hemorrhage, *Dev Med Child Neurol* 31:435-439, 1989.

177. Bongers-Schokking CJ, Colon EJ, Hoogland RA, de Groot CJ, et al: Somatosensory evoked potentials in neonates with primary congenital hypothyroidism during the first week of therapy, *Pediatr Res* 30:34-39, 1991.

178. White CP, Cooke RWI: Maturation of the cortical evoked response to posterior nerve stimulation in the preterm neonate, *Dev Med Child Neurol* 31:657-664, 1989.

179. de Vries LS, Pierrat V, Minami T, Smet M, et al: The role of short latency somatosensory evoked responses in infants with rapidly progressive ventricular dilatation, *Neuropediatrics* 21:136-139, 1990.

180. Majnemer A, Rosenblatt B, Riley PS: Prognostic significance of multimodality evoked response testing in high-risk newborns, *Pediatr Neurol* 6:367-374, 1990.

181. Dreyfus-Brisac C: The bioelectrical development of the central nervous system during early life. In Falkner F, editor: *Human Development*, Philadelphia: 1966, Saunders.

182. Dreyfus-Brisac C: Neonatal electroencephalography, *Rev Perinatal Pediatr* 3:397, 1979.

183. Parmelee AH Jr, Schulte FJ, Akiyama Y, Wenner WH, et al: Maturation of EEG activity during sleep in premature infants, *Electroencephalogr Clin Neurophysiol* 24:319-329, 1968.

184. Anderson CM, Torres F, Faoro A: The EEG of the early premature, *Electroencephalogr Clin Neurophysiol* 60:95-105, 1985.

185. Parmelee AH Jr, Wenner WH, Akiyama Y, Schultz M, et al: Sleep states in premature infants, *Dev Med Child Neurol* 9:70-77, 1967.

186. Dreyfus-Brisac C: Sleep ontogenesis in early human prematurity from 24 to 27 weeks of conceptional age, *Dev Psychobiol* 1:162, 1968.

187. Dreyfus-Brisac C: Ontogenesis of sleep in human prematures after 32 weeks of conceptional age, *Dev Psychobiol* 3:91-121, 1970.

188. Guilleminault C, Souquet M: Sleep states and related pathology. In Korobkin R, Guilleminault C, editors: *Advances in Perinatal Neurology*, New York: 1979, Spectrum.

189. Tharp BR: Unique EEG pattern (comb-like rhythm) in neonatal maple syrup urine disease, *Pediatr Neurol* 8:65-68, 1992.

190. Pedley TA, Lombroso CT, Hanley JW: Introduction to neonatal electroencephalography: Interpretation, *Am J EEG Technol* 21:15-22, 1981.

191. Scher MS, Barmada MA: Estimation of gestational age by electrographic, clinical, and anatomic criteria, *Pediatr Neurol* 3:256-262, 1987.

192. Scher MS, Aso K, Painter MJ: Comparisons between preterm and full-term neonates with seizures [abstract], *Ann Neurol* 24:244, 1988.

193. Scher MS, Kosaburou A, Painter MJ: Comparisons between preterm and full-term neonates with seizures [abstract], *Ann Neurol* 24:A344, 1988.

194. Kohyama J, Iwakawa Y: Interrelationships between rapid eye body movements during sleep: Polysomnographic examinations of infants including premature neonates, *Electroencephalogr Clin Electrophysiol* 79:277-280, 1991.

195. Watanabe K: The neonatal electroencephalogram and sleep cycle patterns. In Eyre JA, editor: *The Neurophysiological Examination of the Newborn Infant*, New York: 1992, MacKeith Press.

196. Shimada M, Segawa M, Higurashi M, Akamatsu H: Development of the sleep and wakefulness rhythm in preterm infants discharged from a neonatal care unit, *Pediatr Res* 33:159-163, 1993.

197. Goto K, Wakayama K, Sonoda H, Ogawa T: Sequential changes in electroencephalogram continuity in very premature infants, *Electroencephalogr Clin Neurophysiol* 82:197-202, 1992.

198. Van Sweden B, Koenderink M, Windau G, Van de Bor M, et al: Long-term EGG monitoring in the early premature: Developmental and chronobiological aspects, *Electroencephalogr Clin Electrophysiol* 79:94-100, 1991.

199. Hahn JS, Tharp BR: A characteristic electroencephalographic pattern in infants with bronchopulmonary dysplasia and its prognostic implications [abstract], *Ann Neurol* 26:471-472, 1989.

200. Hrachovy RA, Mizrahi EM, Kellaway P: Electroencephalography of the newborn. In Daly DD, Pedley TA, editors: *Current Practice of Clinical Electroencephalography*, 2nd ed, New York: 1990, Raven Press.

201. Wakayama K, Ogawa T, Goto K, Sonoda H: Development of ultradian rhythm of EEG activities in premature babies, *Early Hum Dev* 32:11-30, 1993.

202. Ferrari F, Torricelli A, Giustardi A, Benatti A, et al: Bioelectric brain maturation in full-term infants and in healthy and pathological preterm infants at term post-menstrual age, *Early Hum Dev* 28:37-63, 1992.

203. Scher MS, Martin JG, Steppe DA, Banks DL: Comparative estimates of neonatal gestational maturity by electrographic and fetal ultrasonographic criteria, *Pediatr Neurol* 11:214-218, 1994.

204. Scher MS, Steppe DA, Dokianakis SG, Sun M, et al: Cardiorespiratory behavior during sleep in full-term and preterm neonates at comparable postconceptional term ages, *Pediatr Res* 36:738-744, 1994.

205. Scher MS, Steppe DA, Banks DL, Guthrie RD, et al: Maturational trends of EEG-sleep measures in the healthy preterm neonate, *Pediatr Neurol* 12:314-322, 1995.

206. Scher MS, Steppe DA, Banks DL: Prediction of lower developmental performances of healthy neonates by neonatal EEG-sleep measures, *Pediatr Neurol* 14:137-144, 1996.

207. Scher MS: Neurophysiological assessment of brain function and maturation. I. A measure of brain adaptation in high risk infants, *Pediatr Neurol* 16:191-198, 1997.

208. Scher MS: Neurophysiological assessment of brain function and maturation. II. A measure of brain dysmaturity in healthy preterm neonates, *Pediatr Neurol* 16:287-295, 1997.

209. Scher MS: Understanding sleep ontogeny to assess brain dysfunction in neonates and infants, *J Child Neurol* 13:467-474, 1998.

210. Scher MS, Sun M, Steppe Da, Guthrie RD, et al: Comparisons of EEG spectral and correlation measures between healthy term and preterm infants, *Pediatr Neurol* 10:104-108, 1994.

211. Holthausen K, Breidbach O, Scheidt B, Frenzel J: Brain dysmaturity index for automatic detection of high-risk infants, *Pediatr Neurol* 22:187-191, 2000.

212. Hayakawa M, Okumura A, Hayakawa F, Watanabe K, et al: Background electroencephalographic (EEG) activities of very preterm infants born at less than 27 weeks gestation: A study on the degree of continuity, *Arch Dis Child Fetal Neonatal Ed* 84:F163-F167, 2001.

213. Mizrahi EM, Hrachovy RA, Kellaway P: *Atlas of Neonatal Electroencephalography*, 3rd ed, Philadelphia: 2004, Lippincott Williams & Wilkins.

214. Conde JR, de Hoyos AL, Martinez ED, Campo CG, et al: Extrauterine life duration and ontogenic EEG parameters in preterm newborns with and without major ultrasound brain lesions, *Clin Neurophysiol* 116:2796-2809, 2005.

215. Watanabe K, Hayakawa F, Okumura A: Neonatal EEG: A powerful tool in the assessment of brain damage in preterm infants, *Brain Dev* 21:361-372, 1999.

216. Biagioni E, Bartalena L, Boldrini A, Cioni G, et al: Background EEG activity in preterm infants: Correlation of outcome with selected maturational features, *Electroencephalogr Clin Neurophysiol* 91:154-162, 1994.

217. Biagioni E, Bartalena L, Biver P, Pieri R, et al: Electroencephalographic dysmaturity in preterm infants: A prognostic tool in the early postnatal period, *Neuropediatrics* 27:311-316, 1996.

218. Hayakawa F, Okumura A, Kato T, Kuno K, et al: Dysmature EEG pattern in EEGs of preterm infants with cognitive impairment: Maturation arrest caused by prolonged mild CNS depression, *Brain Dev* 19:122-125, 1997.

219. Selton D, Andre M: Prognosis of hypoxic-ischaemic encephalopathy in full-term newborns: Value of neonatal electroencephalography, *Neuropediatrics* 28:276-280, 1997.

220. Holmes G, Rowe J, Hafford J, Schmidt R, et al: Prognostic value of the electroencephalogram in neonatal asphyxia, *Electroencephalogr Clin Neurophysiol* 53:60-72, 1982.

221. Scher MS: Neonatal encephalopathies as classified by EEG-sleep criteria: Severity and timing based on clinical/pathologic correlations, *Pediatr Neurol* 11:189-200, 1994.

222. Holmes GL, Rowe J, Hafford J: Significance of reactive burst suppression following asphyxia in full term infants, *Electroencephalography* 14:138-141, 1983.

223. Douglas LM, Wu JY, Rosman NP, Stafstrom CE: Burst suppression electroencephalography in the newborn predicting the outcome, *Ann Neurol* 44:535, 1998.

224. Biagioni E, Bartalena L, Boldrini A, Pieri R, et al: Constantly discontinuous EEG patterns in full-term neonates with hypoxic-ischaemic encephalopathy, *Clin Neurophysiol* 110:1510-1515, 1999.

225. Douglass LM, Wu JY, Rosman NP, Stafstrom CE: Burst suppression electroencephalogram pattern in the newborn: Predicting the outcome, *J Child Neurol* 17:403-408, 2002.

226. Grigg-Damberger MM, Coker SB, Halsey CL, Anderson CL: Neonatal burst suppression: Its developmental significance, *Pediatr Neurol* 5:84-92, 1989.

227. Menache CC, Bourgeois BFD, Volpe JJ: Prognostic value of neonatal discontinuous EEG, *Pediatr Neurol* 27:93-101, 2002.

228. Volpe JJ: Brain death determination in the newborn, *Pediatrics* 80:293-297, 1987.

229. Moshé SL: Usefulness of EEG in the evaluation of brain death in children: The pros, *Electroencephalogr Clin Neurophysiol* 73:272-275, 1989.

230. Scher MS, Beggarly M: Clinical significance of focal periodic discharges in neonates, *J Child Neurol* 4:175-185, 1989.

231. Chung HJ, Clancy RR: Significance of positive temporal sharp waves in the neonatal electroencephalogram, *Electroencephalogr Clin Neurophysiol* 79:256-263, 1991.

232. Mikati MA, Feraru E, Krishnamoorthy K, Lombroso CT: Neonatal herpes simplex meningoencephalitis: EEG investigations and clinical correlates, *Neurology* 40:1433-1437, 1990.

233. Okumura A, Hayakawa F, Kato T, Maruyama K, et al: Abnormal sharp transients on electroencephalograms in preterm infants with periventricular leukomalacia, *J Biomed Optics* 143:26-30, 2003.

234. Scher MS: A developmental marker of central nervous system maturation. I, *Pediatr Neurol* 4:265-273, 1988.

235. Scher MS: A developmental marker of central nervous system maturation. II, *Pediatr Neurol* 4:329-336, 1988.

236. Bejar R, Coen RW, Merritt TA, Vaucher Y, et al: Focal necrosis of the white matter (periventricular leukomalacia): Sonographic, pathologic, and electroencephalographic features, *AJNR Am J Neuroradiol* 7:1073-1079, 1986.

237. Tharp BR, Scher MS, Clancy RR: Serial EEGs in normal and abnormal infants with birth weights less than 1200 grams: A prospective study with long term follow-up, *Neuropediatrics* 20:64-72, 1989.

238. Novotny EJ Jr, Tharp BR, Coen RW, Bejar R, et al: Positive rolandic sharp waves in the EEG of the premature infant, *Neurology* 37:1481-1486, 1987.

239. Marret S, Parain D, Samson-Dollfus D, Jeannot E, et al: Positive rolandic sharp waves and periventricular leukomalacia in the newborn, *Neuropediatrics* 17:199-202, 1986.

240. Marret S, Parain D, Jeannot E, Eurin D, et al: Positive rolandic sharp waves in the EEG of the premature newborn: A five-year prospective study, *Arch Dis Child* 67:948-951, 1992.

241. Marret S, Parain D, Menard J-F, Blanc T, et al: Prognostic value of neonatal electroencephalography in premature newborns less than 33 weeks of gestational age, *Electroencephalogr Clin Neurophysiol* 102:178-185, 1997.

242. Baud O, D'Allest A-M, Lacaze-Masmonteil T, Zupan V, et al: The early diagnosis of periventricular leukomalacia in premature infants with positive rolandic sharp waves on serial electroencephalography, *J Pediatr* 132:813-817, 1998.

243. Zeinstra E, Fock JM, Begeer JH, Van Weerden T, et al: The prognostic value of serial EEG recordings following acute neonatal asphyxia in full-term infants, *Eur J Paediatr Neurol* 5:155-160, 2001.

244. de Vries LS, Hellstrom-Westas L: Role of cerebral function monitoring in the newborn, *Arch Dis Child Fetal Neonatal Ed* 90:F201-F207, 2005.

245. Connell JA, Ozeer R, Dubowitz V: Continuous 4-channel EEG monitoring: A guide to interpretation, with normal values, in preterm infants, *Neuropediatrics* 18:138-145, 1987.

246. Thornberg E, Thiringer K: Normal pattern of the cerebral function monitor trace in term and preterm neonates, *Acta Paediatr Scand* 79:20-25, 1990.

247. Hellström-Westas L, Rosen I, Svenningsen NW: Cerebral complications detected by EEG-monitoring during neonatal intensive care, *Acta Paediatr Scand* 360:83-86, 1989.

248. Hellström-Westas L, Rosen I, Svenningsen NW: Cerebral function monitoring during the first week of life in extremely small low birthweight (ESLBW) infants, *Neuropediatrics* 22:27-32, 1991.

249. Wertheim DFP, Eaton DGM, Oozeer RC, Connell JA, et al: A new system for cotside display and analysis of the preterm neonatal electroencephalogram, *Dev Med Child Neurol* 33:1080-1086, 1991.

250. Hellström-Westas L: Comparison between tape-recorded and amplitude-integrated EEG monitoring in sick newborn infants, *Acta Paediatr* 81:812-819, 1992.

251. Hellström-Westas L, Rosen I, Svenningsen NW: Predictive value of early continuous amplitude integrated EEG recordings on outcome after severe birth asphyxia in full term infants, *Arch Dis Child Fetal Neonatal Ed* 72:F34-F38, 1995.

252. Hellstrom-Westas L, Rosen I: Continuous brain-function monitoring: State of the art in clinical practice, *Semin Fetal Neonatal Med* 11:503-511, 2006.
253. Hellstrom-Westas L, Rosen I: Amplitude-integrated electroencephalogram in newborn infants for clinical and research purposes, *Acta Paediatr* 91:1028-1030, 2002.
254. Shalak LF, Laptook AR, Velaphi SC, Perlman JM: Amplitude-integrated electroencephalography coupled with an early neurologic examination enhances prediction of term infants at risk for persistent encephalopathy, *Pediatrics* 111:351-357, 2003.
255. Ter Horst HJ, Sommer C, Bergman KA, Fock JM, et al: Prognostic significance of amplitude-integrated EEG during the first 72 hours after birth in severely asphyxiated neonates, *Pediatr Res* 55:1026-1033, 2004.
256. van Rooij LGM, Toet MC, Osredkar D, vanHuffelen AC, et al: Recovery of amplitude integrated electroencephalographic background patterns within 24 hours of perinatal asphyxia, *Arch Dis Child Fetal Neonatal Ed* 90:F245-F251, 2005.
257. Shany E, Goldstein E, Khvatskin S, Friger MD, et al: Predictive value of amplitude-integrated electroencephalography pattern and voltage in asphyxiated term infants, *Pediatr Neurol* 35:335-342, 2006.
258. Toet MC, Hellstrom-Westas L, Groenendaal F, Eken P, et al: Amplitude integrated EEG 3 and 6 hours after birth in full term neonates with hypoxic-ischaemic encephalopathy, *Arch Dis Child Fetal Neonatal Ed* 81:F19-23, 1999.
259. Eken P, Toet MC, Groenendaal F, Devries LS: Predictive value of early neuroimaging, pulsed Doppler and neurophysiology in full term infants with hypoxic-ischaemic encephalopathy, *Arch Dis Child Fetal Neonatal Ed* 73:F75-F80, 1995.
260. Toet MC, Van der Meij W, de Vries LS, Uiterwaal CSPM, et al: Comparison between simultaneously recorded amplitude integrated electroencephalogram (cerebral function monitor) and standard electroencephalogram in neonates, *Pediatrics* 109:772-779, 2002.
261. Rennie JM, Chorley G, Boylan GB, Pressler R, et al: Non-expert use of the cerebral function monitor for neonatal seizure detection, *Arch Dis Child Fetal Neonatal Ed* 89:F37-40, 2004.
262. Shany E: The influence of phenobarbital overdose on aEEG recording, *Eur J Paediatr Neurol* 8:323-325, 2004.
262a. Shellhaas RA, Soaita AI, Clancy RR: Sensitivity of amplitude-integrated electroencephalography for neonatal seizure detection, *Pediatrics* 120:770-777, 2007.
263. ter Horst H, Brouwer O, Bos AF: Burst suppression on amplitude-integrated electroencephalogram may be induced by midazolam: A report on three cases, *Acta Paediatr* 93:559-564, 2004.
264. van Leuven K, Groenendaal F, Toet MC, Schobben AF, et al: Midazolam and amplitude-integrated EEG in asphyxiated full-term neonates, *Acta Paediatr* 93:1221-1227, 2004.
265. Osredkar D, Toet MC, vanRooij LGM, vanHuffelen AC, et al: Sleep-wake cycling on amplitude-integrated electroencephalography in term newborns with hypoxic-ischemic encephalopathy, *Pediatrics* 115:327-332, 2005.
266. Toet MC, Groenendaal F, Osredkar D, van Huffelen AC, et al: Postneonatal epilepsy following amplitude-integrated EEG-detected neonatal seizures, *Pediatr Neurol* 32:241-247, 2005.
267. Burdjalov VF, Baumgart S, Spitzer AR: Cerebral function monitoring: A new scoring system for the evaluation of brain maturation in neonates, *Pediatrics* 112:855-861, 2003.
268. Olischar M, Klebermass K, Kuhle S, Hulek M, et al: Reference values for amplitude-integrated electroencephalographic activity in preterm infants younger than 30 weeks' gestational age, *Pediatrics* 113:61-66, 2004.
269. Sisman J, Campbell DE, Brion LP: Amplitude-integrated EEG in preterm infants: Maturation of background pattern and amplitude voltage with postmenstrual age and gestational age, *J Perinatol* 25:391-396, 2005.
270. Hellstrom-Westas L, Klette H, Thorngren-Jerneck K, Rosen I: Early prediction of outcome with aEEG in preterm infants with large intraventricular hemorrhages, *Neuropediatrics* 32:319-324, 2001.
271. Inder TE, Buckland L, Williams CE, Spencer C, et al: Lowered electroencephalographic spectral edge frequency predicts the presence of cerebral white matter injury in premature infants, *Pediatrics* 111:27-33, 2003.
272. Victor S, Appleton RE, Beirne M, Marson AG, et al: Spectral analysis of electroencephalography in premature newborn infants: Normal ranges, *Pediatr Res* 57:336-341, 2005.
273. Volpe JJ: Anterior fontanel: Window to the neonatal brain, *J Pediatr* 100:395-398, 1982.
274. Rennie JM: *Neonatal Cerebral Ultrasound*, Cambridge: 1997, Cambridge University Press.
275. Rumack CM, Johnson ML: *Perinatal and Infant Brain Imaging*, Chicago: 1984, Year Book.
276. Levene MI, Williams JL, Fawer CL: *Ultrasound of the Infant Brain*, London: 1985, Blackwell Scientific.
277. Fawer CL, Calame A: Ultrasound. In Haddad J, Christmann D, Messer J, editors: *Imaging Techniques of the CNS of the Neonates*, New York: 1991, Springer-Verlag.
278. Fischer AQ, Shuman RM, Anderson JC, Stinson W: *Pediatric Neurosonography. Clinical, Tomographic, and Neuropathologic Correlates*, New York: 1985, John Wiley & Sons.
279. Cohen HL, Haller JO: Advances in perinatal neurosonography, *AJR Am J Roentgenol* 163:801-810, 1994.
280. Correa F, Enriquez G, Rossello J, Lucaya J, et al: Posterior fontanelle sonography: An acoustic window into the neonatal brain, *AJNR Am J Neuroradiol* 25:1274-1282, 2004.
281. Popp RL, Macovski A: Ultrasonic diagnostic instruments, *Science* 210:268-273, 1980.
282. Ferrucci JT Jr: Body ultrasonography. I, *N Engl J Med* 300:538-542, 1979.
283. Birnholz JC: On maps and comparing cross-sectional imaging methods [editorial], *AJR Am J Roentgenol* 129:1133-1134, 1977.
284. Ferrucci JT Jr: Body ultrasonography. II, *N Engl J Med* 300:590-602, 1979.
285. Brown BS: How safe is diagnostic ultrasound? *Nova Scotia Med Bull* 1:3-11, 1984.
286. Huppi PS: MR imaging and spectroscopy of brain development, *Magn Reson Imaging Clin N Am* 9:1-17, 2001.
287. Robertson NJ, Wyatt JS: The magnetic resonance revolution in brain imaging: Impact on neonatal intensive care, *Arch Dis Child Fetal Neonatal Ed* 89:F193-F197, 2004.
288. Rutherford M: *MRI of the Neonatal Brain*, Philadelphia: 2002, Saunders.
289. Barkovich AJ: *Pediatric Neuroimaging*, 4th ed, Philadelphia: 2005, Lippincott Williams & Wilkins.
290. Brownell GL, Budinger TF, Lauterbur PC, McGeer PL: Positron tomography and nuclear magnetic resonance imaging, *Science* 215:619, 1982.
291. James AE Jr, Price RR, Rollo FD, Patton JA, et al: Nuclear magnetic resonance imaging: A promising technique, *JAMA* 247:1331-1334, 1982.
292. Pykett IL: NMR imaging in medicine, *Sci Am* 246:78-88, 1982.
293. Bradbury EM, Radda GK, Allen PS: Nuclear magnetic resonance techniques in medicine, *Ann Intern Med* 98:514-529, 1983.
294. Koutcher JA, Burt CT: Principles of imaging by nuclear magnetic resonance, *J Nucl Med* 25:371-382, 1984.
295. Dubowitz LM, Bydder GM: Nuclear magnetic resonance imaging in the diagnosis and follow-up of neonatal cerebral injury, *Clin Perinatol* 12:243-260, 1985.
296. Kramer DM: Basic principles of magnetic resonance imaging, *Radiol Clin North Am* 22:765-778, 1984.
297. Leonard JC, Younkin DP, Chance B, Subramanian VH, et al: Nuclear magnetic resonance: An overview of its spectroscopic and imaging applications in pediatric patients, *J Pediatr* 106:756-761, 1985.
298. Wolpert SM, Barnes PD: *MRI in Pediatric Neuroradiology*, St. Louis: 1992, Mosby Year Book.
299. Edelman RR, Warach S: Medical progress. I. Magnetic resonance imaging, *N Engl J Med* 328:708-716, 1993.
300. Bydder GM: Principles of magnetic resonance imaging. In Haddad J, Christmann D, Messer J, editors: *Imaging Techniques of the CNS of the Neonates*, New York: 1991, Springer-Verlag.
301. Barkovich AJ: *Pediatric Neuroimaging*, 3rd ed, New York: 2000, Raven Press.
302. Johnson MA, Pennock JM, Bydder GM, Steiner RE, et al: Clinical NMR imaging of the brain in children: Normal and neurologic disease, *AJR Am J Roentgenol* 141:1005-1018, 1983.
303. Barkovich AJ: *Pediatric Neuroimaging*, New York: 1990, Raven Press.
304. Christmann D, Haddad J: Magnetic resonance imaging: Application to the neonatal period. In Haddad J, Christmann D, Messer J, editors: *Imaging Techniques of the CNS of the Neonates*, New York: 1991, Springer-Verlag.
305. Konishi Y, Kuriyama M, Hayakawa K, Konishi K, et al: Magnetic resonance imaging in preterm infants, *Pediatr Neurol* 7:191-195, 1991.
306. van der Knaap MS, Valk J: MR imaging of the various stages of normal myelination during the first year of life, *Neuroradiology* 31:459-470, 1990.
307. Barkovich AJ, Kjos BO, Jackson DE, Norman D: Normal maturation of the neonatal and infant brain: MR imaging at 1.5 T, *Radiology* 166:173-180, 1988.
308. Bird CR, Hedberg M, Drayer BP, Keller PJ, et al: MR assessment of myelination in infants and children: Usefulness of marker sites, *AJNR Am J Neuroradiol* 10:731-740, 1989.
309. McArdle CB, Richardson CJ, Nicholas DA, Mirfakhrace M, et al: Developmental features of the neonatal brain: MR imaging. II. Ventricular size and extracerebral space, *Radiology* 162:230-234, 1987.
310. McArdle CB, Richardson CJ, Nicholas DA, Mirfakhraee M, et al: Developmental features of the neonatal brain: MR imaging. I. Gray-white matter differentiation and myelination, *Radiology* 162:223-229, 1987.
311. van de Bor M, Guit GL, Schreuder AM, van Bel F, et al: Does very preterm birth impair myelination of the central nervous system? *Neuropediatrics* 21:37-39, 1990.
312. Barnes PD: Imaging of the central nervous system in pediatrics and adolescence, *Pediatr Clin North Am* 39:743-776, 1992.
313. Klucznik RP, Wolpert SM, Anderson MJ: Congenital and developmental abnormalities of the brain. In Patterson AS, editor: *MRI in Pediatric Neuroradiology*, St. Louis: 1992, Mosby.
314. van Wezel-Mejiler G, van der Knaap MS, Sie LTL, Oosting J, et al: Magnetic resonance imaging of the brain in premature infants during the neonatal period: Normal phenomena and reflection of mild ultrasound abnormalities, *Neuropediatrics* 29:89-96, 1998.
315. Battin MR, Maalouf EF, Counsell SJ, Herlihy AH, et al: Magnetic resonance imaging of the brain in very preterm infants: Visualization of the germinal matrix, early myelination, and cortical folding, *Pediatrics* 101:957-962, 1998.
316. Counsell SJ, Maalouf EF, Fletcher AM, Duggan PJ, et al: MR imaging assessment of myelination in the very preterm brain, *AJNR Am J Neuroradiol* 23:872-881, 2002.

317. Huppi PS, Warfield S, Kikinis R, Barnes PD, et al: Quantitative magnetic resonance imaging of brain development in premature and mature newborns, *Ann Neurol* 43:224-235, 1998.
318. Isaacs E, Lucas A, Chong WK, wood SJ, et al: Hippocampal volume and everyday memory in children of very low birth weight, *Pediatr Res* 47:713-720, 2000.
319. Peterson BS, Vohr B, Staib LH, Cannistraci CJ, et al: Regional brain volume abnormalities and long-term cognitive outcome in preterm infants, *JAMA* 284:1939-1947, 2000.
320. Nosarti C, Al-Asady MHS, Frangou S, Stewart AL, et al: Adolescents who were born very preterm have decreased brain volumes, *Brain* 125:1616-1623, 2002.
321. Abernethy LJ, Cooke RW, Foulder-Hughes L: Caudate and hippocampal volumes, intelligence, and motor impairment in 7-year-old children who were born preterm, *Pediatr Res* 55:884-893, 2004.
322. Reiss AL, Kesler SR, Vohr B, Duncan CC, et al: Sex differences in cerebral volumes of 8-year-olds born preterm, *J Pediatr* 145:242-249, 2004.
323. Kesler SR, Ment LR, Vohr B, Pajot SK, et al: Volumetric analysis of regional cerebral development in preterm children, *Pediatr Neurol* 31:318-325, 2004.
324. Lin Y, Okumura A, Hayakawa F, Kato T, et al: Quantitative evaluation of thalami and basal ganglia in infants with periventricular leukomalacia, *Dev Med Child Neurol* 43:481-485, 2001.
325. Lodygensky GA, Rademaker KJ, Zimine S, Gex-Fabry M, et al: Structural and functional brain developmental after hydrocortisone treatment for neonatal chronic lung disease, *Pediatrics* 116:1-7, 2005.
325a. Nosarti C, Giouroukou E, Healy E, Rifkin L, et al: Grey and white matter distribution in very preterm adolescents mediates neurodevelopmental outcome, *Brain* 131:205-217, 2008.
326. Inder TE, Huppi PS, Warfield S, Kikinis R, et al: Periventricular white matter injury in the premature infant is associated with a reduction in cerebral cortical gray matter volume at term, *Ann Neurol* 46:755-760, 1999.
327. Ajayi-Obe M, Saeed N, Cowan FM, Rutherford MA, et al: Reduced development of cerebral cortex in extremely preterm infants, *Lancet* 356:1162-1163, 2000.
328. Peterson BS, Anderson AW, Ehrenkranz RA, Staib LH, et al: Regional brain volumes and their later neurodevelopmental correlates in term and preterm infants, *Pediatrics* 111:939-948, 2003.
329. Inder TE, Warfield SK, Wang H, Huppi PS, et al: Abnormal cerebral structure is present at term in premature infants, *Pediatrics* 115:286-294, 2005.
330. Woodward LJ, Edgin JO, Thompson D, Inder TE: Object working memory deficits predicted by early brain injury and development in the preterm infant, *Brain* 128:2578-2587, 2005.
331. Thompson DK, Warfield SK, Carlin JB, Pavlovic M, et al: Perinatal risk factors altering regional brain structure in the preterm infant, *Brain* 130:667-677, 2007.
332. Murphy BP, Inder TE, Huppi PS, Warfield S, et al: Impaired cerebral cortical gray matter growth after treatment with dexamethasone for neonatal chronic lung disease, *Pediatrics* 107:217-221, 2001.
332a. Parikh N, Lasky RE, Kennedy KA, Moya FR, et al: Postnatal dexamethasone therapy and cerebral tissue volumes in extremely low birth weight infants, *Pediatrics* 119:265-272, 2007.
333. Inder TE, Huppi PS: In vivo studies of brain development by magnetic resonance techniques, *Ment Retard Dev Disabil Res Rev* 6:59-67, 2000.
334. Takeda K, Nomura Y, Sakuma H, Tagami TA, et al: MR assessment of normal brain development in neonates and infants: Comparative study of T1- and diffusion-weighted images, *J Comput Assist Tomogr* 21:1-7, 1997.
335. Ono J, Harada K, Mano T, Sakurai K, et al: Differentiation of dys- and demyelination using diffusional anisotrophy, *Pediatr Neurol* 16:63-66, 1997.
336. Toft PB, Leth H, Peitersen B, Lou HC, et al: The apparent diffusion coefficient of water in gray and white matter of the infant brain, *J Comput Assist Tomogr* 20:1006-1011, 1996.
337. Pierpaoli C, Jezzard P, Basser PJ, Barnett A, et al: Diffusion tensor MR imaging of the human brain, *Radiology* 201:637-648, 1996.
338. Neil JJ, Shiran SI, McKinstry RC, Schefft GL, et al: Normal brain in human newborns: Apparent diffusion coefficient and diffusion anisotropy measured by using diffusion tensor MR imaging, *Radiology* 209:57-66, 1998.
339. Huppi PS, Maier SE, Peled S, Zientara GP, et al: Microstructural development of human newborn cerebral white matter assessed in vivo by diffusion tensor magnetic resonance imaging, *Pediatr Res* 44:584-590, 1998.
340. Huppi PS, Murphy B, Maier SE, Zientara GP, et al: Microstructural brain development after perinatal cerebral white matter injury assessed by diffusion tensor magnetic resonance imaging, *Pediatrics* 107:455-460, 2001.
341. Neil JJ, Miller JH, Mukherjee P, Huppi PS: Diffusion tensor imaging of normal and injured developing human brain: A technical review, *NMR Biomed* 15:543-552, 2002.
342. Miller JH, McKinstry RC, Philip JV, Mukherjee P, et al: Diffusion-tensor MR imaging of normal brain maturation: A guide to structural development and myelination, *AJR Am J Roentgenol* 180:851-859, 2003.
343. Yoo SS, Park HJ, Soul JS, Mamata H, et al: In vivo visualization of white matter fiber tracts of preterm- and term-infant brains with diffusion tensor magnetic resonance imaging, *Invest Radiol* 40:110-115, 2005.
344. Berman JI, Mukherjee P, Partridge SC, Miller SP, et al: Quantitative diffusion tensor MRI fiber tractography of sensorimotor white matter development in premature infants, *Neuroimage* 27:862-871, 2005.
345. Huppi PS, Dubois J: Diffusion tensor imaging of brain development, *Semin Fetal Neonatal Med* 11:489-497, 2006.
345a. Counsell SJ, Dyet LE, Larkman DJ, Nunes RG, et al: Thalamo-cortical connectivity in children born preterm mapped using probabilistic magnetic resonance tractography, *Neuroimage* 34:896-904, 2007.
345b. Rose J, Mirmiran M, Butler EE, Lin CY, et al: Neonatal microstructural development of the internal capsule on diffusion tensor imaging correlates with severity of gait and motor deficits, *Dev Med Child Neurol* 49:745-750, 2007.
346. Kroenke CD, Bretthorst GL, Inder TE, Neil JJ: Diffusion MR imaging characteristics of the developing primate brain, *Neuroimage* 25:1205-1213, 2005.
347. Drobyshevsky A, Song SK, Gamkrelidze G, Wyrwicz AM, et al: Developmental changes in diffusion anisotropy coincide with immature oligodendrocyte progression and maturation of compound action potential, *J Neurosci* 25:5988-5997, 2005.
348. Kapellou O, Counsell SJ, Kennea NL, Dyet L, et al: Abnormal cortical development after premature birth shown by altered allometric scaling of brain growth, *PLoS Med* 3:e265, 2006.
349. Gothelf D, Furfaro JA, Penniman LC, Glover GH, et al: The contribution of novel brain imaging techniques to understanding the neurobiology of mental retardation and developmental disabilities, *Ment Retard Dev Disabil Res Rev* 11:331-339, 2005.
350. Battin M, Maalouf EF, Counsell S, Herlihy A, et al: Physiological stability of preterm infants during magnetic resonance imaging, *Early Hum Dev* 52:101-110, 1998.
351. Levene MI, Evans DH: Continuous measurement of subarachnoid pressure in the severely asphyxiated newborn, *Arch Dis Child* 58:1013-1015, 1983.
352. Levene MI, Evans DH: Medical management of raised intracranial pressure after severe birth asphyxia, *Arch Dis Child* 60:12-16, 1985.
353. Salmon JH, Hajjar W, Bada HS: The fontogram: A noninvasive intracranial pressure monitor, *Pediatrics* 60:721-725, 1977.
354. Bada HS, Chua C, Salmon JH, Hajjar W: Changes in intracranial pressure during exchange transfusion, *J Pediatr* 94:129-132, 1979.
355. Vidyasagar D, Raju TN, Chiang J: Clinical significance of monitoring anterior fontanel pressure in sick neonates and infants, *Pediatrics* 62:996-999, 1978.
356. Vidyasagar D, Raju TN: A simple noninvasive technique of measuring intracranial pressure in the newborn, Pediatrics:957–961 1977.
357. Donn SM, Philip AG: Early increase in intracranial pressure in preterm infants, *Pediatrics* 61:904-907, 1978.
358. Philip AG: Noninvasive monitoring of intracranial pressure: A new approach for neonatal clinical pharmacology, *Clin Perinatol* 6:123-137, 1979.
359. Hill A, Volpe JJ: Measurement of intracranial pressure using the Ladd intracranial pressure monitor, *J Pediatr* 98:974-976, 1981.
360. Emery JR, Peabody JL: Head position affects intracranial pressure in newborn infants, *J Pediatr* 103:950-953, 1983.
361. Menke JA, Miles R, McIlhany M, Bashiru M, et al: The fontanelle tonometer: A noninvasive method for measurement of intracranial pressure, *J Pediatr* 100:960-963, 1982.
362. Easa D, Tran A, Bingham W: Noninvasive intracranial pressure measurement in the newborn, *Am J Dis Child* 137:332-335, 1983.
363. Horbar JD, Yeager S, Philip AG, Lucey JF: Effect of application force on noninvasive measurements of intracranial pressure, *Pediatrics* 66:455-457, 1980.
364. Walsh P, Logan WJ: Continuous and intermittent measurement of intracranial pressure by Ladd monitor, *J Pediatr* 102:439-442, 1983.
365. Robinson RO, Rolfe P, Sutton P: Non-invasive method for measuring intracranial pressure in normal newborn infants, *Dev Med Child Neurol* 19:305-308, 1977.
366. Lacey L, John E, McDevitt M, Cassady G, et al: Effect of application pressure and gestational age on transfontanel pressure in healthy neonates, *Biol Neonate* 50:136-140, 1986.
367. Bunegin L, Albin MS, Rauschhuber R, Marlin AE: Intracranial pressure measurement from the anterior fontanelle utilizing a pneumoelectronic switch, *Neurosurgery* 20:726-731, 1987.
368. Rochefort MJ, Rolfe P, Wilkinson AR: New fontanometer for continuous estimation of intracranial pressure in the newborn, *Arch Dis Child* 62:152-155, 1987.
369. Kaiser AM, Whitlaw AGL: Non-invasive monitoring of intracranial pressure: Fact or fancy? *Dev Med Child Neurol* 29:320-326, 1987.
370. Mehta A, Wright BM, Shore C: Clinical fontanometry in the newborn, *Lancet* 1:754-756, 1988.
371. Wayenberg JL, Raftopoulos C, Vermeylen D, Pardou A: Non-invasive measurement of intracranial pressure in the newborn and the infant: The Rotterdam teletransducer, *Arch Dis Child* 69:493-497, 1993.
372. Peters R, Hanlo PW, Gooskens R, Braun K, et al: Non-invasive ICP monitoring in infants: The Rotterdam teletransducer revisited, *Child Nerv Syst* 11:207-213, 1995.
373. Welch K: The intracranial pressure in infants, *J Neurosurg* 52:693-699, 1980.
374. Strassburg HM, Bogner K, Klemm HJ: Alterations of intracranial pressure and cerebral blood flow velocity in healthy neonates and their implication in the origin of perinatal brain damage, *Eur J Pediatr* 147:30-35, 1988.
375. Kaiser AM, Whitelaw AGL: Normal cerebrospinal fluid pressure in the newborn, *Neuropediatrics* 17:100-102, 1986.

376. Levinson A: Cerebrospinal fluid in infants and children, *Am J Dis Child* 36:799, 1928.

377. Munro D: Cerebrospinal fluid pressure in the newborn, *JAMA* 90:1688, 1928.

378. Perlman JM, Volpe JJ: Seizures in the preterm infant: Effects on cerebral blood flow velocity, intracranial pressure, and arterial blood pressure, *J Pediatr* 102:288-293, 1983.

379. Hill A, Perlman JM, Volpe JJ: Relationship of pneumothorax to occurrence of intraventricular hemorrhage in the premature newborn, *Pediatrics* 69:144-149, 1982.

380. Kreusser KL, Tarby TJ, Taylor D, Kovnar E, et al: Rapidly progressive posthemorrhagic hydrocephalus: Treatment with external ventricular drainage, *Am J Dis Child* 138:633-637, 1984.

381. Kreusser KL, Tarby TJ, Kovnar E, Taylor DA, et al: Serial lumbar punctures for at least temporary amelioration of neonatal posthemorrhagic hydrocephalus, *Pediatrics* 75:719-724, 1985.

382. Lupton BA, Hill A, Roland EH, Whitfield MF, et al: Brain swelling in the asphyxiated term newborn: Pathogenesis and outcome, *Pediatrics* 82:139-146, 1988.

383. Pourcelot L: Diagnostic ultrasound for cerebrovascular disease. In Donald J, Levi S, editors: *Present and Future Diagnostic Ultrasound*, New York: 1976, Wiley.

384. Bada HS, Hajjar W, Chua C, Sumner DS: Noninvasive diagnosis of neonatal asphyxia and intraventricular hemorrhage by Doppler ultrasound, *J Pediatr* 95:775-779, 1979.

385. Raju TN: Cerebral Doppler studies in the fetus and newborn infant, *J Pediatr* 119:165-174, 1991.

386. Perlman JM, Hill A, Volpe JJ: The effect of patent ductus arteriosus on flow velocity in the anterior cerebral arteries: Ductal steal in the premature newborn infant, *J Pediatr* 99:767-771, 1981.

387. Hill A, Volpe JJ: Decrease in pulsatile flow in the anterior cerebral arteries in infantile hydrocephalus, *Pediatrics* 69:4-7, 1982.

388. Perlman JM, Volpe JJ: Suctioning in the preterm infant: Effects on cerebral blood flow velocity, intracranial pressure, and arterial blood pressure, *Pediatrics* 72:329-334, 1983.

389. Kehrer M, Goelz R, Krageloh-Mann I, Schoning M: Measurement of volume of cerebral blood flow in healthy preterm and term neonates with ultrasound, *Lancet* 360:1749-1750, 2002.

390. Kehrer M, Krageloh-Mann I, Goelz R, Schoning M: The development of cerebral perfusion in healthy preterm and term neonates, *Neuropediatrics* 34:281-286, 2003.

391. Hansen NB, Stonestreet BS, Rosenkrantz TS, Oh W: Validity of Doppler measurements of anterior cerebral artery blood flow velocity: Correlation with brain blood flow in piglets, *Pediatrics* 72:526-531, 1983.

392. Batton DG, Hellmann J, Hernandez MJ, Maisels MJ: Regional cerebral blood flow, cerebral blood velocity, and pulsatility index in newborn dogs, *Pediatr Res* 17:908-912, 1983.

393. Sonesson S-E, Herin P: Intracranial arterial blood flow velocity and brain blood flow during hypocarbia and hypercarbia in newborn lambs: A validation of range-gated Doppler ultrasound flow velocimetry, *Pediatr Res* 24:423-426, 1988.

394. Greisen G, Johansen K, Ellison PH, Fredriksen PS, et al: Cerebral blood flow in the newborn infant: Comparison of Doppler ultrasound and [133]xenon clearance, *J Pediatr* 104:411-418, 1984.

395. Perlman JM, Herscovitch P, Corriveau S: The relationship of cerebral blood flow velocity, determined by Doppler, to regional cerebral blood flow, determined by positron emission tomography [abstract], *Pediatr Res* 19:357, 1985.

396. Kontos HA: Validity of cerebral arterial blood flow calculations from velocity measurements, *Stroke* 20:1-3, 1989.

397. Abboud FM: Special characteristics of the cerebral circulation, *Fed Proc* 40:2296-2300, 1981.

398. Heistad DD, Marcus MI, Abboud FM: Role of large arteries in regulation of cerebral blood flow in dogs, *J Clin Invest* 62:761-768, 1978.

399. Kontos HA, Wei EP, Navari RM, Levasseur JE, et al: Responses of cerebral arteries and arterioles to acute hypotension and hypertension, *Am J Physiol* 3:H371-H383, 1978.

400. Kuban KC, Gilles FH: Human telencephalic angiogenesis, *Ann Neurol* 17:539-548, 1985.

401. Calvert SA, Ohlsson A, Hosking MC, Erskine L, et al: Serial measurements of cerebral blood flow velocity in preterm infants during the first 72 hours of life, *Acta Paediatr Scand* 77:625-631, 1988.

402. Sonesson S-E, Winberg P, Lundell BPW: Early postnatal changes in intracranial arterial blood flow velocities in term infants, *Pediatr Res* 22:461-464, 1987.

403. Raju TNK, Kin SY: Cerebral artery flow velocity acceleration and deceleration characteristics in newborn infants, *Pediatr Res* 26:588-592, 1989.

404. Raju TNK, Go M, Ryva JC, Schmidt DJ: Common carotid artery flow velocity measurements in the newborn period with pulsed Doppler technique, *Biol Neonate* 52:241-249, 1987.

405. Grant EG, White EM, Schellinger D, Choyke PL, et al: Cranial duplex sonography of the infant, *Radiology* 163:177-185, 1987.

406. Ando Y, Takashima S, Takeshita K: Postnatal changes of cerebral blood flow velocity in normal term neonates, *Brain Dev* 5:525-528, 1983.

407. van Bel F, den Ouden L, van de Bor M, Stijnen T, et al: Cerebral blood-flow velocity during the first week of life of preterm infants and neurodevelopment at two years, *Dev Med Child Neurol* 31:320-328, 1989.

408. Ramaekers VT, Casaer P, Daniels H, Smet M, et al: The influence of behavioural states on cerebral blood flow velocity patterns in stable preterm infants, *Early Hum Dev* 20:229-246, 1989.

409. Bode H, Wais U: Age dependence of flow velocities in basal cerebral arteries, *Arch Dis Child* 63:606-611, 1988.

410. Bode H: *Pediatric Applications of Transcranial Doppler Sonography*, New York: 1988, Springer-Verlag.

411. Bode H, Eden A: Transcranial Doppler sonography in children, *J Child Neurol* 4:S68-S76, 1989.

412. Winberg P, Sonesson SE, Lundell PW: Postnatal changes in intracranial blood flow velocity in preterm infants, *Acta Paediatr Scand* 79:1150-1155, 1990.

413. Fenton AC, Shortland DB, Papathoma E, Evans DH, et al: Normal range for blood flow velocity in cerebral arteries of newly born term infants, *Early Hum Dev* 22:73-79, 1990.

414. Yoshida H, Yasuhara A, Kobayashi Y: Transcranial Doppler sonographic studies of cerebral blood flow velocity in neonates, *Pediatr Neurol* 7:105-110, 1991.

415. Kurmanavichius J, Karrer G, Hebisch G, Huch R, et al: Fetal and preterm newborn cerebral blood flow velocity, *Early Hum Dev* 26:113-120, 1991.

416. Connors G, Hunse C, Gagnon R, Richardson B, et al: Perinatal assessment of cerebral flow velocity wave forms in the human fetus and neonate, *Pediatr Res* 31:649-652, 1992.

417. Horiuchi I, Sanada S, Ohtahara S: Development and physiologic changes in cerebral blood flow velocity, *Pediatr Res* 34:385-388, 1993.

418. Kempley ST, Gamsu HR: Arterial blood pressure and blood flow velocity in major cerebral and visceral arteries. II. Effects of colloid infusion, *Early Hum Dev* 35:25-30, 1993.

419. Ferrari F, Kelsall AW, Rennie JM, Evans DH: The relationship between cerebral blood flow velocity fluctuations and sleep state in normal newborns, *Pediatr Res* 35:50-54, 1994.

420. Mires GJ, Patel NB, Forsyth JS, Howie PW: Neonatal cerebral Doppler flow velocity waveforms in the uncomplicated pre-term infant: Reference values, *Early Hum Dev* 36:205-212, 1994.

421. Mires GJ, Patel NB, Forsyth JS, Howie PW: Neonatal cerebral Doppler flow velocity waveforms in the pre-term infant with cerebral pathology, *Early Hum Dev* 36:213-222, 1994.

422. Cheung YF, Lam PKL, Yeung CY: Early postnatal cerebral Doppler changes in relation to birth weight, *Early Hum Dev* 37:57-66, 1994.

423. Ozek E, Koroglu TF, Karakoc F, Kilic T, et al: Transcranial Doppler assessment of cerebral blood flow velocity in term newborns, *Eur J Pediatr* 154:60-63, 1995.

424. Kempley ST, Vyas S, Bower S, Nicolaides KH, et al: Cerebral and renal artery blood flow velocity before and after birth, *Early Hum Dev* 46:165-175, 1996.

425. Weir FJ, Ohlsson A, Myhr TL, Fong K, et al: A patent ductus arteriosus is associated with reduced middle cerebral artery blood flow velocity, *Eur J Pediatr* 158:484-487, 1999.

426. Chang BL, Santillan G, Bing RJ: Red cell velocity and autoregulation in the cerebral cortex of the cat, *Brain Res* 308:15-24, 1984.

427. McMenamin JB, Volpe JJ: Doppler ultrasonography in the determination of neonatal brain death, *Ann Neurol* 14:302-307, 1983.

428. McMenamin JB, Volpe JJ: Bacterial meningitis in infancy: Effects on intracranial pressure and cerebral blood flow velocity, *Neurology* 34:500-504, 1984.

429. Perlman JM, McMenamin JB, Volpe JJ: Fluctuating cerebral blood-flow velocity in respiratory-distress syndrome: Relation to the development of intraventricular hemorrhage, *N Engl J Med* 309:204-209, 1983.

430. Rosenkrantz TS, Oh W: Cerebral blood flow velocity in infants with polycythemia and hyperviscosity: Effects of partial exchange transfusion with Plasmanate, *J Pediatr* 101:94-98, 1982.

431. Bada HS, Miller JE, Menke JA, Menten TG, et al: Intracranial pressure and cerebral arterial pulsatile flow measurement in neonatal intraventricular hemorrhage, *J Pediatr* 100:291-296, 1982.

432. Lipman B, Serwer GA, Brazy JE: Abnormal cerebral hemodynamics in preterm infants with patent ductus arteriosus, *Pediatrics* 69:778-781, 1982.

433. Menke J, Rabe MH, Bresser BW, Grohs B, et al: Simultaneous influence of blood pressure, PCO2, and PO2 on cerebral blood flow velocity in preterm infants of less than 33 weeks' gestation, *Pediatr Res* 34:173-177, 1993.

434. van Bel F, van de Bor M, Baan J, Ruys JH: The influence of abnormal blood gases on cerebral blood flow velocity in the preterm newborn, *Neuropediatrics* 19:27-32, 1988.

435. Archer LN, Evans DH, Paton JY, Levene MI: Controlled hypercapnia and neonatal cerebral artery Doppler ultrasound waveforms, *Pediatr Res* 20:218-221, 1986.

436. Daven JR, Milstein JM, Guthrie RD: Cerebral vascular resistance in premature infants, *Am J Dis Child* 137:328-331, 1983.

437. Bada HS, Korones SB, Kolni HW: Partial exchange transfusion improves cerebral hemodynamics in symptomatic neonatal polycythemia, *Am J Med Sci* 291:157-163, 1986.

438. Powers AD, Graeber MC, Smith RR: Transcranial Doppler ultrasonography in the determination of brain death, *Neurosurgery* 24:884-889, 1989.

439. Ahmann PA, Carrigan TA, Carlton D, Wyly B, et al: Brain death in children: Characteristic common carotid arterial velocity patterns measured with pulsed Doppler ultrasound, *J Pediatr* 110:723-728, 1987.

440. van Bel F, van de Bor M, Bann J, Stijnen T, et al: Blood flow velocity pattern of the anterior cerebral arteries before and after drainage of posthemorrhagic hydrocephalus in the newborn, *J Ultrasound Med* 7:553-559, 1988.

441. Huang C-C, Chio C-C: Duplex color ultrasound study of infantile progressive ventriculomegaly, *Childs Nerv Syst* 7:251-256, 1991.
442. van Bel F, van de Bor M, Stijnen T, Baan J, et al: Cerebral blood flow velocity pattern in healthy and asphyxiated newborns: A controlled study, *Eur J Pediatr* 146:461-467, 1987.
443. Haddad J, Constantinesco A, Brunot B: Single photon emission computed tomography of the brain perfusion in neonates. In Haddad J, Christmann D, Messer J, editors: *Imaging Techniques of the CNS of the Neonates*, New York: 1991, Springer-Verlag.
444. Archer LN, Levene MI, Evans DH: Cerebral artery Doppler ultrasonography for prediction of outcome after perinatal asphyxia, *Lancet* 2:1116-1118, 1986.
445. Mardoum R, Bejar R, Merritt TA, Berry C: Controlled study of the effects of indomethacin on cerebral blood flow velocities in newborn infants, *J Pediatr* 118:112-115, 1991.
446. Jorch G, Woike H, Rabe H, Reinhold P: Influence of anesthetic induction with halothane and isoflurane on internal carotid blood flow velocity in early infancy, *Dev Parmacol Ther* 13:150-158, 1989.
447. van Bel F, van de Bor M, Stijnen T, Baan J, et al: Does caffeine affect cerebral blood flow in the preterm infant? *Acta Paediatr Scand* 78:205-209, 1989.
448. Saliba E, Autret E, Gold F, Bloc D, et al: Effect of caffeine on cerebral blood flow velocity in preterm infants, *Biol Neonate* 56:198-203, 1989.
449. Ghai V, Raju TNK, Kim SY, McCulloch KM: Clinical and laboratory observations, *J Pediatr* 114:870-873, 1989.
450. Rosenkrantz TS, Oh W: Aminophylline reduces cerebral blood flow velocity in low-birth-weight infants, *Am J Dis Child* 138:489-491, 1984.
451. Deeg KH, Scharf J: Colour Doppler imaging of arteriovenous malformation of the vein of Galen in a newborn, *Neuroradiology* 32:60-63, 1990.
452. Tessler FN, Dion J, Vinuela F, Perrella RR, et al: Cranial arteriovenous malformations in neonates: Color Doppler imaging with angiographic correlation, *AJR Am J Roentgenol* 153:1027-1030, 1989.
453. Shortland DB, Gibson NA, Levene MI, Archer LN, et al: Patent ductus arteriosus and cerebral circulation in preterm infants, *Dev Med Child Neurol* 32:386-393, 1990.
454. Messer J, Haddad J, Casanova R: Transcranial Doppler evaluation of cerebral infarction in the neonate, *Neuropediatrics* 22:147-151, 1991.
455. Yoshida-Shuto H, Yasuhara A, Kobayashi Y: Cerebral blood flow velocity and failure of autoregulation in neonates: Their relation to outcome of birth asphyxia, *Neuropediatrics* 23:241-244, 1992.
456. Nelle M, Hocker C, Zilow EP, Linderkamp O: Effects of red cell transfusion on cardiac output and blood flow velocities in cerebral and gastrointestinal arteries in premature infants, *Arch Dis Child Fetal Neonatal Ed* 71:F45-F48, 1994.
457. Dean LM, Taylor GA: The intracranial venous system in infants: Normal and abnormal findings on duplex and color Doppler sonography, *AJR Am J Roentgenol* 164:151-156, 1995.
458. Hoecker C, Nelle M, Poeschl J, Beedgen B, et al: Caffeine impairs cerebral and intestinal blood flow velocity in preterm infants, *Pediatrics* 109:784-787, 2002.
459. Roll C, Horsch S: Effect of doxapram on cerebral blood flow velocity in preterm infants, *Neuropediatrics* 35:126-129, 2004.
460. Ilves P, Lintrop M, Metsvaht T, Vaher U, et al: Cerebral blood-flow velocities in predicting outcome of asphyxiated newborn infants, *Acta Paediatr* 93:523-528, 2004.
461. Bode H, Sauer M, Pringsheim W: Diagnosis of brain death by transcranial Doppler sonography, *Arch Dis Child* 63:1474-1478, 1988.
462. Jobsis FF: Noninvasive, infrared monitoring of cerebral and myocardial oxygen sufficiency and circulatory parameters, *Science* 198:1264-1267, 1977.
463. Wyatt JS, Delpy DT: Near infrared spectroscopy. In Haddad J, Christmann D, Messer J, editors: *Imaging Techniques of the CNS of the Neonates*, New York: 1991, Springer-Verlag.
464. Reynolds EOR, Wyatt JS, Axxopardi D, Delpy DT, et al: New nonivasive methods for assessing brain oxygenation and haemodynamics, *Br Med Bull* 44:1052-1075, 1988.
465. du Plessis AJ: Near-infrared spectroscopy for the in vivo study of cerebral hemodynamics and oxygenation, *Curr Opin Pediatr* 7:632-639, 1995.
466. du Plessis AJ, Volpe JJ: Cerebral oxygenation and hemodynamic changes during infant cardiac surgery: Measurements by near infreared spectroscopy, *J Biomed Optics* 1:373-386, 1996.
467. Nicklin SE, Hassan IA-A, Wickramasinghe YA, Spencer SA: The light still shines, but not that brightly? The current status of perinatal near infrared spectroscopy, *Arch Dis Child Fetal Neonatal Ed* 88:F263-F268, 2003.
468. Tamura M, Hazeki O, Nioka S, Chance B, et al: The simultaneous measurements of tissue oxygen concentration and energy state by near-infrared and nuclear magnetic resonance spectroscopy, *Adv Exp Med Biol* 222:359-363, 1987.
469. Wickramasinghe YABD, Palmer KS, Houston R, Spencer SA, et al: Effect of fetal hemoglobin on the determination of neonatal cerebral oxygenation by near-infrared spectroscopy, *Pediatr Res* 34:15-17, 1993.
470. Takashima S, Ando Y: Reflectance spectrophotometry, cerebral blood flow and congestion in young rabbit brain, *Brain Dev* 10:20-23, 1988.

471. Hampson NB, Piantadosi A: Near-infrared optical responses in feline brain and skeletal muscle tissues during respiratory acid-base imbalance, *Brain Res* 519:249-254, 1990.
472. Mito T, Koyama K, Houdou S, Takashima S, et al: Response on near-infrared spectroscopy and of cerebral blood flow to hypoxemia induced by N2 and CO2 in young rabbits, *Brain Dev* 12:408-411, 1990.
473. Koyama K, Mito T, Takashima S, Suzuki S: The effects of prostaglandin E1 and nicardipine on cerebral blood flow, blood volume and oxygenation in young rabbits, *Brain Dev* 13:32-35, 1991.
474. Hasegawa M, Houdou S, Takashima S, Tatsuno M, et al: Monitoring of immature rabbit brain during hypoxia with near-infrared spectroscopy, *Pediatr Neurol* 8:47-50, 1991.
475. Wray S, Cope M, Delpy T, Wyatt JS, et al: Characterization of the near infrared absorption spectra of cytochrome aa3 and haemoglobin for the non-invasive monitoring of cerebral oxygenation, *Biochim Biophys Acta* 933:184-192, 1988.
476. Wyatt JS, Cope M, Delpy DT, Wray S, et al: Quantification of cerebral oxygenation and haemodynamics in sick newborn infants by near infrared spectrophotometry, *Lancet* 2:1063-1066, 1986.
477. Delpy DT, Cope MC, Cady EB: Cerebral monitoring in newborn infants by magnetic resonance and near infrared spectroscopy, *Scand J Clin Lab Invest* 47:9-17, 1987.
478. Edwards AD, Wyatt JS, Richardson C, Delpy DT, et al: Cotside measurement of cerebral blood flow in ill newborn infants by near infrared spectroscopy, *Lancet* 2:770-771, 1988.
479. Edwards AD, Wyatt JS, Richardson C, Potter A, et al: Effects of indomethacin on cerebral haemodynamics in very preterm infants, *Lancet* 335:1491-1495, 1990.
480. Wyatt JS, Cope M, Delpy DT, Richardson CE, et al: Quantitation of cerebral blood volume in human infants by near-infrared spectroscopy, *J Appl Physiol* 68:1086-1091, 1990.
481. Wyatt JS, Edwards AD, Cope M, Delpy DT, et al: Response of cerebral blood volume to changes in arterial carbon dioxide tension in preterm and term infants, *Pediatr Res* 29:553-557, 1991.
482. Cope M, Delpy DT, Wyatt JS, Wray SC, et al: A CDD spectrometer to quantitate the concentration of chromophores in living tissue utilizing the absorption peak of water at 975 nm., *Adv Exp Med Biol* 247:33-41, 1989.
483. Wyatt JS, Cope M, Delpy DT, van der Zee P, et al: Measurement of optical path length for cerebral near-infrared spectroscopy in newborn infants, *Dev Neurosci* 12:140-144, 1990.
484. Delpy DT, Cope M, van der Zee P: Estimation of optical pathlength through tissue from direct time of flight measurement, *Phys Med Biol* 33:1433-1442, 1988.
485. Edwards AD, Brown GC, Cope M, Wyatt JS, et al: Quantification of concentration changes in neonatal human cerebral oxidized cytochrome oxidase, *J Appl Physiol* 71:1907-1913, 1991.
486. Skov L, Hellström-Westas L, Jacobsen T, Greisen G, et al: Acute changes in cerebral oxygenation and cerebral blood volume in preterm infants during surfactant treatment, *Neuropediatrics* 23:126-130, 1992.
487. Edwards AD, McCormick DC, Roth SC, Elwell CE, et al: Cerebral hemodynamic effects of treatment with modified natural surfactant investigated by near infrared spectroscopy, *Pediatr Res* 32:532-536, 1992.
488. von Siebenthal K, Bernert G, Casaer P: Near-infrared spectroscopy in newborn infants, *Brain Dev* 14:135-143, 1992.
489. McCormick DC, Edwards AD, Brown GC, Wyatt JS, et al: Effects of indomethacin on cerebral oxidized cytochrome oxidase in preterm infants, *Pediatr Res* 33:603-608, 1993.
490. Hirtz DG: Report of the National Institute of Neurological Disorders and Stroke Workshop on Near Infrared Spectroscopy, *Pediatrics* 91:414-417, 1993.
491. Hirano S, Hasegawa M, Kamei A, Ozaki T, et al: Responses of cerebral blood volume and oxygenation to carotid ligation and hypoxia in young rabbits: Near-infrared spectroscopy study, *J Child Neurol* 8:237-241, 1993.
492. Takei Y, Edwards AD, Lorek A, Peebles DM, et al: Effects of N-omega-nitro-l-arginine methyl ester on the cerebral circulation of newborn piglets quantified in vivo by near-infrared spectroscopy, *Pediatr Res* 34:354-359, 1993.
493. van Bel F, Dorrepaal C, Benders M, van de Bor M, et al: Changes in cerebral hemodynamics and oxygenation in the first 24 hours following birth asphyxia, *Pediatrics* 92:365-372, 1993.
494. Brun NC, Greisen G: Cerebrovascular responses to carbon dioxide as detected by near-infrared spectrophotometry: Comparison of three different measures, *Pediatr Res* 36:20-24, 1994.
495. van de Bor M, Benders MJ, Dorrepaal CA, van Bel F, et al: Cerebral blood volume changes during exchange transfusions in infants born at or near term, *J Pediatr* 125:617-621, 1994.
496. Duncan A, Meek JH, Clemence M, Elwell CE, et al: Measurement of cranial optical path length as a function of age using phase resolved near infrared spectroscopy, *Pediatr Res* 39:889-894, 1996.
497. Wickramasinghe YABD, Rolfe P, Palmer K, Spencer SA: Investigation of neonatal brain cytochrome redox by NIRS, *Brain Res Dev Brain Res* 89:307-308, 1995.
498. Tsuji M, Naruse H, Volpe JJ, Holtzman D: Reduction of cytochrome aa3 measured by near-infrared spectroscopy predicts cerebral energy loss in hypoxic piglets, *Pediatr Res* 37:253-259, 1995.

499. du Plessis AJ, Newburger J, Jonas RA, Hickey P, et al: Cerebral oxygen supply and utilization during infant cardiac surgery, *Ann Neurol* 37:488-497, 1995.

500. Liem KD, Hopman JCW, Osenburg B, de Haan AFJ, et al: Cerebral oxygenation and hemodynamics during induction of extracorporeal membrane oxygenation as investigated by near infrared spectrophotometry, *Pediatrics* 95:555-561, 1995.

501. Nomura F, Naruse H, du Plessis A, Hiramatsu T, et al: Cerebral oxygenation measured by near infrared spectroscopy during cardiopulmonary bypass and deep hypothermic circulatory arrest in piglets, *Pediatr Res* 40:790-796, 1996.

502. Meek JH, Tyszczuk L, Elwell CE, Wyatt JS: Cerebral blood flow increases over the first three days of life in extremely preterm neonates, *Arch Dis Child Fetal Neonatal Ed* 78:F33-F37, 1998.

503. Yoxall CW, Weindling M: Measurement of cerebral oxygen consumption in the human neonate using near infrared spectroscopy: Cerebral oxygen consumption increases with advancing gestational age, *Pediatr Res* 44:283-290, 1998.

504. Meek JH, Firbank M, Elwell CE, Atkinson J, et al: Regional hemodynamic responses to visual stimulation in awake infants, *Pediatr Res* 43:840-843, 1998.

505. Tsuji M, du Plessis A, Taylor G, Crocker R, et al: Near infrared spectroscopy detects cerebral ischemia during hypotension in piglets, *Pediatr Res* 44:591-595, 1998.

506. Barfield C, Yu VYH, Noma O, Kukita J, et al: Cerebral blood volume measures using near-infrared spectroscopy and radiolabels in the immature lamb brain, *Pediatr Res* 46:50-56, 1999.

507. Chang YS, Park WS, Lee M, Kim KS, et al: Near infrared spectroscopic monitoring of secondary cerebral energy failure after transient global hypoxia-ischemia in the newborn piglet, *Neurol Res* 21:216-224, 1999.

508. Benaron DA, Hintz SR, Villringer A, Boas D, et al: Noninvasive functional imaging of human brain using light, *J Cereb Blood Flow Metab* 20:469-477, 2000.

509. Tsuji M, Saul JP, du Plessis A, Eichenwald E, et al: Cerebral intravascular oxygenation correlates with mean arterial pressure in critically ill premature infants, *Pediatrics* 106:625-632, 2000.

509a. Soul JS, Hammer PE, Tsuji M, Saul P, et al: Fluctuating pressure-passivity is common in the cerebral circulation of sick premature infants, *Pediatr Res* 61:467-473, 2007.

510. Naulaers G, Morren G, VanHuffel S, Casaer P, et al: Cerebral tissue oxygenation index in very premature infants, *Arch Dis Child* 87:189-192, 2002.

511. Urlesberger B, Pichler G, Gradnitzer E, Reiterer F, et al: Changes in cerebral blood volume and cerebral oxygenation during periodic breathing in term infants, *Neuropediatrics* 31:75-81, 2000.

512. Baserga MC, Gregory GA, Sola A: Cerebrovascular response in small preterm infants during routine nursery gavage feedings, *Biol Neonate* 83:12-18, 2003.

513. Naulaers G, Delanghe G, Allegaert K, Debeer A, et al: Ibuprofen and cerebral oxygenation and circulation, *Arch Dis Child Fetal Neonatal Ed* 90:F75-F76, 2005.

514. Peeters-Scholte C, vandenTweel E, Groenendaal F, vanBel F: Redox state of near infrared spectroscopy-measured cytochrome aa(3) correlates with delayed cerebral energy failure following perinatal hypoxia-ischaemia in the newborn pig, *Exp Brain Res* 156:20-26, 2004.

515. Altman DI, Perlman JM, Volpe JJ, Powers WJ: Cerebral oxygen metabolism in newborn infants measured with positron emission tomography, *J Cereb Blood Flow Metab* 9:525, 1989.

516. Skov LO, Pryds O, Greisen G: Estimating cerebral blood flow in newborn infants: Comparison of near infrared spectroscopy and ^{133}Xe clearance, *Pediatr Res* 27:445-449, 1991.

517. Altman DI, Powers WJ, Perlman JM, Herscovitch P, et al: Cerebral blood flow requirement for brain viability in newborn infants is lower than in adults, *Ann Neurol* 24:218-226, 1988.

518. Pryds O, Greisen G, Skov LL, Friis-Hansen B: Carbon dioxide-related changes in cerebral blood volume and cerebral blood flow in mechanically ventilated preterm neonates: Comparison of near infrared spectrophotometry and ^{133}xenon clearance, *Pediatr Res* 27:445-449, 1990.

519. Bucher HU, Edwards AD, Lipp AE, Duc G: Comparison between near infrared spectroscopy and ^{133}xenon clearance for estimation of cerebral blood flow in critically ill preterm infants, *Pediatric Res* 33:56-60, 1993.

520. Kuebler WM, Sckell A, Habler O, Kleen M, et al: Noninvasive measurement of regional cerebral blood flow by near-infrared spectroscopy and indocyanine green, *J Cereb Blood Flow Metab* 18:445-456, 1998.

521. Roberts IG, Fallon P, Kirkham FJ, Kirshbom PM, et al: Measurement of cerebral blood flow during cardiopulmonary bypass with near-infrared spectroscopy, *J Thorac Cardiovasc Surg* 115:94-102, 1998.

522. Patel J, Marks K, Roberts I, Azzopardi D, et al: Measurement of cerebral blood flow in newborn infants using near infrared spectroscopy with indocyanine green, *Pediatr Res* 43:34-39, 1988.

523. Soul JS, Taylor GA, Wypij D, du Plessis AJ, et al: Noninvasive detection of changes in cerebral blood flow by near-infrared spectroscopy in a piglet model of hydrocephalus, *Pediatr Res* 48:445-449, 2000.

524. Bassan H, Gauvreau K, Newburger JW, Tsuji M, et al: Identification of pressure passive cerebral perfusion and its mediators after infant cardiac surgery, *Pediatr Res* 57:35-41, 2005.

525. Livera LN, Spencer SA, Thorniley MS, Wickramasinghe YA, et al: Effects of hypoxaemia and bradycardia on neonatal cerebral haemodynamics, *Arch Dis Child* 66:376-380, 1991.

526. Perlman JM, Hersovitch P, Corriveau S, Raichle ME, et al: Cerebral blood flow velocity as determined by Doppler is related to regional cerebral blood flow as determined by positron emission tomography, *Ann Neurol* 18:407-408, 1985.

527. Shah AR, Kurth CD, Gwiazdowski SG, Chance B, et al: Fluctuations in cerebral oxygenation and blood volume during endotracheal suctioning in premature infants, *J Pediatr* 120:769-774, 1992.

528. Perlman JM, Volpe JJ: Are venous circulatory abnormalities important in the pathogenesis of hemorrhagic and/or ischemic cerebral injury? *Pediatrics* 80:705-711, 1987.

529. Kissack CM, Garr R, Wardle SP, Weindling AM: Postnatal changes in cerebral oxygen extraction in the preterm infant are associated with intraventricular hemorrhage and hemorrhagic parenchymal infarction but not periventricular leukomalacia, *Pediatr Res* 56:111-116, 2004.

530. Ijichi S, Kusaka T, Isobe K, Okubo K, et al: Developmental changes of optical properties in neonates determined by near-infrared time-resolved spectroscopy, *Pediatr Res* 58:568-573, 2005.

531. Meek JH, Elwell CE, Khan MJ, Romaya J, et al: Regional changes in cerebral haemodynamics as a result of a visual stimulus measured by near infrared spectroscopy, *Proc Biol Sci* 261:351-356, 1995.

532. Sakatani K, Chen S, Lichty W, Zuo H, et al: Cerebral blood oxygenation changes induced by auditory stimulation in newborn infants measured by near infrared spectroscopy, *Early Hum Dev* 55:229-236, 1999.

533. Zaramella P, Freato F, Amigoni A, Salvadori S, et al: Brain auditory activation measured by near-infrared spectroscopy (NIRS) in neonates, *Pediatr Res* 49:213-219, 2001.

534. Bartocci M, Winberg J, Papendieck G, Mustica T, et al: Cerebral hemodynamic response to unpleasant odors in the preterm newborn measured by near-infrared spectroscopy, *Pediatr Res* 50:324-330, 2001.

535. Taga G, Asakawa K, Maki A, Konishi Y, et al: Brain imaging in awake infants by near-infrared optical topography, *Proc Natl Acad Sci U S A* 100:10722-10727, 2003.

536. Bartocci M, Bergqvist LL, Lagercrantz H, Anand KJ: Pain activates cortical areas in the preterm newborn brain, *Pain* 122:109-117, 2006.

537. Slater R, Cantarella A, Gallella S, Worley A, et al: Cortical pain responses in human infants, *J Neurosci* 26:3662-3666, 2006.

538. Bartocci M, Winberg J, Ruggiero C, Bergqvist LL, et al: Activation of olfactory cortex in newborn infants after odor stimulation: A functional near-infrared spectroscopy study, *Pediatr Res* 48:18-23, 2000.

539. Hoshi Y, Kohri S, Matsumoto Y, Cho K, et al: Hemodynamic responses to photic stimulation in neonates, *Pediatr Neurol* 23:323-327, 2000.

540. Isobe K, Kusaka T, Nagano K, Okubo K, et al: Functional imaging of the brain in sedated newborn infants using near infrared topography during passive knee movement, *Neurosci Lett* 299:221-224, 2001.

541. Austin T, Gibson AP, Branco G, Yusof RM, et al: Three dimensional optical imaging of blood volume and oxygenation in the neonatal brain, *Neuroimage* 31:1426-1433, 2006.

542. Hebden JC, Gibson A, Austin T, Yusof RM, et al: Imaging changes in blood volume and oxygenation in the newborn infant brain using three-dimensional optical tomography, *Phys Med Biol* 49:1117-1130, 2004.

543. Gibson AP, Austin T, Everdell NL, Schweiger M, et al: Three-dimensional whole-head optical tomography of passive motor evoked responses in the neonate, *Neuroimage* 30:521-528, 2006.

544. Cady EB, Costello AM, Dawson MJ, Delpy DT, et al: Non-invasive investigation of cerebral metabolism in newborn infants by phosphorus nuclear magnetic resonance spectroscopy, *Lancet* 1:1059-1062, 1983.

545. Younkin DP, Delivoria-Papadopoulos M, Leonard JC, Subramanian VH, et al: Unique aspects of human newborn cerebral metabolism evaluated with phosphorus nuclear magnetic resonance spectroscopy, *Ann Neurol* 16:581-586, 1984.

546. Hope PL, Costello AM, Cady EB, Delpy DT, et al: Cerebral energy metabolism studied with phosphorus NMR spectroscopy in normal and birth-asphyxiated infants, *Lancet* 2:366-370, 1984.

547. Tofts PS, Cady EB, Delpy DT, Costello AM, et al: Surface coil NMR spectroscopy of brain, *Lancet* 1:459, 1984.

548. Hamilton PA, Hope PL, Cady EB, Delpy DT, et al: Impaired energy metabolism in brains of newborn infants with increased cerebral echodensities, *Lancet* 1:1242-1246, 1986.

549. Younkin DP, Delivoria-Papadopoulos M, Maris J, Donlon E, et al: Cerebral metabolic effects of neonatal seizures measured with in vivo ^{31}P NMR spectroscopy, *Ann Neurol* 20:513-519, 1986.

550. Lawson B, Anday E, Guileet R, Wagerle LC, et al: Brain oxidative phosphorylation following alteration in head position in preterm and term neonates, *Pediatr Res* 22:302-305, 1987.

551. Corbett RJT, Laptook AR, Nunnally RL: The use of the chemical shift of the phosphomonoester P-31 magnetic resonance peak for the determination of intracellular pH in the brains of neonates, *Neurology* 37:1771-1779, 1987.

552. Boesch C, Martin E: Combined application of MR imaging and spectroscopy in neonates and children: Installation and operation of a 2.35-T system in a clinical setting, *Radiology* 168:481-488, 1988.

553. Younkin D, Medoff-Cooper B, Guillet R: In vivo ^{31}P nuclear magnetic resonance measurement of chronic changes in cerebral metabolites following neonatal intraventricular hemorrhage, *Pediatrics* 82:331-336, 1988.

554. Young IR, Hall AS, Bryant DJ: Assessment of brain perfusion with MR imaging, *J Comput Assist Tomogr* 12:721-727, 1988.

555. Ives NK, Blackledge MJ, Hope PL: Inhomogeneity of cerebral energy metabolism in asphyxiated neonates demonstrated by spatially resolved phosphorus magnetic resonance spectroscopy [abstract], *Neonat Soc* 228, 1988.

556. Azzopardi D, Wyatt JS, Hamilton PA, Cady EB, et al: Phosphorus metabolites and intracellular pH in the brains of normal and small for gestational age infants investigated by magnetic resonance, *Pediatr Res* 25:440-444, 1989.

557. Azzopardi D, Wyatt JS, Cady EB, Delpy DT, et al: Prognosis of newborn infants with hypoxic-ischemic brain injury assessed by phosphorus magnetic resonance spectroscopy, *Pediatr Res* 25:445-451, 1989.

558. Laptook AR, Corbett RJ, Uauy R, Mize C, et al: Use of ^{31}P magnetic resonance spectroscopy to characterize evolving brain damage after perinatal asphyxia, *Neurology* 39:709-712, 1989.

559. Boesch C, Grütter R, Martin E, Duc G, et al: Variations in the in-vivo 31-phosphorus magnetic resonance spectra of the developing human brain during postnatal life, *Radiology* 172:197-199, 1989.

560. Cady EB, Hennig J, Martin E: Magnetic resonance spectroscopy. In Haddad J, Christmann D, Messer J, editors: *Imaging Techniques of the CNS of the Neonates*, New York: 1991, Springer-Verlag.

561. Hüppi PS, Posse S, Lazeyras F, Boesch C, et al: 1H-spectroscopy in preterm and term newborns: Regional developmental changes in human brain, *Pediatr Res* 34:205A, 1993.

562. Huppi PS, Posse S, Lazeyras F, Burri R, et al: Magnetic resonance in preterm and term newborns: 1H-spectroscopy in developing human brain, *Pediatr Res* 30:574-578, 1991.

563. Moorcraft J, Bolas NM, Ives NK, Ouwerkerk R, et al: Global and depth resolved phosphorus magnetic resonance spectroscopy to predict outcome after birth asphyxia, *Arch Dis Child* 66:1119-1123, 1991.

564. Peden CJ, Cowan FM, Bryant DJ, Sargentoni J, et al: Proton spectroscopy of the brain in infants, *J Comput Assist Tomogr* 14:886-894, 1990.

565. Moorcraft J, Bolas NM, Ives NK, Sutton P, et al: Spatially localized magnetic resonance spectroscopy of the brains of normal and asphyxiated newborns, *Pediatrics* 87:273-282, 1991.

566. Tzika AA, Ball WS, Vigneron DB, Dunn RS, et al: Clinical proton MR spectroscopy of neurodegenerative disease in childhood, *AJNR Am J Neuroradiol* 14:1267-1281, 1993.

567. Groenendaal F, Veenhoven RH, Van Der Grond J, Jansen GH, et al: Cerebral lactate and N-acetyl-aspartate/choline ratios in asphyxiated full-term neonates demonstrated in vivo using proton magnetic resonance spectroscopy, *Pediatr Res* 35:148-151, 1994.

568. Kimura H, Fujii Y, Itoh S, Matsuda T, et al: Metabolic alterations in the neonate and infant brain during development: Evaluation with proton MR spectroscopy, *Radiology* 194:483-489, 1995.

569. Hashimoto T, Tayama M, Miyazaki M, Fujii E, et al: Developmental brain changes investigated with proton magnetic resonance spectroscopy, *Dev Med Child Neurol* 37:398-405, 1995.

570. Kreis R, Ernst T, Ross BD: Development of the human brain: In vivo quantification of metabolite and water content with proton magnetic resonance spectroscopy, *Magn Reson Med* 30:424-437, 1993.

571. Huppi PS, Fusch C, Boesch C, Burri R, et al: Regional metabolic assessment of human brain during development by proton magnetic resonance spectroscopy in vivo and by high-performance liquid chromatography/gas chromatography in autopsy tissue, *Pediatr Res* 37:145-150, 1995.

572. Huppi PS, Schuknecht B, Boesch C, Bossi E, et al: Structural and neurobehavioral delay in postnatal brain development of preterm infants, *Pediatr Res* 39:895-901, 1996.

573. Peden CJ, Rutherford MA, Sargentoni J, Cox IJ, et al: Proton spectroscopy of the neonatal brain following hypoxic-ischaemic injury, *Dev Med Child Neurol* 35:502-510, 1993.

574. Hanrahan JD, Sargentoni J, Azzopardi D, Manji K, et al: Cerebral metabolism within 18 hours of birth asphyxia: A proton magnetic resonance spectroscopy study, *Pediatr Res* 39:584-590, 1996.

575. Penrice J, Cady EB, Lorek A, Wylezinska M, et al: Proton magnetic resonance spectroscopy of the brain in normal preterm and term infants, and early changes after perinatal hypoxia-ischemia, *Pediatr Res* 40:6-14, 1996.

576. Shu SK, Ashwal S, Holshouser BA, Nystrom G, et al: Prognostic value of 1H-MRS in perinatal CNS insults, *Pediatr Neurol* 17:309-318, 1997.

577. Roth SC, Baudin J, Cady E, Johal K, et al: Relation of deranged neonatal cerebral oxidative metabolism with neurodevelopmental outcome and head circumference at 4 years, *Dev Med Child Neurol* 39:718-725, 1997.

578. Novotny E, Ashwal S, Shevell M: Proton magnetic resonance spectroscopy: An emerging technology in pediatric neurology research, *Pediatr Res* 44:1-10, 1998.

579. Hanaoka S, Takashima S, Morooka K: Study of the maturation of the child's brain using ^{31}P-MRS, *Pediatr Neurol* 18:305-310, 1998.

580. Amess PN, Penrice J, Wylezinska M, Lorek A, et al: Early brain proton magnetic resonance spectroscopy and neonatal neurology related to neurodevelopmental outcome at 1 year in term infants after presumed hypoxic-ischaemic brain injury, *Dev Med Child Neurol* 41:436-445, 1999.

581. Vigneron DB, Barkovich AJ, Noworolski SM, vondemBussche M, et al: Three-dimensional proton MR spectroscopic imaging of premature and term neonates, *AJNR Am J Neuroradiol* 22:1424-1433, 2001.

582. Kreis R, Hofmann L, Kuhlmann B, Boesch C, et al: Brain metabolite composition during early human brain development as measured by quantitative in vivo H-1 magnetic resonance spectroscopy, *Magn Reson Med* 48:949-958, 2002.

583. Groenendaal F, RoelantsvanRijn AM, vanderGrond J, Toet MC, et al: Glutamate in cerebral tissue of asphyxiated neonates during the first week of life demonstrated in vivo using proton magnetic resonance spectroscopy, *Biol Neonate* 79:254-257, 2001.

584. Huppi PS, Lazeyras F: Proton magnetic resonance spectroscopy (1H-MRS) in neonatal brain injury, *Pediatr Res* 49:317-319, 2001.

585. Barkovich AJ, Westmark KD, Bedi HS, Partridge JC, et al: Proton spectroscopy and diffusion imaging on the first day of life after perinatal asphyxia: Preliminary report, *AJNR Am J Neuroradiol* 22:1786-1794, 2001.

586. Zarifi MK, Astrakas LG, Young Poussaint T, du Plessis AJ, et al: Prediction of adverse outcome with cerebral lactate level and apparent diffusion coefficient in infants with perinatal asphyxia, *Radiology* 225:859-870, 2002.

587. Miller SP, Newton N, Ferriero DM, Partridge C, et al: Predictors of 30-month outcome after perinatal depression: Role of proton MRS and socioeconomic factors, *Pediatr Res* 52:71-77, 2002.

588. Khong PL, Tse C, Wong IYC, Lam BCC, et al: Diffusion-weighted imaging and proton magnetic resonance spectroscopy in perinatal hypoxic-ischemic encephalopathy: Association with neuromotor outcome at 18 months of age, *J Child Neurol* 19:872-881, 2004.

589. Bartha AI, Foster-Barber A, Miller SP, Vigneron DB, et al: Neonatal encephalopathy: Association of cytokines with MR spectroscopy and outcome, *Pediatr Res* 56:960-966, 2004.

590. L'Abee C, deVries LS, vanderGrond J, Groenendaal F: Early diffusion-weighted MRI and H-1–magnetic resonance spectroscopy in asphyxiated full-term neonates, *Biol Neonate* 88:306-312, 2005.

591. da Silva LF, Filho JR, Anes M, Nunes ML: Prognostic value of (1)H-MRS in neonatal encephalopathy, *Pediatr Neurol* 34:360-366, 2006.

592. Pi RB, Li WM, Lee NTK, Chan HHN, et al: Minocycline prevents glutamate-induced apoptosis of cerebellar granule neurons by differential regulation of p38 and Akt pathways, *J Neurochem* 91:1219-1230, 2004.

593. van der Knaap MS, Van der Ground J, Van Rijen PC, Faber JAJ: Age-dependent changes in localized proton and phosphorus spectroscopy on the brain, *Radiology* 176:509-515, 1990.

594. Tofts P, Wray S: Changes in brain phosphorous metabolites during the post natal development of the rat, *J Physiol* 359:417-429, 1985.

595. Gyulai L, Bolinger L, Leigh JS Jr, Barlow C, et al: Phosphorylethanolamine: The major constituent of the phosphomonoester peak observed by ^{31}P-NMR on developing dog brain, *FEBS Lett* 178:137-142, 1984.

596. Girard N, Gouny SC, Viola A, Le Fur Y, et al: Assessment of normal fetal brain maturation in utero by proton magnetic resonance spectroscopy, *Magn Reson Med* 56:768-775, 2006.

597. Bhakoo KK, Pearce D: In vivo expression of N-acetyl aspartate by oligodendrocytes: Implications for proton magnetic resonance spectroscopy signal in vivo, *J Neurochem* 74:254-262, 2000.

598. Bjartmar C, Battistuta J, Terada N, Dupree E, et al: N-acetylaspartate is an axon-specific marker of mature white matter in vivo: A biochemical and immunohistochemical study on the rat optic nerve, *Ann Neurol* 51:51-58, 2002.

599. Kirmani BF, Jacobowitz DM, Namboodiri MAA: Developmental increase of aspartoacylase in oligodendrocytes parallels CNS myelination, *Dev Brain Res* 140:105-115, 2003.

600. Raichle ME: Positron emission tomography, *Annu Rev Neurosci* 6:249-267, 1983.

601. Volpe JJ: Positron emission tomography (PET scanning), *Pediatr Rev* 6:121-127, 1984.

602. Altman DI, Volpe JJ: Positron emission tomography in the study of the neonatal brain. In Haddad J, Christmann D, Messer J, editors: *Imaging Techniques of the CNS of the Neonates*, New York: 1991, Springer-Verlag.

603. Chugani HT: Functional brain imaging in pediatrics, *Pediatr Clin North Am* 39:777-799, 1992.

604. Sundaram SK, Chugani HT, Chugani DC: Positron emission tomography methods with potential for increased understanding of mental retardation and developmental disabilities, *Ment Retard Dev Disabil Res Rev* 11:325-330, 2005.

605. Volpe JJ, Herscovitch P, Perlman JM, Kreusser KL, et al: Positron emission tomography in the asphyxiated term newborn: Parasagittal impairment of cerebral blood flow, *Ann Neurol* 17:287-296, 1985.

606. Borch K, Greisen G: Blood flow distribution in the normal human preterm brain, *Pediatr Res* 41:28-33, 1998.

607. Cavazzuti M, Duffy TE: Regulation of local cerebral blood flow in normal and hypoxic newborn dogs, *Ann Neurol* 11:247-257, 1982.

608. Kennedy C, Grave GD, Juhle JW, Sokoloff L: Changes in blood flow in the component structures of the dog brain during postnatal maturation, *J Neurochem* 19:2423-2433, 1972.

609. Tuor UI: Local cerebral blood flow in the newborn rabbit: An autoradiographic study of changes during development, *Pediatr Res* 29:517-523, 1991.

610. Chugani HT, Phelps ME: Maturational changes in cerebral function in infants determined by 18FDG positron emission tomography, *Science* 231:840-843, 1986.

611. Doyle LW, Nahmias C, Firnau G, Kenyon DB, et al: Regional cerebral glucose metabolism of newborn infants measured by positron emission tomography, *Dev Med Child Neurol* 25:143-151, 1983.

612. Thorp PS, Levin SD, Garnett ES, Firnau G, et al: Patterns of cerebral glucose metabolism using ^{18}FDG and positron tomography in the neurologic investigation of the full term newborn infant, *Neuropediatrics* 19:146-153, 1988.

613. Altman DI, Perlman JM, Volpe JJ, Powers WJ: Cerebral oxygen metabolism in newborns, *Pediatrics* 92:99-104, 1993.

614. Suhonen-Polvi H, Kero P, Korvenranta H, Ruotsalainen U, et al: Repeated fluorodeoxyglucose positron emission tomography of the brain in infants with suspected hypoxic-ischaemic brain injury, *Eur J Nucl Med* 20:759-765, 1993.

615. Kinnala A, Suhonen-Polvi H, Aarimaa T, Kero P, et al: Cerebral metabolic rate for glucose during the first six months of life: An FDG positron emission tomography study, *Arch Dis Child Fetal Neonatal Ed* 74:F153-F157, 1996.

616. Powers WJ, Rosenbaum JL, Dence CS, Markham J, et al: Cerebral glucose transport and metabolism in preterm human infants, *J Cereb Blood Flow Metab* 18:632-638, 1998.

617. Rosenbaum JL, Almli CR, Yundt KD, Altman DI, et al: Higher neonatal cerebral blood flow correlates with worse childhood neurologic outcome, *Neurology* 49:1035-1041, 1997.

618. Pryds O, Greisen G, Friis-Hansen B: Compensatory increase of CBF in preterm infants during hypoglycaemia, *Acta Paediatr Scand* 77:632-637, 1988.

619. Pryds O, Greisen G, Lou H, Friis-Hansen B: Heterogeneity of cerebral vasoreactivity in preterm infants supported by mechanical ventilation, *J Pediatr* 115:638-645, 1989.

620. Pryds O, Christensen NJ, Friis HB: Increased cerebral blood flow and plasma epinephrine in hypoglycemic, preterm neonates, *Pediatrics* 85:172-176, 1990.

621. Greisen G, Trojaborg W: Cerebral blood flow, PaCO2 changes, and visual evoked potentials in mechanically ventilated, preterm infants, *Acta Paediatr Scand* 76:394-400, 1987.

622. Greisen G, Pryds O: Low CBF, discontinuous EEG activity, and periventricular brain injury in ill, preterm neonates, *Brain Dev* 11:164-168, 1989.

623. Lipp-Zwahlen AE, Müller A, Tuchschmid P, Duc G: Oxygen affinity of haemoglobin modulates cerebral blood flow in premature infants: A study with the non-invasive xenon-133 method, *Acta Paediatr Scand Suppl* 360:26-32, 1989.

624. Lundstrom KE, Larsen PB, Brendstrup L, Skov L, et al: Cerebral blood flow and left ventricular output in spontaneously breathing, newborn preterm infants treated with caffeine or aminophylline, *Acta Pediatr* 84:6-9, 1995.

625. Baenziger O, Jaggi JL, Mueller AC, Morales CG, et al: Cerebral blood flow in preterm infants affected by sex, mechanical ventilation, and intrauterine growth, *Pediatr Neurol* 11:319-324, 1994.

626. Baenziger O, Jaggi JL, Mueller AC, Morales CG, et al: Regional differences of cerebral blood flow in the preterm infant, *Eur J Pediatr* 154:919-924, 1995.

627. Leech PJ, Miller JD, Fitch W, Barker J: Cerebral blood flow, internal carotid artery pressure and the EEG as a guide to the safety of carotid ligation, *J Neurol Neurosurg Psychiatry* 37:854-862, 1973.

628. Trojaborg W, Boysen G: Relation between EEG, regional cerebral blood flow and internal carotid artery pressure during carotid endarterectomy, *EEG Clin Neurophysiol* 35:62-69, 1973.

629. Sundt TM, Sharbrough FS, Anderson RE, Michenfelder JD: Cerebral blood flow measurements and electroencephalograms during carotid endarterectomy, *J Neurosurg* 41:310-320, 1974.

630. Powers WJ, Grubb RL, Darriet D, Raichle ME: Cerebral blood flow and cerebral metabolic rate of oxygen requirements for cerebral function and viability in humans, *J Cereb Blood Flow Metab* 5:600-608, 1985.

631. Baron JC, Rougemont D, Bousser MG: Local CBF, oxygen extraction and CMRO2: Prognostic value in recent supratentorial infarction, *J Cereb Blood Flow Metab* 3:S1-S2, 1983.

632. Baron JC, Rougemont D, Lebrun-Grandie P: Measurement of local blood flow and oxygen consumption in evolving cerebral infarction: An in vivo

633. study in man. In Meyer JS, Lechner H, Reivich M, et al, editors: *Cerebral Vascular Disease*, Princeton, NJ: 1983, Excerpta Medica.

633. Jones MD, Rosenberg AA, Simmons MA, Molteni RA, et al: Oxygen delivery to the brain before and after birth, *Science* 216:324-325, 1982.

634. Gleason CA, Short BL, Jones MD Jr: Cerebral blood flow and metabolism during and after prolonged hypocapnia in newborn lambs, *J Pediatr* 115:309-314, 1989.

635. Kreisman NR, Olson JE, Horne DS, Holtzman D: Cerebral oxygenation and blood flow in infant and young adult rats, *Am J Physiol* 256:R78-R85, 1989.

636. Abrams RM, Hutchinson AA, Yat TM, Sokoloff L, et al: Local cerebral glucose utilization non-selectively elevated in rapid eye movement sleep of the fetus, *Dev Brain Res* 40:65-70, 1988.

637. Nehlig A, Pereira De Vasconcelos A, Bopyet S: Quantitative autoradiographic measurement of local cerebral glucose utilization in freely moving rats during postnatal development, *J Neurosci* 8:2321-2333, 1988.

638. Himwich HE, Sykowski P, Fazekas JF: A comparative study of excised cerebral tissues of adult and infant rats, *Am J Physiol* 132:293-296, 1941.

639. Tyler DB, Van Harreveld A: The respiration of the developing brain, *Am J Physiol* 136:600-603, 1942.

640. Hernandez MJ, Brennan RW, Vannucci RC, Bowman GS: Cerebral blood flow and oxygen consumption in the newborn dog, *Am J Physiol* 234:R209-R215, 1978.

641. Booth RF, Patel TB, Clark JB: The development of enzymes of energy metabolism in the brain of a precocial (guinea pig) and non-precocial (rat) species, *J Neurochem* 34:17-25, 1980.

642. Bilger A, Nehlig A: Quantitative histochemical changes in enzymes involved in energy metabolism in the rat brain during postnatal development. I. Cytochrome oxidase and lactate dehydrogenase, *Int J Dev Neurosci* 9:545-553, 1991.

643. Diebler ME, Farkas-Bargeton E, Wehrle R: Developmental changes in enzymes associated with energy metabolism and the synthesis of some neurotransmitters in discrete areas of human neocortex, *J Neurochem* 32:429-435, 1979.

644. Patel MS, Johnson CA, Rajan R, Owen OE: The metabolism of ketone bodies in developing human brain: Development of ketone-body–producing enzymes and ketone bodies as precursors for lipid synthesis, *J Neurochem* 25:905-908, 1975.

645. Chugani HT, Phelps ME, Mazziotta JC: Positron emission tomography study of human brain functional development, *Ann Neurol* 22:487-497, 1987.

646. Chugani HT, Hovda DA, Villablanca JR, Phelps ME, et al: Metabolic maturation of the brain: A study of local cerebral glucose utilization in the developing cat, *J Cereb Blood Flow Metab* 11:35-47, 1991.

647. Volpe JJ, Herscovitch P, Perlman JM, Raichle ME: Positron emission tomography in the newborn: Extensive impairment of regional cerebral blood flow with intraventricular hemorrhage and hemorrhagic intracerebral involvement, *Pediatrics* 72:589-601, 1983.

648. Thorngren-Jerneck K, Ohlsson T, Sandell A, Erlandsson K, et al: Cerebral glucose metabolism measured by positron emission tomography in term newborn infants with hypoxic ischemic encephalopathy, *Pediatr Res* 49:495-501, 2001.

649. Thorngren-Jerneck K, Hellstrom-Westas L, Ryding E, Rosen I: Cerebral glucose metabolism and early EEG/aEEG in term newborn infants with hypoxic-ischemic encephalopathy, *Pediatr Res* 54:854-860, 2003.

650. Born AP, Miranda MJ, Rostrup E, Toft PB, et al: Functional magnetic resonance imaging of the normal and abnormal visual system in early life, *Neuropediatrics* 31:24-32, 2000.

651. Yamada H, Sadato N, Konishi Y, Muramoto S, et al: A milestone for normal development of the infantile brain detected by functional MRI, *Neurology* 55:218-223, 2000.

652. Sie LTL, Rombouts SAR, Valk J, Hart SAM, et al: Functional MRI of visual cortex in sedated 18 month-old infants with or without periventricular leukomalacia, *Dev Med Child Neurol* 43:486-490, 2001.

653. Marcar VL, Strassle AE, Loenneker T, Schwarz U, et al: The influence of cortical maturation on the BOLD response: An fMRI study of visual cortex in children, *Pediatr Res* 56:967-974, 2004.

654. Seghier ML, Lazeyras F, Zimine S, Maier SE, et al: Combination of event-related fMRI and diffusion tensor imaging in an infant with perinatal stroke, *Neuroimage* 21:463-472, 2004.

655. Seghier ML, Lazeyras F, Huppi PS: Functional MRI of the newborn, *Semin Fetal Neonatal Med* 11:479-488, 2006.

656. Muramoto S, Yamada H, Sadato N, Kimura H, et al: Age-dependent change in metabolic response to photic stimulation of the primary visual cortex in infants: Functional magnetic resonance imaging study, *J Comput Assist Tomogr* 26:394-901, 2002.

657. Dehaene-Lambertz G, Dehaene S, Hertz-Pannier L: Functional neuroimaging of speech perception in infants, *Science* 298:2013-2015, 2002.

Chapter 5

Neonatal Seizures

Seizures represent the most distinctive signal of neurological disease in the newborn period. The convulsive phenomena are the most *frequent* of the overt manifestations of neonatal neurological disorders. The precise frequency of neonatal seizures is difficult to delineate from available information, for reasons discussed later. Population-based studies using a clinical definition of seizures indicate sharp differences in incidence as a function of birth weight, with values as high as 57.5 per 1000 in infants with birth weights lower than 1500 g, but only 2.8 per 1000 for infants with birth weights of 2500 to 3999 g.[1-3] It is critical to recognize neonatal seizures, to determine their origin, and to treat them, for three major reasons. First, the seizures are usually related to significant illness, sometimes requiring specific therapy. Second, neonatal seizures may interfere with important supportive measures, such as alimentation and assisted respiration for associated disorders. Third, experimental data provide reason for concern that, under certain circumstances, seizures themselves may cause brain injury.

In this chapter, the pathophysiology and clinical aspects of neonatal seizures are reviewed. Particular emphasis is placed on the influence of the developmental characteristics of the perinatal brain on these aspects. Viewed in this context, the otherwise puzzling manifestations, causes, and effects of neonatal seizures become more understandable.

PATHOPHYSIOLOGY

Basic Mechanisms

A seizure results from an excessive synchronous electrical discharge (i.e., depolarization) of neurons within the central nervous system.[4-9] Depolarization is produced by the inward migration of sodium (Na^+), and repolarization is produced by the efflux of potassium (K^+). Maintenance of the potential across the membrane requires an energy (adenosine triphosphate, or ATP)–dependent pump, which extrudes Na^+ and takes in K^+. Although the fundamental mechanisms of neonatal seizures are not entirely understood, current data suggest that the excessive depolarization may result for at least the following reasons (Table 5-1). First, a disturbance in energy production can result in a failure of the ATP-dependent Na^+-K^+ pump. Hypoxemia-ischemia and hypoglycemia can cause sharp decreases in energy production. Second, a

relative excess of excitatory versus inhibitory neurotransmitters can result in an excessive rate of depolarization. Under conditions of hypoxia-ischemia and hypoglycemia, extracellular levels of glutamate (the principal excitatory neurotransmitter in cortex) increase because of excessive synaptic release and diminished reuptake by energy-dependent transport in both presynaptic nerve endings and glia. The result is excessive excitation (see Chapters 6 and 12 and later discussion).[9,10] Third, a relative deficiency of inhibitory versus excitatory neurotransmitters can result in an excessive rate of depolarization. The brain concentration of gamma-aminobutyric acid (GABA), the major inhibitory neurotransmitter, is decreased when the activity of its synthetic enzyme, glutamic acid decarboxylase, is depressed. A disturbance in binding of the critical cofactor of this enzyme, that is, the active form of pyridoxine, pyridoxal-5-phosphate, which is required for the action of this decarboxylase, would be expected to cause a relative decrease in GABA and an excess of excitatory transmitter. This state of *pyridoxine dependency*, in fact, is accompanied by decreased brain and cerebrospinal fluid (CSF) levels of pyridoxal-5-phosphate and GABA.[11-14] A similar basic mechanism for the genesis of seizures (i.e., relative decrease of inhibitory neurotransmitter) could develop if inhibitory synapses were blocked or not well developed. (The importance of insufficient inhibition in neonatal epileptogenesis is discussed in the next section.) Fourth, calcium and magnesium interact with the neuronal membrane to inhibit Na^+ movement; thus, hypocalcemia or hypomagnesemia would be expected to cause an increase in Na^+ influx and depolarization. As more detailed data concerning the biochemical properties of neurons of the perinatal brain are obtained, further insight into the molecular mechanisms underlying neonatal seizures can be expected.

Neuroanatomical and Neurophysiological Substrates

Seizure phenomena in newborns differ considerably from those observed in older infants, and the phenomena in premature infants differ from those in full-term infants.[6,15-29] Unlike older infants, newborns rarely have well-organized, generalized tonic-clonic seizures. Premature infants have even less well-organized spells than do full-term infants. The precise reasons for these differences must relate to the status of neuroanatomical

TABLE 5-1 Probable Mechanisms of Some Neonatal Seizures

Probable Mechanism	Disorder
Failure of sodium-potassium pump secondary to decreased adenosine triphosphate	Hypoxemia, ischemia, and hypoglycemia
Excess of excitatory neurotransmitter	Hypoxemia, ischemia, and hypoglycemia
Deficit of inhibitory neurotransmitter (i.e., relative excess of excitatory neurotransmitter)	Pyridoxine dependency
Membrane alteration: increased sodium permeability	Hypocalcemia and hypomagnesemia

and neurophysiological development in the perinatal period (Table 5-2).

Neuroanatomical Features

The most critical, neuroanatomical developmental processes that occur in the perinatal period are the organizational events (see Table 5-2 and Chapter 2). The relevant events in this context are as follows: the attainment of proper orientation, alignment, and layering (i.e., lamination of cortical neurons); the elaboration of axonal and dendritic ramifications; and the establishment of synaptic connections. Only the first of these processes is well developed in the human newborn. The latter two events (i.e., neurite outgrowth and synaptogenesis) must be highly significant in providing the cortical connectivity to propagate and sustain a generalized seizure. Such a degree of cortical organization is not present in the human newborn. In the newborn monkey, the spread of seizure discharges is relatively

TABLE 5-2 Perinatal Anatomical and Physiological Features of Importance in Determining Neonatal Seizure Phenomena

Anatomical
Neurite outgrowth: dendritic and axonal ramifications (in process)
Active synaptogenesis
Deficient myelination in cortical efferent systems
Physiological
In limbic and neocortical regions, development of excitatory mechanisms before inhibitory mechanisms:
  NMDA receptors overexpressed and exhibit multiple properties that enhance excitation
  AMPA receptors overexpressed and have a subunit composition (deficient GluR2) that enhances excitation
  GABA$_A$ receptors excitatory rather than inhibitory
Deficient development of substantia nigra system for inhibition of seizures
Impaired propagation of electrical seizures, and resulting lack of correlation of synchronous discharges recorded from surface electroencephalogram with behavioral seizure phenomena

AMPA, alpha-amino-3-hydroxy-5-methyl-4-isoxazolepropionic acid; GABA, gamma-aminobutyric acid; NMDA, N-methyl-D-aspartate.

rapid, and well-organized, synchronous, generalized seizures are readily apparent clinically and electroencephalographically.[30] Such propagation and spread may be related to the more advanced cerebral cortical organization and to the myelination of cortical efferent systems and interhemispheric commissures that is present in the neonatal monkey[31,32] but absent in the human (see Chapter 2). The relatively advanced cortical development apparent in human limbic structures[6,9,33,34] and the connections of these structures to diencephalon and brain stem may underlie the frequency and dominance, as clinical manifestations of neonatal seizures, of oral-buccal-lingual movements (e.g., sucking, chewing, or drooling), oculomotor phenomena, and apnea.

Neurophysiological Features

The relation of excitatory to inhibitory synapses is important in determining the capacity of a focal discharge to spread to contiguous and distant areas. Strong evidence indicates that the rates at which excitatory and inhibitory synaptic activities develop in neonatal mammalian cerebral cortex differ (see Table 5-2). A growing body of data indicates that early in development in hippocampus and neocortex, excitatory activity, mediated primarily by glutamate (especially N-methyl-D-aspartate [NMDA]) and alpha-amino-3-hydroxy-5-methyl-4-isoxazolepropionic acid [AMPA]) receptors, predominates, and inhibitory systems are relatively underdeveloped.[6-10,35-52] Indeed, these two excitatory amino acid receptors are expressed in the perinatal period at levels *exceeding* those observed in adult cortical neurons, with the NMDA receptor peaking shortly before the AMPA receptor. Moreover, certain properties of these two glutamate receptors enhance their excitatory function. Thus, the NMDA receptor in the neonatal period exhibits prolonged duration of the NMDA-mediated excitatory postsynaptic potential, reduced ability of magnesium to block NMDA receptor activity, diminished (inhibitory) polyamine binding sites, greater sensitivity to glycine enhancement, and higher density of NMDA receptors.[9,47,48,51,53,54] Similarly, AMPA receptors are deficient in the GluR2 subunit responsible for rendering the AMPA channel impermeable to calcium; thus, these immature AMPA receptors are permeable to calcium and, as a consequence, enhance excitation.[48-50b] In addition, early in development, the principal inhibitory neurotransmitter, GABA, acts at the major postsynaptic GABA$_A$ receptor (GABA$_A$) to produce excitation rather than inhibition, as occurs later in development (see later).[9,47,52,55] Moreover, only the proconvulsant projection network of the substantia nigra (and not the later developing anticonvulsant network) functions early in brain development.[6,56-58] Consistent with these physiological phenomena, various convulsants and hypoxia produce epileptic activity much more readily in the early developing animal than in the adult (Fig. 5-1).[9,59-62] Finally, the electrical discharges that are so readily generated in neonatal brain, particularly in hippocampus, may not propagate sufficiently to be observed by surface electroencephalographic (EEG) findings, and even when synchronous

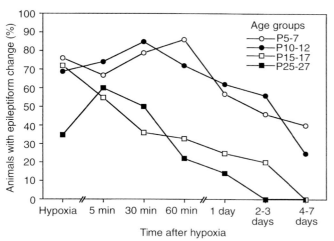

Figure 5-1 Frequency of epileptiform electroencephalographic changes in animals from four age groups sampled at 5, 30, and 60 minutes, and 1 to 7 days following oxygen deprivation. Data are represented as frequency of epileptiform change across all levels of oxygen exposure. *P* is the age in postnatal days. Note the markedly higher frequency of epileptiform changes after hypoxia in the youngest animals studied. *(From Jensen FE, Applegate CD, Holtzman D, Belin TR, et al: Epileptogenic effect of hypoxia in the immature rodent brain, Ann Neurol 29:629-637, 1991.)*

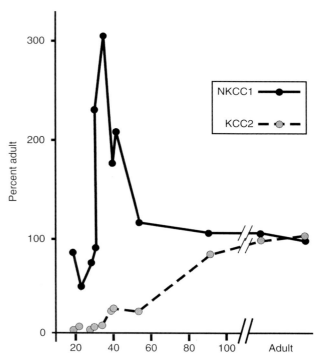

Figure 5-2 Developmental profiles of expression (protein levels) of **NKCC1 (chloride importer) and KCC2 (chloride exporter) in human parietal cortex.** Protein levels, expressed as percentage of adult, are shown as a function of postconceptional weeks. Note the developmental mismatch, such that in the newborn period levels of NKCC1 exceed adult values, whereas levels of KCC2 are markedly lower than adult values. The expected result is elevation of intracellular chloride levels (see text). *(Redrawn from Dzhala VI, Talos DM, Sdrulla DA, Brumback AC, et al: NKCC1 transporter facilitates seizures in the developing brain, Nat Med 11:1205-1213, 2005.)*

discharges do appear at the surface near the end of the seizure, behavioral phenomena may not correlate well because of deficient myelination of cerebral efferent systems (see Table 5-2).

More recent insights into the critical developmental relationship between neuronal chloride (Cl^-) levels and Cl^- transport in the perinatal period have major implications for understanding *the basis of GABA excitation and key clinical and therapeutic aspects of neonatal seizures* (Table 5-3). Thus, GABA activation of the major postsynaptic $GABA_A$ receptor causes Cl^- flux, which, in the mature neuron, occurs as influx down an electrochemical gradient. However, in developing brain, at maturational stages comparable to the human perinatal period, GABA activation causes Cl^- efflux and thereby is excitatory, as noted earlier. Research shows that the basis for this paradoxical effect relates to a *developmental mismatch between the two Cl^- transporters that determine neuronal Cl^- levels.* Thus, in the perinatal period, in human cerebral cortex the expression of the Na^+-K^+-Cl^- cotransporter (NKCC1) responsible for Cl^- influx reaches a developmental peak, whereas the expression of the K^+-Cl^- cotransporter (KCC2) responsible for Cl^- efflux is

relatively low (Fig. 5-2).[52,63-66] The result is a high neuronal level of Cl^- and *efflux* of Cl^- (rather than influx) when the $GABA_A$ receptor is activated. Depolarization/excitation follows. The later developmental up-regulation of the KCC2 cotransporter extruding Cl^- lowers the neuronal Cl^- level, and Cl^- influx with hyperpolarization/inhibition occurs with $GABA_A$ receptor activation. These findings may explain the therapeutic inconsistency regarding neonatal seizures of such GABA agonists as phenobarbital and benzodiazepines (see later). This imperfect anticonvulsant response is particularly apparent after neonatal hypoxic-ischemic insults, which, in an experimental model, are associated with up-regulation of NKCC1.[67] *The NKCC1 inhibitor,*

TABLE 5-3	**Critical Development Relationships of Neuronal Chloride Levels and Chloride Transport in Excitation of Gamma-Aminobutyric Acid**

GABA is excitatory rather inhibitory in perinatal neurons because of elevated neuronal Cl^-.

$GABA_A$ receptor activation therefore causes Cl^- *efflux* and depolarization (excitation) rather than *influx* and hyperpolarization (inhibition).

Elevated neuronal Cl^- levels result in the perinatal period because of exuberant development of NKCC1, which mediates Cl^- *influx*, in the presence of developmentally low levels of KCC2, which mediates Cl^- efflux.

With development, NKCC1 declines, KCC2 increases, and thus neuronal Cl^- levels decrease; $GABA_A$ receptor activation then results in Cl^- influx and hyperpolarization (inhibition).

These developmental changes may explain the imperfect response of neonatal seizures to GABA-agonist anticonvulsant drugs.

Cl^-, chloride; GABA, gamma-aminobutyric acid; KCC2, potassium-chloride cotransporter; NKCC1, sodium-potassium-chloride cotransporter.

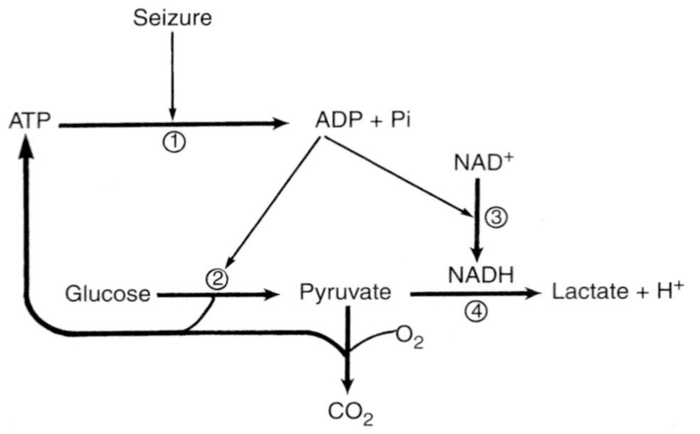

Figure 5-3 Biochemical effects of seizure. The major effects are numbered. ADP, adenosine diphosphate; ATP, adenosine triphosphate; NAD, nicotinamide adenine dinucleotide; NADH, reduced form of nicotinamide adenine dinucleotide; P_i, inorganic phosphate. See text for details.

bumetanide, has potent anticonvulsant properties by enhancing GABA-mediated inhibition through blockage of Cl^- uptake and lowering of neuronal Cl^- levels (see later).[52] Moreover, because the maturation of the two cotransporters and neuronal Cl^- levels occurs in a caudal-rostral direction, spinal cord and brain stem motor neurons would be expected to exhibit GABA-mediated inhibition before cerebral cortical areas. *This feature could explain the frequent occurrence of electroclinical dissociation (i.e., suppression of motor manifestations of seizure but not cortical EEG manifestations), after treatment with GABA agonists such as phenobarbital or benzodiazepines.*

Biochemical Effects

Energy Metabolism

This discussion focuses on the *acute* biochemical effects of neonatal seizures. In the section following, I describe the mechanisms of brain injury with seizures; many of the mechanistic pathways are initiated by the biochemical effects described next.

The most prominent *acute* biochemical effects of seizures involve energy metabolism (Fig. 5-3).[68-78] Thus, seizures are associated with a greatly increased rate of energy-dependent ion pumping, which is accompanied by a fall in concentration of ATP and the storage form of high-energy phosphate in brain, phosphocreatine. The resulting rise in adenosine diphosphate (ADP) has two major effects. The first is stimulation of glycolysis at the rate-limiting, phosphofructokinase step,[79] which ultimately results in accelerated production of pyruvate (see Fig. 5-3). In the first minutes after the onset of seizure, a sharp increase in the rate of glucose utilization can be demonstrated.[71,80] In the absence of seizure, a major proportion of the pyruvate formed from glycolysis enters the mitochondrion, is oxidized to carbon dioxide, and is associated with the production of ATP. With seizure activity, however, a considerable proportion of pyruvate is converted in the cytoplasm to lactate in the presence of elevated levels of the reduced form of nicotinamide adenine dinucleotide (NADH). The latter occurs as the second

TABLE 5-4 Seizure-Induced Changes in Brain Energy Metabolites in the Newborn Monkey*

Metabolite	Cerebral Cortex	Thalamus
Glucose utilization	424%–598%	261%–411%
Glucose	4%	1%
Lactate	267%–650%	308%
Phosphocreatine	23%–28%	28%
Adenosine triphosphate	56%–77%	60%

*Values are expressed as a percentage of control.
Data from Fujikawa DG, Vannucci RC, Dwyer BE, Wasterlain CG: *Brain Res* 454:51-59, 1988; and Fujikawa DG, Dwyer BE, Lake RR, Wasterlain CG: *Am J Physiol* 256:C1160-1167, 1989.

consequence of elevated levels of ADP relative to ATP, that is, a shift of the redox state in the cytoplasm toward reduction (i.e., NADH; see Fig. 5-3). The excess of lactate, specifically the associated hydrogen ion,[81] has the beneficial effect of causing local vasodilation and a consequent increase in local blood supply and substrate influx.[72,82-84] In addition, seizures are associated with elevated blood pressure, which contributes to increased cerebral blood flow (CBF) and substrate influx.[72,83,85,86] This pressor effect is presumed to be a central autonomic component of the seizure because it can be interrupted by section of the spinal cord or by administration of sympathetic ganglion-blocking agents.[68] An impairment of cerebrovascular autoregulation with seizure causes the pressor response to result in increased CBF.[83,84,86-88]

Despite these important compensatory factors, neonatal seizures in experimental animals are accompanied by a distinct *fall in brain glucose concentrations*.[69-71,77,82,89-91] Thus, in the neonatal rat, rabbit, dog, and monkey, despite normal or slightly elevated blood glucose concentrations, brain glucose concentrations fall dramatically within 5 minutes of onset of seizure to nearly undetectable levels after 30 minutes (Table 5-4 and Fig. 5-4). Concomitant with the fall in brain glucose is a rise in brain lactate, which is used readily as a metabolic fuel in neonatal brain (see Chapter 6).[74,78] This fall in brain glucose concentration and rise in brain lactate are directly reminiscent of hypoxic-ischemic brain insult (see Chapter 6) and presumably relate to the accelerated rate of glucose utilization in an attempt to preserve supplies of phosphocreatine and ATP. In this regard, it should be recalled that glucose conversion to lactate, which is accelerated with neonatal seizures, results in only two molecules of ATP for each molecule of glucose, as opposed to the 38 molecules of ATP generated when pyruvate enters the mitochondrion and is oxidized to carbon dioxide. In keeping with these considerations, in vivo studies by magnetic resonance (MR) spectroscopy of cerebral metabolites in newborn dogs subjected to convulsant drug-induced seizures demonstrated a prominent decrease in phosphocreatine (with which ATP is in equilibrium) and in intracellular pH.[72,74,75,82,92] Results of studies with MR spectroscopy in the human newborn demonstrate the relevance of these experimental data to the clinical situation (Fig. 5-5).[93] These observations have important implications for prognosis and therapy, as discussed subsequently.

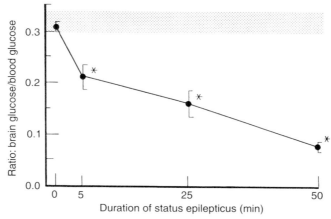

Figure 5-4 **Decline in brain glucose concentration with seizure.** Ratio of brain glucose to blood glucose levels in convulsing neonatal rats as a function of duration of seizure activity. The *shaded area* represents mean control values ± SE. The *asterisks* indicate difference from controls at *P* < .01. *(From Wasterlain CG, Duffy TE: Status epilepticus in immature rats, Arch Neurol 33:821, 1976.)*

Mechanisms of Brain Injury with Seizures

The deleterious effects of seizures are divided best into those related to single prolonged seizures and those related to briefer recurrent seizures. The most prominent feature of the former is cell loss, and of the latter, altered development. Data in human infants are scant and are described; experimental studies, primarily in developing rodent models, are very abundant. Before reviewing the mechanistic details next, note that, in general, although the threshold for seizure generation is lower in the developing brain than in the mature brain, developing neurons are less vulnerable to injury from single prolonged seizures than are mature neurons.[94] This difference may relate to a lower density of active synapses, lower energy consumption, and immaturity of relevant biochemical cascades to cell death.[94]

Prolonged Seizures

The *best-documented* mechanisms by which a prolonged seizure (e.g., status epilepticus) may cause brain injury are depicted in Figure 5-6. Repeated seizures in newborns may be accompanied by serious hypoventilation and apnea, which result in hypercapnia and hypoxemia. The latter is an important potential cause of brain injury, particularly in an infant whose brain already has been compromised by a serious insult. Hypoxemia, if severe, may also result in cardiovascular collapse and ischemic injury to brain. Accentuation of the disturbance in cerebral energy metabolism when hypoxemia or hypoxemia-ischemia is combined with seizures has been shown in several animal models.[73,75,95-97] Hypercapnia may combine with two other events, the adaptive rise in arterial blood pressure that occurs with seizures (see the earlier section

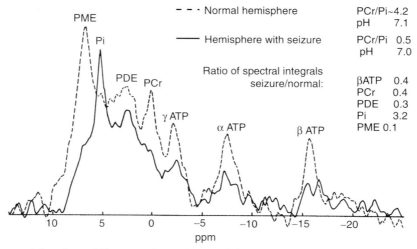

Figure 5-5 **Magnetic resonance (phosphorus-31) spectra from a full-term infant during subtle seizure activity (oral-buccal-lingual movements, i.e., lip smacking and chewing).** The electroencephalogram demonstrated seizure activity emanating from the left temporal region. The magnetic resonance spectrum from the nonictal hemisphere *(dotted line)* is normal. The spectrum from the ictal hemisphere *(solid line)* exhibits a marked decrease in phosphocreatine (PCr) and adenosine triphosphate (ATP) and a corresponding increase in inorganic phosphate (Pi). PDE, phosphodiesters; PME, phosphomonoesters. *(Courtesy of Dr. Donald Younkin.)*

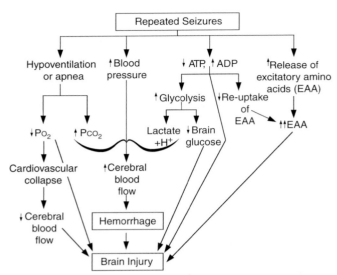

Figure 5-6 Best-documented mechanisms for the occurrence of brain injury consequent to repeated seizures. See text for details. ADP, adenosine diphosphate; ATP, adenosine triphosphate, Po2, oxygen pressure; Pco2, carbon dioxide pressure, EAA, excitatory amino acids (especially glutamate).

"Biochemical Effects") and the increase in lactate, to cause an abrupt increase in CBF. Evidence supporting this increase in flow with seizures is derived from studies in a variety of animal models, as well as in human adults and infants.[72,73,75,82-84,86-88,92,98-106] The importance of this increase in CBF to maintain substrate supply to brain and thereby to preserve energy supplies is shown by the deleterious effect of hypotension when added to seizure. Accentuation of the disturbance in cerebral energy metabolism when hypotension is combined with seizure has been shown in the neonatal dog.[73] Because cardiac dysfunction and diminished cardiac output are late complications of seizures, hypotension, diminished CBF, impaired energy metabolism, and brain injury are major threats of repeated prolonged seizures (see Fig. 5-6).[85] Indeed, because the impairment of cerebrovascular autoregulation persists into the *postictal* period, later decreases in blood pressure may also lead to potentially dangerous decreases in CBF.[87,88]

Several lines of evidence indicate that *elevations of arterial blood pressure and of CBF* also occur in *the human newborn* as in the neonatal animal models. Studies using continuous monitoring of arterial blood pressure demonstrated sharp increases in mean arterial blood pressure during neonatal seizures, including subtle seizures (Fig. 5-7), even in paralyzed patients.[100,107,108] The possibility that such increases in blood pressure in the newborn could lead to increases in CBF is suggested by the mechanisms outlined in Figure 5-6. Additionally, the impairment of cerebrovascular autoregulation with seizures is relevant in this context. Thus, the possibility of increases in CBF with seizure has been shown to be real in the newborn. Studies involving the use of the Doppler ultrasound technique at the anterior fontanelle demonstrated a sharp increase in CBF velocity in 12 newborns during seizures, most of which were subtle in type.[100] Moreover, the likelihood

that this increase in flow velocity is related to an increase in volemic flow was shown by the direct documentation of an increase in regional CBF by positron emission tomography during a subtle seizure in an infant.[101] Indeed, in a study of 12 term infants with seizures, *ictal* measurements of regional CBF by single photon emission computed tomography showed a 50% to 150% increase, and this increase occurred in infants with subtle seizures or subclinical electrical seizures.[103] Although the increase in CBF with seizure is, at least initially, an adaptive response to increase substrate supply to the brain at a time of excessive metabolic demand, this response could become *maladaptive in the newborn infant.* Thus, the newborn with seizures, depending on such factors as the gestational age of the infant or the neuropathological substrate for the seizures, has certain highly vulnerable capillary beds, such as the germinal matrix in the premature infant (see Chapter 11) or the margins of ischemic lesions in the premature infant or the asphyxiated term infant (see Chapter 8). Under these circumstances, an increase in CBF could rupture these capillary beds and, as a consequence, could cause intraventricular hemorrhage, hemorrhagic periventricular leukomalacia, or hemorrhagic infarction (see Fig. 5-6).

Repeated prolonged seizures *may be deleterious* for the brain, *even in the absence of prominent disturbances of ventilation or perfusion* (see Fig. 5-6). The deleterious effects of hypoventilation and apnea can be controlled by prompt and vigorous support of ventilation. However, studies of paralyzed, primarily adult animals subjected to repeated seizures demonstrated that a point is

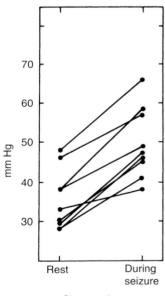

Changes in mean systemic blood pressure with seizures

Figure 5-7 Increase in blood pressure with neonatal seizures. Nine infants with subtle seizure phenomena were monitored during ictal episodes. Note the consistent increases in systemic blood pressure. In each infant, a simultaneous increase in cerebral blood flow velocity was documented by the Doppler ultrasound technique at the anterior fontanelle (not shown).

reached when the factors that increase substrate supply to convulsing brain (see the earlier section "Biochemical Effects") can no longer compensate adequately for the fall in energy reserves. Thus, decreases in brain ATP and phosphocreatine concentrations become progressive, and the EEG discharges become self-sustaining. Irreparable injury may be the end result.[5,61,68,76,77,109-118] Nevertheless, *most studies indicate that the newborn brain is more resistant to seizure-induced neuronal necrosis than is the adult brain.*[94,119-125]

Changes in high-energy phosphate compounds comparable to those observed in animal models were demonstrated by MR spectroscopy during subtle seizures in the human newborn (see Fig. 5-5).[93] Prevention of the changes in high-energy phosphate levels that appear to be important in causation of brain injury by pharmacological treatment of seizure was shown by MR spectroscopy in the neonatal dog.[92] Similarly, the immediately beneficial response to treatment of the seizure with phenobarbital also was demonstrated in the human newborn (Fig. 5-8).[93]

Work with newborn animals showed that *glucose administration* just before the seizures prevents the fall in brain glucose level that occurs with status epilepticus and markedly reduces mortality and brain cell loss.[69,89] This protective effect of glucose was distinctly greater in newborn than in older animals (Fig. 5-9). The precise beneficial effect of the glucose did not seem to relate to brain ATP and phosphocreatine concentrations because neither concentration in whole brain was altered in these experiments. (Neuronal concentrations in selected brain regions could not be measured in this work.) The glucose did appear to serve as a carbon source, because DNA, RNA, protein, and cholesterol concentrations were relatively spared in the glucose-treated animals. In a study with potential clinical relevance, in which status epilepticus was induced in the neonatal rat subjected to hypoxia-ischemia,

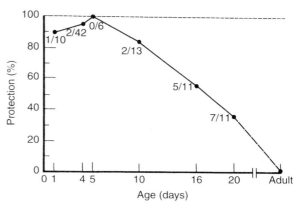

Figure 5-9 **Age-dependent protective effect of glucose on mortality from repetitive seizures in the rat.** The percentage of protection by glucose equals the number of saline-treated rats minus the number of glucose-treated rats: number of saline treated, dead × 100. *(Courtesy of Dr. Claude Wasterlain.)*

glucose administered early during the seizures led to decreased mortality but no change in the extent of ischemic brain injury.[91] The potential for important interactions between glucose homeostasis and seizures is raised further by MR spectroscopic studies of brain of neonatal dogs, which showed that levels of hypoglycemia that do not result in alterations in levels of high-energy phosphates are accompanied by distinct decreases in such levels when seizure is added to hypoglycemia.[72] The data indicate the importance of careful attention to glucose homeostasis in the management of the infant with seizures and raise the possibility that judicious administration of glucose may be a useful adjunct to the therapy of severe neonatal seizures.

An additional mechanism for the genesis of brain injury with severe seizures relates to excitatory amino acids and is based on results of experimental studies.[5,9,10,48,49,61,76,77,110-114,126-139a] Injury to dendrites and cell body of neurons, the most prominent acute manifestation of injury from seizures, occurs particularly in limbic structures (e.g., hippocampus) *and in distant* sites intimately connected with limbic structures (e.g., selected areas of thalamus and cerebellum). The predilection of the limbic system of the newborn for seizure discharges (see earlier discussion) is highly relevant in this regard. The experimental data suggest that the mechanism of neuronal injury in these structures involves *excessive synaptic release of excitatory amino acids*, particularly glutamate, the principal neurotransmitter for the regions that exhibit injury (see Fig. 5-6). When diminution of energy supplies is added, the energy-dependent reuptake systems for excitatory amino acids in presynaptic nerve endings and astrocytes are impaired, and the local accumulation of the neurotransmitters is accentuated (see Fig. 5-6). The result is postsynaptic damage at the axodendritic and axosomatic sites. The evidence that indicates a major role of excitatory amino acids as mediators of neuronal death with prolonged seizures is summarized in Table 5-5. A *particular vulnerability of the developing brain* of the newborn may relate to the rich expression in the developing brain of glutamate receptors, which appear to play an important role in neuronal differentiation and

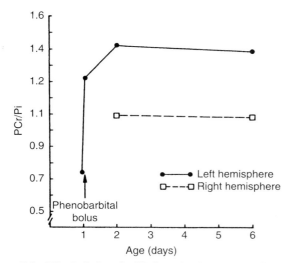

Figure 5-8 **Effect of phenobarbital on the depressed ratio of phosphocreatine (PCr) to inorganic phosphorus (Pi) in an infant with seizure emanating from the left hemisphere.** Note the immediate and then sustained improvement in cerebral energy state (i.e., increase in PCr/Pi ratio) after treatment with phenobarbital. *(Courtesy of Dr. Donald Younkin.)*

TABLE 5-5	Evidence Supportive of Major Role of Excitatory Amino Acids as Mediators of Neuronal Death with Prolonged Seizures

Prolonged seizures cause excessive release of glutamate and aspartate at excitatory amino acid synapses.

The topography of seizure-related neuronal damage corresponds to the topography of postsynaptic sites innervated by glutamate-aspartate transmitters.

Cytopathological features of seizure-related neuronal death are indistinguishable from those of glutamate-induced neuronal death.

Specific blockers of glutamate receptors prevent neuronal death with prolonged seizures in vivo, even without preventing seizure activity per se.

TABLE 5-6	Major Effects of Recurrent Neonatal Seizures*

Impaired cognitive functions

No definite cell loss

Synaptic reorganization of axons and terminals in hippocampus (sprouting of mossy fibers)

Decreased neurogenesis in hippocampus

Loss of dendritic spines in hippocampus

Increased susceptibility to later epilepsy because of increased NMDA and AMPA receptors and decreased GABA receptors, altered AMPA receptors (decreased GluR2), imbalance of excitatory and inhibitory systems, and altered intrinsic neuronal membrane properties, all favoring excitation

*Based on studies of experimental models developmentally comparable to human perinatal brain.
AMPA, alpha-amino-3-hydroxy-5-methyl-4-isoxazolepropionic acid; GABA, gamma-aminobutyric acid; NMDA, N-methyl-D-aspartate.

plasticity.[9,10,50a,50b,131] This rich expression of glutamate receptors, important for normal development, may become a source of overexcitation and neuronal death with repeated or prolonged seizures. Thus, in summary, the data suggest that severe seizures can induce a pathological extension of a normal synaptic event and that excitotoxic amino acids may thereby mediate cellular injury, not only at the site of the epileptic discharge but also at distant sites excited by the epileptic discharge.

Not unexpectedly, *no controlled clinical data in human infants* are available regarding the possibility of neonatal brain injury resulting from seizures per se, although data can be marshalled to show that prolonged or multiple neonatal seizures are associated with a much poorer outlook than are seizures that are readily controlled (see later discussion).[27,140-147] In one study, among 63 infants with seizures secondary to perinatal hypoxia-ischemia, approximately 35% of infants with seizures for 1 to 3 days exhibited moderate or severe neurological sequelae or died, whereas fully 90% of infants with seizures for 4 or more days had such an unfavorable outcome.[141] In a careful study based on electrographic quantitation of the number, duration, and intensity of electrical seizures, the occurrence of electrographic seizures correlated with the later development of microcephaly and severe cerebral palsy.[146] The relationships were particularly notable in the infants with "asphyxia." In a report of 90 term infants with "perinatal asphyxia," each increase in a seizure severity score was independently associated with an increase in lactate and a decrease in *N*-acetylaspartate, assessed by MR spectroscopy.[147] Obviously, the severity of the underlying neurological disease may account for *both* the poorly controlled seizures *and* the poor outcome, but the most recent studies are of major interest. *Clearly, resolution of the question of the deleterious effect of neonatal seizures will require careful prospective studies of well-defined populations.*

Recurrent Seizures

Although most evidence does not suggest serious structural or functional defects from a single prolonged neonatal seizure, *recurrent* seizures, not necessarily prolonged, are associated with long-term functional, morphological, and physiological deficits.[94,125] This

clinically important conclusion is based on a variety of studies in experimental models developmentally comparable to the human perinatal brain (Table 5-6).

The *most consistent functional disturbance* involves deficits in *cognition*.[94,125,148,149] Visual-spatial memory and learning have been particularly involved and are consistent with the locus of the principal structural deficits in the hippocampus (see later).

The *morphological correlates* of the functional disturbances involve *neuronal developmental abnormalities rather than neuronal cell loss*. The most severe disturbances occur in the hippocampus and include dendritic spine loss in CA3 pyramidal cells and a distinctive pattern of synaptic reorganization of axons and terminals of the dentate granule cells (i.e., mossy fibers).[94,148] The degree of this "sprouting" of mossy fibers correlates with the severity of the cognitive deficits. Additionally, dentate granule cell neurogenesis, which, unlike in other cortical areas, persists in the neonatal period, is impaired after recurrent seizures.[150]

Recurrent seizures also lead to *physiological and molecular alterations that favor subsequent neuronal excitability and therefore epileptogenesis*, as well as the occurrence of neuronal injury with subsequent insults.[49-51,94,139,151,151a] Those alterations include increases in excitatory amino acid receptors (NMDA and AMPA/kainate) and decreases in GABA receptors, molecular alterations in AMPA receptors (decrease in the GluR2 subunit) that render them permeable to calcium, imbalance in excitatory and inhibitory systems, and altered intrinsic neuronal membrane properties, all favoring excitation (see Table 5-6).

The critical question, of course, is whether these changes occur in the human infant who experiences recurrent neonatal seizures. This question remains unanswered, but the mounting data are cause for major concern and have implications for the criteria for the onset of anticonvulsant therapy and the type of agent used.

CLINICAL ASPECTS

In nearly all neonatal intensive care units, seizures in the newborn are identified by direct clinical observation. Moreover, much of what we think that we know about neonatal seizures is based on studies of infants whose seizures were identified in this manner. However, the findings of a series of studies, performed largely by techniques of prolonged EEG monitoring with simultaneous observation either by video recorder or by direct inspection, raise two important possibilities about clinically identified neonatal seizures. First, some clinically identified motor and behavioral phenomena characterized as seizures do not have a simultaneous EEG seizure correlate; this finding suggests that the number of certain neonatal seizures may have been overestimated in the past. Second, many electrographic seizures are not accompanied by clinically observable alterations in neonatal motor or behavioral function; this finding suggests that the total number of neonatal seizures may have been underestimated in the past.

These findings have led to some refinement of our current concepts of neonatal seizures and have raised important new questions for future research. Moreover, the observations underscore the importance of bedside EEG recording, preferably with simultaneous video, in the continual management of newborns with seizures (see later). In the following, I present a classification of neonatal seizure types, address the clinical distinction of epileptic from nonepileptic phenomena, and discuss the pathophysiology of the clinical phenomena of neonatal seizures.

Classification

Seizure Types

A *seizure* is defined clinically as a paroxysmal alteration in neurological function (i.e., behavioral, motor, or autonomic function). Such a definition includes clinical phenomena that are associated temporally with (surface-recorded) EEG seizure activity and therefore are clearly epileptic (i.e., related to hypersynchronous electrical discharges that may spread and activate other brain structures). The definition also includes paroxysmal clinical phenomena that are not consistently associated temporally with EEG seizure activity; how many of these clinical phenomena may also be epileptic (e.g., related to hypersynchronous electrical discharges from subcortical structures and not detected by surface EEG) is not entirely resolved (see later discussion). The classification of neonatal seizures that I present here categorizes clinical seizures and designates those clinical seizures likely to be associated with EEG seizure activity.

The classification is altered slightly from my previous scheme (Table 5-7).[152,153] However, the aim is to maintain a relatively simple classification and a framework that allows alterations as further information is gathered from research. Four essential seizure types can be recognized: subtle, clonic, tonic, and myoclonic. The meaning of the additional descriptors shown in Table 5-7 generally is obvious. However, the terms *multifocal* and *generalized* are best defined here: *multifocal* refers to clinical activity that involves more than one site, is asynchronous, and, usually, is migratory,

TABLE 5-7 Classification of Neonatal Seizures		
	ELECTROENCEPHALOGRAPHIC SEIZURE	
Clinical Seizure	**Common**	**Uncommon**
Subtle	+*	
Clonic		
Focal	+	
Multifocal	+	
Tonic		
Focal	+	
Generalized		+
Myoclonic		
Focal, multifocal		+
Generalized	+	

*Only specific varieties of subtle seizures are commonly associated with simultaneous electroencephalographic seizure activity; see text and Table 5-8 for details.

whereas *generalized* refers to clinical activity that is diffusely bilateral, synchronous, and nonmigratory.

Subtle. Because the clinical manifestations of certain neonatal seizures are readily and frequently overlooked, I continue to characterize those paroxysmal alterations in neonatal behavior and motor or autonomic function that are not clearly clonic, tonic, or myoclonic as *subtle* (Table 5-8).[15,152] Available information from studies using EEG recording simultaneously with video recording or direct observation suggests that (1) subtle seizures are more common in premature than in full-term infants,[154] and (2) some subtle clinical phenomena in full-term infants are not consistently associated with EEG seizure activity.[28,29,155-157] Thus, Dreyfus-Brisac and collaborators (Radvanyi-Bouvet and co-workers[154]) indicated that common ictal clinical manifestations, confirmed by "simultaneous abnormal EEG discharges" in a group of premature infants of 26 to 32 weeks of gestation, included sustained opening of eyes, ocular movements, chewing, pedaling motions, and a variety of autonomic phenomena. That similar

TABLE 5-8 Selected Major Manifestations of Subtle Seizures
Ocular phenomena
Tonic horizontal deviation of eyes with or without jerking of eyes*
Sustained eye opening with ocular fixation†
Oral-buccal-lingual movements
Chewing†
Other manifestations (see text and Table 5-9)
Limb movements (see text and Table 5-9)
Autonomic phenomena‡
Apneic spells*

*Documented with simultaneous electroencephalographic seizure activity most commonly in term infants.
†Documented with simultaneous electroencephalographic seizure activity most commonly in premature infants.
‡Documented with simultaneous electroencephalographic seizure activity as a prominent isolated seizure manifestation most commonly in the premature infant, but autonomic phenomena (e.g., increase in blood pressure) are common accompaniments of seizures in term infants as well.

TABLE 5-9	Major Ictal Clinical Manifestations of Electroencephalographic Seizures in Premature Infants
Scher and Co-workers* (N = 12; Mean Birth Weight, 1358 g)	**Radvanyi-Bouvet and Co-workers† (N = 21; Mean Birth Weight, 1220 g)**
Clonic movements (6)	Sustained eye opening with fixed gaze (15)
Myoclonic movements (2)	Tonic, often with facial "wincing" (8)
Staring (2)	Myoclonic movements (7)
Nystagmus (1)	"Jerks" (1)
Apnea (1)	Pedaling movements (2)
Hiccough (1)	Cry-grimace (3)
Chewing (7)	
Ocular movements (4)	
Apnea (4)	
Tachypnea (3)	
Bradycardia (6)	
Tachycardia (1)	

*Data from Scher MS, Painter MJ, Bergman I, Barmada MA, et al: EEG diagnoses of neonatal seizures: Clinical correlations and outcome, *Pediatr Neurol* 5:17-24, 1989.
†Data from Radvanyi-Bouvet MF, Vallecalle MH, Morel-Kahn F, Relier JP, et al: Seizures and electrical discharges in premature infants, *Neuropediatrics* 16:143-148, 1985.

subtle clinical phenomena occur in association with EEG seizure activity in full-term infants (although slightly less commonly than in preterm infants) has been shown by several investigators.[19,25,27,29,158-160b] Thus, eye opening, ocular movements, peculiar extremity movements (e.g., resembling "boxing" or "hooking" movements), mouth movements, and apnea have been documented in association with EEG seizure activity, usually in temporal leads (Table 5-9). In my experience, the most common manifestations of subtle seizure in both premature and full-term infants are ocular phenomena. In premature infants, the dominant ocular phenomenon is sustained eye opening with ocular fixation; in term infants, it is horizontal deviation of the eyes.

The frequency with which subtle clinical seizure phenomena are associated with concomitant EEG seizure activity is controversial. In one study, 22 infants,[155] approximately 85% of whom were of greater than 36 weeks of gestation, exhibited paroxysms of such ocular abnormalities as eye opening or blinking, oral-buccal-lingual movements, pedaling or stepping movements, or rotary arm movements with an "inconsistent association" with EEG seizure activity. Only tonic horizontal deviation of the eyes was consistently associated with EEG seizure activity in that study.[155] In another report of 44 infants (28 premature), subtle clinical phenomena, defined as outlined in Table 5-8, accounted for fully 70% to 75% of all clinical seizures with simultaneous EEG correlates.[25]

Taken together, the data indicate that some caution should be used in attributing an epileptic origin to some subtle clinical phenomena, particularly when these phenomena are the only manifestation of seizure in the infant. Certain observations can be made at the bedside to help determine whether such subtle clinical

phenomena are likely to be epileptic versus nonepileptic (see later). Nevertheless, conventional surface EEG recordings may not detect the epileptic nature of the event (see later discussion).

The issue of *apnea as a seizure manifestation* in the newborn deserves special consideration. Although apnea has been demonstrated as a seizure manifestation in the premature newborn,[19,154,161] most apneic episodes in the premature infant are not epileptic in origin.[154,162-165] However, apnea has been documented with electrical seizure activity more commonly in the full-term newborn.[27,29,158,160b,166-170a] In 14 of the 21 infants studied by Watanabe and co-workers,[158] the infants exhibited other subtle phenomena during the apneic seizure (e.g., eye opening, "staring," deviation of the eyes, and mouth movements). Of additional value in clinical identification of apnea as a seizure is the observation that apnea accompanied by EEG seizure activity (i.e., convulsive apnea) is less likely to be associated with bradycardia than is nonconvulsive apnea.[167] Convulsive apnea that is prolonged (e.g., 60 seconds) may be complicated ultimately by bradycardia, perhaps secondary to cerebral hypoxia.[158,166] Other, rarer clinical phenomena observed in infants with apneic seizures (and occasionally in isolation) include episodic *vertical* deviation of eyes (usually downward) with or without eye jerking, hyperpnea, vasomotor phenomena, and abnormal cardiac rhythm (usually with bradycardia).[28,158,160,160b,168,170-175]

Clonic. *Clonic seizures* represent the seizure type associated most consistently with time-synchronized EEG seizure activity.[28,155,176] Clonic movements in the newborn are rhythmic and usually rather slow (approximately one to three jerks per second at the onset, with the rate progressively declining with the seizure). I categorize clonic seizures in the newborn as focal or multifocal (see Table 5-7). *Focal clonic seizures* involve the face, upper or lower extremities on one side of the body, or axial structures (neck or trunk) on one side of the body (Table 5-10). Infants commonly are not clearly unconscious during or after the focal seizure, and the neuropathological condition often is focal (e.g., cerebral infarction). However, focal clonic seizures may occur with metabolic encephalopathies in the newborn.

Multifocal clonic seizures involve several body parts, often in a migrating fashion, although the migration most often "marches" in a nonjacksonian manner (e.g., left arm jerking may be followed by right leg jerking) (Table 5-11). Generalized clonic seizures (i.e., diffusely bilateral, generally symmetrical, and synchronous movements) are rarely, if ever, observed in the newborn.

Tonic. *Tonic seizures* are clinical episodes, the most common of which are unassociated with

TABLE 5-10	Focal Clonic Seizures
Well-localized clonic jerking	
Infant usually not unconscious	

TABLE 5-11	Multifocal Clonic Seizures

Multifocal clonic movements: simultaneous or in sequence
Nonordered (nonjacksonian) migration

TABLE 5-12	Focal Tonic Seizures

Sustained posturing of a limb
Asymmetrical posturing of trunk or neck

| TABLE 5-14 | Relation of Myoclonic Seizures to Electroencephalographic Seizure Discharges |

Type of Myoclonic Seizure	Consistent EEG Seizure	Inconsistent or No EEG Seizure
Generalized	35	23
Focal	3	38
Multifocal	0	5

EEG, electroencephalographic.
Data from Mizrahi EM, Kellaway P: Characterization and classification of neonatal seizures, *Neurology* 37:1837-1844, 1987; n = 17.

| TABLE 5-15 | Focal and Multifocal Myoclonic Seizures |

Well-localized, single or multiple, migrating jerks, usually of limbs
Usually not accompanied by electroencephalographic seizure discharges

| TABLE 5-16 | Generalized Myoclonic Seizures |

Single or several bilateral synchronous jerks of flexion, more in upper than in lower limbs
May presage infantile spasms with suppression-burst electroencephalographic pattern and typical or atypical hypsarrhythmia

time-synchronized EEG discharges.[28,155] Two categories of tonic seizures should be distinguished: focal and generalized (see Table 5-7). The latter are much more common than the former. I have not observed multifocal (i.e., migrating, asynchronous) tonic seizures in the newborn. *Focal tonic seizures* consist of sustained posturing of a limb or asymmetrical posturing of trunk or neck (Table 5-12). Mizrahi and Kellaway[155] also classified horizontal eye deviation as a focal tonic seizure; I prefer to refer to this clinical seizure as subtle. In contrast to generalized tonic seizures, focal tonic seizures are associated consistently with EEG seizure discharges.[155]

A rare source of confusion with focal tonic seizure is the focal tonic episodes that may occur as the initial manifestation of *alternating hemiplegia of childhood*.[177,178] EEG findings are normal, and after the first weeks of life, the tonic episodes are followed by prolonged hemiparesis characteristic of the disease. Similarly, *hemifacial spasm*, a rare disorder in the newborn with a posterior fossa lesion (e.g., cerebellar tumor, facial nerve trauma), is not accompanied by abnormal EEG features.[179,180]

Generalized tonic seizures are characterized most commonly by tonic extension of both upper and lower extremities (mimicking "decerebrate" posturing) but also by tonic flexion of upper extremities with extension of lower extremities (mimicking "decorticate" posturing) (Table 5-13). The possibility that such clinical seizures usually do represent posturing and not epileptic seizure was raised previously because of the frequent association with severe intraventricular hemorrhage and the often poor response to anticonvulsant therapy.[153,181] Indeed, approximately 85% of such clinical seizures in one careful study were not accompanied by electrical seizure activity or, interestingly, by autonomic phenomena.[157] The 15% of generalized tonic seizures that were accompanied by electrical seizure activity were also accompanied by autonomic

TABLE 5-13	Generalized Tonic Seizures

Tonic extension of upper and lower limbs mimics decerebrate posturing.
Tonic flexion of upper limbs and extension of lower limbs mimic decorticate posturing.
Most generalized tonic seizures are not accompanied by electroencephalographic seizure discharges; in the minority of generalized tonic seizures that do have electroencephalographic seizure correlates, *autonomic phenomena* are prominent clinical features.

phenomena.[29,157] A rarer source of confusion with generalized tonic seizures is the episode of generalized hypertonia provoked by minor tactile or other stimuli and characteristic of *hyperekplexia*, also known as *startle disease* or *congenital stiff-man syndrome* (see later discussion and Chapter 3).[182-187]

Myoclonic. *Myoclonic seizures*, like tonic seizures, are clinical episodes that as a group are most commonly unassociated with time-synchronized EEG discharges (Table 5-14).[28,155] Myoclonic movements are distinguished from clonic movements particularly because of the faster speed of the myoclonic jerk and the particular predilection for flexor muscle groups. Three categories of myoclonic seizures should be distinguished: focal, multifocal, and generalized (see Table 5-7; Tables 5-15 and 5-16). *Focal myoclonic seizures* typically involve flexor muscles of an upper extremity, and of 41 focal myoclonic seizures studied by Mizrahi and Kellaway,[155] only 3 were associated with EEG seizure discharges (see Table 5-14). *Multifocal myoclonic seizures* are characterized by asynchronous twitching of several parts of the body; in five episodes studied by Mizrahi and Kellaway,[155] none had associated EEG seizure discharges. *Generalized myoclonic seizures* are characterized by bilateral jerks of flexion of upper and occasionally of lower limbs (see Table 5-16). These seizures may appear identical to the infantile spasms observed in older infants. Generalized myoclonic seizures are more likely to be associated with EEG seizure discharges than are focal or multifocal myoclonic seizures.[28,155] Of 58 generalized myoclonic seizures studied by Mizrahi and Kellaway,[155] 35 had associated EEG seizure discharges (see Table 5-14). All three varieties of myoclonic seizures may occur as a feature of severe neonatal epileptic and nonepileptic syndromes (see later discussion).

Seizures versus Jitteriness and Other Nonepileptic Movements

Jitteriness, although not a type of seizure, is a movement disorder that is often confused with a convulsion. It is characteristically a disorder of the newborn and is seen rarely, if ever, in similar form at a later age. Jitteriness is characterized by movements with qualities primarily of tremulousness but occasionally of clonus. Distinguishing jitteriness from seizure is readily done at the bedside, if the following five points are remembered (Table 5-17). Jitteriness is not accompanied by ocular phenomena (i.e., eye fixation or deviation); seizures usually are. Jitteriness is exquisitely stimulus sensitive; seizures generally are not. The dominant movement in jitteriness is tremor (i.e., the alternating movements are rhythmic and of equal rate and amplitude), whereas the dominant movement in seizure is clonic jerking (i.e., movements with a fast and slow component). The rhythmic movements of limbs in jitteriness usually can be stopped by gentle passive flexion of the affected limb; convulsive movements do not cease with this maneuver. Finally, jitteriness is not accompanied by autonomic changes (e.g., tachycardia, increase in blood pressure, apnea, cutaneous vasomotor phenomena, pupillary change, salivation or drooling); seizures often are accompanied by one or more of these changes. The most consistently defined causes of jitteriness are hypoxic-ischemic encephalopathy, hypocalcemia, hypoglycemia, and drug withdrawal.

The distinguishing clinical features described are useful in the clinical distinction of episodic movements other than jitteriness that may be confused with an epileptic seizure. Of particular importance is the increase of nonepileptic movements with sensory stimulation, their suppression with gentle restraint, and their lack of accompaniment by autonomic changes.

Finally, newborns exhibit normal motor activity that could be mistaken for seizure (Table 5-18). Moreover, certain unusual but benign paroxysmal neonatal motor phenomena (e.g., paroxysmal downward gaze or upward gaze) also should be readily distinguishable

TABLE 5-18	Normal Neonatal Motor Activity Commonly Mistaken for Seizure Activity

Awake or Drowsy
Roving, sometimes dysconjugate eye movements, with occasional nonsustained nystagmoid jerks at the extremes of horizontal movement (contrast with fixed, tonic horizontal deviation of eyes with or without jerking, characteristic of subtle seizure)
Sucking, puckering movements not accompanied by ocular fixation or deviation
Asleep
Fragmentary myoclonic jerks, may be multiple
Isolated, generalized myoclonic jerk as infant wakes from sleep

from seizure (see Chapter 3).[188-191] Awareness of such motor activity and of the clinical points described in the previous paragraphs should allow ready distinction from seizure at the bedside.

Neonatal Clinical Seizures Not Accompanied by Electroencephalographic Seizure Activity

Pathophysiology

As shown in Table 5-5, certain clinical seizures in the newborn are not consistently accompanied by EEG seizure activity. Such seizures include certain subtle seizures, most generalized tonic seizures, and the focal and multifocal examples of myoclonic seizures. Concerning the pathophysiology of these three seizure types, it is well established that myoclonic jerks may originate as isolated events from several levels of the nervous system (i.e., brain stem and spinal cord, as well as cerebral cortex).[192] Thus, it is not surprising that many of these seizures do not have an EEG correlate.

The pathophysiology of the subtle seizures and generalized tonic seizures that are not consistently accompanied by EEG seizure activity is not clear. Mizrahi and Kellaway[28,155-157] termed the subtle phenomena *motor automatisms*, which include oral-buccal-lingual movements, ocular signs, and such limb and axial movements as swimming or rotatory movements of upper extremities, stepping and pedaling movements of lower extremities, and struggling movements of the head and trunk. The possibility is raised that "tonic posturing and motor automatisms may be primitive brain stem and spinal motor patterns released from the tonic inhibition normally exerted by forebrain structures," that is, "brain stem release phenomena."[28,155] Analogies are drawn between the clinical phenomena in the human newborn and those in animal models of decortication,[155-157] clinical phenomena that include tonic posturing, certain limb movements, and characteristic responses to sensory stimuli. Thus, it is apparent that, as with release phenomena, some of the limb movements and posturing observed in the human newborn, like their counterparts in animal models, are exquisitely stimulus sensitive in that these movements and postures exhibit

TABLE 5-17 Jitteriness versus Seizure		
Clinical Feature	**Jitteriness**	**Seizure**
Abnormality of gaze or eye movement	0	+
Movements exquisitely stimulus sensitive	+	0
Predominant movement	Tremor	Clonic jerking
Movements cease with passive flexion	+	0
Autonomic changes	0	+

spatial summation, radiation, and temporal summation (magnitude and extent of movement greater with more intense stimuli, a larger number of stimuli, or with more frequent stimuli) and can be suppressed by physical restraint. Also compatible with the notion of brain stem release phenomena, among infants with subtle seizures termed motor automatisms by Mizrahi and Kellaway[155-157] or with generalized tonic seizures characterized by decerebrate or decorticate posturing, is the often strong indication of severe cerebral cortical disturbance (and therefore, perhaps functional decortication) manifested by marked EEG suppression and structural evidence of severe cerebral injury. Clearly, the hypothesis raised by Mizrahi and Kellaway[155-157] that many subtle seizures and generalized tonic seizures represent brain stem release phenomena is an important one to test by creating suitable models in developing animals. The findings would have major implications concerning the value, or lack thereof, of treatment of such phenomena with anticonvulsant medication.

Does Absence of Electroencephalographic Seizure Activity Indicate that a Clinical Seizure is Nonepileptic?

Clearly, central to the concept that certain neonatal clinical seizures are nonepileptic (e.g., brain stem release phenomena) is the lack of consistent EEG seizure accompaniment. Does the absence of EEG seizure activity in a newborn rule out an epileptic origin for the clinical activity? The answer vis à vis the newborn is not known unequivocally. However, a large body of information in older children and adults, as well as in newborns, indicates that *epileptic phenomena can occur in the absence of surface-recorded EEG discharges*, and *such phenomena can be generated at subcortical (i.e., deep limbic, diencephalic, brain stem) levels*, as summarized in Table 5-19.[27,193-206]

Particularly strong support for the notion that neonatal seizures may originate from brain stem structures specifically is provided by studies in the rat.[203] Thus, investigators showed that stimulation of inferior colliculus of the adult rat causes a persistent electrical discharge accompanied by wild running behavior. However, stimulation of this midbrain region in the neonatal animal also produced less complex movement (i.e., "forelimb paddling, hindlimb treading, and rolling-curling movements of the torso").[203] The relation to the "boxing," "bicycling," and similar movements of the human newborn is obvious. Moreover, the sensitivity of the inferior colliculus for development of the electrical and clinical seizure activity was considerably greater in the newborn than in the older animal. Thus, these data show that at least one brain stem structure, the inferior colliculus, can generate an electrical seizure that is accompanied by clinical activity highly reminiscent of the subtle seizure of the human newborn. It is perhaps of related interest that neurons of the inferior colliculus of the newborn are particularly sensitive to injury by hypoxic-ischemic insults (see Chapter 8), the most common cause of neonatal seizures (see later discussion).

TABLE 5-19	Epileptic Phenomena in the Absence of Electroencephalographic (Surface-Recorded) Seizure Discharges*

Simple partial seizures in older children and adults have been accompanied by no ictal seizure discharges recorded from surface electrodes in as many as 80% to 90% of episodes.
Complex partial seizures in older children and adults, emanating from the temporal lobe, particularly the hippocampus, may be undetectable on EEG recordings obtained from surface electrodes and even from subdural electrodes; depth electrodes may be required to detect the ictal hippocampal discharges; many subtle seizure phenomena in the newborn suggest complex partial seizures; subtle seizures have been documented in congenital maldevelopment of the hippocampus, and the hippocampus is a frequent site of neuronal disease in neonatal encephalopathies, especially hypoxic-ischemic encephalopathy.
Clinical seizure phenomena can occur in the infant with hydranencephaly in the absence of (surface-recorded) EEG discharges.
Bilateral, synchronous, and rhythmic myoclonic movements can occur in benign neonatal sleep myoclonus and in benign myoclonus of early infancy, always without seizure discharges from surface-recorded EEG.

*See text for references.
EEG, electroencephalographic.

Several particularly careful studies of more than 100 infants with electrographically confirmed seizures helped to clarify further the relation of subtle clinical seizures and electrographic seizures. The proportion of infants who exhibited subtle clinical seizures (characterized by motor phenomena involving ocular, oral, or facial structures) was nearly identical among infants who either did or did not exhibit simultaneous electrographic discharge.[25,29,176] Thus, there was no overrepresentation of subtle clinical seizures in the infants who did not exhibit an EEG correlate. Moreover, the groups with and without electrographic accompaniments of the subtle seizures were clinically similar and had similar neurological outcomes (i.e., no indication that the infants who did not have consistent EEG correlates were more likely to have cerebral destruction and thereby "release" phenomena than were the infants who had consistent EEG correlates). Further, infants with similar subtle clinical phenomena sometimes exhibited a concomitant electrographic seizure discharge and sometimes did not. Finally, in such infants, the clinical phenomena were more likely to begin seconds *before* the electrographic discharge than in infants with consistent coupling of clinical and electrical seizure. These data led to the conclusion that in infants without consistent EEG correlates, subtle clinical seizures may originate from subcortical structures, and at any given particular EEG sampling, propagation of the seizure to the surface either may not occur (thus accounting for the inconsistent electroclinical correlation) or occurs seconds after the motor efferent activation by the subcortical origin of the seizure (thus accounting for the onset of clinical before electrographic seizure).[25,176]

These observations in animals and humans raise the strong possibility that certain clinical seizures in the human newborn originate from electrical seizures in deep cerebral structures (e.g., limbic regions) or in diencephalic or brain stem structures and thereby are either not detectable by surface-recorded EEG or are only inconsistently propagated to the surface. Clearly, more data are needed. Of particular importance is whether such "surface EEG–silent" seizures in the newborn have the potential to result in brain injury and whether they can be eliminated by conventional anticonvulsant therapy.

Etiology

Of the many causes of neonatal seizures, relatively few account for most cases, and these causes should be emphasized. Determination of the origin is highly critical, because it affords the opportunity to treat specifically and also to make a meaningful prognostic statement (see "Prognosis"). The most important causes, their usual time of onset, and their relative frequency as the major cause of seizures in premature or full-term infants are shown in Table 5-20. In my experience, the first four of the categories depicted in Table 5-20 (hypoxic-ischemic encephalopathy, intracranial hemorrhage, intracranial infection, and developmental defects) account for 80% to 85% of all cases. The following discussion of causes emphasizes the characteristics of the accompanying seizures; more detailed discussions of the specific clinical entities may be found in the appropriate chapters of this book.

Hypoxic-Ischemic Encephalopathy

Hypoxic-ischemic encephalopathy, usually secondary to perinatal asphyxia, is the single most common cause of neonatal seizures in both full-term and premature infants (see Chapter 9).[3,17,25,29,207-219] In my experience, approximately 60% of patients have this encephalopathy as the primary cause. Seizures occur in the majority of patients with significant hypoxic-ischemic encephalopathy, and characteristically the spells occur *in the first 24 hours*. In fact, 60% of our infant patients with seizures secondary to this type of encephalopathy experience the onset of spells within 12 hours of birth. The seizures usually become very severe and frequent from 12 to 24 hours after birth, and overt status epilepticus is not unusual. Urgent therapy is then required. (The other clinical features of hypoxic-ischemic encephalopathy are discussed in Chapter 9.) In cases that I have followed, virtually every infant with seizures exhibited subtle seizures. Multifocal clonic or focal clonic seizures are also particularly common. The latter are characteristic of the infant with focal cerebral ischemic injury (i.e., stroke; see Chapter 9). In my experience, approximately 30% of term infants with hypoxic-ischemic disease and seizures (i.e., 20% of all term infants with seizures) exhibit focal cerebral infarction. Often these infants exhibit relatively few other overt signs of encephalopathy, a helpful clinical point.

Intracranial Hemorrhage

Intracranial hemorrhage may be difficult to establish conclusively as a cause of seizures distinct from hypoxic-ischemic or traumatic injury because of the frequent association of one or both of these factors with the hemorrhage (see Chapters 10 and 11). Nevertheless, certain conclusions seem justified on the basis of current information. In my experience, approximately 15% of term infants have intracranial hemorrhage as the primary cause of their spells. This value is approximately double in populations that include large proportions of premature infants with seizures.[25,218]

Primary Subarachnoid Hemorrhage. As discussed in Chapter 10, primary subarachnoid hemorrhage, although very common, is usually not of major clinical significance. Nevertheless, seizures can occur secondary to subarachnoid hemorrhage in the full-term infant, and in that context the spells most often have their onset on the second postnatal day.[220]

TABLE 5-20	**Major Causes of Neonatal Seizures in Relation to Time of Seizure Onset and Relative Frequency**			
	TIME OF ONSET*		**RELATIVE FREQUENCY†**	
Cause	**0–3 Days**	**>3 Days**	**Premature**	**Full Term**
Hypoxic-ischemic encephalopathy	+		+++	+++
Intracranial hemorrhage‡	+	+	++	+
Intracranial infection§	+	+	++	++
Developmental defects	+	+	++	++
Hypoglycemia	+		+	+
Hypocalcemia‖	+	+	+	+
Other metabolic¶	+			+
Epileptic syndromes#	+	+		+

*Postnatal age when seizures most commonly begin.
†Relative frequency of seizures among all causes: +++, most common; ++, less common; +, least common.
‡Hemorrhages are principally germinal matrix intraventricular, often with periventricular hemorrhagic infarction, in the premature infant and subarachnoid or subdural in the term infant. See text concerning time of onset.
§Early seizures occur usually with intrauterine nonbacterial infections (e.g., toxoplasmosis, cytomegalovirus infection), and later seizures usually occur with herpes simplex encephalitis or bacterial meningitis.
‖Two varieties of hypocalcemia are included (see text).
¶See text for types.
#Five different syndromes are included (see text).

Infants with subarachnoid hemorrhage in association with hypoxic-ischemic encephalopathy usually exhibit seizures on the first postnatal day, probably as a result of the encephalopathy rather than the hemorrhage. In the interictal period, the infant with seizures secondary to uncomplicated subarachnoid hemorrhage often appears remarkably well; I have used the appellation "well baby with seizures" to characterize these unusual cases.

Germinal Matrix-Intraventricular Hemorrhage. This type of hemorrhage, emanating from small blood vessels in the subependymal germinal matrix, is principally a lesion of the premature infant, occurring in the first 3 days of life. Seizures in association with this type of hemorrhage usually occur with severe lesions or with accompanying parenchymal involvement or both (see Chapter 11). In one series of EEG-confirmed seizures, 28 of 62 (45%) of preterm infants had severe intraventricular hemorrhage with or without periventricular hemorrhagic infarction.[25] With severe intraventricular hemorrhage, the most prominent seizure type is the generalized tonic variety, often a part of a catastrophic deterioration evolving to coma and respiratory arrest in minutes to hours (see Chapter 11). Subtle seizure phenomena are usual accompaniments. Germinal matrix-intraventricular hemorrhage most often is accompanied by a less prominent neurological syndrome and is only uncommonly accompanied by seizures. This fact and the aforementioned difficulty of distinguishing generalized tonic seizure from decerebrate posturing probably account for the wide range (15% to 50%) of frequencies recorded for seizures with intraventricular hemorrhage. Nevertheless, in one interesting older study, generalized tonic phenomena, whether they represented seizure or posturing, were present in approximately 50% of infants who died of severe intraventricular hemorrhage that was timed with chromium-50–labeled red blood cells; importantly, the tonic episodes constituted the clinical finding that correlated best with the time of occurrence of the intraventricular hemorrhage (accurate within 4 hours in 70% of cases with such tonic phenomena).[221]

Premature infants, particularly those of very low birth weight, who develop periventricular hemorrhagic infarction in association with severe intraventricular hemorrhage most often develop the parenchymal lesion and the seizures in the latter part of the first week of life (see Chapter 11). Thus, this important subgroup of premature infants with hemorrhage experiences the onset of seizures *after* 3 days of age, unlike in other forms of germinal matrix-intraventricular hemorrhage (see Table 5-18).

Subdural Hemorrhage. Subdural hemorrhage is often associated with a traumatic event, and it is probably the associated cerebral contusion that results in the convulsive phenomena. The most common variety of subdural hemorrhage is the convexity type (see Chapter 10), and the seizures in this setting are often focal. In one large series, convulsive phenomena occurred in 50% of newborns with subdural hemorrhage and appeared in the first 48 hours of life.[222]

Intracranial Infection

Intracranial bacterial and nonbacterial infections are not uncommon causes of neonatal seizures, and they account for 5% to 10% of our cases. Of the *bacterial infections*, meningitides secondary to group B streptococci and *Escherichia coli* are the most common substrates (see Chapter 21). The onset of seizures in these instances is usually in the latter part of the first week and subsequent to that period. The relevant *nonbacterial infections* include the various neonatal encephalitides: toxoplasmosis, herpes simplex, coxsackievirus B infection, rubella, and cytomegalovirus infection (see Chapter 20). In intrauterine toxoplasmosis or cytomegalovirus infection that is severe enough to result in neonatal seizures, the episodes occur in the first 3 days of life. Seizures associated with herpes simplex encephalitis tend to occur later. Whether neonatal seizures occur with septicemia only, as in adults,[223] is unclear, although I believe that the presumption in such a clinical setting should be that bacterial meningitis is also present (see Chapter 21).

Developmental Defects

Many aberrations of brain development can result in seizures, which begin at any time during the neonatal period. In my experience, developmental defects account for 5% to 10% of cases. The common denominator of virtually all these aberrations is cerebral cortical dysgenesis, related most commonly to a disturbance of neuronal migration. Thus, the disorders most frequently responsible are lissencephaly, pachygyria, and polymicrogyria (see Chapter 2).

Metabolic Disturbances

In this general category I include the following: disturbances in the levels of glucose, calcium, magnesium, electrolytes, amino acids, organic acids, blood ammonia, and other metabolites; certain intoxications, especially with local anesthetics; mitochondrial or peroxisomal disturbance; pyridoxine and folinic acid responsive seizures; and glucose transporter deficiency (Table 5-21). The aberrations in levels of glucose and divalent cations are the most frequent.

Hypoglycemia. Hypoglycemia is most frequent in small infants, most of whom are small for gestational age, and in infants of mothers who are diabetic or prediabetic (see Chapter 12). The most critical determinants for the occurrence of neurological symptoms in neonatal hypoglycemia are the *duration* of the hypoglycemia and, as a corollary, the amount of time elapsed before treatment is begun.[224] Neurological symptoms consist most commonly of jitteriness, stupor, hypotonia, apnea, and seizures. In a review of infants who were small for gestational age and who had hypoglycemia, approximately 80% exhibited neurological symptoms, and more than 50% of symptomatic infants who were small for gestational age experienced seizures.[225] The onset is usually the second postnatal day. In these

TABLE 5-21 **Major Metabolic Disturbances Associated with Neonatal Seizures**

Hypoglycemia
Hypocalcemia and hypomagnesemia
Local anesthetic intoxication
Hyponatremia
Hypernatremia, especially during correction
Amino acidopathy, especially nonketotic hyperglycinemia
Organic acidopathy
Hyperammonemia, often associated with acidopathies
Mitochondrial disturbance (pyruvate dehydrogenase, cytochrome-*c* oxidase)
Peroxisomal disturbance (Zellweger syndrome, neonatal adrenoleukodystrophy)
Pyridoxine dependency
Folinic acid–responsive seizures
Glucose transporter deficiency

infants, it is often particularly difficult to establish that hypoglycemia is the cause of the neurological syndrome, because perinatal asphyxia, hemorrhage, hypocalcemia, and infection are frequently associated. In our earlier series, although 9% of infants with seizures experienced hypoglycemia, in none was the metabolic defect the only potential etiological factor.[226] In our more recent series, only 3% of neonatal seizures were related to hypoglycemia.[207,209,219]

In contrast to the situation with small infants, neurological symptoms, including seizures, are much less frequent in hypoglycemic infants of diabetic mothers (10% to 20%), possibly because the duration of hypoglycemia in the latter infants is relatively brief.[225] This and related issues are discussed in more detail in Chapter 12.

Hypocalcemia. Hypocalcemia has two major peaks of incidence in the newborn. The first peak, which takes place in the *first 2 to 3 days of life*, occurs most often in low-birth-weight infants, both of average and below-average weight for gestational age, and in infants of diabetic mothers; this peak frequently accompanies the hypoxic-ischemic encephalopathy of perinatal asphyxia. Thus, seizures in this context are usually not accompanied solely by hypocalcemia. In our earlier series, 13% of the infants with seizures exhibited hypocalcemia, but as with hypoglycemia, the metabolic defect was not the *only* major etiological possibility.[226] In our later series, hypocalcemia was the cause of 3% of neonatal seizures.[207,219] A therapeutic response to intravenous calcium is of major value in determining whether the low serum calcium is related etiologically to the seizures. In our experience, it is *much more common* for early hypocalcemia to be a condition associated with neonatal seizures rather than the cause.[209]

When hypocalcemia appears *later in the neonatal period*, without the complicated associated factors of early onset hypocalcemia, delineation of hypocalcemia as the major etiological factor in the convulsive phenomena is easier. Classically, these hypocalcemic babies are large, full-term infants who avidly consume a milk preparation with a suboptimal ratio of

phosphorus to calcium and phosphorus to magnesium (e.g., cow's milk or a high-phosphorus synthetic formula). Hypomagnesemia is a frequent accompaniment or, indeed, may be present without hypocalcemia.[227-229] The neurological syndrome is consistent and distinctive, involving primarily the following: hyperactive tendon reflexes; knee, ankle, and jaw clonus; jitteriness; and seizures. The convulsive phenomena are often focal, both clinically and electroencephalographically.[227,230] Later-onset hypocalcemia of the nutritional type now is very unusual in the United States. Later-onset hypocalcemic seizures are associated more commonly with endocrinopathy (maternal hyperparathyroidism, neonatal hypoparathyroidism) or with congenital heart disease (with or without DiGeorge syndrome.[231,231a] Primary hypomagnesemia, a rare defect of magnesium absorption, may produce a syndrome similar to that just described for late-onset hypocalcemia.[229,232,233] The onset of seizures is most commonly between 2 and 6 weeks of age. Because calcium levels may also be low, the mistaken diagnosis of primary hypocalcemia may be made. Parenteral administration of magnesium prevents the seizures and early infantile death.

Local Anesthetic Intoxication. Seizures are a prominent feature of neonatal intoxication with local anesthetics, inadvertently injected, usually into the infant's scalp, at the time of placement of paracervical, pudendal, or epidural block or local anesthesia for episiotomy.[209,234-245] Although direct injection into the fetus is the usual mode of administration, transplacental transmission is possible. Paracervical and pudendal blocks have been the most common forms of maternal analgesia involved in the well-documented cases of fetal injection.

The *major clinical features* (Table 5-22) are characteristic and should be recognized, particularly because confusion with asphyxia is not uncommon and may delay appropriate therapy, with dire consequences.[246] In one series of seven infants, seizures occurred in each infant within the first 6 hours and were tonic in all but one. This very early occurrence of seizures is mimicked consistently by only one other *major* cause of neonatal seizures, hypoxic-ischemic encephalopathy, which is further suggested by the often low Apgar scores. However, two distinguishing features of local anesthetic intoxication aid in the differential diagnosis:

TABLE 5-22 **Major Features of Neonatal Intoxication with Local Anesthetic (Mepivacaine, Lidocaine)**

Type of maternal analgesia: paracervical > pudendal > epidural > episiotomy (local infiltration)
Apgar scores depressed at 1 and 5 minutes
Bradycardia
Apnea
Hypotonia
Seizures: onset in the first 6 hours, usually tonic
Pupils: dilated and fixed to light
Eyes: fixed to oculocephalic (doll's eyes) reflex

(1) *pupils fixed to light and often dilated* and (2) *eye movements fixed to the oculocephalic (doll's eyes) reflex.* These latter signs are unusual in hypoxic-ischemic disease in the first 12 hours. The finding that infants with intoxication *improve* over the first 24 to 48 hours (if properly supported) further distinguishes the disorder from serious hypoxic-ischemic encephalopathy. Clinical signs suggestive of local anesthetic intoxication should alert the physician to a particularly careful inquiry into the obstetrical history and to a search for needle marks on the infant's scalp. Determination of local anesthetic levels in blood and CSF establishes the diagnosis.

Management depends on prompt recognition. Vigorous support, especially of ventilation, is essential. Therapy required depends in part on the time of recognition of the intoxication; the half-life of the drug in blood is approximately 8 to 10 hours.[246] Removal of the drug is accomplished more effectively by diuresis with acidification of the urine than by exchange transfusion.[246] Anticonvulsant drugs are of questionable value, and control of seizures is effected best by removal of the local anesthetic. The outcome is good, if hypoxic complications do not occur.

Other Metabolic Disturbances. Metabolic disturbances other than hypoglycemia and deficiency of divalent cations are uncommon causes of seizures in the newborn (see Table 5-21). Worthy of note are hyponatremia and hypernatremia, hyperammonemia, other amino acid and organic acid abnormalities, mitochondrial disturbances, peroxisomal disorders, pyridoxine dependency, folinic acid responsive seizures, and glucose transporter deficiency.

Hyponatremia may result in seizures and occurs most commonly in my experience with inappropriate antidiuretic hormone secretion, associated with bacterial meningitis, intracranial hemorrhage, hypoxic-ischemic encephalopathy, or excessive intake of water. The latter may occur in a child with minor gastrointestinal difficulties when an inexperienced mother administers diluted formula or water only or both.[247] *Hypernatremia* occurs primarily in severely dehydrated infants or as a complication of overly vigorous use of sodium bicarbonate for correction of acidosis. Seizures often result during correction of hypernatremia if markedly hypotonic solutions are used, perhaps secondary to the development of intracellular edema.[248,249]

Disturbances of *amino acid* or *organic acid* metabolism may result in neonatal seizures, virtually always in the context of other neurological features (see Chapters 14 and 15). In my experience, the most common of these associated with neonatal seizures are nonketotic hyperglycinemia, sulfite oxidase deficiency, multiple carboxylase deficiency, multiple acyl-coenzyme A dehydrogenase deficiency (glutaric aciduria, type II), and urea cycle defect. *Hyperammonemia* or acidosis, or both, most commonly accompanies these disturbances. *Transient* disturbance of the glycine cleavage enzyme may cause neonatal seizures; the diagnosis can be missed if CSF glycine levels are not determined because plasma glycine levels may be normal (see Chapter 14).

The process resolves spontaneously after approximately 6 weeks of age.[250]

Additional unusual causes of neonatal seizures in this context include *mitochondrial* or *peroxisomal* disturbance. Of the former, pyruvate dehydrogenase deficiency and cytochrome *c* oxidase deficiency, with elevated lactate in blood and CSF, are the most common (see Chapter 15). Although not strictly a "metabolic" disturbance, peroxisomal disease, especially Zellweger syndrome or neonatal adrenoleukodystrophy, associated with elevations of blood levels of very-long-chain fatty acids and other biochemical changes, is associated with severe neonatal seizures, caused principally by associated cerebral neuronal migrational defects (see Chapters 2 and 16).

Pyridoxine dependency, a defect in pyridoxine metabolism, may produce severe seizures, recalcitrant to all therapy.[11,14,251-277a] The usual time of onset is the first hours of life, but intrauterine seizures as well as onset after the neonatal period have been observed (see later discussion). Seizures are usually multifocal clonic and recalcitrant to all therapeutic modalities. Generalized tonic-clonic seizures, a rare form of neonatal seizure, have been described in newborns with pyridoxine dependency. Diagnosis may be suspected from the EEG that, in the majority of infants, shows an unusual paroxysmal pattern consisting of generalized bursts of bilaterally synchronous high-voltage 1- to 4-Hz activity with intermixed spikes or sharp waves (Fig. 5-10).[258] Diagnosis has been suspected most commonly by documentation of cessation of seizures and normalization of the EEG findings within minutes after intravenous injection of 50 to 100 mg of pyridoxine. The EEG findings may not normalize for several hours, even when a prompt clinical response is observed. Subsequently complete control of seizures on pyridoxine monotherapy and recurrence on withdrawal have established the diagnosis. Most infants have exhibited subsequent mental retardation despite therapy from the first days of life. Nevertheless, early therapy may decrease the likelihood or severity, or both, of intellectual deficit; indeed, 8 of the 10 reported infants with normal intellect were identified and treated in the first month of life. However, many infants treated in the first month still exhibit cognitive deficits later. Intrauterine therapy by maternal pyridoxine supplementation may be necessary to prevent fetal brain injury.[273] The major structural features include evidence for both neuronal and white matter injury, with diffuse cortical atrophy, callosal thinning, and impaired cerebral myelination. These findings may relate to the elevation in CSF and brain of glutamate, caused by the molecular defect (see later). Glutamate may lead to neuronal injury by excitotoxic mechanisms and to oligodendroglial injury by free radical mechanisms (see Chapters 6 and 8). Intrauterine onset of anatomic disturbance is suggested by the fetal imaging finding of partial hypoplasia of the corpus callosum. Clinical studies also indicate that the disorder may begin after days or weeks, that the seizures may respond initially to anticonvulsant drugs, and that doses of pyridoxine greater than 100 mg may be necessary to stop the seizures.[254-258,263,273,278] Any suspicion of the

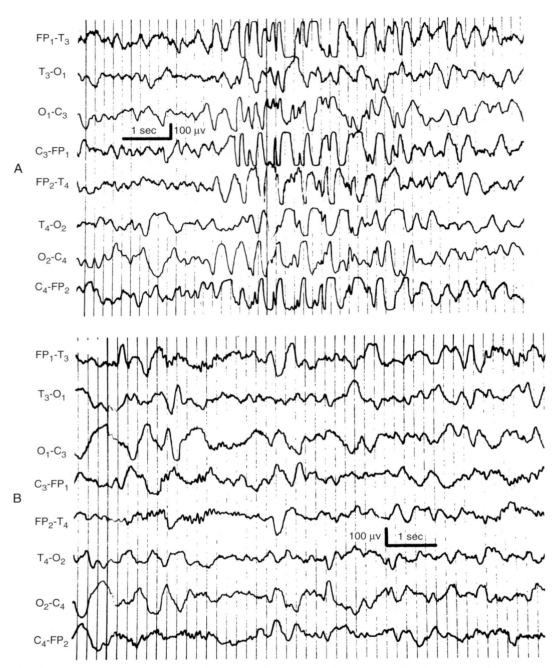

Figure 5-10 **Pyridoxine response in an infant with pyridoxine dependency. A,** Before injection of pyridoxine, the electroencephalogram shows disorganized background with generalized bursts of irregular spikes and sharp-slow wave complexes without clinical accompaniments. Vitamin B6 was injected 30 seconds later. **B,** Ten minutes after vitamin B6 injection. The discharges have subsided (4 minutes earlier), and the patient shows normal sleep background with early sleep spindles appearing in the tracing. *(From Mikati MA, Trevathan E, Krishnamoorthy KS, Lombroso CT: Pyridoxine-dependent epilepsy: EEG investigations and long-term follow-up,* Electroencephalogr Clin Neurophysiol *78:215-221, 1991.)*

disorder should lead to a *therapeutic trial of pyridoxine* (see later), intravenous if the infant is convulsing and has an abnormal EEG, or oral (100 mg or more daily for several days) if seizures are intermittent. Other means of diagnosis include the demonstration of an increase in concentration of pipecolic acid in plasma or of alpha-aminoadipic semialdehyde levels in urine.[275,275a] The probable *molecular defect* involves the active form of pyridoxine, pyridoxal phosphate, necessary for the action of glutamic acid decarboxylase, which leads to the synthesis of the inhibitory neurotransmitter GABA (see "Basic Mechanisms").[13,263,264,279] This formulation is supported by the finding of low GABA levels as well as elevated glutamate levels in CSF.[14] Recent work reveals a defect in cerebral lysine degradation.[280] The accumulating compound inactivates pyridoxal-5-phosphate. In one study, investigators showed that the dose of pyridoxine (5 mg/kg/day) that led to cessation of seizures was not sufficient to lead to normalization of CSF glutamate levels, which required a dose of 10 mg/kg/day.[14] Moreover, an increased dose of pyridoxine led to improvement in psychometric tests in another study.[261] The demonstration of progression of cerebral abnormalities in inadequately treated infants[264,265] further suggests the possibility of continuing injury by glutamate. Thus, it is possible that a dose of pyridoxine sufficient not only to prevent seizures but also to normalize CSF glutamate levels is important in therapy of this disorder. A rare neonatal disorder involving synthesis of pyridoxal-5-phosphate and a requirement for treatment with the active cofactor rather than pyridoxine has also been reported.[280a]

Folinic acid–responsive seizures refer to a clinical syndrome of neonatal seizures with onset as early as the first hours of life, responsiveness to oral administration of folinic acid, and the presence on CSF analysis for monamine neurotransmitters of two unknown metabolic peaks.[281-285] Approximately 10 cases have been identified; I have seen one case. The disorder is accompanied by a discontinuous EEG pattern with multifocal sharp waves and progressive cerebral cortical and white matter atrophy. The seizures respond to oral folinic acid at doses ranging from 2 to 20 mg twice daily; the lowest doses have been used in the neonatal period. At least 50% of the infants have had subsequent cognitive deficits. The nature of the disorder remains unclear, although a disturbance of folate metabolism is suspected.

A *disorder of glucose transport* from blood to brain (often termed *De Vivo's syndrome*) is important to recognize because prompt treatment can lead to cessation of seizures and improved neurological development.[286-295b] Approximately 25% of cases have had onset of seizures in the first 2 months of life. The mean age of onset of seizures is 5 months. The striking metabolic findings are low glucose concentrations in CSF with normal blood glucose concentration. The mean ratio of CSF to blood glucose has been 37%. That the hypoglycorrhachia was not the result of increased glycolysis, but rather of impaired glucose transport, is shown by the consistent finding of a low (rather than high) lactate level in CSF. The impaired glucose transport is related to a defect of the glucose transporter (Glut1) responsible for the facilitative diffusion of glucose across the blood-brain endothelial barrier and across the neuronal plasma membrane. Treatment with a ketogenic diet, which supplies usable metabolic fuel for brain energy metabolism not transported by the glucose transporter, is generally effective in leading to seizure control and may blunt the impaired neurological development that is a consistent feature of the disease. However, in general, the beneficial effect of the ketogenic diet is most apparent vis à vis seizure control. A potentially transient form of the disorder was described in three infants with onset of seizures and hypoglycorrhachia at 2, 4, and 6 weeks of age.

In older writings, hyperbilirubinemia was reported to be accompanied by seizures when kernicterus occurred.[222] More recent observations indicate that seizures are a feature of *marked* hyperbilirubinemia and acute bilirubin encephalopathy (see Chapter 13).

Drug Withdrawal

A rare cause of seizures in most medical centers, but a not infrequent cause of neurological signs (which may include seizures) in certain urban centers, is passive addiction of the newborn and drug withdrawal. The drugs particularly involved are narcotic-analgesics (e.g., methadone), sedative-hypnotics (e.g., shorter-acting barbiturates), propoxyphene, tricyclic antidepressants, cocaine, alcohol, and "T's and Blues" (see Chapter 24). The usual time of onset of seizures in this setting is the first 3 days of life (see Chapter 24).

Miscellaneous Neonatal Seizure Syndromes

Several syndromes of neonatal seizures are distinguished principally according to their distinctive clinical features (see Table 5-20; Table 5-23). Two of these syndromes, benign neonatal sleep myoclonus and hyperekplexia, are not associated with abnormalities of surface-recorded EEG and thus are termed "nonepileptic" (see later discussion) These disorders are important to recognize to ensure appropriate management and family counseling. The five epileptic syndromes are discussed first. Two are benign, and three are very serious (see later discussion).

Benign Familial Neonatal Seizures. A familial syndrome of idiopathic neonatal seizures, termed *benign familial neonatal seizures*, has been described in several hundred cases.[296-318] Onset of seizures is usually on the second or third postnatal day, and in the interictal period the infants appear well. Seizures may occur with a frequency of 10 to 20 per day or even higher. The episodes most often are focal clonic or focal tonic. The electroclinical characteristics are typical and consist of an initial brief period of EEG flattening, accompanied by apnea and tonic motor activity, followed by a bilateral discharge of spikes and slow waves, accompanied by clonic activity. The disorder is usually self-limited, with cessation of seizures in 1 to 6 months. Diagnostic studies, including therapeutic trials of pyridoxine, have been negative. Because of the benign course of the disorder, the history of previously affected family members may be overlooked unless specifically sought by direct questioning. Approximately 10% to

TABLE 5-23	Idiopathic Syndromes of Clinical Seizures in the Newborn

Epileptic Syndromes
Benign familial neonatal seizures
Benign idiopathic neonatal seizures (fifth-day fits)
Early myoclonic encephalopathy
Early infantile epileptic encephalopathy (Ohtahara syndrome)
Malignant migrating partial seizures
Nonepileptic Syndromes
Benign neonatal sleep myoclonus
Hyperekplexia

TABLE 5-24 Two Neonatal Epileptic Syndromes Characterized by Persistence (or Appearance) of Burst Suppression Beyond 1 to 2 Weeks of Age

Clinical Features	Early Myoclonic Encephalopathy	Early Infantile Epileptic Encephalopathy
Major clinical seizure types at onset	Myoclonic and focal clonic seizures → "tonic spasms"	"Tonic spasms"
Electroencephalographic interictal pattern	Suppression burst	Suppression burst
Relation to sleep	Enhanced by sleep	None
Evolution	Persistent suppression burst	Transition to hypsarrhythmia
Most common cause	Metabolic disturbance >> cryptogenic > structural	Bilateral structural cerebral lesions (dysgenetic >> encephaloclastic) >> metabolic or cryptogenic
Outcome	Poor	Poor

15% of infants exhibit subsequent nonfebrile seizures and may require long-term anticonvulsant therapy. Neurological development is normal. Family histories indicate autosomal dominant inheritance with incomplete penetrance. Two separate chromosomal loci have been identified (i.e., chromosome 20q13.3 and chromosome 8q24). Approximately 90% of reported families are linked to the chromosome 20 locus. Both genes encode voltage-gated K^+ channels (KCNQ2 on chromosome 20 and KCNQ3 on chromosome 8), which may function in the same heteromeric complex to regulate the threshold for neuronal excitability. In two reports of a syndrome with the age of onset of seizures at a mean age of 11 weeks, but *occasionally* in the neonatal period, the syndrome was shown to be related to a defect in an Na^+ channel (SCN2A).[319,320]

Benign Idiopathic Neonatal Seizures (Fifth-Day Fits). An interesting syndrome, described initially in Australia[321-323] and France,[324] and subsequently elsewhere,[209,307,325-328] termed *benign idiopathic neonatal seizures*, or *fifth-day fits*, is characterized by the onset of seizures in the latter part of the first week of life in apparently healthy full-term infants. Approximately 200 cases have been reported. The peak time of onset is the fifth day, and approximately 80% to 90% have had their onset between the fourth and sixth days of life. The seizures are usually multifocal clonic, often with apnea, and last less than 24 hours in the majority of cases. However, status epilepticus has occurred during that interval in approximately 80% of cases. All seizures cease generally within 15 days. The role of anticonvulsant therapy in promoting remission is not yet clear, but the outlook has been consistently favorable. The demonstration of low zinc levels in the CSF of affected patients[329] raises the possibility of an acute zinc deficiency syndrome,[207] but the origin of the zinc deficiency and confirmation thereof have not been defined. The possibility that some cases of benign idiopathic neonatal seizures are related to de novo mutations of KCNQ2, the K^+ channel most commonly affected in benign familial neonatal seizures, is suggested by a description of four infants.[318] Examples of benign idiopathic neonatal seizures, not unreasonably, probably have been considered in other series as infants with seizures of "unknown" origin.

Early Myoclonic Encephalopathy and Early Infantile Epileptic Encephalopathy. Two severe epileptic syndromes, *early myoclonic encephalopathy* (EME) and *early infantile epileptic encephalopathy* (EIEE) or *Ohtahara syndrome*, are characteristically present clinically in the first weeks of life.[27,271,330-347] Intrauterine onset has been documented.[338] These disorders are characterized by *severe recurrent seizures*, principally myoclonic and clonic at the onset in EME and "tonic spasms" at the onset in EIEE, and a striking *suppression-burst EEG pattern* (Table 5-24). The characteristics of the suppression-burst EEG pattern differ: in EME, this feature is enhanced by sleep, whereas in EIEE, the pattern is not altered by sleep or waking. The evolution of the EEG pattern is generally to hypsarrhythmia and West syndrome in EIEE, whereas in EME the suppression-burst pattern persists beyond 1 year of age. The responsible *causes* have been multiple, primarily metabolic in EME (especially nonketotic hyperglycinemia but also other amino acid and organic acid disorders) and primarily structural in EIEE (primarily dysgenetic, i.e., migrational defects, micrencephaly or hemimegalencephaly, but also encephaloclastic, i.e., hypoxic-ischemic, disorders). Definition of an etiological mechanism is possible in most cases of EIEE, whereas as many as 50% of cases of EME are cryptogenic. Of the structural bases for EIEE, the rare lesion, dentato-olivary dysplasia, is the most difficult to identify in vivo.[336,342,348,349] Several reports have described infants with EIEE and CSF monamine findings mimicking aromatic acid decarboxylase deficiency (but without an apparent defect of this enzyme).[271,345,346] This disorder is important to detect because a beneficial response to administration of pyridoxal-5-phosphate (the cofactor of aromatic acid decarboxylase) has been shown. *Management* of seizures is difficult and usually involves multiple anticonvulsant drugs, including adrenocorticotropic hormone. One report describes an excellent response of seizures in an infant with EIEE with chloral hydrate.[343] The *outcome* for both EME and EIEE is poor, with death or serious neurological disability nearly the rule.

Malignant Migrating Partial Seizures of Infancy. Approximately 50 cases of a striking epileptic syndrome, often termed *malignant migrating partial seizures*

of infancy, have been reported.[347,350-356] Although the usual time of onset of the seizure disorder is at 1 to 3 months, onset in the first days of life has been reported, and approximately one half of cases have had onset in the first month of life. The seizures are focal clonic at the onset and over the ensuing weeks become multifocal, extremely frequent, and intractable to anticonvulsant drugs. A recent report describes a good therapeutic response to levetiracetam in a single case.[355] EEG findings show striking multifocal epileptic activity. Detailed metabolic studies have been negative, and MR imaging (MRI) has been normal. Neuropathological study has shown no abnormality in neocortex but pronounced hippocampal neuronal loss. The outcome has been poor, with death or moderate to severe mental retardation in most affected infants. However, a more recent report of six cases showed mild deficits in two infants.[354] More data are needed.

Benign Neonatal Sleep Myoclonus. A striking *nonepileptic* syndrome with clinical myoclonic seizures occurring only during sleep, termed *benign neonatal sleep myoclonus*, is well recognized (see Table 5-23).[204-206,357-360a] The onset is in the first week of life, and the clinical episodes include myoclonic jerks that are usually bilateral, synchronous, and repetitive and involve upper or lower extremities, or both. Focal onset may occur. The episodes usually last for several minutes or more and occur only during sleep, particularly quiet (non–rapid eye movement) sleep. They can be provoked by gentle rocking of the crib mattress in a head-to-toe direction and cease abruptly with arousal. The EEG pattern during the episodes does not show an ictal correlate, and interictal EEG findings are either normal or show minor, nonspecific abnormalities. The episodes can be exacerbated or provoked by treatment with benzodiazepines and resolve within approximately 2 months. Neurological outcome is normal.

Hyperekplexia. Also known as *startle disease*, *hyperekplexia* is a *nonepileptic* disorder characterized principally by two abnormal forms of response to unexpected auditory, visual, and somesthetic stimuli, namely, exaggerated startle response and sustained tonic spasm (see earlier discussion of generalized tonic seizures).[182-187,361-367] Additional features are generalized hypertonia and prominent nocturnal myoclonus. The hypertonia and exaggerated startle are apparent from the first hours of life, and sudden jerky movements even have been noted in utero. The typical clinical picture is a hyperalert infant who responds to sudden external stimulus, auditory, visual, or somesthetic (simple handling, nose tap, air blow over face) with recurrent startles, increasing rigidity, jittery movements that become rhythmic and mimic seizure, and occasionally apnea. The stiffness may interfere with bathing and diaper changes. Feeding difficulties and spasms can prevent adequate nutrition. Indeed, the tonic spasms may mimic generalized tonic seizures and can be dangerous, because they may lead to apnea and death. The EEG pattern does not show epileptic discharges. Forced truncal flexion has proven effective in terminating the episodes. Treatment with clonazepam leads to a decrease in the number of apneic episodes, the hypertonicity, and the startle responses. The episodes disappear spontaneously by approximately the age of 2 years. The disorder is inherited in an autosomal dominant fashion, and the responsible gene, on chromosome 5, encodes the alpha-1 subunit of the glycine receptor. Neurophysiological studies suggest that the primary physiological abnormality is related to increased excitability of reticular neurons in brain stem.[184] The alpha-1 subunit of the glycine receptor is critical for Cl^- influx and thereby inhibitory interneuron function in spinal cord and brain stem.[186,365,368-370]

Unknown Cause. A few cases of neonatal seizures are of unknown cause. The proportion of such cases varies inversely with the diligence of the diagnostic evaluation. In our experience, approximately 5% to 10% of cases cannot be assigned a definite or highly probable cause.

Diagnosis

Appropriate diagnostic procedures in the newborn with seizures can be surmised from the discussion of causes. However, the diagnostic evaluation is often made unnecessarily complicated, and many diagnoses can be established nearly conclusively by such uncomplicated maneuvers as obtaining a complete prenatal and natal *history* and completing a careful *physical examination*. The first *laboratory tests* to be performed are directed against the two diseases that are especially dangerous but readily treated when recognized promptly: hypoglycemia and bacterial meningitis. Thus, lumbar puncture and blood glucose determination are performed on an urgent basis. In addition, blood should be drawn for determinations of Na^+, K^+, calcium, phosphorus, and magnesium levels. Other metabolic determinations and radiological and other studies are indicated by the specific clinical features. For example, in the infant without a clearly recognized cause of seizures, the following apply: the presence of low CSF glucose but normal blood glucose should suggest glucose transporter defect (and appropriate therapy; see earlier discussion); the presence of elevated CSF glycine despite normal blood amino acids should suggest transient or true nonketotic hyperglycinemia (see earlier discussion); and the presence of elevated CSF lactate should suggest a mitochondrial disorder (see earlier discussion). In addition, focal seizures should lead to computed tomography or preferably, MRI scanning because of the frequency of focal ischemic cerebral lesions, many of which may not be detected by cranial ultrasound scanning.

Electroencephalogram

The EEG tracing is usually obtained in the interictal period in the evaluation of the infant with clinical seizures. Tracings *during* suspected seizures provide valuable information regarding the presence of true epileptic phenomena, but, as discussed earlier, strong evidence indicates that some epileptic discharges may not be detectable by surface EEG studies. More importantly, diagnostic and, particularly, therapeutic maneuvers should *not* be deferred for the purpose of obtaining an ictal tracing. We consider the major values of the initial EEG tracing in the evaluation of neonatal seizures to be (1) to help determine whether the infant with subtle clinical phenomena is experiencing electrographic seizures, (2) to determine whether the paralyzed infant is experiencing convulsive phenomena,[27-29,107,144,145,215,322,371] and (3) to define the interictal background features, which are of value in estimating *prognosis* (see "Prognosis"). Delineation of seizure phenomena by EEG findings requires awareness of the normal development of EEG features in the newborn (see Chapter 4), skilled technicians, and experienced readers of the EEG tracings. Numerous reviews of the EEG accompaniments of neonatal seizures are available.[17,19,23,27-29,372-380]

Electroclinical Dissociation. A major issue with implications for management is the relative frequency of *electroclinical dissociation* in newborns with seizures. This phenomenon of electrographic seizures not accompanied by clinical seizure phenomena is well documented (Table 5-25).[18,19,25,27-29,145,155,156,381-383] This dissociation is especially common in the most immature infants and in those treated with anticonvulsant drugs. The reasons for electroclinical dissociation are probably multiple, but data concerning the development of Cl^- transporters in perinatal human brain provide a rational explanation. Thus, as discussed earlier, a developmental mismatch occurs between the transporter responsible for Cl^- influx (NKCC1) and that responsible for Cl^- efflux (KCC2), such that in human perinatal brain, neuronal Cl^- levels are likely high, and GABA activation results in Cl^- efflux, depolarization, and thus excitation rather than inhibition. Therefore, with treatment with the usual anticonvulsant drugs, which are principally GABA agonists, electrographic seizures are not consistently diminished. However, because the maturation of the transporters occurs in a caudal-to-rostral direction,[52,384] neuronal Cl^- levels in motor systems in the brain stem and spinal cord would be expected to decrease to normal levels before cortical neuronal levels. The result would be that GABA activation induced by anticonvulsant drugs would eliminate the motor phenomena of the seizure but not the cortical electrographic component, thus resulting in electroclinical dissociation.

In part, because of the phenomenon of electroclinical dissociation, I recommend *continuous video EEG monitoring* of any infant with documented electrographic seizures or who is at very high risk for such seizures (e.g., asphyxiated infant who is paralyzed). Some clinicians have used less complex systems, such as the amplitude-integrated EEG approach. This latter method, discussed in detail in Chapter 4, is of some value in monitoring electrocortical background but is less effective in detection of neonatal seizures, especially the common focal and relatively brief events so common in newborns. However, an intermediate approach between the conventional 10/20 montage and the single-channel amplitude-integrated EEG approach, a reduced montage with only 9 electrodes, may have some promise. In a careful study, 90% of 187 neonatal seizures detected by the full 10/20 electrode montage were detected by the reduced montage.[385]

Major Electroencephalographic Correlates of Neonatal Seizures. Two general points concerning identification of electrical seizure activity in the newborn should be recognized. First, neonatal seizures tend to be brief, usually lasting less than 2 minutes (Fig. 5-11).[386] This point is not inconsistent with the finding that status epilepticus is by no means rare in critically ill infants. Second, neonatal electrical seizures tend to be focal and well localized, arising most commonly from temporal and central regions, less commonly from occipital regions, and least commonly from frontal regions. The characteristics of the interictal EEG pattern that suggest an epileptic basis for clinical seizures are summarized in Table 5-26.[387]

TABLE 5-25	Proportion of Electroencephalographic Seizures Unaccompanied by Clinical Seizures*			
Reference	No. of Infants with EEG Seizures or No. of EEG Seizures	Maturity	Percentage with Absent Clinical Seizure	Percentage Treated with Anticonvulsants
Mizrahi[156]	32 infants	85% >36 wk	34%	36%
Clancy et al[381]	393 seizures	Mean gestational age 40.1 wk	79%	88%
Scher et al[19]	33 infants	62% <36 wk	33%	72%
Connell et al[145]†	23 infants	<37 wk	52%	0%
	17 infants	>37 wk	12%	4%
Scher et al[25]	30 infants	≤30 wk	57%	84% (of total group of infants)
	22 infants	31–37 wk	27%	
	24 infants	>37 wk	33%	
Scher et al[382]	26 infants	25–43 wk	58%	100%

*Paralyzed patients excluded.
†Used two-channel electroencephalogram only.
EEG, electroencephalographic.

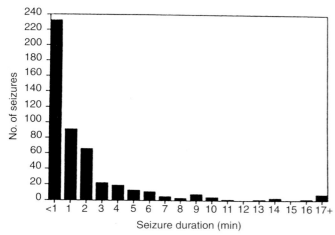

Figure 5-11 Seizure duration. Histogram depicting the distribution of seizure duration among 487 seizures recorded from 42 newborns with seizures. *(From Clancy RR, Legido A: The exact ictal and interictal duration of electroencephalographic neonatal seizures,* Epilepsia *28:537-541, 1987.)*

The major EEG correlates of neonatal seizures thus consist of *focal or multifocal spikes or sharp waves or both* and *focal monorhythmic discharges,* occurring as a distinct change from background. Focal spike discharges are repetitive, localized, and usually followed by some degree of suppression of background voltage activity. These discharges may spread to adjacent cortical regions or to homotypic areas of the contralateral hemisphere (Fig. 5-12). Such discharges are distinguished from normal sharp "transients," which are random rather than localized, are not rhythmic, do not spread, and are not followed by voltage suppression. Multifocal spikes have characteristics similar to those of focal spikes, except for their more widespread distribution (Fig. 5-13). These discharges tend to behave in an autonomous fashion and are more likely to occur on an abnormal background than are focal spike discharges. Monorhythmic discharges (Fig. 5-14), especially rhythmic alpha but also theta and delta discharges, are particularly characteristic of seizures in the newborn. Rhythmic alpha discharges have been observed frequently with subtle seizures with prominent respiratory abnormalities. Bilateral cerebral disease and an unfavorable outcome have been common with this so-called alpha seizure pattern.

TABLE 5-26	**Characteristics of Interictal Electroencephalogram Suggestive of Epileptic Mechanism for Clinical Seizures**

Moderately to markedly abnormal background

Excessive SETS or spikes, especially recurring in short runs or bursts

Nonrandom distribution of SETS in temporal and central regions

Data from Clancy RR: Interictal sharp EEG transients in neonatal seizures, *J Child Neurol* 4:30-38, 1989.
SETS, sharp electroencephalographic transients.

The ictal discharges previously described occur on a *background* of EEG activity, the nature of which is a particularly important determinant of outcome (see "Prognosis"). The background EEG findings consist essentially of either a normal tracing or a variety of abnormalities. The latter include mild to moderate abnormalities (e.g., voltage asymmetries and delayed maturation) and severe abnormalities (e.g., markedly discontinuous activity, severely decreased voltage, the burst-suppression pattern, or electrocerebral silence). The *burst-suppression pattern* (termed *tracé paroxystique* by Monod and Dreyfus-Brisac) [388] is particularly typical of the infant with severe bilateral cerebral disease and is characterized by relatively long periods of voltage suppression ($<5\ \mu V$) or by no electrical activity at all in the intervals between the bursts of activity. The bursts are usually synchronous with high-voltage spikes, sharp waves, and slow activity (Fig. 5-15) (see Chapter 4). This prominent tracing is distinguished from the *tracé alternant* of quiet sleep in the normal term infant (Fig. 5-16) by the occurrence in the latter tracing of at least some low-amplitude activity between bursts and shorter interburst intervals (6 to 10 seconds versus > 20 seconds in burst suppression), which exhibit more nearly regular periodicity (see Chapter 4). Moreover, the tracing in tracé alternant exhibits normal "reactivity" (i.e., the EEG pattern becomes continuous with stimulation, and behavioral states change normally), in contrast to the "nonreactive" fixed EEG pattern in typical burst suppression. As noted later and described in detail in Chapter 4, a discontinuous tracing with a prolonged interburst interval, not as severe as in typical burst suppression, is a more common finding than burst suppression and is similarly ominous.

Prognosis

Overall

The prognosis for infants with seizures in the neonatal period has improved over the past several decades. This is not surprising, because seizures are but a manifestation of neurological disease, and, in general, neonatal neurological diseases have been accompanied by improvements in outlook during this interval. These improvements relate in large part to improved obstetrical management and to modern neonatal intensive care. Thus, in more than 2000 cases of neonatal seizure, predominantly in full-term infants, gathered in a composite series from published reports and patients studied before and after 1969, mortality decreased from approximately 40% to 15% (personal unpublished data).* The incidence of neurological sequelae (mental retardation, motor deficits, and seizures) in survivors changed much less, if at all, and has been approximately 25% to 35%. Mental retardation and

---

*See references 25,28,140,141,143,147,158,171,208,210,211,213-217,219,220,222,227,298,389-397a.

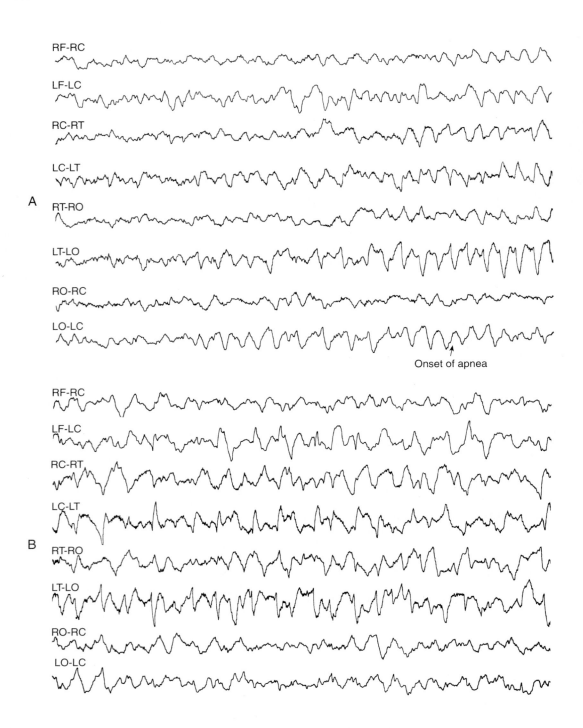

Figure 5-12 Electroencephalogram in neonatal seizures, focal sharp waves. The infant exhibited apnea and tonic deviation of the eyes to the right as the manifestations of seizure. **A**, Onset of apnea is indicated by the *arrow* at the bottom of the tracing. Focal sharp wave discharges originated in the left hemisphere (especially temporal) several seconds before the onset of apnea. **B**, Sharp wave discharges have become generalized. *(Courtesy of Dr. Arthur Prensky.)*

motor deficits are more common sequelae than are seizures, which develop in approximately 15% to 20% of surviving infants with neonatal seizures. However, since the late 1980s, with the increasing survival rates for small premature infants, it has become clear that the overall outcome of infants with seizures varies considerably as a function of gestational age (Table 5-27). Clearly, the outcome is poorest among the smallest infants, who have the most serious, life-threatening illnesses. Indeed, in one population-based study of premature infants who weighed less than 1500 g at birth, of 368 infants with clinical seizures, nearly 40% had

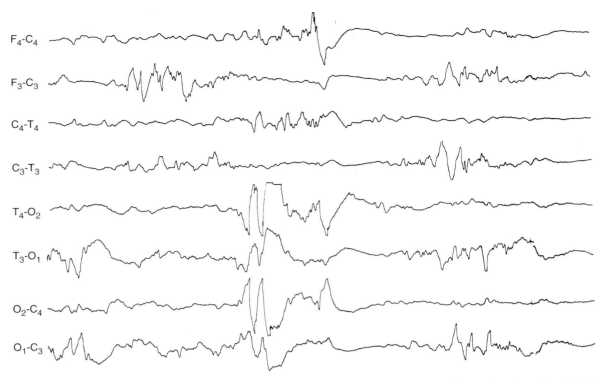

Figure 5-13 Electroencephalogram in neonatal seizures, multifocal sharp waves and spikes. The infant exhibited multifocal clonic seizures. Note the striking multifocal sharp waves and spikes in the central, temporal, and occipital regions. *(Courtesy of Dr. Lawrence Coben.)*

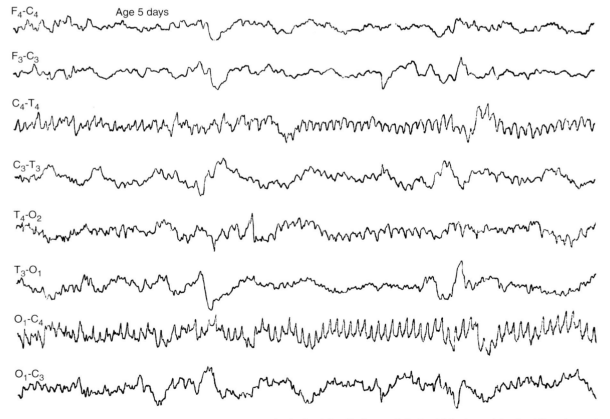

Figure 5-14 Electroencephalogram in neonatal seizures, monorhythmic alpha discharge. Infant exhibited a variety of subtle seizure phenomena. Note the striking, rhythmic, alpha-like pattern in the right central leads. *(Courtesy of Dr. Arthur Prensky.)*

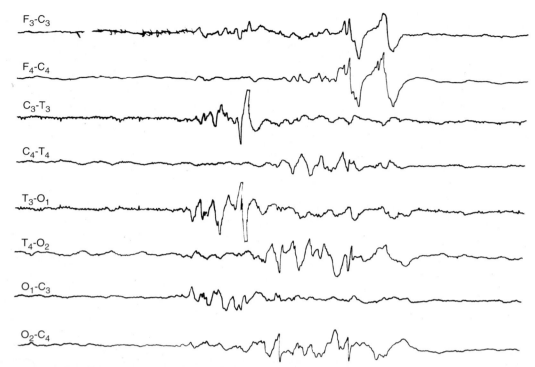

Figure 5-15   **Electroencephalogram in neonatal seizures, burst-suppression pattern.** Background electroencephalogram in a severely asphyxiated infant with neonatal seizures. Note the interruption of the run of very-low-voltage activity by a burst of higher-voltage slow waves and sharp activity. *(Courtesy of Dr. Arthur Prensky.)*

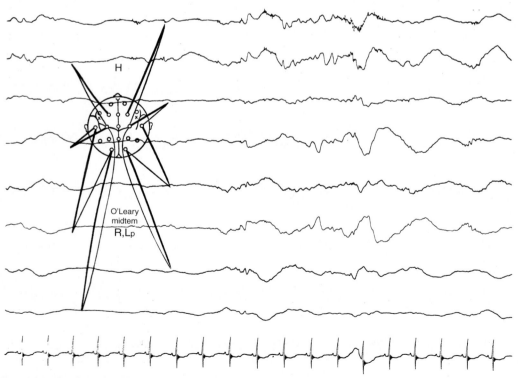

Figure 5-16   **Electroencephalogram of a normal term infant during sleep, tracé alternant.** Note the interruption of the run of relatively low-voltage activity by a burst of higher-voltage slow waves. No spikes are present. Contrast with Fig. 5-15. *(Courtesy of Dr. Arthur Prensky.)*

TABLE 5-27	Prognosis of Neonatal Seizures: Relation to Maturity			
		OUTCOME*		
Maturity		**Normal**	**Dead**	**Sequelae**
Term (>2500 g)[†]		60%	10%	30%
Premature (<2500 g)[†]		35%	35%	30%
Premature (<1500 g)[‡]		20%	40%	40%

*Numbers are rounded off to nearest 5%.
[†]Data from personal experience (approximately 200 term and 100 premature [<2500-g] infants) and from references 25, 147, 208, 216, 217, 219, and 397a.
[‡]Data from references 210, 395, and 217.

severe intraventricular hemorrhage, and approximately 20% had cystic periventricular leukomalacia.[218] *These overall figures, however, do not answer the question that is most critical to the physician responsible for the care of the convulsing newborn:* "How can I predict the outcome in my patient?" The two most useful approaches for estimating outcome are the EEG pattern and recognition of the underlying neurological disease.

Relation to the Electroencephalogram

The interictal EEG pattern is of value in establishing prognosis of infants with seizures.* This conclusion must be made with the qualification that evaluations of neonatal EEG findings are sometimes difficult and may vary significantly among different interpreters. Nevertheless, in several careful studies, the *background* EEG pattern was found to correlate especially well with outcome in both full-term and premature infants with seizures (Table 5-28). Thus, when the EEG correlates of seizures (as described previously) occur on a *background that is normal*, neurological sequelae are unusual. *Severe background abnormalities*, such as a burst-suppression pattern, a prolonged (>20-second) interburst interval, marked voltage suppression, and electrocerebral silence, are associated with neurological sequelae in 90% or more of cases. *Moderate background abnormalities*, which generally account for approximately 15% to 30% of the tracings,[402] are associated with an intermediate likelihood of sequelae.

Despite the frequently documented relationship between the burst-suppression background pattern or the more common excessively discontinuous tracing with a prolonged (>20-second) interburst interval (see Chapter 4) and poor neurological outcome,[†] some caution must be used in attributing a grave prognosis to abnormal paroxysmal patterns with long silent periods in young infants (see Chapter 4). This caveat applies especially to premature infants less than 33 to 34 weeks of conceptional age, in part because of the normal periodicity and relatively lower interburst voltage in the EEG pattern of the premature infant (see Chapter 4).

TABLE 5-28	Prognosis of Neonatal Seizures: Relation to Electroencephalogram*
EEG Background	**Neurological Sequelae**
Normal	≤10%
Severe abnormalities[†]	≥90%
Moderate abnormalities[‡]	~50%

*Based primarily on data reported in references 401, 402, and 404 *and* includes both full-term and premature infants.
[†]Burst-suppression pattern, prolonged (>20-second) interburst interval, marked voltage suppression, and electrocerebral silence.
[‡]Voltage asymmetries and "immaturity."
EEG, electroencephalographic.

Systematic studies of serial EEG examinations are needed to determine whether the *rate of improvement of the EEG pattern* may be a useful indicator of subsequent outcome. Some initial information supporting this suggestion is available, at least regarding hypoxic-ischemic encephalopathy (see Chapter 9).

Certain *electrographic seizures* correlate directly with an unfavorable prognosis.[143,145,146,211,214] Similarly, detection of electrographic status epilepticus (duration > 30 minutes) was followed by death or severe neurological deficits in 90% of infants in one careful study.[211]

Relation to the Neurological Disease

It is nearly self-evident that the most important determinant of neurological prognosis is the nature of the neuropathological process that underlies the seizures. The relationship of prognosis with the underlying disease producing the seizures, based on my experience and that recorded by others, is summarized in Table 5-29.*

---

*See references 28,141,143,146,158,171,181,208-211,213,214,217, 219,220,227,391,393-396,397a,408.

TABLE 5-29	Prognosis of Neonatal Seizures: Relation to Neurological Disease
Neurological Disease*	**Normal Development[†]**
Hypoxic-ischemic encephalopathy	50%
Intraventricular hemorrhage[‡]	10%
Primary subarachnoid hemorrhage	90%
Hypocalcemia	
Early-onset	50%[§]
Later-onset	100%[#]
Hypoglycemia	50%
Bacterial meningitis	50%
Developmental defect	0%

*Prognosis is for those cases with the stated neurological disease *when seizures are a manifestation* (thus, value usually differs from *overall* prognosis for the disease).
[†]Values are rounded off to nearest 5%.
[‡]Usually, severe intraventricular hemorrhage is associated with major periventricular hemorrhagic infarction.
[§]Represents primarily the prognosis of complicating illness; prognosis approaches that of later-onset hypocalcemia of the nutritional type if no or only minor neurological illness is present.
[#]Later-onset hypocalcemia of the nutritional type.

---

*See references 27,28,141,143,146,158,208,209,211,214,215,219, 220,396,397a,398-404.

[†]See references 27,28,141,158,211,214,219,220,339,401,402,404-407.

Unfortunately, nearly all the data are based on periods of follow-up that do not extend to school age; thus, the incidence of subtle but potentially important intellectual deficits is largely unknown. Additionally, in many studies, premature and term infants are considered together. Moreover, the outlook for several of the disorders continues to improve. Infants with hypoxic-ischemic encephalopathy, when accompanied by seizures, currently have an approximately 50% chance for normal development. Primary subarachnoid hemorrhage with seizures is clearly associated with a favorable outlook, whereas intraventricular hemorrhage severe enough to result in seizures is associated with a significantly poorer outlook, primarily because most cases are complicated by periventricular hemorrhagic infarction (see Chapter 11). Nearly all infants with later-onset hypocalcemia (nutritional type) with seizures, *appropriately recognized and treated*, are normal on follow-up, whereas those infants with hypocalcemia of early onset have only approximately a 50% chance for normal development, a finding reflecting the associated complicating illnesses. Infants with early hypocalcemia and no or only minor complicating illness have a prognosis nearly as favorable as that of infants with later-onset cases. Hypoglycemia that continues long enough to result in seizures is associated with approximately a 50% chance for normal development. Those infants with bacterial meningitis and seizures have approximately a 50% chance for a favorable outcome. Infants with developmental anomalies serious enough to cause neonatal seizures have essentially no chance for normal development.

These data indicate that the major task of the physician is to determine as precisely as possible the neurological disease producing the seizures. The purpose of this task is not only to institute appropriate therapy but also to ensure as meaningful a prognostic statement as possible.

Management

Before discussing the usual sequence of therapy in the infant with seizures, I briefly review the selection of the infant to treat and the criteria to determine adequacy of therapy.

Selection of Whom To Treat

Selection of the infant to treat with anticonvulsant or related medication depends, of course, on identification of the infant with epileptic seizures. Particular attention must be paid to the clinical means of distinguishing epileptic seizures from nonepileptic phenomena (see earlier discussion and Table 5-17). However, the particular value of prolonged EEG monitoring with simultaneous observation by video recording or direct inspection was discussed earlier. Indeed, in view of the recent demonstrations of the high frequency of clinically silent electrographic seizures in the newborn (see earlier), I now believe that *prolonged EEG monitoring is extremely important in the evaluation and management of the newborn with documented or suspected seizures*. With advances in the development of digitally based EEG techniques and the wide availability and approachable cost of modern instruments, the goal of continual EEG monitoring seems generally achievable. The possibility of using primarily amplitude-integrated EEG for continuous monitoring, currently in wide use in many centers outside the United States, is worthy of serious consideration. However, detection of all electrographic seizure activity with this and related techniques is somewhat problematic with this approach (see earlier). Moreover, even with EEG examination, recall that the lack of consistent electrical correlates from surface-recorded EEG findings does not rule out an epileptic process.

Why should the infant with epileptic seizures be treated with anticonvulsant medication at all? The answer relates to the potential adverse effects of seizure on ventilatory function, circulation, cerebral metabolism, and subsequent brain development (see earlier). The potential mechanisms of brain injury with repeated seizures include disturbances in CBF, energy metabolism, homeostasis of excitotoxic amino acids, neurogenesis, and subsequent synaptic reorganization and were reviewed earlier. Although not unequivocally established in the human infant, the balance of information indicates that repeated epileptic seizures should be stopped because of the threats of brain injury and impaired subsequent development from the electrical seizures themselves.

Adequacy of Treatment

More controversial than the issue of whom to treat with anticonvulsant medication is the identification of criteria for determination of adequacy of therapy. It now seems clear that elimination or near elimination of all electrical seizure activity should be the goal of therapy. Reliance on elimination of *clinical* seizures no longer can be viewed as the appropriate goal. This conclusion, of course, relates to the finding that elimination of clinical seizure manifestations does not guarantee elimination of electrophysiological seizure manifestations (see earlier discussion). Administration of anticonvulsant drugs often leads to cessation of clinical seizures despite persistence of EEG evidence of seizures. In the careful study of Clancy and co-workers,[381] approximately 80% of 393 electrical seizures recorded were not accompanied by clinical seizure activity monitored by simultaneous, direct observation; 88% of the total population of patients had been treated with one or more anticonvulsant medications. Moreover, the problem of clinically silent electrical seizures also is important in the pharmacologically paralyzed infant.

Conclusive data concerning potentially harmful effects of seizures, abundant in experimental studies (see earlier), are relatively few in *human infants*. Several earlier reports, published primarily in the 1980s, showed a poorer outcome in asphyxiated infants who exhibited seizures than in those who did not (see earlier discussion). The independent effect of seizures, in addition to the severity of the pathological features, was not clear from the earlier work. However, two more recent reports, characterized by quantitation of electrographic seizures and multivariate analyses, suggest that seizures may accentuate brain injury, especially in asphyxiated infants (see earlier).[146,147]

Although the goal of therapy should be total or near-total elimination of electrographic seizures, in some infants, the doses of anticonvulsant medications required lead to dangerous disturbances of cardiac function. Some critically ill infants with multiorgan dysfunction may be even more susceptible to the dangerous side effects of high-dose therapy. Thus, in this setting careful systemic monitoring, frequent assessment of electrographic status, and reconsideration of therapeutic plan as necessary are crucial.

Usual Sequence of Therapy

The infant exhibiting repeated seizure activity should be treated promptly. My usual sequence of therapy for the infant who is actively convulsing is reviewed in the following discussion and in Table 5-30; maintenance therapy is outlined later in Table 5-33.

Before reviewing the individual aspects of the sequence of therapy, it is important to emphasize that before instituting any therapy with drugs or metabolites, the physician should be sure that *ventilation* and *perfusion* are adequate. Disturbances of ventilation and often of perfusion may complicate repeated neonatal seizures, and these life-threatening disturbances must be dealt with first. Moreover, because the administration of certain anticonvulsant drugs may impair ventilation, the necessary equipment for support of ventilation should be immediately available, with the expectation that the need for intubation is highly likely.

Glucose

An intravenous line is established, and a blood glucose (Dextrostix) determination is performed on the first drops of blood. If hypoglycemia is present and if the infant is convulsing, 10% dextrose is given intravenously in a dose of 2 mL/kg (0.2 g/kg), and the baby is maintained on intravenous dextrose at a rate as high as 0.5 g/kg/hour (8 mg/kg/minute) if necessary. (This is approximately the maximum usable dose of glucose in the newborn.) Although constant infusion of glucose at 8 mg/kg/minute corrects hypoglycemia in less than 10 minutes in most patients[409] and is appropriate if the infant is not convulsing, the faster approach of bolus infusion is indicated for the convulsing infant. The initial bolus dose can be repeated if the infant continues to convulse. The possibility of maintaining supranormal levels of blood glucose in newborns with frequent seizures should be considered, in view of the experimental demonstrations of a decline in brain glucose concentration with seizures and the protective effect of pretreatment with glucose (see Figs. 5-3 and 5-9). The potential hazards of this approach, especially in the premature infant, however, must be recognized (see Chapter 12). This remains an important topic for future clinical research.

Anticonvulsant Drugs

Phenobarbital. If hypoglycemia is not present, I administer phenobarbital intravenously in a loading dose of 20 mg/kg, delivered over approximately 10 to 15 minutes. Careful surveillance of respiratory effort is important under these circumstances. The work of Painter and co-workers[142] clearly showed that this dose is necessary to achieve a blood level of approximately 20 µg/mL (Fig. 5-17). This level is necessary to achieve a clearly measurable anticonvulsant effect in the newborn.[24,142,410-414] Weight or gestational age does not appear to influence the dose-blood level relationship appreciably,[142,410,415] although infants less than 30 weeks of gestation may require slightly lower doses to achieve the same blood level.[416] To achieve the same blood level, the intramuscular dose must be approximately 10% to 15% greater than the

TABLE 5-30 **Acute Therapy of Neonatal Seizures**
Hypoglycemia
Glucose, 10% solution: 2 mL/kg, IV
No Hypoglycemia
Phenobarbital: 20 mg/kg, IV (1–2 mg/kg/min)
If necessary:
Additional phenobarbital: 5 mg/kg IV to a maximum of 20 mg/kg (consider omission of this additional phenobarbital if infant is severely "asphyxiated")
Phenytoin*: 20 mg/kg, IV (0.5–1.0 mg/kg/min)
Lorazepam: 0.05–0.10 mg/kg, IV
Midazolam: 0.2 mg/kg, IV; then, 0.1–0.4 mg/kg/hr, IV
Other (as Indicated)
Calcium gluconate, 5% solution: 4 mL/kg, IV
Magnesium sulfate, 50% solution: 0.2 mL/kg, IM
Pyridoxine: 50–100 mg, IV; repeat to maximum of 500 mg if needed
Pyridoxal-5-phosphate, 30 mg/kg/day, PO
Folinic acid, 4 mg/kg/day, PO

*Fosphenytoin is the preferred form of phenytoin (see text); dose shown is in phenytoin equivalents.
IM, intramuscularly; IV, intravenously; PO, by mouth.

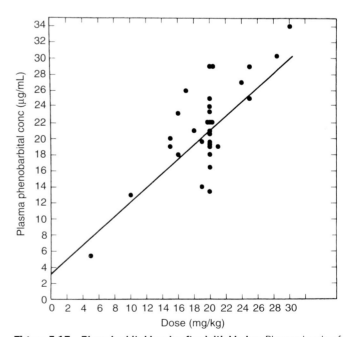

Figure 5-17   **Phenobarbital levels after initial bolus.** Plasma levels of phenobarbital achieved following the initial intravenous dose in human newborns with seizures. *(From Painter MJ, Pippenger C, MacDonald H, Pitlick W: Phenobarbital and diphenylhydantoin levels in neonates with seizures, J Pediatr 92:315-319, 1978.)*

TABLE 5-31 Expected Response of Neonatal *Clinical* Seizures to Sequence of Therapy

Anticonvulsant Drug* (Cumulative Dose)	Cessation of Seizures (Cumulative Percentage)
Phenobarbital, 20 mg/kg	40%
Phenobarbital, 40 mg/kg	70%
Phenytoin, 20 mg/kg	85%
Lorazepam, 0.05–0.10 mg/kg	95%–100%

*All drugs administered intravenously.
Based largely on data of Gilman JT, Gal P, Duchowny MS, Weaver RL, et al: Rapid sequential phenobarbital treatment of neonatal seizures, *Pediatrics* 83:674-678, 1989, and on personal experience.

intravenous dose.[410] I strongly prefer the intravenous route because of the faster onset of action and the more reproducible effect on the blood level of phenobarbital.

If the initial 20 mg/kg dose of phenobarbital is not effective in controlling the seizures, I administer additional doses of 5 mg/kg until seizures have ceased or a total dose of 40 mg/kg has been reached (see Table 5-30). The goal is to achieve a phenobarbital concentration of 40 to 50µg/mL. Using phenobarbital in approximately this manner, Gilman and co-workers[413] and Gal and co-workers[417] attained control of *clinical* seizures in approximately 70% of 71 infants (Table 5-31). Approximately similar doses were used in a later controlled study of 59 infants, and the drug completely controlled the *electrographic* seizures in only 43% (Table 5-32).[418] These data illustrate the difficulty of using only clinical seizures as a measure of anticonvulsant response and the failure of phenobarbital monotherapy in approximately half of all cases of neonatal seizures. This difficulty presumably relates to the likelihood that many cortical neurons contain GABA-excitatory receptors, as described earlier.

In my experience, total loading doses of phenobarbital in excess of 40 mg/kg generally do not provide additional anticonvulsant benefit. Moreover, I have

TABLE 5-32 Response of Neonatal *Electrographic* Seizures to Phenobarbital and Phenytoin*

	EXTENT OF CONTROL	
	Complete	≥80% Reduction*
Phenobarbital[†]	43%	
plus phenytoin	57%	80%
Phenytoin[†]	45%	
plus phenobarbital	62%	72%

*Value includes infants with complete control of seizures and those with 80% or greater reduction (albeit not complete reduction) in seizures.
[†]Blood levels of *free* phenobarbital were 25 µg/mL, and blood levels of *free* phenytoin were 3 µg/mL.
Data from Painter MJ, Scher MS, Stein AD, Armatti S, et al: Phenobarbital compared with phenytoin for the treatment of neonatal seizures, *N Engl J Med* 341:485-489, 1999; the study involved 59 term infants with electrographic seizures, and randomly assigned to receive phenobarbital (n = 30) or phenytoin (n = 29), followed by the two drugs in combination if complete control of electrographic seizures was not attained.

been impressed in severely asphyxiated infants, often with evidence for accompanying hepatic or renal dysfunction, or both, that a total loading dose of phenobarbital of 40 mg/kg may result in blood levels of approximately 50 µg/mL or more. These levels appreciably sedate the infant for several days, thereby impairing neurological analysis, and may lead to toxic effects on the cardiovascular system. Thus, such infants should be monitored carefully, and *consideration should be given to proceeding to phenytoin before a full loading dose of phenobarbital is administered.*

Certain pharmacological properties of phenobarbital are beneficial in the treatment of neonatal seizures. Thus, the drug enters CSF (and presumably brain) rapidly and with high efficiency (e.g., in one series, 30 minutes after an intravenous loading dose was administered, the CSF to blood ratio was 0.58 ± 0.07); the blood level is largely predictable from the dose administered; the agent can be administered intramuscularly as well as intravenously (preferably the latter) for acute therapy; and maintenance therapy is accomplished easily with oral therapy (see later discussion).[411,416] Moreover, experimental data suggest that entrance of phenobarbital into brain is accelerated by the local acidosis associated with seizure.[102] Protein binding is lower in the newborn (33%) than in the older child and adult (41%), and thus free levels of the drug are relatively higher. Because binding may be decreased further by hyperbilirubinemia and apparently other factors, still to be defined,[411] routine monitoring of free phenobarbital levels is optimal for management of the infant with seizures.

Phenytoin-Fosphenytoin. In the infant who continues to exhibit electrographic or clinical seizures after as much as 40 mg/kg of phenobarbital, or in the severely asphyxiated infant in whom less than the full loading dose is deemed appropriate, phenytoin is administered intravenously in a loading dose of 20 mg/kg. When this approach is used in infants who continue to exhibit electrographic seizures after 40 mg/kg of phenobarbital, approximately 15% more respond with cessation (i.e., to a total of nearly 60%; see Table 5-32). The cumulative response to the combined therapy is similar if phenytoin is administered before phenobarbital (see Table 5-32).[418] If *clinical* seizure is the response endpoint, nearly 85% of infants respond (see Table 5-31). However, as noted earlier, clinical seizure is not a suitable parameter for measuring seizure response. If 80% or more reduction of *electrographic* seizure is considered a favorable response, *the combination of phenobarbital and phenytoin achieves this level of benefit in fully 80% of infants* (see Table 5-32).[418] The dose of phenytoin should be administered at a rate of no more than 1 mg/kg/minute to avoid disturbance of cardiac function, particularly cardiac rhythm. Cardiac rate and rhythm should be monitored during the infusion. The drug should be administered directly into the intravenous line, because it is relatively insoluble in aqueous solutions and precipitates in standard dextrose intravenous solutions. The pH of the parenteral solution is 12 and is irritating to the vein and surrounding tissue; thus, the dose should be

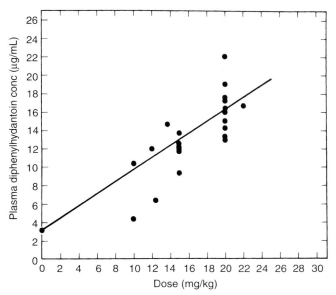

Figure 5-18 Phenytoin levels after initial bolus. Plasma levels of phenytoin achieved following the initial intravenous dose in human newborns with seizures. *(From Painter MJ, Pippenger C, MacDonald H, Pitlick W: Phenobarbital and diphenylhydantoin levels in neonates with seizures,* J Pediatr *92:315-319, 1978.)*

followed by a few milliliters of normal saline solution. These characteristics may lead to serious soft tissue injury and clearly make fosphenytoin the preferred form for use in the newborn (see next). The 20 mg/kg loading dose of phenytoin results in a therapeutic blood level of approximately 15 to 20 µg/kg (Fig. 5-18).

Fosphenytoin, a phosphate ester prodrug of phenytoin, has proved to be a major advance in therapy of status epilepticus in newborns, children, and adults.[419-424] The drug's advantages include high water solubility and a pH value closer to neutral, ease of preparation in standard intravenous solutions, safe intramuscular administration, absence of tissue injury with intravenous infiltration, and a faster allowable rate of intravenous administration. The drug is converted to phenytoin, primarily by plasma phosphatases, in approximately 8 minutes. The effective dose, in phenytoin equivalents (i.e., 1.5 mg of fosphenytoin yields approximately 1.0 mg of phenytoin), is essentially identical to that just described for phenytoin. The rate of conversion of fosphenytoin to phenytoin appears similar in newborns, infants, and older children.[421,423,424] Fosphenytoin is clearly the preferred form of phenytoin for use in the newborn.

Lorazepam. Approximately 20% or more of newborns with electrographic seizures do not respond to the sequential administration of phenobarbital and phenytoin (see Table 5-32). In this situation, I have used lorazepam. Some clinicians prefer to use lorazepam *before* fosphenytoin.

Lorazepam is a benzodiazepine anticonvulsant of proven efficacy in older infants and children.[425-427] The drug is usually compared to the other major benzodiazepine used as an anticonvulsant, diazepam (see next section). Lorazepam, like diazepam, enters brain

rapidly and produces a pronounced anticonvulsant effect in less than 5 minutes. Of importance, however, is that lorazepam is less lipophilic than diazepam and thus does not redistribute from brain as rapidly. The duration of action is generally 6 to 24 hours. Moreover, lorazepam appears less likely to produce respiratory depression or hypotension. This agent has been investigated in the newborn in three separate studies.[428-430] The drug has been very effective in treatment of neonatal *clinical* seizures, whether as a second drug, after phenobarbital, or as a third drug, after phenobarbital and phenytoin. The onset of effect has been in 2 to 3 minutes, and the duration has extended to 24 hours. The effective dose is 0.05 to 0.10 mg/kg, administered intravenously in 0.05 mg/kg increments over several minutes. The half-life of lorazepam, studied in asphyxiated newborns only, is approximately 40 hours (i.e., two- to threefold higher values than in the adult).[430] This prolonged half-life could relate to decreased hepatic glucuronidation activity, a normal neonatal finding perhaps accentuated by asphyxial injury to liver.

Although *diazepam*, like lorazepam, is an effective anticonvulsant in the newborn, I do not use this agent for several reasons. First, diazepam is a poor drug for maintenance because of extremely rapid clearance from brain (minutes after intravenous administration),[431,432] and barbiturate usually must be used. Second, when used with barbiturate, diazepam carries an increased risk of severe circulatory collapse with respiratory failure.[433] Third, the therapeutic dose is extremely variable and is not necessarily less than the toxic dose (doses of 0.30 and 0.36 mg/kg have led to respiratory arrest).[434,435] Fourth, the vehicle for intravenous diazepam, in many preparations, contains sodium benzoate, which is a very effective uncoupler of the bilirubin-albumin complex[436] and theoretically could increase the risk of kernicterus. Results of studies in Gunn rats suggested that the amount of benzoate in the usual diazepam preparation is not high enough to be a serious risk, but the work did not include intravenous administration or measurement of levels of bilirubin in brain.[437] Fifth, although lorazepam shares the previous potential problem, this benzodiazepine appears to be at least as effective, has a longer duration of action, and exhibits less risk of serious side effects (see previous section).

Diazepam has been most effective as a continuous intravenous infusion. Thus, one report described the complete control of seizures in eight term newborns with severe perinatal asphyxia by continuous intravenous infusion of diazepam.[438] Doses of approximately 0.3 mg/kg/hour were required. No patient was said to require assisted ventilation, although stupor and need for gavage feeding were present consistently.

Midazolam. Midazolam, like lorazepam, is a short-acting benzodiazepine in common use in the treatment of status epilepticus in older infants and children. This drug has the advantage of less respiratory depression and sedation than lorazepam (or diazepam).[439] Reports in the past decade suggest that this agent may be useful in refractory neonatal seizures.[440,441,441a] In a recent study of 13 infants with electrographic seizures nonresponsive to phenobarbital with or without phenytoin, 8 responded to midazolam administered as a 0.15 mg/kg bolus followed by infusion of 0.4 mg/kg/hour.[441] The remaining 5 nonresponders responded after an additional bolus and somewhat higher infusion rates (maximum of 1.1 mg/kg/hour). Control of seizures generally was rapid (<2 hours), especially when treatment was begun promptly after failure of phenobarbital. In recent years, I have used midazolam in a bolus dose of 0.2 mg/kg, followed by infusion of 0.1 to 0.4 mg/kg/hour, and I have tended to use this agent promptly in those infants whom I consider likely to require continuous infusion of anticonvulsant to control electrographic seizures. Such infants include those with serious hypoxic-ischemic or dysgenetic cerebral disease, with status epilepticus at the onset, and with a severely disordered background EEG pattern.

Lidocaine. Several reports from Europe indicate value for lidocaine as an adjunctive agent in the treatment of neonatal seizures.[411,442-445] Data on approximately 100 infants treated primarily because of failure of phenobarbital and diazepam indicated cessation of seizures, usually within 10 minutes of the start of intravenous infusion, in approximately 75%. Dosage schedules varied, but most commonly a starting infusion of approximately 2 to 6 mg/kg/hour, with or without a bolus infusion at the onset, was used. In the most recent series, a bolus dose of 4 mg/kg was followed by an infusion rate of 2 mg/kg/hour.[445] The drug was tapered over several days. Doses required in premature infants are somewhat lower than in term infants. Accumulation of lidocaine can be a problem, and diminishing infusion rates are recommended. Of the side effects observed in older patients infused with lidocaine (e.g., arrhythmias, seizures, and hypotension), only recrudescence of seizures on decrease of dosage has been observed (and observed only rarely). More data are needed on this promising therapy.

Other Anticonvulsant Drugs. The potential value of *primidone* as an anticonvulsant drug in the neonatal period is suggested by several reports.[411,439,446,447] In the initial study, primidone was administered orally to 24 infants with neonatal seizures in whom the seizures had recurred despite high levels of phenobarbital (15 to 40 μg/mL) and phenytoin (10 to 20 μg/mL). Seizure control was achieved within 48 hours in 50% of patients, but 34% of infants required up to 9 days for seizure control. The minimum primidone level at which a response occurred was approximately 6 μg/mL. However, marked interpatient variability was noted in blood levels of primidone, and phenobarbital clearance was prolonged after addition of primidone. In a second report, 10 infants were treated with oral primidone after discontinuation of previously ineffective anticonvulsant drugs (primarily phenobarbital or phenytoin, or both). Eight patients achieved seizure control within 1 to 5 days of onset of therapy. Blood levels varied between 5 and 16 μg/mL. Because this agent can be administered only orally, it is unlikely to be very useful in acute therapy.

Thiopental was reported to be highly effective in the treatment of seizures in nine asphyxiated term newborns who continued to convulse despite mean phenobarbital levels of 28 μg/mL.[448] The dose was 10 mg/kg, administered intravenously over 2 minutes, and response occurred "promptly." However, a 27% decrease (mean) of arterial blood pressure occurred in six of the nine infants, and each child was treated with pressor agents or volume expansion. The adjunctive value of this mode of therapy remains to be established conclusively.

Paraldehyde, administered as an intravenous bolus and then a continuous infusion, was effective as adjunctive therapy in approximately 50% of the infants studied.[411,439,449,450] However, the intravenous form of this drug is no longer available in the United States. Moreover, the potential side effects of respiratory disturbance, secondary to pulmonary excretion of paraldehyde, and of hypotension make this drug not highly desirable in the newborn.

Valproic acid, administered orally as adjunctive therapy, led to control of neonatal seizures recalcitrant to phenobarbital (mean blood level > 40 μg/mL) in five of six cases.[451] However, elevation of blood ammonia required cessation of therapy in three infants. Because of the uncertain risk of valproate hepatotoxicity in this age group, the value of this drug in the treatment of neonatal seizures is uncertain.

Carbamazepine was reported to be effective as an initial agent in the treatment of neonatal seizures in a study of 10 full-term infants with hypoxic-ischemic encephalopathy.[452] All patients showed an "excellent" clinical response. Therapeutic levels were achieved within 2 to 4 hours after a loading dose of 10 mg/kg administered by nasogastric tube. However, variability in blood levels suggests that more data are needed to determine the value of this agent.

Toward More Rational Therapy: Promising Future Drugs. As discussed earlier, anticonvulsant drugs with GABA agonist properties (e.g., phenobarbital, benzodiazepines) may not be ideal agents because $GABA_A$ receptors are likely to be excitatory rather than inhibitory in most cerebral cortical neurons. Moreover, as noted later, studies in developing rats suggested that even with short-term exposure, these drugs can be neurotoxic. More rational approaches would be directed either at inhibition of excitation at excitatory amino acid receptors or, perhaps, conversion of $GABA_A$ receptors from excitatory to inhibitory. Two drugs are promising in these regards. *Topiramate* is a blocker of the AMPA type of glutamate receptor and was shown in the neonatal rat to have potent anticonvulsant effects versus hypoxia-induced seizures, to have protective properties versus neuronal or premyelinating oligodendrocyte injury, and *not* to exhibit neurotoxicity to developing neurons.[48,51,139,453-456] Unfortunately, an intravenous preparation of topiramate is not yet available.

Bumetanide is a second agent of potential value as rational anticonvulsant therapy. Thus, this drug inhibits NKCC1, the Cl⁻ cotransporter responsible for the elevated neuronal Cl⁻ levels and the depolarizing (excitation) rather than hyperpolarizing (inhibitory) response on $GABA_A$ receptor activation (see earlier). Blockade of NKCC1 decreases neuronal Cl⁻ levels and restores the inhibitory response of $GABA_A$ receptor activation.[52] Bumetanide suppresses epileptiform activity in neonatal rat hippocampal slices in vitro and in neonatal rat brain in vivo.[52] This drug has been used as a diuretic in the newborn, and an intravenous preparation is available.[457,458] A reasonable speculation is that bumetanide used concurrently with phenobarbital (or benzodiazepines) could be particularly effective, because the former would allow the $GABA_A$ receptor activation produced by phenobarbital to lead to inhibition. Perhaps the 35% to 40% of neonatal seizures that are not totally eliminated by phenobarbital (see earlier) would be eliminated when the drug is combined with bumetanide.

Maintenance Therapy

For *maintenance* of anticonvulsant action, I use phenobarbital in a dose of 3 to 4 mg/kg/day (Table 5-33). If phenytoin is also needed for the acute episode, this drug (fosphenytoin) is also used for maintenance, initially in a similar dose (see Table 5-33). The maintenance doses are begun 12 hours following administration of the loading dose and are given in divided doses every 12 hours. Intravenous, intramuscular, or oral administration is adequate for phenobarbital, although the parenteral routes should be used in the seriously ill infant. Although intravenous administration is preferred, fosphenytoin can be administered intramuscularly effectively. Oral administration of phenytoin is less desirable than intravenous, although pharmacokinetic data have corrected the prior notion that phenytoin absorption is poor in the newborn.[459-462]

Drug accumulation results within 5 to 10 days when maintenance doses of *phenobarbital* of 5 mg/kg/day are used (Fig. 5-19).[142,411] This effect may depress the infant significantly and relates to relatively slow elimination rates in the first 1 to 2 weeks of therapy (Fig. 5-20). These rates are particularly slow in some asphyxiated infants, presumably secondary to hepatic involvement, renal involvement, or both, and lead more readily to drug accumulation than in nonasphyxiated infants.[417,463] However, elimination rates do increase with increasing duration of therapy, and dose requirements may increase.

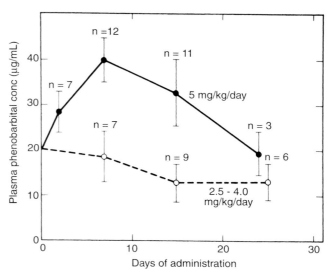

Figure 5-19 **Phenobarbital levels achieved on maintenance therapy of 5 mg/kg/day or 2.5 to 4 mg/kg/day as a function of duration of therapy in human newborns.** Note the accumulation of drug at the end of the first week of therapy with the higher dose. *(From Painter MJ, Pippenger C, MacDonald H, Pitlick W: Phenobarbital and diphenylhydantoin levels in neonates with seizures,* J Pediatr *92:315-319, 1978.)*

Maintenance administration of *phenytoin* in the newborn is particularly difficult because of its nonlinear kinetics and rapid decrease in elimination rates in the first weeks of life.[459-462] Thus, the apparent half-life of the drug decreases from 57 hours in the first week of life to 20 hours in the fourth week.[459] Careful attention to blood levels is particularly necessary when this drug is used for maintenance, including as the preferred agent fosphenytoin.[422]

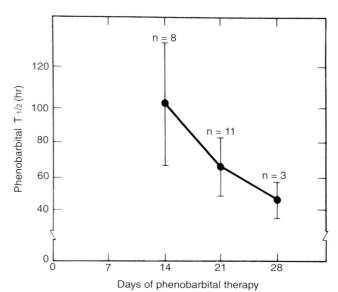

Figure 5-20 **Half-life ($T_{1/2}$) of phenobarbital as a function of duration of therapy in human newborns.** The elimination rate is relatively slow initially and then increases considerably with longer duration of therapy. *(From Painter MJ, Pippenger C, MacDonald H, Pitlick W: Phenobarbital and diphenylhydantoin levels in neonates with seizures,* J Pediatr *92:315-319, 1978.)*

TABLE 5-33	Maintenance Therapy of Neonatal Seizures

Glucose: ≤8 mg/kg/min, IV
Phenobarbital: 3–4 mg/kg/24 hr, IV, IM, or PO
Phenytoin (as fosphenytoin): 3–4 mg/kg/24 hr, IV
Calcium gluconate: 500 mg/kg/24 hr, PO
Magnesium sulfate (50%): 0.2 mL/kg/24 hr, IM

IM, intramuscularly; IV, intravenously, PO, by mouth.

Two reports suggested that carbamazepine may be a useful alternative to phenobarbital or phenytoin in maintenance therapy.[439,452,464] Oral doses of 10 to 15 mg/kg/day were associated with good seizure control. More data are needed.

Overly vigorous maintenance therapy can cause as many problems as undertreatment and must be avoided. Correlations of clinical, EEG, and blood level determinations are necessary for rational therapy of the newborn with seizures.

Duration of Therapy

Optimal duration of therapy of the infant with seizures in the newborn period relates principally to the *likelihood of recurrence of seizure* if the drugs are discontinued. *What is the risk of subsequent epilepsy in infants with neonatal seizures?* The overall incidence of subsequent epilepsy in survivors has varied from study to study between approximately 10% and 30%.* This overall range can be refined in the individual patient if one considers (1) the neonatal neurological examination, (2) the cause of the neonatal seizures, and (3) the EEG pattern (Table 5-34). The first of these is a very critical determinant. For example, in two studies of asphyxiated infants, the risk of recurrence of seizures was approximately 50% when the neurological examination at discharge was abnormal.[158,469] The infants with normal neurological findings did *not* develop subsequent recurrent seizures. The second determinant (i.e., the cause of seizures) is similarly important. Thus, the risk of subsequent epilepsy after neonatal seizures secondary to perinatal asphyxia is approximately 30 to 50%, and after seizures secondary to cortical dysgenesis, the risk is essentially 100%. However, simple, late-onset hypocalcemia has essentially no associated risk. Finally, the third determinant, the EEG tracing, may be particularly useful. Of the 54 asphyxiated infants studied by Watanabe and co-workers,[158] none developed subsequent epilepsy when the results of the neonatal interictal EEG tracing were normal or showed only "minimal" or "mild" depression. In contrast, 41% of infants with "marked" depression developed subsequent epilepsy. The value of EEG patterns in determining the risk of subsequent epilepsy has been shown in other studies.[211,468,470]

I *recommend* that these three factors be assessed carefully in each newborn with seizures to determine duration of therapy (Table 5-35). If the neonatal neurological examination becomes normal, I discontinue all therapy. If the neurological examination is persistently abnormal, I consider the cause and obtain an EEG tracing. (If phenytoin has been used, it is discontinued when intravenous lines are removed, even if the examination is abnormal.) In general I continue phenobarbital unless the EEG pattern shows no paroxysmal activity or the cause is a transient metabolic disturbance. If the infant is given phenobarbital when discharged from the hospital, I reassess the neurological examination and

*See references 25,27,141,146,158,211,214,216,219,397a,404,465-468.

TABLE 5-34 Determinants of Duration of Anticonvulsant Drug Therapy for Neonatal Seizures

Neonatal neurological examination
Cause of the neonatal seizure
Electroencephalogram

development at 1 month of age; if the neurological status has become normal, I discontinue the phenobarbital (over 2 weeks). If the infant's neurological state is not normal, an EEG tracing is obtained; if the study is not *overtly paroxysmal*, I taper and discontinue the phenobarbital. If the EEG pattern is overtly paroxysmal, I reassess in the same manner at 3 months of age. My goal is to discontinue phenobarbital as soon as I can.

The question of a *deleterious effect of phenobarbital* on the developing brain was raised by earlier data obtained with rats and cultured cells of neural origin.[471-475] The relation of these data to the human infant is unclear. The time period of the experiments in the rat corresponded to a period in the human from approximately the sixth month of gestation to years postnatally. The deleterious effects in cell culture require many days of exposure, and thus extrapolation to the human cortex in vivo is difficult. A deleterious effect of phenobarbital on cognitive development of infants treated for febrile seizures raised further questions concerning potential toxicity of phenobarbital.[476] Whether this deleterious effect persists or is related to phenobarbital administration per se or to confounding factors is unclear. In one study, deleterious effects of phenobarbital on neurocognitive behavior in older children were shown to be reversible after discontinuation of therapy.[477]

Particularly concerning are studies in neonatal rats that showed pronounced apoptotic neurodegeneration within 24 hours after administration of phenobarbital, phenytoin, diazepam, clonazepam, and valproate.[478,479] Combinations of drugs produced greater effects. Doses and blood levels attained were generally comparable to those

TABLE 5-35 Duration of Anticonvulsant Therapy: Guidelines

Neonatal Period
If neonatal neurological examination becomes normal, discontinue therapy.
If neonatal neurological examination is persistently abnormal, consider the cause and obtain an EEG.
In most such cases (see text for exceptions):
  Continue phenobarbital.
  Discontinue phenytoin.
  Reevaluate in 1 month.
At 1 Month After Discharge
If neurological examination has become normal, discontinue phenobarbital.
If neurological examination is persistently abnormal, obtain an EEG.
If no seizure activity is noted on the EEG, discontinue phenobarbital.

EEG, electroencephalogram.

used in human infants. The neuronal death was associated with reduced expression of neurotrophins and survival-promoting proteins in brain. Topiramate and levetiracetam did not produce these effects.[456,480] These observations accentuate the importance of finding other agents for treatment of neonatal seizures and of discontinuing these drugs as soon as the threat of seizures diminishes.

Calcium and Magnesium

I do not administer calcium routinely to all newborns during the initial seizure, except in the unusual instance of a classic presentation for later-onset hypocalcemia. If hypocalcemia is present, 5% calcium gluconate is given intravenously at a dose of 4 mL/kg (200 mg/kg) (see Table 5-30). The electrocardiogram, or at least cardiac rhythm by auscultation, should be monitored during administration. Phenobarbital can sometimes suppress the seizures of hypocalcemia,[220] and, thus, a decrease in seizures after phenobarbital administration does not rule out hypocalcemia as cause. If hypomagnesemia is present, magnesium sulfate is best given intramuscularly as a 50% solution in a dose of 0.2 mL/kg (see Table 5-30). Approximately half of all newborns with seizures secondary to later-onset hypocalcemia also have hypomagnesemia.[227] The importance of treating these hypocalcemic infants with magnesium is emphasized by the following: (1) the administration of calcium to such infants may increase renal excretion of magnesium, aggravate the hypomagnesemia, and maintain the convulsive state; and (2) the administration of magnesium has been shown to correct *both* the hypocalcemia and the hypomagnesemia, perhaps by increasing movement of calcium from bone to plasma.[227] However, magnesium cannot be administered with abandon because magnesium can produce neuromuscular blockade. Transient weakness and hypotonia (without concentrations of plasma magnesium out of the normal range) are often noted in infants who are given magnesium.[227] Moreover, the maintenance doses of magnesium and calcium shown in Table 5-33 should be administered only as long as needed to avoid hypomagnesemia or hypocalcemia.

Other Modes of Therapy

Seizures related to other metabolic disturbances or infection require therapeutic approaches that are better discussed in relation to these specific problems (see later chapters). Specific therapy sometimes must be supplemented with administration of anticonvulsant drugs, at least during the neonatal period.

Recurrent seizures that are not accompanied by any obvious associated findings to aid in diagnosis should raise the possibility of *pyridoxine dependency*. As noted previously, the best means of diagnosis is a therapeutic trial of pyridoxine, administered intravenously in a dose of 50 to 100 mg, accompanied by simultaneous monitoring of the EEG pattern (see Table 5-30). In the true case, this trial is accompanied by cessation of seizure within minutes and normalization of the EEG pattern within minutes or hours. In evaluating the response to pyridoxine, one should not consider significant a

transient attenuation of seizure discharges that may accompany infusion of essentially any material. This "arousal" response should last only a few seconds.[172] Any question should provoke repeated 100-mg infusions of pyridoxine (to a maximum of 500 mg), a trial of oral pyridoxine, or both. In addition, infants with pyridoxine dependency may exhibit hypotonia or even apnea after pyridoxine infusion,[258,259] perhaps because of an abrupt increase of synthesis of GABA in brain and activation of inhibitory GABA receptors in brain stem. As noted earlier, some infants not responsive to pyridoxine may require pyridoxal phosphate.[280a] Other therapies include a trial of *folinic acid* (2.5 mg twice daily, to a total of 4 mg/kg/day) for the rare patient with folinic acid–responsive seizures and the *ketogenic diet* for the unusual patient with glucose transporter defect with onset of seizures in the neonatal period (see earlier).

REFERENCES

1. Lanska MJ, Lanska DJ: Neonatal seizures in the United States: Results of the National Hospital Discharge Survey, 1980–1991, *Neuroepidemiology* 15:117-125, 1996.
2. Lanska MJ, Lanska DJ, Baumann RJ, Kryscio RJ: A population-based study of neonatal seizures in Fayette County, Kentucky, *Neurology* 45:724-732, 1995.
3. Ronen GM, Penney S, Andrews W: The epidemiology of clinical neonatal seizures in Newfoundland: A population-based study, *J Pediatr* 134:71-75, 1999.
4. Freeman JM, Lietman PS: A basic approach to the understanding of seizures and the mechanism of action and metabolism of anticonvulsants, *Adv Pediatr* 20:291-321, 1973.
5. Collins RC, Olney JW, Lothman EW: Metabolic and pathological consequences of focal seizures. In Ward AA Jr, Penry JK, Purpura D, editors: *Epilepsy*, New York: 1983, Raven Press.
6. Moshé SL: Epileptogenesis and the immature brain, *Epilepsia* 28:S3-S15, 1987.
7. Lothman EW: Pathophysiology of seizures and epilepsy in the mature and immature brain: Cells, synapses and circuits. In Dodson WE, Pellock JM, editors: *Pediatric Epilepsy: Diagnosis and Therapy*, New York: 1993, Demos Publications.
8. Johnston MV: Developmental aspects of epileptogenesis, *Epilepsia* 37:S2-S9, 1996.
9. Silverstein FS, Jensen FE: Neonatal seizures, *Ann Neurol* 62:112-120, 2007.
10. Johnston MV, McDonald JW: Metabolic and pharmacologic consequences of seizures. In Dodson WE, Pellock JM, editors: *Pediatric Epilepsy: Diagnosis and Therapy*, New York: 1993, Demos Publications.
11. Lott IT, Coulombe T, Di Paolo RV, Richardson EP Jr, et al: Vitamin B₆–dependent seizures: Pathology and chemical findings in brain, *Neurology* 28:47-54, 1978.
12. Kurlemann G, Löscher W, Dominick HC, Palm GD: Disappearance of neonatal seizures and low CSF GABA levels after treatment with vitamin B₆, *Epilepsy Res* 1:152-154, 1987.
13. Kurlemann G, Ziegler R, Gruneberg M, Bomelburg T, et al: Disturbance of GABA metabolism in pyridoxine-dependent seizures, *Neuropediatrics* 23:257-259, 1992.
14. Baumeister FAM, Gsell W, Shin YS, Egger J: Glutamate in pyridoxine-dependent epilepsy: Neurotoxic glutamate concentration in the cerebrospinal fluid and its normalization by pyridoxine, *Pediatrics* 94:318-321, 1994.
15. Volpe JJ: Neonatal seizures, *Clin Perinatol* 4:43-63, 1977.
16. Camfield PR, Camfield CS: Neonatal seizures: A commentary on selected aspects, *J Child Neurol* 2:244-251, 1987.
17. Kellaway P, Mizrahi EM, Hrachovy RA: Seizures of newborns and infants. In Wada FA, Ellingson RE, editors: *Clinical Neurophysiology of Epilepsy EEG Handbook Revised Series*, Rotterdam: 1990, Elsevier Science.
18. Scher MS, Painter MJ: Controversies concerning neonatal seizures, *Pediatr Clin North Am* 36:281-310, 1989.
19. Scher MS, Painter MJ, Bergman I, Barmada MA, et al: EEG diagnoses of neonatal seizures: Clinical correlations and outcome, *Pediatr Neurol* 5:17-24, 1989.
20. Scher MS, Beggarly M: Clinical significance of focal periodic discharges in neonates, *J Child Neurol* 4:175-185, 1989.
21. Legido A, Clancy RR, Berman PH: Recent advances in the diagnosis, treatment, and prognosis of neonatal seizures, *Pediatr Neurol* 4:79-86, 1988.
22. Volpe JJ: Neonatal seizures: Current concepts and revised classification, *Pediatrics* 84:422-428, 1989.
23. Shewmon DA: What is a neonatal seizure? Problems in definition and quantification for investigative and clinical purposes, *J Clin Neurophysiol* 7:315-368, 1990.

24. Painter MJ, Gaus LM: Neonatal seizures: Diagnosis and treatment, *J Child Neurol* 6:101-108, 1991.

25. Scher MS, Aso K, Beggarly ME, Hamid MY, et al: Electrographic seizures in preterm and full-term neonates: Clinical correlates, associated brain lesions, and risk for neurologic sequelae, *Pediatrics* 91:128-134, 1993.

26. Scher MS, Hamid MY, Steppe DA, Beggarly ME, et al: Ictal and interictal electrographic seizure durations in preterm and term neonates, *Epilepsia* 34:284-288, 1993.

27. Lombroso CT: Neonatal seizures: A clinician's overview, *Brain Dev* 18:1-28, 1996.

28. Mizrahi EM, Kellaway P: *Diagnosis and Management of Neonatal Seizures*, Philadelphia: 1998, Lippincott-Raven.

29. Biagioni E, Ferrari F, Boldrini A, Roversi MF, et al: Electroclinical correlation in neonatal seizures, *Eur J Paediatr Neurol* 2:117-125, 1998.

30. Caveness WF, Nielsen KC, Yakovlev PI, Adams RD: Electroencephalographic and clinical studies of epilepsy during the maturation of the monkey, *Epilepsia* 3:137, 1962.

31. Yakovlev PI: Maturation of cortical substrata of epileptic events, *World Neurol* 3:299, 1962.

32. Yakovlev PI, Lecours AR: The myelogenetic cycles of regional maturation of the brain. In Minkowski A, editor: *Regional Development of the Brain in Early Life*, Philadelphia: 1967, Davis.

33. Conel J: *The Postnatal Development of the Human Cerebral Cortex: The Cortex of the Newborn*, Cambridge, MA: 1941, Harvard University Press.

34. Yakovlev PI: Morphological criteria of growth and maturation of the nervous system in man, *Ment Retard* 39:3, 1962.

35. Schwartzkroin PA, Kunkel DD, Mathers LH: Development of rabbit hippocampus: Anatomy, *Dev Brain Res* 2:452-468, 1982.

36. Schwartzkroin PA: Development of rabbit hippocampus, *Dev Brain Dev* 2:469-486, 1982.

37. Swann JW, Smith KL, Brady RJ: Extracellular K+ accumulation during penicillin induced epileptogenesis in the CA3 region of immature rat hippocampus, *Dev Brain Res* 30:243-255, 1986.

38. Swann JW, Brady RJ: Penicillin induced epileptogenesis in immature rat CA3 hippocampal pyramidal cells, *Dev Brain Res* 12:243-254, 1984.

39. Luhmann HJ, Prince DA: Transient expression of polysynaptic NMDA receptor-mediated activity during neocortical development, *Neurosci Lett* 111:109-115, 1990.

40. Haas KZ, Sperber EF, Moshé SL: Kindling in developing animals: Expression of severe seizures and enhanced development of bilateral foci, *Brain Res Dev Brain Res* 56:275-280, 1990.

41. Lee W-L, Hablitz JJ: Excitatory synaptic involvement in epileptiform bursting in the immature rat neocortex, *J Neurophysiol* 66:1894-1901, 1991.

42. Muller D, Oliver M, Lynch G: Developmental changes in synaptic properties in hippocampus of neonatal rats, *Dev Brain Res* 49:105-114, 1989.

43. Pierson M, Snyder-Keller A: NMDA receptor-dependent epileptogenesis in developing inferior colliculus. *Epilepsy Res Suppl* 9:371-382, 1992.

44. Avanzini G, Franceschetti S, Panzica F, Buzio S, et al: Age-dependent changes in excitability of rat neocortical neurons studied in vitro. *Epilepsy Res Suppl* 9:95-104, 1992.

45. Hablitz JJ, Lee WL, Prince DA, Benari Y: NMDA receptor involvement in epileptogenesis in the immature neocortex. *Epilepsy Res Suppl* 8:139-145, 1992.

46. Litzinger MJ, Mouritsen L, Grover BB, Esplin MS, et al: Regional differences in the critical period neurodevelopment in the mouse: Implications for neonatal seizures, *J Child Neurol* 9:77-80, 1994.

47. Holmes GL, Ben-Ari Y: The neurobiology and consequences of epilepsy in the developing brain, *Pediatr Res* 49:320-325, 2001.

48. Sanchez RM, Jensen FE: Maturational aspects of epilepsy mechanisms and consequences for the immature brain, *Epilepsia* 42:577-585, 2001.

49. Sanchez RM, Koh S, Rio C, Wang C, et al: Decreased glutamate receptor 2 expression and enhanced epileptogenesis in immature rat hippocampus after perinatal hypoxia-induced seizures, *J Neurosci* 21:8154-8163, 2001.

50. Sanchez RM, Dai WM, Levada RE, Lippman JJ, et al: AMPA/kainate receptor-mediated downregulation of GABAergic synaptic transmission by calcineurin after seizures in the developing rat brain, *J Neurosci* 25:3442-3451, 2005.

50a. Talos DM, Fishman RE, Park H, Folkerth RD, et al: Developmental regulation of alpha-amino-3-hydroxy-5-methyl-4-isoxazole-propionic acid receptor subunit expression in forebrain and relationship to regional susceptibility to hypoxic/ischemic injury. I. Rodent cerebral white matter and cortex, *J Comp Neurol* 497:42-60, 2006.

50b. Talos DM, Follett PL, Folkerth RD, Fishman RE, et al: Developmental regulation of alpha-amino-3-hydroxy-5-methyl-4-isoxazole-propionic acid receptor subunit expression in forebrain and relationship to regional susceptibility to hypoxic/ischemic injury. II. Human cerebral white matter and cortex, *J Comp Neurol* 497:61-77, 2006.

51. Sanchez RM, Jensen FE: Modeling hypoxia-induced seizures and hypoxic encephalopathy in the neonatal period. In Pitanken A, Schwartzkroin PA, Moshe SL, editors: *Models of Seizures and Epilepsy*, San Diego, 2006, Elsevier.

52. Dzhala VI, Talos DM, Sdrulla DA, Brumback AC, et al: NKCC1 transporter facilitates seizures in the developing brain, *Nat Med* 11:1205-1213, 2005.

53. Tremblay E, Roisin MP, Represa A, Charriaut-Marlangue C, et al: Transient increased density of NMDA binding sites in the developing rat hippocampus, *Brain Res* 461:393-396, 1988.

54. McDonald JW, Johnston MV, Young AB: Differential ontogenic development of three receptors comprising the NMDA receptor/channel complex in the rat hippocampus, *Exp Neurol* 110:237-247, 1990.

55. Cherubini E, Gaiarsa JL, Ben-Ari Y: GABA: An excitatory transmitter in early postnatal life, *Trends Neurosci* 14:515-519, 1991.

56. Moshé SL: Seizures in the developing brain, *Neurology* 43:S3-S7, 1993.

57. Moshe SL, Brown LL, Kubova H, Veliskova J, et al: Maturation and segregation of brain networks that modify seizures, *Brain Res* 665:141-146, 1994.

58. Moshe SL, Garant DS, Sperber EF, Veliskova J, et al: Ontogeny and topography of seizure regulation by the substantia nigra, *Brain Dev* 17:61-72, 1995.

59. Baram TZ, Snead OC 3rd: Bicuculline induced seizures in infant rats: Ontogeny of behavioral and electrocortical phenomena, *Brain Res Dev Brain Res* 57:291-295, 1990.

60. Sperber EF, Haas KZ, Stanton PK, Moshé SL: Resistance of the immature hippocampus to seizure-induced synaptic reorganization, *Brain Res Dev Brain Res* 60:88-93, 1991.

61. Jensen FE, Applegate CD, Holtzman D, Belin TR, et al: Epileptogenic effect of hypoxia in the immature rodent brain, *Ann Neurol* 29:629-637, 1991.

62. Romijn HJ, Voskuyl RA, Coenen AML: Hypoxic-ischemic encephalopathy sustained in early postnatal life may result in permanent epileptic activity and an altered cortical convulsive threshold in rat, *Epilepsy Res* 17:31-42, 1994.

63. Staley K, Smith R, Schaack J, Wilcox C, et al: Alteration of GABA$_A$ receptor function following gene transfer of the CLC-2 chloride channel, *Neuron* 17:543-551, 1996.

64. Yamada J, Okabe A, Toyoda H, Kilb W, et al: Cl− uptake promoting depolarizing GABA actions in immature rat neocortical neurones is mediated by NKCC1, *J Physiol* 557:829-841, 2004.

65. Clayton GH, Owens GC, Wolff JS, Smith RL: Ontogeny of cation-Cl− cotransporter expression in rat neocortex, *Brain Res Dev Brain Res* 109:281-292, 1998.

66. Rivera C, Voipio J, Payne JA, Ruusuvuori E, et al: The K+/Cl− co-transporter KCC2 renders GABA hyperpolarizing during neuronal maturation, *Nature* 397:251-255, 1999.

67. Dai Y, Tang J, Zhang JH: Role of Cl− in cerebral vascular tone and expression of Na+-K+-2Cl− co-transporter after neonatal hypoxia-ischemia, *Can J Physiol Pharmacol* 83:767-773, 2005.

68. Plum F, Howse DC, Duffy TE: Metabolic effects of seizures. In Plum F, editor: *Brain Dysfunction in Metabolic Disorders*, New York: 1974, Raven Press.

69. Dwyer BE, Wasterlain CG: Neonatal seizures in monkeys and rabbits: Brain glucose depletion in the face of normoglycemia, prevention by glucose loads, *Pediatr Res* 19:992-995, 1985.

70. Fujikawa DG, Vannucci RC, Dwyer BE, Wasterlain CG: Generalized seizures deplete brain energy reserves in normoxemic newborn monkeys, *Brain Res* 454:51-59, 1988.

71. Fujikawa DG, Dwyer BE, Lake RR, Wasterlain CG: Local cerebral glucose utilization during status epilepticus in newborn primates, *Am J Physiol* 256:C1160-1167, 1989.

72. Young RS, Cowan BE, Petroff OA, Novotny E, et al: In vivo 31P and in vitro 1H nuclear magnetic resonance study of hypoglycemia during neonatal seizure, *Ann Neurol* 22:622-628, 1987.

73. Cowan BE, Young RS, Briggs RW, Lu D, et al: The effect of hypotension on brain energy state during prolonged neonatal seizure, *Pediatr Res* 21:357-361, 1987.

74. Young RS, Petroff OA, Chen B, Gore JC, et al: Brain energy state and lactate metabolism during status epilepticus in the neonatal dog: In vivo 31P and 1H nuclear magnetic resonance study, *Pediatr Res* 29:191-195, 1991.

75. Young RS, Briggs RW, Yagel SK, Gorman I: 31P nuclear magnetic resonance study of the effect of hypoxemia on neonatal status epilepticus, *Pediatr Res* 20:581-586, 1986.

76. Wasterlain CG, Shirasaka Y: Seizures, brain damage and brain development, *Brain Dev* 16:279-295, 1994.

77. Wasterlain CG: Recurrent seizures in the developing brain are harmful, *Epilepsia* 38:728-734, 1997.

78. Thoresen M, Hallstrom A, Whitelaw A, Puka-Sundvall M, et al: Lactate and pyruvate changes in the newborn gray and white matter during posthypoxic seizures in newborn pigs, *Pediatr Res* 44:746-754, 1998.

79. Lowry OH, Passonneau JV: Kinetic evidence for multiple binding sites on phosphofructokinase, *J Biol Chem* 241:2268-2279, 1966.

80. Borgstrom L, Chapman AG, Siesjö BK: Glucose consumption in the cerebral cortex of rat during bicuculline-induced status epilepticus, *J Neurochem* 27:971-973, 1976.

81. Lassen NA: Brain extracellular pH: The main factor controlling cerebral blood flow, *Scand J Clin Lab Invest* 22:247-251, 1968.

82. Young RS, Osbakken MD, Briggs RW, Yagel SK, et al: 31P NMR study of cerebral metabolism during prolonged seizures in the neonatal dog, *Ann Neurol* 18:14-20, 1985.

83. Fujikawa DG, Dwyer BE, Wasterlain CG: Preferential blood flow to brainstem during generalized seizures in the newborn marmoset monkey, *Brain Res* 397:61-72, 1986.

84. Clozel M, Daval JL, Monin P, Dubruc C, et al: Regional cerebral blood flow during bicuculline-induced seizures in the newborn piglet: Effect of phenobarbital, *Dev Pharmacol Ther* 8:189-199, 1985.

85. Young RS, Fripp RR, Yagel SK, Werner JC, et al: Cardiac dysfunction during status epilepticus in the neonatal pig, *Ann Neurol* 18:291-297, 1985.

86. Pourcyrous M, Leffler CW, Bada HS, Korones SB, et al: Effects of pancuronium bromide on cerebral blood flow changes during seizures in newborn pigs, *Pediatr Res* 31:636-639, 1992.

87. Hascoet JM, Monin P, Vert P: Persistence of impaired autoregulation of cerebral blood flow in the postictal period in piglets, *Epilepsia* 29:743-747, 1988.

88. Monin P, Stonestreet BS, Oh W: Hyperventilation restores autoregulation of cerebral blood flow in postictal piglets, *Pediatr Res* 30:294-298, 1991.

89. Wasterlain CG, Duffy TE: Status epilepticus in immature rats, *Arch Neurol* 33:821, 1976.

90. Vannucci RC, Vasta F: Energy state of the brain in experimental neonatal status epilepticus, *Pediatr Res* 19:396, 1985.

91. Cataltepe O, Vannucci RC, Heitjan DF, Towfighi J: Effect of status epilepticus on hypoxic-ischemic brain damage in the immature rat, *Pediatr Res* 38:251-257, 1995.

92. Young RS, Chen B, Petroff OA, Gore JC, et al: The effect of diazepam on neonatal seizure: In vivo 31P and ¹H NMR study, *Pediatr Res* 25:27-31, 1989.

93. Younkin D, Maris JE: The effect of seizures on cerebral metabolites in children, *Pediatr Res* 19:397, 1985.

94. Holmes GL: Effects of seizures on brain development: Lessons from the laboratory, *Pediatr Neurol* 33:1-11, 2005.

95. Wirrell EC, Armstrong EA, Osman LD, Yager JY: Prolonged seizures exacerbate perinatal hypoxic-ischemic brain damage, *Pediatr Res* 50:445-454, 2001.

96. Dzhala V, Ben-Ari Y, Khazipov R: Seizures accelerate anoxia-induced neuronal death in the neonatal rat hippocampus, *Ann Neurol* 48:632-640, 2000.

97. Yager JY, Armstrong EA, Jaharus C, Saucier DM, et al: Preventing hyperthermia decreases brain damage following neonatal hypoxic-ischemic seizures, *Brain Research* 1011:48-57, 2004.

98. Gado MH, Phelps ME, Hoffman EJ, Raichle ME: Changes in cerebral blood volume and vascular mean transit time during induced cerebral seizures, *Radiology* 121:105-109, 1976.

99. Kuhl DE, Engel J Jr, Phelps ME, Selin C: Epileptic patterns of local cerebral metabolism and perfusion in humans determined by emission computed tomography of 18FDG and 13NH3, *Ann Neurol* 8:348-360, 1980.

100. Perlman JM, Volpe JJ: Seizures in the preterm infant: Effects on cerebral blood flow velocity, intracranial pressure, and arterial blood pressure, *J Pediatr* 102:288-293, 1983.

101. Perlman JM, Herscovitch P, Kreusser KL, Raichle ME, et al: Positron emission tomography in the newborn: Effect of seizure on regional cerebral blood flow in an asphyxiated infant, *Neurology* 35:244-247, 1985.

102. Monin P, Clozel M, Morselli PL, Dubruc C, et al: Effect of seizures on brain phenobarbital concentration in newborn piglets, *Epilepsia* 28:179-183, 1987.

103. Borch K, Pryds O, Holm S, Lou H, et al: Regional cerebral blood flow during seizures in neonates, *J Pediatr* 132:431-435, 1998.

104. Alfonso I. Papazian O, Villalobos R, Acosta JI: Similar brain SPECT findings in subclinical and clinical seizures in two neonates with hemimegalencephaly, *Pediatr Neurol* 19:132-134, 1998.

105. Takei Y, Takashima S, Ohyu J, Takami T, et al: Effects of nitric oxide synthase inhibition on the cerebral circulation and brain damage during kainic acid–induced seizures in newborn rabbits, *Brain Dev* 21:253-259, 1999.

106. Boylan GB, Panerai RB, Rennie JM, Evans DH, et al: Cerebral blood flow velocity during neonatal seizures, *Arch Dis Child Fetal Neonatal Ed* 80:105-110, 1999.

107. Eyre JA, Oozeer RC, Wilkinson AR: Continuous electroencephalographic recording to detect seizures in paralysed newborn babies, *BMJ (Clin Res Ed)* 286:1017-1018, 1983.

108. Lou HC, Friis HB: Arterial blood pressure elevations during motor activity and epileptic seizures in the newborn, *Acta Paediatr Scand* 68:803-806, 1979.

109. Meldrum B: Physiological changes during prolonged seizures and epileptic brain damage, *Neuropadiatrie* 9:203-212, 1978.

110. Lowenstein DH, Shimosaka S, So YT, Simon RP: The relationship between electrographic seizure activity and neuronal injury, *Epilepsy Res* 10:49-54, 1991.

111. Corsellis JA, Bruton CJ: Neuropathology of status epilepticus in humans. *Adv Neurol* 34:129-139, 1983.

112. Nevander G, Ingvar M, Auer R, Siesjö BK: Status epilepticus in well-oxygenated rats causes neuronal necrosis, *Ann Neurol* 18:281-290, 1985.

113. Meldrum B: Excitotoxicity and epileptic brain damage, *Epilepsy Res* 10:55-61, 1991.

114. Meldrum BS: The role of glutamate in epilepsy and other CNS disorders, *Neurology* 44(Suppl 8):S14-S23, 1994.

115. Hussenet F, Boyet S, Nehlig A: Long-term metabolic effects of pentylenetetrazol-induced status epilepticus in the immature rat, *Neuroscience* 67:455-461, 1995.

116. Sankar R, Shin DH, Liu HT, Mazarati A, et al: Patterns of status epilepticus-induced neuronal injury during development and long-term consequences, *J Neurosci* 18:8382-8393, 1998.

117. Sankar R, Shin DH, Wasterlain CG: Serum neuron-specific enolase is a marker for neuronal damage following status epilepticus in the rat, *Epilepsy Res* 28:129-136, 1997.

118. Towfighi J, Housman C, Brucklacher R, Vannucci RC: Neuropathology of seizures in the immature rabbit, *Dev Brain Res* 152:143-152, 2004.

119. Nitecka L, Tremblay E, Charton G, Bouillot JP, et al: Maturation of kainic acid-brain damage syndrome in the rat. II. Histopathological sequela, *Neurosci* 13:1073-1094, 1984.

120. Holmes GL: The long-term effects of seizures on the developing brain: Clinical and laboratory issues, *Brain Dev* 13:393-409, 1991.

121. Fujikawa DG, Söderfeldt B, Wasterlain CG: Neuropathological changes during generalized seizures in newborn monkeys, *Epilepsy Res* 12:243-251, 1992.

122. Sperber EF, Stanton PK, Haas K, Ackermann RF, et al: Developmental differences in the neurobiology of epileptic brain damage, *Epilepsy Res Suppl* 9:67-80, 1992.

123. Owens J, Robbins CA, Wenzel J, Schwartzkroin PA: Acute and chronic effects of hypoxia on the developing hippocampus, *Ann Neurol* 41:187-199, 1997.

124. Yang YL, Tandon P, Liu Z, Sarkisian MR, et al: Synaptic reorganization following kainic acid–induced seizures during development, *Dev Brain Res* 107:169-177, 1998.

125. Baram TZ: Long-term neuroplasticity and functional consequences of single versus recurrent early-life seizures, *Ann Neurol* 54:701-705, 2003.

126. Olney JW: Neurotoxicity of excitatory amino acids. In McGeer E, Olney JW, McGeer PL, editors: *Kainic Acid as a Tool in Neurobiology*, New York: 1978, Raven Press.

127. Ben-Ari Y, Tremblay E, Ottersen OP, Meldrum BS: The role of epileptic activity in hippocampal and "remote" cerebral lesions induced by kainic acid, *Brain Res* 191:79-97, 1980.

128. Ben-Ari Y, Cherubini E: Zinc and GABA in developing brain [letter], *Nature* 353:220, 1991.

129. Collins RC, Olney JW: Focal cortical seizures cause distant thalamic lesions, *Science* 218:177-179, 1982.

130. Collins RC, Lothman EW, Olney JW: Status epilepticus in the limbic system: Biochemical and pathological changes, *Adv Neurol* 34:277-288, 1983.

131. McDonald JW, Johnston MV: Physiological and pathophysiological roles of excitatory amino acids during central nervous system development, *Brain Res Brain Res Rev* 15:41-70, 1990.

132. Meldrum B: Protection against ischaemic neuronal damage by drugs acting on excitatory neurotransmission, *Cerebrovasc Brain Metab Rev* 2:27-57, 1990.

133. Meldrum B, Garthwaite J: Excitatory amino acid neurotoxicity and neurodegenerative disease, *Trends Pharmacol Sci* 11:379-387, 1990.

134. Clifford DB, Zorumski CF, Olney JW: Ketamine and MK-801 prevent degeneration of thalamic neurons induced by focal cortical seizures, *Exp Neurol* 105:272-279, 1989.

135. Furshpan EJ, Potter DD: Seizure-like activity and cellular damage in rat hippocampal neurons in cell culture, *Neuron* 3:199-207, 1989.

136. Millan MH, Chapman AG, Meldrum BS: Extracellular amino acid levels in hippocampus during pilocarpine-induced seizures, *Epilepsy Res* 14:139-148, 1993.

137. During MJ, Spencer DD: Extracellular hippocampal glutamate and spontaneous seizure in the conscious human brain, *Lancet* 341:1607-1610, 1993.

138. Chang D, Baram TZ: Status epilepticus results in reversible neuronal injury in infant rat hippocampus: Novel use of a marker, *Dev Brain Res* 77:133-136, 1994.

139. Koh S, Tibayan FD, Simpson JN, Jensen TE: NBQX or topiramate treatment after perinatal hypoxia-induced seizures prevents later increases in seizure-induced neuronal injury, *Epilepsia* 45:569-575, 2004.

139a. Cornejo BJ, Mesches MH, Coultrap S, Browning MD, et al: A single episode of neonatal seizures permanently alters glutamatergic synapses, *Ann Neurol* 61:411-426, 2007.

140. Mellits ED, Holden KR, Freeman JM: Neonatal seizures. II. A multivariate analysis of factors associated with outcome, *Pediatrics* 70:177-185, 1982.

141. Bergman I, Painter MJ, Hirsch RP, Crumrine PK, et al: Outcome in neonates with convulsions treated in an intensive care unit, *Ann Neurol* 14:642-647, 1983.

142. Painter MJ, Pippenger C, MacDonald H, Pitlick W: Phenobarbital and diphenylhydantoin levels in neonates with seizures, *J Pediatr* 92:315-319, 1978.

143. Legido A, Clancy RR, Berman PH: Neurologic outcome after electroencephalographically proven neonatal seizures, *Pediatrics* 88:583-596, 1991.

144. Connell J, Oozeer R, de Vries L, Dubowitz LM, et al: Clinical and EEG response to anticonvulsants in neonatal seizures, *Arch Dis Child* 64:459-464, 1989.

145. Connell J, Oozeer R, de Vries L, Dubowitz LM, et al: Continuous EEG monitoring of neonatal seizures: Diagnostic and prognostic considerations, *Arch Dis Child* 64:452-458, 1989.

146. McBride MC, Laroia N, Guillet R: Electrographic seizures in neonates correlate with poor neurodevelopmental outcome, *Neurology* 55:506-513, 2000.

147. Miller SP, Weiss J, Barnwell A, Ferriero DM, et al: Seizure-associated brain injury in term newborns with perinatal asphyxia, *Neurology* 58:542-548, 2002.

148. Sogawa Y, Monokoshi M, Silveira DC, Cha BH, et al: Timing of cognitive deficits following neonatal seizures: Relationship to histological changes in the hippocampus, *Dev Brain Res* 131:73-83, 2001.

149. Bo T, Jiang YW, Cao HY, Wang JM, et al: Long-term effects of seizures in neonatal rats on spatial learning ability and *N*-methyl-D-aspartate receptor expression in the brain, *Dev Brain Res* 152:137-142, 2004.

150. McCabe BK, Silveira DC, Cilio MR, Cha BH, et al: Reduced neurogenesis after neonatal seizures, *J Neurosci* 21:2094-2103, 2001.

151. Villeneuve N, Ben-Ari Y, Holmes GL, Gaiarsa J-L: Neonatal seizures induced persistent changes in intrinsic properties of CA1 rat hippocampal cells, *Ann Neurol* 47:729-738, 2000.

151a. Holmes GL, Ben-Ari Y: A single episode of neonatal seizures permanently alters glutamatergic synapses, *Ann Neurol* 61:379-381, 2007.

152. Volpe J: Neonatal seizures, *N Engl J Med* 289:413-416, 1973.

153. Volpe JJ: *Neurology of the Newborn,* 2nd ed, Philadelphia: 1987, WB Saunders.

154. Radvanyi-Bouvet MF, Vallecalle MH, Morel-Kahn F, Relier JP, et al: Seizures and electrical discharges in premature infants, *Neuropediatrics* 16:143-148, 1985.

155. Mizrahi EM, Kellaway P: Characterization and classification of neonatal seizures, *Neurology* 37:1837-1844, 1987.

156. Mizrahi EM: Neonatal seizures: Problems in diagnosis and classification, *Epilepsia* 28:S46-S55, 1987.

157. Kellaway P, Mizrahi EM: Neonatal seizures. In Luders H, Lesser RP, editors: *Epilepsy: Electroclinical Syndromes,* London, 1987, Springer-Verlag.

158. Watanabe K, Hara K, Miyazaki S, Hakamada S, et al: Apneic seizures in the newborn, *Am J Dis Child* 136:980-984, 1982.

159. Duchowny MS: Complex partial seizures of infancy, *Arch Neurol* 44:911-914, 1987.

160. Pratap RC, Gururaj AK: Clinical and electroencephalographic features of complex partial seizures in infants, *Acta Neurol Scand* 79:123-127, 1989.

160a. Bauder F, Wohlrab G, Schmitt B: Neonatal seizures: Eyes open or closed?, *Epilepsia* 48:394-396, 2007.

160b. Murray DM, Boylan GB, Ali I, Ryan CA, et al: Defining the gap between electrographic seizure burden, clinical expression, and staff recognition of neonatal seizure, *Arch Dis Child Fetal Neonatal Ed* 2007.

161. Donati F, Schaffler L, Vassella F: Prolonged epileptic apneas in a newborn: A case report with ictal EEG recording, *Neuropediatrics* 26:223-225, 1995.

162. Schulte FJ: Neonatal convulsions and their relation to epilepsy in early childhood, *Dev Med Child Neurol* 8:381-392, 1966.

163. Henderson SD, Pettigrew AG, Campbell DJ: Clinical apnea and brain-stem neural function in preterm infants, *N Engl J Med* 308:353-357, 1983.

164. Henderson SD: Regulation of breathing rhythm in the newborn: The role of brainstem immaturity and inhibition, *J Dev Physiol* 6:83-92, 1984.

165. Eichenwald EC, Aina A, Stark AR: Apnea frequently persists beyond term gestation in infants delivered at 24 to 28 weeks, *Pediatrics* 100:354-359, 1997.

166. Coulter DL: Partial seizures with apnea and bradycardia, *Arch Neurol* 41:173-174, 1984.

167. Fenichel GM, Olson BJ, Fitzpatrick JE: Heart rate changes in convulsive and nonconvulsive neonatal apnea, *Ann Neurol* 7:577-582, 1980.

168. Willis J, Gould JB: Periodic alpha seizures with apnea in a newborn, *Dev Med Child Neurol* 22:214-222, 1980.

169. Kreisman NR, Sick TJ, Rosenthal M: Importance of vascular responses in determining cortical oxygenation during recurrent paroxysmal events of varying duration and frequency of repetition, *J Cereb Blood Flow Metab* 3:330-338, 1983.

170. Helmers SL, Weiss MJ, Holmes GL: Apneic seizures with bradycardia in a newborn, *J Epilepsy* 4:173-180, 1991.

170a. Sirsi D, Nadiminti L, Packard MA, Engel M, et al: Apneic seizures: A sign of temporal lobe hemorrhage in full-term neonates, *Pediatr Neurol* 37:366-370, 2007.

171. Dreyfus-Brisac C, Monod N: Electroclinical studies of status epilepticus and convulsions in the newborn. In Kellaway P, Peterson S, editors: *Neurological and Electroencephalographic Correlative Studies in Infancy,* New York: 1964, Grune & Stratton.

172. Lombroso CT: Seizures in the newborn period. In Vinken PJ, Bruyn G, editors: *Handbook of Clinical Neurology,* Amsterdam, 1970, North Holland.

173. Knauss TA, Carlson CB: Neonatal paroxysmal monorhythmic alpha activity, *Arch Neurol* 35:102, 1978.

174. Giroud M, Gouyon JB, Sandre D, Nivelon JL, et al: [Epileptic apneas in the neonatal period], *Arch Fr Pediatr* 40:719-722, 1983.

175. Zelnik N, Nir A, Amit S, Iancu TC: Autonomic seizures in an infant: Unusual cutaneous and cardiac manifestations, *Dev Med Child Neurol* 32:74-78, 1990.

176. Weiner SP, Painter MJ, Geva D, Guthrie RD, et al: Neonatal seizures: Electroclinical dissociation, *Pediatr Neurol* 7:363-368, 1991.

177. Bourgeois M, Alcardi J, Goutieres F: Alternating hemiplegia of childhood, *J Pediatr* 122:673-679, 1993.

178. Mikati MA, Maguire H, Barlow CF, Ozelius L, et al: A syndrome of autosomal dominant alternating hemiplegia: Clinical presentation mimicking intractable epilepsy; chromosomal studies; and physiologic investigations, *Neurology* 42:2251-2257, 1992.

179. Harvey AS, Jayakar P, Duchowny M, Resnick T, et al: Hemifacial seizures and cerebellar ganglioglioma: An epilepsy syndrome of infancy with seizures of cerebellar origin, *Ann Neurol* 40:91-98, 1996.

180. Zafeiriou DI, Mauromatis IV, Hatjisevastou HK, Bostantjopoulou MC, et al: Benign congenital hemifacial spasm, *Pediatr Neurol* 17:174-176, 1997.

181. Seay AR, Bray PF: Significance of seizures in infants weighing less than 2,500 grams, *Arch Neurol* 34:381-382, 1977.

182. Vigevano F, Di Capua M, Dalla Bernardina B: Startle disease: An avoidable cause of sudden infant death [letter], *Lancet* 1:216, 1989.

183. Pascotto A, Coppola G: Neonatal hyperekplexia: A case report, *Epilepsia* 33:817-820, 1992.

184. Matsumoto J, Fuhr P, Nigro M, Hallett M: Physiological abnormalities in hereditary hyperekplexia, *Ann Neurol* 32:41-50, 1992.

185. Nigro MA, Lim HC: Hyperekplexia and sudden neonatal death, *Pediatr Neurol* 8:221-225, 1992.

186. Zhou L, Chillag KL, Nigro MA: Hyperekplexia: A treatable neurogenetic disease, *Brain Dev* 24:669-674, 2002.

187. Shahar E, Raviv R: Sporadic major hyperekplexia in neonates and infants: Clinical manifestations and outcome, *Pediatr Neurol* 31:30-34, 2004.

188. Kleiman MD, DiMario FJ, Leconche DA, Zaineraitis EL: Benign transient downward gaze in preterm infants, *Pediatr Neurol* 10:313-316, 1994.

189. Miller VS, Packard AM: Paroxysmal downgaze in term newborn infants, *J Child Neurol* 13:294-296, 1998.

190. Guerrini R, Belmonte A, Carrozzo R: Paroxysmal tonic upgaze of childhood with ataxia: A benign transient dystonia with autosomal dominant inheritance, *Brain Dev* 20:116-118, 1998.

191. Hayman M, Harvey AS, Hopkins IJ, Kornberg AJ, et al: Paroxysmal tonic upgaze: A reappraisal of outcome, *Ann Neurol* 43:514-520, 1998.

192. Halliday AM: Evolving ideas on the neurophysiology of myoclonus. *Adv Neurol* 43:339-355, 1986.

193. Spencer SS, Spencer DD, Williamson PD, Mattson R: Combined depth and subdural electrode investigation in uncontrolled epilepsy, *Neurology* 40:74-79, 1990.

194. Devinsky O, Kelley K, Porter RJ, Theodore WH: Clinical and electroencephalographic features of simple partial seizures, *Neurology* 38:1347-1352, 1988.

195. Devinsky O, Sato S, Kufta CV, Ito B, et al: Electroencephalographic studies of simple partial seizures with subdural electrode recordings, *Neurology* 39:527-533, 1989.

196. Danner R, Shewmon DA, Sherman MP: Seizures in an atelencephalic infant: Is the cortex essential for neonatal seizures? *Arch Neurol* 42:1014-1016, 1985.

197. Berry-Kravis E, Huttenlocher PR, Wollmann RL: Isolated congenital malformation of hippocampal formation as a cause of intractable neonatal seizures [abstract], *Ann Neurol* 26:485, 1989.

198. Snead OC 3rd: Neonatal seizures [letter], *Neurology* 38:1897-1898, 1988.

199. Engel J Jr, Caldecott-Hazard S, Bandler R: Neurobiology of behavior: Anatomic and physiological implications related to epilepsy, *Epilepsia* 27:S3-S13, 1986.

200. Sussman NM, Jackel RA, Kaplan LR, Harner RN: Bicycling movements as a manifestation of complex partial seizures of temporal lobe origin, *Epilepsia* 30:527-531, 1989.

201. Hamby WB, Krauss RF, Beswick WF: Hydranencephaly: Clinical diagnosis—presentation of seven cases, *Pediatrics* 6:371-377, 1950.

202. Reding MJ, Kader FJ, Pellegrino RJ: Seizures in hydranencephaly: A report of two cases, *Electroencephalogr Clin Neurophysiol* 47:27, 1979.

203. McCown TJ, Breese GR: The developmental profile of seizure genesis in the inferior collicular cortex of the rat: Relevance to human neonatal seizures, *Epilepsia* 33:2-10, 1992.

204. Blennow G: Benign infantile nocturnal myoclonus, *Acta Paediatr Scand* 74:505-507, 1985.

205. Resnick TJ, Moshé SL, Perotta L, Chambers HJ: Benign neonatal sleep myoclonus: Relationship to sleep states, *Arch Neurol* 43:266-268, 1986.

206. Coulter DL, Allen RJ: Benign neonatal sleep myoclonus, *Arch Neurol* 39:191-192, 1982.

207. Calciolari G, Perlman JM, Volpe JJ: Seizures in the neonatal intensive care unit of the 1980s: Types, etiologies, timing, *Clin Pediatr* 27:119-123, 1988.

208. Andre M, Matisse N, Vert P, Debruille C: Neonatal seizures: Recent aspects, *Neuropediatrics* 19:201-207, 1988.

209. Rust RS, Volpe JJ: Neonatal Seizures. In Dodson WE, Pellock JM, editors: *Pediatric Epilepsy: Diagnosis and Therapy,* New York: 1993, Demos Publications.

210. Watkins A, Szymonowicz W, Jin X, Yu VV: Significance of seizures in very low-birthweight infants, *Dev Med Child Neurol* 30:162-169, 1988.

211. Ortibus EL, Sum JM, Hahn JS: Predictive value of EEG for outcome and epilepsy following neonatal seizures, *Electroencephalogr Clin Neurophysiol* 98:175-185, 1996.

212. Leth H, Toft PB, Herning M, Peitersen B, et al: Neonatal seizures associated with cerebral lesions shown by magnetic resonance imaging, *Arch Dis Child Fetal Neonatal Ed* 77:105-110, 1997.

213. Estan J, Hope P: Unilateral neonatal cerebral infarction in full term infants, *Arch Dis Child Fetal Neonatal Ed* 76:88-93, 1997.

214. Bye AME, Cunningham CA, Chee KY, Flanagan D: Outcome of neonates with electrographically identified seizures, or at risk of seizures, *Pediatr Neurol* 16:225-231, 1997.

215. Sheth RD: Electroencephalogram confirmatory rate in neonatal seizures, *Pediatr Neurol* 20:27-30, 1999.

216. Bruquell PJ, Glennon CM, DiMario FJ, Lerer T, et al: Prediction of outcome based on clinical seizure type in newborn infants, *J Pediatr* 140:707-712, 2002.

217. Garcias Da Silva LF, Nunes ML, Da Costa JC: Risk factors for developing epilepsy after neonatal seizures, *Pediatr Neurol* 30:271-277, 2004.

218. Kohelet D, Shochat R, Lusky A, Reichman B: Risk factors for neonatal seizures in very low birthweight infants: Population-based survey, *J Child Neurol* 19:123-128, 2004.

219. Tekgul H, Gauvreau K, Soul J, Murphy L, et al: The current etiologic profile and neurodevelopmental outcome of seizures in term newborn infants, *Pediatrics* 117:1270-1280, 2006.

220. Rose AL, Lombroso CT: A study of clinical, pathological, and electroencephalographic features in 137 full-term babies with a long-term follow-up, *Pediatrics* 45:404-425, 1970.

221. Tsiantos A, Victorin L, Relier JP, Dyer N, et al: Intracranial hemorrhage in the prematurely born infant: Timing of clots and evaluation of clinical signs and symptoms, *J Pediatr* 85:854-859, 1974.

222. Craig WB: Convulsive movements in the first ten days of life, *Arch Dis Child* 35:336-343, 1960.

223. Jackson AC, Gilbert JJ, Young GB, Bolton CF: The encephalopathy of sepsis, *Can J Neurol Sci* 12:303-307, 1985.

224. Koivisto M, Blanco SM, Krause U: Neonatal symptomatic and asymptomatic hypoglycaemia: A follow-up study of 151 children, *Dev Med Child Neurol* 14:603-614, 1972.

225. Cornblath M, Schwarz R: *Disorders of Carbohydrate Metabolism in Infancy*, 2nd ed, Philadelphia: 1976, WB Saunders.

226. Marshall R, Sheehan MM: Seizures in a neonatal intensive care unit: A prospective study, *Pediatr Res* 10:450, 1976.

227. Cockburn F, Brown JK, Belton NR, Forfar JO: Neonatal convulsions associated with primary disturbance of calcium, phosphorus, and magnesium metabolism, *Arch Dis Child* 48:99-108, 1973.

228. Chan GM, Venkataraman P, Tsang RC: The physiology of calcium in the human neonate. In Holick MF, Gray TK, Anast CS, editors: *Perinatal Calcium and Phosphorus Metabolism*, New York: 1983, Elsevier.

229. Visudhiphan P, Visudtibhan A, Chiemchanya S, Khongkhatithum C: Neonatal seizures and familial hypomagnesemia with secondary hypocalcemia, *Pediatr Neurol* 33:202-205, 2005.

230. Oki J, Takedatsu M, Itoh J, Yano K, et al: Hypocalcemic focal seizures in a one-month-old infant of a mother with a low circulating level of vitamin D, *Brain Dev* 13:132-134, 1991.

231. Lynch BJ, Rust RS: Natural history and outcome of neonatal hypocalcemic and hypomagnesemic seizures, *Pediatr Neurol* 11:23-27, 1994.

231a. Gorman MP, Soul JS: Neonatal hypocalcemic seizures in siblings exposed to topiramate in utero, *Pediatr Neurol* 36:274-276, 2007.

232. Abdulrazzaq YM, Smigura FC, Wettrell G: Primary infantile hypomagnesaemia: Report of two cases and review of literature, *Eur J Pediatr* 148:459-461, 1989.

233. Shalev H, Phillip M, Galil A, Carmi R, et al: Clinical presentation and outcome in primary familial hypomagnesaemia, *Arch Dis Child* 78:127-130, 1998.

234. Kim WY, Pomerance JJ, Miller AA: Lidocaine intoxication in a newborn following local anesthesia for episiotomy, *Pediatrics* 64:643-645, 1979.

235. Finster M, Poppers PJ, Sinclair JC: Accidental intoxication of the fetus with local anesthetic drug during caudal anesthesia, *Am J Obstet Gynecol* 92:922, 1965.

236. Sinclair JC, Fox HA, Lentz JF, Fuld GL, et al: Intoxication of the fetus by a local anesthetic: A newly recognized complication of maternal caudal anesthesia, *N Engl J Med* 273:1173-1177, 1965.

237. O'Meara OP, Brazie JV: Neonatal intoxication after paracervical block, *N Engl J Med* 278:1127-1128, 1968.

238. Gordon HR: Fetal bradycardia after paracervical block, *N Engl J Med* 279:910, 1968.

239. Shnider SM, Asling JH, Margolis AJ: High fetal blood levels of mepivacaine and fetal bradycardia, *N Engl J Med* 279:947, 1968.

240. Shnider SM, Way EL: Plasma levels of lidocaine (Xylocaine) in mother and newborn following obstetrical conduction anesthesia: Clinical applications, *Anesthesiology* 29:951-958, 1968.

241. Chase D, Brady JP: Ventricular tachycardia in a neonate with mepivacaine toxicity, *J Pediatr* 90:127-129, 1977.

242. Dodson WE, Hillman RE, Hillman LS: Brain tissue levels in a fatal case of neonatal mepivacaine (Carbocaine) poisoning, *J Pediatr* 86:624-627, 1975.

243. Morishima HO, Daniel SS, Finster M, Poppers PJ, et al: Transmission of mepivacaine hydrochloride (Carbocaine) across the human placenta, *Anesthesiology* 27:147-154, 1966.

244. Lurie AO, Weiss JB: Blood concentration of mepivacaine and lidocaine in mother and baby after epidural anesthesia, *Am J Obstet Gynecol* 106:850-856, 1970.

245. De Praeter C, Vanhaesebrouck P, De PN, Govaert P, et al: Episiotomy and neonatal lidocaine intoxication [letter], *Eur J Pediatr* 150:685-686, 1991.

246. Hillman LS, Hillman RE, Dodson WE: Diagnosis, treatment, and follow-up of neonatal mepivacaine intoxication secondary to paracervical and pudendal blocks during labor, *J Pediatr* 95:472-477, 1979.

247. Vanapruks V, Prapaitrakul K: Water intoxication and hyponatraemic convulsions in neonates, *Arch Dis Child* 64:734-735, 1989.

248. Hogan GR, Dodge PR, Gill SR, Master S, et al: Pathogenesis of seizures occurring during restoration of plasma tonicity to normal in animals previously chronically hypernatremic, *Pediatrics* 43:54-64, 1969.

249. Hogan GR, Dodge PR, Gill SR: The incidence of seizures after rehydration of hypernatremic rabbits with intravenous or ad libitum oral fluids, *Pediatr Res* 18:340, 1983.

250. Schiffmann R, Kaye EM, Willis JK 3rd, Africk D, et al: Transient neonatal hyperglycinemia, *Ann Neurol* 25:201-203, 1989.

251. Bejsovec M, Kulenda Z, Ponca E: Familial intrauterine convulsions in pyridoxine dependency, *Arch Dis Child* 42:201-207, 1967.

252. Scriver CR: Vitamin B$_6$-dependency and infantile convulsions, *Pediatrics* 25:62, 1960.

253. Heeley A, Pugh RJ, Clayton BE, Shepherd J, et al: Pyridoxol metabolism in vitamin B$_6$–responsive convulsions of early infancy, *Arch Dis Child* 53:794-802, 1978.

254. Clarke TA, Saunders BS, Feldman B: Pyridoxine-dependent seizures requiring high doses of pyridoxine for control, *Am J Dis Child* 133:963-965, 1979.

255. Bankier A, Turner M, Hopkins IJ: Pyridoxine-dependent seizures: A wider clinical spectrum, *Arch Dis Child* 58:415-418, 1983.

256. Goutieres F, Aicardi J: Atypical presentations of pyridoxine-dependent seizures: A treatable cause of intractable epilepsy in infants, *Ann Neurol* 17:117-120, 1985.

257. Pettit RE: Pyridoxine dependency seizures: Report of a case with unusual features, *J Child Neurol* 2:38-40, 1987.

258. Mikati MA, Trevathan E, Krishnamoorthy KS, Lombroso CT: Pyridoxine-dependent epilepsy: EEG investigations and long-term follow-up, *Electroencephalogr Clin Neurophysiol* 78:215-221, 1991.

259. Tanaka R, Okumura M, Arima J, Yamakura S, et al: Pyridoxine-dependent seizures: Report of a case with atypical clinical features and abnormal MRI scans, *J Child Neurol* 7:24-28, 1992.

260. Jardin LB, Pires RF, Martins CE, Vargas CR, et al: Pyridoxine-dependent seizures associated with white matter abnormalities, *Neuropediatrics* 25:249-261, 1994.

261. Baxter P, Griffiths P, Kelly T, Gardner-Medwin D: Pyridoxine-dependent seizures: Demographic, clinical, MRI and psychometric features, and effect of dose on intelligence quotient, *Dev Med Child Neurol* 38:998-1006, 1996.

262. Shih JJ, Kornblum H, Shewmon DA: Global brain dysfunction in an infant with pyridoxine dependency: Evaluation with EEG, evoked potentials, MRI, and PET, *Neurology* 47:824-826, 1996.

263. Gordon N: Pyridoxine dependency: An update, *Dev Med Child Neurol* 39:63-65, 1997.

264. Gospe SM: Current perspectives on pyridoxine-dependent seizures, *J Pediatr* 132:919-923, 1998.

265. Gospe SM, Hecht ST: Longitudinal MRI findings in pyridoxine-dependent seizures, *Neurology* 51:74-78, 1998.

266. Hammen A, Wagner B, Berkhoff M, Donati F: A paradoxical rise of neonatal seizures after treatment with vitamin B6, *Eur J Paediatr Neurol* 2:319-322, 1998.

267. Ohtsuka Y, Hattori J, Ishida T, Ogino T, et al: Long-term follow-up of an individual with vitamin B$_6$-dependent seizures, *Dev Med Child Neurol* 41:203-206, 1999.

268. Grillo E, da Silva RJM, Barbato JH: Pyridoxine-dependent seizures responding to extremely low-dose pyridoxine, *Dev Med Child Neurol* 43:413-415, 2001.

269. Baxter P: Pyridoxine-dependent and pyridoxine-response seizures, *Dev Med Child Neurol* 43:416-420, 2001.

270. Goto T, Matsuo N, Takahashi T: CSF glutamate/GABA concentrations in pyridoxine-dependent seizures: Etiology of pyridoxine-dependent seizures and the mechanisms of pyridoxine action in seizure control, *Brain Dev* 23:24-29, 2001.

271. Kuo M-F, Wang H-S: Pyridoxal phosphate-responsive epilepsy with resistance to pyridoxine, *Pediatr Neurol* 25:146-147, 2002.

272. Baynes K, Gospe SM Jr: Pyridoxine-dependent seizures and cognition in adulthood, *Dev Med Child Neurol* 45:782-785, 2003.

273. Gospe SM Jr: Pyridoxine-dependent seizures: Findings from recent studies pose new questions, *Pediatr Neurol* 26:181-186, 2002.

274. Tan H, Kardas F, Buyukavci M, Karakelleoglu C: Pyridoxine-dependent seizures and microcephaly, *Pediatr Neurol* 31:211-213, 2004.

275. Plecko B, Hikel C, Korenke GC, Schmitt B, et al: Pipecolic acid as a diagnostic marker of pyridoxine-dependent epilepsy, *Neuropediatrics* 36:200-205, 2005.

275a. Bok LA, Struys E, Willemsen MA, Been JV, et al: Pyridoxine-dependent seizures in Dutch patients: Diagnosis by elevated urinary alpha-aminoadipic semialdehyde levels, *Arch Dis Child* 92:687-689, 2007.

276. Yoshii A, Takeoka M, Kelly PJ, Krishnamoorthy KS: Focal status epilepticus as atypical presentation of pyridoxine-dependent epilepsy, *J Child Neurol* 20:696-698, 2005.

277. Ramachandrannair R, Parameswaran M: Prevalence of pyridoxine dependent seizures in south Indian children with early onset intractable epilepsy: A hospital based prospective study, *Eur J Paediatr Neurol* 9:409-413, 2005.

277a. Rankin PM, Harrison S, Chong WK, Boyd S, et al: Pyridoxine-dependent seizures: A family phenotype that leads to severe cognitive deficits, regardless of treatment regime, *Dev Med Child Neurol* 49:300-305, 2007.

278. Coker SB: Postneonatal vitamin B$_6$-dependent epilepsy, *Pediatrics* 90:221-223, 1992.

279. Yoshida T, Tada K, Arakawa T: Vitamin B6 dependency of glutamic acid decarboxylase in the kidney from a patient with vitamin B$_6$ dependent convulsion, *Tohoku J Exp Med* 104:195-198, 1971.

280. Plecko B, Paul K, Paschke E, Stoeckler-Ipsiroglu S, et al: Biochemical and molecular characterization of 18 patients with pyridoxine-dependent epilepsy and mutations of the antiquitin (ALDH7A1) gene, *Hum Mutat* 28:19-26, 2007.

280a. Hoffmann GF, Schmitt B, Windfuhr M, Wagner N, et al: Pyridoxal 5′-phosphate may be curative in early-onset epileptic encephalopathy, *J Inherit Metab Dis* 30:96-99, 2007.

281. Hyland K: Folinic acid responsive seizures. In Baxter P, editor: *Vitamin Responsive Conditions in Paediatric Neurology*, London: 2002, MacKeith Press.

282. Hyland K, Buist NR, Powell BR, Hoffman GF, et al: Folinic acid responsive seizures: A new syndrome, *J Inherit Metab Dis* 18:177-181, 1995.

283. Torres OA, Miller VS, Buist NM, Hyland K: Folinic acid–responsive neonatal seizures, *J Child Neurol* 14:529-532, 1999.

284. Frye RE, Donner E, Golja A, Rooney CM: Folinic acid–responsive seizures presenting as breakthrough seizures in a 3-month-old boy, *J Child Neurol* 18:562-569, 2003.

285. Nicolai J, van Kranen-Mastenbroek VH, Wevers RA, Hurkx WA, et al: Folinic acid–responsive seizures initially responsive to pyridoxine, *Pediatr Neurol* 34:164-167, 2006.

286. De Vivo DC, Trifiletti RR, Jacobson RI, Ronen GM, et al: Defective glucose transport across the blood-brain barrier as a cause of persistent hypoglycorrhachia, seizures, and developmental delay, *N Engl J Med* 325:703-709, 1991.

287. Fishman RA: The glucose-transporter protein and glucopenic brain injury, *N Engl J Med* 325:731-732, 1991.

288. Kollros PR, Harik SI: A patient with dysfunction of glucose transport at the blood-brain barrier but normal cytochalasin B binding and immunological reactivity to glucose transporter protein on erythrocyte membranes [abstract], *Ann Neurol* 30:451, 1991.

289. Klepper J, Wang D, Fischbarg J, Vera JC, et al: Defective glucose transport across brain tissue barriers: A newly recognized neurological syndrome, *Neurochem Res* 24:587-594, 1999.

290. Brockmann K, Wang D, Korenke CG, von Moers A, et al: Autosomal dominant Glut-1 deficiency syndrome and familial epilepsy, *Ann Neurol* 2001:50, 2002.

291. Gordon N, Newton N: Glucose transporter type 1 (GLUT-2) deficiency, *Brain Dev* 27:477-480, 2003.

292. Leary LD, Wang T, Nordli DR, Engelstad K, et al: Seizure characterization and electroencephalographic features in Glut-1 deficiency syndrome, *Epilepsia* 44:701-707, 2003.

293. Wang D, Pascual JM, Yang H, Engelstad K, et al: Glut-1 deficiency syndrome: Clinical, genetic, and therapeutic aspects, *Ann Neurol* 57:111-118, 2005.

294. Klepper J, Scheffer H, Leiendecker B, Gertsen E, et al: Seizure control and acceptance of the ketogenic diet in GLUT1 deficiency syndrome: A 2- to 5-year follow-up of 15 children enrolled prospectively, *Neuropediatrics* 36:302-308, 2005.

295. Fujii T, Ho YY, Wang D, De Vivo DC, et al: Three Japanese patients with glucose transporter type 1 deficiency syndrome, *Brain Dev* 29:92-97, 2007.

295a. Pascual JM, Wang D, Hinton V, Engelstad K, et al: Brain glucose supply and the syndrome of infantile neuroglycopenia, *Arch Neurol* 64:507-513, 2007.

295b. Klepper J, Leiendecker B: GLUT1 deficiency syndrome—2007 update, *Dev Med Child Neurol* 49:707-716, 2007.

296. Bjerre I, Corelius E: Benign familial neonatal convulsions, *Acta Paediatr Scand* 57:557-561, 1968.

297. Quattlebaum TG: Benign familial convulsions in the neonatal period and early infancy, *J Pediatr* 95:257-259, 1979.

298. Brown JK, Cockburn F, Forfar JO: Clinical and chemical correlates in convulsions of the newborn, *Lancet* 1:135-139, 1972.

299. Pettit RE, Fenichel GM: Benign familial neonatal seizures, *Arch Neurol* 37:47-48, 1980.

300. Tibbles JA: Dominant benign neonatal seizures, *Dev Med Child Neurol* 22:664-667, 1980.

301. Takebe Y, Chiba C, Kimura S: Benign familial neonatal convulsions, *Brain Dev* 5:319-322, 1983.

302. Zonana J, Silvey K, Strimling B: Familial neonatal and infantile seizures: An autosomal-dominant disorder, *Am J Med Genet* 18:455-459, 1984.

303. Leppert M, Anderson VE, Quattlebaum T, Stauffer D, et al: Benign familial neonatal convulsions linked to genetic markers on chromosome 20, *Nature* 337:647-648, 1989.

304. Webb R, Bobele G: "Benign" familial neonatal convulsions, *J Child Neurol* 5:295-298, 1990.

305. Ryan SG, Wiznitzer M, Hollman C, Torres MC, et al: Benign familial neonatal convulsions: Evidence for clinical and genetic heterogeneity, *Ann Neurol* 29:469-473, 1991.

306. Camfield PR, Dooley J, Gordon K, Orlik P: Benign familial neonatal convulsions are epileptic, *J Child Neurol* 6:340-342, 1991.

307. Miles DK, Holmes GL: Benign neonatal seizures, *J Clin Neurophysiol* 7:369-379, 1990.

308. Malafosse A, Leboyer M, Dulac O, Navelet Y, et al: Confirmation of linkage of benign familial neonatal convulsions to D20S19 and D20S20, *Hum Genet* 89:54-58, 1992.

309. Ronen GM, Rosales TO, Connolly M, Anderson VE, et al: Seizure characteristics in chromosome 20 benign familial neonatal convulsions, *Neurology* 43:1355-1360, 1993.

310. Hirsch E, Velez A, Sellal F, Maton B, et al: Electroclinical signs of benign neonatal familial convulsions, *Ann Neurol* 34:835-841, 1993.

311. Bye AME: Neonate with benign familial neonatal convulsions: Recorded generalized and focal seizures, *Pediatr Neurol* 10:164-165, 1994.

312. Bievert C, Schroeder BC, Kubisch C, Berkovic SF, et al: A potassium channel mutation in neonatal human epilepsy, *Science* 279:403-406, 1998.

313. Lerche H, Bievert C, Alekov AK, Schleithoff L, et al: A reduced K$^+$ current due to a novel mutation in KCNQ2 causes neonatal convulsions, *Ann Neurol* 46:305-312, 1999.

314. Hirose S, Zenri F, Fukuma G, Inoue T, et al: A novel mutation of KCNQ3 (c.925T-C) in a Japanese family with benign familial neonatal convulsions, *Ann Neurol* 47:822-826, 2000.

315. Castaldo P, del Giudice EM, Coppola G, Pascotto A, et al: Benign familial neonatal convulsions caused by altered gating of KCNQ2/KCNQ3 potassium channels, *J Neurosci* 22:1-6, 2002.

316. Coppola G, Castaldo P, del Giudice M, Bellini G, et al: A novel KCNQ2 K$^+$ channel mutation in benign neonatal convulsions and centrotemporal spikes, *Neurology* 61:131-134, 2003.

317. Singh NA, Westenskow P, Charlier C, Pappas C, et al: KCNQ2 and KCNQ3 potassium channel genes in benign familial neonatal convulsions: Expansion of the functional and mutation spectrum, *Brain* 126:2726-2737, 2003.

318. Claes LR, Ceulemans B, Audenaert D, Deprez L, et al: De novo KCNQ2 mutations in patients with benign neonatal seizures, *Neurology* 63:2155-2158, 2004.

319. Berkovic SF, Heron SE, Giordano L, Marini C, et al: Benign familial neonatal-infantile seizures: Characterization of a new sodium channelopathy, *Ann Neurol* 55:550-557, 2004.

320. Heron SE, Crossland KM, Andermann E, Phillips HA, et al: Sodium-channel defects in benign familial neonatal-infantile seizures, *Lancet* 360:851-852, 2002.

321. Pryor DS, Don N, Macourt DC: Fifth day fits: A syndrome of neonatal convulsions, *Arch Dis Child* 56:753-758, 1981.

322. Goldberg RN, Goldman SL, Ramsay RE, Feller R: Detection of seizure activity in the paralyzed neonate using continuous monitoring, *Pediatrics* 69:583-586, 1982.

323. Goldberg HJ: Neonatal convulsions: A 10 year review, *Arch Dis Child* 58:976-978, 1983.

324. Dehan M, Quillerou D, Navelet Y, D'Allest AM, et al: Convulsions in the fifth day of life: A new syndrome? *Arch Fr Pediatr* 34:730-742, 1977.

325. Fabris C, Licata D, Stasiowska B, Lio C, et al: Is type of feeding related to fifth day fits of the newborns? Unexpected outcome of a case-control study, *Acta Paediatr Scand* 77:162, 1988.

326. Plouin P: Benign neonatal convulsions. In Wasterlain CG, Vert P, editors: *Neonatal Seizures*, New York: 1990, Raven Press.

327. Alfonso I, Hahn JS, Papazian O, Martinez YL, et al: Bilateral tonic-clonic epileptic seizures in non-benign familial neonatal convulsions, *Pediatr Neurol* 16:249-251, 1997.

328. Guerra MP, Wilson GA, Boylan GB, Rennie JM: An unusual presentation of fifth-day fits in the newborn, *Pediatr Neurol* 26:398-401, 2002.

329. Goldberg HJ, Sheehy EM: Fifth day fits: An acute zinc deficiency syndrome? *Arch Dis Child* 57:633-635, 1982.

330. Aicardi J, Goutieres F: [Neonatal myoclonic encephalopathy (author's transl)], *Rev Electroencephalogr Neurophysiol Clin* 8:99-101, 1978.

331. Aicardi J: Early myoclonic encephalopathy. In Roger J, Dravet C, Bureau M, et al, editors: *Epileptic Syndromes in Infancy, Childhood and Adolescence*, London, 1985, John Libbey Eurotext.

332. Dalla Bernardina B, Colamaria V, Capovilla G, Bondavalli S: Nosological classification of epilepsies in the first three years of life. In Nistico G, DePerri R, Meinardi H, editors: *Epilepsy: An Update On Research and Therapy*, New York: 1983, Alan R. Liss.

333. Lombroso CT: Early myoclonic encephalopathy, early infantile epileptic encephalopathy, and benign and severe infantile myoclonic epilepsies: A critical review and personal contributions, *J Clin Neurophysiol* 7:380-408, 1990.

334. Ohtahara S, Ohtsuka Y, Yamatogi Y, Oka E: The early-infantile epileptic encephalopathy with suppression-burst: Developmental aspects, *Brain Dev* 9:371-376, 1987.

335. Otani K, Abe J, Futagi Y, Yabuuchi H, et al: Clinical and electroencephalographical follow-up study of early myoclonic encephalopathy, *Brain Dev* 11:332-337, 1989.

336. Robain O, Dulac O: Early epileptic encephalopathy with suppression bursts and olivary-dentate dysplasia, *Neuropediatrics* 23:162-164, 1992.

337. Ogihara M, Kinoue K, Takamiya H, Nemoto S, et al: A case of early infantile epileptic encephalopathy (EIEE) with anatomical cerebral asymmetry and myoclonus, *Brain Dev* 15:133-139, 1993.

338. du Plessis AJ, Kaufmann WE, William MD, Kupsky WJ: Intrauterine-onset myoclonic encephalopathy associated with cerebral cortical dysgenesis, *J Child Neurol* 8:164-170, 1993.

339. Williams AN, Gray RG, Poulton K, Ramani P, et al: A case of Ohtahara syndrome with cytochrome oxidase deficiency, *Dev Med Child Neurol* 40:568-570, 1998.

340. Miller SP, Dilenge M-E, Meagher-Villemure K, O'Gorman AM, et al: Infantile epileptic encephalopathy (Ohtahara syndrome) and migrational disorder, *Pediatr Neurol* 19:50-54, 1998.

341. Wang P-J, Lee W-T, Hwu W-L, Young C, et al: The controversy regarding diagnostic criteria for early myoclonic encephalopathy, *Brain Dev* 20:530-535, 1998.

342. Trinka E, Rauscher C, Nagler M, Moroder T, et al: A case of Ohtahara syndrome with olivary-dentate dysplasia and agenesis of mamillary bodies, *Epilepsia* 42:950-953, 2001.

343. Krsek P, Sebronova V, Prochazka T, Maulisova A, et al: Successful treatment of Ohtahara syndrome with chloral hydrate, *Pediatr Neurol* 27:388-391, 2002.

344. Yamatogi Y, Ohtahara S: Early-infantile epileptic encephalopathy with suppression-bursts, Ohtahara syndrome: Its overview referring to our 16 cases, *Brain Dev* 24:13-23, 2002.

345. Clayton PT, Surtees RAH, DeVile C, Hyland K, et al: Neonatal epileptic encephalopathy, *Lancet* 361:1614, 2003.

346. Brautigam C, Hyland K, Wevers RA, Sharma R, et al: Clinical and laboratory findings in twins with neonatal epileptic encephalopathy mimicking aromatic L-amino acid decarboxylase deficiency, *Neuropediatrics* 33:113-117, 2002.

347. Korff CM, Nordli DR Jr: Epilepsy syndromes in infancy, *Pediatr Neurol* 34:253-263, 2006.

348. Saito Y, Hayashi M, Miyazono Y, Shimogama T, et al: Arthrogryposis multiplex congenita with callosal agenesis and dentato-olivary dysplasia, *Brain Dev* 28:261-264, 2006.

349. Raspall M, Ortega-Aznar A, Del Toro M, Roig M, et al: Neonatal rigid-akinetic syndrome and dentato-olivary dysplasia, *Pediatr Neurol* 34:132-134, 2006.

350. Coppola G, Plouin P, Chiron C, Robain O, et al: Migrating partial seizures in infancy: A malignant disorder with developmental arrest, *Epilepsia* 36:1017-1024, 1995.

351. Wilmshurst JM, Appleton DB, Grattan-Smith PJ: Migrating partial seizures in infancy: Two new cases, *J Child Neurol* 15:717-722, 2000.

352. Ishii K, Oguni H, Hayashi K, Shirakawa S, et al: Clinical study of catastrophic infantile epilepsy with focal seizures, *Pediatr Neurol* 27:369-377, 2002.

353. Gross-Tsur V, Ben-Zeev B, Shalev RS: Malignant migrating partial seizures in infancy, *Pediatr Neurol* 31:287-290, 2004.

354. Marsh E, Melamed SE, Barron T, Clancy RR: Migrating partial seizures in infancy: Expanding the phenotype of a rare seizure syndrome, *Epilepsia* 46:568-572, 2005.

355. Hmaimess G, Kadhim H, Nassogne MC, Bonnier C, et al: Levetiracetam in a neonate with malignant migrating partial seizures, *Pediatr Neurol* 34:55-59, 2006.

356. Coppola G, Veggiotti P, Del Giudice EM, Bellini G, et al: Mutational scanning of potassium, sodium and chloride ion channels in malignant migrating partial seizures in infancy, *Brain Dev* 28:76-79, 2006.

357. Reggin JD, Johnson MI: Exacerbation of benign neonatal sleep myoclonus by benzodiazepines [abstract], *Ann Neurol* 26:455, 1989.

358. Daoustroy J, Seshia SS: Benign neonatal sleep myoclonus: A differential diagnosis of neonatal seizures, *Am J Dis Child* 146:1236-1241, 1992.

359. Alfonso I, Papazian O, Aicardi J, Jeffries HE: A simple maneuver to provoke benign neonatal sleep myoclonus, *Pediatrics* 96:1161-1163, 1995.

360. Ramelli GP, Sozzo AB, Vella S, Bianchetti MG: Benign neonatal sleep myoclonus: An under-recognized, non-epileptic condition, *Acta Paediatr* 94:962-963, 2005.

360a. Cohen R, Shuper A, Straussberg R: Familial benign neonatal sleep myoclonus, *Pediatr Neurol* 36:334-337, 2007.

361. Gordon N: Startle disease or hyperekplexia, *Dev Med Child Neurol* 35:1015-1022, 1993.

362. McAbee GN, Kadakia SK, Sisley KC, Delfiner JS: Complete heart block in nonfamilial hyperekplexia, *Pediatr Neurol* 12:149-151, 1995.

363. Gherpelli JLD, Nogueira AR, Troster EJ, Deutsch AD, et al: Hyperekplexia, a cause of neonatal apnea: A case report, *Brain Dev* 17:114-116, 1995.

364. Leventer RJ, Hopkins IJ, Shield LK: Hyperekplexia as cause of abnormal intrauterine movements, *Lancet* 345:461, 1995.

365. Vergouwe MN, Tijssen MA, Peters CB, Wichard R, et al: Hyperexplexia phenotype due to compound heterozygosity for GLRA1 gene mutations, *Ann Neurol* 46:634-638, 1999.

366. Kimura M, Taketani T, Horie A, Isumi H, et al: Two Japanese families with hyperekplexia who have a Arg271Gln mutation in the glycine receptor alpha 1 subunit gene, *Brain Dev* 28:228-231, 2006.

367. Rivera S, Villega F, de Saint-Martin A, Matis J, et al: Congenital hyperekplexia: Five sporadic cases, *Eur J Pediatr* 165:104-107, 2006.

368. Shiang R, Ryan SG, Zhu Y-Z, Fielder TJ, et al: Mutational analysis of familial and sporadic hyperekplexia, *Ann Neurol* 38:85-91, 1995.

369. Floeter MK, Andermann F, Andermann E, Nigro M, et al: Physiological studies of spinal inhibitory pathways in patients with hereditary hyperekplexia, *Neurology* 46:766-772, 1996.

370. Saul B, Kuner T, Sobetzko D, Brune W, et al: Novel GLRA1 missense mutation (P250T) in dominant hyperekplexia defines an intracellular determinant of glycine receptor channel gating, *J Neurosci* 19:869-877, 1999.

371. Hellström-Westas L, Rosén I, Swenningsen NW: Silent seizures in sick infants in early life. Diagnosis by continuous cerebral function monitoring, *Acta Paediatr Scand* 74:741-748, 1985.

372. Werner SS, Stockard JE, Bickford RG: *Atlas of Neonatal Electroencephalography*, New York: 1977, Raven Press.

373. Lombroso CT: Convulsive disorders in newborns. In Thompson RA, Green R, editors: *Pediatric Neurology and Neurosurgery*, New York: 1978, Spectrum Press.

374. Tharp BR: Neonatal electroencephalography. In Korobkin R, Guilleminault C, editors: *Progress in Perinatal Neurology*, Baltimore: 1981, Williams and Wilkins.

375. Pedley TA, Lombroso CT, Hanley JW: Introduction to neonatal electroencephalography: Interpretation, *Am J EEG Technol* 21:15, 1981.

376. Tharp BR: Pediatric electroencephalography. In Aminoff MJ, editor: *Electrodiagnosis in Clinical Neurology*, New York: 1980, Churchill Livingstone.

377. Stockard-Pope JE, Werner SS, Bickford RG: *Atlas of Neonatal Electroencephalography*, New York: 1992, Raven Press.

378. Hrachovy RA, Mizrahi EM, Kellaway P: Electroencephalography of the newborn. In Daly DD, Pedley TA, editors: *Current Practice of Clinical Electroencephalography*, 2nd ed, New York: 1990, Raven Press.

379. Mizrahi EM, Hrachovy RA, Kellaway P: *Atlas of Neonatal Electroencephalography*, 3rd ed, Philadelphia: 2004, Lippincott Williams & Wilkins.

380. Holmes GL, Moshe SL, Jones HR Jr: *Clinical Neurophysiology of Infancy, Childhood, and Adolescence*, Philadelphia: 2006, Elsevier.

381. Clancy RR, Legido A, Lewis D: Occult neonatal seizures, *Epilepsia* 29:256-261, 1988.

382. Scher MS, Alvin J, Gaus L, Minnigh B, et al: Uncoupling of EEG-clinical neonatal seizures after antiepileptic drug use, *Pediatr Neurol* 28:277-280, 2003.

383. Shany E, Khvatskin S, Golan A, Karplus M: Amplitude-integrated electroencephalography: A tool for monitoring silent seizures in neonates, *Pediatr Neurol* 34:194-199, 2006.

384. Stein V, Hermans-Borgmeyer I, Jentsch TJ, Hubner CA: Expression of the KC1 cotransporter KCC2 parallels neuronal maturation and the emergence of low intracellular chloride, *J Comp Neurol* 468:57-64, 2004.

385. Tekgul H, Bourgeois B, Gauvreau K, Bergin A: EEG in neonatal seizures: Comparison of a reduced and a full 10/20 montage, *Pediatr Neurol* 32:155-161, 2005.

386. Clancy RR, Legido A: The exact ictal and interictal duration of electroencephalographic neonatal seizures, *Epilepsia* 28:537-541, 1987.

387. Clancy RR: Interictal sharp EEG transients in neonatal seizures, *J Child Neurol* 4:30-38, 1989.

388. Monod N, Dreyfus-Brisac C: Le tracé paroxystique chez le nouveau né, *Rev Neurol* 106:129, 1962.

389. Harris R, Tizzard JPM: The electroencephalogram in neonatal convulsions, *J Pediatr* 57:501, 1960.

390. Keith HM: Convulsions in children under three years of age: A study of prognosis, *Mayo Clin Proc* 39:895, 1964.

391. McInery TK, Schubert WK: Prognosis of neonatal seizures, *Am J Dis Child* 117:261, 1969.

392. Dennis J: Neonatal convulsions: Aetiology, late neonatal status and long-term outcome, *Dev Med Child Neurol* 20:143-148, 1978.

393. Eriksson M, Zetterstrom R: Neonatal convulsions: Incidence and causes in the Stockholm area, *Acta Paediatr Scand* 68:807-811, 1979.

394. Holden KR, Mellits ED, Freeman JM: Neonatal seizures. I. Correlation of prenatal and perinatal events with outcomes, *Pediatrics* 70:165-176, 1982.

395. van Zeben ADM, Verloove-Vanhorick SP, den Ouden L, Brand R, et al: Neonatal seizures in very preterm and very low birthweight infants: Mortality and handicaps at two years of age in a nationwide cohort, *Neuropediatrics* 21:62-65, 1990.

396. André M, Vert P, Wasterlain CG: To treat or not to treat: A survey of current medical practice toward neonatal seizures. In Wasterlain CG, Vert P, editors: *Neonatal Seizures*, New York: 1990, Raven Press.

397. Temple CM, Dennis J, Carney R, Sharich J: Neonatal seizures: Long-term outcome and cognitive development among "normal" survivors, *Dev Med Child Neurol* 37:109-118, 1995.

397a. Ronen GM, Buckley D, Penney S, Streiner DL: Long-term prognosis in children with neonatal seizures: A population-based study, *Neurology* 69:1816-1822, 2007.

398. Tibbles JAR, Prichard JS: The prognostic value of the electroencephalogram in neonatal convulsions, *Pediatrics* 35:778, 1965.

399. Dreyfus-Brisac C: Neonatal electroencephalography, *Rev Perinatal Pediatr* 3:397-402, 1979.

400. Tharp BR, Cukier F, Monod N: The prognostic value of the electroencephalogram in premature infants, *Electroencephalogr Clin Neurophysiol* 51:219-236, 1981.

401. Lombroso CT: Prognosis in neonatal seizures. *Adv Neurol* 34:101-113, 1983.

402. Rowe JC, Holmes GL, Hafford J, Baboval D, et al: Prognostic value of the electroencephalogram in term and preterm infants following neonatal seizures, *Electroencephalogr Clin Neurophysiol* 60:183-196, 1985.

403. Boylan GB, Pressier RM, Rennie JM, Morton M, et al: Outcome of electroclinical and clinical seizures in the newborn infant, *Dev Med Child Neurol* 41:819-825, 1999.

404. Menache CC, Bourgeois BFD, Volpe JJ: Prognostic value of neonatal discontinuous EEG, *Pediatr Neurol* 27:93-101, 2002.

405. Grigg-Damberger MM, Coker SB, Halsey CL, Anderson CL: Neonatal burst suppression: Its developmental significance, *Pediatr Neurol* 5:84-92, 1989.

406. Biagioni E, Bartalena L, Boldrini A, Pieri R, et al: Constantly discontinuous EEG patterns in full-term neonates with hypoxic-ischaemic encephalopathy, *Clin Neurophysiol* 110:1510-1515, 1999.

407. Douglass LM, Wu JY, Rosman NP, Stafstrom CE: Burst suppression electroencephalogram pattern in the newborn: Predicting the outcome, *J Child Neurol* 17:403-408, 2002.

408. Sarnat HB, Sarnat MS: Neonatal encephalopathy following fetal distress: A clinical and electroencephalographic study, *Arch Neurol* 33:696-705, 1976.

409. Lilien LD, Grajwer LA, Pildes RS: Treatment of neonatal hypoglycemia with continuous intravenous glucose infusion, *J Pediatr* 91:779-782, 1977.

410. Lockman LA, Kriel R, Zaske D, Thompson T, et al: Phenobarbital dosage for control of neonatal seizures, *Neurology* 29:1445-1449, 1979.

411. Painter MJ, Alvin J: Choice of anticonvulsants in the treatment of neonatal seizures. In Wasterlain CG, Vert P, editors: *Neonatal Seizures*, New York: 1990, Raven Press.

412. Van Orman CB, Darwish HZ: Efficacy of phenobarbital in neonatal seizures, *Can J Neurol Sci* 12:95-99, 1985.

413. Gilman JT, Gal P, Duchowny MS, Weaver RL, et al: Rapid sequential phenobarbital treatment of neonatal seizures, *Pediatrics* 83:674-678, 1989.

414. Gherpelli JLD, Cruz AM, Tsanaclis LM, Costa HPF, et al: Phenobarbital in newborns with neonatal seizures: A study of plasma levels after intravenous administration, *Brain Dev* 15:258-262, 1993.

415. Grasela TH Jr, Donn SM: Neonatal population pharmacokinetics of phenobarbital derived from routine clinical data, *Dev Pharmacol Ther* 8:374-383, 1985.

416. De Carolis MP, Muzii U, Romagnoli C, Zuppa AA, et al: Phenobarbital for treatment of seizures in preterm infant: A new administration scheme, *Dev Pharmacol Ther* 14:84-89, 1990.

417. Gal P, Toback J, Erkan NV, Boer HR: The influence of asphyxia on phenobarbital dosing requirements in neonates, *Dev Pharmacol Ther* 7:145-152, 1984.

418. Painter MJ, Scher MS, Stein AD, Armatti S, et al: Phenobarbital compared with phenytoin for the treatment of neonatal seizures, *N Engl J Med* 341:485-489, 1999.

419. Shirer AE: Fosphenytoin sodium (Cerebyx, Parke-Davis): Where will it fit in? In *Question-of-the-Month*, Westchester, NY: 1996, Drug Intelligence Center.

420. Morton LD, Rizkallah E, Pellock JM: New drug therapy for acute seizure management, *Semin Pediatr Neurol* 4:51-63, 1997.

421. Morton LD: Clinical experience with fosphenytoin in children, *J Child Neurol* 13:S19-S22, 1998.

422. Takeoka M, Krishamoorthy KS, Soman TB, Caviness vs: Fosphenytoin in infants, *J Child Neurol* 13:537-540, 1998.

423. Kriel RL, Cifuentes RF: Fosphenytoin in infants of extremely low birth weight, *Pediatr Neurol* 24:219-221, 2001.

424. Riviello JJ: Drug therapy for neonatal seizures. I, *Pharmacol Rev* 5:e215-e220, 2004.

425. Lacey DJ, Singer WD, Horwitz SJ, Gilmore H: Lorazepam therapy of status epilepticus in children and adolescents, *J Pediatr* 108:771-774, 1986.

426. Giang DW, McBride MC: Lorazepam versus diazepam for the treatment of status epilepticus, *Pediatr Neurol* 4:358-361, 1988.

427. Crawford TO, Mitchell WG, Snodgrass SR: Lorazepam in childhood status epilepticus and serial seizures: Effectiveness and tachyphylaxis, *Neurology* 37:190-195, 1987.

428. Deshmukh A, Wittert W, Schnitzler E, Mangurten HH: Lorazepam in the treatment of refractory neonatal seizures: A pilot study, *Am J Dis Child* 140:1042-1044, 1986.

429. Maytal J, Novak GP, King KC: Lorazepam in the treatment of refractory neonatal seizures, *J Child Neurol* 6:319-323, 1991.

430. McDermott CA, Kowalczyk AL, Schnitzler ER, Mangurten HH, et al: Pharmacokinetics of lorazepam in critically ill neonates with seizures, *J Pediatr* 120:479-483, 1992.

431. Langslet A, Meberg A, Bredesen JE, Lunde PK: Plasma concentrations of diazepam and N-desmethyldiazepam in newborn infants after intravenous, intramuscular, rectal and oral administration, *Acta Paediatr Scand* 67:699-704, 1978.

432. Ramsey RE, Hammond EJ, Perchalski RJ, Wilder J: Brain uptake of phenytoin, phenobarbital, and diazepam, *Arch Neurol* 36:535, 1979.

433. Prensky AL, Raff MC, Moore MJ, Schwab RS: Intravenous diazepam in the treatment of prolonged seizure activity, *N Engl J Med* 276:779-784, 1967.

434. McMorris S, McWilliam PK: Status epilepticus in infants and young children treated with parenteral diazepam, *Arch Dis Child* 44:604-611, 1969.

435. Smith BT, Masotti RE: Intravenous diazepam in the treatment of prolonged seizure activity in neonates and infants, *Dev Med Child Neurol* 13:630-634, 1971.

436. Schiff D, Chan G, Stern L: Fixed drug combinations and the displacement of bilirubin from albumin, *Pediatrics* 48:139-141, 1971.

437. Nathenson G, Cohen MI, McNamara H: The effect of Na benzoate on serum bilirubin of the Gunn rat, *J Pediatr* 86:799-803, 1975.

438. Gamstorp I, Sedin G: Neonatal convulsions treated with continuous, intravenous infusion of diazepam, *Ups J Med Sci* 87:143-149, 1982.

439. Riviello JJ: Drug therapy for neonatal seizures. II, *Pharmacol Rev* 5:e262-e268, 2004.

440. Sheth RD, Buckley DJ, Gutierrez AR, Gingold M, et al: Midazolam in the treatment of refractory neonatal seizures, *Clin Neuropharmacol* 19:165-170, 1996.

441. Castro Conde JR, Hernandez Borges AA, Martinez D, Campo CG, et al: Midazolam in neonatal seizures with no response to phenobarbital, *Neurology* 64:876-879, 2005.

441a. Yamamoto H, Aihara M, Niijima S, Yamanouchi H: Treatments with midazolam and lidocaine for status epilepticus in neonates, *Brain Dev* 29:559-564, 2007.

442. Hellström-Westas L, Westgren U, Rosén I, Svenningsen NW: Lidocaine for treatment of severe seizures in newborn infants. I. Clinical effects and cerebral electrical activity monitoring, *Acta Paediatr Scand* 77:79-84, 1988.

443. Hellström-Westas L, Svenningsen NW, Westgren U, Rosén I, et al: Lidocaine for treatment of severe seizures in newborn infants. II. Blood concentrations of lidocaine and metabolites during intravenous infusion, *Acta Paediatr* 81:35-39, 1992.

444. Radvanyi-Bouvet M-F, Torricelli A, Rey E, Bavoux F, et al: Effects of lidocaine on seizures in the neonatal period: Some electroclinical aspects. In Wasterlain CG, Vert P, editors: *Neonatal Seizures*, New York: 1990, Raven Press.

445. Boylan GB, Rennie JM, Chorley G, Pressler RM, et al: Second-line anticonvulsant treatment of neonatal seizures: A video-EEG monitoring study, *Neurology* 62:486-488, 2004.

446. Powell C, Painter MJ, Pippenger CE: Primidone therapy in refractory neonatal seizures, *J Pediatr* 105:651-654, 1984.

447. Sapin JI, Riviello JJ Jr, Grover WD: Efficacy of primidone for seizure control in neonates and young infants, *Pediatr Neurol* 4:292-295, 1988.

448. Bonati M, Marraro G, Celardo A, Passerini F, et al: Thiopental efficacy in phenobarbital-resistant neonatal seizures, *Dev Pharmacol Ther* 15:16-20, 1990.

449. Koren G, Butt W, Rajchgot P, Mayer J, et al: Intravenous paraldehyde for seizure control in newborn infants, *Neurology* 36:108-111, 1986.

450. Tasker RC, Boyd SG, Harden A, Matthew DJ: EEG monitoring of prolonged thiopentone administration for intractable seizures and status epilepticus in infants and young children, *Neuropediatrics* 20:147-153, 1989.

451. Gal P, Oles KS, Gilman JT, Weaver R: Valproic acid efficacy, toxicity, and pharmacokinetics in neonates with intractable seizures, *Neurology* 38:467-471, 1988.

452. Singh B, Singh P, AlHifzi I, Khan M, et al: Treatment of neonatal seizures with carbamazepine, *J Child Neurol* 11:378-382, 1996.

453. Koh S, Jensen FE: Topiramate blocks perinatal hypoxia-induced seizures in rat pups, *Ann Neurol* 50:366-372, 2001.

454. Follett PL, Deng W, Dai W, Talos DM, et al: Glutamate receptor-mediated oligodendrocyte toxicity in periventricular leukomalacia: A protective role for topiramate, *J Neurosci* 24:4412-4420, 2004.

455. Cha BH, Silveira DC, Liu XZ, Hu YC, et al: Effect of topiramate following recurrent and prolonged seizures during early development, *Epilepsy Res* 51:217-232, 2002.

456. Glier C, Dzietko M, Bittigau P, Jarosz B, et al: Therapeutic doses of topiramate are not toxic to the developing rat brain, *Exp Neurol* 187:403-409, 2004.

457. Sullivan JE, Witte MK, Yamashita TS, Myers CM, et al: Pharmacokinetics of bumetanide in critically ill infants, *Clin Pharmacol Ther* 60:405-413, 1996.

458. Lopez-Samblas AM, Adams JA, Goldberg RN, Modi MW: The pharmacokinetics of bumetanide in the newborn infant, *Biol Neonate* 72:265-272, 1997.

459. Bourgeois BFD, Dodson WE: Phenytoin elimination in newborns, *Neurology* 23:173, 1983.

460. Dodson WE: Antiepileptic drug utilization in pediatric patients, *Epilepsia* 25:S132-S139, 1984.

461. Dodson WE, Bourgeois BF: Changing kinetic patterns of phenytoin in newborns. In Wasterlain CG, Vert P, editors: *Neonatal Seizures*, New York: 1990, Raven Press.

462. Dodson WE: Pharmacokinetic principles of antiepileptic therapy in children. In Dodson WE, Pellock JM, editors: *Pediatric Epilepsy: Diagnosis and Therapy*, New York: 1993, Demos Publications.

463. Donn SM, Grasela TH, Goldstein GW: Safety of a higher loading dose of phenobarbital in the term newborn, *Pediatrics* 75:1061-1064, 1985.

464. MacKintosh DA, Baird-Lampert J, Buchanan N: Is carbamazepine an alternative maintenance therapy for neonatal seizures? *Dev Pharmacol Ther* 10:100-106, 1987.

465. Gillam GL: Convulsions following birth asphyxia/birth trauma: Are long-term anticonvulsants necessary?, *Aust Paediatr J* 18:90-91, 1982.

466. Scarpa P, Chierici R, Tamisari L, Fortini C, et al: Criteria for discontinuing neonatal seizure therapy: A long-term appraisal, *Brain Dev* 5:541-548, 1983.

467. Volpe JJ: Neonatal seizures: Clinical overview. In Wasterlain CG, Vert P, editors: *Neonatal Seizures*, New York: 1990, Raven Press.

468. Toet MC, Groenendaal F, Osredkar D, van Huffelen AC, et al: Postneonatal epilepsy following amplitude-integrated EEG-detected neonatal seizures, *Pediatr Neurol* 32:241-247, 2005.

469. Corsellis JAN, Meldrum BS: Epilepsy. In Blackwood W, Corsellis JAN, editors: *Greenfield's Neuropathology*, London, 1976, Edward Arnold.

470. Brod SA, Ment LR, Ehrenkranz RA, Bridgers S: Predictors of success for drug discontinuation following neonatal seizures, *Pediatr Neurol* 4:13-17, 1988.

471. Diaz J, Schain RJ, Bailey BG: Phenobarbital-induced brain growth retardation in artificially reared rat pups, *Biol Neonate* 32:77-82, 1977.

472. Diaz J, Schain RJ: Phenobarbital: Effects of long-term administration on behavior and brain of artificially reared rats, *Science* 199:90, 1978.

473. Neale EA, Sher PK, Graubard BI, Habig WH, et al: Differential toxicity of chronic exposure to phenytoin, phenobarbital, or carbamazepine in cerebral cortical cell cultures, *Pediatr Neurol* 1:143-150, 1985.

474. Serrano EE, Kunis DM, Ransom BR: Effects of chronic phenobarbital exposure on cultured mouse spinal cord neurons, *Ann Neurol* 24:429-438, 1988.

475. Swaiman KF, Machen VL: Effects of phenobarbital and phenytoin on cortical glial cells in culture, *Brain Dev* 13:242-246, 1991.

476. Farwell JR, Lee YJ, Hirtz DG, Sulzbacher SI, et al: Phenobarbital for febrile seizures: Effects on intelligence and on seizure recurrence, *N Engl J Med* 322:364-369, 1990.

477. Riva D, Devoti M: Discontinuation of phenobarbital in children: Effects on neurocognitive behavior, *Pediatr Neurol* 14:36-40, 1996.

478. Bittigau P, Sifringer M, Genz K, Reith E, et al: Antiepileptic drugs and apoptotic neurodegeneration in the developing brain, *Proc Natl Acad Sci U S A* 99:15089-15094, 2002.

479. Bittigau P, Sifringer M, Ikonomidou C: Antiepileptic drugs and apoptosis in the developing brain, *Ann N Y Acad Sci* 993:103-114, 2003.

480. Manthey D, Asimiadou S, Stefovska V, Kaindl AM, et al: Sulthiame but not levetiracetam exerts neurotoxic effect in the developing rat brain, *Exp Neurol* 193:497-503, 2005.

HYPOXIC-ISCHEMIC ENCEPHALOPATHY

Chapter 6

Hypoxic-Ischemic Encephalopathy: Biochemical and Physiological Aspects

Hypoxic-ischemic encephalopathy in the perinatal period is characterized by neuropathological and clinical features that constitute an important portion of neonatal neurology. To understand those features, which are discussed in Chapters 8 and 9, it is necessary to be cognizant of the biochemical and physiological derangements that lead to the structural and functional manifestations of this encephalopathy. In this chapter, I deal with these derangements in detail, on a background of the normal biochemistry and physiology, the latter largely circulatory, of the perinatal brain. Much of what we know is based on experimental data; however, the advent of improved techniques, particularly in the areas of circulatory physiology and magnetic resonance (MR) spectroscopy, and the application of these techniques to the clinical setting, have provided information demonstrating the relevance of the lessons learned in the laboratory to the human situation.

BIOCHEMICAL ASPECTS

Major Pathogenetic Themes

The unifying disturbance to neural tissue in hypoxic-ischemic encephalopathy is a deficit in oxygen supply. Perinatal brain can be deprived of oxygen by two major pathogenetic mechanisms: *hypoxemia*, which is a diminished amount of oxygen in the blood supply; and *ischemia*, which is a diminished amount of blood perfusing the brain. The balance of experimental and clinical data (see later discussion and Chapter 8) leads to the conclusion that *ischemia is the more important of these two forms of oxygen deprivation*. Thus, deprivation of *glucose as well as oxygen* is crucial in the genesis of injury. Moreover, the period of *reperfusion* now has been shown clearly to be the time of occurrence of many, if not most, of the deleterious consequences of ischemia on brain metabolism and, ultimately, structure (see later discussion). In most instances, during the perinatal period, hypoxemia or ischemia or both occur as a result of *asphyxia*, which refers to impairment in the exchange of respiratory gases, oxygen and carbon dioxide. Thus, in asphyxia, the major additional feature is hypercapnia, which results in other metabolic (e.g., additional acidosis) and physiological (e.g., initial increase in cerebral blood flow [CBF]) effects. In the following sections, I discuss the biochemical changes in brain associated with hypoxemia, ischemia, and asphyxia, initially with an emphasis on carbohydrate and energy metabolism. The manner in which these biochemical changes are affected by other perinatal factors (e.g., the status of carbohydrate metabolism at the time of the insult, the state of brain maturation, and the process of birth) also is described. Subsequent sections synthesize the burgeoning literature on the mechanisms of cell death with oxygen deprivation and focus on the critical importance of biochemical events beyond glucose and energy metabolism. Particular roles for increase in extracellular glutamate, excessive activation of glutamate receptors (excitotoxicity), increase in cytosolic calcium (Ca^{2+}), and generation of free radicals are emphasized.

Normal Carbohydrate and Energy Metabolism

Because glucose and oxygen are the principal driving forces for energy production in brain, the major initial biochemical effects of well-established oxygen deprivation are exerted at the levels of carbohydrate and energy metabolism. A brief review of these areas of metabolism is appropriate here (Fig. 6-1) (see also Chapters 12 and 19). Detailed discussions are available from other, more specialized sources.[1-8]

Glucose Uptake

Glucose from blood is taken up by the brain through a process of carrier-mediated, facilitated diffusion that allows transport of glucose faster than would be expected by simple diffusion. Specific glucose transporter proteins are involved (see Chapter 12). The transport process, however, is not energy dependent and thus differs in that critical fashion from active transport. Glucose transport across the blood-brain barrier uses the heavily glycosylated form of the facilitative glucose transporter protein, GLUT1 (55 kDa). Transport across glial membranes is facilitated by the lower molecular form of GLUT1 (45 kDa), and transport across the neuronal membrane is facilitated by GLUT3. The levels of these proteins are relatively low in the immature brain and are limiting to glucose transport and utilization.[1,2,5-7,9-13] Consistent with the experimental findings, elegant studies of human

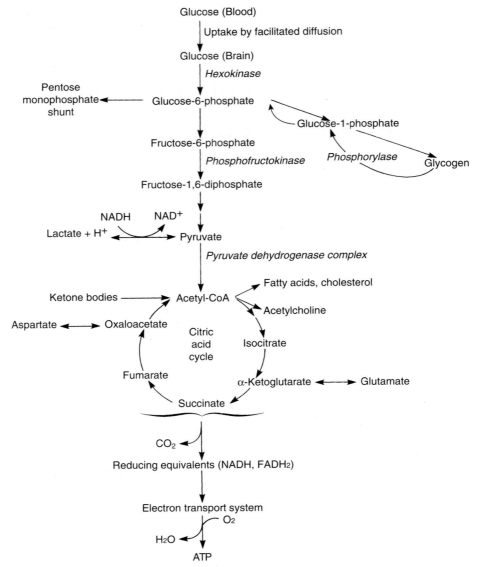

Figure 6-1   Major features of carbohydrate and energy metabolism in brain. See text for details. ATP, adenosine triphosphate; CoA, coenzyme A; FADH$_2$, flavin adenine dinucleotide; NADH, nicotinamide adenine dinucleotide; NAD$^+$, oxidized nicotinamide adenine dinucleotide.

infants by positron emission tomography (PET) show that the cerebral metabolic rate for glucose in brain of preterm newborn infants is approximately one third of that in brain of adults and that this difference relates to a diminished transport capacity rather than a diminished affinity of the transporters for glucose.[14]

Formation of Glucose-6-Phosphate

Glucose in brain is phosphorylated to glucose-6-phosphate; the enzyme involved is hexokinase (see Fig. 6-1). The activity of hexokinase is linked to glucose uptake by the cell and is inhibited by the product of the reaction, glucose-6-phosphate. The activity of this enzyme is also lower in neonatal versus adult rat brain.[1,2,6,7,15] Glucose-6-phosphate is a pivotal metabolite in glucose metabolism, with three major fates: (1) glycolysis and, ultimately, energy production; (2) glycogen synthesis; and (3) the pentose monophosphate shunt for synthesis

of lipids (by formation of reduced nicotinamide adenine dinucleotide phosphate [NADPH]) and nucleic acids.

Glycogen Metabolism

Glycogen is found in relatively small concentrations in brain but represents an important storage form of carbohydrate. Glycogen synthesis and degradation occur primarily in *astrocytes*.[8] Glycogen synthesis proceeds through glucose-1-phosphate and then to glycogen through glycogen synthetase. Glycogen breakdown to glucose-1-phosphate through phosphorylase, and then to glucose-6-phosphate through phosphoglucomutase, is an important mechanism for generating oxidizable substrate by the glycolytic pathway (see Fig. 6-1). Glycogen in astrocytes provides *fuel to neurons* first by conversion to *lactate* and then transport of lactate by specific monocarboxylate transporters to neurons.[8,16] By a similar mechanism astrocytes degrade glycogen to *lactate* that is provided to *developing oligodendrocytes,* primarily for lipid biosynthesis.[17] Brain phosphorylase is activated by cyclic adenosine monophosphate (AMP), and levels of cyclic AMP are elevated by certain hormones, such as epinephrine. Epinephrine release is accentuated sharply with hypoxic, ischemic, and asphyxial insults. Although glycogen is broken down in perinatal brain under certain circumstances, the capacity of the perinatal degradative system, at least in the rodent brain, is considerably less than in the adult.[18,19]

Glycolysis

The major portion of glucose-6-phosphate enters the glycolytic pathway to result ultimately in the formation of pyruvate. The major control step involves the conversion of fructose-6-phosphate to fructose-1,6-diphosphate; the rate-limiting enzyme involved is phosphofructokinase (see Fig. 6-1). The major mechanism of control of this enzyme is through *allosteric* effects—involving conformational changes of component peptides—and thus are very rapid in onset. The activity of phosphofructokinase is inhibited by adenosine triphosphate (ATP), phosphocreatine (PCr), and low pH and activated by adenosine diphosphate (ADP), inorganic phosphorus (Pi), cyclic AMP, and ammonium ion.

Under *aerobic* conditions the major product of glycolysis is pyruvate, which enters the mitochondrion and is converted through the pyruvate dehydrogenase complex to acetyl coenzyme A (acetyl-CoA) (see Fig. 6-1). This mitochondrial enzyme is inhibited by an increase in the ATP/ADP ratio and is activated by a decrease in this ratio. Acetyl-CoA is used for fatty acid and cholesterol biosynthesis and for acetylcholine synthesis but particularly for entry into the citric acid cycle for energy production.

Citric Acid Cycle and Electron Transport Chain

Mitochondrial acetyl-CoA enters the citric acid cycle and undergoes oxidation to carbon dioxide (see Fig. 6-1). The rate-limiting step is the conversion of isocitrate to alpha-ketoglutarate, catalyzed by the enzyme isocitrate dehydrogenase. A critical allosteric regulator of this enzyme is the ratio of ATP to ADP; an increase in the ratio causes a decrease in activity of the cycle, and a decrease in the ratio causes an increase in activity of the cycle. The electrons or reducing equivalents (reduced nicotinamide adenine dinucleotide [NADH], flavin adenine dinucleotide [FADH]) generated by the citric acid cycle next enter the electron transport system.

The transport of electrons takes place through a multimember chain of electron carrier proteins and is associated with release of free energy, which is used to generate ATP from ADP and Pi. The free energy, in essence, is "captured" in this high-energy phosphate bond. ATP is generated at three steps in the scheme, and because the final electron acceptor is oxygen, the process is called *oxidative phosphorylation*. Molecular oxygen is reduced, and water is the final product formed. The ATP generated by the citric acid cycle and the electron transport system is transported from the mitochondrion by a specific carrier and ultimately

is used in brain primarily for *transport processes* (especially of ions and neurotransmitters for impulse transmission and for prevention of dangerous increases thereof, e.g., extracellular glutamate, cytosolic Ca^{2+}) and for *synthetic processes* (especially of neurotransmitters, but also lipids and proteins, particularly in developing brain). The principal ions involved in ATP consumption are sodium (Na^+), potassium (K^+), and Ca^{2+}; in adult brain (under normal conditions), approximately 60% to 75% of ATP is used for maintenance of membrane gradients of these three ions, especially Na^+ and K^+.[6,8]

Summary

The concerted action of glycolysis, the citric acid cycle, and the electron transport system, operative under aerobic conditions, results in the formation of 38 molecules of ATP for each molecule of glucose oxidized (Fig. 6-2). The glycolytic portion of the pathway occurs in the cytosol and generates only 2 of the 38 molecules of ATP; the bulk of the ATP is generated in the mitochondrial portion of the pathway, which begins with pyruvate. The ATP generated is transported from the mitochondrion by a specific carrier and is used in brain for two major purposes: *transport* and *synthetic processes*. Quantitatively, the most important transport processes involve ions in neurons for impulse transmission and maintenance of Ca^{2+} homeostasis. Synthetic processes are important in developing brain and involve neurotransmitters, structural and functional proteins, and membrane lipids.

Effects of Hypoxemia on Carbohydrate and Energy Metabolism

Major Changes

Hypoxemia is accompanied by numerous effects on carbohydrate and energy metabolism in brain[1,2,4,20,21] (Table 6-1), effects that are understandable when viewed in the context of the normal metabolism just reviewed. Although it is likely that lack of oxygen is the major pathogenetic factor in these changes, it is difficult to produce hypoxemia experimentally without also causing other major metabolic changes that either accompany the hypoxemic insult or occur as a consequence of the insult (e.g., hypercapnia, acidosis, and hypotension). In most studies, however, these other changes either are prevented or are documented.

The quantitative and temporal aspects of the biochemical changes associated with a severe hypoxemic

$$Glucose + 2\ NAD^+ + 2\ ADP + 2\ P_i \longrightarrow 2\ Pyruvate + 2\ NADH + 2\ ATP$$

$$2\ Pyruvate + 2\ NADH + 36\ ADP + 36\ P_i + 6\ O_2 \longrightarrow 2\ NAD^+ + 6\ CO_2 + 44\ H_2O + 36\ ATP$$

SUM:
$$Glucose + 38\ ADP + 38\ P_i + 6\ O_2 \longrightarrow 6\ CO_2 + 44\ H_2O + \boxed{38\ ATP}$$

Figure 6-2 Energy production from glucose under aerobic conditions. Contrast with production under anaerobic conditions (see Fig. 6-6). ADP, adenosine diphosphate; ATP, adenosine triphosphate; NADH, reduced nicotinamide adenine dinucleotide; NAD+, oxidized nicotinamide adenine dinucleotide; P_i, inorganic phosphate.

TABLE 6-1	Effects of Hypoxemia on Carbohydrate and Energy Metabolism

↑ Glucose influx to brain
↑ Glycogenolysis
↑ Glycolysis
↓ Brain glucose
↑ Lactate production and tissue acidosis
↓ Phosphocreatine
↓ Adenosine triphosphate

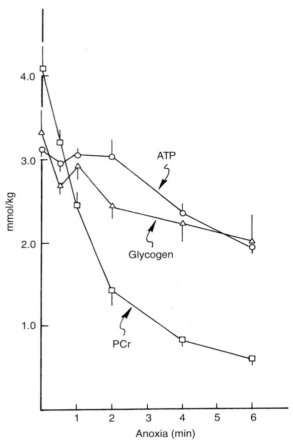

Figure 6-4 **Biochemical effects of hypoxemia.** Concentrations of adenosine triphosphate (ATP), phosphocreatine (PCr), and glycogen in brain of newborn mice as a function of duration of anoxia (nitrogen breathing). *(From Holowach-Thurston J, Hauhart RE, Jones EM: Decrease in brain glucose in anoxia in spite of elevated plasma glucose levels, Pediatr Res 7:691-695, 1973.)*

or anoxic insult (i.e., nitrogen breathing) in the newborn mouse are depicted in Figures 6-3 to 6-5.[22] The earliest significant changes are a decrease in brain glycogen, an elevation in lactate, and a decrease in PCr. These are followed by a decrease in brain glucose and, finally, ATP. The changes appear to reflect principally the impaired production of high-energy phosphate, secondary to failure of the coupled mitochondrial system of the citric acid cycle and electron transport chain, in turn, a consequence of the lack of the ultimate electron acceptor, oxygen. In response to the anaerobic state, glycolysis becomes the sole source of ATP production, and because lactate is the principal product of anaerobic glycolysis, only two molecules of ADP are generated for each molecule of glucose metabolized (Fig. 6-6). This number is clearly a serious difference from the 38 molecules generated under aerobic conditions (see Fig. 6-2). Glycolysis is accelerated five- to 10-fold, and an attempt

to meet this enhanced need for glucose is made by a combination of glycogenolysis and increased net uptake of glucose from blood.[22] (Glycogen contributes approximately one third of the cerebral energy supply under these conditions.[23]) Despite this acceleration, brain energy demands cannot be met, and ATP levels begin to fall after 2 minutes and decrease by 30% after 6 minutes.

The relationship between arterial oxygen delivery and brain PCr levels (expressed as the ratio of PCr to Pi determined by MR spectroscopy) has been clarified in studies of the neonatal dog.[24,25] Thus, a crucial threshold decrease in PCr/Pi ratio of 50% occurred when arterial oxygen pressure decreased to 12 mm Hg (approximate arterial oxygen saturation, 20%).[25] The importance of the 50% decrease in PCr/Pi ratio relates to the finding in the neonatal piglet that at this level, brain lipid peroxidation and impaired Na+/K+-ATPase activity occur.[26] The critical value of arterial partial pressure of oxygen (Pao$_2$) required to lead to the 50% decline in the PCr/Pi ratio in the neonatal dog (12 mm Hg) was higher at 7 to 21 days (17 mm Hg) and higher in the adult (23 mm Hg).[25] This lower threshold

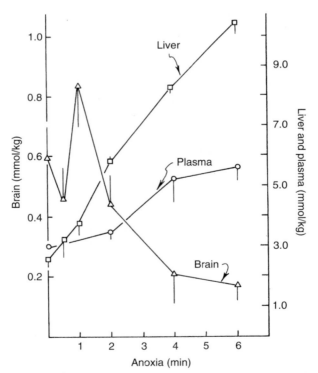

Figure 6-3 **Biochemical effects of hypoxemia.** Concentrations of glucose in brain, liver, and plasma of newborn mice as a function of duration of anoxia (nitrogen breathing). *(From Holowach-Thurston J, Hauhart RE, Jones EM: Decrease in brain glucose in anoxia in spite of elevated plasma glucose levels, Pediatr Res 7:691-695, 1973.)*

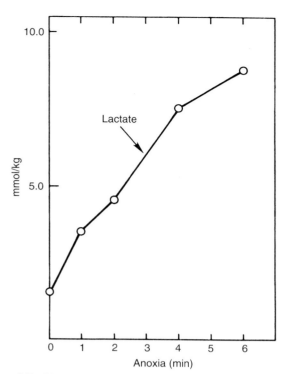

Figure 6-5 Biochemical effects of hypoxemia. Concentrations of lactate in brain of newborn mice as a function of duration of anoxia (nitrogen breathing). *(Redrawn from Holowach-Thurston J, Hauhart RE, Jones EM: Decrease in brain glucose in anoxia in spite of elevated plasma glucose levels, Pediatr Res 7:691-695, 1973.)*

$$\text{Glucose} + 2\,\text{ADP} + 2\,\text{P}_i \longrightarrow 2\,\text{Lactate}^- + 2\,\text{H}^+ + \boxed{2\,\text{ATP}}$$

Figure 6-6 Energy production from glucose under anaerobic conditions. Contrast with production under aerobic conditions (see Fig. 6-2). ADP, adenosine diphosphate; ATP, adenosine triphosphate; P_i, inorganic phosphate.

value of PaO_2 in the neonatal animal correlated with in vitro data showing more efficient oxygen extraction in the neonatal animals (see later discussion). At any rate, it is clear that *marked* hypoxemia is required to produce serious changes in brain energy state in the neonatal animal.

Studies of the effect of hypoxemia on brain energy metabolism in the immature rat brain have delineated a particular window of vulnerability, characterized by *greater* vulnerability in the second postnatal week, comparable to the human brain at term, than in the first postnatal week, comparable to the human premature brain.[27] Thus, the most marked declines in PCr and nucleoside triphosphates, defined by MR spectroscopy, occurred in the second postnatal week. This period of heightened vulnerability corresponds with the period of maximal susceptibility to excitotoxic neuronal injury and to epileptogenic effects of hypoxemia,[28-30] as well as with the period of maximal expression of specific excitatory amino acid receptors, incomplete maturation of inhibitory transmission, relatively low levels of Ca^{2+} binding proteins, and incomplete maturation of Na^+/K^+-ATPase levels (see later discussion).[31] Taken together, these data suggest that the vulnerability of the immature rat in the second versus the first week of life relates to the increased propensity to develop with hypoxia, a hyperexcitable, hypermetabolic state in neurons, which leads to more marked declines in high-energy phosphates because of increased utilization. These considerations could help explain the greater likelihood of *neuronal* injury

with hypoxia in the term brain than in the premature brain of the human.

Studies in the newborn dog defined the *regional* changes in glucose and high-energy metabolism.[32] Thus, animals subjected to acute hypoxemia (oxygen pressure [PO_2] ≈12 mm Hg) and studied by the autoradiographic 2-[^{14}C]deoxyglucose technique exhibited increased glucose utilization in most gray matter structures and every white matter structure. Moreover, the degree of hypoxemia was sufficient to cause accumulation of lactate in brain in both gray and white matter, but only in white matter did a decline in energy state occur (Table 6-2). *Thus, it appears that anaerobic glycolysis with its accelerated glucose utilization was capable of preserving the energy state in gray matter but not in white matter.* Moreover, the finding that glucose levels declined more drastically in white matter than in gray matter (see Table 6-2) suggests that glucose influx could not meet the increased demands for glucose in white matter. That the rate of glucose metabolism, in fact, was *limited by glucose influx from blood* is supported by the demonstration that local CBF increased insignificantly to white matter but dramatically to gray matter.[33] The apparently limited vasodilatory capacity in white matter is discussed in the section on CBF, but *this imbalance between glucose needs and glucose delivery may contribute to the propensity of neonatal cerebral white matter to hypoxic injury.*

Mechanisms

The mechanisms for the biochemical effects relate to several factors (Table 6-3). ATP levels are preserved initially at the expense of PCr. The *initial* fall in PCr, the principal storage form of high-energy phosphate in brain, relates primarily to the shift in the creatine phosphokinase reaction induced by the hydrogen ion (H^+) generated with lactate formation by anaerobic glycolysis (Fig. 6-7). Later, the creatine phosphokinase reaction is driven by elevated concentrations of both ADP and H^+. The *initial acceleration of glycolysis and the glycogenolysis* may relate to primarily a rise in cyclic AMP levels in brain, demonstrated to be approximately threefold in the rat after only 30 seconds of nitrogen breathing.[34] Cyclic AMP leads to activation of phosphorylase for glycogenolysis and of phosphofructokinase (and hexokinase) for glycolysis.[35-37] Further activation of phosphofructokinase and hence glycolysis occurs as ATP levels fall and ADP and Pi levels rise. The fall in brain glucose occurs because the continued excessive utilization of glucose through anaerobic glycolysis, a most inefficient means of generating ATP, outstrips the capacity for glucose delivery from blood. Indeed, after 6 minutes, brain glucose levels had decreased by more than 70%, whereas blood glucose levels had increased by nearly 100% (see Fig. 6-3).[22]

TABLE 6-2   Substrate Concentrations in Brain of Hypoxic Puppies (mmol/kg)

Tissue	Phosphocreatine	Adenosine Triphosphate	Glucose	Lactate
Control				
Parietal cortex	2.74 ± 0.08	2.30 ± 0.08	2.38 ± 0.25	1.08 ± 0.09
Subcortical white matter	1.85 ± 0.22	1.64 ± 0.06	2.14 ± 0.13	1.34 ± 0.07
Hypoxia				
Parietal cortex	2.56 ± 0.06	2.26 ± 0.02	1.64 ± 0.28	12.0 ± 1.4
Subcortical white matter	1.09 ± 0.19	1.40 ± 0.09	0.28 ± 0.04	13.4 ± 1.8

Data from Duffy TE, Cavazzuti M, Cruz NF, Sokoloff L: Local cerebral glucose metabolism in newborn dogs: Effects of hypoxia and halothane anesthesia, *Ann Neurol* 11:233-246, 1982.

Thus, blood glucose level no longer reflected the brain glucose level, an observation of particular clinical relevance.

The accumulation of lactate and the associated H+ is worthy of additional emphasis because this accumulation *initially* is a *beneficial* adaptive response to oxygen deprivation, but *later* it can be a serious *deleterious* factor. Thus, initially, the tissue acidosis leads to the generation of ATP from PCr (because of the shift in the creatine phosphokinase reaction) and also to an increase in CBF (because of the local effect of elevated perivascular H+ concentration on vascular smooth muscle). However, with progression of lactate formation, severe tissue acidosis develops, and three deleterious effects ensue. The first is an impairment of vascular autoregulation and the potential for ischemic injury to brain when cerebral perfusion pressure falls (e.g., secondary to the often associated myocardial injury). Second, phosphofructokinase activity is inhibited by low pH, and thus the brain's remaining source of ATP (i.e., glycolysis) is eliminated. Finally, advanced tissue acidosis leads directly to cellular injury and, ultimately, necrosis. A correlation between brain lactate concentration and cellular injury has been demonstrated in primate brain (see next section).

Effects of Hypoxia-Ischemia on Carbohydrate and Energy Metabolism

Major Changes

Hypoxic-ischemic insults are accompanied by effects on carbohydrate and energy metabolism in brain (Table 6-4) that exhibit important similarities to those observed with hypoxemia. Certain differences occur with the addition of ischemia (see later). In earlier years, the most frequently used models with perinatal animals included decapitation, severe hypotension, or occlusion of blood vessels supplying the cranium.[5,7,18,19,38-46] The most widely used model in the past 20 years has involved the Vannucci adaptation of the Levine model of unilateral carotid artery ligation followed by systemic hypoxemia for generally 1 to 3 hours, a procedure that results in hypoxic-ischemic neuronal and white matter injury.[5,47] I emphasize the studies carried out with this clinically relevant model.

The combination of hypoxemia and ischemia (i.e., *hypoxic-ischemic insult*) is most relevant to the situation in vivo in the human fetus and newborn. The effects of such an insult on carbohydrate and energy metabolism have been studied in detail in experimental models.[1,2,5,7,13,35,46-67]

The biochemical features relative to carbohydrate and energy metabolism bear many similarities to those recorded previously for purely hypoxemic insults (see earlier discussion) (see Table 6-4). In the most commonly used model, the hypoxic-ischemic insult is produced in the 7-day-old rat (approximately

TABLE 6-3   Major Mechanisms for Biochemical Effects of Hypoxemia on Carbohydrate and Energy Metabolism

↑ **Glucose Influx to Brain**
Link to accelerated glucose utilization

↑ **Glycogenolysis**
Phosphorylase activation (↑ cAMP)

↑ **Glycolysis**
Phosphofructokinase activation (↑ cAMP, ↑ ADP, ↑ Pi, ↓ ATP, ↓ phosphocreatine)
Hexokinase activation (↑ cAMP)

↓ **Brain Glucose**
Glucose utilization > glucose influx

↑ **Lactate (and Hydrogen Ion)**
Anaerobic glycolysis
Impaired utilization of pyruvate (through mitochondrial citric acid cycle–electron transport system)

↓ **Phosphocreatine**
↑ Hydrogen ion production through anaerobic glycolysis
↓ ATP, ↑ ADP

↓ **ATP**
↓ Oxidative phosphorylation

ADP, adenosine diphosphate; ATP, adenosine triphosphate; cAMP, cyclic adenosine monophosphate; Pi, inorganic phosphate.

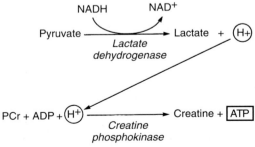

Figure 6-7   Link between lactate production and hydrolysis of phosphocreatine. Adenosine triphosphate (ATP) formation is the result. ADP, adenosine diphosphate; NADH, reduced nicotinamide adenine dinucleotide; NAD+, oxidized nicotinamide adenine dinucleotide; PCr, phosphocreatine.

TABLE 6-4	**Effects of Ischemia on Carbohydrate and Energy Metabolism**

↓ Glucose influx to brain
↑ Glycogenolysis
↑ Glycolysis
↓ Brain glucose
↑ Lactate production and tissue acidosis
↓ Phosphocreatine
↓ Adenosine triphosphate

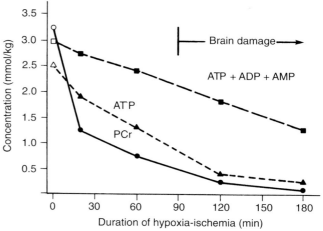

Figure 6-8   Changes in cerebral high-energy phosphate reserves during hypoxia-ischemia in the immature rat. Seven-day-old postnatal rats were subjected to unilateral common carotid artery ligation followed by exposure to hypoxia with 8% oxygen at 37°C. Symbols represent means for adenosine triphosphate (ATP), phosphocreatine (PCr), and total adenine nucleotides (ATP+ADP+AMP). All values are significantly different from control (zero time point). Histological brain damage commences after 90 minutes of hypoxia-ischemia, with increasing severity thereafter. *(From Vannucci RC: Experimental biology of cerebral hypoxia-ischemia: Relation to perinatal brain damage,* Pediatr Res *27:317-326, 1990.)*

analogous to a preterm human newborn brain) by a combination of unilateral carotid occlusion and breathing of a low-oxygen (usually 8%) gas mixture. The *importance of ischemia* in the genesis of the brain injury in this model has been demonstrated by the findings that (1) carotid ligation alone does not lead to a decrease in CBF to the ipsilateral hemisphere, (2) the addition of the hypoxemia leads to marked disturbances in regional blood flow to the ipsilateral hemisphere, and (3) the topography of the injury to this hemisphere correlates closely with the topography of the decreases in regional CBF.[50] Vannucci and co-workers defined the major biochemical changes most clearly.[1,2,5,13,35,48,49,51,52] The initial biochemical changes are compatible with accelerated anaerobic glycolysis with lactate accumulation and glycogenolysis. Particular importance for an increased capacity for glucose uptake in the acceleration of glucose utilization has been shown by the demonstration of elevation in the levels of the glucose transporter proteins, GLUT1 (55 kDa) and GLUT3, for transport of glucose across the blood-brain barrier and the neuronal membrane, respectively, in the brain of hypoxic-ischemic 7-day-old rat pups in the first 4 hours after the insult.[13] As with hypoxemia, a role for cyclic AMP in the induction of the glycolysis and glycogenolysis is suggested by marked rises (13-fold) in the levels of this mononucleotide in the first minutes after the onset of ischemia.[68] Nevertheless, brain glucose concentrations fall more severely than with the anoxia of nitrogen breathing; after 2 minutes of ischemia, glucose had decreased markedly, whereas only a modest decrease occurred with nitrogen breathing after this time. Of course, this difference relates to the impairment of CBF and therefore glucose supply with ischemia. An additional difference between ischemia and hypoxemia is the more drastic increase in lactate and tissue acidosis with ischemia, because the circulation is interrupted.[20] The more severe tissue acidosis obtains because the impaired cerebral circulation results in (1) diminished clearance of accumulated lactate and (2) diminished buffering of tissue carbon dioxide by the bicarbonate buffering system.[20] The increased ratio of lactate to pyruvate in the cytosol is reflected in increased reduction (i.e., decrease) of the $NAD^+/NADH$ ratio. The latter ratio is more oxidized in the mitochondrion because of the limitation in cellular substrate (glucose) supply. (This important limiting role of brain glucose is discussed in more detail later concerning brain carbohydrate status and hypoxic-ischemic injury.) Perhaps most importantly, high-energy phosphate levels begin to decline within minutes, with the reservoir form,

PCr, falling first (Fig. 6-8).[35] Histological evidence of brain injury becomes apparent after approximately 90 minutes.

The particular importance of *ischemia* in the genesis of the deleterious effects of hypoxic-ischemic insults was also shown in the fetal lamb and neonatal piglet.[45,55-57,69,70] In *both animal models, marked hypoxemia did not result in brain injury unless hypotension supervened.* In the piglet, hypotension appeared to be a particular consequence of cardiac dysfunction, and the latter was especially correlated with severe systemic acidosis. In the fetal lamb, pronounced decreases in brain glucose and in high-energy phosphate levels accompanied by an increase in lactate levels to as high as 16 to 24 mM were the principal biochemical effects on carbohydrate and energy metabolism. These effects were particularly pronounced in cerebral white matter (Table 6-5). *This regional predilection may be relevant to the propensity of white matter to exhibit injury with hypotension in the premature newborn* (see Chapter 8).

Secondary Energy Failure

The temporal aspects of the changes in glucose and energy metabolism after hypoxic-ischemic insult in *the living animal* have been identified best by studies of the neonatal piglet with phosphorus and proton MR spectroscopy and have defined a delayed, secondary energy failure.[65-67,70] Thus, immediately after the insult, as expected, a marked increase in cerebral lactate levels and a marked decrease in high-energy phosphate levels were documented (i.e., primary energy failure). High-energy phosphate levels *recovered* to baseline levels in 2 to 3 hours (Fig. 6-9); lactate levels improved but did not recover completely. A second decline in

TABLE 6-5   Brain Metabolites in White Matter of Fetal Sheep Made Hypoxic with or without Hypotension

Fetal Condition	White Matter Injury	BRAIN METABOLITE*		
		Lactate	Phosphocreatine	Adenosine Triphosphate
Normoxic, normotensive	−	3.2	0.7	0.7
Hypoxic, normotensive	−	9.9[†]	0.5	0.9
Hypoxic, hypotensive	+	19.5[†]	0.3[†]	0.1[†]

*Concentrations are mmol/kg; values are rounded off.

[†]$P < .05$ versus normoxic, normotensive.

Data from Wagner KR, Ting P, Westfall MV, Yamaguchi S, et al: Brain metabolic correlates of hypoxic-ischemic cerebral necrosis in mid-gestational sheep fetuses: Significance of hypotension, *J Cereb Blood Flow Metab* 6:425-434, 1986.

high-energy phosphate levels then occurred in the next 24 hours and was especially pronounced at 48 hours (see Fig. 6-9). This *secondary energy failure* and the earlier rise in cerebral lactate levels *have been documented in the human term newborn* subjected to apparent hypoxic-ischemic insult in the context of perinatal asphyxia (see Chapter 9).[71,72] The onset of the secondary decline in high-energy phosphates varies according to species and nature of the insult, but in general the onset is clear by 8 to 16 hours and reaches a nadir at 24 to 48 hours. A *major question has been whether the secondary energy decline causes or accentuates brain injury or whether the decline is a consequence of the injury*.

A particularly informative study of the neonatal rat (unilateral carotid ligation and hypoxemia on postnatal day 7) confirmed the occurrence of secondary energy failure, with onset at approximately 18 to 24 hours and a nadir at 48 hours.[73] However, immunocytochemical studies showed that the loss of neuronal proteins became apparent at 6 hours and was very pronounced at 18 hours (i.e., *before* the onset of the secondary energy failure). The temporal characteristics and the additional finding of a loss of total creatine and adenine nucleotides supported the conclusion that the

secondary energy depletion is a *consequence* rather than a *cause* of cellular destruction. As discussed later, in the hours following the hypoxic-ischemic insult, a cascade of events, which includes accumulation of excitotoxic amino acids, cytosolic Ca^{2+}, activation of phospholipases, generation of free radicals, and a series of related metabolic events, develops and leads to cell death (see later discussion). The crucial mitochondrial disturbance that precipitates this cascade of deleterious events is responsible for the primary energy failure and *persists* into the period *following* the termination of the insult despite initial recovery of high-energy phosphates (see later discussion). The particular vulnerability of the mitochondrion during and following ischemia is supported by biochemical and morphological data.[1,2,4,35,63,74,75] Investigators have suggested that the secondary energy failure *initiates* the cascade of events just noted. However, the work just described[73] appears to favor the notion that the secondary energy depletion is a *consequence* of the cascade of events and the resulting cell death.

Effects of Asphyxia on Carbohydrate and Energy Metabolism

Asphyxia, rather than hypoxemia or ischemia or both, is the most common *clinical* insult in the perinatal period that results in the brain injury under discussion. Although hypoxemia and ischemia usually occur concurrently or in sequence with perinatal asphyxia, certain additional metabolic effects, particularly hypercapnia, are prominent. Most experimental studies of perinatal asphyxia have involved lambs and monkeys and have been concerned with changes in CBF and with the neuropathology (see later sections on CBF and Chapter 8). Some work has provided useful information regarding the biochemical (as well as the physiological) effects in brain with neonatal asphyxia and is reviewed next.[69,76-82]

Major Changes

Striking changes in biochemical, cardiovascular, cerebrovascular, and electrophysiological parameters were observed in neonatal dogs subjected to ventilatory standstill after paralysis with succinylcholine or curare.[83] *Survival* occurred in all animals after 10 minutes of asphyxia, in two thirds after 15 minutes of asphyxia, but in only one fourth after 20 minutes of asphyxia. Changes in *arterial blood gas levels and*

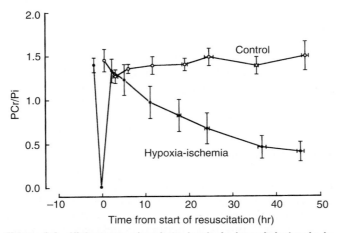

Figure 6-9 High-energy phosphate levels in hypoxia-ischemia in brain of neonatal piglets. Note the sharp decline with the insult, followed by a recovery to baseline in 2 to 3 hours. A few hours later, a second decline ensues and constitutes "secondary energy failure" (see text). PCr, phosphocreatine; Pi, inorganic phosphate. *(From Lorek A, Takei Y, Cady EB, Wyatt JS, et al: Delayed ("secondary") cerebral energy failure after acute hypoxia-ischemia in the newborn piglet: Continuous 48-hour studies by phosphorus magnetic resonance spectroscopy, Pediatr Res 36:699-706, 1994.)*

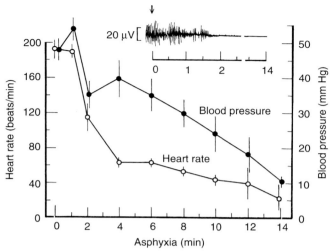

Figure 6-10 Cardiovascular and electroencephalographic effects of asphyxia (respiratory arrest) in newborn dogs. A representative electroencephalogram during 14 minutes of asphyxia is shown in the *upper right*; the *arrow* indicates the onset of respiratory arrest. *(From Vannucci RC, Duffy TE: Cerebral metabolism in newborn dogs during reversible asphyxia, Ann Neurol 1:528-534, 1977.)*

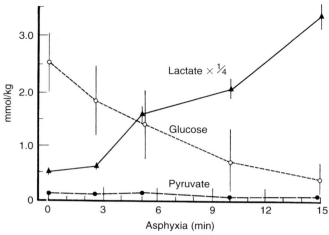

Figure 6-11 Biochemical effects of asphyxia. Concentrations of glucose, pyruvate, and lactate in brain of newborn dogs as a function of duration of asphyxia (respiratory arrest). *(From Vannucci RC, Duffy TE: Cerebral metabolism in newborn dogs during reversible asphyxia, Ann Neurol 1:528-534, 1977.)*

acid-base status were dramatic. Thus, after 2½ minutes of respiratory arrest, Pao_2 had fallen to 4 mm Hg, partial pressure of carbon dioxide ($Paco_2$) had risen to 51 mm Hg (from control value of 35), and pH had fallen to 7.18 (from control value of 7.38). After 10 minutes, $Paco_2$ was 100 mm Hg, and pH was 6.79. *Cardiovascular* effects were also marked (Fig. 6-10); mean arterial blood pressure declined gradually to a low of 10 mm Hg after 14 minutes, and bradycardia was marked after only 4 minutes. *Cerebral perfusion*, assessed qualitatively by carbon black infusion, overall appeared to decline *pari passu* with mean arterial blood pressure, although diminutions were greatest in cerebral cortex and least in brain stem. This more severe affection of *cerebral* flow has been reproduced in other neonatal models of asphyxia (see later discussion). The *electroencephalogram (EEG)* demonstrated rapid deterioration (see Fig. 6-10); between 1 and 2 minutes after the onset of asphyxia, a distinct reduction in the amplitude and frequency occurred, and by 2½ minutes, the EEG was isoelectric. The occurrence of the isoelectric EEG did *not* correlate with any marked change in cerebral perfusion or with any measurable change in brain lactate or ATP levels. In the asphyxiated fetal sheep, this suppression of EEG, initially an energy-conserving protective effect, is mediated by adenosine, an inhibitory neurotransmitter.[82]

Biochemical effects were qualitatively similar to those observed with hypoxemia or ischemia or both (Figs. 6-11 and 6-12). Thus, brain glucose level declined rapidly (despite normal blood glucose level), lactate concentration rose (after a 2½-minute delay), and PCr concentration decreased markedly (to values ≈20% of control within 5 minutes). However, ATP levels were maintained for 6 minutes of asphyxia but then declined by 10 minutes. The changes in high-energy phosphates have been documented in the living animal by MR spectroscopy.[76]

Thus, after 5 minutes of asphyxia, in which electrocerebral silence occurred after 3 minutes, a 40% decrease in the PCr/Pi ratio and a 30% decrease in the ATP/Pi ratio occurred. Despite these changes, on reinstitution of ventilatory support, cerebral metabolism returned to normal within 20 to 30 minutes. However, studies in neonatal piglets showed that during a similar recovery period after an even less severe asphyxial insult (2 to 3 minutes), evidence for lipid peroxidation and altered membrane function (depressed Na^+/K^+-ATPase activity) was demonstrable.[78] Production of *intrauterine* asphyxia by impairment of placental blood flow also decreases cerebral high-energy phosphate levels, as measured by MR spectroscopy in the living animal.[84]

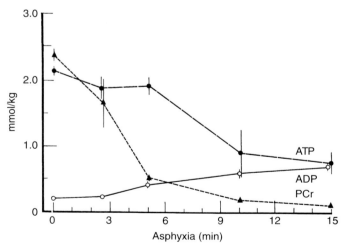

Figure 6-12 Biochemical effects of asphyxia. Concentrations of adenosine triphosphate (ATP), adenosine diphosphate (ADP), and phosphocreatine (PCr) in brain of newborn dogs as a function of duration of asphyxia (respiratory arrest). *(From Vannucci RC, Duffy TE: Cerebral metabolism in newborn dogs during reversible asphyxia, Ann Neurol 1:528-534, 1977.)*

Additional Effects of Asphyxia (versus Solely Hypoxemia or Ischemia or Both)

At least four major factors are added to the constellation of biochemical features controlling the outcome of asphyxia, with its attendant increase in $Paco_2$. The first three of these factors appear to be beneficial, at least initially, and the fourth of these, deleterious. *First,* the hypercapnia acts to maintain or even augment CBF through an increase in perivascular H^+ concentration in brain, which may be beneficial early in asphyxia. *Second,* the hypercapnia may be associated with a diminution in cerebral metabolic rate. Moderate hypercapnia has been shown to cause a diminution in cerebral metabolic rate in adult rat brain, adult monkey brain, and developing rat brain.[12,85-87] *Third,* an increase in $Paco_2$ leads to acidemia, which is accompanied by a shift in the oxygen-hemoglobin dissociation curve such that the affinity of hemoglobin for oxygen is decreased. The result is an increase in the delivery of oxygen to cells. The operation of one or more of these three factors could underlie the protective effect of moderate hypercapnia in immature rats subjected to hypoxia-ischemia.[5,88] The *fourth* important factor relative to hypercapnia and the outcome with asphyxia may be deleterious; intracellular pH falls more drastically for a given amount of lactate formed when the effect of elevated Pco_2 is added by asphyxia.[20,77] Thus, extreme acidosis and consequent tissue injury could result. Future studies directed at defining the relative roles of these four factors in the genesis of the biochemical and physiological derangements associated with asphyxia in the perinatal animal will be of great interest.

Influence of Carbohydrate Status on Hypoxic-Ischemic Brain Injury

Deleterious Role of Low Brain Glucose in Perinatal Animals

A series of older studies with immature animals suggests a beneficial effect of prior administration of glucose and a deleterious effect of hypoglycemia on the survival response to anoxic insult (i.e., nitrogen breathing).[89-92] The effects of glucose appeared to be exerted on the central nervous system rather than on the heart, because time to last gasp was altered before cardiac function. This observation is compatible with data indicating the particular resistance of immature heart to combined hypoxia and hypoglycemia, presumably because of rich carbohydrate stores and high glycogenolytic and glycolytic capacities.[93-95] Later work on the survival and neuropathological response to hypoxia and ischemia of neonatal animals also has demonstrated a beneficial effect of pretreatment with glucose and a deleterious effect of hypoglycemia (Fig. 6-13; see also Chapter 12).[1,2,39,96-99] One study of 185 term human infants who had sustained apparent intrapartum asphyxia (markedly low cord pH) showed a deleterious effect of initial *hypoglycemia* on neurological outcome.[100] Thus, of infants who had initial blood glucose values lower than 40 mg/dL, 56% had an

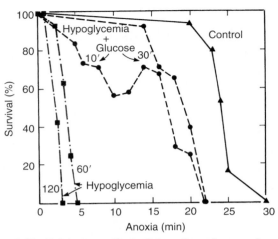

Figure 6-13 **Deleterious effect of hypoglycemia on vulnerability to anoxia (nitrogen breathing).** The percentage of survival of newborn rats was determined as a function of duration of anoxia. Hypoglycemia was produced by insulin injection 1 to 2 hours before onset of anoxia; some hypoglycemic animals were pretreated with glucose (1.8 g/kg subcutaneously) either 10 or 30 minutes before anoxia. *(From Vannucci RC, Vannucci SJ: Cerebral carbohydrate metabolism during hypoglycemia and anoxia in newborn rats,* Ann Neurol 4:73-79, 1978.)

abnormal neurological outcome, versus only 16% among those with initial blood glucose values higher than 40 mg/dL.

Importance of Endogenous Brain Glucose Reserves. The biochemical mechanisms for the relation between carbohydrate status and resistance to hypoxic-ischemic insult relate to glycolytic capacity. Thus, with hypoxic-ischemic states, replenishment of brain high-energy phosphate levels depends on anaerobic glycolysis. Because of the 19-fold reduction in ATP production per molecule of glucose when the brain is forced to oxidize glucose anaerobically, glycolytic rate must be enhanced greatly. The adaptive mechanisms that come into play for this purpose are summarized in previous sections. The greatly enhanced glycolytic rate leads to a decline of brain glucose levels.[1,2,5,19,22,39,83] If this decline is prevented (e.g., by prior administration of glucose), glycolytic rate and, hence, ATP production are increased, and the biochemical and clinical outcome for animals rendered hypoxic or partially ischemic is improved considerably.[1,2,39,96,97,101-103] Indeed, the careful studies of Vannucci and co-workers[1,2,98] indicated that the major factor accounting for the difference in outcome between normoglycemic and hypoglycemic animals rendered hypoxic is the amount of *endogenous brain glucose reserves* at the time of the insult. In hypoglycemic animals, a 10- to 20-fold reduction in endogenous brain glucose resulted and correlated best with the impaired glycolytic rate and the decline in high-energy phosphate levels in brain with nitrogen breathing. Brain glycogen levels seemed less important. Thus, the capacity for surviving hypoxemia was reduced fivefold in hypoglycemic animals at a time (i.e., 60 minutes after insulin injection) when brain glycogen level was reduced by only 20%, but brain glucose level was reduced by more than 10-fold (Fig. 6-14).

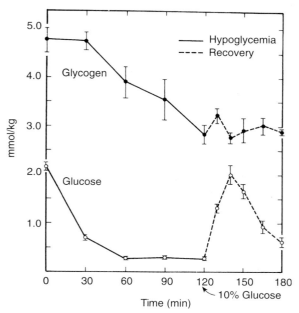

Figure 6-14 **Greater importance of brain glucose reserves than glycogen in effects of hypoglycemia on vulnerability to anoxia (nitrogen breathing).** Brain glucose and glycogen levels in newborn rats were determined as a function of duration of anoxia. Hypoglycemia was produced by insulin injection at the onset of the experiment. At 60 minutes, survival was fivefold lower in hypoglycemic versus control animals (data not shown). At this 60-minute point, glucose was reduced much more severely than was glycogen. The *arrow* indicates subcutaneous administration of 10% glucose (1.8 g/kg). This resulted in a marked improvement in survival (data not shown) and a normalization of brain glucose, but not of glycogen. *(From Vannucci RC, Vannucci SJ: Cerebral carbohydrate metabolism during hypoglycemia and anoxia in newborn rats, Ann Neurol 4:73-79, 1978.)*

Similarly, reversal of the vulnerability correlated with a rapid normalization of brain glucose levels but no significant change in brain glycogen levels.

Summary. Taken together, these data on immature animals (principally rodents) indicate that carbohydrate status plays an important role in determining the biochemical and clinical responses to hypoxemic and ischemic insults. Hypoglycemia is deleterious, and pretreatment with glucose is beneficial. The mechanism of the effect appears to relate to changes in endogenous, readily mobilized brain glucose reserves, which lead to the enhanced glycolytic rate required to slow the decline of, or even maintain the levels of, high-energy phosphate in brain.

Deleterious Role of Abundant Brain Glucose in Adult Animals

A potentially deleterious role for abundant brain glucose in the clinical, pathological, and biochemical responses to hypoxemia and ischemia was suggested initially by studies with juvenile rhesus monkeys.[104-107] In a series of experiments with animals routinely food deprived for 12 to 24 hours before subjection to circulatory arrest, investigators showed that a period of circulatory arrest as long as 14 minutes was compatible with apparently good neurological recovery and "minimal" neuropathological abnormalities,

restricted principally to brain stem nuclei, hippocampus, and Purkinje cells.[104] However, animals that were administered an infusion of 1.5 to 3 g/kg of glucose (5% dextrose in saline) that terminated 10 minutes before the 14-minute period of circulatory arrest did very poorly. The clinical course was characterized by seizures, hypertonia, and ultimately, decerebrate rigidity, evolving over hours. On sacrifice, these glucose-pretreated monkeys, in contrast to the food-deprived monkeys, exhibited "changes indicative of widespread injury to tissue ... and diffuse cytologic injury" with widespread involvement of cerebral cortex. In a subsequent study, glucose was administered as a 50% solution in a dose of 2.5 to 5 g/kg 15 minutes before circulatory arrest, and similar clinical and neuropathological consequences were observed.[106]

Importance of Severe Lactic Acidosis in Brain. The biochemical mechanism for the deleterious effect of pretreatment with glucose in the previously mentioned juvenile monkeys may relate to the greater accumulation of lactic acid in the glucose-pretreated than in the food-deprived (control) monkeys (Table 6-6).[105,108] ATP levels declined approximately 10-fold in food-deprived animals subjected to circulatory arrest, and only a minimal difference in the magnitude of that decline was observed in animals pretreated with glucose. However, whereas lactate levels increased approximately fourfold in the food-deprived animals subjected to circulatory arrest, the levels increased more than 10-fold in those pretreated with glucose. The greater increases in brain lactate levels in the glucose-pretreated animals presumably reflected higher endogenous brain glucose reserves and, as a consequence, enhanced lactate production by anaerobic glycolysis. These experiments and related observations with animals rendered severely hypoxemic led Myers and Yamaguchi[109] to suggest that the accumulation of brain lactate to concentrations of approximately 20 mmol/kg or greater leads to tissue destruction and brain edema. This approximate threshold level is supported by the observations that accumulation of lactate to higher than this level occurs in the brain of monkeys rendered ischemic in those regions that have been shown to be particularly vulnerable to neuronal injury.[108]

TABLE 6-6	Effect of Carbohydrate Status on Biochemical Response to Circulatory Arrest (10 Minutes) in Juvenile Monkeys	
	BRAIN CONCENTRATION (μmmol/g)	
Experimental Condition	**Adenosine Triphosphate**	**Lactate**
Control	2.2	3.0
Circulatory arrest	0.2	13.0
Circulatory arrest and glucose pretreatment	0.3	33.0

Data from references 104, 107, 108, and 109.

Considerable support for the concept of a deleterious effect of abundant glucose and resulting lactic acidosis in brain in the pathogenesis of hypoxic-ischemic brain injury in the adult was provided by further studies in a variety of experimental models in *mature animals*.[109-124] A threshold value of lactate of approximately 20 mmol/kg, above which major tissue injury occurs, can be suggested from the data. The apparent mechanism for the principal injury from these high levels of lactate is injury to endothelial cells, and perhaps also to perivascular astrocytes, with resulting disturbance of cerebral perfusion. Direct neuronal injury is likely, but widespread, secondary ischemic injury appears to develop primarily because of the vascular changes.

Beneficial(?) Role of Abundant Brain Glucose in Perinatal Animals

In contrast to the deleterious role for glucose in hypoxic-ischemic injury in adult animals (see previous section), considerable data in the immature rat suggest a beneficial role for abundant glucose administered primarily during or at the termination of the insult.[1,2,10,97,99,101,103,125-130] Hattori and Wasterlain,[129] using a model of bilateral carotid occlusion and ventilation with 8% oxygen for 1 hour, showed marked reduction of neuropathological injury in animals treated with supplemental glucose at the termination of the hypoxic breathing (Fig. 6-15). Supplementation 1 hour after termination of the hypoxia had no beneficial effect. In a neonatal lamb model of asphyxia, glucose supplementation prevented the prolonged postasphyxial impairment in cerebral oxygen consumption observed in control (or hypoglycemic) animals (Fig. 6-16).[126] Moreover, neonatal rats breathing 8% oxygen survived twice as long when they were treated with 50% glucose; 50% survival was approximately 4 hours in saline-treated animals versus 8 hours in glucose-treated animals.

The *mechanism* for any beneficial effect of glucose in these perinatal models of hypoxia-ischemia is not conclusively known but probably relates to preservation of mitochondrial energy production. Thus, Yager and co-workers[48] showed that glucose supply becomes limiting in hypoxia-ischemia (unilateral carotid occlusion and 8% oxygen breathing) in the neonatal rat, a conclusion based on the relatively oxidized state of mitochondrial NAD$^+$/NADH. Brain glucose levels clearly increase after glucose supplementation, in several models of hypoxia-ischemia.[2,103] With the model of carotid occlusion and 8% oxygen breathing, brain levels of high-energy phosphates were clearly higher in glucose-treated versus saline-treated animals (Table 6-7).[103] In addition, brain lactate levels in the hypoxic-ischemic neonatal rats were considerably higher in the glucose-treated animals.[103] Indeed, after 2 hours of hyperglycemia, brain lactate levels reached 25.5 mmol/kg. However, no evidence for tissue injury caused by the elevated brain lactate levels was reported. Moreover, in other perinatal models (in near-term fetal sheep, newborn lamb, and newborn dog), brain lactate levels did not rise to such levels with hypoxia-ischemia or asphyxia.[40,41,44,131] Increase in brain lactate levels in neonatal brain relative to adult brain is limited by the lower capacity for glucose uptake by the glucose transporter proteins, especially GLUT1 (55 kDa), and by

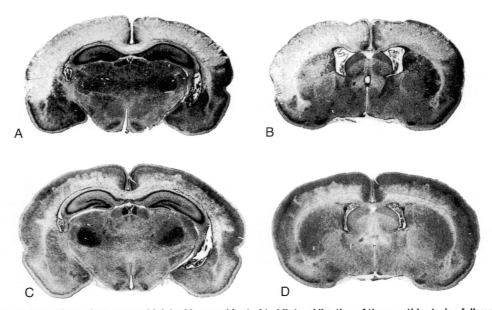

Figure 6-15 Coronal brain sections of rat pups, which had been subjected to bilateral ligation of the carotid arteries followed by exposure to an 8% oxygen atmosphere for 1 hour at the age of 7 days and were sacrificed 72 hours later. Note gross infarction in, **A**, neocortex and, **B**, lateral part of the striatum in a saline-injected pup. **C** and **D**, Immediate (0 hour) posthypoxic glucose supplement reduced neocortical and striatal infarction. (Hematoxylin and eosin ×2.5 before 52% reduction.) *(From Hattori H, Wasterlain CG: Posthypoxic glucose supplement reduces hypoxic-ischemic brain damage in the neonatal rat, Ann Neurol 28:122-128, 1990.)*

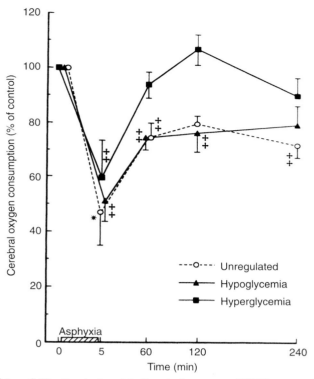

Figure 6-16 Cerebral metabolic rate for oxygen (CMRO$_2$; percentage of control) over time in the unregulated glucose, hyperglycemic, and hypoglycemic groups of newborn lambs during and following asphyxia. Zero (0) time represents the control measurement that is followed by the 75-minute period of asphyxia. Measurements were then made at 5 minutes and at 1, 2, and 4 hours after asphyxia. All values are means ± SEM. Note the highest CMRO$_2$ in animals rendered hyperglycemic. [++], $P <.05$ compared with control; [*], $P <.005$ compared with control. (From Rosenberg AA, Murdaugh E: The effect of blood glucose concentration on postasphyxia cerebral hemodynamics in newborn lambs, Pediatr Res 27:454-459, 1990.)

TABLE 6-7	Effect of Glucose or Saline Treatment on Brain Adenosine Triphosphate in Hypoxic-Ischemic Rats (Unilateral Carotid Ligation and Hypoxemia)[*]		
Experimental Condition	**Phosphocreatine**[*]	**ATP**[*]	**Lactate**[*]
Control	3.00	2.41	1.6
Ligation-hypoxemia[†]			
Saline (60 min)	1.00	1.25	11.1
Glucose (60 min)	1.80	2.31	15.2
Saline (120 min)	0.35	0.43	9.4
Glucose (120 min)	1.00	1.80	25.5

[*]Values are mean concentrations (mmol/kg) in hemisphere ipsilateral to carotid ligation.
[†]All values for ligated-hypoxemic animals different from controls ($P <.05$), and all values for glucose-treated animals different from saline-treated animals ($P <.05$).
ATP, adenosine triphosphate.
Data from Vannucci RC, Brucklacher RM, Vannucci SJ: The effect of hyperglycemia on cerebral metabolism during hypoxia-ischemia in the immature rat, J Cereb Blood Flow Metab 16:1026-1033, 1996.

lower hexokinase activity, the rate-limiting enzyme for glucose utilization.[1,2,5,9,13,15] Indeed, the possibility should be considered that any increase in lactate that may occur in the glucose-treated animal is used for energy production (by oxidation to pyruvate and entrance into the tricarboxylic acid cycle), because lactate is a preferred fuel in neonatal brain.[5,103,132-134] Moreover, lactate is transported rapidly across the blood-brain barrier in the immature animal, and, at least in the rat, brain pH normalizes by 10 minutes of recovery and tissue lactate levels normalize by 4 hours, unlike the prolonged tissue acidosis that occurs in adult rats subjected to hypoxia-ischemia and glucose treatment.[103] Indeed, the combination of rapid utilization of lactate by brain and rapid efflux from brain may explain the lack of serious tissue injury by levels of lactate that lead to injury in adult brain.

Enthusiasm for supplementation with glucose during or after hypoxic-ischemic insults in the immature brain must be tempered by the results of four other studies of young animals.[135-137] Thus, in a model of focal ischemia in the 7-day-old rat, glucose administration *following* hypoxia-ischemia led to more severe neuronal injury (although no increase in infarct size) than did saline administration.[135] Moreover, in a model of global hypoxia-ischemia in 1- to 3-day-old piglets, glucose administration *during* the insult led to accentuated neuronal injury.[136] Glucose administration *following* the insult did not ameliorate the injury, as such therapy accomplished in the immature rat (see earlier.)[137] Finally, studies of fetal sheep at 80 days of gestation subjected to bilateral carotid occlusion show no effect on degree of brain injury of prolonged *moderate* hyperglycemia before ischemia and during reperfusion but a clear detrimental effect when an acute and *marked* increase in plasma glucose concentration (approximately sevenfold greater than control values) was added to the moderate hyperglycemia just before ischemia.[138] Brain lactate levels were not measured. The reasons for the differences in results obtained in the several perinatal models (see earlier discussion) are unclear but may relate to methodological differences.

Summary. Current experimental data allow several tentative conclusions to be made about the effects of glucose administration with perinatal hypoxic-ischemic insults (Table 6-8). On balance, the findings favor maintenance of blood glucose concentrations in the normal range in infants who have sustained hypoxic-ischemic insults or who are at risk for sustaining such insults.

Influence of Maturation on Glucose and Energy Metabolism with Hypoxia-Ischemia

The influence of the maturational state of the brain on the severity and topography of the brain injury caused by hypoxia-ischemia is complex. It is now clear that the long-held general notion that the perinatal brain is more resistant than the adult brain is too simplistic. Evidence indicates that cerebral glucose

TABLE 6-8   Tentative Conclusions Concerning Effects of Glucose Administration with Perinatal Hypoxic-Ischemic Insults*

Glucose transport into brain and glucose concentration in brain are increased. Lactate levels are increased, and intracellular pH values are decreased but recover promptly.

Decrease in cerebral metabolic rate of oxygen is prevented, perhaps reflecting improved mitochondrial function.

Improvement in high-energy phosphate levels is usual but has not reached statistical significance in all studies.

Neuropathological injury may be prevented, ameliorated, or accentuated, according to the model of hypoxia-ischemia and the species and state of maturation of the animal.

Improved survival occurs and may relate at least partially to improvement in cardiorespiratory function.

Determinations of cerebral lactate and high-energy phosphates, as a function of blood glucose, are needed in asphyxiated human newborns for definitive recommendations concerning glucose supplementation.

*See text for references.

and energy metabolism are *more resistant* to perturbation by hypoxia-ischemia in the immature than in the adult brain.[1,2,18,19,23,25,35,44,96,97,139-146] Some of the mechanisms underlying the resistance of energy metabolism in the immature brain are summarized in Table 6-9. However, neuropathological studies indicate that many critical neuronal groups are *more vulnerable* to hypoxic-ischemic injury in the immature animal.[147-149] This vulnerability of immature neurons relates particularly to enhanced density and function of excitatory amino acid receptors and enhanced vulnerability to attack by reactive oxygen species (ROS) and reactive nitrogen species (RNS), as discussed later. A particular vulnerability of immature oligodendrocytes to hypoxic-ischemic, excitatory amino acid and free radical injury is discussed later but also is relevant in this context. The various influences of maturation on the regional aspects of hypoxic-ischemic brain injury and on the responses to interventions are highlighted in appropriate subsequent sections of this chapter.

Birth as an Additive or Potentiating Factor in Hypoxic Injury

Perinatal hypoxic-ischemic injury occurs in the setting of a profound alteration of biochemical and physiological homeostasis (i.e., the process of birth). Transient hypoxemia and hypercapnia, variable in severity and duration, are consistent occurrences.[150-152] Transient disturbances in CBF may also occur (see Chapter 4).[153,154] It is appropriate to ask whether the biochemical state of the brain is affected by the major systemic alterations that take place at birth.

Careful studies of perinatal rat brain indicate that *spontaneous vaginal delivery* is associated with the *signs of hypoxemic or ischemic insult to brain*.[155,156] Alterations in glycogen, certain glycolytic intermediates, and high-energy compounds after spontaneous vaginal delivery

are shown in Table 6-10. Evidence for glycogenolysis, enhanced lactate production, PCr conversion to ATP, and a decline in ATP concentrations is apparent in the first minute after birth. Simultaneous elevation of the concentrations of glucose-6-phosphate and glucose-1-phosphate and decline of the concentration of glycogen are consistent with the occurrence of glycogenolysis.[156] The elevation of lactate level and of the lactate/pyruvate ratio indicates enhanced anaerobic glycolysis. The sharp decline of PCr is not adequate in the first minute to preserve ATP concentrations, and in fact the small persisting deficit in ATP levels 10 minutes after birth is statistically significant.[155] Not shown, but accompanying these changes, is a decline in brain glucose concentrations relative to blood glucose, a finding reflecting further the enhanced glycolysis. By 1 hour after delivery, high-energy phosphate concentrations were no longer depressed, and the ratio of lactate to pyruvate was considerably improved. The latter was normal by 8 hours after delivery. Determinations of identical parameters after cesarean section showed very transient and much smaller changes; indeed, no significant change in ATP levels was observed at any time after delivery by cesarean section.[155]

TABLE 6-9   Resistance of High-Energy Phosphate Levels in Perinatal (versus Adult) Brain to Hypoxic Injury: Probable Mechanisms

Lower rate of energy utilization
Lower rate of accumulation of toxic products (i.e., lactate)
Utilization of lactate and ketone bodies for energy

TABLE 6-10   Effect of Spontaneous Vaginal Delivery on Glycogen, Glycolytic Metabolites, and High-Energy Compounds in Rat Brain

Metabolic Compound	TIME AFTER DELIVERY (MIN)		
	1	10	60
	PERCENTAGE OF TERM FETAL VALUES		
Glycogen	88	74	90
Lactate	367	408	230
Lactate-pyruvate	425	181	157
Phosphocreatine	38	105	170
Adenosine triphosphate	67	92	96

Data from Vannucci RC, Duffy TE: Influence of birth on carbohydrate and energy metabolism in rat brain, *Am J Physiol* 226:933-940, 1974; and Kohle SJ, Vannucci RC: Glycogen metabolism in fetal and postnatal rat brain: Influence of birth, *J Neurochem* 28:441-443, 1977.

These data indicate that the process of birth through the vaginal route in a neonatal animal model is associated with the biochemical signs of hypoxic insult to brain. The influence of this phenomenon on the impact of hypoxic-ischemic insults occurring before or immediately following birth is not known. An intuitive conclusion would be that the insult at birth may be additive. However, it is possible that the insult at birth may play a protective role in relation to a subsequent insult. Thus, a degree of protection to hypoxic-ischemic neuronal injury has been shown in the immature rat by prior exposure to hypoxia.[157-160] This *hypoxic preconditioning* appears to be related to induction of multiple genes, particularly the transcription factor hypoxia-inducing-factor 1 (HIF1) and its target genes, that blunt the adverse effects of hypoxia-ischemia by induction of vasodilation, glucose transport, glycolysis, and antiexcitotoxic, antioxidant, antiapoptotic, and other mechanisms.

Biochemical Mechanisms of Neuronal Death with Hypoxia-Ischemia: Beyond Glucose and Energy Metabolism

The principal biochemical mechanisms of cell death with hypoxia-ischemia and asphyxia are presumably very similar, if not identical, and are initiated by oxygen (and glucose) deprivation and an impairment in energy supplies. Because all the principal, currently considered mechanisms for cell death with oxygen deprivation at least begin with the disturbances of brain glucose and energy metabolism, it is appropriate to synthesize current concepts concerning the mechanisms for cell death immediately following the preceding sections, which emphasize these disturbances. Nevertheless, it is now clear that the mechanisms of cell death with oxygen deprivation are not simply the result of energy failure and, indeed, extend beyond glucose and energy metabolism. An enormous amount of literature attests to the complexity of the mechanisms. In the following section, I attempt to synthesize the essential data and to isolate the most critical mechanisms. The emphasis is on mechanisms of *neuronal* death. Although mechanisms of white matter injury, *especially oligodendroglial death*, bear many similarities, sufficient differences warrant *separate consideration in the next major section.*

General Themes: Importance of the Reperfusion Period and Mode of Cell Death (Necrosis-Apoptosis)

Importance of the Reperfusion Period. As discussed in the next section, the cascade of deleterious events that lead to cell death after insults that result in oxygen deprivation and energy failure appears to occur *primarily following termination of the insult.* Careful studies in animal models and in human patients provide strong support for this notion.[161-170] The phenomena are initiated particularly by energy depletion, accumulation of extracellular excitatory amino acids (particularly glutamate), increase in cytosolic Ca^{2+}, and generation of free radicals. The importance of this "delayed" death of brain in the hours following termination of the insult is related in largest part to the possibility that intervention during the postinsult period could be beneficial. Data to support this possibility are now available, as discussed later.

Importance of the Mode of Cell Death (Necrosis-Apoptosis). Two fundamental modes of cell death in the nervous system, as in other tissues, are distinguished: *necrosis* and *apoptosis*. It is now clear that hypoxic-ischemic insults may lead to necrosis or apoptosis, or both, dependent principally on the severity of the insult and the maturational state of the cell. Certain characteristics readily distinguish these two forms of cell death (Table 6-11).[171-183] Thus, *necrotic cell death* is characterized by cell swelling, membrane disintegration, cell rupture, release of intracellular contents, and, as a consequence, inflammation and phagocytosis. By contrast, *apoptosis* is characterized by condensation and margination of chromatin, cell shrinkage, relative preservation of cellular membranes, and death without inflammation. Apoptotic cell death is difficult to detect in tissue because of the lack of inflammation and the rapid removal of the cell debris. Apoptotic cell death requires activation of specific death genes, ATP, and new protein synthesis, which result particularly in a

TABLE 6-11 Necrosis and Apoptosis: Distinguishing Characteristics*		
Distinguishing Feature	**Necrosis**	**Apoptosis**
Morphology	Cell swelling; dispersed chromatin; membrane fragmentation; inflammatory responses	Cell shrinkage; chromatin condensation; intact membranes; *no* inflammation
DNA fragmentation	Nonspecific	Specific oligonucleosomal cleavage
Involvement of specific death genes/enzymes (e.g., Bax, Bid, p53, AIF, PARP, cytochrome c, caspases)	No	Yes
Adenosine triphosphate required	No	Yes
Protein synthesis required	No	Yes
Temporal characteristics	Usually rapid (minutes to hours)	Slow (hours to days)
Insult characteristics	More severe	Less severe

*See text for references.

series of biochemical changes that include cleavage of DNA at specific sites to result in the characteristic oligonucleosomal fragmentation (see later). Necrotic cell death occurs typically after intense, often relatively brief insults, whereas apoptotic cell death occurs typically after less intense, longer-acting insults. Apoptotic cell death may be the dominant form of so-called delayed cell death, observable after many hours to several days in various experimental neonatal models and human brain. Important intrinsic properties of the cell itself in the determination of the mode of cell death relate particularly to the developmental stage of the cell. Thus, the susceptibility to apoptosis is enhanced in immature versus mature neurons in vitro and in vivo.[176,184-188] Apoptotic cell death was noted to be common in a study of infants who died after intrauterine hypoxic-ischemic insult (see Chapter 8).[181] Moreover, careful studies in the neonatal piglet subjected to hypoxia-ischemia demonstrated in the same paradigm exclusively necrotic cell death in certain neuronal populations, both necrosis and apoptosis in other neuronal populations, but exclusively apoptotic cell death in immature cerebral white matter.[175] Indeed, in many models, electron microscopic study reveals an apoptotic-necrotic continuum in neuronal regions, with clearly apoptotic and necrotic cells present, as well as hybrid cells with "intermediate" characteristics.[189] Often, the early cell death appears necrotic and later cell death appears apoptotic.[190,191]

The *molecular mechanisms involved in apoptosis* associated with *neonatal* hypoxia-ischemia have been clarified considerably, although not completely, in recent years.[183,184,189-198] Although many molecular triggers of apoptosis exist, perhaps most important with hypoxia-ischemia, influx of Ca^{2+} and generation of ROS (see later) are membrane perturbations that involve release of ceramide from sphingomyelin, translocation to the mitochondrion of proapoptotic members of the Bc1-2 family (i.e., Bax, Bid), formation of a mitochondrial permeability pore, release from mitochondrion of cytochrome c and apoptosis-inducing factor, and stimulation of endonucleases by apoptosis-inducing factor and of caspases, especially caspase-3 by cytochrome c. *Both caspase-dependent and caspase-independent mechanisms of apoptotic cell death have been recognized.* Caspases are proteases with cysteine residues in their active sites and catalyze proteolysis at specific aspartate residues, hence the term *caspase.* Caspase-3 is activated within 1 to 3 hours after neonatal hypoxia-ischemia and is a principal executioner of apoptosis. The substrates attacked by caspases include cytoskeletal and associated proteins, nuclear and DNA-associated proteins, signal transduction proteins, ion channel subunits, and other key molecules. One of the results of the process is DNA cleavage, and poly(ADP ribose) polymerase (PARP), involved in DNA repair, is activated. PARP activation is a prominent feature of the caspase-dependent apoptotic cascade. PARP inactivation occurs by caspase-3–mediated cleavage during the early stages of apoptosis. This inactivation facilitates nuclear

disassembly and ensures the completion of the apoptotic process, because PARP activation depletes the cell of ATP, which is essential for apoptosis. The action of apoptosis-inducing factor to cause apoptotic cell death is caspase-*independent* and involves principally translocation to the nucleus and activation of endonucleases. The complex molecular cascades involved in apoptosis occur over many hours and days, thus raising the possibility of interruption of the cascade during a relatively long time window (see later).

Initiating Role of Energy Failure

In earlier years, cell death with oxygen deprivation was explained entirely by reference to the sharply decreased production of high-energy phosphate from anaerobic glycolysis (see Fig. 6-2). The mechanism cited was deficiency of high-energy phosphates that are necessary for synthesis of macromolecules and lipids and thus maintenance of structural integrity. Several decades of research make it clear that this explanation is too simple and that cell death does not require energy depletion severe enough to eliminate synthesis of structural components. However, an initial decrease in high-energy phosphates is capable of *triggering a series of additional mechanisms* that begin with a failure of the ATP-dependent Na^+-K^+ pump (Fig. 6-17). If the insult is very severe, the acute result is Na^+ influx, followed by chloride (Cl^-) and water influx, cell swelling, cell lysis, and thus *early cell death by necrosis* (see Fig. 6-17). In the more typical, less severe insult, membrane depolarization occurs and is followed by extracellular accumulation of glutamate, increased cytosolic Ca^{2+} and a cascade of events leading to a

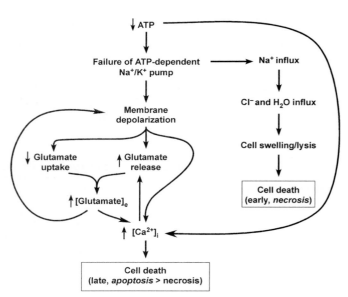

Figure 6-17 Relation between energy depletion and cell death. Early cell death is primarily necrosis, and the more important, later cell death is primarily apoptosis. Concerning the latter, delayed cell death, accumulation of extracellular glutamate with excitotoxicity and elevations of intracellular calcium are important. ATP, adenosine triphosphate; Ca^{2+}, calcium; Cl^-, chloride; K^+, potassium; Na^+, sodium. See text for details.

more delayed cell death, principally apoptotic, although necrosis may also occur by this mechanism. The details are discussed in the ensuing sections. Suffice it to say here that the increased extracellular glutamate results from (1) excessive presynaptic glutamate release (because of membrane depolarization and later increased cytosolic Ca^{2+}) and (2) failure of glutamate uptake mechanisms in presynaptic nerve endings and astrocytes (because of membrane depolarization and failure of high-affinity, Na^+-dependent glutamate transporters). The increase in cytosolic Ca^{2+} is a consequence of (1) failure of energy-dependent Ca^{2+}-pumping mechanisms, (2) opening of voltage-dependent Ca^{2+} channels (secondary to membrane depolarization), and probably most importantly, (3) activation of specific glutamate receptors (see later discussion). The subsequent deleterious events provoked by Ca^{2+} and leading to cell death after these initial events are described next.

Role of Accumulation of Cytosolic Calcium

A large body of information indicates a major role for accumulation of cytosolic Ca^{2+} during and following hypoxia-ischemia in the mediation of cell death.[4,35,146,199-211] In perinatal models of hypoxia-ischemia, increased Ca^{2+} uptake into the insulted brain regions, close correlation within brain regions between increased uptake of Ca^{2+} and subsequent neuronal injury, and some protection from subsequent brain injury by pretreatment with voltage-dependent Ca^{2+} channel antagonists have been documented.[4,52,53,204,205,209,212-216] *Moreover, because a major mechanism of Ca^{2+} influx into the cytosol is through the N-methyl-D-aspartate (NMDA) and alpha-amino-3-hydroxy-5-methyl-4-isoxazolepropionic acid (AMPA) types of glutamate receptors, the protection from brain injury afforded by antagonists of these receptors (see later discussion)* *may be mediated primarily by decreasing accumulation of cytosolic Ca^{2+}.*

Mechanisms. The mechanisms by which increased cytosolic Ca^{2+} leads to cell death are multiple but are best discussed in the context of normal Ca^{2+} homeostasis (Fig. 6-18).[4,35,199-205,209,217,218,218a] The cellular mechanisms for maintenance of low cytosolic Ca^{2+} concentrations (10^{-7} M) relative to high extracellular Ca^{2+} concentrations (10^{-3} M) are located in the *plasma membrane* (voltage-dependent channels; three agonist-dependent, i.e., glutamate-dependent, channels: the NMDA, AMPA [immature, i.e., lacking GluR2 subunit] and metabotropic receptor-activated channels [see later discussion]; an ATP-dependent uniport system and an Na^+-dependent antiport system), the *endoplasmic reticulum* (an ATP-dependent import system and a release mechanism activated by inositol triphosphate), and the *mitochondrion* (a voltage-dependent channel and an Na^+/H^+-dependent antiport system) (see Fig. 6-18).[203-205] The mechanisms for the increased cytosolic Ca^{2+} in neurons subjected to hypoxia-ischemia, and the metabolic and ionic changes caused by ischemia that underlie these mechanisms, are summarized in Table 6-12. *The central roles for ATP depletion, membrane depolarization, and voltage-dependent and glutamate-activated Ca^{2+} channels are apparent.*

The deleterious effects of increased cytosolic Ca^{2+} are multiple and affect the cell in a variety of ways (Table 6-13).[4,35,199-205,209,211,214,218-224] These effects include degradation of cellular lipids by activation of phospholipases, of cellular proteins (especially cytoskeletal elements) by activation of proteases, and of cellular DNA by activation of nucleases, as well as crucial indirect mechanisms of destruction mediated by generation of free radicals and nitric oxide (NO) (Fig. 6-19). The utilization of ATP by ATP-dependent

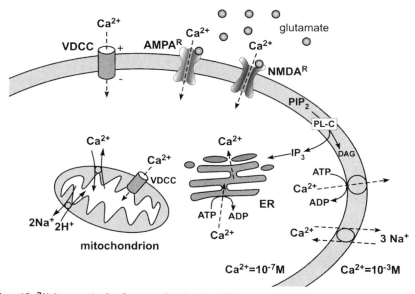

Figure 6-18 **Cellular calcium (Ca^{2+}) homeostasis.** See text for details. ADP, adenosine diphosphate; AMPA, alpha-amino-3-hydroxy-5-methyl-4-isoxazolepropionic acid; ATP; adenosine triphosphate; DAG, diacylglycerol; ER, endoplasmic reticulum; Na^+, sodium; NMDA, *N*-methyl-D-aspartate; PIP_2, phosphatidylinositol-4,5-diphosphate; PL-C, phospholipase C; VDCC, voltage-dependent calcium channel.

TABLE 6-12   Mechanisms for Increased Cytosolic Calcium in Neurons with Hypoxia-Ischemia

Site	Mechanism*
Plasma membrane	↑ Ca^{2+} influx through voltage-dependent Ca^{2+} channels (cell depolarization)
	↑ Ca^{2+} influx through agonist-dependent Ca^{2+} channels (glutamate action at NMDA and immature AMPA receptors)†
	Activation of phospholipase C and liberation of IP_3 (see below) (glutamate action at metabotropic receptor)
	↓ Ca^{2+} efflux through ATP-dependent uniport system (ATP depletion)
	↓ Ca^{2+} efflux through Na^+-dependent antiport system (↓ extracellular Na^+)
Endoplasmic reticulum	↑ Ca^{2+} release to cytosol through effect of IP_3 (see above)
	↓ Ca^{2+} uptake by ATP-dependent uniport system (ATP depletion)
Mitochondrion	↑ Ca^{2+} release to cytosol via Na^+,H^+–dependent antiport system (↑ cytosolic Na^+,H^+)

*The primary effect of ischemia to cause the indicated change in Ca^{2+} homeostasis is shown in parentheses.
†Probably the single most important mechanism.
AMPA, alpha-amino-3-hydroxy-5-methyl-4-isoxazole-propionic acid; ATP, adenosine triphosphate; Ca^{2+}, calcium; H^+, hydrogen; Na^+, sodium; NMDA, N-methyl-D-aspartate; IP_3, inositol triphosphate.

Ca^{2+}-transport systems, attempting to correct the cytosolic Ca^{2+} accumulation, and the Ca^{2+}-mediated uncoupling of oxidative phosphorylation serve to perpetuate the process (see Fig. 6-19).

Role of Free Radicals: Reactive Oxygen and Nitrogen Species

Free Radicals. The crucial role of free radicals, generated in considerable part by Ca^{2+}-activated processes just described, in the mediation of cell death with hypoxia-ischemia has been established by study of a variety of models in vivo, in culture, and in vitro (see later).[35,182,211,225-246] The emphasis in these studies has been neuronal injury. Discussion of the role of free radicals in oligodendroglial injury is contained in a later section. Free radicals are highly reactive compounds with an uneven number of electrons in the outermost orbital. These compounds can react with certain normal cellular components (e.g., unsaturated fatty acids of membrane lipids) and can generate a new free radical

and thereby a chain reaction, which results in irreversible biochemical injury (e.g., peroxidation of the unsaturated fatty acids, membrane injury, and cell necrosis). With less intense insults, free radicals can lead to apoptotic cell death by activation of specific death genes.[231,246-249] Free radicals in mammalian cells exist primarily as ROS (e.g., superoxide anion, hydrogen peroxide, hydroxyl radical) or as RNS (e.g., peroxynitrite [$ONOO^-$]) (see later). When these reactive species are present in excess, the cell is said to be subjected to oxidative stress or nitrative stress, respectively. Although studies have generally focused on ROS or RNS separately, these species usually exist together (e.g., under conditions of hypoxia-ischemia-reperfusion). I discuss the investigations of ROS and RNS in separate sections later.

The principal sources of free radicals with hypoxia-ischemia, the endogenous defenses against such radicals, and their major deleterious effects are summarized in Table 6-14. Of the sources of free radicals with

TABLE 6-13   Deleterious Effects of Calcium in Hypoxia-Ischemia

Calcium Action	Deleterious Effect
Activate phospholipases	Phospholipid hydrolysis and membrane injury
	Generation of arachidonic acid and ultimately free radicals by cyclooxygenase and lipoxygenase pathways
Activate proteases, disassembly of microtubules	Cytoskeletal disruption (caused by microtubular disruption and proteolysis of neurofilaments)
	Proteolysis of other cellular proteins
Activate nucleases	Nuclear injury
Activate calcium-ATPase and other energy-dependent calcium extrusion mechanisms	Consumption of ATP at a time of deficient ATP
Enter mitochondrion and uncouple oxidative phosphorylation	Decrease in ATP production
Increase neurotransmitter release (e.g., glutamate, catecholamines)	Activation of glutamate receptors (e.g., calcium influx)
	Autooxidation of catecholamines with production of free radicals
Activate a protease for transformation of xanthine dehydrogenase to xanthine oxidase	Oxidation of hypoxanthine to xanthine and of xanthine to uric acid with production of free radicals
Activate nitric oxide synthase	Generation of nitric oxide and ultimately peroxynitrite, with toxic effect on neurons

ATP, adenosine triphosphate.

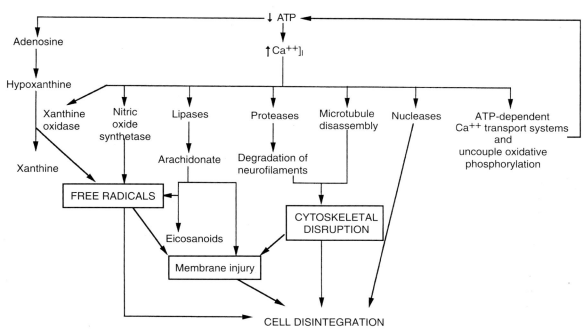

Figure 6-19　Deleterious effects of elevated cytosolic calcium ([Ca⁺⁺]ᵢ). Generation of free radicals is especially important. ATP; adenosine triphosphate. See text for details.

hypoxia-ischemia, the electron transport system is important when oxygen deprivation prevents the complete passage of electrons to cytochrome c oxidase. Free radicals, specifically superoxide anion, then are generated proximal to this terminal enzyme in the electron transport system. The next four sources are directly or indirectly related to cytosolic Ca^{2+} (see Fig. 6-19 and Table 6-13). Arachidonic acid is generated by Ca^{2+}-activated phospholipase A_2, xanthine oxidase is activated by Ca^{2+}, catecholamine release is stimulated by an increase in cytosolic Ca^{2+}, and NO synthase (NOS; see next section) is activated by Ca^{2+}.[35,205,218,221-229,231,242,250-267] Finally, data indicate that early reactive cells at the site of initial insult, especially *microglia*, are potent sources of free radicals (see later discussion).

Reactive Oxygen Species. An important role for ROS in perinatal models of fetal and neonatal hypoxemic, ischemic, hypoxic-ischemic, and asphyxial insults now seems established.[59,182,229,230,240-245,249,265,268-288] Following the insults, generation of ROS or elevations of compounds known to lead to generation of ROS has been found. Moreover, studies principally of asphyxia in the newborn lamb and in the neonatal piglet and of hypoxia-ischemia (carotid ligation and low oxygen breathing) in the immature (7-day-old) rat have shown elevations of free radicals, deleterious effects of free radical attack (e.g., evidence for lipid peroxidation), or a neuroprotective effect of treatment (pretreatment, treatment during the insult, or after termination of the insult) with free radical scavengers (e.g., vitamin E analogues, edaravone, or drugs that inhibit free radical

TABLE 6-14　Free Radicals in Hypoxia-Ischemia

Sources
Mitochondrial electron transport system
Action of cyclooxygenase and lipoxygenase on arachidonic acid
Action of xanthine oxidase on hypoxanthine and xanthine
Autooxidation of catecholamines
Infiltrating reactive microglia
Action of nitric oxide synthase

Endogenous Defenses
Major: superoxide dismutase (generates H_2O_2), catalase (degrades H_2O_2), and glutathione peroxidase (degrades H_2O_2)
Free radical scavengers: vitamin E (alpha-tocopherol), other sterols (21-aminosteroids), vitamin C (ascorbic acid), glutathione, other thiol compounds

Major Deleterious Effects
Peroxidation of PUFAs of membrane phospholipids (PUFAs especially abundant in brain membranes)
Damage to DNA and to proteins containing unsaturated or sulfhydryl groups
Activation of proapoptotic genes

H_2O_2, hydrogen peroxide; PUFAs, polyunsaturated fatty acids.

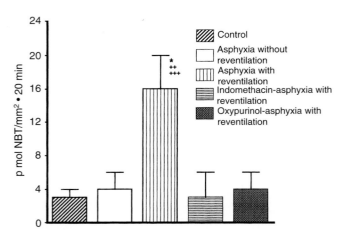

Figure 6-20 **Free radical (superoxide anion) production,** determined as superoxide dismutase-inhibitable nitroblue tetrazolium (NBT) reduction in control (n = 7), asphyxia without reventilation (n = 9), asphyxia-reventilation (n = 11), asphyxia-reventilation after indomethacin 0.2 mg/kg (n = 4), and asphyxia-reventilation after oxypurinol 50.0 mg/kg (n = 10) pretreated piglets. Values are mean ± SEM. *, $P < .05$ compared with control; ++, $P < .05$ compared with asphyxia without reventilation group; +++, $P < .05$ compared with indomethacin and oxypurinol pretreatment groups. Note the production of superoxide anion after (with reventilation) but not during (without reventilation) asphyxia and the prevention by administration of indomethacin or oxypurinol. *(From Pourcyrous M, Leffler CW, Bada HS, Korones SB, et al: Brain superoxide anion generation in asphyxiated piglets and the effect of indomethacin at therapeutic dose, Pediatr Res 34:366-369, 1993.)*

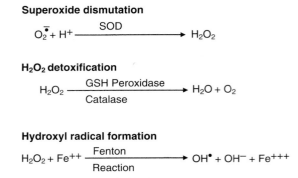

Superoxide dismutation

$$O_2^{\bar{\cdot}} + H^+ \xrightarrow{\text{SOD}} H_2O_2$$

H$_2$O$_2$ detoxification

$$H_2O_2 \xrightarrow[\text{Catalase}]{\text{GSH Peroxidase}} H_2O + O_2$$

Hydroxyl radical formation

$$H_2O_2 + Fe^{++} \xrightarrow[\text{Reaction}]{\text{Fenton}} OH^{\cdot} + OH^- + Fe^{+++}$$

Figure 6-21 **Free radical metabolism.** The upper two reactions, catalyzed respectively by superoxide dismutases (SOD; both copper-zinc SOD [extracellular and cytosol] and manganese SOD [mitochondrion]) and by GSH peroxidase and catalase, are the major antioxidant defense mechanisms. In the presence of hydrogen peroxide (H_2O_2) and iron (Fe^{++}), the Fenton reaction (lowest reaction) generates the highly toxic hydroxyl radical. GSH, glutathione; SOD, superoxide dismutases.

formation (e.g., allopurinol, oxypurinol, indomethacin, superoxide dismutase [SOD], catalase, and iron chelators).* The importance of the reperfusion period, rather than the time of the hypoxic-ischemic insult per se, in the generation of the ROS also has been emphasized (Fig. 6-20).

The *major endogenous antioxidant defense system* is illustrated in Figure 6-21. Thus, the most commonly generated initial oxygen free radical, the superoxide anion, is converted to hydrogen peroxide by the enzyme SOD, the three different forms of which are cytosolic copper-zinc SOD, extracellular copper-zinc SOD, and mitochondrial manganese SOD. The hydrogen peroxide generated is detoxified by catalase and glutathione peroxidase. If this step fails or is overloaded, and if iron is available, the Fenton reaction and the production of the deadly hydroxyl radical occur. Studies of animal models and more recent studies of asphyxiated human infants indicate that after hypoxia-ischemia, iron is released and is therefore relatively abundant.[5,230,239,241,300-305] Studies of hypoxia-ischemia in the neonatal mouse indicate that the detoxification of hydrogen peroxide is deficient in the immature brain. Thus, mice made transgenic for copper-zinc SOD and therefore overexpressing this enzyme, when subjected to hypoxia-ischemia, exhibit decreased brain injury in the adult but *increased* brain injury in the perinatal period.[240,282] This *exacerbation*

of brain injury in the *immature* brain was associated with an accumulation of hydrogen peroxide, because catalase and glutathione peroxidase did not increase in activity in response to the insult (catalase increases after similar hypoxia-ischemia in the adult).[240] Indeed, the levels of glutathione peroxidase decreased after hypoxia-ischemia, and importantly, in the normal animal levels already developmentally low in the perinatal period. Consistent with this, in normally developing rats (P7) rendered hypoxic-ischemic, an accumulation of hydrogen peroxide in cortex was much greater than occurred with hypoxia-ischemia at later ages (P42).[306] The particular importance of glutathione peroxidase was shown in two models derived from transgenic mice overexpressing glutathione peroxidase.[307,308] Thus, in cultured neurons exposed to oxidative stress and in a neonatal hypoxic-ischemic model, glutathione peroxidase overexpression led to neuronal protection. Additional importance for glutathione is suggested by the finding in the hypoxic-ischemic 7-day rat that the crucial mitochondrial fraction of glutathione, necessary for glutathione peroxidase function, was markedly decreased after hypoxia-ischemia, with a nadir after 24 hours.[309] Thus, the data suggest that the normal immature brain has a limited capacity to detoxify hydrogen peroxide and with hypoxia-ischemia accumulates hydrogen peroxide, both because of this developmental lack and because of failure to respond with an adaptive increase in the antioxidant defense enzymes. With the hypoxia-ischemia-induced increase in iron, generation of the hydroxyl radical and brain injury is the result (see Fig. 6-21).

The *propensity for oxidative neuronal injury* in the immature brain relates not only to the deficient antioxidant defenses just described but also to several *pro-oxidant characteristics.* Thus, at baseline, the developing brain has a relatively high concentration of polyunsaturated fatty acids, especially in neuronal membranes, an excellent target for ROS, and a relatively high concentration of nonprotein-bound iron.[245] Therefore, with exposure

---

*See references 59,62,125,182,232-245,249,270,277-279,281, 283-299.

to conditions that lead to an increase in ROS (e.g., hypoxia-ischemia-reperfusion) and available iron, the balance strongly favors oxidative injury. Similar considerations apply to the increased oxidative injury observed after hypoxia-ischemia in developing animals or in asphyxiated infants when resuscitation is carried out with 100% oxygen rather than with room air (see Chapter 9).[267,310-316a]

Nitric Oxide and Reactive Nitrogen Species.

Particular importance for the synthesis of NO by NOS both in normal brain and under conditions of hypoxia-ischemia is now well established.[211,266,317-330] At least three forms of NOS are recognized: a constitutive neuronal form (nNOS), a constitutive endothelial form (eNOS), and an inducible form (iNOS) found in astrocytes and microglia. The constitutive forms are activated by Ca^{2+}, whereas iNOS stimulation appears to be Ca^{2+} independent and is activated especially well by inflammatory stimuli (e.g., cytokines, lipopolysaccharide [LPS], and oxidative stress). Because NO is a diffusible gas, both its normal functions (i.e., cell signaling and neurotransmission) and its deleterious actions (i.e., neurotoxicity) appear to be mediated by synthesis and then diffusion to intracellular sites and to adjacent cells.

Under *normal* conditions, NO has multiple cellular effects.[329] Many of these, but not all, are initiated by guanylate cyclase activation with the subsequent production of cyclic guanosine monophosphate and protein phosphorylation. This activation occurs when NO binds to the heme group of guanylate cyclase. Other biological effects of NO relate to action of its metabolites. Thus, formation of a nitro group (NO_2) allows the *nitration* of proteins, especially at tyrosine residues, to form nitrotyrosine. Formation of nitrosonium ion (NO^+) allows *nitrosylation* of thiol residues on proteins, especially cysteine sulfhydryl group. Formation of $ONOO^-$ and other reactive intermediates, including the hydroxyl radical, leads to *oxidation* of multiple amino acid residues, including formation of nitrotyrosine. The biological effects of these actions of NO include modulation of cell proliferation, apoptosis, mitochondrial energy metabolism, and signal transduction.

Under pathological conditions of *hypoxia-ischemia-reperfusion*, an increase in cytosolic Ca^{2+} is an early event (see earlier). A particularly important effector for the increase in Ca^{2+} is activation of the NMDA receptor (see later). The effects on NO metabolism are multiple and sequential (Fig. 6-22).[211,317-322,328-332] Thus, in the first few minutes, the activity of Ca^{2+}-dependent eNOS in endothelial cells is increased to produce vasodilation and to replenish substrate supply. The activity of Ca^{2+}-dependent nNOS in neurons also is increased, and initially this increase may help to improve blood flow because of the presence of nNOS in perivascular nerves.[329] However, the principal effect of induction of nNOS in neurons is the generation of NO that diffuses to adjacent neurons. Under conditions of oxidative stress with abundant superoxide anion ($O_2^{\bullet-}$), NO reacts quickly with $O_2^{\bullet-}$ to

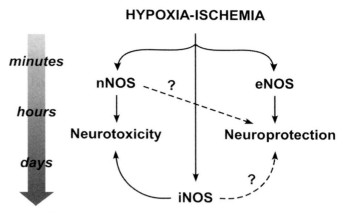

Figure 6-22 **Major effects of the various forms of nitric oxide synthase (NOS) after hypoxia-ischemia**. Effects in the first minutes to hours and in the hours to days after the insult can be distinguished, although these effects overlap. *Dotted lines* indicate neuroprotective effects that appear plausible under certain circumstances but require more study. See text for details. eNOS, endothelial NOS; iNOS, inducible NOS; nNOS, neuronal NOS.

form the particularly toxic RNS, $ONOO^-$. Indeed, the affinity of $O_2^{\bullet-}$ for NO to form $ONOO^-$ greatly exceeds the reaction of $O_2^{\bullet-}$ with SOD, and thus $ONOO^-$ formation is greatly favored. This compound leads to neuronal death by multiple mechanisms, including especially *mitochondrial impairment*, energy depletion, and further failure of Ca^{2+}-homeostasis (see earlier).[325-328,333] Glutamate activation of the NMDA receptor is a major cause of the initial increase of cytosolic Ca^{2+} that activates nNOS and leads to this deleterious cascade. Those NMDA receptor–containing neurons that express nNOS are resistant to the deleterious effects of hypoxia-ischemia and excitotoxicity (see later).

A *later result* of hypoxia-ischemia-reperfusion is the *activation of iNOS*, principally in astrocytes and microglia, with a resulting large, sustained increase in NO production, over many hours to days, depending on the experimental model studied (see Fig. 6-22).[328,329] This activation occurs in parallel with inflammatory responses and is based on the activation of specific cell surface receptors for cytokines (tumor necrosis factor-alpha [TNF-alpha], interferon-gamma, and interleukin-1beta [IL-1beta]) and on the intracellular effects of ROS. The deleterious effects of this increase in NO is mediated primarily through formation of $ONOO^-$, as discussed earlier. The possibility of a neuroprotective role of NO, mediated by NO^+, has been raised, because S-nitrosylation at critical thiols on the NMDA receptor's redox modulatory site leads to down-regulation of channel activity.[331] The biological impact of such a neuroprotective role currently is unclear.

In *perinatal models of asphyxia or hypoxia-ischemia*, evidence for both the neurotoxic effects and the beneficial vascular effects of NO synthesis have been obtained.[211,245,246,266,301,332,334-354] Evidence for neurotoxic effects of NOS activation has consisted particularly of demonstration of neuroprotection by specific inhibitors of the synthase (e.g., nitrosoarginine derivatives). Although the data are not completely consistent, on balance the scheme shown in Figure 6-22 depicts the major effects mediated by stimulation of the several forms of NOS. Particular importance of NO and RNS during development in part is suggested by the observation that the relative resistance of NOS-expressing neurons to NMDA-mediated toxicity is lost after the neonatal period in the developing rat.[245]

Role of Excitatory Amino Acids

A remarkable series of studies primarily from the past 15 to 20 years has revolutionized understanding of the role of excitatory amino acids, particularly glutamate, as the mediators of neuronal death under conditions of hypoxia-ischemia. Before discussion of these studies, the normal aspects of glutamate biology at the excitatory synapse are reviewed.

Normal Features. The relationships at the *glutamate synapse* among the presynaptic nerve ending, the postsynaptic dendrite, and the associated astrocyte are shown in Figure 6-23.[203,204,355-363] Only the ionotropic receptors are shown in Figure 6-23 (see next paragraph). Glutamate release is provoked by influx of Ca^{2+} into the presynaptic nerve ending. Depolarization of the postsynaptic dendrite is related to Na^+ entry. The action of glutamate is terminated by potent, high-affinity, Na^+-dependent reuptake mechanisms in both astrocytes and presynaptic nerve endings. Although the

transporters per se are not energy dependent, energy failure, as with hypoxia-ischemia, leads to disruption of Na^+-K^+ ionic gradients across the plasma membrane because of failure of the ATP-dependent Na^+-K^+ pump; the results are *impairment* of the Na^+-dependent glutamate transporters and ultimately *reversal* of transporter function. In the astrocyte, the ATP-dependent enzyme, glutamine synthetase, uses ammonia and glutamate to form glutamine, which diffuses to the presynaptic nerve ending to regenerate glutamate on removal of this second amino group (see Fig. 6-23). ATP depletion also causes this mechanism to fail, and thus, clearly ATP depletion results in failure of the major reuptake and removal mechanisms and leads to accumulation of extracellular glutamate and to excitotoxicity (see the following discussion).

These mechanisms of reuptake and removal must be highly efficient, because although the intracellular concentration of glutamate is extraordinarily high (i.e., 5 to 10 mmol/kg), the extracellular concentration is approximately 1000-fold less (i.e., in the low micromolar range or perhaps lower).[356,357,362] The high concentration of glutamate in neurons implies a large release of glutamate into the extracellular space when cell death occurs, an occurrence that is relevant not only to amplification of primary excitotoxic cell death, as occurs with hypoxia-ischemia, but also to the development of secondary excitotoxic cell death from other types of injury to neurons (e.g., trauma). In addition,

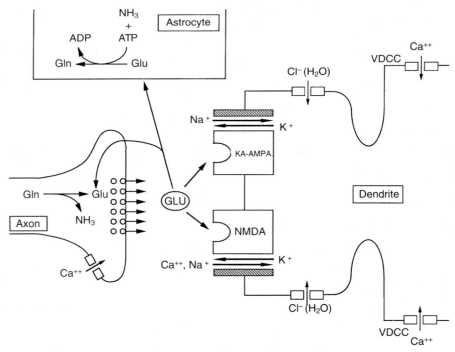

Figure 6-23 **Relationships at the glutamate synapse among the presynaptic axonal terminal, the postsynaptic dendrite, and the associated astrocyte.** See text for details. In this figure, the non–*N*-methyl-D-aspartate (NMDA) (kainate-alpha-amino-3-hydroxy-5-methyl-4-isoxazole-propionic acid (KA-AMPA)) receptors are shown together; see text regarding calcium (Ca^{++}) permeability of the AMPA receptor in developing neurons. ADP, adenosine diphosphate; ATP, adenosine triphosphate; Cl^-, chloride; Gln, glutamine; Glu, glutamate; Na^+, sodium; NH_3, ammonia; VDCC, voltage-dependent calcium channel. (*Modified from Siesjö BK: Calcium in the brain under physiological and pathological conditions, Eur Neurol 30:3-9, 1990.*)

TABLE 6-15	Glutamate Receptors*
Type	**Function**
Ionotropic	
NMDA	Ca^{2+} entry, Na^+ entry
AMPA	Na^+ entry, Ca^{2+} entry (*immature neurons*)†
Kainate	Na^+ entry
Metabotropic	
Ibotenate	Phosphoinositide hydrolysis; protein kinase C activation; Ca^{2+} mobilization from endoplasmic reticulum; multiple downstream effects

*The receptors are named according to the glutamate analogue most potent in activation of the individual receptor.
†In immature neurons AMPA receptors lack the GluR2 subunit, the subunit which renders the receptor Ca^{2+} impermeable, thus resulting in Ca^{2+}-permeable receptors.
AMPA, alpha-amino-3-hydroxy-5-methyl-4-isoxazolepropionic acid; Ca^{2+}, calcium; Na^+, sodium; NMDA, N-methyl-D-aspartate.

release of glutamate from astrocytes may be even more marked than from neurons, under ischemic conditions.[364]

Glutamate acts at both *ionotropic and metabotropic receptors* (Table 6-15).[357,359,361-363,365-379] Three of these are *ionotropic* (i.e., are linked to ion channels). The NMDA receptor is linked to an ion channel for Ca^{2+}, the AMPA receptor is linked to a channel for Na^+ entry, and the kainate receptor is linked to a channel for Na^+ entry. The AMPA receptor is rendered Ca^{2+} impermeable by the presence of one of its four subunits, namely the GluR2 subunit. This subunit is relatively sparse during early development both in rodent and human neurons, and this feature renders the AMPA receptor in immature neurons Ca^{2+} permeable.[361,362,380-383] This feature may underlie the involvement of AMPA receptors in hypoxic-ischemic or glutamate-induced death of immature neurons (see later discussion). Although the NMDA receptor often is considered the most crucial for the excitotoxic effects of glutamate in developing neurons, data suggest comparable importance for the AMPA receptor (see later). Agents that increase or decrease glutamate activation at the synapse mediated by the NMDA receptor-channel complex are shown in Table 6-16.

TABLE 6-16	Excitation at Glutamate Synapse of *N*-Methyl-D-Aspartate Type	
	EFFECT ON EXCITATION	
Site	**Increase**	**Decrease**
Presynaptic (glutamate release)	Calcium Theophylline	Magnesium Adenosine
Receptor	Glutamate Glycine	APV/CPP Kynurenate
Channel		MK-801/ketamine/ dextromethorphan Magnesium/memantine

APV, 2-amino-5-phosphonovalerate; CPP, 3-(2-carboxypiperazine-4-yl)-propyl-1-phosphoric acid.

A fourth glutamate receptor type is *metabotropic* (i.e., is coupled through a guanosine triphosphate binding protein [G protein] to an enzyme producing a second messenger, phospholipase C, for phosphoinositide hydrolysis). The resulting products, diacylglycerol and inositol triphosphate, function as second messengers, the former activating protein kinase C, which has many cellular effects, and the latter promoting Ca^{2+} mobilization from the endoplasmic reticulum (see Fig. 6-19).

The normal *ontogeny of glutamate receptors* is relevant to normal brain development and to the vulnerability of immature brain regions to excitotoxic cell death with hypoxia-ischemia. Detailed earlier studies of the development of binding sites for NMDA and non-NMDA receptor agonists in the rat showed a striking increase in the early phases of brain development.[359-361,379,384-390] Later work, largely based on immunocytochemical and in situ hybridization studies, demonstrated the marked developmental increase more clearly, with peak values for the NMDA and AMPA receptors that *exceed* those in adult brain.[245,381,382] The peak values for NMDA and AMPA receptors were reached at only slightly different ages, with the NMDA peak preceding the AMPA peak. *The timing of these peaks in the rat correlated with the perinatal period for human brain.*

The *molecular characteristics of the NMDA and AMPA receptors* also are developmentally regulated, and the major characteristics of the developing receptors indicate enhanced Ca^{2+} influx.[381,382] Thus, regarding the NMDA receptor, the relative expression of the NR2B subunit compared with that of the NR2A subunit is increased in the immature brain versus the adult. *NMDA receptors containing predominately NR2B exhibit increased duration of NMDA receptor-mediated excitation and increased Ca^{2+} influx.* With regard to the AMPA receptor, in the immature brain the expression of the *GluR2 subunit*, which renders the AMPA receptor Ca^{2+} impermeable, as in the mature brain, is relatively *low*. *Thus, the large numbers of AMPA receptors in developing neurons are largely permeable to Ca^{2+}.*

The transient, dense expressions of these ionotropic glutamate receptors of enhanced functional capabilities have implications not only for their role in normal development, but also in determining neuronal death with hypoxia-ischemia (see later). The role of glutamate receptor activation and Ca^{2+} influx relates to such processes as regulation of neurite outgrowth, synapse formation, cell death, selective elimination of neuronal processes, and functional organization of neuronal systems.[359-361,374,381,386,391] *However, in addition, these transient dense expressions of glutamate receptors of enhanced functional capabilities may become the unintended mediators of neuronal death with hypoxia-ischemia (see later).* Moreover, the likelihood that these principles apply to *developing* human brain is supported by the demonstration of *early overexpression* of glutamate receptors in human hippocampus, cerebral cortex, deep nuclear structures (i.e., basal ganglia and thalamus), and certain brain stem nuclei, regions vulnerable to hypoxic-ischemic injury in the newborn (see Chapter 8).[359-361,381,383,387,392-396]

TABLE 6-17 **Major Evidence Supporting a Critical Role for Glutamate in Hypoxic-Ischemic Neuronal Death in Developing Brain***

In developing neurons in cell culture, excitatory synaptic activity is necessary for hypoxia to lead to neuronal death.

Nonspecific blockade of this synaptic activity prevents hypoxic neuronal death in culture.

Specific glutamate receptor channel blockers also prevent hypoxic neuronal death in culture and in brain slices.

Glutamate accumulates extracellularly in vivo with hypoxic-ischemic insult.

Topography of hypoxic-ischemic neuronal death in vivo is similar to the topography of glutamate synapses.

Increased vulnerability of certain brain structures to hypoxic-ischemic injury during early development correlates, in those structures, with transiently increased concentration of glutamate receptors, which also have molecular characteristics associated with increased calcium influx.

Ontogeny of hypoxic-ischemic neuronal death in vivo is similar to the ontogeny of glutamate-induced neuronal death.

Delayed neuronal death after glutamate exposure in cell culture has a correlate in delayed neuronal death after hypoxia-ischemia in vivo, and both can be prevented by specific glutamate receptor channel blockers, some administered after termination of the insult.

*See text for references.

Role of Glutamate in Hypoxic-Ischemic Cell Death in Cultured Neurons.

The critical role for glutamate in the mediation of hypoxic-ischemic neuronal death is established by a large body of experimental information, as summarized in Table 6-17.* The essential neurotoxicity of glutamate was shown initially in cultured neurons and subsequently in other in vitro and in vivo models (see later).

The crucial initial observation was that cultured hippocampal neurons, obtained from the fetal rat, were *resistant to prolonged anoxia before synapse formation* occurred in the cultures, but they were very sensitive to the same anoxic insult after synaptogenesis was well developed. Thus, such mature cultures markedly deteriorated in the absence of oxygen.[405] However, when synaptic activity in these mature cultures was blocked by addition of high concentrations of magnesium, no effect of anoxia on the cultured neurons occurred (Fig. 6-24). Thus, the data demonstrated that *synaptic activity resulted in neuronal death* with oxygen deprivation. This protection by synaptic blockage with magnesium was shown later in a hippocampal slice preparation in which neuronal death could be produced in the CA1 region under anoxic conditions.[406]

Because glutamate (as in hippocampus in vivo) was presumed to be the neurotransmitter mediating the synaptic activity in the experiments with the cultured hippocampal neurons and the slice preparation, a nonspecific postsynaptic blocker of glutamate was investigated to prevent the hypoxic neuronal death in culture. This agent protected neurons dramatically from anoxia (Fig. 6-25).[407] The particular role of glutamate synapses in hippocampal neuronal death was supported further shortly thereafter by the demonstration that hypoxic-ischemic neuronal injury could be prevented in vivo by prior section of glutamatergic afferents to the CA1 region.[408]

*See references 129,209,211,355-362,376,378,381,386,387,389, 397-404.

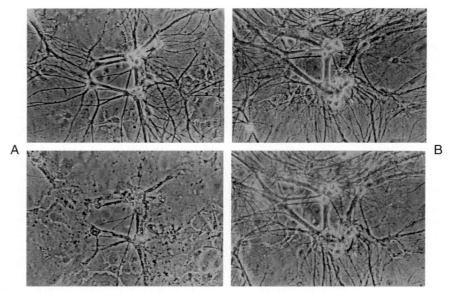

Figure 6-24 **Effect of blockade of synaptic activity on anoxic cell death in hippocampal neuronal cultures.** **A,** Phase contrast micrograph (*top*) shows normoxic culture with abundant neurons; *bottom,* cultures rendered anoxic for 24 hours show extensive neuronal destruction provoked by anoxia. **B,** Micrograph shows cultures treated with magnesium chloride to block synaptic activity before *(top)* and after *(bottom)* anoxia. Note the lack of neuronal destruction. *(From Rothman SM: Synaptic activity mediates death of hypoxic neurons,* Science *220:536-537, 1983.)*

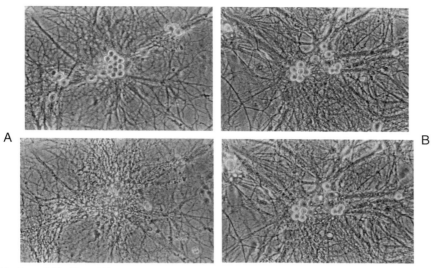

Figure 6-25 **Effect of a blocker of the *N*-methyl-ᴅ-aspartate (NMDA)–type glutamate receptor on cell death in hippocampal neuronal cultures.** **A,** Phase contrast micrographs show cultures before *(top)* and 8 hours after *(bottom)* anoxia. Note neuronal destruction after anoxia. **B,** Micrographs show cultures treated with the NMDA receptor blocker, gamma-ᴅ-glutamylglycine. The appearance before *(top)* and 8 hours after *(bottom)* anoxia are shown. Note the prevention of neuronal destruction in the presence of the blocker. *(From Rothman SM: Synaptic release of excitatory amino acid neurotransmitter mediates anoxic neuronal death,* J Neurosci *4:1884, 1984.)*

The *mechanisms of glutamate-induced neuronal death* in cultured neurons were elucidated next.* Two basic mechanisms were identified. One of these is rapid cell death that occurs in minutes and is initiated by glutamate receptor activation, Na^+ entry through all three ionotropic receptors, passive influx of Cl^- down its electrochemical gradient with water following, and ultimately cell swelling and lysis. A second variety, so-called delayed cell death, occurring over many hours, is initiated principally by activation of the NMDA and immature (GluR2-deficient) AMPA receptors, with influx of Ca^{2+} (as well as Na^+) and a series of Ca^{2+}-mediated events to cell death (see Table 6-13). *Delayed cell death* appears to be the crucial form of neuronal death in vivo, and the importance of the NMDA and GluR2-deficient AMPA receptors and Ca^{2+} influx is well established by studies of specific blockers of these receptors in cultured cells, brain slices, and in vivo models (see later discussion).† The data support the scheme shown in Figure 6-26. Note the particular involvement of the NMDA and immature GluR2-deficient AMPA receptors. Not shown in the figure is the *accentuation of the increase in cytosolic Ca^{2+}* by Na^+ influx through all three ionotropic receptors, membrane depolarization, and opening of voltage-dependent Ca^{2+} channels. Sustained membrane depolarization also leads to *failure of glutamate uptake mechanisms* and to *sustained glutamate release.* Thus, cyclical internal amplification with multiple vicious cycles likely becomes operative.

Relevance of Glutamate-Induced Excitotoxicity to Hypoxic-Ischemic Injury In Vivo. Relevance of the *glutamate excitotoxic mechanisms* to the in vivo situation is now clear.* The first body of evidence establishing this relevance showed that *extracellular glutamate concentrations in vivo increase* manyfold with hypoxic-ischemic insults.[356] Such increases have been documented in *perinatal* animal models as well as in adults, although glutamate increases tend to be somewhat less in the

---

*See references 209,211,336,355,356,374,376,378,380,381,386,387, 389,403,418-428,430-433.

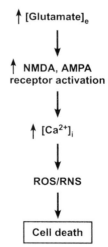

Figure 6-26 Mechanisms of glutamate-induced neuronal death. Note the involvement of the *N*-methyl-ᴅ-aspartate (NMDA) and alpha-amino-3-hydroxy-5-methyl-4-isoxazole-propionic acid (AMPA) receptors, the increase in intracellular calcium ([Ca^{2+}]ᵢ) the generation of reactive oxygen (ROS) and reactive nitrogen (RNS) species, and the resulting cell death.

---

*See references 209,211,355,356,358,360-362,374,376,378,386,387, 389,397-401,409.

†See references 129,209,211,293,336,355,356,376,378,386,387,397-399,401,410-429.

former models than in the latter.[386,422,424,425,427,434-439] However, studies using microdialysis have documented accumulation of extracellular glutamate in brain of asphyxiated fetal sheep and of hypoxic-ischemic immature rats to concentrations of approximately 500 µmmol/L,[434,437,440] concentrations easily sufficient to cause neuronal death in cultured cells. *Moreover, glutamate concentrations in the cerebrospinal fluid of asphyxiated human newborns are markedly greater than concentrations in normal newborns.*[441,442] The reasons for the increase of extracellular glutamate with hypoxic-ischemic insults relate to *impaired uptake of glutamate and to excessive release. The impaired uptake* is related to defective operation of the high-affinity, Na+-dependent glutamate transporters in neurons and astrocytes (because of the failure of the ATP-dependent Na+-K+ pump and loss of the Na+-K+ ionic gradient across the plasma membrane) and to defective function of the ATP-using glutamine synthetase reaction in astrocytes).[211,362,439,443-446] Transporter function also is disrupted by ROS and RNS and by cytokines (e.g., TNF-alpha), released by activated microglia.[447,448] The *excessive release of glutamate* relates to at least five factors. The first of these is the persistent membrane depolarization resulting from failure of the ATP-dependent Na+-K+ pump.[449] (Destruction of gamma-aminobutyric acid neurons by hypoxia also may contribute to the excessive excitation and release of glutamate.)[450] The second factor of critical importance is *reversal* of glutamate transport because of the loss of the Na+-K+ ionic gradient and elevated intracellular Na+ levels. Indeed, this factor may be most important for the sustained release of glutamate into the extracellular space.[451] A third factor is the rapid blockade of inhibitory synaptic transmission with relative preservation of excitatory synaptic transition with anoxia in the immature versus adult animal.[452] A fourth factor promoting excessive release of glutamate is the acute development of epileptic phenomena after hypoxia in the immature (but not mature) animal.[30] A fifth factor is glutamate release from microglia, a process enhanced in an autocrine manner by TNF-alpha released by microglia with diverse inflammatory stimuli.[453]

The second body of evidence delineating the relevance of glutamate to the in vivo situation is the demonstration in a wide variety of *perinatal models* of hypoxia-ischemia that *glutamate is toxic to neurons in vivo* and that this *toxicity is particularly marked* in the *immature* versus the mature animal.* In general, in the immature animal, the most toxic glutamate analogue is NMDA; AMPA is slightly less toxic, and kainate is least toxic.[336,358-361,386,387,401,455-457] The approximate time of peak sensitivity in the rat is 6 days for NMDA and 9 to 10 days for AMPA. The especial vulnerability of the brain of the immature animal to hypoxia-ischemia and the importance of the NMDA receptor in this ontogeny of vulnerability are illustrated by the similar developmental profiles of hypoxic-ischemic neuronal death

and NMDA-mediated neuronal death (Fig. 6-27). A similar relationship has been shown for the GluR2-deficient AMPA receptor for the rat.[382] Presumably, these particular vulnerabilities of the immature animal relate at least in part to the transient dense expression of NMDA and GluR2-deficient AMPA receptors during brain development (see earlier discussion).

The third body of evidence linking glutamate to hypoxic-ischemic injury relates to the finding that the topography of glutamate receptors, particularly NMDA and AMPA receptors, corresponds closely to the topography of hypoxic-ischemic neuronal injury observed in vivo.[336,358-361,379,381,382,386,389,390,458] Although more data are needed concerning the perinatal human, the overwhelming balance of evidence indicates a close relationship between regional neuronal vulnerability to hypoxia-ischemia and regional distribution of glutamate receptors (see Chapter 8).

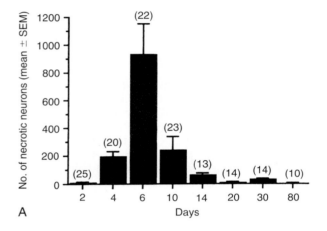

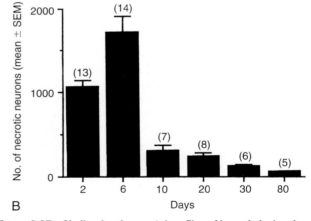

Figure 6-27 Similar developmental profiles of hypoxic-ischemic and *N*-methyl-D-aspartate (NMDA)–mediated neuronal death. Mean number of neurons destroyed in rat brain under conditions of, **A**, hypoxia-ischemia and, **B**, intrastriatal injection of NMDA (9 nmol). Pups at the age of 6 days show the highest number of necrotic neurons under either condition. The numbers on top of each column represent the number of animals studied for each group. SEM, standard error of the mean. *(From Ikonomidou C, Mosinger JL, Salles KS, Labruyere J, et al: Sensitivity of the developing rat brain to hypobaric/ischemic damage parallels sensitivity to N-methyl-aspartate neurotoxicity, J Neurosci 9:2809-2818, 1989.)*

---

*See references 28,211,245,358,360,361,381,386,401,404,454.

Finally, perhaps the strongest evidence of the relevance of the glutamate excitotoxic mechanism to the in vivo situation has been the demonstration of *protection from neuronal death in a variety of perinatal hypoxic-ischemic models by treatment with glutamate receptor blockers.*[394,418,419,423,426,428,430-433,457,459-474] Most experiments used compounds with effects on the NMDA receptor-channel complex, and in nearly all, benefit was achieved. AMPA antagonists, however, also have been neuroprotective. Benefit was manifested as prevention of morphological, biochemical, or electrophysiological evidence of injury. Although in most studies the antagonists were administered at the onset or during the insult, most striking has been the marked, though not complete, protection in experiments in which the antagonists were administered *after termination of the insult* (Fig. 6-28). Available data suggest that treatment within 1 to 2 hours is highly effective. This response is compatible with the concepts that delayed cell death is the operative mechanism and that treatment in the clinical situation after termination of the insult ultimately may be beneficial.

Role of Inflammation

The relationship between the brain inflammatory response after hypoxia-ischemia-reperfusion and cell death is discussed in detail later in relation to oligodendroglial injury, as in periventricular leukomalacia (PVL). Similarly, the potentiation of the deleterious effects of hypoxia-ischemia by infection also is emphasized later. Nevertheless, it is important in this context of neuronal death to introduce these concepts, especially in relation to experimental models that focus particularly on gray matter injury rather than white matter injury.

Adult Models of Hypoxic-Ischemic Injury. A series of studies in adult models of hypoxic-ischemic injury, especially models of stroke, initially indicated that inflammatory mechanisms, although important in subsequent reparative processes, also are important in the final common biochemical pathway to hypoxic-ischemic neuronal death.[475-489] The principal sequence of events is activation of microglia in the first hours after the insult, with release of a variety of neurotoxic products, including excitatory amino acids, ROS, NO, and certain cytokines. Most important among the cytokines appear to be IL-1beta and TNF-alpha. IL-1beta is particularly important in the activation of endothelial-leukocyte adhesion molecules, especially intercellular adhesion molecule-1 (ICAM-1). The leukocytes involved include not only polymorphonuclear cells but also mononuclear cells, especially of the monocytic-phagocytic series. The leukocytes are important in release of deleterious compounds, especially ROS and cytokines. The particular importance of activated microglia is supported by the demonstration of neuroprotection by minocycline, a tetracycline analogue that has antimicroglial effects, in several models of hypoxic-ischemic neuronal death.[490-492]

Perinatal Models of Hypoxic-Ischemic Injury. That the sequence of events just explained appears to be operative in *perinatal hypoxia-ischemia* is supported by study of perinatal experimental models (Table 6-18) and human epidemiological data.[482-486,493-503] Thus, studies in perinatal rats have shown *activation of microglia* after hypoxia-ischemia that proceeds more rapidly than in adult animals.[484] Activated microglia begin to accumulate in the first 4 hours after reperfusion and continue to increase over the next 48 hours. *Neutrophil accumulation in brain blood vessels* has been documented on reperfusion after hypoxia-ischemia in the neonatal rat and piglet.[485,494] In the rat model, the accumulation peaked at 4 to 8 hours after reperfusion, although much less infiltration of brain parenchyma was apparent than that occurring in adult animals.[485,504] However, the neutrophilic accumulation

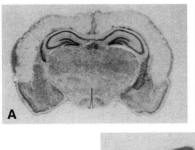
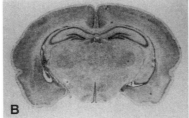
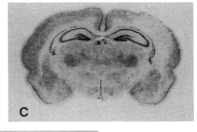
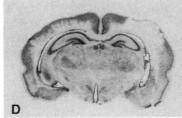
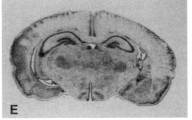

Figure 6-28 **Coronal brain sections from rat pups. A** is from a saline-injected control, and **B** through **E** are from rat pups that were given MK-801 intraperitoneally: **B**, 0.5 hour before and, **C**, immediately, **D**, 1 hour, and, **E**, 4 hours after the hypoxic-ischemic insult. Note the sharply demarcated hypoxic-ischemic infarction in **A**. The neuroprotective effects of MK-801 are seen in **B, C,** and **D** in a time-dependent fashion. (Hematoxylin and eosin stain, original magnification ×2.5 before 31% reduction.) *(From Hattori H, Morin AM, Schwartz PH, Fujikawa DG, et al: Posthypoxic treatment with MK-801 reduces hypoxic-ischemic damage in the neonatal rat, Neurology 39:713-718, 1989.)*

TABLE 6-18 Inflammation in Experimental Models of Perinatal Hypoxic-Ischemic Brain Injury

Microglial activation occurs promptly and briskly after hypoxia-ischemia.
Microglial cells release neurotoxic products (e.g., cytokines and reactive oxygen and nitrogen species).
Cytokines (especially IL-1beta and TNF-alpha) increase promptly in brain after hypoxia-ischemia, and IL-1 receptor antagonist
   ameliorates hypoxic-ischemic brain injury when it is administered either before or at the termination of hypoxia-ischemia.
Antimicroglial agents (e.g., minocycline) are neuroprotective in several experimental paradigms of perinatal hypoxia-ischemia.
Inflammatory mechanisms provoked by prior exposure to molecular products of infection (e.g., lipopolysaccharide) potentiate
   subthreshold hypoxic-ischemic insults to lead to severe brain injury.

IL, interleukin; TNF, tumor necrosis factor.

in blood vessels was shown to be important in the genesis of the brain injury by the marked reduction in cerebral edema and subsequent cerebral atrophy in animals made neutropenic before the hypoxic-ischemic insult. Whether the deleterious effect of the neutrophils is related to adherence to endothelium and obstruction of flow or to vascular injury secondary to release of ROS, or to both, remains to be established. Finally, a burst of *cytokine expression*, presumably principally from activated microglia, has been documented in the first 6 hours after cerebral hypoxic-ischemic insult in the immature rat.[482,483,486] Both IL-1beta and TNF-alpha have been shown to increase markedly in brain in the first 4 to 6 hours after the insult, and notably intracerebral injection of IL-1 receptor antagonist has been shown to ameliorate the brain injury.[483,495] Moreover, pentoxifylline, which inhibits TNF-alpha production, is neuroprotective when administered before hypoxia-ischemia in the 7-day old rat.[496] Additionally, the key role of activated microglia in the genesis of neuronal death has been shown by neuroprotection with minocycline in several models of hypoxic-ischemic injury in the neonatal rat as in adult animals.[505,506] Finally, the potentially deleterious role of the inflammatory cascade is suggested by the partial neuroprotection provided by dexamethasone administered before hypoxia-ischemia in the neonatal rat.[507-509]

Potentiation of Perinatal Hypoxic-Ischemic Brain Injury by Inflammation Provoked by Infection. Potentiation of perinatal hypoxic-ischemic brain injury by inflammation provoked by infection is particularly important in relation to oligodendroglial or white matter injury and is discussed in detail in the next section. However, this situation is likely also important in the genesis of hypoxic-ischemic neuronal injury. Thus, several studies showed a potentiation of hypoxic-ischemic brain injury after pretreatment with LPS.[510-515b] The most common paradigm has been application of a hypoxic-ischemic insult itself not sufficient to produce brain injury, after short-term (several hours) exposure to LPS, itself not sufficient to produce brain injury. In one report, the effect of LPS was shown to depend on the presence on brain microglia of Toll-like receptor 4 (TLR4), a specific microglial receptor for LPS activation of microglia (see later) (Fig. 6-29).[513] The particular involvement in this combined insult paradigm of an inflammatory cascade, initiated by activated microglia, is suggested by

the finding of neuroprotection by pretreatment with dexamethasone.[509] In a related experiment, use of a glucocorticoid receptor blocker resulted in accentuation of the combined LPS and hypoxic-ischemic injury.[516]

The influence of preceding infection or inflammation on hypoxic-ischemic injury varies according to the timing of the LPS pretreatment. Thus, in the experiments just described, LPS exposure 4 hours before hypoxia-ischemia accentuated injury. A similar potentiation was observed when LPS was administered 72 hours earlier.[517] However, when LPS was administered 24 hours before hypoxia-ischemia, injury was *reduced*. This beneficial effect of LPS preconditioning at 24 hours versus 4 and 72 hours illustrates the potential complexity of the interaction between preceding infection or inflammation and hypoxia-ischemia (see discussion later of oligodendroglial injury).

Inflammation and Brain Injury in Human Infants. Initial clinical support for a role for inflammation in the genesis of neonatal brain injury emanated especially from epidemiological studies relating *neonatal levels of cytokines in term infants* with brain injury, manifested usually by cerebral palsy defined later in infancy.[518-524] In a minority of these reports the cytokine evidence of inflammation was a component of an apparent perinatal hypoxic-ischemic insult.[519,522,524] Consistent with these observations is the increased likelihood of later cerebral palsy in newborns who had evidence of chorioamnionitis at birth.[525,526] In the largest case-control study (N = 231,582), chorioamnionitis led to a 3.8-fold increased risk for cerebral palsy.[526] The nature of the relationship between perinatal evidence of inflammation and poorer neurological outcome, both in infants with apparent perinatal asphyxial events and in those with no overt hypoxic-ischemic insult, is not entirely clear. The earlier discussion of the potentiating effect of infection or inflammation on subthreshold hypoxic-ischemic insults may be relevant in this context. Further data will be of great interest.

Interventions for Prevention of Neurons from Hypoxic-Ischemic Injury

The insights into the biochemical and cellular mechanisms of neuronal and glial injury with perinatal hypoxic-ischemic-reperfusion insults, as just discussed, provide a rational basis for formulation of

BALB/cJ   Ips^d

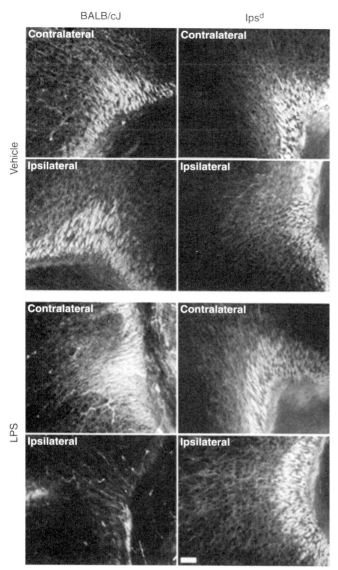

Figure 6-29 **Activation of microglia by Toll-like receptor 4 (TLR4) is necessary for the prominent neuronal injury in immature mice treated with lipopolysaccharide (LPS) before a subthreshold hypoxic-ischemic insult**. The latter insult was produced by unilateral carotid ligation and hypoxemia in normal (BALB/cJ) and TLR4-lacking (Lps^d) mice. Coronal sections of cerebrum were stained for neurofilament protein. No vehicle-treated animal developed a lesion. By contrast, LPS-pretreated normal animals (BALB/cJ) developed a clear (ipsilateral) hypoxic-ischemic lesion, whereas TLR4-lacking (Ips^d) animals did not. *(From Lehnardt S, Massillon L, Follett P, Jensen FE, et al: Activation of innate immunity in the CNS triggers neurodegeneration through a Toll-like receptor 4-dependent pathway, Proc Natl Acad Sci U S A 100: 8514-8519, 2003.)*

interventions to interrupt those mechanisms and thereby prevent or ameliorate the injury. The general sequence of operation of these mechanisms (Fig. 6-30) provides the framework for this discussion of such interventions as outlined in Table 6-19. The following information is derived almost exclusively from data obtained in *perinatal* models of hypoxia-ischemia, *with an emphasis on neuronal injury (see later for oligodendroglial injury)*.

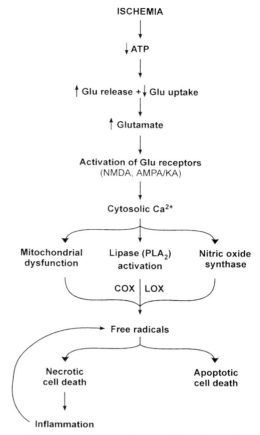

Figure 6-30 **General sequence of mechanisms leading to apoptotic and necrotic neuronal death with hypoxia-ischemia**. AMPA, alpha-amino-3-hydroxy-5-methyl-4-isoxazole-propionic acid; ATP, adenosine triphosphate; COX, cyclooxygenase; Glu, glutamine; KA, kainate; LOX, lipoxygenase; NMDA, *N*-methyl-ᴅ-aspartate; PLA$_2$, phospholipase A$_2$. See text for details.

Decrease in Energy Depletion. Depletion of high-energy phosphate, not necessarily severe, almost certainly initiates the cascade of events leading to neuronal death (see Fig. 6-30). The most potent and promising intervention to prevent energy depletion is *mild hypothermia* (see Table 6-19; Fig. 6-31).[527-534] In some models, this effect has been correlated with the neuroprotective benefit of this approach. Moreover, mild hypothermia ameliorates the secondary energy failure that follows many hours of reperfusion.[535,536] Nevertheless, the beneficial effects of mild hypothermia occur at *multiple sites* in the cascade to cell death, and the relative importance of each effect remains to be clarified (see Table 6-19; Table 6-20). A preventive-ameliorative effect of mild hypothermia has been documented in a wide variety of perinatal animal models of hypoxia-ischemia.[527,528,530-535,537-558a] In earlier studies, hypothermia was instituted during hypoxia-ischemia or immediately on reperfusion, or both. In the most recent studies, hypothermia was instituted on reperfusion, to model the usual clinical situation (see Table 6-20). Of particular importance, hypothermia must be commenced before the onset of delayed energy failure and particularly excitatory features, especially seizures.

TABLE 6-19 Potentially Valuable Interventions in Prevention or Amelioration of Perinatal Hypoxic-Ischemic Neuronal Injury[*]

Decrease of Energy Depletion
Hypothermia
Glucose
Barbiturates
Hypercapnia (mild)
Amiloride

Inhibition of Glutamate Release
Hypothermia
Calcium channel blockers
Magnesium
Adenosine or adenosine agonists
Free radical scavengers
Lamotrigine
Phenytoin
Cannabinoids

Amelioration of Impairment in Glutamate Uptake
Hypothermia

Blockade of Glutamate Receptors
NMDA receptor antagonists (MK-801, xenon, memantine, magnesium, ketamine, dextrorphan)
Non-NMDA receptor antagonists (NBQX, CNQX, topiramate)

Blockade of Free Radical Generation
Hypothermia
Inhibitors of cyclooxygenases (e.g., indomethacin)
Inhibitors of lipoxygenases (e.g., AA-861)
Nitric oxide synthase inhibitors (e.g., nitroarginine derivatives, 2-iminobiotin)
Allopurinol
Iron chelators
Fructose-1,6-biphosphate

Removal of Free Radicals
Free radical scavengers (vitamin E and analogues, edaravone, N-acetylcysteine)
Antioxidant enzyme mimetics

Blockade of Downstream Effects
Hypothermia
Erythropoietin
Growth factors (insulin-like growth factor-I, brain-derived neurotrophic factor, nerve growth factor)
Caspase inhibitors

Inhibition of Inflammatory Effects
Hypothermia
Minocycline
Anti–Toll-like receptor agents
Interleukin-1 receptor antagonists
Platelet-activating factor antagonists
Neutropenia

[*]See text for references.
CNQX, 6-cyano-7-nitroquinoxaline-2,3-dione; NBQX, 2,3-dihydroxy-6-nitro-7-sulfamoyl-benzo[f]quinoxaline-2,3-dione; NMDA, N-methyl-D-aspartate.

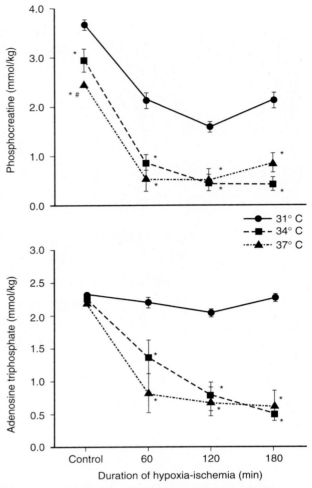

Figure 6-31 Preservation of high-energy phosphate levels in brain of the immature (P7) rat subjected to hypoxia-ischemia at the temperatures shown. With mild hypothermia (31°C), the decline in brain phosphocreatine level was partially prevented, and the decline in ATP levels was completely prevented. *(From Yager JY, Asselin J: Effect of mild hypothermia on cerebral energy metabolism during the evolution of hypoxic-ischemic brain damage in the immature rat, Stroke 27:919-926, 1996.)*

TABLE 6-20 Mild Hypothermia as Neuroprotective Therapy[*]

Principal Features
Timing: commence before delayed energy failure and excitatory features such as seizures (i.e., ≈6 hr)
Degree: decrease body temperature 3°–4° C
Duration: ≈72 hr

Mechanisms of Benefit
Decrease energy consumption
Decrease accumulation of glutamate
Decrease synthesis of reactive oxygen and nitrogen species
Block downstream molecular cascade to apoptosis
Inhibit inflammatory mechanisms

Synergistic Neuroprotective Combinations
Hypothermia and xenon
Hypothermia and topiramate
Hypothermia and N-acetylcysteine
Hypothermia and caspase inhibitor

[*]See text for references.

In the experimental models, the onset of the delayed energy failure and seizures is approximately 6 hours after reperfusion. In one especially informative study of ischemic fetal sheep, mild cooling of the cranium *instituted 5.5 hours after the insult* resulted in reduction of injury assessed electrophysiologically and

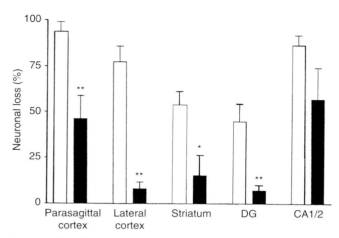

Figure 6-32 Effect of selective cerebral cooling (extradural temperature, 30.4°C) from 6 to 72 hours after ischemia in near-term fetal sheep on neuronal loss in different brain regions 5 days after the ischemia. A significant overall reduction (P <.001) in neuronal loss was observed in fetuses treated with selective cerebral cooling (black bars), compared with sham-cooled fetuses (white bars), except in the most severely affected field of the hippocampus (CA1/2). *, P <.05; **, P <.01; mean ± SEM. *(From Gunn AJ, Gunn TR, Gunning MI, Williams CE, et al: Neuroprotection with prolonged head cooling started before postischemic seizures in fetal sheep, Pediatrics 102:1098-1106, 1998.)*

neuropsychologically (Fig. 6-32). (This beneficial effect did not occur in the fetal sheep when hypothermia was instituted at 8.5 hours, just after the occurrence of seizures at 6 to 8 hours.[559]) *Of all the interventions discussed in this section, mild hypothermia shows the greatest potential, and indeed preliminary data to support its value in human infants are available* (see Chapter 9).

Depletion of high-energy phosphates and its initiation of the cascade of events leading to neuronal death can be counteracted in several other ways. The importance of maintenance of glucose at physiological levels was discussed earlier, and data in this regard are summarized in Table 6-8. Barbiturates administered in high doses can lead to decreased cerebral metabolic rate and thereby energy preservation (see Chapter 9).[4] The apparent protective effect of mild hypercapnia, at least in part, may be mediated by decreasing energy utilization.[88] Amiloride, an inhibitor of the Na^+/H^+ transporter, has been shown to be neuroprotective in perinatal hypoxic-ischemic models in vitro and in vivo, and one of the effects of this drug is preservation of energy supplies.[554,560] The Na^+/H^+ transporter is activated with hypoxia-ischemia and leads to sustained intracellular alkalosis, observed in vivo by MR spectroscopy of asphyxiated infants (see Chapter 9). The alkaline pH has multiple effects, including exacerbation of excitotoxicity and impairment of ATP synthesis. Excessive utilization of ATP also can supervene when the increase in intracellular Na^+ concentration leads to activation of the ATP-dependent Na^+/K^+-ATPase.

Inhibition of Glutamate Release. Because glutamate is important in neuronal death, inhibition of the

enhanced glutamate release with hypoxia-ischemia is important (see Fig. 6-30 and Table 6-19). Hypothermia is beneficial at this level both by inhibiting glutamate release and by blunting the disturbance of glutamate transporters that contributes significantly to the accumulation of extracellular glutamate (see earlier).[530,534,561,562] Because Ca^{2+} influx is necessary for glutamate release and because magnesium blocks the former process, part of the beneficial effect of Ca^{2+} channel blockers or of magnesium could occur at this step.[215,563,564] However, Ca^{2+} channel blockers have adverse cardiovascular effects, and magnesium administration in a variety of hypoxic-ischemic models has not been clearly beneficial.[565-567] Adenosine, adenosine agonists, and adenosine antagonists have been studied because activation of the adenosine receptor inhibits glutamate release. Although in some perinatal models adenosine agonists have been beneficial, the available data do not show clearly consistent effects.[568-571]

The neuroprotective effect of free radical scavengers may be exerted partially at the level of glutamate release because free radicals increase neuronal glutamate release in some models.[572] Moreover, phenytoin has partial neuroprotective effects in cultured neurons and in hypoxic-ischemic models in neonatal rats and fetal guinea pigs, perhaps by blocking Na^+ channels and thereby action potential-induced glutamate release.[573-576] The beneficial effect of lamotrigine in an adult model of ischemic neuronal injury probably relates to this anticonvulsant's inhibition of glutamate release.[577] Finally, the recently described neuroprotective effect of cannabinoid agonists in in vitro and in vivo models of neonatal hypoxic-ischemic neuronal injury is mediated in part at the level of glutamate release.[578,578a]

Amelioration of Impairment in Glutamate Uptake. As noted earlier, hypothermia may exert some of its neuroprotective effect by decreasing the impairment in astrocytic Na^+-dependent, high-affinity glutamate uptake related to ischemia (see Table 6-19). This conclusion is based primarily on studies of neonatal piglets and cultured astrocytes.[562,579]

Blockade of Glutamate Receptors. The neuroprotective effect of NMDA receptor antagonists, especially MK-801 but also xenon, magnesium, ketamine, and dextrorphan, in various models of ischemic neuronal injury, both in culture and in vivo, was discussed earlier concerning glutamate neurotoxicity (see Table 6-17). More often, neuroprotection is achieved when the agents are administered at the termination of the insult or from up to several hours afterward. *Xenon* appears to be particularly efficacious in concentrations likely to be clinically safe.[580,581] Indeed in one study of hypoxia-ischemia in neonatal rats, *xenon and mild hypothermia acted synergistically* to provide neuroprotection (see Table 6-20). The benefit was greatest when xenon was commenced with the insult, but it was still significant when xenon was used 4 hours after the insult.

Similarly, neuroprotective effects have been apparent in several perinatal models of hypoxia-ischemia by the use of non-NMDA antagonists, especially AMPA antagonists (2,3-dihydroxy-6-nitro-7-sulfamoyl-benzo [f]quinoxaline-2,3-dione [NBQX], 6-cyano-7-nitroqui-noxaline-2,3-dione [CNQX], topiramate).[431-433,472-474,582,583] Particularly noteworthy is the *synergistic* neuroprotective effect of *topiramate and mild hypothermia* in a perinatal model (P7 rat) in which neither intervention alone produced appreciable benefit (Fig. 6-33). *Topiramate* is of particular interest because postinsult treatment with this drug *also protects developing oligodendrocytes from injury* (see later). Moreover, unlike many other excitatory amino acid antagonists, topiramate, in clinically used doses, does *not* lead to apoptotic neuronal death in developing brain.[584-586]

Blockade of Free Radical Generation. The downstream intracellular biochemical events leading to cell death include the large series of Ca^{2+}-activated processes, leading to generation of ROS and RNS, and apoptotic and necrotic cell death (see Table 6-13). *Hypothermia* probably acts at multiple levels in this cascade, but prominent among these effects are reductions in free radical production and NO synthesis (see Tables 6-19 and 6-20).[336,531,532,534,587-590] Inhibitors of free radical production of demonstrated neuroprotective value in various models of hypoxia-ischemia include allopurinol (inhibits xanthine oxidase step), indomethacin (inhibits cyclooxygenase), iron chelation (diminishes hydroxyl radical production by the Fenton reaction), fructose-1,6-biphosphate (preserves intracellular glutathione), and magnesium (inhibits lipid peroxidation) (see earlier discussions and references cited herein).[4,229,230,243,294,295,591-594]

Inhibitors of NO synthesis have been shown to be beneficial in a variety of perinatal models (see earlier discussion). Because of the temporal characteristics of activation of, first, nNOS and, later, iNOS (see Fig. 6-22), specific inhibitors of each isoform have been used in perinatal models.[353,354,594-596] Particularly promising results have been obtained with inhibitors of *both* nNOS and iNOS. Hypothermia also appears to decrease NO generation.[534]

Removal of Free Radicals. A deficiency in antioxidant defenses is an important determinant of neuronal vulnerability in the immature brain (see earlier discussion). Thus, accumulation of free radicals occurs, and an important protective intervention involves removal of these injurious components (see Table 16-19). Two major approaches employed have been administration of either free radical scavengers or antioxidant enzyme mimetics. *Free radical scavengers* shown to be effective in perinatal models of hypoxia-ischemia have included vitamin E and its analogues, edaravone, and *N*-acetylcysteine (see Fig. 6-20).[286,296,298,299,597a] Of particular interest is the recent demonstration in a hypoxic-ischemic model in the neonatal rat of *synergistic* protection by mild to moderate (30° C) hypothermia (2 hours) and *N*-acetylcysteine (daily) begun following the insult.[597] *N*-Acetylcysteine has been shown not only to scavenge free radicals but also to restore intracellular glutathione levels.

Antioxidant enzyme mimetics may prove to be an important advance in the removal of free radicals. Thus, these low-molecular-weight, nonpeptidyl molecules mimic the activity of SOD, catalase, or glutathione peroxidase and have the capacity to penetrate the blood-brain barrier.[285,598] Most available data concerning neuroprotective effects have been obtained in adult models, but protection in neonatal hypoxia-ischemia also has been shown.[285]

Blockade of Downstream Effects. Because a substantial proportion of injury to developing neurons with hypoxia-ischemia is apoptotic (see earlier), *inhibitors of apoptotic cell death* have been studied for neuroprotective

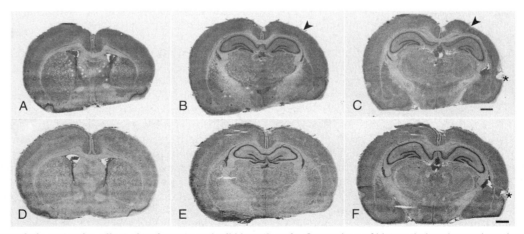

Figure 6-33 **Synergistic protective effect of topiramate and mild hypothermia.** Comparison of histopathology (coronal sections, cresyl violet) in two P35 rats subjected at P7 to unilateral carotid ligation and hypoxemia, followed by delayed (3 hours) hypothermia with vehicle (**A** to **C**) or topiramate (**D** to **F**). In the vehicle-treated hypothermic animals, a major lesion (*arrowheads*) is apparent, whereas minimal injury is apparent in the topiramate-treated hypothermic animals. *(From Liu Y, Barks JD, Xu G, Silverstein FS: Topiramate extends the therapeutic window for hypothermia-mediated neuroprotection after stroke in neonatal rats, Stroke 25;1460-1465, 2004.)*

effects (see Table 6-19). *Hypothermia* has been shown to protect neonatal rat brain against hypoxia-ischemia by reducing both apoptosis and necrosis (see Table 6-20).[534,557,599,600] The modality may be especially useful against apoptosis, a particularly important mode of neuronal death in neonatal hypoxia-ischemia.[534] Postischemic hypothermia blocks the intense activation of caspase-3, critical for apoptotic cell death after ischemia.[601] Indeed, in the P7 rat model of hypoxia-ischemia, a combination of systemic hypothermia and administration of a pan-caspase inhibitor *synergistically* led to reductions of both caspase-3 activation and neuronal injury in hippocampus (see Table 6-20).[602]

Erythropoietin (EPO), a glycoprotein originally recognized for its role in erythropoiesis, has been shown to be involved in the adaptive response to perinatal hypoxia-ischemia and to exhibit neuroprotective properties (Table 6-21).[603-607b] Thus, hypoxia-ischemia leads to an increase in expression of EPO and the EPO receptor, beginning within hours initially in neurons (as well as endothelial cells) and after days, especially in astrocytes.[608-610] The resulting beneficial effects include upstream mechanisms (i.e., antiexcitotoxic effects: attenuation of glutamate release), antioxidant actions (up-regulation of glutathione peroxidase, decrease of lipid peroxidation), inhibition of NO production, and downstream mechanisms (i.e., antiapoptotic and survival-promoting effects, as well as stimulation of angiogenesis and neurogenesis) (see Table 6-21).[160,603,607,610,611] Although not yet shown in perinatal hypoxia-ischemia, EPO may also serve to preserve cerebrovascular autoregulation and to blunt injurious inflammatory responses.[603] Neuroprotective effects have been shown by treatment *after* as well as before neonatal hypoxia-ischemia. Moreover, although EPO is a 34-kDa glycoprotein, it has been beneficial after *systemic* administration. The principal initiating stimulus for EPO expression is the hypoxia-induced up-regulation of hypoxia-inducible factor (HIF1), a transcription factor whose target genes are involved in such key physiological responses as energy metabolism, angiogenesis, and cell proliferation, in addition to EPO expression. Iron is required for degradation

of HIF1, and at least part of the neuroprotective benefit of desferrioxamine after hypoxia-ischemia relates to its stabilization of HIF1 and preservation of up-regulation of EPO.[610] Up-regulation of HIF1 and induction of these adaptive responses underlie the neuroprotection observed in experimental models of *hypoxic-ischemic preconditioning.*[159,160,612-618] EPO produces its key antiapoptotic effects by binding to its receptor, with subsequent activation of the Jak-Stat pathway. The latter involves translocation of Stat-5 to the nucleus, binding to DNA and promoting Bcl-x2 and Bcl2-2 expression, and finally inhibition of caspase-3 activation.[603,607] Additionally, NF-kappaB is activated, and the latter ultimately promotes expression of such protective genes as inhibitor of apoptotic protein and SOD. Although *EPO shows great promise as a potential neuroprotective agent,*[603,619] one report indicated *enhanced* neuronal injury when cultured neurons or immature rats were subjected to moderate hypoxia-ischemia *after* treatment with EPO.[620] Clinical situations in which hypoxia-ischemia may occur after treatment with EPO include the asphyxiated fetus or critically ill premature newborn. More data are needed concerning this critical issue.

Because *growth factors and other neurotrophic substances* generally prevent apoptotic cell death, many have been investigated for neuroprotection (see Table 6-19). Those with demonstrated value in various neonatal models of hypoxia-ischemia have included insulin-like growth factor-I (IGF-I), nerve growth factor (NGF), brain-derived neurotrophic factor (BDNF), and growth hormone.[192,600,621-631] Reductions of caspase-3 activation and thus an antiapoptotic effect have been observed after administration of BDNF and IGF-I.[192,629] Additionally, IGF-I activates a major pathway mediating neuronal survival involving activation of the serine/threonine kinase AKt.[629] Because in neuronal cultures, both BDNF and IGF-I potentiate necrotic cell death with free radical attack, concern exists that, at least under certain circumstances, growth factors may prevent apoptosis but accentuate necrosis.[171] More data are needed.

Inhibition of Inflammatory Effects. As noted earlier, inflammatory mechanisms, initiated after hypoxia-ischemia severe enough to cause tissue necrosis, are important in generating a cascade of deleterious effects that can be cyclical. Thus, tissue injury causes inflammation, which, in turn, causes more tissue injury (see Fig. 6-30). A critical aspect of the inflammatory cascade is activation of microglia. Other events include release of cytokines and ROS and RNS, accentuation of excitotoxicity, and induction of leucocyte adhesion molecules.

Hypothermia exerts a portion of its neuroprotective effects by suppression of the inflammatory response (see Table 6-19).[534] The responses blunted include microglial activation, generation of free radicals, release of cytokines, and neutrophil accumulation. The first of these effects may be the most important.

Minocycline, a tetracycline derivative, has been shown to be neuroprotective in perinatal models of

---

TABLE 6-21 Major Neuroprotective Mechanisms of Erythropoietin in Hypoxia-Ischemia

Upstream Initiating Mechanisms
Antiexcitotoxic (attenuation of glutamate release)
Antioxidant effects
Inhibition of nitric oxide production
Preservation of autoregulation (?)

Downstream Mechanisms
Antiapoptotic effects
Survival promoting effects
Stimulation of angiogenesis
Stimulation of neurogenesis
Anti-inflammatory effects (?)

Adapted from Sola A, Wen TC, Hamrick SE, Ferriero DM: Potential for protection and repair following injury to the developing brain: A role for erythropoietin? *Pediatr Res* 57:110R-117R, 2005.

hypoxia-ischemia, when it is administered either before or immediately after the insult (see Table 6-19; Fig. 6-34).[505,506] The beneficial effects of minocycline have been shown in a variety of other models, including excitotoxicity, oxidative stress, and cytokine attack.[490-492,632-636] The bases for the neuroprotective effects of minocycline are likely multiple, although inhibition of microglial activation appears to be most important. In one careful experimental study of neonatal hypoxia-ischemia, minocycline *accentuated* neuronal injury.[637] The negative effect was observed in a neonatal mouse model, whereas the beneficial effects have been shown in neonatal rat models. However, a beneficial effect was documented in an adult mouse model of hypoxia-ischemia.[492] Moreover, minocycline was shown to be protective to white matter in perinatal models (see later). Thus, this agent, or related antimicroglial agents, show considerable promise for hypoxic-ischemic neuroprotection (see Table 6-19).

The beneficial effect of *induced neutropenia* before hypoxia-ischemia was discussed earlier.[485] Platelet-activating factor (PAF), the levels of which increase with ischemia-reperfusion, is important in induction of leukocyte adhesion molecules and thereby subsequent events in the inflammatory cascade. In the immature rat, administration of a *PAF antagonist* has been shown to decrease infarct size with both pretreatment and post-treatment regimens (i.e., begun on reperfusion).[496,638-641] Finally, a critical product of

microglia-macrophages is IL-1beta, which, in turn, induces formation of other proinflammatory cytokines, including TNF-alpha. Notably, use of an antagonist of the IL-1 receptor both preinsult and on reperfusion has had protective effects in hypoxic-ischemic brain injury in the neonatal rat.[483] These and related issues are discussed further later concerning white matter injury.

Biochemical Mechanisms of Oligodendroglial Death with Hypoxia-Ischemia

Intrinsic Vulnerability of Early Differentiating Oligodendroglia to Hypoxic-ischemic Injury

The principal form of brain injury in the premature infant involves cerebral white matter and, particularly, early differentiating, premyelinating oligodendrocytes (pre-OLs) (see Chapter 8). Pre-OL death is an important characteristic of PVL. As for neuronal death, the most important initiating event is *ischemia* to cerebral white matter (Fig. 6-35). The premature infant has a particular propensity for ischemia to cerebral white matter because of the presence of (1) vascular end zones and border zones in that region and (2) impairment of cerebrovascular autoregulation (see Chapter 8). The latter leads readily to cerebral ischemia and affection of cerebral white matter vascular border and end

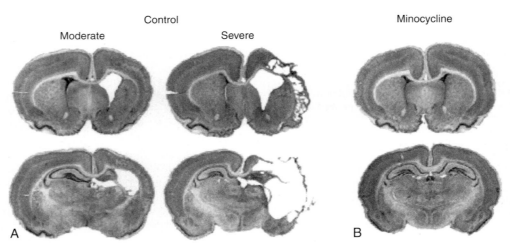

Figure 6-34 **Neuroprotective effect of minocycline in hypoxia-ischemia.** Representative coronal sections of postnatal day (P) 14 rat brains are shown 1 week after unilateral (*left*) carotid ligation and exposure to hypoxia for 2.5 hours at P7. In a typical example of animals given intraperitoneal injections of minocycline (**B**) immediately before or after hypoxia, there was little to no damage in almost all brains in comparison with the characteristic moderate or severe injury seen in the hemisphere ipsilateral to carotid ligation in most animals treated with phosphate-buffered saline alone (control) (**A**). (*From Arvin KL, Han BH, Du Y, Lin S-Z, et al: Minocycline markedly protects the neonatal brain against hypoxic-ischemic injury,* Ann Neurol *52;54;61, 2002.*)

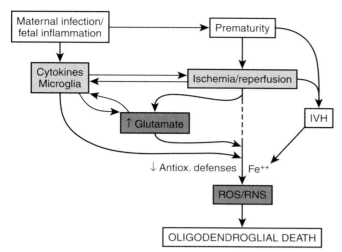

Figure 6-35 **Sequence of mechanisms leading to oligodendroglial death.** See text for details. The two major upstream mechanisms are ischemia and infection or inflammation (*lighter shading*), and the two principal downstream mechanisms are excitotoxicity and free radical attack by reactive oxygen species (ROS) and reactive nitrogen species (RNS) (*darker shading*). IVH, intraventricular hemorrhage.

zones (see Chapter 8). The importance of cerebral ischemia in pathogenesis of cerebral white matter injury (i.e., PVL) is illustrated in many models in developing animals (primarily sheep, piglet, rat) in which ischemia has been shown to lead to selective or predominant cerebral white matter injury.[80,175,642-672] The principal cellular target has been identified as the preoligodendrocyte (O4+) and the immature oligodendrocyte (O1+), especially the former,[647,662,668,669,673] which, together, I refer to as pre-OLs. (Recall from Chapter 2 that the sequence of oligodendroglial development is the A2B5+ [or NG2+] oligodendrocyte precursor, the O4+ preoligodendrocyte, the O1+ immature oligodendrocyte, and the mature, myelin basic protein [MBP+] oligodendrocyte.) Indeed, in one careful study in fetal sheep, under conditions of ischemia, the regional distribution of pre-OLs correlated closely with the regional distribution of the cerebral white matter injury.[669] As discussed in Chapter 8, the pre-OL is the predominant phase of the oligodendroglial lineage observed in human cerebral white matter in the third trimester during the peak period of vulnerability to PVL. In some of the ischemic models, other cellular elements in cerebral white matter (e.g., axons, subplate neurons) or in adjacent neuronal structures (e.g., basal ganglia, cerebral cortex) have been variably affected, but overall the principal cellular target has been the pre-OL.

Infection or Inflammation as an Additional or Potentiating Mechanism

Although ischemia has been the dominant initiating upstream mechanism in the experimental models of white matter injury, infection or inflammation has been shown to lead to injury to pre-OLs in developing brain (see later). Because a relationship is strongly suspected between maternal intrauterine infection with a systemic fetal inflammatory response and PVL in the

human infant, these findings suggest that infection or inflammation is a second important initiating mechanism in cerebral white matter injury (see Fig. 6-35).

Gram-Negative Infection, Endotoxin (Lipopolysaccharide), and White Matter Injury. A role for maternal/fetal and perhaps neonatal infection in the pathogenesis of PVL was suggested initially by neuropathological studies of human brain and related experimental studies of developing kittens in the 1970s.[674-676] A particular focus on endotoxin (LPS) characterized this earlier work. Subsequent studies have documented varying degrees of white matter injury, including oligodendroglial loss, hypomyelination, ventriculomegaly, and, to a lesser extent, cyst formation after systemic or intracerebral injection of LPS to pregnant rats, fetal sheep, and neonatal rats or after induction of gram-negative infection in pregnant rats or pregnant rabbits.[515a,515b,659,677-692] Although the neuropathological findings often are not marked and all findings are not consistent among studies, prominent observations, in addition to white matter injury, include infiltration with activated microglia and up-regulation of several inflammatory cytokines. These findings are reminiscent of the human lesion (see Chapter 8). Because LPS may cause systemic hypotension, hypoglycemia, a microvascular procoagulant effect, and diminished CBF, cerebral hypoxia-ischemia could complicate these experiments.[693-696] However, some studies of LPS-induced white matter injury in fetal sheep do not demonstrate prominent systemic vascular effects.[659]

Because the experimental studies just noted support a relationship between maternal/fetal infection or inflammation and white matter injury, elucidation of the major mechanisms underlying this relation would be critical. Currently data are inconsistent regarding whether LPS, or any related microbial molecular product, may enter the fetus.[697-699] Moreover, it is unclear whether LPS can enter the fetal or neonatal brain from blood (see next section). However, striking responses in brain have been well documented following systemic LPS exposure (i.e., up-regulation of a variety of cytokines, Fas, NF-kappaB, SOD, ornithine decarboxylase, BDNF, NGF, lipid peroxidation, and, of particular importance, the TLRs TLR4 and TLR2, as well as CD14).[700-715] In a study using gene microarray techniques, more than a thousand genes were shown to be regulated in immature rat brain after systemic LPS administration, with a substantial number of cell death-associated genes represented.[715] *Nearly all the responses involve brain microglia, and at least two of these (i.e., up-regulation of TLR4 and CD14) are of particular interest because these molecules are the microglial receptors for LPS that mediate innate immunity (see next section). Activation of these receptors on microglia results in death of pre-OLs.*[685]

Innate Immunity and the Relation of Systemic Inflammation to the Brain. Activation of microglia in the context of infection is postulated to occur in considerable part by way of a relatively small number of specific cell surface receptors (i.e., TLRs) that respond to specific molecular motifs shared by the products of multiple microorganisms (so-called pathogen-associated molecular patterns or PAMPs).[714,716-720b] Because similar molecular motifs are shared by many microbial products, the relatively small number of specific TLRs is the basis for an immediate response to many different organisms (i.e., the mechanism of *innate immunity*). Relevance of this system to the link between maternal/fetal infection and PVL is suggested by the demonstrations that brain microglia contain TLR4, the specific receptor for LPS, the key molecular product of many gram-negative microorganisms, and that when activated by LPS, these microglia secrete diffusible products, perhaps principally NO/ONOO⁻, that are highly toxic to pre-OLs (Fig. 6-36).[685,721a] The mechanisms by which *systemic* LPS produces these responses *in brain* are unclear. The possibilities include the following: (1) penetration by LPS of a blood-brain barrier still "immature" in the developing animal or the human premature infant; (2) passage of LPS across a blood-brain barrier compromised by the action of cytokines or by hypoxia-ischemia, or both; (3) passage of LPS into brain across areas devoid of a blood-brain barrier (i.e., circumventricular organs, with subsequent propagation of immune signals into brain parenchyma); (4) stimulation by LPS of brain endothelial

cells with subsequent propagation of immune signals (e.g., cytokines) into brain parenchyma; (5) passage of peripheral LPS-stimulated cytokines across an intact or compromised blood-brain barrier; or (6) penetration of an intact or compromised blood-brain barrier by LPS-stimulated peripheral monocytes.[707,711,714,717,722-732] Experimental data are available to support all these possibilities, although relevance to the human premature infant remains unclear.

Central Role of Microglia. Although the mechanisms by which maternal/fetal infection and inflammation initiate deleterious molecular and structural events in the brain are not fully understood, *it is clear that microglial cells play a central role.* Moreover, studies in a variety of systems indicate that ROS, RNS, cytokines, and glutamate are important in mediating the actions of these cells (see later). Because mechanisms of ROS/RNS toxicity and excitotoxicity are central to the intrinsic maturation-dependent vulnerability of pre-OLs to both hypoxia-ischemia and infection or inflammation, I discuss the microglial downstream roles further later. However, *it is important here to reemphasize the finding in study of human PVL of the marked microgliosis discovered in the diffuse component of the lesion* (see Chapter 8).[733] This seminal observation supports their involvement in the human lesion.

The particular involvement of microglia, supported by both human neuropathological observations and by experimental studies, in such an apparently diffuse process as exposure to microbial products or to cytokines raises the important question of why PVL is confined to the cerebral white matter and spares the overlying cerebral cortex. One potential answer is that hypoxia-ischemia *initiates* the activation of microglia, and the resulting selectivity of cerebral white matter relates to the cerebral hemodynamic and vascular anatomical factors leading to hypoxia-ischemia, as described earlier and in Chapter 8. Additionally, however, microglial cells can be identified in normal human brain very early in development, become abundant in forebrain from 16 to 22 weeks of gestation, and *notably are concentrated in cerebral white matter, with a deep to superficial gradient.*[707,729,734-736] Relatively few microglial cells are found in cerebral cortex at this time. *Thus, a maturation-dependent population of cells (i.e., microglia) is concentrated in cerebral white matter at the right time and in the right place to contribute to white matter injury when activated.*

Hypoxia-Ischemia and Maternal/Fetal Infection: Potentiating Insults

Deleterious interactions between maternal/fetal infection or inflammation and hypoxia-ischemia could occur at several steps in the pathway to oligodendroglial death (see Fig. 6-35). Thus, such potentiation could develop at the level of the major upstream initiating events of hypoxia-ischemia and infection or inflammation or at the level of the major downstream events of ROS/RNS toxicity and excitotoxicity, or both (see later). Not unexpectedly, most current evidence supporting a potentiating interaction of hypoxia-ischemia and infection or inflammation emanates

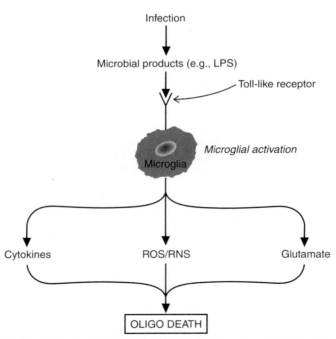

Figure 6-36 **Innate immunity in the pathogenesis of oligodendroglial death.** Activation of specific Toll-like receptors (TLRs) by specific molecular motifs of microbial products (e.g., TLR4 for lipopolysaccharide [LPS] of gram-negative organisms) causes microglial activation and secretion of toxic products, especially reactive oxygen species (ROS) and reactive nitrogen species (RNS). This immediate response to infection (i.e., innate immunity) can cause "innocent bystander" injury to developing oligodendrocytes (OLIGO).

from experimental studies. However, clinical and neuropathological studies of human PVL also support the notion of a potentiating interaction of these two insults (see Chapter 8).

Potentiation of Adverse Systemic and Cerebral Circulatory Effects by Combined Infection or Inflammation and Hypoxia-Ischemia. The combination of infection or inflammation and hypoxia-ischemia could result in deleterious circulatory effects, ultimately affecting the cerebral circulation (see Fig. 6-35). Thus, as noted earlier, in some experimental studies, deleterious systemic hemodynamic effects were shown to accompany fetal or neonatal infection or exposure to LPS or cytokines. That a similar interaction could occur in the premature infant is suggested by several reports (see Chapter 8). Moreover, because several cytokines stimulated by infection, especially TNF-alpha and IL-1beta, exhibit vasoactive properties, it is reasonable to postulate that these inflammatory molecules could contribute to the impaired cerebrovascular autoregulation shown to be important in the pathogenesis of PVL (see Chapter 8).[737,738] Under such circumstances, modest decreases in arterial blood pressure could result in decreases in CBF. Indeed, major disturbances in the regulation of CBF and cerebral oxygen delivery have been observed in fetal sheep after relatively low doses of LPS.[694] Finally, it is well established that hypoxia-ischemia also leads to both systemic and cerebral elevations of vasoactive proinflammatory cytokines (e.g., TNF-alpha and IL-1beta) derived from peripheral monocytes and brain microglia (see earlier).[739-742] *Thus, the possibility of amplifying or at least additive effects on the systemic and cerebral circulations is considerable in the presence of both infection or inflammation and hypoxia-ischemia.*

Microglia as a Convergence Point in the Potentiation of White Matter Injury by Infection or Inflammation and Hypoxia-Ischemia. Potentiation of the deleterious effects of infection or inflammation and hypoxia-ischemia could also occur downstream of the initiating insults and the effects on the systemic and cerebral circulations (see Fig. 6-35). As discussed earlier concerning neuronal injury, *several studies of immature animals demonstrated that pretreatment with LPS, at doses insufficient alone to cause brain injury, caused a hypoxic-ischemic insult, also insufficient alone to result in appreciable injury, to produce marked degrees of injury, including white matter injury.*[510-515b,743] In most of these experimental models, injury to both neurons and differentiating oligodendroglia were observed. Notably, the potentiation of hypoxic-ischemic injury by LPS involved pretreatment in the several hours before hypoxia-ischemia. However, tolerance rather than potentiation was observed when the LPS pretreatment occurred 24 hours before hypoxia-ischemia.[517] The latter effect was shown to be mediated by up-regulation of corticosterone after the LPS administration.[516] No benefit was observed when dexamethasone was administered after the hypoxic-ischemic insult. Among the potential beneficial effects of the

endogenous glucocorticoids is inhibition of phospholipase A_2 with liberation of arachidonic acid; LPS activates cyclooxygenase 2 expression, involved in arachidonate metabolism, and thereby generation of injurious ROS.[509]

Importance for innate immunity in the genesis of the potentiation of white matter injury by hypoxia-ischemia and infection or inflammation is suggested by the following observations: (1) CD-14, essential for the action of TLR4, the TLR for LPS, was up-regulated following LPS treatment[510]; and (2) in parallel experiments with mice lacking TLR4, the combination of LPS and hypoxia-ischemia produced *no* injury.[513] *These data strongly suggest that microglial cells are central to the sensitizing effect of LPS and that the two potent activators of microglia, infection* (with its associated pathogen-associated molecular patterns, i.e., PAMPs) *and hypoxia-ischemia, may converge on the microglial cell to provoke a deleterious series of effects* (Fig. 6-37). The downstream molecular events involved in the potentiation of hypoxic-ischemic injury by LPS likely involve ROS and, particularly, RNS, cytokines, and glutamate (see Fig. 6-37). These events are discussed next in relation to the maturation-dependent vulnerability of pre-OLs.

Perhaps additional indications of the potentiating interaction of infection or inflammation and hypoxia-ischemia are the demonstrations of the *exacerbation of excitotoxic white matter and gray matter lesions by proinflammatory cytokines.*[497,744] Excitotoxicity, of course, is a well-established mediator of hypoxic-ischemic death to both pre-OLs and to neurons (see earlier). A central role for *microglia* in this potentiation of excitotoxicity by cytokines is likely because the pretreatment with proinflammatory cytokines increased microglial density in the white matter areas that developed excitotoxic

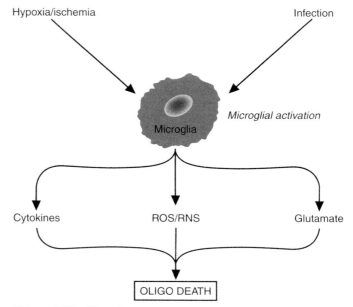

Figure 6-37 Microglia as a central convergence point in the mechanisms of cell death with hypoxia-ischemia and infection. OLIGO, oligodendrocytes; RNS, reactive nitrogen species; ROS, reactive oxygen species. See text for details.

injury.[497] Moreover, TNF-alpha, released from microglia, has been shown to lead, in turn, to release of glutamate from microglia in an autocrine manner.[453] Also of relevance in this context is the inhibition of glutamate uptake in astrocytes and oligodendrocytes by proinflammatory cytokines (see later).[745-748]

Maturation-Dependent Intrinsic Vulnerability of Premyelinating Oligodendrocytes in Cerebral White Matter

An intrinsic vulnerability of pre-OLs in the cerebral white matter of the human premature infant is suggested by the experimental studies, by the rarity of the lesion at later ages, by the concentration of these cells in human cerebral white matter during the peak time period for occurrence of PVL, and by their specific involvement in the lesion. To address and to clarify the issue of the maturation-dependent vulnerability of oligodendroglial precursors, we and others studied this cell lineage, identified by immunocytochemical criteria (see Chapter 2), in experimental systems, both in culture and in vivo, and in human postmortem brain. Within this lineage, as stated earlier, the data indicate that the principal cellular target in PVL is the *pre-OL, a term that includes both the O4+ pre-oligodendrocyte and the O1+ immature oligodendrocyte.* The data indicate that these cells are particularly vulnerable to the *two principal downstream events* in PVL (i.e., *ROS/RNS toxicity* and *excitotoxicity;* see Fig. 6-35), as discussed next.

Reactive Oxygen and Nitrogen Species Toxicity

The most compelling direct evidence that ROS/RNS toxicity is involved in the injury to pre-OLs in PVL emanates from our study of the human lesion reported by Haynes and associates (see Chapter 8).[733] Thus, using immunocytochemical markers for oxidative (hydroxynonenal) and nitrative (nitrotyrosine) attack, abundant staining was documented in both pre-OLs and reactive astrocytes in PVL. The free radical attack appeared to lead to death of the former but not the latter. This key discovery of oxidative and nitrative attack in PVL is consistent with experimental data indicative of oxidative and nitrative cellular injury with both hypoxic-ischemic and inflammatory insults to brain (see later), the two likely key upstream mechanisms in PVL (see Fig. 6-35). The bases for the maturation-dependent sensitivity of pre-OLs to ROS and RNS toxicity are discussed next.

Reactive Oxygen Species Toxicity. A particular maturation-dependent vulnerability of pre-OLs to both endogenous and exogenous ROS is now well established in both cultured cells and in vivo models (Fig. 6-38).[668,749-754] Thus, pre-OLs are killed under conditions of ROS attack that do not harm mature oligodendrocytes. Moreover, the mechanism of cell death is principally apoptotic (Fig. 6-39). In addition, in cultured pre-OLs, a potent protective effect of clinically safe free radical scavengers (e.g., vitamin E) was shown, even when it was added *after the onset* of ROS

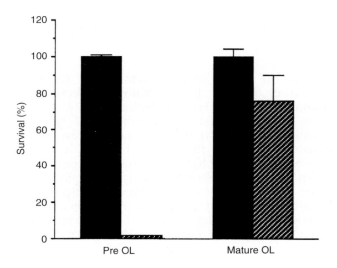

Figure 6-38 Developing preoligodendrocytes (PreOL) are exquisitely vulnerable to free radical attack (produced by the use of cystine-depleted medium, which leads to decreased intracellular glutathione and oxidative stress), whereas mature oligodendrocytes (Mature OL) are resistant. Solid bars are control cells in cystine-containing medium, and hatched bars are cells undergoing free radical attack in cystine-depleted medium. *(From Back SA, Gan X, Li Y, Rosenberg PA, et al: Maturation-dependent vulnerability of oligodendrocytes to oxidative stress-induced death caused by glutathione depletion,* J Neurosci *18:6241-6253, 1998.)*

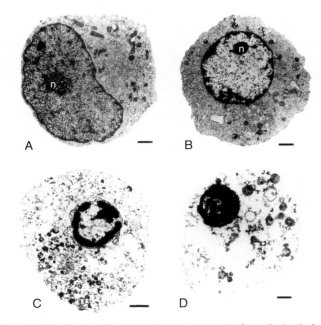

Figure 6-39 Free radical attack causes apoptotic cell death in developing oligodendrocytes. The ultrastructural characteristics of, **A,** a control cell and, **B** through **D,** cells undergoing progressive free radical attack in cystine-depleted medium over 14 hours are shown. Note in **B,** the margination and clumping of chromatin; in **C,** the condensed marginated chromatin but intact nuclear and plasma membranes; and in **D,** the shrunken nucleus with very condensed chromatin but still-intact nuclear and plasma membranes. These features are characteristic of apoptosis (see Table 6-11). n, nucleolus. *(From Back SA, Gan X, Li Y, Rosenberg PA, et al: Maturation-dependent vulnerability of oligodendrocytes to oxidative stress-induced death caused by glutathione depletion,* J Neurosci *18:6241-6253, 1998.)*

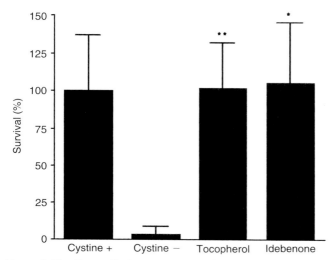

Figure 6-40 **Free radical scavengers, alpha-tocopherol and idebenone, protect developing oligodendrocytes in culture from free radical attack.** Free radical attack was produced by the use of cystine-depleted medium, which leads to oxidative stress by provoking glutathione depletion, and survival was determined at 24 hours. Note the minimal survival in cystine-depleted medium. When alpha-tocopherol or idebenone was added to the cystine-depleted medium, total protection from free radical-mediated death was observed. The protective effect was observed even when the agents were added as long as 15 hours *after* the onset of cystine depletion. *(From Back SA, Gan X, Li Y, Rosenberg PA, et al: Maturation-dependent vulnerability of oligodendrocytes to oxidative stress-induced death caused by glutathione depletion,* J Neurosci *18:6241-6253, 1998.)*

attack (Fig. 6-40).[751] Moreover, vitamin K has been shown to be extraordinarily potent in preventing oxidative injury to developing oligodendrocytes.[753] The mechanism of the protection by vitamin K was not established, although the vitamin prevented accumulation of ROS in one model of oxidative stress. Moreover, the protective effect occurred even when vitamin K was added hours after the onset of the insult. An important clue to the basis of the particular vulnerability of pre-OLs versus mature cells to ROS toxicity was the discovery that, under conditions of identical exposure to ROS, pre-OLs accumulated ROS, whereas mature cells did not.[751] The importance of *ROS accumulation in pre-OLs versus mature oligodendrocytes*, despite a similar degree of exposure to ROS, suggested that the intrinsic vulnerability of pre-OLs to oxidation related in part to a *deficit in antioxidant defenses.*

The mechanisms underlying the maturation-dependent vulnerability of developing oligodendrocytes to ROS attack have been addressed in both human brain and in cell culture. The findings in human brain indicate a delay in development of enzymes at the SOD and catalase steps (see Chapter 8), and the findings in cultured pre-OLs show an additional disturbance at the glutathione peroxidase/catalase steps (see Fig. 6-21).[755-757] Additionally, the possibility that hydrogen peroxide accumulates and is converted to the hydroxyl radical by the Fenton reaction is suggested by the observations of others of the early appearance of iron in devel-oping human white matter,[758,759] as well as by the acquisition of iron by

developing oligodendrocytes for differentiation.[760] In addition, non–protein-bound iron increases prominently in cerebral white matter after hypoxia-ischemia.[761,762] Supportive of a relationship between iron and PVL are observations in a mouse model that iron pretreatment increases the amount of white matter injury,[763] and that for many weeks after human intraventricular hemorrhage, a disorder that sharply increases the risk of PVL,[764-766] cerebrospinal fluid levels of nonprotein-bound iron are markedly increased (see Fig. 6-35).[767] Taken together, the findings indicate a maturation-dependent window of vulnerability to oxidative attack during oligodendroglial development related principally to delayed development of antioxidant enzymes and acquisition of iron for differentiation (see Fig. 6-35).

Multiple reports suggest that the vulnerability to oxidative attack in the premature white matter shares similarities with features in the periphery. Thus, studies of plasma of human premature infants indicate a propensity to generate free radicals, including the hydroxyl radical, increases in plasma non–protein-bound iron, accentuated by hypoxia or blood transfusion, and impaired antioxidant defenses.[310,768-777]

As for hypoxia-ischemia, experimental studies relevant to maternal/fetal infection and inflammation also indicate a link to oxidative stress. Thus, research based primarily on cellular systems indicate that ROS, produced largely by microglia activated by cytokines, LPS, or other factors, are important mediators of oligodendroglial (and neuronal) toxicity in many paradigms.[778-787] The critical sequence for killing of pre-OLs by LPS-activated microglia is LPS activation of the TLR4 receptor, generation of superoxide anion, NO, and then ONOO⁻, the final mediator of pre-OL death.[685,721]

Reactive Nitrogen Species Toxicity. As with oxidative stress, experimental studies in a variety of models demonstrated the importance of RNS in the cascade to cell death induced by hypoxia-ischemia-reperfusion (see earlier). The presence of NOS in neurons (including subplate neurons), astrocytes, activated microglia, endothelial cells, and perhaps pre-OLs (see later) provides abundant sources for NO. NO toxicity to oligodendrocytes was shown in primary cultures, oligodendroglial-derived cell lines, and isolated rat optic nerve.[327,788-794] The work of my colleagues and I showed that NO toxicity to oligodendrocytes is maturation dependent, with pre-OLs much more vulnerable than mature MBP-expressing oligodendrocytes.[788] The mechanisms of the NO toxicity to pre-OLs are likely multiple. Thus, in the presence of activated microglia, formation of superoxide anion and NO and then ONOO⁻ is important.[721] However, NO can lead to pre-OL death directly and without formation of ONOO⁻. Thus, in the latter instance, NO acts as a mitochondrial poison with subsequent translocation of apoptosis-inducing factor from mitochondria to nuclei and caspase-independent cell death.[788] *Relevance of these mechanisms to human PVL is indicated* by the finding of a significant increase in the number of iNOS-positive astrocytes in the diffuse component of PVL (see Chapter 8). The data suggest that a key source of NO in the human lesion, potentially leading to a major portion of the nitrative stress identified previously in diffuse PVL,[733] is the reactive astrocyte (see Chapter 8).

As for hypoxia-ischemia, experimental studies relevant to maternal/fetal infection and inflammation also indicate a link to RNS toxicity. Thus, research based primarily on cellular systems indicate that RNS, produced largely by microglia activated by cytokines, LPS, or other factors, but also probably produced by astrocytes, are important mediators of oligodendroglial (and neuronal) toxicity in a variety of models.[721,795-799] Interferon-gamma is of particular importance in this context for several reasons. First, induction of iNOS, particularly in microglia but also in astrocytes, appears to be the principal mode of killing induced by this cytokine.[795,796,798-801] Second, of proinflammatory cytokines thus far studied, interferon-gamma appears to be the most toxic to oligodendrocytes, and particularly developing oligodendrocytes.[802-805] Third, although data are not entirely consistent concerning toxicity of TNF-alpha to oligodendrocytes,[791,805-813] it is clear that TNF-alpha potentiates the oligodendroglial toxicity of interferon-gamma.[802,806,814] Moreover, in one careful study of the entire oligodendroglial lineage, the toxicity of TNF-alpha decreased as maturation progressed.[815] Fourth, interferon-gamma levels increase in neonatal piglet brain after systemic LPS treatment.[740] Fifth, mice made transgenic for cerebral expression of interferon-gamma exhibit marked hypomyelination and impaired remyelination.[816,817] Finally, our studies of human PVL showed in the diffuse component of the lesion abundant interferon-gamma expression in astrocytes and interferon-gamma receptor expression in pre-OLs (see Chapter 8).[818] Taken together, the data suggest that RNS toxicity is involved in cell death with infection or inflammation and that interferon-gamma especially, through induction of iNOS and thereby NO production, may be a critical mediator of pre-OL death in PVL. TNF-alpha likely plays a critical role as well.

Excitotoxicity

An intrinsic maturation-dependent vulnerability of pre-OLs to excitotoxicity was shown by experimental studies and by related observations of developing human brain (see Chapter 8). Indeed, with free radical toxicity, excitotoxicity may be considered one of the two major downstream mechanisms in the cascade to oligodendroglial death (see Fig. 6-35). Glutamate is capable of inducing maturation-dependent death of pre-OLs by nonreceptor and receptor-mediated mechanisms. The *nonreceptor-mediated mechanism* involves glutamate competition for the cystine transporter and promotion of cystine efflux under conditions of high extracellular levels of glutamate.[749] The results are depletion of intracellular glutathione (which requires cysteine for biosynthesis) and cell death by oxidative stress.[749-751] However, the substantial levels (millimolar) of glutamate required for this effect suggest that this mechanism may operate in vivo only under extreme pathological conditions.

By contrast, the *receptor-mediated mechanism*, which requires micromolar levels of glutamate, is more likely to occur in vivo, as shown directly in animal models by us and others (see later). In the following discussion, I review evidence for glutamate elevations in white matter in vivo, the sources of glutamate, the receptors involved, and the interaction of excitotoxicity and ROS/RNS toxicity.

Elevated Glutamate Levels In Vivo. Although elevation of brain glutamate levels in vivo with hypoxia-ischemia and inflammation has been recognized in cerebral neuronal structures,[439] only recently have such elevations been documented in cerebral white matter.[819] Thus, in an established model of cerebral white matter injury produced by umbilical cord occlusion in near-term fetal sheep, marked increases in extracellular glutamate were detected in white matter by microdialysis in the hours following occlusion. The extent of the increase in extracellular glutamate correlated directly with the ultimate extent of white matter injury. The *delayed* increase in glutamate over the *hours* after the insult was much greater than the increase during the insult and is considered to be the more important increase in the genesis of the injury. This delayed and large increase has been observed in other models in which an effect on glutamate transport systems occurs (see next section).

Sources of Glutamate. The sources of glutamate in cerebral white matter after hypoxia-ischemia appear to be principally glutamate transporters.[820,821] Glutamate levels in white matter are regulated by high-affinity, Na^+-dependent glutamate transporters on oligodendroglia, astrocytes, axons, and, probably, microglia.[820,821] The two principal transporters, GLAST and GLT-1, are involved. When ATP levels fall and the energy-dependent Na^+-K^+ cellular gradient is lost, the glutamate transporters fail and operate in reverse. This fact may underlie the potentiation of pre-OL excitotoxicity by impaired mitochondrial function.[822] Oligodendrocytes are quantitatively important cells for glutamate transport in white matter, and *both pre-OLs and axons appear to be the major sources for extracellular glutamate with hypoxia-ischemia, oxygen-glucose deprivation, or inflammation.*[673,746,820,821,823-826] Recently described vesicular release from axons also could be involved.[826a,826b] With ischemia, astrocytes also are important sources.[827,828] Although a portion of this latter effect is reversal of transport, another mechanism involves ischemic activation of the Na^+/K^+/Cl^- cotransporter, with Cl^- and water import, astrocyte swelling, and, ultimately, lysis, with release of intracellular glutamate. Microglial cells, activated by inflammatory stimuli, also release glutamate by varied mechanisms that may include reversal of an Na^+-dependent transporter, operation of the cystine-glutamate antiporter, and vesicular release.[453,821,829-833] Additional links of altered glutamate homeostasis to inflammation include the potent inhibition of glutamate transport in oligodendrocytes by TNF-alpha and in astrocytes by IL-1beta.[745-748]

Relevance of this work on glutamate transport and thereby excitotoxicity to the other major downstream mechanism of pre-OL death initiated by hypoxia-ischemia or inflammation (see Fig. 6-35) (i.e., ROS/RNS toxicity) is suggested by the demonstration that ROS disrupts glutamate transport in astrocytes.[447] Because excitotoxicity to pre-OLs is mediated in considerable part by generation of ROS (see later), the possibilities of amplification of the two downstream mechanisms of excitotoxicity and ROS/RNS attack through effects on glutamate transport are real.

Involvement of glutamate transport in the maturation-dependence of pre-OL toxicity and in the genesis of human PVL is suggested by the demonstration of overexpression of glutamate transporters in cerebral white matter in the fetal sheep and in the human infant during the time period of peak vulnerability to PVL (see Chapter 8).[834,835] Our studies of the human brain demonstrate also that the glutamate transporter is overexpressed in the pre-OL.[834]

Glutamate Receptors. Only in the past decade has it become clear that oligodendrocytes contain glutamate receptors, which, when excessively activated, can lead to cell injury. The most widely studied type of glutamate receptor, the AMPA/KA type, concentrated in cell somata, leads to cell death when excessively activated (see later). The more recently discovered type, the NMDA receptor, concentrated in oligodendroglial processes, leads to loss of cell processes when excessively activated. I discuss each of these in sequence next.

Oligodendrocytes express *AMPA/kainate (AMPA/KA)–type glutamate receptors*, the activation of which results in cell death.[754,820,822,836-844] Our study of excitotoxicity to the major phases of the oligodendroglial lineage showed that the toxicity is maturation dependent and that both functional activity and subunit expression of AMPA/KA receptors are down-regulated in mature oligodendrocytes versus pre-OLs.[845] Relevance of these findings to hypoxia-ischemia was suggested by the demonstration in culture by others and by us that receptor-mediated excitotoxicity was the principal mechanism for pre-OL death with oxygen-glucose deprivation.[754,823,838,843,846-848] Relevance to hypoxia-ischemia in vivo was shown after the development of a rodent model of hypoxia-ischemia-induced PVL (P7 rat subjected to unilateral carotid ligation and hypoxemia).[849] This white matter injury could be prevented by *systemic* administration, beginning immediately *after insult*, of NBQX, an AMPA/KA antagonist (Fig. 6-41).[849] Because NBQX may not be clinically safe, in subsequent work, topiramate, a clinically safe anticonvulsant drug with AMPA blocking properties, was shown to also have a similar protective effect.[850] Additionally supportive of a relationship among hypoxia-ischemia, excitotoxicity, and PVL is the observation that AMPA receptors are overexpressed (relative to the mature brain) in white matter of developing rats during the peak period of vulnerability of this species for selective, hypoxic-ischemic white matter injury (see earlier).[382]

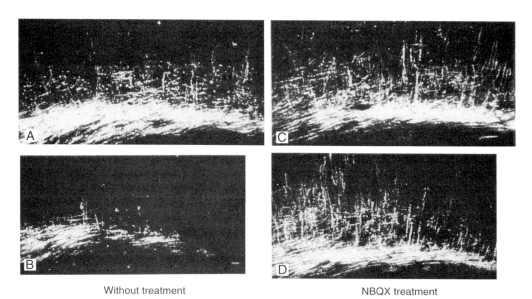

Without treatment   NBQX treatment

Figure 6-41 **Protection from hypoxic-ischemic cerebral white matter injury in the immature (P7) rat by systemic administration of the non–N-methyl-D-aspartate (NMDA) receptor blocker, NBQX, after the termination of the insult.** A through D show myelin basic protein (MBP) staining in cerebral white matter at P11, 4 days after cerebral hypoxia-ischemia produced by unilateral carotid ligation and hypoxemia at P7. Developing oligodendrocytes at P7 normally differentiate into MBP-positive oligodendrocytes by P11. At the termination of the insult on P7, animals received either injection of, **A** and **B**, vehicle or, **C** and **D**, NBQX, the non-NMDA receptor blocker. **A** and **C** show MBP staining contralateral to the ligation, and **B** and **D** show staining ipsilateral to the ligation. Note the marked disturbance in the hypoxic-ischemic (ipsilateral) hemisphere in the nontreated animal (**B** compared with **A**) and the protection afforded by NBQX in the hypoxic-ischemic hemisphere in the treated animal (**D** compared with **C**). *(From Follett P, Rosenberg PA, Volpe JJ, Jensen FE: NBQX attenuates excitotoxic injury in developing white matter. J Neurosci 20:9235-9241, 2000.)*

The mechanism of the receptor-mediated toxicity appears to involve Ca²⁺ influx.[382,754,823,836,843,845,851,852] The basis for the Ca²⁺ influx relates to the expression in developing versus mature oligodendrocytes of AMPA receptors that lack the GluR2 subunit, the subunit that renders the receptor Ca²⁺ impermeable.[754,836,850] *Relevance of these observations to PVL is suggested by the demonstration that pre-OL killing induced by* oxygen-glucose deprivation *occurs by Joro spider toxin–sensitive Ca²⁺ permeable AMPA/KA receptors.*[754] Moreover, of potential clinical relevance is the additional finding that *sublethal* oxygen-glucose deprivation *resulted in enhanced toxicity to subsequent exposure to* oxygen-glucose deprivation *(or to kainate)* because of down-regulation of the GluR2 subunit and an increase in Ca²⁺ influx.[754] Studies of cerebral hemodynamics in the premature infant suggest that infants with a pressure-passive cerebral circulation experience *multiple,* but usually not severe, declines in CBF (see later discussion). Finally, and perhaps most importantly, in developing white matter of the rat brain and, critically, the *human brain,* not only are AMPA receptors *overexpressed* during the peak period of vulnerability to PVL, but also these receptors are relatively deficient in the GluR2 subunit and are thereby Ca²⁺ permeable. [382,383,850]

A major advance in the understanding of oligodendroglial excitotoxicity was the recent discovery of *NMDA receptors on processes of oligodendrocytes,* from the developing to the mature, myelin-producing stages.[844,853-856] When activated by ischemic conditions or exposure to agonists, loss of processes occurs. Moreover, NMDA receptors are permeable to Ca²⁺, and it is likely that the downstream mechanisms related to Ca²⁺ influx, generation of ROS/RNS, account for the deleterious effects. Because axons can release glutamate, the findings suggest that the presence of NMDA receptors on oligodendrocytes provides a mechanism of axonal-oligodendroglial signaling important for myelination. However, with excessive glutamate, as occurs with ischemia, this normal mechanism becomes pathological. The data suggest an additional site for protection of pre-OLs from ischemic injury. Indeed, in preliminary data, we showed a potent protective effective of memantine, a specific NMDA antagonist, in a neonatal rat model of hypoxic-ischemic white matter injury. Moreover, preliminary studies of human brain showed, analogous to the findings with AMPA receptors, a marked expression of NMDA receptors in pre-OLs in human cerebral white matter during the peak period of vulnerability to PVL.[857] The findings of NMDA receptors on pre-OLs may help explain the white matter injury produced in developing mice and rabbits by intracerebral injection of ibotenic acid and NMDA, both agonists of the NMDA receptor.[497,858-860] However, because NMDA receptors are also present on microglia and astrocytes, secondary effects involving pre-OLs could account for some of the white matter injury in these models. At any rate, the findings of an overexpression of both Ca²⁺-permeable AMPA receptors and NMDA receptors on pre-OLs suggest a particularly maturation-dependent vulnerability of these cells to excitotoxicity (Table 6-22).

TABLE 6-22	Maturation-Dependent Vulnerability of Differentiating Oligodendrocytes to Excitotoxicity

AMPA receptors (GluR2-deficient) are concentrated on pre-oligodendrocyte somata, and NMDA receptors are concentrated on preoligodendrocyte processes.

These receptors are overexpressed in cerebral white matter during the peak period of vulnerability to hypoxic-ischemic white matter injury.

Both GluR2-deficient AMPA receptors and NMDA receptors are permeable to calcium.

Ischemia leads to calcium influx through activation of these receptors with either cell death (AMPA activation) or loss of processes (NMDA activation), or both.

Both receptors can be blocked by specific antagonists and lead to protection.

AMPA, alpha-amino-3-hydroxy-5-methyl-4-isoxazolepropionic acid; NMDA, *N*-methyl-ᴅ-aspartate

The findings concerning AMPA and NMDA receptors on pre-OL cell bodies and processes, respectively, suggest the possibility of differential effects and temporal aspects of excessive activation of these receptors (Fig. 6-42). Thus, activation of the NMDA receptor, which can flux Ca²⁺ more readily and more vigorously

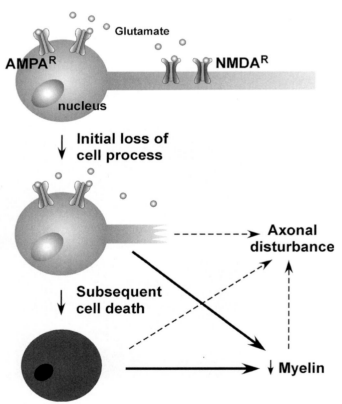

Figure 6-42 Potential differential effects and temporal aspects of excitotoxicity to developing oligodendrocytes. The intact cell *(top)* has alpha-amino-3-hydroxy-5-methyl-4-isoxazole-propionic acid (AMPA) receptors primarily on the cell soma and *N*-methyl-ᴅ-aspartate (NMDA) receptors primarily on the cell processes. Initially with excess extracellular glutamate, activation of NMDA receptors could lead to loss of cell processes, and if excitotoxicity continues, to activation of AMPA receptors and cell death. Either event could lead to impaired myelination *(solid arrows)* and potentially also to axonal disturbance *(dotted lines).*

than even GluR2-deficient AMPA receptors, would lead initially to loss of oligodendroglial processes but not cell death. By contrast, more pronounced or prolonged exposure to glutamate may be required to activate the AMPA receptors to lead to cell death. The consequence of both could be subsequent hypomyelination, although perhaps the possibilities of recovery would be greater if only cell processes were lost and the cell body were spared (see Chapter 8). Additionally possible are secondary axonal disturbances, caused by a failure of both ensheathment by pre-OLs and subsequent myelination (see Fig. 6-42).

Relation of Excitotoxicity to Reactive Oxygen Species/ Reactive Nitrogen Species Toxicity. A direct relationship between the two downstream mechanisms leading to death of pre-OLs (i.e., excitotoxicity and ROS/RNS toxicity; see Fig. 6-35) is suggested by the demonstrations that AMPA/KA receptor toxicity to oligodendroglial precursors is accompanied by generation of ROS and RNS.[843,852,861] The occurrence of nitrotyrosine immunoreactivity in pre-OLs suggested that, under these conditions, $ONOO^-$ is the key RNS. This deadly compound is likely formed from NO, produced by Ca^{2+}-activated iNOS in the oligodendrocytes and superoxide anion, produced by one or more of several Ca^{2+}-inducible enzymes resulting in ROS formation.[861] The oxidative stress associated with AMPA receptor activation in oligodendrocytes is greater than that associated with activation in neurons.[409] The use of an SOD/catalase mimetic, Euk, protected pre-OLs from excitotoxicity.[843] This nonpeptidyl molecule has neuroprotective properties in vivo (see earlier discussion of neuronal death). Thus, the data indicate how multiple maturation-dependent characteristics of pre-OLs interact in an amplifying manner to produce a highly vulnerable cell, with the

upstream mechanisms (hypoxia-ischemia and inflammation) converging on two interacting downstream mechanisms (excitotoxicity and free radical attack) (see Fig. 6-35).

Interventions for Prevention of Oligodendrocytes from Hypoxic-Ischemic and Inflammatory Injury

As for the earlier discussion of neuronal death, the insights into the biochemical and cellular mechanisms of injury to differentiating oligodendrocytes by hypoxia-ischemia and inflammation, as just discussed, provide a rational basis for formulation of mechanisms to interrupt those mechanisms and thereby to prevent or ameliorate the injury. The sequence just described and the best candidates for intervention are shown in Figure 6-43. Some of the interventions have been shown to be effective against neuronal death (see earlier) and thus will be particularly promising as an approach to dual neuronal-oligodendroglial protection, a feature of some perinatal human hypoxic-ischemic lesions (see Chapter 8).

Prevention of Hypoxia-Ischemia. Prevention of hypoxia-ischemia is discussed in detail in Chapter 8. Prevention requires detection of the infant with impaired cerebrovascular autoregulation, and this requirement may be possible with *near-infrared spectroscopy*, with subsequent correction of the cerebrovascular disturbance. Progress in these areas has been accomplished in recent years (see Chapter 8).

Prevention of Infection or Inflammation. Prevention of the infection or inflammation upstream mechanism appears most promising at the level of interventions to *blunt or prevent microglial activation, cytokine action, or related inflammatory cascades* (see Fig. 6-43). Most promising in experimental models has been the use of

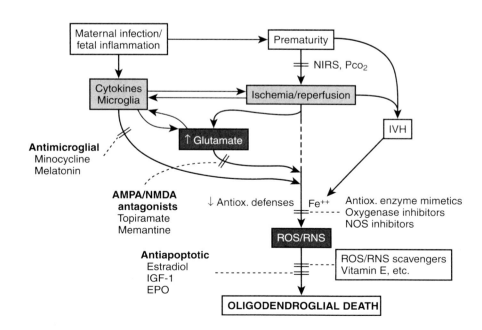

Figure 6-43 Interventions for prevention of injury to developing oligodendrocytes resulting from hypoxic-ischemic and inflammatory insults. AMPA, alpha-amino-3-hydroxy-5-methyl-4-isoxazole-propionic acid; Fe^{++}, iron; IVH, intraventricular hemorrhage; NIRS, near-infrared spectroscopy; NMDA, N-methyl-D-aspartate; NOS, nitric oxide synthase; RNS, reactive nitrogen species; ROS, reactive oxygen species. See text for details.

minocycline (see earlier discussion regarding neuronal protection).[862-866] Melatonin may exert some of its white matter protection at this level.[866a] Thus, these agents or related antimicroglial compounds could be useful against both gray matter (neuronal) and white matter (oligodendroglial) injury.

Antenatal administration of corticosteroids is associated with a decreased incidence of cerebral white matter injury in the premature newborn (see Chapter 8). Whether this effect relates to the well-documented anti-inflammatory properties of the drug is unclear. Whether other targets (e.g., TLRs or their downstream molecules) would be suitable for interventions remains unclear. Such approaches are in the early phases of development.[867]

Prevention of Excitotoxicity. Concerning the two major downstream mechanisms, excitotoxicity and free radical attack, *blockade of non-NMDA, particularly AMPA receptors*, appears very promising to prevent pre-OL death (see earlier discussion) (see Fig. 6-43).[849,850] The apparently clinically safe agent, *topiramate*, is very effective in a well-characterized animal model.[584,850]

Blockade of NMDA receptors appears similarly promising to prevent loss of pre-OL processes (see Fig. 6-43) (see earlier). *Memantine* may be the most clinically safe NMDA receptor antagonist in this setting.[850a] More data are needed. The potentially beneficial effect of *melatonin* on white matter injury in an animal model involving direct injection of an NMDA agonist may occur in part at this level.[868]

Combination therapy with non-NMDA and NMDA antagonists could be particularly useful in two ways. This approach may provide optimal protection for pre-OLs and may also combine an important neuronal protective effect (see the discussion of neuronal protection).

Prevention of Free Radical Generation. *ROS and RNS attack* is a critical area because the deleterious effects of both upstream mechanisms *and* the major portion of excitotoxicity occur through the actions of ROS/RNS (see Fig. 6-43). *Counteraction of the impaired antioxidant defenses in pre-OLs* and thereby prevention of free radical accumulation by the use of mimetics of antioxidant enzymes may be of particular value,[843] because nonpeptidyl agents can enter the brain. *Prevention of free radical generation* by vitamin K may be a particularly powerful approach because available data indicate high potency for this intervention and effectiveness even hours *after* the onset of free radical accumulation (see earlier).[753] This agent should be safe in premature infants because vitamin K is administered routinely in newborns for blood coagulation in vivo and is protective in vitro in very low concentrations. *Inhibition of enzymes that are crucial in genesis of oxygen free radicals* (e.g., oxygenase inhibitors, especially 12-lipoxygenase) by specific agents also may be valuable, based on published data.[869] Whether these agents are useful in vivo remains to be determined. Because of the important role of

nitrative mechanisms, the use of *inhibitors of NO synthesis* may be particularly valuable (see earlier). More data are needed.

Scavenging of Free Radicals. Scavengers of ROS/RNS may be particularly useful against pre-OL death because these agents also would be useful against neuronal death (see earlier) (see Fig. 6-43). Vitamin E and related scavengers have been effective, especially in cultured models.[597a,751] One *free-radical scavenging* agent, the spin-trapping agent alpha-phenyl-*N*-tert-butyl-nitrone (PBN), administered systemically following the hypoxic-ischemic insult, attenuated white matter injury in the immature rat.[870]

Blockade of Downstream Effects. The principal downstream effects in the cascade to pre-OL cell death involve progression to apoptosis. Thus, studies of pre-OLs undergoing free radical attack,[751] hypoxic-ischemic white matter injury in the neonatal piglet,[175] and human neuropathology (see Chapter 8) indicate that apoptosis is the principal mechanism of pre-OL death in PVL. Thus, antiapoptotic interventions, as discussed for neuronal protection (see earlier), are relevant in this context.

Of the agents that block apoptotic mechanisms and shown to be protective to neurons (see earlier), *several growth factors* have been most effective versus pre-OL death. Thus, *IGF-I* has been shown to be protective to pre-OLs in the hypoxic-ischemic neonatal rat[871] and in near-term fetal sheep.[872] In both paradigms, IGF-I suppressed apoptotic death and promoted oligodendroglial precursor proliferation. The antiapoptotic effect involves activation of Akt and prevention of both mitochondrial cytochrome c release and caspase activation.[872-874] Administration of the peptide was by the intracerebral or intraventricular route, and thus clinical application could be problematic. However, a report in hypoxic-ischemic *adult* rats suggested appreciable neuroprotection after intravenous administration of the N-terminal tripeptide of IGF-I.[875]

Other growth factors may also be protective against pre-OL death. In separate animal models involving excitotoxic or inflammatory mechanisms, BDNF and ciliary neurotrophic factor (CNTF) have shown benefit.[630,876] Finally, the recently described protective effect of *estradiol* in neonatal white matter injury appears to be primarily antiapoptotic.[876a]

Among other interventions discussed in relation to neuronal protection, *mild hypothermia* was shown to decrease postischemic white matter injury sharply in the near-term fetal sheep.[877,877a] Protection was associated with reduced caspase-3 activation. However, hypothermia was not effective when it was delayed until 5.5 hours after reperfusion. Moreover, because, unlike in hypoxic-ischemic *neuronal* injury, the insults that lead to white matter injury in the human infant are likely to be mild, multiple, and protracted, hypothermia does not appear to be an ideal intervention.

EPO, discussed earlier as particularly promising with regard to neuronal protection, may be predicted to be promising against white matter injury as well, in view of several of its molecular effects (e.g., antiapoptotic, antioxidant, antiexcitotoxic). However, at the time of this writing, no reports are available regarding EPO in models of selective white matter injury.

PHYSIOLOGICAL ASPECTS

Importance of Cerebral Blood Flow and Regulation

Extensive clinical and neuropathological data emphasize the major role of ischemia in the genesis of brain injury associated with adverse perinatal events (see earlier discussion and Chapter 8). Thus, alterations in CBF are of prime importance for understanding the neuropathological and neurological consequences of all varieties of perinatal asphyxial and hypoxic-ischemic insults, as well as the pathogenesis, prevention, and treatment of these consequences. In the following discussion, I review CBF, its regulation, and the changes associated with asphyxia and related hypoxic-ischemic insults. By necessity, the discussion involves studies with experimental animals. However, growing experience with the human newborn, described in the final sections, indicates that the lessons learned from animal research are largely relevant to the perinatal human.

Cerebral Blood Flow: Knowledge from Experimental Studies

Fetal Circulation

The essential features of the fetal circulation, based principally on work with large animals (e.g., sheep, goats, and nonhuman primates) begin with events at the placenta.[878-903] Gas exchange occurs efficiently at the placenta, although oxygen diffusion is somewhat restricted, and fetal arterial oxygen tension values are considerably lower than maternal values. Compensatory responses to this lower oxygen tension in the fetus include hemoglobin F, with its favorable oxygen affinity curve, polycythemia, and a relatively high cardiac output. Oxygenated blood from the placenta is carried through the umbilical vein, which empties into the inferior vena cava. This well-oxygenated blood enters the right atrium and is preferentially shunted through the patent foramen ovale ultimately to the aortic arch and then to the coronary and cerebral circulations.[884] Poorly oxygenated blood from the superior vena cava is preferentially shunted into the right ventricle and the pulmonary artery. Because of the high pulmonary vascular resistance, this blood primarily enters the ductus arteriosus and the descending aorta and returns to the placenta through the umbilical arteries.

Regulation of Cerebral Blood Flow: General Principles

CBF in experimental animals has been measured principally by techniques based on the clearance of an inert gas (e.g., xenon and nitrous oxide), carotid artery flow determinations, [^{14}C]antipyrine infusion with autoradiography, and infusion of radioactive microspheres with subsequent tissue sampling. In recent years, near-infrared spectroscopy, sometimes combined with infusion of indocyanine green, has been used. Because considerable variability in absolute values of CBF is observed with different techniques, species, modes of anesthesia, preparation of animals, and so forth, I place most emphasis in this discussion on the major conclusions of the many studies rather than on the absolute values of CBF recorded. The focus of this section is on general principles of cerebral hemodynamics, primarily in mature animals; immature animals are discussed subsequently in a separate section.

Autoregulation. *Autoregulation* of CBF refers to the maintenance of a constant CBF over a broad range of perfusion pressures.[885,886,904,905] This constancy of CBF results from arteriolar vasoconstriction with increased perfusion pressure and vasodilation with decreased perfusion pressure.[887,888,904] Autoregulation is operative in brain of the later fetal and neonatal lamb as well as the neonatal puppy and piglet (discussed later). The mechanisms underlying autoregulation are not entirely understood. Currently, the balance of data suggests that autoregulation is mediated primarily by an interplay between endothelial-derived constricting and relaxing factors (see discussion later of perinatal CBF).[906-908] Autoregulation in the adult human is operative over a range of mean blood pressure between approximately 60 and 150 mm Hg,[904] and the response time is approximately 3 to 15 seconds.[905,909]

Coupling of Cerebral Function, Metabolism, and Blood Flow. Tight coupling of cerebral function, metabolism, and blood flow is well established and can be demonstrated by a variety of correlative physiological, biochemical, and even clinical studies.[885,897,904,910,911] This coupling appears to be mediated by regulation of CBF by one or more local chemical factors that are vasoactive. Vasoactive factors

TABLE 6-23	**Local Chemical Factors: Change in Brain Extracellular Fluid and Effect on Cerebral Blood Vessels**[*]			
	CHANGE IN BRAIN EXTRACELLULAR FLUID		**EFFECT ON CEREBRAL VESSELS**	
Local Chemical Factor	**Hypoxia**	**Cortical Activity**[†]	**Increase**	**Decrease**
Hydrogen ion	Increase	Increase	Dilate	Constrict
Potassium ion	Increase	Increase	Dilate	Constrict
Adenosine	Increase	Increase	Dilate	Constrict
Prostaglandins	Increase	Increase	Dilate	Constrict
Osmolarity	?	?	Dilate	Constrict
Calcium ion	Decrease	Decrease	Constrict	Dilate

[*]See text for references.
[†]Includes seizures.

of importance in brain include H^+, K^+, adenosine, prostaglandins, osmolarity, and Ca^{2+} (Table 6-23). (NO is an induced vasoactive factor discussed earlier.) Increase in the perivascular H^+ concentration (i.e., decrease in local pH) is associated with arteriolar vasodilation. Greater neuronal metabolic activity can decrease local pH and therefore increase substrate supply. The effect of perivascular H^+ concentration mediates the vasodilating action of arteriolar carbon dioxide[898-900,904,912] and is important under a variety of other physiological and pathological conditions (see later discussion). This vascular response is well established in perinatal brain (see later section). K^+ has a vasoactive effect.[901,902,904,913-915] Vasodilation increases linearly with extracellular K^+ levels to 10 mmol/kg (levels >20 mmol/kg induce vasoconstriction). The vasodilation is mediated by a Ca^{2+}-activated K^+ channel on vascular smooth muscle. Because K^+ is released from nerve cells with electrical activity or a variety of insults, including oxygen deprivation (see earlier discussion), this ion may play a role in the regulation of CBF under certain pathological conditions. *Adenosine*, administered on the perivascular side of pial arteries, results in a concentration-dependent vasodilation.[904,911,915-917] Changes in adenosine also accompany certain pathological states with changes in CBF, including oxygen deprivation (see later section). Adenosine may be important in regulation of CBF in perinatal animals (see later discussion). *Prostaglandins*, particularly prostaglandins E and F_2, lead to cerebral vasodilation. The concentrations of these compounds increase in response to cerebral ischemia, and agents that inhibit prostaglandin biosynthesis (e.g., indomethacin) have cerebral vasoconstrictive effects. Prostaglandins appear to be of cerebral hemodynamic importance in immature animals (see later discussion). Increases in perivascular *osmolarity* have a vasodilating effect, and decreases have a vasoconstricting effect.[918] These data may bear on such effects on CBF as the vasodilation associated with infusion of hypertonic solutions.[919] Ca^{2+} may also play a role in the control of CBF (e.g., high perivascular concentrations of Ca^{2+} lead to vasoconstriction, and low concentrations lead to dilation of cerebral vessels).[904,920] The ability of Ca^{2+} channel blockers to lead to increases in CBF relates to the prevention of the vasoconstricting effects of Ca^{2+}.[921] Extracellular Ca^{2+} concentrations decline with hypoxia (see earlier discussion) and status epilepticus.[910,922] Other chemical factors (e.g., renin-angiotensin, vasopressin, endogenous opioids, other neuropeptides, adrenergic compounds, acetylcholine, and endothelium-derived relaxing and constricting factors) may play important roles in regulation of CBF, but more data are needed on these issues.[906-908,911,923,924] Limited data are available on these agents in immature animals. One report shows that morphine infusions in neonatal piglets result in an up-regulation of the vasoconstrictor, endothelin-1, and its receptors.[925]

Cerebral Blood Flow in the Perinatal Period

Ontogenetic Effects. Total and regional CBF changes significantly with maturation. In general, CBF overall

increases with postnatal age,[38,881,926–929] and this increase correlates well with similar increases in cerebral metabolic rates and energy demands and with neuroanatomical development (see Chapter 4). Changes in regional CBF with maturation also reflect *coupling with metabolic and anatomical development.* The most dramatic short-term ontogenetic change in CBF occurs around the time of birth. In the lamb, CBF decreases by approximately threefold in the first 24 hours after birth.[930] This decrease correlates well with the postnatal increase in oxygen content (Fig. 6-44), consistent with the importance of oxygen delivery in regulation of CBF.[929,931]

Regional Effects. Impressive regional differences in CBF are apparent in the perinatal animal, and these differences relate in considerable part to regional differences in metabolic activity. Using the microsphere technique to study regional CBF in term fetal sheep, Ashwal and co-workers[932] initially noted (1) higher flows in brain stem than in cerebrum and (2) higher values in cortical gray matter than in subcortical white matter.[932] Using the 4-iodo-[14C]antipyrine technique, Cavazutti and Duffy[33] amplified these findings in a study of blood flow to 32 brain regions in the newborn dog. Blood flows were highest in cerebral gray matter, nuclear structures of brain stem, and diencephalon and were lowest in cerebral white matter. Blood flows to cerebral cortex were approximately five- to 10-fold of those to subcortical white matter. These regional differences were confirmed in studies of the perinatal rabbit, lamb, piglet, and puppy.[928,929,933-939] Parallel studies of regional CBF and cerebral glucose metabolism ([2-14C]deoxyglucose method) demonstrated a close correlation with CBF, thus indicating that *coupling of blood flow and metabolism* is present in the neonatal and adult animal.[32] (The correlation of blood flow and glucose metabolism in the newborn animals was not as strong as it is in adult animals, presumably because a greater proportion of glucose in the newborn animal enters the pentose monophosphate

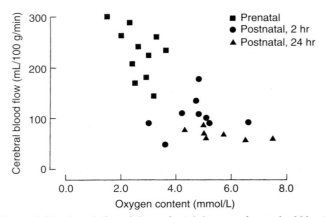

Figure 6-44 Correlation of the perinatal decrease in cerebral blood flow with the increase in arterial oxygen content in the lamb. *(From Richardson BS, Carmichael L, Homan J, Tanswell K, et al: Regional blood flow change in the lamb during the perinatal period, Am J Obstet Gynecol 160:919-925, 1989.)*

shunt for synthetic purposes.[32,33]) Finally, studies of blood flow to various regions of primate cerebrum indicate that the *parasagittal regions*, especially in the posterior aspects of the cerebral hemispheres, have significantly lower flow than other cerebral regions.[940] This finding may have major implications for the distribution of brain injury with perinatal ischemic insults (see the section on parasagittal cerebral injury in Chapter 8).

Regulation. CBF in perinatal brain has been shown clearly to be regulated by the major factors summarized in the previous section on general principles of regulation. The major features are described briefly next.

Autoregulation appears to be operative over a broad range of arterial blood pressure in the preterm and term fetal lamb, the neonatal lamb, and the neonatal dog.[889-894,911,934,936,941-953] The principal stimulus for the autoregulatory change in vascular diameter appears to be induced largely by deformation of endothelial cells and generation of endothelial-derived signals that act on the vascular smooth muscle.[947,949,950,954-956] With a decrease in transmural pressure, NO and Ca^{2+}-activated K^+ channels are important in the vasodilation response, and with an increase in transmural pressure, endothelin-1 is critical in mediation of the vasoconstriction response. The autoregulatory range of blood pressures varies slightly among species and experimental conditions. The curve for the preterm lamb at approximately 80% gestation is shown in Figure 6-45. The curve for the preterm lamb differs from that for the term or neonatal lamb in two respects.[893] First, the *autoregulatory range in the preterm lamb is narrower*, especially at the upper limit of the curve. Second, and perhaps more strikingly, the *normal arterial blood pressure in the preterm lamb is very*

near or at the lower autoregulatory limit. Indeed, in the preterm lamb at 80% of gestation, normal arterial blood pressure is only 5 to 10 mm Hg above the lower limit of the curve, in contrast to the situation in older animals. Thus, in term neonatal animals, the normal blood pressure is 30 to 40 mm Hg above the lower autoregulatory limit, and in term fetal animals, the margin of normal arterial blood pressure above the lower limit is intermediate, approximately 15 to 25 mm Hg. In a subsequent study that included preterm fetal lambs at approximately 65% gestation (i.e., the onset of the third trimester), the lower autoregulatory limit was *essentially identical* to the normal resting arterial blood pressure.[936] More recent data indicate that the range of blood pressure over which autoregulation is operative decreases with lower gestational age.[952,953] *These data indicate that with decreasing gestational age, resting mean arterial blood pressure values approach the lower limit of the autoregulatory plateau, and the range of blood pressure over which CBF remains constant narrows.* Stated in another way, the observations suggest that the margin of safety, at least in the preterm fetus, and to a lesser extent in the term fetus, is small at the lower end of the autoregulatory curve and point to *vulnerability to ischemic brain injury with modest hypotension*, particularly in the preterm animal. *Vulnerability to hypertension* also may result because little change occurs in the upper limit of the autoregulatory range during a brief developmental period (third trimester in the lamb and the human) when normal arterial blood pressure increases markedly.[943] Thus, normal arterial blood pressure shifts precariously close to the upper autoregulatory limit and renders capillary beds (e.g., germinal matrix) vulnerable to hemorrhage with modest hypertension.

Autoregulation in the term fetal lamb and in the newborn lamb has been shown to be *sensitive to hypoxia*.[892,894,948,951] Changes in PaO_2 from 20 to 16 mm Hg in the fetal animal and from approximately 70 to 30 mm Hg in the newborn animal abolished autoregulation.[892,894] These decreases in PaO_2 resulted in decreases in arterial oxygen saturation of less than 50%, which can be considered a hypoxic threshold for impairment of cerebrovascular autoregulation. The impairment of autoregulation required only a 20-minute exposure to hypoxia, and autoregulation *did not recover until 7 hours after restoration of normoxia*.[894] Studies in adult animals showed that autoregulation is *abolished in the presence of hypercarbia*,[904,957] and a similar phenomenon was observed in the perinatal animal[958] and in the human preterm newborn.[959] In a single study of the newborn lamb, *systemic acidosis* also was shown to cause a *loss in cerebrovascular autoregulation*.[960]

Regional variation in the decrease in CBF provoked by hypotension to blood pressure values below the lower limit of the autoregulatory plateau has been described in the neonatal piglet, puppy, and lamb.[936,942,943,961-963] In the neonatal piglet, the percentage of reduction in blood flow was least to the brain stem and greatest to the cerebrum.[961,962] In a more detailed regional study in the newborn puppy, *flow to cerebral white matter was most vulnerable to hypotension*.[942] Similarly, in the preterm lamb, the lower autoregulatory limit with

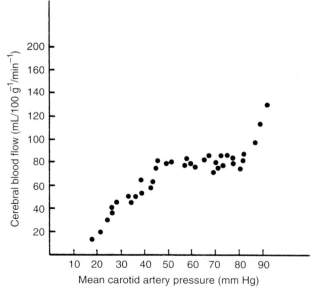

Figure 6-45 **Autoregulation of cerebral blood flow in the preterm lamb**. See text for details. *(From Papile LA, Rudolph AM, Heymann MA: Autoregulation of cerebral blood flow in the preterm fetal lamb,* Pediatr Res *19:159-161, 1985.)*

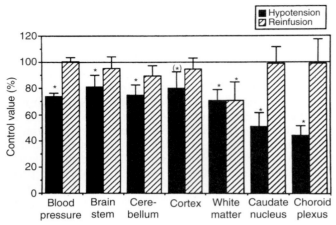

Figure 6-46 Mean arterial blood pressure and regional cerebral blood flow (CBF; percentage of control values, mean ± SE) after hemorrhagic hypotension and reinfusion in the preterm lamb. The approximately 25% reduction in blood pressure resulted in significant lowering of CBF in all regions. However, only in cerebral white matter CBF failed to return to baseline levels on reinfusion. *(From Szymonowicz W, Walker AM, Yu VY, Stewart ML, et al: Regional cerebral blood flow after hemorrhagic hypotension in the preterm, near-term, and newborn lamb, Pediatr Res 28:361-366, 1990.)*

hypotension was lower in brain stem than in cerebrum.[936,943] Perhaps even more importantly, in the preterm lamb at the start of the third trimester, blood flow to cerebral white matter not only was particularly vulnerable to hypotension but also did not recover under conditions of reinfusion that restored blood flow to all other brain regions (Figs. 6-46 and 6-47).[936] The latter observations may have implications for the topography of the brain injury with hypoxic-ischemic insults (see following discussion and Chapter 8).

Changes in *arterial* P_{CO_2} (i.e., Pa_{CO_2}) have marked effects on CBF in perinatal as in adult animals.[4,33,152,933,958,964-981] In a study of blood flow to 32 brain regions of the newborn dog, a positive linear correlation was obtained in each structure examined.[33] However, the response to carbon dioxide varied widely among brain regions, ranging from an increase of only 0.15 mL/100 g/minute/mm Hg in P_{CO_2} in subcortical white matter to an increase of 4.8 in the vestibular and superior olivary nuclei. The *limited vasodilatory response in cerebral white matter* may have implications for the vulnerability of this region to hypoxic-ischemic injury (see later section and Chapter 8). In general, the higher the blood flow to a particular structure, the greater the vasodilatory response to increasing P_{CO_2} (Fig. 6-48). A similar conclusion can be derived from a less detailed study of regional CBF in the newborn piglet.[969]

The effects of profound hypocarbia on CBF are of particular importance because hyperventilation is one means of induction of *pulmonary* vasodilation in infants with persistent pulmonary hypertension. Studies in neonatal lambs indicated an abrupt decrease in CBF with hypocarbia induced by hyperventilation.[933,978,982] The decrease was nonlinear, such that the vasoconstricting effect of hypocarbia declined at lower Pa_{CO_2} tensions. Moreover, the decline in CBF became less prominent with time, such that CBF was no longer statistically different in hypocarbic animals ($Pa_{CO_2} = 15$ mm Hg) compared with control animals ($Pa_{CO_2} = 36$ mm Hg) after 6 hours (Table 6-24). Perhaps most importantly, the declines in CBF did *not* cause any change in cerebral metabolic rate for oxygen because cerebral oxygen extraction fraction increased. The attenuation of the decline in CBF with increasing duration of hypocarbia

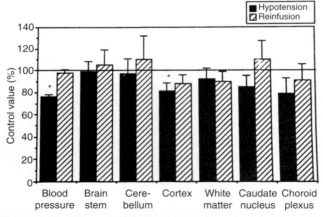

Figure 6-47 Mean arterial blood pressure and regional cerebral blood flow (CBF; percentage of control values, mean ± SE) after hemorrhagic hypotension and reinfusion in the near-term lamb. In contrast to the effect on CBF of a similar decrease in blood pressure in the preterm lamb (see Fig. 6-46), during hypotension a significant decline occurred only in cerebral cortex, and on reinfusion all values returned to baseline levels. *(From Szymonowicz W, Walker AM, Yu VY, Stewart ML, et al: Regional cerebral blood flow after hemorrhagic hypotension in the preterm, near-term, and newborn lamb, Pediatr Res 28:361-366, 1990.)*

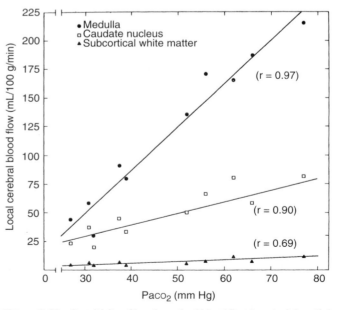

Figure 6-48 Sensitivity of local cerebral blood flow to arterial partial pressure of carbon dioxide (Pa_{CO_2}). Note that regions with the higher normocapnic blood flow exhibit the highest sensitivities to Pa_{CO_2}. *(From Cavazutti M, Duffy TE: Regulation of local cerebral blood flow in normal and hypoxic newborn dogs, Ann Neurol 11:247-257, 1982.)*

TABLE 6-24	Effect of Hyperventilation and Abrupt Termination Thereof on Cerebral Blood Flow in Newborn Lamb[*]	
Condition	**Cerebral Blood Flow[*][†] (Percentage of Change)**	
Hyperventilation		
30 min	−36%	
6 hr	−12%[‡]	
After Hyperventilation		
30 min	+210%	
6 hr	+226%	

[*]No effect on cerebral metabolic rate for oxygen was observed at any time.

[†]Blood flow to cerebral hemispheres and midbrain.

[‡]Not significantly different from zero; all other numbers different from control at $P < .05$ level.

Data from Gleason CA, Short BL, Jones MD Jr: Cerebral blood flow and metabolism during and after prolonged hypocapnia in newborn lambs, *J Pediatr* 115:309-314, 1989.

probably relates to an increase in perivascular H^+ concentration, primarily secondary to an increase in lactate levels. This formulation is supported by *the marked increase in CBF above baseline levels* on restoration of normocarbia.[933] This marked cerebral hyperemia could be of pathogenetic importance for development of hemorrhage in the clinical circumstance in which the infant with severe pulmonary hypertension first is hyperventilated and then is restored to normocarbia by extracorporeal membrane oxygenation (see Chapter 10).

The effects of *modest hypocarbia* (e.g., $Pa_{CO_2} = 26$ mm Hg) interact adversely with hypoxic-ischemic insults in the 7-day-old animal.[88,958,980,981] Thus, animals exposed to hypoxia-ischemia sustained a greater decline in CBF and a greater degree of brain injury when they were simultaneously rendered modestly hypocarbic and compared with CBF and brain injury in animals who were normocarbic ($Pa_{CO_2} = 39$ mm Hg) or rendered mildly hypercarbic ($Pa_{CO_2} = 54$ mm Hg). The latter two groups had better preserved CBF, less severe cerebral metabolic deficits, and less severe brain injury. The modestly hypercarbic animals had the most favorable hemodynamic, biochemical, and neuropathological outcomes. However, more marked hypercarbia accentuated brain injury, because of marked decrease in CBF.[958] The latter effect is presumably related to impaired autoregulation and cardiovascular depression.

Alterations in *arterial* P_{O_2} (Pa_{O_2}) also cause distinct changes in CBF.[32,33,152,743,931,951,967,983-989] Decreases in oxygen tension result in increases in flow and vice versa. Jones and co-workers[931,984,985] demonstrated that cerebral oxygen delivery is maintained by this increase in CBF over a wide range of arterial oxygen content. In a study of 32 brain regions of the newborn dog, as with Pa_{CO_2}, the magnitude of the vasodilatory response to hypoxia varied.[33] Hypoxia caused the largest percentage increases in regional blood flow in brain stem structures, moderate increases in cortical and diencephalic structures, and smallest increases in cerebral white matter. These observations again suggest that

cerebral white matter has limited vasodilatory capacity, and they have implications for the vulnerability of this region to hypoxic-ischemic injury (see later discussion and Chapter 8). The *mechanisms* of the increase in CBF with hypoxia are likely to be related to local metabolic factors and to vascular factors per se.[911,986] Thus, with hypoxia, rapid local increases in vasodilatory metabolic factors (e.g., perivascular H^+, K^+, adenosine, and prostaglandins) and decreases in vasoconstricting factors (e.g., Ca^{2+}) occur. Additionally, strikingly rapid decreases in isometric tension generated by the major cerebral arteries isolated from near-term fetal lambs and studied in vitro as isolated segments have been shown with P_{O_2} lowered to 15 mm Hg.[986] The relaxation was much faster than that observed in adult cerebral arterial segments. Whether this effect is related to local release of NO or another factor remains to be determined. However, the findings indicate that the myogenic properties of the major cerebral vessels themselves must be considered in the evaluation of mechanisms of changes in cerebral hemodynamics. Importance for the large cerebral vessels in regulation of CBF in the preterm human is suggested further by the presence in their vascular wall of a muscularis, in distinct contrast to the absence of a muscularis in the smaller penetrating cerebral arteries and arterioles.[990]

The role of *acidemia* in the regulation of CBF in the perinatal animal requires further study. Whether produced by hypoxemia, lactate infusion, or respiratory means, acidemia caused a sharp increase in CBF in perinatal goats.[991] However, effects were most impressive when acidemia was induced by elevation in Pa_{CO_2}, a potent effector of CBF (as described earlier). Moreover, a subsequent study of the fetal lamb did not report an alteration in regional CBF over an arterial pH range from 6.9 to 7.5 produced by infusions of lactate or bicarbonate.[967] Studies of newborn dogs and piglets showed inconsistent effects of lactate infusions or other changes in arterial pH on CBF.[992-994]

A role for *adenosine* in regulation of CBF in the immature brain is suggested by observations primarily in the neonatal piglet.[995,996] Studies correlated CBF with parallel measurements of interstitial concentrations of adenosine and have used specific agonists and antagonists of the A_2 receptor (the adenosine receptor on vascular smooth muscle; the A_1 receptor, the adenosine receptor on neurons, is involved in decreasing glutamate release and Ca^{2+} influx). The data suggest that adenosine has a vasodilatory effect and that it is involved in the cerebrovascular response to decreases in blood pressure and thereby cerebrovascular autoregulation. Recall that brain adenosine concentrations increase with hypoxia and seizures; both conditions require increases in substrate influx to brain. Finally, in addition to its vasodilatory effect, adenosine may influence CBF by inhibitions of platelet aggregation and activation of neutrophils (implicated in endothelial dysfunction), events shown to be important in the postischemic impairment of CBF in adult models.[996,997]

Prostaglandins are important regulators of CBF in the perinatal period.[269,911,937,938,949,950,998-1013] Prostanoids may exhibit vasodilator or vasoconstrictor properties, depending on the specific prostanoid, and they appear to be important in the setting of both the upper and lower limits of autoregulation. However, *in neonatal animals*, prostanoids exert effects that are different from those observed in the adult. In general, these compounds function as cerebral vasodilators and are important in regulation of CBF with decreases in blood pressure within and below the autoregulatory range, with changes in blood PCO_2 and perivascular H^+ concentrations and following ischemia, asphyxia, and seizures (conditions characterized by increases in cerebral prostaglandin biosynthesis). Prostaglandins also attenuate the vasoconstrictor responses of norepinephrine and are the apparent mediators of the vasodilatory responses of endogenous opiates. As a consequence of these important roles, indomethacin, through its inhibition of cyclooxygenase and thereby prostanoid biosynthesis, may have a variety of important cerebral hemodynamic effects that are vasoconstrictive. Such vasoconstrictor effects may be potentially beneficial (e.g., concerning prevention of intraventricular hemorrhage; see Chapter 11), or potentially deleterious (e.g., under conditions requiring maintenance or increase in CBF, as with hypotension, asphyxia, or seizures).

Cerebral Blood Flow during and after Perinatal Asphyxia or Other Hypoxic-Ischemic Insults

Important cerebral circulatory effects of perinatal asphyxia and related hypoxic-ischemic insults have been defined by studies of a variety of experimental models, some based on techniques that result in impaired gas exchange between mother and fetus or postnatally and others based on controlled manipulation of only specific blood gases or of blood pressure.* *During asphyxia*, three of these circulatory effects occur initially, and two occur with more prolonged episodes. The effects include, initially, (1) an alteration in the fetal circulation such that a larger proportion of the cardiac output is distributed to the brain, (2) an increase in total and regional CBF, and (3) a loss of vascular autoregulation, and, later, (4) a diminution in cardiac output with the occurrence of systemic hypotension, and, largely as a consequence, (5) a decrease in CBF (Table 6-25). *Following asphyxia*, critical additional circulatory effects develop, and, indeed, from the clinical standpoint, these postinsult effects are as important, if not more so, than those occurring during asphyxia (Table 6-26). These phenomena during and following the insult are discussed next.

Redistribution of Fetal Circulation. Promptly after the onset of asphyxia in the term fetal primate or lamb, cardiac output is redistributed such that a

---

*See references 32,33,74,152,154,238,289,290,342,345,669,891,897, 931,932,938,939,942,951,952,962,963,967,979,998,1014-1032.

TABLE 6-25	Major Circulatory Effects *During* Perinatal Asphyxia
Initially	
Redistribution of cardiac output so larger proportion enters brain	
Increase in cerebral blood flow	
Loss of cerebral vascular autoregulation	
Later	
Diminution of cardiac output; hypotension	
Decrease in cerebral blood flow	

significantly larger proportion enters the brain, the coronary circulation, and the adrenals, at the expense of blood flow to other regions.[154,884,932,1017,1033,1034] Approximately twofold increases in the proportion of cardiac output to brain were noted in studies of term fetal primates. This redistribution of blood flow is reminiscent of the diving reflex observed in aquatic animals and appears designed to protect the most critical and vulnerable organs. The response requires an intact sympathoadrenal system.[878] The important afferent components of the response include particularly the oxygen chemoreceptors.[884,1034] Moreover, to be effective, circulation must be maintained, hence the hypertension noted shortly after the onset of fetal asphyxia is particularly important.[878,1015,1016]

Increase in Cerebral Blood Flow. The major purpose of the circulatory changes as outlined is to maintain CBF in the presence of impending tissue oxygen debt. In experiments with fetal and neonatal lambs, puppies, and primates, CBF in perinatal asphyxia increased generally by 50% to 500%.* In severe and prolonged asphyxia, CBF eventually falls as a consequence of decreasing cardiac output (secondary to myocardial failure and hypoxic-induced bradycardia) and the loss of vascular autoregulation (see next section).

The *mechanisms* underlying the initial increase in CBF relate in part to cerebral vasodilation, secondary to hypoxemia or hypercapnia, or both, presumably with increased perivascular H^+ concentration.[1035,1036] Roles for elevated extracellular fluid concentrations of K^+,

---

*See references 32,33,152,154,289,932,967,1014,1016,1017, 1019-1022.

TABLE 6-26	Major Circulatory Effects *Following* Perinatal Asphyxia
Increase in cerebral blood flow beginning within minutes after the insult and lasting for up to several hours	
Decline in cerebral blood flow toward baseline or lower, with hypotension, following initial hyperemia	
"Delayed" increase in cerebral blood flow ("delayed" hyperemia) beginning between 12 and 24 hours and lasting many hours and attenuated by nitric oxide synthase inhibitors	
Delayed cerebral hyperemia correlating with impaired mitochondrial oxygenation, "secondary" energy failure, and neuropathological injury	

adenosine, and prostaglandins, all of which increase markedly in brain with hypoxemia and ischemia, are likely.[269,911,995,996,1037-1041] The particular importance of a rise or at least maintenance of blood pressure in the increase of CBF with asphyxia was indicated by several studies.[1015-1017] In term fetal sheep subjected to asphyxia by cord compression, the initial increase in mean arterial blood pressure persisted for 60 minutes before decreasing to normal values.[1015] Carefully controlled experiments with the same animal suggested that fetal blood pressure may be even more critical than local chemical factors, which lead to cerebral vasodilation, in the enhancement of CBF.[1016]

Although blood flow to various regions of brain increases generally in concert with the increase in total CBF, *distinct regional differences* in this increase are apparent. In general, the increase in blood flow is most marked in brain stem structures and is least apparent in cerebral white matter. This general pattern was documented in the fetal lamb, neonatal lamb, and neonatal puppy.[32,33,126,891,938,967,1016,1019-1021,1042] This effect has been interpreted as an attempt to maintain integrity of vital brain stem centers. The mechanism for the heterogeneity in regulation of CBF is unknown; an endogenous opioid-mediated mechanism appears likely.[1020,1043] Thus, administration of naloxone results in an increase in telencephalic blood flow and oxygen metabolism, and, consequently, a decrease in the fraction of CBF to the brain stem. This decrease in fraction of flow to brain stem may negate the attempt to preserve vital brain stem centers. A likely conclusion from this work is that with hypoxia or asphyxia, the role of endogenous opiates is to suppress *cerebral* rate of oxygen consumption, with the associated decrease in telencephalic blood flow serving to preserve brain stem by an increase in fraction of total brain blood flow to brain stem. The burst in release of endogenous opiates with hypoxia and asphyxia and the well-known suppression of cerebral neural activity and oxygen consumption by endogenous opiates support this notion.[1044-1046] In this context, administration of naloxone during asphyxia may be deleterious to brain stem.

Loss of Vascular Autoregulation. A serious impairment of cerebral vascular autoregulation develops with perinatal asphyxia. Using the radioactive microsphere technique and producing asphyxia (pH 6.8 to 7.0) in term fetal sheep by partial occlusion of umbilical vessels, Lou and co-workers[1015] demonstrated a striking pressure-passive CBF. Marked hyperemia, with CBF values up to six times normal, occurred when mean arterial blood pressure was raised to 60 to 70 mm Hg, whereas CBF declined to close to zero in large cortical areas when mean arterial blood pressure was lowered to 30 mm Hg. Vascular autoregulation in these term fetal animals appeared to be very sensitive to asphyxia. The likely mechanism relates most probably to the hypoxemia and hypercapnia that are the hallmarks of perinatal asphyxia. The sensitivity of the autoregulatory system in fetal and neonatal brain to these alterations in blood gas levels was described earlier (see section on

autoregulation). The implications of these data for ischemic injury to perinatal brain are obvious. In one study of near-term fetal sheep, autoregulation of CBF was lost within 4 minutes of cord occlusion, and overt cerebral injury occurred by 10 minutes secondary to decreased CBF in the presence of hypotension.[951]

Hypotension and Diminished Cerebral Blood Flow. Although the initial response to asphyxia is hypertension, this response is followed by hypotension.[878,951] The rapidity and severity of this occurrence depend on the duration and severity of the asphyxial insult. In large part, this effect is related to a diminution in cardiac output,[38,154] probably secondary to an effect on the myocardium. The consequence for the brain may be devastating, because the impairment of vascular autoregulation leaves CBF at the mercy of perfusion pressure. Deficits in CBF may be marked, with relatively modest changes in mean arterial blood pressure. Impressive deficits in CBF (20% to 80%) have been demonstrated, particularly in the parasagittal regions of the cerebral hemispheres and especially posteriorly, in the term fetal monkey subjected to severe and prolonged asphyxia.[940] A similar parasagittal distribution of cerebral cortical injury was demonstrated in near-term fetal sheep subjected to cerebral ischemia.[342,1047] Detailed regional study of newborn dogs demonstrated that cerebral white matter also is particularly likely to exhibit diminished blood flow with hypotension.[942] In the preterm sheep (0.65 gestation) cerebral white matter was particularly affected with ischemia, with white matter injury then determined by the topographic distribution within the ischemic regions of vulnerable differentiating oligodendrocytes.[669] These observations correlate well with the neuropathological and clinical observations made of asphyxiated human infants (see Chapters 8 and 9).

A summary of the major relationships between perinatal asphyxia and CBF *during asphyxia* is shown graphically in Figure 6-49. The initial effects leading to increased CBF are considered best as compensatory, adaptive responses (which could become maladaptive by leading to hemorrhage in vulnerable capillary beds). The later effects represent a decompensation of these responses and a cascade that leads to diminished CBF and brain injury.

Postasphyxial-Postischemic Effects. The period *following termination of the asphyxial-ischemic insult* is critical because, during this interval, progression to brain injury occurs (see earlier discussion) and, in the clinical setting, this time represents a window of opportunity for therapeutic intervention. The principal experimental models used have been near-term fetal sheep and neonatal piglets and rat pups, and the insults have primarily consisted of hypoxia-ischemia and, less commonly, asphyxia.* The major circulatory effects

---

*See references 42,43,74,126,238,289,290,342,345,938,939,978,998, 999,1014,1022-1025,1029,1030,1047.

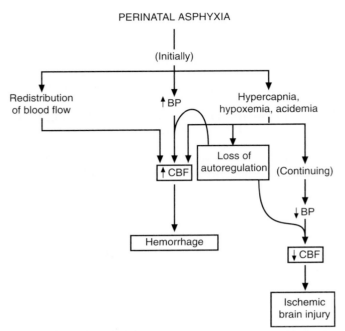

Figure 6-49 **Major relationships between perinatal asphyxia and cerebral blood flow (CBF).** The major consequences of the changes in cerebral blood flow (i.e., hemorrhage and ischemic brain injury) are shown. BP, blood pressure.

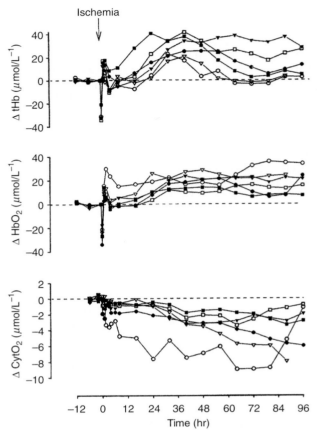

Figure 6-50 **Cerebral hemodynamic changes after transient cerebral ischemia in the late-gestation fetal lamb.** Changes in total cerebral hemoglobin (tHb), oxygenated hemoglobin (HbO2), and cytochrome oxidase (CytO2) were measured by near-infrared spectroscopy. In each graph, different symbols represent data from separate fetuses. Note the two phases of cerebral vasodilation and increased cerebral blood flow, as assessed by the hemoglobin signals; the early increase occurs in the first 2 to 3 hours after ischemia, and the delayed increase occurs from 12 to 48 hours. The delayed increase in flow is accompanied by a decline in CytO2, consistent with impaired mitochondrial oxygenation. *(From Marks KA, Mallard EC, Roberts I, Williams CE, et al: Delayed vasodilation and altered oxygenation after cerebral ischemia in fetal sheep, Pediatr Res 39:48-54, 1996.)*

identified are summarized in Table 6-26. A consistent observation has been a marked increase in CBF on reperfusion, hyperemia that continues for up to several hours (Fig. 6-50). This *early increase in CBF* is presumably related to the same mechanism operative for the initial increase in CBF during asphyxia noted earlier (i.e., the accumulation of such vasodilating factors as H^+, K^+, adenosine, and prostaglandins). Moreover, superoxide anion, a consequence of reperfusion after asphyxia (see earlier), may lead to a disturbance of cerebrovascular autoregulation through stimulation of vasodilation.[1048] This early increase in cerebral perfusion is followed by a decline toward baseline. In some models, especially if associated with hypotension, CBF declines below normal with the threat of cerebral ischemia. This postasphyxial cerebral hypoperfusion has not been a consistent feature in all experimental models. It is likely that hypotension could lead to cerebral ischemia in this period, *because autoregulation is not operative* (Fig. 6-51).

Importantly, a second (i.e., "delayed") increase in CBF develops, with onset generally between 12 to 24 hours and with a duration of many hours or a day or more (see Fig. 6-50). This increase is associated with evidence of impaired mitochondrial oxygenation (as assessed by brain levels of oxidized cytochrome c), with the energy failure described earlier, and with neuropathological evidence for neuronal and white matter injury. The delayed hyperemia, its association with energy failure, and its correlation with severity of brain injury have also been observed in asphyxiated human infants (see later discussion and Chapter 9). The mechanisms underlying the vasodilation and hyperemia are not established but may relate in part

to NO. Because NO synthesis in endothelial cells (eNOS) is activated after hypoxic-ischemic insults, an attempt to reduce the delayed cerebral hyperemia with an NOS inhibitor was attempted in the fetal sheep model of ischemia.[342,345] The inhibitor did attenuate the delayed hyperemia, but, surprisingly, inhibition of NO synthesis *increased* histological injury.[342] This combination of findings suggests that NO synthesis has a protective effect either because of the vasodilatory effect or because of a biochemical effect. Concerning the latter, as noted in the earlier discussion of NO, when NO exists as NO^+, the nitrosonium ion, a protective effect on neurons occurs because of S-nitrosylation of the NMDA receptor and resulting decline in Ca^{2+} influx. NO also may act as a scavenger of superoxide anion, although injurious $ONOO^-$ results from the combination of superoxide anion and NO. Finally, under conditions of free radical attack, NO donors

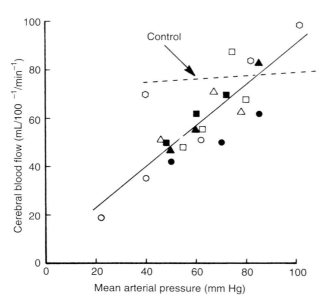

Figure 6-51 Postasphyxial impairment of cerebrovascular autoregulation. Cerebral blood flow versus mean arterial blood pressure following asphyxia. Symbols (n = 7) represent responses to changes in blood pressure in individual asphyxiated lambs (n = 7). The *regression line* is derived from pooled data of all lambs. The *dashed line* represents data from nonasphyxiated (control) lambs. *(From Rosenberg AA: Regulation of cerebral blood flow after asphyxia in neonatal lambs, Stroke 19:239-244, 1988.)*

are initially protective for differentiating oligodendroglia.[793] Further data concerning the molecular basis of the delayed hyperemia will be of great interest.

Cerebral Blood Flow in the Human Newborn

Methodology

In approximately the past 25 to 30 years, considerable insight into CBF in the human newborn has been provided by application of one or more of several techniques (Table 6-27). The largest amount of information has been provided by the *xenon-133 clearance*

TABLE 6-27	Methods for Determination of Cerebral Blood Flow in the Newborn

Xenon-133 clearance techniques (intravenous, intra-arterial, or inhalation administration)
Xenon computed tomography
Positron emission tomography (intravenous administration of $H_2^{15}O$)
Single photon emission computed tomography
Near-infrared spectroscopy (continuous measurement of hemoglobin D [oxyhemoglobin − deoxyhemoglobin] or intermittent inhalation of oxygen)
Doppler ultrasonic techniques
Venous occlusion plethysmography
Electrical impedance techniques
Magnetic resonance techniques* (utilization of motion-sensitizing gradient pulses or paramagnetic contrast agent, e.g., gadolinium)

*Not yet applied to the newborn.

technique.[1049–1075] The technique uses administration of xenon-133, either by intraarterial or intravenous injection or by inhalation (preferably intravenous injection), and detection of the brain clearance of xenon-133, specifically the gamma radiation thereof, by external detectors. The particular advantage of the xenon-133 clearance technique is the ability to provide quantitative data with relatively low radiation exposure and portable equipment. *Xenon computed tomography* has the advantage of providing regional data, but the technique requires transport to a specialized suite.

PET has been valuable in demonstration in the premature and term newborn of normal values of regional CBF, coupling to oxygen consumption, increases of flow with seizure, and characteristic changes in premature infants with periventricular hemorrhagic infarction and intraventricular hemorrhage, as well as in term asphyxiated infants with parasagittal cerebral injury (see Chapters 4, 5, 9, and 11). The particular advantage of PET is the ability to provide not only quantitative data but also regional information. *Single photon emission tomography* also provides regional data but is nonquantitative. *Near-infrared spectroscopy*, a noninvasive optical technique, has the capability to provide serial quantitative measurements of CBF and is discussed in detail in Chapter 4. With *venous occlusion plethysmography*, changes in intracranial volume after brief occlusion of the jugular veins are determined by a strain-gauge instrument placed around the compliant infant skull.[1076–1080] This technique cannot provide quantitative information and has the disadvantage of causing a transient rise in intracranial pressure. Application of this method is discussed briefly later. The *Doppler ultrasonic technique* for measurement of CBF velocity, a noninvasive method, can provide serial information about cerebrovascular resistance and flow velocity in the insonated cerebral vessels. Determination of changes in volemic flow from the velocity data is complicated by the inability to determine cross-sectional diameter of the insonated vessel; this method is discussed in Chapter 4. *Electrical impedance techniques* are noninvasive but have not proven sufficiently sensitive to be consistently useful.[1081-1083] *MR* techniques for determination of CBF, either after administration of a paramagnetic contrast agent (e.g., gadolinium) or by use of gradients, are under intensive study but have not yet been applied to the newborn.

In the following section, I review information concerning, first, normal values and development of CBF in the human newborn, second, regulation of flow, and, finally, alterations in flow following perinatal asphyxia.

Development and Normal Values of Cerebral Blood Flow in the Human Newborn

Changes Immediately after Delivery. A sharp decrease in "apparent" CBF ("apparent" because the plethysmographic method is only semiquantitative) occurs in the term infant in the first hours after delivery (Fig. 6-52).[1076] The decrease in the first 3 hours is nearly twofold, and, over the ensuing hours, CBF is relatively stable. The reason for the relatively higher

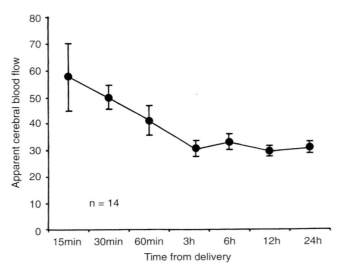

Figure 6-52 **Apparent cerebral blood flow in term infants following delivery, as estimated by the jugular venous occlusion plethysmographic technique**. Note the decline in the first several hours, followed by stable flow. *(From Cooke RW, Rolfe P, Howat P: Apparent cerebral blood-flow in newborns with respiratory disease,* Dev Med Child Neurol *21:154, 1979.)*

value shortly after delivery is not known, although a relationship with higher $Paco_2$ levels immediately after birth has been suggested.[1076] Alternatively, it is possible that a reflex activity, mediated by vagal afferents, is operative because the relatively higher CBF near the time of birth requires intact vagus nerves in the sheep.[152] Both factors may be relevant in the human newborn, when $Paco_2$ levels may be elevated and vagal activity from lung expansion may be considerable.[1076] A third factor may involve arterial oxygen content, because, as noted earlier, a similar sharp decline in CBF after birth has been observed in the lamb and correlates well with the increase in arterial oxygen content in the newborn versus fetal state. The relatively enhanced CBF in the first minutes to hours after delivery may provide a margin of safety for cerebral metabolic needs in the period of adaptation to birth.

Changes Beyond the Immediate Postpartum Period. Detailed ontogenetic data are limited concerning CBF in the human newborn. Data obtained by PET suggest that CBF is approximately 20% of the adult value in the premature infant of approximately 28 weeks of gestation and approximately 40% of the adult value in the term newborn.[1084] These data and their relation to changes in cerebral oxygen consumption are discussed in Chapter 4. Serial studies of CBF in normal preterm infants show an approximately twofold increase in flow over the first 3 days of life, perhaps related to an increase in cardiac output.[1085] One study of preterm infants by spatially resolved near-infrared spectroscopy showed a sharp increase in cerebral oxygenation during this period, most consistent with an increase in CBF.[1086] Doppler studies of CBF velocity also are consistent with this postnatal increase in CBF (see Chapter 4).[1087]

Normal Values. Values for CBF reported in the human premature newborn, studied by xenon clearance and shown in Table 6-28, are generally between 10 and 20 mL/100 g/minute. A similar range is apparent in studies by PET and near-infrared spectroscopy (see Chapter 4). The relationship of these relatively low values of CBF and of oxygen consumption with the state of immaturity of neuronal and oligodendroglial development is described in Chapter 4. The analogies with findings in developing animals, described earlier, are obvious. Regional values for CBF are notable for higher flows in cerebral gray matter structures than in cerebral white matter (see Chapter 4).

Regulation in the Human Newborn. The major established regulatory mechanisms for CBF in the human newborn include autoregulation, $Paco_2$, oxygen delivery, blood glucose, and neuronal activity (e.g., seizure). Certain pharmacological agents also have been shown to exert regulatory effects. These various regulatory factors and their effects on CBF are summarized in Table 6-29 and are reviewed briefly next.

Autoregulation. Autoregulation appears to be operative in both the normal human preterm and full-term infants.[1061,1063,1069,1070,1072-1074,1088-1097] *Although the actual limits of the autoregulatory plateau cannot be established with certainty*, the *approximate* autoregulatory range appears to be from 25 to 50 mm Hg mean arterial blood pressure. Both the size of this range and its actual upper and lower limits vary according to gestational age (Fig. 6-53) and, likely, postnatal age and multiple other factors. Autoregulation in mature animals and adult humans is rendered inoperative by factors that lead to pronounced vasodilation (e.g., hypercarbia, hypoxia, hypoglycemia, seizure, postasphyxial state, and selected cytokines), and available data suggest that these factors also impair autoregulation in the human infant, particularly the seriously asphyxiated full-term infant and in the sick, mechanically ventilated preterm infant (see Chapters 8 and 9 and Table 6-29).[1063,1067,1072,1074,1075,1090-1092,1094,1095,1098]

The problem of a persistent pressure-passive cerebral circulation is particularly important in sick premature infants. Thus, initial studies employing the invasive technique of radioactive xenon clearance initially showed that certain premature infants, mechanically ventilated and usually clinically unstable, appeared to exhibit pressure-passive cerebral circulation.[1015,1063] This fundamental initial observation has been confirmed by less invasive methods multiple times.[1090-1092,1095,1097] Thus, in such sick premature infants with pressure-passive cerebral circulation, it would be expected that when blood pressure falls, as occurs commonly in such infants, so would CBF, with the consequence of cerebral ischemia. The presence of arterial end zones and border zones and vulnerable early differentiating oligodendroglia in developing cerebral white matter would render this region especially vulnerable (see Chapter 8). Moreover, the particular danger is compounded by the very low normal blood flow to cerebral white matter in the premature infant,

TABLE 6-28 Cerebral Blood Flow in the Newborn as Determined by the Intravenous Xenon-133 Clearance Technique*

Birth Weight/ Gestational Age (Mean or Range)	No. of Infants	Age at Study (Mean or Range)	Conditions	Mean Cerebral Blood Flow (mL/100 g/min)	Reference (First Author/Year)
33.4 wk	16	5 days	Stable	29.7	Greisen, 1984[1056]
29–34 wk	15	15–17 days	Quiet sleep	17.4	Greisen, 1985[1113]
			Active sleep	17.0	
			Wakeful	21.8	
			Unclassified	16.8	
1510 g/31 wk	42	0–5 days	Nonventilatory support	19.8	Greisen, 1986[1057]
			Continuous positive airway pressure	21.3	
			Mechanical ventilation (IMV <20)	12.4	
			Mechanical ventilation (IMV >20)	11.0	
			Entire group	15.5	
1340 g/31 wk	15	3.7 wk	Stable	F_1–87.5[†] F_2–17.2	Younkin, 1987[1061]
<33 wk	25	1.6 days	Mechanical ventilation	12.3	Greisen, 1987[1058]
1420 g/30.9 wk	14	3 hr	Glucose ≥ 1.7 mmol/L	11.8	Pryds, 1988[1060]
1210 g/30.5 wk	10	3 hr	Glucose ≤ 1.7 mmol/L	26.0	
1569 g/31.7 wk	21	31 days	Stable	35.4–41.3[†]	Younkin, 1988[1061]
1050 g/29.2 wk	18	12.6 hr	Stable	13.1	Lipp-Zwahlen, 1989[1106]
1540 g/30.4 wk	18	6.4 hr	Mechanical ventilation	8.4	Pryds, 1989[1063]
1380 g/30.4 wk	8	16.9 hr	Mechanical ventilation	10.2	
1470 g/30.3 wk	12	34.3 hr	Mechanical ventilation	11.5	
27-33 wk	20	48 hr	Mechanical ventilation	10.0	Greisen, 1987[1058]
1310 g/29.5 wk	12	2 hr	Glucose ≥30 mg/dL	12.0	Pryds, 1990[1065]
1500 g/31.2 wk	13	2 hr	Glucose ≤30 mg/dL	18.6	
1175 g/29 wk	20	<12 hr	Mechanical ventilation	8.7 (total group) 9.2 (9 infants with normal outcome)	Pryds, 1990[1065]
1300 g/28.0 wk	16	4 days	Before aminophylline	13.2	Pryds, 1991[1071]
			After (1 hr) aminophylline	10.9	
1060 g/28 wk	10	<36 hr	Mechanical ventilation	10.4	Muller, 1997[1075]

*Excludes studies based on administration of xenon-133 by inhalation or intra-arterial injection and values obtained from infants with documented major brain lesions.
†Calculation of cerebral blood flow employed partition coefficients derived from studies of adults, which may result in overestimation of cerebral blood flow in the newborn.
IMV, intermittent mandatory ventilation.

TABLE 6-29 Regulation of Cerebral Blood Flow in the Human Newborn*

Increase in Regulatory Factor	Change in Cerebral Blood Flow
BP: normal preterm or term infant	0 (autoregulation)
BP: severely asphyxiated term infant	↑
BP: before severe intracranial hemorrhage or periventricular leukomalacia, or both—in preterm infant	↑
$Paco_2$: normal preterm or term infant	↑
$Paco_2$: severely asphyxiated term infant	0
$Paco_2$: before severe intracranial hemorrhage in preterm infant	0
Total hemoglobin concentration	↓
Proportion of fetal hemoglobin	↑
Glucose (blood)	↓
Seizure	↑
Indomethacin	↓
Ibuprofen	0
Aminophylline	↓

*See text for references.
BP, blood pressure; $Paco_2$, arterial partial pressure of carbon dioxide in arterial blood.

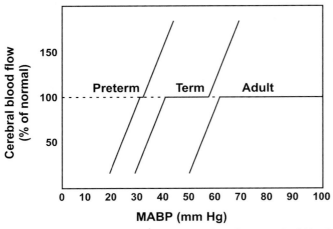

Figure 6-53 An *approximation* of the relationship of cerebral blood flow as a function of mean arterial blood pressure (MABP) with maturation. See text for details.

a feature suggesting that a minimal margin of safety may exist. In one serial study of 32 mechanically ventilated premature infants from the first hours, near-infrared spectroscopy was used to demonstrate a pressure-passive cerebral circulation in 53%.[1092] The example shown in Figure 9-47 is typical (i.e., an infant with mean arterial blood pressures that fluctuate gradually over minutes and are accompanied by parallel changes in the cerebral circulation; see Chapter 9). *The nadirs of blood pressure often are not markedly low and thus may be readily overlooked.* However, the cumulative effect of many repeated modest declines in CBF is likely to be considerable (see Chapter 8). In this regard, both neuropathological and imaging studies show that the incidence of PVL increases with advancing postnatal age. Importantly, nearly all the cases of PVL (and severe germinal matrix hemorrhage/intraventricular hemorrhage) later identified in the series of 32 infants were in the pressure-passive group.[1092] These findings were critical because they suggested that (1) infants with a pressure-passive cerebral circulation could be identified by near-infrared spectroscopy before the occurrence of white matter injury, (2) that the circulatory abnormality is related strongly to the occurrence of white matter injury, and (3) if the pressure-passive state could be corrected, perhaps the white matter injury could be prevented. However, this study involved a relatively small number of infants.

A subsequent study of 90 premature infants used a frequency-based assessment of autoregulation and quantitated the degree and duration of altered autoregulation over the first 5 days of life.[1097] The findings were striking. *Pressure-passive epochs were documented in 95% of the infants.* The overall mean proportion of the pressure-passive time was 20%, although some infants had a pressure-passive state more than 50% of the time. The likelihood of a pressure-passive state increased with decreasing gestational age and periods of hypotension.

The *lower limit of the autoregulatory curve in newborns* obviously is of great importance, particularly for management purposes and especially in sick premature infants. The precise lower limit is unknown, and it is likely that this value varies not only with gestational age but also with postnatal age and with factors that alter the concentration of vasoactive molecules in brain (e.g., blood gases, cytokines, seizures, hypoxia-ischemia). In one report, blood pressure values in the first day of life in infants 24 to 30 weeks of gestation of less than 31 mm Hg were associated with impaired EEG continuity on the EEG, a finding raising the possibility of decreased CBF at such values.[1099] Similarly, in a study of extremely low-birth-weight infants (mean birth weight 772 g, mean gestational age 26 weeks) by near-infrared spectroscopy, a pressure-passive cerebral circulation resulted when mean arterial blood pressures were lower than 30 mm Hg (see Fig. 9-48 and Chapter 9).[1100] However, to what extent, if any, arterial blood pressures lower than 30 mm Hg are clearly dangerous is unclear. Thus, a careful study of cerebral electrical activity and cerebral fractional oxygen extraction, presumably a reflection of CBF, in 35 23- to 30-week premature infants showed no electrical abnormality at mean blood pressure levels higher than 23 mm Hg. [1101] Clearly, more data combining cerebral hemodynamic and functional parameters are needed.

Carbon Dioxide. $Paco_2$ is a potent regulator of CBF in the human newborn.* The marked reactivity of CBF to $Paco_2$ is present in the first hours of life in spontaneously breathing preterm infants but does not appear until the second day in mechanically ventilated preterm infants (Table 6-30).[1063,1064,1070] The reason for the attenuated reactivity of CBF to $Paco_2$ in the first day of life in mechanically ventilated infants is unclear, although the same phenomenon has been

---

*See references 959,1050,1051,1058,1063,1064,1069,1070,1074-1076, 1078,1101.

TABLE 6-30	Relation of Cerebral Blood Flow to Partial Pressure of Carbon Dioxide in Arterial Blood in the Human Preterm Infant in the First 2 Days of Life	
Age	**Ventilation**	**Change in CBF (%)/ Change in $Paco_2$ (mm Hg)**
2–3 hr	Spontaneously breathing	3.85
2–12 hr	Mechanically ventilated	1.50
12–24 hr	Mechanically ventilated	1.57
24–48 hr	Mechanically ventilated	4.35

CBF, cerebral blood flow; $Paco_2$, arterial partial pressure of carbon dioxide in arterial blood.

Data for mechanically ventilated infants from Pryds O, Greisen G, Lou H, Friis-Hansen B: Heterogeneity of cerebral vasoreactivity in preterm infants supported by mechanical ventilation, *J Pediatr* 115:638-645, 1989, and derived from 38 preterm infants (mean birth weight 1470 g) with persistently normal neonatal ultrasound scans; data for spontaneously breathing infants from Pryds O, Andersen GE, Friis-Hansen B: Cerebral blood flow reactivity in spontaneously breathing, preterm infants shortly after birth, *Acta Paediatr Scand* 79:391-396, 1990.

observed in the newborn monkey, rat, dog, and lamb.[966,982,1072,1102] A state of attenuated or absent reactivity to $Paco_2$, as with blood pressure (see earlier discussion), has been observed both in seriously asphyxiated full-term infants and in mechanically ventilated preterm infants before severe intracranial hemorrhage (Table 6-31; see Chapters 8, 9, and 11). In general, the loss of reactivity to $Paco_2$ follows the loss of autoregulation (but precedes loss of reactivity to hypoxemia).[1072] In one report, a progressive loss of cerebrovascular autoregulation was noted with increasing $Paco_2 \geq 45$ mm Hg.[959]

The *mechanism* for the vasodilating effect of carbon dioxide relates to the increase in *perivascular H+ concentration*, as observed in experimental models (see earlier discussion). The observation of a 50% decrease in CBF after sodium bicarbonate administration to term and premature infants with acidosis also supports the important role of perivascular H^+ concentration.[1050] The mechanism proposed for a decrease in the latter situation was enhanced movement of bicarbonate across the blood-brain barrier "because of vasodilation caused by the asphyxia" in these infants.[1050] The demonstration of a decrease in CBF after sodium bicarbonate administration in acidotic postasphyxial infants may have important implications for management.

Oxygen. Arterial oxygen concentration is an important effector of CBF in the human infant, as it is in the perinatal animal.[931,984,1061,1062,1064,1103-1110] A vivid demonstration of the vasoconstrictive effect of oxygen is the observation that preterm infants administered 80% oxygen during stabilization at birth had a 23% lower value for CBF than did infants administered room air during stabilization, when measured by xenon-133 clearance at 2 hours of life.[1110] This finding may have implications concerning the use of high concentrations of inspired oxygen at the time of birth (see Chapters 8 and 9). Arterial oxygen concentration is related not only to Pao_2 but also to hemoglobin concentration and the oxygen affinity of hemoglobin. In preterm infants studied in the first day of life, Pryds and Greisen[1064] observed a mean increase in CBF of 11.9% per 1 mmol/kg decrease in hemoglobin

concentration. In a separate series of preterm infants studied at a mean postnatal age of 3.7 weeks, a mean increase in CBF of 5% per percentage point of decrease in hematocrit was documented.[1061]

Oxygen delivery to brain may be affected not only by hemoglobin concentration, but also by the viscosity of blood, at which point the inverse relationship of CBF with hemoglobin concentration becomes more pronounced. However, in general, hematocrit does not alter blood viscosity in the newborn at levels lower than approximately 60% (and perhaps somewhat higher).[1074,1111,1112]

Finally, a direct relationship of CBF (determined by xenon-133 clearance) with the relative proportion of fetal hemoglobin has been shown,[1106] presumably reflecting the stronger affinity of fetal hemoglobin for oxygen. This conclusion had been suggested by a prior study of CBF velocity.[1109]

Glucose. A striking observation by Pryds and co-workers[1060,1065] established an important role for glucose in regulation of CBF in the human newborn (see Table 6-29). As discussed in more detail in Chapter 12, an increase in CBF became apparent as blood glucose concentration decreased to less than approximately 30 mg/dL (1.7 mmol/L). Increases in CBF of two- to threefold then occurred in proportion to the decline in blood glucose. The mechanism for this vasodilatory effect of glucose is not clear, but stimulation of beta-receptors by the increased compensatory secretion of epinephrine is suggested by data in human adults.[1072] The clinical significance of this effect of glucose could be appreciable (see Chapter 12).

Neuronal Activity (Seizure). The coupling of neuronal activity to CBF is apparent in at least two situations, sleep states and seizure. A decrease in CBF during *sleep* has been shown by xenon-133 clearance.[1113] The effect is not striking. A striking increase ($\approx$50%) in CBF with the excessive neuronal activity of *seizure* has been documented in the human newborn by PET (see Chapter 5).[1114] This effect had been suggested by earlier studies of CBF velocity by Doppler.[1115]

TABLE 6-31 **Relation of Outcome in Term Infants to Mean Cerebral Blood Flow in the First 12 Hours After Asphyxia***

Clinical Group	Neurological Outcome	Mean CBF (mL/100 g/min)	MABP Reactivity[†]	Carbon Dioxide Reactivity[‡]
Asphyxiated	Death or severe brain injury	30.6	−	−
Asphyxiated	Moderate to severe brain injury	15.1	−	+
Asphyxiated	Normal	9.2	+	+
Nonasphyxiated	Normal	11.9	+	+

*CBF determined in three groups of asphyxiated infants at mean age of 9 hours and in a group of nonasphyxiated infants at the age of 1–5 days.
[†]MABP reactivity: −, CBF fluctuates directly with MABP (i.e., autoregulation not operating); +, CBF does not change with MABP (i.e., autoregulation normal).
[‡]Carbon dioxide reactivity: −, CBF does not change directly with changes in $Paco_2$ (i.e., lack of normal reactivity of CBF); +, CBF changes directly with changes in $Paco_2$ (i.e., normal reactivity of CBF).
CBF, cerebral blood flow; MABP, mean arterial blood pressure; $Paco_2$, arterial partial pressure of carbon dioxide.
Data from Pryds O, Greisen G, Lou H, Friis-Hansen B: Vasoparalysis associated with brain damage in asphyxiated term infants, *J Pediatr* 117:119-125, 1990.

Pharmacological Agents. Indomethacin and aminophylline are the two pharmacological agents shown to have a clear effect on CBF in the human newborn. *Indomethacin* administration in doses used for closure of the ductus arteriosus led to a 20% to 40% decrease in CBF in the premature infant, as studied by xenon-133 clearance and near-infrared spectroscopy.[1012,1059,1116] Notably, however, no change in CBF, assessed by Doppler, was observed after continuous versus bolus infusion of indomethacin.[1117] The vasoconstrictive effect is mediated by the inhibition of synthesis of vasodilatory prostaglandins at the cyclooxygenase step, as shown in experimental models and studies of isolated neonatal human cerebral artery.[1118,1119] An increase in cerebrovascular resistance was shown by Doppler studies of very low-birth-weight infants after indomethacin administration.[1120] Interestingly, by contrast with indomethacin, *ibuprofen* does not lead to a decline in CBF.[1074]

Administration of *aminophylline*, an antagonist of adenosine, led to only a small decrease (10% to 15%) in CBF in the human premature infant within 1 hour of intravenous administration.[1071] No alteration of visual evoked potentials accompanied this modest decrease in blood flow. *Dopamine* administered to treat hypotension was reported in two studies to increase CBF as well as arterial blood pressure.[1074,1100]

Perinatal Asphyxia, Autoregulation of Cerebral Blood Flow, and Cerebral Hyperemia

Impaired Autoregulation. A xenon-133 study of CBF in a group of 19 term and preterm infants first suggested that autoregulation in the human newborn is very sensitive to perinatal asphyxia.[1051] Thus, 19 infants were examined with the xenon clearance technique "a few hours after birth."[1051] Eleven of the infants weighed less than 2000 g. Although most of the infants were considered "distressed," Apgar scores at 5 minutes were less than 7 in only 4 of the 19 infants. At the time of study, pH was less than 7.20 in only 4 infants. For the total group of 19 infants, a linear relationship existed between CBF and systolic blood pressure (Fig. 6-54). This pressure-passive relationship suggests inoperative vascular autoregulation and was seen to a similar degree in the infants less than or more than 2000 g body weight. This apparent impairment of vascular autoregulation is directly reminiscent of the data obtained with fetal and neonatal animals after asphyxia (see earlier section).

Impaired Vascular Reactivity and Cerebral Hyperemia. Subsequent work clarified the relationship between perinatal asphyxia and impairment of vascular reactivity, particularly autoregulation. In a systematic study of 19 term infants (mean birth weight, 3200 g) with perinatal asphyxia defined by a 5-minute Apgar score of 5 or lower and umbilical cord pH lower than 7.0, or both, a striking relationship among the severity of brain injury, the absolute value of CBF, and the reactivity to changes in blood pressure and $Paco_2$ was defined (see Table 6-31).[1067] Thus, infants with the poorest neurological outcome (isoelectric amplitude-integrated

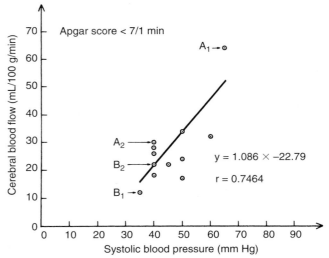

Figure 6-54   Linear relationship between cerebral blood flow (CBF) and systolic blood pressure in 10 newborns with Apgar scores of less than 7 at 1 minute. CBF was measured by the xenon clearance technique. A_1 and A_2 represent measurements of CBF in one patient before and after a spontaneous decrease in blood pressure. B_1 and B_2 represent measurements in another patient before and after a spontaneous increase in blood pressure. *(From Lou HC, Lassen NA, Friis-Hansen B: Low cerebral blood flow in hypotensive perinatal distress, J Pediatr 94:118, 1979.)*

EEG, death) had the highest values for CBF and no autoregulation or carbon dioxide reactivity (see Table 6-31). Infants with a burst-suppression EEG and moderate to severe brain injury had slightly elevated values for CBF and impaired autoregulation, but retained reactivity to $Paco_2$ (see Table 6-31). Infants without evidence of brain injury had normal values for CBF, intact autoregulation, and reactivity to $Paco_2$. A later study of 16 term infants with hypoxic-ischemic encephalopathy used PET to determine CBF primarily at 1 to 4 days of life and found higher flows in those infants with abnormal neurological outcome (35.6 mL/100 g/minute) than in those with normal neurological outcome (18.3 mL/100 g/minute).[1121]

The pronounced, sustained *cerebral hyperemia* observed in the human infant has been shown by less invasive techniques, such as Doppler ultrasound and near-infrared spectroscopy. Thus, determinations of CBF velocity in term infants with hypoxic-ischemic encephalopathy from approximately 6 to 130 hours after the insult showed an increase in mean flow velocity with decreased resistance indices (i.e., vasodilation).[1122-1133] Similarly, studies of asphyxiated human infants on the first day of life by near-infrared spectroscopy are consistent with a loss of vascular reactivity and an increase in cerebral blood volume and CBF, with temporal characteristics similar to those observed in fetal sheep, described earlier.[74,1134] The mechanism for this hyperemia is unclear. An increase in neuronal excitability, although documented following hypoxic-ischemic insults, seems unlikely in view of the relation of highest flows to isoelectric EEG. It appears more likely that an accumulation of vasodilatory compounds or vascular injury, or both, occurs and that this accumulation or injury in many ways may be similar in the human newborn and the perinatal animal. Delineation of the mechanisms underlying this vasoparalytic state and cerebral hyperemia following perinatal asphyxia in the human infant will be of major importance.

The aforementioned data thus define in the postasphyxial human newborn a state of *vasoparalysis* and *cerebral hyperemia* that is correlated with the degree of brain injury and presumably the severity of the asphyxial insult. The altered vascular reactivity, with autoregulation impaired more readily than carbon dioxide reactivity, is similar to observations made in the postasphyxial state in perinatal animal models (see earlier discussion). Presumably, a state of maximal vasodilation exists, related perhaps to the effects of elevated perivascular H^+ concentration, prostaglandins, adenosine, free radicals, or NO, or all these factors. Whether this hyperemic state is caused by the same factors that lead to the brain injury, is an adaptive mechanism to preserve brain tissue, or in some way causes additional brain injury remains to be clarified. It does appear likely that the loss of vascular reactivity renders the infant vulnerable to systemic hypotension and resulting cerebral ischemia.

REFERENCES

1. Vannucci RA: Cerebral carbohydrate and energy metabolism in perinatal hypoxic-ischemic brain damage, *Brain Pathol* 2:229-234, 1992.
2. Vannucci RC, Yager JY: Glucose, lactic acid and perinatal hypoxic-ischemic brain damage, *Pediatr Neurol* 8:3-12, 1992.
3. Clark JB, Bates TE, Cullingford T, Land JM: Development of enzymes of energy metabolism in the neonatal mammalian brain, *Dev Neurosci* 15:174-180, 1993.
4. Vannucci RC: Interventions for perinatal hypoxic-ischemic encephalopathy, *Pediatrics* 100:1004-1014, 1997.
5. Vannucci RC, Connor JR, Mauger DT, Palmer C, et al: Rat model of perinatal hypoxic-ischemic brain damage, *J Neurosci Res* 55:158-163, 1999.
6. Erecinska M, Cherian S, Silver IA: Energy metabolism in mammalian brain during development, *Prog Neurobiol* 73:397-445, 2004.
7. Vannucci RC, Brucklacher RM, Vannucci SJ: Glycolysis and perinatal hypoxic-ischemic brain damage, *Dev Neurosci* 27:185-190, 2005.
8. McKenna MC, Gruetter R, Sonnewald U, Waagepetersen HS, et al: Energy metabolism of the brain. In Siegel GJ, Albers RW, Brady ST, et al, editors: *Basic Neurochemistry: Molecular, Cellular and Medical Aspects,* 7th ed, New York: 2006, Elsevier.
9. Moore TJ, Lione AP, Regen DM, Tarpley HL, et al: Brain glucose metabolism in the newborn rat, *Am J Physiol* 221:1746-1753, 1971.
10. Vannucci RC, Vasta F, Vannucci SJ: Cerebral metabolic responses of hyperglycemic immature rats to hypoxia-ischemia, *Pediatr Res* 21:524-529, 1987.
11. Hawkins RA, Miller AL, Cremer JE, Veech RL: Measurement of the rate of glucose utilization by rat brain in vivo, *J Neurochem* 23:917-923, 1974.
12. Miller AL, Corddry DH: Brain carbohydrate metabolism in developing rats during hypercapnia, *J Neurochem* 36:1202-1210, 1981.
13. Vannucci SJ, Seaman LB, Vannucci RC: Effects of hypoxia-ischemia on GLUT1 and GLUT3 glucose transporters in immature rat brain, *J Cereb Blood Flow Metab* 16:77-81, 1996.
14. Powers WJ, Rosenbaum JL, Dence CS, Markham J, et al: Cerebral glucose transport and metabolism in preterm human infants, *J Cereb Blood Flow Metab* 18:632-638, 1998.
15. Booth RF, Patel TB, Clark JB: The development of enzymes of energy metabolism in the brain of a precocial (guinea pig) and non-precocial (rat) species, *J Neurochem* 34:17-25, 1980.
16. Tekkok SB, Brown AM, Westenbroek R, Pellerin L, et al: Transfer of glycogen-derived lactate from astrocytes to axons via specific monocarboxylate transporters supports mouse optic nerve activity, *J Neurosci Res* 81:644-652, 2005.
17. Sanchez-Abarca LI, Tabernero A, Medina JM: Oligodendrocytes use lactate as a source of energy and as a precursor of lipids, *Glia* 36:321-329, 2001.
18. Duffy TE, Kohle SJ, Vannucci RC: Carbohydrate and energy metabolism in perinatal rat brain: Relation to survival in anoxia, *J Neurochem* 24:271-276, 1975.
19. Holowach-Thurston J, McDougal DB Jr: Effect of ischemia on metabolism of the brain of the newborn mouse, *Am J Physiol* 216:348-352, 1969.
20. Siesjö BK, Plum F: Pathophysiology of anoxic brain damage. In Gaull GE, editor: *Biology of Cerebral Dysfunction,* New York: 1973, Plenum Press.
21. Van Cappellen Van Walsum A-M, Rijpkema M, Heerschap A, Oeseburg B, et al: Cerebral ^{31}P magnetic resonance spectroscopy and system acid-base balance during hypoxia in fetal sheep, *Pediatr Res* 54:747-752, 2003.
22. Holowach-Thurston J, Hauhart RE, Jones EM: Decrease in brain glucose in anoxia in spite of elevated plasma glucose levels, *Pediatr Res* 7:691-695, 1973.
23. Vannucci SJ, Vannucci RC: Glycogen metabolism in neonatal rat brain during anoxia and recovery, *J Neurochem* 34:1100-1105, 1980.
24. Mayevsky A, Nioka S, Subramanian VH, Chance B: Brain oxidative metabolism of the newborn dog: Correlation between ^{31}P NMR spectroscopy and pyridine nucleotide redox state, *J Cereb Blood Flow Metab* 8:201-207, 1988.
25. Nioka S, Chance B, Smith DS, Mayevsky A, et al: Cerebral energy metabolism and oxygen state during hypoxia in neonate and adult dogs, *Pediatr Res* 28:54-62, 1990.
26. DiGiacomo JE, Pane CR, Gwiazdowski S, Mishra OP, et al: Effect of graded hypoxia on brain cell membrane injury in newborn piglets, *Biol Neonate* 61:25-32, 1992.
27. Jensen F, Tsuji M, Offutt M, Firkusny I, et al: Profound, reversible energy loss in the hypoxic immature rat brain, *Brain Res Dev* 73:99-105, 1993.
28. Ikonomidou C, Mosinger JL, Salles KS, Labruyere J, et al: Sensitivity of the developing rat brain to hypobaric/ischemic damage parallels sensitivity to N-methyl-aspartate neurotoxicity, *J Neurosci* 9:2809-2818, 1989.
29. McDonald JW, Trescher WH, Johnston MV: The selective ionotropic-type quisqualate receptor agonist AMPA is a potent neurotoxin in immature rat brain, *Brain Res* 526:165-168, 1990.
30. Jensen FE, Applegate CD, Holtzman D, Belin TR, et al: Epilepto-genic effect of hypoxia in the immature rodent brain, *Ann Neurol* 29:629-637, 1991.
31. Wasterlain CG, Hattori H, Yang C, Schwartz PH, et al: Selective vulnerability of neuronal subpopulations during ontogeny reflects discrete molecular events associated with normal brain development. In Wasterlain CG, Vert P, editors: *Neonatal Seizures,* New York: 1991, Raven Press.
32. Duffy TE, Cavazzuti M, Cruz NF, Sokoloff L: Local cerebral glucose metabolism in newborn dogs: Effects of hypoxia and halothane anesthesia, *Ann Neurol* 11:233-246, 1982.
33. Cavazzuti M, Duffy TE: Regulation of local cerebral blood flow in normal and hypoxic newborn dogs, *Ann Neurol* 11:247-257, 1982.
34. Stefanovich V, John JP: The increase of cyclic AMP in rat's brain during anoxia, *Res Commun Chem Pathol Pharmacol* 9:591-593, 1974.
35. Vannucci RC: Experimental biology of cerebral hypoxia-ischemia: Relation to perinatal brain damage, *Pediatr Res* 27:317-326, 1990.
36. Maker HS, Clarke DD, Lajtha AL: Intermediary metabolism of carbohydrates and amino acids. In Siegel GJ, Albers RW, Katzman R, et al, editors: *Basic Neurochemistry,* Boston: 1976, Little, Brown.
37. Lowry OH: Energy metabolism in brain and its control. In Ingvar WH, Lassen NA, editors: *Brain Work,* Copenhagen, 1975, Munksgaard.
38. Vannucci RC, Plum F: Pathophysiology of perinatal hypoxic-ischemic brain damage. In Gaull GE, editor: *Biology of Brain Dysfunction,* New York: 1975, Plenum Press.
39. Holowach-Thurston J, Hauhart RE, Jones EM: Anoxia in mice: Reduced glucose in brain with normal or elevated glucose in plasma and increased survival after glucose treatment, *Pediatr Res* 8:238-243, 1974.
40. Chao CR, Hohimer AR, Bissonnette JM: The effect of elevated blood glucose on the electroencephalogram and cerebral metabolism during short-term brain ischemia in fetal sheep, *Am J Obstet Gynecol* 161:221-228, 1989.
41. Chao CR, Hohimer AR, Bissonnette JM: Cerebral carbohydrate metabolism during severe ischemia in fetal sheep, *J Cereb Blood Flow Metab* 9:53-57, 1989.
42. Hope PL, Cady EB, Chu A, Delpy DT, et al: Brain metabolism and intracellular pH during ischaemia and hypoxia: An in vivo ^{31}P and ^1H nuclear magnetic resonance study in the lamb, *J Neurochem* 49:75-82, 1987.
43. Corbett RJ, Laptook AR: Acid homeostasis following partial ischemia in neonatal brain measured in vivo by ^{31}P and ^1H nuclear magnetic resonance spectroscopy, *J Neurochem* 54:1208-1217, 1990.
44. Young RS, Petroff OA, Aquila WJ, Cheung A, et al: Hyperglycemia and the rate of lactic acid accumulation during cerebral ischemia in developing animals: In vivo proton MRS study, *Biol Neonate* 61:235-242, 1992.
45. Bunt JEH, Gavilanes AWD, Reulen JPH, Blanco CE, et al: The influence of acute hypoxemia and hypovolemic hypotension of neuronal brain activity measured by the cerebral function monitor in newborn piglets, *Neuropediatrics* 27:260-264, 1996.
46. Laptook AR, Corbett RJT, Burns DK, Sterett R: A limited interval of delayed modest hypothermia for ischemic brain resuscitation is not beneficial in neonatal swine, *Pediatr Res* 46:383-389, 1999.
47. Vannucci RC, Vannucci SJ: Perinatal hypoxic-ischemic brain damage: Evolution of an animal model, *Dev Neurosci* 27:81-86, 2005.
48. Yager JY, Brucklacher RM, Vannucci RC: Cerebral oxidative metabolism and redox state during hypoxia-ischemia and early recovery in immature rats, *Am J Physiol* 261:H1102-H1108, 1991.
49. Vannucci RC, Christensen MA, Stein DT: Regional cerebral glucose utilization in the immature rat: Effect of hypoxia-ischemia, *Pediatr Res* 26:208-214, 1989.
50. Vannucci RC, Lyons DT, Vasta F: Regional cerebral blood flow during hypoxia-ischemia in immature rats, *Stroke* 19:245-250, 1988.

51. Welsh FA, Vannucci RC, Brierley JB: Columnar alterations of NADH fluorescence during hypoxia-ischemia in immature rat brain, *J Cereb Blood Flow Metab* 2:221-228, 1982.

52. Stein DT, Vannucci RC: Calcium accumulation during the evolution of hypoxic-ischemic brain damage in the immature rat, *J Cereb Blood Flow Metab* 8:834-842, 1988.

53. Silverstein FS, Buchanan K, Hudson C, Johnston MV: Flunarizine limits hypoxia-ischemia induced morphologic injury in immature rat brain, *Stroke* 17:477-482, 1986.

54. Schwartz PH, Massarweh WF, Vinters HV, Wasterlain CG: A rat model of severe neonatal hypoxic-ischemic brain injury, *Stroke* 23:539-546, 1992.

55. de Courten-Myers GM, Fogelson HM, Kleinholz M, Myers RE: Hypoxic brain and heart injury thresholds in piglets, *Biomed Biochim Acta* 48:S143-148, 1989.

56. Wagner KR, Ting P, Westfall MV, Yamaguchi S, et al: Brain metabolic correlates of hypoxic-ischemic cerebral necrosis in mid-gestational sheep fetuses: Significance of hypotension, *J Cereb Blood Flow Metab* 6:425-434, 1986.

57. Ting P, Yamaguchi S, Bacher JD, Killens RH, et al: Hypoxic-ischemic cerebral necrosis in midgestational sheep fetuses: Physiopathologic correlations, *Exp Neurol* 80:227-245, 1983.

58. Williams GD, Palmer C, Roberts RL, Heitjan DF, et al: ^{31}P NMR spectroscopy of perinatal hypoxic-ischemic brain damage: A model to evaluate neuroprotective drugs in immature rats, *NMR Biomed* 5:145-153, 1992.

59. Williams GD, Palmer C, Heitjan DF, Smith MB: Allopurinol preserves cerebral energy metabolism during perinatal hypoxia-ischemia: A P-31 NMR study in unanesthetized immature rats, *Neurosci Lett* 144:103-106, 1992.

60. Palmer C, Brucklacher RM, Christensen MA, Vannucci RC: Carbohydrate and energy metabolism during the evolution of hypoxic-ischemic brain damage in the immature rat, *J Cereb Blood Flow Metab* 10:227-235, 1990.

61. Vannucci RC, Yager JY, Vannucci SJ: Cerebral glucose and energy utilization during the evolution of hypoxic-ischemic brain damage in the immature rat, *J Cereb Blood Flow Metab* 14:279-288, 1994.

62. De Haan HH, Ijzermans AC, De Haan J, Van Belle H, et al: Effects of surgery and asphyxia on levels of nucleosides, purine bases, and lactate in cerebrospinal fluid of fetal lambs, *Pediatr Res* 36:595-600, 1994.

63. Nelson C, Silverstein FS: Acute disruption of cytochrome oxidase activity in brain in a perinatal rat stroke model, *Pediatr Res* 36:12-19, 1994.

64. Blumberg RM, Cady EB, Wigglesworth JS, McKenzie JE, et al: Relation between delayed impairment of cerebral energy metabolism and infarction following transient focal hypoxia-ischaemia in the developing brain, *Exp Brain Res* 113:130-137, 1997.

65. Lorek A, Takei Y, Cady EB, Wyatt JS, et al: Delayed ("secondary") cerebral energy failure after acute hypoxia-ischemia in the newborn piglet: Continuous 48-hour studies by phosphorus magnetic resonance spectroscopy, *Pediatr Res* 36:699-706, 1994.

66. Penrice J, Lorek A, Cady EB, Amess PN, et al: Proton magnetic resonance spectroscopy of the brain during acute hypoxia-ischemia and delayed cerebral energy failure in the newborn piglet, *Pediatr Res* 41:795-802, 1997.

67. Amess PN, Penrice J, Cady EB, Lorek A, et al: Mild hypothermia after severe transient hypoxia-ischemia reduces the delayed rise in cerebral lactate in the newborn piglet, *Pediatr Res* 41:803-808, 1997.

68. Kobayashi M, Lust WD, Passonneau JV: Concentrations of energy metabolites and cyclic nucleotides during and after bilateral ischemia in the gerbil cerebral cortex, *J Neurochem* 29:53-59, 1977.

69. De Haan HH, Gunn AJ, Williams CE, Gluckman PD: Brief repeated umbilical cord occlusions cause sustained cytotoxic cerebral edema and focal infarcts in near-term fetal lambs, *Pediatr Res* 41:96-104, 1997.

70. Kusaka T, Matsuura S, Fujikawa Y, Okubo K, et al: Relationship between cerebral interstitial levels of amino acids and phosphorylation potential during secondary energy failure in hypoxic-ischemic newborn piglets, *Pediatr Res* 55:273-279, 2004.

71. Martin E, Buchli R, Ritter S, Schmid R, et al: Diagnostic and prognostic value of cerebral ^{31}P magnetic resonance spectroscopy in neonates with perinatal asphyxia, *Pediatr Res* 40:749-758, 1996.

72. Hanrahan JD, Sargentoni J, Azzopardi D, Manji K, et al: Cerebral metabolism within 18 hours of birth asphyxia: A proton magnetic resonance spectroscopy study, *Pediatr Res* 39:584-590, 1996.

73. Vannucci RC, Towfighi J, Vannucci SJ: Secondary energy failure after cerebral hypoxia-ischemia in the immature rat, *J Cereb Blood Flow Metab* 24:1090-1097, 2004.

74. Marks KA, Mallard EC, Roberts I, Williams CE, et al: Delayed vasodilation and altered oxygenation after cerebral ischemia in fetal sheep, *Pediatr Res* 39:48-54, 1995.

75. Puka-Sundvall M, Wallin C, Gilland E, Hallin U, et al: Impairment of mitochondrial respiration after cerebral hypoxia-ischemia in immature rats: Relationship to activation of caspase-3 and neuronal injury, *Dev Brain Res* 125:43-50, 2000.

76. Ment LR, Stewart WB, Gore JC, Duncan CC: Beagle puppy model of perinatal asphyxia: Alterations in cerebral blood flow and metabolism, *Pediatr Neurol* 4:98-104, 1988.

77. Yoshioka H, Fujiwara K, Ishimura K, Iino S, et al: Brain energy metabolism in two kinds of total asphyxia: An in vivo phosphorus nuclear magnetic resonance spectroscopic study, *Brain Dev* 10:88-91, 1988.

78. Goplerud JM, Mishra OP, Delivoria-Papadopoulos M: Brain cell membrane dysfunction following acute asphyxia in newborn piglets, *Biol Neonate* 61:33-41, 1992.

79. Rose VC, Shaffner DH, Gleason CA, Koehler RC, et al: Somatosensory evoked potential and brain water content in post-asphyxic immature piglets, *Pediatr Res* 37:661-666, 1995.

80. Ikeda T, Murata Y, Quilligan EJ, Choi BH, et al: Physiologic and histologic changes in near-term fetal lambs exposed to asphyxia by partial umbilical cord occlusion, *Am J Obstet Gynecol* 178:24-32, 1998.

81. Van Cappellen Van Walsum A-M, Jongma HW, Wevers RA, Nuhuis JG, et al: ^{1}H-NMR spectroscopy of cerebrospinal fluid of fetal sheep during hypoxia-induced acidemia and recovery, *Pediatr Res* 52:56-63, 2002.

82. Hunter CJ, Bennet L, Power GG, Roelfsema V, et al: Key neuroprotective role for endogenous adenosine A(1) receptor activation during asphyxia in the fetal sheep, *Stroke* 34:2240-2245, 2003.

83. Vannucci RC, Duffy TE: Cerebral metabolism in newborn dogs during reversible asphyxia, *Ann Neurol* 1:528-534, 1977.

84. O'Shaughnessy CT, Lythgoe DJ, Butcher SP, Kendall L, et al: Effects of hypoxia on fetal rat brain metabolism studied in utero by ^{31}P-NMR spectroscopy, *Brain Res* 551:334-337, 1991.

85. Kogure K, Busto R, Scheinberg P, Reinmuth O: Dynamics of cerebral metabolism during moderate hypercapnia, *J Neurochem* 24:471-478, 1975.

86. Des Rosiers MH, Kennedy C, Sakurada O: Effects of hypercapnia on cerebral oxygen and glucose consumption in the conscious rat, *Stroke* 9:98-104, 1978.

87. Kliefoth AB, Grubb RL Jr, Raichle ME: Depression of cerebral oxygen utilization by hypercapnia in the rhesus monkey, *J Neurochem* 32:661-663, 1979.

88. Vannucci RC, Towfighi J, Heitjan DF, Brucklacher RM: Carbon dioxide protects the perinatal brain from hypoxic-ischemic damage: An experimental study in the immature rat, *Pediatrics* 95:868-874, 1995.

89. Stafford A, Weatherall AC: The survival of young rats in nitrogen, *J Physiol* 153:457-474, 1960.

90. Britton SW, Kline RF: Age, sex, carbohydrate, adrenal cortex and other factors in anoxia, *Am J Physiol* 145:190, 1945-1946.

91. Himwich HE, Bernstein AO, Herlich H: Mechanisms for the maintenance of life in the newborn during anoxia, *Am J Physiol* 135:387, 1942.

92. Selle WA: Influence of glucose on the gasping pattern of young animals subjected to acute anoxia, *Am J Physiol* 141:297-311, 1944.

93. Dawes GS, Mott JC, Shelley HJ: The importance of cardiac glycogen for the maintenance of life in fetal lambs and newborn animals during anoxia, *J Physiol* 152:271-298, 1960.

94. Shelley HJ: Glycogen reserves and their changes at birth and in anoxia, *BMJ* 17:137, 1961.

95. Su JY, Friedman WF: Comparison of the responses of fetal and adult cardiac muscle to hypoxia, *Am J Physiol* 224:1249-1253, 1973.

96. Vannucci RC, Vasta F, Vannucci SJ: Glucose supplementation does not accentuate hypoxic-ischemic brain damage in immature rats: Biochemical mechanisms, *Pediatr Res* 19:396, 1985.

97. Voorhies TM, Rawlinson D, Vannucci RC: Glucose and perinatal hypoxic-ischemic brain damage in the rat, *Neurology* 36:1115-1118, 1986.

98. Vannucci RC, Vannucci SJ: Cerebral carbohydrate metabolism during hypoglycemia and anoxia in newborn rats, *Ann Neurol* 4:73-79, 1978.

99. Yager JY, Heitjan DF, Towfighi J, Vannucci RC: Effect of insulin-induced and fasting hypoglycemia on perinatal hypoxic-ischemic brain damage, *Pediatr Res* 31:138-142, 1992.

100. Salhab WA, Wyckoff MH, Laptook AR, Perlman JM: Initial hypoglycemia and neonatal brain injury in term infants with severe fetal acidemia, *Pediatrics* 114:361-366, 2004.

101. Laptook AR, Corbett RJT, Arencibiamireles O, Ruley J: Glucose-associated alterations in ischemic brain metabolism of neonatal piglets, *Stroke* 23:1504-1511, 1992.

102. Corbett RJ, Laptook AR, Sterett R, Tollefsbol G, et al: Effect of hypoxia on glucose-modulated cerebral lactic acidosis, agonal glycolytic rates, and energy utilization, *Pediatr Res* 39:477-486, 1996.

103. Vannucci RC, Brucklacher RM, Vannucci SJ: The effect of hyperglycemia on cerebral metabolism during hypoxia-ischemia in the immature rat, *J Cereb Blood Flow Metab* 16:1026-1033, 1996.

104. Myers RE, Yamaguchi S: Nervous system effects of cardiac arrest in monkeys: Preservation of vision, *Arch Neurol* 34:65-74, 1977.

105. Myers RE: Lactic acid accumulation as cause of brain edema and cerebral necrosis resulting from oxygen deprivation. In Korobkin C, Guilleminault C, editors: *Advances in Perinatal Neurology*, New York: 1979, Spectrum.

106. Myers RE: Anoxic brain pathology and blood glucose, *Neurology* 26:345-356, 1976.

107. Myers RE: Brain damage due to asphyxia: Mechanism of causation, *J Perinat Med* 9:78-86, 1981.

108. Wagner KR, Myers RE: Topographic aspects of lactic acid accumulation in brain tissue during circulatory arrest, *Neurology* 29:546-554, 1979.

109. Yamaguchi M, Myers RE: Comparison of brain biochemical changes produced by anoxia and hypoxia, *J Neuropathol Exp Neurol* 35:302, 1976.

110. Kagstrom E, Smith ML, Siesjö BK: Recirculation in the rat brain following incomplete ischemia, *J Cereb Blood Flow Metab* 3:183-192, 1983.

111. DeCourten GM, Yamaguchi S, Myers RE: Influence of serum glucose concentration upon rapidity of circulatory failure during hypoxia and brain injury in cats. In Meyer JS, Lechner H, Reivich M, editors: *International Congress Series No 532, Cerebral Vascular Disease*, Amsterdam: 1980, Excerpta Medica.
112. Ginsberg MD, Welsh FA, Budd WW: Deleterious effect of glucose pretreatment on recovery from diffuse cerebral ischemia in the cat. I. Local cerebral blood flow and glucose utilization, *Stroke* 11:347-354, 1980.
113. Rehncrona S, Rosen I, Siesjö BK: Excessive cellular acidosis: An important mechanism of neuronal damage in the brain? *Acta Physiol Scand* 110:435-437, 1980.
114. Kalimo H, Rehncrona S, Soderfeldt B, Olsson Y, et al: Brain lactic acidosis and ischemic cell damage. II. Histopathology, *J Cereb Blood Flow Metab* 1:313-327, 1981.
115. Rehncrona S, Rosen I, Siesjö BK: Brain lactic acidosis and ischemic cell damage. I. Biochemistry and neurophysiology, *J Cereb Blood Flow Metab* 1:297-311, 1981.
116. Pulsinelli WA, Waldman S, Rawlinson D, Plum F: Moderate hyperglycemia augments ischemic brain damage: A neuropathologic study in the rat, *Neurology* 32:1239-1246, 1982.
117. Siemkowicz E, Hansen AJ, Gjedde A: Hyperglycemic ischemia of rat brain: The effect of post-ischemic insulin on metabolic rate, *Brain Res* 243:386-390, 1982.
118. Paljarvi L, Rehncrona S, Soderfeldt B, Olsson Y, et al: Brain lactic acidosis and ischemic cell damage: Quantitative ultrastructural changes in capillaries of rat cerebral cortex, *Acta Neuropathol (Berl)* 60:232-240, 1983.
119. Plum F: What causes infarction in ischemic brain? The Robert Wartenberg Lecture, *Neurology* 33:222-233, 1983.
120. Pulsinelli WA, Kraig RP, Plum F: Hyperglycemia, cerebral acidosis, and ischemic brain damage. In Plum F, Pulsinelli W, editors: *Cerebrovascular Diseases*, New York: 1985, Raven Press.
121. Wagner KR, Kleinholz M, Myers RE: Delayed decreases in specific brain mitochondrial electron transfer complex activities and cytochrome concentrations following anoxia/ischemia, *J Neurol Sci* 100:142-151, 1990.
122. Wagner KR, Kleinholz M, de Courten-Myers GM, Myers RE: Hyperglycemic versus normoglycemic stroke: Topography of brain metabolites, intracellular pH, and infarct size, *J Cereb Blood Flow Metab* 12:213-222, 1992.
123. Marie C, Bralet J: Blood glucose level and morphological brain damage following cerebral ischemia, *Cerebrovasc Brain Metab Rev* 3:29-38, 1991.
124. de Courten-Myers GM, Kleinholz M, Wagner KR, Myers RE: Normoglycemia (not hypoglycemia) optimizes outcome from middle cerebral artery occlusion, *J Cereb Blood Flow Metab* 14:227-236, 1994.
125. Palmer C, Vannucci RC, Towfighi J: Reduction of perinatal hypoxic-ischemic brain damage with allopurinol, *Pediatr Res* 27:332-336, 1990.
126. Rosenberg AA, Murdaugh E: The effect of blood glucose concentration on postasphyxia cerebral hemodynamics in newborn lambs, *Pediatr Res* 27:454-459, 1990.
127. Corbett RJ, Laptook AR, Ruley JI, Garcia D: The effect of age on glucose-modulated cerebral agonal glycolytic rates measured in vivo by ¹H NMR spectroscopy, *Pediatr Res* 30:579-586, 1991.
128. Laptook AR, Corbett RJ, Nunnally RL: Effect of plasma glucose concentration on cerebral metabolism during partial ischemia in neonatal piglets, *Stroke* 21:435-440, 1990.
129. Hattori H, Wasterlain CG: Posthypoxic glucose supplement reduces hypoxic-ischemic brain damage in the neonatal rat, *Ann Neurol* 28:122-128, 1990.
130. Callahan DJ, Engle MJ, Volpe JJ: Hypoxic injury to developing glial cells: Protective effect of high glucose, *Pediatr Res* 27:186-190, 1990.
131. Hope PL, Cady EB, Delpy DT, Ives NK, et al: Brain metabolism and intracellular pH during ischaemia: Effects of systemic glucose and bicarbonate administration studied by ³¹P and ¹H nuclear magnetic resonance spectroscopy in vivo in the lamb, *J Neurochem* 50:1394-1402, 1988.
132. Young RS, Petroff OA, Chen B, Aquila WJ Jr, et al: Preferential utilization of lactate in neonatal dog brain: In vivo and in vitro proton NMR study, *Biol Neonate* 59:46-53, 1991.
133. Vicario C, Arizmendi C, Malloch G, Clark JB, et al: Lactate utilization by isolated cells from early neonatal rat brain, *J Neurochem* 57:1700-1707, 1991.
134. Dombrowski GJ Jr, Swiatek KR, Chao KL: Lactate, 3-hydroxybutyrate, and glucose as substrates for the early postnatal rat brain, *Neurochem Res* 14:667-675, 1989.
135. Sheldon RA, Partridge JC, Ferriero DM: Postischemic hyperglycemia is not protective to the neonatal rat brain, *Pediatr Res* 32:489-493, 1992.
136. LeBlanc MH, Huang M, Vig V, Patel D, et al: Glucose affects the severity of hypoxic-ischemic brain injury in newborn pigs, *Stroke* 24:1055-1062, 1993.
137. Leblanc MH, Huang M, Patel D, Smith EE, et al: Glucose given after hypoxic ischemia does not affect brain injury in piglets, *Stroke* 25:1443-1447, 1994.
138. Petersson KH, Pinar H, Stopa EG, Sadowska GB, et al: Effects of exogenous glucose on brain ischemia in ovine fetuses, *Pediatr Res* 56:621-629, 2004.
139. Fazekas JF, Alexander FAD, Himwich HE: Tolerance of the newborn to anoxia, *Am J Physiol* 134:281-290, 1941.
140. Glass HG, Snyder FF, Webster E: The rate of decline in resistance to anoxia of rabbits, dogs, and guinea pigs from the onset of viability to adult life, *Am J Physiol* 140:609-614, 1944.
141. Himwich HE, Alexander FAD, Fazekas JF: Tolerance of the newborn to hypoxia and anoxia, *Am J Physiol* 133:327-339, 1941.
142. Kabat H: The greater resistance of very young animals to arrest of the brain circulation, *Am J Physiol* 130:588-595, 1940.
143. Jilek L, Fischer J, Kruligh L, Trojan S: The reaction of the brain to stagnant hypoxia and anoxia during ontogeny: The developing brain, *Prog Brain Res* 9:113, 1964.
144. Lowry OH, Passonneau JV, Hasselberger FX, Schulz D: Effect of ischemia on known substrates and cofactors of the glycolytic pathway in brain, *J Biol Chem* 239:18-30, 1964.
145. Samson FE Jr, Balfour WM, Dahl NA: Rate of cerebral ATP utilization in rats, *Am J Physiol* 198:213-216, 1960.
146. Bickler PE, Gallego SM, Hansen BM: Developmental changes in intracellular calcium regulation in rat cerebral cortex during hypoxia, *J Cereb Blood Flow Metab* 13:811-819, 1993.
147. Yager JY, Shuaib A, Thornhill J: The effect of age on susceptibility to brain damage in a model of global hemispheric hypoxia-ischemia, *Develop Br Res* 93:143-154, 1996.
148. Yager JY, Thornhill JA: The effect of age on susceptibility to hypoxic-ischemic brain damage, *Neurosci Biobehav Rev* 21:167-174, 1997.
149. Towfighi J, Mauger D, Vannucci RC, Vannucci SJ: Influence of age on the cerebral lesions in an immature rat model of cerebral hypoxia-ischemia: A light microscopic study, *Dev Brain Res* 100:149-160, 1997.
150. Weisbrot IM, James LS, Prince CE: Acid-base homeostasis of the newborn infant during the first 24 hours of life, *J Pediatr* 52:395-403, 1958.
151. Comline RS, Silver M: The composition of foetal and maternal blood during parturition in the ewe, *J Physiol* 222:233-256, 1972.
152. Purves MJ, James IM: Observations on the control of cerebral blood flow in the sheep fetus and newborn lamb, *Circ Res* 25:651-667, 1969.
153. Lucas W, Kirschbaum T, Assali NS: Cephalic circulation and oxygen consumption before and after birth, *Am J Physiol* 210:287-292, 1966.
154. Behrman RE, Lees MH, Peterson EN, De Lannoy CW, et al: Distribution of the circulation in the normal and asphyxiated fetal primate, *Am J Obstet Gynecol* 108:956-969, 1970.
155. Vannucci RC, Duffy TE: Influence of birth on carbohydrate and energy metabolism in rat brain, *Am J Physiol* 226:933-940, 1974.
156. Kohle SJ, Vannucci RC: Glycogen metabolism in fetal and postnatal rat brain: Influence of birth, *J Neurochem* 28:441-443, 1977.
157. Gidday JM, Fitzgibbons JC, Shah AR: Neuroprotection from ischemic brain injury by hypoxic preconditioning in the neonatal rat, *Neurosci Lett* 1768:221-224, 1994.
158. Vannucci RC, Towfighi J, Vannucci SJ: Hypoxic preconditioning and hypoxic-ischemic brain damage in the immature rat: Pathologic and metabolic correlates, *J Neurochem* 71:1215-1220, 1998.
159. Brucklacher RM, Vannucci RC, Vannucci SJ: Hypoxic preconditioning increases brain glycogen and delays energy depletion from hypoxia-ischemia in the immature rat, *Dev Neurosci* 24:411-417, 2002.
160. Gidday JM: Cerebral preconditioning and ischaemic tolerance, *Nat Rev Neurosci* 7:437-448, 2006.
161. Pulsinelli WA, Levy DE, Duffy TE: Regional cerebral blood flow and glucose metabolism following transient forebrain ischemia, *Ann Neurol* 11:499-509, 1982.
162. Pulsinelli WA, Brierley JB, Plum F: Temporal profile of neuronal damage in a model of transient forebrain ischemia, *Ann Neurol* 11:491-498, 1982.
163. Pulsinelli WA, Duffy TE: Regional energy balance in rat brain after transient forebrain ischemia, *J Neurochem* 40:1500-1503, 1983.
164. Petito CK, Pulsinelli WA: Delayed neuronal recovery and neuronal death in rat hippocampus following severe cerebral ischemia: Possible relationship to abnormalities in neuronal processes, *J Cereb Blood Flow Metab* 4:194-205, 1984.
165. Arai H, Passonneau JV, Lust WD: Energy metabolism in delayed neuronal death of CA1 neurons of the hippocampus following transient ischemia in the gerbil, *Metab Brain Dis* 1:263-278, 1986.
166. Petito CK, Feldmann E, Pulsinelli WA, Plum F: Delayed hippocampal damage in humans following cardiorespiratory arrest, *Neurology* 37:1281-1286, 1987.
167. Kuroiwa T, Bonnekoh P, Hossmann KA: Therapeutic window of CA1 neuronal damage defined by an ultrashort-acting barbiturate after brain ischemia in gerbils, *Stroke* 21:1489-1493, 1990.
168. Horn M, Schlote W: Delayed neuronal death and delayed neuronal recovery in the human brain following global ischemia, *Acta Neuropathol* 85:79-87, 1992.
169. Abe K, Aoki M, Kawagoe J, Yoshida T, et al: Ischemic delayed neuronal death: A mitochondrial hypothesis, *Stroke* 26:1478-1489, 1995.
170. Petito CK, Olarte J-P, Roberts B, Nowak TS, et al: Selective glial vulnerability following transient global ischemia in rat brain, *J Neuropathol Exp Neurol* 57:231-238, 1998.
171. Gwag BJ, Koh JY, Chen MM, Dugan LL, et al: BDNF or IGF-1 potentiates free radical-mediated injury in cortical cell cultures, *Neuroreport* 7:93-96, 1995.

172. Bruck Y, Bruck W, Kretzschmar HA, Lassmann H: Evidence for neuronal apoptosis in pontosubicular neuron necrosis, *Neuropathol Appl Neurobiol* 22:23-29, 1996.
173. Edwards AD, Mehmet H: Apoptosis in perinatal hypoxic-ischaemic cerebral damage, *Neuropathol Appl Neurobiol* 22:482-503, 1996.
174. Choi DW: Ischemia-induced neuronal apoptosis, *Curr Opin Neurobiol* 6:667-672, 1996.
175. Yue X, Mehmet H, Penrice J, Cooper C, et al: Apoptosis and necrosis in the newborn piglet brain following transient cerebral hypoxia-ischemia, *Neuropathol Appl Neurobiol* 23:16-25, 1997.
176. McDonald JW, Behrens MI, Chung C, Bhattacharyya T, et al: Susceptibility to apoptosis is enhanced in immature cortical neurons, *Brain Res* 759:228-232, 1997.
177. Kato H, Kanellopoulos GK, Matsuo S, Wu YJ, et al: Neuronal apoptosis and necrosis following spinal cord ischemia in the rat, *Exp Neurol* 148:464-474, 1997.
178. Pulera MR, Adams LM, Liu HT, Santos DG, et al: Apoptosis in a neonatal rat model of cerebral hypoxia-ischemia, *Stroke* 29:2622-2629, 1998.
179. Mazarakis ND, Edwards AD, Mehmet H: Apoptosis in neural development and disease, *Arch Dis Child Fetal Neonatal Ed* 77:F165-F170, 1997.
180. Datta SR, Greenberg ME: Molecular mechanisms of neuronal survival and apoptosis, *Horm Signaling* 1:257-306, 1998.
181. Edwards AD, Yue X, Cox P, Hope PL, et al: Apoptosis in the brains of infants suffering intrauterine cerebral injury, *Pediatr Res* 42:684-689, 1997.
182. Taylor DL, Edwards AD, Mehmet H: Oxidative metabolism, apoptosis and perinatal brain injury, *Brain Pathol* 9:93-117, 1999.
183. Mattson MP, Bazan NG: Apoptosis and necrosis. In Siegel GJ, Albers RW, Brady ST, et al, editors: *Basic Neurochemistry: Molecular, Cellular and Medical Aspects*, 7th ed, New York: 2006, Elsevier.
184. Zhu CL, Xu FL, Wang XY, Shibata M, et al: Different apoptotic mechanisms are activated in male and female brains after neonatal hypoxia-ischaemia, *J Neurochem* 96:1016-1027, 2006.
185. Gill R, Soriano M, Blomgren K, Hagberg H, et al: Role of caspase-3 activation in cerebral ischemia-induced neurodegeneration in adult and neonatal brain, *J Cereb Blood Flow Metab* 22:420-430, 2002.
186. Hu BR, Liu CL, Ouyang Y, Blomgren K, et al: Involvement of caspase-3 in cell death after hypoxia-ischemia declines during brain maturation, *J Cereb Blood Flow Metab* 20:1294-1300, 2000.
187. Liu CL, Siesjo BK, Hu BR: Pathogenesis of hippocampal neuronal death after hypoxia-ischemia changes during brain development, *Neuroscience* 127:113-123, 2004.
188. Zhu C, Wang X, Xu F, Bahr BA, et al: The influence of age on apoptotic and other mechanisms of cell death after cerebral hypoxia-ischemia, *Cell Death Differ* 12:162-176, 2005.
189. Nakajima W, Ishida A, Lange MS, Gabrielson KL, et al: Apoptosis has a prolonged role in the neurodegeneration after hypoxic ischemia in the newborn rat, *J Neurosci* 20:7994-8004, 2000.
190. Northington FJ, Ferriero DM, Flock DL, Martin LJ: Delayed neurodegeneration in neonatal rat thalamus after hypoxia-ischemia is apoptosis, *J Neurosci* 21:1931-1938, 2001.
191. Northington FJ, Ferriero DM, Graham EM, Traystman RJ, et al: Early neurodegeneration after hypoxia-ischemia in neonatal rat is necrosis while delayed neuronal death is apoptosis, *Neurobiol Dis* 8:207-219, 2001.
192. Han BH, D'Costa A, Back SA, Parsadanian M, et al: BDNF blocks caspase-3 activation in neonatal hypoxia-ischemia, *Neurobiol of Disease* 7:38-53, 2000.
193. Manabat C, Han BH, Wendland M, Derugin MA, et al: Reperfusion differentially induces caspase-3 activation in ischemic core and penumbra after stroke in immature brain, *Stroke* 34:207-213, 2003.
194. Aito H, Aalto KT, Raivio KO: Biphasic ATP depletion caused by transient oxidative exposure is associated with apoptotic cell death in rat embryonal cortical neurons, *Pediatr Res* 52:40-45, 2002.
195. Joly L-M, Benjelloun N, Plotkine M, Charriaut-Marlangue C: Distribution of poly-ADP-ribosyl)ation and cell death after cerebral ischemia in the neonatal rat, *Pediatr Res* 53:776-782, 2003.
196. Wang XY, Karlsson JO, Zhu CL, Bahr BA, et al: Caspase-3 activation after neonatal rat cerebral hypoxia-ischemia, *Biol Neonate* 79:172-179, 2001.
197. Daval JL, Pourie G, Grojean S, Lievre V, et al: Neonatal hypoxia triggers transient apoptosis followed by neurogenesis in the rat CA1 hippocampus, *Pediatr Res* 55:561-567, 2004.
198. Malagelada C, Xifro X, Minano A, Sabria J, et al: Contribution of caspase-mediated apoptosis to the cell death caused by oxygen-glucose deprivation in cortical cell cultures, *Neurobiol Dis* 20:27-37, 2005.
199. Siesjo BK, Wieloch T: Molecular mechanisms of ischemic brain damage: Ca^{2+}-related events. In Plum F, Pulsinelli W, editors: *Cerebrovascular Diseases*, New York: 1985, Raven Press.
200. Cheung JY, Bonventre JV, Malis CD, Leaf A: Calcium and ischemic injury, *N Engl J Med* 314:1670-1676, 1986.
201. Siesjo BK: Calcium and cell death, *Magnesium* 8:223-237, 1989.
202. Meyer FB: Calcium, neuronal hyperexcitability and ischemic injury, *Brain Res Brain Res Rev* 14:227-243, 1989.
203. Siesjo BK: Calcium in the brain under physiological and pathological conditions, *Eur Neurol* 30:3-9, 1990.
204. Siesjö BK: Pathophysiology and treatment of focal cerebral ischemia. I. Pathophysiology, *J Neurosurg* 77:169-184, 1992.
205. Siesjö BK: Pathophysiology and treatment of focal cerebral ischemia. II. Mechanisms of damage and treatment, *J Neurosurg* 77:337-354, 1992.
206. Goldberg MP, Choi DW: Intracellular free calcium increases in cultured cortical neurons deprived of oxygen and glucose, *Stroke* 21(Suppl):III75-III77, 1990.
207. Amagasa M, Ogawa A, Yoshimoto T: Effects of calcium and calcium antagonists against deprivation of glucose and oxygen in guinea pig hippocampal slices, *Brain Res* 526:1-7, 1990.
208. Hashimoto K, Kikuchi H, Ishikawa M, Kobayashi S: Changes in cerebral energy metabolism and calcium levels in relation to delayed neuronal death after ischemia, *Neurosci Lett* 137:165-168, 1992.
209. Choi DW, Hartley DM: Calcium and glutamate-induced cortical neuronal death. In Waxman SG, editor: *Molecular and Cellular Approaches to the Treatment of Neurological Disease*, New York: 1993, Raven Press.
210. Morley P, Hogan MJ, Hakim AM: Calcium-mediated mechanisms of ischemic injury and protection, *Brain Pathol* 4:37-47, 1994.
211. Calvert JW, Zhang JH: Pathophysiology of an hypoxic-ischemic insult during the perinatal period, *Neurol Res* 27:246-260, 2005.
212. Gunn AJ, Mydlar T, Bennet L, Faull RL, et al: The neuroprotective actions of a calcium channel antagonist, flunarizine, in the infant rat, *Pediatr Res* 25:573-576, 1989.
213. De Haan HH, Van Reempts JLH, Borgers M, De Haan J, et al: Possible neuroprotective properties of flunarizine infused after asphyxia in fetal lambs are not explained by effects on cerebral blood flow or systemic blood pressure, *Pediatr Res* 34:379-384, 1993.
214. Ostwald K, Hagberg H, Andine P, Karlsson JO: Upregulation of calpain activity in neonatal rat brain after hypoxic-ischemia, *Brain Res* 630:289-294, 1993.
215. Gunn aJ, Williams CE, Mallard EC, Tan WK, et al: Flunarizine, a calcium channel antagonist is partially prophylactically neuroprotective in hypoxic-ischemic encephalopathy in the fetal sheep, *Pediatr Res* 35:657-663, 1994.
216. Berger R, Lehmann T, Karcher J, Garnier Y, et al: Low dose flunarizine protects the fetal brain from ischemic injury in sheep, *Pediatr Res* 44:277-282, 1998.
217. Fisher SK, Heacock AM, Agranoff BW: Inositol lipids and signal transduction in the nervous system: An update, *J Neurochem* 58:18-38, 1992.
218. Dugan LL, Kim-Han JS: Hypoxic-ischemic brain injury and oxidative stress. In Siegel GJ, Albers RW, Brady ST, et al, editors: *Basic Neurochemistry: Molecular, Cellular and Medical Aspects*, 7th ed, New York: 2006, Elsevier.
218a. Annunziato L, Cataldi M, Pignataro G, Secondo A, et al: Glutamate-independent calcium toxicity: Introduction, *Stroke* 38:661-664, 2007.
219. Louis JC, Magal E, Yavin E: Protein kinase C alterations in the fetal rat brain after global ischemia, *J Biol Chem* 263:19282-19285, 1988.
220. Huang KP: The mechanism of protein kinase C activation, *Trends Neurosci* 12:425-432, 1989.
221. Dawson TM, Bredt DS, Fotuhi M, Hwang PM, et al: Nitric oxide synthase and neuronal NADPH diaphorase in brain and peripheral tissues, *Proc Natl Acad Sci U S A* 88:7797-7801, 1991.
222. Dawson VL, Dawson TM, London ED, Bredt DS, et al: Nitric oxide mediates glutamate neurotoxicity in primary cortical cultures, *Proc Natl Acad Sci U S A* 88:6368-6371, 1991.
223. Vincent SR, Hope BT: Neurons that say NO, *Trends Neurosci* 15:108-113, 1992.
224. Bredt DS, Snyder SH: Nitric oxide, a novel neuronal messenger, *Neuron* 8:3-11, 1992.
225. Siesjö BK, Agardh CD, Bengtsson F: Free radicals and brain damage, *Cerebrovasc Brain Metab Rev* 1:165-211, 1989.
226. Monyer H, Hartley DM, Choi DW: 21-aminosteroids attenuate excitotoxic neuronal injury in cortical cell cultures, *Neuron* 5:121-126, 1990.
227. Sies H: Oxidative stress: From basic research to clinical application, *Am J Med* 91:S31-S38, 1991.
228. Traystman RJ, Kirsch JR, Koehler RC: Oxygen radical mechanisms of brain injury following ischemia and reperfusion, *Am J Physiol* 71:1185-1195, 1991.
229. Fellman V, Raivio KO: Reperfusion injury as the mechanism of brain damage after perinatal asphyxia, *Pediatr Res* 41:599-606, 1997.
230. Palmer C: Iron and oxidative stress in neonatal hypoxic-ischemic brain injury: Directions for therapeutic intervention. In Connor JR, editor: *Metal and Oxidative Damage in Neurological Disorders*, New York: 1997, Plenum Press.
231. Chan PH: Oxygen radical mechanisms in cerebral ischemia and reperfusion. In Hsu CY, editor: *Ischemic Stroke: From Basic Mechanisms to New Drug Development*, Basel: 1998, Karger.
232. Oillett J, Koziel V, Vert P, Daval J-L: Influence of post-hypoxia reoxygenation conditions on energy metabolism and superoxide production in cultured neurons from the rat forebrain, *Pediatr Res* 39:598-603, 1996.
233. Saugstad OD: Role of xanthine oxidase and its inhibitor in hypoxia: Reoxygenation injury, *Pediatrics* 98:103-107, 1996.
234. Bagenholm R, Nilsson UA, Kjellmer I: Formation of free radicals in hypoxic ischemic brain damage in the neonatal rat, assessed by an endogenous spin trap and lipid peroxidation, *Brain Res* 773:132-138, 1997.

235. Bagenholm R, Nilsson A, Gotborg CW, Kjellmer I: Free radicals are formed in the brain of fetal sheep during reperfusion after cerebral ischemia, *Pediatr Res* 43:271-275, 1998.
236. Ikeda T, Murata Y, Quiligan EJ, Parer JT, et al: Brain lipid peroxidation and antioxidant levels in fetal lambs 72 hours after asphyxia by partial umbilical cord occlusion, *Am J Obstet Gynecol* 178:474-478, 1998.
237. Maulik D, Numagami Y, Ohnishi ST, Mishra O, et al: Direct measurement of oxygen free radicals during in utero hypoxia in the fetal guinea pig brain, *Brain Res* 798:166-172, 1998.
238. Shadid M, Moison R, Steenduk P, Hiltermann L, et al: The effect of antioxidative combination therapy on post hypoxic-ischemic perfusion, metabolism, and electrical activity of the newborn brain, *Pediatr Res* 44:119-124, 1998.
239. Shadid M, Buonocore G, Groenendaal F, Moison R, et al: Effect of deferoxamine and allopurinol on non–protein-bound iron concentrations in plasma and cortical brain tissue of newborn lambs following hypoxia-ischemia, *Neurosci Lett* 248:5-8, 1998.
240. Fullerton HJ, Ditelberg JS, Chen SF, Sarco DP, et al: Copper/zinc superoxide dismutase transgenic brain accumulates hydrogen peroxide after perinatal hypoxia ischemia, *Ann Neurol* 44:357-364, 1998.
241. Palmer C, Menzies SL, Roberts RL, Pavlick G, et al: Changes in iron histochemistry after hypoxic-ischemic brain injury in the neonatal rat, *J Neurosci Res* 56:60-71, 1999.
242. Wakatsuki A, Izumiya C, Okatani Y, Sagara Y: Oxidative damage in fetal rat brain induced by ischemia and subsequent reperfusion: Relation to arachidonic acid peroxidation, *Biol Neonate* 76:84-91, 1999.
243. Nakai A, Asakura H, Taniuchi Y, Koshino T, et al: Effect of α-phenyl-N-tert-butyl nitrone (PBN) on fetal cerebral energy metabolism during intrauterine ischemia and reperfusion in rats, *Pediatr Res* 47:451-456, 2000.
244. Tan S, Zhou F, Nielsen VG, Wang ZW, et al: Increased injury following intermittent fetal hypoxia-reoxygenation is associated with increased free radical production in fetal rabbit brain, *J Neuropathol Exp Neurol* 58:972-981, 1999.
245. McQuillen PS, Ferriero DM: Selective vulnerability in the developing central nervous system, *Pediatr Neurol* 30:227-235, 2004.
246. Blomgren K, Hagberg H: Free radicals, mitochondria, and hypoxia-ischemia in the developing brain, *Free Radic Biol Med* 40:388-397, 2006.
247. Gardner AM, Xu FH, Fady C, Jacoby FJ, et al: Apoptotic vs nonapoptotic cytotoxicity induced by hydrogen peroxide, *Free Radic Biol Med* 22:73-83, 1997.
248. Bhat NR, Zhang PS: Hydrogen peroxide activation of multiple mitogen-activated protein kinases in an oligodendrocyte cell line: Role of extracellular signal-regulated kinase in hydrogen peroxide-induced cell death, *J Neurochem* 72:112-119, 1999.
249. Castillo-Melendez M, Chow JA, Walker DW: Lipid peroxidation, caspase-3 immunoreactivity, and pyknosis in late-gestation fetal sheep brain after umbilical cord occlusion, *Pediatr Res* 55:864-871, 2004.
250. Chan PH, Fishman RA: Free fatty acids, oxygen free radicals, and membrane alterations in brain ischemia and injury. In Plum F, Pulsinelli W, editors: *Cerebrovascular Diseases*, New York: 1985, Raven Press.
251. Chan PH, Fishman RA: Transient formation of superoxide radicals in polyunsaturated fatty acid-induced brain swelling, *J Neurochem* 35:1004-1007, 1980.
252. Chan PH, Fishman RA: Alterations of membrane integrity and cellular constituents by arachidonic acid in neuroblastoma and glioma cells, *Brain Res,* 248:151-157, 1982.
253. McCord JM: Oxygen-derived free radicals in postischemic tissue injury, *N Engl J Med* 312:159-163, 1985.
254. Chan PH, Yurko M, Fishman RA: Phospholipid degradation and cellular edema induced by free radicals in brain cortical slices, *J Neurochem* 38:525-531, 1982.
255. Chan PH, Schmidley JW, Fishman RA, Longar SM: Brain injury, edema, and vascular permeability changes induced by oxygen-derived free radicals, *Neurology* 34:315-320, 1984.
256. Demopoulos H, Flamm E, Seligman M: Molecular pathology of lipids in CNS membranes. In Jobsis FF, editor: *Oxygen and Physiological Function*, Dallas: 1977, Professional Information Library.
257. Flamm ES, Demopoulos HB, Seligman ML, Poser RG, et al: Free radicals in cerebral ischemia, *Stroke* 9:445-447, 1978.
258. Yoshida S, Abe K, Busto R, Watson BD, et al: Influence of transient ischemia on lipid-soluble antioxidants, free fatty acids and energy metabolites in rat brain, *Brain Res* 245:307-316, 1982.
259. Chan PH, Chu L, F. CS, Carlson EJ, et al: Reduced neurotoxicity in transgenic mice overexpressing human copper-zinc-superoxide dismutase, *Stroke* 21 (Suppl):III80-III82, 1990.
260. Kitagawa K, Matsumoto M, Oda T, Niinobe M, et al: Free radical generation during brief period of cerebral ischemia may trigger delayed neuronal death, *Neuroscience* 35:551-558, 1990.
261. Kinouchi H, Epstein CJ, Mizui T, Carlson E, et al: Attenuation of focal cerebral ischemic injury in transgenic mice overexpressing CuZn superoxide dismutase, *Proc Natl Acad Sci U S A* 88:11158-11162, 1991.
262. Bast A, Haenen GR, Doelman CJ: Oxidants and antioxidants: State of the art, *Am J Med* 91:2S-13S, 1991.
263. Shimizu T, Wolfe LS: Arachidonic acid cascade and signal transduction, *J Neurochem* 55:1-15, 1990.
264. Dawson TM, Dawson VL, Solomon H, Snyder MD: A novel neuronal messenger molecule in brain: The free radical nitric oxide, *Ann Neurol* 32:297-311, 1992.
265. Halliwell B: Free radicals, antioxidants, and human disease: Curiosity, cause, or consequence?, *Lancet* 344:721-724, 1995.
266. Murphy S: Production of nitric oxide by glial cells: Regulation and potential roles in the CNS, *Glia* 29:1-4, 2000.
267. Saugstad OD: Oxidative stress in the newborn: A 30-year perspective, *Biol Neonate* 88:228-236, 2005.
268. Thiringer K, Blomstrand S, Hrbek A, Karlsson K, et al: Cerebral arteriovenous difference for hypoxanthine and lactate during graded asphyxia in the fetal lamb, *Brain Res* 239:107-117, 1982.
269. Pourcyrous M, Leffler C, Busija D: Postasphyxial increases in prostanoids in cerebrospinal fluid of piglets, *Pediatr Res* 24:229-232, 1988.
270. Kjellmer I, Andiné P, Hagberg H, Thiringer K: Extracellular increase of hypoxanthine and xanthine in the cortex and basal ganglia of fetal lambs during hypoxia-ischemia, *Brain Res* 478:241-247, 1989.
271. Mishra OP, Delivoria-Papadopoulos M: Lipid peroxidation in developing fetal guinea pig brain during normoxia and hypoxia, *Brain Res Dev Brain Res* 45:129-135, 1989.
272. Pourcyrous M, Leffler CW, Mirro R, Busija DW: Brain superoxide anion generation during asphyxia and reventilation in newborn pigs, *Pediatr Res* 28:618-621, 1990.
273. Yavin E, Goldin E, Harel S: Hypoxic-ischemic episodes in the developing brain during intrauterine life. In Braquet P, Robinson L, editors: *New Trends in Lipid Mediators Research*, Basel: 1990, Karger.
274. Goldin E, Harel S, Tomer A, Yavin E: Thromboxane and prostacyclin levels in fetal rabbit brain and placenta after intrauterine partial ischemic episodes, *J Neurochem* 54:587-591, 1990.
275. Hasegawa K, Yoshioka H, Sawada T, Nishikawa H: Lipid peroxidation in neonatal mouse brain subjected to two different types of hypoxia, *Brain Dev* 13:101-103, 1991.
276. Razdan B, Marro PJ, Tammela O, Goel R, et al: Selective sensitivity of synaptosomal membrane function to cerebral cortical hypoxia in newborn piglets, *Brain Res* 600:308-314, 1993.
277. Palmer C, Towfighi J, Roberts RL, Heitjan DF: Allopurinol administered after inducing hypoxia-ischemia reduces brain injury in 7-day-old rats, *Pediatr Res* 33:405-411, 1993.
278. Thordstein M, Bagenholm R, Thiringer K, Kjellmer I: Scavengers of free oxygen radicals in combination with magnesium ameliorate perinatal hypoxic-ischemic brain damage in the rat, *Pediatr Res* 34:23-26, 1993.
279. Pourcyrous M, Leffler CW, Bada HS, Korones SB, et al: Brain superoxide anion generation in asphyxiated piglets and the effect of indomethacin at therapeutic dose, *Pediatr Res* 34:366-369, 1993.
280. Stoltenberg L, Rootwelt T, Oyasaeter S, Rognum TO, et al: Hypoxanthine, xanthine, and uric acid concentrations in plasma, cerebrospinal fluid, vitreous humor, and urine in piglets subjected to intermittent versus continuous hypoxemia, *Pediatr Res* 34:767-771, 1993.
281. Kirsch JR, Helfaer MA, Haun SE, Koehler RC, et al: Polyethylene glycol-conjugated superoxide dismutase improves recovery of postischemic hypercapnic cerebral blood flow in piglets, *Pediatr Res* 34:530-537, 1993.
282. Ditelberg JS, Sheldon RA, Epstein CJ, Ferriero DM: Brain injury after perinatal hypoxia-ischemia is exacerbated in copper/zinc superoxide dismutase transgenic mice, *Pediatr Res* 39:204-208, 1996.
283. Capani F, Loidl CF, Aguirre F, Piehl L, et al: Changes in reactive oxygen species (ROS) production in rat brain during global perinatal asphyxia: An ESR study, *Brain Res* 914:204-207, 2001.
284. Ortega-Gutierrez S, Garcia JJ, MartinezBallarin E, Reiter RJ, et al: Melatonin improves deferoxamine antioxidant activity in protecting against lipid peroxidation caused by hydrogen peroxide in rat brain homogenates, *Neurosci Lett* 323:55-59, 2002.
285. Shimizu K, Rajapakse N, Horiguchi T, Payne RM, et al: Neuroprotection against hypoxia-ischemia in neonatal rat brain by novel superoxide dismutase mimetics, *Neurosci Lett* 346:41-44, 2003.
286. Nakai A, Shibazaki Y, Taniuchi Y, Oya A, et al: Vitamins ameliorate secondary mitochondrial failure in neonatal rat brain, *Pediatr Neurol* 27:30-35, 2002.
287. Sanchez-Alvarez R, Almeida A, Medina JM: Oxidative stress in preterm rat brain is due to mitochondrial dysfunction, *Pediatr Res* 51:34-39, 2002.
288. Calamandrei G, Venerosi A, Valazano A, De Berardinis MA, et al: Increased brain levels of F2-isoprostane are an early marker of behavioral sequels in a rat model of global perinatal asphyxia, *Pediatr Res* 55:85-92, 2004.
289. Rosenberg AA, Murdaugh E, White CW: The role of oxygen free radicals in postasphyxia cerebral hypoperfusion in newborn lambs, *Pediatr Res* 26:215-219, 1989.
290. Rosenberg AA, Parks JK, Murdaugh E, Parker WD Jr: Mitochondrial function after asphyxia in newborn lambs, *Stroke* 20:674-679, 1989.
291. Mcgowan JE, Mcgowan JC, Mishra OP, Delivoria-Papadopoulos M: Effect of cyclooxygenase inhibition on brain cell membrane lipid peroxidation during hypoxia in newborn piglets, *Biol Neonate* 66:367-375, 1994.
292. Goplerud JM, Kim S, Delivoria-Papadopoulos M: The effect of postasphyxial reoxygenation with 21% vs 100% oxygen on Na+,K+-ATPase activity in striatum of newborn piglets, *Brain Res* 696:161-164, 1995.

293. Almli LM, Hamrick SEG, Koshy AA, Tauber MG, et al: Multiple pathways of neuroprotection against oxidative stress and excitotoxic injury in immature primary hippocampal neurons, *Dev Brain Res* 132:121-129, 2001.

294. Peeters-Scholte CP, Braun K, Koster J, Kops N, et al: Effects of allopurinol and deferoxamine on reperfusion injury of the brain in newborn piglets after neonatal hypoxia-ischemia, *Pediatr Res* 54:516-522, 2003.

295. Sarco DP, Becker J, Palmer C, Sheldon RA, et al: The neuroprotective effect of deferoxamine in the hypoxic-ischemic immature mouse brain, *Neurosci Lett* 282:113-116, 2000.

296. Osakada F, Hashino A, Kume T, Katsuki H, et al: alpha-Tocotrienol provides the most potent neuroprotection among vitamin E analogs on cultured striatal neurons, *Neuropharmacology* 47:904-915, 2004.

297. Nakajima Y, Masaoka N, Hayakawa Y, Watanabe M, et al: The production of hydroxyl radicals in the fetal lamb brain resulting from occlusion of the umbilical circulation and the transplacental effect of MCI-186 to inhibit hydroxyl radical production, *Pediatr Res* 59:216-220, 2006.

298. Noor JI, Ikeda T, Ueda Y, Ikenoue T: A free radical scavenger, edaravone, inhibits lipid peroxidation and the production of nitric oxide in hypoxic-ischemic brain damage of neonatal rats, *Am J Obstet Gynecol* 193:1703-1708, 2005.

299. Yasuoka N, Nakajima W, Ishida A, Takada G: Neuroprotection of edaravone on hypoxic-ischemic brain injury in neonatal rats, *Dev Brain Res* 151:129-139, 2004.

300. Dorrepaal CA, Berger HM, Benders MJ, van Zoeren-Grobben D, et al: Nonprotein-bound iron in postasphyxial reperfusion injury of the newborn, *Pediatrics* 98:883-889, 1996.

301. Dorrepaal CA, Van Bel F, Moison RM, Shadid M, et al: Oxidative stress during post-hypoxic-ischemic reperfusion in the newborn lamb: The effect of nitric oxide synthesis inhibition, *Pediatr Res* 41:321-326, 1997.

302. Adcock LM, Yamashita Y, Goddard-Finegold J, Smith CV: Cerebral hypoxia-ischemia increases microsomal iron in newborn piglets, *Metab Brain Dis* 11:359-367, 1996.

303. Lipscomb DC, Gorman LG, Traystman RJ, Hurn PD: Low molecular weight iron in cerebral ischemic acidosis in vivo, *Stroke* 29:487-493, 1998.

304. Ogihara T, Hirano K, Ogihara H, Misaki K, et al: Non–protein-bound transition metals and hydroxyl radical generation in cerebrospinal fluid of newborn infants with hypoxic ischemic encephalopathy, *Pediatr Res* 53:594-599, 2003.

305. Yu T, Kui LQ, Ming QZ: Effect of asphyxia on non–protein-bound iron and lipid peroxidation in newborn infants, *Dev Med Child Neurol* 45:24-27, 2003.

306. Lafemina MJ, Sheldon RA, Ferriero DM: Acute hypoxia-ischemia results in hydrogen peroxide accumulation in neonatal but not adult mouse brain, *Pediatr Res* 59:680-683, 2006.

307. Sheldon RA, Jiang X, Francisco C, Christen S, et al: Manipulation of antioxidant pathways in neonatal murine brain, *Pediatr Res* 56:656-662, 2004.

308. McLean CW, Mirochnitchenko O, Claus CP, Noble-Haeusslein LJ, et al: Overexpression of glutathione peroxidase protects immature murine neurons from oxidative stress, *Dev Neurosci* 27:169-175, 2005.

309. Wallin C, Puka-Sundvall M, Hagberg H, Weber SG, et al: Alterations in glutathione and amino acid concentrations after hypoxia-ischemia in the immature rat brain, *Dev Brain Res* 125:51-60, 2000.

310. Lubec G, Widness JA, Hayde M, Menzel D, et al: Hydroxyl radical generation in oxygen-treated infants, *Pediatrics* 100:700-704, 1997.

311. Temesvari P, Karg E, Bodi I, Nemeth I, et al: Impaired early neurologic outcome in newborn piglets reoxygenated with 100% oxygen compared with room air after pneumothorax-induced asphyxia, *Pediatr Res* 49:812-815, 2001.

312. Munkeby BH, Borke WB, Bjornland K, Sikkeland LI, et al: Resuscitation with 100% O_2 increases cerebral injury in hypoxemic piglets, *Pediatr Res* 56:783-790, 2004.

313. Maniscalco WM, Watkins RH, Roper JM, Staversky R, et al: Hyperoxic ventilated premature baboons have increased p53, oxidant DNA damage and decreased VEGF expression, *Pediatr Res* 58:549-556, 2005.

314. Dohlen G, Carlsen H, Blomhoff R, Thaulow E, et al: Reoxygenation of hypoxic mice with 100% oxygen induces brain nuclear factor-kappa B, *Pediatr Res* 58:941-945, 2005.

315. Shimabuku R, Ota A, Pereyra S, Veliz B, et al: Hyperoxia with 100% oxygen following hypoxia-ischemia increases brain damage in newborn rats, *Biol Neonate* 88:168-171, 2005.

316. Fugelseth D, Borke WB, Lenes K, Matthews I, et al: Restoration of cardiopulmonary function with 21% versus 100% oxygen after hypoxaemia in newborn pigs, *Arch Dis Child Fetal Neonatal Ed* 90:F229-F234, 2005.

316a. Solberg R, Andresen JH, Escrig R, Vento M, et al: Resuscitation of hypoxic newborn piglets with oxygen induces a dose-dependent increase in markers of oxidation, *Pediatr Res* 62:559-563, 2007.

317. Dawson TM, Snyder SH: Gases as biological messengers: Nitric oxide and carbon monoxide in the brain, *J Neurosci* 14:5147-5159, 1994.

318. Dalkara T, Moskowitz MA: The complex role of nitric oxide in the pathophysiology of focal cerebral ischemia, *Brain Pathol* 4:49-57, 1994.

319. Dawson TM, Dawson VL: Nitric oxide: Actions and pathological roles, *Neuroscientist* 1:7-18, 1995.

320. Murphy S, Grzybicki D: Glial NO: Normal and pathological roles, *Neuroscientist* 2:90-99, 1996.

321. Ergenekon E, Gucuyener K: Nitric oxide in developing brain, *Eur J Paediatr Neurol* 2:297-301, 1998.

322. Dalkara T, Moskowitz MA: Nitric oxide in cerebrovascular regulation and ischemia. In Hsu CY, editor: *Ischemic Stroke: From Basic Mechanisms to New Drug Development*, Basel: 1998, Karger.

323. Ohyu J, Takashima S: Developmental characteristics of neuronal nitric oxide synthase (nNOS) immunoreactive neurons in fetal to adolescent human brains, *Dev Brain Res* 110:193-202, 1998.

324. Beckman JS, Viera L, Estevez AG, Teng R: Nitric oxide and peroxynitrite in the perinatal period, *Semin Perinatol* 24:37-41, 2000.

325. Kindler DD, Thiffault C, Solenski NJ, Dennis J, et al: Neurotoxic nitric oxide rapidly depolarizes and permeabilizes mitochondria by dynamically opening the mitochondrial transition pore, *Mol Cellular Neurosci* 23:559-573, 2003.

326. Waxman SG: Nitric oxide and the axonal death cascade, *Ann Neurol* 53:150-153, 2003.

327. Garthwaite G, Goodwin DA, Batchelor AM, Leeming K, et al: Nitric oxide toxicity in CNS white matter: An in vitro study using rat optic nerve, *Neuroscience* 109:145-155, 2002.

328. Ischiropoulos H, Beckman JS: Oxidative stress and nitration in neurodegeneration: Cause, effect, or association? *J Clin Invest* 111:163-169, 2003.

329. Guix FX, Uribesalgo I, Coma M, Munoz FJ: The physiology and pathophysiology of nitric oxide in the brain, *Prog Neurobiol* 76:126-152, 2005.

330. Wainwright MS, Grundhoefer D, Sharma S, Black SM: A nitric oxide donor reduces brain injury and enhances recovery of cerebral blood flow after hypoxia-ischemia in the newborn rat, *Neurosci Lett* 415:124-129, 2007.

331. Lipton SA, Choi Y-B, Pan Z-H, Lei SZ, et al: A redox-based mechanism for the neuroprotective and neurodestructive effects of nitric oxide and related nitroso-compounds, *Nature* 364:626-632, 1993.

332. Tsuji M, Higuchi Y, Shiraishi K, Kume T, et al: Protective effect of aminoguanidine on hypoxic-ischemic brain damage and temporal profile of brain nitric oxide in neonatal rat, *Pediatr Res* 47:79-83, 2000.

333. Araujo IM, Verdasca MJ, Ambrosio AF, Carvalho CM: Nitric oxide inhibits complex I following AMPA receptor activation via peroxynitrite, *Neuroreport* 15:2007-2011, 2004.

334. Brown GC, Cooper CE: Nanomolar concentrations of nitric oxide reversibly inhibit synaptosomal respiration by competing with oxygen at cytochrome oxidase, *FEBS Lett* 356:295-298, 1994.

335. Ferriero DM, Sheldon RA, Black SM, Chuai J: Selective destruction of nitric oxide synthase neurons with quisqualate reduces damage after hypoxia-ischemia in the neonatal rat, *Pediatr Res* 38:912-918, 1995.

336. Tan WKM, Williams CE, During MJ, Mallard CE, et al: Accumulation of cytotoxins during the development of seizures and edema after hypoxic-ischemic injury in late gestation fetal sheep, *Pediatr Res* 39:791-797, 1996.

337. Higuchi Y, Hattori H, Hattori R, Furusho K: Increased neurons containing neuronal nitric oxide synthase in the brain of a hypoxic-ichemic neonatal rat model, *Brain Dev* 18:369-375, 1996.

338. Bolanos JP, Almeida A, Medina JM: Nitric oxide mediates brain mitochondrial damage during perinatal anoxia, *Brain Res* 787:117-122, 1998.

339. Groenendaal F, Mishra P, McGowan JE, Hoffman DJ, et al: Function of cell membranes in cerebral cortical tissue of newborn piglets after hypoxia and inhibition of nitric oxide synthase, *Pediatr Res* 42:174-179, 1997.

340. Numagami Y, Zubrow AB, Mishra OP, Delivoria Papadopoulos M: Lipid free radical generation and brain cell membrane alteration following nitric oxide synthase inhibition during cerebral hypoxia in the newborn piglet, *J Neurochem* 69:1542-1547, 1997.

341. van Bel F, Sola A, Roman C, Rudolph AM: Role of nitric oxide in the regulation of the cerebral circulation in the lamb fetus during normoxemia and hypoxemia, *Biol Neonate* 68:200-210, 1995.

342. Marks KA, Mallard CE, Roberts I, Williams CE, et al: Nitric oxide synthase inhibition attenuates delayed vasodilation and increases injury after cerebral ischemia in fetal sheep, *Pediatr Res* 40:185-191, 1996.

343. van Bel F, Sola A, Roman C, Rudolph AM: Perinatal regulation of the cerebral circulation: Role of nitric oxide and prostaglandins, *Pediatr Res* 42:299-304, 1997.

344. Ioroi T, Yonetani M, Nakamura H: Effects of hypoxia and reoxygenation on nitric oxide production and cerebral blood flow in developing rat striatum, *Pediatr Res* 43:733-737, 1998.

345. Beasley TC, Bari F, Thore C, Thrikawala N, et al: Cerebral ischemia/reperfusion increases endothelial nitric oxide synthase level by an indomethacin-sensitive mechanism, *J Cereb Blood Flow Metab* 18:88-96, 1998.

346. Blumberg RM, Taylor DL, Yue X, Aguan K, et al: Increased nitric oxide synthesis is not involved in delayed cerebral energy failure following focal hypoxic-ischemic injury to the developing brain, *Pediatr Res* 46:224-231, 1999.

347. Marks KA, Mallard CE, Roberts I, Williams CE, et al: Nitric oxide synthase inhibition and delayed cerebral injury after severe cerebral ischemia in fetal sheep, *Pediatr Res* 46:8-13, 1999.

348. Groenendaal F, De Graaf, RA Van, Vliet G, Nicolay K: Effects of hypoxia-ischemia and inhibition of nitric oxide synthase on cerebral energy metabolism in newborn piglets, *Pediatr Res* 45:827-833, 1999.

349. Ashwal S, Tone B, Tian HR, Cole DJ, et al: Core and penumbral nitric oxide synthase activity during cerebral ischemia and reperfusion in the rat pup, *Pediatr Res* 46:390-400, 1999.

350. Gidday JM, Shah AR, Maceren RG, Wang QO, et al: Nitric oxide mediates cerebral ischemic tolerance in a neonatal rat model of hypoxic preconditioning, *J Cereb Blood Flow Metab* 19:331-340, 1999.

351. Mishra OP, Zanelli S, Ohnishi ST, Delivoria-Papadopoulos M: Hypoxia-induced generation of nitric oxide free radicals in cerebral cortex of newborn guinea pigs, *Neurochem Res* 25:1559-1565, 2000.

352. Pryor EC, Zhang J, Massmann A, Figueroa JP: Prolonged mild fetal hypoxia up-regulates type I nitric oxide synthase expression in discrete areas of the late-gestation fetal sheep brain, *Am J Obstet Gynecol* 187:164-170, 2002.

353. Peeters-Scholte CP, Koster J, Veldhuis W, van den Tweel E, et al: Neuroprotection by selective nitric oxide synthase inhibition at 24 hours after perinatal hypoxia-ischemia, *Stroke* 33:2304-2310, 2002.

354. Feng Y, Piletz JE, LeBlanc MH: Agmatine suppresses nitric oxide production and attenuates hypoxic-ischemic brain injury in neonatal rats, *Pediatr Res* 52:606-611, 2002.

355. Siesjö BK, Memezawa H, Smith ML: Neurocytotoxicity: Pharmacological implications, *Fundam Clin Pharmacol* 5:755-767, 1991.

356. Beneveniste H: The excitotoxin hypothesis in relation to cerebral ischemia, *Cerebrovasc Metab Rev* 3:213-245, 1991.

357. Greenamyre JT, Porter RHP: Anatomy and physiology of glutamate in the CNS, *Neurology* 44(Suppl):S7-S13, 1994.

358. Johnston MV, Ishiwa S: Ischemia and excitotoxins in development, *Ment Retard Dev Disabil Res Rev* 1:193-200, 1995.

359. Johnston MV: Neurotransmitters and vulnerability of the developing brain, *Brain Dev* 17:301-306, 1995.

360. Johnston MV: Hypoxic and ischemic disorders of infants and children: Lecture for 38th meeting of Japanese Society of Child Neurology, Tokyo, Japan, July 1996, *Brain Dev* 19:235-239, 1997.

361. Bittigau P, Ikonomidou C: Glutamate in neurologic diseases, *J Child Neurol* 12:471-485, 1997.

362. Choi DW, Lobner D, Dugan LL: Glutamate receptor-mediated neuronal death in the ischemic brain. In Hsu CY, editor: *Ischemic Stroke: From Basic Mechanisms to New Drug Development*, Basel: 1998, Karger.

363. Hassel B, Dingledine R: Glutamate. In Siegel GJ, Albers RW, Brady ST, et al, editors: *Basic Neurochemistry: Molecular, Cellular and Medical Aspects*, 7th ed, New York: 2006, Elsevier.

364. Ogata T, Nakamura Y, Shibata T, Kataoka K: Release of excitatory amino acids from cultured hippocampal astrocytes induced by a hypoxic-hypoglycemic stimulation, *J Neurochem* 58:1957-1959, 1992.

365. Young AB, Penney JB: Benzodiazepine, GABA, and glutamate receptors in cerebral cortex, hippocampus, basa ganglia, and cerebellum, *Receptors in the Human Nervous System*. In New York: 1991, Academic Press.

366. Sladeczek F, Récasens M, Bockaert J: A new mechanism for glutamate receptor action: Phosphoinositide hydrolysis, *Trends Neurosci* 11:545-549, 1988.

367. Young AB, Fagg GE: Excitatory amino acid receptors in the brain: Membrane binding and receptor autoradiographic approaches, *Trends Pharmacol Sci* 11:126-133, 1990.

368. Schoepp D, Bockaert J, Sladeczek F: Pharmacological and functional characteristics of metabotropic excitatory amino acid receptors, *Trends Pharmacol Sci* 11:508-515, 1990.

369. Meldrum B: Protection against ischaemic neuronal damage by drugs acting on excitatory neurotransmission, *Cerebrovasc Brain Metab Rev* 2:27-57, 1990.

370. Baskys A: Metabotropic receptors and 'slow' excitatory actions of glutamate agonists in the hippocampus, *Trends Neurosci* 15:92-96, 1992.

371. Gasic GP, Hollmann M: Molecular neurobiology of glutamate receptors, *Annu Rev Physiol* 54:507-536, 1992.

372. Blackstone CD, Levey AI, Martin LJ, Price DL, et al: Immunological detection of glutamate receptor subtypes in human central nervous system, *Ann Neurol* 31:680-683, 1992.

373. Barnes JM, Henley JM: Molecular characteristics of excitatory amino acid receptors, *Prog Neurobiol* 39:113-133, 1992.

374. Zorumski CF, Thio LL: Properties of vertebrate glutamate receptors: Calcium mobilization and desensitization, *Prog Neurobiol* 39:295-336, 1992.

375. Choi DW: Excitotoxic cell death, *J Neurobiol* 23:1261-1276, 1992.

376. Ginsberg MD: Emerging strategies for the treatment of ischemic brain injury. In Waxman SG, editor: *Molecular and Cellular Approaches to the Treatment of Neurological Disease*, New York: 1993, Raven Press.

377. Schoepp DD, Conn PJ: Metabotropic glutamate receptors in brain function and pathology, *Trends Pharmacol Sci* 14:13-20, 1993.

378. Westbrook GL: Glutamate receptors and excitotoxicity. In Waxman SG, editor: *Molecular and Cellular Approaches to the Treatment of Neurological Disease*, New York: 1993, Raven Press.

379. Young AB, Sakurai SY, Albin RL, Makowiec R, et al: Excitatory amino acid receptor distribution: Quantitative autoradiographic studies. In *Excitatory Amino Acids and Synaptic Function*, Ann Arbor, MI: 1991, Academic Press.

380. Sanchez RM, Koh S, Rio C, Wang C, et al: Decreased glutamate receptor 2 expression and enhanced epileptogenesis in immature rat hippocampus after perinatal hypoxia-induced seizures, *J Neurosci* 21:8154-8163, 2001.

381. Sanchez RM, Jensen FE: Maturational aspects of epilepsy mechanisms and consequences for the immature brain, *Epilepsia* 42:577-585, 2001.

382. Talos DM, Fishman RE, Park H, Folkerth RD, et al: Developmental regulation of alpha-amino-3-hydroxy-5-methyl-4-isoxazole-propionic acid receptor subunit expression in forebrain and relationship to regional susceptibility to hypoxic/ischemic injury. I. Rodent cerebral white matter and cortex, *J Comp Neurol* 497:42-60, 2006.

383. Talos DM, Follett PL, Folkerth RD, Fishman RE, et al: Developmental regulation of alpha-amino-3-hydroxy-5-methyl-4-isoxazole-propionic acid receptor subunit expression in forebrain and relationship to regional susceptibility to hypoxic/ischemic injury. II. Human cerebral white matter and cortex, *J Comp Neurol* 497:61-77, 2006.

384. Tremblay E, Roisin MP, Represa A, Charriaut-Marlangue C, et al: Transient increased density of NMDA binding sites in the developing rat hippocampus, *Brain Res* 461:393-396, 1988.

385. Erdö SL, Wolff JR: Transient increase in ligand binding to quisqualate and kainate sites in cerebral cortex of immature rats, *Neurosci Lett* 104:161-166, 1989.

386. McDonald JW, Johnston MV: Physiological and pathophysiological roles of excitatory amino acids during central nervous system development, *Brain Res Brain Res Rev* 15:41-70, 1990.

387. Hattori H, Wasterlain CG: Excitatory amino acids in the developing brain: Ontogeny, plasticity, and excitotoxicity, *Pediatr Neurol* 6:219-228, 1990.

388. McDonald JW, Johnston MV, Young AB: Differential ontogenic development of three receptors comprising the NMDA receptor/channel complex in the rat hippocampus, *Exp Neurol* 110:237-247, 1990.

389. Barks JDE, Silverstein FS: Excitatory amino acids contribute to the pathogenesis of perinatal hypoxic-ischemic brain injury, *Brain Pathol* 2:235-243, 1992.

390. Piggott MA, Perry EK, Perry RH, Scott D: N-Methyl-D-aspartate (NMDA) and non-NMDA binding sites in developing human frontal cortex, *Neurosci Res Commun* 12:9-16, 1993.

391. Parnavelas JG, Cavanagh ME: Transient expression of neurotransmitters in the developing neocortex, *Trends Neurosci* 11:92-93, 1988.

392. Barks JD, Silverstein FS, Sims K, Greenamyre JT, et al: Glutamate recognition sites in human fetal brain, *Neurosci Lett* 84:131-136, 1988.

393. Represa A, Tremblay E, Ben-Ari Y: Transient increase of NMDA-binding sites in human hippocampus during development, *Neurosci Lett* 99:61-66, 1989.

394. McDonald JW, Silverstein FS, Cardona D, Hudson C, et al: Systemic administration of MK-801 protects against N-methyl-D-aspartate– and quisqualate-mediated neurotoxicity in perinatal rats, *Neuroscience* 36:589-599, 1990.

395. Ritter LM, Unis AS, Meador-Woodruff JH: Ontogeny of ionotropic glutamate receptor expression in human fetal brain, *Dev Brain Res* 127:123-133, 2001.

396. Panigrahy A, Rosenberg PS, Assmann S, Foley EC, et al: Differential expression of glutamate receptor subtypes in human brainstem sites involved in perinatal hypoxia-ischemia, *J Comp Neurol* 437:196-208, 2001.

397. Choi DW: Glutamate neurotoxicity and diseases of the nervous system, *Neuron* 1:623-634, 1988.

398. Choi DW, Rothman SN: The role of glutamate neurotoxicity in hypoxic-ischemic neuronal death, *Annu Rev Neurosci* 12:171-182, 1990.

399. Choi DW: Methods for antagonizing glutamate neurotoxicity, *Cerebrovasc Brain Metab Rev* 2:105-147, 1990.

400. Garthwaite G, Williams GD, Garthwaite J: Glutamate toxicity: An experimental and theoretical analysis, *Eur J Neurosci* 4:353-360, 1992.

401. McDonald JW, Trescher WH, Johnston MV: Susceptibility of brain to AMPA induced excitotoxicity transiently peaks during early postnatal development, *Brain Res* 583:54-70, 1992.

402. Hirose K, Chan PH: Blockade of glutamate excitotoxicity and its clinical applications, *Neurochem Res* 18:479-483, 1993.

403. McDonald JW, Fix AS, Tizzano JP, Schoepp D: Seizures and brain injury in neonatal rats induced by 1S,3R-ACPD, a metabotropic glutamate receptor agonist, *J Neurosci* 13:4445-4455, 1993.

404. Seo SY, Kim EY, Kim H, Gwag BJ: Neuroprotective effect of high glucose against NMDA, free radical, and oxygen-glucose deprivation through enhanced mitochondrial potentials, *J Neurosci* 19:8849-8855, 1999.

405. Rothman SM: Synaptic activity mediates death of hypoxic neurons, *Science* 220:536-537, 1983.

406. Clark GD, Rothman SM: Blockade of excitatory amino acid receptors protects anoxic hippocampal slices, *Neuroscience* 21:665-671, 1987.

407. Rothman S: Synaptic release of excitatory amino acid neurotransmitter mediates anoxic neuronal death, *J Neurosci* 4:1884-1891, 1984.

408. Pulsinelli WA: Deafferentation of the hippocampus protects CA1 pyramidal neurons against ischemic injury, *Stroke* 16:144-152, 1985.

409. Ibarretxe G, Sanchez-Gomez MV, Campos-Esparza MR, Alberdi E, et al: Differential oxidative stress in oligodendrocytes and neurons after excitotoxic insults and protection by natural polyphenols, *Glia* 53:201-211, 2006.

410. Ellrén K, Lehmann A: Calcium dependency of N-methyl-D-aspartate toxicity in slices from the immature rat hippocampus, *Neuroscience* 32:371-379, 1989.

411. Pellegrini-Giampietro DE, Cherici G, Alesiani M, Carla V, et al: Excitatory amino acid release and free radical formation may cooperate in the genesis of ischemia-induced neuronal damage, *J Neurosci* 10:1035-1041, 1990.

412. Sacaan AI, Schoepp DD: Activation of hippocampal metabotropic excitatory amino acid receptors leads to seizures and neuronal damage, *Neurosci Lett* 139:77-82, 1992.

413. Randall RD, Thayer SA: Glutamate-induced calcium transient triggers delayed calcium overload and neurotoxicity in rat hippocampal neurons, *J Neurosci* 12:1882-1895, 1992.

414. Michaels RL, Rothman SM: Glutamate neurotoxicity in vitro: Antagonist pharmacology and intracellular calcium concentrations, *J Neurosci* 10:283-292, 1990.

415. Harada K, Yoshimura T, Nakajima K, Ito H, et al: *N*-Methyl-D-aspartate increases cytosolic Ca²⁺ via G proteins in cultured hippocampal neurons, *Am J Physiol* 262:C870-C875, 1992.

416. Levy DI, Lipton SA: Comparison of delayed administration of competitive and uncompetitive antagonists in preventing NMDA receptor-mediated neuronal death, *Neurology* 40:852-855, 1990.

417. Lipton SA: Prospects for clinically tolerated NMDA antagonists: Open-channel blockers and alternative redox states of nitric oxide, *Trends Neurosci* 16:527-532, 1993.

418. Hagberg H, Gilland E, Diemer NH, Andine P: Hypoxia-ischemia in the neonatal rat brain: Histopathology after post-treatment with NMDA and non-NMDA receptor antagonists, *Biol Neonate* 66:205-213, 1994.

419. Taylor GA, Trescher WH, Johnston MV, Traystman RJ: Experimental neuronal injury in the newborn lamb: A comparison of *N*-methyl-D-aspartic acid receptor blockade and nitric oxide synthesis inhibition on lesion size and cerebral hyperemia, *Pediatr Res* 38:644-651, 1995.

420. Ciani E, Groneng L, Voltattorni M, Rolseth V, et al: Inhibition of free radical production or free radical scavenging protects from the excitotoxic cell death mediated by glutamate in cultures of cerebellar granule neurons, *Brain Res* 728:1-6, 1996.

421. Gressens P, Marret S, Evrard P: Developmental spectrum of the excitotoxic cascade induced by ibotenate: A model of hypoxic insults in fetuses and neonates, *Neuropathol Appl Neurobiol* 22:498-502, 1996.

422. Puka-Sundvall M, Sandberg M, Hagberg H: Brain injury after hypoxia-ischemia in newborn rats: Relationship to extracellular levels of excitatory amino acids and cysteine, *Brain Res* 750:325-328, 1997.

423. Laroia N, McBride L, Baggs R, Guillet R: Dextromethorphan ameliorates effects of neonatal hypoxia on brain morphology and seizure threshold in rats, *Dev Brain Res* 100:29-34, 1997.

424. Henderson JL, Reynolds JD, Dexter F, Atkins B, et al: Chronic hypoxemia causes extracellular glutamate concentration to increase in the cerebral cortex of the near-term fetal sheep, *Dev Brain Res* 105:287-293, 1998.

425. Puka-Sundvall M, Gilland E, Bona E, Lehmann A, et al: Development of brain damage after neonatal hypoxia-ischemia: Excitatory amino acids and cysteine, *Metab Brain Dis* 11:109-123, 1996.

426. Gilland E, Puka-Sundvall M, Hillered L, Hagberg H: Mitochondrial function and energy metabolism after hypoxia-ischemia in the immature rat brain: Involvement of NMDA-receptors, *J Cereb Blood Flow Metab* 18:297-304, 1998.

427. Feet BA, Gilland E, Groenendaal F, Brun NC, et al: Cerebral excitatory amino acids and Na⁺, K⁺-ATPase activity during resuscitation of severely hypoxic newborn piglets, *Acta Paediatr* 87:889-895, 1998.

428. Marret S, Bonnier C, Raymackers J-M, Delpech A, et al: Glycine antagonist and NO synthase inhibitor protect the developing mouse brain against neonatal excitotoxic lesions, *Pediatr Res* 45:337-342, 1999.

429. Poulsen CF, Simeone TA, Maar TE, Smith-Swintosky V, et al: Modulation by topiramate of AMPA and kainate mediated calcium influx in cultured cerebral cortical, hippocampal and cerebellar neurons, *Neurochem Res* 29:275-282, 2004.

430. Spandou E, Karkavelas G, Soubasi V, Avgovstides-Savvopoulou P, et al: Effect of ketamine on hypoxic-ischemic brain damage in newborn rats, *Brain Res* 819:1-7, 1999.

431. Koh S, Jensen FE: Topiramate blocks perinatal hypoxia-induced seizures in rat pups, *Ann Neurol* 50:366-372, 2001.

432. Koh S, Tibayan FD, Simpson JN, Jensen TE: NBQX or topiramate treatment after perinatal hypoxia-induced seizures prevents later increases in seizure-induced neuronal injury, *Epilepsia* 45:569-575, 2004.

433. Yoneda S, Tanaka E, Goto W, Ota T, et al: Topiramate reduces excitotoxic and ischemic injury in the rat retina, *Brain Res* 967:257-266, 2003.

434. Hagberg H, Andersson P, Kjellmer I, Thiringer K, et al: Extracellular overflow of glutamate, aspartate, GABA and taurine in the cortex and basal ganglia of fetal lambs during hypoxia-ischemia, *Neurosci Lett* 78:311-317, 1987.

435. Silverstein FS, Naik B, Simpson J: Hypoxia-ischemia stimulates hippocampal glutamate efflux in perinatal rat brain: An in vivo microdialysis study, *Pediatr Res* 30:587-590, 1991.

436. Gordon KE, Simpson J, Statman D, Silverstein FS: Effects of perinatal stroke on striatal amino acid efflux in rats studied with in vivo microdialysis, *Stroke* 22:928-932, 1991.

437. Andiné P, Sandberg M, Bågenholm R, Lehmann A, et al: Intra- and extracellular changes of amino acids in the cerebral cortex of the neonatal rat during hypoxic-ischemia, *Brain Res Dev Brain Res* 64:115-120, 1991.

438. Cataltepe O, Towfighi J, Vannucci RC: Cerebrospinal fluid concentrations of glutamate and GABA during perinatal cerebral hypoxia-ischemia and seizures, *Brain Res* 709:326-330, 1996.

439. Hagberg H, Peebles D, Mallard C: Models of white matter injury: Comparison of infectious, hypoxic-ischemic, and excitotoxic insults, *Ment Retard Dev Disabil Res Rev* 8:30-38, 2002.

440. Hagberg H: Personal communication, Goteborg, Goteborg University, 1992.

441. Hagberg H, Thornberg E, Blennow M, Kjellmer I, et al: Excitatory amino acids in the cerebrospinal fluid of asphyxiated infants: Relationship to hypoxic ischemic encephalopathy, *Acta Paediatr* 82:925-929, 1993.

442. Groenendaal F, Roelantsvan-Rijn AM, van der, Grond J, Toet MC, et al: Glutamate in cerebral tissue of asphyxiated neonates during the first week of life demonstrated in vivo using proton magnetic resonance spectroscopy, *Biol Neonate* 79:254-257, 2001.

443. Swanson RA, Farrell K, Simon RP: Acidosis causes failure of astrocyte glutamate uptake during hypoxia, *J Cereb Blood Flow Metab* 15:417-424, 1995.

444. Martin LJ, Brambrink AM, Lehmann C, Portera-Cailliau C, et al: Hypoxia-ischemia causes abnormalities in glutamate transporters and death of astroglia and neurons in newborn striatum, *Ann Neurol* 42:335-345, 1997.

445. Szatkowski M, Attwell D: Triggering and execution of neuronal death in brain ischaemia: Two phases of glutamate release by different mechanisms, *Trends Neurosci* 17:359-366, 1994.

446. Krajnc D, Neff NH, Hadjiconstantinou M: Glutamate, glutamine and glutamine synthetase in the neonatal rat brain following hypoxia, *Brain Res* 707:134-137, 1996.

447. Rao SD, Yin HZ, Weiss JH: Disruption of glial glutamate transport by reactive oxygen species produced in motor neurons, *J Neurosci* 23:2627-2633, 2003.

448. Zou JY, Crews FT: TNF alpha potentiates glutamate neurotoxicity by inhibiting glutamate uptake in organotypic brain slice cultures: Neuroprotection by NF kappa B inhibition, *Brain Res* 1034:1-4, 2005.

449. Schiff SJ, Somjen GG: Hyperexcitability following moderate hypoxia in hippocampal tissue slices, *Brain Res* 337:337-340, 1985.

450. Romijn HJ, Ruijter JM, Wolters PS: Hypoxia preferentially destroys GABAergic neurons in developing rat neocortex explants in culture, *Exp Neurol* 100:332-340, 1988.

451. Rossi DJ, Oshima T, Attwell D: Glutamate release in severe brain ischaemia is mainly by reversed uptake, *Nature* 403:316-321, 2000.

452. Cherubini E, Ben-Ari Y, Krnjevic K: Anoxia produces smaller changes in synaptic transmission, membrane potential, and input resistance in immature rat hippocampus, *J Neurophysiol* 62:882-895, 1989.

453. Takeuchi H, Jin S, Wang J, Zhang G, et al: Tumor necrosis factor-alpha induces neurotoxicity via glutamate release from hemichannels of activated microglia in an autocrine manner, *J Biol Chem* 281:21362-21368, 2006.

454. Ikonomidou C, Price MT, Mosinger JL, Frierdich G, et al: Hypobaric-ischemic conditions produce glutamate-like cytopathology in infant rat brain, *J Neurosci* 9:1693-1700, 1989.

455. Stewart GR, Olney JW, Pathikonda M, Snider WD: Excitotoxicity in the embryonic chick spinal cord, *Ann Neurol* 30:758-766, 1991.

456. Young RS, Petroff OA, Aquila WJ, Yates J: Effects of glutamate, quisqualate, and *N*-methyl-D-aspartate in neonatal brain, *Exp Neurol* 111:362-368, 1991.

457. Hattori H, Morin AM, Schwartz PH, Fujikawa DG, et al: Posthypoxic treatment with MK-801 reduces hypoxic-ischemic damage in the neonatal rat, *Neurology* 39:713-718, 1989.

458. Engelsen B: Neurotransmitter glutamate: Its clinical importance, *Acta Neurol Scand* 74:337-355, 1986.

459. Simon RP, Young RS, Stout S, Cheng J: Inhibition of excitatory neurotransmission with kynurenate reduces brain edema in neonatal anoxia, *Neurosci Lett* 71:361-364, 1986.

460. McDonald JW, Silverstein FS, Johnston MV: MK-801 protects the neonatal brain from hypoxic-ischemic damage, *Eur J Pharmacol* 140:359-361, 1987.

461. McDonald JW, Silverstein FS, Johnston MV: Neurotoxicity of *N*-methyl-D-aspartate is markedly enhanced in developing rat central nervous system, *Brain Res* 459:200-203, 1988.

462. McDonald JW, Johnston MV: Pharmacology of *N*-methyl-D-aspartate-induced brain injury in an in vivo perinatal rat model, *Synapse* 6:179-188, 1990.

463. Andiné P, Lehmann A, Ellrén K, Wennberg E, et al: The excitatory amino acid antagonist kynurenic acid administered after hypoxic-ischemia in neonatal rats offers neuroprotection, *Neurosci Lett* 90:208-212, 1988.

464. Ford LM, Sanberg PR, Norman AB, Fogelson MH: MK-801 prevents hippocampal neurodegeneration in neonatal hypoxic-ischemic rats, *Arch Neurol* 46:1090-1096, 1989.

465. Uckele JE, McDonald JW, Johnston MV, Silverstein FS: Effect of glycine and glycine receptor antagonists on NMDA-induced brain injury, *Neurosci Lett* 107:279-283, 1989.

466. Ment LR, Stewart WB, Petroff OA, Duncan CC, et al: Beagle puppy model of perinatal asphyxia: Blockade of excitatory neurotransmitters, *Pediatr Neurol* 5:281-286, 1989.

467. McDonald JW, Uckele J, Silverstein FS, Johnston MV: HA-966 (1-hydroxy-3-aminopyrrolidone-2) selectively reduces *N*-methyl-D-aspartate (NMDA)-mediated brain damage, *Neurosci Lett* 104:167-170, 1989.

468. Olney JW, Ikonomidou C, Mosinger JL, Frierdich G: MK-801 prevents hypobaric-ischemic neuronal degeneration in infant rat brain, *J Neurosci* 9:1701-1704, 1989.

469. LeBlanc MH, Vig V, Smith B, Parker CC, et al: MK-801 does not protect against hypoxic-ischemic brain injury in piglets, *Stroke* 22:1270-1275, 1991.

470. Miller VS: Pharmacologic management of neonatal cerebral ischemia and hemorrhage: Old and new directions, *J Child Neurol* 8:7-18, 1993.

471. McDonald JW, Silverstein FS, Johnston MV: Magnesium reduces *N*-methyl-D-aspartate (NMDA)-mediated brain injury in perinatal rats, *Neurosci Lett* 109:234-238, 1990.

472. Schubert S, Brandl U, Brodhun M, Ulrich C, et al: Neuroprotective effects of topiramate after hypoxia-ischemia in newborn piglets, *Brain Res* 1058:129-136, 2005.

473. Sfaello I, Baud O, Arzimanoglou A, Gressens P: Topiramate prevents excitotoxic damage in the newborn rodent brain, *Neurobiol Dis* 20:87-848, 2005.

474. Noh MR, Kim SK, Sun W, Park SK, et al: Neuroprotective effect of topiramate on hypoxic ischemic brain injury in neonatal rats, *Exp Neurol* 201:470-478, 2006.

475. Wood PL: Microglia as a unique cellular target in the treatment of stroke: Potential neurotoxic mediators produced by activated microglia, *Neurol Res* 17:242-248, 1995.

476. Gehrmann J, Banati RB, Wiessnert C, Hossmann KA, et al: Reactive microglia in cerebral ischaemia: An early mediator of tissue damage, *Neuropathol Appl Neurobiol* 21:277-289, 1995.

477. Soriano SG, Lipton SA, Wang YF, Xiao M, et al: Intercellular adhesion molecule 1–deficient mice are less susceptible to cerebral ischemia: Reperfusion injury, *Ann Neurol* 39:618-624, 1996.

478. Probert L, Akassoglou K, Kassiotis G, Pasparakis M, et al: TNF-α transgenic and knockout models of CNS inflammation and degeneration, *J Neuroimmunol* 72:137-141, 1997.

479. Zhai QH, Futrell N, Chen FJ: Gene expression of IL-10 in relationship to TNF-alpha, IL-1 beta and IL-2 in the rat brain following middle cerebral artery occlusion, *J Neurol Sci* 152:119-124, 1997.

480. Botchkina GI, Meistrell ME, III. Botchkina IL, Tracey KJ: Expression of TNF and TNF receptors (p55 and p75) in the rat brain after focal cerebral ischemia, *Mol Med* 3:675-681, 1997.

481. Smith ME, van der Maesen K, Somera FP: Macrophage and microglial responses to cytokines in vitro: Phagocytic activity, proteolytic enzyme release, and free radical production, *J Neurosci Res* 54:68-78, 1998.

482. Szaflarski J, Burtrum D, Silverstein FS: Cerebral hypoxia-ischemia stimulates cytokine gene expression in perinatal rats, *Stroke* 26:1093-1100, 1995.

483. Hagberg H, Gilland E, Bona E, Hanson LA, et al: Enhanced expression of interleukin (IL)-1 and IL-6 messenger RNA and bioactive protein after hypoxia-ischemia in neonatal rats, *Pediatr Res* 40:603-609, 1996.

484. Ivacko JA, Sun R, Silverstein FS: Hypoxic-ischemic brain injury induces an acute microglial reaction in perinatal rats, *Pediatr Res* 39:39-47, 1995.

485. Hudome S, Palmer C, Roberts RL, Mauger D, et al: The role of neutrophils in the production of hypoxic-ischemic brain injury in the neonatal rat, *Pediatr Res* 41:607-616, 1997.

486. Bona E, Andersson A-L, Blomgren K, Gilland E, et al: Chemokine and inflammatory cell response to hypoxia-ischemia in immature rats, *Pediatr Res* 45:500-509, 1999.

487. Zhang Z, Chopp M, Powers C: Temporal profile of microglial response following transient (2h) middle cerebral artery occlusion, *Brain Res* 744:189-198, 1997.

488. Danton GH, Dietrich WD: Inflammatory mechanisms after ischemia and stroke, *J Neuropathol Exp Neurol* 62:127-136, 2003.

489. Uno H, Matsuyama T, Akita H, Nishimura H, et al: Induction of tumor necrosis factor-α in the mouse hippocampus following transient forebrain ischemia, *J Cereb Blood Flow Metab* 17:4910-4999, 1997.

490. Yrjanheikki J, Tikka T, Keinanen R, Goldsteins G, et al: A tetracycline derivative, minocycline, reduces inflammation and protects against focal cerebral ischemia with a wide therapeutic window, *Proc Natl Acad Sci U S A* 96:13496-13500, 1999.

491. Lee SM, Yune TY, Kim SJ, Kim YC, et al: Minocycline inhibits apoptotic cell death via attenuation of TNF-alpha expression following iNOS/NO induction by lipopolysaccharide in neuron/glia co-cultures, *J Neurochem* 91:568-578, 2004.

492. Morimoto N, Shimazawa M, Yamashima T, Nagai H, et al: Minocycline inhibits oxidative stress and decreases in vitro and in vivo ischemic neuronal damage, *Brain Res* 1044:8-15, 2005.

493. Hara H, Friedlander RM, Gagliardini V, Ayata C, et al: Inhibition of interleukin 1 beta converting enzyme family proteases reduces ischemic and excitotoxic neuronal damage, *Proc Natl Acad Sci U S A* 94:2007-2012, 1997.

494. Gidday JM, Park TS, Gonzales ER, Beetsch JW: CD18-dependent leukocyte adherence and vascular injury in pig cerebral circulation after ischemia, *Am J Physiol* 272:H2622-H2629, 1997.

495. Hagan P, Barks JDE, Yabut M, Davidson BL, et al: Adenovirus-mediated over-expression of interleukin-1 receptor antagonist reduces susceptibility to excitotoxic brain injury in perinatal rats, *Neuroscience* 75:1033-1045, 1996.

496. Eun B-L, Liu X-H, Barks JDE: Pentoxifylline attenuates hypoxic-ischemic brain injury in immature rats, *Pediatr Res* 47:73-78, 2000.

497. Dommergues M-A, Patkai J, Renauld J-C, Evrard P, et al: Proinflammatory cytokines and interleukin-9 exacerbate excitotoxic lesions of the newborn murine neopallium, *Ann Neurol* 47:54-63, 2000.

498. Dammann O, Leviton A: Role of the fetus in perinatal infection and neonatal brain damage, *Curr Opin Pediatr* 12:99-104, 2000.

499. Dammann O, Leviton A: Brain damage in preterm newborns: Biological response modification as a strategy to reduce disabilities, *J Pediatr* 136:433-438, 2000.

500. Hedtjarn M, Leverin AL, Eriksson K: Interleukin-18 involvement in hypoxic-ischemic brain injury, *J Neurosci* 22:5910-5919, 2002.

501. Cowell RM, Xu HY, Galasso JM, Silverstein FS: Hypoxic-ischemic injury induces macrophage inflammatory protein-1α expression in immature rat brain, *Stroke* 33:795-801, 2002.

502. Chock VY, Giffard RG: Development of neonatal murine microglia in vitro: Changes in response to lipopolysaccharide and ischemia-like injury, *Pediatr Res* 57:475-480, 2005.

503. Van Den, Tweel ER, Kavelaars A, Lombardi MS, Nijboer CH, et al: Bilateral molecular changes in a neonatal rat model of unilateral hypoxic-ischemic brain damage, *Pediatr Res* 59:434-439, 2006.

504. Palmer C, Roberts RL, Young PI: Timing of neutrophil depletion influences long-term neuroprotection in neonatal rat hypoxic-ischemic brain injury, *Pediatr Res* 55:549-556, 2004.

505. Arvin KL, Han BH, Du Y, Lin S-Z, et al: Minocycline markedly protects the neonatal brain against hypoxic-ischemic injury, *Ann Neurol* 52:54-61, 2002.

506. Fan LW, Pang Y, Lin SY, Tien LT, et al: Minocycline reduces lipopolysaccharide-induced neurological dysfunction and brain injury in the neonatal rat, *J Neurosci Res* 82:71-82, 2005.

507. Tuor UI, Yager JY, Bascaramurty S, Del Bigio MR: Dexamethasone prevents hypoxia/ischemia-induced reductions in cerebral glucose utilization and high-energy phosphate metabolites in immature brain, *J Neurochem* 69:1954-1963, 1997.

508. Felszeghy K, Banisadr G, Rostene W, Nyakas C, et al: Dexamethasone downregulates chemokine receptor CXCR4 and exerts neuroprotection against hypoxia/ischemia-induced brain injury in neonatal rats, *Neuroimmunomodulation* 11:404-413, 2004.

509. Ikeda T, Mishima K, Aoo N, Liu AX, et al: Dexamethasone prevents long-lasting learning impairment following a combination of lipopolysaccharide and hypoxia-ischemia in neonatal rats, *Am J Obstet Gynecol* 192:719-726, 2005.

510. Eklind S, Mallard C, Leverin A-L, Gilland E, et al: Bacterial endotoxin sensitizes the immature brain to hypoxic-ischaemic injury, *Eur J Neurosci* 13:1101-1106, 2001.

511. Eklind S, Arvidsson P, Hagberg H, Mallard C: The role of glucose in brain injury following the combination of lipopolysaccharide or lipoteichoic acid and hypoxia-ischemia in neonatal rats, *Dev Neurosci* 26:61-67, 2004.

512. Coumans ABC, Middelanis J, Garnier Y, Vaihinger H-M, et al: Intracisternal application of endotoxin enhances the susceptibility to subsequent hypoxic-ischemic brain damage in neonatal rats, *Pediatr Res* 53:770-775, 2003.

513. Lehnardt S, Massillon L, Follett P, Jensen FE, et al: Activation of innate immunity in the CNS triggers neurodegeneration through a Toll-like receptor 4-dependent pathway, *Proc Natl Acad Sci U S A* 100:8514-8519, 2003.

514. Ikeda T, Mishima K, Aoo N, Egashira N, et al: Combination treatment of neonatal rats with hypoxia-ischemia and endotoxin induces long-lasting memory and learning impairment that is associated with extended cerebral damage, *Am J Obstet Gynecol* 191:2132-2141, 2004.

515. Larouche A, Roy M, Kadhim H, Tsanaclis AM, et al: Neuronal injuries induced by perinatal hypoxic-ischemic insults are potentiated by prenatal exposure to lipopolysaccharide: Animal model for perinatally acquired encephalopathy, *Dev Neurosci* 27:134-142, 2005.

515a. Wang X, Hagberg H, Nie C, Zhu C, et al: Dual role of intrauterine immune challenge on neonatal and adult brain vulnerability to hypoxia-ischemia, *J Neuropathol Exp Neurol* 66:552-561, 2007.

515b. Wang X, Hagberg H, Zhu C, Jacobsson B, et al: Effects of intrauterine inflammation on the developing mouse brain, *Brain Res* 1144:180-185, 2007.

516. Ikeda T, Yang L, Ikenoue T, Mallard C, et al: Endotoxin-induced hypoxic-ischemic tolerance is mediated by up-regulation of corticosterone in neonatal rat, *Pediatr Res* 59:56-60, 2006.

517. Eklind S, Mallard C, Arvidsson P, Hagberg H: Lipopolysaccharide induces both a primary and a secondary phase of sensitization in the developing rat brain, *Pediatr Res* 58:112-116, 2005.

518. Nelson KB, Dambrosia JM, Grether JK, Phillips TM: Neonatal cytokines and coagulation factors in children with cerebral palsy, *Ann Neurol* 44:665-675, 1998.

519. Martin-Ancel A, Carcia-Alix A, Pascual-Salcedo D, Cabanas F, et al: Interleukin-6 in the cerebrospinal fluid after perinatal asphyxia is related to early and late neurological manifestations, *Pediatrics* 100:789-794, 1997.

520. Grether JK, Nelson KB, Dambrosia JM, Phillips TM: Interferons and cerebral palsy, *J Pediatr* 134:324-332, 1999.

521. Rouse DJ, Landon M, Leveno KJ, Leindecker S, et al: The Maternal-Fetal Medicine Units cesarean registry: Chorioamnionitis at term and its duration-relationship to outcomes, *Am J Obstet Gynecol* 191:211-216, 2004.

522. Foster-Barber A, Dickens B, Ferriero DM: Human perinatal asphyxia: Correlation of neonatal cytokines with MRI and outcome, *Dev Neurosci* 23:213-218, 2002.

523. Foster-Barber A, Ferriero DM: Neonatal encephalopathy in the term infant: Neuroimaging and inflammatory cytokines, *Ment Retard Dev Disabil Res Rev* 8:20-24, 2002.

524. Bartha AI, Foster-Barber A, Miller SP, Vigneron DB, et al: Neonatal encephalopathy: Association of cytokines with MR spectroscopy and outcome, *Pediatr Res* 56:960-966, 2004.

525. Shalak LF, Perlman JM: Infection markers and early signs of neonatal encephalopathy in the term infant, *Ment Retard Dev Disabil Res Rev* 8:14-19, 2002.

526. Wu YW, Escobar GJ, Grether JK, Croen LA, et al: Chorioamnionitis and cerebral palsy in term and near-term infants, *JAMA* 290:2677-2684, 2003.

527. Laptook AR, Corbett RJT, Sterett R, Garcia D, et al: Quantitative relationship between brain temperature and energy utilization rate measured in vivo using ^{31}P and ^{1}H magnetic resonance spectroscopy, *Pediatr Res* 38:919-925, 1995.

528. Yager JY, Asselin J: Effect of mild hypothermia on cerebral energy metabolism during the evolution of hypoxic-ischemic brain damage in the immature rat, *Stroke* 27:919-925, 1996.

529. Williams GD, Dardzinski BJ, Buckalew AR, Smith MB: Modest hypothermia preserves cerebral energy metabolism during hypoxia-ischemia and correlates with brain damage: A ^{31}P nuclear magnetic resonance study in unanesthetized neonatal rats, *Pediatr Res* 42:700-708, 1997.

530. Edwards AD, Wyatt JS, Thoresen M: Treatment of hypoxic-ischaemic brain damage by moderate hypothermia, *Arch Dis Child Fetal Neonatal Ed* 78:F85-F88, 1998.

531. Wagner CL, Eicher DJ, Katikaneni LD, Barbosa E, et al: The use of hypothermia: A role in the treatment of neonatal asphyxia? *Pediatr Neurol* 21:429-443, 1999.

532. Thoresen M: Cooling the newborn after asphyxia: Physiological and experimental background and its clinical use, *Semin Neonatol* 5:61-73, 2000.

533. Thoresen M, Whitelaw A: Therapeutic hypothermia for hypoxic-ischaemic encephalopathy in the newborn infant, *Curr Opin Neurol* 18:111-116, 2005.

534. Gunn AJ, Thoresen M: Hypothermic neuroprotection, *NeuroRx* 3:154-169, 2006.

535. Thoresen M, Penrice J, Lorek A, Cady EB, et al: Mild hypothermia after severe transient hypoxia-ischemia ameliorates delayed cerebral energy failure in the newborn piglet, *Pediatr Res* 37:667-670, 1995.

536. O'Brien FE, Iwata O, Thornton JS, De Vita E, et al: Delayed whole-body cooling to 33 or 35 degrees C and the development of impaired energy generation consequential to transient cerebral hypoxia-ischemia in the newborn piglet, *Pediatrics* 117:1549-1559, 2006.

537. dwards AD, Yue X, Squier MV, Thoresen M, et al: Specific inhibition of apoptosis after cerebral hypoxia-ischaemia by moderate post-insult hypothermia, *Biochem Biophys Res Commun* 217:1193-1199, 1995.

538. Laptook AR, Corbett R, Burns D, Sterett R: Neonatal ischemic neuroprotection by modest hypothermia is associated with attenuated brain acidosis, *Stroke* 26:1240-1246, 1995.

539. Thoresen M, Haaland K, Loberg EM, Whitelaw A, et al: A piglet survival model of posthypoxic encephalopathy, *Pediatr Res* 40:738-748, 1996.

540. Sirimanne ES, Blumberg RM, Bossano D, Gunning M, et al: The effect of prolonged modification of cerebral temperature on outcome after hypoxic-ischemic brain injury in the infant rat, *Pediatr Res* 39:591-597, 1996.

541. Thoresen M, Bagenholm R, Loberg EM, Apricena F, et al: Posthypoxic cooling of neonatal rats provides protection against brain injury, *Arch Dis Child Fetal Neonatal Ed* 74:F3-F9, 1996.

542. Trescher WH, Ishiwa S, Johnston MV: Brief post-hypoxic-ischemic hypothermia markedly delays neonatal brain injury, *Brain Dev* 19:326-338, 1997.

543. Haaland K, Loberg EM, Steen PA, Thoresen M: Posthypoxic hypothermia in newborn piglets, *Pediatr Res* 41:505-512, 1997.

544. Thoresen M, Wyatt J: Keeping a cool head, post-hypoxic hypothermia: An old idea revisited, *Acta Paediatr* 86:1029-1033, 1997.

545. Laptook AR, Corbett RJT, Sterett R, Burns DK, et al: Modest hypothermia provides partial neuroprotection when used for immediate resuscitation after brain ischemia, *Pediatr Res* 42:17-23, 1997.

546. Bona E, Hagberg H, Loberg EM, Bagenholm R, et al: Protective effects of moderate hypothermia after neonatal hypoxia-ischemia: Short- and long-term outcome, *Pediatr Res* 41:738-745, 1998.

547. Gunn AJ, Gunn TR, Gunning MI, Williams CE, et al: Neuroprotection with prolonged head cooling started before postischemic seizures in fetal sheep, *Pediatrics* 102:1098-1106, 1998.

548. Taylor DL, Mehmet H, Cady EB, Edwards AD: Improved neuroprotection with hypothermia delayed by 6 hours following cerebral hypoxia-ischemia in the 14-day-old rat, *Pediatr Res* 51:13-19, 2002.

549. Thoresen M, Simmonds M, Satas S, Tooley JR, et al: Effective selective head cooling during posthypoxia hypothermia in newborn piglets, *Pediatr Res* 49:594-599, 2001.

550. Tooley JR, Satas S, Eagle R, Silver IA, et al: Significant selective head cooling can be maintained long-term after global hypoxia ischemia in newborn piglets, *Pediatrics* 109:643-649, 2002.

551. Tomimatsu T, Fukuda H, Endoh M, Mu JW, et al: Long-term neuroprotective effects of hypothermia on neonatal hypoxic-ischemic brain injury in rats, assessed by auditory brainstem response, *Pediatr Res* 53:57-61, 2003.

552. Agnew DM, Koehler RC, Guerguerian A-M, Shaffner DH, et al: Hypothermia for 24 hours after asphyxic cardiac arrest in piglets provides striatal neuroprotection that is sustained 10 days after rewarming, *Pediatr Res* 54:253-262, 2003.

553. Tooley JR, Satas S, Porter H, Silver IA, et al: Head cooling with mild systemic hypothermia in anesthetized piglets is neuroprotective, *Ann Neurol* 53:65-72, 2003.

554. Robertson NJ, Bhakoo K, Puri BK, Edwards AD, et al: Hypothermia and amiloride preserve energetics in a neonatal brain slice model, *Pediatr Res* 58:288-296, 2005.

555. Iwata O, Thornton JS, Sellwood MW, Iwata S, et al: Depth of delayed cooling alters neuroprotection pattern after hypoxia-ischemia, *Ann Neurol* 58:75-87, 2005.

556. Tooley JR, Eagle RC, Satas S, Thoresen M: Significant head cooling can be achieved while maintaining normothermia in the newborn piglet, *Arch Dis Child Fetal Neonatal Ed* 90:F262-F266, 2005.

557. Zhu C, Wang X, Xu F, Qiu L, et al: Intraischemic mild hypothermia prevents neuronal cell death and tissue loss after neonatal cerebral hypoxia-ischemia, *Eur J Neurosci* 23:387-393, 2006.

558. George S, Scotter J, Dean JM, Bennet L, et al: Induced cerebral hypothermia reduces post-hypoxic loss of phenotypic striatal neurons in preterm fetal sheep, *Exp Neurol* 203:137-147, 2007.

558a. Iwata O, Iwata S, Thornton JS, De Vita E, et al: "Therapeutic time window" duration decreases with increasing severity of cerebral hypoxia-ischaemia under normothermia and delayed hypothermia in newborn piglets, *Brain Res* 1154:173-180, 2007.

559. Gunn AJ, Bennet L, Gunning MI, Gluckman PD, et al: Cerebral hypothermia is not neuroprotective when started after postischemic seizures in fetal sheep, *Pediatr Res* 46:274-280, 1999.

560. Kendall GS, Robertson NJ, Iwata O, Peebles D, et al: N-Methyl-isobutyl-amiloride ameliorates brain injury when commenced before hypoxia ischemia in neonatal mice, *Pediatr Res* 59:227-231, 2006.

561. Bruno V, Goldberg MP, Dugan LL, Giffard RG, et al: Neuroprotective effect of hypothermia in cortical cultures exposed to oxygen-glucose deprivation or excitatory amino acids, *J Neurochem* 63:1398-1406, 1994.

562. Thoresen M, Satas S, Puka-Sundvall M: Post-hypoxic hypothermia reduces cerebrocortical release of NO and excitotoxins, *Neuroreport* 8:3359-3362, 1997.

563. Hirtz DG, Nelson K: Magnesium sulfate and cerebral palsy in premature infants, *Curr Opin Pediatr* 10:131-137, 1998.

564. Zhu HD, Meloni BP, Bojarski C, Knuckey MW, et al: Post-ischemic modest hypothermia (35 degrees C) combined with intravenous magnesium is more effective at reducing CA1 neuronal death than either treatment used alone following global cerebral ischemia in rats, *Exp Neurol* 193:361-368, 2005.

565. Penrice J, Amess PN, Punwani S, Wylezinska M, et al: Magnesium sulfate after transient hypoxia-ischemia fails to prevent delayed cerebral energy failure in the newborn piglet, *Pediatr Res* 41:443-447, 1997.

566. Galvin KA, Oorschot DE: Postinjury magnesium sulfate treatment is not markedly neuroprotective for striatal medium spiny neurons after perinatal hypoxia/ischemia in the rat, *Pediatr Res* 44:740-745, 1998.

567. de Haan HH, Gunn AJ, Williams CE, Heymann MA, et al: Magnesium sulfate therapy during asphyxia in near-term fetal lambs does not compromise the fetus but does not reduce cerebral injury, *Am J Obstet Gynecol* 176:18-27, 1997.

568. Bona E, Aden U, Fredholm BB, Hagberg H: The effect of long term caffeine treatment on hypoxic-ischemic brain damage in the neonate, *Pediatr Res* 38:312-318, 1995.

569. Gidday JM, Fitzgibbons JC, Shah AR, Kraujalis MJ, et al: Reduction in cerebral ischemic injury in the newborn rat by potentiation of endogenous adenosine, *Pediatr Res* 38:306-311, 1995.

570. Bona E, Aden U, Gilland E, Fredholm BB, et al: Neonatal cerebral hypoxia-ischemia: The effect of adenosine receptor antagonists, *Neuropharmacology* 36:1327-1338, 1997.

571. Halle JN, Kasper CE, Gidday JM, Koos BJ: Enhancing adenosine A(1) receptor binding reduces hypoxic-ischemic brain injury in newborn rats, *Brain Res* 759:309-312, 1997.

572. Rosenberg PA: Potential therapeutic intervention following hypoxic-ischemic insult, *Ment Retard Dev Disabil Res Rev*:1-9, 1997.

573. Boehm FH, Liem LK, Stanton PK, Potter PE, et al: Phenytoin protects against hypoxia-induced death of cultured hippocampal neurons, *Neurosci Lett* 175:171-174, 1994.

574. Hayakawa T, Hamada Y, Maihara T, Hattori H, et al: Phenytoin reduces neonatal hypoxic-ischemic brain damage in rats, *Life Sci* 54:387-392, 1994.

575. Lampley EC, Mishra OP, Graham E, Delivoriapapadopoulos M: Neuroprotective effect of phenytoin against in utero hypoxic brain injury in fetal guinea pigs, *Neurosci Lett* 186:192-196, 1995.

576. Vartanian MG, Cordon JJ, Kupina NC, Schielke GP, et al: Phenytoin pretreatment prevents hypoxic-ischemic brain damage in neonatal rats, *Dev Brain Res* 95:169-175, 1996.

577. Crumrine RC, Bergstrand K, Cooper AT, Faison WL, et al: Lamotrigine protects hippocampal CA1 neurons from ischemic damage after cardiac arrest, *Stroke* 28:2230-2236, 1997.

578. Fernandez-Lopez D, Martinez-Orgado J, Nunez E, Romero J, et al: Characterization of the neuroprotective effect of the cannabinoid agonist WIN-55212 in an in vitro model of hypoxic-ischemic brain damage in newborn rats, *Pediatr Res* 60:169-173, 2006.

578a. Fernandez-Lopez D, Pazos MR, Tolon RM, Moro MA, et al: The cannabinoid agonist Win55212 reduces brain damage in an in vivo model of hypoxic-ischemic encephalopathy in newborn rats, *Pediatr Res* 62:255-260, 2007.

579. Huang R, Shuaib A, Hertz L: Glutamate uptake and glutamate content in primary cultures of mouse astrocytes during anoxia, substrate of deprivation and simulated ischemia under normothermic and hyperthermic conditions, *Brain Res* 618:346-351, 1993.

580. Ma D, Hossain M, Chow A, Arshad M, et al: Xenon and hypothermia combine to provide neuroprotection from neonatal asphyxia, *Ann Neurol* 58:182-193, 2005.

581. Dingley J, Tooley J, Porter H, Thoresen M: Xenon provides short-term neuroprotection in neonatal rats when administered after hypoxia-ischemia, *Stroke* 37:501-506, 2006.

582. Liu Y, Barks JD, Xu G, Silverstein FS: Topiramate extends the therapeutic window for hypothermia-mediated neuroprotection after stroke in neonatal rats, *Stroke* 35:1460-1465, 2004.

583. Choi JW, Kim WK: Is topiramate a potential therapeutic agent for cerebral hypoxic/ischemic injury? *Exp Neurol* 203:5-7, 2007.

584. Glier C, Dzietko M, Bittigau P, Jarosz B, et al: Therapeutic doses of topiramate are not toxic to the developing rat brain, *Exp Neurol* 187:403-409, 2004.

585. Bittigau P, Sifringer M, Genz K, Reith E, et al: Antiepileptic drugs and apoptotic neurodegeneration in the developing brain, *Proc Natl Acad Sci U S A* 99:15089-15094, 2002.

586. Ikonomidou C, Stefovska V, Turski L: Neuronal death enhanced by N-methyl-D-aspartate antagonists, *Proc Natl Acad Sci U S A* 97:12885-12890, 2000.

587. Kil HY, Zhang J, Piantadosi CA: Brain temperature alters hydroxyl radical production during cerebral ischemia reperfusion in rats, *J Cereb Blood Flow Metab* 16:100-106, 1996.

588. Dietrich WD, Busto R, Globus MY, Ginsberg MD: Brain damage and temperature: Cellular and molecular mechanisms, *Adv Neurol* 71:177-194, 1996.

589. Brooks KJ, Hargreaves I, Bhakoo K, Sellwood M, et al: Delayed hypothermia prevents decreases in N-acetylaspartate and reduced glutathione in the cerebral cortex of the neonatal pig following transient hypoxia-ischaemia, *Neurochem Res* 27:1599-1604, 2002.

590. McManus T, Sadgrove M, Pringle AK, Chad JE, et al: Intraischaemic hypothermia reduces free radical production and protects against ischaemic insults in cultured hippocampal slices, *J Neurochem* 91:327-336, 2004.

591. Regan RF, Jasper E, Guo YP, Panter SS: The effect of magnesium on oxidative neuronal injury in vitro, *J Neurochem* 70:77-85, 1998.

592. Domoki F, Perciaccante JV, Puskar M, Bari F, et al: Cyclooxygenase-2 inhibitor NS398 preserves neuronal function after hypoxia/ischemia in piglets, *Neuropharmacol Neurotoxicol* 12:4065-4068, 2001.

593. Vexler ZS, Wong A, Francisco C, Manabat C, et al: Fructose-1,6-bisphosphate preserves intracellular glutathione and protects cortical neurons against oxidative stress, *Brain Res* 960:90-98, 2003.

594. Tutak E, Satar M, Zorludemir S, Erdogan S, et al: Neuroprotective effects of indomethacin and aminoguanidine in the newborn rats with hypoxic-ischemic cerebral injury, *Neurochem Res* 30:937-942, 2005.

595. Muramatsu K, Sheldon RA, Black SM, Tauber M, et al: Nitric oxide synthase activity and inhibition after neonatal hypoxia ischemia in the mouse brain, *Dev Brain Res* 123:119-127, 2000.

596. van den Tweel ER, van Bel F, Kavelaars A, Peeters-Scholte CM, et al: Long-term neuroprotection with 2-iminobiotin, an inhibitor of neuronal and inducible nitric oxide synthase, after cerebral hypoxia-ischemia in neonatal rats, *J Cereb Blood Flow Metab* 25:67-74, 2005.

597. Jatana M, Singh I, Singh AK, Jenkins D: Combination of systemic hypothermia and N-acetylcysteine attenuates hypoxic-ischemic brain injury in neonatal rats, *Pediatr Res* 59:684-689, 2006.

597a. Wang X, Svedin P, Nie C, Lapatto R, et al: N-acetylcysteine reduces lipopolysaccharide-sensitized hypoxic-ischemic brain injury, *Ann Neurol* 61:263-271, 2007.

598. Lapchak PA, Zivin JA: Ebselen, a seleno-organic antioxidant, is neuroprotective after embolic strokes in rabbits: Synergism with low-dose tissue plasminogen activator, *Stroke* 34:2013-2018, 2003.

599. Ohmura A, Nakajima W, Ishida A, Yasuoka N, et al: Prolonged hypothermia protects neonatal rat brain against hypoxia-ischemia by reducing both apoptosis and necrosis, *Brain Dev* 27:517-526, 2005.

600. Bossenmeyer-Pourie C, Koziel V, Daval J-L: Effects of hypothermia on hypoxia-induced apoptosis in cultured neurons from developing rat forebrain: Comparison with preconditioning, *Pediatr Res* 47:385-391, 2000.

601. Fukuda H, Tomimatsu T, Watanabe N, Mu JW, et al: Post-ischemic hypothermia blocks caspase-3 activation in the newborn rat brain after hypoxia-ischemia, *Brain Res* 910:187-191, 2001.

602. Adachi M, Sohma O, Tsuneishi S, Takada S, et al: Combination effect of systemic hypothermia and caspase inhibitor administration against hypoxic-ischemic brain damage in neonatal rats, *Pediatr Res* 50:590-595, 2001.

603. Sola A, Wen TC, Hamrick SE, Ferriero DM: Potential for protection and repair following injury to the developing brain: A role for erythropoietin? *Pediatr Res* 57:110R-117R, 2005.

604. Wang XY, Zhu CL, Wang XH, Gerwien JG, et al: The nonerythropoietic asialoerythropoietin protects against neonatal hypoxia-ischemia as potently as erythropoietin, *J Neurochem* 91:900-910, 2004.

605. Chang YS, Mu D, Wendland M, Sheldon RA, et al: Erythropoietin improves functional and histological outcome in neonatal stroke, *Pediatr Res* 58:106-111, 2005.

606. Spandou E, Papadopoulou Z, Soubasi V, Karkavelas G, et al: Erythropoietin prevents long-term sensorimotor deficits and brain injury following neonatal hypoxia-ischemia in rats, *Brain Res* 1045:22-30, 2005.

607. Sola A, Rogido M, Lee BH, Genetta T, et al: Erythropoietin after focal cerebral ischemia activates the Janus kinase-signal transducer and activator of transcription signaling pathway and improves brain injury in postnatal day 7 rats, *Pediatr Res* 57:481-487, 2005.

607a. Kellert BA, McPherson RJ, Juul SE: A comparison of high-dose recombinant erythropoietin treatment regimens in brain-injured neonatal rats, *Pediatr Res* 61:451-455, 2007.

607b. Statler PA, McPherson RJ, Bauer LA, Kellert BA, et al: Pharmacokinetics of high-dose recombinant erythropoietin in plasma and brain of neonatal rats, *Pediatr Res* 61:671-675, 2007.

608. Castillo-Melendez M, Yan E, Walker DW: Expression of erythropoietin and its receptor in the brain of late-gestation fetal sheep, and responses to asphyxia caused by umbilical cord occlusion, *Dev Neurosci* 27:220-227, 2005.

609. Spandou E, Papoutsopoulou S, Soubasi V, Karkavelas G, et al: Hypoxia-ischemia affects erythropoietin and erythropoietin receptor expression pattern in the neonatal rat brain, *Brain Res* 1021:167-172, 2004.

610. Mu DZ, Chang YS, Vexler ZS, Feniero DM: Hypoxia-inducible factor 1 alpha and erythropoietin upregulation with deferoxamine salvage after neonatal stroke, *Exp Neurol* 195:407-415, 2005.

611. Kumral A, Gonenc S, Acikgoz O, Sonmez A, et al: Erythropoietin increases glutathione peroxidase enzyme activity and decreases lipid peroxidation levels in hypoxic-ischemic brain injury in neonatal rats, *Biol Neonate* 87:15-18, 2005.

612. Wang X, Deng J, Boyle DW, Zhong J, et al: Potential role of IGF-I in hypoxia tolerance using a rat hypoxic-ischemic model: Activation of hypoxia-inducible factor 1 alpha, *Pediatr Res* 55:385-394, 2004.

613. Mu DZ, Jiang XN, Sheldon RA, Fox CK, et al: Regulation of hypoxia-inducible factor 1 alpha and induction of vascular endothelial growth factor in a rat neonatal stroke model, *Neurobiol Dis* 14:524-534, 2003.

614. Bergeron MG, Gidday JM, Yu AY, Semenza GL, et al: Role of hypoxia-inducible factor-1 in hypoxia-induced ischemic tolerance in neonatal rat brain, *Ann Neurol* 48:285-296, 2000.

615. Gustavsson M, Anderson MF, Mallard C, Hagberg H: Hypoxic preconditioning confers long-term reduction of brain injury and improvement of neurological ability in immature rats, *Pediatr Res* 57:305-309, 2005.

616. Hagberg H, Dammann O, Mallard C, Leviton A: Preconditioning and the developing brain, *Semin Perinatol* 28:388-395, 2004.

617. Puisieux F, Deplanque D, Bulckaen H, Maboudou P, et al: Brain ischemic preconditioning is abolished by antioxidant drugs but does not up-regulate superoxide dismutase and glutathion peroxidase, *Brain Res* 1027:30-37, 2004.

618. Liu J, Narasimhan P, Yu F, Chan PH: Neuroprotection by hypoxic preconditioning involves oxidative stress-mediated expression of hypoxia-inducible factor and erythropoietin, *Stroke* 36:1264-1269, 2005.

619. Strunk T, Hartel C, Schultz C: Does erythropoietin protect the preterm brain? *Arch Dis Child Fetal Neonatal Ed* 89:F364-F366, 2004.

620. Weber A, Dzietko M, Berns M, Felderhoff-Mueser U, et al: Neuronal damage after moderate hypoxia and erythropoietin, *Neurobiol Dis* 20:594-600, 2005.

621. Gluckman P, Klempt N, Guan J, Mallard C, et al: A role for IGF-1 in the rescue of CNS neurons following hypoxic-ischemic injury, *Biochem Biophys Res Commun* 182:593-599, 1992.

622. Johnston BM, Mallard EC, Williams CE, Gluckman PD: Insulin-like growth factor-1 is a potent neuronal rescue agent after hypoxic-ischemic injury in fetal lambs, *J Clin Invest* 97:300-308, 1996.

623. Holtzman DM, Sheldon RA, Jaffe W, Cheng Y, et al: Nerve growth factor protects the neonatal brain against hypoxic-ischemic injury, *Ann Neurol* 39:114-122, 1996.

624. Cheng Y, Gidday JM, Yan Q, Shah AR, et al: Marked age-dependent neuroprotection by brain-derived neurotrophic factor against neonatal hypoxic-ischemic brain injury, *Ann Neurol* 41:521-529, 1997.

625. Gustafson K, Hagberg H, Bengtsson B-A, Brantsing C, et al: Possible protective role of growth hormone in hypoxia-ischemia in neonatal rats, *Pediatr Res* 45:318-323, 1999.

626. Johnston MV, Trescher WH, Ishida A, Nakajima W: Novel treatments after experimental brain injury, *Semin Neonatol* 5:75-86, 2000.

627. Guan J, Gunn AJ, Sirimanne ES, Tuffin J, et al: The window of opportunity for neuronal rescue with insulin-like growth factor-1 after hypoxia-ischemia in rats is critically modulated by cerebral temperature during recovery, *J Cereb Blood Flow Metab* 20:513-519, 2000.

628. Guan J, Bennet L, George S, Waldvogel HJ, et al: Selective neuroprotective effects with insulin-like growth factor-1 in phenotypic striatal neurons following ischemic brain injury in fetal sheep, *Neuroscience* 95:831-839, 2000.

629. Brywe KG, Mallard C, Gustavsson M, Hedtjarn M, et al: IGF-I neuroprotection in the immature brain after hypoxia-ischemia, involvement of Akt and GSK3beta? *Eur J Neurosci* 21:1489-1502, 2005.

630. Husson I, Rangon CM, Lelievre V, Bemelmans AP, et al: BDNF-induced white matter neuroprotection and stage-dependent neuronal survival following a neonatal excitotoxic challenge, *Cereb Cortex* 15:250-261, 2005.

631. Bemelmans AP, Husson I, Jaquet M, Mallet J, et al: Lentiviral-mediated gene transfer of brain-derived neurotrophic factor is neuroprotective in a mouse model of neonatal excitotoxic challenge, *J Neurosci Res* 83:50-60, 2006.

632. Tikka T, Fiebich BL, Goldsteins G, Keinanen R, et al: Minocycline, a tetracycline derivative, is neuroprotective against excitotoxicity by inhibiting activation and proliferation of microglia, *J Neurosci* 21:2580-2588, 2001.

633. Song Y, Wei EQ, Zhang WP, Zhang L, et al: Minocycline protects PC12 cells from ischemic-like injury and inhibits 5-lipoxygenase activation, *Neuroreport* 15:2181-2184, 2004.

634. Pi RB, Li WM, Lee NTK, Chan HHN, et al: Minocycline prevents glutamate-induced apoptosis of cerebellar granule neurons by differential regulation of p38 and Akt pathways, *J Neurochem* 91:1219-1230, 2004.

635. Kraus RL, Pasieczny R, Lariosa-Willingham K, Turner MS, et al: Antioxidant properties of minocycline: Neuroprotection in an oxidative stress assay and direct radical-scavenging activity, *J Neurochem* 94:819-827, 2005.

636. Ryu JK, Franciosi S, Sattayaprasert P, Kim SU, et al: Minocycline inhibits neuronal death and glial activation induced by beta-amyloid peptide in rat hippocampus, *Glia* 48:85-90, 2004.

637. Tsuji M, Wilson MA, Lange MS, Johnston MV: Minocycline worsens hypoxic-ischemic brain injury in a neonatal mouse model, *Exp Neurol* 189:58-65, 2004.

638. Liu X-H, Eun B-L, Silverstein S, Barks JD: The platelet-activating factor antagonist BN 52021 attenuates hypoxic-ischemic brain injury in the immature rat, *Pediatr Res* 6:797-803, 1996.

639. Zhang RI, Chopp M, Li Y, Zalonga C, et al: Anti-ICAM-1 antibody reduces ischemic cell damage after transient middle cerebral artery occlusion in the rat, *Neurology* 44:1747-1751, 1994.

640. Zhang ZG, Chopp M, Tang WX, Jiang N, et al: Postischemic treatment (2–4 h) with anti-CD11b and anti-CD18 monoclonal antibodies are neuroprotective after transient (2 h) focal cerebral ischemia in the rat, *Brain Res* 698:79-85, 1995.

641. Jiang N, Moyle M, Soule HR, Rote WE, et al: Neutrophil inhibitory factor is neuroprotective after focal ischemia in rats, *Ann Neurol* 38:935-942, 1995.

642. Rees S, Stringer M, Just Y, Hooper SB, et al: The vulnerability of the fetal sheep brain to hypoxemia at mid-gestation, *Brain Res Dev Brain Res* 103:103-118, 1997.

643. Mallard EC, Rees S, Stringer M, Cock MI, et al: Effects of chronic placental insufficiency on brain development in fetal sheep, *Pediatr Res* 43:262-270, 1998.

644. Reddy K, Mallard C, Guan J, Marks K, et al: Maturational change in the cortical response to hypoperfusion injury in the fetal sheep, *Pediatr Res* 43:674-682, 1998.

645. Jelinski SE, Yager JY, Juurlink BHJ: Preferential injury of oligodendroblasts by a short hypoxic-ischemic insult, *Brain Res* 815:150-153, 1999.

646. Uehara H, Yoshioka H, Kawase S, Nagai H, et al: A new model of white matter injury in neonatal rats with bilateral carotid artery occlusion, *Brain Res* 837:213-220, 1999.

647. Follett P, Rosenberg P, Volpe JJ, Jensen F: NBQX attenuates excitotoxic injury in developing white matter, *J Neurosci*, 20:9235-9241, 2000.

648. Matsuda T, Okuyama K, Cho K, Hoshi N, et al: Induction of antenatal periventricular leukomalacia by hemorrhagic hypotension in the chronically instrumented fetal sheep, *Am J Obstet Gynecol* 181:725-730, 1999.

649. Rees S, Breen S, Loeliger M, McCrabb G, et al: Hypoxemia near midgestation has long-term effects on fetal brain development, *J Neuropathol Exp Neurol* 58:932-945, 1999.

650. Duncan JR, Cock ML, Harding R, Rees SM: Relation between damage to the placenta and the fetal brain after late-gestation placental embolization and fetal growth restriction in sheep, *Am J Obstet Gynecol* 183:1013-1022, 2000.

651. Kohlhauser C, Mosgoller W, Hoger H, Lubec B: Myelination deficits in brain of rats following perinatal asphyxia, *Life Sci* 67:2355-2368, 2000.

652. Skoff RP, Bessert DA, Barks JDE, Song DK, et al: Hypoxic-ischemic injury results in acute disruption of myelin gene expression and death of oligodendroglial precursors in neonatal mice, *Int J Dev Neurosci* 19:197-208, 2001.

653. Levison SW, Rothstein RP, Romanko MJ, Snyder MJ, et al: Hypoxia-ischemia depletes the rat perinatal subventricular zone of oligodendrocyte progenitors and neural stem cells, *Dev Neurosci* 23:234-247, 2001.

654. Ness JK, Romanko MJ, Rothstein RP, Wood TL, et al: Perinatal hypoxia-ischemia induces apoptotic and excitotoxic death of periventricular white matter oligodendrocyte progenitors, *Dev Neurosci* 23:203-208, 2001.

655. Liu Y, Silverstein FS, Skoff R, Barks JD: Hypoxic-ischemic oligodendroglial injury in neonatal rat brain, *Pediatr Res* 51:25-33, 2002.

656. Cai ZW, Pang Y, Xiao F, Rhodes PG: Chronic ischemia preferentially causes white matter injury in the neonatal rat brain, *Brain Res* 898:126-135, 2001.

657. Kusaka T, Matsuda T, Okuyama K, Cho K, et al: Analyses of factors contributing to vulnerability to antenatal periventricular leukomalacia induced by hemorrhagic hypotension in chronically instrumented fetal sheep, *Pediatr Res* 51:20-24, 2002.

658. Petersson KH, Pinar H, Stopa EG, Faris RA, et al: White matter injury after cerebral ischemia in ovine fetuses, *Pediatr Res* 51:768-776, 2002.

659. Mallard C, Welin A-K, Peebles D, Hagberg H, et al: White matter injury following systemic endotoxemia or asphyxia in the fetal sheep, *Neurochem Res* 28:215-223, 2003.

660. Sizonenko SV, Sirimanne E, Mayall Y, Gluckman PD, et al: Selective cortical alteration after hypoxic-ischemic injury in the very immature rat brain, *Pediatr Res* 54:263-269, 2003.

661. Wakita H, Tomimoto H, Akiguchi I, Matsuo A, et al: Axonal damage and demyelination in the white matter after chronic cerebral hypoperfusion in the rat, *Brain Res* 924:63-70, 2002.

662. Back SA, Han BH, Luo NL, Chricton CA, et al: Selective vulnerability of late oligodendrocyte progenitors to hypoxia-ischemia, *J Neurosci* 22:455-463, 2002.

663. McQuillen PS, Sheldon RA, Shatz CJ, Ferriero DM: Selective vulnerability of subplate neurons after early neonatal hypoxia-ischemia, *J Neurosci* 23:3308-3315, 2003.

664. Zaidi AU, Bessert DA, Ong JE, Xu H, et al: New oligodendrocytes are generated after neonatal hypoxic-ischemic brain injury in rodents, *Glia* 46:380-390, 2004.

665. Baud O, Daire JL, Dalmaz Y, Fontaine RH, et al: Gestational hypoxia induces white matter damage in neonatal rats: A new model of periventricular leukomalacia, *Brain Pathol* 14:1-10, 2004.

666. Robinson S, Petelenz K, Li Q, Cohen ML, et al: Developmental changes induced by graded prenatal systemic hypoxic-ischemic insults in rats, *Neurobiol Dis* 18:568-581, 2005.

667. Welin AK, Sandberg M, Lindblom A, Arvidsson P, et al: White matter injury following prolonged free radical formation in the 0.65 gestation fetal sheep brain, *Pediatr Res* 58:100-105, 2005.

668. Back SA, Luo NL, Mallinson AR, O'Malley JP, et al: Selective vulnerability of preterm white matter to oxidative damage defined by F(2)-isoprostanes, *Ann Neurol* 58:108-120, 2005.

669. Riddle A, Luo NL, Manese M, Beardsley DJ, et al: Spatial heterogeneity in oligodendrocyte lineage maturation and not cerebral blood flow predicts fetal ovine periventricular white matter injury, *J Neurosci* 26:3045-3055, 2006.

670. Meng S, Qiao M, Scobie K, Tomanek B, et al: Evolution of magnetic resonance imaging changes associated with cerebral hypoxia-ischemia and a relatively selective white matter injury in neonatal rats, *Pediatr Res* 59:554-559, 2006.

671. Olivier P, Baud O, Evrard P, Gressens P, et al: Prenatal ischemia and white matter damage in rats, *J Neuropathol Exp Neurol* 64:998-1006, 2005.

672. Biran V, Joly LM, Heron A, Vernet A, et al: Glial activation in white matter following ischemia in the neonatal P7 rat brain, *Exp Neurol* 199:103-112, 2006.

673. Back SA, Craig A, Kayton RJ, Luo NL, et al: Hypoxia-ischemia preferentially triggers glutamate depletion from oligodendroglia and axons in perinatal cerebral white matter, *J Cereb Blood Flow Metab* 27:334-347, 2007.

674. Gilles FH, Averill DR Jr, Kerr CS: Neonatal endotoxin encephalopathy, *Ann Neurol* 2:49-56, 1977.

675. Gilles FH, Leviton A, Kerr CS: Susceptibility of the neonatal feline telencephalic white matter to a lipopolysaccharide, *J Neurol Sci* 27:183-191, 1976.

676. Leviton A, Gilles FH: Acquired perinatal leukoencephalopathy, *Ann Neurol* 16:1-10, 1984.

677. Debillon T, Gras-Leguen C, Verielle V, Winer N, et al: Intrauterine infection induces programmed cell death in rabbit periventricular white matter, *Pediatr Res* 47:736-742, 2000.

678. Yoon BH, Kim CJ, Romero R, Jun JK, et al: Experimentally induced intrauterine infection causes fetal brain white matter lesions in rabbits, *Am J Obstet Gynecol* 177:797-802, 1997.

679. Bell MJ, Hallenbeck JM: Effects of intrauterine inflammation on developing rat brain, *J Neurosci* 70:570-579, 2002.

680. Cai Z, Pan Z-L, Pang Y, Evans OB, et al: Cytokine induction in fetal rat brains and brain injury in neonatal rats after maternal lipopolysaccharide administration, *Pediatr Res* 47:64-72, 2000.

681. Cai Z, Pang Y, Lin S, Rhodes PG: Differential roles of tumor necrosis factor-α and interleukin-1β in lipopolysaccharide-induced brain injury in the neonatal rat, *Brain Res* 975:37-47, 2003.

682. Debillon T, Gras-Le Guen C, Leroy S, Caillon J, et al: Patterns of cerebral inflammatory response in a rabbit model of intrauterine infection-mediated brain lesion, *Dev Brain Res* 145:39-48, 2003.

683. Duncan JR, Cock ML, Scheerlinck JP, Westcott KT, et al: White matter injury after repeated endotoxin exposure in the preterm ovine fetus, *Pediatr Res* 52:941-949, 2002.

684. Pang Y, Cai ZW, Rhodes PG: Disturbance of oligodendrocyte development, hypomyelination and white matter injury in the neonatal rat brain after intracerebral injection of lipopolysaccharide, *Dev Brain Res* 140:205-214, 2003.

685. Lehnardt S, Lachance C, Patrizi S, Lefebvre S, et al: The toll-like receptor TLR4 is necessary for lipopolysaccharide-induced oligodendrocyte injury in the CNS, *J Neurosci* 22:2478-2486, 2002.

686. Poggi SH, Park J, Toso L, Abebe D, et al: No phenotype associated with established lipopolysaccharide model for cerebral palsy, *Am J Obstet Gynecol* 192:727-733, 2005.

687. Paintlia MK, Paintlia AS, Barbosa E, Singh I, et al: N-Acetylcysteine prevents endotoxin-induced degeneration of oligodendrocyte progenitors and hypomyelination in developing rat brain, *J Neurosci Res* 78:347-361, 2004.

688. Rodts-Palenik S, Wyatt-Ashmead J, Pang Y, Thigpen B, et al: Maternal infection-induced white matter injury is reduced by treatment with interleukin-10, *Am J Obstet Gynecol* 191:1387-1392, 2004.

689. Stolp HB, Dziegielewska KM, Ek CJ, Potter AM, et al: Long-term changes in blood-brain barrier permeability and white matter following prolonged systemic inflammation in early development in the rat, *Eur J Neurosci* 22:2805-2816, 2005.

690. Toso L, Poggi S, Park J, Einat H, et al: Inflammatory-mediated model of cerebral palsy with developmental sequelae, *Am J Obstet Gynecol* 193:933-941, 2005.

691. Svedin P, Kjellmer I, Welin AK, Blad S, et al: Maturational effects of lipopolysaccharide on white-matter injury in fetal sheep, *J Child Neurol* 20:960-964, 2005.

692. Rousset CI, Chalon S, Cantagrel S, Bodard S, et al: Maternal exposure to LPS induces hypomyelination in the internal capsule and programmed cell death in the deep gray matter in newborn rats, *Pediatr Res* 59:428-433, 2006.

693. Ando M, Takashima S, Mito T: Endotoxin, cerebral blood flow, amino acids and brain damage in young rabbits, *Brain Dev* 10:365-370, 1988.

694. Garnier Y, Coumans ABC, Berger R, Jensen A, et al: Endotoxemia severely affects circulation during normoxia and asphyxia in immature fetal sheep, *J Soc Gynecol Invest* 8:134-142, 2003.

695. Moller K, Strauss GI, Qvist J, Fonsmark L, et al: Cerebal blood flow and oxidative metabolism during human endotoxemia, *J Cereb Blood Flow Metab* 22:1262-1270, 2002.

696. Young RS, Yagel SK, Towfighi J: Systemic and neuropathologic effects of E. coli endotoxin in neonatal dogs, *Pediatr Res* 17:349-353, 1983.

697. Goto M, Yoshioka T, Ravindranath T, Battelino T, et al: LPS injected into the pregnant rat late in gestation does not induce fetal endotoxemia, *Mol Pathol Pharmacol* 85:109-112, 1994.

698. Kohmura Y, Kirikae t, Kirikae F, Nakano M, et al: Lipopolysaccharide (LPS)-induced intra-uterine fetal death (IUFD) in mice is principally due to maternal cause but not fetal sensitivity to LPS, *Microbiol Immunol* 44:897-904, 2000.

699. Romero R, Lafreniere D, Duff GW, Kadar N, et al: Failure of endotoxin to cross the chorioamniotic membranes in vitro, *Am J Perinatol* 4:360-362, 1987.

700. Bordet R, Deplanque D, Maboudou P, Puisieux F, et al: Increase in endogenous brain superoxide dismutase as a potential mechanism of lipopolysaccharide-induced brain ischemic tolerance, *J Cereb Blood Flow Metab* 20:1190-1196, 2000.

701. Descamps L, Coisne C, Dehouck B, Cecchelli R, et al: Protective effect of glial cells against lipopolysaccharide-mediated blood-brain barrier injury, *Glia* 42:46-58, 2003.

702. Gatti S, Bartfai T: Induction of tumor necrosis factor-α mRNA in the brain after peripheral endotoxin treatment: Comparison with interleukin-1 family and interleukin-6, *Brain Res* 624:291-294, 1993.

703. Gilmore JH, Jarskog LF, Vadlamudi S: Maternal infection regulates BDNF and NGF expression in fetal and neonatal brain and maternal-fetal unit of the rat, *J Neuroimmunol* 138:49-55, 2003.

704. Glezer I, Munhoz CD, Kawamoto EM, Marcourakis T, et al: MK-801 and 7-Ni attenuate the activation of brain NF-kappa B induced by LPS, *Neuropharmacology* 45:1120-1129, 2003.

705. Laflamme N, Echchannaoul H, Landmann R, Rivest S: Cooperation between Toll-like receptor 2 and 4 in the brain of mice challenged with cell wall components derived from gram-negative and gram-positive bacteria, *Eur J Immunol* 33:1127-1138, 2003.

706. Laflamme N, Rivest S: Toll-like receptor 4: The missing link of the cerebral innate immune response triggered by circulating gram-negative bacterial cell wall components, *FASEB J* 15:155-163, 2001.

707. Rivest S: Molecular insights on the cerebral innate immune system, *Brain Behav Immun* 17:13-19, 2003.

708. Soulet D, Rivest S: Polyamines play a critical role in the control of the innate immune response in the mouse central nervous system, *J Cell Biol* 162:257-268, 2003.

709. Terrazzino S, Bauleo A, Baldan A, Leon A: Peripheral LPS administrations up-regulate Fas and FasL on brain microglial cells: A brain protective or pathogenic event? *J Neuroimmunol* 124:45-53, 2002.

710. Turrin NP, Gayle D, Ilyin SE, Flynn MC, et al: Pro-inflammatory and anti-inflammatory cytokine mRNA induction in the periphery and brain following intraperitoneal administration of bacterial lipopolysaccharide, *Brain Res Bull* 54:443-453, 2001.

711. Hagberg H, Mallard C: Effect of inflammation on central nervous system development and vulnerability, *Curr Opin Neurol* 18:117-123, 2005.

712. Bell MJ, Hallenbeck JM, Gallo V: Determining the fetal inflammatory response in an experimental model of intrauterine inflammation in rats, *Pediatr Res* 56:541-546, 2004.

713. Lynch AM, Walsh C, Delaney A, Nolan Y, et al: Lipopolysaccharide-induced increase in signalling in hippocampus is abrogated by IL-10: A role for IL-1 beta? *J Neurosci* 88:635-646, 2004.

714. Chakravarty S, Herkenham M: Toll-like receptor 4 on nonhematopoietic cells sustains CNS inflammation during endotoxemia, independent of systemic cytokines, *J Neurosci* 25:1788-1796, 2005.

715. Eklind S, Hagberg H, Wang X, Savman K, et al: Effect of lipopolysaccharide on global gene expression in the immature rat brain, *Pediatr Res* 60:161-168, 2006.

716. Hallman M, Ramet M, Ezekowitz RA: Toll-like receptors as sensors of pathogens, *Pediatr Res* 50:315-321, 2001.

717. Nguyen MD, Julien J-P, Rivest S: Innate immunity: The missing link in neuroprotection and neurodegeneration? *Nat Rev Neurosci* 3:216-227, 2002.

718. Zhang GL, Ghosh S: Toll-like receptor-mediated NF-kappa B activation: A phylogenetically conserved paradigm in innate immunity, *J Clin Invest* 107:13-19, 2001.

719. Abreu MT, Arditi M: Innate immunity and Toll-like receptors: Clinical implications of basic science research, *J Pediatr* 144:421-429, 2004.

720. Rifkin IR, Leadbetter EA, Busconi L, Viglianti G, et al: Toll-like receptors, endogenous ligands, and systemic autoimmune disease, *Immunol Rev* 204:27-42, 2005.

720a. Konat GW, Kielian T, Marriott I: The role of Toll-like receptors in CNS response to microbial challenge, *J Neurochem* 99:1-12, 2006.

720b. Miyake K: Innate immune sensing of pathogens and danger signals by cell surface Toll-like receptors, *Semin Immunol* 19:3-10, 2007.

721. Li J, Baud O, Vartanian T, Volpe JJ, et al: Peroxynitrite generated by inducible nitric oxide synthase and NADPH oxidase mediates microglial toxicity to oligodendrocytes, *Proc Natl Acad Sci U S A* 102:9936-9941, 2005.

721a. Barger SW, Goodwin ME, Porter MM, Beggs ML: Glutamate release from activated microglia requires the oxidative burst and lipid peroxidation, *J Neurochem* 101:1205-1213, 2007.

722. Banks WA, Kastin AJ, Gutierrez EG: Penetration of interleukin-6 across the murine blood-brain barrier, *Neurosci Lett* 179:53-56, 1994.

723. Banks WA, Kastin AJ, Gutierrez EG: Interleukin-1α in blood has direct access to cortical brain cells, *Neurosci Lett* 163:41-44, 1993.

724. Banks WA, Ortiz L, Plotkin SR, Kastin AJ: Human interleukin (IL) 1α, murine IL-1α and murine IL-1β are transported from blood to brain in the mouse by a shared saturable mechanism, *J Pharmacol Exp Ther* 159:988-996, 1991.

725. Brett FM, Mizisin AP, Powell HC, Campbell IL: Evolution of neuropathologic abnormalities associated with blood-brain barrier breakdown in transgenic mice expressing interleukin-6 in astrocytes, *J Neuropathol Exp Neurol* 54:766-775, 1995.

726. Gutierrez EG, Banks WA, Kastin AJ: Murine tumor necrosis factor alpha is transported from blood to brain in the mouse, *J Neuroimmunol* 47:169-176, 1993.

727. Monje ML, Toda H, Palmer TD: Inflammatory blockade restores adult hippocampal neurogenesis, *Science* 302:1760-1765, 2003.

728. Pachter JS, De Vries HE, Fabry Z: The blood-brain barrier and its role in immune privilege in the central nervous system, *J Neuropathol Exp Neurol* 62:593-604, 2003.

729. Rezaie P, Dean A: Periventricular leukomalacia, inflammation and white matter lesions within the developing nervous system, *Neuropathology* 22:106-132, 2002.

730. Saija A, Princi P, Lanza M, Scalese M, et al: Systemic cytokine administration can affect blood-brain barrier permeability in the rat, *Life Sci* 56:775-784, 1995.

731. Trembovler V, Beit-Yannai E, Younis F, Gallily R, et al: Antioxidants attenuate acute toxicity of tumor necrosis factor-alpha induced by brain injury in rat, *J Interferon Cytokine Res* 19:791-795, 1999.

732. Wright JL, Merchant RE: Blood-brain barrier changes following intracerebral injection of human recombinant tumor necrosis factor-a in the rat, *J Neurooncol* 20:17-25, 1994.

733. Haynes RL, Folkerth RD, Keefe R, Sung I, et al: Nitrosative and oxidative injury to premyelinating oligodendrocytes in periventricular leukomalacia, *J Neuropathol Exp Neurol* 62:441-450, 2003.

734. Andjelkovic AV, Nikolic B, Pachter JS, Zecevic N: Macrophages/microglial cells in human central nervous system during development: An immunohistochemical study, *Brain Res* 814:13-25, 1998.

735. Rezaie P, Cairns NJ, Male DK: Expression of adhesion molecules on human fetal cerebral vessels: Relationship to microglial colonisation during development, *Dev Brain Res* 104:175-189, 1997.

736. Billiards SS, Haynes RL, Folkerth RD, Trachtenberg FL, et al: Development of microglia in the cerebral white matter of the human fetus and infant, *J Comp Neurol* 497:199-208, 2006.

737. Brian JE, Faraci FM: Tumor necrosis factor-a-induced dilatation of cerebral arterioles, *Stroke* 29:509-515, 1998.

738. Sibson NR, Blamire AM, Perry VH, Gauldie J, et al: TNF-alpha reduces cerebral blood volume and disrupts tissue homeostasis via an endothelin-and TNFR2-dependent pathway, *Brain* 125:2446-2459, 2002.

739. Berti R, Williams AJ, Moffett JR, Hale SL, et al: Quantitative real-time RT-PCR analysis of inflammatory gene expression associated with ischemia-reperfusion brain injury, *J Cereb Blood Flow Metab* 22:1068-1079, 2002.

740. Froen JF, Munkeby BH, Stray-Pedersen B, Saugstad OD: Interleukin-10 reverses acute detrimental effects of endotoxin-induced inflammation on perinatal cerebral hypoxia-ischemia, *Brain Res* 942:87-94, 2002.

741. Ghezzi P, Cimarello CA, Bianchi M, Rosandich ME, et al: Hypoxia increases production of interleukin-1 and tumor necrosis factor by human mononuclear cells, *Cytokine* 3:189-194, 1991.

742. Okuma Y, Uehara T, Miyazaki H, Miyasaka T, et al: The involvement of cytokines, chemokines and inducible nitric oxide synthase (iNOS) induced by a transient ischemia in neuronal survival/death in rat brain, *Folia Pharmacol* 111:37-44, 1998.

743. Lyng K, Braakhuis M, Froen JF, Stray-Pedersen B, et al: Inflammation increases vulnerability to hypoxia in newborn piglets: Effect of reoxygenation with 21% and 100% O_2, *Am J Obstet Gynecol* 192:1172-1178, 2005.

744. Stroemer RP, Rothwell NJ: Exacerbation of ischemic brain damage by localized striatal injection of interleukin-1β in the rat, *J Cereb Blood Flow Metab* 18:833-839, 1998.

745. Hu S, Sheng WS, Ehrlich LC: Cytokine effects on glutamate uptake by human astrocytes, *Neuroimmunomodulation* 7:153-159, 2000.

746. Pitt D, Nagelmeier IE, Wilson HC, Raine CS: Glutamate uptake by oligodendrocytes. Implications for excitotoxicity in multiple sclerosis, *Neurology* 61:1113-1120, 2003.

747. Ye ZC, Sontheimer H: Cytokine modulation of glial glutamate uptake: A possible involvement of nitric oxide, *Neuroreport* 7:2181-2185, 1996.

748. Takahashi JL, Giuliani F, Power C, Imai Y, et al: Interleukin-1β promotes oligodendrocyte death through glutamate excitotoxicity, *Ann Neurol* 53:588-595, 2003.

749. Oka A, Belliveau MJ, Rosenberg PA, Volpe JJ: Vulnerability of oligodendroglia to glutamate: Pharmacology, mechanisms and prevention, *J Neurosci* 13:1441-1453, 1993.

750. Yonezawa M, Back SA, Gan X, Rosenberg PA, et al: Cystine deprivation induces oligodendroglial death: Rescue by free radical scavengers and by a diffusible glial factor, *J Neurochem* 67:566-573, 1996.

751. Back SA, Gan X, Li Y, Rosenberg PR, et al: Maturation-dependent vulnerability of oligodendrocytes to oxidative stress-induced death caused by glutathione depletion, *J Neurosci* 18:6241-6253, 1998.

752. Fragoso G, MartinezBermudez AK, Liu HN, Khorchid A, et al: Developmental differences in H_2O_2-induced oligodendrocyte cell death: Role of glutathione, mitogen-activated protein kinases and caspase 3, *J Neurochem* 90:392-404, 2004.

753. Li J, Lin JC, Wang H, Peterson JW, et al: Novel role of vitamin K in preventing oxidative injury to developing oligodendrocytes and neurons, *J Neurosci* 23:5816-5826, 2003.

754. Deng W, Rosenberg PA, Volpe JJ, Jensen FE: Calcium-permeable AMPA/kainate receptors mediate toxicity and preconditioning by oxygen-glucose deprivation in oligodendrocyte precursors, *Proc Natl Acad Sci U S A* 100:6801-6806, 2003.

755. Baud O, Greene A, Li J, Wang H, et al: Glutathione peroxidase-catalase cooperativity is required for resistance to hydrogen peroxide by mature rat oligodendrocytes, *J Neurosci* 26:1531-1549, 2004.

756. Baud O, Haynes RF, Wang H, Folkerth RD, et al: Developmental up-regulation of MnSOD in rat oligodendrocytes confers protection against oxidative injury, *Eur J Neurosci* 20:29-40, 2004.

757. Folkerth RD, Haynes RL, Borenstein NS, Belliveau RA, et al: Developmental lag in superoxide dismutases relative to other antioxidant enzymes in premyelinated human telencephalic white matter, *J Neuropathol Exp Neurol* 63:990-999, 2004.

758. Iida K, Takashima S, Ueda K: Immunohistochemical study of myelination and oligodendrocyte in infants with periventricular leukomalacia, *Pediatr Neurol* 13:296-304, 1995.

759. Ozawa H, Nishida A, Mito T, Takashima S: Development of ferritin-positive cells in cerebrum of human brain, *Pediatr Neurol* 10:44-48, 1994.

760. Connor JR, Menzies SL: Relationship of iron to oligodendrocytes and myelination, *Glia* 17:83-93, 1996.

761. Savman K, Nilsson UA, Thoresen M, Kjellmer I: Non–protein-bound iron in brain interstitium of newborn pigs after hypoxia, *Dev Neurosci* 27:176-184, 2005.

762. Cheepsunthorn P, Palmer C, Menzies S, Roberts RL, et al: Hypoxic/ischemic insult alters ferritin expression and myelination in neonatal rat brains, *J Comp Neurol* 431:382-396, 2001.

763. Dommergues M-A, Gallego J, Evrard P, Gressens P: Iron supplementation aggravates periventricular cystic white matter lesions in newborn mice, *Eur J Paediatr Neurol* 2:313-318, 1998.

764. Armstrong DL, Sauls CD, Goddard-Finegold J: Neuropathologic findings in short-term survivors of intraventricular hemorrhage, *Am J Dis Child* 141:617-621, 1987.

765. Leviton A, Gilles F: Ventriculomegaly, delayed myelination, white matter hypoplasia, and "periventricular" leukomalacia. How are they related? *Pediatr Neurol* 15:127-136, 1996.

766. Takashima S, Mito T, Houdou S, Ando Y: Relationship between periventricular hemorrhage, leukomalacia and brainstem lesions in prematurely born infants, *Brain Dev* 11:121-124, 1989.

767. Savman K, Nilsson UA, Blennow M, Kjellmer I, et al: Non–protein-bound iron is elevated in cerebrospinal fluid from preterm infants with posthemorrhagic ventricular dilation, *Pediatr Res* 49:208-212, 2001.

768. Ciccoli L, Rossi V, Leoncini S, Signorini C, et al: Iron release in erythrocytes and plasma non protein-bound iron in hypoxic and non hypoxic newborns, *Free Radic Res* 37:51-58, 2003.

769. Hirano K, Morinobu T, Kim H, Hiroi M, et al: Blood transfusion increases radical promoting non-transferrin bound iron in preterm infants, *Arch Dis Child Fetal Neonatal Ed* 84:F188-F193, 2001.

770. Inder TE, Darlow BA, Winterbourn SKB, Graham CC, et al: The correlation of elevated levels of an index of lipid peroxidation (MDA-TBA) with adverse outcome in the very low birthweight infant, *Acta Paediatr* 85:1116-1122, 1996.

771. Lackmann GM, Hesse L, Tollner U: Reduced iron-associated antioxidants in premature newborns suffering intracerebral hemorrhage, *Free Radic Biol Med* 20:407-409, 1996.

772. Saugstad OD: Bronchopulmonary dysplasia and oxidative stress: Are we closer to an understanding of the pathogenesis of BPD? *Acta Paediatr* 86:1277-1282, 1997.

773. Varsila E, Pitkanen O, Hallman M, Andersson S: Immaturity-dependent free radical activity in premature infants, *Pediatr Res* 36:55-59, 1994.

774. Wardle SP, Drury J, Garr R, Weindling AM: Effect of blood transfusion on lipid peroxidation in preterm infants, *Arch Dis Child Fetal Neonatal Ed* 86:F46-F48, 2002.

775. Buonocore G, Perrone S, Longini M, Terzuoli L, et al: Total hydroperoxide and advanced oxidation protein products in preterm hypoxic babies, *Pediatr Res* 47:221-224, 2000.

776. Buonocore G, Perrone S, Longini M, Vezzosi P, et al: Oxidative stress in preterm neonates at birth and on the seventh day of life, *Pediatr Res* 52:46-49, 2002.

777. Ochoa JJ, Ramirez-Tortosa MC, Quiles JL, Palomino N, et al: Oxidative stress in erythrocytes from premature and full-term infants during their first 72h of life, *Free Radic Res* 37:317-322, 2003.

778. Bartnik BL, Juurlink BHJ, Devon RM: Macrophages: Their myelinotrophic or neurotoxic actions depend upon tissue oxidative stress, *Mult Scler* 6:37-42, 2000.

779. Mehindate K, Sahlas DJ, Frankel D, Mawal Y, et al: Proinflammatory cytokines promote glial heme oxygenase-1 expression and mitochondrial iron deposition: Implications for multiple sclerosis, *J Neurochem* 77:1386-1395, 2001.

780. Qin LY, Liu YX, Cooper C, Liu B, et al: Microglia enhance beta-amyloid peptide-induced toxicity in cortical and mesencephalic neurons by producing reactive oxygen species, *J Neurochem* 83:973-983, 2002.

781. Sauer H, Wefer K, Vetrugno V, Pocchiari M, et al: Regulation of intrinsic prion protein by growth factors and TNF-alpha: The role of intracellular reactive oxygen species, *Free Radic Biol Med* 35:586-594, 2003.

782. Wilde GJC, Pringle AK, Sundstrom LE, Mann DA, et al: Attenuation and augmentation of ischaemia-related neuronal death by tumour necrosis factor-alpha in vitro, *Eur J Neurosci* 12:3863-3870, 2000.

783. Yoshida T, Tanaka M, Sotomatsu A, Hirai S: Activated microglia cause superoxide-mediated release of iron from ferritin, *Neurosci Lett* 190:21-24, 1995.

784. Didion SP, Kinzenbaw DA, Fegan PE, Didion LA, et al: Overexpression of CuZn-SOD prevents lipopolysaccharide-induced endothelial dysfunction, *Stroke* 35:1963-1967, 2004.

785. Yoshida T, Tanaka M, Suzuki Y, Sohmiya M, et al: Antioxidant properties of cabergoline: Inhibition of brain auto-oxidation and superoxide anion production of microglial cells in rats, *Neurosci Lett* 330:1-4, 2002.

786. Godbout JP, Berg BM, Kelley KW, Johnson RW: alpha-Tocopherol reduces lipopolysaccharide-induced peroxide radical formation and interleukin-6 secretion in primary murine microglia and in brain, *J Neuroimmunol* 149:101-109, 2004.

787. Block ML, Hong JS: Microglia and inflammation-mediated neurodegeneration: Multiple triggers with a common mechanism, *Prog Neurobiol* 76:77-98, 2005.

788. Baud O, Li J, Zhang Y, Neve RL, et al: Nitric oxide-induced cell death in developing oligodendrocytes is associated with mitochondrial dysfunction and apoptosis-inducing factor translocation, *Eur J Neurosci* 20:1713-1726, 2004.

789. Boullerne AI, Nedelkoska L, Benjamins JA: Role of calcium in nitric oxide-induced cytotoxicity: EGTA protects mouse oligodendrocytes, *J Neurosci Res* 63:124-135, 2001.

790. Mackenzie-Graham aJ, Mitrovic B, Smoll A, Merrill JE: Differential sensitivity to nitric oxide in immortalized, cloned murine oligodendrocyte cell lines, *Dev Neurosci* 16:162-171, 1994.

791. Merrill JE, Ignarro LJ, Sherman MP, Melinek J, et al: Microglial cell cytotoxicity of oligodendrocytes is mediated through nitric oxide, *J Immunol* 151:2132-2141, 1993.

792. Mitrovic B, Ignarro L, Vinters HV, Akers MA, et al: Nitric oxide induces necrotic but not apoptotic cell death in oligodendrocytes, *Neuroscience* 65:531-539, 1995.

793. Rosenberg PA, Li Y, Back SA, Volpe JJ: Intracellular redox state determines whether nitric oxide is toxic or protective to rat oligodendrocytes in culture, *J Neurochem* 73:476-484, 1999.

794. Scott GS, Virag L, Szabo C, Hooper DC: Peroxynitrite-induced oligodendrocyte toxicity is not dependent on poly(ADP-ribose) polymerase activation, *Glia* 41:105-116, 2003.

795. Choi J-J, Kim W-K: Potentiated glucose deprivation-induced death of astrocytes after induction of iNOS, *J Neurosci Res* 54:870-875, 1998.

796. Possel H, Noack H, Putzke J, Wolf G, et al: Selective upregulation of inducible nitric oxide synthase (INOS) by lipopolysaccharide (LPS) and cytokines in microglia: In vitro and in vivo studies, *Glia* 32:51-59, 2000.

797. Simard JM, Tewari K, Kaul A, Nowicki B, et al: Early signaling events by endotoxin in PC12 cells: Involvement of tyrosine kinase, constitutive nitric oxide synthase, cGMP-dependent protein kinase, and Ca²⁺ channels, *J Neurosci Res* 45:216-225, 1996.

798. Sola A, Casal C, Tusell JM, Serratosa J: Astrocytes enhance lipopolysaccharide-induced nitric oxide production by microglial cells, *Eur J Neurosci* 16:1275-1283, 2002.

799. Xie Z, Wei M, Morgan TE, Fabrizio P, et al: Peroxynitrite mediates neurotoxicity of amyloid β-peptide 1-42- and lipopolysaccharide-activated microglia, *J Neurosci* 22:3484-3492, 2002.

800. Molina-Holgado E, Vela JM, Arevalo-Martin A, Guaza C: LPS/IFN-gamma cytotoxicity in oligodendroglial cells: Role of nitric oxide and protection by the anti-inflammatory cytokine IL-10, *Eur J Neurosci* 13:493-502, 2001.

801. Gendron F-P, Chalimoniuk M, Strosznajder J, Shen S, et al: P2X₇ nucleotide receptor activation enhances IFNγ-induced type II nitric oxide synthase activity in BV-2 microglial cells, *J Neurochem* 87:344-352, 2003.

802. Andrews T, Zhang P, Bhat NR: TNFα potentiates IFNγ-induced cell death in oligodendrocyte progenitors, *J Neurosci Res* 54:574-583, 1998.

803. Baerwald KD, Popko B: Developing and mature oligodendrocytes respond differently to the immune cytokine interferon-gamma, *J Neurosci Res* 52:230-239, 1998.

804. Popko B, Baerwald KD: Oligodendroglial response to the immune cytokine interferon gamma, *Neurochem Res* 24:331-338, 1999.

805. Vartanian T, Li Y, Zhao MJ, Stefansson K: Interferon-γ–induced oligodendrocyte cell death: Implications for the pathogenesis of multiple sclerosis, *Mol Med* 1:732-743, 1995.

806. Agresti C, D'Urso D, Levi G: Reversible inhibitory effects of interferon-γ and tumour necrosis factor-α on oligodendroglial lineage cell proliferation and differentiation in vitro, *Eur J Neurosci* 8:1106-1116, 1996.

807. Jurewicz A, Matysiak M, Tybor K, Selmaj K: TNF-induced death of adult human oligodendrocytes is mediated by c-jun NH2-terminal kinase-3, *Brain* 126:1358-1370, 2003.

808. Louis JC, Magal E, Takayama S, Varon S: CNTF protection of oligodendrocytes against natural and tumor necrosis factor–induced death, *Science* 259:689-692, 1993.

809. Mayer M, Noble M: N-Acetyl-L-cysteine is a pluripotent protector against cell death and enhancer of trophic factor-mediated cell survival in vitro, *Proc Natl Acad Sci U S A* 91:7496-7500, 1994.

810. Selmaj K, Raine CS, Farooq M: Cytokine cytotoxicity against oligodendrocytes: Apoptosis induced by lymphotoxin, *J Immunol* 147:1522-1529, 1991.

811. Jurewicz A, Matysiak M, Tybor K, Kilianek L, et al: Tumour necrosis factor–induced death of adult human oligodendrocytes is mediated by apoptosis inducing factor, *Brain* 128:2675-2688, 2005.

812. Zhang X, Haaf M, Todorich B, Grosstephan E, et al: Cytokine toxicity to oligodendrocyte precursors is mediated by iron, *Glia* 52:199-208, 2005.

813. Sherwin C, Fern R: Acute lipopolysaccharide-mediated injury in neonatal white matter glia: Role of TNF-α, IL-1β, and calcium, *J Immunol* 175:155-161, 2005.

814. Buntinx M, Moreels M, Vandenabeele F, Lambrichts N, et al: Cytokine-induced cell death in human oligodendroglial cell lines. I. Synergistic effects of IFN-gamma and TNF-alpha on apoptosis, *J Neurosci Res* 76:834-845, 2004.

815. Pang Y, Cai ZW, Rhodes PG: Effect of tumor necrosis factor-alpha on developing optic nerve oligodendrocytes in culture, *J Neurosci Res* 80:226-234, 2005.

816. LaFerla FM, Sugarman MC, Lane TE, Leissring MA: Regional hypomyelination and dysplasia in transgenic mice with astrocyte-directed expression of interferon-gamma, *J Mol Neurosci* 15:45-59, 2000.

817. Lin W, Kemper A, Dupree JL, Harding HP, et al: Interferon-gamma inhibits central nervous system remyelination through a process modulated by endoplasmic reticulum stress, *Brain* 129:1306-1318, 2006.

818. Folkerth RD, Keefe RJ, Haynes RL, Trachtenberg FL, et al: Interferon-gamma expression in periventricular leukomalacia in the human brain, *Brain Pathol* 14:265-274, 2004.

819. Loeliger M, Watson CS, Reynolds JD, Penning DH, et al: Extracellular glutamate levels and neuropathology in cerebral white matter following repeated umbilical cord occlusion in the near term fetal sheep, *Neuroscience* 116:705-714, 2003.

820. Matute C, Alberdi E, Domercq M, Sanchez-Gomez MV, et al: Excitotoxic damage to white matter, *J Anat* 210:693-702, 2007.

821. Matute C, Domercq M, Sanchez-Gomez MV: Glutamate-mediated glial injury: Mechanisms and clinical importance, *Glia* 53:212-224, 2006.

822. Deng W, Yue Q, Rosenberg PA, Volpe JJ, et al: Oligodendrocyte excitotoxicity determined by local glutamate accumulation and mitochondrial function, *J Neurochem* 96:213-222, 2006.

823. Fern R, Moller T: Rapid ischemic cell death in immature oligodendrocytes: A fatal glutamate release feedback loop, *J Neurosci* 20:34-42, 2000.

824. Pitt D, Werner P, Raine CS: Glutamate excitotoxicity in a model of multiple sclerosis, *Nat Med* 6:67-70, 2000.

825. Werner P, Pitt D, Raine CS: Multiple sclerosis: Altered glutamate homeostasis in lesions correlates with oligodendrocyte and axonal damage, *Ann Neurol* 50:169-180, 2001.

826. Domercq M, Etxebarria E, Perez-Samartin A, Matute C: Excitotoxic oligodendrocyte death and axonal damage induced by glutamate transporter inhibition, *Glia* 52:36-46, 2005.

826a. Kukley M, Capetillo-Zarate E, Dietrich D: Vesicular glutamate release from axons in white matter, *Nat Neurosci* 10:311-320, 2007.

826b. Ziskin JL, Nishiyama A, Rubio M, Fukaya M, et al: Vesicular release of glutamate from unmyelinated axons in white matter, *Nat Neurosci* 10:321-330, 2007.

827. Wilke SR, Thomas R, Allcock N, Fern R: Mechanism of acute ischemic injury of oligodendroglia in early myelinating white matter: The importance of astrocyte injury and glutamate release, *J Neuropathol Exp Neurol* 63:872-881, 2004.

828. Thomas R, Salter MG, Wilke S, Husen A, et al: Acute ischemic injury of astrocytes is mediated by Na-K-Cl cotransport and not Ca²⁺ influx at a key point in white matter development, *J Neuropathol Exp Neurol* 63:856-871, 2004.

829. Barger SW, Basile AS: Activation of microglia by secreted amyloid precursor protein evokes release of glutamate by cystine exchange and attenuates synaptic function, *J Neurochem* 76:846-854, 2001.

830. Ikezu T, Luo X, Weber GA, Zhao J, et al: Amyloid precursor protein-processing products affect mononuclear phagocyte activation: Pathways for sAPP- and Ab-mediated neurotoxicity, *J Neurochem* 85:925-934, 2003.

831. Kingham PJ, Cuzner ML, Pocock JM: Apoptotic pathways mobilized in microglia and neurones as a consequence of chromogranin A–induced microglial activation, *J Neurochem* 73:538-547, 1999.

832. Rimaniol A-C, Haik S, Martin M, Le Grand R, et al: Na⁺-dependent high-affinity glutamate transport in macrophages, *J Immunol* 164:5430-5438, 2000.

833. Miller BA, Sun F, Christensen RN, Ferguson AR, et al: A sublethal dose of TNF alpha potentiates kainate-induced excitotoxicity in optic nerve oligodendrocytes, *Neurochem Res* 30:867-875, 2005.

834. DeSilva TM, Kinney HC, Borenstein NS, Trachtenberg F, et al: The glutamate transporter EAAT2 is transiently expressed in developing human cerebral white matter, *J Comp Neurol* 501:879-890, 2007.

835. Northington FJ, Traystman RJ, Koehler RC, Martin LJ: GLT1, glial glutamate transporter, is transiently expressed in neurons and develops astrocyte specificity only after midgestation in the ovine fetal brain, *J Neurobiol* 39:515-526, 2001.

836. Itoh T, Beesley J, Itoh A, Cohen AS, et al: AMPA glutamate receptor-mediated calcium signaling is transiently enhanced during development of oligodendrocytes, *J Neurochem* 81:390-402, 2002.

837. Matute C, Sanchez-Gomez MV, Martinez-Millan L, Miledi R: Glutamate receptor-mediated toxicity in optic nerve oligodendrocytes, *Proc Natl Acad Sci U S A* 94:8830-8835, 1997.

838. McDonald JW, Althomsons SP, Hyrc KL, Choi DW, et al: Oligodendrocytes from forebrain are highly vulnerable to AMPA/kainate receptor-mediated excitotoxicity, *Nat Med* 4:291-297, 1998.

839. Rosenberg PA, Dai W, Gan XD, Ali S, et al: Mature myelin basic protein expressing oligodendrocytes are insensitive to kainate toxicity, *J Neurosci Res* 71:237-245, 2003.

840. Sanchez-Gomez MV, Alberdi E, Ibarretxe G, Torre I, et al: Caspase-dependent and caspase-independent oligodendrocyte death mediated by AMPA and kainate receptors, *J Neurosci* 23:9519-9528, 2003.

841. Sanchez-Gomez MV, Matute C: AMPA and kainate receptors each mediate excitotoxicity in oligodendroglial cultures, *Neurobiol Dis* 6:475-485, 1999.

842. Yoshioka A, Bacskai B, Pleasure D: Pathophysiology of oligodendroglial excitotoxicity, *J Neurosci Res* 46:427-438, 1996.

843. Deng W, Wang H, Rosenberg PA, Volpe JJ, et al: Role of metabotropic glutamate receptors in oligodendrocyte excitotoxicity and oxidative stress, *Proc Natl Acad Sci U S A* 101:7751-7756, 2004.

844. Karadottir R, Attwell D: Neurotransmitter receptors in the life and death of oligodendrocytes, *Neuroscience* 145:1426-1438, 2007.

845. Jensen FE: Role of glutamate receptors in periventricular leukomalacia, *J Child Neurol* 20:950-959, 2005.

846. Tekkok SB, Goldberg MP: AMPA/kainate receptor activation mediates hypoxic oligodendrocyte death and axonal injury in cerebral white matter, *J Neurosci* 21:4237-4248, 2001.

847. Yoshioka A, Yamaya Y, Saiki S, Kanemoto M, et al: Non–*N*-methyl-D-aspartate glutamate receptors mediate oxygen-glucose deprivation-induced oligodendroglial injury, *Brain Res* 854:207-215, 2000.

848. Deng W, Neve RL, Rosenberg PA, Volpe JJ, et al: alpha-Amino-3-hydroxy-5-methyl-4-isoxazole propionate receptor subunit composition and cAMP-response element-binding protein regulate oligodendrocyte excitotoxicity, *J Biol Chem* 281:36004-36011, 2006.

849. Follett PL, Rosenberg PA, Volpe JJ, Jensen FE: NBQX attenuates excitotoxic injury in developing white matter, *J Neurosci* 20:9235-9241, 2000.

850. Follett PL, Deng W, Dai W, Talos DM, et al: Glutamate receptor-mediated oligodendrocyte toxicity in periventricular leukomalacia: A protective role for topiramate, *J Neurosci* 24:4412-4420, 2004.

850a. Manning SM, Talos DM, Zhou C, Selip DR, et al: NMDA receptor blockade with memantine attenuates white matter deficits in a rat model of periventricular leukomalacia, 2007 submitted.

851. Alberdi E, Sanchez-Gomez MV, Marino A, Matute C: Ca(2+) influx through AMPA or kainate receptors alone is sufficient to initiate excitotoxicity in cultured oligodendrocytes, *Neurobiol Dis* 2:234-243, 2002.

852. Liu H-N, Giasson BI, Mushynski WE, Almazan G: AMPA receptor-mediated toxicity in oligodendrocyte progenitors involves free radical generation and activation of JNK, *calpain and caspase 3, J Neurochem* 82:398-409, 2002.

853. Salter MG, Fern R: NMDA receptors are expressed in developing oligodendrocyte processes and mediate injury, *Nature* 438:1167-1171, 2005.

854. Karadottir R, Cavelier P, Bergersen LH, Attwell D: NMDA receptors are expressed in oligodendrocytes and activated in ischaemia, *Nature* 438:1162-1166, 2005.

855. Micu I, Jiang Q, Coderre E, Ridsdale A, et al: NMDA receptors mediate calcium accumulation in myelin during chemical ischaemia, *Nature* 439:988-992, 2006.

856. Matute C: Oligodendrocyte NMDA receptors: A novel therapeutic target, *Trends Mol Med* 12:289-292, 2006.

857. Talos DM, Numis A, Sucher NJ, Folkerth RD, et al: Maturational profile of NR1, NR2 and NR3 subunit expression in human parietal white matter (in preparation, 2007).

858. Hennebert O, Marret S, Carmeliet P, Gressens P, et al: Role of tissue-derived plasminogen activator (T-PA) in an excitotoxic mouse model of neonatal white matter lesions, *J Neuropathol Exp Neurol* 63:53-63, 2004.

859. Tahraoui SL, Marret S, Bodenant C, Leroux P, et al: Central role of microglia in neonatal excitotoxic lesions of the murine periventricular white matter, *Brain Pathol* 11:56-71, 2001.

860. Sfaello I, Daire JL, Husson I, Kosofsky B, et al: Patterns of excitotoxin-induced brain lesions in the newborn rabbit: A neuropathological and MRI correlation, *Dev Neurosci* 27:160-168, 2005.

861. Martinez-Palma L, Pehar M, Cassina P, Peluffo H, et al: Involvement of nitric oxide on kainate-induced toxicity in oligodendrocyte precursors, *Neurotox Res* 5:385-394, 2003.

862. Stirling DP, Khodarahmi K, Liu J, McPhail LT, et al: Minocycline treatment reduces delayed oligodendrocyte death, attenuates axonal dieback, and improves functional outcome after spinal cord injury, *J Neurosci* 24:2182-2190, 2004.

863. Cho KO, La HO, Cho YJ, Sung KW, et al: Minocycline attenuates white matter damage in a rat model of chronic cerebral hypoperfusion, *J Neurosci Res* 83:285-291, 2006.

864. Fan LW, Pang Y, Lin S, Rhodes PG, et al: Minocycline attenuates lipopolysaccharide-induced white matter injury in the neonatal rat brain, *Neuroscience* 133:159-168, 2005.

865. Cai Z, Lin S, Fan LW, Pang Y, et al: Minocycline alleviates hypoxic-ischemic injury to developing oligodendrocytes in the neonatal rat brain, *Neuroscience* 137:425-435, 2006.

866. Lechpammer M, Manning SM, Samonte F, Nelligan J, et al: Minocycline treatment following hypoxic-ischemic injury attenuates white matter injury in a rodent model of periventricular leukomalacia, *Neuropathol Appl Neurobiol*: in press, 2008.

866a. Welin AK, Svedin P, Lapatto R, Sultan B, et al: Melatonin reduces inflammation and cell death in white matter in the mid-gestation fetal sheep following umbilical cord occlusion, *Pediatr Res* 61:153-158, 2007.

867. Andreakos E, Foxwell B, Feldmann M: Is targeting Toll-like receptors and their signaling pathway a useful therapeutic approach to modulating cytokine-driven inflammation? *Immunol Rev* 202:250-265, 2004.

868. Husson I, Mesples B, Bac P, Vamecq J, et al: Melatoninergic neuroprotection of the murine periventricular white matter against neonatal excitotoxic challenge, *Ann Neurol* 51:82-92, 2002.

869. Wang H, Li J, Follett PL, Zhang Y, et al: 12-Lipoxygenase plays a key role in cell death caused by glutathione depletion and arachidonic acid in rat oligodendrocytes, *Eur J Neurosci* 20:2049-2058, 2004.

870. Lin S, Cox HJ, Rhodes PG, Cai Z: Neuroprotection of alpha-phenyl-*N*-tert-butyl-nitrone on the neonatal white matter is associated with anti-inflammation, *Neurosci Lett* 405:52-56, 2006.

871. Lin SY, Fan LW, Pang Y, Rhodes PG, et al: IGF-1 protects oligodendrocyte progenitor cells and improves neurological functions following cerebral hypoxia-ischemia in the neonatal rat, *Brain Res* 1063:15-26, 2005.

872. Cao Y, Gunn AJ, Bennet L, Wu D, et al: Insulin-like growth factor (IGF)-1 suppresses oligodendrocyte caspase-3 activation and increases glial proliferation after ischemia in near-term fetal sheep, *J Cereb Blood Flow Metab* 23:739-747, 2003.

873. Ness JK, Wood TL: Insulin-like growth factor I, but not neurotrophin-3, sustains Akt activation and provides long-term protection of immature oligodendrocytes from glutamate-mediated apoptosis, *Mol Cell Neurosci* 20:476-488, 2002.

874. Ness JK, Scaduto RC, Wood TL: IGF-I prevents glutamate-mediated Bax translocation and cytochrome C release in O4(+.) oligodendrocyte progenitors, *Glia* 46:183-194, 2004.

875. Guan J, Thomas GB, Lin H, Mathai S, et al: Neuroprotective effects of the N-terminal tripeptide of insulin-like growth factor-1, glycine-proline-glutamate (GPE) following intravenous infusion in hypoxic-ischemic adult rats, *Neuropharmacology* 47:892-903, 2004.

876. Linker RA, Maurer M, Gaupp S, Martini R, et al: CNTF is a major protective factor in demyelinating CNS disease: A neurotrophic cytokine as modulator in neuroinflammation, *Nat Med* 8:620-624, 2002.

876a. Gerstner B, L. J. M, Lee J, DeSilva TM, et al: 17β Estradiol protects against hypoxic-ischemic white matter damage in the neonatal rat brain., *Eur J Neurosci*: in press, 2007.

877. Roelfsema V, Bennet L, George S, Wu D, et al: Window of opportunity of cerebral hypothermia for postischemic white matter injury in the near-term fetal sheep, *J Cereb Blood Flow Metab* 24:877-886, 2004.

877a. Bennet L, Roelfsema V, George S, Dean JM, et al: The effect of cerebral hypothermia on white and grey matter injury induced by severe hypoxia in preterm fetal sheep, *J Physiol* 578:491-506, 2007.

878. Dawes CS: *Foetal and Neonatal Physiology.* Chicago: 1968, Year Book.

879. Young M: The fetal and neonatal circulation. In *Handbook of Physiology: Circulation,* Baltimore: 1963, Waverly Press.

880. Rudolph AM, Heymann MA: The fetal circulation, *Annu Rev Med* 19:195, 1958.

881. Rudolph AM, Heymann MA: The circulation of the fetus in utero. Methods for studying distribution of blood flow, *cardiac output and organ blood flow, Circ Res* 21:163-184, 1967.

882. Barclay AE, Barcroft J, Barron DH, Franklin KJ: A radiographic demonstration of the circulation through the heart in the adult and in the fetus and the identification of the ductus arteriosus, *Brit J Radiol* 12:505, 1939.

883. Kaplan S, Assali NS: Fetal circulation. In Assali NS, Brinkman CR, editors: *Pathophysiology of Gestation III Fetal and Neonatal Disorders,* New York: 1972, Academic Press.

884. Rudolph AM: The fetal circulation and its response to stress, *J Dev Physiol* 6:11-19, 1984.

885. Kuschinsky W, Wahl M: Local chemical and neurogenic regulation of cerebral vascular resistance, *Physiol Res* 58:656, 1978.

886. Lassen NA, Christensen MS: Physiology of cerebral blood flow, *Br J Anaesth* 48:719-734, 1976.

887. MacKenzie ET, Strandgaard S, Graham DI, Jones JV, et al: Effects of acutely induced hypertension in cats on pial arteriolar caliber, local cerebral blood flow, and the blood-brain barrier, *Circ Res* 39:33-41, 1976.

888. Mchedlishvili GI, Nikolaishvili LS, Antia RV: Are the pial arterial responses dependent on the direct effect of intravascular pressure and extravascular and intravascular pO_2, pCO_2, and pH? *Microvascular Res* 10:298, 1976.

889. Hernandez MJ, Brennan RW, Bowman GS, Vannucci RC: Autoregulation of cerebral blood flow in the newborn dog, *Ann Neurol* 6:177, 1979.

890. Camp D, Kotagal UR, Kleinman LI: Preservation of cerebral autoregulation in the unanesthetized hypoxemic newborn dog, *Brain Res* 241:207-213, 1982.

891. Tweed WA, Cote J, Wade JG, Gregory G, et al: Preservation of fetal brain blood flow relative to other organs during hypovolemic hypotension, *Pediatr Res* 16:137-140, 1982.

892. Tweed WA, Cote J, Pash M, Lou H: Arterial oxygenation determines autoregulation of cerebral blood flow in the fetal lamb, *Pediatr Res* 17:246-249, 1983.

893. Papile LA, Rudolph AM: Autoregulation of cerebral blood flow in the preterm fetal lamb, *Pediatr Res* 19:159-161, 1985.

894. Tweed A, Cote J, Lou H, Gregory G, et al: Impairment of cerebral blood flow autoregulation in the newborn lamb by hypoxia, *Pediatr Res* 20:516-519, 1986.

895. Beausang-Linder M, Bill A: Cerebral circulation in acute arterial hypertension: Protective effects of sympathetic nervous activity, *Acta Physiol Scand* 111:193-199, 1981.

896. Heistad DD, Busija DW, Marcus ML: Neural effects on cerebral vessels: Alteration of pressure-flow relationship, *Fed Proc* 40:2317-2321, 1981.

897. Busija DW, Heistad DD: Factors involved in the physiological regulation of the cerebral circulation, *Rev Physiol Biochem Pharmacol* 101:161-211, 1984.

898. Kontos HA, Wei EP, Raper AJ, Patterson JL Jr: Local mechanism of CO_2 action of cat pial arterioles, *Stroke* 8:227-229, 1977.

899. Kontos HA, Raper AJ, Patterson JL: Analysis of vasoactivity of local pH, P_{CO_2} and bicarbonate on pial vessels, *Stroke* 8:358-360, 1977.

900. Pannier JL, Leusen I: Circulation to the brain of the rat during acute and prolonged respiratory changes in the acid-base balance, *Pflugers Arch* 338:347-359, 1973.

901. Betz E, Enzenross HG, Vlahov V: Interactions of ionic mechanisms in the regulation of the resistance of pial vessels. In Langfitt TW, McHenry LC, Reivich M, et al, editors: *Cerebral Circulation and Metabolism*, New York: 1975, Springer.

902. Knabe U, Betz E: The effect of varying extracellular K^{+-}, Mg^{++} and CA^{++} on the diameter of pial arterioles. In Betz E, editor: *Vascular Smooth Muscle*, Berlin: 1972, Springer.

903. Rudolph AM: Distribution and regulation of blood flow in the fetal and neonatal lamb, *Circ Res* 57:811-821, 1985.

904. Paulson OB, Strandgaard S, Edvinsson L: Cerebral autoregulation, *Cerebrovasc Brain Metab Rev* 2:161-192, 1990.

905. Florence G, Seylaz J: Rapid autoregulation of cerebral blood flow: A laser-Doppler flowmetry study, *J Cereb Blood Flow Metab* 12:674-680, 1992.

906. Rubanyi GM, Botelho LH: Endothelins, *FASEB J* 5:2713-2720, 1991.

907. Faraci FM: Role of endothelium-derived relaxing factor in cerebral circulation: Large arteries vs. microcirculation, *Am J Physiol* 26:H1038-H1042, 1991.

908. Greenberg DA, Chan J, Sampson HA: Endothelins and the nervous system, *Neurology* 42:25-31, 1992.

909. Aaslid R, Lindegaard KF, Sorteberg W, Nornes H: Cerebral autoregulation dynamics in humans, *Stroke* 20:45-52, 1989.

910. Siesjö BK: Cerebral circulation and metabolism, *J Neurosurg* 60:883-908, 1984.

911. Armstead WM, Leffler CW: Neurohumoral regulation of the cerebral circulation, *Proc Soc Exp Biol Med* 199:149-157, 1992.

912. Faraci FM, Heistad DD: Regulation of large cerebral arteries and cerebral microvascular pressure, *Circ Res* 66:8-17, 1990.

913. Kuschinsky W, Wahl M, Bosse O, Thurau K: Perivascular potassium and pH as determinants of local pial arterial diameter in cats: A microapplication study, *Circ Res* 31:240-247, 1972.

914. Moskalenk YY: Regional cerebral blood flow and its control at rest during increased functional activity. In Ingvar DH, Lassen NA, editors: *Brain Work*, Copenhagen: 1975, Munksgaard.

915. Berne RM, Rubio R, Curnish RR: Release of adenosine from ischemic brain: Effect on cerebral vascular resistance and incorporation into cerebral adenine nucleotides, *Circ Res* 35:262, 1974.

916. Wahl M, Kuschinsky W: The dilatatory action of adenosine on pial arteries of cats and its inhibition by theophylline, *Pflugers Arch* 362:55-59, 1976.

917. O'Regan M: Adenosine and the regulation of cerebral blood flow, *Neurol Res* 27:175-181, 2005.

918. Wahl M, Kuschinsky W, Bosse O, Thurau K: Dependency of pial arterial and arteriolar diameter on perivascular osmolarity in the cat: A microapplication study, *Circ Res* 32:162-169, 1973.

919. Grubb RL Jr, Hernandez-Perez MJ, Raichle ME, Phelps ME: The effects of iodinated contrast agents on autoregulation of cerebral blood flow, *Stroke* 5:155-160, 1974.

920. Betz E: Ionic interaction in pial vascular smooth muscles. In Betz E, editor: *Ionic Actions on Vascular Smooth Muscle*, Berlin: 1976, Springer.

921. Mogilner M, Ashwal S, Dale PS, Longo LD: Effect of nimodipine on newborn lamb cerebral blood flow, *Biol Neonate* 53:279-289, 1988.

922. Siesjö BK: Cell damage in the brain: A speculative synthesis, *J Cereb Blood Flow Metab* 1:155-185, 1981.

923. Iadecola C: Does nitric oxide mediate the increases in cerebral blood flow elicited by hypercapnia? *Proc Natl Acad Sci U S A* 89:3913-3916, 1992.

924. Hallenbeck JM, Dutka AJ: Background review and current concepts of reperfusion injury, *Arch Neurol* 47:1245-1254, 1990.

925. Van Woerkom R, Beharry KDA, Modanlou HD, Parker J, et al: Influence of morphine and naloxone on endothelin and its receptors in newborn piglet brain vascular endothelial cells: Clinical implications in neonatal care, *Pediatr Res* 55:147-151, 2004.

926. Sokoloff L, Grave GD, Jehle JW, Kennedy C: Postnatal development of the local cerebral blood flow in the dog, *Eur Neurol* 6:269-273, 1971.

927. Tuor UI: Local cerebral blood flow in the newborn rabbit: An autoradiographic study of changes during development, *Pediatr Res* 29:517-523, 1991.

928. Nehlig A, Pereira de Vasconcelos A, Boyet S: Postnatal changes in local cerebral blood flow measured by the quantitative autoradiographic [^{14}C]iodoantipyrine technique in freely moving rats, *J Cereb Blood Flow Metab* 9:579-588, 1989.

929. Gleason CA, Hamm C, Jones MD Jr: Cerebral blood flow, oxygenation, and carbohydrate metabolism in immature fetal sheep in utero, *Am J Physiol* 256:R1264-1268, 1989.

930. Richardson BS, Carmichael L, Joman J, Tanswell K, et al: Regional blood flow change in the lamb during the perinatal period, *Am J Obstet Gynecol* 160:919-925, 1989.

931. Jones MD Jr, Traystman RJ: Cerebral oxygenation of the fetus, newborn, and adult, *Semin Perinatol* 8:205-216, 1984.

932. Ashwal S, Majcher JS, Vain N, Longo LD: Patterns of fetal lamb regional cerebral blood flow during and after prolonged hypoxia, *Pediatr Res* 14:1104-1110, 1980.

933. Gleason CA, Short BL, Jones MD Jr: Cerebral blood flow and metabolism during and after prolonged hypocapnia in newborn lambs, *J Pediatr* 115:309-314, 1989.

934. Pasternak JF, Groothuis DR: Autoregulation of cerebral blood flow in the newborn beagle puppy, *Biol Neonate* 48:100-109, 1985.

935. Lyons DT, Vasta F, Vannucci RC: Autoradiographic determination of regional cerebral blood flow in the immature rat, *Pediatr Res* 21:471-476, 1987.

936. Szymonowicz W, Walker AM, Yu VY, Stewart ML, et al: Regional cerebral blood flow after hemorrhagic hypotension in the preterm, near-term, and newborn lamb, *Pediatr Res* 28:361-366, 1990.

937. DeGiulio PA, Roth RA, Mishra OP, Delivoria-Papadopoulos M, et al: Effect of indomethacin on the regulation of cerebral blood flow during respiratory alkalosis in newborn piglets, *Pediatr Res* 26:593-597, 1989.

938. Leffler CW, Busija DW, Mirro R, Armstead WM, et al: Effects of ischemia on brain blood flow and oxygen consumption of newborn pigs, *Am J Physiol* 257:H1917-H1926, 1989.

939. Ringel M, Bryan RM, Vannucci RC: Regional cerebral blood flow during hypoxia-ischemia in the immature rat: Comparison of iodoantipyrine and iodoamphetamine as radioactive tracers, *Brain Res Dev Brain Res* 59:231-235, 1991.

940. Reivich M, Brann AW Jr, Shapiro HM, Myers RE: Regional cerebral blood flow during prolonged partial asphyxia. In Meyer JS, Reivich M, Lechner H, et al, editors: *Research on the Cerebral Circulation*, Springfield, IL: 1972, Charles C Thomas.

941. Hohimer AR, Bissonnette JM: Effects of cephalic hypotension, hypertension, and barbiturates on fetal cerebral flood flow and metabolism, *Am J Obstet Gynecol* 161:1344-1351, 1989.

942. Young RS, Hernandez MJ, Yagel SK: Selective reduction of blood flow to white matter during hypotension in newborn dogs: A possible mechanism of periventricular leukomalacia, *Ann Neurol* 12:445-448, 1982.

943. Arnold BW, Martin CG, Alexander BJ, Chen T, et al: Autoregulation of brain blood flow during hypotension and hypertension in infant lambs, *Pediatr Res* 29:110-115, 1991.

944. Monin P, Stonestreet BS, Oh W: Hyperventilation restores autoregulation of cerebral blood flow in postictal piglets, *Pediatr Res* 30:294-298, 1991.

945. Hascoet JM, Monin P, Vert P: Persistence of impaired autoregulation of cerebral blood flow in the postictal period in piglets, *Epilepsia* 29:743-747, 1988.

946. Del Toro J, Louis PT, Goddard-Finegold J: Cerebrovascular regulation and neonatal brain injury, *Pediatr Neurol* 7:3-12, 1991.

947. Meadow W, Rudinsky B, Bell A, Lozon M, et al: The role of prostaglandins and endothelium-derived relaxation factor in the regulation of cerebral blood flow and cerebral oxygen utilization in the piglet: Operationalizing the concept of an essential circulation, *Pediatr Res* 35:649-656, 1994.

948. Odden JP, Farstad T, Roll EB, Hall C, et al: Cerebral blood flow autoregulation after moderate hypoxemia in the newborn piglet, *Biol Neonate* 65:367-377, 1994.

949. Chemtob S, Li DY, Abran D, Hardy P, et al: The role of prostaglandin receptors in regulating cerebral blood flow in the perinatal period, *Acta Paediatr* 85:517-524, 1996.

950. Martinez-Orgado J, Gonzalez R, Alonso MJ, Rodriguez-Martinez MA, et al: Endothelial factors and autoregulation during pressure changes in isolated newborn piglet cerebral arteries, *Pediatr Res* 44:161-167, 1998.

951. Lotgering FK, Bishai JM, Struijk PC, Blood AB, et al: Ten-minute umbilical cord occlusion markedly reduces cerebral blood flow and heat production in fetal sheep, *Am J Obstet Gynecol* 189:233-238, 2003.

952. van Os S, Liem D, Hopman J, Klaessens J, et al: Cerebral O_2 supply thresholds for the preservation of electrocortical brain activity during hypotension in near-term-born lambs, *Pediatr Res* 57:358-362, 2005.

953. van Os S, Klaessens J, Hopman J, Liem D, et al: Cerebral oxygen supply during hypotension in near-term lambs: A near-infrared spectroscopy study, *Brain Dev* 28:115-121, 2006.

954. Eidson TH, Edrington JL, Luiza M, Albuquerque C, et al: Light/dye microvascular injury eliminates pial arteriolar dilation in hypotensive piglets, *Pediatr Res* 37:10-14, 1995.

955. Shimoda LA, Norins NA, Jeutter DC, Madden JA: Flow-induced responses in piglet isolated cerebral arteries, *Pediatr Res* 39:574-583, 1996.

956. Shimoda LA, Norins NA, Madden JA: Responses to pulsatile flow in piglet isolated cerebral arteries, *Pediatr Res* 43:514-520, 1998.

957. Haggendal E, Johansson B: Effects of arterial carbon dioxide tension and oxygen saturation on cerebral blood flow autoregulation in dogs, *Acta Physiol Scand Suppl* 258:27-53, 1965.

958. Vannucci RC, Towfighi J, Brucklacher R, Vannucci SJ: Effect of extreme hypercapnia on hypoxic-ischemic brain damage in the immature rate, *Pediatr Res* 49:799-803, 2001.

959. Kaiser JR, Gauss CH, Williams DK: The effects of hypercapnia on cerebral autoregulation in ventilated very low birth weight infants, *Pediatr Res* 58:931-935, 2005.

960. Ong BY, Greengrass R, Bose D, Gregory G, et al: Acidemia impairs autoregulation of cerebral blood flow in newborn lambs, *Can Anaesth Soc J* 33:5-9, 1986.

961. Laptook A, Stonestreet BS, Oh W: Autoregulation of brain blood flow in the newborn piglet: Regional differences in flow reduction during hypotension, *Early Hum Dev* 6:99-107, 1982.

962. Laptook AR, Stonestreet BS, Oh W: Brain blood flow and O_2 delivery during hemorrhagic hypotension in the piglet, *Pediatr Res* 17:77-80, 1983.

963. Hilario E, Rey-Santano MC, Goni-de-Cerio F, Alvarez FJ, et al: Cerebral blood flow and morphological changes after hypoxic-ischaemic injury in preterm lambs, *Acta Paediatr* 94:903-911, 2005.

964. Dunnihoo DR, Quilligan EJ: Carotid blood flow distribution in the in utero sheep fetus, *Am J Obstet Gynecol* 116:648-656, 1973.

965. Mann LI: Developmental aspects and the effect of carbon dioxide tension on fetal cephalic blood flow, *Exp Neurol* 26:136-147, 1970.

966. Shapiro HM, Greenberg JH, Naughton KV, Reivich M: Heterogeneity of local cerebral blood flow– $Paco_2$ sensitivity in neonatal dogs, *J Appl Physiol* 49:113-118, 1980.

967. Ashwal S, Dale PS, Longo LD: Regional cerebral blood flow: Studies in the fetal lamb during hypoxia, hypercapnia, acidosis, and hypotension, *Pediatr Res* 18:1309-1316, 1984.

968. Cartwright D, Gregory GA, Lou H, Heyman MA: The effect of hypocarbia on the cardiovascular system of puppies, *Pediatr Res* 18:685-690, 1984.

969. Hansen NB, Brubakk AM, Bratlid D, Oh W, et al: The effects of variations in $Paco_2$ on brain blood flow and cardiac output in the newborn piglet, *Pediatr Res* 18:1132-1136, 1984.

970. Rosenberg AA, Koehler RC, Jones MD Jr: Distribution of cardiac output in fetal and neonatal lambs with acute respiratory acidosis, *Pediatr Res* 18:731-735, 1984.

971. Young RS, Yagel SK: Cerebral physiological and metabolic effects of hyperventilation in the neonatal dog, *Ann Neurol* 16:337-342, 1984.

972. Brubakk AM, Oh W, Stonestreet BS: Prolonged hypercarbia in the awake newborn piglet: Effect on brain blood flow and cardiac output, *Pediatr Res* 21:29-33, 1987.

973. Reuter JH, Disney TA: Regional cerebral blood flow and cerebral metabolic rate of oxygen during hyperventilation in the newborn dog, *Pediatr Res* 20:1102-1106, 1986.

974. Rosenberg AA: Response of the cerebral circulation to profound hypocarbia in neonatal lambs, *Stroke* 19:1365-1370, 1988.

975. Stiris T, Odden JP, Hansen TW, Hall C, et al: The effect of arterial Pco_2-variations on ocular and cerebral blood flow in the newborn piglet, *Pediatr Res* 25:205-208, 1989.

976. Yamashita N, Kamiya K, Nagai H: CO_2 reactivity and autoregulation in fetal brain, *Childs Nerv Syst* 7:327-331, 1991.

977. Leffler CW, Mirro R, Shibata M, Parfenova H, et al: Effects of indomethacin on cerebral vasodilator responses to arachidonic acid in hypercapnia in newborn pigs, *Pediatr Res* 33:609-614, 1993.

978. Rosenberg AA: Response of the cerebral circulation to hypocarbia in postasphyxia newborn lambs, *Pediatr Res* 32:537-541, 1992.

979. Mirro R, Lowerysmith L, Armstead WM, Shibata M, et al: Cerebral vasoconstriction in response to hypocapnia is maintained after ischemia reperfusion injury in newborn pigs, *Stroke* 23:1613-1616, 1992.

980. Vannucci RC, Brucklacher RM, Vannucci SJ: Effect of carbon dioxide on cerebral metabolism during hypoxia-ischemia in the immature rat, *Pediatr Res* 42:24-29, 1997.

981. Greisen G, Vannucci RC: Is periventricular leucomalacia a result of hypoxic-ischaemic injury? Hypocapnia and the preterm brain, *Biol Neonate* 79:194-200, 2001.

982. Rosenberg AA, Jones MD Jr, Traystman RJ, Simmons MA, et al: Response of cerebral blood flow to changes in Pco_2 in fetal, newborn, and adult sheep, *Am J Physiol* 242:H862-H866, 1982.

983. Hasegawa M, Tatsuno M, Houdou S, Takashima S, et al: Continuous comparison of cerebral blood flow velocity and volume on hypoxia, *Brain Dev* 13:433-437, 1991.

984. Jones MD Jr, Sheldon RE, Peeters LL, Makowski EL, et al: Regulat of cerebral blood flow in the ovine fetus, *Am J Physiol* 235:H162-H166, 1978.

985. Koehler RC, Jones MD Jr, Traystman RJ: Cerebral circulatory response to carbon monoxide and hypoxic hypoxia in the lamb, *Am J Physiol* 243:H27-H32, 1982.

986. Gilbert RD, Pearce WJ, Ashwal S, Longo LD: Effects of hypoxia on contractility of isolated fetal lamb cerebral arteries, *J Dev Physiol* 13:199-203, 1990.

987. Suguihara C, Bancalari E, Hehre D: Brain blood flow and ventilatory res-ponse to hypoxia in sedated newborn piglets, *Pediatr Res* 27:327-331, 1990.

988. Suguihara C, Bancalari E, Hehre D, Osiovich H: Effect of alpha adrenergic blockade on brain blood flow and ventilation during hypoxia in newborn piglets, *J Dev Physiol* 15:289-295, 1991.

989. Fumagalli M, Mosca F, Knudsen GM, Greisen G: Transient hyperoxia and residual cerebrovascular effects in the newborn rat, *Pediatr Res* 55:380-384, 2004.

990. Kuban KC, Gilles FH: Human telencephalic angiogenesis, *Ann Neurol* 17:539-548, 1985.

991. Bucciarelli RL, Eitzman DV: Cerebral blood flow during acute acidosis in perinatal goats, *Pediatr Res* 13:178-180, 1979.

992. Laptook AR, Peterson J, Porter AM: Effects of lactic acid infusions and pH on cerebral blood flow and metabolism, *J Cereb Blood Flow Metab* 8:193-200, 1988.

993. Hermansen MC, Kotagal UR, Kleinman LI: The effect of metabolic acidosis upon autoregulation of cerebral blood flow in newborn dogs, *Brain Res* 324:101-105, 1984.

994. Laptook AR: The effects of sodium bicarbonate on brain blood flow and O_2 delivery during hypoxemia and acidemia in the piglet, *Pediatr Res* 19:815-819, 1985.

995. Laudignon N, Beharry K, Farri E, Aranda JV: The role of adenosine in the vascular adaptation of neonatal cerebral blood flow during hypotension, *J Cereb Blood Flow Metab* 11:424-431, 1991.

996. Park TS, Van Wylen DGL, Rubio R, Berne RM: Brain interstitial fluid adenosine and autoregulation of cerebral blood flow in the neonatal piglet. In Marlin AE, editor: *Concepts in Pediatric Neurosurgery*, Basel: 1990, Karger.

997. Palluy O, Morliere L, Gris JC, Bonne C, et al: Hypoxia/reoxygenation stimulates endothelium to promote neutrophil adhesion, *Free Radic Biol Med* 13:21-30, 1992.

998. Leffler CW, Busija DW, Beasley DG, Armstead WM, et al: Postischemic cerebral microvascular responses to norepinephrine and hypotension in newborn pigs, *Stroke* 20:541-546, 1989.

999. Leffler CW, Busija DW, Armstead WM, Mirro R, et al: Ischemia alters cerebral vascular responses to hypercapnia and acetylcholine in piglets, *Pediatr Res* 25:180-183, 1989.

1000. Mirro R, Armstead W, Busija D, Green R, et al: Increasing ventilation pressure increases cortical subarachnoid cerebrospinal fluid prostanoids in newborn pigs, *Pediatr Res* 22:647-650, 1987.

1001. Leffler CW, Busija DW, Fletcher AM, Beasley DG, et al: Effects of indomethacin upon cerebral hemodynamics of newborn pigs, *Pediatr Res* 19:1160-1164, 1985.

1002. Leffler CW, Busija DW, Beasley DG, Fletcher AM: Maintenance of cerebral circulation during hemorrhagic hypotension in newborn pigs: Role of prostanoids, *Circ Res* 59:562-567, 1986.

1003. Leffler CW, Busija DW: Prostanoids and pial arteriolar diameter in hypotensive newborn pigs, *Am J Physiol* 252:H687-H691, 1987.

1004. Busija DW, Leffler CW: Eicosanoid synthesis elicited by norepinephrine in piglet parietal cortex, *Brain Res* 403:243-248, 1987.

1005. Wagerle LC, Mishra OP: Mechanism of CO_2 response in cerebral arteries of the newborn pig: Role of phospholipase, cyclooxygenase, and lipoxygenase pathways, *Circ Res* 62:1019-1026, 1988.

1006. Armstead WM, Mirro R, Busija DW, Leffler CW: Permissive role of prostanoids in acetylcholine-induced cerebral vasoconstriction, *J Pharmacol Exp Ther* 251:1012-1019, 1989.

1007. Busija DW, Leffler CW: Role of prostanoids in cerebrovascular responses during seizures in piglets, *Am J Physiol* 256:H120-H125, 1989.

1008. Armstead WM, Mirro R, Busija DW, Leffler CW: Prostanoids modulate opioid cerebrovascular responses in newborn pigs, *J Pharmacol Exp Ther* 255:1083-1089, 1990.

1009. Chemtob S, Beharry K, Rex J, Varma DR, et al: Prostanoids determine the range of cerebral blood flow autoregulation of newborn piglets, *Stroke* 21:777-784, 1990.

1010. Armstead WM, Mirro R, Busija DW, Leffler CW: Opioids and the prostanoid system in the control of cerebral blood flow in hypotensive piglets, *J Cereb Blood Flow Metab* 11:380-387, 1991.

1011. Pourcyrous M, Busija DW, Shibata M, Bada HS, et al: Cebrovascular responses to therapeutic dose of indomethacin in newborn pigs, *Pediatr Res* 45:582-587, 1999.

1012. Patel J, Roberts I, Azzopardi D, Hamilton P, et al: Randomized double-blind controlled trial comparing the effects of ibuprofen with indomethacin on cerebral hemodynamics in preterm infants with patent ductus arteriosus, *Pediatr Res* 47:36-42, 2000.

1013. Brown DW, Lee D, Kumaran VS, Lee T-Y: Age-dependent cerebral hemodynamic effects of indomethacin in the newborn piglet, *J Appl Physiol* 97:1880-1887, 2004.

1014. Rosenberg AA: Regulation of cerebral blood flow after asphyxia in neonatal lambs, *Stroke* 19:239-244, 1988.

1015. Lou HC, Lassen NA, Tweed WA, Johnson G, et al: Pressure passive cerebral blood flow and breakdown of the blood-brain barrier in experimental fetal asphyxia, *Acta Paediatr Scand* 68:57-63, 1979.

1016. Johnson GN, Palahniuk RJ, Tweed WA, Jones MV, et al: Regional cerebral blood flow changes during severe fetal asphyxia produced by slow partial umbilical cord compression, *Am J Obstet Gynecol* 135:48-52, 1979.

1017. Cohn HE, Sacks EJ, Heymann MA, Rudolph AM: Cardiovascular responses to hypoxemia and acidemia in fetal lambs, *Am J Obstet Gynecol* 120:817-824, 1974.

1018. Mann LI: Effect of hypoxia on fetal cephalic blood flow, cephalic metabolism and the electroencephalogram, *Exp Neurol* 29:336-348, 1970.

1019. Ashwal S, Majcher JS, Longo LD: Patterns of fetal lamb regional cerebral blood flow during and after prolonged hypoxia: Studies during the posthypoxic recovery period, *Am J Obstet Gynecol* 139:365-372, 1981.

1020. Lou HC, Tweed WA, Davies JM: Preferential blood flow increase to the brain stem in moderate neonatal hypoxia: Reversal by naloxone, *Eur J Pediatr* 144:225-227, 1985.

1021. McPhee AJ, Kotagal UR, Kleinman LI: Cerebrovascular hemodynamics during and after recovery from acute asphyxia in the newborn dog, *Pediatr Res* 19:645-650, 1985.

1022. Rosenberg AA: Cerebral blood flow and O$_2$ metabolism after asphyxia in neonatal lamb, *Pediatr Res* 20:778-782, 1986.

1023. Takashima S, Ando Y, Takeshita K: Hypoxic-ischemic brain damage and cerebral blood flow changes in young rabbits, *Brain Dev* 8:274-277, 1986.

1024. Odden JP, Stiris T, Hansen TW, Bratlid D: Cerebral blood flow during experimental hypoxaemia and ischaemia in the newborn piglet, *Acta Paediatr Scand Suppl* 360:13-19, 1989.

1025. Mujsce DJ, Christensen MA, Vannucci RC: Cerebral blood flow and edema in perinatal hypoxic-ischemic brain damage, *Pediatr Res* 27:450-453, 1990.

1026. Laptook AR, Corbett R, Ruley J, Olivares E: Blood flow and metabolism during and after repeated partial brain ischemia in neonatal piglets, *Stroke* 23:380-387, 1992.

1027. Leffler CW, Thompson CC, Armstead WM, Mirro R, et al: Superoxide scavengers do not prevent ischemia-induced alteration of cerebral vasodilation in piglets, *Pediatr Res* 33:164-170, 1993.

1028. Ball RH, Espinoza MI, Parer JT, Alon E, et al: Regional blood flow in asphyxiated fetuses with seizures, *Am J Obstet Gynecol* 170:156-161, 1994.

1029. Takashima S, Hirano S, Kamei S, Hasegawa M, et al: Cerebral hemodynamics on near-infrared spectroscopy in hypoxia and ischemia in young animal studies, *Brain Dev* 17:312-316, 1995.

1030. Pourcyrous M, Parfenova H, Bada HS, Dorones SB, et al: Changes in cerebral cyclic nucleotides and cerebral blood flow during prolonged asphyxia and recovery in newborn pigs, *Pediatr Res* 41:617-623, 1997.

1031. Giussani DA, Thakor AS, Frulio R, Gazzolo D: Acute hypoxia increases S100beta protein in association with blood flow redistribution away from peripheral circulations in fetal sheep, *Pediatr Res* 58:179-184, 2005.

1032. van Os S, van den Tweel E, Egberts H, Hopman J, et al: Cerebral cortical tissue damage after hemorrhagic hypotension in near-term born lambs, *Pediatr Res* 59:221-226, 2006.

1033. Friedman WF, Kirkpatrick SE: Fetal cardiovascular adaptation to asphyxia. In Gluck L, editor: *Intrauterine Asphyxia and the Developing Fetal Brain*, Chicago: 1977, Year Book.

1034. Davies JM, Tweed WA: The regional distribution and determinants of myocardial blood flow during asphyxia in the fetal lamb, *Pediatr Res* 18:764-767, 1984.

1035. Johannsson H, Siesjö BK: Cerebral blood flow and oxygen consumption in the rat in hypoxic hypoxia, *Acta Physiol Scand* 93:269-276, 1975.

1036. Lassen NA: Brain extracellular pH: The main factor controlling cerebral blood flow, *Scand J Clin Lab Invest* 22:247-251, 1968.

1037. Kirshner HS, Blank WF Jr, Myers RE: Brain extracellular potassium activity during hypoxia in the cat, *Neurology* 25:1001-1005, 1975.

1038. Kirshner HS, Blank WF Jr, Myers RE: Changes in cortical subarachnoid fluid potassium concentrations during hypoxia, *Arch Neurol* 33:84-90, 1976.

1039. Morris ME: Hypoxia and extracellular potassium activity in the guinea-pig cortex, *Can J Physiol Pharmacol* 52:872-882, 1974.

1040. Rubio R, Berne RM, Bockman EL, Curnish RR: Relationship between adenosine concentration and oxygen supply in rat brain, *Am J Physiol* 228:1896-1902, 1975.

1041. Phillis JW, Preston G, DeLong RE: Effects of anoxia on cerebral blood flow in the rat brain: Evidence for a role of adenosine in autoregulation, *J Cereb Blood Flow Metab* 4:586-592, 1984.

1042. Hernandez MJ, Brennan RW, Hawkins RA: Regional cerebral blood flow during neonatal asphyxia. In Passonneau RA, Hawkins WD, Lust WD, et al, editors: *Cerebral Metabolism and Neural Function*, Baltimore: 1980, Williams & Wilkins.

1043. Lou HC, Tweed WA, Davis JM: Endogenous opioids may protect the perinatal brain in hypoxia, *Dev Pharmacol Ther* 13:129-133, 1989.

1044. Wardlaw SL, Stark RI, Daniel S, Frantz AG: Effects of hypoxia on beta-endorphin and beta-lipotropin release in fetal, newborn, and maternal sheep, *Endocrinology* 108:1710-1715, 1981.

1045. Ruth V, Pohjavuori M, Rovamo L, Salminen K, et al: Plasma beta-endorphin in perinatal asphyxia and respiratory difficulties in newborn infants, *Pediatr Res* 20:577-580, 1986.

1046. Martinez AM, Padbury JF, Burnell EE, Thio SL, et al: The effects of hypoxia on (methionine) enkephalin peptide and catecholamine release in fetal sheep, *Pediatr Res* 27:52-55, 1990.

1047. Williams CE, Gunn AJ, Synek B, Gluckman PD: Delayed seizures occurring with hypoxic-ischemic encephalopathy in the fetal sheep, *Pediatr Res* 27:561-565, 1990.

1048. Zagorac D, Yamaura K, Zhang C, Roman RJ, et al: The effect of superoxide anion on autoregulation of cerebral blood flow, *Stroke* 36:2589-2594, 2005.

1049. Lou HC, Lassen NA, Friis-Hansen B: Low cerebral blood flow in hypotensive perinatal distress, *Acta Neurol Scand* 56:343-352, 1977.

1050. Lou HC, Lassen NA, Fris-Hansen B: Decreased cerebral blood flow after administration of sodium bicarbonate in the distressed newborn infant, *Acta Neurol Scand* 57:239-247, 1978.

1051. Lou HC, Lassen NA, Friis-Hansen B: Impaired autoregulation of cerebral blood flow in the distressed newborn infant, *J Pediatr* 94:118-121, 1979.

1052. Lou HC, Skov H, Pedersen H: Low cerebral blood flow: A risk factor in the neonate, *J Pediatr* 95:606-609, 1979.

1053. Ment LR, Ehrenkranz RA, Lange RC, Rothstein PT, et al: Alterations in cerebral blood flow in preterm infants with intraventricular hemorrhage, *Pediatrics* 68:763-769, 1981.

1054. Younkin DP, Reivich M, Jaggi J, Obrist W, et al: Noninvasive method of estimating human newborn regional cerebral blood flow, *J Cereb Blood Flow Metab* 2:415-420, 1982.

1055. Greiss FC: A clinical concept of uterine blood flow during pregnancy, *Obstet Gynecol* 40:595, 1967.

1056. Greisen G, Friis-Hansen B: CBF in the preterm infant. In Second International Conference, Fetal and Neonatal Physiological Measurements, 1984; Oxford: 1984.

1057. Greisen G: Cerebral blood flow in preterm infants during the first week of life, *Acta Paediatr Scand* 75:43-51, 1986.

1058. Greisen G, Trojaborg W: Cerebral blood flow, Paco$_2$ changes, and visual evoked potentials in mechanically ventilated, preterm infants, *Acta Paediatr Scand* 76:394-400, 1987.

1059. Pryds O, Greisen G, Johansen KH: Indomethacin and cerebral blood flow in premature infants treated for patent ductus arteriosus, *Eur J Pediatr* 147:315-316, 1988.

1060. Pryds O, Greisen G, Friis-Hansen B: Compensatory increase of CBF in preterm infants during hypoglycaemia, *Acta Paediatr Scand* 77:632-637, 1988.

1061. Younkin DP, Reivich M, Jaggi JL, Obrist WD, et al: The effect of hematocrit and systolic blood pressure on cerebral blood flow in newborn infants, *J Cereb Blood Flow Metab* 7:295-299, 1987.

1062. Younkin J, Delivoria-Papadopoulos M, Reivich M, Jaggi J, et al: Regional variations in human newborn cerebral blood flow, *J Pediatr* 112:104-108, 1988.

1063. Pryds O, Greisen G, Lou H, Friis-Hansen B: Heterogeneity of cerebral vasoreactivity in preterm infants supported by mechanical ventilation, *J Pediatr* 115:638-645, 1989.

1064. Pryds O, Greisen G: Effect of Paco$_2$ and haemoglobin concentration on day to day variation of CBF in preterm neonates, *Acta Paediatr Scand Suppl* 360:33-36, 1989.

1065. Pryds O, Christensen NJ, Friis HB: Increased cerebral blood flow and plasma epinephrine in hypoglycemic, *preterm neonates, Pediatrics* 85:172-176, 1990.

1066. Obrist WD, Wilkinson WE: Regional cerebral blood flow measurement in humans by xenon-133 clearance, *Cerebrovasc Brain Metab Rev* 2:283-327, 1990.

1067. Pryds O, Greisen G, Lou H, Friis-Hansen B: Vasoparalysis associated with brain damage in asphyxiated term infants, *J Pediatr* 117:119-125, 1990.

1068. Pryds O, Greisen G: Preservation of single-flash visual evoked potentials at very low cerebral oxygen delivery in preterm infants, *Pediatr Neurol* 6:151-158, 1990.

1069. Pryds O, Greisen G, Skov LL, Friis-Hansen B: Carbon dioxide-related changes in cerebral blood volume and cerebral blood flow in mechanically ventilated preterm neonates: Comparison of near infrared spectrophotometry and ^{133}xenon clearance, *Pediatr Res* 27:445-449, 1990.

1070. Pryds O, Andersen GE, Friis-Hansen B: Cerebral blood flow reactivity in spontaneously breathing, preterm infants shortly after birth, *Acta Paediatr Scand* 79:391-396, 1990.

1071. Pryds O, Schneider S: Aminophylline reduces cerebral blood flow in stable, preterm infants without affecting the visual evoked potential, *Eur J Pediatr* 150:366-369, 1991.

1072. Pryds O: Control of cerebral circulation in the high-risk neonate, *Ann Neurol* 30:321-329, 1991.

1073. Greisen G: Effect of cerebral blood flow and cerebrovascular autoregulation on the distribution, type and extent of cerebral injury, *Brain Pathol* 2:223-228, 1992.

1074. Pryds O, Edwards AD: Cerebral blood flow in the newborn infant, *Arch Dis Child Fetal Neonatal Ed* 74:F63-F69, 1996.

1075. Muller AM, Morales C, Briner J, Baenziger O, et al: Loss of CO$_2$ reactivity of cerebral blood flow is associated with severe brain damage in mechanically ventilated very low birth weight infants, *Eur J Paediatr Neurol* 5:157-163, 1997.

1076. Cooke RW, Rolfe P, Howat P: Apparent cerebral blood-flow in newborns with respiratory disease, *Dev Med Child Neurol* 21:154-159, 1979.

1077. Milligan DW, Bryan MH: Failure of autoregulation of the cerebral circulation in the sick newborn infant, *Pediatr Res* 13:527-531, 1979.

1078. Leahy F, Sankaran K, Cates D: Changes in cerebral blood flow (CBF) in preterm infants during inhalation of CO$_2$ and 100% O$_2$, *Pediatr Res* 13:526, 1979.

1079. Rahilly PM: Effects of sleep state and feeding on cranial blood flow of the human neonate, *Arch Dis Child* 55:265-270, 1980.

1080. Mukhtar AI, Cowan FM, Stothers JK: Cranial blood flow and blood pressure changes during sleep in the human neonate, *Early Hum Dev* 6:59-64, 1982.

1081. Rolfe P, Persson B, Zetterstrom R: An appraisal of techniques for studying cerebral circulation in the newborn: Report of a mini-symposium held in September 1982, *Acta Paediatr Scand Suppl* 311:5-13, 1983.

1082. Colditz P, Greisen G, Pryds O: Comparison of electrical impedance and ^{133}xenon clearance for the assessment of cerebral blood flow in the newborn infant, *Pediatr Res* 24:461-464, 1988.

1083. Colditz PB, Valimaki IA, Murphy D, Rolfe P, et al: Continuous cerebral electrical impedance monitoring in sick preterm infants, *Eur J Pediatr* 149:428-431, 1990.

1084. Altman DI, Powers WJ, Perlman JM, Herscovitch P, et al: Cerebral blood flow requirement for brain viability in newborn infants is lower than in adults, *Ann Neurol* 24:218-226, 1988.

1085. Meek JH, Tyszczuk L, Elwell CE, Wyatt JS: Cerebral blood flow increases over the first three days of life in extremely preterm neonates, *Arch Dis Child Fetal Neonatal Ed* 78:F33-F37, 1998.

1086. Naulaers G, Morren G, VanHuffel S, Casaer P, et al: Cerebral tissue oxygenation index in very premature infants, *Arch Dis Child* 87:189-192, 2002.

1087. Fukuda S, Kato T, Kakita H, Yamada Y, et al: Hemodynamics of the cerebral arteries of infants with periventricular leukomalacia, *Pediatrics* 117:1-8, 2006.

1088. Panerai RB, Kelsall A, Rennie JM, Evans DH: Cerebral autoregulation dynamics in premature newborns, *Stroke* 26:74-80, 1995.

1089. Tsuji M, Saul JP, du Plessis A, Eichenwald E, et al: Cerebral intravascular oxygenation correlates with mean arterial pressure in critically ill premature infants, *Pediatrics* 106:625-632, 2000.

1090. von Siebenthal K, Beran J, Wolf M, Keel M, et al: Cyclical fluctuations in blood pressure, *heart rate and cerebral blood volume in preterm infants, Brain Dev* 21:529-534, 1999.

1091. Boylan GB, Young K, Panerai RB, Rennie JM, et al: Dynamic cerebral autoregulation in sick newborn infants, *Pediatr Res* 48:12-17, 2000.

1092. Tsuji M, Saul JP, du Plessis A, Eichenwald E, et al: Cerebral intravascular oxygenation correlates with mean arterial pressure in critically ill premature infants, *Pediatrics* 106:625-632, 2000.

1093. Jayasinghe DJ, Gill AB, Levene M: CBF reactivity in hypotensive and normotensive preterm infants, *Pediatr Res* 54:848-853, 2003.

1094. Bassan H, Gauvreau K, Newburger JW, Tsuji M, et al: Identification of pressure passive cerebral perfusion and its mediators after infant cardiac surgery, *Pediatr Res* 57:35-41, 2005.

1095. Lemmers PM, Toet M, van Schelven LJ, van, Bel F: Cerebral oxygenation and cerebral oxygen extraction in the preterm infant: The impact of respiratory distress syndrome, *Exp Brain Res* 173:458-467, 2006.

1096. Victor S, Appleton RE, Beirne M, Marson AG, et al: The relationship between cardiac output, cerebral electrical activity, cerebral fractional oxygen extraction and peripheral blood flow in premature newborn infants, *Pediatr Res* 60:456-460, 2006.

1097. Soul JS, Hammer PE, Tsuji M, Saul P, et al: Fluctuating pressure-passivity is common in the cerebral circulation of sick premature infants, *Pediatr Res* 61:467-473, 2007.

1098. Menke J, Michel E, Hillebrand S, Von Twickel J, et al: Cross-spectral analysis of cerebral autoregulation dynamics in high risk preterm infants during the perinatal period, *Pediatr Res* 42:690-699, 1997.

1099. West CR, Groves AM, Williams CE, Harding JE, et al: Early low cardiac output is associated with compromised electroencephalographic activity in very preterm infants, *Pediatr Res* 59:610-615, 2006.

1100. Munro MJ, Barfield CP, Walker AM: Hypotensive extremely low birth weight infants have reduced cerebral blood flow, *Pediatrics* 114:1591-1596, 2004.

1101. Victor S, Marson AG, Appleton RE, Beirne M, et al: Relationship between blood pressure, cerebral electrical activity, cerebral fractional oxygen extraction, and peripheral blood flow in very low birth weight newborn infants, *Pediatr Res* 59:314-319, 2006.

1102. Reivich M, Brann AW Jr, Shapiro H, Rawson J, et al: Reactivity of cerebral vessels to CO_2 in the newborn rhesus monkey, *Eur Neurol* 6:132-136, 1971.

1103. Rosenberg AA, Harris AP, Koehler RC, Hudak ML, et al: Role of O_2-hemoglobin affinity in the regulation of cerebral blood flow in fetal sheep, *Am J Physiol* 251:H56-H62, 1986.

1104. Jones MD Jr, Traystman RJ, Simmons MA, Molteni RA: Effects of changes in arterial O_2 content on cerebral blood flow in the lamb, *Am J Physiol* 240:H209-H215, 1981.

1105. Rosenkrantz TS, Stonestreet BS, Hansen NB, Nowicki P, et al: Cerebral blood flow in the newborn lamb with polycythemia and hyperviscosity, *J Pediatr* 104:276-280, 1984.

1106. Lipp-Zwahlen AE, Müller A, Tuchschmid P, Duc G: Oxygen affinity of haemoglobin modulates cerebral blood flow in premature infants. A study with the non-invasive xenon-133 method, *Acta Paediatr Scand Suppl* 360:26-32, 1989.

1107. Rahilly PM: Effects of 2% carbon dioxide, 0.5% carbon dioxide, and 100% oxygen on cranial blood flow of the human neonate, *Pediatrics* 66:685-689, 1980.

1108. Leahy FA, Cates D, MacCallum M, Rigatto H: Effect of CO_2 and 100% O_2 on cerebral blood flow in preterm infants, *J Appl Physiol* 48:468-472, 1980.

1109. Ramaekers VT, Casaer P, Marchal G, Smet M, et al: The effect of blood transfusion on cerebral blood-flow in preterm infants: A Doppler study, *Dev Med Child Neurol* 30:334-341, 1988.

1110. Lundstrom KE, Pryds O, Greisen G: Oxygen at birth and prolonged cerebral vasoconstriction in preterm infants, *Arch Dis Child Fetal Neonatal Ed* 73:F81-F86, 1995.

1111. Rosenkrantz TS, Oh W: Cerebral blood flow velocity in infants with polycythemia and hyperviscosity: Effects of partial exchange transfusion with Plasmanate, *J Pediatr* 101:94-98, 1982.

1112. Riopel L, Fouron JC, Bard H: Blood viscosity during the neonatal period: The role of plasma and red blood cell type, *J Pediatr* 100:449-453, 1982.

1113. Greisen G, Hellström-Vestas L, Lou H, Rosen I, et al: Sleep-walking shifts and cerebral blood flow in stable preterm infants, *Pediatr Res* 19:1156-1159, 1985.

1114. Perlman JM, Herscovitch P, Kreusser KL, Raichle ME, et al: Positron emission tomography in the newborn: Effect of seizure on regional cerebral blood flow in an asphyxiated infant, *Neurology* 35:244-247, 1985.

1115. Perlman JM, Volpe JJ: Seizures in the preterm infant: Effects on cerebral blood flow velocity, intracranial pressure, and arterial blood pressure, *J Pediatr* 102:288-293, 1983.

1116. Edwards AD, Wyatt JS, Richardson C, Potter A, et al: Effects of indomethacin on cerebral haemodynamics in very preterm infants, *Lancet* 335:1491-1495, 1990.

1117. Christmann V, Liem KD, Semmekrot BA, vandeBor M: Changes in cerebral, renal and mesenteric blood flow velocity during continuous and bolus infusion of indomethacin, *Acta Paediatr* 91:440-446, 2002.

1118. Bevan R, Dodge J, Nichols P, Poseno T, et al: Responsiveness of human infant cerebral arteries to sympathetic nerve stimulation and vasoactive agents, *Pediatr Res* 44:730-739, 1998.

1119. Bevan RD, Vijayakumaran E, Gentry A, Wellman T, et al: Intrinsic tone of cerebral artery segments of human infants between 23 weeks of gestation and term, *Pediatr Res* 43:20-27, 1998.

1120. Yanowitz TD, Yao AC, Werner JC, Pettigrew KD, et al: Effects of prophylactic low-dose indomethacin on hemodynamics in very low birth weight infants, *J Pediatr* 132:28-34, 1998.

1121. Rosenbaum JL, Almli CR, Yundt KD, Altman DI, et al: Higher neonatal cerebral blood flow correlates with worse childhood neurologic outcome, *Neurology* 49:1035-1041, 1997.

1122. Archer LN, Levene MI, Evans DH: Cerebral artery Doppler ultrasonography for prediction of outcome after perinatal asphyxia, *Lancet* 2:1116-1118, 1986.

1123. Archer LN, Evans DH, Paton JY, Levene MI: Controlled hypercapnia and neonatal cerebral artery Doppler ultrasound waveforms, *Pediatr Res* 20:218-221, 1986.

1124. van Bel F, Hirasing RA, Grimberg MT: Can perinatal asphyxia cause cerebral edema and affect cerebral blood flow velocity? *Eur J Pediatr* 142:29-32, 1984.

1125. van Bel F, van de Bor M: Cerebral edema caused by perinatal asphyxia: Detection and follow-up, *Helv Paediatr Acta* 40:361-369, 1985.

1126. Sankaran K: Hypoxic-ischemic encephalopathy: Cerebrovascular carbon dioxide reactivity in neonates, *Am J Perinatol* 1:114-117, 1984.

1127. Bada HS, Hajjar W, Chua C, Sumner DS: Noninvasive diagnosis of neonatal asphyxia and intraventricular hemorrhage by Doppler ultrasound, *J Pediatr* 95:775-779, 1979.

1128. Levene MI, Fenton AC, Evans DH, Archer LN, et al: Severe birth asphyxia and abnormal cerebral blood-flow velocity, *Dev Med Child Neurol* 31:427-434, 1989.

1129. Ramaekers VT, Casaer P: Defective regulation of cerebral oxygen transport after severe birth asphyxia, *Dev Med Child Neurol* 32:56-62, 1990.

1130. Morrison FK, Patel NB, Howie PW, Mires GJ, et al: Neonatal cerebral arterial flow velocity waveforms in term infants with and without metabolic acidosis at delivery, *Early Hum Dev* 42:155-168, 1995.

1131. Ilves P, Talvik R, Talvik T: Changes in Doppler ultrasonography in asphyxiated term infants with hypoxic-ischaemic encephalopathy, *Acta Paediatr* 87:680-684, 1998.

1132. Meek JH, Elwell CE, McCormick DC, Edwards AD, et al: Abnormal cerebral haemodynamics in perinatally asphyxiated neonates related to outcome, *Arch Dis Child Fetal Neonatal Ed* 81:F110-F115, 1999.

1133. Ilves P, Lintrop M, Metsvaht T, Vaher U, et al: Cerebral blood-flow velocities in predicting outcome of asphyxiated newborn infants, *Acta Paediatr* 93:523-528, 2004.

1134. Wyatt JS: Near infrared spectroscopy in asphyxiated brain injury, *Clin Perinatol* 20:369-378, 1993.

Chapter 7

Hypoxic-Ischemic Encephalopathy: Intrauterine Assessment

Identification of an intrauterine disturbance in gas exchange between the human fetus and mother (i.e., asphyxia) or the likelihood that such a disturbance will occur during labor or delivery is critical, in view of the large body of data that intrauterine asphyxia occurs in a large proportion of infants with hypoxic-ischemic encephalopathy. (In this context, *hypoxic-ischemic encephalopathy* refers to the entire spectrum of neuropathological processes described in Chapters 8 and 9.) Moreover, attempts at prevention of the brain injury caused by intrauterine asphyxia, antepartum and intrapartum, demand precise awareness of when such injury is imminent. Although the most definitive information concerning detection of hypoxic-ischemic insult to the fetus still applies primarily to the intrapartum period, major advances in antepartum assessment have been made in recent years. In this chapter, the major current means of antepartum assessment of the fetus and then the approach to intrapartum assessment are reviewed.

My focus in this chapter is hypoxic-ischemic disease. Therefore, I specifically do not discuss such issues as prenatal diagnosis of genetic disorders affecting the nervous system, imaging of the fetal brain for structural abnormalities by ultrasonography or magnetic resonance imaging (MRI), evaluation of fetal brain biochemistry by proton MR spectroscopy, study of fetal brain function by functional MRI or magnetoencephalography, or percutaneous fetal blood sampling for various metabolic and infectious disorders that affect the brain. Such issues are discussed in standard sources and are beyond the scope of this book.[1-10]

ANTEPARTUM ASSESSMENT

Although quantitative conclusions are not entirely established, it is clear that some hypoxic-ischemic insults affect the brain before labor and delivery (i.e., during the antepartum period). The search for means of assessing such disturbances, acute or chronic, has been the subject of a vast amount of obstetrical research. In this section, a brief review of the current means of evaluating the fetus during the antepartum period is provided. The techniques are best divided into those based on measurement of fetal movement, fetal heart rate, a combination of factors that include fetal movement and heart rate (biophysical profile), fetal growth, and blood flow velocity in uterine and fetal blood vessels (Table 7-1).

Fetal Movement and Behavioral States

Fetal movement is a useful indicator of fetal health.[11-22] Techniques for monitoring fetal movement have included systematic maternal recording of perceived activity, electromechanical devices (tocodynamometry), and real-time ultrasonography (see Table 7-1). The first of these methods is the most convenient and widely used, the second is primarily an investigative tool, and the third has received increasingly wide clinical and investigational use because of the diversity of information that it can provide.

Fetal movements are one aspect of the determination of fetal behavioral states (i.e., states analogous to those described postnatally as sleep states; see Chapter 4). Most commonly, fetal behavioral states are defined according to the quantitative and qualitative aspects of fetal body movements, eye movements, and fetal heart rate.[19,22-29] Distinct fetal states are definable by 36 to 38 weeks of gestation. Recognizable behavioral states at that time are summarized in Table 7-2. These states approximate *neonatal* behavioral states, that is, quiet sleep (1F), REM sleep (2F), quiet waking (3F), and active waking (4F). Active sleep (2F) is the most frequently observed, followed by quiet sleep (1F).[22] The waking states are either infrequent (4F) or rare (3F).

Maturational Changes

Distinct maturational changes in fetal movement can be identified (Fig. 7-1).[12,21,22] Although with ultrasonography it is possible to detect movement as early as the second month of gestation,[30-32] maternal perception of movement ("quickening") occurs at approximately 16 weeks. Thereafter, the movements increase in strength and reach a plateau from 26 to 32 weeks of gestation, when an abrupt fall to a second plateau occurs between 32 and 36 weeks. No appreciable change occurs thereafter until delivery.

Prechtl and others[15,17,20,33-37] emphasized the *quality* of fetal movements and the striking maturational changes in the variety and complexity of these movements. Certain fetal movements increase in incidence gradually with advancing gestation (e.g., breathing, sucking, and swallowing), other movements increase in incidence to a plateau (e.g., general movements, isolated arm movements), and still others increase in incidence and then decrease (e.g., startles, hiccups).

TABLE 7-1	Major Means of Antepartum Assessment of the Human Fetus
Fetal Movement	
Detection by maternal perception or by real-time ultrasonography	
Fetal Heart Rate	
Nonstress test: response of fetal heart rate to movement	
Contraction stress test: response of fetal heart rate to stimulated (oxytocin and nipple stimulation) or spontaneous uterine contraction	
Fetal Biophysical Profile	
Combination of fetal breathing, movement, tone, heart rate reactivity, and amniotic fluid volume	
Fetal Growth	
Detection of intrauterine growth retardation	
Fetal Blood Flow Velocity	
Detection by the Doppler technique of flow velocity in umbilical and fetal systemic and cerebral vessels	

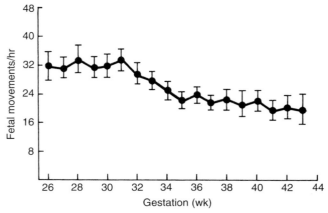

Figure 7-1 **Relation of quantity of fetal movement to gestational age.** Movements were quantitated by maternal perception. *(From Rayburn WF: Antepartum fetal assessment: Monitoring fetal activity, Clin Perinatol 9:231-240, 1982.)*

Relation to Fetal Well-Being

The relation of quantity and quality of fetal movement to fetal well-being is illustrated by the study summarized in Figure 7-2. Decreased fetal movements perceived by the mother over the 7 days before delivery could be documented in a series of pregnancies with "unfavorable perinatal outcome" (i.e., abnormal intrapartum fetal heart rate patterns, depressed Apgar scores, and antepartum or intrapartum stillbirth).[12] The most common denominator of fetal inactivity was *chronic uteroplacental insufficiency*. In another study in which pregnant women were instructed to report to the delivery unit if 2 hours elapsed without 10 fetal movements perceived, further evaluations and any indicated interventions for fetal compromise were performed.[17] During the study period, fetal mortality among women with such decreased fetal movement was 10 per 1000; in the control period immediately before onset of the study, fetal mortality with such decreased fetal movement was 44 per 1000. Subsequent work also indicates the value of assessment of fetal movements in the evaluation of fetal condition.[18,21,38-40] Overall, the data show the value of this approach in identifying the infant who may be exhibiting signs of cerebral dysfunction and who may be vulnerable to injury imminently or by the processes of later labor and vaginal delivery, or both.

Fetal Neurological Examination

The observations described in the preceding paragraphs are reminiscent of many of those made during the neonatal neurological examination. The utilization of fetal movements as part of a detailed analysis of fetal behavior by real-time ultrasonography led to the identification of *distinct behavioral states*, as noted earlier. These analyses include assessment of a large variety of specific body movements (e.g., yawning, stretching, and startle), as well as fetal eye movements, posture, breathing, and heart rate. The analogy of these phenomena to those observed after birth in the premature infant (see Chapter 3) is obvious, and, indeed, to a major extent, one can consider these observations *a kind of fetal neurological examination*. When amplified by such assessments as habituation of the fetus to vibrotactile stimuli or response to acoustical stimuli, the analogy to neurological assessment becomes even more impressive.[21,22,41-47] Finally, detailed analysis of the *quantity and quality of fetal breathing* can provide still further information about the fetal nervous system.[15,21,34,36,48,49] With the wide use of real-time ultrasonography, the standardization of the neurological phenomena observable, and, most important and still most difficult, the correlation of aberrations with the topography of neuropathology, highly valuable evaluation of the fetal central nervous system and dysfunction thereof should be possible. The design of appropriate interventions for disturbances then would be an appropriate next step.

Fetal Heart Rate: Nonstress and Stress Tests

The evaluation of fetal well-being by *antepartum* fetal heart rate testing is a standard obstetrical practice in

TABLE 7-2	Fetal Behavioral States at 38 Weeks of Gestation*		
State†	**Body Movements**	**Eye Movements**	**Fetal Heart Rate Pattern**
1F	Absent (occasional startle)	Absent	Narrow variability, isolated acceleration
2F	Present (frequent bursts)	Present	Wide variability, acceleration with movement
3F	Absent	Present	Wide variability, no accelerations
4F	Present (almost continuous)	Present (continuous)	Long accelerations or sustained tachycardia

*See text for references.
†These fetal states approximate neonatal behavioral states, that is, quiet sleep (1F), active sleep (2F), quiet waking (3F), and active waking (4F).

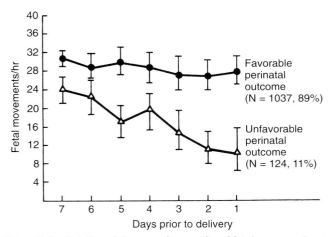

Figure 7-2 **Relation of decrease in quantity of fetal movement over 7 days before delivery to unfavorable perinatal outcome.** See text for details. *(From Rayburn WF: Antepartum fetal assessment: Monitoring fetal activity,* Clin Perinatol *9:231-240, 1982.)*

high-risk pregnancies. The two commonly used techniques determine fetal heart rate changes with either stimulated (or spontaneous) uterine contractions (contraction stress test) or spontaneous fetal events (e.g., fetal movement test, or nonstress test) (see Table 7-1).

Nonstress Test

Of the two techniques, the so-called *nonstress test* is the approach used as an initial evaluation.[50-53] In general, the particular value of the technique is the determination of a healthy fetus,[50,51,53-55] based on the demonstration of at least two accelerations of fetal heart rate during the period of observation (usually ≈40 minutes), generally in association with fetal movement or vibroacoustical stimulation. The accelerations must exceed 15 beats/minute and last at least 15 seconds, and the normal result is called a *reactive* nonstress test. A *nonreactive* test is characterized by the failure to note such accelerations over the observation period. The demonstration of accelerations of fetal heart rate with acoustical stimulation and the correlation of a reactive acoustical stimulation test with the conventional nonstress test have led to use of such stimulation as part of the nonstress test in many centers.[21,47,51-53]

Concerning the *predictive value* of nonstress testing, the incidence of fetal distress leading to cesarean delivery increases from about 1% to 20% when antepartum reactive and nonreactive patterns are compared.[47,50,51] It is clear, however, that most "abnormal" or nonreactive tests are not followed by difficulties with labor and delivery. A normal, reactive nonstress test is highly predictive of fetal well-being. *Thus, as with most other modes of fetal evaluation, both antepartum and intrapartum, the prediction of a normal fetus and the relative lack of need for intervention are the greatest values of the test.* However, the test does not detect such important maternal-fetal problems as oligohydramnios, umbilical cord or placental abnormalities, growth disorders, and twin demise. When suspicion or concern for such problems exists, another approach, using ultrasonography, as in fetal biophysical profile, is essential.[53]

Contraction Stress Test

The so-called *contraction stress test* in the past was most commonly used as a follow-up evaluation after a nonreactive stress test. Experimental data suggest that the occurrence of late decelerations with contractions, the basis for a *positive (abnormal) stress test,* is an early warning sign of uteroplacental insufficiency.[53-56] The established clinical as well as experimental premise of the stress test is that chronic uteroplacental insufficiency results in late decelerations of the fetal heart rate, a sign of fetal hypoxia (see following discussion), in response to uterine contractions, which can be stimulated by breast stimulation or oxytocin infusion.[53,57-60] In approximately 10% of women, spontaneous uterine contractions obviate the need to stimulate uterine contractions. A *positive (abnormal) result* is indicated by persistent late decelerations over several or more contractions; these positive tests can be subdivided further as *reactive,* when accompanied by accelerations at some time during the test, or *nonreactive,* when not accompanied by accelerations. An *equivocal result* refers to the occurrence of nonpersistent *late decelerations.* A *negative stress test* is defined as absence of any late decelerations with the contractions.

As with nonstress testing and other fetal assessments, a negative stress test is a reliable indicator of fetal well-being. Concerning the predictive value of a positive stress test, in one multi-institutional study of high-risk pregnancies, a negative test was followed by perinatal death in less than 1% of cases versus 5% to 20% of infants with positive contraction tests (the lower value was for infants with reactive positive tests, and the higher value was for those with nonreactive positive tests).[58-60] Thus, the stress test is of value in predicting the infant at risk for intrapartum disturbances.

Currently, the contraction stress test is no longer the principal method for follow-up in most centers.[53] This change relates to logistical and interpretive difficulties and relatively low positive predictive values. The fetal biophysical profile is now favored as the primary means of fetal surveillance for high-risk pregnancies, identified by a nonreactive nonstress test or other evidence.[53]

Fetal Biophysical Profile

In view of the relatively high incidence of false-positive assessments with the tests of fetal heart rate just described, *a series of fetal measures,* termed a *composite biophysical profile,* has been used to refine antepartum evaluation.[52,53,61-69] These measures include quantitation *not only of fetal heart rate reactivity* (see the earlier discussion of the nonstress test), but also of *fetal breathing movements, gross body movements, fetal tone (as assessed by posture and flexor-extensor movements), and amniotic fluid volume* (see Table 7-1). Each item is graded, usually on a score of 0 to 2. The use of *real-time ultrasonography* has made such an assessment possible, and the relative ease of this methodology in modern obstetrical centers has led to widespread use. The rationale of using such a profile is entirely reasonable (i.e., the various measures reflect

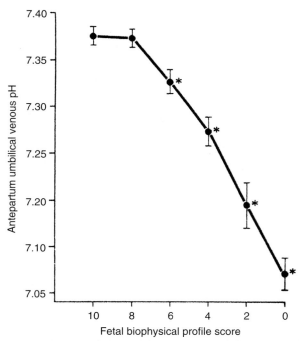

Figure 7-3 Relation of fetal biophysical profile (BPP) score to mean umbilical vein pH (±2 SD) in fetal blood obtained by cordocentesis. A progressive and highly significant direct linear relationship exists between abnormal BPP scores (≤6) and umbilical vein pH (P <.01). *Asterisks* denote a significantly lower mean pH compared with the value recorded for the immediately higher BPP score. *(From Manning FA: Fetal assessment by evaluation of biophysical variables. In Creasy RK, Resnik R, editors:* Maternal-Fetal Medicine, *4th ed, Philadelphia: 1999, WB Saunders.)*

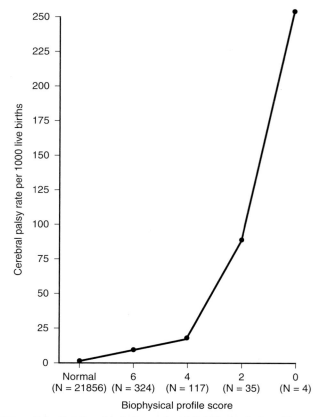

Figure 7-4 Relationship between last fetal biophysical profile score and incidence of cerebral palsy. An inverse, exponential, and highly significant relationship is apparent (P <.001). *(From Harman CR: Assessment of fetal health. In Creasy RK, Resnik R, Iams JD, editors:* Maternal-Fetal Medicine: Principles and Practice, *5th ed, Philadelphia: 2004, WB Saunders.)*

activity of several levels of the central nervous system, including cerebrum, diencephalon, and brain stem). The predictive value of the score is demonstrated by the data in Figure 7-3, which illustrate the relation of the fetal biophysical score to umbilical venous pH determined by cordocentesis.[40] Similar correlations are available regarding incidence of meconium passage during labor, signs of intrapartum fetal distress, and perinatal mortality.[53,64] Of particular importance, the degree of abnormality of the fetal biophysical score has been shown to correlate with the occurrence of brain injury that results in cerebral palsy (Fig. 7-4).[53,69] Data from a single center suggested that alterations in obstetrical management provoked by the results of the score could lead to a three- to fourfold decline in cerebral palsy rates.[69] Although the procedure requires expertise in ultrasonography and experience in recognition of the phenomena, the value of the profile is striking. The role of this technique in the detection of acute and chronic intrauterine asphyxia and in the prevention of further injury by appropriate management of the remainder of the pregnancy and the delivery can be substantial (Table 7-3).

Fetal Growth

As with other antepartum assessments, advances in ultrasound technology have provided the capability of accurate quantitative assessment of fetal growth.[7,70] The particular value of this assessment is in the detection of intrauterine growth retardation (see Table 7-1), although other aberrations of growth (e.g., large body size and large head) have important implications for management of labor and delivery and the neonatal period, as discussed elsewhere in this book. Detection of intrauterine growth retardation is important, principally because significant management decisions follow. Most such fetuses are "constitutionally small," are not at increased perinatal risk, and do not require aggressive intervention.[7] However, some such infants (≈5% to 10%) exhibit a major developmental anomaly, including chromosomal aberration, that may require further intrauterine assessment (e.g., amniocentesis and chromosomal or other genetic analyses). Moreover, of greatest importance, particularly in this context, is that approximately 10% to 15% of infants with intrauterine growth retardation are growth retarded because of uteroplacental failure and are *at risk for intrapartum asphyxia.*[7,71-77] In one series from a single high-risk service, 35% of growth-retarded fetuses exhibited intrapartum fetal heart rate abnormalities indicative of fetal distress.[72] A significant increase in fetal asphyxia, as judged by cord acid-base studies, was apparent even when growth-retarded infants were compared with other high-risk groups.[73] Moreover, growth-retarded infants with intrapartum fetal heart decelerations demonstrate considerably

TABLE 7-3 **Fetal Biophysical Score: Relation to Outcome and Recommended Management**

Biophysical Profile Score*	Interpretation	Predicted Perinatal Mortality	Recommended Management
0/10	Severe acute asphyxia	60/100	Immediate delivery by cesarean section
2/10	Acute fetal asphyxia, most likely with chronic decompensation	125/100	Delivery for fetal indications (usually cesarean section)
4/10	Acute fetal asphyxia likely; if oligohydramnios present, chronic asphyxia also very likely	9.1/100	Delivery by obstetrically appropriate method with continuous monitoring
10/10	No evidence of fetal asphyxia	<0.1/100	No acute intervention

*Values intermediate between 4/10 and 10/10 not shown; see Harman CR: Assessment of fetal health. In Creasy RK, Resnik R, Iams JD, editors: *Maternal-Fetal Medicine: Principles and Practice*, 5th ed, Philadelphia: WB Saunders, 2004.

Adapted from Harman CR: Assessment of fetal health. In Creasy RK, Resnik R, Iams JD, editors: *Maternal-Fetal Medicine: Principles and Practice*, 5th ed, Philadelphia: WB Saunders, 2004.

higher umbilical artery lactate levels than do normally grown infants with similar decelerations.[74] Thus, growth-retarded infants tolerate labor less well than do normally grown infants, perhaps in part because of deficient stores of glycogen in liver, heart, and, possibly, brain. Therefore, antepartum detection of such infants is important in formulating rational decisions concerning further assessment of the fetus (e.g., fetal biophysical profile, Doppler blood flow velocity studies) and optimal management of labor and delivery (see next section).

Doppler Measurements of Blood Flow Velocity in Umbilical and Fetal Cerebral Vessels

The application of the Doppler technique to the study of blood flow velocity in umbilical vessels has led to an enormous literature. The potential value of determination of blood flow and vascular resistance in elucidation of a wide variety of disease processes in both the pregnant woman and her fetus clearly is great. The basic principles of the Doppler technique are reviewed in Chapter 4 in relation to neonatal studies of the cerebral circulation and are not reiterated here. In the following section, I review separately studies of umbilical and fetal cerebral vessels, particularly the umbilical artery and the fetal middle cerebral artery.

Umbilical Artery

Most studies based on the use of Doppler in pregnancy have focused on the umbilical artery.[18,53,71,75,76,78-93] The principal quantitative parameters of the Doppler waveform used have been the *pulsatility index of Gosling* (peak systolic velocity [S] − end diastolic velocity [D]/ mean velocity), the *resistance index of Pourcelot* (S − D/S), and the *S/D ratio*. The values of these ratios, in general, are not affected by the angle of insonation, clearly difficult to maintain constant in the clinical situation. The pulsatility index and the resistance index reflect, in largest part, vascular resistance. The principal change in umbilical artery blood flow velocity with progression of *normal pregnancy* is a decline in the resistance parameters.[53,79,81,87,94] Although the decline is gradual, a more pronounced decrease occurs after 30 weeks of gestation. This decrease is considered secondary to a decrease in placental vascular resistance, related particularly to increased numbers of small vessels. A similar phenomenon was documented in the fetal lamb.[95] The decrease in placental vascular resistance with advancing pregnancy is accompanied by an increase in volemic placental blood flow, calculated in human fetuses by simultaneous measurements of the blood flow velocity in the umbilical vein and the cross-sectional area of that vessel by combined Doppler and imaging ultrasonography (Fig. 7-5).[96]

The major application of Doppler studies of blood flow velocity in the umbilical artery has been in the investigation of the fetus with intrauterine growth retardation and the complications associated with this fetal state.* In intrauterine growth retardation, the principal finding is an increase in the resistance measures.† With progression of this disturbance in resistance measures in the umbilical artery, marked impairment of the end diastolic flow or even loss or reversal of diastolic flow (an ominous sign) may occur. In one study, the changes in resistance indices *preceded* antepartum late heart rate decelerations in more than 90% of fetuses who developed such decelerations, and the median duration of the interval between the severe abnormality of resistance measure and decelerations was 17 days.[103] The importance of the rising placental vascular resistance to the fetus is shown by the striking curvilinear relationship between the pulsatility index in the umbilical artery and the lactate concentration in fetal blood, a measure of fetal hypoxia (Fig. 7-6).[104] The clinical predictive value of the diastolic flow in the umbilical artery was apparent in a study of 459 high-risk pregnancies.[94] Thus, the rate of fetal or neonatal death in the presence of end diastolic flow was 4% and increased to 41% with absence of flow and to 75% with reversal of flow. With prompt and detailed further fetal assessments and appropriate interventions, the unfavorable outlook with absence of diastolic flow has not been so marked.[53,107] However, reversal of flow is associated with a considerable risk of fetal compromise, perinatal mortality, neonatal neurological disturbances, and

---

*See references 18,53,71,75,76,78-80,82,83,85-87,89-94,97-107a.
†See references 18,71,75,76,79,80,86,87,89-94,97,99,106.

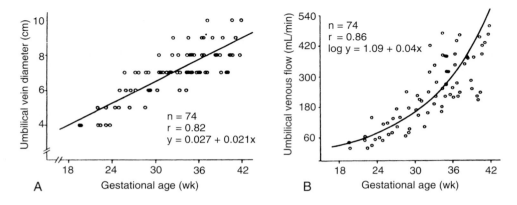

Figure 7-5   Relationship between umbilical vein diameter and umbilical venous flow in human pregnancy. A, umbilical vein diameter. **B,** Umbilical venous flow. Note the linear increase in venous diameter and the exponential increase in blood flow. *(From Sutton MS, Theard MA, Bhatia SJ, et al: Changes in placental blood flow in the normal human fetus with gestational age, Pediatr Res 28:383-387, 1990.)*

subsequent neurodevelopmental disability, with the magnitude of risk varying considerably with the selection of the population studied.

The central abnormality in the growth-retarded fetus leading to the increase in placental vascular resistance is a disturbance in placental vessels.[108] The major features include loss of small blood vessels, decreased vascular diameter because of media and intima thickening, and thrombosis. Placental vascular obstruction produced by a variety of experimental techniques in pregnant sheep reproduced the changes in the resistance measures observed in the human fetus.[109] Indeed, elevated umbilical artery resistance measures have been observed in a variety of pathological conditions of the placenta, including partial abruption, placental scarring from intervillous thrombosis, and inflammatory villitis secondary to bacterial or viral infection.[53] Thus, the value of this

technique in the evaluation of a wide variety of high-risk pregnancies is very high.

Fetal Cerebral Vessels

Following soon after the initial applications of Doppler for study of umbilical blood flow velocity was the successful study of blood flow velocity in fetal cerebral vessels, particularly the middle cerebral artery. This now widely used methodology allows monitoring during pregnancy of cerebral hemodynamics, perhaps the most crucial physiological process with regard to fetal brain injury.

During *normal pregnancy*, in contrast to the decreasing values for resistance measures defined in the umbilical circulation, values in the cerebral circulation change little until approximately the last 5 weeks, when a distinct decline is apparent (Fig. 7-7).[53,87,94,110-115] Additionally, mean cerebral blood flow velocity has been shown to increase during the same period that resistance appears to decrease.[111] This combination of findings suggests an increase in cerebral blood flow

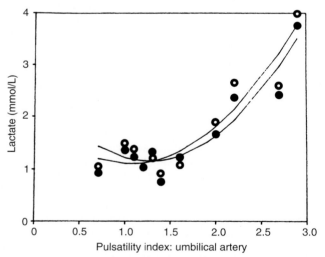

Figure 7-6   Relationship between lactate concentration of fetal blood (sampled from the umbilical vein [*solid circles*] or artery [*open circles*] at the time of cesarean section) and pulsatility index obtained from the umbilical artery before delivery. Note the marked increase in fetal blood lactate with increasing pulsatility index (i.e., increasing placental vascular resistance). *(From Ferrazzi E, Pardi G, Bauscaglia M, et al: The correlation of biochemical monitoring versus umbilical flow velocity measurements of the human fetus, Am J Obstet Gynecol 159:1081-1087, 1988.)*

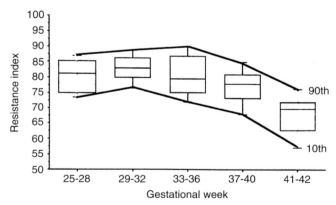

Figure 7-7   Resistance index values of fetal intracranial arterial velocity waveforms in normal pregnancies. The framed areas represent the values between the 25th and 75th percentiles for each gestational age period. The medians (*horizontal lines within the framed areas*) and the 10th and 90th percentiles are indicated. Note the sharp decline in the last month of pregnancy. *(From Kirkinen P, Müller R, Huch R, Huch A: Blood flow velocity waveforms in human fetal intracranial arteries, Obstet Gynecol 70:617-621, 1987.)*

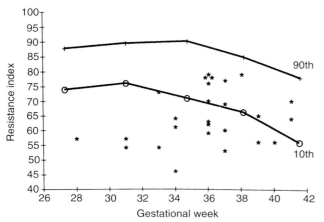

Figure 7-8 Resistance index values in fetal intracranial arteries of small-for-dates newborns (*asterisks*). The 10th and 90th percentiles for normal pregnancy are indicated by the lines. Note the lower resistance values in the small-for-dates newborns. *(From Kirkinen P, Müller R, Huch R, Huch A: Blood flow velocity waveforms in human fetal intracranial arteries,* Obstet Gynecol *70:617-621, 1987.)*

TABLE 7-4	Neonatal Outcome as a Function of Ratio of Cerebral-Umbilical Pulsatility Index	
	Ratio* <1.08 (n = 18)	Ratio* >1.08 (n = 72)
Small for gestational age	100%	38%
Cesarean section (for fetal distress)	89%	12%
Umbilical vein pH (mean)	7.25	7.33
Five-minute Apgar score <7	17%	3%
Neonatal complications[†]	33%	1%

*Ratio of pulsatility index from cerebral circulation to index from umbilical artery; normal mean value is approximately 2.0.
[†]Intracerebral hemorrhage, seizures, respiratory distress syndrome.
Data from Gramellini D, Folli MC, Raboni S, et al: Cerebral-umbilical Doppler ratio as a predictor of adverse perinatal outcome, *Obstet Gynecol* 79:416-420, 1992.

during the last trimester of pregnancy, perhaps related to cerebral vasodilation or development of vascular beds, or both. A particular role for the development of cerebrovascular reactivity to relatively low oxygen tension in the fetus is suggested by the findings that cerebral resistance indices in the fetus have been shown to be more responsive to blood oxygen tension than to carbon dioxide tension, and that in the immediate postnatal period, when blood oxygen tensions rise dramatically, cerebral mean flow velocity transiently declines markedly (consistent with an increase in cerebrovascular resistance).[111,116]

As with Doppler studies of the umbilical vessels, study of cerebral blood flow velocity has been directed most commonly at the growth-retarded fetus. The dominant abnormality has been a diminished value of cerebral resistance indices, in contrast to the elevated value in the umbilical artery (Fig. 7-8).[53,71,90,92-94,107a, 110,114,117-123] This apparent vasodilation in the cerebrum at a time of decreasing umbilical flow has been interpreted as an adaptive response, perhaps mediated by hypoxia, and has been termed *fetal brain sparing*. It seems reasonable to suggest that, with severe impairment of umbilical flow and hypoxia, such an adaptive response could become insufficient. Indeed, the decline in cerebral resistance indices and the increase in umbilical resistance indices have been quantitatively combined as a cerebral-to-umbilical ratio. This ratio has been predictive of such subsequent disturbances as fetal distress requiring cesarean section, fetal acidosis, and early neonatal complications (Table 7-4).[124]

The potential value of Doppler study of the cerebral circulation in other fetal states is suggested by the demonstration of increased values for pulsatility index in the presence of hydrocephalus.[110,125] This observation is identical to that made postnatally with posthemorrhagic hydrocephalus (see Chapters 4 and 11), and it raises the possibility of the use of Doppler in determination of the need for intervention in fetal hydrocephalus. Changes in cerebral blood flow velocity have also been documented with changes in fetal behavioral states and after administration of indomethacin to the mother.[119,126]

INTRAPARTUM ASSESSMENT

The occurrence of injury to brain during the birth process has been the focus of clinical research for more than a century. In my view, work has shown that brain injury in the intrapartum period does occur, affects a large absolute number of infants worldwide, is obscure in most cases in terms of exact timing and precise mechanisms, awaits more sophisticated means of detection in utero, and represents a large source of potentially preventable neurological morbidity. Among the many adverse consequences of the explosion in obstetrical litigation has been a tendency in some quarters of the medical profession to deny the importance or even the existence of intrapartum brain injury. *Although it is unequivocally clear that true obstetrical malpractice is a rare occurrence* and that the obstetrician is called on to deal with perhaps the most dangerous period in an individual's life with *inadequate methods*, this tendency is particularly unfortunate. With the recognition from experimental studies that much of hypoxic-ischemic brain injury evolves *after* cessation of the insult and can be interrupted to a considerable extent by several approaches (see Chapters 6 and 8), the ultimate possibility of intervention both in utero and in the early postnatal period is strongly suggested. Denial that intrapartum injury occurs may impair development and application of such brain-saving intervention.

In general, the hallmark of intrapartum asphyxia has been the occurrence of specific fetal heart rate abnormalities. The passage of meconium in utero is an often-cited but far less useful indicator of serious fetal distress. The alterations in fetal heart rate that occur with disturbances to fetal well-being have been defined in great detail in the past several decades with the widespread use of electronic fetal monitoring, sometimes supplemented with fetal blood sampling to assess acid-base status. In the following sections, I review the basic elements of intrapartum assessment of the

TABLE 7-5	Major Means of Intrapartum Assessment of the Fetus

Meconium passage
Fetal heart rate
Fetal acid-base status
Other techniques
   Transcutaneous monitoring of blood gases and pH
   Near-infrared spectroscopy
   Doppler measurements of fetal blood flow velocity
   Fetal electroencephalogram

human fetus (Table 7-5), namely, the implications of meconium passage in utero, the important fetal heart rate patterns, and the relation of fetal heart rate alterations to fetal acidosis and to neurological morbidity in the newborn period. Finally, I briefly discuss certain other measures of fetal surveillance. In the first section that follows, the relationship between intrapartum asphyxia and cerebral palsy is reviewed.

Relationship between Intrapartum Asphyxia and Cerebral Palsy

Numerous epidemiological studies have shown that most cases of cerebral palsy observed in children are *not* related to intrapartum asphyxia.[127-136] Related clinical epidemiological data also support this conclusion.[69,136-148] The epidemiological data have been derived from studies of many thousands of infants born over the past 3 to 4 decades, including the era of modern perinatology and neonatology (Table 7-6). Thus, if one excludes premature infants, in whom the overwhelming balance of data shows that timing of injury is primarily postnatal (see Chapters 8 and 9), approximately 12% to 24% of cases of cerebral palsy can be related to intrapartum asphyxia. Indeed, if one considers the six large-scale studies of term infants born in the last 3 decades, the data are remarkably consistent in showing that 17% to 24% of cases of cerebral palsy are related to intrapartum asphyxia. A careful MRI study of 40 individuals with cerebral palsy also led to the conclusion that 17% to 24% of term infants sustained their injury from "perinatal" events.[149,150]

Although the data just described indicate that the majority of children examined later with the diagnosis

TABLE 7-6	Relationship between Intrapartum Asphyxia and Cerebral Palsy: Term Infants*

Country	Years of Infants' Births	Percentage Related to "Asphyxia"
United States	1959-1966	12%
Australia	1975-1980	17%
Finland	1978-1982	24%
Ireland	1981-1983	23%
England	1984-1987	17%
Sweden	1987-1990	17%
Sweden	1991-1994	24%

*See text for references.

of cerebral palsy did not sustain intrapartum asphyxia, the findings have been interpreted by some clinicians to mean that intrapartum brain injury is rare or nonexistent and therefore unimportant. As noted in the introduction to this section, such a conclusion is incorrect. A large body of clinical and brain imaging data shows that brain injury occurs intrapartum in a large absolute number of infants. Indeed, in view of the relatively high prevalence of cerebral palsy, in most countries, generally 2 to 3 cases per 1000 children born, even a relatively small percentage of cases caused by intrapartum events translates into a very large absolute number. (Consider the approximately 4 million live births and the 8000 to 9000 new cases of cerebral palsy in the United States yearly.) These points were stated eloquently in an exchange of communications in *The Lancet* (Table 7-7).[151] *The tasks for the future are to devise technologies that can aid in definition of the exact timing and mechanisms of this intrapartum brain injury and to develop interventions both during and after the insult that will prevent brain injury in the affected infants.*

Meconium Passage In Utero

Fetal hypoxia may lead to meconium passage in utero secondary to increased intestinal peristalsis and perhaps also relaxation of the anal sphincter. However, the increased vagal tone associated with fetal maturation may lead to meconium passage; approximately

TABLE 7-7	Interesting Exchanges Published in *The Lancet* Concerning Intrapartum Events and Cerebral Palsy

Editorial (Anonymous), November 25, 1989
"In light of the evidence reviewed above, the continued willingness of doctors to reinforce the fable that intrapartum care is an important determinant of cerebral palsy can only be regarded as shooting the specialty of obstetrics in the foot."

Letter to *The Lancet*
"However medicolegally comforting the new epidemiological orthodoxy you espouse may be, most of us will continue to believe that severe hypoxia/ischemia is deleterious to the brain, that the longer it goes on the worse the effect, and that delayed, inefficient, or inappropriate treatment can be disastrous. It is no longer a matter for conjecture whether asphyxia and cerebral damage are causally related, or merely occur in the same antenatally imperfect individual. Ultrasonography, and many other objective tests of cerebral structure and function allow us to follow the time course of evolving neuronal damage in the postnatal period following severe asphyxia."

"You suggest that by accepting '...the fable that intrapartum care is an important determinant of cerebral palsy,' the specialty of obstetrics is shooting itself in the foot, and that it is time to look elsewhere. We are concerned that by ignoring the 23% of cerebral palsy that *is* related to intrapartum asphyxia, obstetricians and their colleagues will take the advice too literally and shoot themselves somewhere else."

*From Hope PL, Moorcraft J: Cerebral palsy in infants born during trial of intrapartum monitoring, *Lancet* 335:238, 1990.

10% to 20% of apparently normal pregnancies at term and 25% to 50% of postdate pregnancies are accompanied by meconium-stained amniotic fluid. Thus, although the presence of meconium-stained amniotic fluid during labor is a potentially ominous sign concerning fetal well-being, controversy exists over the relative importance of this sign.[152-169] The discrepancy in conclusions may relate in part to the failure to assess *the timing and quantity of meconium passed*. In a prospective study of 2923 pregnancies, Meis and co-workers[161] observed the presence of meconium-stained amniotic fluid in 646 (22%) of cases. Meconium passage was classified as either early (light or heavy) or late. "Early" passage referred to meconium noted on rupture of the fetal membranes before or during the active phase of labor; "light" or "heavy" designations were made on the basis of quantity (and color). "Late" passage referred to meconium-stained amniotic fluid passed in the second stage of labor, after clear fluid had been noted previously. Patients with "early-light" meconium-stained amniotic fluid constituted approximately 54% of the total group with stained fluid and were no more likely to be depressed at birth than were control patients. Patients with "late" passage of meconium constituted approximately 21% of the total group with stained fluid and exhibited 1- and 5-minute Apgar scores lower than 7 two to three times more often than did control patients, but this difference was not statistically significant. (In a subsequent study, the same investigators demonstrated that the presence of *both* "late" passage of meconium *and* certain intrapartum fetal heart rate abnormalities, i.e., loss of beat-to-beat variability and variable decelerations [see next section], sharply increased the likelihood of depressed Apgar scores.[163]) Finally, however, patients with "early-heavy" meconium-stained amniotic fluid, which constituted 25% of the total group, had a sharply increased likelihood of neonatal depression as well as intrapartum and neonatal death. Indeed, of this group 33% exhibited Apgar scores lower than 7 at 1 minute, and 6.3% had scores lower than 7 at 5 minutes. Early-heavy meconium-stained amniotic fluid was also associated with other signs of fetal distress (e.g., *fetal heart rate abnormalities*) and with antecedent obstetrical conditions that lead to neonatal morbidity. Thus, the data suggest that the timing and quantity of meconium passage are critical variables in attempting to assess the significance of this occurrence for fetal well-being. Presumably, these two aspects of meconium passage correlate with the duration and severity of the intrauterine insult. Clinical estimation of the timing of meconium passage in utero is aided by examination of placental membranes or the newborn (Table 7-8).[170] In general, *in most cases*, the finding of meconium-stained amniotic fluid is not of serious import concerning intrauterine asphyxia. Moreover, in view of the high rate of meconium passage without serious perinatal complications, the most prevalent current view is that "the presence of meconium per se does not imply fetal distress during labor until other parameters, e.g., fetal heart rate abnormalities, support such a contention."[169]

TABLE 7-8 **Timing of Meconium Passage before Birth**	
Clinical-Pathological Feature	**Probable Duration before Birth**
Pigment-laden macrophages in amnion	>1 hr
Pigment-laden macrophages in chorion	>3 hr
Meconium-stained fetal nails	>4-6 hr

Data from Miller PW, Coen RW, Benirschke K: Dating the time interval from meconium passage to birth, *Obstet Gynecol* 66:459-462, 1985.

Fetal Heart Rate Alterations

In most medical centers, the central means of the intrapartum assessment of fetal well-being is electronic fetal monitoring.[164,168,171-188] Evaluation of fetal heart rate, particularly in relation to uterine contractions, is the most widely used form of electronic fetal monitoring. Although the necessity and relative merits of electronic fetal heart rate monitoring have been the subjects of disagreement,[164,168,171,174,175,181,184-201a] utilization of such monitoring during labor has been standard obstetrical practice in the United States. The bases for the major controversy concerning the value of electronic monitoring of the fetal heart rate are that (1) the abnormalities are detected in labor in a large number of infants who are normal at birth and on follow-up, and (2) the increase in operative deliveries provoked by the finding of such abnormalities has had little or no impact on adverse neurological outcome, particularly cerebral palsy. It is beyond the scope of this book to discuss in detail the relative merits of the use of electronic fetal monitoring in all pregnancies versus use in high-risk pregnancies only. It is perhaps worthy of emphasis only that in the so-called Dublin trial of nearly 13,000 women, a study generally acknowledged to be among the best designed of all trials, the use of electronic fetal monitoring was followed by a decrease in the incidence of neonatal seizures, and the presence of certain heart rate patterns (see subsequent discussion) was an important predictor of abnormal neonatal neurological examinations.[135,196] A decrease in neonatal seizures was documented in a meta-analysis of 12 studies involving 59,324 infants.[185] In another well-designed study, 27% of the 78 patients with cerebral palsy who had intrapartum fetal monitoring exhibited multiple late decelerations or decreased beat-to-beat variability of the heart rate.[186]

The major aspects of the fetal heart rate pattern evaluated are divided into *baseline features* (i.e., rate and beat-to-beat variability) and *periodic features* (i.e., accelerations or decelerations), usually in relation to uterine contractions (Fig. 7-9 and Table 7-9). The significance of these aspects of the fetal heart rate is discussed in detail in standard writings on maternal-fetal medicine. A brief overview is provided next.

Rate

Assessment of the fetal heart rate begins with the finding that the normal heart rate (±2 standard deviations) is 120 to 160 beats/minute (see Fig. 7-9).[164,202]

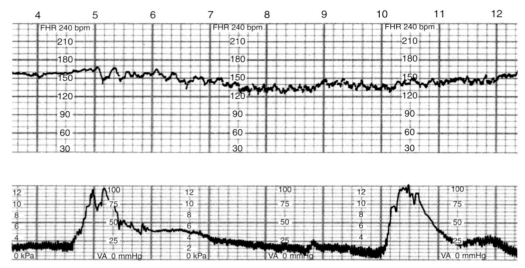

Figure 7-9 Fetal heart rate tracing, normal pattern. The *upper trace* represents the fetal heart rate, and the *lower trace* represents uterine activity. The fetal heart rate ranges generally between 130 and 150 beats/minute, with normal beat-to-beat variability of approximately 10 to 15 beats/minute. The uterine contractions shown are approximately 5 minutes apart. (*Courtesy of Dr. Barry Schifrin.*)

Abnormalities of baseline fetal heart rate are suspicious, but in the absence of disturbances of beat-to-beat variability or decelerations (see later discussions), these abnormalities usually do not reflect an ominous event, such as severe fetal hypoxia.[164,188] The most common cause of baseline tachycardia in the fetus is maternal fever secondary to amnionitis. Other causes include fetal infection, certain drugs (e.g., atropine and beta-sympathomimetics), arrhythmia, and maternal anxiety. Fixed tachycardia with loss of beat-to-beat variability may be observed with fetal hypoxia and has been observed in infants before intrapartum or early neonatal death.[203]

Baseline bradycardia with average beat-to-beat variability and no sign of fetal compromise is observed most commonly in the postmature fetus.[164] Bradycardia may be observed with fetal heart block, as a drug effect and with hypothermia. Baseline bradycardia as a feature of fetal hypoxia is accompanied by loss of beat-to-beat variability and decelerations.

Beat-to-Beat Variability

Normal fetal heart rate exhibits fluctuations of approximately 6 to 25 beats/minute (see Fig. 7-9).[188,204,205]

TABLE 7-9	Fetal Heart Rate Patterns: Major Causes and Usual Significance	
Fetal Heart Rate Pattern	**Major Cause**	**Usual Significance**
Loss of beat-to-beat variability	Multiple	Variable
Early decelerations	Head compression	Benign
Late decelerations	Uteroplacental insufficiency	Ominous
Variable decelerations	Umbilical cord compression	Variable

This beat-to-beat variability reflects the modulation of heart rate by autonomic, particularly parasympathetic, input and especially depends on inputs from cerebral cortex, diencephalon, and upper brain stem to the cardiac centers in the medulla and then to the vagus nerve.[164,172,188,206-208] Of the autonomic input, parasympathetic influences are more important than sympathetic influences.[188,209-211] *The presence of normal beat-to-beat variability is considered the best single assessment of fetal well-being.*[164,188,202,208] Indeed, the presence of normal variability is a reassuring finding in the presence of the mild variable decelerations common in the second stage of labor.[164] Loss of or diminished beat-to-beat variability may be observed not only with significant fetal hypoxia but also with prematurity, fetal sleep, drugs (e.g., sedative-hypnotics, narcotic-analgesics, benzodiazepines, atropine, and local anesthetics), congenital malformations (e.g., anencephaly), and intrauterine, antepartum cerebral destruction.[164,172,188,202,208,212-214] *The loss of beat-to-beat variability coupled with variable or late decelerations (see subsequent sections) significantly enhances the likelihood that the fetus is undergoing significant hypoxia.*[164,172,188,202,208] Indeed, ample documentation has shown the association between decreased fetal heart rate variability and decelerations, fetal acidosis, intrauterine fetal death, and low Apgar scores.[164,188,208,209]

Accelerations

Increases or decreases in fetal heart rate associated particularly with contractions are designated *accelerations* or *decelerations* and constitute the periodic features of the fetal heart rate. Accelerations during the uterine contractions of labor, as in the case of antepartum contractions (see previous discussion) or with fetal movement, are not of concern and in fact are generally considered a sign of fetal well-being.[164,215,216] Uncommonly, heart rate accelerations may be an early sign of compression of the umbilical vein.[164,217]

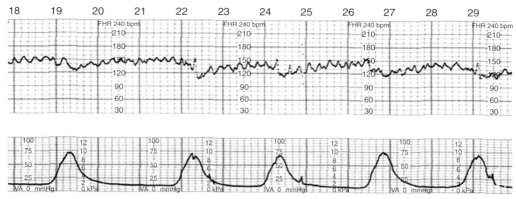

Figure 7-10 **Fetal heart rate tracing, early deceleration.** Note the typical early deceleration (i.e., the deceleration begins with the onset of the contraction, reaches its peak with the peak of the contraction, and returns to a normal baseline as the contraction ends). Variability is preserved. (*Courtesy of Dr. Barry Schifrin.*)

Maintenance of fetal heart rate variability is a reassuring sign of fetal well-being in the presence of such accelerations.

Decelerations

Decelerations are of three major types: early, late, and variable (Figs. 7-10 to 7-12; see Table 7-9). These decreases in heart rate associated with uterine contraction have significantly different mechanisms and implications for outcome.

Early Type. An *early deceleration* is one that begins with the onset of a contraction, reaches its peak with the peak of the contraction, and then returns to normal baseline levels as the contraction ends (see Fig. 7-10).[164,188,218,219] These decelerations appear to be related to compression of the fetal head and are mediated by vagal input to the heart.[220-222] The mechanism of this effect of head compression may relate to a transient increase in intracranial pressure with secondary hypertension and bradycardia through the Cushing reflex. Early decelerations are not associated with fetal hypoxia, as reflected in fetal acid-base measurements or in neonatal depression.[164,196,223]

Late Type. A *late deceleration* is one that begins after a contraction starts but reaches a peak well after the peak of contraction is reached and does not return to baseline

until 30 to 60 seconds after the contraction is completed (see Fig. 7-11).[164,188,201a,224] These decelerations are related primarily to *uteroplacental insufficiency* (e.g., placental disorder, uterine hyperactivity, and maternal hypotension) and are mediated by fetal hypoxia (see Table 7-9).[164,180,188,201a,208,225-230] Such decelerations are unusual with fetal scalp pressure of oxygen (PO_2) greater than 20 mm Hg but appear in more than 50% of infants with fetal scalp PO_2 less than 10 mm Hg.[231] It is understandable that fetal hypoxia occurs after the onset of a uterine contraction when uteroplacental insufficiency is present, because uterine contractions normally reduce uterine blood flow and thereby oxygen delivery to the fetus.[180,232] Fetal hypoxia causes bradycardia by a multifactorial mechanism that primarily includes initially a chemoreceptor-mediated vagal response and then a direct effect on myocardial function.[180,229,230,233] The initial reflex vagally mediated response is accompanied by normal fetal heart rate variability and thus "normal CNS integrity," whereas the nonreflex myocardial late deceleration is observed without heart rate variability and thus "inadequate fetal cerebral and myocardial oxygenation."[188]

The *causal relationship* between fetal hypoxia and late decelerations has been shown in several ways. First, as just noted, the decelerations have been correlated temporally with fetal hypoxia, identified with fetal capillary blood sampling and tissue oxygen electrodes.[225,231]

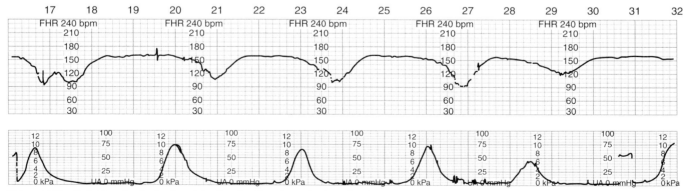

Figure 7-11 **Fetal heart rate tracing, late deceleration.** Note the late decelerations (i.e., the peak of the deceleration is reached well after the peak of the contraction). The absent variability is consistent with decreased cerebral oxygenation. (*Courtesy of Dr. Barry Schifrin.*)

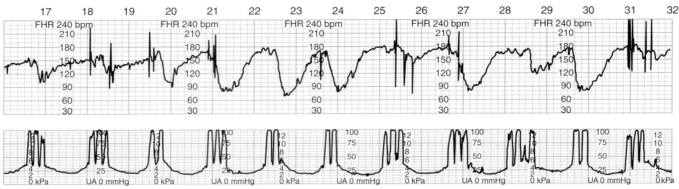

Figure 7-12 **Fetal heart rate tracing, variable deceleration.** Note the recurrent variable decelerations, as described in the text, associated here with maternal pushing, evidenced by the spikes in uterine activity (*lower trace*). The decreasing variability is concerning for recurrent ischemia and fetal compromise. (*Courtesy of Dr. Barry Schifrin.*)

Second, when fetal oxygenation is improved by the administration of 100% oxygen to the normotensive mother or of intravenous fluids and pressors to the hypotensive mother, the bradycardia may cease. Third, a strong correlation exists between the occurrence of late decelerations and alterations in fetal acid-base status secondary to fetal hypoxia.[227]

The possibility that the *late decelerations* may have *secondary deleterious effects* was suggested by studies in subhuman primates that showed that late decelerations are accompanied not only by fetal hypoxia and acidosis but also by hypotension. The bradycardia per se appeared to cause the hypotension.[226] Moreover, studies with fetal sheep documented decreased cardiac output with bradycardia, particularly at rates lower than 60 beats/minute.[47,230,234,235] Data on cerebral blood flow are lacking, however.

The *duration of asphyxia* with late decelerations required to produce brain injury is not entirely clear, although experiments with fetal monkeys suggested that time periods less than 1 hour are not generally sufficient.[236] Studies of human infants also suggested that a time period of less than 1 hour is not likely to be harmful.[237,238] However, *this conclusion must be made very cautiously* because the *severity of the insult* is critical and has not been studied systematically with regard to the timing required to produce fetal brain injury. Indeed, in the case of severe, abrupt, terminal insults (i.e., acute "total" asphyxia just before delivery), brain injury appears to occur after insults of less than 1 hour.[239,240]

Variable Type. The most commonly observed fetal heart rate deceleration is *variable deceleration*,[164,202] which occurs in a substantial minority of all fetuses (see Fig. 7-12).[181,241] This characteristically abrupt slowing of the fetal heart rate may begin before, with, or after the onset of the uterine contraction and is variable in duration. The deceleration pattern is principally the result of varying degrees of umbilical cord compression (see Table 7-9).[47,164,172,219,227] Thus, this periodic pattern is more common with nuchal, short, or prolapsed umbilical cord or decreased amniotic fluid volume (oligohydramnios, ruptured membranes). The *mechanism* of the bradycardia is considered to be an increase in peripheral resistance, which leads to fetal hypertension

that, in turn, causes baroreceptor-stimulated, vagally mediated bradycardia.[242] Occasionally, the umbilical cord compression with each contraction can be prevented by alteration of maternal position. Distinction of early from late cord compression can be made on the basis of determinations of fetal carbon dioxide pressure (PcO_2) and base excess; thus, respiratory acidosis reflects early umbilical cord compression with impaired umbilical blood flow, and metabolic acidosis indicates late cord compression with fetal tissue hypoxia.[243] When variable decelerations are accompanied by or evolve into late decelerations, or *when beat-to-beat variability is diminished or lost* (even without late decelerations), the likelihood of significant fetal hypoxia is markedly enhanced.[164,188,200,227,241]

Relation of Fetal Heart Rate Abnormalities to Neonatal Neurological Course and Subsequent Outcome

A distinct relationship has been demonstrated between intrapartum abnormalities of fetal heart rate, sometimes with documented fetal acidosis, and neurological morbidity in the neonatal period and after 1 year of follow-up.[188,196,201a,237,238,244-248] In a prospective study, 50 infants of high-risk mothers who were provided intrauterine fetal heart rate monitoring during labor were examined by a pediatric neurologist in the neonatal period and then were subsequently evaluated periodically (Table 7-10).[188,244,246-248] Thirty-eight of

TABLE 7-10	Neonatal Neurological Course and Subsequent Development in Electronically Monitored Infants		
	FETAL HEART RATE PATTERNS[*]		
Time of Evaluation	**Normal**	**Moderate to Severe Variable Decelerations**	**Severe Variable and/or Late Decelerations**
Neonatal (48-72 hr)	16%[*]	63%	73%
1 yr	0%	6%	27%
6-9 yr	0%	0%	10%

[*]Percentage of patients with fetal heart rate pattern and *abnormal neurological evaluation.*

the infants exhibited *clearly abnormal fetal heart rate patterns*. These were categorized as *moderate to severe variable decelerations* (defined as decelerations to 70 to 80 beats/minute for >60 seconds with three contractions or to a rate of <70 beats/minute for 30 to 60 seconds), *severe variable decelerations* (decelerations to a rate <70 beats/minute for ≥ 60 seconds), and *late decelerations* (a uniform deceleration of the fetal heart rate of any magnitude that occurred consistently in the late phase of each contraction). A striking relationship of these patterns with the occurrence of neonatal neurological signs was apparent (see Table 7-10). The most consistent sign was hypotonia. By 1 year of age, many fewer abnormalities were apparent, although approximately 25% of the infants with severe variable decelerations or late decelerations or both exhibited neurological disturbances (see Table 7-10). Of the abnormal infants at 1 year of age, approximately 30% exhibited severe deficits. Only 10% of the group with abnormal fetal heart rate patterns had abnormal neurological evaluations at 6 to 9 years of age.[246] These data demonstrate that certain abnormal intrapartum fetal heart rate patterns alone can be valuable indicators of intrauterine insults, presumably hypoxic-ischemic, that result in neurological injury. Further support for this notion is provided by the demonstration of markedly elevated levels of brain-specific creatine phosphokinase in umbilical cord blood of infants with similarly ominous fetal heart rate alterations.[249] In the latter study, approximately 29% of this group exhibited poor neurological outcome. *However, the disappearance of a large portion of the neurological disturbance by 6 to 9 years of age, as shown by Painter and co-workers,[246,247] suggests that the plasticity of the developing human brain is capable of overcoming much of the injury apparent earlier in life, if that injury is not severe.*

Fetal Electrocardiogram

The possibility that analysis of the fetal electrocardiogram could add appreciably to the identification of fetal compromise secondary to intrapartum hypoxia was suggested by studies in the United Kingdom and Sweden.[250-254] The parameters of greatest apparent value are elevation of the ST segment and shortening of the QT interval, which become progressively worse with fetal hypoxia. The mediator of these effects on the myocardium appears to be the surge in catecholamines provoked by hypoxia.[254] Clearly, such information about myocardial insufficiency is relevant to the central nervous system because, ultimately, with asphyxia myocardial insufficiency results in the ischemia that causes brain injury. In a multicenter randomized trial in Sweden involving 4966 women with term fetuses, women were monitored either with fetal heart rate monitoring alone or with fetal heart rate monitoring in addition to evaluation of the electrocardiogram (for elevated ST segment).[252,253] In those women managed according to fetal heart rate monitoring in addition to evaluation of the electrocardiogram, the investigators noted less umbilical cord metabolic acidosis, fewer 1-minute Apgar scores lower than 4, less neonatal encephalopathy, and no neonatal seizures. Subsequent work suggests that in the distressed acidotic fetus, the

QT interval is shortened irrespective of changes in heart rate.[254] Thus, this approach appears to add significantly to the information gained from assessment of the fetal heart rate. However, the method requires *placement of a fetal scalp electrode* and thereby is more invasive than fetal heart rate monitoring. The particular role of fetal electrocardiographic evaluation in fetal monitoring is promising but remains to be established.

Fetal Acid-Base Status

As alluded to in the previous section, certain fetal heart rate patterns are indicative of (or ultimately productive of) fetal hypoxia and the biochemical correlate of tissue oxygen debt, fetal acidosis. Fetal acidemia may occur as a consequence of accumulation of (1) carbon dioxide and thereby carbonic acid, (2) "metabolic" acids, particularly lactate but also ketone bodies, or (3) both the carbonic and noncarbonic acids. Carbon dioxide, which is highly diffusible and thereby subject to rapid changes, can lead to alterations in fetal pH that occur and resolve quickly. By contrast, metabolic acids, which accumulate usually as a consequence of oxygen deprivation and thus anaerobic glycolysis (or incomplete oxidation of fatty acids), increase in tissue and blood more slowly and thus cause slower and more sustained alterations in fetal pH. More detailed consideration of the relevant biochemical aspects is presented in Chapter 6.

Although most studies of "fetal acidosis" are assessed by measurements from the umbilical artery at delivery, the intrapartum use of fetal scalp blood samples provides more nearly real-time information. However, the need for fetal scalp access prevents this approach from being widely used.[255] *Indeed, more commonly used than scalp sampling as an adjunct to fetal heart rate monitoring is assessment of acceleration of fetal heart rate to vibroacoustical (or tactile) stimulation; the presence of acceleration is a reliable indicator of fetal pH higher than 7.2 (normal fetal scalp pH is greater than 7.25; values lower than 7.20 are considered concerning).*[255]

Normal values for fetal blood gas and acid-base measures, obtained from umbilical artery at delivery, are shown in Table 7-11.[238,256,257] In one large series, the 2.5th percentile values for umbilical artery pH and base deficit were 7.10 and 11, respectively.[257] The value of

TABLE 7-11 **Mean Fetal Blood Gas and Acid-Base Data as Measured in Umbilical Artery at Delivery**

Variable	Mean Value
pH	7.26
Partial pressure of oxygen	15 mm Hg
Oxygen saturation	25%
Partial pressure of carbon dioxide	48 mm Hg
Base deficit*	5 mmol/L

Base deficit is concentration of bicarbonate lower than normal. When the term *base excess* is used, the concentration value is expressed as a negative number.

Data from Low JA: Fetal acid-base status and outcome. In Hill A, Volpe JJ, editors: *Fetal Neurology*, New York: 1989, Raven Press.

fetal acid-base measurements as an *adjunct* to fetal heart rate monitoring in the assessment of fetal well-being is well established, although the extent of that value is not without controversy.[168,195,238,255,258-280] Results of several studies showed a strong correlation between the duration and severity of fetal heart rate deceleration patterns of the variable and late types and the occurrence of fetal acidosis or acidosis at delivery.[154,180,181,238,255,261,272,275,281-287]

Alterations in Fetal Acid-Base Measurements and Neonatal Outcome

Alterations in fetal acid-base measurements, particularly when combined with fetal heart rate assessment, are effective predictors of the *condition of the infant at birth*. An early, careful study of 587 high-risk pregnancies, in which fetal heart rate patterns and fetal acid-base data were combined, showed a strong correlation between biochemically documented fetal asphyxia and subnormal Apgar scores at 1 and 5 minutes and abnormal neurological signs in the first hour.[238,264] A later study showed the particular predictive value of the measurement of base deficit in umbilical arterial blood (Table 7-12).[272] Thus, *deficits less than 12 mmol/L very rarely resulted in moderate or severe neurological signs*. Fully 41% of infants with umbilical artery base deficits in excess of 16 mmol/L exhibited such signs. The particular importance of the *base deficit* may relate to the measure's reflection of the accumulation of metabolic acids and thereby not only the severity but also the *duration* of the hypoxic-ischemic insult (see earlier). The severity of fetal acidosis at delivery has been studied most commonly in relation to umbilical artery pH, and although valuable data have been obtained, a relatively high incidence of neonatal neurological complications after presumed prolonged partial asphyxia is not observed until markedly low pH values are obtained (see next section). This difficulty may relate in part to the finding that umbilical artery pH may decline rapidly and may recover promptly with transient changes in Pco_2.

As just noted, the relation of neonatal neurological features to the *severity of fetal acidosis*, as manifested by umbilical arterial pH values at delivery, was delineated in several large-scale studies.[255,267,270,271,273-278,280]

TABLE 7-12 Relation between Fetal Acidemia and Neonatal Encephalopathy

Neonatal Encephalo-pathy*	UMBILICAL ARTERY BASE DEFICIT		
	4-12 mmol/L (n = 116)	12-16 mmol/L (n = 58)	>16 mmol/L (n = 59)
None	89%	72%	39%
Minor	10%	19%	20%
Moderate	1%	7%	29%
Severe	0%	2%	12%

*Minor encephalopathy, "irritability or jitteriness"; moderate, "profound lethargy or abnormal tone"; severe, "coma or abnormal tone and seizures."

Data from Low JA, Lindsay BG, Derrick EJ: Threshold of metabolic acidosis associated with newborn complications, *Am J Obstet Gynecol* 177:1391-1394, 1997.

TABLE 7-13 Relation between Severity of Fetal Acidosis and Neonatal Neurological and Systemic Features

Clinical Dysfunction	UMBILICAL ARTERY pH			
	6.61-6.70	6.71-6.79	6.80-6.89	6.90-6.99
Hypoxic-ischemic encephalopathy*	80%	60%	33%	12%
Renal dysfunction	60%	53%	26%	16%
Cardiac dysfunction	60%	60%	30%	18%
Pulmonary dysfunction	80%	47%	30%	12%
None	20%	40%	48%	75%

*Manifested as seizures and hypotonia in 76%, seizures only in 6%, and hypotonia only in 18%.

Data from Goodwin TM, Belai I, Hernandez P, Durand M, et al: Asphyxial complications in the term newborn with severe umbilical acidemia, *Am J Obstet Gynecol* 167:1506-1512, 1992; derived from study of 129 term infants with umbilical arterial pH <7.00.

Thus, in a study of 129 term, singleton infants with umbilical pH less than 7.00,[267] a distinct relationship between severity of the acidosis and neonatal neurological and systemic manifestations of presumed hypoxic-ischemic insult was observed (Table 7-13). As stated earlier, despite the high incidence of neonatal neurological phenomena, overall, 78% of the infants with umbilical pH less than 7.00 were normal on follow-up examinations. In a later report, 62% of term infants with pH of or less than 7.00 had no neonatal clinical abnormalities.[276]

Alterations in Fetal Acid-Base Measurements and Later Neurological Outcome

The relationship between fetal acidemia and later neurological outcome was studied particularly well by Low and co-workers.[262] These investigators defined the *neurological outcome* at 1 year of age of 37 term infants identified prospectively by detection of fetal asphyxia in term infants derived from a high-risk obstetrical population (Table 7-14). Fourteen percent of the infants with fetal asphyxia had major deficits at 1 year, and a relationship between outcome and severity of acidosis in the asphyxiated group was apparent. However, approximately 85% of the asphyxiated infants either were normal or exhibited only minor deficits at 1 year of age (see Table 7-14). In the relatively

TABLE 7-14 Relationship between Fetal Asphyxia (Defined by Fetal Acidemia) in Term Infants and Neurological Outcome at 1 Year of Age

	NEUROLOGICAL OUTCOME		
	Normal	Minor Deficit	Major Deficit
Control (n = 76)	93%	6%	1%
Fetal asphyxia (n = 37)	61%	25%	14%

Data from Low JA, Galbraith RS, Muir DW, Killen HL, et al: Motor and cognitive deficits after intrapartum asphyxia in the mature fetus, *Am J Obstet Gynecol* 158:356-361, 1988.

uncommon circumstance of severe, abrupt, terminal insults (i.e., acute "total" asphyxia), umbilical cord blood pH most often is *not* markedly depressed; in one large series (N = 47), 60% of such infants (who later exhibited major neurological deficits) had umbilical cord pH higher than 7.00, and in this and other series, cord pH in the normal range was documented.[239,240]

Supporting the value of fetal acid-base assessment *in conjunction with* fetal heart rate monitoring was a study of 60 children with intrapartum fetal hypoxia documented by fetal acid-base studies after detection of fetal heart rate abnormalities.[237] Of the 60 infants, 29% exhibited neurological deficits at age 1 year; the deficits included motor abnormalities in approximately one third. Of the infants with deficits, approximately one half were marked. The severity of deficits correlated closely with the severity of the intrapartum hypoxia as judged by the associated acidosis (Fig. 7-13). Moreover, analysis of the intrapartum obstetrical and biochemical data in the usual case of prolonged partial asphyxia suggested that *the likelihood of neurological deficits correlated with duration of the insult and that approximately 1 hour was a critical time period.* In the infants without deficits, the data indicated that metabolic acidosis developed during the hour before delivery. In the children with minor deficits, the data indicated that acidosis had been developing over at least the hour before delivery. In the children with major deficits, the data indicated that acidosis had developed over a period "in excess of one hour."[237] The results of a later study by the same group also were consistent with the duration of 1 hour as an important threshold.[168]

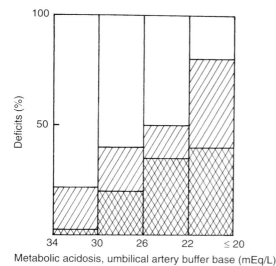

Figure 7-13 **Relation of intrapartum fetal hypoxia to neurological outcome, derived from a study of 60 infants, 42 of whom were full term.** Intrapartum fetal hypoxia is expressed as the degree of acidosis, assessed by umbilical artery buffer base values. "Significant" metabolic acidosis in this laboratory is considered to be a buffer base level of less than 34 mEq/L (base deficit >12 mmol/L). Major (*hatched areas*) and minor (*diagonal lines*) deficits are motor or cognitive (or both) in type. See text for details. (*From Low JA, Galbraith RS, Muir DW, Killen HL, et al: Factors associated with motor and cognitive deficits in children after intrapartum fetal hypoxia, Am J Obstet Gynecol 148:533-539, 1984.*)

As noted earlier, the circumstance of severe, abrupt, terminal asphyxia may lead to brain injury with durations of less than 1 hour.[239,240]

Thus, current observations demonstrate the predictive value of intrapartum monitoring of fetal acid-base status. Moreover, the observations provide major insight into the importance not only of *severity* but also of a critical threshold of *duration* of the hypoxic insult. The latter observations are compatible with experimental data obtained with the fetal monkey that suggest that several hours of "partial asphyxia" result in serious neurological deficits.[288]

Other Techniques for Monitoring Fetal Well-Being Intrapartum

Fetal Pulse Oximetry

Although intermittent measurements of fetal pH, Po_2, and Pco_2 by sampling of fetal scalp blood have provided useful information, *continuous* intrauterine assessment would be of great value. Indeed, as noted earlier, the role of fetal scalp blood sampling is limited by difficulties with access, safety, and accuracy of information.[188] With pulse oximetry, continuous measurements of arterial oxygen saturation can be achieved by application of the oximeter sensor on the infant's cheek. The principle of oximetry relates to the differential absorption of red-infrared (735 nm) and near-infrared (890 nm) by oxyhemoglobin and deoxyhemoglobin. Oximeters in newborns placed on the fingers or toes are based on transmission of light through an emitting optode and reception of light after absorption by the two chromophores by a receiving optode. In fetal oximetry, the optode on the fetal cheek both emits the light and receives the reflected light after absorption.

Initial studies showed that the method is feasible and capable of reproducibly monitoring oxygen saturation.[289-293] Large-scale studies showed that an arterial oxygen saturation of 30% is an apparent threshold for detection of fetal acidosis, as demonstrated by simultaneous fetal scalp blood sampling or umbilical artery blood sampling at delivery. In one study, the use of fetal pulse oximetry in conjunction with fetal heart rate monitoring of high-risk pregnancies led to a 50% reduction in operative deliveries.[293] However, in a randomized trial of more than 5000 women, the use of fetal pulse oximetry and knowledge of intrapartum fetal oxygen saturation had no significant effect on the rates of cesarean delivery overall or specifically for the indication of nonreassuring fetal heart rate.[294] Thus, to what extent this promising methodology will serve as an adjunct to fetal heart rate monitoring remains to be established.

Fetal Electroencephalogram

Although the value of monitoring of fetal heart rate and fetal acid-base status is apparent from the data available, a more direct means of assessing the status of the central nervous system in utero obviously would be preferred. One attempt in this direction was the earlier study of the *fetal electroencephalogram* (*EEG*) during labor by Rosen and co-workers.[295-302] By correlating the fetal patterns on the EEG with fetal heart rate tracings, neonatal assessment, and neurological evaluation at age 1 year, these investigators were able to demonstrate that brain injury is incurred in utero during labor in selected high-risk patients. Late decelerations of the fetal heart rate and traction of the head with forceps were among the factors shown to be associated with voltage suppression on the EEG.[296] Prolonged voltage suppression and persistent sharp waves were shown to be associated with neurological abnormality in the neonatal period and at 1 year of age.[301-303] The relevant abnormalities on the EEG were adapted to a system of computer interpretation, and investigators showed that the fetal EEG accurately predicted 63% of infants found to be abnormal (primarily delayed neurological development) at 1 year of age.[301-303] When data related to fetal heart rate, Apgar scores, and neonatal neurological examination were considered in addition to the findings on the fetal EEG, the accuracy of prediction increased to 80%. These observations, with a physiological measure of central nervous system function during labor, indicated that the brain injury occurring in utero often can be detected at that time. The possibility of identifying such patients has major implications for interventions at the time of or immediately following the injurious insult in utero as well as shortly after birth.

Because of methodological difficulties, use of the fetal EEG has not reached the level of clinical applicability, despite attempts to develop electrodes more easily used in clinical obstetrics.[304,305] Certainly, evaluation of fetal cerebral electrical activity has provided insight into timing of disturbance to fetal central nervous system during labor, but technological advances are required before application to clinical practice is feasible. One potential solution is a more simplified system based on real-time spectral analysis of the fetal EEG obtained from two leads embedded in a single probe that can be applied to the fetal scalp by suction cups.[306] The spectral analysis of the signal on the fetal EEG determines the frequency and amplitude of the signal. The most useful measure is the spectral edge frequency, the frequency lower than which 90% of the power of the power spectrum resides. Changes in spectral edge frequency correlate with changes in behavioral state, and during episodes of variable decelerations, a decrease in spectral edge frequency has been observed. Whether this limited measure of the fetal EEG will prove clinically useful remains to be established.

Doppler Measurements of Blood Flow Velocity

The value of measurements of blood flow velocity in the umbilical and fetal cerebral arteries in antepartum monitoring was described earlier. The feasibility of measurements of umbilical arterial blood flow velocity intrapartum has been demonstrated.[307-311] Although application of the technique has provided useful pathophysiological information, the method has not proven applicable for widespread clinical use.

Measurement of uterine blood flow velocity has been correlated with uterine contractions during labor (Table 7-15).[310] A linear decrease in velocity was shown with the increase in intrauterine pressure with contractions.

Of particular interest has been the determination of blood flow velocity during labor in the fetal anterior and middle cerebral arteries, insonated either through the anterior fontanelle by transvaginal Doppler ultrasound or through the transabdominal approach with duplex Doppler.[312,313] An approximately 40% decrease in resistance index in the middle cerebral artery was observed between contractions during active labor in one study.[313] One of several explanations for this observation is the occurrence of vasodilation caused by accumulation of vasoactive molecules (e.g., hydrogen ion, adenosine, prostaglandins) provoked by intermittent ischemia. Further studies would be of interest, although technical difficulties in obtaining reproducible measurements have proved substantial.

Near-Infrared Spectroscopy

An approach to intrapartum fetal monitoring of potential value involves the use of near-infrared spectroscopy for the study of *fetal cerebral hemodynamics and oxygenation*. As described in Chapter 4, by application of a near-infrared light source and a photon-counting device to the cranium of the newborn and appropriate selection of light wavelengths, information concerning intracranial concentrations of oxygenated and deoxygenated hemoglobin can be obtained. With such data, information concerning cerebral hemoglobin oxygen saturation, cerebral oxygen delivery, and cerebral blood volume can be determined. This method, like intrapartum Doppler study, has provided useful pathophysiological information, but the method has not proven applicable for widespread clinical use.

Peebles and co-workers[314-318] designed a rubber probe that incorporates the two fiberoptic bundles containing the near-infrared light source and the photon counter, separated by approximately 3 to 4 cm. This probe can be attached to the fetal head after membranes have ruptured and when cervical dilation is sufficient to attach the probe. Initial studies showed that with normal uterine contractions, the cerebral content of both oxygenated and deoxygenated hemoglobin, and thereby total hemoglobin, decreased. The data

TABLE 7-15	Decrease in Uterine Blood Flow Velocity as a Function of Increase in Intrauterine Pressure with Contractions	
Pressure Increase (mm Hg)	**Velocity Decrease (Median)**
10	8%
20	23%
30	30%
40	44%
50	65%
60	60%

Data from Janbu T, Nesheim BI: Uterine artery blood velocities during contractions in pregnancy and labour related to intrauterine pressure, *Br J Obstet Gynaecol* 94:1150-1155, 1987.

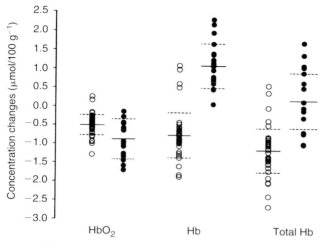

Figure 7-14 **Near-infrared spectroscopic findings obtained from human fetuses during normal uterine concentrations (*left: open circles*) and those accompanied by fetal heart rate decelerations (*right: solid circles*).** Mean values ± standard deviations are indicated. Note the lower oxyhemoglobin (HbO₂) and higher deoxyhemoglobin (Hb), indicative of cerebral hemoglobin oxygen desaturation, in contractions complicated by fetal heart rate decelerations. *(From Peebles DM, Edwards AD, Wyatt JS, Bishop AP, et al: Changes in human fetal cerebral hemoglobin concentration and oxygenation during labor measured by near-infrared spectroscopy, Am J Obstet Gynecol 166:1369-1373, 1992.)*

suggested a decline in cerebral blood volume with contractions. With late fetal heart rate decelerations, a different pattern emerged. Oxygenated hemoglobin declined, whereas deoxygenated hemoglobin increased, a finding indicating cerebral hemoglobin oxygen desaturation (Fig. 7-14). This observation suggests a decrease in cerebral oxygen delivery with the decelerations. One possible reason for this decrease would be a reduction in cerebral blood flow. Another study of 14 women under epidural analgesia during uncomplicated labor at term showed that the supine position was associated with a decline in mean cerebral oxygenated hemoglobin concentration sufficient to produce an 8.3% decrease in mean cerebral oxygen saturation.[317] This finding may reflect a decrease in uterine blood flow, secondary to maternal aortocaval obstruction by the gravid uterus, and resulting in fetal hypoxemia. Further studies would be of interest, but the expense of the instrumentation and the technical difficulties in obtaining reproducible measurements in the clinical setting have proved substantial.

REFERENCES

1. Kok RD, van den Bergh AJ, Heerschap A, Nijland R, et al: Metabolic information from the human fetal brain obtained with proton magnetic resonance spectroscopy, *Am J Obstet Gynecol* 185:1011-1015, 2001.
2. Levine D, Barnes PD, Robertson RR, Wong G, et al: Fast MR imaging of fetal central nervous system abnormalities, *Radiology* 229:51-61, 2003.
3. Eswaran H, Wilson JD, Preissl H, Robinson SE, et al: Magneto-encephalographic recordings of visual evoked brain activity in the human fetus, *Lancet* 360:779-780, 2002.
4. Fulford J, Vadeyar SH, Dodampahala SH, Moore RJ, et al: Fetal brain activity in response to a visual stimulus, *Hum Brain Mapp* 20:239-245, 2003.
5. Righini A, Bianchini E, Parazzini C, Gementi P, et al: Apparent diffusion coefficient determination in normal fetal brain: A prenatal MR imaging study, *AJNR Am J Neuroradiol* 24:799-804, 2003.
6. Gowland P, Fulford J: Initial experiences of performing fetal fMRI, *Exp Neurol* 190(Suppl):S22-S27, 2004.
7. Manning FA: General principles and applications of ultrasonography. In Creasy RK, Resnik R, Iams JD, editors: *Maternal-Fetal Medicine: Principles and Practice*, 5th ed, Philadelphia: 2004, WB Saunders.
8. Milunsky A: *Genetic Disorders and the Fetus: Diagnosis, Prevention, and Treatment*, 5th ed, Baltimore: 2004, Johns Hopkins University Press.
9. Roelants-van Rijn AM, Groenendaal F, Stoutenbeek P, van der Grond J: Lactate in the foetal brain: Detection and implications, *Acta Paediatr* 93:937-940, 2004.
10. Bijma HH, Schoonderwaldt EM, van der Heide A, Wildschut HIJ, et al: Ultrasound diagnosis of fetal anomalies: An analysis of perinatal management of 318 consecutive pregnancies in a multidisciplinary setting, *Prenat Diagn* 24:890-895, 2004.
11. Harper RG, Greenberg M, Farahani G, Glassman I, et al: Fetal movement, biochemical and biophysical parameters, and the outcome of pregnancy, *Am J Obstet Gynecol* 141:39-42, 1981.
12. Rayburn WF: Antepartum fetal assessment: Monitoring fetal activity, *Clin Perinatol* 9:231-243, 1982.
13. Neldam S: Fetal movements as an indicator of fetal well-being, *Dan Med Bull* 30:274-278, 1983.
14. Sadovsky E, Ohel G, Havazeleth H, Steinwell A, et al: The definition and the significance of decreased fetal movements, *Acta Obstet Gynecol Scand* 62:409-413, 1983.
15. Rayburn WF: Antepartum fetal monitoring: Fetal movement. In Hill A, Volpe JJ, editors: *Fetal Neurology*, New York: 1989, Raven Press.
16. McNay MB: Fetal movements, *Dev Med Child Neurol* 30:821-824, 1988.
17. Moore TR, Piacquadio K: A prospective evaluation of fetal movement screening to reduce the incidence of antepartum fetal death, *Am J Obstet Gynecol* 160:1075-1080, 1989.
18. Ribbert LSM, Visser GHA, Mulder EJH, Zonneveld MF, et al: Changes with time in fetal heart rate variation, movement incidences and haemodynamics in intrauterine growth retarded fetuses: A longitudinal approach to the assessment of fetal well being, *Early Hum Dev* 31: 195-208, 1993.
19. Romanini C, Rizzo G: Fetal behaviour in normal and compromised fetuses: An overview, *Early Hum Dev* 43:117-131, 1995.
20. Prechtl HFR: State of the art of a new functional assessment of the young nervous system: An early predictor of cerebral palsy, *Early Hum Dev* 50:1-11, 1997.
21. Richardson BS, Gagnon R: Fetal breathing and body movements. In Creasy RK, Resnik R, Iams JD, editors: *Maternal-Fetal Medicine: Principles and Practice*, 5th ed, Philadelphia: 2004, WB Saunders.
22. Dipietro JA: Neurobehavioral assessment before birth, *Ment Retard Dev Disabil Res Rev* 11:4-13, 2005.
23. Pillai M, James D: Are the behavioural states of the newborn comparable to those of the fetus?, *Early Hum Dev* 22:39-49, 1990.
24. Pillai M, James D: Behavioural states in normal mature human fetuses, *Arch Dis Child* 65:39-43, 1990.
25. Griffin RL, Caron FJ, van Geijn HP: Behavioral states in the human fetus during labor, *Am J Obstet Gynecol* 152:828-833, 1985.
26. Drogtrop AP, Ubels R, Nijhuis JG: The association between fetal body movements, eye movements and heart rate patterns in pregnancies between 25 and 30 weeks of gestation, *Early Hum Dev* 23:67-73, 1990.
27. Swartjes JM, van Geijn HP, Mantel R, van Woerden EE, et al: Coincidence of behavioural state parameters in the human fetus at three gestational ages, *Early Hum Dev* 23:75-83, 1990.
28. Nijhuis JG, Martin CB Jr, Prechtl HFR: Behavioural states of the human fetus. In Prechtl HFR, editor: *Continuity of Neural Functions*, London: 1984, Spastics International Medical Publications.
29. van Vliet MA, Martin CB Jr, Nijhuis JG, Prechtl HF: Behavioural states in the fetuses of nulliparous women, *Early Hum Dev* 12:121-135, 1985.
30. Birnholz JC, Farrell EE: Ultrasound images of human fetal development, *Am Sci* 72:608-612, 1984.
31. Birnholz JC, Stephens JC, Faria M: Fetal movement patterns: A possible means of defining neurologic developmental milestones in utero, *AJR Am J Roentgenol* 130:537-540, 1978.
32. Natsuyama E: In utero behavior of human embryos at the spinal-cord stage of development, *Biol Neonate* 60:11-29, 1991.
33. Prechtl HFR: Prenatal motor development. In Wade MG, Whiting HTA, editors: *Motor Development in Children: Aspects of Coordination and Control*, Dordrecht: 1986, Martinus Nijhoff.
34. Prechtl HFR: Fetal behavior. In Hill A, Volpe JJ, editors: *Fetal Neurology*, New York: 1989, Raven Press.
35. de Vries JI, Visser GH, Prechtl HF: The emergence of fetal behaviour. II. Quantitative aspects, *Early Hum Dev* 12:99-120, 1985.
36. Roodenburg PJ, Wladimiroff JW, van Es A, Prechtl HF: Classification and quantitative aspects of fetal movements during the second half of normal pregnancy, *Early Hum Dev* 25:19-35, 1991.
37. Prechtl HF: Qualitative changes of spontaneous movements in fetus and preterm infant are a marker of neurological dysfunction [editorial], *Early Hum Dev* 23:151-158, 1990.
38. Koyanagi T, Horimoto N, Maeda H, Kukita J, et al: Abnormal behavioral patterns in the human fetus at term: Correlation with lesion sites in the central nervous system after birth, *J Child Neurol* 8:19-26, 1993.
39. Horimoto N, Koyanagi T, Maeda H, Satoh S, et al: Can brain impairment be detected by in utero behavioural patterns?, *Arch Dis Child* 69:3-9, 1993.

40. Manning FA: Fetal assessment by evaluation of biophysical variables. In Creasy RK, Resnik R, editors: *Maternal-Fetal Medicine*, 4th ed, Philadelphia: 1999, WB Saunders.

41. Leader LR, Baillie P, Martin B, Vermeulen E: The assessment and significance of habituation to a repeated stimulus by the human fetus, *Early Hum Dev* 7:211-219, 1982.

42. Serafini P, Lindsay MB, Nagey DA, Pupkin MJ, et al: Antepartum fetal heart rate response to sound stimulation: The acoustic stimulation test, *Am J Obstet Gynecol* 148:41-45, 1984.

43. Divon MY, Platt LD, Cantrell CJ, Smith CV, et al: Evoked fetal startle response: A possible intrauterine neurological examination, *Am J Obstet Gynecol* 153:454-456, 1985.

44. Visser GH, Mulder HH, Wit HP, Mulder EJ, et al: Vibro-acoustic stimulation of the human fetus: Effect on behavioural state organization, *Early Hum Dev* 19:285-296, 1989.

45. Kisilevsky BS, Muir DW, Low JA: Human fetal responses to sound as a function of stimulus intensity, *Obstet Gynecol* 73:971-976, 1989.

46. Parkes MJ, Moore PJ, Moore DR, Fisk NM, et al: Behavioral changes in fetal sheep caused by vibroacoustic stimulation: The effects of cochlear ablation, *Am J Obstet Gynecol* 164:1336-1343, 1991.

47. Parer JT: Fetal heart rate. In Creasy RK, Resnik R, editors: *Maternal-Fetal Medicine*, 4th ed, Philadelphia: 1999, WB Saunders.

48. Jansen AH, Chernick V: Development of respiratory control, *Physiol Rev* 63:437-483, 1983.

49. Walker DW: Brain mechanisms, hypoxia and fetal breathing, *J Dev Physiol* 6:225-236, 1984.

50. Paul RH: The evaluation of antepartum fetal well-being using the nonstress test, *Clin Perinatol* 9:253-263, 1982.

51. Smith CV, Phelan JP: Antepartum fetal assessment: The nonstress test. In Hill A, Volpe JJ, editors: *Fetal Neurology*, New York: 1989, Raven Press.

52. Platt LD, Paul RH, Phelan J, Walla CA, et al: Fifteen years of experience with antepartum fetal testing, *Am J Obstet Gynecol* 156:1509-1515, 1987.

53. Harman CR: Assessment of fetal health. In Creasy RK, Resnik R, Iams JD, editors: *Maternal-Fetal Medicine: Principles and Practice*, 5th ed, Philadelphia: 2004, WB Saunders.

54. Devoe LD: Clinical implications of prospective antepartum fetal heart rate testing, *Am J Obstet Gynecol* 137:983-990, 1980.

55. Beischer NA, Drew JH, Ashton PW, Oats JN, et al: Quality of survival of infants with critical fetal reserve detected by antenatal cardiotocography, *Am J Obstet Gynecol* 146:662-670, 1983.

56. Murata Y, Ikenoue T, Hashimoto T: Fetal heart rate acceleration and late deceleration during a course of intrauterine death in chronically catheterized rhesus monkeys. In Twenty-eighth Annual Meeting of the Society for Gynecologic Investigation, 1981, St. Louis, MO, 1981.

57. Freeman RK: Contraction stress testing for primary fetal surveillance in patients at high risk for uteroplacental insufficiency, *Clin Perinatol* 9:265-270, 1982.

58. Freeman RK, Anderson G, Dorchester W: A prospective multi-institutional study of antepartum fetal heart rate monitoring. I. Risk of perinatal mortality and morbidity according to antepartum fetal heart rate test results, *Am J Obstet Gynecol* 143:771-777, 1982.

59. Freeman RK, Anderson G, Dorchester W: A prospective multi-institutional study of antepartum fetal heart rate monitoring. II. Contraction stress test versus nonstress test for primary surveillance, *Am J Obstet Gynecol* 143:778-781, 1982.

60. Phelan PP, Smith CV: Antepartum fetal assessment: The contraction stress test. In Hill A, Volpe JJ, editors: *Fetal Neurology*, New York: 1989, Raven Press.

61. Manning FA, Morrison I, Lange IR, Harman C: Antepartum determination of fetal health: Composite biophysical profile scoring, *Clin Perinatol* 9:285-296, 1982.

62. Platt LD, Eglinton GS, Sipos L, Broussard PM, et al: Further experience with the fetal biophysical profile, *Obstet Gynecol* 61:480-485, 1983.

63. Vintzileos AM, Campbell WA, Ingardia CJ, Nochimson DJ: The fetal biophysical profile and its predictive value, *Obstet Gynecol* 62:271-278, 1983.

64. Brar HS, Platt LD: Fetal biophysical score and fetal well being. In Hill A, Volpe JJ, editors: *Fetal Neurology*, New York: 1989, Raven Press.

65. Vintzileos AM, Gaffney SE, Salinger LM, Kontopoulos VG, et al: The relationships among the fetal biophysical profile, umbilical cord pH, and Apgar scores, *Am J Obstet Gynecol* 157:627-631, 1987.

66. Vintzileos AM, Campbell WA, Nochimson DJ, Weinbaum PJ: The use and misuse of the fetal biophysical profile, *Am J Obstet Gynecol* 156:527-533, 1987.

67. Johnson JM, Harman CR, Lange IR, Manning FA: Biophysical profile scoring in the management of the postterm pregnancy: An analysis of 307 patients, *Am J Obstet Gynecol* 154:269-273, 1986.

68. Platt LD, Walla CA, Paul RH, Trujillo ME, et al: A prospective trial of the fetal biophysical profile versus the nonstress test in the management of high-risk pregnancies, *Am J Obstet Gynecol* 153:624-633, 1985.

69. Manning FA, Bondaji N, Harman CR, Casiro O, et al: Fetal assessment based on fetal biophysical profile scoring. VIII. The incidence of cerebral palsy in tested and untested perinates, *Am J Obstet Gynecol* 178:696-906, 1998.

70. Tropper PJ, Fox HE: Evaluation of antepartum fetal well-being by measuring growth, *Clin Perinatol* 9:271-284, 1982.

71. Creasy RK, Resnik R: Intrauterine growth restriction. In Creasy RK, Resnik R, editors: *Maternal-Fetal Medicine*, 4th ed, Philadelphia: 1999, WB Saunders.

72. Cetrulo CL, Freeman R: Bioelectric evaluation in IUGR, *Clin Obstet Gynecol* 20:979, 1977.

73. Low JA, Boston RW, Pancham SR: Fetal asphyxia during the intrapartum period in intrauterine growth retarded infants, *Am J Obstet Gynecol* 113:351-357, 1972.

74. Lin CC, Moawad AH, Rosenow PJ, River P: Acid-base characteristics of fetuses with intrauterine growth retardation during labor and delivery, *Am J Obstet Gynecol* 137:553-559, 1980.

75. Gazzolo D, Visser GH, Santi F, Magliano CP, et al: Behavioural development and Doppler velocimetry in relation to perinatal outcome in small for dates fetuses, *Early Hum Dev* 43:185-195, 1995.

76. Steiner H, Staudach A, Spitzer D, Schaffer KH, et al: Growth deficient fetuses with absent or reversed umbilical artery end-diastolic flow are metabolically compromised, *Early Hum Dev* 41:1-9, 1995.

77. Resnik R, Creasy RK: Intrauterine growth restriction. In Creasy RK, Resnik R, Iams JD, editors: *Maternal-Fetal Medicine: Principles and Practice*, 5th ed, Philadelphia: 2004, WB Saunders.

78. Schulman H: The clinical implications of Doppler ultrasound analysis of the uterine and umbilical arteries, *Am J Obstet Gynecol* 156:888-893, 1987.

79. van Vugt JM, Ruissen CJ, Hoogland HJ, de Haan J: A prospective study of the umbilical artery waveform in appropriate-for-date and growth-retarded fetuses, *Gynecol Obstet Invest* 23:217-225, 1987.

80. van Vugt JM, Ruissen CJ, Hoogland HJ, de Haan J: Prospective study of velocity waveforms in the fetal descending thoracic and abdominal aorta in fetuses appropriate for gestational age and in growth-retarded fetuses, *Gynecol Obstet Invest* 24:14-22, 1987.

81. Hendricks SK, Sorensen TK, Wang KY, Bushnell JM, et al: Doppler umbilical artery waveform indices: Normal values from fourteen to forty-two weeks, *Am J Obstet Gynecol* 161:761-765, 1989.

82. McParland P, Pearce JM: Doppler blood flow in pregnancy, *Placenta* 9:427-450, 1988.

83. Carroll BA: Duplex Doppler systems in obstetric ultrasound, *Radiol Clin North Am* 28:189-203, 1990.

84. Newnham JP, Patterson LL, James IR, Diepeveen DA, et al: An evaluation of the efficacy of Doppler flow velocity waveform analysis as a screening test in pregnancy, *Am J Obstet Gynecol* 162:403-410, 1990.

85. Ritchie JW: Use of Doppler technology in assessing fetal health, *J Dev Physiol* 15:121-123, 1991.

86. Fitzgerald DE, Stuart BT: Fetoplacental and uteroplacental blood flow in pregnancy. In Hill A, Volpe JJ, editors: *Fetal Neurology*, New York: 1989, Raven Press.

87. Raju TN: Cerebral Doppler studies in the fetus and newborn infant, *J Pediatr* 119:165-174, 1991.

88. Oosterhof H, Dijkstra K, Aarnoudse JG: Fetal Doppler velocimetry in the internal carotid and umbilical artery during Braxton-Hicks' contractions, *Early Hum Dev* 30:33-40, 1992.

89. Pattison RC, Odendaal HJ, Kirsten G: The relationship between absent end-diastolic velocities of the umbilical artery and perinatal mortality and morbidity, *Early Hum Dev* 33:61-69, 1993.

90. Chan FY, Pun TC, Lam P, Lam C, et al: Fetal cerebral Doppler studies as a predictor of perinatal outcome and subsequent neurologic handicap, *Obstet Gynecol* 87:981-988, 1996.

91. Adiotomre PNA, Johnstone FD, Laing IA: Effect of absent end diastolic flow velocity in the fetal umbilical artery on subsequent outcome, *Arch Dis Child Fetal Neonatal Ed* 76:F35-F38, 1997.

92. Dubiel M, Sudmundsson S, Gunnarsson G, Marsal K: Middle cerebral artery velocimetry as a predictor of hypoxemia in fetuses with increased resistance to blood flow in the umbilical artery, *Early Hum Dev* 47:177-184, 1997.

93. Harrington K, Thompson MO, Carpenter RG, Nguyen M, et al: Doppler fetal circulation in pregnancies complicated by pre-eclampsia or delivery of a small for gestational age baby. II. Longitudinal analysis, *Br J Obstet Gynaecol* 106:453-466, 1999.

94. Trudinger B: Doppler ultrasound assessment of blood flow. In Creasy RK, Resnik R, editors: *Maternal-Fetal Medicine*, 4th ed, Philadelphia: 1999, WB Saunders.

95. Newnham JP, Kelly RW, Roberts RV, MacIntyre M, et al: Fetal and maternal Doppler flow velocity waveforms in normal sheep pregnancy, *Placenta* 8:467-476, 1987.

96. Sutton MS, Theard MA, Bhatia SJ, Plappert T, et al: Changes in placental blood flow in the normal human fetus with gestational age, *Pediatr Res* 28:383-387, 1990.

97. Laurin J, Marsal K, Persson PH, Lingman G: Ultrasound measurement of fetal blood flow in predicting fetal outcome, *Br J Obstet Gynaecol* 94:940-948, 1987.

98. Divon MY, Girz BA, Lieblich R, Langer O: Clinical management of the fetus with markedly diminished umbilical artery end-diastolic flow, *Am J Obstet Gynecol* 161:1523-1527, 1989.

99. Laurin J, Lingman G, Marsal K, Persson PH: Fetal blood flow in pregnancies complicated by intrauterine growth retardation, *Obstet Gynecol* 69:895-902, 1987.

100. Reuwer PJ, Sijmons EA, Rietman GW, van Tiel MW, et al: Intrauterine growth retardation: Prediction of perinatal distress by Doppler ultrasound, *Lancet* 2:415-418, 1987.
101. Rochelson B, Schulman H, Farmakides G, Bracero L, et al: The significance of absent end-diastolic velocity in umbilical artery velocity waveforms, *Am J Obstet Gynecol* 156:1213-1218, 1987.
102. Rightmire DA, Campbell S: Fetal and maternal Doppler blood flow parameters in postterm pregnancies, *Obstet Gynecol* 69:891-894, 1987.
103. Bekedam DJ, Visser GH, van der Zee AG, Snijders RJ, et al: Abnormal velocity waveforms of the umbilical artery in growth retarded fetuses: Relationship to antepartum late heart rate decelerations and outcome, *Early Hum Dev* 24:79-89, 1990.
104. Ferrazzi E, Pardi G, Bauscaglia M, Marconi AM, et al: The correlation of biochemical monitoring versus umbilical flow velocity measurements of the human fetus, *Am J Obstet Gynecol* 159:1081-1087, 1988.
105. Soothill PW, Nicolaides KH, Bilardo CM, Campbell S: Relation of fetal hypoxia in growth retardation to mean blood velocity in the fetal aorta, *Lancet* 2:1118-1120, 1986.
106. Hawdon JM, Ward Platt MP, McPhail S, Cameron H, et al: Prediction of impaired metabolic adaptation by antenatal Doppler studies in small for gestational age fetuses, *Arch Dis Child* 67:789-792, 1992.
107. Schreuder AM, McDonnell M, Gaffney G, Johnson A, et al: Outcome at school age following antenatal detection of absent or reversed end diastolic flow velocity in the umbilical artery, *Archives of Disease in Childhood* 86:108-114, 2002.
107a. Maunu J, Ekholm E, Parkkola R, Palo P, et al: Antenatal Doppler measurements and early brain injury in very low birth weight infants, *J Pediatr* 150:51-56 e51, 2007.
108. Fok RY, Pavlova Z, Benirschke K, Paul RH, et al: The correlation of arterial lesions with umbilical artery Doppler velocimetry in the placentas of small-for-dates pregnancies, *Obstet Gynecol* 75:578-583, 1990.
109. van Huisseling H, Hasaart TH, Muijsers GJ, de Haan J: Umbilical artery flow velocity waveforms and placental vascular resistance during maternal placental outflow obstruction in sheep, *J Dev Physiol* 13:93-97, 1990.
110. Kirkinen P, Müller R, Huch R, Huch A: Blood flow velocity waveforms in human fetal intracranial arteries, *Obstet Gynecol* 70:617-621, 1987.
111. Meerman RJ, van Bel F, van Zwieten PH, Oepkes D, et al: Fetal and neonatal cerebral blood velocity in the normal fetus and neonate: A longitudinal Doppler ultrasound study, *Early Hum Dev* 24:209-217, 1990.
112. Kurmanavichius J, Karrer G, Hebisch G, Huch R, et al: Fetal and preterm newborn cerebral blood flow velocity, *Early Hum Dev* 26:113-120, 1991.
113. Satoh S, Koyanagi T, Hara K, Shimokawa H, et al: Developmental characteristics of blood flow in the middle cerebral artery in the human fetus in utero, assessed using the linear-array pulsed Doppler method, *Early Hum Dev* 17:195-203, 1988.
114. Chandran R, Serrasserra V, Sellers SM, Redman C: Fetal cerebral Doppler in the recognition of fetal compromise, *Br J Obstet Gynaecol* 100:139-144, 1993.
115. Veille JC, Hanson R, Tatum K: Longitudinal quantitation of middle cerebral artery blood flow in normal human fetuses, *Am J Obstet Gynecol* 169:1393-1398, 1993.
116. Simonazzi E, Wladimiroff JW, van Eyck J: Flow velocity waveforms in the fetal internal carotid artery relative to fetal blood gas and acid-base measurements in normal pregnancy, *Early Hum Dev* 19:111-115, 1989.
117. Wladimiroff JW, Tonge HM, Stewart PA: Doppler ultrasound assessment of cerebral blood flow in the human fetus, *Br J Obstet Gynaecol* 93:471-475, 1986.
118. Satoh S, Koyanagi T, Fukuhara M, Hara K, et al: Changes in vascular resistance in the umbilical and middle cerebral arteries in the human intrauterine growth-retarded fetus, measured with pulsed Doppler ultrasound, *Early Hum Dev* 20:213-220, 1989.
119. Mari G, Moise KJ Jr, Deter RL, Kirshon B, et al: Doppler assessment of the pulsatility index in the cerebral circulation of the human fetus, *Am J Obstet Gynecol* 160:698-703, 1989.
120. Wladimiroff JW, Noordam MJ, van den Wijngaard JA, Hop WC: Fetal internal carotid and umbilical artery blood flow velocity waveforms as a measure of fetal well-being in intrauterine growth retardation, *Pediatr Res* 24:609-612, 1988.
121. Veille JC, Cohen I: Middle cerebral artery blood flow in normal and growth-retarded fetuses, *Am J Obstet Gynecol* 162:391-396, 1990.
122. Scherjon SA, Smoldersdehaas H, Kok JH, Zondervan HA: The brain-sparing effect: Antenatal cerebral Doppler findings in relation to neurologic outcome in very preterm infants, *Am J Obstet Gynecol* 169:169-175, 1993.
123. Scherjon SA, Oosting H, Kok JH, Zondervan HA: Effect of fetal brain-sparing on the early neonatal cerebral circulation, *Arch Dis Child Fetal Neonatal Ed* 71:F11-F15, 1994.
124. Gramellini D, Folli MC, Raboni S, Vadora E, et al: Cerebral-umbilical Doppler ratio as a predictor of adverse perinatal outcome, *Obstet Gynecol* 79:416-420, 1992.
125. Degani S, Lewinsky R, Shapiro I, Sharf M: Decrease in pulsatile flow in the internal carotid artery in fetal hydrocephalus, *Br J Obstet Gynaecol* 95:138-141, 1988.
126. Connors G, Gillis S, Hunse C, Gagnon R, et al: The interaction of behavioural state, heart rate and resistance index in the human fetus, *J Dev Physiol* 15:331-336, 1991.
127. Hagberg B, Hagberg G, Zetterstrom R: Decreasing perinatal mortality: Increase in cerebral palsy morbidity, *Acta Paediatr Scand* 78:664-670, 1989.
128. Hagberg B, Hagberg G, Olow I, von Wendt L: The changing panorama of cerebral palsy in Sweden. V. The birth year period 1979-82, *Acta Paediatr Scand* 78:283-290, 1989.
129. Hagberg B, Hagberg G: The changing panorama of infantile hydrocephalus and cerebral palsy over forty years: A Swedish survey, *Brain Dev* 11:368-373, 1989.
130. Hagberg B, Hagberg G, Olow I: The changing panorama of cerebral palsy in Sweden. VI. Prevalence and origin during the birth year period 1983-1986, *Acta Paediatr Scand* 82:387-393, 1993.
131. Riikonen R, Raumavirta S, Sinivuori E, Seppala T: Changing pattern of cerebral palsy in the southwest region of Finland, *Acta Paediatr Scand* 78:581-587, 1989.
132. Nelson KB, Ellenberg JH: Antecedents of cerebral palsy: Multivariate analysis of risk, *N Engl J Med* 315:81-86, 1986.
133. Blair E, Stanley FJ: Intrapartum asphyxia: A rare cause of cerebral palsy, *J Pediatr* 112:515-519, 1988.
134. Grant A, O'Brien N, Joy MT, Hennessy E, et al: Cerebral palsy among children born during the Dublin randomised trial of intrapartum monitoring, *Lancet* 2:1233-1236, 1989.
135. MacDonald D, Grant A, Sheridan-Pereira M, Boylan P, et al: The Dublin randomized controlled trial of intrapartum fetal heart rate monitoring, *Am J Obstet Gynecol* 152:524-539, 1985.
136. Kuban KCK, Leviton A: The epidemiology of cerebral palsy, *N Engl J Med* 330:188-195, 1994.
137. Nelson KB: What proportion of cerebral palsy is related to birth asphyxia? [editorial], *J Pediatr* 112:572-574, 1988.
138. Nelson KB: Perspective on the role of perinatal asphyxia in neurologic outcome, *CMAJ* 53(Suppl):3-10, 1988.
139. Naeye RL, Peters EC, Bartholomew M, Landis JR: Origins of cerebral palsy, *Am J Dis Child* 143:1154-1161, 1989.
140. Torfs CP, van den Berg B, Oechsli FW, Cummins S: Prenatal and perinatal factors in the etiology of cerebral palsy, *J Pediatr* 116:615-619, 1990.
141. Melone PJ, Ernest JM, O'Shea MD Jr, Klinepeter KL: Appropriateness of intrapartum fetal heart rate management and risk of cerebral palsy, *Am J Obstet Gynecol* 165:272-276, 1991.
142. Nelson KB, Leviton A: How much of neonatal encephalopathy is due to birth asphyxia, *Am J Dis Child* 145:1325-1331, 1991.
143. Stanley FJ, Blair E: Why have we failed to reduce the frequency of cerebral palsy? *Med J Aust* 154:623-626, 1991.
144. Gaffney G, Flavell V, Johnson A, Squier MV, et al: Model to identify potentially preventable cerebral palsy of intrapartum origin, *Arch Dis Child Fetal Neonatal Ed* 73:F106-F108, 1995.
145. Hagberg B, Hagberg G, Olow I, von Wendt L: The changing panorama of cerebral palsy in Sweden. VII. Prevalence and origin in the birth year period 1987-90, *Acta Paediatr Scand* 85:954-960, 1996.
146. Goldenberg RL, Nelson KG: Cerebral palsy. In Creasy RK, Resnik R, editors: *Maternal-Fetal Medicine*, 4th ed, Philadelphia: 1999, WB Saunders.
147. Hagberg B, Hagberg G, Beckung E, Uvebrant P: Changing panorama of cerebral palsy in Sweden. VIII. Prevalence and origin in the birth year period 1991-94, *Acta Paediatr Scand* 90:271-277, 2001.
148. Clark SL, Hankins GDV: Temporal and demographic trends in cerebral palsy: Fact and fiction, *Am J Obstet Gynecol* 188:628-633, 2003.
149. Truwit CL, Barkovich AJ, Koch TK, Ferriero DM: Cerebral palsy: MR findings in 40 patients, *AJNR Am J Neuroradiol* 13:67-78, 1992.
150. Volpe JJ: Value of MR in definition of the neuropathology of cerebral palsy in vivo, *AJNR Am J Neuroradiol* 13:79-83, 1992.
151. Hope PL, Moorcraft J: Cerebral palsy in infants born during trial of intrapartum monitoring [letter], *Lancet* 335:238, 1990.
152. Hobel CJ: Intrapartum clinical assessment of fetal distress, *Am J Obstet Gynecol* 110:336-342, 1971.
153. Spellacy WN, Buhi WC, Birk SA, Holsinger KK: Human placental lactogen levels and intrapartum fetal distress: Meconium-stained amniotic fluid, fetal heart rate patterns, and Apgar scores, *Am J Obstet Gynecol* 114:803-808, 1972.
154. Low JA, Pancham SR, Piercy WN, Worthington D, et al: Intrapartum fetal asphyxia: Clinical characteristics, diagnosis, and significance in relation to pattern of development, *Am J Obstet Gynecol* 129:857-872, 1977.
155. Saldana LR, Schulman H, Yang WH: Electronic fetal monitoring during labor, *Obstet Gynecol* 47:706-710, 1976.
156. Fujikura T, Klionsky B: The significance of meconium staining, *Am J Obstet Gynecol* 212:45-50, 1975.
157. Gregory GA, Gooding CA, Phibbs RH, Tooley WH: Meconium aspiration in infants: A prospective study, *J Pediatr* 85:848-852, 1974.
158. Wood C, Pinkerton J: Foetal distress, *Br J Obstet Gynaecol* 68:427-437, 1961.
159. Miller FC, Sacks DA, Yeh SY, Paul RH, et al: Significance of meconium during labor, *Am J Obstet Gynecol* 122:573-580, 1975.
160. Abramovich H, Brandes JJ, Fuchs K, Timor-Tritsch I: Meconium during delivery: A sign of compensated fetal distress, *Am J Obstet Gynecol* 118:251-260, 1974.

161. Meis PJ, Hall MD, Marshall JR, Hobel CJ: Meconium passage: A new classification for risk assessment during labor, *Am J Obstet Gynecol* 131:509-513, 1978.

162. Krebs HB, Petres RE, Dunn LJ, Jordaan HV, et al: Intrapartum fetal heart rate monitoring. III. Association of meconium with abnormal fetal heart rate patterns, *Am J Obstet Gynecol* 137:936-943, 1980.

163. Meis PJ, Hobel CJ, Ureda JR: Late meconium passage in labor: A sign of fetal distress, *Obstet Gynecol* 59:332-335, 1982.

164. Schifrin BS: The diagnosis and treatment of fetal distress. In Hill A, Volpe JJ, editors: *Fetal Neurology*, New York: 1989, Raven Press.

165. Nathan L, Leveno KJ, Carmody TJ, Kelly MA, et al: Meconium: A 1990s perspective on an old obstetric hazard, *Obstet Gynecol* 83:329-332, 1994.

166. Spinillo A, Capuzzo E, Orcesi S, Stronati M, et al: Antenatal and delivery risk factors simultaneously associated with neonatal death and cerebral palsy in preterm infants, *Early Hum Dev* 48:81-91, 1997.

167. Glantz JC, Woods JR: Significance of amniotic fluid meconium. In Creasy RK, Resnik R, editors: *Maternal-Fetal Medicine*, 4th ed, Philadelphia: 1999, WB Saunders.

168. Low JA, Victory R, Derrick EJ: Predictive value of electronic fetal monitoring for intrapartum fetal asphyxia with metabolic acidosis, *Obstet Gynecol* 93:285-291, 1999.

169. Glantz JC, Woods JR: Significance of amniotic fluid meconium. In Creasy RK, Resnik R, Iams JD, editors: *Maternal-Fetal Medicine: Principles and Practice*, 5th ed, Philadelphia: 2004, WB Saunders.

170. Miller PW, Coen RW, Benirschke K: Dating the time interval from meconium passage to birth, *Obstet Gynecol* 66:459-462, 1985.

171. Haverkamp AD, Orleans M, Langendoerfer S, McFee J, et al: A controlled trial of the differential effects of intrapartum fetal monitoring, *Am J Obstet Gynecol* 134:399-412, 1979.

172. Hon EH, Zannini D, Quilligan EJ: The neonatal value of fetal monitoring, *Am J Obstet Gynecol* 122:508-519, 1975.

173. Hobbins JC, Freeman R, Queenan JT: The fetal monitoring debate, *Pediatrics* 63:942-951, 1979.

174. Hobbins JC, Freeman R, Queenan JT: Reply [letter], *Pediatrics* 65:367, 1980.

175. Zuspan FP, Quilligan EJ, Iams JD, van Geijn HP: NICHD Consensus Development Task Force report: Predictors of intrapartum fetal distress—the role of electronic fetal monitoring, *J Pediatr* 95:1026-1030, 1979.

176. Krebs HB, Petres RE, Dunn LJ, Jordaan HV, et al: Intrapartum fetal heart rate monitoring. I. Classification and prognosis of fetal heart rate patterns, *Am J Obstet Gynecol* 133:762-772, 1979.

177. Mueller-Heubach E, MacDonald HM, Joret D, Portman MA, et al: Effects of electronic fetal heart rate monitoring on perinatal outcome and obstetric practices, *Am J Obstet Gynecol* 137:758-763, 1980.

178. Paul RH, Gauthier RJ, Quilligan EJ: Clinical fetal monitoring: The usage and relationship to trends in cesarean delivery and perinatal mortality, *Acta Obstet Gynecol Scand* 59:289-295, 1980.

179. Ingemarsson E, Ingemarsson I, Svenningsen NW: Impact of routine fetal monitoring during labor on fetal outcome with long-term follow-up, *Am J Obstet Gynecol* 141:29-38, 1981.

180. Gimovsky ML, Caritis SN: Diagnosis and management of hypoxic fetal heart rate patterns, *Clin Perinatol* 9:313-324, 1982.

181. Schifrin BS: The fetal monitoring polemic, *Clin Perinatol* 9:399-408, 1982.

182. Yeh SY, Diaz F, Paul RH: Ten-year experience of intrapartum fetal monitoring in Los Angeles County/University of Southern California Medical Center, *Am J Obstet Gynecol* 143:496-500, 1982.

183. Douvas SG, Meeks GR, Graves G, Walsh DA, et al: Intrapartum fetal heart rate monitoring as a predictor of fetal distress and immediate neonatal condition in low-birth weight (less than or equal to 1,800 grams) infants, *Am J Obstet Gynecol* 148:300-302, 1984.

184. Vintzileos AM, Nochimson DJ, Knuppel RA, Schifrin BS: Intrapartum electronic fetal heart rate monitoring versus intermittent auscultation: A meta-analysis, *Obstet Gynecol* 85:149-155, 1995.

185. Thacker SB, Stroup DF, Peterson HB: Efficacy and safety of intrapartum electronic fetal monitoring: An update, *Obstet Gynecol* 86:613-620, 1995.

186. Nelson KB, Dambrosia JM, Ting TY, Grether JK: Uncertain value of electronic fetal monitoring in predicting cerebral palsy, *N Engl J Med* 334:613-618, 1996.

187. MacDonald D: Cerebral palsy and intrapartum fetal monitoring, *N Engl J Med* 334:659-660, 1996.

188. Parer JT, Nageotte MP: Intrapartum fetal surveillance. In Creasy RK, Resnik R, Iams JD, editors: *Maternal-Fetal Medicine: Principles and Practice*, 5th ed, Philadelphia: 2004, WB Saunders.

189. Thacker SB: The efficacy of intrapartum electronic fetal monitoring, *Am J Obstet Gynecol* 156:24-30, 1987.

190. Jenkins HM: Thirty years of electronic intrapartum fetal heart rate monitoring: Discussion paper, *J R Soc Med* 82:210-214, 1989.

191. Steer PJ, Eigbe F, Lissauer TJ, Beard RW: Interrelationships among abnormal cardiotocograms in labor, meconium staining of the amniotic fluid, arterial cord blood pH, and Apgar scores, *Obstet Gynecol* 74:715-721, 1989.

192. Colditz PB, Henderson-Smart DJ: Electronic fetal heart rate monitoring during labour: Does it prevent perinatal asphyxia and cerebral palsy? *Med J Aust* 153:88-90, 1990.

193. Shy KK, Luthy DA, Bennett FC, Whitfield M, et al: Effects of electronic fetal-heart-rate monitoring, as compared with periodic auscultation, on the neurologic development of premature infants, *N Engl J Med* 322:588-593, 1990.

194. Freeman R: Intrapartum fetal monitoring: A disappointing story, *N Engl J Med* 322:624-626, 1990.

195. Anthony MY, Levene MI: An assessment of the benefits of intrapartum fetal monitoring, *Dev Med Child Neurol* 32:547-553, 1990.

196. Ellison PH, Foster M, Sheridan-Pereira M, MacDonald D: Electronic fetal heart monitoring, auscultation, and neonatal outcome, *Am J Obstet Gynecol* 164:1281-1289, 1991.

197. Morrison JC, Chez BF, Davis ID, Martin RW, et al: Intrapartum fetal heart rate assessment: Monitoring by auscultation or electronic means, *Am J Obstet Gynecol* 168:63-66, 1993.

198. Vintzileos AM, Antsaklis A, Varvarigos I, Papas C, et al: A randomized trial of intrapartum electronic fetal heart rate monitoring versus intermittent auscultation, *Obstet Gynecol* 81:899-907, 1993.

199. Albers LL, Krulewitch CJ: Electronic fetal monitoring in the United States in the 1980s, *Obstet Gynecol* 82:8-10, 1993.

200. Williams KP, Galerneau F: Intrapartum fetal heart rate patterns in the prediction of neonatal acidemia, *Am J Obstet Gynecol* 188:820-823, 2003.

201. Althaus JE, Petersen SM, Fox HE, Holcroft CJ, et al: Can electronic fetal monitoring identify preterm neonates with cerebral white matter injury? *Obstet Gynecol* 105:458-465, 2005.

201a. Schifrin BS, Ater S: Fetal hypoxic and ischemic injuries, *Curr Opin Obstet Gynecol* 18:112-122, 2006.

202. Petrie RH: Intrapartum fetal status, *Perinat Care* 2:32-39, 1978.

203. Cibils LA: Clinical significance of fetal heart rate patterns during labor. IV. Agonal patterns, *Am J Obstet Gynecol* 129:833-844, 1977.

204. Paul RH, Suidan AK, Yeh S, Schifrin BS, et al: Clinical fetal monitoring. VII. The evaluation and significance of intrapartum baseline FHR variability, *Am J Obstet Gynecol* 123:206-210, 1975.

205. Boehm FJ: FHR variability: Key to fetal well-being, *Contemp Obstet Gynecol* 9:57-61, 1977.

206. Gellhorn E: *Anatomic Imbalance and the Hypothalamus*, Minneapolis: 1957, University of Minnesota Press.

207. Vallbona C, Cardus D, Spencer WA, Hoff HE: Patterns of sinus arrhythmia in patients with lesions of the central nervous system, *Am J Cardiol* 16:379-389, 1965.

208. Parer JT, Livingston EG: What is fetal distress? *Am J Obstet Gynecol* 162:1421-1425, 1990.

209. Martin C Jr: Physiology and clinical use of fetal heart rate variability, *Clin Perinatol* 9:339-352, 1982.

210. Dalton KJ, Dawes GS, Patrick JE: The autonomic nervous system and fetal heart rate variability, *Am J Obstet Gynecol* 146:456-462, 1983.

211. Yu Z-Y, Lumbers ER: Measurement of baroreceptor-mediated effects on heart rate variability in fetal sheep, *Pediatr Res* 47:233-239, 2000.

212. Adams RD, Prod'hom LS, Rabinowicz T: Intrauterine brain death: Neuraxial reticular core necrosis, *Acta Neuropathol (Berl)* 40:41-49, 1977.

213. van der Moer PE, Gerretsen G, Visser GH: Fixed fetal heart rate pattern after intrauterine accidental decerebration, *Obstet Gynecol* 65:125-127, 1985.

214. Nijhuis JG, Kruyt N, van Wijck JA: Fetal brain death: Two case reports, *Br J Obstet Gynaecol* 95:197-200, 1988.

215. Powell OH, Melville A, MacKenna J: Fetal heart rate acceleration in labor: Excellent prognostic indicator, *Am J Obstet Gynecol* 134:36-38, 1979.

216. Krebs HB, Petres RE, Dunn LJ, Smith PJ: Intrapartum fetal heart rate monitoring. VI. Prognostic significance of accelerations, *Am J Obstet Gynecol* 142:297-305, 1982.

217. James LS, Yeh MN, Morishima HO, Daniel SS, et al: Umbilical vein occlusion and transient acceleration of the fetal heart rate: Experimental observations in subhuman primates, *Am J Obstet Gynecol* 126:276-283, 1976.

218. In Hon EH, editor: *An Atlas of Fetal Heart Rate Patterns*, New Haven, CT: Harty Press, 1968.

219. Hutson JM, Mueller-Heubach E: Diagnosis and management of intrapartum reflex fetal heart rate changes, *Clin Perinatol* 9:325-337, 1982.

220. Austt EG, Ruggia R, Caldeyro-Barcia R: Effects of intrapartum uterine contractions on the EEG of the human fetus. In Angle CR, Bering EA Jr, editors: *Physical Trauma as an Etiologic Agent in Mental Retardation*, Washington, DC: 1970, U.S. Government Printing Office.

221. Aramburu G, Althabe O, Caldeyro-Barcia R: Obstetrical factors influencing intrapartum compression of the fetal head and the incidence of dips I in fetal heart rate. In Angle CR, Bering EA Jr, editors: *Physical Trauma as an Etiologic Agent in Mental Retardation*, Washington, DC: 1970, U.S. Government Printing Office.

222. Schwarcz RL, Strada-Saenz G, Althabe O: Compression received by the head of the fetus during labor. In Angle CR, Bering EA Jr, editors: *Physical Trauma as an Etiologic Agent in Mental Retardation*, Washington, DC: 1970, U.S. Government Printing Office.

223. Hon EH: Detection of asphyxia in utero: Fetal heart rate. In Gluck L, editor: *Intrauterine Asphyxia and the Developing Fetal Brain*, Chicago: 1977, Year Book.

224. Hon EH: Observation on pathologic fetal bradycardia, *Am J Obstet Gynecol* 77:1084, 1959.

225. Althabe O Jr, Schwarcz RL, Pose SV, Escarcena L, et al: Effects on fetal heart rate and fetal pO$_2$ of oxygen administration to the mother, *Am J Obstet Gynecol* 98:858-870, 1967.

226. James LS, Morishima HO, Daniel SS, Bowe ET, et al: Mechanism of late deceleration of the fetal heart rate, *Am J Obstet Gynecol* 113:578-582, 1972.

227. Cibils LA: Clinical significance of fetal heart rate patterns during labor. V. Variable decelerations, *Am J Obstet Gynecol* 132:791-805, 1978.

228. Mueller-Heubach E, Myers RE, Adamsons K: Fetal heart rate and blood pressure during prolonged partial asphyxia in the rhesus monkey, *Am J Obstet Gynecol* 137:48-52, 1980.

229. Parer JT, Krueger TR, Harris JL: Fetal oxygen consumption and mechanisms of heart rate response during artificially produced late decelerations of fetal heart rate in sheep, *Am J Obstet Gynecol* 136:478-482, 1980.

230. Harris JL, Krueger TR, Parer JT: Mechanisms of late decelerations of the fetal heart rate during hypoxia, *Am J Obstet Gynecol* 144:491-496, 1982.

231. Aarnoudse JG, Huisjes HJ, Gordon H, Oeseburg B, et al: Fetal subcutaneous scalp Po$_2$ and abnormal heart rate during labor, *Am J Obstet Gynecol* 153:565-566, 1985.

232. Greiss FC: A clinical concept of uterine blood flow during pregnancy, *Obstet Gynecol* 40:595-603, 1967.

233. LaGamma EF, Itskovitz J, Rudolph AM: Effects of naloxone on fetal circulatory responses to hypoxemia, *Am J Obstet Gynecol* 143:933-940, 1982.

234. Cohn HE, Piasecki GJ, Jackson BT: The effect of fetal heart rate on cardiovascular function during hypoxemia, *Am J Obstet Gynecol* 138:1190-1199, 1980.

235. Ikeda T, Murata Y, Quilligan EJ, Parer JT, et al: Fetal heart rate patterns in postasphyxiated fetal lambs with brain damage, *Obstet Gynecol* 179:1329-1337, 1998.

236. Adamsons K, Myers RE: Late decelerations and brain tolerance of the fetal monkey to intrapartum asphyxia, *Am J Obstet Gynecol* 128:893-900, 1977.

237. Low JA, Galbraith RS, Muir DW, Killen HL, et al: Factors associated with motor and cognitive deficits in children after intrapartum fetal hypoxia, *Am J Obstet Gynecol* 148:533-539, 1984.

238. Low JA: Fetal acid-base status and outcome. In Hill A, Volpe JJ, editors: *Fetal Neurology*, New York: 1989, Raven Press.

239. Pasternak JF, Gorey MT: The syndrome of acute near-total intrauterine asphyxia in the term infant, *Pediatr Neurol* 18:391-398, 1998.

240. Korst LM, Phelan JP, Wang YM, Martin GI, et al: Acute fetal asphyxia and permanent brain injury: A retrospective analysis of current indicators, *J Matern Fetal Med* 8:101-106, 1999.

241. Krebs HB, Petres RE, Dunn LJ: Intrapartum fetal heart rate monitoring. VIII. Atypical variable decelerations, *Am J Obstet Gynecol* 145:297-305, 1983.

242. Goodlin RC, Haesslein HC: Fetal reacting bradycardia, *Am J Obstet Gynecol* 129:845-856, 1977.

243. Finster M, Petrie RH: Monitoring of the fetus, *Anesthesiology* 45:198-215, 1976.

244. Painter MJ, Depp R, O'Donoghue PD: Fetal heart rate patterns and development in the first year of life, *Am J Obstet Gynecol* 132:271-277, 1978.

245. Keegan KA Jr, Waffarn F, Quilligan EJ: Obstetric characteristics and fetal heart rate patterns of infants who convulse during the newborn period, *Am J Obstet Gynecol* 153:732-737, 1985.

246. Painter MJ, Scott M, Hirsch RP, O'Donoghue P, et al: Fetal heart rate patterns during labor: Neurologic and cognitive development at six to nine years of age, *Am J Obstet Gynecol* 159:854-858, 1988.

247. Painter MJ: Fetal heart rate patterns, perinatal asphyxia, and brain injury, *Pediatr Neurol* 5:134-144, 1989.

248. Low JA, Killen H, Derrick EJ: The prediction and prevention of intrapartum fetal asphyxia in preterm pregnancies, *Am J Obstet Gynecol* 186:279-282, 2002.

249. Feldman RC, Tabsh KM, Shields WD: Correlation of ominous fetal heart rate patterns and brain-specific creatine kinase, *Obstet Gynecol* 65:476-480, 1985.

250. Westgate J, Harris MC, Gurnow JSH, Greene KR: Plymouth randomized trial of cardiotocogram only versus ST waveforms plus cardiotocogram for intrapartum monitoring in 2400 cases, *Am J Obstet Gynecol* 169:1151-1160, 1993.

251. Rosen KG: Fetal electrocardiogram waveform analysis in labour, *Curr Opin Obstet Gynecol* 13:137-140, 2001.

252. Amer-Wahlin I, Hellsten C, Noren H, Hagberg H, et al: Cardiotocography only versus cardiotocography plus ST analysis of fetal electrocardiogram for intrapartum fetal monitoring: A Swedish randomised controlled trial, *Lancet* 358:534-538, 2001.

253. Noren H, Amer-Wahlin I, Hagberg H, Herbst A, et al: Fetal electrocardiography in labor and neonatal outcome: Data from the Swedish randomized controlled trial on intrapartum fetal monitoring, *Am J Obstet Gynecol* 188:183-192, 2003.

254. Oudijk MA, Kwee A, Visser GHA, Blad S, et al: The effects of intrapartum hypoxia on the fetal QT interval, *Br J Obstet Gynaecol* 111:656-660, 2004.

255. Gilstrap LC: Fetal acid-base balance. In Creasy RK, Resnik R, Iams JD, editors: *Maternal-Fetal Medicine: Principles and Practice*, 5th ed, Philadelphia: 2004, WB Saunders.

256. Gilstrap LC: Fetal acid-base balance. In Creasy RK, Resnik R, editors: *Maternal-Fetal Medicine:*, 4th ed, Philadelphia: 1999, WB Saunders.

257. Helwig JT, Parer JT, Kilpatrick SJ, Laros RK: Umbilical cord blood acid-base state: What is normal?, *Am J Obstet Gynecol* 174:1807-1814, 1996.

258. Gilstrap LD, Leveno KJ, Burris J, Williams ML, et al: Diagnosis of birth asphyxia on the basis of fetal pH, Apgar score, and newborn cerebral dysfunction, *Am J Obstet Gynecol* 161:825-830, 1989.

259. Dijxhoorn MJ, Visser GH, Huisjes HJ, Fidler V, et al: The relation between umbilical pH values and neonatal neurological morbidity in full term appropriate-for-dates infants, *Early Hum Dev* 11:33-42, 1985.

260. Ruth VJ, Raivio KO: Perinatal brain damage: Predictive value of metabolic acidosis and the Apgar score, *BMJ* 297:24-27, 1988.

261. Low JA: The role of blood gas and acid-base assessment in the diagnosis of intrapartum fetal asphyxia, *Am J Obstet Gynecol* 159:1235-1240, 1988.

262. Low JA, Galbraith RS, Muir DW, Killen HL, et al: Motor and cognitive deficits after intrapartum asphyxia in the mature fetus, *Am J Obstet Gynecol* 158:356-361, 1988.

263. Fee SC, Malee K, Deddish R, Minogue JP, et al: Severe acidosis and subsequent neurologic status, *Am J Obstet Gynecol* 162:802-806, 1990.

264. Low JA, Muir DW, Pater EA, Karchmar EJ: The association of intrapartum asphyxia in the mature fetus with newborn behavior, *Am J Obstet Gynecol* 163:1131-1135, 1990.

265. Hibbard JU, Hibbard MC, Whalen MP: Umbilical cord blood gases and mortality and morbidity in the very low birth weight infant, *Obstet Gynecol* 78:768-773, 1991.

266. Tejani N, Verma UL: Correlation of Apgar scores and umbilical artery acid-base status to mortality and morbidity in the low birth weight neonate, *Obstet Gynecol* 73:597-600, 1989.

267. Goodwin TM, Belai I, Hernandez P, Durand M, et al: Asphyxial complications in the term newborn with severe umbilical acidemia, *Am J Obstet Gynecol* 167:1506-1512, 1992.

268. Gaudier FL, Goldenberg RL, Nelson KG, Peraltacarcelen M, et al: Acid-base status at birth and subsequent neurosensory impairment in surviving 500 to 1000 gm infants, *Am J Obstet Gynecol* 170:48-53, 1994.

269. Low JA, Panagiotopoulos C, Derrick EJ: Newborn complications after intrapartum asphyxia with metabolic acidosis in the preterm fetus, *Am J Obstet Gynecol* 172:805-810, 1995.

270. van den Berg PP, Nelen WL, Jongsma HW, Nijland R, et al: Neonatal complications in newborns with an umbilical artery pH <7.00, *Am J Obstet Gynecol* 175:1152-1157, 1996.

271. Belai YI, Goodwin TM, Durand M, Greenspoon JS, et al: Umbilical arteriovenous Po$_2$ and Pco$_2$ differences and neonatal morbidity in term infants with severe acidosis, *Am J Obstet Gynecol* 178:13-19, 1998.

272. Low JA, Lindsay BG, Derrick EJ: Threshold of metabolic acidosis associated with newborn complications, *Am J Obstet Gynecol* 177:1391-1394, 1997.

273. Sehdev HM, Stamilio DM, Macones GA, Graham E, et al: Predictive factors for neonatal morbidity in neonates with an umbilical arterial cord pH less than 7.00, *Am J Obstet Gynecol* 177:1030-1034, 1997.

274. Shankaran S: Identification of term infants at risk for neonatal morbidity, *J Pediatr* 132:571-572, 1998.

275. Carter BS, McNabb F, Merenstein GB: Prospective validation of a scoring system for predicting neonatal morbidity after acute perinatal asphyxia, *J Pediatr* 132:619-623, 1998.

276. King TA, Jackson GL, Josepy AS, Vedro DA, et al: The effect of profound umbilical artery acidemia in term neonates admitted to a newborn nursery, *J Pediatr* 132:624-629, 1998.

277. da Silva S, Hennebert N, Denis R, Wayenberg JL: Clinical value of a single postnatal lactate measurement after intrapartum asphyxia, *Acta Paediatr* 89:320-323, 2000.

278. Toh VC: Early predictors of adverse outcome in term infants with post-asphyxial hypoxic ischaemic encephalopathy, *Acta Paediatr* 89:343-347, 2000.

279. Williams KP, Singh A: The correlation of seizures in newborn infants with significant acidosis at birth with umbilical artery cord gas values, *Obstet Gynecol* 100:557-560, 2002.

280. Ross MG, Gala R: Use of umbilical artery base excess: Algorithm for the timing of hypoxic injury, *Am J Obstet Gynecol* 187:1-9, 2002.

281. Low JA, Galbraith RS, Sauerbrei EE, Muir DW, et al: Motor and cognitive development of infants with intraventricular hemorrhage, ventriculomegaly, or periventricular parenchymal lesions, *Am J Obstet Gynecol* 155:750-756, 1986.

282. Hon EH, Khazin AF: Observations on fetal heart rate and fetal biochemistry. I. Base deficit, *Obstet Gynecol* 105:721, 1969.

283. Kubli FW, Hon EH, Khazin AF, Takemura H: Observations on heart rate and pH in the human fetus during labor, *Am J Obstet Gynecol* 104:1190-1206, 1969.

284. Khazin AF, Hon EH, Yeh S: Observations on fetal heart rate and fetal biochemistry. III. Base deficit of umbilical cord blood, *J Pediatr* 79:406-412, 1971.

285. Low JA, Cox MJ, Karchmar EJ, McGrath MJ, et al: The prediction of intrapartum fetal metabolic acidosis by fetal heart rate monitoring, *Am J Obstet Gynecol* 139:299-305, 1981.

286. Miller FC: Prediction of acid-base values from intrapartum fetal heart rate data and their correlation with scalp and funic values, *Clin Perinatol* 9:353-361, 1982.

287. Westgren M, Hormquist P, Ingemarsson I, Svenningsen N: Intrapartum fetal acidosis in preterm infants: Fetal monitoring and long-term morbidity, *Obstet Gynecol* 63:355-359, 1984.

288. Brann AW Jr, Myers RE: Central nervous system findings in the newborn monkey following severe in utero partial asphyxia, *Neurology* 25:327-338, 1975.

289. Dildy GA, Thorp JA, Yeast JD, Clark SL: The relationship between oxygen saturation and pH in umbilical blood: Implications for intrapartum fetal oxygen saturation monitoring, *Am J Obstet Gynecol* 175:682-687, 1996.

290. Kuhnert M, Seelbach-Goebel B, Butterwegge M: Predictive agreement between the fetal arterial oxygen saturation and fetal scalp pH: Results of the German multicenter study, *Am J Obstet Gynecol* 178:330-335, 1998.

291. Seelbach-Gobel B, Heupel M, Kuhnert M, Butterwegge M: The prediction of fetal acidosis by means of intrapartum fetal pulse oximetry, *Am J Obstet Gynecol* 180:73-81, 1999.

292. Garite TJ, Dildy GA, McNamara H, Nageotte MP, et al: A multicenter controlled trial of fetal pulse oximetry in the intrapartum management of nonreassuring fetal heart rate patterns, *Am J Obstet Gynecol* 183:1049-1058, 2000.

293. Kuhnert M, Schmidt S: Intrapartum management of nonreassuring fetal heart rate patterns: A randomized controlled trial of fetal pulse oximetry, *Am J Obstet Gynecol* 191:1989-1995, 2004.

294. Bloom SL, Spong CY, Thom E, Varner MW, et al: Fetal pulse oximetry and cesarean delivery, *N Engl J Med* 355:2195-2202, 2006.

295. Rosen MG, Scibetta JJ, Hochberg CJ: Human fetal electroencephalogram. III. Pattern changes in presence of fetal heart rate alterations and after use of maternal medications, *Obstet Gynecol* 36:132-140, 1970.

296. Rosen MG, Scibetta JJ, Hochberg CJ: Fetal electroencephalography. IV. The FEEG during spontaneous and forceps births, *Obstet Gynecol* 42:283-289, 1973.

297. Rosen MG, Scibetta J, Chik L, Borgstedt AD: An approach to the study of brain damage: The principles of fetal electroencephalography, *Am J Obstet Gynecol* 115:37-47, 1973.

298. Borgstedt AD, Rosen MG, Chik L, Sokol RJ, et al: Fetal electroencephalography: Relationship to neonatal and one-year developmental neurological examinations in high-risk infants, *Am J Dis Child* 129:35-38, 1975.

299. Chik L, Sokol RJ, Rosen MG, Borgstedt AD: Computer interpreted fetal electroencephalogram. I. Relative frequency of patterns, *Am J Obstet Gynecol* 125:537-540, 1976.

300. Chik L, Sokol RJ, Rosen MG, Borgstedt AD: Computer interpreted fetal electroencephalogram. II. Patterns in infants who were neurologically abnormal at 1 year of age, *Am J Obstet Gynecol* 125:541-544, 1976.

301. Chik L, Sokol RJ, Rosen MG: Computer interpreted fetal electroencephalogram: Sharp wave detection and classification of infants for one year neurological outcome, *Electroencephalogr Clin Neurophysiol* 42:745-753, 1977.

302. Chik L, Sokol RJ, Rosen MG, Regula GA, et al: Computer interpreted fetal monitoring data: Discriminant analysis or perinatal data as a model for prediction of neurologic status at one year of age, *J Pediatr* 90:985-989, 1977.

303. Sokol RJ, Rosen MG, Chik L: Fetal electroencephalographic monitoring related to infant outcome, *Am J Obstet Gynecol* 127:329-330, 1977.

304. Maynard DE, Cohen RJ, Viniker DA: Intrapartum fetal monitoring with the cerebral function monitor, *Br J Obstet Gynaecol* 86:941-947, 1979.

305. Weller C, Dyson RJ, McFadyen IR: Fetal electroencephalography using a new, flexible electrode, *Am J Obstet Gynecol* 88:983-986, 1981.

306. Thaler I, Boldes R, Timor-Tritsch I: Real-time spectral analysis of the fetal EEG: A new approach to monitoring sleep states and fetal condition during labor, *Pediatr Res* 48:340-345, 2000.

307. Feinkind L, Abulafia O, Delke I, Feldman J, et al: Screening with Doppler velocimetry in labor, *Am J Obstet Gynecol* 161:765-770, 1989.

308. Sarno AP Jr, Ahn MO, Brar HS, Phelan JP, et al: Intrapartum Doppler velocimetry, amniotic fluid volume, and fetal heart rate as predictors of subsequent fetal distress. I. An initial report, *Am J Obstet Gynecol* 161:1508-1514, 1989.

309. Mansouri H, Gagnon R, Hunse C: Relationship between fetal heart rate and umbilical blood flow velocity in term human fetuses during labor, *Am J Obstet Gynecol* 160:1007-1012, 1989.

310. Janbu T, Nesheim BI: Uterine artery blood velocities during contractions in pregnancy and labour related to intrauterine pressure, *Br J Obstet Gynaecol* 94:1150-1155, 1987.

311. Ogunyemi D, Stanley R, Lynch C, Edwards D, et al: Umbilical artery velocimetry in predicting perinatal outcome with intrapartum fetal distress, *Obstet Gynecol* 80:377-380, 1992.

312. Mirro R, Gonzalez A: Perinatal anterior cerebral artery Doppler flow indexes: Methods and preliminary results, *Am J Obstet Gynecol* 156:1227-1231, 1987.

313. Yagel S, Anteby E, Lavy Y, Ben Chetrit A, et al: Fetal middle cerebral artery blood flow during normal active labour and in labour with variable decelerations, *Br J Obstet Gynaecol* 99:483-485, 1992.

314. Peebles DM, Edwards AD, Wyatt JS, Bishop AP, et al: Changes in human fetal cerebral hemoglobin concentration and oxygenation during labor measured by near-infrared spectroscopy, *Am J Obstet Gynecol* 166:1369-1373, 1992.

315. Peebles DM, Spencer JA, Edwards AD, Wyatt JS, et al: Relation between frequency of uterine contractions and human fetal cerebral oxygen saturation studied during labour by near infrared spectroscopy, *Br J Obstet Gynaecol* 101:44-48, 1994.

316. Aldrich CJ, Wyatt JS, Spencer JAD, Reynolds EOR, et al: The effect of maternal oxygen administration on human fetal cerebral oxygenation measured during labour by near infrared spectroscopy, *Br J Obstet Gynaecol* 101:509-513, 1994.

317. Aldrich CJ, D'Antona D, Spencer JAD, Wyatt JS, et al: The effect of maternal posture on fetal cerebral oxygenation during labour, *Br J Obstet Gynaecol* 102:14-19, 1995.

318. Aldrich CJ, Dantona D, Spencer J, Wyatt JS, et al: Late fetal heart decelerations and changes in cerebral oxygenation during the first stage of labour, *Br J Obstet Gynaecol* 102:9-13, 1995.

Chapter 8

Hypoxic-Ischemic Encephalopathy: Neuropathology and Pathogenesis

Hypoxic-ischemic brain injury is a very important neurological problem of the perinatal period. This importance relates to the general gravity of the lesions and to the relatively large number of affected infants. In the premature infant, this encephalopathy is often accompanied by intraventricular hemorrhage and its concomitants, which contribute to the neurological morbidity (see Chapter 11). Thus, it is apparent that a basic understanding of hypoxic-ischemic brain injury provides insight into a major portion of neonatal neurology. The subsequent neurological deficits of concern are, principally, a variety of motor deficits, especially spasticity, but also choreoathetosis, dystonia, and ataxia, often grouped together as "cerebral palsy," with or without accompanying cognitive deficits and seizures.

In this chapter, I review the neuropathology and pathogenesis of neonatal hypoxic-ischemic encephalopathy. The major lesions are discussed separately, although commonly there is overlap in the occurrence of each lesion. In Chapter 9, I review the clinical features of neonatal hypoxic-ischemic encephalopathy and use the same framework of neuropathological lesions discussed in this chapter.

NEUROPATHOLOGY

The neuropathological features of neonatal hypoxic-ischemic encephalopathy vary considerably with the gestational age of the infant, the nature of the insult, the types of interventions, and other factors, most still to be defined. Nevertheless, certain basic lesions can be recognized, and recognition of these lesions provides a useful framework for discussion of clinical aspects. The major neuropathological varieties are shown in Table 8-1 and are discussed subsequently. Readers of previous editions of this book should note that I have deleted status marmoratus from this list; the reasons for this change are apparent in the later section "Selective Neuronal Necrosis." Initially, the relationship between brain swelling and brain necrosis is reviewed.

Brain Swelling and Brain Necrosis

Brain swelling is discussed separately from the recognized neuropathological disorders associated with perinatal hypoxic-ischemic insults because some workers have suggested that brain swelling is a separate and dominant lesion that may lead to additional brain injury. This view is derived principally from experience with adult patients and from experimental data (see later discussion). Indeed, it is well known in standard neuropathological writings concerning adult patients that severe hypoxic-ischemic insults are associated with a major degree of brain swelling and increased intracranial pressure, and the latter may accentuate neurological morbidity. Extrapolation of such data to the neonatal brain cannot be made a priori, as I illustrate. Earlier work with neonatal kittens and rats indicated a relative resistance of immature brain to the development of prominent edema produced by hypoxic-ischemic or cold-induced injury; similar insults regularly produce pronounced brain edema in adult animals.[1,2] Therefore, it is reasonable to ask whether brain swelling with hypoxic-ischemic injury is a consistent feature in the human newborn with perinatal asphyxia.

Pathological Aspects in Human Infants

Pathological studies of neonatal hypoxic-ischemic encephalopathy do not provide decisive support for the occurrence of brain swelling as a separate and dominant lesion, without comparable degrees of tissue necrosis.[3-8] Several older reports do emphasize brain swelling in asphyxiated newborn infants.[9-12] However, often the definition of swelling is not precise, the degree of associated brain injury is not clearly quantitated, the duration of time spent on ventilatory and circulatory support before death is not defined, and the type of postinsult management is not described. These factors have major bearing on the questions whether edema, in fact, was present and, if so, whether it was simply the *consequence* of brain necrosis or was a predominant lesion per se. Moreover, because fetal and neonatal human brain contains more water than myelinated, mature brain, and because the immature brain swells considerably during fixation, Gilles and associates[13] suggested that "much of what has been called edema in the fixed brain may well reflect the initial high water content of this tissue plus the water accumulated during fixation." The absence of external signs of swelling and of necrosis caused by transtentorial (hippocampal) or transmagnal (cerebellar) herniation in the huge autopsy population of the National Collaborative Perinatal Project has been emphasized.[13]

Several clinical studies also indicated that primary brain swelling (i.e., in the absence of marked brain

TABLE 8-1	Major Neuropathological Varieties of Neonatal Hypoxic-Ischemic Encephalopathy
Selective neuronal necrosis	
Parasagittal cerebral injury	
Periventricular leukomalacia	
Focal (and multifocal) ischemic brain necrosis, stroke	

necrosis) is not a prominent feature of hypoxic-ischemic encephalopathy in the human newborn.[14-18] In one study, clearly increased intracranial pressure (i.e., >10 mm Hg) was observed in only 22% of 32 asphyxiated term newborns, it did not compromise cerebral perfusion pressure, it reached a maximum at 36 to 72 hours, and it correlated with computed tomography evidence for early brain necrosis.[17] In a second systematic study, intracranial pressure reached a maximum at a mean age of 29 hours and was not correlated with clinical or electroencephalographic evidence for neurological deterioration.[16] Changes in cerebral perfusion pressure most often reflected decreases in arterial blood pressure rather than increases in intracranial pressure.[16] Moreover, administration of mannitol in a single dose to asphyxiated infants in a controlled study had no beneficial clinical effect.[18] These observations support the conclusion that early brain edema is a *consequence of, rather than a causative factor in*, hypoxic-ischemic brain injury (Table 8-2).[14-18]

Experimental Aspects in Perinatal Animals

Intrauterine Partial Asphyxia in the Fetal Monkey. The notion that brain swelling is an important *early* feature with perinatal hypoxic-ischemic insults and the *cause* of subsequent tissue necrosis is based on studies with term fetal monkeys by Myers and co-workers.[19-25] In these experiments, in association with "prolonged partial asphyxia" of the term fetal monkey (produced by a variety of procedures that impair placental gas exchange, e.g., maternal hypotension, maternal hypoxemia, and umbilical cord compression), a pattern of cerebral injury characterized by necrosis and edema was observed. The topography of the necrosis was typical of the parasagittal cerebral injury observed in the asphyxiated human term infant (see later discussion).

TABLE 8-2	Evidence Against Early Brain Edema as a Causative Factor in Hypoxic-Ischemic Brain Injury*
Intracranial pressure higher than 10 mm Hg is uncommon in asphyxiated term infants.	
When intracranial pressure greater than 10 mm Hg occurs, timing is relatively late (i.e., 24 to 72 hours).	
Marked decreases in cerebral perfusion pressure are uncommon, and decreases in cerebral perfusion pressure that do occur are usually caused by decreases in blood pressure rather than by increases in intracranial pressure.	

*See text for references.

Associated with the cerebral injury in the monkeys was *brain swelling*, defined primarily by gyral flattening. The edema was considered to be intracellular on the basis of electron microscopic observations in related experiments.[25] In similar experiments, statistically significant changes in brain water content could not be demonstrated.[24] On balance, the brain swelling in these experiments appears most likely to be secondary to the pronounced tissue injury (with cytotoxic edema), rather than a primary event leading to the injury. This possibility would be compatible with conclusions derived from human pathological material (see earlier discussion).

Intrauterine Partial Asphyxia in the Fetal Lamb. Studies of the fetal lamb subjected to intrauterine partial asphyxia do not support the notion of brain edema, at least of the vasogenic variety, as an important consequence of acute hypoxic-ischemic brain injury in this model.[26,27] Extravascular plasma volume was quantitated by the iodine-125–labeled albumin method with asphyxia and was found not to be significantly increased in cerebrum, brain stem, or cerebellum.[26] Moreover, the postasphyxial delayed cerebral hypoperfusion observed in this model occurred in the absence of brain edema.[27] In later studies of near-term fetal lambs subjected to hypoxia-ischemia, findings indicative of *cytotoxic* edema correlated with documented neuronal injury were obtained, a correlation consistent with the observations in human infants (see earlier).[28]

Hypoxic-Ischemic Insult in the Neonatal Rat and Piglet. Careful morphological, physiological, and biochemical studies of the neonatal rat and piglet subjected to a combination of ischemia (carotid ligation) and hypoxemia also fail to support the notion of brain edema as a primary or injury-causing result of hypoxic-ischemic insult.[29-38] In the studies of neonatal rats, although the water content of brain increased, a close correlation was defined between the degree of tissue necrosis and the increase in brain water. No sign of transtentorial or cerebellar herniation was observed, *unlike in adult animals similarly studied*. No inverse correlation of cerebral blood flow (CBF) and brain water content could be identified over the 6 days following the hypoxic-ischemic insult. Moreover, administration of four doses of mannitol over 2 days following the insult did not ameliorate the incidence, distribution, or severity of the extensive tissue injury, despite reduction in the increase in brain water content in the hypoxic-ischemic hemisphere.[30] Additionally, the spatial relationships between this increase in brain volume and the tissue injury did not suggest that the apparent edema caused or contributed to the cerebral injury.[33] The conclusion is that the brain "edema" is a "consequence rather than a cause of major ischemic damage in the immature animal."[29-31,33-35,37]

Selective Neuronal Necrosis

Selective neuronal necrosis is the most common variety of injury observed in neonatal hypoxic-ischemic encephalopathy. The term refers to necrosis of neurons in a characteristic, although often widespread, distribution. Neuronal necrosis often coexists with other distinctive manifestations of neonatal hypoxic-ischemic encephalopathy (see later sections), and in fact it is very unusual to observe one of the other varieties of neonatal hypoxic-ischemic encephalopathy without some degree of selective neuronal injury as well. The topography of the neuronal injury depends in considerable part on the severity and temporal characteristics of the insult and on the gestational age of the infant. Three basic patterns derived primarily from correlative clinical and brain imaging findings, and observed best in term infants, can be distinguished (Table 8-3). *Diffuse* neuronal injury occurs with very severe and very prolonged insults in both term and premature infants. A *cerebral cortical–deep nuclear* neuronal predominance occurs in primarily term infants with moderate to severe, relatively prolonged insults. The deep nuclear involvement includes basal ganglia (especially putamen) and thalamus. *Deep nuclear–brain stem* neuronal predominance occurs in primarily term infants with severe, relatively abrupt insults. Two other patterns, *pontosubicular* neuronal injury and *cerebellar* injury, occur particularly in premature infants with a still-to-be-defined temporal pattern of insult (see later discussion), but these patterns are usually accompanied by other features of selective neuronal injury and are discussed in this overall context. Thus, overall five patterns are described. In the discussion that follows, I review the cellular aspects of selective neuronal injury, the regions of predilection, and the current concepts of pathogenesis.

Cellular Aspects

As the name implies, the neuron is the primary site of injury.[4-6,8] Experimental studies indicate that the first observable change in the neuron is cytoplasmic vacuolation, caused by mitochondrial swelling, occurring within 5 to 30 minutes after the onset of hypoxia.[39-42] In contrast to the rapid onset of *neuronal* changes in tissue cultures of neonatal mouse cerebellum exposed to hypoxia, no structural alteration was observed in astrocytes.[42] However, as discussed later, studies of a variety of developing models suggest that differentiating oligodendrocytes exhibit approximately the same sensitivity to glucose and oxygen deprivation as do neurons. On balance, the data suggest that in the immature and mature brain, the order of vulnerability is neuron $\geq$ oligodendroglia > astrocyte > microglia. In the context of the present discussion, the neuron is the cellular element most vulnerable to hypoxia-ischemia.

The *temporal features* of neuronal and related changes in neonatal human brain have been well documented.[3-8,43,44] The major changes seen by classic light microscopy occur after 24 to 36 hours and are characterized by marked eosinophilia of neuronal cytoplasm, loss of Nissl substance (endoplasmic reticulum), condensation (pyknosis) or fragmentation (karyorrhexis) of nuclei, and breakdown of nuclear and plasma membranes, often with observable cell swelling (Fig. 8-1). Two factors alter the ability to identify such neuronal changes early after perinatal asphyxia: (1) the gestational age of the infant and (2) the nature of the survival period. Thus, recognition of neuronal changes in premature infants is difficult because of the close packing of immature cortical neurons and their relative lack of Nissl substance. Moreover, the brain of any infant who has been maintained on a respirator for several days, with compromised ventilation or perfusion, may have undergone enough autolysis to obscure early cellular changes. When these factors are not taken into account, the presence and magnitude of neuronal injury may be misjudged and may lead to spurious conclusions about the nature of the neuropathology.

The early neuronal changes are followed in several days by overt signs of cell necrosis (Fig. 8-2). Associated with this cell necrosis is the appearance of microglial cells and, by 3 to 5 days after the insult, hypertrophic astrocytes. Foamy macrophages consume the necrotic

TABLE 8-3	Major Patterns of Selective Neuronal Injury and Characteristics of Usual Insult in Term Newborns	
Pattern*	**Usual Insult**
Diffuse	Very severe, very prolonged
Cerebral cortex–deep nuclear[†]	Moderate to severe, prolonged
Deep nuclear[†]–brain stem	Severe, abrupt

*The patterns reflect areas of *predominant* neuronal injury; considerable overlap is common. Two additional patterns of selective neuronal necrosis (i.e., *pontosubicular* and *cerebellar*), which occur predominantly in premature newborns (see text), are not listed here because the temporal characteristics of the insult are unknown.

[†]Deep nuclear: basal ganglia (especially putamen) and thalamus.

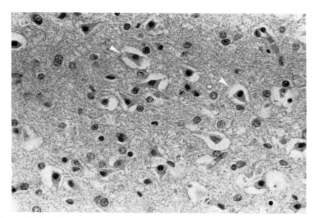

Figure 8-1 **Ischemic neuronal injury (*arrowheads*) within the hippocampus of an asphyxiated term infant.** Note shrinkage of cytoplasm and pyknotic nuclei with irregular nuclear membranes, loss of nucleoli, and nuclear hyperchromasia. (Hematoxylin and eosin stain, ×500.) In typical hematoxylin and eosin sections, the shrunken neuron is eosinophilic, and thus this appearance is the classic "red, dead" neuron of ischemic injury. (*From Clancy RR, Sladky JT, Rorke LB: Hypoxic-ischemic spinal cord injury following perinatal asphyxia, Ann Neurol 25:185-189, 1989.*)

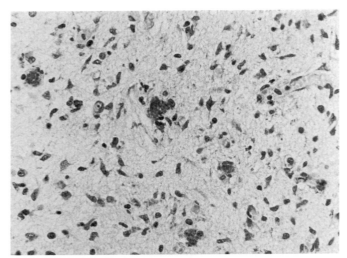

Figure 8-2 **Selective neuronal necrosis.** Note the "encrusted" necrotic neuron in the center of the figure. Most of the other cells in this brain stem nucleus are reactive astrocytes and microglial cells. *(Courtesy of Dr. Margaret G. Norman.)*

debris, and a glial mat forms over the next several weeks. Severe lesions may result in cavity formation, especially in the cerebral cortex.[3,5-8]

Apoptotic as well as *necrotic* cell death is observed in hypoxic-ischemic disease in human infants, as in neonatal animal models.[8,43,45-52] In one study of neuronal injury after "birth asphyxia," the mean fractions of apoptotic and necrotic cells in cerebral cortex were 8.3% and 20.8%, respectively.[43] In a study of the neonatal piglet subjected to hypoxia-ischemia, apoptotic neuronal death predominated among immature neurons and necrotic cell death predominated among mature neurons.[45] A similar susceptibility of immature neurons to apoptosis has been shown in *N*-methyl-D-aspartate (NMDA)–treated neurons in culture.[50] In one specific form of human neonatal injury, pontosubicular necrosis (see later), the predominant form of cell death appears to be apoptosis.[47,53]

Regional Aspects

As noted earlier, three major regional patterns of selective neuronal necrosis can be delineated in the human newborn, especially the term infant (see Table 8-3). In *diffuse* disease, certain neurons at essentially all levels of the neuraxis are affected. In predominantly *cerebral–deep nuclear* disease, the prominent involvement is of cerebral neocortex, hippocampus, and basal ganglia-thalamus. In predominantly *deep nuclear–brain stem* disease, *basal ganglia–thalamus–brain stem* is the topography. A fourth pattern, more commonly observed in the preterm infant, *pontosubicular necrosis*, is characterized by involvement of neurons of the base of the pons and the subiculum of the hippocampus (see later). A fifth pattern, observed particularly in the small premature infant but to a different degree in the term infant, involves the *cerebellum* (see later). Given that *overlap among these groups is the rule rather than the exception*, I discuss diffuse disease first, because all the vulnerable groups are involved.

Diffuse Neuronal Injury. The major sites of predilection for diffuse neuronal necrosis in the term and preterm newborn infant are shown in Table 8-4.[2-6,8,43,47,54-75]

Cerebral Cortex. Neurons of the cerebral cortex in the term infant are particularly vulnerable, most notably the hippocampus (pyramidal cells) among the cerebral cortical regions. Sommer's sector (and contiguous areas) in the term newborn and the subiculum of the hippocampus in the premature newborn (see later discussion) are especially prone to injury (see Table 8-4). With more severe injury in the term infant, the better differentiated neurons of the calcarine (visual) cortex and of the precentral and postcentral cortices (i.e., perirolandic cortex) may be injured. In very severe injury, diffuse involvement of cerebral cortex occurs. Neurons in deeper cortical layers and, particularly, in the depths of sulci are especially affected. A role for patterns of blood flow in the determination of the topography is apparent from the more severe neuronal injury consistently observed in border zones between the major cerebral arteries, especially in the posterior cerebrum, and in depths of sulci. Perhaps reflecting the relative immaturity of cerebral cortical neurons in premature infants, involvement of cerebral cortex is uncommon,[75] particularly in comparison with neurons of deep nuclear structures and brain stem (see later). However, sophisticated brain imaging studies of *premature infants at term equivalent age and later in childhood show impressive abnormalities of cerebral cortex* (see Chapter 9). Thus, diminutions of cerebral cortical volumes

TABLE 8-4   **Sites of Predilection for the Diffuse Form of Hypoxic-Ischemic Selective Neuronal Injury in Premature and Term Newborns***

Brain Region	Premature	Term Newborn
Cerebral neocortex		+
Hippocampus		
Sommer's sector		+
Subiculum	+	
Deep nuclear structures		
Caudate-putamen	+	+
Globus pallidus	+	+
Thalamus	+	+
Brain stem		
Cranial nerve nuclei	+	+
Pons (ventral)	+	+
Inferior olivary nuclei	+	+
Cerebellum		
Purkinje cells		+
Granule cells (internal, external)	±	±
Spinal cord		
Anterior horn cells (alone)		±
Anterior horn cells and contiguous cells (? infarction)	±	

+, common; ±, less common.
*See text for references.

and gyral development have been documented. The disturbances may reflect abnormalities of cerebral cortical *development* and may be related to concomitant cerebral white matter injury (see later). The important point in this context is that the abnormalities of cerebral cortex do not appear to reflect direct cortical neuronal necrosis, at least as evidenced by histological criteria.

Deep Nuclear Structures. Involvement of deep nuclear structures, *principally thalamus and basal ganglia,* is particularly characteristic of hypoxic-ischemic neuronal injury in both preterm and term newborns. With diffuse disease, *thalamus* is particularly vulnerable. As discussed later, a particular pattern of injury in term newborns involves a combination of affection of neurons of thalamus, basal ganglia, and brain stem, with relative sparing of cerebral cortical neurons. Hypothalamic neurons and those of the lateral geniculate nuclei also are especially vulnerable. In preterm newborns, involvement of deep nuclear structures is a major form of gray matter injury.[75] Injury to thalamus and basal ganglia was apparent in 40% to 50% of one series of 41 premature infants studied at autopsy (see later).[75] Of the *basal ganglia,* neurons of the caudate, putamen, and globus pallidus are often injured, in both term and premature newborns (see Table 8-4). Neurons of the putamen (and head of the caudate nucleus) are somewhat more likely to be affected in the term infant, whereas neurons of the globus pallidus are more likely to be affected in the premature infant.[5,6] This distinction is subtle, however. Neuronal injury to basal ganglia usually is accompanied by thalamic neuronal injury. Indeed, the combination of putaminal and thalamic neuronal injury in my experience is typical of neonatal hypoxic-ischemic disease, especially in the term infant.

Brain Stem. Particularly characteristic of hypoxic-ischemic encephalopathy in the newborn is involvement of the brain stem.[4,6-8,54-67,69-72,74-88] In general, hypoxic-ischemic injury to the brain stem in the term newborn tends to be more or less restricted to neurons. With premature infants, although neurons are involved primarily, injury may be so marked as to result in cystic necrosis.[65] As discussed later, involvement of neurons of brain stem may occur in combination with basal ganglia and thalamic involvement.

In *midbrain,* the inferior colliculus stands out in terms of vulnerability. This finding is in keeping with the studies of Ranck, Windle, Faro[89,90] of asphyxiated fetal monkeys, particularly with total asphyxia. Neuronal injury is also found frequently in the neurons of the oculomotor and trochlear nuclei, substantia nigra, and reticular formation.

In *pons,* particularly frequently involved are the motor nuclei of the fifth and seventh cranial nerves, the reticular formation, the dorsal cochlear nuclei, and the pontine nuclei. Striking involvement of the nuclei in ventral pons and of the neurons of the subicular portion of the hippocampus in some cases led Friede[6] to the term *pontosubicular neuronal necrosis.* This pattern of injury is discussed later.

In *medulla,* particularly vulnerable are the dorsal nuclei of the vagus, nucleus ambiguus (ninth and tenth cranial nerves), inferior olivary nuclei, and the cuneate and gracilis nuclei. Involvement of neurons of the inferior olivary nuclei is the single most common brain stem neuronal lesion in both term and preterm infants.[8,72,75] In one series of 41 premature infants studied at autopsy, fully 90% had evidence of inferior olivary injury.[75] Important clinical correlates of many of these brain stem lesions are discussed in Chapter 9.

Cerebellum. The cerebellum is especially vulnerable to hypoxic-ischemic neuronal injury, and the Purkinje cells in the term infant and the granule cell neurons (of both the internal and external granule cell layers) in both the term and premature infant are the most vulnerable cerebellar neurons (see Table 8-4). Neurons of the vermis may be especially easily injured in the term infant.[91,91a] Neurons of the dentate nucleus (and other roof nuclei) are also somewhat susceptible to injury, more so in the preterm newborn than at later ages. In the term infant, a subsequent disturbance of cerebellar growth, especially involving the vermis, has been observed by magnetic resonance imaging (MRI).[91,91a] In this setting, frequent concomitant injury to thalamus and basal ganglia also raises the possibility of transsynaptic effects.[91,91a,92] Involvement of the cerebellum, especially cerebellar hemispheres, and subsequently impaired cerebellar growth are particular features of very premature infants and are sufficiently distinctive to be discussed as a separate form of selective neuronal necrosis (see later).

Spinal Cord. Affection of anterior horn cells by hypoxic-ischemic injury has been identified.[5,93,94] This involvement is accompanied clinically by hypotonia and weakness and electrophysiologically by signs of anterior horn cell disturbance and may underlie at least some cases of so-called atonic cerebral palsy (see Chapter 9). The neuronal injury occurs in typical form in the term infant and is similar cytopathologically to that observed in other regions. When present in the premature infant, the lesion, as with hypoxic-ischemic injury to brain stem, often also involves contiguous cellular elements that may have the histological appearance of infarction and may be accompanied by hemorrhage.[93]

Cerebral–Deep Nuclear Neuronal Injury. Although systematic data are difficult to gather, MRI studies of "asphyxiated" term infants suggest that approximately 35% to 85% exhibit predominantly cerebral–deep nuclear neuronal involvement.[95-101] Among neurons of cerebral cortex, those in the parasagittal areas of perirolandic cortex are especially likely to be affected. Involvement of the hippocampus and of other neocortical areas was described earlier. The most common additional neuronal lesion affects basal ganglia, especially putamen, and thalamus. The pathogenesis appears usually to involve a *moderate or moderate-to-severe insult that evolves in a gradual manner* (i.e., a "prolonged, partial" insult; see "Pathogenesis").

Deep Nuclear–Brain Stem Neuronal Injury.
Although involvement of neurons of basal ganglia
and thalamus occurs in approximately two thirds of
"asphyxiated" term infants, in approximately 15% to
20% of infants with hypoxic-ischemic disease, involvement of deep nuclear structures (i.e., basal ganglia, thalamus, and tegmentum of brain stem) is the *predominant*
lesion.[6,70,71,79,85,102-104] Until the advent of MRI,
detection of this deep gray matter predominance in
the living infant had not been accomplished readily,
and thus the relative frequency of this pattern of neuronal injury was not recognized. However, studies
based on MRI and careful clinical pathological correlations have delineated this pattern as a distinct
entity.[70,71,85] The topography of the neuropathology
is illustrated in Figure 8-3.

At least some cases of this predominantly deep gray
matter form of selective neuronal injury may evolve to
status marmoratus, a disorder of basal ganglia and thalamus not seen in its complete form until the latter part
of the first year of life, despite the perinatal timing of
the insult. The basic initiating role of hypoxia-ischemia
is demonstrated not only by clinical data in human
infants (see later discussion) but also by the reproduction of the lesion in the newborn rat subjected to
hypoxic-ischemic insult,[105,106] as well as in the term
fetal monkey subjected to intrauterine asphyxia.[19]

Status marmoratus has three major features:
neuronal loss, gliosis, and hypermyelination.[5-7,107]
Hypermyelination is the characteristic feature of the
lesion; this term refers to an apparent increase in
amount and an abnormal distribution of myelinated
fibers within the affected nuclear structures, especially
the putamen (Fig. 8-4). The hypermyelination has been
noted at as early as 8 months of life.[6] The abnormal
myelin pattern provides a *marbled appearance* to the basal
ganglia, hence the term *status marmoratus* or *état marbré*.
Previous observations by light microscopy had led to
the suggestion that the many myelinated fibers in status
marmoratus were axons, and the idea that such apparent overgrowth was a result of aberrant myelination of
nerve fibers was accepted for many years. However,
electron microscopic techniques were used to show
that the abnormal myelinated fibers, at least in part,
are astrocytic processes.[108] It appears that the very
young brain, at the time of normal myelination, may
myelinate fibers that are not axonal in origin. Thus, this
distinctive response to injury appears to depend on the
time of occurrence of the insult as well as the locus of the
injury. Nevertheless, the proportion of infants with
hypoxic-ischemic involvement of basal ganglia and
thalamus who develop status marmoratus and the
determinants for the occurrence of this relatively
specific pathological response to injury versus that of
only gliosis and atrophy remain to be determined.
Concerning the sequela of gliosis and atrophy alone,
a reasonable speculation is that injury that is so
severe as to eliminate oligodendrocytes as well as
neurons may prevent the occurrence of the typical
hypermyelination of status marmoratus. As discussed
later (see "Pathogenesis"), the hypoxic-ischemic insult
associated with the occurrence of predominant

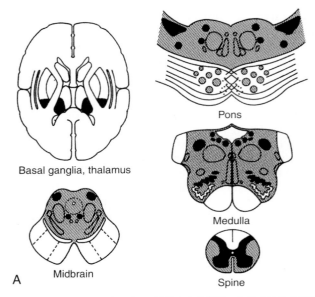

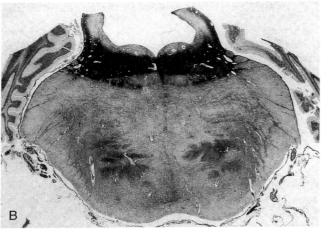

Figure 8-3 Neuropathology of the deep nuclear–brain stem form of
selective neuronal necrosis. **A,** Schematic depiction of the topography
of the lesions in a typical case of a term newborn subjected to severe,
terminal asphyxia. The *dark areas* indicate nuclei with neuronal loss,
and the *diagonally striped areas* represent regions of marked gliosis.
B, Holzer stain of the pons for gliosis in a typical case. The tegmentum
is atrophied and deeply stained because of gliosis; the base of the
pons is nearly normal. *(From Natsume J, Watanabe K, Kuno K,
Hayakawa F, et al: Clinical, neurophysiologic, and neuropathological
features of an infant with brain damage of total asphyxia type
(Myers), Pediatr Neurol 13:61-64, 1995.)*

involvement of deep gray matter structures typically is
severe and *abrupt* in evolution (i.e., an "acute, total"
insult).

Pontosubicular Neuronal Necrosis. Pontosubicular
neuronal necrosis is a fourth type of selective neuronal
injury with predominant involvement of neurons of the
basis pontis (i.e., not the tegmentum, as described ear-
lier) and the subiculum of hippocampus.[47,66,67,74,78,80-83,109-111] Among all types of selective neuronal injury,
pontosubicular neuronal necrosis is by far the least
common. The lesion is characteristic of the premature

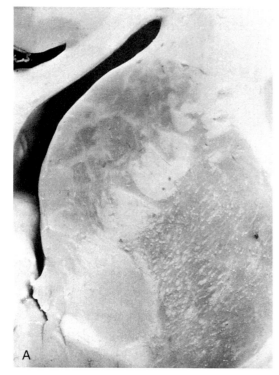

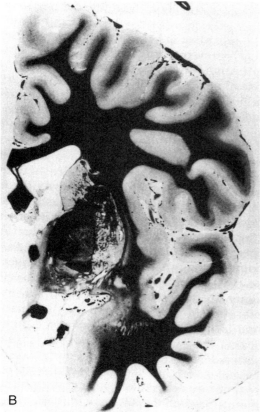

Figure 8-4   Status marmoratus. Coronal sections of cerebrum from two infants who died several years after the perinatal insult. **A,** Formalin fixed and unstained; note the marbled appearance of the caudate nucleus and putamen. **B,** Stained for myelin; note the black-staining myelin, particularly in the putamen. *(Courtesy of Dr. E. P. Richardson, Jr.)*

infant but occurs in infants up to 1 to 2 months beyond term (Table 8-5).[66,67,78,80-83,109,112] A strong association exists with periventricular leukomalacia (PVL). Although the disorder is characterized principally by affection of neurons of ventral pons and of subiculum of hippocampus, neuronal death in the fascia dentata of the hippocampus was observed in 60% of cases in one series.[67] In several neuropathological studies that included electron microscopy, labeling of oligonucleosomal fragments, and detection of Fas receptor and activated caspase-3, the neuronal death in pontosubicular neuronal necrosis appeared to be predominantly apoptotic.[47,53,110,111,113]

Cerebellar Injury. *Cerebellar injury is particularly characteristic of premature infants, especially those of extremely low birth weights,* and it is sufficiently distinctive to be considered a fifth type of selective neuronal necrosis (Table 8-6). This injury has occurred primarily in premature infants with serious respiratory disease, although single major hypoxic-ischemic insults typical of asphyxiated term infants have not been present. Cerebellar disturbance has been identified most often by the finding by MRI of bilateral, generally symmetric decreases of cerebellar hemispheric volumes at term equivalent or later in infancy or childhood.[114-126] Although a few cases have been focal and asymmetric, suggestive of infarction, nearly all abnormalities have consisted of bilateral and symmetric diminutions in size. The possibility of a trophic disturbance, perhaps related to supratentorial white matter injury, is suggested by a strong association with *cerebral* white matter injury (see later).[122,124,125] Moreover, the high frequency of injury to neurons of brain stem cerebellar relay nuclei (see earlier) also raises the possibility of impaired trophic interactions at the transsynaptic level.

Pathogenesis

Cerebral Ischemia, Impaired Cerebrovascular Autoregulation, and Pressure-Passive Cerebral Circulation. *Cerebral ischemia,* with deprivation of oxygen and glucose, followed by reperfusion and the cascade of metabolic events described in Chapter 6, is the likely pathogenetic sequence in selective neuronal necrosis (Table 8-7). Although the causative relationship between cerebral ischemia and both selective neuronal necrosis and parasagittal cerebral injury (see later) has been established in several excellent perinatal animal models (see previous section), studies in *human infants* also provide excellent support for the role of

TABLE 8-5	Pontosubicular Neuronal Necrosis in the Premature Newborn*

Pons and subiculum common sites of neuronal injury in premature newborns

Strong association with periventricular leukomalacia

Clinically associated with hypoxia-ischemia, hypocarbia, and hyperoxia (reproducible in newborn rat by hyperoxia alone)

*See text for references.

TABLE 8-6	Cerebellar Injury in the Premature Newborn

Cerebellar injury, especially involving the cerebellar hemispheres, is generally bilateral and symmetric, especially in very small premature infants.

Microscopic features include cerebellar neuronal injury, cerebellar white matter necrosis/gliosis, and neuronal injury to brain stem relay nuclei to cerebellum.

Diminished cerebellar volume is the most common structural sequela.

Cerebellar injury is often associated with supratentorial injury, especially to cerebral white matter, and with relay nuclei in brain stem, both principally hypoxic-ischemic.

The cause may reflect a combination of transsynaptic trophic disturbances and direct neuronal injury.

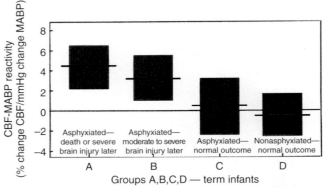

Figure 8-5 Cerebrovascular autoregulation. This is expressed as reactivity of cerebral blood flow (CBF) to changes in mean arterial blood pressure (MABP), in a group of 19 asphyxiated term newborns and 12 control infants. Note the normal reactivity in the control infants *(D)* and the loss of reactivity in the infants with the poorest outcomes *(A and B)*. *(Data from Pryds O, Greisen G, Lou H, Friis-Hansen B: Vasoparalysis associated with brain damage in asphyxiated term infants, J Pediatr 117:119-125, 1990.)*

diminished CBF secondary to systemic hypotension. Thus, as discussed in detail in Chapter 6, because of the *impaired vascular autoregulation* in asphyxiated infants, CBF becomes passively related to arterial blood pressure (Fig. 8-5; see Table 8-7). The impaired vascular autoregulation has been documented in the hours to days after the insult and, by extrapolation from experimental data (see Chapter 6), is presumed to begin during the insult, when hypotension is most pronounced. This situation makes the infant exquisitely vulnerable to the diminutions in blood pressure characteristic of severe asphyxia, and those regions most vulnerable are in the distribution of selective neuronal necrosis as well as the watershed (i.e., parasagittal) distributions of the cerebrum; see later. The data of Pryds and Greisen and their co-workers[127,128] clearly show that those asphyxiated term infants with impaired autoregulation have the poorest neurological outcome (see Fig. 8-5). The *causes of the pressure-passive circulation* in the asphyxiated newborn could relate to the following factors: (1) the hypoxemia or hypercarbia, or both, of the primary asphyxial insult; (2) the postasphyxial impairment in vascular reactivity observed in experimental models of perinatal asphyxia and presumably related to the effect of one or more of the vasodilatory compounds that accumulate secondary to ischemia-reperfusion (see Chapter 6); (3) an "immature"

TABLE 8-7	Selective Neuronal Necrosis: Pathogenesis

Cerebral ischemia
    Impaired cerebrovascular autoregulation with pressure-passive cerebral circulation
    Systemic hypotension
Regional vascular factors
Regional metabolic factors
Regional distribution of excitatory (glutamate) receptors on neurons*
Factors related to the hypoxic-ischemic insult
    Severity and temporal characteristics
    Preceding/concomitant infection/inflammation

*Single most important factor for determining regional distribution of selective neuronal necrosis.

autoregulatory system with limited capacity for reactivity because of the deficient arteriolar muscular lining of penetrating cerebral arteries and arterioles in the third trimester[129,130]; (4) an autoregulatory system with a lower limit so close to the range of "normal" blood pressure that even slight hypotension places CBF on the down slope of the curve (see later discussion of PVL); or (5) a combination of these factors. Whatever the mechanisms, the clinical implications are enormous. Falls in arterial blood pressure lead to decreases in CBF and injury to certain vulnerable brain *cells* (i.e., neurons in the distribution of selective neuronal necrosis), and *regions* (i.e., parasagittal cerebrum; see later).

Regional Vascular Factors. The reasons for the *selective vulnerability* of neuronal groups in the central nervous system have become increasingly clear. *Regional vascular factors* certainly can play a role because neuronal injury is more marked in vascular border zones (e.g., depths of sulci and parasagittal cerebral cortex; see Table 8-7). Moreover, the relationship of pontosubicular necrosis with hypocarbia and hyperoxemia (often following hypoxic-ischemic insult) suggests a role for cerebral vasoconstriction in pathogenesis of this specific type of neuronal necrosis of the premature infant (see Table 8-5).[6,66,112] However, the finding that most of selective neuronal injury is not in strictly vascular distributions suggests that other factors are operative. For example, the rapid neuronal maturation in the pons and subiculum during the time of occurrence of this lesion suggests that vulnerability of this region may relate in part to the simultaneous occurrence of neuronal differentiation, the insults that impair brain blood flow, and a propensity of these neurons to undergo apoptosis.[47,109-111]

Regional Metabolic Factors. *Regional metabolic factors* must play a central role (see Table 8-7). Those factors that lead to hypoxic cell death in experimental systems (see Chapter 6) raise the possibilities of regional differences in anaerobic glycolytic capacity, energy requirements, lactate accumulation, mitochondrial function, calcium (Ca^{2+}) influx, nitric oxide synthesis, and free radical formation and scavenging capacity. For example, the high metabolic rate and energy use of deep gray matter may render these neurons particularly vulnerable to the severe, abrupt ischemic insults that lead to particular injury to these neuronal structures (see later). Similarly, a particular regional vulnerability of mitochondrial cytochrome oxidase activity to hypoxic-ischemic insult may play a role in determining the regional vulnerability of certain neurons to injury.[131] However, little is known about these issues in human brain.

Regional Distribution of Excitatory (Glutamate) Receptors. The *regional distribution of glutamate receptors, particularly of the N-methyl-D-aspartate (NMDA) and alpha-amino-3-hydroxy-5-methyl-4-isoxazole-propionic acid* (AMPA) types, now appears to be the single most important determinant of the distribution of selective neuronal injury (see Table 8-7). As discussed in detail in Chapter 6, the topography of hypoxic-ischemic neuronal death in vivo is similar to the topography of glutamate synapses; the particular vulnerability of certain neuronal groups in the perinatal period correlates with a transient, maturation-dependent density of glutamate receptors; extracellular glutamate increases dramatically at such receptors with hypoxia-ischemia; and hypoxic-ischemic neuronal death in vivo can be prevented by administration of blockers of the NMDA receptor-channel complex and, to a considerable extent also, of non-NMDA receptors, especially Ca^{2+}-permeable AMPA receptors (see Chapter 6). The demonstrations that the molecular mechanisms by which activation of the glutamate receptors leads to cell death operate over hours after termination of the insult and that prevention or amelioration of such excitotoxic injury can be effected by glutamate receptor blockers also administered after termination of the insult have profound and obvious clinical implications (see Chapters 6 and 9).

The importance of the regional distribution of glutamate receptors in the determination of regional selectivity of neuronal injury is particularly apparent in basal ganglia. Thus, first, it is clear that a transient, dense glutamatergic innervation of the basal ganglia occurs in the perinatal period, both in the rat (see Chapter 6) and in the human.[132-136] Second, the development of vulnerability of striatum to hypoxic-ischemic injury parallels the expression of glutamate receptors and the vulnerability to direct injections of glutamate (see Chapter 6). Third, extracellular glutamate levels have been shown to rise in perinatal models of hypoxic-ischemic striatal injury (see Chapter 6). Fourth, a highly effective blocker of perinatal hypoxic-ischemic striatal injury is MK-801, a specific blocker of the NMDA receptor-channel complex (see Chapter 6). Fifth, a specific hierarchy of potency of glutamate receptor agonists exists for the production of striatal injury, and this potency parallels the expression of

receptor subtypes and the inhibitory capabilities of specific receptor antagonists (see Chapter 6).

As noted earlier, neuronal injury in the brain stem often accompanies such injury in basal ganglia. Notably, studies of the developmental profiles of glutamate receptor subtype binding in the human brain stem have shown transient elevations in inferior olive and basis pontis of NMDA and kainate receptors in early infancy.[72,137]

Perhaps related to the role of glutamate receptors of the NMDA type in pathogenesis of selective striatal neuronal injury is a *relative sparing of the reduced form of nicotinamide-adenine dinucleotide phosphate (NADPH)–diaphorase neurons* in hypoxia-ischemia.[138,139] *NADPH diaphorase* has been shown to be identical to nitric oxide synthase, and generation of nitric oxide has been shown to be one mechanism whereby activation of NMDA receptors (expressed by NADPH-diaphorase neurons) leads to striatal neuronal death (see also Chapter 6). Because nitric oxide synthase is activated by Ca^{2+}, and Ca^{2+} influx follows activation of the NMDA receptor (see Chapter 6), the data suggest a sequence of NMDA receptor activation, activation of nitric oxide synthase, generation of nitric oxide, and diffusion of nitric oxide (a highly reactive molecule that can generate free radicals) to adjacent neurons, and free radical–mediated cell death. The peak period of vulnerability of striatal neurons in the immature rat corresponds to the peak periods of sparing of NADPH-diaphorase neurons and of hypoxic-ischemic vulnerability.[138,139] The reason for the relative sparing of NADPH-diaphorase neurons remains unclear, but this sparing may contribute importantly to perinatal striatal neuronal death. Currently, it is not known whether a similar sparing of nitric oxide–synthesizing neurons contributes to selective neuronal injury in cerebral cortical and other areas vulnerable in hypoxia-ischemia in the neonatal human. However, the potential importance for neuronal nitric oxide synthase in mediation of such hypoxic-ischemic neuronal injury is suggested by the results of a study of the development of neuronal expression of the enzyme in human brain.[140] The striking findings were a higher density of nitric oxide synthase–positive neurons in late fetal human brain than in adult brain and a concentration of such neurons in areas known to be injured in selective neuronal necrosis (i.e., deeper layers of cerebral cortex, striatum, and brain stem tegmentum).

Studies of glutamate receptors in developing *human* cerebral cortex suggest that a transient expression of Ca^{2+}-permeable AMPA receptors and NMDA receptors occurs around the time of term birth (Fig. 8-6).[141] Thus, the theme is similar to that for basal ganglia and brain stem (i.e., a maturation-dependent exuberant expression of Ca^{2+}-permeable glutamate receptors becomes lethal to neurons with excessive activation, as occurs with cerebral ischemia).

Factors Related to the Hypoxic-Ischemic Insult. Factors related to the *severity and the temporal characteristics* of the insult appear to be of particular importance in determining the major pattern of selective neuronal injury in the newborn (see Table 8-3). Severe and prolonged insults result in diffuse and marked neuronal necrosis, involving the many levels of the neuraxis described earlier as the *diffuse pattern* of injury. The *cerebral–deep nuclear pattern* of neuronal injury appears to be related to insults that are less severe and prolonged, often termed *partial, prolonged asphyxia*. The *deep nuclear–brain stem* pattern of injury to basal ganglia–thalamus–brain stem has been described in human infants with a severe, abrupt event, often termed *total asphyxia* (see earlier discussion). It is postulated that the severe, abrupt event prevents the operation of major adaptive mechanisms normally operative with asphyxial events (see Chapter 6). The most important of these may be the diversion of blood from the cerebral hemispheres to the "vital" deep nuclear structures. Because the latter have high rates of energy use (and also a high content of glutamate receptors), these nuclei are particularly likely to be injured. In the more prolonged and less severe insults, the diversion of blood to deep nuclear structures occurs at least to a degree, and the cerebral regions are more likely to be affected. Studies in the near-term fetal lamb indicate that the severe terminal insult that results in injury to deep nuclear structures especially may be likely to occur after brief, repeated hypoxic-ischemic insults *first* cause a cumulative deleterious effect on cardiovascular function that presumably *then* can result in a severe late insult.[28,142-144]

As discussed in detail in Chapter 6, experimental data demonstrate the *potentiation of hypoxic-ischemic insults by preceding or concomitant infection/inflammation*. Thus, hypoxic-ischemic insults not severe enough to cause injury alone can be rendered seriously injurious if the fetus or infant is exposed to inflammatory factors associated with intrauterine or postnatal infection. This phenomenon could underlie, at least in part, the accentuated risk of apparent hypoxic-ischemic brain injury observed in infants who sustain their insults in association with chorioamnionitis or who have elevated levels of cytokines in blood or cerebrospinal fluid (CSF).[145-155] However, most term infants who are exposed to chorioamnionitis have an uncomplicated neonatal course and neurological outcome, and histological chorioamnionitis does not appear to increase the risk of adverse outcome even in infants with hypoxic-ischemic encephalopathy.[156] The presence or absence of a *fetal inflammatory response* may be most critical, and the determinants of such a response in the presence of chorioamnionitis require clarification.

Parasagittal Cerebral Injury

Cellular and Regional Aspects

Parasagittal cerebral injury refers to a lesion of the cerebral cortex and subcortical white matter with a characteristic distribution (i.e., parasagittal, superomedial aspects of the cerebral convexities) (Figs. 8-7 and 8-8). The injury is bilateral and, although usually symmetrical, may be more striking in one hemisphere than the other. The posterior aspect of the cerebral hemispheres, especially the parietal-occipital regions, is more impressively affected than the anterior aspect. The term *watershed infarct* has been used to describe the lesion and to emphasize its ischemic nature (see later discussion). I prefer the more descriptive term *parasagittal cerebral injury*.

Parasagittal cerebral injury is characterized by necrosis of the cortex and the immediately subjacent white

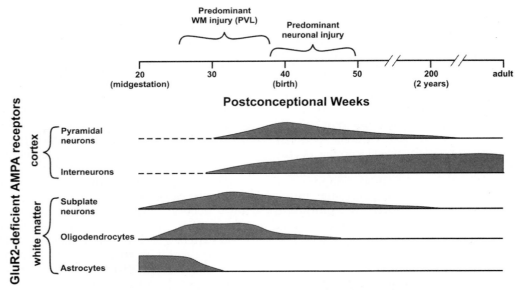

Figure 8-6 Transient expression of calcium-permeable (GluR2-deficient) alpha-amino-3-hydroxy-5-methyl-4-isoxazole-propionic acid (AMPA) receptors in cerebral cortex and cerebral white matter (WM) in developing human brain. Note the transient dense expression of GluR2-deficient AMPA receptors in cortical pyramidal neurons around the time of term. *N*-Methyl-D-aspartate receptors show a similar time course (data not shown). The changes in cerebral white matter are discussed later in relation to periventricular leukomalacia (PVL). *(From Talos DM, Follett PL, Folkerth RD, Fishman RE, et al: Developmental regulation of alpha-amino-3-hydroxy-5-methyl-4-isoxazole-propionic acid receptor subunit expression in forebrain and relationship to regional susceptibility to hypoxic/ischemic injury. II. Human cerebral white matter and cortex, J Comp Neurol 497:61-77, 2006.)*

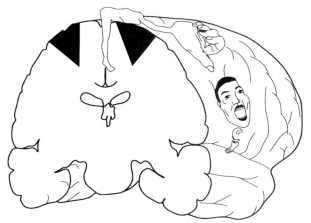

Figure 8-7   Parasagittal cerebral injury, coronal view. Schematic diagram of the distribution of the injury, which is indicated by symmetrical *black areas* in the superomedial aspects of cerebrum.

the necrosis extends to a large proportion of the lateral cerebral convexity (see Fig. 8-8B), especially in the parietal-occipital regions, the most vulnerable regions of the cerebrum. The precise pathological evolution of parasagittal cerebral injury in the newborn is not known, but atrophic gyri or ulegyria, or both, are the chronic neuropathological correlates. Parasagittal cerebral injury is characteristic of the full-term infant with perinatal asphyxia; it is unlikely, in fact, that cerebral necrosis in the parasagittal distribution occurs in the premature infant to a major degree for reasons outlined in the section "Periventricular Leukomalacia."

Parasagittal cerebral injury has been well documented in classic neuropathological writings (e.g., the work of Friede,[157] Courville,[158] and Norman and colleagues[159]), particularly those concerned with older survivors with cerebral palsy. However, the lesion has been more difficult to define as *an isolated entity* in neuropathological studies of infants dying in the neonatal period, although examples are apparent (see Fig. 8-8). I believe that the difficulty in pathological identification of the discrete lesion in the neonatal period relates to the severe nature of the cases in *newborns who die*. Thus, the neuropathological findings are most often diffuse

matter; neuronal elements are most severely affected. Although usually nonhemorrhagic, the areas of infarction may be hemorrhagic. In particularly severe cases,

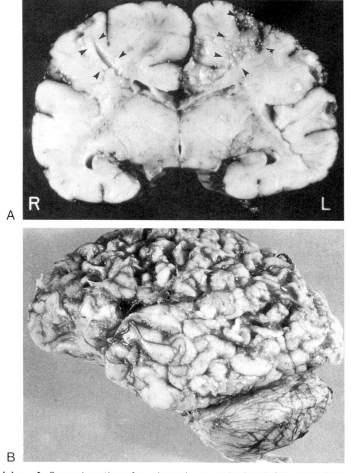

Figure 8-8   Parasagittal cerebral injury. A, Coronal section of cerebrum in an asphyxiated, full-term infant who died on the third postnatal day. Areas of necrosis of cerebral cortex and subcortical white matter in the parasagittal regions are marked by *arrowheads*. **B,** Lateral view of cerebral convexity of a 6-month-old infant who had experienced severe perinatal asphyxia. Note the cortical atrophy in parasagittal distribution (compare with Fig. 8-9). *(B, Courtesy of Dr. Alan Hill.)*

TABLE 8-8	Parasagittal Cerebral Injury: Pathogenesis

Cerebral ischemia
Impaired cerebrovascular autoregulation with pressure-passive cerebral circulation
Systemic hypotension
Parasagittal vascular factors
Arterial border zones and end zones
Excitatory (glutamate) receptors on neurons (and premyelinating oligodendrocytes)

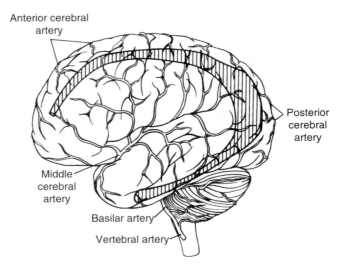

Figure 8-9 **Parasagittal cerebral injury, lateral view.** Schematic diagram of cerebral convexity, lateral view, showing distribution of major cerebral arteries. The distribution of injury, shown by the *line-marked area*, is in the border zones and end fields of these arteries.

and severe, very frequently complicated by autolytic changes related to survival for many hours or days on life support. These diffuse changes obscure elemental lesions, such as parasagittal cerebral injury, which, however, is identifiable in those less severely affected infants who *survive*. In keeping with this explanation is the observation of a high frequency in asphyxiated term newborns (≈90% of whom survive) of parasagittal cerebral injury identifiable by radionuclide brain scanning,[160,161] positron emission tomography,[162] and MRI[98,163,164] (see the section in Chapter 9 on diagnosis). Indeed, in an MRI study of 173 term infants with neonatal encephalopathy, fully 45% (n = 78) had watershed injury as the predominant lesion.[164] The computed tomography scan, still often used in evaluation of such infants, is not particularly sensitive for detection of this lesion because the axial images frequently fail to detect the superficial cortical-subcortical lesions of parasagittal injury. The advent of MRI scanning, with coronal and lateral views, has proved more effective in identification of parasagittal cerebral injury in vivo and has provided further documentation of its frequency (see Chapter 9).

Pathogenesis

The pathogenesis of parasagittal cerebral injury relates principally to a disturbance in cerebral perfusion. The two factors underlying the propensity of the parasagittal region to ischemic injury relate to parasagittal vascular anatomical factors and cerebral ischemia with a pressure-passive state of the cerebral circulation (Table 8-8). The reasons that one infant with ischemia may develop primarily parasagittal cerebral injury and another may have the various patterns of selective neuronal necrosis are not entirely clear. As discussed in the section "Selective Neuronal Necrosis," the severity and the temporal characteristics of the insult are likely to be very important. Indeed, some degree of concomitant selective neuronal injury, particularly involving basal ganglia and thalamus, is common in my experience.

Cerebral Ischemia, Impaired Cerebrovascular Autoregulation, and Pressure-Passive Cerebral Circulation. The importance of the asphyxial and postasphyxial impairment of cerebrovascular autoregulation (see Chapter 6) in the genesis of cerebral ischemia with associated systemic circulatory failure is apparent for parasagittal cerebral injury, as described earlier for selective neuronal necrosis (see earlier discussion).

Parasagittal Vascular Anatomical Factors. The likely areas of greatest ischemia relate to parasagittal vascular anatomical factors (see Table 8-8). Thus, the areas of necrosis in parasagittal cerebral injury are in the *border zones* between the end fields of the major cerebral arteries (Fig. 8-9).[165,166] These border zones are the brain regions most susceptible to a fall in cerebral perfusion pressure. Meyer,[165] who defined the characteristic topography of the cerebral lesions in 30 infants in the 1950s, related the injury to systemic hypotension. This watershed concept is based on the analogy with an irrigation system supplying a series of fields with water and emphasizes the vulnerability of the "last fields" when the head of pressure falls.[167,168] Experimental support for this concept initially was provided in the monkey by Brierley and co-workers,[169,170] who produced rapid, profound systemic hypotension and prevented hypoxemia when respiratory failure developed. Typical watershed lesions were produced in the cerebral cortex (and cerebellum) and were ascribed to the sharply reduced CBF. As my colleagues and I[160,162] observed in asphyxiated human infants, more marked injury was demonstrated in the *posterior* cerebrum in the experimental animals, as well as in the adult human.[166,169,170] The more marked injury in posterior cerebrum presumably relates to the finding that this region represents the watershed of all three major cerebral vessels (see Fig. 8-9).

The border zone concept has received ample additional experimental support in several developing animal models. Parasagittal cerebral cortical-subcortical injury has been documented in the perinatal monkey, sheep, rabbit, and mouse subjected to a variety of insults complicated by hypotension and

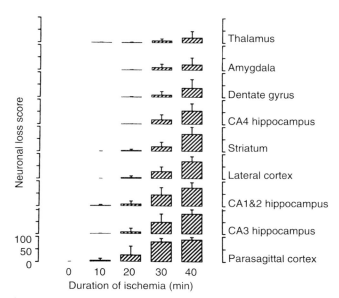

Figure 8-10 **Neuronal damage in nine brain regions following increasing durations of ischemia.** These regions are ranked in inverse order of total damage scores: the parasagittal cortex was the most severely and earliest damaged *(bottom)*, whereas the thalamus *(top)* showed the least damage. The damage scores are on a linearized scale from 0 to 100: 0, no neuronal loss; 100, total necrosis. *(From Williams CE, Gunn AJ, Mallard C, Gluckman PD: Outcome after ischemia in the developing sheep brain: An electroencephalographic and histological study, Ann Neurol 31:14-21, 1992.)*

presumed or documented cerebral ischemia.[20,28,171-176] Studies of the near-term sheep fetus showed particularly clearly the greater vulnerability of the parasagittal regions versus more laterally placed cerebrum with less than maximal insults (Fig. 8-10). Moreover, the cellular pattern of laminar necrosis of cortical pyramidal neurons was similar to the pattern observed in the asphyxiated human infant.[3] Although parasagittal cerebral cortex was most vulnerable, with prolonged ischemia (e.g., 40 minutes), many other regions became affected and the parasagittal predilection was less apparent (see Fig. 8-10). The latter situation is reminiscent of findings with severely asphyxiated human infants who die. A vivid example of the occurrence of parasagittal cerebral injury in a *primate model* of intrauterine asphyxia and fetal cerebral ischemia is provided by elegant studies of the term fetal monkey (Fig. 8-11).[20]

Although vascular border zones are the most vulnerable to drops in perfusion pressure, other "distal fields," not necessarily border zones (e.g., posterior occipital regions), are particularly vulnerable and are especially affected by systemic hypotension. Moreover, certain border zones supplied by larger *proximal* branches of cerebral vessels (e.g., temporal region between middle and posterior cerebral arteries) would be expected to be less vulnerable and, indeed, tend to be relatively less affected in parasagittal cerebral injury, whether in the asphyxiated infant (see Fig. 8-8B), hypotensive adult human, or monkey.[169,170]

In addition to the recognized vascular border zones and end zones just described, a factor related to *vascular development* appears to predispose the human newborn to ischemic injury of the cortex and subcortical white matter. Takashima and co-workers[177] showed that as sulci form and deepen near term in the human brain, the penetrating vessels from the meningeal arteries are forced to bend acutely at the cortical-white matter junction. This bending results in a triangular area at the depth of the sulcus (the site of particular predilection for ischemic cerebral injury), which represents a border zone of relative avascularity between the penetrating vessels (Fig. 8-12). This relatively avascular region presumably is even more vulnerable to a fall in perfusion pressure within the border zone regions between the major cerebral vessels. Thus, we are dealing with a border zone within a border zone, which results during a specific phase of gyral and vascular development in the human brain. These observations may explain why the cerebral injury in the parasagittal vascular border zones is more severe in the depths of sulci and why the atrophic gyri have their subsequent characteristic "mushroom" appearance (Fig. 8-13).[98,178-189] In the living infant, these localized border zones in the depths of sulci may be the regions involved in the unusual *subcortical leukomalacia* identified by brain imaging studies in parasagittal areas (see Chapter 9).[190-192]

Excitatory (Glutamate) Receptors on Neurons (and Premyelinating Oligodendrocytes). The final pathway to cell death occurs both in neurons of cerebral cortex and premyelinating oligodendrocytes (pre-OLs) of subcortical white matter involved in the parasagittal lesions (see Table 8-8). The pathogenetic mechanisms operative in both neurons and pre-OLs involve principally excitatory (glutamate) receptors. The details for neurons were noted earlier concerning selective neuronal necrosis and are described next for pre-OLs (see the following section).

Periventricular Leukomalacia

PVL, by literal definition, refers to necrosis ("softening") of white matter in a characteristic distribution (i.e., in the white matter dorsal and lateral to the external angles of the lateral ventricles) and less severe injury to the white matter peripheral to these focal necroses (see later). Virchow[193] described the periventricular locus of the lesion in 1867; several years later, Parrott[194] noted that the injury often affected premature infants; in 1932, Rydberg[195] suggested that the injury was related in some way to circulatory insufficiency at delivery; and in 1961, Schwartz[196] postulated that venous stasis caused by parturitional events played a role in pathogenesis. The most lucid and complete pathological description of PVL was that of Banker and Larroche[197] in 1962, who described the characteristic topography of the lesion and its cellular evolution and suggested a relation to vascular border zones. Subsequent work has refined the pathology and pathogenesis of PVL further (see later discussion).

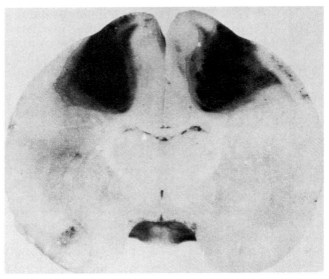

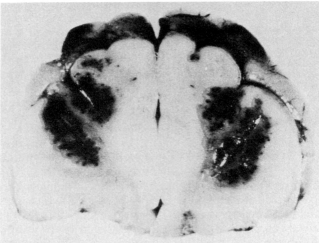

Figure 8-11 **Cerebral lesions after prolonged partial asphyxia of the term fetal monkey.** Coronal sections of cerebrum. Note the symmetrical, parasagittal distribution of necrosis, and observe the similarity to the topography of the injury in asphyxiated infants (see Fig. 8-8A). *(From Brann AW Jr, Myers RE: Central nervous system findings in the newborn monkey following severe in utero partial asphyxia, Neurology 25:327-338, 1975.)*

As I discuss in more detail (see the section "Cellular and Regional Aspects"), PVL consists of two basic components: focal necrosis (with subsequent cyst formation or glial scarring) and a more diffuse gliosis, involving both astrocytes and microglia. The characteristics of the focal necrotic component determine the basic nomenclature. Thus, *cystic PVL* refers to the classic lesion in which the focal necrotic component is *macroscopic* and evolves to *cystic formation* (Fig. 8-14). *Noncystic PVL* refers to the more common current lesion (Fig. 8-15) in which the focal necrotic component is *microscopic* and evolves to a *small glial* scar, rather than a cyst. Both cystic and noncystic PVL exhibit the diffuse gliosis (see Figs. 8-14 and 8-15) surrounding and peripheral to the necrosis. Many premature infants (see later) exhibit *diffuse white matter gliosis alone* (i.e., without focal necrosis). These cases currently are difficult to classify (see later). This abnormality could represent the mildest end of a continuum of white matter disease, with cystic PVL at the most severe end and

noncystic PVL as intermediate. This issue is unresolved. For the moment, I prefer to restrict the term *noncystic PVL* to those cases with *microscopic* areas of necrosis or glial scars, and I use the term *diffuse white matter gliosis* of uncertain pathological significance only for those cases without necrosis or glial scars.

The incidence of PVL *at autopsy* varies considerably from one medical center to another (i.e., from ≈25% to 80%) (Table 8-9). The variability in incidence relates in considerable part to the characteristics of the population studied. In the most recent detailed neuropathological study, involving 41 premature infants from a modern neonatal intensive care unit, none had classic cystic PVL, whereas 41% had noncystic PVL (41% had diffuse white matter gliosis alone).[75] Several facts are clear concerning PVL from the neuropathological studies: the lesion is observed particularly (1) in premature infants, (2) in infants with postnatal survival of more than a few days, (3) in infants who also have intraventricular hemorrhage, (4) in infants with evidence of

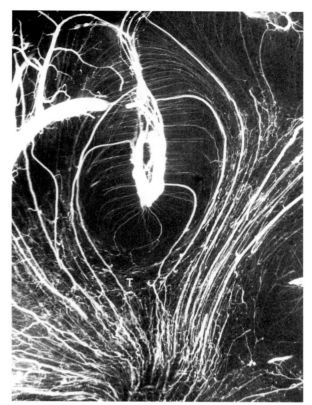

Figure 8-12 **Vascular supply to depth of sulcus in full-term newborn.** Postmortem microarteriography demonstrates the relatively avascular, triangular area (T) at the depth of the sulcus. *(From Takashima S, Armstrong DL, Becker LE: Subcortical leukomalacia: Relationship to development of the cerebral sulcus and its vascular supply,* Arch Neurol *35:470-472, 1978.)*

cardiorespiratory disturbance (e.g., cardiac arrest, severe hypotension, cardiac surgery, extracorporeal membrane oxygenation [ECMO]), and (5) in infants with evidence of antenatal maternal-placental-fetal infection and inflammation.[3,72,75,78,80,197-218]

Although the lesion is most common in premature infants, PVL is not uncommon in term infants subjected to hypoxic-ischemic insults (see later).

The incidence of PVL reported in *living infants* varies particularly according to the imaging modality used. For example, cranial ultrasonography, the most widely used modality in premature infants, is effective at detection of the classic focal necrotic/cystic component of PVL but is ineffective at detection of the diffuse component (see earlier and Chapter 9). However, MRI is valuable for detection of both overt necrotic/cystic and noncystic white matter disease (see later). Large-scale studies of the incidence of cystic PVL detected by cranial ultrasonography in the 1980s and 1990s ranged generally from 6% to 10%.[210,219,220] Currently, the *incidence of cystic PVL* is only approximately 3% or less.[221-224] In a recent series of 167 premature infants studied by MRI, cystic PVL was observed in only 3 infants.[225]

The *incidence of noncystic PVL* is difficult to establish conclusively because the microscopic areas of necrosis and subsequent glial scars of noncystic PVL are likely below the resolution of ultrasonography.[220,226-228] In marked contrast to the paucity of the finding of focal necrotic/cystic PVL in premature infants in modern neonatal intensive care units has been the high frequency of the MRI demonstration of diffuse white matter abnormality.[217,222-226,229-232] The abnormality consists principally of MRI signal change, usually accompanied by ventricular dilation. The *frequency of the abnormality on MRI, as with PVL at autopsy, increases as a function of postnatal age.* In one well-studied series, the finding of diffuse MRI signal abnormality in premature infants increased from 21% in the first postnatal week, to 53% in the next several weeks, to 79% at term equivalent (see later and Chapter 9).[229] It is likely that at least a major proportion of these cases reflects noncystic PVL, as described earlier. However, the proportion of infants with the diffuse MRI signal abnormality with diffuse white matter gliosis *alone*

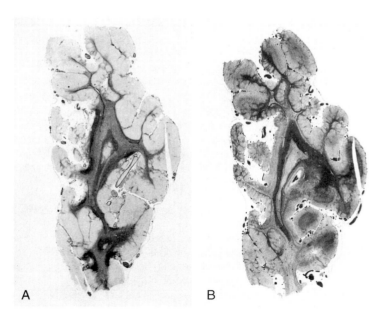

Figure 8-13 **Ulegyria.** Coronal section of cerebrum, stained for, **A**, glial fibers and, **B**, myelin. Note the mushroom-shaped gyri, especially in parasagittal areas. *(From Norman MG: Perinatal brain damage. In Rosenberg HS, Bolande RP, editors:* Perspectives in Pediatric Pathology, *Chicago: 1978, Mosby.)*

A   B

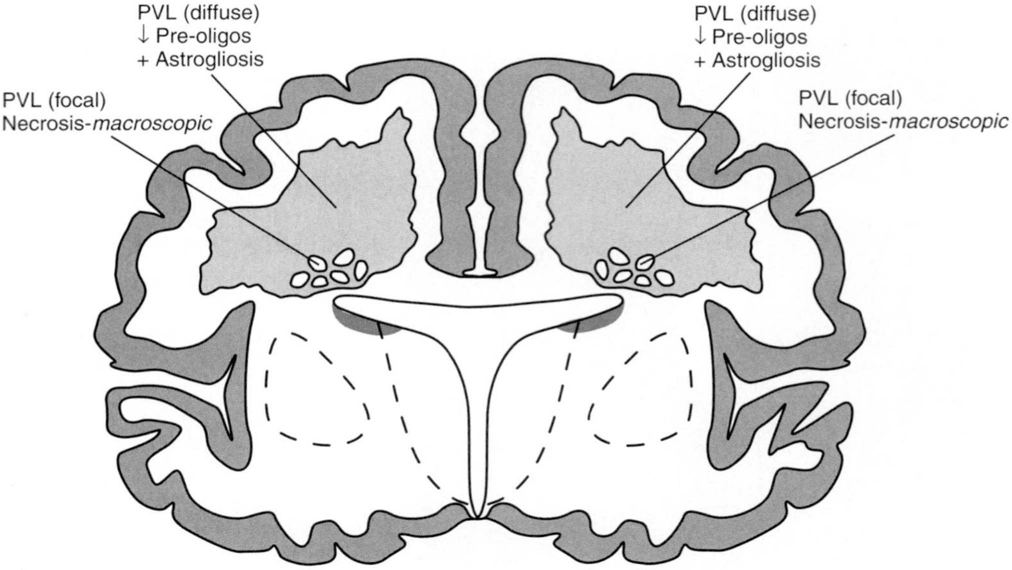

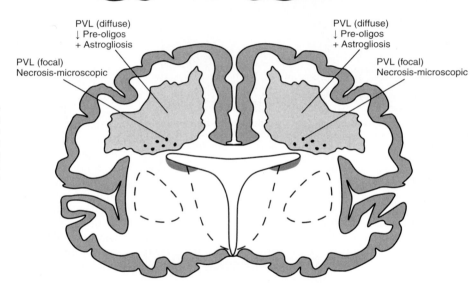

Figure 8-14 Cystic periventricular leukomalacia (PVL), coronal view. Schematic diagram of severe PVL, characterized by macroscopic focal necrotic lesions that become cystic and by diffuse astrogliosis and deficiency of premyelinating oligodendrocytes (pre-oligos).

Figure 8-15 Noncystic periventricular leukomalacia (PVL), coronal view. Schematic diagram shows the two components of the lesion (see Fig. 8-14), but in this less severe form, the focal necrotic lesions are *microscopic* and evolve principally to small glial scars rather than cysts. Pre-oligos, premyelinating oligodendrocytes.

TABLE 8-9	Incidence of Neuropathologically Proven Periventricular White Matter Injury in Premature Infants			
Population Studied	**No.**	**Incidence of White Matter Injury**	**Other Lesions**	**First Author of Report**
Gestational age <38 wk	96	24%	Pontosubicular necrosis: 87% IVH: 74%	Skullerud[80]
Birth weight <1500 g with IVH and survival ≥1 wk	24	75%	Pontine necrosis: 50%	Armstrong[82]
Gestational age ≤34 wk	68	26%		de Vries[200]
Gestational age <33 wk	56	38%		Hope[201]
Birth weight ≤1500 g	86	45% (20% if IVH absent) (53% if IVH present)	IVH: 77%	Takashima[78]
Birth weight <2000 g with ≥6 days (mean, 948 g)	22	68%	Basal ganglia necrosis: 60%	Paneth[202]
"Gestational age" at time of death ≤34 wk	22	32%	IVH: 50%	Carson[203]
Gestational age <37 wk	41	42%	Neuronal loss or gliosis or both: thalamus and basal ganglia 40%–55%, cerebral cortex 10%–30%	Pierson[75]

IVH, intraventricular hemorrhage.

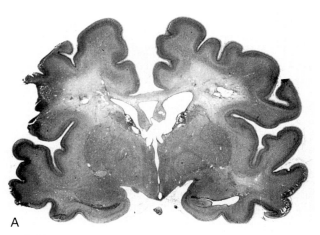 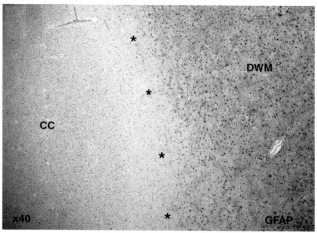

Figure 8-16 Periventricular leukomalacia. A, Coronal section of cerebrum in a premature infant who died with periventricular leukomalacia several weeks after a cardiac arrest. Note the two components of the lesion (i.e., deep *focal* areas of cystic necrosis and more *diffuse* cerebral white matter pallor consistent with loss of developing oligodendrocytes). Note also the diffuse gliosis more peripherally in the cerebral white matter. **B,** Microscopic section showing cerebral cortex (CC), subcortical white matter *(asterisks),* and deeper cerebral white matter (DWM) stained for glial fibrillary acidic protein (GFAP), characteristic of astrocytes. Note the marked astrogliosis in deeper white matter. *(From Haynes RL, Folkerth RD, Keefe R, Sung I, et al: Nitrosative and oxidative injury to premyelinating oligodendrocytes is accompanied by microglial activation in periventricular leukomalacia in the human premature infant,* J Neuropathol Exp Neurol *62:441-450, 2003.)*

(i.e., without microscopic areas of necrosis/glial scars) is unknown and requires clarification.

Cellular and Regional Aspects

Concerning the *gross and regional neuropathology of PVL,* the features of *classic necrotic/cystic PVL* are distinctive and, as just noted, consist primarily of both *focal macroscopic periventricular necrosis* and more *diffuse* cerebral white matter injury (Fig. 8-16).* The focal necrotic lesions occur deep in the cerebral white matter,

---

*See references 3,4,8,78,80,82,197,199-203,206,233-241.

primarily in the distribution of the end zones of the long penetrating arteries (Fig. 8-17). The two most common sites for the focal necroses of PVL are at the level of the cerebral white matter near the trigone of the lateral ventricles and around the foramen of Monro.[199] The predilection for these sites may relate to periventricular vascular anatomical factors and to a concentration of vulnerable pre-OLs, as discussed later. The more diffuse regions of cerebral white matter injury (see Fig. 8-16) have been emphasized particularly in studies with larger numbers of smaller infants with longer periods of postnatal survival.[78,201,202,205,236,238,240-243] In *noncystic PVL* the focal lesions are microscopic and thus are likely to be undetected by cranial ultrasonography during life (see Chapter 9).[201]

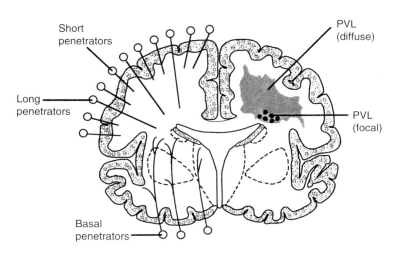

Figure 8-17 Coronal section of cerebrum (schematic) depicting the vascular supply in one hemisphere and the two components (focal and diffuse) of periventricular leukomalacia (PVL) in the other. See text for details. *(Vessels redrawn from Rorke LB: Anatomical features of the developing brain implicated in pathogenesis of hypoxic-ischemic injury,* Brain Pathol *2:211-221, 1992.)*

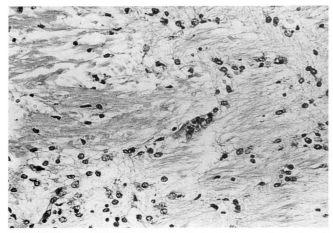

Figure 8-18 Periventricular leukomalacia. (Hematoxylin and eosin stain of region of necrosis ×36.) Note the smudgy area of coagulation necrosis with dark pyknotic nuclei to the *left* and nearly normal white matter to the *right*. *(Courtesy of Dr. Margaret G. Norman.)*

Evolution of the *cellular aspects* of the focal and diffuse components of PVL provides clues to pathogenesis (see later). The *cellular neuropathology of the focal component of classic necrotic/cystic PVL* is characterized in the first 6 to 12 hours after an acute hypoxic-ischemic

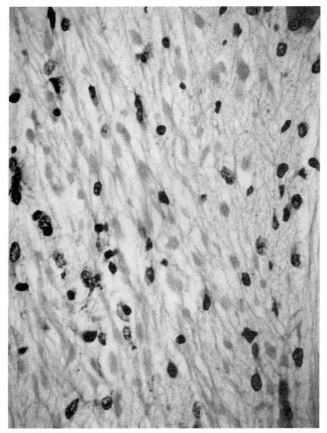

Figure 8-19 Periventricular leukomalacia. (Hematoxylin and eosin stain of region of necrosis ×400.) Note the lighter-stained neuroaxonal swellings ("retraction clubs and balls"). *(Courtesy of Dr. Margaret G. Norman.)*

insult by coagulation necrosis at the sites of the focal periventricular lesion. This lesion appears as a loss of normal architecture and a homogeneous periodic acid–Schiff–positive area of necrosis of all cellular elements (i.e., the acute appearance of a localized infarction) (Fig. 8-18).[197] Round neuroaxonal swellings (retraction clubs and balls) (Fig. 8-19) are prominent, especially at the periphery of the lesion, and immunocytochemical studies have confirmed the abundance of such axonal injury.[244,245] Thus, both within the center of the focal lesion and around its periphery, evidence indicates axonal rupture and, potentially therefore, extravasation of substantial amounts of glutamate, present in millimolar concentrations in neurons, into the periventricular white matter (see later discussion). The cellular response that follows over subsequent days includes infiltration by microglia, proliferation of hypertrophic astrocytes, endothelial hyperplasia, and appearance of foamy macrophages. Subsequent tissue dissolution and cavity formation occur over 1 to 3 weeks. These multiple small cysts are generally large enough (≥3 mm) to be demonstrable by cranial ultrasonography.

The *cellular neuropathology of the diffuse component of classic necrotic/cystic PVL* was emphasized initially particularly by Gilles and co-workers.[13] The cellular hallmarks are pyknotic glial nuclei (i.e., "acutely damaged glia") and hypertrophic astrocytes.[5,13,205] Thus, unlike the focal necroses, this less severe, although more widespread, lesion does not affect all cellular elements. That these cells are early differentiating pre-OLs is suggested by the following observations. First, the neuropathological sequelae of the diffuse injury are hypomyelination and ventriculomegaly.[5,201,202,206] Second, in surviving infants, the principal finding on subsequent brain imaging, particularly MRI, in premature infants with previous imaging evidence for PVL is ventriculomegaly, with diminished cerebral white matter volume (see Chapter 9). Third, and most important, careful immunocytochemical studies show a diminution in pre-OLs in cerebral white matter of infants with PVL (Fig. 8-20).[243,246,247] Whether *surviving* pre-OLs have sustained *nonlethal injury, with loss of processes required for axonal wrapping and myelination*, is unknown. However, this is a critical point because of experimental evidence that NMDA receptors are present in pre-OL processes and, when activated with ischemia, can lead to process destruction (see Chapter 6). Taken together, these findings suggest that the diffuse component of PVL is largely a cell-specific lesion and that the cellular target is the pre-OL.

The cellular pathology of the *diffuse component in noncystic PVL (i.e., without overt macroscopic focal necroses)* is similar to that just described. Studies with modern immunocytochemical techniques and double labeling have provided detailed insight into the nature of diffuse noncystic PVL.[243] Thus, using modern immunocytochemical techniques and double labeling to study autopsy brain tissue from 17 infants with PVL and 28 controls, Haynes and associates made several key observations.[243] First, *the injury to cerebral white matter was regionalized*, with the microscopic areas of necrosis localized in deep periventricular white matter, and less

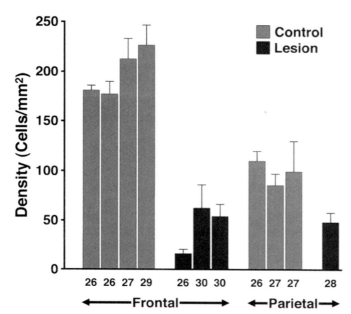

Figure 8-20 Premyelinating oligodendrocytes (pre-OLs) are depleted in early periventricular white matter injury. The density of pre-OLs in three cases *(black bars)* is shown relative to age- and region-matched control cases. *(From Back SA, Luo NL, Mallinson RA, O'Malley JP, et al: Selective vulnerability of preterm white matter to oxidative damage defined by F(2)-isoprostanes, Ann Neurol 58:108-120, 2005.)*

severe, more cell-specific injury present more diffusely in central white matter. The areas of necrosis were followed by small glial scars but not cysts. These regional characteristics are consistent with, although not proof of, the presence of vascular end zones and border zones, more marked in periventricular white matter, and less marked more diffusely in central white matter. Second, in the *diffuse injury, preferential death of pre-OLs occurred;* these cells were identified by specific immunocytochemical markers and were previously shown to be the dominant cell in the oligodendroglial lineage in the cerebral white matter during the period of particular predilection for PVL.[248,249] This observation identifies the pre-OL as the key cellular target in the diffuse white matter injury. Death of these cells likely contributes importantly to the subsequent failure of white matter development, identified by diffusion-based MRI at term, and of myelination, identified by volumetric MRI and conventional brain imaging (see Chapter 9). As noted earlier, even surviving pre-OLs may be unable to wrap axons and carry out myelination because of a loss of processes related to pathological NMDA receptor activation (see "Pathogenesis"). Third, *the diffuse white matter injury contained a marked prominence of astrocytes and activated microglia,* identified by a specific immunocytochemical marker. The prominent activated microglial cells strongly raise the possibility of a role for these cells in the origin of the diffuse injury to pre-OLs (see later). Fourth, specific markers identified *striking evidence in pre-OLs for lipid peroxidation and protein nitration in the diffuse white matter injury.* Evidence of lipid peroxidation in diffuse PVL was also obtained by Back and co-workers.[246] These findings

suggest that the mode of killing of these cells is attack by reactive oxygen species (ROS) and reactive nitrogen species (RNS). Consistent with these direct observations of brain, a study of premature infants found elevated neonatal levels of markers of lipid peroxidation and oxidative protein products in CSF of those who had PVL documented at term by MRI.[250] These several observations have major implications concerning pathogenesis, as discussed later.

Diffuse white matter gliosis alone, without microscopic areas of necrosis and glial scars, is a common finding at postmortem examination of premature infants. In the most recent study, fully 41% of infants had this so-called diffuse white matter gliosis.[75] This white matter finding obviously bears some similarities to the diffuse component of noncystic (and cystic) PVL (see earlier). It remains to be determined whether this diffuse gliosis alone is a mild form of white matter injury on a continuum with PVL (see earlier). Cases with diffuse white matter gliosis alone may contribute to the very frequent finding of abnormal white matter signal on MRI, as noted earlier and discussed in Chapter 9.

Hemorrhage. A not uncommon and occasionally serious complication of classic PVL is hemorrhage into the lesion.[251] This hemorrhage has been observed in approximately 25% of cases of periventricular infarcts studied post mortem.[202,251] Most commonly, the hemorrhage is petechial and circumscribed (Fig. 8-21). However, the hemorrhages within the areas of severe PVL may be massive and, if associated with severe intraventricular hemorrhage, may be difficult to distinguish from the periventricular hemorrhagic venous infarction that can complicate severe intraventricular

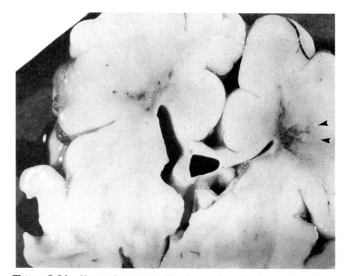

Figure 8-21 Hemorrhage complicating periventricular leukomalacia. Coronal section of cerebrum. Note streaky hemorrhages into the area of periventricular leukomalacia on the *right.* The white spots of the leukomalacia are still visible at the periphery of the lesion *(arrowheads).* This hemorrhagic lesion occurs in the centrum semiovale, dorsal and lateral to the usual site of germinal matrix hemorrhage (see Chapter 11). *(From Armstrong D, Norman MG: Periventricular leucomalacia in neonates: Complications and sequelae, Arch Dis Child 49:367-375, 1974.)*

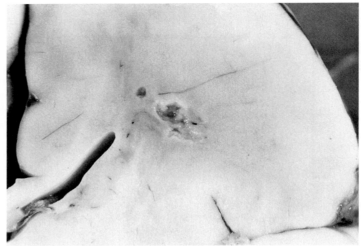

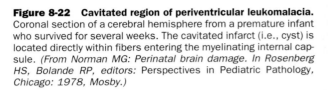

Figure 8-22   Cavitated region of periventricular leukomalacia. Coronal section of a cerebral hemisphere from a premature infant who survived for several weeks. The cavitated infarct (i.e., cyst) is located directly within fibers entering the myelinating internal capsule. *(From Norman MG: Perinatal brain damage. In Rosenberg HS, Bolande RP, editors:* Perspectives in Pediatric Pathology, *Chicago: 1978, Mosby.)*

hemorrhage (see Chapter 11). Microscopically, the distinction is possible because the hemorrhage in PVL occurs on a background of coagulation necrosis, not observed with the venous infarction that can complicate intraventricular hemorrhage.

More importantly, intraventricular hemorrhage is a common accompaniment of PVL (see Table 8-9). Indeed, PVL is more than twice as likely to be found in the presence intraventricular hemorrhage than in its absence. This observation may be relevant to a potential role of iron in the generation of ROS (see "Pathogenesis" later).

Neuropathological Sequelae. The end result of PVL, of course, depends on the size of the initial lesion and the time after the acute insult. With large *focal periventricular lesions*, as noted earlier, some degree of tissue dissolution is often apparent macroscopically after 1 to 3 weeks (Fig. 8-22). These small *cavities* are usually multiple and are visualized readily by cranial ultrasonography, if of sufficient size, also as noted earlier (see Chapter 9). With progression of gliosis, these cavities usually constrict, and some may no longer be visualizable by ultrasonography (Fig. 8-23). Subsequently, *deficient myelin* and *focal ventricular dilation*, usually in the region of the trigone of the lateral ventricles, are the chronic sequelae. With more *diffuse involvement of cerebral white matter, deficient myelin* with more *diffuse ventricular dilation*, but almost always with a predominant involvement of the trigone, provides macroscopic evidence of the lesion.

Gray Matter Disease. Although cerebral white matter disease with subsequently impaired myelination classically has been considered the principal result of PVL of the premature infant, more recent findings, initially and principally from quantitative MRI studies, suggested that *gray matter disease is a common and important accompaniment*. In the following subsections, I discuss first the imaging findings and next the anatomical data.

Quantitative Magnetic Resonance Imaging Studies. Advanced MRI techniques applied to *premature infants*

as early as term equivalent suggest that gray matter abnormalities are important features of the neuropathology of prematurity, especially in the presence of cerebral white matter injury.

The first clear indication from advanced MRI of a disturbance in the cerebral cortex in premature infants emanated from the study of Inder and associates.[252] Thus, when compared with cerebral cortical gray matter volume in healthy term infants, a 28% reduction in cortical gray matter was observed at term in 10 premature infants who had earlier MRI evidence for PVL, defined as either cystic (n = 5) or noncystic (n = 5). A small (n = 14) later series of premature infants without overt white matter lesions showed at term a quantitative deficit in the complexity of cortical folding,[253] a finding raising the possibility of a disturbance of cerebral cortical development in the absence of *major* white matter injury. Apparent deficits in volume of several cerebral cortical regions, especially parieto-occipital cortex, were identified in 10 premature infants studied at 35 weeks' postmenstrual age by Peterson and associates.[254] The most decisive demonstrations of a disturbance of gray matter in premature infants as early as term equivalent were obtained more recently in reports of approximately 200 consecutively studied premature infants and 36 normal term-born infants.[223,225,255] Infants with MRI-defined white matter injury had 33% lower cerebral cortical gray matter volume, consistent with the earlier findings by Inder and associates in a much smaller cohort (see Chapter 2, Fig. 2-52).[223] However, unlike the earlier report of 10 preterm infants with white matter injury, in the larger study of 119 infants, 80% of the infants with white matter injury exhibited apparent *noncystic* disease. The region of brain most affected was the parieto-occipital region, a site of predilection for PVL.[255] Additionally, overall the volume of deep nuclear structures was significantly lower in the preterm than in the term-born infants, and this significant volumetric deficit was greatest not only in infants with white matter injury but also in the most immature infants. Moreover, the neuronal deficits in both cerebral cortex and deep nuclear structures correlated with moderate to severe neurodevelopmental

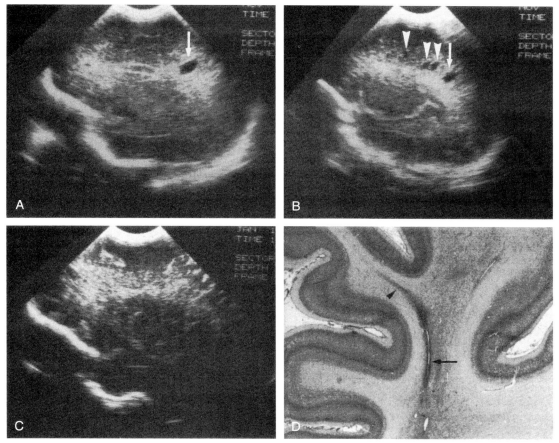

Figure 8-23 **Ultrasonographic-pathological study of constriction of cavities in periventricular leukomalacia. A** and **B**, Parasagittal ultrasound scans at 7 weeks of age at two angles show periventricular echolucencies *(arrows* and *arrowheads)* with an echogenic background, consistent with cystic periventricular leukomalacia. **C**, At 15 weeks of age, no cavities are visible on the ultrasound scan. **D**, Post mortem (at 18 weeks of age), a coronal section through the left parietal lobe shows only a slitlike cavity *(arrow)* in the center of thin glial bands extending from the corona radiata into the paracentral white matter *(arrowhead).* (Cresyl violet ×10.) *(From Rodriguez J, Claus D, Verellen G, Lyon G: Periventricular leukomalacia: Ultrasonic and neuropathological correlations,* Dev Med Child Neurol *32:347-352, 1990.)*

disability at 1 and 2 years of age.[223,225] Taken together, the volumetric findings at term equivalent show pronounced deficits in cerebral cortical and deep nuclear gray matter volumes. The deficits are unequivocal in infants with white matter disease that is not necessarily severe. The white matter disease is consistent with noncystic PVL, although to what extent MRI can distinguish the latter from diffuse white matter gliosis alone is unknown. Whether less pronounced neuronal deficits are also present in infants with *no* MRI-demonstrable white matter disease also remains to be clarified.

The disturbances of gray matter identified in the neonatal period at term equivalent appear to presage long-term structural disturbances. Thus, advanced MRI techniques applied to *children and adults who were born prematurely* have shown distinct abnormalities in cerebral gray matter.[256-264b] Decreased cerebral cortical gray matter volumes have been shown most consistently.[256-262] However, abnormalities of cortical thickness and fiber tract development also have been found. Regional differences in the cerebral cortical volumetric deficits have been shown, with the most pronounced decreases generally in sensorimotor, parieto-occipital,

temporal, and hippocampal cortices.[256-258,261] In addition to decreases in cerebral cortical volumes, decreases in volumes of deep nuclear structures (e.g., basal ganglia and thalamus, usually studied in combination) have been documented.[257,259-261,265] The functional significance of these various neuronal disturbances in former premature infants is suggested by correlations of the cortical or deep nuclear deficits with abnormal cognitive measures.[256,257,259,261,266] *The extent to which these findings in children and adolescents relate to neonatal white matter injury is not entirely clear*, because the infants were evaluated in the neonatal period by imaging modalities (e.g., ultrasonography) generally ineffective for detection of noncystic white matter disease.

Neuropathological Studies. Delineation of the neuropathological substrate underlying the deficits in cerebral cortical and deep nuclear volumes defined by imaging, especially in premature infants with white matter disease, is critical to help define the mechanisms leading to the deficits. The cellular elements of particular concern are cerebral cortical neurons, underlying subplate neurons, white matter axons (ascending thalamocortical, descending corticofugal, commissural

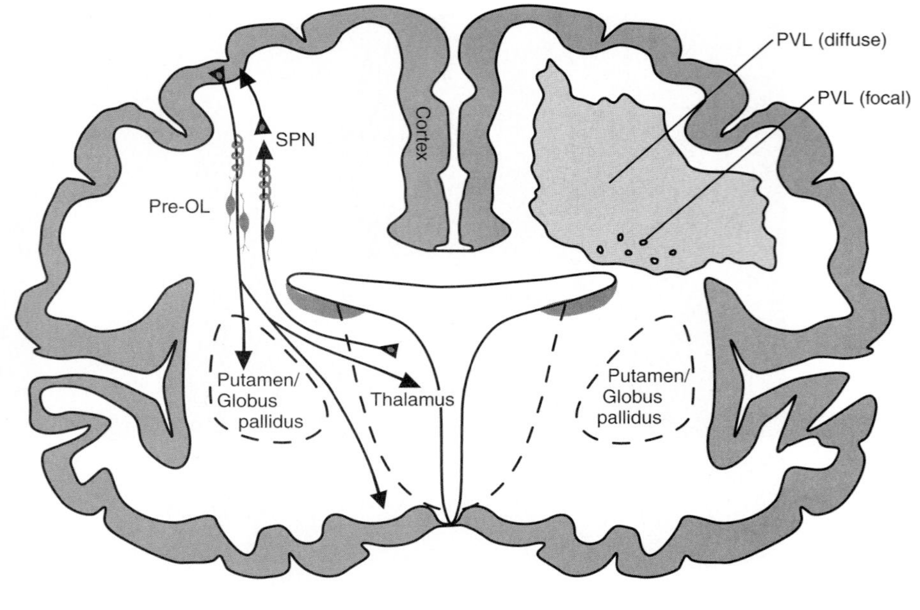

Figure 8-24 Schematic diagram of the developing thalamocortical connections. Thalamic afferents in the early third trimester synapse transiently on subplate neurons (SPNs) (see Chapter 2). The connections of SPNs to cortex are important for cortical development. The wrapping of premyelinating oligodendrocytes (pre-OLs) around white matter axons also is active during this developmental period (see Chapter 2). PVL, periventricular leukomalacia. See text for details.

and corticocortical association fibers), and deep nuclear neurons, especially those of the thalamus. These elements comprise an interacting corticothalamic unit, as described later (Fig. 8-24). The key question in premature infants is whether one or more of the components of this neuronal-axonal unit sustain changes that are destructive or dysgenetic, or both.

Neuropathological studies of *cerebral cortical or thalamic neuronal* structures in premature infants are relatively few. Earlier work indicated that neuronal injury may accompany severe forms of PVL.[82,197,239,267,268] The most detailed neuropathological analysis of premature infants in a modern neonatal intensive care unit involved 41 premature infants (Fig. 8-25).[75] The findings were noted earlier concerning *selective neuronal necrosis.* Thus, the major findings were evidence of neuronal loss or gliosis, or both, in thalamus and basal ganglia in 40% to 55% of infants, in cerebral cortex in 10% to 30% of infants, and in brain stem (basis

pontis, inferior olivary nuclei) in nearly 90%. Notably, *nearly all the involvement of thalamus/basal ganglia and cerebral cortex occurred in the infants with PVL, and virtually all the PVL was noncystic.* Infants with diffuse white matter gliosis alone had minimal gray matter disease. Whether the findings in deep nuclear structures and cortex reflect direct injury or retrograde or anterograde transsynaptic effects is unclear.

Neuropathological evidence of *axonal* injury in premature infants is limited to studies of infants dying with classic cystic PVL.[74,241,244,245,247,269,269a] Early descriptions of PVL included the observation that axonal swellings or spheroids, indicative of acute axonal injury, are present in the necrotic foci.[197,267] More extensive axonal injury around necrotic foci was detected by immunocytochemical staining for beta-amyloid precursor protein, a marker of axonal damage.[74,241,244,245,269,269a] However, neuropathological investigation of possible axonal injury in the more

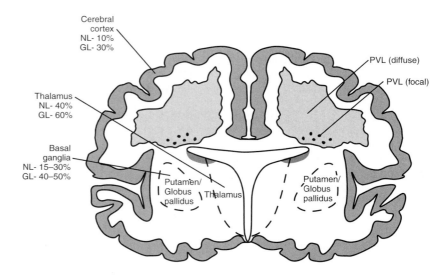

Figure 8-25 Neuronal loss and gliosis in cerebral cortex, thalamus, and basal ganglia in premature infants with PVL (periventricular leukomalacia). The schematic diagram is in coronal section. GL, gliosis; NL, neuronal loss. See text for details.

common noncystic white matter injury characteristic of most of the living premature infants studied by quantitative volumetric MRI is lacking (see Fig. 8-24). Thus, the role of this key component of the neuronal-axonal unit in the genesis of the cortical or thalamic volumetric deficits is a key topic for future work.

The pivotal intermediary neuronal component in the corticothalamic unit is the *subplate neuron*, the only neuronal element of developing cerebral white matter (see Fig. 8-24). This component is central to both cortical and thalamic development (see later). The neuropathological changes of this white matter neuronal constituent in human premature infants have not been delineated. Subplate neurons contain excitatory amino acid receptors and have been shown in a developing animal model to be selectively vulnerable to hypoxia-ischemia.[270] Indeed, a recent preliminary study of developing *human* brain showed that subplate neurons exhibit an exuberant overexpression of Ca^{2+}-permeable AMPA receptors during the peak period of vulnerability to PVL (see Fig. 8-6).[271] Because hypoxia-ischemia and excitotoxicity are important in the pathogenesis of white matter injury (see next), and the presence of white matter injury is associated with the cortical and deep nuclear volumetric deficits, a potential role for concomitant injury to subplate neurons in this situation is raised. Initial data support this possibility.[247] More detailed study is needed.

Thus, it is clear that the neuropathology of neuronal-axonal elements in the human infant largely remains to be defined. Currently, available data indicate that neuronal and axonal injury per se is relatively common in overt necrotic/cystic PVL. However, application of modern immunocytochemical techniques to detect sublethal injury to neurons or axons and perhaps subsequently impaired development to these structures is needed to assess the large proportion of infants with noncystic PVL.

Potential Mechanisms Underlying the Relationship of PVL to Neuronal Deficits. The cerebral cortical and deep nuclear neuronal deficits just described could relate to a variety of mechanisms, in basic nature principally either destructive or developmental, or both. These potential mechanisms are discussed briefly next.

Regarding *neurons of deep nuclear structures and cerebral cortex,* evidence of *acute destructive disease (i.e., overt neuronal necrosis)* is generally lacking.[75,243] However, *neuronal loss and gliosis* are common, especially in the thalamus and basal ganglia. Involvement of these deep nuclear structures is apparent in approximately one half of the infants (see earlier). Whether this injury reflects a direct effect or is a secondary trophic disturbance is unclear. A *developmental or trophic effect* on thalamic neurons could occur secondary to interruption of afferent or efferent axonal connections (see Fig. 8-24). This mechanism ultimately could affect the cerebral cortex, as suggested by the anatomical studies of severe PVL by Marin-Padilla,[239] who demonstrated distinct alterations in morphology and organization of neurons and neuronal processes in the cerebral cortex

overlying relatively severe necrotic/cystic PVL weeks and months after the neonatal period. Whether these secondary developmental effects could occur in living infants with the less severe noncystic white matter injury seems possible but remains to be proven. Relevant in this context is the probable trophic disturbance that underlies the *diminished cerebellar growth* in premature infants with cerebral white matter injury (see earlier).[121,122,124,272,273]

Subplate neurons are crucial for cortical and thalamic neuronal *development* and, if injured, could lead to profound neuronal abnormalities.[274-279] Thus, subplate neurons reach their peak abundance in the human infant during the gestational period of human prematurity, particularly the period of peak vulnerability to PVL (i.e., 22 to 34 weeks).[274,276,280] These cells, which serve as transient sites for connections by awaiting afferents to the developing cerebral cortex (thalamocortical and corticocortical axonal projections), may guide axons to cortical and subcortical targets and are involved in the structural and functional maturation of the cerebral cortex and the thalamus (see Fig. 8-24).[217,274-289] As noted earlier, in a neonatal rat model, subplate neurons exhibit a selective vulnerability to hypoxia-ischemia.[270] The exuberant expression of excitatory amino acid receptors in the human subplate during the peak period of vulnerability to PVL suggests a similar vulnerability (see Fig. 8-6 and earlier discussion). Initial neuropathological data in human premature infants are also consistent with such vulnerability.[247] The critical issue of the status of subplate neurons in the human premature infant is a key topic for future research.

Axonal disturbance could have a profound impact on cortical and thalamic neuronal *development* by retrograde and anterograde effects and potentially thereby on the volumetric measures detected by MRI (see Fig. 8-24). Very little is known about the status of axons in human premature infants. To elucidate axonal development during this period, our group undertook a study of cerebral white matter by immunocytochemical and Western blot analysis in 46 normative cases beginning at 20 postconceptional weeks.[290] The findings were unexpected and dramatic (see Chapter 2). Thus, although axons were clearly detectable as early as 23 weeks, specific markers indicated that these axons were clearly immature. Importantly, GAP-43, a marker of axonal growth and elongation, showed high levels of expression (four- to fivefold greater than the adult) throughout the premature period, a finding indicating that these *immature axons are in a phase of very active development*. These data appear to define the *human premature period as a critical period in axonal development*. As such, it is likely that these immature axons are highly vulnerable to injurious insults (e.g., ischemia, inflammation). Indeed, axons are known to be vulnerable to ischemia.[291,292,292a] Additionally, oligodendroglial-axonal interactions are critical for axonal survival, maturation, and function.[293-297] Thus, in the diffuse component of PVL, the injury to pre-OLs[243] could ultimately contribute to impaired axonal number or maturation, or both (see Fig. 8-24). Potentially supportive of a

TABLE 8-10 **Periventricular Leukomalacia: Pathogenesis***

Periventricular Vascular Anatomical and Physiological Factors
Arterial end zones and border zones
Very low physiological blood flow to cerebral white matter
Cerebral Ischemia, Impaired Cerebrovascular Autoregulation, and Pressure-Passive Cerebral Circulation
Danger of systemic hypotension
Danger of marked hypocarbia
Infection and Inflammation
Propensity for maternal/intrauterine infection and for fetal systemic inflammatory response
Propensity for postnatal infection
Presence of Toll-like receptors on microglia capable of producing pre-OL death on activation by release of ROS, RNS, and
    cytokines
Maturation-dependent concentration of microglia in cerebral white matter during the peak period of vulnerability to PVL
Interferon-gamma expression in astrocytes of human cerebral white matter, especially in diffuse PVL
Interferon-gamma receptor expression on pre-OLs
TNF-alpha in cerebrospinal fluid and brain in PVL
Interferon-gamma toxicity potentiated by TNF-alpha and greater to pre-OLs than to mature cells
Potentiating Relationship of Infection/Inflammation and Ischemia
Infection/inflammation leading to impaired cerebral perfusion
Microglia as a convergence point for both infection/inflammation and ischemia
Intrinsic Vulnerability of Cerebral White Matter of Premature Newborn
Vulnerability of pre-OLs to free radical attack
  Production of both ROS and RNS
  Deficient antioxidant defenses
  Acquisition of iron
Vulnerability of pre-OLs to excitotoxicity
  Exuberant expression of glutamate transporter
  Exuberant expression of AMPA receptors, which also are deficient in the GluR2 subunit and therefore calcium permeable
  Exuberant expression of NMDA receptors, which are calcium permeable
Presence of other potentially vulnerable, rapidly differentiating cellular elements
  Subplate neurons
  Axons

*Includes those factors shown in *human* premature brain (see Chapter 6 for *additional factors* based on *experimental* studies).
AMPA, alpha-amino-3-hydroxy-5-methyl-4-isoxazolepropionic acid; NMDA, *N*-methyl-D-aspartate; pre-OLs, premyelinating oligodendrocytes; PVL, peri-
    ventricular leukomalacia; RNS, reactive nitrogen species; ROS, reactive oxygen species; TNF, tumor necrosis factor.

disturbance in axonal development in premature infants are diffusion-based MRI studies that show white matter abnormalities consistent with (though not specific for) impaired axonal development.[231,264b,298-303,303a] *Thus, taken together, these data raise the possibility that axonal disturbance is present in premature infants and could be related, perhaps causally, to deficits in cerebral cortical and deep nuclear (especially thalamic) neuronal development.* More data clearly are needed.

Pathogenesis

The pathogenesis of PVL is related to a remarkable confluence of maturation-dependent pathogenetic factors that conspire to render the cerebral white matter of the human premature infant vulnerable to injury (Table 8-10). The result is a propensity to injury initiated by two major *upstream mechanisms,* especially *ischemia* but also *infection/inflammation* (see Table 8-10) (Fig. 8-26). These mechanisms may operate in concert to potentiate each other. The critical *downstream mechanisms* are *excitotoxicity* and *free radical attack* by both ROS and RNS (see later).

Ischemia. Premature infants appear to have a propensity for the development of cerebral ischemia, especially to white matter. The likely reasons for this propensity include (1) the presence of vascular end zones and

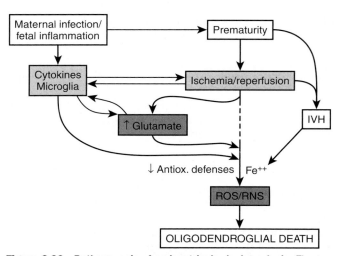

Figure 8-26 **Pathogenesis of periventricular leukomalacia.** The two major upstream mechanisms are ischemia and infection/inflammation *(lighter shading).* The two major downstream mechanisms are excitotoxicity and free radical attack by reactive oxygen and nitrogen species *(darker shading).* Antiox., antioxidant; Fe++, iron; IVH, intraventricular hemorrhage. See Chapter 6 for details.

border zones in cerebral white matter and (2) an impairment of regulation of CBF. These two factors are discussed next.

Periventricular Vascular Anatomical and Physiological Factors. The *deep focal necrotic lesions* of PVL occur in areas that are considered *arterial end zones.*[3,7,304-309] (The earlier concept that the deep periventricular region also contained arterial border zones involving so-called ventriculofugal arteries[304,306] is not supported by the later studies of Gilles and co-workers.[129,130]) The periventricular arterial end zones have been described best by Rorke,[7] Larroche,[3] and Takashima and co-workers.[307,309] The vessels penetrating the cerebral wall from the pial surface, the long penetrators, are derived from the middle cerebral artery, and, to a lesser extent, the anterior or posterior cerebral artery, and they terminate in the deep periventricular white matter (see Fig. 8-17). The end zones that result appear to be the sites for the focal necroses of PVL (see Fig. 8-17). These arterial end zones are essentially *distal fields*, and, as such, these periventricular zones would be expected to be most susceptible to a fall in perfusion pressure and CBF. The period over the last 16 weeks of human gestation has been shown to be one of active development of this periventricular vasculature.[7,307,308,310,311] Indeed, this development could be used as an index of cerebrovascular maturity.[307] Infants with PVL exhibited avascular areas at the periventricular site of focal necrosis of white matter (Fig. 8-27).[307,308] In a series of infants with PVL, Takashima and co-workers[307,308] distinguished two groups: one in which the deep periventricular branches were relatively well developed and one in which they were not. The latter infants, usually more premature, more often had no history of neonatal clinical complications, whereas the former infants did. *The data suggest that the degree of ischemia required to produce the focal necrotic*

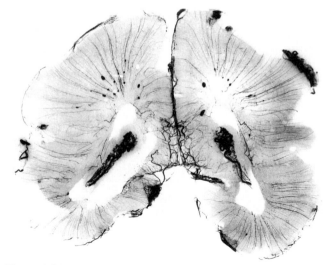

Figure 8-27 **Microangiography of the occipital region in a premature infant with periventricular leukomalacia.** Note the avascular areas at the sites of leukomalacia. *(From Takashima S, Tanaka K: Development of cerebrovascular architecture and its relationship to periventricular leukomalacia, Arch Neurol 35:11-16, 1978.)*

lesions of PVL may vary depending on the state of development of the periventricular vessels and that this state of development is primarily a function of gestational age.

The pathogenesis of *the more diffuse white matter injury*, similarly, may relate in part to the *development* of the *penetrating* cerebral vasculature more peripherally.[7,305,307,308,311] Thus, as emphasized by Rorke,[7] the penetrating cerebral arteries can be divided into the long penetrators that terminate deep in periventricular white matter, as just discussed in relation to the periventricular focal necroses, and the short penetrators that extend only into subcortical white matter (see Fig. 8-17). At 24 to 28 weeks of gestation, the long penetrators have relatively few side branches and infrequent intraparenchymal anastomoses with each other and with the short penetrators, which importantly also are relatively sparse.[7] Thus, end zones and border zones may exist at this time in the cerebral white matter relatively distant from the periventricular region. From 32 weeks to term, increases in the development of the short penetrators and in anastomoses between the long and short penetrators occur and perhaps thereby lead to a decrease in vulnerable end zones and border zones in the subcortical and central cerebral white matter.

A *physiological correlate of these vascular anatomical factors appears to be the extremely low blood flow to cerebral white matter in the human premature newborn*, first shown by our work with positron emission tomography.[312] The likelihood of extremely low white matter flows was suggested initially by the results of xenon clearance studies that documented mean global CBF values in ventilated human premature infants of only approximately 10 to 12 mL/100 g/minute.[313] Subsequent xenon studies confirmed these very low mean global values (see Chapter 6).[127,314-319] Our studies of *regional* CBF by positron emission tomography confirmed the low global values, but, more important, they showed that values in cerebral white matter in surviving preterm infants with normal or nearly normal neurological outcome ranged from only 1.6 to 3.0 mL/100 g/minute.[312] These remarkably low values in white matter were approximately 25% of those in cortical gray matter, a regional difference confirmed in a study using single photon emission tomography.[320] Our blood flow values of less than 5.0 mL/100 g/minute in normal or nearly normal cerebral white matter in the preterm infant are markedly less than the threshold value for viability in adult human brain of 10 mL/100 g/minute (*normal* CBF in the adult is ≈50 mL/100 g/minute).[321] *The very low values of volemic flow in cerebral white matter in the human premature infant suggest a minimal margin of safety for blood flow to cerebral white matter in such infants.*

Thus, these maturation-dependent cerebrovascular factors, coupled with the neuropathology of PVL discussed earlier, suggest that the focal necroses, affecting all cellular elements and localized to deep cerebral white matter, are related to relatively severe ischemia. The more peripheral diffuse cerebral white matter injury, affecting principally early differentiating oligodendroglia or oligodendroglial precursor cells,

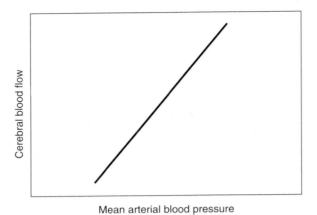

Figure 8-28 Pressure-passive relationship of cerebral blood flow and mean arterial blood pressure. See text for details.

although relatively sparing of other cellular elements, may be related to less severe ischemia.

Cerebral Ischemia, Impaired Cerebrovascular Autoregulation, and Pressure-Passive Cerebral Circulation. The vascular end zones and border zones just described would render the premature infant's brain particularly vulnerable to injury in the presence of cerebral ischemia. Perhaps of particular importance in the genesis of impaired CBF and thereby cerebral ischemia is an apparent impairment of cerebrovascular regulation in sick premature infants. Thus, earlier seminal studies employing the invasive technique of radioactive xenon clearance showed that certain premature infants, mechanically ventilated and often clinically unstable, appear to exhibit a pressure-passive cerebral circulation (Fig. 8-28).[322-325] This fundamental observation has been confirmed by less invasive methods multiple times.[326-330] Thus, in such sick premature infants with a pressure-passive cerebral circulation, it would be expected that when blood pressure falls, as occurs commonly in such infants, so would CBF, with the consequence of ischemia in the distribution of the arterial end zones and border zones in cerebral white matter. Moreover, the particular danger is compounded by the demonstration that blood flow to cerebral white matter of the infant is very low (see earlier), and a minimal margin of safety may thereby exist.

The proportion of infants with a pressure-passive cerebral circulation and the duration of the abnormality are substantial (see Chapter 6). In a serial study of 32 mechanically ventilated premature infants from the first hours, near-infrared spectroscopy was used to demonstrate a pressure-passive cerebral circulation in 53% (see Chapter 9, Fig. 9-47).[328] The nadirs of blood pressure often are not markedly low and thus could be readily overlooked with routine monitoring. However, the cumulative effects of repeated modest declines in CBF, including potentiation of excitotoxicity and free radical accumulation, could be considerable. This concern is accentuated by the repeated finding from neuropathological and imaging studies that the incidence of PVL increases with advancing postnatal age (see earlier). In the study of Tsuji and colleagues, nearly all the

cases of PVL (and severe intraventricular hemorrhage) were in the pressure-passive group.[328] Although the numbers were small, the observations suggested that (1) infants with impaired cerebrovascular autoregulation and a pressure-passive cerebral circulation could be identified by near-infrared spectroscopy before the occurrence of white matter injury, (2) the circulatory abnormality was related to the occurrence of such injury, and (3) if the pressure-passive state could be corrected, perhaps the white matter injury could be prevented. Clearly more data are needed.

In a later, more detailed study of a larger number of infants (N = 90), pressure-passive periods were identified in 95% of the infants, and the overall mean proportion of the pressure-passive time was 20%.[330] Some infants had a pressure-passive circulation more than 50% of the time. The likelihood of a pressure-passive state increased with decreasing gestational age and periods of hypotension.

Clinically stable premature infants seem less likely to exhibit this apparent lack of cerebrovascular autoregulation.[313,314,324,331,332] With intact cerebrovascular autoregulation, CBF is not pressure passive but rather remains constant over a wide range of blood pressure because of arteriolar dilation with decreases in blood pressure and arteriolar constriction with increases in blood pressure (see the curve for the mature "child" in Fig. 8-29). However, experimental studies indicate that during the maturation of cerebrovascular autoregulation, an early phase occurs in which the range of blood pressure over which CBF is maintained constant, although present, is narrow, and the normal blood pressure is near the downslope of the autoregulatory curve (see the curve for "premature" in Fig. 8-29, and see also Chapter 6). Such a situation would render even the premature infant with intact autoregulation vulnerable to less than severe declines in blood pressure.

The propensity to a pressure-passive abnormality in premature infants may relate in part to an absent muscularis around penetrating cerebral arteries and arterioles in the third trimester in the human brain.[129,130] Additional potential reasons for a pressure-passive cerebral

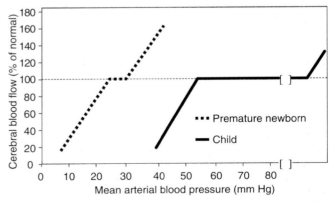

Figure 8-29 Probable relationships between cerebral blood flow and mean arterial blood pressure in the healthy premature newborn and the mature child. See text for details.

circulation in such infants include hypercarbia or hypoxemia related to respiratory disease, the mechanical trauma of labor or vaginal delivery to the easily deformed cranium of the premature infant, and, as just noted, the occurrence of normal blood pressures that are dangerously close to the downslope of a normal "immature" autoregulatory curve (see Fig. 8-29).[220,324,326-329,333] A combination of these factors or still-to-be-defined perturbants (e.g., cytokine vascular effects) could be operative.

Finally, *even in the presence of intact cerebrovascular autoregulation*, marked cerebral vasoconstriction or severe systemic hypotension could lead to sufficiently impaired CBF to the cerebral vascular end zones and border zones to result in cerebral white matter injury. This explanation may account for the demonstrated relationships between marked hypocarbia or hypotension and PVL.[198,314,334-340] Moreover, hypotension and related models of cerebral hypoperfusion have been shown to lead to selective or predominant cerebral white matter injury in *many* experimental models involving developing animals (see Chapter 6). A recent study of 905 infants (birth weight, 501 to 1249 g) evaluated a *cumulative* index of hypocarbia over the first 7 days of life and found a strong association with the occurrence of PVL (identified as echolucencies on cranial ultrasonography) (Fig. 8-30). Infants with the highest quartile of cumulative index of exposure to hypocarbia had more than a fivefold increased risk of PVL, when compared with those infants in the lowest quartile.[340]

Additional evidence supportive of a relationship between impaired CBF and the occurrence of PVL includes the association of the lesion with markers of hypoxic-ischemic events (e.g., neonatal acidosis, elevations of plasma uric acid on the first day of life), episodes of mean arterial

TABLE 8-11	**Prominence at Autopsy of Periventricular White Matter Injury among Hypoxic-Ischemic Lesions in Infants Treated with Extracorporeal Membrane Oxygenation***
Lesion	**No. (Percentage of Total)[†]**
Periventricular leukomalacia	18 (78%)
Diffuse white matter injury	8 (35%)
Selective neuronal necrosis	
Thalamus	9 (39%)
Inferior olivary nucleus	8 (35%)
Cerebral infarction[‡]	7 (30%)

*Derived from 23 infants (born at 35–41 weeks of gestation) treated with extracorporeal membrane oxygenation at Boston Children's Hospital from 1984 to 1991.[360] Nine infants (39%) also sustained subdural, subarachnoid, or intraparenchymal hemorrhage (see Chapter 10).

[†]Infants often had more than one lesion; thus, percentages exceed 100%.

[‡]Four infarcts were hemorrhagic.

blood pressure less than 30 mm Hg, hypovolemia, oliguria, abrupt decreases in blood pressure in chronically hypertensive premature newborns (in whom cerebrovascular autoregulation may be present but with the curve shifted to the right), patent ductus arteriosus, congenital heart disease, and severely ill infants treated with ECMO, or cardiac surgery.[72,333,341-353b] The adverse effect of patent ductus arteriosus on the cerebral circulation, documented by earlier studies,[354-356] as well as subsequently,[347,357-359] supports a direct link between cerebral ischemia and PVL. Thus, infants with the most severe derangement of CBF (i.e., retrograde flow in diastole) had a 36% incidence of PVL (ultrasonographic criteria) versus a 15% incidence in those infants with no retrograde flow.[347] The high frequency of the lesion in the hypoxemic and hypotensive infants treated with ECMO also demonstrates a striking relationship with apparent cerebral ischemia (Table 8-11).[360] Other pathological evidence for generalized ischemic insults (e.g., selective neuronal necrosis) also was present in these infants (see Table 8-11). The occurrence of focal cerebral infarction in this patient group probably relates to other factors (i.e., carotid ligation, embolus, and thrombus; see later discussion and Chapter 10). Similarly, in the largest autopsy series of infants dying after cardiac surgery, PVL was the dominant lesion (nearly 80% of cases).[72] Finally, a relationship of cerebral ischemia with PVL may be operative in infants with apneic spells. A relationship of apnea and bradycardia with PVL has been suspected for many years because earlier work, carried out before the era of cranial ultrasonography, showed an association between spastic diplegia and apneic-bradycardic episodes.[361] Studies of CBF velocity by Doppler showed an impairment in cerebral flow velocity with mild to moderate bradycardia (80 to 100 beats/minute) and a marked impairment with severe bradycardia (<80 beats/minute) (Fig. 8-31).[362] Studies with near-infrared spectroscopy documented a sharp decrease in cerebral oxygenated hemoglobin and cerebral blood volume in association with apneic spells

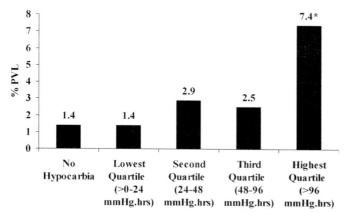

Figure 8-30 Cumulative index of hypocarbia in the first week of life and the occurrence of periventricular leukomalacia (PVL). The study involved 925 infants with a range of birth weights of 501 to 1249 g. PVL was identified by the occurrence of echolucencies on cranial ultrasonography at approximately 28 days of age. Hypocarbia was defined as an arterial partial pressure of carbon dioxide ($Paco_2$) lower than 35 mm Hg, and the cumulative index of exposure to hypocarbia was calculated as ($35 - Paco_2$) multiplied by the time interval in hours for each 6-hour block in a 24-hour day. The frequency of PVL in the highest quartile of the cumulative index of exposure differed from that with no hypocarbia ($P < .03$). (From Shankaran S, Langer JC, Kazzi SN, Laptook AR, et al: Cumulative index of exposure to hypocarbia and hyperoxia as risk factors for periventricular leukomalacia in low birth weight infants, Pediatrics 118:1654-1659, 2006.)

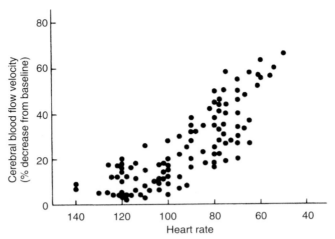

Figure 8-31 **Effect of apnea and bradycardia on cerebral blood flow velocity.** Cerebral blood flow velocity, quantitated as area under the velocity curve, is shown as a function of heart rate with apnea in premature infants. Individual values for 101 separate episodes of apnea and bradycardia are shown. *(From Perlman JM, Volpe JJ: Episodes of apnea and bradycardia in the preterm newborn: Impact on cerebral circulation,* Pediatrics *76:333-338, 1985.)*

with bradycardia,[363-366] and findings were consistent with the likelihood of a decrease in CBF with such spells.

These anatomical, pathological, and physiological data indicate that PVL is strongly related etiologically to ischemia. It remains to be explained, however, why ischemia in the premature infant does not result in the parasagittal cerebral injury observed in the full-term infant with ischemia (see previous section). The *relative sparing of parasagittal cerebral cortex and subcortical white matter* is apparently the result of the presence of many meningeal interarterial anastomoses among the anterior, middle, and posterior cerebral arteries, anastomoses characteristic of the fetal brain, which do not regress until approximately term.[7,305,367,368] This explanation is supported by the observation that, in the mature cat, which has interarterial anastomoses comparable to those in the human fetal brain, PVL, and not parasagittal watershed infarcts, is produced by generalized cerebral ischemia associated with experimental occlusion of the basilar artery and subsequent narrowing of one or both carotid arteries.[369] The nature and temporal characteristics of the ischemic insult(s) for PVL also likely are quite different from the more acute insult that leads to parasagittal cerebral injury in the term infant.

Infection/Inflammation. Infection/inflammation is the second major upstream event in pathogenesis (see Table 8-10 and Fig. 8-26). Thus, an important series of clinical/epidemiological, neuropathological, and experimental studies suggested that maternal intrauterine infection and fetal systemic inflammation were involved in the pathogenesis of a proportion of cases of PVL. Postnatal infection may be a previously underestimated factor. The magnitude of the role of infection/inflammation and especially the potential mechanisms thereof are still unresolved issues.

Clinical/Epidemiological Observations. Clinical and epidemiological studies suggest a link between maternal and fetal infection and inflammation and the occurrence of PVL.[370,371] The most commonly held view is that maternal intrauterine infection causes a fetal systemic inflammatory response that results in injury to cerebral white matter. The fetal systemic inflammatory response, recognized for many years, is defined in considerable part by detection of proinflammatory cytokines in blood. A relationship with PVL or associated cerebral palsy in premature infants is suggested by the finding of increased incidence of these outcomes in the presence of (1) evidence for maternal and fetal infection/inflammation (e.g., chorioamnionitis, funisitis, premature rupture of membranes),[209,210,370-380] (2) elevated levels of proinflammatory cytokines, especially interleukin-6 (IL-6) and IL-1beta, in amniotic fluid[212] or umbilical cord blood,[211,370,380-382] and (3) evidence for intrauterine T-cell activation.[381] However, nearly all these studies used for the diagnosis of PVL the ultrasonographic finding of echolucencies (i.e., apparent *cystic* PVL). As noted earlier, cystic PVL now is recognized to account for less than 5% of white matter injury, and thus the likely presence of noncystic PVL in the "controls" makes the interpretation of these data difficult. Moreover, two studies of former preterm infants showed no significant relationship between levels of proinflammatory cytokines in early neonatal blood and the later diagnosis of cerebral palsy,[383,384] and a study of 126 infants showed no correlation between clinical chorioamnionitis and ultrasonographically demonstrated white matter injury.[385] Finally, in a careful study of 100 consecutive premature infants studied by MRI at term, no significant relationship was noted between the occurrence of chorioamnionitis or prolonged rupture of membranes and moderate to severe white matter injury.[223]

A potential role for *postnatal* infection and white matter injury should be considered. Thus, in the aforementioned MRI study of 100 premature infants, a weak relationship was noted between neonatal sepsis and white matter injury identified at term.[230] Other reports have shown an increased rate of cerebral palsy and other neurodevelopmental disabilities in preterm infants after neonatal sepsis.[386,387] This relationship is particularly apparent among infants of extremely low birth weight (401 to 1000 g), of whom 65% exhibit at least one infection during the postnatal period.[386] Moreover, because as many as 25% of all infants who weigh less than 1500 g at birth experience neonatal sepsis,[388-391] the contributory role of postnatal infection/inflammation could be considerable. More data are needed.

Human Neuropathological Observations. A potential role for inflammation and, specifically, cytokines in the pathogenesis of PVL is supported by the neuropathological finding of proinflammatory cytokines in the human lesion.[241,392-396] The principal cytokines observed have been tumor necrosis factor-alpha (TNF-alpha), IL-2, IL-6, and interferon-gamma.

In most studies, the cellular origin of the cytokines has not been characterized unequivocally, but by morphological criteria, microglia/macrophages appear to be the most common originating cells. A similar observation concerning microglia/macrophages has been made in multiple sclerosis, another disorder associated with destruction of oligodendrocytes.[397] However, in the diffuse component of PVL, abundant interferon-gamma expression has been shown in *astrocytes*.[396] Moreover, the interferon-gamma *receptor* was shown to be present on pre-OLs, and the degree of oxidative injury identified in the diffuse lesion correlated with the degree of interferon-gamma expression.[396] These observations are of major interest because interferon-gamma is particularly toxic to pre-OLs in cell culture, and this toxicity is both maturation dependent and potentiated by TNF-alpha (see Chapter 6). *Taken together, the neuropathological findings indicate that cytokines are present in human PVL, and their likely sources are most commonly microglia and astrocytes.* It remains possible that systemic cytokines or systemic activated monocytic cells enter the brain through an intact or damaged blood-brain barrier to contribute importantly to the brain cytokine response (see Chapter 6). Perhaps related to these findings are the demonstrations in living premature infants of a relationship between elevated levels of interferon-gamma in blood or CSF and ultrasonographically defined white matter injury[398,398a] and of TNF-alpha in *CSF* and *MRI-defined* white matter injury.[399]

Delineation of the insult leading to the brain cytokine response in PVL would be of major value in the understanding of pathogenesis. Identification of the initiating insult is difficult in neuropathological studies, but available data *suggest a role both for hypoxia-ischemia and systemic infection/inflammation.* In the neuropathological series of Kadhim and associates,[394] the 19 cases with PVL and cytokines in the lesion had "asphyxia" in the background. *Thus, the possibility that hypoxia-ischemia could have led to the inflammatory response in these cases of human PVL is important to consider.* It is well established in animal models and to some extent in human adult stroke that ischemia/reperfusion is associated with a brisk inflammatory response, characterized by activation of microglial cells, secretion of cytokines, mobilization, adhesion and migration of macrophages and inflammatory cells, and reactive astrocytosis.[400-415] Persistence of this response, with activated microglia and astrocytes, for many *weeks* following the insult has been documented in hypoxic-ischemic models in immature animals and in human stroke.[400,410,415]

An important interacting role for systemic infection/inflammation with hypoxia-ischemia in a portion of the 19 cases of PVL well studied by Kadhim and colleagues[394] is suggested by the finding that 8 of the 19 cases with "asphyxia" were complicated by either fetal inflammation (chorioamnionitis) or neonatal infection. *Importantly, brain cytokine immunoreactivity (TNF-alpha, IL-1beta) in the PVL cases with infection was at least double the immunoreactivity in the PVL cases without infection. Thus, the possibility of a potentiating interaction between a hypoxic-ischemic insult and systemic infection/inflammation in the inflammatory*

response in brain is suggested (see later). Moreover, activated microglial cells and perhaps astrocytes, both shown by Kinney and co-workers to be key features of the diffuse component of human PVL,[243] may be central to this interaction (see later).

As discussed later, activated microglial cells secrete toxic diffusible products (e.g., ROS and RNS) that are likely more important than cytokines in the genesis of white matter injury. Moreover, the means of activation of microglia by the molecular products of infection is crucial to the cascade to injury (see Chapter 6). Few data are available for the human brain, but involvement of the innate immune system in brain through Toll-like receptors on microglia and the results of the activation of these receptors are likely to be relevant, as in experimental studies described in Chapter 6.

Central Role of Microglia. Although the mechanisms by which maternal and fetal infection/inflammation initiate deleterious molecular and structural events in the brain are not fully understood, *it is clear that microglial cells play a central role* (see Fig. 8-26 and Chapter 6). Moreover, studies principally of other systems indicate that ROS and RNS and perhaps glutamate are important in mediating the actions of these cells (see later). Because the mechanisms of ROS/RNS toxicity and excitotoxicity are central to the intrinsic maturation-dependent vulnerability of pre-OLs to both hypoxia-ischemia and infection/inflammation, I discuss the microglial downstream roles further later. However, *it is important here to reemphasize the finding in our study of human PVL of the marked microgliosis discovered in the diffuse component of the lesion.*[243] This seminal observation supports the involvement of these cells in the human lesion.

The particular involvement of microglia in the pathogenesis of cerebral white matter disease in the premature infant may also relate to a maturation-dependent feature. Thus, microglial cells can be identified in normal human brain very early in development, become abundant in forebrain from 16 to 22 weeks of gestation, and *are concentrated in cerebral white matter, with a deep-to-superficial gradient.*[416-420b] Relatively few microglial cells are found in cerebral cortex at this time. In the largest longitudinal study of human postmortem brain, density of microglia reached a *peak* during the period of greatest vulnerability to PVL (third trimester of gestation) and declined markedly in white matter after 37 weeks of gestation.[420] As density declined in cerebral white matter, it increased in cerebral cortex. This observation suggests that a wave of migrating microglia is apparent in cerebral white matter at the optimum time for activation by hypoxia-ischemia or infection or both. *Thus, although more data on these developmental features are needed, a maturation-dependent population of cells (i.e., microglia) may be concentrated in cerebral white matter at the right time and in the right place to contribute to white matter injury when activated.*

Infection and Hypoxia-Ischemia-Potentiating Insults. Deleterious interactions between maternal or fetal and postnatal infection/inflammation and hypoxia-ischemia could occur at several steps in the pathway to oligodendroglial death (see Table 8-10 and Fig. 8-26). Thus, such potentiation could develop at the level of the major upstream initiating events of hypoxia-ischemia and infection/inflammation or at the level of the major downstream events of ROS/RNS toxicity and excitotoxicity. Not unexpectedly, most current evidence supporting a potentiating interaction of infection/inflammation and hypoxia-ischemia emanates from experimental studies (see Chapter 6). However, clinical and neuropathological studies of human PVL also support the notion of a potentiating interaction.

Potentiation of Adverse Systemic and Cerebral Circulatory Effects by Combined Infection/Inflammation and Hypoxia-Ischemia. The combination of infection/inflammation and hypoxia-ischemia could result in deleterious circulatory effects, ultimately affecting the cerebral circulation (see Fig. 8-26). Thus, as noted earlier, in some experimental studies, deleterious systemic hemodynamic effects have been shown to accompany fetal or neonatal infection or exposure to lipopolysaccharide or cytokines. That a similar interaction could occur in the premature infant is suggested from three important studies of premature infants by Yanowitz and co-workers. Thus, in one report of 55 premature infants (25 to 32 weeks of gestation), chorioamnionitis was evident in 22 placentas and was associated both with elevated blood IL-6 concentrations and with decreased mean arterial blood pressures in the first hours of life.[421] In a later report, the decreased blood pressures were shown to persist for the entire first week of life.[422] In a more recent report, near-infrared spectroscopy was used to show an apparent impairment in cerebrovascular autoregulation, thereby raising the possibility that the decreased blood pressure could result in diminished CBF.[423] Moreover, because several cytokines stimulated by infection, especially TNF-alpha and IL-1beta, exhibit vasoactive properties, it is reasonable to postulate that these inflammatory molecules could contribute to impaired cerebrovascular autoregulation, likely important in pathogenesis of PVL (see earlier).[424-426] *Under such circumstances, modest decreases in arterial blood pressure could result in decreases in CBF.* Indeed, major disturbances in the regulation of CBF and cerebral oxygen delivery have been observed in fetal sheep after relatively low doses of lipopolysaccharide.[427] Finally, it is well established that hypoxia-ischemia (without infection) also leads to both systemic and cerebral elevations of vasoactive proinflammatory cytokines (e.g., TNF-alpha and IL-1beta) derived from peripheral monocytes and brain microglia (see earlier).[428-431] *Thus, the possibility of amplifying or at least additive effects on the systemic and cerebral circulations is considerable in the presence of both infection/inflammation and hypoxia-ischemia.*

Human Disease: Evidence Supporting Potentiation by Infection/Inflammation and Hypoxia-Ischemia. Neuropathological and clinical findings in human PVL are consistent with the notion of a potentiating relationship between maternal or fetal infection/inflammation and hypoxia-ischemia. Thus, *from the neuropathological perspective,* in human PVL, microgliosis is a consistent and prominent feature of the lesion.[243] Moreover, a resident population of microglia, presumably capable of the same sensitizing relationship between the two insults shown in the experimental models, is concentrated in human cerebral white matter at the correct time and in the correct distribution to be activated and become injurious (see earlier).[420] Finally, as noted earlier, in a study of 19 cases of PVL, all were stated to have "asphyxia" in the background, and cytokine immunoreactivity was detected in microglia/macrophages.[394] However, *this immunoreactivity was at least double in PVL cases with systemic fetal infection* (e.g., chorioamnionitis) in the background versus PVL cases without infection. Taken together, these neuropathological data suggest *clear potential for a potentiating relationship between infection/inflammation and hypoxia-ischemia in human PVL.*

From the clinical perspective, our studies with near-infrared spectroscopy of cerebral hemodynamics in premature infants (see earlier) showed frequent but often not marked declines in CBF (see Chapter 9, Fig. 9-47). These declines were associated with an increased risk for PVL. These observations suggest that PVL may develop as a result of *accumulation of hypoxic-ischemic insults.* The latter possibility is supported by the demonstration both by neuropathological studies and by MRI studies that white matter injury in premature infants increases markedly in frequency with increasing duration of survival.[75,220,226] Moreover, in our neuropathological studies of PVL, lesions of multiple ages (i.e., acute, subacute and chronic) typically are present.[75,243] Does the lesion become more frequent during the neonatal period because of (1) an additive effect of many small decreases in CBF, (2) alterations in excitatory amino acid receptor subunit composition caused by the initial insult and thereby rendering the receptors more sensitive to subsequent insults, as shown in cultured pre-OLs and in an animal model of PVL,[432] or, in this context, (3) a sensitizing effect of maternal/fetal infection, not severe enough to produce injury alone, on subsequent or concomitant hypoxic-ischemic insults, perhaps also not severe enough to produce injury alone? *These possibilities, of course, are not mutually exclusive.*

Additional support for a potentiating relationship for infection/inflammation and hypoxia-ischemia vis-à-vis PVL is suggested by a recent study of 61 consecutively born preterm infants (<32 weeks of gestation). Thus, the risk of white matter injury, identified by MRI and ultrasonography, was enhanced with a history of histological chorioamnionitis *only in the presence* of *concurrent* placental vascular disturbances consistent with a placental perfusion defect.[433] Whether the latter was caused by intrauterine infection was not clear, although such a relationship has been shown.[434] Histological chorioamnionitis without placental perfusion defect was not associated with white matter disease.

Thus, taken together, a rapidly growing body of experimental (see Chapter 6), neuropathological, and clinical evidence suggests that infection/inflammation and hypoxia-ischemia may potentiate each other to produce PVL. Such potentiation would have major implications concerning the means of surveillance of infants at risk and the

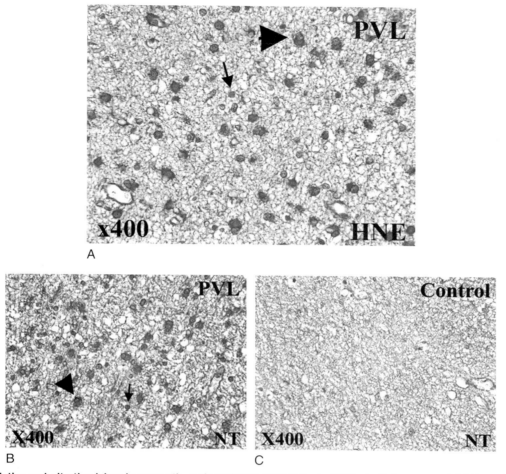

Figure 8-32 Oxidative and nitrative injury in noncystic periventricular leukomalacia (PVL). A, Hydroxynonenal (HNE) staining, a marker for attack by reactive oxygen species, is abundant in cerebral white matter in both premyelinating oligodendrocytes *(arrow)* and astrocytes *(arrowhead).* **B,** Nitrotyrosine (NT) staining, a marker for attack by reactive nitrogen species, is abundant in cerebral white matter in similar cells. **C,** Age-matched control section of white matter shows no staining with NT; a similar lack of staining was apparent for HNE (not shown). *(From Haynes RL, Folkerth RD, Keefe R, Sung I, et al: Nitrosative and oxidative injury to premyelinating oligodendrocytes is accompanied by microglial activation in periventricular leukomalacia in the human premature infant,* J Neuropathol Exp Neurol *62:441-450, 2003.)*

approaches to prevention. Clearly, the mechanisms involved in and the means to ameliorate the deleterious interaction of the two key upstream mechanisms in PVL are critical for future research.

Intrinsic Vulnerability of Cerebral White Matter of the Premature Newborn. A maturation-dependent *intrinsic* vulnerability of the cerebral white matter, particularly the differentiating pre-OL, in diffuse PVL of the premature infant is suggested by experimental studies (see Chapter 6), by the rarity of the lesion at later ages, by the concentration of these vulnerable cells during the peak time period of occurrence of the lesion, and by their specific involvement in the diffuse injury. The intrinsic vulnerability relates principally to the two major downstream mechanisms in PVL (i.e., free radical attack by ROS and RNS and excitotoxicity; see Table 8-10). The details of the intrinsic vulnerabilities, as derived from experimental studies, are described in Chapter 6. Here I emphasize studies performed on human premature brain. Relevance of

the cascade to pre-OL death described in Chapter 6 to the human infant is strikingly apparent.

Vulnerability to Free Radical Attack. The most compelling direct evidence that free radical attack by both ROS and RNS is involved in the injury to pre-OLs in PVL emanates from study of the human lesion.[243,246] In our study of 17 cases, in which immunocytochemical markers for oxidative (hydroxynonenal) and nitrative (nitrotyrosine) attack were used, abundant staining was documented in both pre-OLs and reactive astrocytes in the diffuse lesion (Fig. 8-32). The free radical attack appeared to lead to death of the former but not the latter. This key discovery of oxidative and nitrative attack in PVL is consistent with experimental data indicative of oxidative and nitrative cellular injury with both hypoxic-ischemic and inflammatory insults to the brain (see Chapter 6), the two likely key upstream mechanisms in PVL (see Fig. 8-26).

Studies of CSF in *living premature infants also supported toxicity of ROS in PVL.* Thus, in a longitudinal study of premature infants, those with MRI evidence for PVL at

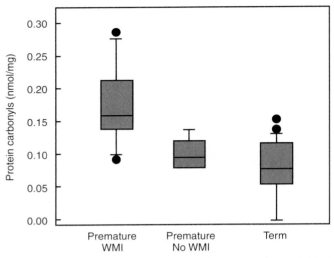

Figure 8-33 **Markers of protein oxidation in cerebrospinal fluid of premature infants in the neonatal period as a function of subsequent documentation of white matter injury (WMI) at term by magnetic resonance imaging.** Twenty-two premature infants with a mean gestational age of 27.4 weeks had cerebrospinal fluid samples obtained at 5 to 8 days of life and magnetic resonance imaging scans performed at term. The 26 healthy term infants were similarly studied. *(Data from Inder TE, Mocatta T, Darlow B, Spencer C, et al: Elevated free radical products in the cerebrospinal fluid of VLBW infants with cerebral white matter injury, Pediatr Res 52:213-218, 2002.)*

term exhibited, earlier in the neonatal period, sharply elevated CSF levels of oxidative products, detected as protein carbonyls (Fig. 8-33), when compared with CSF levels in premature infants without MRI evidence for PVL.[250]

The mechanisms underlying the maturation-dependent vulnerability of developing oligodendrocytes to ROS attack have been addressed in both human brain and experimental studies

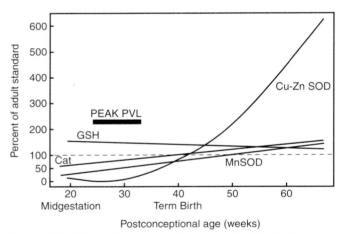

Figure 8-34 **Regression curves of analyses of antioxidant enzyme expressions (Western blots) in cerebral white matter from midgestation to 60 postnatal weeks, relative to the adult standard (100% value).** Immunocytochemical studies showed similar temporal changes in premyelinating oligodendrocytes. Cat, catalase; Cu, copper; GSH, glutathione; Mn, manganese; PVL, periventricular leukomalacia; SOD, superoxide dismutase; Zn, zinc. See text for details. *(From Folkerth RD, Haynes RL, Borenstein NS, Belliveau RA, et al: Developmental lag in superoxide dismutases relative to other antioxidant enzymes in premyelinated human telencephalic white matter, J Neuropathol Exp Neurol 63:990-999, 2004.)*

(see Chapter 6). The findings in human brain indicate a delay in development of enzymes at the superoxide dismutase step, both manganese superoxide dismutase and copper-zinc superoxide dismutase, and catalase (Fig. 8-34).[435] Additionally, the possibility that hydrogen peroxide accumulates and is converted to the hydroxyl radical by the Fenton reaction is suggested by the observations of others of the early appearance of iron in developing human white matter,[206,436] as well as by the acquisition of iron by developing oligodendrocytes for differentiation.[437] Supportive of a relationship between iron and PVL is the observation that, for many weeks after human intraventricular hemorrhage, a disorder that sharply increases the risk of PVL,[78,82,438] CSF levels of non–protein-bound iron are markedly increased.[439] *Taken together, the findings indicate a maturation-dependent window of vulnerability to oxidative attack during oligodendroglial development* (see Chapter 6 and Table 8-10).

Several reports suggested that the vulnerability to oxidative attack in the premature white matter shares similarities with features in the periphery. Thus, studies of plasma of human premature infants indicated a propensity to generate free radicals, including the hydroxyl radical, increases in plasma non–protein-bound iron, accentuated by hypoxia or blood transfusion, and impaired antioxidant defenses.[440-447]

The mechanisms underlying the maturation-dependent vulnerability of pre-OLs to RNS attack have been addressed especially in studies of cultured cells (see Chapter 6).[448,449] Relevance of these mechanisms to human PVL is provided by our preliminary data, which show a significant increase in the number of inducible nitric oxide synthase–positive glia in the diffuse component of PVL. Moreover, inducible nitric oxide synthase was expressed strongly in the reactive astrocytes in the diffuse lesion, but not prominently in the activated microglia. The data suggest that a key source of nitric oxide in the human lesion, potentially leading to a major portion of the nitrative stress identified previously in diffuse PVL,[243] is the reactive astrocyte. Our preliminary data also suggest that pre-OLs and subplate neurons also contain inducible nitric oxide synthase and thereby could be additional sources of nitric oxide. It is likely that the superoxide anion necessary for generation of the injurious RNS, peroxynitrite, is derived from both the abundance of activated microglia in diffuse PVL and the pre-OL itself (see Chapter 6). Recall the relative deficiency of both superoxide dismutases in cerebral white matter of the human premature infant (see Fig. 8-34).

Vulnerability to Excitotoxicity. An intrinsic maturation-dependent vulnerability of pre-OLs to excitotoxicity was suggested by experimental studies (see Chapter 6) and, more recently, by related observations of developing human brain (see later). As detailed in Chapter 6, glutamate is capable of inducing maturation-dependent death of pre-OLs by non–receptor-mediated and receptor-mediated mechanisms. The *non–receptor-mediated mechanism* involves glutamate competition for the cystine transporter and promotion of cystine efflux under conditions of high extracellular levels of glutamate.[450-452] The results are depletion of intracellular glutathione (which requires cysteine for biosynthesis) and cell death by oxidative stress. However, the substantial levels (millimolar) of glutamate required for this effect suggest that this mechanism may not operate in vivo under most pathological conditions. By contrast, the *receptor-mediated mechanism*, which requires micromolar levels of glutamate, is more likely to occur in vivo, as shown directly in animal models by us and by others (see Chapter 6). Both AMPA and NMDA receptors appear to be involved. Several studies indicate that such receptor-mediated toxicity is involved in human PVL.

The *principal sources of elevated extracellular glutamate* in cerebral white matter with hypoxia-ischemia are glutamate transporters (see Chapter 6). Failure of glutamate uptake and actual reversal of transport occur in the setting of energy failure because of the failure of the sodium-potassium ion pump. These transporters are high-affinity, sodium-dependent systems. That this situation may occur in the *human infant* is suggested by the recent discovery of maturation-dependent overexpression in cerebral white matter of the principal glutamate transporter during the peak period of PVL.[453] The principal locus for this transporter is the pre-OL.[453]

The critical initiators of excitotoxic cell death are *glutamate receptors*. As described in Chapter 6, oligodendrocytes express AMPA/kainate (AMPA/KA)-type glutamate receptors, the activation of which results in cell death.[432,454-463] The experimental data show an overexpression of AMPA receptors on the cell somata of pre-OLs versus mature oligodendroglia. Moreover, these pre-OL receptors are deficient in the GluR2 subunit, which renders them Ca^{2+} permeable and thereby capable of toxicity. The overexpression of the Ca^{2+}-permeable receptors in immature rat cerebral white matter correlates with the period of vulnerability to hypoxic-ischemic white matter injury (see Chapter 6). *Relevance of the experimental work to human PVL* is apparent by the demonstration in human cerebral white matter pre-OLs of a similar overexpression of AMPA receptors that also are GluR2 deficient and presumably Ca^{2+} permeable *during the peak period of occurrence of PVL* (see Fig. 8-6).[141]

Studies in experimental systems show that a *second type of glutamate receptor, an NMDA receptor*, is present on the processes of pre-OLs, and that excessive activation of these receptors, as in models of ischemia, leads to Ca^{2+}-influx, generation of ROS/RNS, and loss of processes (see Chapter 6). These observations led us to study developing *human brain*, and a marked expression of NMDA receptors on pre-OLs was defined during the peak period of vulnerability to PVL.[271] Thus, the data indicated that excessive glutamate in human cerebral white matter during the peak period of PVL could lead both to death of pre-OLs by activation of AMPA receptors on the cell soma and to loss of oligodendroglial processes by activation of NMDA receptors on cell processes. These events could result in impaired myelination and perhaps axonal function or structure, or both (see Chapter 6, Fig. 6-42).

Presence of Other Potentially Vulnerable Rapidly Differentiating Cellular Elements. Other potentially vulnerable rapidly differentiating cellular elements in cerebral white matter during the peak period of PVL are subplate neurons. *Subplate neurons* were shown in experimental systems to be exquisitely vulnerable to hypoxia-ischemia (see Chapter 6), and these transient cells were noted to reach their peak in human brain during the peak PVL period (see Chapters 2 and 6).[218] Currently, no data are available concerning their status in human PVL. Similarly, *axons* are in a state of very active development in cerebral white matter of the human premature infant.[290,464] The confluence of developing ascending and descending projection fibers, commissural fibers, and sagittal corticocortical association fibers in the peritrigonal region is particularly prominent at this time and is a particular site of predilection for PVL. Currently, no data are available concerning the status of axons in human PVL. These two rapidly developing elements, subplate neurons and axons, could be especially vulnerable, and injury thereof could have secondary deleterious effects on development and function of cerebral cortex and thalamus (see Chapter 9).

Focal and Multifocal Ischemic Brain Necroses

Cellular and Regional Aspects

In this category, I include the localized areas of necrosis that occur *within the distribution of single (or multiple) major cerebral vessel or vessels*. Involvement of *specific vascular distributions* thus is the distinguishing hallmark of this lesion. *The term* arterial stroke *is often (and appropriately) used for the lesion*. Distinction from the ischemic lesions associated with a generalized decrease in CBF (i.e., parasagittal cerebral injury and PVL, discussed previously) is sometimes difficult; indeed, overlap is apparent.

The *relative frequency* of these ischemic lesions at autopsy was emphasized by a neuropathological review of 592 infants examined over a 4-year period.[465] Cerebral infarcts with arterial occlusion were seen in 5.4% of infants. The incidence as a function of gestational age was 0% for infants less than 28 weeks, approximately 5% for those between 28 and 32 weeks, 10% for those between 32 and 37 weeks, and 15% for those between 37 and 40 weeks. Involvement of the middle cerebral artery occurred in approximately one half of the affected infants (Fig. 8-35). Multiple smaller vessels were the sites of occlusion in the remaining cases. The predominance of middle cerebral artery distribution has been more marked in infants identified in vivo by brain imaging modalities (see later discussion).

The *cellular aspects of the neuropathology* of these lesions are dominated by necrosis of all cellular elements, within specific arterial distributions (i.e., an infarction). The cellular features relate primarily to the time after the insult.[6,7,466-469] After 18 to 24 hours, anoxic neuronal change is apparent by light microscopy; earlier, no change may be detectable.

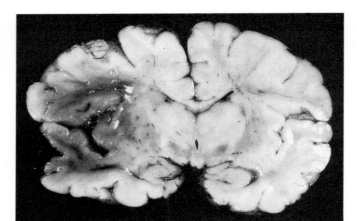

Figure 8-35 Focal ischemic brain injury. Coronal section of the cerebrum from a full-term infant with thrombosis of the left middle cerebral artery and a large ischemic infarct. The infant died 2 days after birth complicated by meconium aspiration. *(From Barmada MA, Moossy J, Shuman RM: Cerebral infarcts with arterial occlusion in neonates, Ann Neurol 6:495-502, 1979.)*

Shortly thereafter, activated cells of the monocyte-macrophage type migrate from vessels and enter the lesion as elongated and pleomorphic microglial cells. These cells become foamy macrophages by 36 to 48 hours. Astrocytic hypertrophy, with the characteristically large, eosinophilic, sail-like cytoplasm of the gemistocytic astrocyte, becomes apparent by 3 to 5 days. Astrocytic proliferation, with prominent staining of glial fibrillary acidic protein in astrocytic fibers, then forms a dense mat of glial fibrillary processes. This process occurs over weeks to months. Mineralization of neurons, sometimes with more diffuse calcification, may occur. Cavity formation is common and is discussed later.

The *topography of infarction in arterial distribution*, occurring in the perinatal period and identified in the newborn by brain imaging, is distinctive (Table 8-12).[98,178-188,470-482a] Approximately 75% of lesions are unilateral, and nearly all the unilateral lesions involve the middle cerebral artery. Of all *unilateral* middle cerebral artery infarcts, approximately 65% involve the distribution of the left artery.

TABLE 8-12 Focal and Multifocal Ischemic Cerebral Necrosis: Topography of Infarction*

Topography of Infarction	Percentage of Total
Laterality	
Unilateral	75%
Bilateral	25%
Vascular Distribution	
Left MCA	55%
Right MCA	30%
Bilateral MCA	10%
Other arteries	5%

*Data derived from 244 infants (90% full term) studied primarily by computed tomography and magnetic resonance imaging (see references in text); 45 are personal cases. Numbers are rounded off.
MCA, middle cerebral artery.

TABLE 8-13 Neonatal Cerebral Venous Thrombosis*

Superior sagittal sinus involvement in ≈65% of patients; thrombosis of lateral sinus in ≈50% or deep venous system in ≈50%; multiple site involvement in ≈50%
Infarction present in 40%-60% and hemorrhagic in most; intraventricular hemorrhage present in 20%-35%
Seizures initial presentation in 60%-70% of cases
Diagnosis by computed tomography or magnetic resonance imaging (preferable); cerebrospinal fluid often hemorrhagic
Pathogenesis often involving *multiple* factors, most often preeclampsia, maternal diabetes, perinatal "distress," dehydration, congenital cardiac disease, ECMO, sepsis, or prothrombotic coagulation defect

*See text for references; also includes unpublished personal experience. ECMO, extracorporeal membrane oxygenation.

Venous thrombosis, recognized best in the neonatal period by MRI, is more common than previously expected in the era before MRI (Table 8-13).[483-498] Approximately 65% of the thromboses affect the superior sagittal sinus, especially the posterior portion, and the remainder involve the lateral sinus (50%) or deep veins (e.g., straight sinus and Galenic system [50%]). Infarction is present in 40% to 60% of cases; brain edema is the principal finding in those without infarction. The infarcts characteristically are hemorrhagic. MRI often demonstrates hemorrhagic infarction in the parasagittal regions bilaterally with sagittal sinus thrombosis and hemorrhagic infarction in the region of the striatum and internal capsule with deep venous thrombosis (involving internal cerebral and terminal veins). Intraventricular hemorrhage is present in 20% to 35% of cases and is often associated with infarction involving the thalamus and internal capsule.

When these focal and multifocal necroses of brain of the prenatal and early postnatal periods are associated with dissolution of tissue and cavity formation, the terms *porencephaly, hydranencephaly*, and *multicystic encephalomalacia* are used to describe the lesions.[7,8,499,500] In this discussion, I use the term *porencephaly* to refer to a single unilateral cavity within the cerebral hemisphere that may or may not communicate with the lateral ventricle (Fig. 8-36).[501] When related to ischemia (rather than intracerebral hemorrhage or infection), porencephaly is the sequela of an infarction with involvement of both cortex and cerebral white matter in the distribution of a single major cerebral vessel. *Hydranencephaly* refers to massive bilateral lesions, in which most or all of both hemispheres are reduced to CSF-filled sacs. When related to ischemia, hydranencephaly most commonly is the sequela of bilateral cerebral infarction, with involvement of both cortex and cerebral white matter in the distribution of both internal carotid arteries (i.e., the anterior circulation). Because the posterior cerebral artery may have its origin from the anterior circulation in nearly 25% of newborns, the posterior cerebral artery distribution may also be affected.[502] *Multicystic encephalomalacia* refers to *multiple* cavitated foci of cerebral necrosis,

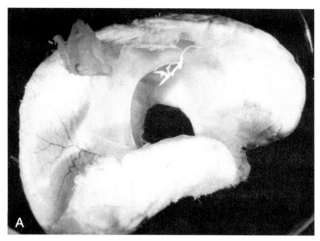

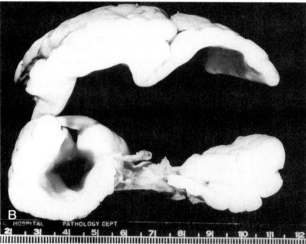

Figure 8-36   Focal ischemic brain injury with porencephaly. The infant, who died after 2 months, also exhibited a large head. **A**, Lateral view of cerebrum floating in water. **B**, Coronal section of cerebrum. Note the destruction in the distribution of the right middle cerebral artery; no lesion of the right internal carotid or middle cerebral artery could be demonstrated. Associated hydrocephalus was related to aqueductal obstruction; the cause was unknown. *(From Norman MG: Perinatal brain damage. In Rosenberg HS, Bolande RP, editors: Perspectives in Pediatric Pathology, Chicago: 1978, Mosby.)*

TABLE 8-14	**Major Causes of Ischemic Focal and Multifocal Brain Necrosis**

Focal and Multifocal Cerebrovascular Occlusion-Insufficiency
Vascular Abnormality (Prenatal)
Vascular maldevelopment
Vasculopathy
Familial, proliferative
Isoimmune thrombocytopenia
Vasospasm
Cocaine
Vascular distortion
Embolus (Prenatal or Postnatal)
Placental thromboses or tissue fragments, detritus (twin pregnancy with dead co-twin)
Involuting fetal vessels (thrombi)
Catheterized vessels (thrombi or air)
Cardiac: atrial myxoma, rhabdomyoma (tuberous sclerosis), congenital heart disease with right-to-left shunt, patent foramen ovale
Thrombus (Arterial or Venous) (Prenatal or Postnatal)
Meningitis with arteritis or phlebitis
Trauma
Dissection
Fibromuscular dysplasia
Vascular ligation-manipulation: extracorporeal membrane oxygenation
Hypernatremia-dehydration
Disseminated intravascular coagulation (e.g., sepsis, twin pregnancy with dead co-twin)
Polycythemia
Prothrombotic/hypercoagulable, endogenous factors: factor V Leiden mutation, protein C deficiency, protein S deficiency, prothrombin mutation, antithrombin III deficiency, antiphospholipid antibodies, *MTHFR* mutation, elevated lipoprotein *a*, elevated factor VIIIc

Generalized Systemic Circulatory Insufficiency
Prenatal
Maternal hypotension or cardiac arrest
Maternal trauma
Twin pregnancy (fetofetal transfusion [see Table 8-18])
Umbilical cord or placental catastrophe
Postnatal
Systemic hypotension or cardiac arrest (usually with "perinatal asphyxia")
Persistent pulmonary hypertension
Congenital heart disease with cardiac failure (exclusive of thromboembolic phenomena)

MTHFR, methylene tetrahydrofolate reductase.

usually bilateral in distribution. Most examples of this lesion, when related to ischemia, are the sequelae of predominantly cerebral white matter destruction caused by generalized ischemia (i.e., more analogous to severe PVL than to affection of single or several vessels).

Although the emphasis of this section is the ischemic type of these pathological states, various other fetal and neonatal insults may cause necrosis and similar disease. The tendency of immature human brain to undergo dissolution and cavitation is not principally a function of the nature of the insult but rather the *timing* of the insult (see the later "Pathogenesis" section). Thus, any major destructive insult (e.g., ischemic, hemorrhagic, infectious, or traumatic) may result in large cavitated lesions in the cerebrum if the insult strikes from approximately the second trimester of gestation to the early postnatal period.

In this section, I discuss the *ischemic* causes of focal and multifocal brain destruction (i.e., stroke) (Table 8-14). Those disorders related to other insults are discussed in Chapters 10, 11, 20, 21, and 22. (Not listed in Table 8-14 are major disturbances of brain *development*, schizencephalies, which also may lead to large cavities in the cerebral hemispheres [see Chapter 2]. These disorders are to be distinguished from the destructive [i.e., encephaloclastic] lesions that result in formation of porencephaly, hydranencephaly, and multicystic encephalomalacia.)

Pathogenesis

Factors Determining the Propensity to Cavitation. The time period involved in the propensity to cavitation

TABLE 8-15	Factors Determining the Propensity of Immature Cerebrum to Undergo Dissolution

High content of water
Relative paucity of tightly packed, myelinated fiber bundles
Deficient astroglial response

is from approximately the second trimester of gestation to the first postnatal weeks or months. The major factors determining the propensity of human brain to undergo dissolution and cavitation with necrosis during this time are primarily threefold (Table 8-15). The relatively *high water content* is characteristic of unmyelinated tissue and approaches 90% of wet weight in fetal brain. In contrast, myelinated white matter in the mature human brain is composed of approximately 70% water.[503] The deposition of myelin lipids occurs principally postnatally pari passu with the diminution of water content and the development of tightly packed fiber bundles. This axonal fiber development is reflected in the increasing anisotropic diffusion demonstrated in human brain of 28 to 40 postconceptional weeks by diffusion tensor MRI.[300] Thus, the first two factors, high water content and relative paucity of tightly packed myelinated fibers, are complementary and result in a tissue that is quite different from the relatively dense, mature cerebrum. Therefore, dissolution of tissue is prone to occur with ischemic or other types of necrosis. The additional evolution from dissolution to cavitation relates importantly to the deficient astroglial response to injury.[6] This deficient response is both quantitative and qualitative. As discussed in Chapter 2, rapid proliferation of glia in human cerebrum does not begin until the last half of gestation and continues for many months postnatally; therefore, the number of astrocytes to respond to injury may be relatively less than at later ages. In addition, some deficiency in the astrocytic response per se (i.e., the proliferation and hypertrophy of the cell and the development of glial fibers important for the formation of a tight glial scar) does appear to occur. As a consequence, areas of necrosis become areas of cavitation with deficient glial lining. The glial components in multicystic encephalomalacia are more obvious than in most cases of porencephaly and hydranencephaly, at least in part because of the less complete destruction of entire regions of brain and relative sparing of some glial cells in the former lesion, as opposed to the latter two lesions.

The importance of *timing* of ischemic injury in the development of porencephaly and hydranencephaly is well demonstrated by experiments with fetal monkeys.[504,505] Animals whose carotid arteries were ligated in the second trimester of gestation (latter part of the second trimester) developed cavitated areas of necrosis, similar to those in hydranencephaly or porencephaly and observable at term. Hydranencephaly resulted especially with early second trimester ligation, and porencephaly resulted from late second trimester ligations. An example of porencephaly produced experimentally in the fetal monkey by unilateral carotid ligation in the

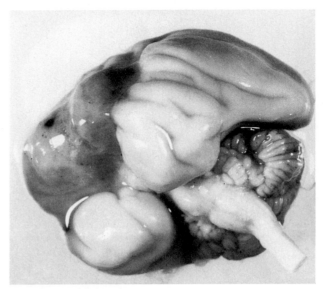

Figure 8-37   Porencephaly produced experimentally by vascular occlusion in the fetal monkey. At 90 days of gestation (term is approximately 160 days), the fetus was exposed surgically, and the carotid artery was ligated in the neck. The pregnancy was allowed to continue until term, when the fetus was delivered by cesarean section. This right lateral view demonstrates a sharply circumscribed area of infarction with a membrane-covered cyst. *(Courtesy of Dr. Philip R. Dodge.)*

latter part of the second trimester is shown in Figure 8-37. Vascular ligation before the early to middle second trimester of gestation resulted in cerebral "dysgenesis," characterized by gyral abnormalities that were not further defined.[251,505] A combination of destructive and dysgenetic features occurred with middle second trimester ligations in the monkey. The analogy in the human is the finding of polymicrogyria in the margins of porencephalies of prenatal origin in the human fetus.[3,469]

Prenatal ultrasonographic studies followed by postnatal imaging and neuropathology clearly demonstrated the human correlates of the studies with monkeys concerning the importance of timing of the insult for the occurrence of cavitation.[6,469,506-515] Porencephaly and hydranencephaly have been documented to develop after insults as early as 20 to 27 weeks, and multicystic encephalomalacia has occurred after insults as early as 30 weeks. Causes of the fetal ischemia in these well-studied cases have included severe maternal hypotension secondary to cardiac failure, anaphylaxis, attempted maternal suicide with butane gas, maternal abdominal trauma, placental and umbilical cord catastrophes, and death of one twin (see later discussion).

Major Causes of Ischemic Focal and Multifocal Brain Destruction. Of the four major categories of disease leading to large focal and multifocal brain lesions—ischemia, hemorrhage, infection, and trauma—the ischemic phenomena are the subject of this section, and the causes of this form of brain injury are discussed next. The other three categories are discussed in other chapters (see Chapters 10, 11, and 20

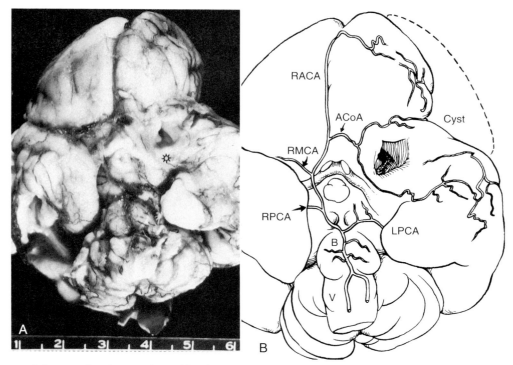

Figure 8-38   Porencephaly secondary to vascular maldevelopment. The specimen is from a small-for-gestational-age infant with multiple congenital anomalies who died 1 hour after birth. **A,** Ventral surface of the brain illustrating the defect in the left frontal lobe *(asterisk)* on its ventral surface. A meningeal cyst, which arose from the margins of the defect, was disrupted on removal of the brain. **B,** Drawing of the ventral surface of the brain to illustrate the abnormal configuration of the circle of Willis. ACoA, anterior communicating artery; B, basilar artery; LPCA, left posterior cerebral artery; RACA, right anterior cerebral artery; RMCA, right middle cerebral artery; RPCA, right posterior cerebral artery; V, vertebral artery. *(From Stewart RM, Williams RS, Lukl P, Schoenen J: Ventral porencephaly: A cerebral defect associated with multiple congenital anomalies,* Acta Neuropathol (Berl) *42:231-235, 1978.)*

through 22). I find it most useful to distinguish causes that are characterized by focal or multifocal cerebrovascular occlusion-insufficiency or by generalized systemic circulatory insufficiency.

Focal and Multifocal Cerebrovascular Insufficiency. The pathogeneses of impaired or absent blood flow in a major cerebral vessel (or vessels) are multiple (see Table 8-14). In most cases, the anterior circulation, and particularly the middle cerebral artery distribution (see Table 8-12), is involved, although occasionally necrosis is observed in the distribution of the vertebral-basilar circulation (see earlier discussion and Table 8-12). Such clear associations with a vascular distribution appropriately have led to the conclusion that the disorders occur secondary to vascular occlusion or maldevelopment. However, documentation of the structural basis for the vascular insufficiency often is lacking, especially in lesions occurring prenatally. Thus, when the cerebral lesions are examined at later stages even by neuropathological examination, often years after the lesion has been established, only attenuated vessels without recognizable occlusion are apparent. In such cases, it is usually difficult to determine conclusively whether an intravascular occlusion (e.g., embolus that subsequently moved distally, thrombus that recanalized) or a vascular maldevelopment (easily suggested by *secondary* changes in vessels after massive necrosis) caused the lesion. The advent of MRI and noninvasive means of imaging cerebral vessels (e.g., MR angiography) has provided major insight into

the structural causes of focal cerebrovascular insufficiency. The distribution of causes identified in approximately 250 neonatal cases of cerebral infarction identified by brain imaging and derived from personal experience and reports of others in the 1980s and 1990s included approximately 50% "idiopathic" and 35% related to "perinatal asphyxia."[178-189,470-478,493,516-532] Major changes in pathogenetic concepts have developed in the past few years (see later).

Prenatal stroke has been increasingly identified in utero with advances in fetal imaging. Many of these disorders are related to *vascular abnormalities* (see Table 8-14). A particularly well-documented case of a prenatal focal parenchymal defect with porencephaly, secondary to *vascular maldevelopment* (see Table 8-14), involved the lenticulostriate branches of the middle cerebral artery and the anterior choroidal arteries.[533] An infant with multiple somatic anomalies had an anomalous configuration of the circle of Willis, with absence of proximal branches of the anterior cerebral, middle cerebral, anterior choroidal, and posterior communicating arteries on the side of the lesion (Fig. 8-38). Of additional interest in this case was the occurrence of polymicrogyric cortex in the margins of the porencephalic defect, compatible with a destructive process in the sixth month of gestation. The similarity to the experiments involving second trimester carotid occlusion in fetal monkeys discussed earlier is interesting.

Intrauterine focal or multifocal *ischemic injury secondary to vasculopathy* (see Table 8-14) has been shown in several disorders. A multifocal vascular disorder in association with hydranencephaly in utero was observed in association with a proliferative vasculopathy.[466,534-537] The likelihood of a genetic disorder was supported by the occurrence of multiple affected siblings in three families. It is not yet clear whether the proliferative vasculopathy caused the hydranencephaly directly or is an associated disturbance. In two cases, a mitochondrial disorder was suspected because of the finding of low levels of complexes III and IV of the electron transport chain.[536,537] Microangiopathy related to a *mutation in collagen IV A1* appeared to underlie another familial disorder with congenital porencephaly.[538,539] In a second disorder, *neonatal isoimmune thrombocytopenia*, intrauterine multifocal cystic lesions have been described and are generally considered to represent a sequela of intracerebral hemorrhage.[540-545] However, the apparent relation to vascular territories suggests an ischemic lesion (perhaps with secondary hemorrhage).[541,542,546] I observed a fetus with isoimmune thrombocytopenia and a cystic lesion in the distribution of the middle cerebral artery identified in utero by ultrasonography 5 weeks after a normal sonogram; no ultrasonic echogenicity on the second sonogram to suggest hemorrhage could be identified. Endothelial injury and even thrombosis have been observed in other types of immune thrombocytopenia.[547-549]

Vasospasm may underlie the focal cerebral infarctions observed with intrauterine exposure to cocaine (see Chapter 24).[520,550,551] The vasospasm is postulated to occur secondary to transplacentally acquired cocaine as well as to the surge of catecholamines caused by the systemic and local cerebral effects of cocaine, as detailed in Chapter 24.

Vascular distortion is a potential cause of intrauterine stroke. I raise this possibility because extremes of neck extension or rotation have the potential to produce impairment of blood flow in the vertebrobasilar system or in the carotid system, respectively. Precedent for such occurrences in older patients is available.[552-558] The vertebrobasilar system may be particularly vulnerable in the fetus and newborn because of poorly developed ligamentous structures of the upper cervical spine that allow sliding and slipping movements between the atlanto-occipital and atlanto-axial articulations.[7,559,560] Hyperextension of the head may cause inversion of the atlas through the foramen magnum and may impair flow coursing through the vertebral arteries.[13] In a careful postmortem study, cerebral artery compression was shown in three of five infants with neck extension and in three of nine cases of neck rotation.[560]

Arterial occlusion by embolus or thrombus (see Table 8-14) is a well-documented cause of focal and multifocal parenchymal defects, with or without cavitation.* Often, it has been difficult by clinical imaging or even pathological criteria to distinguish between a

thrombotic and embolic process. As noted earlier, the lesions have been observed principally in the regions of the middle (and sometimes anterior) cerebral arteries (see Figs. 8-35 and 8-36), although thrombi in the basilar artery causing infarcts involving isolated cranial nerve nuclei and more severe involvement of the vertebrobasilar system causing essentially total pontine destruction have also been described.[55,572,573] The cerebral lesions have varied from small infarcts to the large unilateral or bilateral cavitations of porencephaly and hydranencephaly.[3] Both prenatal and neonatal origins have been defined.

Sources of emboli (see Table 8-13) most commonly have included placental fragments or clots (e.g., with placental infarcts), thrombi in involuting fetal vessels (e.g., umbilical vein, portal vein, or ductus arteriosus), and thrombi or air in punctured or catheterized vessels. The *placenta* has been recognized increasingly as a potential source of emboli and cerebral infarction.[522,571a,574-576] The principal placental lesions have involved fetal vessels (fetal thrombotic vasculopathy or fetal vasculitis) and have been associated with intrauterine infection with chorioamnionitis and maternal and, perhaps, fetal coagulopathies. Related placental lesions could underlie in part the increased risk of perinatal stroke with preeclampsia, ovarian-hyperstimulating treatments in women with a history of infertility, and severe intrauterine growth retardation.[480,522,571] Emboli from the fetal or neonatal venous circulation could enter the arterial circulation by passage across the foramen ovale. In 50% to 90% of normal newborns at rest, interatrial left-to-right shunting is documented readily, and in approximately 60% of healthy newborns studied at 24 hours of age, right-to-left blood flow could be demonstrated across the foramen ovale.[577,578]

Other sources of emboli include, as noted earlier, thrombi in the internal carotid artery, portal vein, central venous catheter-related thromboses, and the heart.[579-581] Cardiac sources of emboli are relatively uncommon in the newborn period, although infants with congenital heart disease, especially with right-to-left shunts, may exhibit thromboembolic phenomena of cerebral arteries.[4,521] I have observed single cases of atrial myxoma and rhabdomyoma (infant with tuberous sclerosis) as sources of emboli. My suspicion has been that emboli may be more common causes of cerebral infarction than currently recognized. Cerebral emboli at later ages more commonly affect the left hemisphere (perhaps because of the direct route from the aorta of the left common carotid artery), and the left hemisphere predominance in neonatal middle cerebral artery stroke is striking (see Table 8-12). Additionally, transient right-to-left shunting through the ductus arteriosus also may favor the occurrence of left hemispheral emboli. Further support for a relative frequency of embolic infarction is the finding by serial Doppler studies of four infants with focal middle cerebral artery strokes of an ipsilateral decrease in CBF velocity at the time of diagnosis of the infarct and a reemergence of blood flow in the ensuing days, consistent with embolic occlusion with subsequent

---

*See references 3,6,7,55,180-189,465,470-476,478,480,497,516,517, 520-522,524,525,527,530,545-548,561-571a.

fragmentation and distal migration of embolic fragments.[520]

Thrombosis may involve arteries or veins (see Table 8-14). The most common cause of infarction related to an abnormality of the artery or vein per se is the vasculitis associated with *bacterial meningitis* (see Chapter 21). Cases of apparent occlusion caused by extremes of neck movement or cranial *trauma* may relate to vascular injury and resulting thrombosis (see earlier discussion of vascular distortion).[470,546,559,560,582,583] Intrauterine trauma, secondary to blunt trauma to the maternal abdomen, has resulted in intrauterine stroke.[544,545,545a] The mechanism of this effect is not clear. Neonatal stroke has also been described in relation to carotid artery *dissection* and to *fibromuscular dysplasia* affecting multiple intracranial vessels.[584,585]

ECMO may lead to focal cerebral infarction (see Table 8-14 and Chapter 10). In one series of 180 infants subjected to serial brain imaging studies, 16 (9%) exhibited a major brain lesion; 6 of the 16 infants exhibited focal ischemic lesions, and 10 exhibited hemorrhagic lesions.[586] Of the 6 ischemic lesions, 5 were in the right hemisphere (i.e., ipsilateral to the carotid artery ligation). Of the 10 hemorrhagic lesions, 7 were in the left hemisphere, and only 3 were in the right hemisphere; the origin of the hemorrhages in the infants treated with ECMO is discussed in Chapter 10. A preponderance of right hemispheric *ischemic* phenomena has been observed by others.[587-589] The mechanisms for the right hemispheral infarcts include the following: (1) prior ischemic injury, secondary to persistent pulmonary hypertension and the associated systemic hypotension and impaired cerebrovascular autoregulation (secondary to hypoxemia or hypercarbia or both), partially compensated by cerebral vasodilation before institution of carotid ligation and ECMO; (2) ischemia caused by the carotid artery ligation because of insufficient collateral circulation through the circle of Willis; (3) ischemia caused by impaired cerebrovascular autoregulation during ECMO with disproportionate decrease in CBF with hypotension in the right hemisphere because of the ligated carotid artery; and (4) thrombosis propagated into the anterior cerebral circulation from the ligated carotid artery.[586-588,590] The occurrence of ischemic lesions in the left hemisphere could relate to emboli emanating from the ECMO circuit or to a steal phenomenon caused by the strong collateral flow from the left cerebral circulation to the right.[591,592]

Abnormalities of blood volume and coagulability account for most of the remaining cases of thrombosis. *Hypernatremia-dehydration*, which leads to thrombosis probably by a combination of vascular and hypovolemic causes, is among the unusual causes of neonatal thrombosis, affecting either arteries or veins, most commonly veins (see Table 8-13). *Disseminated intravascular coagulation* in association with sepsis or twin pregnancy with dead co-twin (see later discussion) is among the most commonly documented cause for thrombosis in many *neuropathological series*. For example, in the study of 29 newborns with cerebral infarcts and arterial occlusions by Barmada and co-workers,[465]

disseminated intravascular coagulation, usually with sepsis, was present in approximately two thirds. *Polycythemia* has been associated with neonatal ischemic lesions, often complicated by hemorrhage.[593-595] Polycythemia may lead to arterial or venous thrombosis, and the nature of the disease in neonatal cases is rarely clear. Impaired cognitive outcome, possibly related to ischemic cerebral phenomena, has been documented in infants with polycythemia and hyperviscosity.[596-598] Increased cerebrovascular resistance and diminished CBF velocity, determined by Doppler studies, also have been observed in polycythemic infants with hyperviscosity,[598-601] and decreased CBF and oxygen delivery have been shown directly by studies of neonatal piglets with hyperviscosity produced by infusion of cryoprecipitate.[602] The hemodynamic factors are probably important in genesis of the overt ischemic lesions associated with polycythemia, but such lesions are very unusual even among polycythemic infants with neurological symptoms (see Chapter 9).

Prothrombotic and hypercoagulable endogenous factors are now recognized to be of extreme importance in the genesis of perinatal arterial stroke (see Table 8-14; Table 8-16).[73,529,565-568,571a,603-610] Similarly, these factors are frequent contributing factors in sinovenous thrombosis in newborns (see earlier and Table 8-13).[494-496,611-613] The most commonly implicated factor in neonatal arterial stroke has been the factor V Leiden mutation; other factors implicated include prothrombin mutation, methylene tetrahydrofolate reductase (MTHFR) deficiency (with resulting hyperhomocysteinemia), protein C deficiency, protein S deficiency, antithrombin III deficiency, antiphospholipid antibodies, elevated lipoprotein *a*, and elevated factor VIIIc (see later). Although present in 30% to 70% of cases of neonatal stroke, *these factors are usually combined with other pathogenetic factors* that favor thrombosis or embolus (i.e., preeclampsia, placental vasculopathy, chorioamnionitis, signs of "perinatal asphyxia," sepsis, and congenital heart disease; see later). Indeed, although I classify these disorders here under thrombosis, the likely mechanism of cerebral stroke in these disorders probably relates less to thrombosis in situ in cerebral vessels but rather to embolus from thrombi in

---

TABLE 8-16 **Prothrombotic Factors in Neonatal Arterial Stroke***
Prothrombotic factors associated with neonatal arterial stroke in 30%–70% of cases
Most common factors: factor V Leiden mutation, prothrombin mutation, *MTHFR* mutation, protein C deficiency, protein S deficiency, antithrombin III deficiency, antiphospholipid antibodies, elevated lipoprotein *a*, elevated factor VIIIc
Usually (50%–80%) associated with other pathogenetic factors (i.e., preeclampsia, gestational diabetes, placental vasculopathy, chorioamnionitis, signs of "perinatal asphyxia," sepsis, congenital heart disease)

*See text for references.
MTHFR, methylene tetrahydrofolate reductase.

other sites, such as placenta, involuting fetal vessels or the heart.

The potential importance of the inherited deficiencies was suggested initially by the detection of a syndrome of multiple thromboses, primarily venous, and particularly associated with hemorrhagic, ischemic skin lesions termed *purpura fulminans*, in newborns with inherited deficiencies principally of protein C or protein S.[546,614-621] In general, in these two disorders thromboses were predominantly systemic, although cerebral ischemic lesions in arterial distributions were observed. Several newborns with isolated cerebral ischemic lesions have been described.[530-532] The mechanism is related to failure of the protein C regulatory system to limit coagulation and to augment fibrinolysis. This system is composed of protein C, the pivotal regulatory vitamin K–dependent protein, protein S, a cofactor of activated protein C, and two additional proteins. Of particular interest, protein C and protein S levels are low in the neonatal period, although the activity of protein S is less impaired than that of protein C because of low levels of a protein that inactivates protein S.[622,623] Indeed, protein C activity is extremely low in approximately 30% of preterm twin gestations and in approximately 35% of preterm infants with respiratory distress syndrome.[621,622]

Probably the single most important of the prothrombotic factors is the factor V Leiden mutation or so-called resistance to activated protein C.[568-570,605] In this disorder, a defect in factor V, a procoagulant molecule, occurs such that the factor cannot be inactivated by activated protein C. This so-called factor V Leiden mutation thus causes a "resistance" to the normal inactivating property of activated protein C. The result is an excess of the procoagulant, factor V. The newborn may have a particular propensity for thrombosis with the factor V Leiden mutation because, unlike the relatively low levels of protein C in the newborn, factor V levels are similar to adult values. Therefore, the capacity of protein C to inactivate the factor V, even without the Leiden

mutation, is diminished.[526] This defect has been described in association with neonatal cerebral infarction in approximately 100 infants.[478,480,493,523-528,568,605,609,610,624] Careful examination of the placenta has led to detection of placental thromboses,[525,605] a finding suggesting that one mechanism of stroke in this setting is embolus originating in the placenta and reaching the fetal cerebral circulation through the foramen ovale. (Approximately 60% of fetal cardiac output enters brain from this right-to-left shunt.) In approximately 50% of cases, other risk factors (e.g., perinatal complications, infection, cardiac disease, or the presence of another endogenous prothrombotic factor) were present.

The importance of multiple risk factors and the nature of these factors in the genesis of perinatal arterial stroke are illustrated by the data shown in Table 8-17.[571] In this careful study of 37 cases, although data on endogenous prothrombotic factors were not available, the importance of such factors as preeclampsia, chorioamnionitis, prolonged rupture of membranes, and cord abnormality (tight nuchal cord, umbilical cord knot, body cord) is shown (see Table 8-17). Moreover, the markedly increased risk related to *multiple* rather than single risk factors is apparent. The data further illustrate that the pathogenesis of perinatal arterial stroke is very often multifactorial.

Twin gestation deserves special consideration as a cause of focal and multifocal ischemic brain injury, often related to *thromboembolic* phenomena (Table 8-18).[6,465,482a,551,625-666] As discussed, generalized as well as focal disturbance of CBF is involved in the origin of the neuropathology. Most of the clinically significant brain injury observed with twin gestation occurs in monozygotic *monochorionic* (i.e., a single placenta) twin gestations. Approximately 70% of twin gestations are dizygotic, diamniotic, dichorionic, and generally not associated with brain injury (except for a modest risk related to prematurity or the rare occurrence of stroke). Approximately 30% of twin gestations

TABLE 8-17 **Risk of Perinatal Arterial Stroke as a Function of Risk Factors Present before Delivery**

A. Risk Factors	Odds Ratio (95% Confidence Interval)	P Value
Preeclampsia	5.3 (1.3-22.0)	.02
Oligohydramnios	5.4 (0.9-31.3)	.06
Cord abnormality	3.6 (1.0-12.7)	.05
Primiparity	2.5 (1.0-6.4)	.05
Prolonged rupture of membranes	3.8 (1.1-12.8)	.03
Chorioamnionitis	3.4 (1.1-10.5)	.03

B. Numbers of Risk Factors*	Percentage of Cases (N = 37)	Odds Ratio (95% Confidence Interval)
≥1	86%	4.2 (1.4-14.8)
≥2	69%	6.5 (2.6-16.5)
≥3	60%	25.3 (7.9-87.1)
≥4	31%	24.1 (4.7-230.0)

*Includes risk factors shown in A, and in addition, decreased fetal movement, prolonged second stage of labor, fetal heart rate abnormalities, and history of infertility (treated with ovarian-stimulating drugs, which are prothrombotic).

Data from Lee J, Croen LA, Backstrand KH, Yoshida CK, et al: Maternal and infant characteristics associated with perinatal arterial stroke in the infant, *JAMA* 293:723-729, 2005.

TABLE 8-18 Brain Injury in Monochorionic Twins*
General Features
Incidence of brain injury overall ≈30%
Occurrence of brain injury associated with placental vascular anastomoses, particularly artery to vein, with twin-twin transfusion syndrome; incidence of death or brain injury in untreated severe twin-twin transfusion syndrome >80%
Intrauterine death of one twin commonly associated with brain injury in the surviving twin, but most twin gestations with brain injury in one or both twins *not* complicated by fetal death
Neuropathology
Injury in First Half of Pregnancy
Porencephaly-microcephaly
Polymicrogyria
Rarely, anencephaly, exencephaly, encephalocele
Injury in Second Half of Pregnancy
Isolated or multiple infarcts
Porencephaly with or without polymicrogyria
Hydranencephaly
Multicystic encephalomalacia
Periventricular leukomalacia
Rarely, venous thrombosis with hemorrhagic infarct
Pathogenesis
With Death of Co-twin
Disseminated intravascular coagulation (thromboplastin material from dead fetus)
Thromboembolic (placental material, detritus from dead fetus)
Severe hypotension with cerebral ischemia (hemorrhage into dead fetus)
With or without Death of Co-twin
Fetofetal transfusion leading to, in *the donor*, hypovolemia, hypotension, severe anemia, resulting in oligohydramnios ("stuck twin") and cerebral hypoxic-ischemic injury, and in *the recipient*, hypervolemia, polycythemia, hyperviscosity, cardiac failure, resulting in polyhydramnios, premature delivery, and cerebral hypoxic-ischemic injury
Mechanical factors: transient disturbance of umbilical blood flow by compression or distortion, placental circulatory stasis with thromboembolism

*See text for references.

are monozygotic. Of the latter, approximately 30% are diamniotic, dichorionic (if the zygote splits early before blastocyst formation). However, approximately 70% of monozygotic twin gestations are diamniotic but *monochorionic* (when the zygote splits after blastocyst formation). In the latter group, in which each fetus shares the single placenta, the risk of brain injury approaches 30% (see Table 8-18). In this context occur *placental vascular anastomoses*, especially arteriovenous connections, in which placental tissue perfused by an artery from one fetus is drained by a vein from the other.[667] In most situations, the anastomoses are balanced, but in 10% to 15%, they are unbalanced, and the twin-twin transfusion syndrome (TTTS) results. The TTTS is the setting for most of the brain injury associated with twin gestations. Although this brain injury may occur consequent to the fetal death of a co-twin, most such injury occurs without such fetal death.

The *neuropathology* of brain injury associated with twin gestations relates particularly to the timing of the injury, as outlined in Table 8-18. Disturbances in early brain development (e.g., anencephaly and encephalocele) occur only rarely, and such early lesions are considered to be caused by vascular insufficiency. Also of presumed vascular basis are the somewhat more common occurrences of microcephaly with multiple porencephalies and of polymicrogyria. The polymicrogyria may contain features both of a disorder of neuronal migration (nonlayered cortex, heterotopias) and of a postmigrational encephaloclastic process (cortical laminar necrosis). The most characteristic lesions are associated with insults in the second trimester and later and consist of the full range of focal, multifocal, and generalized ischemic lesions (i.e., isolated infarction, porencephaly, hydranencephaly, multicystic encephalomalacia, and PVL). Concerning the most serious of the ischemic lesions (i.e., hydranencephaly and severe porencephaly), twin gestations accounted for 11% of all cases in one series.[630] In most such cases, a deceased co-twin is identified.[630,662,664] (The incidence of deceased co-twin in these most severe cases could be higher because the remnants of such a co-twin are easily missed without careful examination of the placenta. In addition, the prenatal mortality in twins is high [i.e., approximately 20% to 80% of twins detected in the first trimester of gestation were singletons by the time of birth].[649,668,669])

Pathogeneses of the brain injuries are best divided into those associated with *a dead co-twin* and those associated with *severe TTTS* but not necessarily fetal demise. Pathogenesis in cases with *death of a co-twin* includes the following: (1) thrombosis caused primarily by transfer of thromboplastin material from the dead twin, with disseminated intravascular coagulation resulting; (2) embolus from the placenta or the dead fetus through the fetal vascular anastomoses; and (3), considered most common, fetal exsanguination from the surviving to the dead fetus through placental anastomoses, resulting in severe hypotension and cerebral ischemia (see Table 8-18).[640] Pathogenesis in the more common situation of *severe TTTS* relates principally to the cerebral hemodynamic consequences of TTTS (see Table 8-18). Thus, the donor fetus experiences hypovolemia, hypotension, and severe anemia, with diminished CBF and cerebral hypoxic-ischemic injury the consequence. Because of decreased renal blood flow, oliguria leads to oligohydramnios with the additional potential for umbilical cord disturbance or placental compression. The recipient fetus experiences hypervolemia, polycythemia, hyperviscosity, and cardiac failure and thereby risks generalized and focal (thrombotic) cerebral circulatory insufficiency. Polyhydramnios and resulting premature delivery may contribute to risk. These hemodynamic factors may be complicated by or conceivably superseded by mechanical factors (e.g., disturbances by compression or distortion of umbilical blood flow or of placental flow, with risk of thrombosis; see Table 8-18).

Therapy has been directed toward the pregnancies complicated by severe TTTS (Table 8-19).

TABLE 8-19 Survival and Neurological Outcome in Severe Twin-Twin Transfusion Syndrome as a Function of Treatment*			
	None	**Amnioreduction**	**Laser**
Survival at 28 days	20%-30%	55%	75%
Normal neurological outcome	20%-30%[†]	50%-60%	85%
Cystic PVL	20%-30%	15%	5%

*Data for amnioreduction and intrauterine laser surgery largely from a large clinical trial (N = 142), (Senat MV, Deprest J, Boulvain M, Paupe A, et al: Endoscopic laser surgery versus serial amnioreduction for severe twin-to-twin transfusion syndrome, *N Engl J Med* 351:136-144, 2004), and from a separate cohort followed for a median of 3 years and 2 months (Graef C, Ellenrieder B, Hecher K, Hackeloer BJ, et al: Long-term neurodevelopmental outcome of 167 children after intrauterine laser treatment for severe twin-twin transfusion syndrome, *Obstet Gynecol* 194:303-308, 2006). See text for references for no treatment.

[†]Long-term follow-up data are limited.

Two fundamental approaches (i.e., serial amnioreduction and fetoscopic laser occlusion of the vascular anastomoses) have been used.[670-673a] Diagnosis of severe TTTS in the second trimester of gestation and institution of therapy shortly thereafter have comprised the usual protocol. The basis for any benefit from serial amnioreduction is unknown, but reduction of polyhydramnios, and consequently the risk for premature delivery, and improvement of placental hemodynamics seem most likely. The benefit of laser therapy relates to the reduction of the vascular anastomoses (a single amnioreduction to reduce polyhydramnios is carried out at the time of the laser surgery). Available data suggest benefit from both approaches, with laser therapy the better intervention (see Table 8-19).

Generalized Systemic Circulatory Insufficiency. An apparently *generalized* disturbance of systemic circulation with impaired perfusion of brain in the past has been considered to account for a substantial proportion of ischemic cerebral lesions, occurring either in utero or in the neonatal period. Indeed, the frequent occurrence of "prolonged second stage of labor," "fetal heart rate abnormalities," "signs of perinatal asphyxia," placental and cord "complications," and related features have suggested that generalized circulatory insufficiency could *contribute* to the pathogenesis of neonatal stroke.[482a,570,571,674,675] However, it is unclear how the strikingly unilateral predominance, in the distribution often of only a single vessel, could occur in the presence of an *apparently* generalized disturbance of perfusion. The phenomenon has been observed in the fetal and neonatal monkey.[676] Possible explanations include variations in the development of the cerebral vessels or their responses to regulatory effectors. The vessels of the anterior circulation, unlike those of the vertebrobasilar circulation, have a dense sympathetic innervation.[677] Thus, asphyxia, a potent sympathetic stimulator, may be particularly likely to induce vasoconstriction in the anterior circulation and may thereby favor the preponderance of focal cerebral ischemic lesions in the distribution of the middle cerebral artery.

A speculation would be that this innervation may exhibit asymmetries during development, and this developmental feature could explain some of the unilateral lesions seen with this apparently generalized insult.

REFERENCES

1. Spector RG: Water content of the immature rat brain following cerebral anoxia and ischaemia, *Br J Exp Pathol* 43:472-479, 1962.
2. Streicher E, Wisniewski H, Klatzo I: Resistance of immature brain to experimental cerebral edema, *Neurology* 15:833-836, 1965.
3. Larroche JC: *Developmental Pathology of the Neonate*, New York: 1977, Excerpta Medica.
4. Norman MG: Perinatal brain damage, *Perspect Pediatr Pathol* 4:41-92, 1978.
5. Rorke LB: *Pathology of Perinatal Brain Injury*, New York: 1982, Raven Press.
6. Friede RL: *Developmental Neuropathology*, 2nd ed, New York: 1989, Springer-Verlag.
7. Rorke LB: Anatomical features of the developing brain implicated in pathogenesis of hypoxic-ischemic injury, *Brain Pathol* 2:211-221, 1992.
8. Folkerth RD, Kinney HC: Perinatal neuropathology. In Louis DN, Love S, Ellison D, editors: *Greenfield's Neuropathology*, London: 2006, Arnold Publishers.
9. Clifford SH: The effects of asphyxia on the newborn infant, *J Pediatr* 18:567-579, 1941.
10. Thorn K: Cerebral symptoms in the newborn, *Acta Paediatr Scand* 195(Suppl):1, 1969.
11. Pryse-Davies J, Beard RW: A necropsy study of brain swelling in the newborn with special reference to cerebellar herniation, *J Pathol* 109:51-73, 1973.
12. Anderson JM, Belton NR: Water and electrolyte abnormalities in the human brain after severe intrapartum asphyxia, *J Neurol Neurosurg Psychiatry* 37:514-520, 1974.
13. Gilles FH, Leviton A, Dooling EC: *The Developing Human Brain: Growth and Epidemiologic Neuropathology*, Boston: 1983, John Wright.
14. Levene MI, Evans DH: Medical management of raised intracranial pressure after severe birth asphyxia, *Arch Dis Child* 60:12-16, 1985.
15. Levene MI, Evans DH, Forde A, Archer LN: Value of intracranial pressure monitoring of asphyxiated newborn infants, *Dev Med Child Neurol* 29:311-319, 1987.
16. Clancy R, Legido A, Newell R, Bruce D, et al: Continuous intracranial pressure monitoring and serial electroencephalographic recordings in severely asphyxiated term neonates, *Am J Dis Child* 142:740-747, 1988.
17. Lupton BA, Hill A, Roland EH, Whitfield MF, et al: Brain swelling in the asphyxiated term newborn: Pathogenesis and outcome, *Pediatrics* 82:139-146, 1988.
18. Adhikari M, Moodley M, Desai PK: Mannitol in neonatal cerebral oedema, *Brain Dev* 12:349-351, 1990.
19. Myers RE: Four patterns of perinatal brain damage and their conditions of occurrence in primates, *Adv Neurol* 10:223-234, 1975.
20. Brann AW, Jr, Myers RE: Central nervous system findings in the newborn monkey following severe in utero partial asphyxia, *Neurology* 25:327-338, 1975.
21. Myers RE: Two patterns of perinatal brain damage and their conditions of occurrence, *Am J Obstet Gynecol* 112:246-276, 1972.
22. Myers RE: Fetal asphyxia due to umbilical cord compression: Metabolic and brain pathologic consequences, *Biol Neonate* 26:21-43, 1975.
23. Myers RE: Two classes of dysergic brain abnormality and their conditions of occurrence, *Arch Neurol* 29:394-399, 1973.
24. Selzer ME, Myers RE, Holstein SB: Prolonged partial asphyxia: Effects on fetal brain water and electrolytes, *Neurology* 22:732-737, 1972.
25. Bondareff W, Myers RE, Brann AW: Brain extracellular space in monkey fetuses subjected to prolonged partial asphyxia, *Exp Neurol* 28:167-178, 1970.
26. Tweed WA, Pash M, Doig G: Cerebrovascular mechanisms in perinatal asphyxia: The role of vasogenic brain edema, *Pediatr Res* 15:44-46, 1981.
27. Rosenberg AA: Regulation of cerebral blood flow after asphyxia in neonatal lambs, *Stroke* 19:239-244, 1988.
28. De Haan HH, Gunn AJ, Williams CE, Gluckman PD: Brief repeated umbilical cord occlusions cause sustained cytotoxic cerebral edema and focal infarcts in near-term fetal lambs, *Pediatr Res* 41:96-104, 1997.
29. Rice JE, III, Vannucci RC, Brierley JB: The influence of immaturity on hypoxic-ischemic brain damage in the rat, *Ann Neurol* 9:131-141, 1981.
30. Mujsce DJ, Christensen MA, Vannucci RC: Cerebral blood flow and edema in perinatal hypoxic-ischemic brain damage, *Pediatr Res* 27:450-453, 1990.
31. Mujsce DJ, Towfighi J, Stern D, Vannucci RC: Mannitol therapy in perinatal hypoxic-ischemic brain damage in rats, *Stroke* 21:1210-1214, 1990.
32. Stonestreet BS, Burgess GH, Cserr HF: Blood-brain barrier integrity and brain water and electrolytes during hypoxia/hypercapnia and hypotension in newborn piglets, *Brain Res* 590:263-270, 1992.

33. Vannucci RC, Christensen MA, Yager JY: Nature, time-course, and extent of cerebral edema in perinatal hypoxic-ischemic brain damage, *Pediatr Neurol* 9:29-34, 1993.

34. Vannucci RC, Christensen MA, Yager JY: Cerebral edema and perinatal hypoxic-ischemic (H-1) brain damage, *Pediatr Res* 33:355A, 1993.

35. Rose VC, Shaffner DH, Gleason CA, Koehler RC, et al: Somatosensory evoked potential and brain water content in post-asphyxic immature piglets, *Pediatr Res* 37:661-666, 1995.

36. Rumpel H, Buchli R, Gehrmann J, Aguzzi A, et al: Magnetic resonance imaging of brain edema in the neonatal rat: A comparison of short and long term hypoxia-ischemia, *Pediatr Res* 38:113-118, 1995.

37. Nedelcu J, Klein MA, Aguzzi A, Boesiger P, et al: Biphasic edema after hypoxic-ischemic brain injury in neonatal rats reflects early neuronal and late glial damage, *Pediatr Res* 46:297-304, 1999.

38. Dijkhuizen RM, deGraaf RA, Tulleken KAF, Nicolay K: Changes in the diffusion of water and intracellular metabolites after excitotoxic injury and global ischemia in neonatal rat brain, *J Cereb Blood Flow Metab* 19:341-349, 1999.

39. Levy DE, Brierley JB, Silverman DG, Plum F: Brief hypoxia-ischemia initially damages cerebral neurons, *Arch Neurol* 32:450-456, 1975.

40. Brown AW, Brierley JB: The earliest alterations in rat neurones and astrocytes after anoxia-ischaemia, *Acta Neuropathol (Berl)* 23:9-22, 1973.

41. Salford LG, Plum F, Brierley JB: Graded hypoxia-oligemia in rat brain. II. Neuropathological alterations and their implications, *Arch Neurol* 29:234-238, 1973.

42. Kim SU: Brain hypoxia studied in mouse central nervous system cultures. I. Sequential cellular changes, *Lab Invest* 33:658-669, 1975.

43. Edwards AD, Yue X, Cox P, Hope PL, et al: Apoptosis in the brains of infants suffering intrauterine cerebral injury, *Pediatr Res* 42:684-689, 1997.

44. Becher JC, Bell JE, Keeling JW, et al: The Scottish perinatal neuropathology study: Clinicopathological correlation in early neonatal deaths, *Arch Dis Child Fetal Neonatal Ed* 89:F399-407, 2004.

45. Yue X, Mehmet H, Penrice J, Cooper C, et al: Apoptosis and necrosis in the newborn piglet brain following transient cerebral hypoxia-ischemia, *Neuropathol Appl Neurobiol* 23:16-25, 1997.

46. Edwards AD, Mehmet H: Apoptosis in perinatal hypoxic-ischaemic cerebral damage, *Neuropathol Appl Neurobiol* 22:482-503, 1996.

47. Bruck Y, Bruck W, Kretzschmar HA, Lassmann H: Evidence for neuronal apoptosis in pontosubicular neuron necrosis, *Neuropathol Appl Neurobiol* 22:23-29, 1996.

48. Mazarakis ND, Edwards AD, Mehmet H: Apoptosis in neural development and disease, *Arch Dis Child Fetal Neonatal Ed* 77:F165-F170, 1997.

49. Pulera MR, Adams LM, Liu HT, Santos DG, et al: Apoptosis in a neonatal rat model of cerebral hypoxia-ischemia, *Stroke* 29:2622-2629, 1998.

50. McDonald JW, Behrens MI, Chung C, Bhattacharyya T, et al: Susceptibility to apoptosis is enhanced in immature cortical neurons, *Brain Res* 759:228-232, 1997.

51. Taylor DL, Edwards AD, Mehmet H: Oxidative metabolism, apoptosis and perinatal brain injury, *Brain Pathol* 9:93-117, 1999.

52. Bossenmeyer-Pourie C, Koziel V, Daval J-L: Effects of hypothermia on hypoxia-induced apoptosis in cultured neurons from developing rat forebrain: Comparison with preconditioning, *Pediatr Res* 47:385-391, 2000.

53. Van Landeghem FKH, Felderhoff-Mueser U, Moysich, Stadelmann C, et al: Fas (CD95/Apo-1)/Fas ligand expression in neonates with pontosubicular neuron necrosis, *Pediatr Res* 51:129-135, 2002.

54. Leech RW, Alvord EC, Jr: Anoxic-ischemic encephalopathy in the human neonatal period: The significance of brain stem involvement, *Arch Neurol* 34:109-113, 1977.

55. Norman MG: Unilateral encephalomalacia in cranial nerve nuclei in neonates: Report of two cases, *Neurology* 24:424-427, 1974.

56. Norman MG: Antenatal neuronal loss and gliosis of the reticular formation, thalamus, and hypothalamus: A report of three cases, *Neurology* 22:910-916, 1972.

57. Schneider H, Ballowitz L, Schachinger H, Hanefeld F, et al: Anoxic encephalopathy with predominant involvement of basal ganglia, brain stem and spinal cord in the perinatal period: Report on seven newborns, *Acta Neuropathol (Berl)* 32:287-298, 1975.

58. Griffiths AD, Laurence KM: The effect of hypoxia and hypoglycaemia on the brain of the newborn human infant, *Dev Med Child Neurol* 16:308-319, 1974.

59. Grunnet ML, Curless RG, Bray PF, Jung AL: Brain changes in newborns from an intensive care unit, *Dev Med Child Neurol* 16:320-328, 1974.

60. Schneck SA, Neubuerger KT: Lesions of the brain in hyaline membrane disease of infants, *Acta Neuropathol (Berl)* 2:11-19, 1962.

61. Buckingham S, Sommers SC, Sherwin RP: Lesions of the dorsal vagal nucleus in the respiratory distress syndrome, *Am J Clin Pathol* 48:269-276, 1967.

62. Hall JG: A histological investigation of the auditory pathways in neonatal asphyxia: A preliminary report, *Acta Otolaryngol* 54:369-375, 1962.

63. Hall JG: On the neuropathological changes in the central nervous system following neonatal asphyxia, with special reference to the auditory system in man, *Acta Otolaryngol* 188(Suppl):331, 1963.

64. Leech RW, Brumback RA: Massive brain stem necrosis in the human neonate: Presentation of three cases with review of the literature, *J Child Neurol* 3:258-262, 1988.

65. Pindur J, Capin DM, Johnson MI, Rance NE: Cystic brain stem necrosis in a premature infant after prolonged bradycardia, *Acta Neuropathol (Berl)* 83:667-669, 1992.

66. Hashimoto K, Takeuchi Y, Takashima S: Hypocarbia as a pathogenic factor in pontosubicular necrosis, *Brain Dev* 13:155-157, 1991.

67. Torvik A, Skullerud K, Andersen SN, Hurum J, et al: Affection of the hippocampal granule cells in pontosubicular neuron necrosis, *Acta Neuropathol (Berl)* 83:535-537, 1992.

68. Galloway PG, Roessmann U: Neuronal karyorrhexis in Sommer's sector in a 22-week stillborn, *Acta Neuropathol (Berl)* 70:343-344, 1986.

69. Becker LE, Takashima S: Chronic hypoventilation and development of brain stem gliosis, *Neuropediatrics* 16:19-23, 1985.

70. Natsume J, Watanabe K, Kuno F, Hayakawa F, et al: Clinical, neurophysiologic, and neuropathological features of an infant with brain damage of total asphyxia type (Myers), *Pediatr Neurol* 13:61-64, 1995.

71. Roland EH, Poskitt K, Rodriguez E, Lupton BA, et al: Perinatal hypoxic-ischemic thalamic injury: Clinical features and neuroimaging, *Ann Neurol* 44:161-166, 1998.

72. Kinney HC, Panigrahy A, Newburger JW, Jonas RA, et al: Hypoxic-ischemic brain injury in infants with congenital heart disease dying after cardiac surgery, *Acta Neuropathol (Berl)* 110:563-578, 2005.

73. Cowan F, Rutherford M, Groenendaal F, Eken P, et al: Origin and timing of brain lesions in term infants with neonatal encephalopathy, *Lancet* 361:736-742, 2003.

74. Bell JE, Becher JC, Wyatt B, Keeling JW, et al: Brain damage and axonal injury in a Scottish cohort of neonatal deaths, *Brain* 128:1070-1081, 2005.

75. Pierson CR, Folkerth RD, Billards SS, Trachtenberg FL, et al: Gray matter injury associated with periventricular leukomalacia in the premature infant, *Acta Neuropathol* 114:619-631, 2007.

76. Roland EH, Hill A, Norman MG, Flodmark O, et al: Selective brainstem injury in an asphyxiated newborn, *Ann Neurol* 23:89-92, 1988.

77. Takashima S: Olivocerebellar lesions in infants born prematurely, *Brain Dev* 4:361-366, 1982.

78. Takashima S, Mito T, Houdou S, Ando Y: Relationship between periventricular hemorrhage, leukomalacia and brainstem lesions in prematurely born infants, *Brain Dev* 11:121-124, 1989.

79. Kreusser KL, Schmidt RE, Shackelford GD, Volpe JJ: Value of ultrasound for identification of acute hemorrhagic necrosis of thalamus and basal ganglia in an asphyxiated term infant, *Ann Neurol* 16:361-363, 1984.

80. Skullerud K, Westre B: Frequency and prognostic significance of germinal matrix hemorrhage, periventricular leukomalacia, and pontosubicular necrosis in preterm neonates, *Acta Neuropathol (Berl)* 70:257-261, 1986.

81. Skullerud K, Skjaeraasen J: Clinicopathological study of germinal matrix hemorrhage, pontosubicular necrosis, and periventricular leukomalacia in stillborn, *Childs Nerv Syst* 4:88-91, 1988.

82. Armstrong DL, Sauls CD, Goddard-Finegold J: Neuropathologic findings in short-term survivors of intraventricular hemorrhage, *Am J Dis Child* 141:617-621, 1987.

83. Scher MS, Painter MJ: Electroencephalographic diagnosis of neonatal seizures: Issues of diagnostic accuracy, clinical correlation, and survival. In Wasterlain CG, Vert P, editors: *Neonatal Seizures*, New York: 1990, Raven Press.

84. Gilles FH: Hypotensive brain stem necrosis: Selective symmetrical necrosis of tegmental neuronal aggregates following cardiac arrest, *Arch Pathol* 88:32-41, 1969.

85. Pasternak JF, Gorey MT: The syndrome of acute near-total intrauterine asphyxia in the term infant, *Pediatr Neurol* 18:391-398, 1998.

86. Sugama S, Ariga M, Hoashi E, Eto Y: Brainstem cranial-nerve lesions in an infant with hypoxic cerebral injury, *Pediatr Neurol* 29:256-259, 2003.

87. Sugama S, Eto Y: Brainstem lesions in children with perinatal brain injury, *Pediatr Neurol* 28:212-215, 2003.

88. Sarnat HB: Watershed infarcts in the fetal and neonatal brainstem: An aetiology of central hypoventilation, dysphagia, Mobius syndrome and micrognathia, *Eur J Pediatr Neurol* 8:71-87, 2004.

89. Ranck JB, Windle WF: Brain damage in the monkey, *Macaca mulatta*, by asphyxia neonatorum, *Exp Neurol* 1:130, 1959.

90. Faro MD, Windle WF: Transneuronal degeneration in brains of monkeys asphyxiated at birth, *Exp Neurol* 24:38-53, 1969.

91. Sargent MA, Poskitt KJ, Roland EH, Hill A, et al: Cerebellar vermian atrophy after neonatal hypoxic-ischemic encephalopathy, *AJNR Am J Neuroradiol* 25:1008-1015, 2004.

91a. Connolly DJ, Widjaja E, Griffiths PD: Involvement of the anterior lobe of the cerebellar vermis in perinatal profound hypoxia, *AJNR Am J Neuroradiol* 28:16-19, 2007.

92. LeStrange E, Saeed N, Cowan FM, Edwards AD, et al: MR imaging quantification of cerebellar growth following hypoxic-ischemic injury to the neonatal brain, *AJNR Am J Neuroradiol* 25:463-468, 2004.

93. Sladky JT, Rorke LB: Perinatal hypoxic-ischemic spinal cord injury, *Pediatr Pathol* 6:87-101, 1986.

94. Clancy RR, Sladky JT, Rorke LB: Hypoxic-ischemic spinal cord injury following perinatal asphyxia, *Ann Neurol* 25:185-189, 1989.

95. Martin E, Barkovich AJ: Magnetic resonance imaging in perinatal asphyxia, *Arch Dis Child Fetal Neonatal Ed* 72:F62-F70, 1995.

96. Barkovich AJ, Hallam D: Neuroimaging in perinatal hypoxic-ischemic injury, *Ment Retard Dev Disabil Res Rev* 3:1-14, 1997.

97. Rutherford M, Pennock J, Schwieso J, Cowan F, et al: Hypoxic-ischaemic encephalopathy: Early and late magnetic resonance imaging findings in relation to outcome, *Arch Dis Child Fetal Neonatal Ed* 75:F145-F151, 1996.

98. Kuenzle C, Baenziger O, Martin E, Thun-Hohenstein L, et al: Prognostic value of early MR imaging in term infants with severe perinatal asphyxia, *Neuropediatrics* 25:191-200, 1994.

99. Rutherford MA, Pennock JM, Schwieso JE, Cowan FM, et al: Hypoxic ischaemic encephalopathy: Early magnetic resonance imaging findings and their evolution, *Neuropediatrics* 26:183-191, 1995.

100. Mercuri E, Ricci D, Cowan FM, Lessing D, et al: Head growth in infants with hypoxic-ischemic encephalopathy: Correlation with neonatal magnetic resonance imaging, *Pediatrics* 106:235-243, 2000.

101. Rutherford MA, Azzopardi D, Whitelaw A, Cowan F, et al: Mild hypothermia and the distribution of cerebral lesions in neonates with hypoxic-ischemic encephalopathy, *Pediatrics* 116:1001-1006, 2005.

102. Wilson ER, Mirra SS, Schwartz JF: Congenital diencephalic and brain stem damage: Neuropathologic study of three cases, *Acta Neuropathol (Berl)* 57:70-74, 1982.

103. Parisi JE, Collins GH, Kim RC, Crosley CJ: Prenatal symmetrical thalamic degeneration with flexion spasticity at birth, *Ann Neurol* 13:94-97, 1983.

104. Cohen M, Roessmann U: In utero brain damage: Relationship of gestational age to pathological consequences, *Dev Med Child Neurol* 36:263-270, 1994.

105. Johnston MV: Neurotransmitter alterations in a model of perinatal hypoxic-ischemic brain injury, *Ann Neurol* 13:511-518, 1983.

106. McDonald JW, Johnston MV: Physiological and pathophysiological roles of excitatory amino acids during central nervous system development, *Brain Res Brain Res Rev* 15:41-70, 1990.

107. Malamud N: Status marmoratus: A form of cerebral palsy following either birth injury or inflammation of the central nervous system, *J Pediatr* 37:610, 1950.

108. Borit A, Herndon RM: The fine structure of plaques fibromyeliniques in ulegyria and in status marmoratus, *Acta Neuropathol (Berl)* 14:304-311, 1970.

109. Mito T, Kamei A, Takashima S, Becker LE: Clinicopathological study of pontosubicular necrosis, *Neuropediatrics* 24:204-207, 1993.

110. Stadelmann C, Mews I, Srinivasan A, Deckwerth TL, et al: Expression of cell death-associated proteins in neuronal apoptosis associated with pontosubicular neuron necrosis, *Brain Pathol* 11:273-281, 2001.

111. Rossiter JP, Anderson LI, Yang F, Cote GM: Caspase-3 activation and caspase-like proteolytic activity in human perinatal hypoxic-ischemic brain injury, *Acta Neuropathol (Berl)* 103:66-73, 2002.

112. Ahdab-Barmada M, Moossy J, Nemoto EM, Lin MR: Hyperoxia produces neuronal necrosis in the rat, *J Neuropathol Exp Neurol* 45:233-246, 1986.

113. Takizawa Y, Takashima S, Itoh M: A histopathological study of premature and mature infants with pontosubicular neuron necrosis: Neuronal cell death in perinatal brain damage, *Brain Res* 1095:200-206, 2006.

114. Allin M, Matsumoto H, Santhouse AM, Nosarti C, et al: Cognitive and motor function and the size of the cerebellum in adolescents born very pre-term, *Brain* 124:60-66, 2001.

115. Johnsen SD, Tarby TJ, Lewis KS, Bird R, et al: Cerebellar infraction: An unrecognized complication of very low birthweight, *J Child Neurol* 17:320-324, 2002.

116. Peterson BS, Vohr B, Staib LH, Cannistraci CJ, et al: Regional brain volume abnormalities and long-term cognitive outcome in preterm infants, *JAMA* 284:1939-1947, 2000.

117. Mercuri E, Atkinson J, Braddick O, Anker S, et al: Visual function in full-term infants with hypoxic-ischaemic encephalopathy, *Neuropediatrics* 28:155-161, 1997.

118. Argyropoulou MI, Xydis V, Drougia A, Argyropoulou PI, et al: MRI measurements of the pons and cerebellum in children born preterm; associations with the severity of periventricular leukomalacia and perinatal risk factors, *Neuroradiology* 45:730-734, 2003.

119. Bodensteiner JB, Johnsen SD: Cerebellar injury in the extremely premature infant: Newly recognized but relatively common outcome, *J Child Neurol* 20:139-142, 2005.

120. Johnsen SD, Bodensteiner JB, Lotze TE: Frequency and nature of cerebellar injury in the extremely premature survivor with cerebral palsy, *J Child Neurol* 20:60-64, 2005.

121. Limperopoulos C, Soul JS, Gauvreau K, Huppi PS, et al: Late gestation cerebellar growth is rapid and impeded by premature birth, *Pediatrics* 115:688-695, 2005.

122. Limperopoulos C, Soul JS, Haidar H, Huppi PS, et al: Impaired trophic interactions between the cerebellum and the cerebrum among preterm infants, *Pediatrics* 116:844-850, 2005.

123. Miall LS, Cornette LG, Tanner SF, Arthur RJ, et al: Posterior fossa abnormalities seen on magnetic resonance brain imaging in a cohort of newborn infants, *J Perinatol* 23:396-403, 2003.

124. Srinivasan L, Allsop J, Counsell SJ, Boardman JP, et al: Smaller cerebellar volumes in very preterm infants at term-equivalent age are associated with the presence of supratentorial lesions, *AJNR Am J Neuroradiol* 27:573-579, 2006.

125. Shah DK, Anderson PJ, Carlin JB, Pavlovic M, et al: Reduction in cerebellar volumes in preterm infants: Relationship to white matter injury and neurodevelopment at two years of age, *Pediatr Res* 60:97-102, 2006.

126. Bodensteiner JB, Johnsen SD: Magnetic resonance imaging (MRI) findings in children surviving extremely premature delivery and extremely low birthweight with cerebral palsy, *J Child Neurol* 21:743-747, 2006.

127. Pryds O, Greisen G, Lou H, Friis-Hansen B: Vasoparalysis associated with brain damage in asphyxiated term infants, *J Pediatr* 117:119-125, 1990.

128. Greisen G: Effect of cerebral blood flow and cerebrovascular autoregulation on the distribution, type and extent of cerebral injury, *Brain Pathol* 2:223-228, 1992.

129. Kuban KC, Gilles FH: Human telencephalic angiogenesis, *Ann Neurol* 17:539-548, 1985.

130. Nelson MD, Gonzalez-Gomez I, Gilles FH: The search for human telencephalic ventriculofugal arteries, *AJNR Am J Neuroradiol* 12:215-222, 1991.

131. Nelson C, Silverstein FS: Acute regionally specific reductions in cytochrome oxidase activity predict selective vulnerability to ischemic injury in perinatal rodent brain [abstract], *Ann Neurol* 30:482, 1991.

132. Barks JD, Silverstein FS, Sims K, Greenamyre JT, et al: Glutamate recognition sites in human fetal brain, *Neurosci Lett* 84:131-136, 1988.

133. McDonald JW, Trescher WH, Johnston MV: The selective ionotropic-type quisqualate receptor agonist AMPA is a potent neurotoxin in immature rat brain, *Brain Res* 526:165-168, 1990.

134. Lee HS, Choi BH: Density and distribution of excitatory amino acid receptors in the developing human fetal brain: A quantitative autoradiographic study, *Exp Neurol* 118:284-290, 1992.

135. Piggott MA, Perry EK, Perry RH, Scott D: N-Methyl-D-aspartate (NMDA) and non-NMDA binding sites in developing human frontal cortex, *Neurosci Res Commun* 12:9-16, 1993.

136. Johnston MV: Neurotransmitters and vulnerability of the developing brain, *Brain Dev* 17:301-306, 1995.

137. Panigrahy A, Rosenberg PS, Assmann S, Foley EC, et al: Differential expression of glutamate receptor subtypes in human brainstem sites involved in perinatal hypoxia-ischemia, *J Comp Neurol* 437:196-208, 2001.

138. Ferriero DM, Arcavi LJ, Sagar SM, McIntosh TK, et al: Selective sparing of NADPH-diaphorase neurons in neonatal hypoxia-ischemia, *Ann Neurol* 24:670-676, 1988.

139. Ferriero DM, Arcavi LJ, Simon RP: Ontogeny of excitotoxic injury to nicotinamide adenine dinucleotide phosphate diaphorase reactive neurons in the neonatal rat striatum, *Neuroscience* 36:417-424, 1990.

140. Downen M, Zhao ML, Lee P, Weidenheim KM, et al: Neuronal nitric oxide synthase expression in developing and adult human CNS, *J Neuropathol Exp Neurol* 58:12-21, 1999.

141. Talos DM, Follett PL, Folkerth RD, Fishman RE, et al: Developmental regulation of alpha-amino-3-hydroxy-5-methyl-4-isoxazole-propionic acid receptor subunit expression in forebrain and relationship to regional susceptibility to hypoxic/ischemic injury. II. Human cerebral white matter and cortex, *J Comp Neurol* 497:61-77, 2006.

142. Mallard EC, Williams CE, Gunn AJ, Gunning MI, et al: Frequent episodes of brief ischemia sensitize the fetal sheep brain to neuronal loss and induce striatal injury, *Pediatr Res* 33:61-65, 1993.

143. Mallard EC, Waldvogel HJ, Williams CE, Faull R, et al: Repeated asphyxia causes loss of striatal projection neurons in the fetal sheep brain, *Neuroscience* 65:827-836, 1995.

144. Mallard EC, Williams CE, Johnston BM, Gunning MI, et al: Repeated episodes of umbilical cord occlusion in fetal sheep lead to preferential damage to the striatum and sensitize the heart to further insults, *Pediatr Res* 37:707-713, 1995.

145. Martin-Ancel A, Carcia-Alix A, Pascual-Salcedo D, Cabanas F, et al: Interleukin-6 in the cerebrospinal fluid after perinatal asphyxia is related to early and late neurological manifestations, *Pediatrics* 100:789-794, 1997.

146. Grether JK, Nelson KB: Maternal infection and cerebral palsy in infants of normal birth weight, *JAMA* 287:207-211, 1997.

147. Nelson KB, Dambrosia JM, Grether JK, Phillips TM: Neonatal cytokines and coagulation factors in children with cerebral palsy, *Ann Neurol* 44:665-675, 1998.

148. Grether JK, Nelson KB, Dambrosia JM, Phillips TM: Interferons and cerebral palsy, *J Pediatr* 134:324-332, 1999.

149. Foster-Barber A, Dickens B, Ferriero DM: Human perinatal asphyxia: Correlation of neonatal cytokines with MRI and outcome, *Dev Neurosci* 23:213-218, 2002.

150. Shalak LF, Perlman JM: Infection markers and early signs of neonatal encephalopathy in the term infant, *Ment Retard Dev Disabl Res Rev* 8:14-19, 2002.

151. Shalak LF, Laptook AR, Jafri HS, Ramilo O, et al: Clinical chorioamnionitis, elevated cytokines, and brain injury in term infants, *Pediatrics* 110:673-680, 2002.

152. Wu YW, Escobar GJ, Grether JK, Croen LA, et al: Chorioamnionitis and cerebral palsy in term and near-term infants, *JAMA* 290:2677-2684, 2003.

153. Silveira RC, Procianoy RS: Interleukin-6 and tumor necrosis factor-α levels in plasma and cerebrospinal fluid of term newborn infants with hypoxic-ischemic encephalopathy, *J Pediatr* 143:625-629, 2003.

154. Bartha AI, Foster-Barber A, Miller SP, Vigneron DB, et al: Neonatal encephalopathy: Association of cytokines with MR spectroscopy and outcome, *Pediatr Res* 56:960-966, 2004.

155. Rouse DJ, Landon M, Leveno KJ, Leindecker S, et al: The Maternal-Fetal Medicine Units cesarean registry: Chorioamnionitis at term and its duration—relationship to outcomes, *Am J Obstet Gynecol* 191:211-216, 2004.

156. Shalak L, Johnson-Welch S, Perlman JM: Chorioamnionitis and neonatal encephalopathy in term infants with fetal acidemia: Histopathologic correlations, *Pediatr Neurol* 33:162-165, 2005.

157. Friede RL: *Developmental Neuropathology*, New York: 1975, Springer-Verlag.

158. Courville CB: *Birth and Brain Damage*, Pasadena: 1971, MF Courville.

159. Norman RM, Urich H, McMenemey WH: Vascular mechanisms of birth injury, *Brain* 80:49-58, 1957.

160. Volpe JJ, Pasternak JF: Parasagittal cerebral injury in neonatal hypoxic-ischemic encephalopathy: Clinical and neuroradiologic features, *J Pediatr* 91:472-476, 1977.

161. O'Brien MJ, Ash JM, Gilday DL: Radionuclide brain-scanning in perinatal hypoxia/ischemia, *Dev Med Child Neurol* 21:161-169, 1979.

162. Volpe JJ, Herscovitch P, Perlman JM, Kreusser KL, et al: Positron emission tomography in the asphyxiated term newborn: Parasagittal impairment of cerebral blood flow, *Ann Neurol* 17:287-296, 1985.

163. Yokochi K, Fujimoto S: Magnetic resonance imaging in children with neonatal asphyxia: Correlation with developmental sequelae, *Acta Paediatr* 85:88-95, 1996.

164. Miller SP, Ramaswamy V, Michelson D, Barkovich AJ, et al: Patterns of brain injury in term neonatal encephalopathy, *J Pediatr* 146:453-460, 2005.

165. Meyer JE: Uber die Lokalisation fruhkindlicher Hirschaden in arteriellen Grenzgebieten, *Arch Psychiatr Nervenkr Z Gesamte Neurol Psychiatr* 190:328-341, 1953.

166. Adams JH, Brierley JB, Connor RC, Treip CS: The effects of systemic hypotension upon the human brain: Clinical and neuropathological observations in 11 cases, *Brain* 89:235-268, 1966.

167. Zulch KJ: Die Pathogenese von Massenblutung und Erweichung unter besonderer berucksichtigung klinischer Gesichtspunkte, *Acta Neurochir* 7(Suppl):51, 1961.

168. Torvik A: The pathogenesis of watershed infarcts in the brain, *Stroke* 15:221-223, 1984.

169. Brierley JB, Excell BJ: The effects of profound systemic hypotension upon the brain of *M. rhesus*: Physiological and pathological observations, *Brain* 89:269-298, 1966.

170. Brierley JB, Brown AW, Excell BJ, Meldrum BS: Brain damage in the rhesus monkey resulting from profound arterial hypotension. I. Its nature, distribution and general physiological correlates, *Brain Res* 13:68-100, 1969.

171. Takashima S, Ando Y, Takeshita K: Hypoxic-ischemic brain damage and cerebral blood flow changes in young rabbits, *Brain Dev* 8:274-277, 1986.

172. Yoshioka H, Iino S, Sato N, Osamura T, et al: New model of hemorrhagic hypoxic-ischemic encephalopathy in newborn mice, *Pediatr Neurol* 5:221-225, 1989.

173. Williams CE, Gunn AJ, Synek B, Gluckman PD: Delayed seizures occurring with hypoxic-ischemic encephalopathy in the fetal sheep, *Pediatr Res* 27:561-565, 1990.

174. Williams CE, Gunn AJ, Mallard C, Gluckman PD: Outcome after ischemia in the developing sheep brain: An electroencephalographic and histological study, *Ann Neurol* 31:14-21, 1992.

175. Gunn AJ, Parer JT, Mallard EC, Williams CE, et al: Cerebral histologic and electrocorticographic changes after asphyxia in fetal sheep, *Pediatr Res* 31:486-491, 1992.

176. Marks KA, Mallard CE, Roberts I, Williams CE, et al: Nitric oxide synthase inhibition attenuates delayed vasodilation and increases injury after cerebral ischemia in fetal sheep, *Pediatr Res* 40:185-191, 1996.

177. Takashima S, Armstrong DL, Becker LE: Subcortical leukomalacia: Relationship to development of the cerebral sulcus and its vascular supply, *Arch Neurol* 35:470-472, 1978.

178. Rutherford MA, Pennock JM, Dubowitz L: Cranial ultrasound and magnetic resonance imaging in hypoxic-ischaemic encephalopathy: A comparison with outcome, *Dev Med Child Neurol* 36:813-825, 1994.

179. Rollins NK, Morriss MC, Evans D, Perlman JM: The role of early MR in the evaluation of the term infant with seizures, *AJNR Am J Neuroradiol* 15:239-248, 1994.

180. Mercuri E, Rutherford M, Cowan F, Pennock J, et al: Early prognostic indicators of outcome in infants with neonatal cerebral infarction: A clinical, electroencephalogram, and magnetic resonance imaging study, *Pediatrics* 103:103-139, 1999.

181. de Vries LS, Groenendaal F, Eken P, van Haastert IC, et al: Infarcts in the vascular distribution of the middle cerebral artery in preterm and full-term infants, *Neuropediatrics* 28:88-96, 1997.

182. Trauner DA, Mannino FL: Neurodevelopmental outcome after neonatal cerebrovascular accident, *J Pediatr* 108:459-461, 1986.

183. Bode H, Strassburg HM, Pringsheim W, Kunzer W: Cerebral infarction in term neonates: Diagnosis by cerebral ultrasound, *Childs Nerv Syst* 2:195-199, 1986.

184. Filipek PA, Krishnamoorthy KS, Davis KR, Kuehnle K: Focal cerebral infarction in the newborn: A distinct entity, *Pediatr Neurol* 3:141-147, 1987.

185. Coker SB, Beltran RS, Myers TF, Hmura L: Neonatal stroke: Description of patients and investigation into pathogenesis, *Pediatr Neurol* 4:219-223, 1988.

186. Hernanz-Schulman M, Cohen W, Genieser NB: Sonography of cerebral infarction in infancy, *AJR Am J Roentgenol* 150:897-902, 1988.

187. Roodhooft AM, Parizel PM, Van Acker KJ, Deprettere AJ, et al: Idiopathic cerebral arterial infarction with paucity of symptoms in the full-term neonate, *Pediatrics* 80:381-385, 1987.

188. Sran SK, Baumann RJ: Outcome of neonatal strokes, *Am J Dis Child* 142:1086-1088, 1988.

189. Fujimoto S, Yokochi K, Togari H, Nishimura Y, et al: Neonatal cerebral infarction: Symptoms, CT findings and prognosis, *Brain Dev* 14:48-52, 1992.

190. Trounce JQ, Levene MI: Diagnosis and outcome of subcortical cystic leucomalacia, *Arch Dis Child* 60:1041-1044, 1985.

191. Houdou S, Takashima S, Takeshita K, Ohta S: Infantile subcortical leukohypodensity demonstrated by computed tomography, *Pediatr Neurol* 4:165-167, 1988.

192. Yokochi K: Clinical profiles of subjects with subcortical leukomalacia and border-zone infarction revealed by MR, *Acta Paediatr* 87:879-883, 1998.

193. Virchow R: Zur pathologischen Anatomie des Gehirns. I. Congenitale Encephalitis und Myelitis, *Virchow Arch Pathol Anat* 38:129, 1867.

194. Parrot J: Etude sur le ramollissement de l'encephale chez le nouveau-né, *Arch Physiol Norm Pathol* 5:59, 1873.

195. Rydberg E: Cerebral injury in newborn children, consequent on birth trauma: With an inquiry into the normal and pathological anatomy of the neuroglia, *Acta Pathol Microbiol Scand Suppl* 19:1, 1932.

196. Schwartz P: *Birth Injuries of the Newborn: Morphology, Pathogenesis, Clinical Pathology and Prevention*, New York: 1961, Hafner Publishing.

197. Banker BQ, Larroche JC: Periventricular leukomalacia of infancy: A form of neonatal anoxic encephalopathy, *Arch Neurol* 7:386-410, 1962.

198. Volpe JJ: *Neurology of the Newborn*, 3rd ed, Philadelphia: 1995, WB Saunders.

199. Shuman RM, Selednik LJ: Periventricular leukomalacia: A one-year autopsy study, *Arch Neurol* 37:231-235, 1980.

200. de Vries LS, Wigglesworth JS, Regev R, Dubowitz LM: Evolution of periventricular leukomalacia during the neonatal period and infancy: Correlation of imaging and postmortem findings, *Early Hum Dev* 17:205-219, 1988.

201. Hope PL, Gould SJ, Howard S, Hamilton PA, et al: Precision of ultrasound diagnosis of pathologically verified lesions in the brains of very preterm infants, *Dev Med Child Neurol* 30:457-471, 1988.

202. Paneth N, Rudelli R, Monte W, Rodriguez E, et al: White matter necrosis in very low birth weight infants: Neuropathologic and ultrasonographic findings in infants surviving six days or longer, *J Pediatr* 116:975-984, 1990.

203. Carson SC, Hertzberg BS, Bowie JD, Burger PC: Value of sonography in the diagnosis of intracranial hemorrhage and periventricular leukomalacia: A postmortem study of 35 cases, *AJNR Am J Neuroradiol* 155:595-601, 1990.

204. Barth PG, Stam FC, Oosterkamp RF, Bezemer PD, et al: On the relationship between germinal layer haemorrhage and telencephalic leucoencephalopathy in the preterm infant, *Neuropediatrie* 11:17-26, 1980.

205. Golden JA, Gilles FH, Rudewlli R, Leviton A: Frequency of neuropathological abnormalities in very low birth weight infants, *J Neuropathol Exp Neurol* 56:472-478, 1997.

206. Iida K, Takashima S, Ueda K: Immunohistochemical study of myelination and oligodendrocyte in infants with periventricular leukomalacia, *Pediatr Neurol* 13:296-304, 1995.

207. Takashima S, Iida K, Deguchi K: Periventricular leukomalacia, glial development and myelination, *Early Hum Dev* 43:177-184, 1995.

208. Leviton A, Gilles FH: Acquired perinatal leukoencephalopathy, *Ann Neurol* 16:1-10, 1984.

209. Perlman JM, Risser R, Broyles RS: Bilateral cystic periventricular leukomalacia in the premature infant: Associated risk factors, *Pediatrics* 97:822-827, 1996.

210. Zupan V, Gonzalez P, Lacaze-Masmonteil T, Boithias C, et al: Periventricular leukomalacia: Risk factors revisited, *Dev Med Child Neurol* 38:1061-1067, 1996.

211. Yoon BH, Romero R, Yang SH, Jun JK, et al: Interleukin-6 concentrations in umbilical cord plasma are elevated in neonates with white matter lesions associated with periventricular leukomalacia, *Am J Obstet Gynecol* 174:1433-1440, 1996.

212. Yoon BH, Jun JK, Romero R, Park KH, et al: Amniotic fluid inflammatory cytokines (interleukin-6, interleukin-1β, and tumor necrosis factor-α), neonatal brain white matter lesions, and cerebral palsy, *Am J Obstet Gynecol* 177:19-26, 1997.

213. Dammann O, Leviton A: Maternal intrauterine infection, cytokines, and brain damage in the preterm newborn, *Pediatr Res* 42:1-8, 1997.

214. Kuban K, Sanocka U, Leviton A, Allred EN, et al: White matter disorders of prematurity: Association with intraventricular hemorrhage and ventriculomegaly, *J Pediatr* 134:539-546, 1999.

215. Dammann O, Leviton A: Brain damage in preterm newborns: Biological response modification as a strategy to reduce disabilities, *J Pediatr* 136:433-438, 2000.

216. Volpe JJ: Neurobiology of periventricular leukomalacia in the premature infant, *Pediatr Res* 50:553-562, 2001.
217. Volpe JJ: Cerebral white matter injury of the premature infant: More common than you think, *Pediatrics* 112:176-179, 2003.
218. Volpe JJ: Encephalopathy of prematurity includes neuronal abnormalities, *Pediatrics* 116:221-225, 2005.
219. Bejar RF, Vaucher YE, Benirschke K, Berry CC: Postnatal white matter necrosis in preterm infants, *J Perinatol* 12:3-8, 1992.
220. Volpe JJ: *Neurology of the Newborn,* 4th ed, Philadelphia: 2001, WB Saunders.
221. Larroque B, Marret S, Ancel PY, Arnaud C, et al: White matter damage and intraventricular hemorrhage in very preterm infants: The EPIPAGE study, *J Pediatr* 143:477-483, 2003.
222. Miller SP, Cozzio CC, Goldstein RB, Ferriero DM, et al: Comparing the diagnosis of white matter injury in premature newborns with serial MR imaging and transfontanel ultrasonography findings, *AJNR Am J Neuroradiol* 24:1661-1669, 2003.
223. Inder TE, Warfield SK, Wang H, Huppi PS, et al: Abnormal cerebral structure is present at term in premature infants, *Pediatrics* 115:286-294, 2005.
224. Miller SP, Ferriero DM, Leonard C, Piecuch R, et al: Early brain injury in premature newborns detected with magnetic resonance imaging is associated with adverse early neurodevelopmental outcome, *J Pediatr* 147:609-616, 2005.
225. Woodward LJ, Anderson PJ, Austin NC, Howard K, et al: Neonatal MRI to predict neurodevelopmental outcomes in preterm infants, *N Engl J Med* 355:685-694, 2006.
226. Maalouf EF, Duggan PJ, Counsell S, Rutherford MA, et al: Comparison of findings on cranial ultrasound and magnetic resonance imaging in preterm infants, *Pediatrics* 107:719-727, 2001.
227. Inder TE, Anderson NJ, Spencer C, Wells SJ, et al: White matter injury in the premature infant: A comparison between serial cranial ultrasound and MRI at term, *AJNR Am J Neuroradiol* 24:805-809, 2003.
228. Debillon T, Guyen SN, Muet A, Quere MP, et al: Limitations of ultrasonography for diagnosing white matter damage in preterm infants, *Arch Dis Child Fetal Neonatal Ed* 88:F275-F279, 2003.
229. Maalouf EF, Duggan PJ, Rutherford MA, Counsell SJ, et al: Magnetic resonance imaging of the brain in a cohort of extremely preterm infants, *J Pediatr* 135:351-357, 1999.
230. Inder TE, Wells SJ, Mogridge N, Spencer C, et al: Defining the nature of the cerebral abnormalities in the premature infant: A qualitative magnetic resonance imaging study, *J Pediatr* 143:171-179, 2003.
231. Counsell SJ, Allsop JM, Harrison MC, Larkman DJ, et al: Diffusion weighted imaging of the brain in preterm infants with focal and diffuse white matter abnormality, *Pediatrics* 112:1-7, 2003.
232. Dyet LE, Kennea N, Counsell SJ, Maalouf EF, et al: Natural history of brain lesions in extremely preterm infants studied with serial magnetic resonance imaging from birth and neurodevelopmental assessment, *Pediatrics* 118:536-548, 2006.
233. Leech RW, Alvord EC, Jr: Morphologic variations in periventricular leukomalacia, *Am J Pathol* 74:591-602, 1974.
234. Pape KE, Wigglesworth JS: *Haemorrhage, Ischaemia and the Perinatal Brain,* Philadelphia: 1979, JB Lippincott.
235. Fawer CL, Calame A, Perentes E, Anderegg A: Periventricular leukomalacia: A correlation study between real-time ultrasound and autopsy findings—periventricular leukomalacia in the neonate, *Neuroradiology* 27:292-300, 1985.
236. Dambska M, Laure-Kamionowska M, Schmidt-Sidor B: Early and late neuropathological changes in perinatal white matter damage, *J Child Neurol* 4:291-298, 1989.
237. Leviton A, Paneth N: White matter damage in preterm newborns: An epidemiologic perspective, *Early Hum Dev* 24:1-22, 1990.
238. Iida K, Takashima S, Takeuchi Y, Ohno T, et al: Neuropathologic study of newborns with prenatal-onset leukomalacia, *Pediatr Neurol* 9:45-48, 1993.
239. Marin-Padilla M: Developmental neuropathology and impact of perinatal brain damage. II. White matter lesions of the neocortex, *J Neuropathol Exp Neurol* 56:219-235, 1997.
240. Kinney HC, Back SA: Human oligodendroglial development: Relationship to periventricular leukomalacia, *Semin Pediatr Neurol* 5:180-189, 1998.
241. Deguchi K, Oguchi K, Takashima S: Characteristic neuropathology of leukomalacia in extremely low birth weight infants, *Pediatr Neurol* 16:296-300, 1997.
242. Rodriguez J, Claus D, Verellen G, Lyon G: Periventricular leukomalacia: Ultrasonic and neuropathological correlations, *Dev Med Child Neurol* 32:347-352, 1990.
243. Haynes RL, Folkerth RD, Keefe R, Sung I, et al: Nitrosative and oxidative injury to premyelinating oligodendrocytes is accompanied by microglial activation in periventricular leukomalacia in the human premature infant, *J Neuropathol Exp Neurol* 62:441-450, 2003.
244. Arai Y, Deguchi K, Mizuguchi M, Takashima S: Expression of β-amyloid precursor protein in axons of periventricular leukomalacia brains, *Pediatr Neurol* 13:161-163, 1995.
245. Meng SZ, Arai Y, Deguchi K, Takashima S: Early detection of axonal and neuronal lesions in prenatal-onset periventricular leukomalacia, *Brain Dev* 19:480-484, 1997.
246. Back SA, Luo NL, Mallinson RA, O'Malley JP, et al: Selective vulnerability of preterm white matter to oxidative damage defined by F(2)-isoprostanes, *Ann Neurol* 58:108-120, 2005.
247. Robinson S, Li Q, Dechant A, Cohen ML: Neonatal loss of gamma-aminobutyric acid pathway expression after human perinatal brain injury, *J Neurosurg* 104:396-408, 2006.
248. Back SA, Luo NL, Borenstein NS, Levine JM, et al: Late oligodendrocyte progenitors coincide with the developmental window of vulnerability for human perinatal white matter injury, *J Neurosci* 21:1302-1312, 2001.
249. Back SA, Luo NL, Borenstein NS, Volpe JJ, et al: Arrested oligodendrocyte lineage progression during human cerebral white matter development: Dissociation between the timing of progenitor differentiation and myelinogenesis, *J Neuropathol Exp Neurol* 61:197-211, 2002.
250. Inder TE, Mocatta T, Darlow B, Spencer C, et al: Elevated free radical products in the cerebrospinal fluid of VLBW infants with cerebral white matter injury, *Pediatr Res* 52:213-218, 2002.
251. Armstrong D, Norman MG: Periventricular leucomalacia in neonates: Complications and sequelae, *Arch Dis Child* 49:367-375, 1974.
252. Inder TE, Huppi PS, Warfield S, Kikinis R, et al: Periventricular white matter injury in the premature infant is associated with a reduction in cerebral cortical gray matter volume at term, *Ann Neurol* 46:755-760, 1999.
253. Ajayi-Obe M, Saeed N, Cowan FM, Rutherford MA, et al: Reduced development of cerebral cortex in extremely preterm infants, *Lancet* 356:1162-1163, 2000.
254. Peterson BS, Anderson AW, Ehrenkranz RA, Staib LH, et al: Regional brain volumes and their later neurodevelopmental correlates in term and preterm infants, *Pediatrics* 111:939-948, 2003.
255. Thompson DK, Warfield SK, Carlin JB, Pavlovic M, et al: Perinatal risk factors altering regional brain structure in the preterm infant, *Brain* 130:667-677, 2007.
256. Isaacs E, Lucas A, Chong WK, Wood SJ, et al: Hippocampal volume and everyday memory in children of very low birth weight, *Pediatr Res* 47:713-720, 2000.
257. Peterson BS, Vohr B, Staib LH, Cannistraci CJ, et al: Regional brain volume abnormalities and long-term cognitive outcome in preterm infants, *JAMA* 284:1939-1947, 2000.
258. Nosarti C, Al-Asady MHS, Frangou S, Stewart AL, et al: Adolescents who were born very preterm have decreased brain volumes, *Brain* 125:1616-1623, 2002.
259. Abernethy LJ, Cooke RW, Foulder-Hughes L: Caudate and hippocampal volumes, intelligence, and motor impairment in 7-year-old children who were born preterm, *Pediatr Res* 55:884-893, 2004.
260. Reiss AL, Kesler SR, Vohr B, Duncan CC, et al: Sex differences in cerebral volumes of 8-year-olds born preterm, *J Pediatr* 145:242-249, 2004.
261. Kesler SR, Ment LR, Vohr B, Pajot SK, et al: Volumetric analysis of regional cerebral development in preterm children, *Pediatr Neurol* 31:318-325, 2004.
262. Lodygensky GA, Rademaker KJ, Zimine S, Gex-Fabry M, et al: Structural and functional brain developmental after hydrocortisone treatment for neonatal chronic lung disease, *Pediatrics* 116:1-7, 2005.
263. Thomas B, Eyssen M, Peeters R, Molenaers G, et al: Quantitative diffusion tensor imaging in cerebral palsy due to periventricular white matter injury, *Brain* 128:2562-2577, 2005.
264. Kraus RL, Pasieczny R, Lariosa-Willingham K, Turner MS, et al: Antioxidant properties of minocycline: Neuroprotection in an oxidative stress assay and direct radical-scavenging activity, *J Neurochem* 94:819-827, 2005.
264a. Nosarti C, Giouroukou E, Healy E, Rifkin L, et al: Grey and white matter distribution in very preterm adolescents mediates neurodevelopmental outcome, *Brain* 131:205-217, 2008.
264b. Skranes J, Vangberg TR, Kulseng S, Indredavik MS, et al: Clinical findings and white matter abnormalities seen on diffusion tensor imaging in adolescents with very low birth weight, *Brain* 130:654-666, 2007.
265. Lin Y, Okumura A, Hayakawa F, Kato T, et al: Quantitative evaluation of thalami and basal ganglia in infants with periventricular leukomalacia, *Dev Med Child Neurol* 43:481-485, 2001.
266. Peterson BS, Vohr B, Kane MJ, Whalen DH, et al: A functional magnetic resonance imaging study of language processing and its cognitive correlates in prematurely born children, *Pediatrics* 110:1153-1162, 2002.
267. Kinney HC, Armstrong DL: Perinatal neuropathology. In Graham DI, Lantos PE, editors: *Greenfield's Neuropathology* 7, London: 2002, Arnold Publishers.
268. Paneth N, Rudelli R, Monte W, Rodriguez E, et al: White matter necrosis in very low birth weight infants: Neuropathologic and ultrasonographic findings in infants surviving six days or longer, *J Pediatr* 116:975-984, 1990.
269. Deguchi K, Oguchi K, Matsuura N, Armstrong DD, et al: Periventricular leukomalacia: Relation to gestational age and axonal injury, *Pediatr Neurol* 20:370-374, 1999.
269a. Bell JE, Becher JC, Wyatt B, Keeling JW, et al: Brain damage and axonal injury in a Scottish cohort of neonatal deaths, *Brain* 128:1070-1081, 2005.
270. McQuillen PS, Sheldon RA, Shatz CJ, Ferriero DM: Selective vulnerability of subplate neurons after early neonatal hypoxia-ischemia, *J Neurosci* 23:3308-3315, 2003.

271. Talos DM, Numis A, Sucher NJ, Folkerth RD, et al: Maturational profile of NR1, NR2 and NR3 subunit expression in human parietal white matter (in preparation).
272. Limperopoulos C, Benson CB, Bassan H, DiSalvo DN, et al: Cerebellar hemorrhage in the preterm infant: Ultrasonographic findings and risk factors, *Pediatrics* 116:717-724, 2005.
273. Shah DK, Lavery S, Doyle LW, Wong C, et al: Use of 2-channel bedside electroencephalogram monitoring in term-born encephalopathic infants related to cerebral injury defined by magnetic resonance imaging, *Pediatrics* 118:47-55, 2006.
274. Kostovic I, Lukinovic N, Judas M, Bogdanovic N, et al: Structural basis of the developmental plasticity in the human cerebral cortex: The role of the transient subplate zone, *Metab Brain Dis* 4:17-23, 1989.
275. Kostovic I, Judas M: Correlation between the sequential ingrowth of afferents and transient patterns of cortical lamination in preterm infants, *Anat Rec* 267:1-6, 2002.
276. Kostovic I, Rakic P: Developmental history of the transient subplate zone in the visual and somatosensory cortex of the macaque monkey and human brain, *J Comp Neurol* 297:441-454, 1990.
277. Kanold PO, Kara P, Reid RC, Shatz CJ: Role of subplate neurons in functional maturation of visual cortical columns, *Science* 301:521-525, 2003.
278. Volpe JJ: Subplate neurons: Missing link in brain injury of the premature infant?, *Pediatrics* 97:112-113, 1996.
279. Kostovic I, Judas M: Prolonged coexistence of transient and permanent circuitry elements in the developing cerebral cortex of fetuses and preterm infants, *Dev Med Child Neurol* 48:388-393, 2006.
280. Kostovic I, Jovanov-Milosevic N: The development of cerebral connections during the first 20-45 weeks' gestation, *Semin Fetal Neonatal Med* 11:415-422, 2006.
281. Friauf E, McConnell SK, Shatz CJ: Functional synaptic circuits in the subplate during fetal and early postnatal development of cat visual cortex, *J Neurosci* 10:2601-2613, 1990.
282. Antonini A, Shatz CJ: Relation between putative transmitter phenotypes and connectivity of subplate neurons during cerebral cortical development, *Eur J Neurosci* 2:744-761, 1990.
283. Ghosh A, Antonini A, McConnell SK, Shatz CJ: Requirement for subplate neurons in the formation of thalamocortical connections, *Nature* 347:179-181, 1990.
284. Friauf E, Shatz CJ: Changing patterns of synaptic input to subplate and cortical plate during development of visual cortex, *J Neurophysiol* 66:2059-2071, 1991.
285. Ghosh A, Shatz CJ: Involvement of subplate neurons in the formation of ocular dominance columns, *Science* 255:1441-1443, 1992.
286. Ghosh A, Shatz CJ: A role for subplate neurons in the patterning of connections from thalamus to neocortex, *Development* 117:1031-1047, 1993.
287. Allendoerfer KL, Shatz CJ: The subplate, a transient neocortical structure: Its role in the development of connections between thalamus and cortex, *Annu Rev Neurosci* 17:185-218, 1994.
288. O'Leary DDM, Schlagger BL, Tuttle R: Specification of neocortical areas and thalamocortical connections, *Annu Rev Neurosci* 17:419-439, 1994.
289. Braisted JE, Catalano SM, Stimac R, Kennedy TE, et al: Netrin-1 promotes thalamic axon growth and is required for proper development of the thalamocortical projection, *J Neurosci* 20:5792-5801, 2000.
290. Haynes RL, Borenstein NS, DeSilva TM, Folkerth RD, et al: Axonal development in the cerebral white matter of the human fetus and infant, *J Comp Neurol* 484:156-167, 2005.
291. Tekkok SB, Goldberg MP: AMPA/kainate receptor activation mediates hypoxic oligodendrocyte death and axonal injury in cerebral white matter, *J Neurosci* 21:4237-4248, 2001.
292. Wakita H, Tomimoto H, Akiguchi I, Matsuo A, et al: Axonal damage and demyelination in the white matter after chronic cerebral hypoperfusion in the rat, *Brain Res* 924:63-70, 2002.
292a. McCarran WJ, Goldberg MP: White matter axon vulnerability to AMPA/kainate receptor-mediated ischemic injury is developmentally regulated, *J Neurosci* 27:4220-4229, 2007.
293. Bjartmar C, Yin X, Trapp BD: Axonal pathology in myelin disorders, *J Neurocytol* 28:383-395, 1999.
294. Biffiger K, Bartsch S, Montag D, Aguzzi A, et al: Severe hypomyelination of the murine CNS in the absence of myelin-associated glycoprotein and fyn tyrosin kinase, *J Neurosci* 20:7430-7437, 2000.
295. Gotow T, Leterrier JF, Ohsawa Y, Watanabe T, et al: Abnormal expression of neurofilament proteins in dysmyelinating axons located in the central nervous system of jimpy mutant mice, *Eur J Neurosci* 11:3893-3903, 1999.
296. Lappe-Siefke C, Goebbels S, Gravel M, Nicksch E, et al: Disruption of Cnp1 uncouples oligodendroglial functions in axonal support and myelination, *Nat Genet* 33:366-374, 2003.
297. Rasband MN, Tayler R, Kaga Y, Yang Y, et al: CNP is required for maintenance of axon-glia interactions at nodes of Ranvier in the CNS, *Glia* 50:86-90, 2005.
298. Miller SP, Vigneron DB, Henry RG, Bohland MA, et al: Serial quantitative diffusion tensor MRI of the premature brain: Development in newborns with and without injury, *J Magn Reson Imaging* 16:621-632, 2002.
299. Huppi PS, Murphy B, Maier SE, Zientara GP, et al: Microstructural brain development after perinatal cerebral white matter injury assessed by diffusion tensor magnetic resonance imaging, *Pediatrics* 107:455-460, 2001.
300. Huppi PS, Maier SE, Peled S, Zientara GP, et al: Microstructural development of human newborn cerebral white matter assessed *in vivo* by diffusion tensor magnetic resonance imaging, *Pediatr Res* 44:584-590, 1998.
301. Martinussen M, Fischl B, Larsson HB, Skranes J, et al: Cerebral cortex thickness in 15-year-old adolescents with low birth weight measured by an automated MRI-based method, *Brain* 128:2588-2596, 2005.
302. Vangberg TR, Skranes J, Dale AM, Martinussen M, et al: Changes in white matter diffusion anisotropy in adolescents born prematurely, *Neuroimage* 32:1538-1548, 2006.
303. Anjari M, Srinivasan L, Allsop JM, Hajnal JV, et al: Diffusion tensor imaging with tract-based spatial statistics reveals local white matter abnormalities in preterm infants, *Neuroimage* 35:1021-1027, 2007.
303a. Counsell SJ, Dyet LE, Larkman DJ, Nunes RG, et al: Thalamo-cortical connectivity in children born preterm mapped using probabilistic magnetic resonance tractography, *Neuroimage* 34:896-904, 2007.
304. De Reuck J: The human periventricular arterial blood supply and the anatomy of cerebral infarctions, *Eur Neurol* 5:321-334, 1971.
305. De Reuck JL: Cerebral angioarchitecture and perinatal brain lesions in premature and full-term infants, *Acta Neurol Scand* 70:391-395, 1984.
306. De Reuck J, Chattha AS, Richardson EP, Jr: Pathogenesis and evolution of periventricular leukomalacia in infancy, *Arch Neurol* 27:229-236, 1972.
307. Takashima S, Tanaka K: Development of cerebrovascular architecture and its relationship to periventricular leukomalacia, *Arch Neurol* 35:11-16, 1978.
308. Takashima S: Pathology on neonatal hypoxic brain damage and intracranial hemorrhage. Factors important in their pathogenesis. In Fukuyama Y, Arima M, Maekawa K, et al, editors: *International Congress Series No. 579: Child Neurology*, Amsterdam: 1982, Excerpta Medica.
309. Inage YW, Itoh M, Takashima S: Correlation between cerebrovascular maturity and periventricular leukomalacia, *Pediatr Neurol* 22:204-208, 2000.
310. Miyawaki T, Matsui K, Takashima S: Developmental characteristics of vessel density in the human fetal and infant brains, *Early Hum Dev* 53:65-72, 1998.
311. Ballabh P, Braun A, Nedergaard M: Anatomic analysis of blood vessels in germinal matrix, cerebral cortex, and white matter in developing infants, *Pediatr Res* 56:117-124, 2004.
312. Altman DI, Powers WJ, Perlman JM, Herscovitch P, et al: Cerebral blood flow requirement for brain viability in newborn infants is lower than in adults, *Ann Neurol* 24:218-226, 1988.
313. Greisen G: Cerebral blood flow in preterm infants during the first week of life, *Acta Paediatr Scand* 75:43-51, 1986.
314. Greisen G, Trojaborg W: Cerebral blood flow, Paco$_2$ changes, and visual evoked potentials in mechanically ventilated, preterm infants, *Acta Paediatr Scand* 76:394-400, 1987.
315. Pryds O, Greisen G, Friis-Hansen B: Compensatory increase of CBF in preterm infants during hypoglycaemia, *Acta Paediatr Scand* 77:632-637, 1988.
316. Pryds O, Greisen G: Effect of Paco$_2$ and haemoglobin concentration on day to day variation of CBF in preterm neonates, *Acta Paediatr Scand Suppl* 360:33-36, 1989.
317. Greisen G: Cerebral blood flow in mechanically ventilated, preterm neonates. University of Copenhagen, thesis, 1989.
318. Pryds O, Greisen G: Low CBF, discontinuous EEG activity, and periventricular brain injury in ill, preterm neonates, *Brain Dev* 11:164-168, 1989.
319. Pryds O, Greisen G: Preservation of single-flash visual evoked potentials at very low cerebral oxygen delivery in preterm infants, *Pediatr Neurol* 6:151-158, 1990.
320. Borch K, Greisen G: Blood flow distribution in the normal human preterm brain, *Pediatr Res* 41:28-33, 1998.
321. Powers WJ, Grubb RL, Darriet D, Raichle ME: Cerebral blood flow and cerebral metabolic rate of oxygen requirements for cerebral function and viability in humans, *J Cereb Blood Flow Metab* 5:600-608, 1985.
322. Lou HC, Lassen NA, Tweed WA, Johnson G, et al: Pressure passive cerebral blood flow and breakdown of the blood-brain barrier in experimental fetal asphyxia, *Acta Paediatr Scand* 68:57-63, 1979.
323. Pryds O, Greisen G, Lou H, Friis-Hansen B: Heterogeneity of cerebral vasoreactivity in preterm infants supported by mechanical ventilation, *J Pediatr* 115:638-645, 1989.
324. Pryds O, Edwards AD: Cerebral blood flow in the newborn infant, *Arch Dis Child Fetal Neonatal Ed* 74:F63-F69, 1996.
325. Muller AM, Morales C, Briner J, Baenziger O, et al: Loss of CO$_2$ reactivity of cerebral blood flow is associated with severe brain damage in mechanically ventilated very low birth weight infants, *Eur J Paediatr Neurol* 5:157-163, 1997.
326. Boylan GB, Young K, Panerai RB, Rennie JM, et al: Dynamic cerebral autoregulation in sick newborn infants, *Pediatr Res* 48:12-17, 2000.

327. von Siebenthal K, Beran J, Wolf M, Keel M, et al: Cyclical fluctuations in blood pressure, heart rate and cerebral blood volume in preterm infants, *Brain Dev* 21:529-534, 1999.

328. Tsuji M, Saul JP, du Plessis A, Eichenwald E, et al: Cerebral intravascular oxygenation correlates with mean arterial pressure in critically ill premature infants, *Pediatrics* 106:625-632, 2000.

329. Lemmers PM, Toet M, van Schelven LJ, van Bel F: Cerebral oxygenation and cerebral oxygen extraction in the preterm infant: The impact of respiratory distress syndrome, *Exp Brain Res* 173:458-467, 2006.

330. Soul JS, Hammer PE, Tsuji M, Saul JP, et al: Fluctuating pressure-passivity is common in the cerebral circulation of sick premature infants, *Pediatr Res* 61:467-473, 2007.

331. Pryds O: Control of cerebral circulation in the high-risk neonate, *Ann Neurol* 30:321-329, 1991.

332. Younkin DP, Reivich M, Jaggi JL, Obrist WD, et al: The effect of hematocrit and systolic blood pressure on cerebral blood flow in newborn infants, *J Cereb Blood Flow Metab* 7:295-299, 1987.

333. Bassan H, Gauvreau K, Newburger JW, Tsuji M, et al: Identification of pressure passive cerebral perfusion and its mediators after infant cardiac surgery, *Pediatr Res* 57:35-41, 2005.

334. Graziani IJ, Spitzer AR, Mitchell DG: Mechanical ventilation in preterm infants: Neurosonographic and developmental studies, *Pediatrics* 90:515-522, 1993.

335. Calvert SA, Hoskins EM, Fong KW, Forsyth SC: Periventricular leukomalacia: Ultrasonic diagnosis and neurological outcome, *Acta Paediatr Scand* 75:489-496, 1986.

336. Fujimoto S, Togari H, Yamaguchi N, Mizutani F, et al: Hypocarbia and cystic periventricular leukomalacia in premature infants, *Arch Dis Child Fetal Neonatal Ed* 71:F107-F110, 1994.

337. Wiswell TE, Graziani LJ, Kornhauser MS, Stanley C, et al: Effects of hypocarbia on the development of cystic periventricular leukomalacia in premature infants treated with high-frequency jet ventilation, *Pediatrics* 98:918-924, 1996.

338. Graziani LJ, Baumgart S, Desai S, Stanley C, et al: Clinical antecedents of neurologic and audiologic abnormalities in survivors of neonatal extracorporeal membrane oxygenation, *J Child Neurol* 12:415-422, 1997.

339. Okumura A, Hayakawa F, Kato T, Itomi K, et al: Hypocarbia in preterm infants with periventricular leukomalacia: The relation between hypocarbia and mechanical ventilation, *Pediatrics* 107:469-475, 2001.

340. Shankaran S, Langer JC, Kazzi SN, Laptook AR, et al: Cumulative index of exposure to hypocarbia and hyperoxia as risk factors for periventricular leukomalacia in low birth weight infants, *Pediatrics* 118:1654-1659, 2006.

341. Low JA, Froese AF, Galbraith RS, Sauerbrei EE, et al: The association of fetal and newborn metabolic acidosis with severe periventricular leukomalacia in the preterm newborn, *Am J Obstet Gynecol* 162:977-981, 1990.

342. Greisen G, Munck H, Lou H: May hypocarbia cause ischaemic brain damage in the preterm infant? *Lancet* 2:460, 1986.

343. Miall-Allen VM, de Vries LS, Whitelaw AG: Mean arterial blood pressure and neonatal cerebral lesions, *Arch Dis Child* 62:1068-1069, 1987.

344. Greisen G, Pryds O, Rosen I, Lou H: Poor reversibility of EEG abnormality in hypotensive, preterm neonates, *Acta Paediatr Scand* 77:785-790, 1988.

345. Glauser TA, Rorke LB, Weinberg PM, Clancy RR: Acquired neuropathologic lesions associated with the hypoplastic left heart syndrome, *Pediatrics* 85:991-1000, 1990.

346. Perlman JM, Volpe JJ: Neurologic complications of captopril treatment of neonatal hypertension, *Pediatrics* 83:47-52, 1989.

347. Shortland DB, Gibson NA, Levene MI, Archer LN, et al: Patent ductus arteriosus and cerebral circulation in preterm infants, *Dev Med Child Neurol* 32:386-393, 1990.

348. Low JA, Froese AB, Galbraith RS, Smith JT, et al: The association between preterm newborn hypotension and hypoxemia and outcome during the first year, *Acta Paediatr* 82:433-437, 1993.

349. Jarjour IT, Ahdab-Barmada A: Cerebrovascular lesions in infants and children dying after extracorporeal membrane oxygenation, *Pediatr Neurol* 10:13-19, 1994.

350. Perlman JM, Risser R: Relationship of uric acid concentrations and severe intraventricular hemorrhage/leukomalacia in the premature infant, *J Pediatr* 132:436-439, 1998.

351. Pladys P, Beuchee A, Wodey E, Treguier C, et al: Patent ductus arteriosus and cystic periventricular leucomalacia in preterm infants, *Acta Paediatr* 90:309-315, 2001.

352. Galli KK, Zimmerman RA, Jarvik GP, Wernovsky G, et al: Periventricular leukomalacia is common after neonatal cardiac surgery, *J Thorac Cardiovasc Surg* 127:692-704, 2004.

353. Kaltman JR, Di H, Tian Z, Rychik J: Impact of congenital heart disease on cerebrovascular blood flow dynamics in the fetus, *Ultrasound Obstet Gynecol* 25:32-36, 2005.

353a. Kidokoro H, Okumura A, Kato T, Hayakawa F, et al: Mild oliguria in preterm infants who later developed periventricular leukomalacia, *Brain Dev* 29:142-146, 2007.

353b. Miller SP, McQuillen PS, Hamrick SE, Xu D, et al: Abnormal brain development in newborns with congenital heart disease, *N Engl J Med* 357:1928-1938, 2007.

354. Perlman JM, Hill A, Volpe JJ: The effect of patent ductus arteriosus on flow velocity in the anterior cerebral arteries: Ductal steal in the premature newborn infant, *J Pediatr* 99:767-771, 1981.

355. Lipman B, Serwer GA, Brazy JE: Abnormal cerebral hemodynamics in preterm infants with patent ductus arteriosus, *Pediatrics* 69:778-781, 1982.

356. Serwer GA, Armstrong BE, Anderson PA: Continuous wave Doppler ultrasonographic quantitation of patent ductus arteriosus flow, *J Pediatr* 100:297-299, 1982.

357. Mellander M, Larsson LE: Effects of left-to-right ductus shunting on left ventricular output and cerebral blood flow velocity in 3-day-old preterm infants with and without severe lung disease, *J Pediatr* 113:101-109, 1988.

358. Kurtis PS, Rosendrantz TS, Zalneraitis EL: Cerebral blood flow and EEG changes in preterm infants with patent ductus arteriosus, *Pediatr Neurol* 12:114-119, 1995.

359. Weir FJ, Ohlsson A, Myhr TL, Fong K, et al: A patent ductus arteriosus is associated with reduced middle cerebral artery blood flow velocity, *Eur J Pediatr* 158:484-487, 1999.

360. Kupsky W: Personal communication, 1992.

361. McDonald A: *Children of Very Low Birthweight*, M.E.I.U. research monograph no.1, London: 1967, Spastic Society and Heinemann.

362. Perlman JM, Volpe JJ: Episodes of apnea and bradycardia in the preterm newborn: Impact on cerebral circulation, *Pediatrics* 76:333-338, 1985.

363. Livera LN, Spencer SA, Thorniley MS, Wickramasinghe YA, et al: Effects of hypoxaemia and bradycardia on neonatal cerebral haemodynamics, *Arch Dis Child* 66:376-380, 1991.

364. Urlesberger B, Kaspirek A, Pichler G, Muller W: Apnea of prematurity and changes in cerebral oxygenation and cerebral blood volume, *Neuropediatrics* 30:29-33, 1999.

365. Payer C, Urlesberger B, Pauger M, Muller W: Apnea associated with hypoxia in preterm infants: Impact on cerebral blood volume, *Brain Dev* 25:25-31, 2003.

366. Pichler G, Urlesberger B, Muller W: Impact of bradycardia on cerebral oxygenation and cerebral blood volume during apnoea in preterm infants, *Physiol Meas* 24:671-680, 2003.

367. Vander Eecken H, Adams RD: The anatomy and functional significance of the meningeal arterial anastomoses of the human brain, *J Neuropathol Exp Neurol* 12:132-157, 1953.

368. Vander Eecken H: *Anastomoses Between the Leptomeningeal Arteries of the Brain: Their Morphology, Pathological and Clinical Significance*, Springfield, IL: 1959, Charles C Thomas.

369. Abramowicz A: The pathogenesis of experimental periventricular cerebral necrosis and its possible relation to the periventricular leukomalacia of birth trauma, *J Neurol Neurosurg Psychiatry* 27:85-95, 1964.

370. Dammann O, Kuban KCK, Leviton A: Perinatal infection, fetal inflammatory response, white matter damage, and cognitive limitations in children born preterm, *Ment Retard Dev Disabil Res Rev* 8:46-50, 2002.

371. Wu YW: Systematic review of chorioamnionitis and cerebral palsy, *Ment Retard Dev Disabil Res Rev* 8:25-29, 2002.

372. De Felice C, Toti P, Laurini RN, Stumpo M, et al: Early neonatal brain injury in histologic chorioamnionitis, *J Pediatr* 138:101-104, 2001.

373. Grether JK, Nelson KB, Emery ES, Cummins SK: Prenatal and perinatal factors and cerebral palsy in very low birth weight infants, *J Pediatr* 128:407-414, 1996.

374. Jacobsson B, Hagberg G, Hagberg B, Ladfors L, et al: Cerebral palsy in preterm infants: A population-based case-control study of antenatal and intrapartal risk factors, *Acta Paediatr* 91:946-951, 2002.

375. Leviton A, Paneth N, Reuss ML, Susser M, et al: Maternal infection, fetal inflammatory response, and brain damage in very low birth weight infants, *Pediatr Res* 46:566-575, 1999.

376. Mittendorf R, Montag AG, MacMillan W, Janeczek S, et al: Components of the systemic fetal inflammatory response syndrome as predictors of impaired neurologic outcomes in children, *Am J Obstet Gynecol* 188:1436-1438, 2003.

377. O'Shea TM, Klinepeter KL, Meis PJ, Dillard RG: Intrauterine infection and the risk of cerebral palsy in very low-birthweight infants, *Pediatr Perinatal Epidemiol* 12:72-83, 1998.

378. Resch B, Vollaard E, Maurer U, Haas J, et al: Risk factors and determinants of neurodevelopmental outcome in cystic periventricular leucomalacia, *Eur J Pediatr* 159:663-670, 2000.

379. Wu YW, Colford JM: Chorioamnionitis as a risk factor for cerebral palsy: A meta-analysis, *JAMA* 284:1417-1424, 2000.

380. Yoon BH, Romero R, Park JS, Kim CJ, et al: Fetal exposure to an intra-amniotic inflammation and the development of cerebral palsy at the age of three years, *Am J Obstet Gynecol* 182:675-681, 2000.

381. Duggan PJ, Maalouf EF, Watts TL, Sullivan MHF, et al: Intrauterine T-cell activation and increased proinflammatory cytokine concentrations in preterm infants with cerebral lesions, *Lancet* 358:1699-1700, 2001.

382. Minagawa K, Tsuji Y, Ueda H, Koyama K, et al: Possible correlation between high levels of IL-18 in the cord blood of pre-term infants and neonatal development of periventricular leukomalacia and cerebral palsy, *Cytokine* 17:164-170, 2002.

383. Nelson KB, Grether JK, Dambrosia JM, Walsh E, et al: Neonatal cytokines and cerebral palsy in very preterm infants, *Pediatr Res* 53:600-607, 2003.

384. Kaukola T, Saryaraj E, Patel DD, Tchernev V, et al: Cerebral palsy is characterized by protein mediators in cord serum, *Ann Neurol* 55:186-194, 2004.

385. Locatelli A, Vergani P, Ghidini A, Assi F, et al: Duration of labor and risk of cerebral white-matter damage in very preterm infants who are delivered with intrauterine infection, *Am J Obstet Gynecol* 193:928-932, 2005.

386. Stoll BJ, Hansen NI, Adams-Chapman I, Fanaroff AA, et al: Neurodevelopmental and growth impairment among extremely low-birth-weight infants with neonatal infection, *JAMA* 292:2357-2365, 2004.

387. Greenwood C, Yudkin P, Sellers S, Impey L, et al: Why is there a modifying effect of gestational age on risk factors for cerebral palsy? *Arch Dis Child Fetal Neonatal Ed* 90:F141-F146, 2005.

388. Stoll BJ, Hansen N, Fanaroff AA, Wright LL, et al: Late-onset sepsis in very low birth weight neonates: The experience of the NICHD neonatal research network, *Pediatrics* 110:285-291, 2002.

389. Stoll BJ, Hansen N, Fanaroff AA, Wright LL, et al: Changes in pathogens causing early onset sepsis in very low birth weight infants, *N Engl J Med* 347:240-247, 2002.

390. Makhoul IR, Sujov P, Smolkin T, Lusky A, et al: Pathogen-specific early mortality in very low birth weight infants with late-onset sepsis: A national survey, *Clin Infect Dis* 40:218-224, 2005.

391. Bizzarro MJ, Raskind C, Baltimore RS, Gallagher PG: Seventy-five years of neonatal sepsis at Yale: 1928-2003, *Pediatrics* 116:595-602, 2005.

392. Deguchi K, Mizuguchi M, Takashima S: Immunohistochemical expression of tumor necrosis factor α in neonatal leukomalacia, *Pediatr Neurol* 14:13-16, 1996.

393. Yoon BH, Romero R, Kim CJ, Koo JN, et al: High expression of tumor necrosis factor-alpha and interleukin-6 in periventricular leukomalacia, *Am J Obstet Gynecol* 177:406-411, 1997.

394. Kadhim HJ, Tabarki B, Verellen G, De Prez C, et al: Inflammatory cytokines in the pathogenesis of periventricular leukomalacia, *Neurology* 56:1278-1284, 2001.

395. Kadhim HJ, Tabarki B, De Prez C, Rona A-M, et al: Interleukin-2 in the pathogenesis of perinatal white matter damage, *Neurology* 58:1125-1128, 2002.

396. Folkerth RD, Keefe RJ, Haynes RL, Trachtenberg FL, et al: Interferon-gamma expression in periventricular leukomalacia in the human brain, *Brain Pathol* 14:265-274, 2004.

397. Cannella B, Raine CS: Multiple sclerosis: Cytokine receptors on oligodendrocytes predict innate regulation, *Ann Neurol* 55:46-57, 2004.

398. Hansen-Pupp I, Harling S, Berg AC, Cilio C, et al: Circulating interferon-gamma and white matter brain damage in preterm infants, *Pediatr Res* 58:946-952, 2005.

398a. Schmitz T, Heep A, Groenendaal F, Huseman D, et al: Interleukin-1-beta, interleukin-18, and interferon-gamma expression in the cerebrospinal fluid of premature infants with posthemorrhagic hydrocephalus—markers of white matter damage?, *Pediatr Res* 61:722-726, 2007.

399. Ellison VJ, Mocatta TJ, Winterbourn CC, Darlow BA, et al: The relationship of CSF and plasma cytokine levels to cerebral white matter injury in the premature newborn, *Pediatr Res* 57:282-286, 2005.

400. Bona E, Andersson A-L, Blomgren K, Gilland E, et al: Chemokine and inflammatory cell response to hypoxia-ischemia in immature rats, *Pediatr Res* 45:500-509, 1999.

401. Botchkina GI, Meistrell ME, III, Botchkina IL, Tracey KJ: Expression of TNF and TNF receptors (p55 and p75) in the rat brain after focal cerebral ischemia, *Mol Med* 3:675-681, 1997.

402. Cowell RM, Xu HY, Galasso JM, Silverstein FS: Hypoxic-ischemic injury induces macrophage inflammatory protein-1α expression in immature rat brain, *Stroke* 33:795-801, 2002.

403. Danton GH, Dietrich WD: Inflammatory mechanisms after ischemia and stroke, *J Neuropathol Exp Neurol* 62:127-136, 2003.

404. del Zoppo GJ, Becker KJ, Hallenbeck JM: Inflammation after stroke: Is it harmful? *Arch Neurol* 58:669-672, 2001.

405. Eun B-L, Liu X-H, Barks JDE: Pentoxifylline attenuates hypoxic-ischemic brain injury in immature rats, *Pediatr Res* 47:73-78, 2000.

406. Fellman V, Raivio KO: Reperfusion injury as the mechanism of brain damage after perinatal asphyxia, *Pediatr Res* 41:599-606, 1997.

407. Hedtjarn M, Leverin AL, Eriksson K: Interleukin-18 involvement in hypoxic-ischemic brain injury, *J Neurosci* 22:5910-5919, 2002.

408. Hudome S, Palmer C, Roberts RL, Mauger D, et al: The role of neutrophils in the production of hypoxic-ischemic brain injury in the neonatal rat, *Pediatr Res* 41:607-616, 1997.

409. Ivacko JA, Sun R, Silverstein FS: Hypoxic-ischemic brain injury induces an acute microglial reaction in perinatal rats, *Pediatr Res* 39:39-47, 1995.

410. Sairanen T, Carpen O, Karjalainen-Lindsberg ML, Paetau A, et al: Evolution of cerebral tumor necrosis factor-alpha production during human ischemic stroke, *Stroke* 32:1750-1757, 2001.

411. Schroeter M, Jander S, Huitinga I, Stoll G: CD8+ phagocytes in focal ischemia of the rat brain: Predominant origin from hematogenous macrophages and targeting to areas of pannecrosis, *Acta Neuropathol (Berl)* 101:440-448, 2001.

412. Uno H, Matsuyama T, Akita H, Nishimura H, et al: Induction of tumor necrosis factor-alpha in the mouse hippocampus following transient forebrain ischemia, *J Cereb Blood Flow Metab* 17:491-499, 1997.

413. Wood PL: Microglia as a unique cellular target in the treatment of stroke: Potential neurotoxic mediators produced by activated microglia, *Neurol Res* 17:242-248, 1995.

414. Zhang Z, Chopp M, Powers C: Temporal profile of microglial response following transient (2h) middle cerebral artery occlusion, *Brain Res* 744:189-198, 1997.

415. Biran V, Joly LM, Heron A, Vernet A, et al: Glial activation in white matter following ischemia in the neonatal P7 rat brain, *Exp Neurol* 199:103-112, 2006.

416. Andjelkovic AV, Nikolic B, Pachter JS, Zecevic N: Macrophages/microglial cells in human central nervous system during development: An immunohistochemical study, *Brain Res* 814:13-25, 1998.

417. Rezaie P, Cairns NJ, Male DK: Expression of adhesion molecules on human fetal cerebral vessels: Relationship to microglial colonisation during development, *Dev Brain Res* 104:175-189, 1997.

418. Rezaie P, Dean A: Periventricular leukomalacia, inflammation and white matter lesions within the developing nervous system, *Neuropathology* 22:106-132, 2002.

419. Rivest S: Molecular insights on the cerebral innate immune system, *Brain Behav Immun* 17:13-19, 2003.

420. Billiards SS, Haynes RL, Folkerth RD, Trachtenberg FL, et al: Development of microglia in the cerebral white matter of the human fetus and infant, *J Comp Neurol* 497:199-208, 2006.

420a. Monier A, Evrard P, Gressens P, Verney C: Distribution and differentiation of microglia in the human encephalon during the first two trimesters of gestation, *J Comp Neurol* 499:565-582, 2006.

420b. Monier A, Adle-Biassette H, Delezoide AL, Evrard P, et al: Entry and distribution of microglial cells in human embryonic and fetal cerebral cortex, *J Neuropathol Exp Neurol* 66:372-382, 2007.

421. Yanowitz TD, Jordan JA, Gilmour CH, Towbin R, et al: Hemodynamic disturbances in premature infants born after chorioamnionitis: Association with cord blood cytokine concentrations, *Pediatr Res* 51:310-316, 2002.

422. Yanowitz TD, Baker RW, Roberts JM, Brozanski BS: Low blood pressure among very-low-birth-weight infants with fetal vessel inflammation, *J Perinatol* 24:299-304, 2004.

423. Yanowitz TD, Potter DM, Bowen A, Baker RW, et al: Variability in cerebral oxygen delivery is reduced in premature neonates exposed to chorioamnionitis, *Pediatr Res* 59:299-304, 2006.

424. Brian JE, Faraci FM: Tumor necrosis factor-α-induced dilatation of cerebral arterioles, *Stroke* 29:509-515, 1998.

425. Sibson NR, Blamire AM, Perry VH, Gauldie J, et al: TNF-alpha reduces cerebral blood volume and disrupts tissue homeostasis via an endothelin- and TNFR2-dependent pathway, *Brain* 125:2446-2459, 2002.

426. Cheranov SY, Jaggar JH: TNF-alpha dilates cerebral arteries via NAD(P)H oxidase-dependent Ca2+ spark activation, *Am J Physiol* 290:C964-C971, 2006.

427. Garnier Y, Coumans ABC, Berger R, Jensen A, et al: Endotoxemia severely affects circulation during normoxia and asphyxia in immature fetal sheep, *J Soc Gynecol Invest* 8:134-142, 2003.

428. Berti R, Williams AJ, Moffett JR, Hale SL, et al: Quantitative real-time RT-PCR analysis of inflammatory gene expression associated with ischemia-reperfusion brain injury, *J Cereb Blood Flow Metab* 22:1068-1079, 2002.

429. Froen JF, Munkeby BH, Stray-Pedersen B, Saugstad OD: Interleukin-10 reverses acute detrimental effects of endotoxin-induced inflammation on perinatal cerebral hypoxia-ischemia, *Brain Res* 942:87-94, 2002.

430. Ghezzi P, Cimarello CA, Bianchi M, Rosandich ME, et al: Hypoxia increases production of interleukin-1 and tumor necrosis factor by human mononuclear cells, *Cytokine* 3:189-194, 1991.

431. Okuma Y, Uehara T, Miyazaki H, Miyasaka T, et al: The involvement of cytokines, chemokines and inducible nitric oxide synthase (iNOS) induced by a transient ischemia in neuronal survival/death in rat brain, *Folia Pharmacol* 111:37-44, 1998.

432. Deng W, Rosenberg PA, Volpe JJ, Jensen FE: Calcium-permeable AMPA/kainate receptors mediate toxicity and preconditioning by oxygen-glucose deprivation in oligodendrocyte precursors, *Proc Natl Acad Sci U S A* 100:6801-6806, 2003.

433. Kaukola T, Herva R, Perhomaa M, Paakko E, et al: Population cohort associating chorioamnionitis, cord inflammatory cytokines and neurologic outcome in very preterm, extremely low birth weight infants, *Pediatr Res* 59:478-483, 2006.

434. Wang X, Athayde N, Trudinger B: Placental vascular disease and Toll-like receptor 4 gene expression, *Am J Obstet Gynecol* 192:961-966, 2005.

435. Folkerth RD, Haynes RL, Borenstein NS, Belliveau RA, et al: Developmental lag in superoxide dismutases relative to other antioxidant enzymes in premyelinated human telencephalic white matter, *J Neuropathol Exp Neurol* 63:990-999, 2004.

436. Ozawa H, Nishida A, Mito T, Takashima S: Development of ferritin-positive cells in cerebrum of human brain, *Pediatr Neurol* 10:44-48, 1994.

437. Connor JR, Menzies SL: Relationship of iron to oligodendrocytes and myelination, *Glia* 17:83-93, 1996.

438. Leviton A, Gilles F: Ventriculomegaly, delayed myelination, white matter hypoplasia, and "periventricular" leukomalacia: How are they related? *Pediatr Neurol* 15:127-136, 1996.

439. Savman K, Nilsson UA, Blennow M, Kjellmer I, et al: Non–protein-bound iron is elevated in cerebrospinal fluid from preterm infants with posthemorrhagic ventricular dilation, *Pediatr Res* 49:208-212, 2001.

440. Varsila E, Pitkanen O, Hallman M, Andersson S: Immaturity-dependent free radical activity in premature infants, *Pediatr Res* 36:55-59, 1994.

441. Inder TE, Darlow BA, Winterbourn SKB, Graham CC, et al: The correlation of elevated levels of an index of lipid peroxidation (MDA-TBA) with adverse outcome in the very low birthweight infant, *Acta Paediatr* 85:1116-1122, 1996.

442. Lubec G, Widness JA, Hayde M, Menzel D, et al: Hydroxyl radical generation in oxygen-treated infants, *Pediatrics* 100:700-704, 1997.

443. Lackmann GM, Hesse L, Tollner U: Reduced iron-associated antioxidants in premature newborns suffering intracerebral hemorrhage, *Free Radic Biol Med* 20:407-409, 1996.

444. Saugstad OD: Bronchopulmonary dysplasia and oxidative stress: Are we closer to an understanding of the pathogenesis of BPD? *Acta Paediatr* 86:1277-1282, 1997.

445. Hirano K, Morinobu T, Kim H, Hiroi M, et al: Blood transfusion increases radical promoting non-transferrin bound iron in preterm infants, *Arch Dis Child Fetal Neonatal Ed* 84:F188-F193, 2001.

446. Wardle SP, Drury J, Garr R, Weindling AM: Effect of blood transfusion on lipid peroxidation in preterm infants, *Arch Dis Child Fetal Neonatal Ed* 86:F46-F48, 2002.

447. Ciccoli L, Rossi V, Leoncini S, Signorini C, et al: Iron release in erythrocytes and plasma non protein-bound iron in hypoxic and non hypoxic newborns, *Free Radic Res* 37:51-58, 2003.

448. Baud O, Li J, Zhang Y, Neve RL, et al: Nitric oxide-induced cell death in developing oligodendrocytes is associated with mitochondrial dysfunction and apoptosis-inducing factor translocation, *Eur J Neurosci* 20:1713-1726, 2004.

449. Li J, Baud O, Vartanian T, Volpe JJ, et al: Peroxynitrite generated by inducible nitric oxide synthase and NADPH oxidase mediates microglial toxicity to oligodendrocytes, *Proc Natl Acad Sci U S A* 102:9936-9941, 2005.

450. Oka A, Belliveau MJ, Rosenberg PA, Volpe JJ: Vulnerability of oligodendroglia to glutamate: Pharmacology, mechanisms and prevention, *J Neurosci* 13:1441-1453, 1993.

451. Yonezawa M, Back SA, Gan X, Rosenberg PA, et al: Cystine deprivation induces oligodendroglial death: Rescue by free radical scavengers and by a diffusible glial factor, *J Neurochem* 67:566-573, 1996.

452. Back SA, Gan X, Li Y, Rosenberg PR, et al: Maturation-dependent vulnerability of oligodendrocytes to oxidative stress-induced death caused by glutathione depletion, *J Neurosci* 18:6241-6253, 1998.

453. De Silva TM, Kinney HC, Borenstein NS, Trachtenberg F, et al: The glutamate transporter EAAT2 is transiently expressed in developing human cerebral white matter, *J Comp Neurol* 501:879-890, 2007.

454. Yoshioka A, Bacskai B, Pleasure D: Pathophysiology of oligodendroglial excitotoxicity, *J Neurosci Res* 46:427-438, 1996.

455. Matute C, Sanchez-Gomez MV, Martinez-Millan L, Miledi R: Glutamate receptor-mediated toxicity in optic nerve oligodendrocytes, *Proc Natl Acad Sci U S A* 94:8830-8835, 1997.

456. McDonald JW, Althomsons SP, Hyrc KL, Choi DW, et al: Oligodendrocytes from forebrain are highly vulnerable to AMPA/kainate receptor-mediated excitotoxicity, *Nat Med* 4:291-297, 1998.

457. Matute C, Alberdi E, Domercq M, Perez-Cerda F, et al: The link between excitotoxic oligodendroglial death and demyelinating diseases, *Trends Neurosci* 24:224-230, 2001.

458. Sanchez-Gomez MV, Matute C: AMPA and kainate receptors each mediate excitotoxicity in oligodendroglial cultures, *Neurobiol Dis* 6:475-485, 1999.

459. Itoh T, Beesley J, Itoh A, Cohen AS, et al: AMPA glutamate receptor-mediated calcium signaling is transiently enhanced during development of oligodendrocytes, *J Neurochem* 81:390-402, 2002.

460. Rosenberg PA, Dai W, Gan XD, Ali S, et al: Mature myelin basic protein expressing oligodendrocytes are insensitive to kainate toxicity, *J Neurosci Res* 71:237-245, 2003.

461. Sanchez-Gomez MV, Alberdi E, Ibarretxe G, Torre I, et al: Caspase-dependent and caspase-independent oligodendrocyte death mediated by AMPA and kainate receptors, *J Neurosci* 23:9519-9528, 2003.

462. Deng W, Wang H, Rosenberg PA, Volpe JJ, et al: Role of metabotropic glutamate receptors in oligodendrocyte excitotoxicity and oxidative stress, *Proc Natl Acad Sci U S A* 101:7751-7756, 2004.

463. Deng W, Yue Q, Rosenberg PA, Volpe JJ, et al: Oligodendrocyte excitotoxicity determined by local glutamate accumulation and mitochondrial function, *J Neurochem* 96:213-222, 2006.

464. Judas M, Rados M, Jovanov-Milosevic N, Hrabac P, et al: Structural, immunocytochemical, and MR imaging properties of periventricular crossroads of growing cortical pathways in preterm infants, *AJNR Am J Neuroradiol* 26:2671-2684, 2005.

465. Barmada MA, Moossy J, Shuman RM: Cerebral infarcts with arterial occlusion in neonates, *Ann Neurol* 6:495-502, 1979.

466. Norman MG, McGillivray B: Fetal neuropathology of proliferative vasculopathy and hydranencephaly-hydrocephaly with multiple limb pterygia, *Pediatr Neurosci* 14:301-306, 1988.

467. Norman MG: The pathology of perinatal asphyxia, *CMAJ* 83:(Suppl): 15-20, 1988.

468. Roessmann U, Gambetti P: Pathological reaction of astrocytes in perinatal brain injury. Immunohistochemical study, *Acta Neuropathol (Berl)* 70:302-307, 1986.

469. Larroche JC: Fetal encephalopathies of circulatory origin, *Biol Neonate* 50:61-74, 1986.

470. Mannino FL, Trauner DA: Stroke in neonates, *J Pediatr* 102:605-610, 1983.

471. Ment LR, Duncan CC, Ehrenkranz RA: Perinatal cerebral infarction, *Ann Neurol* 16:559-568, 1984.

472. Olson DM, Shewmon DA: Electroencephalographic abnormalities in infants with hypoplastic left heart syndrome, *Pediatr Neurol* 5:93-98, 1989.

473. Scher MS, Klesh KW, Murphy TF, Guthrie RD: Seizures and infarction in neonates with persistent pulmonary hypertension, *Pediatr Neurol* 2:332-339, 1986.

474. Voorhies TM, Lipper EG, Lee BC, Vannucci RC, et al: Occlusive vascular disease in asphyxiated newborn infants, *J Pediatr* 105:92-96, 1984.

475. Levy SR, Abroms IF, Marshall PC, Rosquete EE: Seizures and cerebral infarction in the full-term newborn, *Ann Neurol* 17:366-370, 1985.

476. Clancy R, Malin S, Laraque D, Baumgart S, et al: Focal motor seizures heralding stroke in full-term neonates, *Am J Dis Child* 139:601-606, 1985.

477. Estan J, Hope P: Unilateral neonatal cerebral infarction in full term infants, *Arch Dis Child Fetal Neonatal Ed* 76:F88-F93, 1997.

478. Govaert P, Matthys E, Zecic A, Roelens F, et al: Perinatal cortical infarction within middle cerebral artery trunks, *Arch Dis Child Fetal Neonatal Ed* 82:F59-F63, 2000.

479. Sreenan C, Bhargava R, Robertson CMT: Cerebral infarction in the term newborn: Clinical presentation and long-term outcome, *J Pediatr* 137:351-355, 2000.

480. Golomb MR, MacGregor DL, Domi T, Armstrong DC, et al: Presumed pre- or perinatal arterial ischemic stroke: Risk factors and outcomes, *Ann Neurol* 50:163-168, 2001.

481. Ramaswamy V, Miller SP, Barkovich AJ, Partridge JC, et al: Perinatal stroke in term infants with neonatal encephalopathy, *Neurology* 62:2088-2091, 2004.

482. Lee J, Croen LA, Lindan C, Nash KB, et al: Predictors of outcome in perinatal arterial stroke: A population-based study, *Ann Neurol* 58:303-308, 2005.

482a. Benders MJNL, Groenendaal F, Uiterwaal CSPM, Nikkels PGJ, et al: Maternal and infant characteristics associated with perinatal arterial stroke in the preterm infant, *Stroke* 38:1759-1765, 2007.

483. Shevell MI, Silver K, O'Gorman AM, Watters GV, et al: Neonatal dural sinus thrombosis, *Pediatr Neurol* 5:161-165, 1989.

484. Hurst RW, Kerns SR, McIlhenny J, Park TS, et al: Neonatal dural venous sinus thrombosis associated with central venous catheterization: CT and MR studies, *J Comput Assist Tomogr* 13:504-507, 1989.

485. Baram TZ, Butler IJ, Nelson MD, Jr, McArdle CB: Transverse sinus thrombosis in newborns: Clinical and magnetic resonance imaging findings, *Ann Neurol* 24:792-794, 1988.

486. Hanigan WC, Tracy PT, Tadros WS, Wright RM: Neonatal cerebral venous thrombosis, *Pediatr Neurosci* 14:177-183, 1988.

487. Wong VK, LeMesurier J, Franceschini R, Heikali M, et al: Cerebral venous thrombosis as a cause of neonatal seizures, *Pediatr Neurol* 3:235-237, 1987.

488. Konishi Y, Kuriyama M, Sudo M, Konishi K, et al: Superior sagittal sinus thrombosis in neonates, *Pediatr Neurol* 3:222-225, 1987.

489. Hanigan WC, Rossi LJ, McLean JM, Wright RM: MRI of cerebral vein thrombosis in infancy: A case report, *Neurology* 36:1354-1356, 1986.

490. Rivkin MJ, Anderson ML, Kaye EM: Neonatal idiopathic cerebral venous thrombosis: An unrecognized cause of transient seizures or lethargy, *Ann Neurol* 32:51-56, 1992.

491. Grossman R, Novak G, Patel M, Maytal J, et al: MRI in neonatal dural sinus thrombosis, *Pediatr Neurol* 9:235-238, 1993.

492. Khurana DS, Buonanno F, Ebb D, Krishnamoorthy KS: The role of anticoagulation in idiopathic cerebral venous thrombosis, *J Child Neurol* 11:248-249, 1996.

493. Pohl M, Zimmerbackl LB, Heinen F, Sutor AH, et al: Bilateral renal vein thrombosis and venous sinus thrombosis in a neonate with factor V mutation (FV Leiden), *J Pediatr* 132:159-161, 1998.

494. deVeber G, Andrew M, Adams C, Bjornson B, et al: Cerebral sinovenous thrombosis in children, *N Engl J Med* 345:417-423, 2001.

495. Wu TW, Miller SP, Chin K, Collins AE, et al: Multiple risk factors in neonatal sinovenous thrombosis, *Neurology* 59:438-440, 2002.

496. Hunt RW, Badawi N, Laing S, Lam A: Pre-eclampsia: A predisposing factor for neonatal venous sinus thrombosis? *Pediatr Neurol* 25:242-246, 2001.

497. Golomb MR, Dick PT, MacGregor DL, Curtis R, et al: Neonatal arterial ischemic stroke and cerebral sinovenous thrombosis are more commonly diagnosed in boys, *J Child Neurol* 19:493-497, 2004.

498. Fitzgerald KC, Williams LS, Garg BP, Carvalho KS, et al: Cerebral sinovenous thrombosis in the neonate, *Arch Neurol* 63:405-409, 2006.

499. Raybaud C: Destructive lesions of the brain, *Neuroradiology* 25:265-291, 1983.

500. Schmitt HP: Multicystic encephalopathy: A polyetiologic condition in early infancy: Morphologic, pathogenetic and clinical aspects, *Brain Dev* 1:1, 1984.
501. Kundrat H: Die porencephalie: Eine anatomische studie, *Graz Leuschlub Lubensky* 80:126, 1882.
502. Fischer CM: The circle of Willis: Anatomical variations, *Vasc Dis* 2:99, 1965.
503. Suzuki K: Chemistry and metabolism of brain lipids. In Siegel GJ, Albers RW, Agranoff BW, et al, editors: *Basic Neurochemistry*, Boston: 1981, Little, Brown.
504. Myers RE: Brain pathology following fetal vascular occlusion: An experimental study, *Invest Ophthalmol* 8:41-50, 1969.
505. Myers RE: Cerebral ischemia in the developing primate fetus, *Biomed Biochim Acta* 48:S137-S142, 1989.
506. Neuburger F: Fall einer intrauterinen Hirnschadigung nach einer Leuchtgasvergiftgung der Mutter, *Beitr Gerichtl Med* 13:85, 1935.
507. Sharpe O, Hall EG: Renal impairment, hypertension, and encephalomalacia in an infant surviving severe intrauterine anoxia, *Proc R Soc Med* 46:1063-1065, 1953.
508. Ferrer I, Navarro C: Multicystic encephalomalacia of infancy: Clinicopathological report of 7 cases, *J Neurol Sci* 38:179-189, 1978.
509. Erasmus C, Blackwood W, Wilson J: Infantile multicystic encephalomalacia after maternal bee sting anaphylaxis during pregnancy, *Arch Dis Child* 57:785-787, 1982.
510. Gosseye S, Golaire MC, Larroche JC: Cerebral, renal and splenic lesions due to fetal anoxia and their relationship to malformations, *Dev Med Child Neurol* 24:510-518, 1982.
511. Greene MF, Benacerraf B, Crawford JM: Hydranencephaly: US appearance during in utero evolution, *Radiology* 156:779-780, 1985.
512. Amato M, Huppi P, Herschkowitz N, Huber P: Prenatal stroke suggested by intrauterine ultrasound and confirmed by magnetic resonance imaging, *Neuropediatrics* 22:100-102, 1991.
513. Fernandez F, Pèrez-Higueras A, Hernàndez R, Verdú A, et al: Hydranencephaly after maternal butane-gas intoxication during pregnancy, *Dev Med Child Neurol* 28:361-363, 1986.
514. Scher MS, Belfar H, Martin J, Painter MJ: Destructive brain lesions of presumed fetal onset: Antepartum causes of cerebral palsy, *Pediatrics* 88:898-906, 1991.
515. Dildy GA, 3d, Smith LG, Jr, Moise KJ, Jr, Cano LE, et al: Porencephalic cyst: A complication of fetal intravascular transfusion, *Am J Obstet Gynecol* 165:76-78, 1991.
516. Klesh KW, Murphy TF, Scher MS, Buchanan DE, et al: Cerebral infarction in persistent pulmonary hypertension of the newborn, *Am J Dis Child* 141:852-857, 1987.
517. Aso K, Scher MS, Barmada MA: Cerebral infarcts and seizures in the neonate, *J Child Neurol* 5:224-228, 1990.
518. Boyce LH, Khandji AG, DeKlerk AM, Nordli DR: Fetomaternal hemorrhage as an etiology of neonatal stroke, *Pediatr Neurol* 11:255-257, 1994.
519. Lien JM, Towers CV, Quilligan EJ, de Veciana M, et al: Term early-onset neonatal seizures: Obstetric characteristics, etiologic classifications, and perinatal care, *Obstet Gynecol* 85:163-169, 1995.
520. Perlman JM, Rollins NK, Evans D: Neonatal stroke: Clinical characteristics and cerebral blood flow velocity measurements, *Pediatr Neurol* 11:281-284, 1994.
521. Pellicer A, Cabanas F, Garciaalix A, Perezhigueras A, et al: Stroke in neonates with cardiac right-to-left shunt, *Brain Dev* 14:381-385, 1992.
522. Burke CJ, Tannenberg AE, Payton DJ: Ischemic cerebral injury, intrauterine growth retardation, and placental infarction, *Dev Med Child Neurol* 39:726-730, 1997.
523. Kohlhase B, Vielhaber H, Kehl HG, Kececioglu D, et al: Thromboembolism and resistance to activated protein C in children with underlying cardiac disease, *J Pediatr* 129:677-679, 1996.
524. Varelas PN, Sleight BJ, Rinder HM, Sze G, et al: Stroke in a neonate heterozygous for factor V Leiden, *Pediatr Neurol* 18:262-264, 1998.
525. Thorarensen O, Ryan S, Hunter J, Younkin DP: Factor V Leiden mutation: An unrecognized cause of hemiplegic cerebral palsy, neonatal stroke, and placental thrombosis, *Ann Neurol* 42:372-375, 1997.
526. Hagstrom JN, Walter J, Bluebond-Langner R, Amatnick JC, et al: Prevalence of the factor V Leiden mutation in children and neonates with thromboembolic disease, *J Pediatr* 133:777-781, 1998.
527. Pipe SW, Schmaier AH, Nichols WC, Ginsburg D, et al: Neonatal purpura fulminans in association with factor V R506Q mutation, *J Pediatr* 128:706-709, 1996.
528. Mandel H, Brenner B, Berant M, Rosenberg N, et al: Coexistence of hereditary homocystinuria and factor V Leiden: Effect on thrombosis, *N Engl J Med* 334:763-768, 1996.
529. deVeber G, Monagle P, Chan A, MacGregor D, et al: Prothrombotic disorders in infants and children with cerebral thromboembolism, *Arch Neurol* 55:1539-1543, 1998.
530. Gould RJ, Black K, Pavlakis SG: Neonatal cerebral arterial thrombosis: Protein C deficiency, *J Child Neurol* 11:250-251, 1996.
531. Kennedy CR, Warner G, Kai M, Chisholm M: Protein C deficiency and stroke in early life, *Dev Med Child Neurol* 37:723-730, 1995.
532. Koh S, Chen LS: Protein C and S deficiency in children with ischemic cerebrovascular accident, *Pediatr Neurol* 17:319-321, 1997.
533. Stewart RM, Williams RS, Lukl P, Schoenen J: Ventral porencephaly: A cerebral defect associated with multiple congenital anomalies, *Acta Neuropathol (Berl)* 42:231-235, 1978.
534. Fowler M, Dow R, White TA, Greer CH: Congenital hydrocephalus-hydrencephaly in five siblings, with autopsy studies: A new disease, *Dev Med Child Neurol* 14:173-188, 1972.
535. Harper C, Hockey A: Proliferative vasculopathy and an hydranencephalic-hydrocephalic syndrome: A neuropathological study of two siblings, *Dev Med Child Neurol* 25:232-239, 1983.
536. Castro-Gago M, Alonso A, Pintos-Martinez E, Beiras-Iglesias A, et al: Congenital hydranencephalic-hydrocephalic syndrome associated with mitochondrial dysfunction, *J Child Neurol* 14:131-135, 1999.
537. Castro-Gago M, Pintos-Martinez E, Forteza-Vila J, Iglesias-Diz M, et al: Congenital hydranencephalic-hydrocephalic syndrome with proliferative vasculopathy: A possible relation with mitochondrial dysfunction, *J Child Neurol* 16:858-862, 2001.
538. Aguglia U, Gambardella A, Breedveld GJ, Oliveri RL, et al: Suggestive evidence for linkage to chromosome 13qter for autosomal dominant type 1 porencephaly, *Neurology* 62:1613-1615, 2004.
539. van der Knaap MS, Smit LM, Barkhof F, Pijnenburg YA, et al: Neonatal porencephaly and adult stroke related to mutations in collagen IV A1, *Ann Neurol* 59:504-511, 2006.
540. Zalneraitis EL, Young RS, Krishnamoorthy KS: Intracranial hemorrhage in utero as a complication of isoimmune thrombocytopenia, *J Pediatr* 95:611-614, 1979.
541. Naidu S, Messmore H, Caserta V, Fine M: CNS lesions in neonatal isoimmune thrombocytopenia, *Arch Neurol* 40:552-554, 1983.
542. Manson J, Speed I, Abbott K, Crompton D: Congenital blindness, porencephaly, and neonatal thrombocytopenia: A report of four cases, *J Child Neurol* 3:120-124, 1988.
543. Forestier F, Hohlfeld P: Management of fetal and neonatal alloimmune thrombocytopenia, *Biol Neonate* 74:395-401, 1998.
544. Corona-Rivera JR, Corona-Rivera E, Romero-Velarde E, Hernandez-Rocha J, et al: Report and review of the fetal brain disruption sequence, *Eur J Pediatr* 160:664-667, 2001.
545. Ozduman K, Pober BR, Barnes P, Copel JA, et al: Fetal stroke, *Pediatr Neurol* 30:151-162, 2004.
545a. Hayes B, Ryan S, King MD: Cerebral palsy after maternal trauma in pregnancy, *Dev Med Child Neurol* 49:700-706, 2007.
546. Smith CD, Baumann RJ: Clinical features and magnetic resonance imaging in congenital and childhood stroke, *J Child Neurol* 6:263-272, 1991.
547. Gross RE: Arterial embolism and thrombosis in infancy, *Am J Dis Child* 70:61, 1945.
548. Prian GW, Wright GB, Rumack CM, O'Meara OP: Apparent cerebral embolization after temporal artery catheterization, *J Pediatr* 93:115-118, 1978.
549. Mueh JR, Herbst KD, Rapaport SI: Thrombosis in patients with lupus anticoagulant, *Ann Intern Med* 92:156-159, 1980.
550. Chasnoff IJ, Bussey ME, Savich R, Stack CM: Perinatal cerebral infarction and maternal cocaine use, *J Pediatr* 108:456-459, 1986.
551. Bejar R, Vigliocco G, Gramajo H, Solana C, et al: Antenatal origin of neurologic damage in newborn infants. II. Multiple gestations, *Am J Obstet Gynecol* 162:1230-1236, 1990.
552. Frisoni GB, Anzola GP: Vertebrobasilar ischemia after neck motion, *Stroke* 22:1452-1460, 1991.
553. Dragon R, Saranchak H, Lakin P, Strauch G: Blunt injuries to the carotid and vertebral arteries, *Am J Surg* 141:497-500, 1981.
554. Beatty RA: Dissecting hematoma of the internal carotid artery following chiropractic cervical manipulation, *J Trauma* 17:248-249, 1977.
555. Nagler W: Vertebral artery obstruction by hyperextension of the neck: Report of three cases, *Arch Phys Med Rehabil* 54:237-240, 1973.
556. Okawara S, Nibbelink D: Vertebral artery occlusion following hyperextension and rotation of the heard, *Stroke* 5:640-642, 1974.
557. Sherman DG, Hart RG, Easton JD: Abrupt change in head position and cerebral infarction, *Stroke* 12:2-6, 1981.
558. Choi KD, Shin HY, Kim JS, Kim SH, et al: Rotational vertebral artery syndrome: Oculographic analysis of nystagmus, *Neurology* 65:1287-1290, 2005.
559. Pamphlett R, Murray N: Vulnerability of the infant brain stem to ischemia: A possible cause of sudden infant death syndrome, *J Child Neurol* 11:181-184, 1996.
560. Pamphlett R, Raisanen J, Kum-Jew S: Vertebral artery compression resulting from head movement: A possible cause of the sudden infant death syndrome, *Pediatrics* 103:460-468, 1999.
561. Clark RM, Linnell EA: Case report: Prenatal occlusion of the internal carotid artery, *J Neurol Neurosurg Psychiatry* 17:295, 1954.
562. Harvey FH, Alvord EC, Jr: Juvenile cerebral arteriosclerosis and other cerebral arteriopathies of childhood: Six autopsied cases, *Acta Neurol Scand* 48:479-509, 1972.
563. Cocker J, George SW, Yates PO: Perinatal occlusions of the middle cerebral artery, *Dev Med Child Neurol* 7:235, 1965.
564. Banker BQ: Cerebral vascular disease in infancy and childhood. I. Occlusive vascular disease, *J Neuropathol Exp Neurol* 20:127, 1961.
565. Silver RK, Macgregor SN, Pasternak JF, Neely SE: Fetal stroke associated with elevated maternal anticardiolipin antibodies, *Obstet Gynecol* 80:497-499, 1992.

566. Gunther G, Junker R, Strater R, Schobess R, et al: Symptomatic ischemic stroke in full-term neonates: Role of acquired and genetic prothrombotic risk factors, *Stroke* 31:2437-2441, 2003.

567. Hogeveen M, Blom HJ, van Amerogen M, Boogmans B, et al: Hyperhomocysteinemia as risk factor for ischemic and hemorrhagic stroke in newborn infants, *J Pediatr* 141:429-431, 2002.

568. Mercuri E, Cowan F, Gupte G, Manning R, et al: Prothrombotic disorders and abnormal neurodevelopmental outcome in infants with neonatal cerebral infarction, *Pediatrics* 107:1400-1404, 2001.

569. Nelson KB, Lynch JK: Stroke in newborn infants, *Lancet* 3:150-158, 2004.

570. Lynch JK, Hirtz DG, De Veber G, Nelson KB: Report of the National Institute of Neurological Disorders and Stroke workshop on perinatal and childhood stroke, *Pediatrics* 109:116-123, 2002.

571. Lee J, Croen LA, Backstrand KH, Yoshida CK, et al: Maternal and infant characteristics associated with perinatal arterial stroke in the infant, *JAMA* 293:723-729, 2005.

571a. Curry CJ, Bhullar S, Holmes J, Delozier CD, et al: Risk factors for perinatal arterial stroke: A study of 60 mother-child pairs, *Pediatr Neurol* 37:99-107, 2007.

572. Robinson RO, Trounce JQ, Janota I, Cox T: Late fetal pontine destruction, *Pediatr Neurol* 9:213-215, 1993.

573. Mamourian AC, Miller G: Neonatal pontomedullary disconnection with aplasia or destruction of the lower brain stem: A case of pontoneocerebellar hypoplasia? *AJNR Am J Neuroradiol* 15:1483-1485, 1994.

574. Kraus FT: Cerebral palsy and thrombi in placental vessels of the fetus: Insights from litigation, *Hum Pathol* 28:246-248, 2003.

575. Kraus FT, Acheen VI: Fetal thrombotic vasculopathy in the placenta: Cerebral thrombi and infarcts, coagulopathies, and cerebral palsy, *Hum Pathol* 30:759-769, 1999.

576. Redline RW: Severe fetal placental vascular lesions in term infants with neurologic impairment, *Am J Obstet Gynecol* 192:452-457, 2005.

577. Hannu H, Pentti K, Henrik E, Markku S, et al: Patency of foramen ovale: Does it influence haemodynamics in newborn infants? *Early Hum Dev* 20:281-287, 1989.

578. Markhorst DG, Rothuis E, Sobotka-Plojhar M, Moene RJ: Transient foramen ovale incompetence in the normal newborn: An echocardiographic study, *Eur J Pediatr* 154:667-671, 1995.

579. Alfonso I, Prieto G, Vasconcellos E, Aref K, et al: Internal carotid artery thrombus: An underdiagnosed source of brain emboli in neonates? *J Child Neurol* 16:446-447, 2001.

580. Filippi L, Palermo L, Pezzati M, Dani C, et al: Paradoxical embolism in a preterm infant, *Dev Child Neurol* 46:713-716, 2004.

581. Parker MJ, Joubert GI, Levin SD: Portal vein thrombosis causing neonatal cerebral infarction, *Arch Dis Child Fetal Neonatal Ed* 87:F125-F127, 2002.

582. Yates PO: Birth trauma to the vertebral arteries, *Arch Dis Child* 34:436, 1959.

583. Roessmann U, Miller RT: Thrombosis of the middle cerebral artery associated with birth trauma, *Neurology* 30:889-892, 1980.

584. Lequin MH, Peeters EA, Holscher HC, De Krijger R, et al: Arterial infarction caused by carotid artery dissection in the neonate, *Eur J Paediatr Neurol* 8:155-160, 2004.

585. Kaneko K, Someya T, Ohtaki R, Yamashiro Y, et al: Congenital fibromuscular dysplasia involving multivessels in an infant with fatal outcome, *Eur J Pediatr* 163:241-244, 2004.

586. Mendoza JC, Shearer LL, Cook LN: Lateralization of brain lesions following extracorporeal membrane oxygenation, *Pediatrics* 88:1004-1009, 1991.

587. Schumacher RE, Barks JDE, Johnston MV, Donn SM, et al: Right-sided brain lesions in infants following extracorporeal membrane oxygenation, *Pediatrics* 82:115-161, 1988.

588. Hahn JS, Vaucher Y, Bejar R, Coen RW: Electroencephalographic and neuroimaging findings in neonates undergoing extracorporeal membrane oxygenation, *Neuropediatrics* 24:19-24, 1993.

589. Park CH, Spitzer AR, Desai HJ, Zhang JJ, et al: Brain SPECT in neonates following extracorporeal membrane oxygenation: Evaluation of technique and preliminary results, *J Nucl Med* 33:1943-1948, 1992.

590. Short BL, Walker K, Bender KS, Traystman RJ: Impairment of cerebral autoregulation during extracorporeal membrane oxygenation in newborn lambs, *Pediatr Res* 33:289-294, 1993.

591. Vogler C, Sotelo-Avila C, Lagunoff D, Braun P, et al: Aluminum-containing emboli in infants treated with extracorporeal membrane oxygenation, *N Engl J Med* 319:75-79, 1988.

592. Fink SM, Bockman DE, Howell C, Falls DG, et al: Bypass circuits as the source of thromboemboli during extracorporeal membrane oxygenation, *J Pediatr* 115:621-624, 1989.

593. Amit M, Camfield PR: Neonatal polycythemia causing multiple cerebral infarcts, *Arch Neurol* 37:109-110, 1980.

594. Miller GM, Black VD, Lubchenco LO: Intracerebral hemorrhage in a term newborn with hyperviscosity, *Am J Dis Child* 135:377-378, 1981.

595. Wiswell TE, Cornish JD, Northam RS: Neonatal polycythemia: Frequency of clinical manifestations and other associated findings, *Pediatrics* 78:26-30, 1986.

596. Black VD, Lubchenco LO, Koops BL, Poland RL, et al: Neonatal hyperviscosity: Randomized study of effect of partial plasma exchange transfusion on long-term outcome, *Pediatrics* 75:1048-1053, 1985.

597. Delaney-Black V, Camp BW, Lubchenco LO, Swanson C, et al: Neonatal hyperviscosity association with lower achievement and IQ scores at school age, *Pediatrics* 83:662-667, 1989.

598. Bada HS, Korones SB, Pourcyrous M, Wong SP, et al: Asymptomatic syndrome of polycythemic hyperviscosity: Effect of partial plasma exchange transfusion, *J Pediatr* 120:579-585, 1992.

599. Maertzdorf WJ, Tangelder GJ, Slaaf DW, Blanco CE: Effects of partial plasma exchange transfusion on cerebral blood flow velocity in polycythaemic preterm, term and small for date newborn infants, *Eur J Pediatr* 148:774-778, 1989.

600. Rosenkrantz TS, Oh W: Cerebral blood flow velocity in infants with polycythemia and hyperviscosity: Effects of partial exchange transfusion with Plasmanate, *J Pediatr* 101:94-98, 1982.

601. Bada HS, Korones SB, Kolni HW, Fitch CW, et al: Partial plasma exchange transfusion improves cerebral hemodynamics in symptomatic neonatal polycythemia, *Am J Med Sci* 291:157-163, 1986.

602. Goldstein M, Stonestreet BS, Brann BS, 4th, Oh W: Cerebral cortical blood flow and oxygen metabolism in normocythemic hyperviscous newborn piglets, *Pediatr Res* 24:486-489, 1988.

603. Chow G, Mellor D: Neonatal cerebral ischaemia with elevated maternal and infant anticardiolipin antibodies, *Dev Med Child Neurol* 42:412-413, 2000.

604. Smith RA, Skelton M, Howard M, Levene M: Is thrombophilia a factor in the development of hemiplegic cerebral palsy? *Dev Med Child Neurol* 43:724-730, 2001.

605. Lynch JK, Nelson KB, Curry CJ, Grether JK: Cerebrovascular disorders in children with the factor V Leiden mutation, *J Child Neurol* 16:735-744, 2001.

606. Aronis S, Bouza H, Pergantou H, Kapsimalis Z, et al: Prothrombotic factors in neonates with cerebral thrombosis and intraventricular hemorrhage, *Acta Paediatr Suppl* 91:87-91, 2002.

607. Ebeling F, Petaja J, Alanko S, Hirvasniemi A, et al: Infant stroke and beta-2-glycoprotein 1 antibodies: Six cases, *Eur J Pediatr* 162:678-681, 2003.

608. Verdu A, Cazorla MR, Moreno JC, Casado LF: Prenatal stroke in a neonate heterozygous for factor V Leiden mutation, *Brain Dev* 27:451-454, 2005.

609. De Haan TR, Van Wezel-Meijler G, Beersma MF, Von Lindern JS, et al: Fetal stroke and congenital parvovirus B19 infection complicated by activated protein C resistance, *Acta Paediatr* 95:863-867, 2006.

610. Reid S, Halliday J, Ditchfield M, Ekert H, et al: Factor V Leiden mutation: A contributory factor for cerebral palsy? *Dev Med Child Neurol* 48:14-19, 2006.

611. Baud O, Picard V, Durand P, Duchemin J, et al: Intracerebral hemorrhage associated with a novel antithrombin gene mutation in a neonate, *J Pediatr* 139:741-743, 2001.

612. Friese S, Muller-Hansen I, Schoning M, Nowak-Gottl U, et al: Isolated internal cerebral venous thrombosis in a neonate with increased lipoprotein (a) level: Diagnostic and therapeutic considerations, *Neuropediatrics* 34:36-39, 2003.

613. Abrantes M, Lacerda AF, Abreu CR, Levy A, et al: Cerebral venous sinus thrombosis in a neonate due to factor V Leiden deficiency, *Acta Paediatr* 91:243-245, 2002.

614. Mahasandana C, Suvatte V, Chuansumrit A, Marlar RA, et al: Homozygous protein S deficiency in an infant with purpura fulminans, *J Pediatr* 117:750-753, 1990.

615. Pegelow CH, Ledford M, Young JN, Zilleruelo G: Severe protein S deficiency in a newborn, *Pediatrics* 89:674-676, 1992.

616. Sills RH, Marlar RA, Montgomery RR, Deshpande GN, et al: Severe homozygous protein C deficiency, *J Pediatr* 105:409-413, 1984.

617. Branson HE, Katz J, Marble R, Griffin JH: Inherited protein C deficiency and coumarin-responsive chronic relapsing purpura fulminans in a newborn infant, *Lancet* 2:1165-1168, 1983.

618. Seligsohn U, Berger A, Abend M, Rubin L, et al: Homozygous protein C deficiency manifested by massive venous thrombosis in the newborn, *N Engl J Med* 310:559-562, 1984.

619. Yuen P, Cheung A, Lin HJ, Ho F, et al: Purpura fulminans in a Chinese boy with congenital protein C deficiency, *Pediatrics* 77:670-676, 1986.

620. Marciniak E, Wilson HD, Marlar RA: Neonatal purpura fulminans: A genetic disorder related to the absence of protein C in blood, *Blood* 65:15-20, 1985.

621. Manco-Johnson MJ, Marlar RA, Jacobson LJ, Hays T, et al: Severe protein C deficiency in newborn infants, *J Pediatr* 113:359-363, 1988.

622. Manco-Johnson MJ, Abshire TC, Jacobson LJ, Marlar RA: Severe neonatal protein C deficiency: Prevalence and thrombotic risk, *J Pediatr* 119:793-798, 1991.

623. Fok TF, Yin JA, Yuen PMP: Comparison of antithrombin-III, protein C and protein S levels in capillary and venous blood of newborn infants, *Acta Paediatr* 81:204-206, 1992.

624. Debus OM, Kosch A, Strater R, Rossi R, et al: The factor V G1691A mutation is a risk for porencephaly: A case-control study, *Ann Neurol* 56:287-290, 2004.

625. Yoshioka H, Kadomoto Y, Mino M, Morikawa Y, et al: Multicystic encephalomalacia in liveborn twin with a stillborn macerated co-twin, *J Pediatr* 95:798-800, 1979.

626. Manterola A, Towbin A, Yakovlev PI: Cerebral infarction in the human fetus near term, *J Neuropathol Exp Neurol* 25:479-488, 1966.

627. Moore CM, McAdams AJ, Sutherland J: Intrauterine disseminated intravascular coagulation: A syndrome of multiple pregnancy with a dead twin fetus, *J Pediatr* 74:523-528, 1969.
628. Aicardi J, Goutieres F, De Verbois AH: Multicystic encephalomalacia of infants and its relation to abnormal gestation and hydranencephaly, *J Neurol Sci* 15:357-373, 1972.
629. Norman MG: Mechanisms of brain damage in twins, *Can J Neurol Sci* 9:339-344, 1982.
630. Jung JH, Graham JMJ, Schultz N, Smith DW: Congenital hydranencephaly/porencephaly due to vascular disruption in monozygotic twins, *Pediatrics* 73:467-469, 1984.
631. Hughes HE, Miskin M: Congenital microcephaly due to vascular disruption: In utero documentation, *Pediatrics* 78:85-87, 1986.
632. Shah DM, Chaffin D: Perinatal outcome in very preterm births with twin-twin transfusion syndrome, *Am J Obstet Gynecol* 161:1111-1113, 1989.
633. Carlson NJ, Towers CV: Multiple gestation complicated by the death of one fetus, *Obstet Gynecol* 73:685-689, 1989.
634. Cherouny PH, Hoskins IA, Johnson TR, Niebyl JR: Multiple pregnancy with late death of one fetus, *Obstet Gynecol* 74:318-320, 1989.
635. Patten RM, Mack LA, Nyberg DA, Filly RA: Twin embolization syndrome: Prenatal sonographic detection and significance, *Radiology* 173:685-689, 1989.
636. Anderson RL, Golbus MS, Curry CJ, Callen PW, et al: Central nervous system damage and other anomalies in surviving fetus following second trimester antenatal death of co-twin. Report of four cases and literature review, *Prenat Diagn* 10:513-518, 1990.
637. Larroche JC, Droulle P, Delezoide AL, Narcy F, et al: Brain damage in monozygous twins, *Biol Neonate* 57:261-278, 1990.
638. Elliott JP, Urig MA, Clewell WH: Aggressive therapeutic amniocentesis for treatment of twin-twin transfusion syndrome, *Obstet Gynecol* 77:537-540, 1991.
639. Scheller JM, Nelson KB: Twinning and neurologic morbidity, *Am J Dis Child* 146:1110-1113, 1992.
640. Benirschke K: The contribution of placental anastomoses to prenatal twin damage, *Hum Pathol* 23:1319-1320, 1992.
641. Bordarier C, Robain O: Microgyric and necrotic cortical lesions in twin fetuses: Original cerebral damage consecutive to twinning, *Brain Dev* 14:174-178, 1992.
642. Sugama S, Kusano K: Monozygous twin with polymicrogyria and normal co-twin, *Pediatr Neurol* 11:62-63, 1994.
643. Perlman J, Burns DK, Twickler DM, Weinberg AG: Fetal hypokinesia syndrome in the monochorionic pair of a triplet pregnancy secondary to severe disruptive cerebral injury, *Pediatrics* 96:521-523, 1995.
644. Weig SG, Marshall PC, Abroms IF, Gauthier NS: Patterns of cerebral injury and clinical presentation in the vascular disruptive syndrome of monozygotic twins, *Pediatr Neurol* 13:279-285, 1995.
645. Van Bogaert P, Donner C, David P, Rodesch F, et al: Congenital bilateral perisylvian syndrome in a monozygotic twin with intrauterine death of the co-twin, *Dev Med Child Neurol* 38:166-171, 1996.
646. Larroche JC, Girard N, Narcy F, Fallet C: Abnormal cortical plate (polymicrogyria), heterotopias and brain damage in monozygous twins, *Biol Neonate* 65:343-352, 1994.
647. Maier RF, Bialobrzeski B, Gross A, Vogel M, et al: Acute and chronic fetal hypoxia in monochorionic and dichorionic twins, *Obstet Gynecol* 86:973-977, 1996.
648. Machin G, Still K, Lalani T: Correlations of placental vascular anatomy and clinical outcomes in 69 monochorionic twin pregnancies, *Am J Med Genet* 61:229-236, 1996.
649. Pharoah POD, Cooke RWI: A hypothesis for the aetiology of spastic cerebral palsy: The vanishing twin, *Dev Med Child Neurol* 39:292-296, 1997.
650. Williams K, Hennessy E, Alberman E: Cerebral palsy: Effects of twinning, birthweight, and gestational age, *Arch Dis Child Fetal Neonatal Ed* 75:F178-F182, 1996.
651. Pharoah POD, Cooke T: Cerebral palsy and multiple births, *Arch Dis Child Fetal Neonatal Ed* 75:F174-F177, 1996.
652. Ulfig N, Nickel J, Saretzki U: Alterations in myelin formation in fetal brains of twins, *Pediatr Neurol* 19:287-293, 1998.
653. Pharoah POD, Adi Y: Consequences of in-utero death in a twin pregnancy, *Lancet* 355:1597-1602, 2000.
654. Pharoah POD: Cerebral palsy in the surviving twin associated with infant death of the co-twin, *Arch Dis Child Fetal Neonatal Ed* 84:F111-F116, 2001.
655. Seng YC, Rajadurai VS: Twin-twin transfusion syndrome: A five year review, *Arch Dis Child Fetal Neonatal Ed* 83:F168-F170, 2000.
656. Scher AI, Petterson B, Blair E, Ellenberg JH, et al: The risk of mortality or cerebral palsy in twins: A collaborative population-based study, *Pediatr Res* 52:671-681, 2002.
657. Duncombe GJ, Dickinson JE, Evans SF: Perinatal characteristics and outcomes of pregnancies complicated by twin-twin transfusion syndrome, *Obstet Gynecol* 101:1190-1196, 2003.
658. Buldini B, Drigo P, Via LD, Calderone M, et al: Symmetrical thalamic calcifications in a monozygotic twin: Case report and literature review, *Brain Dev* 27:66-69, 2005.
659. Mari G, Roberts A, Detti L, Kovanci E, et al: Perinatal morbidity and mortality rates in severe twin-twin transfusion syndrome: Results of the International Amnioreduction Registry, *Am J Obstet Gynecol* 185:708-715, 2001.
660. Lopriore E, Nagel HTC, Vandenbussche FPHA, Walther FJ: Long-term neurodevelopmental outcome in twin-to-twin transfusion syndrome, *Am J Obstet Gynecol* 189:1314-1319, 2003.
661. Chiswick M: Assessing outcomes in twin-twin transfusion syndrome, *Arch Dis Child Fetal Neonatal Ed* 83:F165-F167, 2000.
662. Hahn JS, Lewis AJ, Barries P: Hydranencephaly owing to twin-twin transfusion: Serial fetal ultrasonography and magnetic resonance imaging findings, *J Child Neurol* 18:367-370, 2003.
663. Glinianaia SV, Pharoah POD, Wright C, Rankin JM: Fetal or infant death in twin pregnancy: Neurodevelopmental consequence for the survivor, *Arch Dis Child Fetal Neonatal Ed* 86:F9-F15, 2002.
664. Zankl A, Brooks D, Boltshauser E, Largo R, et al: Natural history of twin disruption sequence, *Am J Med Genet A* 127:133-138, 2004.
665. Dickinson JE, Duncombe GJ, Evans SF, French NP, et al: The long term neurologic outcome of children from pregnancies complicated by twin-to-twin transfusion syndrome, *Br J Obstet Gynecol* 112:63-68, 2005.
666. Golomb MR, Williams LS, Garg BP: Perinatal stroke in twins without co-twin demise, *Pediatr Neurol* 35:75-77, 2006.
667. Redline RW: Nonidentical twins with a single placenta: Disproving dogma in perinatal pathology, *N Engl J Med* 349:111-114, 2003.
668. Levi S: Ultrasonic assessment of the high rate of human multiple pregnancy in the first trimester, *J Clin Ultrasound* 4:3-5, 1976.
669. Landy HJ, Weiner S, Carson S, Batzer FR, et al: The "vanishing twin": Ultrasonographic assessment of fetal disappearance in the first trimester, *Am J Obstet Gynecol* 155:14-19, 1986.
670. Senat MV, Deprest J, Boulvain M, Paupe A, et al: Endoscopic laser surgery versus serial amnioreduction for severe twin-to-twin transfusion syndrome, *N Engl J Med* 351:136-144, 2004.
671. Lopriore E, Sueters M, Middeldorp JM, Oepkes D, et al: Neonatal outcome in twin-to-twin transfusion syndrome treated with fetoscopic laser occlusion of vascular anastomoses, *J Pediatr* 147:597-602, 2005.
672. Graef C, Ellenrieder B, Hecher K, Hackeloer BJ, et al: Long-term neurodevelopmental outcome of 167 children after intrauterine laser treatment for severe twin-twin transfusion syndrome, *Obstet Gynecol* 194:303-308, 2006.
673. Lopriore E, van Wezel-Meijler G, Middeldorp JM, Sueters M, et al: Incidence, origin, and character of cerebral injury in twin-to-twin transfusion syndrome treated with fetoscopic laser surgery, *Am J Obstet Gynecol* 194:1215-1220, 2006.
673a. Norton ME: Evaluation and management of twin-twin transfusion syndrome: Still a challenge, *Am J Obstet Gynecol* 196:419-420, 2007.
674. Wu YW, March WM, Croen LA, Grether JK, et al: Perinatal stroke in children with motor impairment: A population-based study, *Pediatrics* 114:612-619, 2004.
675. Steinlin M, Pfister I, Pavlovic J, Everts R, et al: The first three years of the Swiss Neuropaediatric Stroke Registry (SNPSR): A population-based study of incidence, symptoms and risk factors, *Neuropediatrics* 36:90-97, 2005.
676. Ford L, de Courten-Myers GM, Mandybur T, Myers RE: Cerebral hemiatrophy: Correlation of human with animal experimental data, *Pediatr Neurosci* 14:114-119, 1988.
677. Sheth RD, Bodensteiner JB, Riggs JE, Schochet SS: Differential involvement of the brain in neonatal asphyxia: A pathogenic explanation, *J Child Neurol* 10:464-466, 1995.

Chapter 9

Hypoxic-Ischemic Encephalopathy: Clinical Aspects

The clinical aspects of neonatal hypoxic-ischemic encephalopathy are appropriately discussed following the neuropathology (see Chapter 8), because understanding of the clinical phenomena is facilitated greatly by an awareness of the underlying pathological substrates. Moreover, choices of appropriate diagnostic modalities, formulation of rational prognostic statements, and development of appropriate plans of management are based, in many ways, on awareness of the probable neuropathologies. In this chapter, I discuss the clinical settings for neonatal hypoxic-ischemic encephalopathy, the clinical syndrome, diagnostic studies, clinical correlations, prognosis, and management.

CLINICAL SETTINGS

The clinical settings for neonatal hypoxic-ischemic encephalopathy are dominated by the ultimate occurrence of ischemia (i.e., diminished blood supply to brain), usually but not necessarily preceded or accompanied by hypoxemia (i.e., diminished amount of oxygen in the blood supply). Hypoxemia leads to brain injury principally by causing myocardial disturbance and loss of cerebrovascular autoregulation, with ischemia the major consequence. The temporal characteristics and the severity of the hypoxemia and ischemia, as well as the gestational age of the infant, are the principal determinants of the type of neuropathology that results (see Chapter 8).

The major causes of serious hypoxemia in the perinatal period are (1) asphyxia with intrauterine disturbance of gas exchange across the placenta and with respiratory failure at the time of birth, (2) postnatal respiratory insufficiency secondary to severe respiratory distress syndrome or recurrent apneic spells, and (3) severe right-to-left shunt secondary to persistent fetal circulation or cardiac disease. The major causes of serious ischemia are as follows: (1) intrauterine asphyxia (i.e., hypoxemia, hypercarbia, and acidosis) with cardiac insufficiency and loss of cerebrovascular autoregulation both in utero and at the time of birth; (2) postnatal cardiac insufficiency secondary to severe recurrent apneic spells, large patent ductus arteriosus, or severe congenital heart disease; and (3) postnatal (postcardiac) circulatory insufficiency secondary to patent ductus arteriosus (with "ductal steal") or vascular collapse (e.g., with sepsis).

The relative importance of antepartum, intrapartum, and postnatal hypoxic-ischemic insults in the pathogenesis of neonatal hypoxic-ischemic encephalopathy is difficult to quantitate conclusively. I refer here to the encephalopathic syndrome described later *and* the presence of evidence for intrapartum asphyxia (see "Neurological Syndrome"). Thus, obviously, not all neonatal encephalopathies are related to hypoxic-ischemic disease. Antepartum and postpartum disorders (e.g., infectious, metabolic, dysgenetic) may lead to neonatal encephalopathies, as discussed throughout this book. In one large population-based observational study, the prevalence of moderate to severe encephalopathy was 1.64 per 1000 live term births, and the prevalence of "birth asphyxia" was 0.86 per 1000 term live births.[1] Fully 56% of all cases of newborn encephalopathy were related to intrapartum events. Additionally, although obvious, hypoxic-ischemic injury may affect the brain in the antepartum and postnatal periods, *albeit relatively uncommonly*. On the basis of earlier work,[2-18] approximately 20% of hypoxic-ischemic injury recognized in the newborn period was said to be related primarily to antepartum insults. These data should be interpreted with the awareness that assessment of timing of insults to the fetus is based on imprecise methods, and the variability of findings is considerable.

Data indicate that most infants with neonatal hypoxic-ischemic encephalopathy and intrapartum evidence of asphyxia exhibit on magnetic resonance imaging (MRI) evidence only of acute injury and no clear evidence of long-standing antenatal hypoxic-ischemic disease (Table 9-1).[19,20] In one study of 245 term infants with neonatal encephalopathy and evidence of intrauterine asphyxia, fully 80% had acute lesions consistent with hypoxic-ischemic disease, 16% had normal MRI scans, and only 4% had concomitant evidence of chronic antenatal injury.[19] In another MRI study of 173 term newborns with encephalopathy and signs of intrauterine asphyxia, only acute injury was observed.[20] Related clinical and epidemiological data support the marked preponderance of intrapartum events in the origin of neonatal hypoxic-ischemic encephalopathy, especially in the term infant.[21-23]

The principal *intrapartum events* leading to hypoxic-ischemic fetal insults include acute placental or umbilical cord disturbances, such as abruptio placentae or cord prolapse, prolonged labor with transverse arrest, difficult forceps extractions, or rotational maneuvers (see Chapters 7 and 8). *Postpartum* events alone (e.g., severe persistent fetal circulation, severe recurrent apneic spells, cardiac failure secondary to large patent

TABLE 9-1	Timing of Insults Leading to Hypoxic-Ischemic Encephalopathy

Of 245 infants who had an MRI scan after neonatal neurological signs ("neonatal encephalopathy"), and evidence of intrapartum perinatal asphyxia,

197 (80%) had MRI evidence of *acute* lesions consistent with hypoxic-ischemic insult; only 8 (4%) also had MRI evidence of antenatal injury.

40 (16%) had normal MRI scans.

8 (4%) had other disorders (e.g., neuromuscular or metabolic diseases).

MRI, magnetic resonance imaging.
Data from Cowan F, Rutherford M, Groenendaal F, Eken P, et al: Origin and timing of brain lesions in term infants with neonatal encephalopathy, *Lancet* 361:736–742, 2003.

ductus arteriosus or other congenital heart disease, severe pulmonary disease) may lead to hypoxic-ischemic encephalopathy and may account for approximately 10% of cases.[21] Most of these and related *postnatal* factors are much more important in the pathogenesis of hypoxic-ischemic brain injury in the *premature infant* than in the term infant (see Chapters 8 and 11). Although hypoxic-ischemic injury certainly can occur in the antepartum period (e.g., secondary to maternal trauma, maternal hypotension, uterine hemorrhage), this injury cumulatively accounts for only a small proportion of neonatal hypoxic-ischemic encephalopathy. However, antepartum factors may *predispose* to intrapartum hypoxia-ischemia during the stresses of labor and delivery, especially through threats to placental flow. Such factors include maternal diabetes, preeclampsia, placental vasculopathy, intrauterine growth retardation, and twin gestation (see Chapter 8). In one series, such factors were present in approximately one third of cases of intrapartum asphyxia.[21] Indeed, "perinatal asphyxia" was identified in 27% of infants of diabetic mothers, and its occurrence correlated closely with diabetic vasculopathy (nephropathy) and presumed placental vascular insufficiency.[24] The additional stress of labor would be expected to compromise placental blood flow. Similarly, impaired placental function and an increased risk of perinatal asphyxia in *the infant with intrauterine growth retardation* are recognized and appear to account for some of the increased risk of subsequent neurological disability in such infants.[25-32] Other factors (e.g., dysmorphic syndromes, severe undernutrition, infection) may also lead to increased risk of neurological disability in intrauterine growth retardation.[29,33-37] Studies in fetal and neonatal animals suggest that the mechanisms for the increased vulnerability of the growth-retarded fetus relate not only to placental insufficiency but also to diminished glucose reserves in heart, liver, and brain and to impaired capability to increase substrate supply to brain with the hypoxic stress of vaginal delivery.[38,39] In general, more extensive use of sophisticated techniques for antepartum assessment of the fetus (see Chapter 7) may help determine whether, when, and to what extent hypoxic-ischemic injury to the fetus occurs before labor or delivery.

Although the particular importance of intrauterine asphyxia, especially intrapartum asphyxia with or without antepartum predisposing factors, in the genesis of the clinical syndrome of neonatal hypoxic-ischemic encephalopathy is apparent, most infants who experience intrauterine hypoxic-ischemic insults do *not* exhibit overt neonatal neurological features *or* subsequent neurological evidence of brain injury.[2,3,14,16,18,40-46] The severity and duration of the asphyxia obviously are critical. The elegant studies of Low and others demonstrated a striking relationship among the severity and duration of intrapartum hypoxia, assessed by the use of fetal acid-base studies (see Chapter 7), the subsequent occurrence of a neonatal neurological syndrome, and later neurological deficits. Current data suggest that approximately 1.3 per 1000 live term births experience hypoxic-ischemic encephalopathy,[22,46-48] and approximately 0.3 per 1000 of these live term births have significant neurological residua (see later discussion).

NEUROLOGICAL SYNDROME

The neurological syndrome that accompanies serious intrauterine asphyxia is the prototype for neonatal hypoxic-ischemic encephalopathy. *The occurrence of a neonatal neurological syndrome, indeed, is a sine qua non for attributing subsequent brain injury to intrapartum insult.* Indeed, I consider three features important in considering that intrapartum insult is the likely cause of neonatal brain injury: (1) evidence of fetal distress (e.g., fetal heart rate abnormalities, meconium-stained amniotic fluid), (2) depression at birth, and (3) an overt neonatal neurological syndrome in the first hours and days of life. Important conclusions about a clinically significant neonatal neurological syndrome in this setting are noted in Table 9-2.

Although not discussed here in depth, important *systemic abnormalities*, presumably related to ischemia, often accompany the neonatal neurological syndrome. The relative frequencies of manifestations of organ injury in term infants with evidence of asphyxia were addressed in several studies.[44,45,49-52] The findings varied as a function of the severity of asphyxia and the definitions of organ dysfunction. In combined data from two reports (Table 9-3),[45,49] approximately 20% of infants with apparent fetal asphyxia had no evidence of organ injury. Evidence of involvement of the central nervous system occurred in 62% of infants. Indeed, in 16% of infants, involvement of only the nervous system was apparent. Central nervous system

TABLE 9-2	Neonatal Neurological Syndrome Associated with Clinically Significant Encephalopathy

Not subtle
Indicative of recent (e.g., intrapartum) insult
Prenatal insult (e.g., antepartum) *also* possible
Absence rules out intrapartum insult capable of causing major brain injury

TABLE 9-3 **Manifestations of Organ Injury in Term Asphyxiated Infants***

Organ	Percentage of Total
None	22%
CNS only	16%
CNS and one or more other organs	46%
Other organ(s), no CNS	16%

*Cumulative total of 107 term infants; definition of asphyxia in both series included umbilical cord arterial pH < 7.2.
CNS, central nervous system.
Data from Perlman JM, Tack ED, Martin T, Shackelford G, et al: Acute systemic organ injury in term infants after asphyxia, *Am J Dis Child* 143:617–620, 1989; and Martin-Ancel A, Garcia-Alix A, Gaya F, Cabanas F, et al: Multiple organ involvement in perinatal asphyxia, *J Pediatr* 127:786–793, 1995.

involvement without overt dysfunction of systemic organs is particularly likely after severe, acute, terminal intrapartum insults with resulting injury primarily to deep nuclear structures (see Chapter 8).[50] Systemic organ involvement, without neurological disease, occurred in only 16% of infants. The order of frequency of systemic organ involvement overall has been hepatic > pulmonary > renal > cardiac. In an autopsy series, cardiac involvement was the most common among affection of systemic organs.[53] With careful electrocardiographic and enzymatic studies of living infants after perinatal asphyxia, evidence of myocardial ischemia has been commonly observed.[54]

The following discussion is based primarily on my findings with *term infants* who have sustained *serious* intrauterine asphyxia. A continuum of severity is recognized readily, and various classification schemes have been devised.[8,46,55-57] Certain variations in the syndrome relate to the topography of the neuropathology, as noted later.

Birth to 12 Hours

In the first hours after the insult, signs of presumed bilateral cerebral hemispheral disturbance predominate (Table 9-4).[58,59] The severely affected infant is either deeply stuporous or in coma (i.e., not arousable and minimal or no response to sensory input). Periodic breathing, or respiratory irregularity akin to this pattern, is prominent, and I consider this form of respiratory disturbance to be the neonatal counterpart

TABLE 9-4 **Clinical Features of Severe Hypoxic-Ischemic Encephalopathy: Birth to 12 Hours**

Depressed level of consciousness: usually deep stupor or coma
Ventilatory disturbance: "periodic" breathing or respiratory failure
Intact pupillary responses
Intact oculomotor responses
Hypotonia, minimal movement > hypertonia
Seizures

of Cheyne-Stokes respiration, which is observed in older children and adults with bilateral hemispheral disease. In one series, approximately 80% of asphyxiated infants had abnormal breathing patterns, particularly periodic breathing.[60] Those most severely affected may exhibit marked hypoventilation or respiratory failure. Pupillary responses to light are intact, spontaneous eye movements are present, and eye movements with the oculocephalic response (doll's eye maneuver) are usually full. (Pupillary size is variable, although dilated reactive pupils tend to predominate in the less affected infants, and constricted reactive pupils are common in the more severely affected infants.[55]) Commonly, disconjugate eye movements are apparent. However, only in a few babies are eye signs of major brain stem disturbance seen. Fixed, midposition, or dilated pupils and eye movements fixed to the doll's eyes maneuver and to cold caloric stimulation are unusual at this stage. If either of these signs is evident at this time, especially in the full-term infant, injury to brain stem is likely. Most infants at this stage are markedly and diffusely hypotonic with minimal spontaneous or elicited movement. Less severely affected infants have preserved tone. Others exhibit increased tone, especially with prominent involvement of basal ganglia. Seizures, in my experience, occur by 6 to 12 hours after birth in approximately 50% to 60% of the infants who ultimately have convulsions. Similar data have been recorded by others.[15,46,61] The particular propensity for convulsions in asphyxiated infants is reminiscent of the particular propensity of the immature rat (compared with the adult) to exhibit epileptic phenomena after hypoxia-ischemia.[62]

Virtually every one of the infants with seizures, in my experience, exhibits "subtle seizures," manifested by one or more of the following (see also Chapter 5): (1) ocular phenomena, such as tonic horizontal deviation of eyes with or without accompanying jerking movements of eyes, or sustained eye opening with ocular fixation; (2) sucking, smacking, or other oral-buccal-lingual movements; (3) "swimming" or "rowing" movements of limbs; and (4) apneic spells, usually accompanied by one or more of the foregoing. Premature infants with hypoxic-ischemic encephalopathy often exhibit generalized tonic seizures, which may mimic decerebrate or decorticate posturing. (Indeed, posturing, rather than or in addition to seizure, may be present in such infants, as discussed in Chapter 5.) Full-term infants often also exhibit multifocal clonic seizures, characterized by clonic movements that migrate in a nonordered fashion. Focal seizures are especially common in full-term infants with focal ischemic cerebral lesions. Indeed, approximately 40% to 80% of infants with focal cerebral infarcts exhibit focal seizures.[63-83] Infants with arterial stroke often exhibit focal seizures *without* other major signs of encephalopathy (see later).[19,84,85] In one large series of term infants with neonatal encephalopathy or early seizures, or both, only 8 of 197 with overt neonatal encephalopathy (with or without seizures) had acute focal infarction, whereas fully 35 of the 90 infants with early seizures (first 3 days of life) but without major signs of encephalopathy had focal cerebral infarction.[19]

Recognition of the presence and prominence of the aforementioned abnormal neurological signs presupposes an awareness of the normal neurological findings at various gestational ages (see Chapter 3). Thus, the normal infant of 28 weeks of gestation requires stimulation for arousal from sleep. At 32 weeks of gestation, spontaneous arousal occurs, but vigorous crying during wakefulness is unusual. Only at 40 weeks of gestation should the observer expect to see discrete periods of attention to visual and auditory stimuli. Similarly, periodic breathing in a full-term newborn is much more likely to be an abnormal finding than in a premature infant at 32 weeks of gestation. No pupillary reaction to light is usual at 28 weeks but is unusual at 32 to 34 weeks. However, full extraocular movements with doll's eyes maneuver are present in the youngest normal infants (i.e., 28 weeks of gestation or even younger). Finally, hypotonia in the upper extremities is usual at 28 or 32 weeks of gestation but is abnormal at term. Spontaneous movements also exhibit a progression from lower to upper extremities from 28 weeks of gestation to term, so "weakness" of upper extremities must be defined with caution in the premature infant.

12 to 24 Hours

From approximately 12 to 24 hours, the infant's level of consciousness changes in a variable manner (Table 9-5). Infants with severe disease remain deeply stuporous or in a coma. Infants with less severe disease often begin to exhibit some degree of improvement in alertness. However, in some infants, this *improvement is more apparent than real*, because the appearance of alertness may not be accompanied by visual fixation or following, habituation to sensory stimulation, or other signs of cerebral function. The notion of apparent rather than real improvement in such cases is supported further by the occurrence at this time of severe seizures, apneic spells, jitteriness, and weakness. (Approximately 15% to 20% of infants experience the *onset* of seizures at this time.) Overt status epilepticus is not unusual, and vigorous therapy is needed urgently. Apneic spells appear in approximately 50% of infants (65% in one series).[2,3,60] Jitteriness develops in about one fourth of infants and may be so marked that the

movements are mistaken for seizures. Distinction can usually be made at the bedside (see Chapter 5). Infants with involvement of basal ganglia may exhibit an increase in their hypertonia, especially in response to handling. In my experience, many infants manifest definite albeit not marked weakness (see Table 9-5). Although precise correlation is often difficult, these infants appear from the clinical circumstances surrounding their insult to have sustained particularly marked *ischemic* insults. Full-term infants most often exhibit weakness in the hip-shoulder distribution, with more impressive involvement usually of the proximal extremities. Distinct asymmetry of these latter motor findings is unusual to elicit at this time, although a few full-term infants do exhibit weakness that is confined to or is clearly more severe on one side than on the other. Premature infants may exhibit primarily lower extremity weakness, although it can be very difficult to be certain of such findings in the small, sick baby. This pattern of weakness appears to relate to the topography of the cerebral white matter neuropathology (see later discussion of periventricular leukomalacia [PVL]).

24 to 72 Hours

Between approximately 24 and 72 hours, the severely affected infant's level of consciousness often deteriorates further, and deep stupor or coma may ensue (Table 9-6). Respiratory arrest may occur, often after a period of irregularly irregular ("ataxic") respirations. Brain stem oculomotor disturbances are now more common. These usually consist of skew deviation and loss of responsiveness of the eyes to the doll's eyes maneuver and to cold caloric stimulation. (Rarely, ocular bobbing may appear.) Pupils may become fixed to light in the mid or dilated position. Reactive but constricted pupils are more common in less severely affected infants. Babies who die with hypoxic-ischemic encephalopathy most often do so at this time, particularly if the criterion is "brain death."[86] In one large series of infants who died after perinatal asphyxia and hypoxic-ischemic encephalopathy, the median age of death was 2 days.[53] The cause for the apparent delay in progression to brain death until this period is not known definitely, but delayed cell death has been documented in in vivo models and in neurons in culture (see Chapters 6 and 8). The importance of excitatory amino acids, calcium-mediated deleterious metabolic events, and free radical production has

TABLE 9-5	Clinical Features of Severe Hypoxic-Ischemic Encephalopathy: 12 to 24 Hours

Variable change in level of alertness
More seizures
Apneic spells
Jitteriness
Weakness
    Proximal limbs, upper > lower (full term)
    Hemiparesis (full term)
    Lower limbs (premature)

TABLE 9-6	Clinical Features of Severe Hypoxic-Ischemic Encephalopathy: 24 to 72 Hours

Stupor or coma
Respiratory arrest
Brain stem oculomotor and pupillary disturbances
Catastrophic deterioration with severe intraventricular hemorrhage and periventricular hemorrhagic infarction (premature)

been detailed in Chapters 6 and 8. Indeed, studies by MR spectroscopy in the asphyxiated human infant (see later discussion) have documented a delayed deterioration of cerebral energy state. However, although delayed cell death most probably accounts for this clinical deterioration, consideration should also be given to the occurrence of frequent subclinical electrical seizures as the reason for the deterioration. Although electroencephalography (EEG) is required for this determination, the potential effectiveness of anticonvulsant therapy warrants the procedure.

In my experience, most of the premature infants who die at 24 to 72 hours experience *marked* intraventricular hemorrhage, usually with periventricular hemorrhagic infarction (see Chapter 11). This hemorrhage may be heralded by a characteristic catastrophic clinical syndrome (i.e., evolution in hours of bulging anterior fontanelle, falling hematocrit, hypoventilation proceeding to respiratory arrest, generalized tonic seizure, decerebrate posturing, pupils fixed to light, eyes fixed to all vestibular stimulation, and flaccid quadriparesis; see Chapter 11). In a majority of premature infants, the intraventricular hemorrhage is accompanied by a more saltatory deterioration or by fragments of the aforementioned syndrome; such infants are much less likely to die with their hemorrhage.

The full-term infants who die at this time only uncommonly have significant hemorrhage, although a few exhibit clinical signs of increased intracranial pressure (ICP), for example, bulging anterior fontanelle and split cranial sutures. In the large classic series reported by Brown and co-workers,[2] these signs appeared ultimately in 31% of the infants. In my experience, such infants have sustained severe insults and exhibit major cerebral necrosis at postmortem examination. Thus, signs of brain swelling and increased ICP appear to occur in infants *after*, rather than before, severe cerebral injury has occurred. Systematic studies of increased ICP in asphyxiated human infants support this notion (see Chapter 8).[87,88]

After 72 Hours

Infants who survive to this point usually improve over the next several days to weeks; however, certain neurological features persist (Table 9-7). Although the level of consciousness improves, often dramatically, mild to moderate stupor continues. The persistence of this depression of consciousness may provoke, sometimes unnecessarily, many different diagnostic procedures in an attempt to define a complicating process, such as sepsis. Disturbances of feeding are extremely common and relate to abnormalities of sucking, swallowing, and tongue movements. The power and coordination of the muscles involved (innervated by cranial nerves V, VII, IX, X, and XII) are deranged. A few infants require tube feedings for weeks to months. (In the large series studied by Brown and co-workers,[2,3] 80% of infants required early tube feedings because of feeding difficulty.) The abnormalities of brain stem function are especially dramatic in infants with the form of selective neuronal necrosis involving deep nuclear structures (basal ganglia, thalamus) and brain stem tegmentum (see later discussion and Chapter 8).[50,89,90] Generalized hypotonia of limbs is common, although hypertonia, particularly with passive manipulation of limbs, is frequent on careful examination, especially among infants with prominent involvement of basal ganglia. The patterns of weakness discussed in the previous section become more readily elicited, although the weakness is rarely marked. In the premature infant, demonstration of the lower limb pattern of PVL or the hemiparesis later seen with periventricular hemorrhagic infarction is very difficult. The rate of improvement of each of these clinical features is variable and is not easily predicted, but infants with the fastest initial improvement clearly have the best long-term outlook. Indeed, infants with an essentially normal neurological examination by approximately 1 week of age have an excellent chance for a normal outcome (see "Prognosis").[55,91]

DIAGNOSIS

The recognition of neonatal hypoxic-ischemic encephalopathy depends principally on information gained from a careful history and a thorough neurological examination. The contributing role of certain metabolic derangements requires evaluation. Determination of the site or sites and extent of the injury is made to an appreciable degree by the history and neurological examination, but supplementary evaluations, including especially EEG and brain imaging studies (ultrasonography, computed tomography [CT], MRI), are very important. Certain other neurodiagnostic studies, not yet widely used, may prove particularly valuable, especially in selected instances, as discussed later.

History

Recognition of neonatal hypoxic-ischemic encephalopathy requires awareness of those intrauterine situations that account for most cases. Thus, information should be sought regarding maternal disorders that could lead to uteroplacental insufficiency and disturbances of labor or delivery that could impair placental respiratory gas exchange or fetal blood flow or exert a direct traumatic effect on the fetal central nervous system. The value of electronic fetal monitoring, particularly when supplemented by fetal blood sampling to determine acid-base status, is discussed in Chapter 7.

TABLE 9-7	Clinical Features of Severe Hypoxic-Ischemic Encephalopathy: After 72 Hours

Persistent, yet diminishing stupor
Disturbed sucking, swallowing, gag, and tongue movements
Hypotonia > hypertonia
Weakness
    Proximal limbs, upper > lower (full term)
    Hemiparesis (full term)
    Lower limbs or hemiparesis (premature)

The occurrence of meconium-stained amniotic fluid provides additional information when interpreted appropriately (see Chapter 7).

Neurological Examination

Recognition of the neurological signs outlined previously provides critical information concerning the presence, site, and extent of hypoxic-ischemic injury in the newborn infant. The value of the carefully performed neurological examination was doubted by some clinicians in the past, but a growing body of information now demonstrates conclusively the contributions that the examination can make (see Chapter 3). In addition to critical information about the current state of the infant, the neurological examination provides important information for establishing a prognosis (see "Prognosis").

Metabolic Parameters

Certain metabolic derangements may contribute significantly to the severity and qualitative aspects of the neurological syndrome, and the diagnostic evaluation should include evaluation of such derangements. Hypoglycemia, hyperammonemia, hypocalcemia, hyponatremia (inappropriate secretion of antidiuretic hormone [ADH]), hypoxemia, and acidosis are among the metabolic complications that may occur, often because of associated disorders, and that may exacerbate certain neurological features or add new ones.

Of particular interest in this context is the occurrence of *hypoglycemia* and its potential role in accentuation of brain injury. In a detailed study of 185 infants with evidence of intrauterine asphyxia (cord pH < 7.00), fully 15% exhibited blood glucose concentrations lower than 40 mg/dL in the first 30 minutes of life.[92] The hypoglycemia may relate in large part to enhanced anaerobic glycolysis and thereby glucose use, in an attempt to preserve cellular energy levels (see Chapter 6). By multivariate analysis, the odds ratio for an abnormal neurological outcome was 18.5 when infants with blood glucose levels lower than 40 mg/dL were compared with those with levels higher than 40 mg/dL. These data may have important implications for management (see later).

Hyperammonemia may occur in newborns with severe perinatal asphyxia.[93] Although very uncommon, levels of approximately 300 to 900 μg/mL have been detected in the first 24 hours of life and are usually accompanied by elevated serum glutamic oxaloacetic transaminase levels. Clinical correlates may be difficult to distinguish from those secondary to hypoxic-ischemic encephalopathy, although hyperthermia and hypertension have been frequent additions in patients with hyperammonemia. Clinical improvement is coincident with falling blood ammonia levels. The pathogenesis of the hyperammonemia is unclear, although a combination of increased protein catabolism, secondary to hypoxic "stress,"[94] and impaired liver function, and therefore hepatic urea synthesis, is a good possibility (see Chapter 14). Recall that hepatic disturbance is a common feature of the systemic multiorgan dysfunction observed with intrauterine asphyxia (see earlier).

Other metabolic parameters have been studied and may hold promise as measures of severity of the hypoxic-ischemic insult (Table 9-8), although currently the precise sensitivity and specificity of these determinations require further study before general use is warranted. The metabolites and markers are best considered in terms of their relevance to energy metabolism, excitatory amino acids, free radical metabolism, inflammation, brain-specific proteins, and other compounds (see Table 9-8). Concerning *energy metabolism*, perinatal asphyxia has been associated with hypoglycemia, elevated lactate in blood and cerebrospinal fluid (CSF), elevated lactate/creatinine ratio in urine, and elevated lactate and hydroxybutyrate dehydrogenases in CSF.[92,95-98] Of these, the value of early hypoglycemia was discussed in the preceding paragraph. Of particular interest is the ratio of lactate/creatinine in urine. In a

TABLE 9-8 Potential Adjunctive Determinations in Blood, Urine, or Cerebrospinal Fluid in Assessment of Perinatal Asphyxia*	
Determination	**Body Fluid**
Energy Metabolism	
Glucose	Blood
Lactate	Blood, CSF
Lactate/creatinine ratio	Urine
Lactate dehydrogenase	CSF
Hydroxybutyrate dehydrogenase	CSF
Excitatory Amino Acids	
Glutamate	CSF
Aspartate	CSF
Glycine	CSF
Free Radical Metabolism	
Hypoxanthine	Blood, urine
Uric acid	Blood, urine
Nonprotein-bound iron	Blood
Protein carbonyls	CSF
Isoprostanes	CSF
Ascorbic acid	CSF
Arachidonate metabolites	CSF
Nitric oxide	Blood, CSF
Antioxidant enzymes	CSF
Inflammatory Markers	
Interleukin-6	Blood, CSF
Interleukin-10	CSF
Interleukin-1 beta	Blood
Tumor necrosis factor-alpha	Blood, CSF
Brain-Specific Proteins	
Neuron-specific enolase	Blood, CSF
Neurofilament protein	CSF
Protein S-100	Blood, urine, CSF
Glial fibrillary acidic protein	Blood, CSF
Creatine kinase-BB	Blood, CSF
Other	
Erythropoietin	Blood
Nerve growth factor	CSF
Cyclic adenosine monophosphate	CSF

*See text for references.
CSF, cerebrospinal fluid.

study of 40 infants with evidence of intrapartum asphyxia, the mean (±SD) ratio within 6 hours of life was 16.8 ± 27.4 in the asphyxiated infants who subsequently developed the clinical features of hypoxic-ischemic encephalopathy versus 0.2 ± 0.1 in those who did not develop encephalopathy and 0.09 ± 0.02 in normal infants.[97] Moreover, the ratio was significantly higher in the infants who had neurological sequelae at 1 year (25.4 ± 32.0) than in those with favorable outcomes (0.6 ± 1.5). The degree of elevation of lactate in blood at 30 minutes of life also may be a useful predictor of the severity of perinatal asphyxia.[98]

Concerning *excitatory amino acids*, elevations of the excitotoxic amino acids glutamate, aspartate, and glycine (through the *N*-methyl-D-aspartate [NMDA] receptor) have been observed in CSF in the first day of life (see Table 9-8).[99-102] Correlations with severity of hypoxic-ischemic encephalopathy have been shown.

Concerning *free radical metabolism*, many studies support involvement of reactive oxygen and nitrogen species in the final common pathway to cell death with neonatal hypoxic-ischemic encephalopathy (see Table 9-8).[103-120] These studies have shown elevations in sources of free radicals (e.g., hypoxanthine, non–protein-bound iron, arachidonate metabolites), indicators of lipid peroxidation (e.g., isoprostanes) or oxidized proteins (e.g., protein carbonyls), and markers of free radical use (e.g., ascorbic acid, antioxidant enzymes). Supporting data are relevant to hypoxic-ischemic injury both in term and in preterm infants (see Fig. 8-33).

Concerning *inflammatory markers*, related potentially to hypoxic-ischemic or intrauterine infection or both, elevations of certain cytokines (interleukin-6 [IL-6], IL-10, IL-1beta and tumor necrosis factor-alpha) have been documented in blood and CSF in both term and preterm infants (see Table 9-8).[121-126] The degree to which the elevations in cytokines are primary or secondary is unclear (see Chapter 8).

Concerning *brain-specific proteins*, specific components of neurons (neuron-specific enolase, neurofilament protein, creatine kinase-BB [CK-BB]) and astrocytes (S-100, glial fibrillary acidic protein, CK-BB) have been studied in blood and CSF to detect evidence of neuronal and glial injury.[127-152] In general, elevations of these markers in blood or CSF in the first hours of life after perinatal asphyxia have correlated approximately with severity of clinical and brain imaging findings. However, the value of studies of blood is tempered somewhat by the finding of S-100 and neuron specific enolase in placenta; this suggests that these molecules are not entirely brain specific.[146] Available data suggest that determination of CK-BB is a very sensitive indicator of brain disturbance.[130,132-138,143,148,149] However, the extreme sensitivity of the indicator in blood impairs the specificity of the measure because variable but appreciable proportions of infants with elevated concentrations of CK-BB in cord blood or neonatal blood samples have no evidence of irreversible brain injury and have a normal neurological outcome. However, two studies of the concentrations of CK-BB in *CSF* suggested greater specificity as well as sensitivity concerning identification of hypoxic-ischemic brain

TABLE 9-9	Relation of Neonatal Cerebrospinal Fluid Concentration of Creatine Kinase to Severity of Parenchymal Involvement in Apparent Hypoxic-Ischemic Disorders*
Neurological Disorder	**Creatine Kinase-BB Concentration (Median, µg/L)**
Control Group (total)	2.1
Postasphyxial Encephalopathy	
Normal outcome	10.3
Neurological sequelae	55.6
Periventricular Intraparenchymal Echodensity	
Transient	13.7
Evolution to "cystic leukomalacia"	44.0

*Derived from study of 84 control infants, 10 infants with postasphyxial encephalopathy, and 13 infants with periventricular intraparenchymal echodensity.
Data from De Praeter C, Vanhaesebrouck P, Govaert P, Delanghe J, et al: Creatine kinase isoenzyme BB concentrations in the cerebrospinal fluid of newborns: Relationship to short-term outcome, *Pediatrics* 88:1204–1210, 1991.

injury than with determination of blood CK-BB concentrations (Table 9-9).[138,143]

Concerning *other markers*, elevations of erythropoietin in blood and nerve growth factor and cyclic adenosine monophosphate in CSF have been documented after perinatal asphyxia (see Table 9-8).[153-156] The value of these markers and the significance of their elevations remain to be established.

Currently, none of the markers has been established to be of sufficiently high sensitivity and specificity to be appropriate for general use. However, determinations of the brain-specific isoenzyme, CK-BB, especially in CSF, appear to be most promising.

Lumbar Puncture

Lumbar puncture should be performed on any infant with hypoxic-ischemic encephalopathy in whom the diagnosis is unclear. It is particularly important to rule out other potentially treatable intracranial disorders (e.g., early-onset meningitis) that may mimic the clinical features of hypoxic-ischemic encephalopathy.

Electroencephalogram

The EEG changes in hypoxic-ischemic encephalopathy may provide valuable information concerning the severity of the injury.[55,157-186] Although a considerable variety of tracings may be observed, the most common evolution of EEG changes in severe hypoxic-ischemic encephalopathy is depicted in Figure 9-1. The initial alteration is voltage suppression and a decrease in the frequency (i.e., slowing) into the delta and low theta ranges. Within approximately 1 day and often less, an excessively discontinuous pattern appears, characterized by periods of greater voltage suppression interspersed with bursts, usually asynchronous, of sharp and slow waves. It may be difficult in the premature infant to distinguish this change from normal periodicity, and in the more mature infant, from the tracé

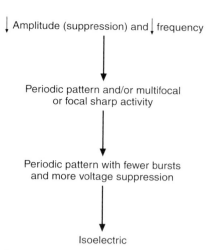

↓ Amplitude (suppression) and ↓ frequency

↓

Periodic pattern and/or multifocal
or focal sharp activity

↓

Periodic pattern with fewer bursts
and more voltage suppression

↓

Isoelectric

Figure 9-1 **Evolution of the electroencephalographic changes in severe hypoxic-ischemic encephalopathy.** See text for temporal aspects.

alternant of normal quiet sleep (see Chapter 4). Some infants exhibit multifocal or focal sharp waves or spikes at this time, often with a degree of periodicity. Over the next day or so, the excessively discontinuous pattern may become very prominent, with more severe voltage suppression and fewer bursts, now characterized by spikes and slow waves. This *burst-suppression pattern* is of ominous significance, especially in the full-term infant (see Chapter 4). However, it is critical to recognize that excessively discontinuous patterns with prolonged interburst intervals (IBIs) that are not as severe as classic burst-suppression patterns nevertheless also are associated with an unfavorable outcome (see "Prognosis" later and Chapter 4). Indeed, in one large series of infants, only 16% of excessively discontinuous tracings (in patients with a generally unfavorable outcome) exhibited burst-suppression patterns by classic definition.[187] Notably, however, as many as 50% of asphyxiated term infants with a burst-suppression pattern identified by amplitude-integrated EEG (aEEG) *in the first hours of life* develop normal or nearly normal tracings within 24 hours (see later).[188] In the severely affected infant, the excessively discontinuous EEG may then evolve into an isoelectric tracing and a hopeless prognosis. Caution in interpretation of apparent isoelectric tracings in the newborn, *especially in the first 10 hours of life*, is indicated by the findings of Pezzani and co-workers,[166] which showed that of

17 asphyxiated newborns with isoelectric or "minimal" background activity in the first 10 hours, one was normal and one exhibited only epilepsy on follow-up (15 of the 17 died in the neonatal period). In general, those asphyxiated infants whose EEG tracings revert to normal within approximately 1 week have favorable outcomes.[55,188]

aEEG, an increasingly common method for continuous monitoring of electrical activity in the newborn (see Chapter 4),[189] has been of considerable value in the assessment of the asphyxiated term newborn.[188-194] This approach has been crucial in the selection of infants for treatment with mild hypothermia (see later). The most useful tracings for detection of severe encephalopathy have been continuous low-voltage, flat, and burst-suppression tracings. Positive predictive values for an unfavorable outcome with such tracings in the first hours of life are 80% to 90% (see "Prognosis" later). Of infants with these marked background abnormalities, 10% to 50% may normalize within 24 hours. Rapid recovery is associated with a favorable outcome in 60% of cases.

Continuous monitoring of conventional EEG with portable equipment has been found to be particularly useful in the identification of *seizure activity* in asphyxiated term infants subjected to muscle paralysis for purposes of ventilation for respiratory failure (see Chapter 4).[168,195] Early detection of the seizures and evaluation of response to anticonvulsant therapy are facilitated by modern portable monitoring systems. Currently, I recommend, when available, continual monitoring with digital EEG of all asphyxiated infants with seizures or other manifestations of severe hypoxic-ischemic disease. This approach provides insight not only into potentially treatable conditions (frequent, clinically silent seizures) but also into the status of the cerebral hemispheres in an infant who is heavily sedated or therapeutically paralyzed.

The *type of EEG abnormality* may indicate a specific pathological variety of hypoxic-ischemic brain injury (Table 9-10). Diffuse and severe abnormalities (excessive discontinuity with prolonged IBI, burst suppression, marked voltage suppression, isoelectric EEG) are observed most commonly with diffuse cortical neuronal necrosis. Excessive sharp waves, especially positive vertex or rolandic sharp waves, positive frontal sharp waves, and negative occipital sharp waves, are particularly suggestive of cerebral white matter injury in the premature infant (see Chapter 4) (Table 9-11).[159,161-164,168,176,180-185] The

TABLE 9-10	Most Frequent Correlations of Electroencephalographic Patterns and Topography of Neonatal Hypoxic-Ischemic Brain Injury*	
EEG Pattern	**Type of Hypoxic-Ischemic Brain Injury**
Excessive discontinuity, burst suppression, persistent marked voltage suppression, isoelectric EEG pattern	Diffuse cortical and thalamic neuronal necrosis
Excessive sharp waves: positive vertex or rolandic, positive frontal, and negative occipital sharp waves	Periventricular leukomalacia (also periventricular hemorrhagic infarction; see Chapter 11)
Focal periodic lateralized epileptiform discharges	Focal cerebral ischemic necrosis (infarction)

*See text for references.
EEG, electroencephalographic.

TABLE 9-11 Value of Electroencephalography in Detection of Cerebral White Matter Injury in Premature Infants*

Abnormal sharp waves of value are positive rolandic or vertex (central), positive frontal, and negative occipital.

Frontal positive or occipital negative sharp waves or both are present in 100% of cases of severe PVL and in 60% to 90% of cases of mild or moderate PVL.

Positive rolandic sharp waves (>0.1/minute) are present in 65% to 90% of cases of severe PVL and in 25% of cases of mild or moderate PVL.

Abnormal sharp waves accompany echodense lesions and *precede* the development of echolucent, presumed cystic change evident on ultrasonography.

The peak period of occurrence of sharp waves is from 5 to 14 days.

*See text for references.
PVL, periventricular leukomalacia.

sensitivity of these abnormal sharp waves increases with the frequency of the waves (>0.1/minute) and the severity of the white matter injury and decreases with the degree of immaturity (especially <28 weeks of gestational age). The EEG abnormalities appear days before the appearance of the most pronounced ultrasonographic abnormalities (see Table 9-11).

The particular value of *serial EEG* in assessment of the asphyxiated infant is pronounced. This caveat holds for both premature and term infants.[161,177,179,180,196] A single EEG study, particularly during the acute phase of the disease, may suggest a more ominous outcome than do subsequent EEG studies (see earlier and Chapter 4, Table 4-11). Focal periodic epileptiform discharges are characteristic of focal cerebral infarction[197,198]; in one series, approximately 90% of infants with such discharges had infarctions.[197]

The role of the EEG in the *assessment of brain death* in the asphyxiated newborn has not been delineated decisively.[86,199-209] Thus, an isoelectric EEG can be observed in infants with *cerebral* neuronal necrosis *but not death of the entire brain* (i.e., brain death). Conversely, persistent EEG activity for many days has been documented in infants with clinical and radionuclide evidence of brain death.[86,204,205,210] Currently, I believe that the guidelines of the Task Force for the Determination of Brain Death in Children are most

appropriate: declaration of brain death in infants between the ages of 7 days and 2 months requires two clinical examinations indicative of loss of all cerebral and brain stem function and two isoelectric EEG tracings carried out according to standardized techniques separated by 48 hours.[211] Although data are limited,[204,205] I favor a 72-hour observation period for term infants less than 7 days of age and only when the cause of the coma is unequivocally established.

Computed Tomography

CT, in medical centers without ready access to MRI, has some value in the initial evaluation of the infant with hypoxic-ischemic encephalopathy. As I discuss later, MRI, in my view, is far preferable. Neverth-less, CT can provide important diagnostic information in identification of diffuse cortical injury in severe selective neuronal necrosis, injury to basal ganglia and thalamus, PVL, and focal and multifocal ischemic brain necrosis (Table 9-12). CT has some value, albeit limited, in identification of parasagittal cerebral injury and venous thrombosis (see later discussion). Hemorrhagic complications of hypoxic-ischemic disease, such as hemorrhagic infarction, are detected readily by CT.

The value of CT in the assessment of *diffuse cortical neuronal injury* is most apparent several weeks after severe asphyxial insults (Fig. 9-2). During the acute period (i.e., the first days of life), the striking, bilateral, diffuse hypodensity that is apparent in clinically more severely affected term infants at least in part reflects marked cortical neuronal injury, perhaps with associated edema (Fig. 9-3).[212-220] The diffuse cerebral hypodensity with loss of gray-white differentiation but with relatively increased density of deep nuclear structures (see Fig. 9-3) has been termed the *reversal sign*.[219]

CT demonstrates hypoxic-ischemic injury to *basal ganglia and thalamus*,[220-222] although MRI is more useful (see subsequent sections). The affected areas exhibit a featureless appearance, with loss of distinction of the deep nuclear structures, and usually clearly decreased attenuation of these structures. Some infants may exhibit increased attenuation, especially in the presence of hemorrhagic necrosis. The subsequent evolution is clearly decreased attenuation over several months (Fig. 9-4). Rarely, the injury develops

TABLE 9-12 Major Techniques for Diagnosis of Specific Neuropathological Types of Neonatal Hypoxic-Ischemic Encephalopathy

	DIAGNOSTIC TECHNIQUE		
Neuropathological Type	**Magnetic Resonance Imaging**	**Computed Tomography**	**Ultrasound**
Selective neuronal necrosis: cerebral cortical	++	+	−
Selective neuronal necrosis: basal ganglia and thalamus	++	+	+
Selective neuronal necrosis: brain stem	++	±	−
Parasagittal cerebral injury	++	+	−
Focal and multifocal ischemic brain injury	++	++	+
Periventricular leukomalacia	++	+	++*

*Very useful for detection of focal component; not useful for detection of diffuse component or "noncystic periventricular leukomalacia" (see text).
++, Very useful; +, useful; ±, questionably useful; −, not useful.

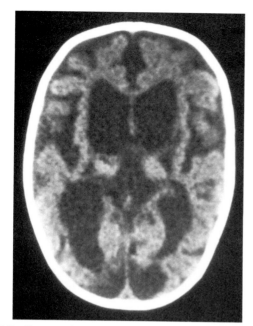

Figure 9-2 Computed tomography scan of residua of diffuse cortical neuronal necrosis from a 6-week-old infant who experienced severe perinatal asphyxia. Note the striking degree of cortical atrophy, manifested by very prominent subarachnoid spaces and shriveled gyri. (Accompanying cerebral white matter injury is apparent from the ventricular enlargement.)

calcification, observable both by CT and by neuropathological study.[223,224]

Parasagittal cerebral injury is more difficult to demonstrate by CT than by MRI (see later), perhaps because the lesion is relatively superficial and interpretation of changes on the most superior CT images may be difficult. However, the lesion in its overt form can be visualized by CT (see example in later section on MRI).[225] I consider MRI to be the imaging modality of choice for the demonstration of parasagittal cerebral injury (see later discussion).

The CT scan is of particular value in the identification of *focal and multifocal ischemic brain injury* (Figs. 9-5 to 9-7; see Table 9-12).[63,65,66,220,226-228] The lesions depicted in Figure 9-5 were of prenatal, antepartum origin. In keeping with the neuropathological data (see Chapter 8), most focal ischemic lesions of perinatal origin involve the distribution of the middle cerebral artery. The timing of the CT scans in the neonatal period for detection is important. For example, lesions with onset near the time of birth, and often heralded by focal seizures on day 1, frequently are difficult to detect by CT (see Fig. 9-6). Only after days to a week or more does the decreased attenuation in a vascular distribution become clearly apparent (see Fig. 9-6). An uncommon complication of neonatal stroke (i.e., secondary hemorrhage into the infarct; see Fig. 9-7), is detected readily by CT.

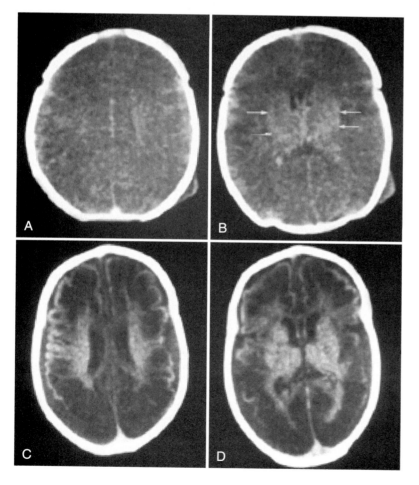

Figure 9-3 Computed tomography (CT) scans of evolution of cortical neuronal necrosis. **A** and **B**, CT slices obtained 5 days after severe perinatal asphyxia show loss of cortical gray-white matter differentiation and, in **B**, relative increase in attenuation of basal ganglia and thalamus (*arrows*). **C** and **D**, CT slices obtained at 4 weeks of age demonstrate evidence of cortical (and white matter) atrophy.

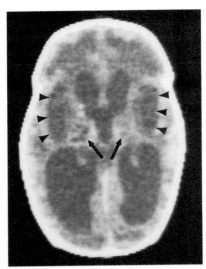

Figure 9-4 **Computed tomography scan of injury to basal ganglia and thalamus**. The scan is from a 2-month-old infant who experienced severe perinatal asphyxia. Note the marked decrease in attenuation in basal ganglia, especially putamen *(arrowheads)*, and the thalamus *(arrows)*. Dilation of the third ventricle reflects the thalamic tissue loss. (Cerebral white matter loss with dilation of lateral ventricles is also apparent.)

CT is only modestly useful for the identification of *PVL* (Fig. 9-8). A propensity for involvement of the anterior and posterior periventricular areas of predilection around the frontal horn and trigone of the lateral ventricles (see Chapter 8 for neuropathology) is apparent. However, considerable caution must be exercised in the interpretation of periventricular hypodensity in asphyxiated preterm infants.[212,220,229] Indeed, low-density periventricular areas are the rule in apparently normal infants, and the gradual increase in density with maturation of the infant has been documented many times.[220,228,230-234] This maturational change is attributed to the decrease in water and increase in lipid and protein in cerebral white matter with myelination. Subsequently, the CT findings of PVL are reduction in quantity of periventricular white matter, particularly at the trigone, ventriculomegaly with irregular outline of the lateral ventricles, and deep sulci that abut the wall of the lateral ventricles (Fig. 9-9).[235] Calcification of the areas of white matter necrosis may occur (Fig. 9-10). In a large neuropathological series of asphyxiated infants, of 29 infants with calcification, 19 (65%) had the mineralization in white matter.[224]

The CT scan may also detect *hemorrhagic lesions* that complicate asphyxia (see Chapters 10 and 11), including subarachnoid, intraventricular, and intracerebral hemorrhage. Although such hemorrhagic lesions are well described in premature infants, 10% to 25% of asphyxiated term infants also exhibit CT evidence of major degrees of intraventricular or intraparenchymal hemorrhage, or both.[212-214]

To summarize, the CT scan is useful in the evaluation of both the premature and full-term infant with hypoxic-ischemic injury (see Table 9-12). The several neuropathological varieties of the injury can be visualized (parasagittal cerebral injury with difficulty, however), as can the associated hemorrhagic complications. However, as noted later, MRI is clearly superior.

Ultrasound

Cranial ultrasonography, the highly effective, noninvasive, portable technique used at the anterior fontanelle (see Chapter 4), is often of value in the urgent initial evaluation of the infant with hypoxic-ischemic brain injury. However, a negative study is not particularly meaningful. In hypoxic-ischemic disease in the term infant, the cranial ultrasound scan initially is negative in as many as 50% of cases.[236] Thus, as with CT, I prefer MRI (see later). Nevertheless, of the major neuropathological lesions, cranial ultrasonography is useful in the identification of injury to basal ganglia and thalamus, focal and multifocal ischemic brain injury, and PVL (see Table 9-12). Ultrasonography is not useful in the definition either of selective cortical or brain stem neuronal injury because the cortical and brain stem lesions are too restricted or too peripherally located to be visualized, or of parasagittal cerebral injury, for similar reasons. (Indeed, in one correlative study of ultrasonography and neuropathology, five cases of cortical neuronal necrosis were observed at postmortem examination without ultrasonographic correlate in any.[237])

Injury to basal ganglia and thalamus, a major accompaniment of selective neuronal injury of the diffuse type and of the two deep nuclear types (see Chapter 8), was demonstrated conclusively by real-time ultrasound when *hemorrhagic necrosis* was present (Fig. 9-11).[238-241] However, the technique can be also effective in demonstration of apparent nonhemorrhagic necrosis, at least as defined by the simultaneous appearance of hypoattenuation, rather than hyperattenuation by CT or abnormal signal on MRI (Fig. 9-12).[241-245]

Ultrasound scanning has demonstrated *focal and multifocal ischemic brain lesions* in the newborn.[70,73,82,237,243,244,246-254] Infarcts, porencephaly, hydranencephaly, and multicystic encephalomalacia have been identified. The evolution of the ultrasonographic appearance of acute infarction consists in the first week of echodensity in a vascular distribution, usually that of the middle cerebral artery (Fig. 9-13). (Doppler ultrasound also may show loss of vascular pulsations in the affected vessel in the acute period.[255]) The CT scan may show relatively little or no abnormality at this stage (see Fig. 9-13). After approximately 1 week, decreased attenuation on CT develops, whereas the echodensity persists on ultrasonography. Over the ensuing 6 to 12 weeks, the echodensity evolves to echolucency, often passing through a stage of heterogeneous appearance termed *checkerboard*.[251] Several long-standing hypoxic-ischemic lesions of prenatal onset (e.g., hydranencephaly) are visualized readily ultrasonographically (Fig. 9-14).

Nevertheless, the sensitivity of ultrasound for detection of focal ischemic injury is not optimal. In two *large* studies, the sensitivity of early ultrasound scan (1 to 3 days) for detection of MRI-proven arterial cerebral

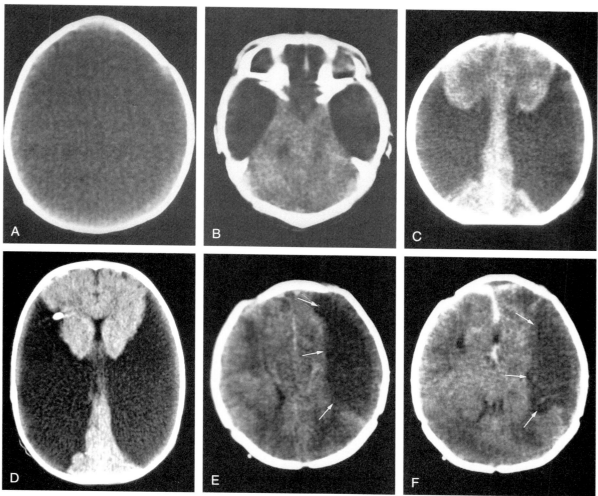

Figure 9-5   Computed tomography scans of ischemic brain injury of prenatal origin. **A** and **B**, Hydranencephaly in a 1-day-old infant; note the symmetrical and diffuse loss of virtually all cerebral tissue. **C** and **D**, Scans obtained from a 1-day-old infant demonstrating bilateral symmetrical loss of cerebral tissue in the distribution of the middle cerebral arteries. **E** and **F**, Scans obtained from a 1-day-old infant demonstrating unilateral loss of cerebral tissue in the distribution of the middle cerebral artery *(arrows)*.

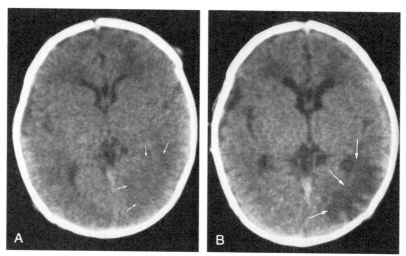

Figure 9-6   Computed tomography scans of focal ischemic brain injury (i.e., stroke). **A**, Scan obtained on the first postnatal day from a full-term infant with right focal seizures. Note the subtle area of decreased attenuation in the left posterior parietal region *(arrows)* and the lack of visualization of the left trigone of the lateral ventricle. **B**, Scan obtained from the same infant at 13 days of age. Note the markedly decreased attenuation in the distribution of the posterior division of the middle cerebral artery *(arrows)*.

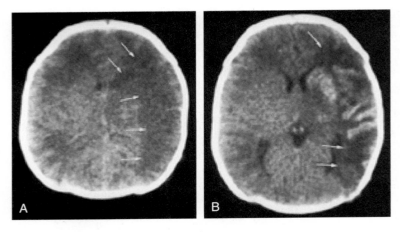

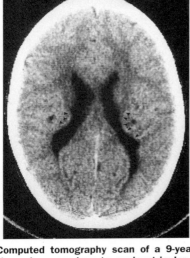

Figure 9-7 Computed tomography scans of secondary hemorrhage into an area of focal ischemic brain injury (i.e., hemorrhagic infarction). **A**, Scan obtained on the third postnatal day in an infant with focal seizures. Note the area of decreased attenuation in the distribution of the middle cerebral artery *(arrows)*. **B**, Scan obtained on the ninth postnatal day shows multiple areas of increased attenuation, consistent with hemorrhage, within the region of decreased attenuation, consistent with infarction *(arrows)*.

infarction in term neonates was 30% to 70%, although scans performed later (4 to 14 days) detected abnormality in 86%.[253,254] However, the findings that the distribution of the middle cerebral artery is affected in most cases and that the region of the sylvian fissure is visualized well on coronal ultrasound scans explain why carefully performed ultrasonography can be useful in this context. After the several days or more required for the development of decreased attenuation, CT becomes more useful than ultrasound in identification of focal ischemic cerebral lesions, particularly the extent of the lesions. However, MRI is the most useful imaging modality (see later discussion).

Ultrasound scanning has been very useful in the evaluation of *periventricular white matter injury*, particularly the focal necrotic/cystic component of PVL (see Chapter 8).[237,243,244,246-249,251,252,256-300] The deep

Figure 9-9 Computed tomography scan of a 9-year-old boy with spastic quadriparesis secondary to periventricular leukomalacia. There is virtual absence of peritrigonal white matter such that cortical gray matter virtually abuts the ventricular wall in that region. *(From Flodmark O, Lupton B, Li D, Stimac GK, et al: MR imaging of periventricular leukomalacia in childhood, AJNR Am J Neuroradiol 10:111–118, 1989.)*

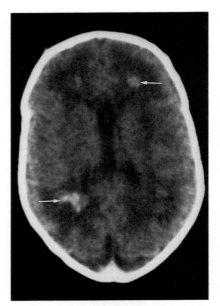

Figure 9-8 Computed tomography scan of periventricular leukomalacia. The scan is from an infant of 33 weeks of gestation and was obtained at 17 days of age. Note the symmetrical, markedly decreased attenuation in frontal and parieto-occipital white matter. The focal areas of increased attenuation *(arrows)* probably reflect secondary hemorrhage into the leukomalacia.

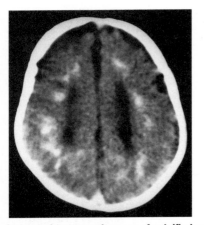

Figure 9-10 Computed tomography scan of calcified periventricular leukomalacia. The scan was obtained at 7 months of age from a premature infant who sustained periventricular leukomalacia. Note the symmetrical calcification in periventricular white matter. Dilated lateral ventricles reflect a degree of white matter atrophy.

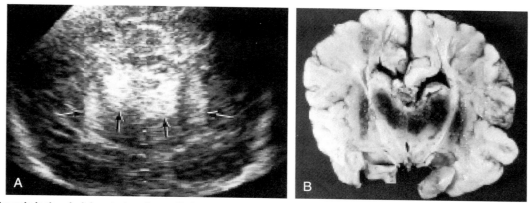

Figure 9-11 **Hypoxic-ischemic injury to basal ganglia in a 24-hour-old full-term infant who experienced severe perinatal asphyxia. A,** Coronal ultrasound scan shows marked bilateral echodensities in the region of basal ganglia and thalamus *(arrows).* The ventricles are not visible. **B,** Coronal section of the cerebrum from the same infant, who died at 80 hours of age. Note the bilateral areas of hemorrhagic necrosis, involving putamen, globus pallidus, and thalamus.

focal necrotic lesions of PVL are visualized especially well when they are hemorrhagic (Fig. 9-15), although nonhemorrhagic focal/necrotic/cystic PVL, proved at postmortem examination, is also demonstrated effectively. Indeed, in one careful study of 12 focal PVL lesions visualized by cranial ultrasonography, 8 were found at postmortem examination to be nonhemorrhagic, and only 4 were hemorrhagic.[261] However, the more diffuse cell-specific component of PVL is *not* visualized well by ultrasonography (see later discussion).

The *evolution of the ultrasonographic appearance* of focal PVL has been defined clearly by studies reported by others[259,261,279-281,283,285,291,298-302] and by approximately 25 years of personal experience with this imaging technique (Table 9-13). In coronal projections, the acute lesions appear on sonograms as bilateral, often linear or "flare" echodensities adjacent to the external angles of the lateral ventricles (Fig. 9-16). In coronal projections angled slightly posteriorly, the echogenic lesions are visualized better because the peritrigonal region is imaged (Fig. 9-17). On parasagittal projections, the echodensities may be diffusely

distributed in periventricular white matter or localized to the sites of predilection for PVL (i.e., the regions adjacent to the trigone of the lateral ventricles or to the frontal horns at the level of the foramen of Monro, particularly the former, or both) (Fig. 9-18; see Chapter 8). Posterior parietal and parieto-occipital echodensities, although at the site of predilection for PVL, should be assessed very carefully, because these are very common findings in premature infants with no neuropathological correlate.[220,303,304] Echodensities may be categorized primarily according to severity (relative to echogenicity of choroid plexus), timing (age of onset), duration (transient or prolonged >7 days), and evolution. Although some data suggest more prognostic importance for echodensities that are severe, appear after the first week, or are prolonged (see "Prognosis" later),[302,305,306] the most consistent correlation of echodensities with MRI-proven abnormality or neurological sequelae occurs with evolution to echolucency (i.e., cyst formation; Table 9-14). The characteristic evolution of the echodensities of PVL is the formation of multiple small echolucent cysts, sometimes rendering a "Swiss cheese" appearance (see Figs.

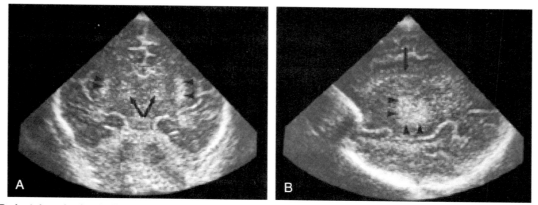

Figure 9-12 **Perinatal asphyxia. A,** Coronal and, **B,** parasagittal ultrasound scans in a 1-day-old full-term infant who experienced perinatal asphyxia. In **A,** note the increased echogenicity in the basal ganglia (putamen) *(arrowheads)* and the thalamus *(arrows).* In **B,** note the increased echogenicity in the region of the thalamus and basal ganglia *(arrowheads);* the slitlike lateral ventricle is indicated by the arrow for orientation. A computed tomography scan on day 6 (not shown) demonstrated decreased attenuation in the echogenic areas.

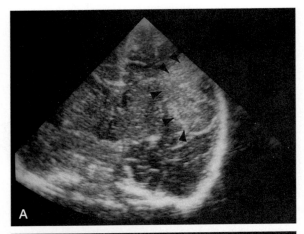

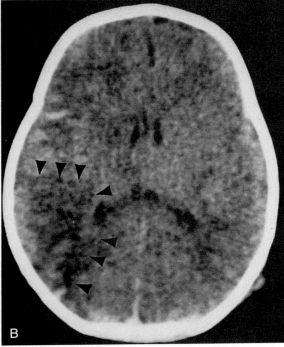

Figure 9-13 **Focal ischemic infarction. A,** Ultrasound and, **B,** computed tomography (CT) scans of focal ischemic infarction. Both scans were obtained from a 7-day-old term infant with focal seizures. On the coronal ultrasound scan, the area of echogenicity *(arrowheads)* is in the distribution of the left middle cerebral artery. The CT scan showed only a subtle area of decreased attenuation in the same region *(arrowheads)* *(left* is to the reader's left).

9-17 and 9-18), after approximately 1 to 3 weeks. A decrease in the echodensities may precede the appearance of the echolucent cysts. With relatively small circumscribed cysts, it is common for the echolucencies to disappear after 1 to 3 months, leaving enlarged ventricles with decreased cerebral myelin (Fig. 9-19). The neuropathological correlate of this disappearance of cysts (i.e., gliosis and collapse of the cyst walls) is illustrated in Chapter 8. *More commonly, cysts are never apparent (i.e., noncystic PVL), and the result is ventriculomegaly, presumably representing a deficit in white matter volume caused by impaired cerebral myelination, in turn a result of the diffuse component of the disease (i.e., the loss of early*

differentiating oligodendrocytes; see Chapter 8). The qualitative demonstration of this occurrence has been the documentation of ventriculomegaly by a variety of imaging techniques in survivors of preterm birth.[286,287,294,299,307-310] Quantitative volumetric MRI studies indicate that this deficiency in subsequent myelination can be detected as early as 40 weeks of postconceptional age in infants born prematurely.[311]

Despite the proven value of ultrasonography in the delineation of focal necrotic/cystic PVL, the incidence of cystic PVL in modern neonatal intensive care units is very low, generally 1% to 4%.[306,312-320] More importantly, cranial ultrasonography is quite insensitive to the detection of the diffuse, more cell-specific component of PVL (see Table 9-14; Table 9-15). Earlier neuropathological studies indicated that cranial ultrasonography did not detect approximately 70% of cerebral white matter injury, especially diffuse gliosis, myelin loss, or even moderate (<1 cm) areas of necrosis.[280,283,285] More recent correlative studies with MRI confirmed that the diffuse noncystic cerebral white matter injury is not detected effectively by cranial ultrasonography (see Tables 9-14 and 9-15).[313] In the largest prospective series (N = 96), cranial ultrasonographic abnormalities (prolonged echodensity, echolucencies) were observed in only approximately 30% of cases of MRI-detected white matter injury. Several other excellent ultrasound-MRI correlative studies also showed poor sensitivity for cranial ultrasonography for detection of noncystic white matter injury.[302,312,314,321]

To summarize, cranial ultrasonography is of particular value in the identification of necrosis (especially hemorrhagic necrosis) of basal ganglia and thalamus, the focal necrotic/cystic component of PVL, and, to a lesser extent, focal and multifocal ischemic brain injury (see Table 9-12). CT is less useful in the study of focal ischemic injury in the very early acute period but is more useful in defining the full topography of the lesion after this time. Cranial ultrasonography is superior to CT in the identification of both the acute and the subacute-chronic manifestations of focal periventricular white matter injury. The role of real-time ultrasound scanning in the identification of the *hemorrhagic* complications of asphyxial injury is discussed in Chapters 10 and 11. MRI is the most useful of the three imaging modalities (see next).

Magnetic Resonance Imaging

MRI is the most accurate imaging modality in the diagnosis of hypoxic-ischemic injury in the newborn (see Chapter 4). The advantage with MRI of superlative anatomical detail is tempered somewhat by the need to study the infant within a magnet and free of the ferromagnetic materials still occasionally found in equipment required for intensive support of the sick infant and by the relatively long time required for data acquisition (e.g., relative to CT). However, advances in monitoring equipment and imaging instrumentation and data processing have allayed these concerns. Indeed, current information indicates that this imaging

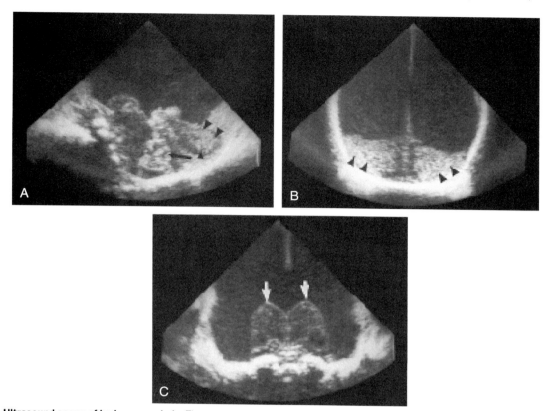

Figure 9-14 **Ultrasound scans of hydranencephaly**. The scans were obtained on the first postnatal day. **A**, In the parasagittal projection, note the near total lack of cerebral tissue. A portion of the occipital poles *(arrowheads)* and the cerebellum *(arrow)* are seen readily. **B** and **C**, In the coronal projections, note the residual occipital tissue *(arrowheads)* and midline diencephalic structure *(arrows)*.

modality has proven to be the most informative of all imaging modalities.

MRI, in my view, is the diagnostic modality of choice in the immediate neonatal period in infants with hypoxic-ischemic injury, and it has been used in a large number of studies[19,20,81-83,236,243,244,262,322-344c] The entire spectrum of hypoxic-ischemic brain injury has been demonstrated (see Table 9-12).

MRI has been of greatest use in the neonatal period in the evaluation of *the term infant* with the neonatal clinical features of hypoxic-ischemic disease (see earlier discussion). The major findings by MRI are outlined in Table 9-16. *Conventional MRI* shows the abnormalities in the first 3 to 4 days, but generally not on the first day. However, diffusion-weighted MRI (DWI), based on the molecular diffusion of water, is not only more sensitive than conventional MRI, but also shows abnormalities earlier, often in the first 24 to 48 hours after birth (see later discussion). The correlates of the MRI findings with the neuropathological states described in Chapter 8 are apparent (Figs. 9-20 to 9-30). Thus, *selective cerebral cortical neuronal injury* is manifested by loss of the cerebral gray-white matter differentiation and by cortical high signal (highlighting) on T1-weighted (T1W) or fluid-attenuated inversion recovery (FLAIR) images at the sites of particular predilection, the parasagittal perirolandic cortex, and the depths of sulci (see Fig. 9-20). Decreased diffusion (increased signal) is seen on DWI (see Fig. 9-21). Selective cerebral cortical

neuronal injury is usually accompanied by involvement of *basal ganglia (especially dorsal putamen) and thalamus (especially lateral thalamus;* see Fig. 9-22). In the unusual cases of principally deep nuclear and brain stem involvement, as with severe, acute asphyxial insults, high signal (T1W or FLAIR) is seen in the brain stem tegmentum as well as basal ganglia. DWI is more sensitive for detection of cerebral cortical and deep nuclear involvement (see Fig. 9-23). In one series of 173 encephalopathic term newborns, predominant involvement of perirolandic cortex and basal ganglia/thalamus was observed in 44 (25%) and in an additional 24 (14%) in association with predominant involvement of parasagittal regions.[345] *Parasagittal cerebral injury* is seen readily as areas of increased signal (T1W and FLAIR) in the parasagittal cerebral cortex and subcortical white matter (see Figs. 9-24 and 9-25). In a series of 173 term newborns, fully 78 (45%) had predominant involvement of the parasagittal areas, and an additional 9 (5%) with predominant involvement of perirolandic cortex and deep nuclear structures also had parasagittal injury.[20] PVL is shown to occur in *30% to 50% of term asphyxiated infants*, a finding not expected from the results of other imaging studies, and it is identified by decreased signal on T1W images (and increased signal on T2W images). *Decreased signal of the posterior limb of the internal capsule* also has been noted in approximately 50% of asphyxiated term infants; whether this abnormality reflects direct

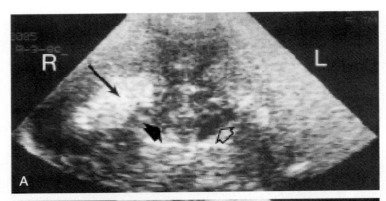

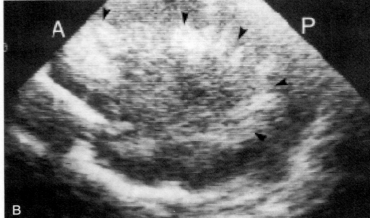

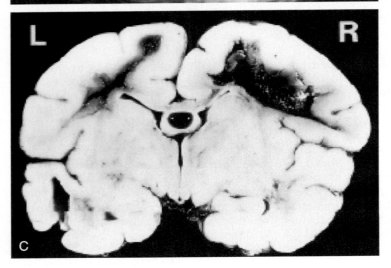

Figure 9-15 Hemorrhagic periventricular leukomalacia in an infant of 33 weeks of gestation who experienced cardiorespiratory arrest at 20 days of age. **A**, Coronal ultrasound scan shows an ovoid echodense area in the right periventricular region *(long arrow)*; a smaller periventricular echodense area is present on the left. The lateral ventricles are marked by *short arrows*. **B**, Right parasagittal ultrasound scan shows an extensive anteroposterior region of periventricular echodensity *(arrowheads)*. **C**, Coronal section of cerebrum from the same infant, who died several days later, shows massive hemorrhagic periventricular leukomalacia on the right and a smaller area on the left.

injury or wallerian degeneration is not clear,[338] but the observation has prognostic importance (see later discussion). *Focal cerebral ischemic lesions*, especially in the distribution of the middle cerebral artery, are visualized as areas of decreased signal on T1W images (see Figs. 9-26 to 9-28). DWI demonstrates such lesions earlier and more effectively than does conventional MRI. MRI also demonstrates the structural sequelae of focal and multifocal cerebral ischemic lesions exceptionally well (see Figs. 9-29 and 9-30).

Another type of focal and multifocal ischemic injury that is particularly well demonstrated by MRI in either the term or the premature infant is *venous sinus*

thrombosis (Fig. 9-31). CT findings may be normal or may show increased attenuation of sinuses (see Fig. 9-31) that is sometimes difficult to distinguish from subarachnoid or subdural hemorrhage or from normal increased attenuation. (On CT, the triangular increased attenuation in the region of the torcular has been termed the *delta sign*, and with clot retraction or partial canalization, the appearance of a rim of increased attenuation with a core of decreased attenuation may give rise to an "empty" delta sign.)

Although many of the lesions just discussed are visualized well by conventional MRI, they are visualized better and, importantly, earlier by *DWI* (Fig. 9-32).

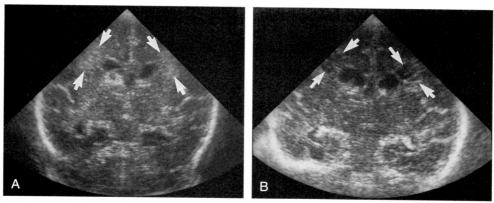

Figure 9-16 **Periventricular leukomalacia**. Coronal ultrasound scans of periventricular leukomalacia in a premature infant on postnatal days, **A**, 5 and, **B**, 24. Note, in **A**, the periventricular echodensities *(arrows)* and, in **B**, the small echolucent foci, consistent with cysts, in the same areas *(arrows)*.

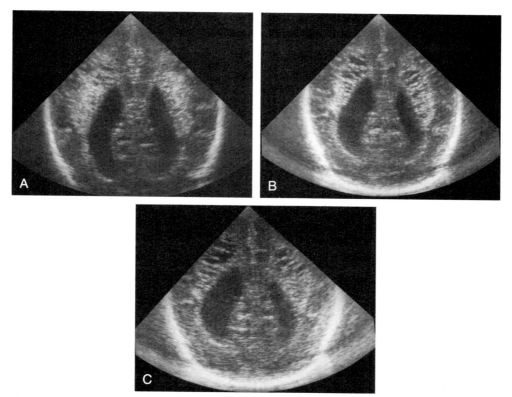

Figure 9-17 **Coronal ultrasound scans angled slightly posteriorly to image the peritrigonal regions in periventricular leukomalacia.** The scans were obtained in a premature infant at, **A**, 10, **B**, 17, and, **C**, 25 days of age. Note the evolution from echodensities to multiple small echolucencies in the periventricular white matter.

TABLE 9-13	**Ultrasonographic Diagnosis of Periventricular Leukomalacia: Appearance, Temporal Features, and Pathological Correlation**	
Ultrasonographic Appearance	**Temporal Features**	**Neuropathological Correlation**
Echogenic foci, bilateral, posterior > anterior	1st wk	Necrosis with congestion or hemorrhage (>1 cm), or both
Echolucent foci ("cysts")	1–3 wk	Cyst formation secondary to tissue dissolution (>3 mm)
Ventricular enlargement, often with disappearance of "cysts"	≥2–3 mo	Deficient myelin formation; gliosis, often with collapse of cyst

Data from references 259, 261, 279 to 281, 283, and 285, as well as from personal unpublished material.

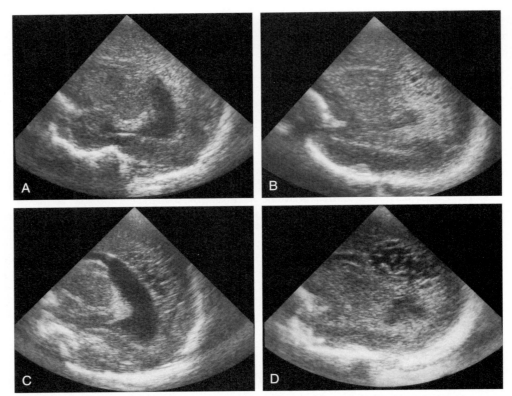

Figure 9-18 **Periventricular leukomalacia**. Parasagittal ultrasound scans of periventricular leukomalacia obtained from a premature infant at **A**, 2, **B**, 13, **C**, 17, and, **D**, 26 days of age. Note the evolution from echodensity to multiple small echolucencies in the periventricular white matter adjacent to the trigone of the lateral ventricles.

TABLE 9-14	Cranial Ultrasonography Not Highly Predictive of Noncystic Periventricular Leukomalacia Identified by Magnetic Resonance Imaging		
	MRI FINDING AT TERM		
Cranial Ultrasound Finding	**Normal**	**White Matter Signal Abnormality**	**Cystic Change**
Normal or transient echodensity (n = 74)	48	25	1
Prolonged echodensity (n = 19)	10	9	0
Echolucencies (n = 3)	0	0	3

MRI, magnetic resonance imaging.
Data from Inder TE, Anderson NJ, Spencer C, Wells SJ, et al: White matter injury in the premature infant: A comparison between serial cranial ultrasound and MRI at term, *AJNR Am J Neuroradiol* 24:805–809, 2003.

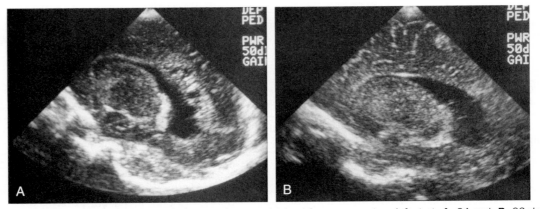

Figure 9-19 **Disappearance of cysts**. Parasagittal ultrasound scans obtained from a premature infant at, **A**, 24 and, **B**, 93 days of age. The echolucent cysts apparent at 24 days disappeared by 93 days of age. The trigonal region of the lateral ventricle at 93 days was dilated because of loss of periventricular white matter and failure of early myelination.

TABLE 9-15	**Cranial Ultrasonography and the Diagnosis of Periventricular Leukomalacia***

Echolucencies on ultrasound scans are sensitive and specific for focal cystic lesions.

Echodensities on ultrasound scans may be transient (<7 days) or prolonged (>7 days), or they may evolve to lucencies.

Transient echodensities are generally not predictive of WM abnormality on MRI at term.

Echodensities that are prolonged (>7 days) or severe or apparent after the first week of life are variably predictive of WM abnormality on MRI at term.

Mild or moderate WM signal abnormalities on MRI at term are poorly predicted by cranial ultrasonography; approximately 70% of noncystic white matter abnormality on MRI at term is not detected by cranial ultrasonography.

*See text for references.
MRI, magnetic resonance imaging; WM, white matter.

Increased signal on DWI, indicative of decreased water diffusion, has been shown in experimental models of focal cerebral ischemia and in adult stroke in the first 1 to 2 hours after the insult.[346-352] Many studies of newborns with hypoxic-ischemic disease have demonstrated the superior sensitivity of DWI versus conventional MRI in delineating the site and extent of tissue injury early in the neonatal period.[83,330,339,340,353-360c] The DWI signal in neonatal hypoxic-ischemic encephalopathy is influenced greatly by the timing of the scan and the region studied. The *timing* of DWI abnormality in asphyxiated term infants with presumed selective

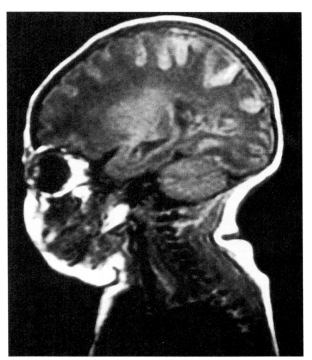

Figure 9-20 Magnetic resonance imaging scan of cortical neuronal injury. The infant had severe apnea on the first day of life, and the scan was performed on the third postnatal day. On this parasagittal fluid-attenuated inversion recovery image, note the striking cortical highlighting, especially marked in depths of sulci.

TABLE 9-16	**Major Aspects of Magnetic Resonance Imaging in the Diagnosis of Hypoxic-Ischemic Encephalopathy in the Term Infant***

Major Conventional MRI Findings in First Week

Cerebral cortical gray-white differentiation lost (on T1W or T2W)

Cerebral cortical high signal (T1W and FLAIR), especially in parasagittal perirolandic cortex

Basal ganglia-thalamus, high signal (T1W and FLAIR, usually associated with the cerebral cortical changes but possibly alone with increased signal in brain stem tegmentum in cases of acute severe insults; see Chapter 8)

Parasagittal cerebral cortex, subcortical white matter, high signal (T1W and FLAIR)

Periventricular white matter, decreased signal (T1W) or increased signal (T2W)

Posterior limb of internal capsule, decreased signal (T1W or FLAIR)

Cerebrum in a vascular distribution, decreased signal (T1W), but much better visualized as decreased diffusion (increased signal) on diffusion-weighted MRI

Diffusion-weighted MRI more sensitive than conventional MRI, especially in first days after birth, when former shows decreased diffusion (increased signal) in injured areas

*See text for references and more details concerning timing of findings.
FLAIR, fluid-attenuated inversion recovery; MRI, magnetic resonance imaging; T1W and T2W, T1- and T2-weighted images.

neuronal necrosis or parasagittal cerebral injury, or both, is shown in Figure 9-33.[358] Thus, although some infants exhibit abnormality on the first day, injury is generally underestimated at that time. The nadir for diffusion occurs between the second and third days. By 7 to 8 days, pseudonormalization is apparent and is probably related to recovery processes that ultimately lead to angiogenesis and other factors causing increased diffusion. *Thus, the optimal time for detection of DWI abnormality in the most common varieties of hypoxic-ischemic disease in the term newborn is approximately 2 to 3 days* (see Fig. 9-33). In *adult human stroke* (i.e., permanent occlusion), diffusion is decreased *in the first hours after the insult and remains* low until pseudonormalization occurs at 7 to 9 days.[361] This time course is similar to that observed in animal models of permanent vascular occlusion. By contrast, in newborns, the insult usually is *transient* and is followed by reperfusion. In animal models of transient occlusion, during the occlusion diffusion decreases, whereas on reperfusion, diffusion recovers before a secondary decline many hours later, as in the usual asphyxiated human infant (see Fig. 9-33). In view of these considerations, it is likely that in *neonatal stroke*, as in adult stroke, DWI would be abnormal on the first postnatal day, perhaps in the first hours, as in adult stroke. My personal experience corroborates this suggestion, but more data are needed.

The importance of the *region injured* is illustrated by the scans shown in Figure 9-34.[355] Thus, in this unusual example of precise knowledge of the timing of the insult (postnatal cardiac arrest), decreased

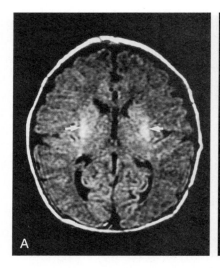
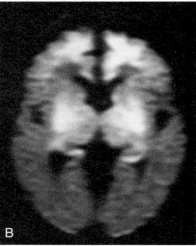

Figure 9-21 Magnetic resonance imaging (MRI) scans of selective neuronal injury. The infant experienced intrapartum asphyxia and had seizures on the first postnatal day. Scans were performed on the fifth postnatal day. **A,** The axial fluid-attenuated inversion recovery image shows increased signal in putamen bilaterally *(arrows)* but no definite abnormality in cerebral cortex. **B,** By contrast, diffusion-weighted MRI (DWI) shows striking increased signal (i.e., decreased diffusion) in frontal cortex (in addition to more pronounced basal ganglia abnormality).

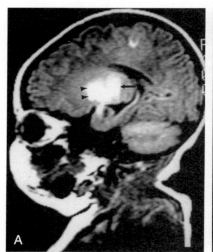
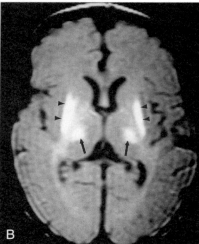

Figure 9-22 Magnetic resonance imaging scans of hypoxic-ischemic injury to basal ganglia and thalamus. Scans were obtained from a 5-day-old infant who experienced severe perinatal asphyxia. **A,** Note in the parasagittal T1-weighted image markedly increased signal in basal ganglia, especially putamen *(arrowheads),* and in thalamus *(arrow).* **B,** The axial proton density image also demonstrates the injury well in the same distribution. *(Courtesy of Dr. Patrick Barnes.)*

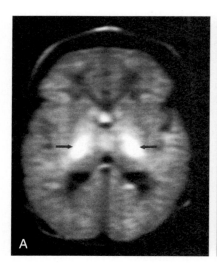
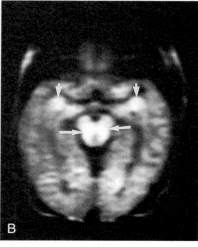

Figure 9-23 Diffusion-weighted magnetic resonance imaging (DWI) of deep nuclear and brain stem injury. This full-term infant experienced a severe late intrapartum asphyxial insult. MRI and DWI scans were carried out late on the first postnatal day. No definite abnormality was discerned by conventional MRI (not shown). However, DWI shows striking decreased diffusion (increased signal) in basal ganglia-thalamus *(arrows in* **A**), hippocampus *(short arrows in* **B**), and midbrain tegmentum *(long arrows in* **B**).

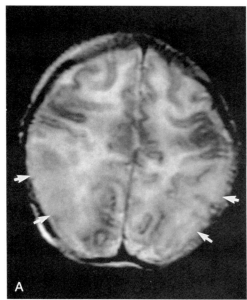

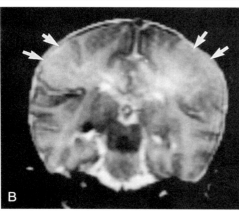

Figure 9-24   Magnetic resonance imaging (MRI) scan of parasagittal cerebral injury. A, Axial T2-weighted MRI scan obtained on postnatal day 5 from an infant with perinatal asphyxia and neonatal seizures shows striking loss of normal cerebral gray-white matter signals symmetrically in parasagittal regions, especially posteriorly *(arrows).* A computed tomography (CT) scan obtained 2 days earlier (not shown) showed much less well-localized decreased attenuation. **B,** Coronal T2-weighted MRI scan obtained on postnatal day 4 from an infant with perinatal asphyxia and neonatal seizures. Note the striking abnormality in parasagittal areas bilaterally *(arrows).* A CT scan performed 1 day before showed equivocal findings (not shown). *(Courtesy of Dr. Patrick Barnes.)*

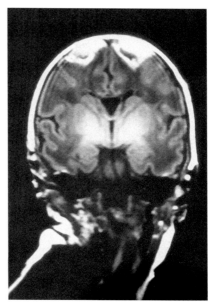

Figure 9-25   Magnetic resonance imaging (MRI) scan of parasagittal cerebral injury. Coronal T1-weighted MRI, obtained on the fifth postnatal day in an asphyxiated term infant, shows striking, triangular lesions in the parasagittal areas bilaterally. Increased signal is also apparent in basal ganglia and thalamus bilaterally. *(Courtesy of Dr. Alan Hill.)*

diffusion in basal ganglia and thalamus was apparent at 6 hours of age, but decreased diffusion did not appear in cerebral cortex until 32 hours. Other investigators showed that although severe white matter injury is associated with early decreased diffusion, with more moderate white matter injury diffusion is normal or slightly increased early and increases in the ensuing days (Fig. 9-35).[359] A similar increase in white matter diffusion was observed in cerebral hypoxia-ischemia in the neonatal rat.[362]

Evaluation of the *premature infant* by MRI in the neonatal period is dominated by the search for *cerebral white matter injury*, although deep nuclear abnormalities can be shown as just described for term infants, albeit less commonly (see Chapter 8). The focal necrotic/cystic

component of PVL, observed well on cranial ultrasonography, is readily demonstrated by MRI (see earlier). However, this component of PVL is now uncommon, and *the much more common diffuse noncystic component is detected by MRI but not by cranial ultrasonography.* Indeed, the high frequency of diffuse noncystic cerebral white matter abnormality, manifested principally as MRI signal change, in the premature infant was unexpected until the application of MRI.[302,312-314,363-370] The *frequency of the abnormality on MRI increases as a function of postnatal age.* In one well-studied series with serial MRI scans, the finding of diffuse MRI signal abnormality in premature infants (median gestational age, 27 weeks) increased from 21% in the first postnatal week, to 53% in the next several weeks, to 79% at term equivalent.[302] In a later prospective study of 100 premature infants, 64 exhibited white matter signal abnormality at term.[364] A summary of the possible relation of MRI findings to the PVL spectrum of white matter disease (see Chapter 8) is shown in Table 9-17.

DWI appears to be even more sensitive than conventional MRI in the detection of PVL (Fig. 9-36).[371] DWI has been used particularly in the study of the common noncystic white abnormality readily detected by conventional MRI. In a particularly important study, Counsell and colleagues[365] used DWI to quantitate at term equivalent the apparent diffusion coefficient (ADC) in cerebral white matter of 50 selected premature infants (median gestational age, 29 weeks).[365] ADC is a measure of the overall diffusion of water in the tissue and has been shown by our group and by others to decline in normal cerebral white matter of premature infants as they approach term.[372-374] In the study of Counsell and associates, 31 of the 50 infants or

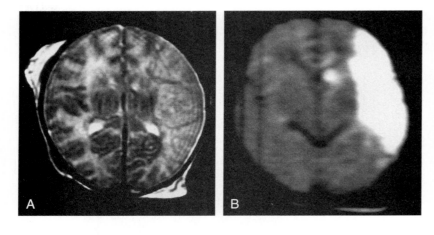

Figure 9-26 Magnetic resonance imaging (MRI) scans of focal ischemic cerebral injury. Scans were performed on the third postnatal day. **A,** Axial T2-weighted MRI scan shows a lesion in the distribution of the main branch of the left middle cerebral artery. **B,** The diffusion-weighted MRI (DWI) scan demonstrates the lesion more strikingly.

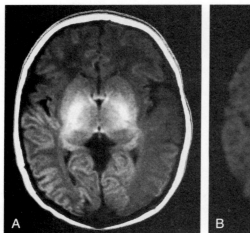
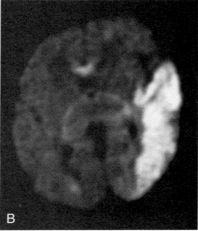

Figure 9-27 Magnetic resonance imaging (MRI) scans of focal ischemic cerebral injury. Scans were formed on the third postnatal day. **A,** Axial T1-weighted MRI scan shows an area of decreased signal in the distribution of the posterior division of the left middle cerebral artery. (The normal increased signal bilaterally in the posterior limb of the internal capsule also is apparent.) **B,** The diffusion-weighted MRI (DWI) scan demonstrates the apparent infarction more strikingly.

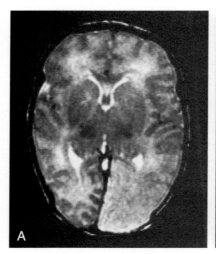
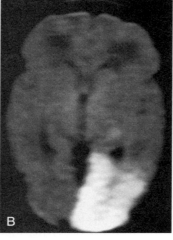

Figure 9-28 Magnetic resonance imaging (MRI) scans of focal ischemic cerebral injury. Scans were performed on the fifth postnatal day. **A,** Axial T2-weighted MRI shows increased signal in the distribution of the left posterior cerebral artery. **B,** The diffusion-weighted MRI (DWI) scan demonstrates the apparent infarction more strikingly.

fully 62% exhibited MRI signal abnormality by term.[365] Notably, when compared with infants with normal white matter, infants with signal abnormality had increased values for ADC in cerebral white matter. *Thus, the finding of this later signal abnormality by conventional MRI was associated with a quantifiable abnormality in a measure of overall water diffusion, and the abnormal values were similar to the values of more immature cerebral white matter.*

The importance of the findings at term of high ADC values in the presence of signal abnormality relates to the likely mechanism for the normal decline in ADC values in the period from 28 to 40 weeks of postconceptional age. As described in Chapter 4, this decline in

Figure 9-29 **Magnetic resonance imaging scans of focal cerebral infarction**. The scan was obtained at 6 months of age in a full-term infant who experienced an infarction in the distribution of the right middle cerebral artery, shown by computed tomography scan, in the neonatal period. Note on these T1-weighted images in the, **A**, coronal and, **B**, axial planes the distinct area of decreased signal in the territory of the right middle cerebral artery and the compensatory dilation of the right lateral ventricle. Note also the smaller cerebral peduncle on the right (*arrow* in **A**) consistent with wallerian degeneration of corticospinal tract fibers.

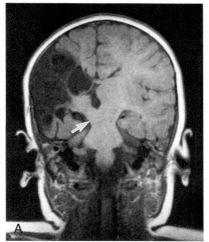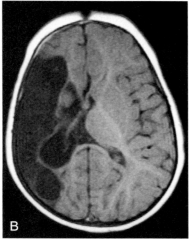

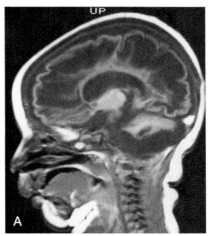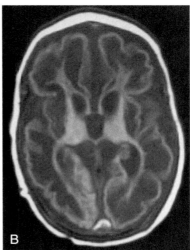

Figure 9-30 **Magnetic resonance imaging scan of multifocal ischemic brain necrosis**. The scan was obtained at 6 weeks of age in an infant who had severe perinatal asphyxia. T1-weighted images in the, **A**, sagittal and, **B**, axial planes show striking changes consistent with multicystic encephalomalacia.

ADC occurs during a period in which *premyelinating oligodendrocytes* are abundant in human cerebral white matter.[375] During this maturational phase, these early differentiating cells are beginning to ensheathe cerebral white matter axons,[376] in preparation for myelination, which occurs primarily after term in the human cerebrum.[377] It is likely that these oligodendroglial changes contribute importantly to the decreases in the extracellular space and water content in cerebral white matter and thus to the normal decline in ADC. Indeed, measurements of relative anisotropy (i.e., an MRI measure of preferred *directionality* of diffusion) normally increase during this time interval, consistent with the notion of ensheathment of axons and consequent restriction of diffusion perpendicular but not parallel to the axons.[372,373] Changes in axon size, axonal membranes, and intracellular axonal constituents accompany these premyelination events and likely contribute to the decline in ADC and the rise in relative anisotropy.[378-382] In this context, a reasonable hypothesis is that the failure of ADC to decline fully from the higher levels of the small premature infant to the lower levels of the term infant in the presence of signal abnormality relates principally to prior injury or destruction of premyelinating oligodendrocytes and subsequent failure of their development and ensheathment of axons. Consistent with this hypothesis is the finding by various imaging modalities, especially MRI, of hypomyelination, signal abnormality, ventricular dilation, and corpus callosal thinning in follow-up studies of premature infants.[262,322,329,331,332,364,368-370,383-402] Neuropathological studies, albeit limited, also have shown the preferential death of premyelinating oligodendrocytes in diffuse PVL (see Chapter 8). However, *both* the neonatal findings of signal and diffusion abnormality in cerebral white matter *and* the subsequent demonstrations of impaired white matter development could reflect concomitant injury to axons, which, in the human premature infant, are in an active phase of development (see Chapter 8). More data are needed.

Two advanced types of MR determinations, *quantitative volumetric MRI and diffusion tensor MRI* (see Chapter 4),

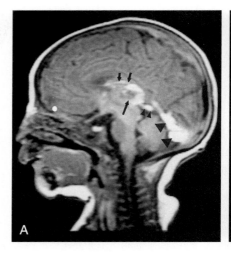
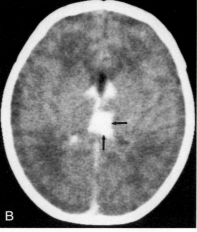

Figure 9-31 Magnetic resonance imaging (MRI) scan of venous thrombosis and hemorrhagic infarction. A, T1-weighted MRI scan was obtained on postnatal day 11 from a full-term infant with antithrombin III deficiency and venous thromboses. Note the increased signal in the torcular *(large arrowhead, bottom),* straight sinus *(large arrowhead, top),* vein of Galen *(small arrowheads),* and internal cerebral vein *(small arrows),* consistent with thrombosis. The mixed signal in the thalamus *(large arrow)* is consistent with venous (hemorrhagic) infarction. **B,** On computed tomography scan, obtained on day 10, the venous thromboses are not apparent, although the increased attenuation in the thalamus *(arrows)* is consistent with the venous infarction delineated better by MRI **(A).** *(Courtesy of Dr. Patrick Barnes.)*

show considerable promise for providing quantitative insights into the impact of cerebral white matter injury on subsequent brain development (see Chapter 8). As discussed in Chapter 4, these approaches provide information about regional brain development and microstructural fiber development in a way that is not possible by any conventional imaging technique. *Concerning white matter development,* our initial studies of 10 premature infants with PVL showed by *volumetric MRI* a nearly 50% lower volume of myelinated white matter in infants as early as 40 weeks of postconceptional age.[311] Approximately one half of these infants exhibited only the diffuse component of PVL, detected only by neonatal MRI and not by cranial ultrasonography. A subsequent prospective study of 119 premature infants studied at term equivalent showed an approximately 35% decrease in myelinated white matter volume.[403] The volumetric deficits were most pronounced in premature infants with earlier evidence of white matter injury (especially signal abnormality), intrauterine growth retardation, and postnatal dexamethasone therapy.[404,405] A later *regional*

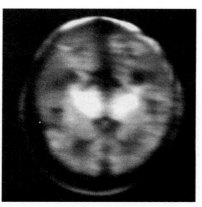

Figure 9-32 Diffusion-weighted magnetic resonance imaging (DWI) scan in selective neuronal injury in deep nuclear structures. This term asphyxiated infant presented with multifocal clonic seizures on the first postnatal day. MRI was performed on the second postnatal day. Conventional MRI scans showed *no* definite abnormality (not shown). The axial DWI scan shows striking increased signal (decreased diffusion) bilaterally in dorsal putamen and ventrolateral thalamus.

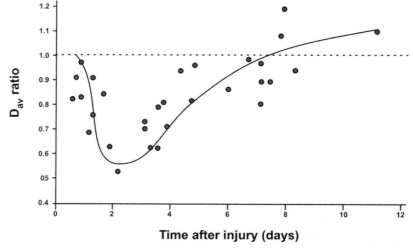

Figure 9-33 Time course of the diffusion abnormality following perinatal hypoxic-ischemic brain injury. Data were derived from study of 10 infants. Diffusion is expressed as a ratio normalized to reference values for newborn infants. Thus, the normal D_{av} ratio is 1.0. Note that in the first day after birth, diffusion is near normal or is only modestly decreased. The nadir occurs after 2 to 3 days. Pseudonormalization is apparent after the seventh day. *(Redrawn from McKinstry RC, Miller JH, Snyder AZ, Mathur A, et al: A prospective, longitudinal diffusion tensor imaging study of brain injury in newborns,* Neurology *59:824–833, 2002.)*

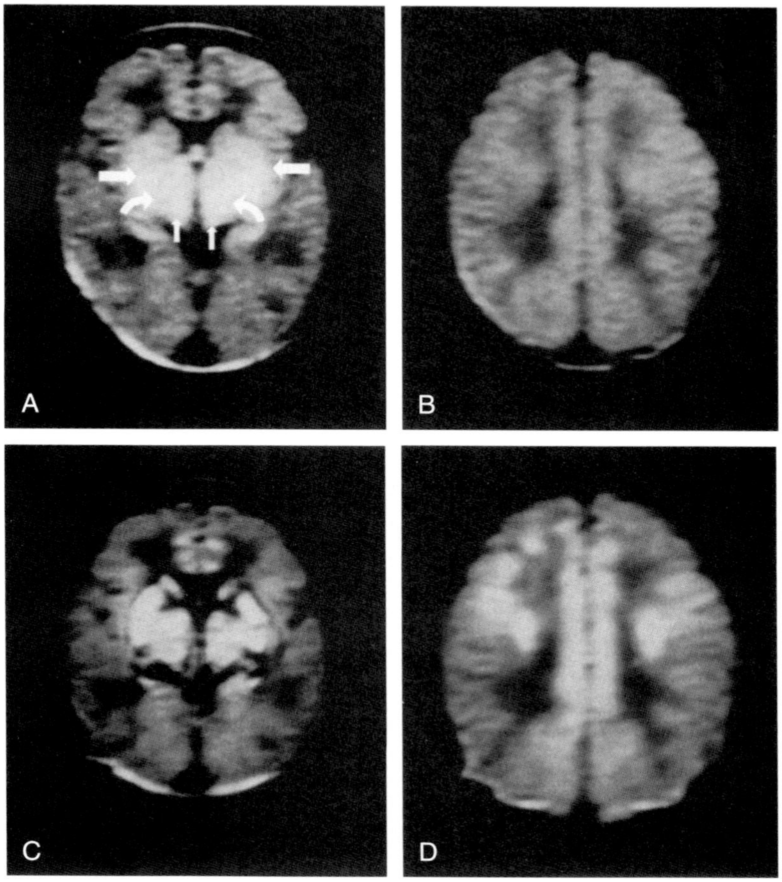

Figure 9-34 **Differential regional decreases in diffusion after neonatal hypoxia-ischemia**. Diffusion-weighted magnetic resonance imaging (DWI) images **A** and **B**, obtained 6 hours after cardiorespiratory arrest, show bright signal (i.e., decreased diffusion) in basal ganglia *(thick arrows)*, thalami *(curved arrows)*, and dorsal brain stem *(thin arrows)*. There is no decrease in diffusion in cerebral cortex. DWI images **C** and **D**, obtained 32 hours after cardiorespiratory arrest, show persistence of the decreased diffusion in deep nuclear structures but also bright signal (decreased diffusion) in cerebral cortex. Conventional magnetic resonance imaging (not shown) at 6 hours was normal but at 32 hours, it was clearly abnormal. *(From Soul JS, Robertson RL, Tzika AA, du Plessis AJ, et al: Time course of changes in diffusion-weighted magnetic resonance imaging in a case of neonatal encephalopathy with defined onset and duration of hypoxic-ischemic insult,* Pediatrics *108:1211–1214, 2001.)*

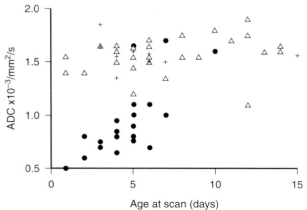

Figure 9-35 **Diffusion abnormalities in cerebral white matter after apparent neonatal hypoxia-ischemia**. The infants were born at term and were control (+), with severe white abnormalities on conventional magnetic resonance imaging (MRI) (●), or with moderate white matter abnormalities (△) on conventional MRI. Note in the infants with severe white matter abnormalities, diffusion was clearly decreased in the first week, whereas in the infants with moderate abnormalities, diffusion was not decreased. A nonsignificant increase in diffusion was noted in the latter infants after the first week. *(From Rutherford M, Counsell S, Allsop J, Boardman J, et al: Diffusion-weighted magnetic resonance imaging in term perinatal brain injury: A comparison with site of lesion and time from birth,* Pediatrics *114:1004–1014, 2004.)*

analysis of volumetric MRI findings in 202 preterm infants at term equivalent showed that changes were most pronounced in sensorimotor and parieto-occipital regions, sites of predilection for PVL.[405] *Diffusion tensor MRI* also has shown abnormalities in cerebral white matter as early as term. The most consistent finding has been diminished relative anisotropy, in areas both of white matter injury and distant from the lesions (e.g., posterior limb of the internal capsule).[373,406-408a] These findings could relate to a failure of ensheathment of axons by developing oligodendrocytes or a primary disturbance of axons or both. Volumetric and diffusion tensor MRI studies of premature infants during childhood or later also have shown diminutions in cerebral white matter volume, thinned corpus callosum, and increased ventricular volume, in varying combinations.[405,409-416] Similarly, a predilection for sensorimotor, parieto-occipital, and premotor regions was observed.[409] Moreover, later disturbances in fiber tract development were documented by diffusion tensor MRI.[417-419] However, these children were not studied by MRI in the neonatal period, and thus the relative role of white matter injury in these subsequent changes could not be assessed as well as in the neonatal studies.

Concerning *gray matter development, volumetric and diffusion tensor MRI* have documented disturbances that are particularly prominent after neonatal cerebral white

TABLE 9-17 **Magnetic Resonance Imaging Correlates of the Periventricular Leukomalacia Spectrum in Premature Infants**

| | NEUROPATHOLOGY* | | | | | MAGNETIC RESONANCE IMAGING† | |
| | Focal | | | Diffuse | | | |
Term Used*	Necrosis	Cyst	Glial Scar	Astrocytosis	Microgliosis	Focal	Diffuse
Cystic periventricular leukomalacia	+ *(macroscopic)*	+	+	+	+	+	+
Noncystic periventricular leukomalacia	+ *(microscopic)*	−	+	+	+	±	+
Diffuse white matter gliosis	−	−	−	+	?	−	?

*See Chapter 8.
†Abnormality: +, detectable; ±, variably detectable; , not detectable; ?, unknown.

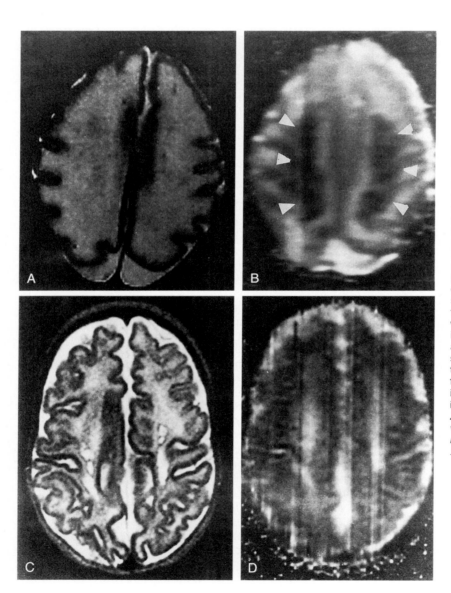

Figure 9-36 **Magnetic resonance imaging (MRI) scans of periventricular leukomalacia.** **A,** Axial T2-weighted MRI and, **B,** diffusion weighted MRI (DWI) scans carried out on postnatal day 5; **C,** axial T2-weighted MRI and, **D,** DWI scans repeated at 10 weeks of age in a premature infant born after 30 weeks of gestation. The initial T2-weighted MRI scan **(A)** at 5 days of age shows no definite abnormality, whereas the DWI scan **(B)** shows a striking area of decreased diffusion in the cerebral white matter *(arrowheads)*. (Note that with this technique [an apparent diffusion coefficient map], the decreased diffusion is manifested as *decreased* signal intensity, unlike the DWI scans shown in earlier figures.) The follow-up T2-weighted MRI scan at 10 weeks of age **(C)** shows increased signal intensity in the cerebral white matter consistent with bilateral apparent cystic change. The DWI scan **(D)** at this time shows increased diffusion (increased signal with this technique) in the cerebral white matter. The evolution from decreased diffusion in the acute period to increased diffusion after weeks is typical of cerebral ischemic lesions in general. *(From Inder T, Huppi PS, Zientara GP, Maier SE, et al: Early detection of periventricular leukomalacia by diffusion-weighted magnetic resonance imaging techniques, J Pediatr 134:631–634, 1999.)*

matter injury. As noted in Chapter 8, the first clear indication of a disturbance in cerebral cortical development associated with cerebral white matter injury was obtained by volumetric MRI analysis of premature infants at term.[311] Subsequent studies confirmed the initial report and also documented diminished volume of deep nuclear structures as well as impaired cerebral cortical gyral development.[368,403-405,420-423a] The disturbances were observed principally in infants with MRI evidence of PVL, nearly exclusively noncystic. Postnatal dexamethasone therapy can play a contributory role in these deficits. These disturbances in gray matter identified in the neonatal period at term equivalent are followed by persistent abnormalities in children and adults who were born prematurely (see Chapter 8).[32,409-412,415,419,424-426a] Decreased cerebral cortical development has been observed most consistently. Additionally, abnormalities of cortical thickness and fiber tract development also have been found.[417-419,426] Regional differences are somewhat similar to those noted for white matter development, with the most pronounced decreases in sensorimotor, parieto-occipital, temporal, and hippocampal cortices.[409,410,412,424] Decreases in volumes of deep nuclear structures, basal ganglia, and thalamus also have been documented consistently.[409,411,412,425,427] These deficits correlate with cognitive disturbances (see later).

MRI techniques have also been valuable in the identification of *cerebellar injury*, especially in premature infants of extremely low birth weight (see Chapter 8). As in PVL, this injury is not attributable to a single hypoxic-ischemic insult but is observed primarily in infants with serious respiratory disease. Cerebellar disturbance has been identified most often by the finding by MRI of decreased cerebellar volume at term equivalent or later in infancy or childhood.[428-439] The possibility of a trophic disturbance, perhaps related to supratentorial white matter injury, is suggested by the strong association with MRI evidence of cerebral white matter injury. However, the high frequency of injury in premature infants of injury to brain stem relay nuclei (see Chapter 8) also raises the possibility of impaired trophic interactions at the transsynaptic level.

To *summarize*, MRI clearly provides superior imaging resolution for delineation of all hypoxic-ischemic lesions, both in the neonatal period and on follow-up (see Tables 9-12, 9-16, and 9-17). DWI provides the capability for identification of injury by 24 to 48 hours after asphyxia in the term infant and probably earlier in cases of neonatal stroke. DWI appears to have a particular capacity to identify most readily the diffuse component of PVL, an important feature of the white matter injury generally invisible to other imaging modalities in the acute period. However, conventional MRI is also especially valuable in detection of the diffuse component of PVL. Thus, major new insights into the prevalence and the clinical aspects of PVL have been obtained. Finally, the advent of quantitative volumetric MRI and diffusion tensor MRI has provided insights into the impact of neonatal hypoxic-ischemic injury, especially white matter injury, on subsequent brain *development*, especially in the premature infant.

Technetium Scan and Single Photon Emission Computed Tomography

Although now used only rarely, two radionuclear procedures provided important insights into the identification of brain injury in newborns with hypoxic-ischemic disease. Thus, I review them briefly here. The first technique, for which the most recorded experience is available, is the so-called *technetium brain scan*, based on uptake of technetium-99m (^{99m}Tc) pertechnetate, which crosses a damaged blood-brain barrier, is detected by an external array of gamma detectors, and provides a coarse image of the topography of the injury. This technique has been replaced in many medical centers by *single photon emission CT (SPECT)*, which is used primarily to measure patterns of regional cerebral perfusion after administration of radiolabeled lipophilic tracers, primarily iodine-123 iodoamphetamine (IMP) or ^{99m}Tc-hexamethylpropyleneamineoxine (HMPAO). Areas of injury are marked by decreased regional perfusion, detected topographically with greater resolution than with conventional technetium brain scans.[440-443] Because the data available concerning the use of SPECT in the evaluation of asphyxiated infants are relatively limited, and because the data largely confirm, although more clearly, the findings reported with technetium brain scanning, I focus the following discussion on the latter findings.

The technetium brain scan has provided valuable information concerning the site and extent of injury.[444,445] The largest reported experience is that of O'Brien and co-workers,[445] involving 85 full-term infants with hypoxic-ischemic encephalopathy primarily related to perinatal asphyxia. The most useful patterns for delineation of topography of injury, in their experience as well as ours, are those associated with increased uptake of the radionuclide on the delayed images (i.e., those obtained 2 to 4 hours after injection of the isotope and therefore more clearly reflecting disturbance of the blood-brain barrier and presumably tissue injury). These abnormal delayed patterns were observed in nearly one half of the total group in the series of O'Brien and co-workers,[445] and approximately 50% were consistent with parasagittal injury. Approximately 20% had findings consistent with middle cerebral artery stroke. A similar spectrum of abnormalities has been defined by SPECT.[440-443] Thus, it appears from these findings of the in vivo neuropathology that ischemic injury, particularly the neuropathological states described in the preceding chapter as parasagittal cerebral injury and focal cerebral ischemic injury, accounts for a large proportion of lesions. Indeed, a study of regional cerebral blood flow (CBF) in full-term asphyxiated infants by positron emission tomography (PET) suggests that parasagittal cerebral injury in the asphyxiated full-term infant may be even more common than is suggested by these data (see later discussion). At any rate, the observations lend further support to the notion that the infant is extremely vulnerable to disturbances of cerebral perfusion pressure and is highly susceptible to cerebral ischemic injury. Moreover, the findings are consistent with those reported from more recent application of MRI (see earlier).

Cerebral Metabolic-Hemodynamic Neurodiagnostic Studies

Neurodiagnostic studies that address changes in metabolism and physiology after perinatal hypoxic-ischemic insults include MR spectroscopy, PET, near-infrared spectroscopy, and other measures of the cerebral circulation (see Chapter 4). Of these, *MR spectroscopy* has proven most useful for diagnostic assessment and is emphasized here. The other approaches have been useful primarily for delineation of pathogenesis and prognosis and thus are discussed primarily in Chapter 8 and later in this chapter.

Magnetic Resonance Spectroscopy

MR spectroscopy has proved to be a diagnostic modality of particular importance in the evaluation of the infant with perinatal hypoxic-ischemic brain injury. Both phosphorus and proton MR spectroscopy are useful, although currently the more readily available proton MR spectroscopy is used most widely. Indeed, over the past few years at Boston Children's Hospital, proton MR spectroscopy has joined DWI as part of the standard evaluation of infants evaluated by MR techniques for hypoxic-ischemic disease. The basic principles of phosphorus and proton MR spectroscopy and the normative data obtainable are described in Chapter 4. The value of these techniques in the assessment of hypoxic-ischemic encephalopathy in the term infant is summarized in Table 9-18.

Phosphorus Magnetic Resonance Spectroscopy.

Multiple studies of infants who sustained perinatal asphyxia, especially intrapartum, have focused on phorphorus-31 (^{31}P) spectra.[446-455] The sequence of findings has been initially normal spectra (concentrations of phosphocreatine [PCr], inorganic phosphate (P$_i$),[456] and adenosine triphosphate [ATP]) in the first hours after birth, followed by a decline in concentration of PCr and a rise in that of P$_i$ (and thus a decline in the PCr/P$_i$ ratio) over approximately the next 24 to 72 hours (Fig. 9-37; see Table 9-18). In the most severely affected infants, ATP concentrations also decline at this time. Subsequently, spectra return to normal over the ensuing weeks, although the total

^{31}P signal may be reduced when marked loss of brain tissue has occurred.[449] *This sequence of events is directly reminiscent of the progression of the "delayed energy failure" described in Chapter 6.* This secondary energy failure correlates directly with the ultimate degree of cell death. Consistent with the experimental data, the severity of this delayed energy failure in human infants correlates closely with the severity of the neonatal neurological syndrome (Fig. 9-38) and with the subsequent occurrence of neurological deficits (see later).[452,453,455] The findings not only demonstrate the value of phosphorus MR spectroscopy in the early delineation of

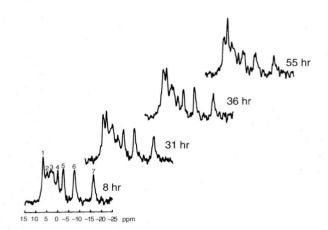

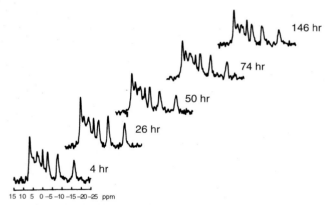

Figure 9-37 **Phosphorus (P)-31 magnetic resonance spectra from two asphyxiated infants born at 37 and 36 weeks of gestation.** Postnatal ages at the time of study are indicated. **A,** Peak assignments (numbers *1* to *7*) are as follows: *1,* phosphomonoester (PME); *2,* inorganic P (P$_i$); *3,* phosphodiester (PDE); *4,* phosphocreatine (PCr); *5, 6,* and *7,* gamma, alpha, and beta nucleotide triphosphate (mainly adenosine triphosphate [ATP]). At 8 hours, spectra were within normal limits (i.e., PCr/P$_i$ was 0.99, ATP/total P was 0.09, and intracellular pH [pH$_i$] was 7.06; pH$_i$ rose to a maximum of 7.28 at 36 hours). Minimum value for PCr/P$_i$ was 0.32 at 55 hours, when ATP/total P was only 0.04 and pH$_i$ was 6.99. The infant died at age 60 hours. **B,** At 4 hours, PCr/P$_i$ and ATP/total P were normal at 0.97 and 0.09, respectively, and pH$_i$ was 7.08 (pH$_i$ rose to a maximum of 7.23 at 26 hours). Minimum value for PCr/P$_i$ was 0.65 at 50 hours, but by 146 hours it was normal. ATP/total P never fell below normal. However, the infant died at age 27 days with cerebral atrophy. *(From Azzopardi D, Wyatt JS, Cady EB, Delpy DT, et al: Prognosis of newborn infants with hypoxic-ischemic brain injury assessed by phosphorus magnetic resonance spectroscopy, Pediatr Res 25:445–451, 1989.)*

TABLE 9-18	Value of Magnetic Resonance Spectroscopy in Assessment of Hypoxic-Ischemic Encephalopathy in the Term Infant*

Phosphorus Magnetic Resonance Spectroscopy

Detects high-energy phosphates (PCr, ATP), inorganic phosphate, and pHi; in first few hours after insult PCr, ATP, and pHi are often normal.

After approximately 8 hours, with development of secondary energy failure, PCr (and later ATP) declines, and pHi increases.

In first 1 to 2 weeks, the severity of decline in PCr and the increase in pHi correlate with the severity of brain injury.

Proton Magnetic Resonance Spectroscopy

Detects multiple compounds, especially lactate, *N*-acetylaspartate, choline, creatine, and glutamate.

Lactate is elevated as early as a few hours after the insult, and it appears to be an earlier indicator of brain injury than is diffusion-weighted magnetic resonance imaging.

In the first days after insult, elevations of lactate (and perhaps glutamate) and declines in *N*-acetylaspartate are identified, and the severity of changes correlates with the severity of brain injury.

*See text for references.

ATP, adenosine triphosphate; PCr, phosphocreatine; pHi, intracellular pH.

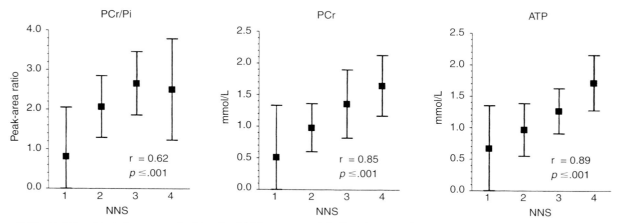

Figure 9-38 **Relationship between cerebral levels of high-energy metabolites (mean ± SD), determined by phosphorus magnetic resonance spectroscopy, and the severity of the neonatal neurological syndrome (NNS) in 23 asphyxiated term newborns.** The numerical scoring was as follows: NNS1, severe; NNS2, moderate; NNS3, mild; and NNS4, normal neurological examination in healthy control infants. ATP, adenosine triphosphate; PCr, phosphocreatine; Pi, inorganic phosphate. *(From Martin E, Buchli R, Ritter S, Schmid R, et al: Diagnostic and prognostic value of cerebral ^{31}P magnetic resonance spectroscopy in neonates with perinatal asphyxia, Pediatr Res 40:749–758, 1996.)*

impairments of energy metabolism in the asphyxiated infant but also provide important prognostic information (see "Prognosis").

Phosphorus MR spectroscopy also is valuable in detection of a paradoxical postischemic increase in intracellular pH (pH$_i$).[455] The evolution of this increase in the days to weeks after hypoxia-ischemia correlates with the degree of brain injury. This *postischemic alkalinization* may lead to cellular injury and appears related in considerable part to postischemic activation of the neuronal and glial sodium-hydrogen transporter. Consistent with this formulation, experimental data indicate a neuroprotective role for amiloride, a sodium-hydrogen exchange blocker, when administered after ischemia (see Chapter 6 and later).

Proton Magnetic Resonance Spectroscopy. Proton MR spectroscopy (see Chapter 4) has been applied extensively to the study of infants with hypoxic-ischemic encephalopathy.[355,454,457-480] Although not all the reported observations are entirely consistent, important and consistent findings can be recognized (see Table 9-18). First, in the acute period, as early as a few hours after birth, *elevation in cerebral lactate*, often expressed as the ratio of lactate to N-acetylaspartate (NAA), creatine, or choline, can be detected (Fig. 9-39A). Indeed, detection of lactate by proton MR spectroscopy is a more consistent indicator of brain injury than is DWI (or other imaging modality) in the first hours after hypoxic-ischemic injury.[471] *Currently, I consider MR spectroscopy the most sensitive modality for detection of neonatal brain disturbance in the acute period.* More data regarding sensitivity and specificity for structural injury are needed. During this early period, ratios of NAA to choline or creatine have been either unchanged or only slightly decreased. The elevated lactate is most pronounced in deep nuclear structures, especially basal ganglia and thalamus, with their high metabolic rate and propensity for hypoxic-ischemic injury. The acutely elevated lactate

correlates with the severity of the neonatal neurological syndrome, the subsequent delayed energy failure (see Fig. 9-39B), and the neurological deficits on follow-up (see "Prognosis"). Lactate levels may remain elevated for weeks, perhaps in part because of enhanced glycolysis and lactate production by astrocytes. Second, after days to weeks, ratios of NAA to choline or creatine decline and reflect tissue injury. Recall from Chapter 4 that NAA is contained in neurons (and presumably axons) and in oligodendroglial precursors. Thus, the declines in NAA in both gray and white matter are not surprising. The severity of the decline in NAA correlates with the severity of subsequent neurological deficits. Glutamate levels also have been shown to be elevated in the first days of life in infants with severe hypoxic-ischemic encephalopathy.[470] This determination is more difficult than that for lactate or NAA and may not be as useful.

Positron Emission Tomography

Although PET is not a routine diagnostic procedure (for the reasons described in Chapter 4), the technique has provided major insight into the frequency, basic nature, and probable pathogenesis of the cerebral injury observed in asphyxiated *term* infants.[481] Because experience with adult patients had indicated that measurements of regional CBF provided critical information concerning the topography of hypoxic-ischemic cerebral injury, my colleagues and I studied a series of 17 asphyxiated term infants with the $H_2^{15}O$ technique to measure regional CBF.[481] The infants had experienced primarily intrapartum asphyxia, exhibited the clinical syndrome described earlier, including proximal limb weakness, and were evaluated by PET during the acute period of their illness (i.e., the first week). The *disturbance of regional CBF in the asphyxiated infants* constituted a continuum of deviation from the normal (or nearly normal) pattern described in Chapter 4. The consistent and apparently unifying abnormality was a relative decrease in CBF to parasagittal regions,

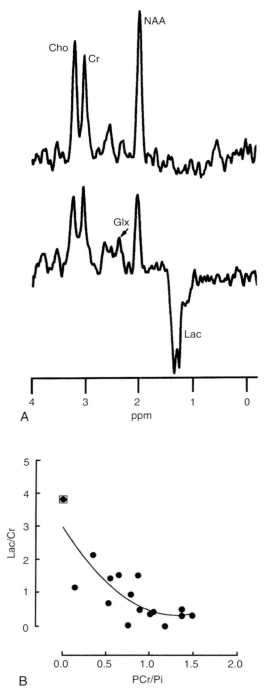

Figure 9-39 **Proton magnetic resonance (MR) spectroscopy from basal ganglia in 16 asphyxiated term newborns. A,** Spectra from a control infant *(upper tracing)* and from a severely asphyxiated infant *(lower tracing),* both obtained at 14 hours of age. Note the striking lactate peak in the asphyxiated infant. **B,** Relationship between lactate/creatine (Lac/Cr) measured by proton MR spectroscopy at 4 to 18 hours of age and phosphocreatine/inorganic phosphate (PCr/Pi) measured by phosphorus MR spectroscopy at 33 to 106 hours. Note the correlation between the severity of the early increase in lactate and the degree of secondary energy failure as manifested by the decreased PCr/Pi ratio. Cho, choline; Glx, glutamic acid; NAA, *N*-acetylaspartate. *(From Hanrahan JD, Sargentoni J, Azzopardi D, Manji K, et al: Cerebral metabolism within 18 hours of birth asphyxia: A proton magnetic resonance spectroscopy study, Pediatr Res 39:584–590, 1996.)*

generally symmetrical and more marked posteriorly than anteriorly. The extent of the relative decreases in parasagittal CBF correlated directly with the severity of clinical manifestations.[481]

The *structural correlates* of the decrease in CBF in parasagittal regions were elucidated in four infants by technetium brain scan and by neuropathology and consisted of parasagittal cerebral injury. Thus, our CBF findings by PET indicated that *parasagittal cerebral injury* is a *common* feature in neonatal hypoxic-ischemic encephalopathy, at least in patients who survive the perinatal insult.[481] This observation has been confirmed and amplified by subsequent studies with MRI (see earlier discussion).

CLINICOPATHOLOGICAL CORRELATIONS

The neurological correlates of hypoxic-ischemic encephalopathy, as observed in the neonatal period and subsequently, are understood when one recalls the topography of the neuropathological lesions. Considerably more is known about the long-term neurological correlates of the several lesions than about the correlates in the newborn period. Indeed, in the latter instance, correlates must be made with some reservation. The reasons for the difficulty in establishing correlations relate primarily to the large degree of overlap in the occurrence of the four basic lesions and to the heretofore imperfect definition of topography by available imaging studies. Although the overlap of the various lesions will be a persistent confounder, improvements in imaging, especially the use of MRI, have allowed better definition of the topography of the brain injury in the neonatal period. The latter now has allowed certain probable correlations to be made. In the following discussion, I review the major neuropathological lesions in terms of the neurological correlates in the newborn period and subsequent periods (i.e., neurological sequelae).

Selective Neuronal Necrosis

Neonatal Correlates

The neurological correlates in the *neonatal period* are diverse, as is the topography of the major neuronal injury (Table 9-19). Of the major varieties of selective neuronal necrosis (diffuse, cerebral cortical–deep nuclear, deep nuclear–brain stem, and pontosubicular necrosis [see Chapter 8]), tentative clinical correlates can be established for the first three. In the *diffuse variety of selective neuronal necrosis,* associated with very severe and prolonged insults, all levels of the neuraxis are affected. With this variety, I have attributed the derangement of the level of consciousness to involvement of bilateral cerebral hemispheres or the reticular activating system in the upper brain stem and diencephalon, including the thalamus. Indeed, in one careful series studied by MRI, involvement of basal ganglia and thalamus was associated strongly with severe encephalopathy, including decreased level of alertness.[482] Seizures appear to relate to cerebral cortical injury,

TABLE 9-19 **Clinical Correlates of Selective Neuronal Necrosis**[*]

	NEUROLOGICAL FEATURES[†]	
Topography of the Major Injury	**Neonatal Period**	**Long-Term Sequelae**
Cerebral cortex; basal ganglia; thalamus; reticular formation; brain stem nuclei, including inferior colliculus, cochlear nuclei, and motor nuclei of cranial nerves; cerebellum; anterior horn cells	Stupor and coma Seizures Hypotonia Hypertonia-dystonia[‡] Oculomotor disturbances[§] Disturbed sucking, swallowing, and tongue movements[§]	Cognitive deficits[‡] Spastic quadriparesis Choreoathetosis[‡] Dystonia[‡] Seizure disorder Ataxia Bulbar and pseudobulbar palsy[§]

[*]As discussed in the text, three major forms of selective neuronal necrosis should be recognized: *diffuse, cerebral cortical–deep nuclear,* and *deep nuclear–brain stem.*
[†]All the neurological features may be seen to varying degrees in the diffuse form of selective neuronal necrosis.
[‡]Common abnormalities in those infants with involvement of basal ganglia and thalamus.
[§]Common additional abnormalities in those infants with involvement of brain stem tegmentum (and usually associated with deep nuclear involvement).

although some of the seizure phenomena, especially some of the tonic phenomena of the premature infant, may emanate from subcortical nuclear structures in basal ganglia, thalamus, or midbrain. The uncommon but dramatic occurrence of the syndrome of inappropriate ADH secretion or diabetes insipidus presumably relates to hypothalamic neuronal involvement. The hypotonia could relate to cerebral cortical or anterior horn cell disturbances or combinations of both. Electrophysiological evidence (e.g., fibrillations), as well as clinical data (hypotonia, absent deep tendon reflexes, weakness), support a role for anterior horn cell involvement.[483,484] The oculomotor abnormalities presumably relate primarily to disturbance of cranial nerve nuclei (III, IV, and VI). The impairments of sucking (V), swallowing (IX and X), and tongue movements (XII) also are probably largely the basis of brain stem cranial nerve nuclear involvement. A contribution of corticobulbar disturbance to these deficits, however, is possible. The facial appearance of an infant with striking brain stem involvement, proven neuropathologically, is shown in Figure 9-40.

With the *cerebral cortical–deep nuclear variety of selective neuronal necrosis,* associated with moderate to severe and relatively prolonged insults, involvement of cerebral cortex and basal ganglia (especially putamen) and thalamus predominates (see Chapter 8). The major clinical difference from the syndrome just described is the occurrence of *increased tone* in many such affected infants. The hypertonia often increases with stimulation, especially manipulation, and has characteristics of dystonia. I have attributed this finding to extrapyramidal involvement, perhaps unmasked by the less severe injury to the pyramidal system than occurs with the diffuse variety of selective neuronal injury.

With the *deep nuclear–brain stem variety of selective neuronal necrosis,* associated with severe and abrupt insults, involvement of basal ganglia, thalamus, and brain stem tegmental neurons occurs, with relative sparing of cerebral cortex. The major additional clinical correlates relate to the brain stem injury and include ptosis, oculomotor disturbances, facial diparesis, ventilatory disturbances, and impaired sucking and swallowing.[50,89,90]

Long-Term Correlates

The *long-term neurological sequelae* depend on the topography of the neuronal injury. With the *diffuse variety of selective neuronal necrosis,* intellectual retardation is nearly uniform and is the consequence principally of cerebral cortical injury (see Table 9-19). However, injury to basal ganglia[485,486] and thalamus and to cerebellum (see later) could play a role. (The possibility of impairment of subsequent cortical neuronal differentiation is raised by experimental data,[487,488] but studies of human infants are lacking.) The spastic motor deficits could relate to cortical injury, although the relative

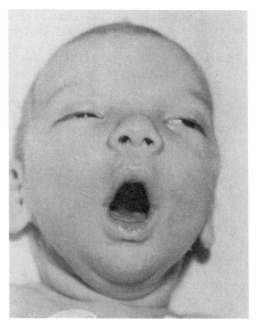

Figure 9-40 **Facial appearance at age 1 month in an infant who experienced perinatal asphyxia.** Note the disconjugate gaze, ptosis, marked facial weakness, and wide-open mouth. The infant also exhibited fasciculations of the tongue on physical examination. *(From Roland EH, Hill A, Norman MG, Flodmark O, et al: Selective brainstem injury in an asphyxiated newborn,* Ann Neurol *23:89–92, 1988.)*

roles of concomitant ischemic parasagittal cerebral injury and PVL have not been elucidated. Seizure disorders, which develop in approximately 10% to 30% of infants with hypoxic-ischemic encephalopathy (see Chapter 5), probably relate to cerebral cortical injury. Impairment of cortical visual functions occurs in severely affected infants, and cerebral cortical atrophy was reported to be the principal finding on CT in approximately 60% of such patients.[489-492] MRI studies have emphasized the association of basal ganglia or thalamic lesions and cerebral white matter injury with impaired visual function in such infants.[493-495] (The improvement of vision in as many as 50% of such infants over the first 2 years of life may reflect the operation of cortical organizational events, i.e., brain plasticity, as outlined in Chapter 2.) Disturbances of hypothalamic neurons presumably underlie the early sexual maturation that occurs in 10% of term asphyxiated infants with other signs of neurological disturbance.[496] Impairments of sucking, swallowing, and facial movement may relate to nuclear injury (i.e., bulbar palsy), although some infants also exhibit the features of upper motor neuron injury (i.e., pseudobulbar palsy), probably cerebral in origin, such as "all-or-none smile" and fixed facial expression with drooling.[497,498] Hyperactivity and impaired attentive capacities, particularly observable (unmasked?) in less affected patients, may relate to involvement of neurons of the reticular activating system, the basal ganglia, or the cerebellum.[499-501] The substantial minority of infants with hearing deficits presumably may have involvement of dorsal cochlear nuclei (which subserve perception of higher frequency sounds) or of cochlea, or both (see Chapters 3 and 4). Involvement of superior olivary nucleus and inferior colliculus may contribute. Finally, involvement of anterior horn cells may explain the characteristic persistence of hypotonia in the first months of life, and when it is severe, this topography of involvement may explain the unusual persistence into childhood of hypotonia and weakness (i.e., atonic quadriparesis or "atonic cerebral palsy").

With the *cerebral cortical–deep nuclear variety of selective neuronal necrosis*, the major clinical features include not only the deficits attributable to cerebral cortical neuronal injury but also those related to the involvement of basal ganglia and thalamus, discussed separately later. With the *deep nuclear–brain stem variety of selective neuronal necrosis*, the additional clinical features relate not only to the basal ganglia-thalamic involvement, discussed separately later, but also to the brain stem injury. All surviving infants with this injury have prolonged difficulties with feeding, usually for many months and often requiring tube feeding.[50,90,502,503] Approximately 20% to 30% require gastrostomy for feeding. However, because of the relative sparing of cerebral cortex with this variety of selective neuronal injury, approximately 50% of these patients have exhibited normal cognition.[50]

With *involvement of basal ganglia and thalamus*, whether as a component of the cerebral–deep nuclear variety of selective neuronal necrosis or the deep nuclear

syndrome with brain stem involvement, subsequent extrapyramidal abnormalities are common. Unknown numbers of such infants undoubtedly develop the neuropathological lesion *status marmoratus* (see Chapter 8), but the fundamental clinicoanatomical correlate is neuronal loss in putamen and thalamus, whether or not the final pathological appearance is that of status marmoratus.[504,505] The essential anatomical combination for choreoathetosis and dystonia appears to be *bilateral* involvement of basal ganglia and *intact* pyramidal tracts because in one neuropathological series the several patients without choreoathetosis had unilateral or bilateral sparing of basal ganglia or degeneration of the pyramidal tracts.[506] The thalamoputaminal involvement is different from the subthalamic nucleus and globus pallidus distribution in bilirubin encephalopathy, the other major neonatal disorder with subsequent choreoathetosis (see Chapter 13). Careful studies employing MRI in infants with "dyskinetic" or "athetoid" cerebral palsy demonstrated the thalamoputaminal predilection in hypoxic-ischemic disease.[392,506a] Indeed, thalamus was affected without putaminal involvement as often as with putaminal involvement and more often than involvement of putamen alone.[392] Of particular interest and not readily explicable is the finding that the onset of the extrapyramidal abnormalities is not clearly apparent until after 6 to 12 months and often much later. Thus, most such infants develop overt choreoathetosis or dystonia, or both, between 1 and 4 years of age.[507-509] Abnormal motor development and hypertonia commonly are obvious before this time (i.e., as early as 6 months of life).[495]

An important minority of children will not develop abnormal movements until as late as 7 to 14 years of age.[509-513] In the largest reported series of the *delayed-onset syndrome*, the mean age of onset of choreoathetosis and dystonia was 12.9 years, and the mean duration of progression was 7 years (Table 9-20).[513] Four of the 10 patients studied had attained early developmental milestones at ages within the normal range. Although the children ultimately had mild to moderate motor disability, all were ambulatory. The only class of drugs with clear benefit was anticholinergic medication, perhaps reflecting that the relatively spared

---

TABLE 9-20 Delayed-Onset Dystonia after Perinatal Asphyxia

The mean age of onset of dystonia, often with choreoathetosis, is 12.9 years.

Nearly 50% of patients have a history of normal neurological development.

Approximately 80% have other neurological signs, but fewer than 50% have overt "cerebral palsy."

Intellect is in normal range in approximately 80%.

Progression of dystonia continues for a mean of 7 years to moderate disability (not wheelchair bound).

Treatment with anticholinergic agents may be beneficial.

Data from Saint-Hilaire MH, Burke RE, Bressman SB, Brin MF, et al: Delayed-onset dystonia due to perinatal or early childhood asphyxia, *Neurology* 41:216–222, 1991.

cholinergic neurons (see Chapter 8) were responsible for the development of the extrapyramidal clinical phenomena.[513]

Intellectual function often is *relatively* preserved in those infants with choreoathetosis. Thus, in the older literature, intellectual function in infants with "athetoid cerebral palsy," presumably many or most of whom had putaminothalamic injury to a varying degree, was not noted to be markedly affected consistently.[514-517] In the largest reported series of the delayed-onset extrapyramidal syndrome, 8 of 10 individuals had a normal intelligence quotient.[513] The pathological substrate for the intellectual failure with injury to basal ganglia and thalamus presumably relates in considerable part to any associated hypoxic-ischemic cerebral cortical neuronal injury; indeed, in the large neuropathological series of Malamud,[506] approximately 50% of patients with severe involvement (i.e., the pathological features of status marmoratus) exhibited neuropathological signs of cerebral cortical injury. However, these latter patients also manifested thalamic injury, and approximately one third of patients with pathologically proven status marmoratus and with impaired intellect exhibited thalamic injury *without* significant involvement of cerebral cortex.[506] This finding suggests that the thalamic injury can play an important role in causing the intellectual deficits. MRI data support this contention (see "Prognosis").[20,518] These observations have major implications for the *role of the thalamus in the development of intellectual function.*

The clinical correlates of the *cerebellar vermian atrophy/hypoplasia* that is a common sequela in term infants with hypoxic-ischemic disease (see Chapter 8) remain to be defined. This abnormality may contribute to varying degrees of motor incoordination, occasionally including overt ataxia. Cognitive and behavioral deficits also could be correlates of the cerebellar involvement (see later). Cerebellar involvement and the likely correlates thereof are most prominent in premature infants with concomitant cerebral white matter injury (see "Periventricular Leukomalacia" later).

Parasagittal Cerebral Injury

Neonatal Correlates

The neurological correlates in the *neonatal period* include particularly weakness of proximal limbs, consistently more prominent in upper than in lower extremities (Table 9-21). This pattern of weakness is readily predicted from the topography of the lesion (Fig. 9-41).

The topographical representation of the homunculus on the motor cortex indicates that the proximal extremities, upper more than lower, lie within the distribution of the necrosis. Other deficits referable to parasagittal cerebral injury are likely, but ready detection of such deficits in the newborn requires specialized clinical techniques. For example, careful analysis of "cortical" somesthetic-visual-auditory associations, functions residing within the areas of posterior cerebrum especially affected in parasagittal necrosis, has not been accomplished in the newborn. This topic is clearly important for future clinical research. The advances in electrophysiological, behavioral, and functional MR techniques for assessing such associative functions in the newborn (see Chapters 3 and 4) could be used effectively in this clinical setting. Indeed, the disturbances of visual- and somatosensory-evoked responses observed in asphyxiated infants appear to correlate with cerebral injury in the parasagittal cerebral distributions, affecting parieto-occipital regions in the former instance (visual-evoked responses) and parietal regions in the latter instance.[489,519]

Long-Term Correlates

The *long-term sequelae* of parasagittal cerebral injury relate primarily to motor and cognitive function. However, in general, subsequent deficits are much less common than in infants who also exhibit deep nuclear injury (see "Prognosis" later.)[20] Our current data indicate that some examples of the lesion result in spastic quadriparesis. The particular involvement of proximal limbs, upper more than lower, is detectable on follow-up, as in the neonatal period (see Table 9-18). Although severely affected infants exhibit multiple cognitive deficits, many infants have exhibited "specific" intellectual deficits, such as disproportionate disturbances in the development of language or of visual-spatial abilities, or both.[520-523a] I believe these discrete intellectual deficits to relate particularly to the larger, posteriorly located lesions (i.e., in posterior parietal-occipital-temporal regions) that reside within areas of critical importance for many associative functions, especially those relating to auditory and visual input and output and to a variety of visual-motor phenomena.

Periventricular Leukomalacia

Neonatal Correlates

The neurological correlates of PVL, both overt necrotic/cystic and more common noncystic forms, in the *neonatal period* have been difficult to establish.

TABLE 9-21 Clinical Correlates of Parasagittal Cerebral Injury		
	NEUROLOGICAL FEATURES	
Topography of the Major Injury	**Neonatal Period**	**Long-Term Sequelae**
Cerebral cortex and subcortical white matter, superomedial (parasagittal) convexities, and posterior > anterior cerebrum	Proximal limb weakness upper > lower	Spastic quadriparesis Intellectual deficits (often "specific")

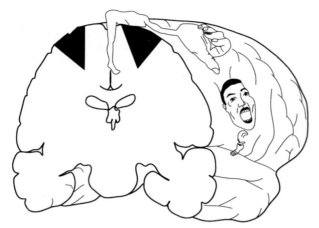

Figure 9-41 Schematic diagram of representation of the homunculus on the motor cortex and the sites of parasagittal cerebral injury (*black triangular areas bilaterally*). Note that the proximal extremities, upper more than lower, are most likely to be affected.

This difficulty relates principally to the problems of carrying out a careful neurological examination in the sick, labile, premature infant and the frequent association of other neurological manifestations related to complicating hemorrhagic and neuronal injury. The ability to identify the focal component of this lesion in the neonatal period by ultrasonography has facilitated identification of the neonatal neurological correlates. Since the early 1980s, I have seen a substantial number of infants with weakness of lower limbs in the first weeks of life and focal periventricular white matter injury documented by ultrasound scan (Table 9-22). In general, the weakness in the neonatal period is not marked, even in the presence of relatively large lesions. The frequent affection of optic radiations[279,282,283,285,524-526] is consistent with electrophysiological studies that indicate a high incidence of disturbance of visual-evoked potentials and with subsequent careful clinical studies that indicate a high incidence of visual perceptual and visual field impairment in affected infants.[160,322,489,491,526-547]

Long-Term Correlates

The *major long-term correlates* of PVL include spastic diplegia, less severe motor deficits, cognitive deficits, visual disturbances, and behavioral and attentional deficits. These neurological disturbances relate in varying degrees directly to the cerebral white matter injury and to associated deficits of cerebral cortex, basal ganglia, thalamus, and cerebellum (see Table 9-22).

The major *long-term motor sequela* of the focal component of PVL is *spastic diplegia* (see Table 9-22), the major prominent motor deficit subsequently observed in premature infants. This motor disturbance has as its central feature spastic paresis of the extremities with greater affection of lower than upper limbs. Three major lines of evidence indicate that focal PVL results in spastic diplegia and its variants. First, the topography of the focal lesions includes the region of cerebral white matter traversed by descending fibers from motor cortex, and those subserving function of lower extremities are more likely to be affected by the periventricular locus of the necrosis (Fig. 9-42). More severe lesions, with lateral extension into the centrum semiovale and corona radiata, would be expected to affect upper extremities and intellectual functions as well. Indeed, patients with spastic diplegia with significant involvement of upper extremities exhibit other manifestations of more severe cerebral disturbance, including intellectual deficits (Table 9-23).[310,548-550]

A second major line of evidence linking spastic diplegia and focal PVL, related to the first, is that the ultrasonographic, CT, and MRI correlates of cystic PVL are associated with spastic diplegia (see Chapter 8, earlier "Diagnosis" and later "Prognosis").[278,282,283,322,383,384,386-394,526,551-556] The severity and extent of injury, as manifested by cystic change or ventricular dilation or both, are correlated with more severe involvement of lower limbs, prominent involvement of upper limbs, and impairment of cognitive function. Although the MRI features of focal PVL in premature infants are nearly consistently followed by spastic diplegia, similar imaging features are present in as many as 30% to 60% of *term* infants who subsequently exhibit similar motor deficits.[394,557-562] Investigators have speculated that the latter infants were injured in utero in the third trimester. The motor deficits in premature infants with mild spastic diplegia may disappear in the first several years of life, especially if the white matter lesions are "noncystic" by ultrasonography.[160]

Premature infants without overt cystic PVL may exhibit *motor deficits without spastic diplegia*. Indeed, the 25% to 50% of infants who weigh less than 1500 g at birth and who have subsequent cognitive, behavioral or attentional, and visual deficits usually exhibit motor dyscoordination without overt spasticity. The principal neuropathological correlate of this less severe motor disease is diffuse noncystic PVL (see Chapter 8 and "Prognosis" later). Whether such motor disturbances relate to the less severe white matter affection or to the commonly associated disturbances of basal ganglia, cortex, or cerebellum, or to all these disturbances (see Chapter 8), is unclear (see later). Notably, diffuse

TABLE 9-22	Clinical Correlates of Periventricular Leukomalacia		
Topography of the Major Injury	**Neonatal Period**		**Long-Term Sequelae**
Periventricular white matter, including descending motor fibers, optic radiations, and association fibers; *and associated deficits of cerebral cortex, basal ganglia, thalamus, and cerebellum*	Probable lower limb weakness		Spastic diplegia Motor deficits (without spastic diplegia) Cognitive deficits Visual deficits Behavioral/attentional deficits

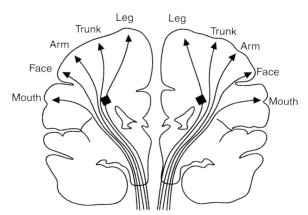

Figure 9-42 Schematic diagram of corticospinal tracts from their origin in the motor cortex, with descent past the periventricular region and into the internal capsule. The locus of periventricular leukomalacia *(marked square areas)* would be expected to affect, particularly, descending fibers for lower extremity more than the laterally placed fibers for upper extremity and face.

cerebral white matter injury is common in the asphyxiated *term infant* (see earlier) and likely contributes to motor disturbances in these infants.[495]

The major *long-term sequela* of infants with PVL is *cognitive disturbance* (see Table 9-22). Indeed, fully 25% to 50% of survivors of birth weight lower than 1500 g exhibit cognitive deficits (see "Prognosis" later). A relation of *severe* cognitive deficits to the white matter involvement is apparent in infants with focal PVL and spastic involvement of both upper and lower extremities, as described earlier (see Table 9-23). However, most infants with noncystic PVL exhibit only minor motor deficits, but prominent cognitive disturbance. Involvement of cerebral white matter fibers subserving visual, auditory, somesthetic, and associative functions may be crucial in this context. Indeed, the peritrigonal region, a site of predilection of PVL, is a region containing a high concentration of interhemispheric callosal commissural fibers, intrahemispheric associative fibers, and ascending (thalamocortical) and descending (cortical to deep nuclear structures and to brain stem/cord) projection fibers.[563,564] The particular role of white matter disturbance in the genesis of cognitive deficits with noncystic PVL is supported by neuroimaging studies. Thus, such deficits are correlated strongly with evidence of diffuse noncystic PVL, manifested by such features as diffuse excessive high MRI signal intensities, multifocal signal abnormalities,

nonhydrocephalic ventriculomegaly, and white matter volume reduction.[367,368,370,397,398,400,401,565,566] As noted earlier, cerebral white matter injury is a common accompaniment of the neuronal injury in asphyxiated *term infants* and may contribute to subsequent cognitive deficits in these infants.

Visual deficits, especially higher-level visual disturbances, are common in infants with PVL and likely relate to involvement of optic radiation (geniculocalcarine tract) and visual association fibers. Impairments include visual perceptual deficits, reduced visual resolution acuity, and visual field impairments.[526,547,567-569] The precise frequency of such deficits remains to be established but appears to include as many as 70% of infants with PVL.[526]

An important role for *gray matter injury* in the genesis of *cognitive deficits* in premature infants with noncystic PVL has been established by advanced MRI (see Chapter 8). Thus, deficits in cerebral cortical and deep nuclear (thalamus and basal ganglia) volumes have been shown conclusively both in the neonatal period[311,367,368,403,405,420,421] and in children and adolescents born prematurely.[409-412,415,419,423a,424,425,570] Regional differences in cortical deficits have involved particularly deficits in sensorimotor, parieto-occipital, temporal, and hippocampal cortices (see Chapter 8). Regional characteristics of the decreases in volume of thalamus and basal ganglia (usually studied in combination) have not yet been delineated. These cortical and deep nuclear neuronal disturbances have correlated with abnormal cognitive measures. The nature of the relationship of these gray matter deficits with PVL is discussed in Chapter 8. The relative roles of the cortical and deep nuclear disturbances in contributing to the cognitive deficits remain to be established, but cortical, thalamic, and basal ganglia all influence cognitive functions (see earlier).

The gray matter abnormalities just described, perhaps especially those of cerebral cortex and thalamus, may contribute to the subsequent occurrence of *seizures* in premature infants. Thus, approximately 5% to 10% of very-low-birth-weight infants subsequently exhibit seizures, including West's syndrome.[571,572] An important role for periventricular hemorrhagic infarction in this context is described in Chapter 11.

Cerebellar disturbance may contribute to *multiple neurological deficits in premature infants with PVL.* As described in Chapter 8, generally bilateral and symmetrical reductions in cerebellar size have been documented subsequently in premature infants, especially those

TABLE 9-23 Intellectual Function in Preterm Infants with Spastic Diplegia and Spastic Quadriplegia

Intellectual Function	Spastic Diplegia[*] (n = 81)	Spastic Quadriplegia[*] (n = 56)
Normal or intelligence quotient ≥70	68%	14%
Moderate mental retardation	15%	21%
Severe mental retardation	17%	54%

Data from Pharoah PO, Cooke T, Rosenbloom L, Cooke RW: *Arch Dis Child* 62:1035–1040, 1987.
[*]Spastic diplegia, lower extremities affected more than upper extremities; spastic quadriplegia, lower and upper extremities equally affected.

TABLE 9-24 Potential Clinical Correlates of Cerebellar Injury in Premature Infants*

Motor disturbances: spectrum from incoordination to overt ataxia
Cognitive deficits: involving visual-spatial abilities, verbal fluency, memory, and learning
Attentional deficits: deficits in shifting attention
Social/affective disturbances: socialization and mood abnormalities, autistic behavior

*See text for references.

TABLE 9-26 Neurological Correlates in Term Infants with Unilateral Cerebral Infarction*

Magnetic resonance imaging is valuable for determining both the extent of the unilateral lesion and the presence of milder injury to the contralateral hemisphere.
Hemiparesis occurs in approximately 25% to 35% of survivors.
Hemiparesis occurs in nearly 100% if the lesion involves the distribution of the *stem* of the middle cerebral artery (cerebral cortex–white matter–basal ganglia–posterior limb of internal capsule).
The presence of concomitant, albeit milder injury to the contralateral hemisphere *sharply increases* the likelihood of hemiparesis.
Cognitive deficits occur in approximately 25% to 50% of survivors, especially if the lesion is large or bilateral.
Epilepsy occurs in approximately 10% to 30% of survivors.

*See text for references; includes unpublished personal cases.

with cerebral white matter injury, particularly PVL.[428-439] (The roles of trophic and transsynaptic effects in the genesis of the cerebellar abnormality are discussed in Chapter 8). The cerebellar disturbance may contribute not only to a broad spectrum of motor deficits, as expected from classical neurology, but as learned from more recent studies, to cognitive, attentional, and social or affective disturbances (Table 9-24).[573-576a]

Focal and Multifocal Ischemic Brain Necrosis: Stroke

Neonatal Correlates

The most prominent *neonatal* neurological correlate is *seizure* (Tables 9-25 and 9-26). Indeed, 80% to 90% of newborns with unilateral cerebral infarction identified in the neonatal period by CT or MRI have had seizure as the presenting sign.* The onset is usually on the first postnatal day, and almost all seizures are clearly and consistently focal, with movements contralateral to the lesion. Other neurological signs often are much less prominent between seizures, when compared with the encephalopathy associated with selective neuronal necrosis.[19]

The *motor correlates* of focal and multifocal ischemic brain necrosis in the *neonatal period* are definite, although often not striking. Infants with major *unilateral lesions*, in my experience, usually exhibit slight but

definite hemiparesis, involving the upper more than the lower extremity and face approximately equal to upper extremities. This pattern is compatible with the locus of the usual disease (i.e., distribution of the middle cerebral artery; Fig. 9-43). Because these are cerebral lesions, it should be recalled that limb movements usually are symmetrical with the Moro reflex; asymmetry of movement is detected most effectively by

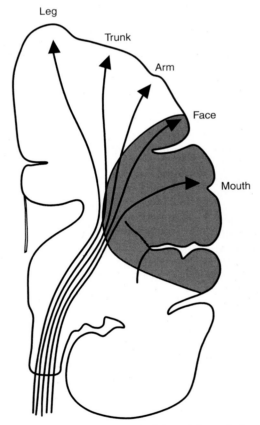

Figure 9-43 Schematic diagram of origin and descent of corticospinal tract fibers and location of the usual infarction in the distribution of the middle cerebral artery (*marked area*). Note that face and upper extremity are more likely to be affected than lower extremity.

TABLE 9-25 Clinical Correlates of Focal (and Multifocal) Ischemic Brain Necrosis

Topography of the Major Injury	NEUROLOGICAL FEATURES	
	Neonatal Period	Long-Term Sequelae
Cerebral cortex and subcortical white matter necrosis, primarily unilateral, in a *vascular distribution*	Seizures, usually focal Hemiparesis (and quadriparesis if bilateral)	Spastic hemiparesis (and quadriparesis if bilateral) Cognitive deficits Seizure disorder

observing the quantity and quality of spontaneous motility or movements elicited after gentle shaking of the infant. In major *bilateral lesions*, the signs vary with the severity of the lesion. A slight but definite degree of quadriparesis is apparent, and neonatal motor reflexes (e.g., Moro and tonic neck reflexes) often do not exhibit evidence of higher level control (i.e., they are elicited with a brief latency, are stereotyped, and do not habituate). Responses to visual and somesthetic stimulation depend on the degrees of involvement of occipital and parietal cortices (see Chapter 3). Infants with involvement of diencephalon (e.g., severe bilateral ischemic brain necrosis with hydranencephaly) may have disordered temperature control and sleep-wake cycles.

The neonatal neurological correlates of *neonatal venous sinus thrombosis* include seizures in approximately 60% to 70% of cases (Table 9-27).[585-596] The seizures are generally not consistently focal and usually are associated with overt parenchymal injury detectable by neurological imaging in approximately 50% of cases (see Chapter 8). Evidence of brain edema may be the only imaging finding concerning the cerebral parenchyma. Modest depression of level of consciousness (i.e., "lethargy") is a common presenting feature.[590,593]

Long-Term Correlates

The *long-term neurological sequelae* of lesions identified in recent years by MRI are less severe and less frequent than was suggested by earlier studies based principally on CT identification.[65,67,69,71,72,77,577,578,597] Thus, more recent work, based primarily on the use of *MRI* in the neonatal period, leads to the conclusions outlined in Table 9-26.[79,82,334,335,562,580,582,583,598-611] Hemiparesis occurs subsequently in 25% to 35% of surviving term infants with apparent unilateral cerebral infarction. When hemiparesis occurs, the motor disturbance becomes overt after approximately 6 months of age. *The likelihood of hemiparesis depends on the extent of the lesion or on the presence of involvement, albeit not severe, of the contralateral hemisphere or both.* Thus, the likelihood of hemiparesis is nearly 100% if the distribution of the stem of the middle cerebral artery is affected (i.e., cerebral cortex, white matter, basal ganglia, and posterior limb of the internal capsule). When the distributions of a cortical branch or only the lenticulostriate vessels are affected, the likelihood of hemiparesis is less than 10%. For example, hemiparesis is rare if the internal capsule is involved together with *either* basal ganglia *or* cerebral

cortical involvement. When the hemisphere contralateral to the infarction is affected, even if not severely, the likelihood of hemiparesis approaches 100%. This occurrence presumably relates to an inability of the opposite hemisphere to reestablish its earlier developed ipsilateral corticospinal tract innervation, the presence of which has been demonstrated in older hemiplegic patients by a variety of functional studies (see discussion of plasticity in Chapter 2).[612-614] This plasticity may require many months to evolve. For example, in one study, both infants with "moderate" hemiparesis at 6 to 8 months of age had no hemiparesis on followup at 2 years of age, and three of nine infants with severe hemiparesis early had only moderate weakness later.[597]

Cognitive function is impaired after *unilateral* infarctions in approximately 25% to 50% of infants (see Table 9-26). In general, the likely involvement of language versus nonlanguage functions bears no consistent relation to location of the injury on the right side or left side, although one study observed spatial deficits more commonly with right hemispheral lesions and language deficits more with left hemispheral lesions.[597,600,602,615,616] When cognitive function is clearly impaired after apparent unilateral infarction, the possibility of injury to the other cerebral hemisphere is high.

Seizure disorders also occur in approximately 10% to 30% of infants on follow-up after *unilateral* infarctions (see Table 9-26). The seizures often are focal but in general are responsive to therapy. In my experience, seizures associated with *prenatal lesions and porencephaly* are more likely to be recalcitrant to therapy than are those related to lesions of perinatal onset. Disorders of *cortical sensory functions* (e.g., stereognosis, two-point discrimination, visual fields, visuospatial functions) have been described in infants with unilateral lesions and could be of more functional significance than has been previously suspected.[431,598,599,617-619] More data are needed on these issues.

Infants with overt *bilateral* ischemic lesions in clear vascular distributions in both hemispheres (i.e., bilateral strokes) generally have severe neurological deficits on follow-up. Thus, the incidence of some degree of quadriparesis and cognitive disturbance approaches 100%. Seizure disorders are present in the majority in my experience, although systematic data are lacking. The sequelae of *major bilateral lesions*, particularly those of prenatal onset (e.g., hydranencephaly) are as dire as one would expect. Spastic quadriparesis and failure of development of higher visual and auditory discriminations, as well as of many other aspects of neurological function, are the rule. (Rarely, infants with apparently severe bilateral cerebral destruction have remarkable preservation of neurological function and subsequent development.[620]) An additional complication frequently observed with hydranencephaly is rapid enlargement of the head in the first months of life. Obstruction of CSF flow at the aqueduct has been demonstrated,[621] but often the source of the disturbance in CSF dynamics is unclear. This event may require a shunt procedure to prevent massive enlargement of the head.

TABLE 9-27	Neonatal and Long-Term Neurological Correlates of Neonatal Venous Sinus Thrombosis	
Neurological Correlates	**Percentage Affected**
Neonatal seizures	60%–70%
Long-term Correlates	
Motor impairment	30%–60%
Cognitive deficits	30%–60%
Seizures	20%–40%

*See text for references; includes unpublished personal cases.

The *long-term neurological correlates* of *neonatal venous sinus thrombosis* remain to be defined clearly.[593,596] Later in infancy, approximately 30% to 60% of infants have exhibited motor impairment and cognitive deficits, and 20% to 40% have had seizures (see Table 9-27). The presence of infarction is associated with the highest likelihoods for these deficits. More data are needed.

PROGNOSIS

Precise determination of the prognosis in the term new-born who sustains a hypoxic-ischemic insult is hindered by the difficulties in determining the severity of the insult. As indicated earlier, most of the primary insults occur in utero, and the difficulties of determining the degree of hypoxemia and ischemia in the fetus are obvious. The value of *electronic fetal monitoring* and associated fetal blood sampling is probably appreciable, but further advances in monitoring the status of the fetal brain clearly are needed (see Chapter 7). Because significant intrauterine (particularly intrapartum) hypoxic-ischemic insult is usually associated with depressed Apgar scores, correlation of outcome with the *Apgar score* also has been used for assessing prognosis. The presence of a *neonatal neurological syndrome* is a crucial indicator of a perinatal insult with the potential to cause neurological injury. Moreover, certain *specific aspects of the neurological syndrome* (e.g., seizures and duration of abnormalities) are useful in estimating outcome. Finally, selected neurodiagnostic studies, such as *EEG, evoked potentials, ultrasound, CT, and MRI* are also of proven prognostic value. Value for *MR spectroscopy* is also indicated by more recent data. In the following discussion, I evaluate the relative value of each of these factors in estimating outcome. Although more emphasis is placed on the asphyxiated full-term infant, it is appropriate initially to consider prematurity as a specific prognostic factor per se.

Prematurity

Prematurity can be considered an important prognostic factor for hypoxic-ischemic brain injury, if it is accepted that PVL and its associated neuronal deficits are particularly common in premature infants, account for most of the subsequent motor and cognitive deficits, and are caused at least in considerable part, by neonatal ischemic events (see earlier discussions and Chapter 8). Large numbers of follow-up studies of very-low-birth-weight infants reported from around the world indicate that survival rates for infants less than 1500 g birth weight are 85% to 90%, and that, of the survivors, approximately 5% to 10% exhibit the overt motor deficits categorized under the rubric "cerebral palsy," and 25% to 50% exhibit a variety of cognitive and behavioral or attentional deficits that result in important school problems.* The rates of cerebral palsy and cognitive disturbances exceed these ranges

if only the smallest infants are considered (see later). The magnitude of the problem of brain injury in the premature infant less than 1500 g birth weight relates in part to the large absolute number of affected infants. For example, in the United States, approximately 60,000 infants are born yearly with a birth weight lower than 1500 g.[764-766] Thus, of the approximately 55,000 survivors yearly, approximately 5000 later exhibit cerebral palsy, and 15,000 to 25,000 have cognitive and behavioral or attentional deficits. Therefore, it is not surprising that although the rate of neurological deficits in such infants has changed little in recent years, in most studies the prevalence and thereby the absolute numbers of infants with disabilities have increased pari passu with the increase in survival rates.

This effect of increased survival rates is particularly noteworthy for the most premature infants, and the overall outcome for infants less than 26 weeks of gestation deserves separate emphasis.[767-783] In one comprehensive study of more than 1000 infants studied during two time periods (period 1, 1982 to 1989; period 2, 1990 to 1998), survival rates increased from period 1 to period 2 from 66% to 85% for birth weights 750 to 999 g and, notably, from 27% to 48% for birth weights 500 to 749 g.[320] Among survivors, most experienced some combination of motor, cognitive, and neurosensory disability (Table 9-28).[320,768,770-772,775-777,783]

As discussed earlier, when follow-up studies of premature infants include prospective analysis of infants evaluated by brain imaging in the neonatal period and on follow-up, a strong relationship with periventricular

TABLE 9-28 Neurological Disability of Extremely Preterm (≤ 23- to 25-Week) Children at 6 Years of Age

Disability	Percentage of Total (n = 241)
Cognitive Disability	
None	28%
Mild	31%
Moderate to severe	41%
Neuromotor Disability	
None	76%
Mild	11%
Moderate to severe	13%
Hearing Disability	
None	90%
Mild	4%
Moderate to severe	6%
Visual Disability	
None	64%
Mild	29%
Moderate to severe	7%
Overall Disability	
None	20%
Mild	34%
Moderate to severe	46%

Data from Marlow N, Wolke D, Bracewell MA, Samara M: Neurologic and developmental disability at six years of age after extremely preterm birth, *N Engl J Med* 352:9–19, 2005.

*See references 306,315,318-321,368,370,398,400,565-566,571-572, 622-763b.

white matter injury is apparent. *However, the frequent associations of gray matter and cerebellar disturbance, discussed earlier, likely play a still to be defined role.* Concerning the specific results of neurological follow-up of premature infants, several general themes are apparent. First, the incidence of cerebral palsy declines modestly during early to middle childhood, especially in infants with milder deficits, presumably secondary to the beneficial effects of plasticity (see Chapter 2). Second, the incidence of cognitive deficits increases with the detail of the analysis (i.e., infants performing in the normal range on overall intellectual measures may exhibit educationally important deficits on specific cognitive measures). Third, attentional and behavioral disturbances and hyperactivity contribute significantly and independently to the risk of academic difficulties. Fourth, many more survivors of preterm birth exhibit cognitive-behavioral deficits without overt cerebral palsy than with such motor deficits. This finding may relate to the relative infrequency of overt necrotic/cystic PVL. Fifth, socioeconomic and presumably environmental factors are important in modulating the effect of neonatal brain injury, particularly regarding language development. (In one study, a *majority* of surviving infants of 501 to 1000 g birth weight, from relatively advantaged environments, completed high school and were gainfully employed.[784]) Sixth, the presence of severe neurosensory disability (e.g., blindness secondary to retinopathy of prematurity) is associated with a markedly worse degree of disability. Seventh, gender differences, often not rigorously addressed, are often apparent and generally indicate that boys are affected more severely than girls.

Apgar Scores, Fetal Acidosis, and Neonatal Resuscitation

Because hypoxic-ischemic injury is one cause of *depressed Apgar scores,* and because depressed Apgar scores imply the possibility of an ongoing hypoxic-ischemic insult, correlation of outcome with such scores has been attempted for many years. This approach is fraught with hazards for several reasons. First, precise quantitation of the Apgar score varies among observers, sometimes considerably. Second, each of the five factors that make up the score is given equal weight, and clearly the importance of each for central nervous system integrity differs greatly. Third, causes of the depressed scores, other than hypoxic-ischemic insult,[785-792] include laryngeal inhibition (e.g., caused by aspiration of a small amount of amniotic fluid or by oronasopharyngeal-laryngeal stimulation from suction catheters), maternal medications or anesthesia, and prematurity and are associated with generally favorable prognoses unless additional postnatal insults occur. In a population-based cohort study of 235,165 term infants, of the 292 with a 5-minute Apgar score of 0 to 3, only 16, or 6.8%, later exhibited cerebral palsy.[793] Similarly, in another series of 1200 consecutive deliveries, only 20% of infants with a 5-minute Apgar score of less than 7 had acidosis with a pH of 7.10 or less (umbilical artery).[794] This tenuous

relationship between apparent fetal asphyxia and low Apgar scores has been confirmed.[44,788,795-800]

The value of the "extended" Apgar score (i.e., the score after 5 minutes) was demonstrated initially by data from the Collaborative Perinatal Project of the National Institutes of Health (Table 9-29).[801] The likelihood of cerebral palsy in infants weighing 2500 g or more increased dramatically with increasing duration of Apgar scores of 3 or less, especially after 15 minutes. Infants with such scores experienced a progressive increase in mortality rate such that almost 60% of those with Apgar scores of 0 to 3 after 20 minutes subsequently died. Similarly, premature infants also exhibited a distinctly worsening prognosis with low "extended" Apgar scores. It is likely that the major determinant of the poor outcome with longer duration of a low Apgar score in both premature and full-term infants was in largest part the severity of the initial intrauterine insult. However, even though low Apgar scores for as long as 15 minutes are associated with high mortality rates, the majority of *survivors* escaped *major* neurological injury (see Table 9-29). A similar conclusion can be derived from other studies.[44,91,792,802,803] Indeed, even with the worst of Apgar scores at 1 minute of age (i.e., 0 or apparent stillbirth), in the largest reported series (N = 93), of the 40% of infants who survived, approximately 60% had a normal outcome.[803] However, of the 58 infants whose Apgar score still was 0 at 10 minutes of age, 57 died, and the sole survivor had an abnormal neurological outcome.

The severity of *fetal acidosis,* as determined by measurement of umbilical arterial pH and base deficit, is a useful reflection of the severity and duration of intrauterine hypoxia-ischemia. The relationship between the severity of fetal acidosis and neonatal neurological features as well as neurological outcome is reviewed in Chapter 7.

Certain aspects of the *neonatal resuscitation,* and particularly the need for positive pressure ventilation and more intensive cardiopulmonary resuscitation efforts (e.g., chest compressions), are predictive of an unfavorable outcome. In one careful study, when the need for cardiopulmonary resuscitation was associated with evidence of fetal acidemia (pH < 7.00), 5 of 5 infants either died in the neonatal period or exhibited neonatal

TABLE 9-29 Relation of Apgar Score to Mortality and Cerebral Palsy*

Apgar Score of 0–3	Death in First Year	Cerebral Palsy in Survivors (with Known Outcome)
1 min	3%	1%
5 min	8%	1%
10 min	18%	5%
15 min	48%	9%
20 min	59%	57%

*For infants ≥2501 g.

Adapted from Nelson KB, Ellenberg JH: Apgar scores as predictors of chronic neurologic disability, *Pediatrics* 68:36–44, 1981.

seizures, whereas of 10 infants requiring such resuscitation measures but without evidence of an appreciable intrauterine insult (cord pH normal), all 10 had normal outcome.[804] In a later study, requirement for intubation in full-term infants with severe fetal acidemia (i.e., umbilical arterial pH $\leq$ 7.0) was associated with a 6.4-fold increase in abnormal neurological outcome.[92] The importance of the duration of delayed onset of breathing, also presumably reflecting the severity of the intrauterine insult, was emphasized by a study of 165 infants who exhibited "postasphyxial encephalopathy."[805] Thus, the rate of death or subsequent neurological deficits was 42% with delayed onset of breathing for 1 to 9 minutes, 56% for 10 to 19 minutes, and 88% for more than 20 minutes. An additional prognostic feature of the first 30 minutes of life in asphyxiated term infants with severe fetal acidemia (umbilical arterial pH $\leq$ 7.0) is the occurrence of hypoglycemia.[92] Thus, the 15% of acidemic infants in this study with an initial blood glucose of 40 mg/dL or lower had an 18.5-fold increased risk for death or moderate to severe encephalopathy than those with a glucose concentration higher than 40 mg/dL.

A recent study of more than 300 term infants with apparent intrapartum asphyxia and hypoxic-ischemic encephalopathy identified three key variables that together provided strong prediction of a serious adverse outcome (death or severe neurological sequelae) (Table 9-30).[806] The data suggested that the combination of need for chest compressions for more than 1 minute, a base deficit of 16 or greater, and age at onset of respiration at 30 minutes or greater was associated with a 93% risk of serious adverse outcome. The findings could be useful not only for early prognostication but perhaps also for decision making concerning neuroprotective therapies. The additions of pH and arterial carbon dioxide pressure (Pco_2) of cord blood gas measurements also provide predictive accuracy.[807]

Neonatal Neurological Syndrome

The occurrence of a recognizable neonatal neurological syndrome after signs of intrauterine asphyxia (see earlier) is the single most useful indicator that a significant hypoxic-ischemic insult to the brain has occurred. Studies completed since the 1970s support this contention and suggest improvements in overall outcome.* In an excellent representative earlier series of 93 patients (most term infants) reported by Brown and co-workers[2] in 1974, perinatal asphyxia was manifested by such features as meconium-stained amniotic fluid, fetal bradycardia, the need for endotracheal intubation and assisted ventilation at birth, and Apgar scores of less than 3 at 1 minute or less than 5 at 5 minutes, *in addition to neurological signs*, such as feeding difficulties, apnea, seizures, and hypotonia. Approximately 20% of the infants died in the neonatal period, approximately

---

*See references 2,5-8,11,14,16,20,46,55,57,214,336,370,468,482, 790,804,805,808-827a.

TABLE 9-30 **Relation of Three Key Early Neonatal Variables to Risk of Severe Adverse Outcome with Neonatal Hypoxic-Ischemic Encephalopathy**

Variables	PROBABILITY OF SEVERE OUTCOME*	
	Percentage of Total	95% Confidence Interval
None	46%	33%–58%
One Variable		
CC	69%	NA
Resp	67%	NA
BD	66%	NA
Overall	64%	54%–73%
Two Variables		
CC and Resp	67%	NA
CC and BD	77%	NA
BD and Resp	81%	NA
Overall	77%	66%–85%
Three Variables		
CC and Resp and BD	93%	81%–99%

*Severe adverse outcome was defined as death or severe neurological disability; total N = 302.
BD, base deficit $\geq$16; CC, chest compression for >1 minute; NA, not applicable; Resp, age at onset of respiration $\geq$30 min.
Data from Shah PS, Beyene J, To T, Ohlsson A, et al: Postasphyxial hypoxic-ischemic encephalopathy in neonates: Outcome prediction rule within 4 hours of birth, *Arch Pediatr Adolesc Med* 160:729–736, 2006.

40% subsequently exhibited neurological sequelae, and approximately 40% were found to be normal. In later series, although direct comparisons are hindered by differences in selection criteria, the outcome was somewhat better. Among term infants, only approximately 10% died in the neonatal period, and approximately 75% (i.e., nearly 85% of survivors) were normal on follow-up. The outcome for premature infants differed from that for term infants primarily in regard to mortality rate ($\approx$30% for asphyxiated premature infants versus $\approx$10% for term infants).

The likelihood of neurological sequelae in infants after hypoxic-ischemic insult *without* a neonatal neurological syndrome is not known absolutely. The regionalization of *both* perinatal and pediatric care in the area served by Brown and co-workers[2] allowed these investigators to conclude that such an occurrence was very unlikely. A similar conclusion can be drawn from a later study.[46] In more than 35 years of study of newborns and children with neurological disorders, I have not encountered a child with documented perinatal asphyxia but no neonatal neurological syndrome and the subsequent development of major neurological abnormalities. Although more data are needed on this issue, the available information suggests that the occurrence of neonatal neurological features provides the best indicator of infants at risk for subsequent neurological deficits.

Specific Aspects

Certain aspects of the neonatal neurological syndrome particularly useful in estimating prognosis include the *severity of the syndrome*, the *presence of seizures*, and the *duration of the abnormalities*.

Before discussing these specific neurological aspects, it is important to recognize that certain aspects of the *non-neurological evaluation* may provide prognostic information. Thus, in a study of asphyxiated infants (defined by depressed Apgar scores or fetal acidosis or both), of the 22 term infants with normal urine output, the mortality rate was approximately 5%, and neurological sequelae occurred in only 10% of survivors, whereas with oliguria persisting beyond 24 hours of life, the mortality rate was 33%, and neurological sequelae occurred in 67% of survivors.[810] A similar relationship between the severity of renal injury and an unfavorable neurological outcome was shown in the preterm infants. However, as also observed by others, neurological abnormalities in the neonatal period and on follow-up can occur in the absence of apparent renal injury (see "Neurological Syndrome" earlier).[44,809,810]

The *severity* of the neonatal neurological syndrome is of major value. Thus, when systematically quantitated, the severity correlated directly with the incidence of neurological sequelae.* The studies of Finer and co-workers,[11,814,815] which involved 226 full-term infants with hypoxic-ischemic encephalopathy, and of Thornberg and co-workers, which involved 65 such infants, demonstrated this point clearly (Table 9-31).[46] Although the overall incidence of death or neurological sequelae was 27%, infants with a mild neonatal syndrome had *no* subsequent deficits, whereas those with a severe syndrome uniformly either died (80%) or

exhibited sequelae (20%). Prolonged follow-up is important; in one report of teenage outcome among term infants with moderate neonatal encephalopathy and considered normal on earlier assessment (n = 28), the majority exhibited some learning problems or behavioral disturbances, or both, at the later evaluation.[827]

The presence of *seizures* as part of the neonatal neurological syndrome increases the risk for neurological sequelae (Table 9-32).* The incidence of neurological sequelae in infants with seizures is as much as 40-fold greater than the incidence in those without seizures. Thus, in one series of 27 infants with hypoxic-ischemic encephalopathy complicated by seizures, death or subsequent neurological deficits occurred in 67%.[46] Moreover, neurological sequelae are more likely if seizures occur in the first 12 hours or are difficult to control. For example, in one series of 45 infants, 76% with seizure onset at 4 hours of age or less died or exhibited neurological sequelae.[805] In one careful study of 68 term newborns with apparent hypoxic-ischemic encephalopathy, the *combination* of a neonatal neurological syndrome and seizures on the first day of life predicted abnormal outcome with 94% specificity and 72% sensitivity.[826] The degree to which the seizures per se *contribute* to the poorer outcome in certain cases (see Chapter 5) or simply reflect a more serious insult is unresolved.

The *duration* of neonatal neurological abnormalities is useful in identifying the infant at greatest risk for sequelae.[11,55,91,816,817,823] In two large series, essentially all infants who exhibited no neurological abnormalities after about 1 week of life (or on "discharge from the hospital") were normal on follow-up.[11,55] In a more recent series of 84 infants, approximately 90% of those with a normal examination at 7 days were normal on follow-up, and 10% had only mild abnormalities.[823] In another careful study of 23 severely asphyxiated infants, all 17 infants who were normal on follow-up exhibited neurological signs for less than 2 weeks.[55] My experience is similar. Thus, the

TABLE 9-31 Outcome of Term Infants with Hypoxic-Ischemic Encephalopathy as a Function of Severity of Neonatal Neurological Syndrome*

| Severity of Neonatal Syndrome[†] | No. of Patients | PERCENTAGE OF TOTAL | | |
		Deaths[‡]	Neurological Sequelae[§]	Normal
Mild	115	0%	0%	100%
Moderate	136	5%	24%	71%
Severe	40	80%	20%	0%
All	291	13%	14%	73%

*Derived from 291 full-term infants with hypoxic-ischemic encephalopathy.
[†]Mild, "hyperalert, hyperexcitable; normal muscle tone, no seizures"; moderate, "hypotonia, decreased movements, and often seizures"; severe, "stuporous, flaccid, and absent primitive reflexes."
[‡]Includes in-hospital and postdischarge deaths.
[§]Principally spastic motor deficits and cognitive disturbances.
Data from Robertson C, Finer N: Term infants with hypoxic-ischemic encephalopathy: Outcome at 3.5 years, *Dev Med Child Neurol* 27:473–484, 1985; and Thornberg E, Thiringer K, Odeback A, Milsom I: Birth asphyxia: Incidence, clinical course and outcome in a Swedish population, *Acta Paediatr* 84:927–932, 1995.

TABLE 9-32 Seizures as an Unfavorable Prognostic Sign in Neonatal Hypoxic-Ischemic Encephalopathy in Term Infants*

Seizures increase the risk of neurological sequelae by as much as 40-fold.
Seizures persistently recalcitrant to anticonvulsant treatment are nearly uniformly associated with death or subsequent neurological deficits.
Early onset of seizures increases the risk of adverse outcome, and the risk is approximately 75% with onset in the first 4 hours.

*See text for references.

*See references 8,14,20,46,57,94,336,468,482,804,805,808,811,813-816,821,823-828.

*See references 5,6,11,20,44,46,55,804,805,809,813,816,819,823, 824,826,829-833.

duration of neurological abnormalities is a good indicator of the severity of hypoxic-ischemic injury, and disappearance of abnormalities by 1 or 2 weeks is an excellent prognostic sign. However, such analyses do not include systematic evaluation at school age, and hence the possibility of learning disturbances cannot be ruled out conclusively.

Results of Neurodiagnostic Techniques

Because outcome clearly relates to the severity of the neuropathology, any specialized technique that defines the extent of brain injury in the newborn period should provide valuable information regarding prognosis. Such techniques include electrophysiological measures, especially EEG, but also evoked potentials, brain imaging methods, and methods to evaluate cerebral hemodynamics and metabolism.

Electroencephalography and Evoked Potentials

As discussed in the "Diagnosis" section, *specific EEG patterns* are indicative of particular types of hypoxic-ischemic brain injury (see Table 9-10). Such information, coupled with imaging data, is valuable for prognostic assessment (see earlier).

The *severity* of EEG abnormalities and their *duration* in the asphyxiated infant also are of prognostic importance (Table 9-33).* Regarding *severity*, in the term infant the most common feature is a continuous or intermittent discontinuity of EEG (see Chapter 4). The most extreme of these discontinuous tracings is the *burst-suppression pattern*, which is associated with a very high likelihood of an unfavorable outcome, especially when the tracing is nonreactive (see Chapter 4). However, burst-suppression tracings account for the *minority* of excessively discontinuous neonatal EEG tracings. We have found that a relatively simple means of quantitation of excessively discontinuous tracings in the term infant (i.e., analysis of the duration, in 10-second blocks, of the predominant IBI) has major prognostic value (Table 9-34).[187] Predominant IBI durations of more than 30 seconds were invariably associated

TABLE 9-34 Predominant Interburst Interval Duration in Prediction of Outcome*

Predominant interburst interval duration is obtained readily by manual measurement of the predominant interval accounting for more than 50% of all interburst interval durations.

A predominant interburst interval duration of more than 30 seconds is associated with an unfavorable outcome in 100% of cases, a duration of more than 20 seconds is associated with an unfavorable outcome in 92% of cases, and an interval lasting longer than 10 seconds is associated with an unfavorable outcome in 72% of cases.

The predominant interburst interval duration is more useful than the burst-suppression periodic pattern because the latter accounts for a small minority of discontinuous tracings.

*See text for details and Chapter 4.

with an unfavorable outcome, and durations of more than 20 seconds were associated with an unfavorable outcome in 92%. Notably, predominant IBI durations of more than 10 seconds still predicted abnormal outcome in 72%. Of the 43 discontinuous tracings studied, only 7 (16%) exhibited a burst-suppression pattern, as defined classically (see Table 9-34 and Chapter 4). Thus, the predominant IBI duration, readily quantitated at the bedside, was highly effective and, critically, applicable to *most* excessively discontinuous tracings in the term newborn with encephalopathy.

Regarding the *duration* of EEG abnormalities, as with the neonatal neurological syndrome, recovery of normal EEG background by day 7 is associated with a favorable outcome (see Table 9-33). In one large series of 77 term infants with apparent hypoxic-ischemic encephalopathy studied at 7 days of age, of 52 with a normal EEG tracing, 83% were later (at 1 year of age) found to be normal, 17% had mild abnormalities, and none had severe abnormalities.[823]

aEEG has been of considerable value in estimation of prognosis in the asphyxiated term newborn (Table 9-35).[188-193,834,836-838] As described earlier in "Diagnosis," the most useful tracings for detection of

TABLE 9-33 Electroencephalographic Patterns of Prognostic Significance in Asphyxiated Term Infants*

Associated with Favorable Outcome
Mild depression (or less) on day 1
Normal background by day 7

Associated with Unfavorable Outcome
Predominant interburst interval >20 sec on any day
Burst-suppression pattern on any day
Isoelectric tracing on any day
Mild (or greater) depression after day 12

*See text for references. Associations with favorable or unfavorable outcome are generally 90% or greater, but the clinical context must be considered.

TABLE 9-35 Value of Amplitude-Integrated Electroencephalography in Assessment of Asphyxiated Term Infants*

Detection of severe abnormalities (i.e., CLV, FT, BSP) in the first hours of life has a positive predictive value of an unfavorable outcome of 80% to 90%.

Severe abnormalities may improve within 24 hours (≈50% of BSP and 10% of CLV/FT).

Rapid recovery of severe abnormalities is associated with a favorable outcome in 60% of cases.

The *combination* of early neonatal neurological examination and early aEEG enhances the positive predictive value and specificity.

*See text for references.
aEEG, amplitude-integrated encephalography; BSP, burst-suppression pattern; CLV, continuous low voltage; FT, flat trace.

*See references 55,157,166,167,170,172,173,175,177-181,184,187, 823,833-835.

severe encephalopathy have been continuous low-voltage, flat, and burst-suppression patterns. Because positive predictive values for such tracings in the first hours of life are 80% to 90%, aEEG has been valuable for early selection of infants for neuroprotective therapies (e.g., hypothermia; see later). Notably, 10% to 15% of infants with these marked background abnormalities may normalize within 24 hours. Rapid recovery is associated with a favorable outcome in 60% (see Table 9-35). Importantly, although aEEG in the first 6 hours is slightly superior to the neonatal neurological examination in identifying infants with an unfavorable outcome, the *combination* of aEEG *and* the neurological examination is more nearly optimal, with a specificity of 94%.[191]

Serial *visual-evoked potentials* carried out in term asphyxiated infants have been shown to provide valuable prognostic information.[491,839,840] In one study of 34 full-term infants with hypoxic-ischemic encephalopathy who were studied *within 6 hours of delivery*, the finding of normal visual-evoked potentials was associated with a normal neurological outcome in 10 of 12 infants, whereas no response to visual input was followed by death in 8 of 8 infants (Table 9-36).[837] However, the 14 infants with delayed latencies had an intermediate outcome.

Serial *somatosensory-evoked potentials* also have been shown to provide valuable prognostic information in assessment of the asphyxiated infant.[837,841-846] In 20 survivors of asphyxia at term, all 13 infants with normal outcome had normal somatosensory evoked response by 4 days of age, whereas the 7 infants with subsequent deficits had abnormal or absent responses beyond 4 days.[843] One study of 34 term infants with hypoxic-ischemic encephalopathy who were studied *within 6 hours of delivery* showed striking predictive value for favorable or unfavorable outcomes with normal potentials or no response, respectively (see Table 9-36).[837] Moreover, compared with the results with visual-evoked potentials, fewer infants had intermediate abnormalities on somatosensory-evoked

potential testing (see Table 9-36).[837] Thus, the data suggest that somatosensory-evoked potentials could be useful for early prognostic formulations. Results with *preterm* infants are not so promising.[844,847] For example, in a study of 126 preterm infants, neonatal somatosensory-evoked potentials were of somewhat limited value in prediction of subsequent cerebral palsy (sensitivity of 44%).[844]

Computed Tomography

Although MRI is more valuable, CT in the neonatal period can provide adjunct information of prognostic value. As noted in the "Diagnosis" section, in infants with major injury to basal ganglia and thalamus and focal or multifocal ischemic lesions, to a considerable extent CT defines the site and extent of the lesion and allows estimation of the neurological sequelae outlined in the "Clinicopathological Correlations" section. More often, however, the CT appearance in the infant with hypoxic-ischemic encephalopathy cannot be so neatly categorized, and the nature of the difficulties in evaluation varies with the gestational age of the infant.

In the *term infant*, several earlier series categorized the CT findings as normal or showing variable degrees of hypoattenuation or hemorrhage, or both.[212,214-218] Infants with normal CT scans rarely exhibit major neurological deficits on follow-up, and infants with scans demonstrating marked diffuse hypodensity, as illustrated in Figure 9-3, rarely are normal on follow-up. Moreover, those infants with major degrees of intracerebral hemorrhage, usually indicative of hemorrhagic infarction, almost always exhibit neurological deficits on follow-up. However, in several reported series, as many as one third of infants with less severe degrees of hypoattenuation had no intraparenchymal hemorrhage; in this group, the outcome is variable and not readily predicted. Nevertheless, it is apparent that in more than one half of term infants with hypoxic-ischemic encephalopathy, the CT scan provides very useful prognostic information. This proportion may be increased by a follow-up CT study at 2 to 6 weeks of age, when initially ambiguous findings may evolve to either a normal or an overtly abnormal scan.[216]

In the *preterm infant*, the CT scan provides some information of prognostic value,[818,848] although ultrasound scanning also is somewhat effective and more convenient. Nevertheless, the demonstration by CT of intraventricular hemorrhage, and especially its concomitants (particularly major degrees of periventricular hemorrhagic infarction and PVL), can be useful in determining outcome (see earlier sections and Chapter 11). The difficulties in interpretation of periventricular hypoattenuation in the premature newborn are discussed earlier (see "Diagnosis" section). I consider ultrasound to be more useful generally than CT in providing adjunct prognostic information in the preterm infant in the neonatal period. MRI, of course, is optimal (see "Diagnosis" earlier). The value of CT in detection *later* in infancy of the degree of peritrigonal white matter atrophy and ventricular dilation, secondary to PVL and correlated closely with the severity of

TABLE 9-36	**Prognostic Value of Visual- and Somatosensory-Evoked Potentials in Term Infants with Hypoxic-Ischemic Encephalopathy (<6 Hours of Age)**			
		OUTCOME		
Rsult of Evoked Potentials	**Total No.**	**Normal**	**Sequelae**	**Death**
Somatosensory				
Normal	12	11	0	1
Delayed	8	4	2	2
No response	14	0	0	14
Visual				
Normal	12	10	2	0
Delayed	14	5	0	9
No response	8	0	0	8

Data from Eken P, Toet MC, Groenendaal F, De Vries LS: Predictive value of early neuroimaging, pulsed Doppler and neurophysiology in full term infants with hypoxic-ischaemic encephalopathy, *Arch Dis Child Fetal Neonatal Ed* 73:F75-F80, 1995.

spastic diplegia or cognitive deficits, or both, has been well documented.[235,552,848]

Ultrasound

The ultrasound scan can provide useful information concerning prognosis, particularly in the premature infant, but to some extent also in the term infant. In the *term infant*, as discussed earlier (see "Diagnosis" section), major injury to basal ganglia and thalamus and focal and multifocal ischemic parenchymal lesions have been identified and have contributed to prediction of outcomes. However, most scans do not show such discrete lesions.[237,247] In one careful study of 40 term infants with hypoxic-ischemic encephalopathy and cranial ultrasonography in the first week, 13 of 14 infants (93%) with either a normal scan or with isolated germinal matrix or intraventricular or subarachnoid hemorrhage were normal on follow-up.[243] Of the remaining infants, the ultrasonographic findings nearly consistently associated with subsequent neurological deficits were *bilateral* abnormalities of basal ganglia in 9 infants, focal parenchymal echodensities or apparent stroke in 8, or a featureless appearance with patchy echodensities in 7. Periventricular echodensities may occur in the asphyxiated term infant, as in the preterm infant, but they are generally observed uncommonly. Confusion sometimes exists concerning the finding in the asphyxiated term infant of small ventricles or those that cannot be visualized. Whereas this observation has been said to be indicative of major brain edema,[247] in another study this finding was present in 62% of control subjects in the first week of life and could not be clearly related to structural disease.[237] In the latter study, the finding of a normal ultrasound scan in 9 of the 32 term infants with hypoxic-ischemic encephalopathy was followed by a normal outcome in 8 of the 9 infants.[237]

In the *preterm infant*, the value of the ultrasound scan in the evaluation of presumed hypoxic-ischemic disease relates primarily to the identification of periventricular white matter injury (i.e., periventricular echodensities, subsequent echolucencies at the sites of periventricular cysts, and ventricular dilation; see "Diagnosis" section). In this discussion, I do not include the large hemorrhagic parenchymal lesions, presumed periventricular hemorrhagic infarction, occurring nearly always in association with germinal matrix-intraventricular hemorrhage, which is addressed in Chapter 11. A large body of literature attests to the prognostic value of detection of periventricular echodensities, echolucencies ("cysts"), and ventricular dilation in premature infants (Table 9-37).* In one large study, the occurrence of *periventricular echodensities* that *persisted* longer than 2 weeks was associated with an approximately 17% risk of later cerebral palsy.[306] Risks have been somewhat lower in other studies.[305,318,854] The degree of echogenicity, especially those lesions with brighter signal than choroid plexus,

TABLE 9-37	**Rates of Cerebral Palsy in Relation to Neonatal Cranial Ultrasound Abnormalities***	
Abnormality	**No.**	**Percentage with Cerebral Palsy**
None	1238	4%
Persistent echodensities[†]	165	17%
Cystic periventricular leukomalacia (echolucencies)		
Unilateral	33	35%
Bilateral	43	75%
Parietal/occipital	60	67%
Other loci	16	25%
Ventricular dilation[‡]	98	10%

*Numbers for the percentage of infants with cerebral palsy are rounded off.
[†]Echodensities present for > 14 days but without cyst formation.
[‡]Isolated ventricular dilation (without intraventricular hemorrhage).
Data from Ancel PY, Livinec F, Larroque B, Marret S, et al: Cerebral palsy among very preterm children in relation to gestational age and neonatal ultrasound abnormalities: The EPIPAGE cohort study, *Pediatrics* 117:828–835, 2006.

may increase the risk of adverse outcome.[284,305] The occurrence of *echolucencies*, indicative of tissue dissolution and cyst formation, is of particular prognostic importance (see Table 9-37). The risk of cerebral palsy is approximately 75% and is enhanced by the location of the lesion, with highest rates of cerebral palsy in patients with more posterior lesions. In one careful study, extensive cystic lesions that included both posterior and anterior periventricular white matter were associated with a 94% risk of cerebral palsy.[318] Optimal detection of echolucencies is achieved with a 7.5-MHz transducer and serial scans. In one series with serial studies, cystic lesions were rarely detected in the first 14 days and generally appeared from 15 to 35 days of life.[318] These data support the notion that PVL is largely a postnatal lesion (see Chapter 8).

Magnetic Resonance Imaging

Because the likelihood, nature, and severity of subsequent neurological deficits in the infant with hypoxic-ischemic encephalopathy are related most decisively to the extent and specific topography of the lesions, MRI should prove to be the best imaging modality for determining prognosis. Studies of *term infants* support this prediction.* Particularly vivid examples of the value of neonatal MRI in establishing prognosis were discussed earlier and include those infants with evidence of selective neuronal necrosis of the major varieties defined in Chapter 8 (i.e., the diffuse type, the cerebral–deep nuclear type, and the deep nuclear–brain stem type) and for focal ischemic brain injury

---

*See references 160,237,247,260,263-280,283,284,286-293,295,297, 299,300,305,306,310,315,318,849-855.

*See references 20,50,79,81,82,90,243,326,328,329,332,334-336, 339,342,344,356,497,518,551,856.

(see "Clinicopathological Correlations" section). Of all imaging modalities currently applied to the newborn, only MRI provides consistent delineation particularly of involvement of specific areas of cerebral cortex, basal ganglia, thalamus, and brain stem, as well as clear demonstration of the full extent of cerebral infarction.

Among the several topographic patterns of neuronal injury (see earlier and Chapter 8), term infants with predominant injury to *basal ganglia and thalamus* (usually with associated injury to perirolandic and other areas of cortex) have an unfavorable neurological outcome.[20,243,342] A particularly interesting study showed that among a group of infants (n = 173) with presumed hypoxic-ischemic encephalopathy, the 25% (n = 44) with *predominantly basal ganglia/thalamic* injury had a poorer outcome than the 45% (n = 78) with predominantly parasagittal watershed pattern or the 30% (n = 51) with a normal neonatal MRI (Fig. 9-44).[20]

An interesting earlier study of 73 term infants with hypoxic-ischemic encephalopathy studied by MRI in the first days of life demonstrated *prognostic value for the single finding of abnormal signal in the posterior limb of the internal capsule*.[334] Of 32 infants with normal signal intensity, on follow-up 28 were normal and only one had severe deficits, whereas of 41 infants with abnormal (including 5 "equivocally" abnormal) signal intensity, all 41 had an abnormal outcome (including 16 deaths). Notably, all 41 infants with abnormal signal intensity also had abnormalities involving basal ganglia and thalamus. Because the signal intensity may be normal in the first few days, before becoming abnormal, the optimal imaging time is after approximately the fourth day. Studies based on measurement of the ADC in the posterior limb of the internal capsule support the notion that the signal abnormality in the posterior limb represents the onset of wallerian degeneration of descending corticospinal tract axons.[356]

MRI is also valuable in estimation of prognosis in pre-term infants. Early studies in this context involved MRI scans carried out many months or several years after birth.[262,307-309,322,383-394,526,551,857-859] The principal findings were a strong relationship between MRI evidence of PVL and subsequent cerebral palsy, cognitive deficits, or visual deficits. The MRI features included primarily increased signal on T2W images in cerebral white matter, especially periventricular, decreased white matter volume, and ventricular dilation, usually most pronounced posteriorly. In one population-based series of preterm infants, all infants with later cerebral palsy had evidence of PVL.[308] Approximately 70% of infants with MRI evidence of PVL had no major neurological deficits but on psychological testing had cognitive and attentional deficits.[858] These initial findings are consistent with later data that cognitive and attentional deficits may be a consequence of the more diffuse cerebral component of PVL (see "Clinicopathological Correlations" earlier). The common finding of ventricular dilation in such infants also supports this notion. Finally, the relationship between visual deficits and MRI evidence of involvement of the optic radiation

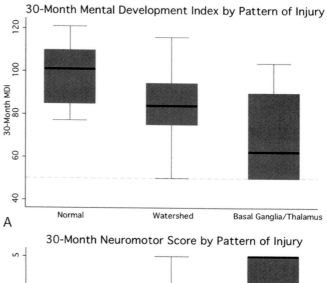

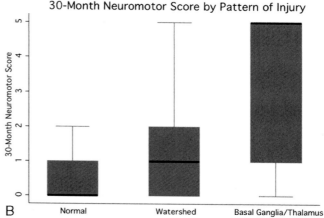

Figure 9-44 **Relationship between predominant regions injured and neurological outcome.** Predominant regional patterns were obtained by magnetic resonance imaging (MRI) in 173 term infants with encephalopathy, most probably resulting from hypoxia-ischemia. The relative distribution of MRI patterns was "parasagittal watershed" (n = 78), "basal ganglia/thalamus" (n = 44), or "normal" (n = 51). **A,** Box plot of the 30-month Mental Development Index (MDI) by the pattern of injury. The MDI was lowest in the infants with the basal ganglia/thalamus predominant pattern, with intermediate scores in infants with the watershed pattern (*P* = .0007). The *thick line* represents the median, with the 25th and 75th percentiles as the lower and upper limits of the box; whiskers indicate the 5th and 95th percentiles. The *dashed line* indicates the lowest attainable MDI score. **B,** Box plot of the 30-month neuromotor score by the pattern of injury. Neuromotor impairments were most severe in the infants with the basal ganglia/thalamus pattern (*P* = .0001). *(From Miller SP, Ramaswamy V, Michelson D, Barkovich AJ, et al: Patterns of brain injury in term neonatal encephalopathy, J Pediatr 146:453–460, 2005.)*

in PVL is discussed earlier (see "Clinicopathological Correlations" section).

The value of *neonatal* MRI in estimation of *prognosis in preterm infants* has been established.[321,368,370,400,565,566] The optimal time for MRI scanning for prognostic assessment is not entirely clear, but the balance of available data suggests that a scan nearest to term equivalent is most useful. For example, the frequency of diffuse excessive high signal intensity (DEHSI), which is related significantly to subsequent developmental quotient (no DEHSI, 111 ± 20; any DEHSI, 94 ± 11.6; severe DEHSI, 92 ± 7.5; *P* =.027), increases from approximately 25% in

TABLE 9-38   **Relation of Cerebral White Matter Abnormalities Identified by Magnetic Resonance Imaging at Term Equivalent to Outcome in Premature Infants at 2 Years of Age***

| | WHITE MATTER ABNORMALITY AT TERM[†] | | | | |
Outcome Measure	None (n = 47)	Mild (n = 85)	Moderate (n = 29)	Severe (n = 6)	*P*
MDI cognitive score	92	85	80	70	<.001
PDI psychomotor score	95	91	80	56	.008
Severe motor delay	4%	5%	26%	67%	<.001
Cerebral palsy	2%	6%	24%	67%	<.001
Neurosensory impairment	4%	9%	21%	50%	.003

*Numbers are rounded off.

[†]Severity of white matter abnormality graded according to a numerical scale based on nature and extent of white matter signal abnormality, white matter volume loss, cystic abnormalities, ventricular dilation, and thinning of the corpus callosum.

MDI, Mental Development Index; PDI, Psychomotor Development Index.

Data from Woodward LJ, Anderson PJ, Austin NC, Howard K, et al: Neonatal MRI to predict neurodevelopmental outcomes in preterm infants, *N Engl J Med* 355:685–694, 2006.

the first week to nearly 80% at term.[302,566] In addition to diffuse signal abnormality, white matter volume loss, ventricular dilation, cystic abnormalities, thinning of corpus callosum, and abnormal signal in the posterior limb of the internal capsule are important prognostic features. The largest available study (N = 167) of very preterm infants (≤30 weeks of gestation) showed clearly the relationship between the frequency and severity of these neonatal MRI measures (obtained at term equivalent) and subsequent cognitive and motor deficits (Table 9-38).[368] The increasing severity of white matter injury was accompanied by such abnormalities of gray matter as impaired gyral maturation and increased size of the cerebral subarachnoid space, both reflecting the volumetric and other cortical abnormalities described in Chapter 8.

Magnetic Resonance Spectroscopy

MR spectroscopy of both the proton and phosphorus types has been valuable in determination of outcome in neonatal hypoxic-ischemic disease in the term newborn. The data should be interpreted in the context of the findings in experimental models of an early increase in cerebral lactate, detectable by proton MR spectroscopy, preceding a "secondary delayed energy failure," characterized by a decline in high-energy phosphate compounds, detectable by phosphorus MR spectroscopy (see Chapter 6). (The primary, initial energy failure occurs close to the time of the initial insult, usually in utero and before any measurements can be made.)

Studies by *proton MR spectroscopy* performed in the first several days of life showed distinctly elevated cerebral lactate in asphyxiated human infants.[454,459-462,464,467-469,471-480] The elevation in lactate is apparent in the first 18 hours of life and, importantly, correlates with the severity of the delayed secondary energy failure observed on subsequent days (see Fig. 9-39B), the neonatal neurological syndrome, and the neurological outcome (Fig. 9-45).[459,467-469,480] Infants with the poorest outcomes have persistently elevated lactate levels (i.e., for several weeks or more[454,455,465]), whereas those with favorable outcomes had resolution of lactate elevations during this interval.

NAA, a marker of the neuronal-axonal unit as well as oligodendroglial precursors and immature oligodendrocytes,[860,861] is usually only variably affected during these early phases.[461,463,466,468-470,473-475,477,479,862] However, a decline in NAA does become apparent after many days to weeks as tissue loss becomes established.

Studies by *phosphorus MR spectroscopy* performed in the first week of life show a delayed secondary decline in high-energy phosphate compounds in asphyxiated human infants.[449,450,452,453] This decline becomes apparent generally on the second day of life and reaches a nadir at 2 to 4 days of life. The severity of this delayed secondary energy failure correlates with the severity of both the neonatal neurological syndrome (see Fig. 9-38) and the subsequent neurological deficits (Fig. 9-46).[452,453] As noted earlier, the sustained

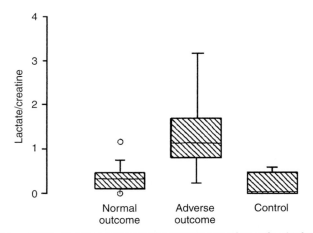

Figure 9-45   Relation between the lactate/creatine ratio obtained by proton magnetic resonance spectroscopy in the first 18 hours of life and neurological outcome. Median, interquartile ranges, and upper and lower adjacent values of the ratios in infants with normal outcome, infants with abnormal outcome, and control infants are shown. The value for infants with adverse outcome was significantly different from the values for both infants with normal outcome and control infants. *(From Hanrahan JD, Cox IJ, Azzopardi D, Cowan FM, et al: Relation between proton magnetic resonance spectroscopy within 18 hours of birth asphyxia and neurodevelopment at 1 year of age, Dev Med Child Neurol 41:76–82, 1999.)*

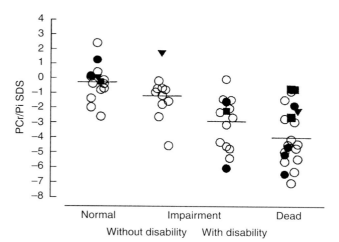

Figure 9-46 Relation between phosphocreatine/inorganic phosphate (PCr/Pi) standard deviation score (SDS), determined by phosphorus magnetic resonance spectroscopy (during the period of secondary energy failure) as number of standard deviations from the mean of control values, and neurodevelopmental outcome, determined by evaluation at 4 years in 62 asphyxiated infants. *Open circles* represent term average for gestational age (AGA) infants, *closed circles* represent term small for gestational age (SGA) infants, *closed triangles* represent preterm AGA infants, and *closed squares* represent preterm SGA infants. *(From Roth SC, Baudin J, Cady E, Johal K, et al: Relation of deranged neonatal cerebral oxidative metabolism with neurodevelopmental outcome and head circumference at 4 years, Dev Med Child Neurol 39:718–725, 1997.)*

alkaline intracellular pH identified by phosphorus MR spectroscopy also correlates with poor neurodevelopmental outcome.[455]

Currently, proton MR spectroscopy is used much more widely than phosphorus MR spectroscopy in the evaluation of newborn infants, because this approach, unlike phosphorus MR spectroscopy, is adapted readily to clinically used MR instruments. Thus, although the data obtained by phosphorus MR spectroscopy have provided important information, it is likely that future work will continue to be carried out primarily with proton MR spectroscopy.

Measurement of Cerebral Blood Flow Velocity, Cerebral Blood Volume, or Cerebral Blood Flow

A series of studies has established that the postasphyxial human newborn exhibits a state of vasoparalysis and cerebral hyperemia, detectable as increased CBF velocity and decreased cerebrovascular resistance by Doppler studies, as increased cerebral blood volume by near-infrared spectroscopy, and as increased CBF by xenon-133 clearance or PET (see Chapter 6). These changes are correlated with the degree of brain injury, as discussed next.

Measurements of *CBF velocity by the Doppler technique* at the anterior fontanelle have provided useful prognostic information in full-term asphyxiated infants studied in the first days of life. Determination of CBF velocity in such infants generally from approximately 1 to 6 days after the insult showed an increase in mean flow velocity with decreased resistance indices (i.e., cerebral vasodilation).[863-872] One large study involved 39 term asphyxiated infants with

"postasphyxial encephalopathy" in whom Doppler measurements from the anterior cerebral artery from the first hour delineated distinct abnormalities at a median age of 26 hours (i.e., increased CBF velocity and decreased Pourcelot resistance index).[868] This constellation suggested a state of cerebral hyperemia with vasodilation, leading to both decreased resistance and increased flow. The mechanism underlying this "delayed hyperemia" is unclear (see Chapter 6). The cerebral hyperemia could account in part for the increase in ICP sometimes observed at this time in severely asphyxiated infants (see Chapter 8). An important point for this discussion is that the changes were correlated with unfavorable outcome. Thus, no infant with CBF velocity greater than 3 standard deviations above the mean survived without severe neurological impairment.[868] One report showed that the increased CBF velocity in infants with an unfavorable outcome is not apparent until 12 to 24 hours of age, and thus earlier measurements do not have appreciable prognostic value.[872]

That the Doppler measurements reflected cerebral vasodilation, at least in part, was shown in studies of similar infants by *near-infrared spectroscopy*.[873-875] Such studies of asphyxiated human infants on the first day of life suggested an increase in both cerebral blood volume and CBF. Moreover, other work with near-infrared spectroscopy showed that the state of cerebral hyperemia is accompanied by evidence of diminished oxygen extraction and elevated cerebral venous oxygen saturation, perhaps reflecting tissue injury.[876] Whether the use of near-infrared spectroscopy could provide valuable information for long-term prognostic estimation is not established by these short-term studies, but it seems likely.

Decisive demonstration of both the prognostic value of direct measurement of CBF and of the likelihood that the studies using Doppler ultrasound and near-infrared spectroscopy reflected cerebral hyperemia was accomplished by such direct measurements in asphyxiated infants *by xenon-133 clearance* and *by PET*.[877,878] In the large series of infants studied by xenon clearance, infants with the poorest outcome had the highest values for CBF in the first day of life (see Table 6-31). Asphyxiated infants who died or had severe brain injury had mean CBF of 30.6 mL/100 g/minute; those who had moderate to severe brain injury had CBF of 15.1 mL/100 g/minute; and those with normal outcome had CBF of 9.2 mL/100 g/minute. That the low Pourcelot resistance index shown by Doppler reflected cerebral vasodilation, presumably secondary to vasoparalysis, also was shown by Pryds and co-workers,[877] who demonstrated no reactivity of flow to arterial blood pressure or arterial carbon dioxide tension ($Paco_2$) in the group with poorest outcome, no reactivity to blood pressure (although retained reactivity to carbon dioxide) in the group with intermediate outcome, and retained reactivity to both pressure and carbon dioxide in the group with normal outcome. A later study of 16 term infants with hypoxic-ischemic encephalopathy used PET to determine CBF primarily at 1 to 4 days of life and found higher flows in those infants with abnormal neurological outcome (35.6 mL/100 g/minute) than in those with normal neurological outcome (18.3 mL/100 g/minute).[878]

That these measures of cerebral hyperemia are *not* related to increased cerebral metabolic rate was shown by a study of 20 infants with hypoxic-ischemic encephalopathy with PET measurements of cerebral metabolic rate for glucose.[879] Thus, the total cerebral metabolic rate for glucose was *inversely* correlated with severity of the encephalopathy and the degree of neurological deficits. Those infants with the most severe deficits later had the lowest neonatal values of cerebral metabolic rate for glucose.

Conclusion

No neurodiagnostic technique is capable of diminishing the importance of the clinical evaluation of the infant in assessment of outcome. Clinical and specialized diagnostic approaches are of value only when they are used *in concert*.

MANAGEMENT

Management requires attention to the involvement of multiple systems. Although I emphasize the neurological aspects of therapy, it is the rule rather than the exception that infants with hypoxic-ischemic encephalopathy have disturbances of pulmonary, cardiovascular, hepatic, and renal functions as well.[45,49,51-53,810,880] Although I do not deal in detail with the specific management of these various disturbances, I touch on several relevant issues in the following discussion. The emphasis is on management in terms of the following: prevention of intrauterine asphyxia; maintenance of adequate ventilation, perfusion, and blood glucose levels; control of seizures; control of brain swelling; and other potential neuroprotective therapies (Table 9-39). Concerning the last of these, the major portion of neuronal death following hypoxic-ischemic insult evolves *after* termination of the insult (i.e., often during the time that the therapeutic maneuvers to be reviewed next are applied).

Prevention of Intrauterine Asphyxia

A critical aspect of management is prevention of the hypoxic-ischemic insult, and because most infants appear to experience the primary insult in utero,

TABLE 9-39	Basic Elements of the Management of Neonatal Hypoxic-Ischemic Encephalopathy
Prevention of intrauterine asphyxia
Maintenance of adequate ventilation
Maintenance of adequate perfusion
Maintenance of adequate blood glucose levels
Control of seizures
Control of brain swelling
Neuroprotective interventions

TABLE 9-40	Prevention of Intrauterine Asphyxia
Antepartum assessment and identification of the high-risk pregnancy
Electronic fetal monitoring
Fetal blood sampling
Appropriate interventions (e.g., cesarean section)

prevention of intrauterine asphyxia is paramount. Detailed discussion of the management of pregnancy, labor, and delivery is beyond the scope of this book, but the basic elements of this aspect of management are summarized in Table 9-40 and are based on the considerations discussed in Chapter 7.

The first goal is identification of the fetus being subjected to or likely to experience hypoxic-ischemic insults with labor and delivery. Thus, antepartum assessment (see Chapter 7) with identification of the high-risk pregnancy is central (see Table 9-40). The fetus should be monitored during the intrapartum period primarily by the electronic techniques described in Chapter 7, supplemented, when necessary, by fetal blood sampling to determine pH and blood gas values. The need for better methods to assess *fetal neurological status*, particularly fetal cerebral hemodynamics and metabolism, was emphasized earlier. The particular mode of intervention for the fetus threatened by hypoxic-ischemic insult depends on a variety of factors related to the fetus and the mother, but often cesarean section is a critical intervention in the prevention of the degree of asphyxia that leads to brain injury. The potential future use of such agents as calcium channel blockers, excitatory amino acid antagonists, and free radical scavengers is based on the principles outlined in Chapter 6. In this context, the agent must have the capability of crossing both the placenta and the fetal blood-brain barrier.

Maintenance of Adequate Ventilation

Maintenance of adequate ventilation is a central aspect of *supportive care*, an imprecise term that refers to the maintenance also of temperature, perfusion, and metabolic status. The importance of these various postnatal aspects of management cannot be overemphasized; although a significant intrauterine insult has occurred in most asphyxiated infants, postnatal disturbances of ventilation and perfusion particularly may play an important role in determining the ultimate severity of neurological injury. In this section, I discuss the particular importance of maintenance of adequate arterial concentrations of oxygen and carbon dioxide.

Oxygen

Hypoxemia. Avoidance of oxygen deprivation clearly is a cornerstone of supportive therapy. Hypoxemia may lead to a disturbance of cerebrovascular autoregulation and, as a consequence, a *pressure-passive circulation* (Table 9-41; see Chapter 6). Under such circumstances, the infant is vulnerable to superimposed ischemic cerebral injury with only moderate decreases

TABLE 9-41	Deleterious Neurological Consequences of Disturbed Oxygenation
Hypoxemia	
Pressure-passive cerebral circulation	
Neuronal and white matter injury	
Hyperoxia	
Neuronal injury (pontosubicular)	
Increased oxidative stress (systemic)	
Retinopathy of prematurity	

in arterial blood pressure. Indeed, this mechanism may be the most important by which hypoxemia leads to parenchymal injury. Provision of adequate oxygen also is necessary to prevent additional *neuronal and white matter injury* (see Table 9-41). The propensity for the white matter injury presumably relates in part to the limited vasodilatory capacity in neonatal cerebral white matter in the presence of anaerobic glycolysis and increased substrate demand (see Chapters 6 and 8).

Concerning *detection and causes of hypoxemia* in the infant with hypoxic-ischemic encephalopathy, very diligent surveillance is critical. The use of pulse oximetry and transcutaneous oxygen monitoring has demonstrated that among infants in neonatal intensive care facilities, especially low-birth-weight infants, episodes of hypoxemia are more frequent than often thought and are readily overlooked by *periodic* sampling of arterial blood. Thus, *continuous* transcutaneous oxygen or pulse oximetry monitoring in sick, low-birth-weight infants has detected some very frequent and, in some cases, previously unsuspected causes of hypoxemia (Table 9-42).[881-897] These causes include feeding procedures that disturb inflow of oxygen, crying (presumably by breath holding), bowel movements (presumably by breath holding), airway manipulations that disturb inflow of oxygen, and diagnostic procedures that cause hypoxemia by a combination of these mechanisms. Careful studies of handling and of ambient noise in the neonatal intensive care unit have led to the

TABLE 9-42	Common Causes of Hypoxemia in Low-Birth-Weight Infants
Feeding Procedures	
Overfeeding with abdominal distention, neck flexion, and hand-under-jaw feeding	
Crying	
Airway Manipulations	
Suctioning, neck flexion, neck hyperextension, and poorly placed nasal mask or endotracheal tube	
Diagnostic Procedures	
Painful procedures and abdominal examination with compression	
Seizures	
Apneic Episodes	
Other	
Handling, excessive noise, active sleep, and ambient temperature out of infant's thermoneutral zone	

discovery of appreciable deleterious effects on oxygen tension and to alterations in care-taking practices and procedures that ameliorate these effects considerably. The hypoxemic effect of apnea is expected, but the episodes of apnea frequently may not be detected by conventional monitoring devices. Moreover, that the hypoxemia with apnea results in *cerebral* deoxygenation has been shown clearly by near-infrared spectroscopy.[898] Finally, seizures may be subtle and may still produce important hypoventilation and hypoxemia.

The causes of hypoxemia outlined in the preceding paragraph generally can be dealt with effectively. The *most common cause of serious persistent hypoxemia* in the *term* infant, persistent fetal circulation, is not so readily managed. This issue is discussed in standard writings on neonatology. Suffice it to say here that the principal therapeutic modalities range from oxygen and assisted ventilation to administration of pulmonary vasodilator drugs (e.g., nitric oxide), passive hyperventilation, and high-frequency ventilation. Extracorporeal membrane oxygenation has been used for the most severe cases, although the advent of nitric oxide therapy decreased the need for this invasive approach considerably.

Hyperoxia. Although hypoxemia is serious and requires prompt reaction, overreaction also may be deleterious if *hyperoxia* is produced (see Table 9-41). The latter may lead to *neuronal injury*. For example, the neuropathological data reviewed in Chapter 8 suggest a role for hyperoxia in the genesis of a specific pattern of neuronal injury, pontosubicular necrosis. In addition, the possibility that hyperoxia may contribute to neuronal injury by causing a reduction in CBF must be considered. Reductions of CBF of 20% to 30% were shown with hyperoxia in newborn puppies, although the arterial oxygen tensions (Pao_2) of approximately 350 mm Hg used were very high.[899] In one study of 218 term infants with "post-asphyxial hypoxic-ischemic encephalopathy," infants who experienced severe hyperoxia (Pao_2 >200 mm Hg) in the first hours of life had an increased risk on multivariate analysis of adverse neurological outcome (odds ratio 3.85, 95% confidence interval 1.67–8.86, $P = .002$).[900] This deleterious effect was accentuated if severe hypocarbia also occurred (see later).

Concern about deleterious effects of hyperoxia has led in recent years to a reconsideration of previous recommendations to use 100% oxygen in resuscitation.[901-905a] Resuscitation with room air versus 100% oxygen has been associated with reduced neonatal mortality and *evidence systemically for increased oxidative stress*. Whether the latter contributes to increased oxidative stress in brain, deleterious for both neurons and differentiating oligodendrocytes (see Chapters 6 and 8), is not yet known, although experimental data support this possibility. Currently, in many European centers, resuscitation is initiated with room air or oxygen concentrations between 21% (room air) and 40%, and 100% oxygen is used after 90 seconds if the response is poor.[905] Notably, in human premature infants, CBF measured by xenon clearance 2 hours after birth was 23% lower in infants who were resuscitated with 80% oxygen versus infants resuscitated with room air.[906]

Finally, although the cause of *retinopathy of prematurity* is now recognized to be complex, hyperoxia remains an important factor.[907,908] Because very-low-birth-weight newborns have red blood cells with high oxygen affinity, the PaO_2 required to achieve adequate saturation of oxygen is lower than often recognized; thus, the value of PaO_2 required to achieve 90% saturation of hemoglobin is only 41 mm Hg.[909] Ultrastructural studies of developing hamsters rendered hyperoxic demonstrate vaso-obliterative changes in brain comparable to those produced in retina and suggest the possibility of a deleterious vascular effect as a source of brain injury.[910]

Carbon Dioxide

Because $PaCO_2$ may have serious metabolic and vascular effects, careful control thereof is critical (Table 9-43). As with oxygen determinations, periodic sampling of arterial blood is not an optimal means to monitor serially and to maintain $PaCO_2$. Experience with continuous transcutaneous monitoring of PCO_2 or serial measurements of end-tidal carbon dioxide pressure indicates that events as frequent as, and often similar to, those recorded in Table 9-42 result in marked changes in $PaCO_2$.[888,891,911-913] Elaboration of this experience is particularly relevant to the management of the infant with hypoxic-ischemic encephalopathy.

Hypercarbia. Marked elevations of $PaCO_2$ are particularly dangerous in such infants because of the resulting increase in tissue PCO_2 and consequent worsening of intracellular acidosis in brain (see Table 9-43). Perhaps more important than the *metabolic* effects and worsening of tissue acidosis are the *vascular* effects of hypercarbia. Thus, hypercarbia results in an impairment of cerebrovascular autoregulation and, as a consequence, a pressure-passive circulation (see Chapter 6). In one careful study of 43 ventilated preterm infants in the first week of life, a progressive loss of vascular autoregulation was observed with $PaCO_2$ values of 45 mm Hg or greater.[914] As noted previously concerning hypoxemia, with hypercarbia the infant becomes especially vulnerable to ischemic cerebral injury with decreases in arterial blood pressure. Moreover, because of the potent vasodilatory effect of hypercarbia, CBF may increase and may cause a risk of hemorrhage in vulnerable capillary beds (e.g., germinal matrix and thereby intraventricular hemorrhage in the preterm infant, margins of an infarct and thereby hemorrhagic infarct in the term infant). Finally, the cerebral vasodilation in uninjured areas may lead to "steal" of blood from those reversibly injured areas in need of maximal substrate supply. (This risk, shown in adult experimental models, has not been studied in a newborn model.) These adverse effects with marked hypercarbia should be contrasted with the apparent *beneficial* effects of *mild* hypercarbia during hypoxia-ischemia (see later discussion).

Hypocarbia. The effect of *hypocarbia* on CBF is pronounced. Although marked diminutions have been documented in adult humans and animals,[915-917] the findings in neonatal animals have not been entirely consistent.[918-928] Differences in results appear to relate in part to species and methodological differences. The following conclusions seem warranted. With hypocarbia to approximately 20 mm Hg, little change in CBF occurs. With lower levels (mean, 17 mm Hg), a definite decline in regional CBF occurs in the puppy,[923] more marked (30% to 60%) in regions with highest basal levels of blood flow and, therefore, highest sensitivity to carbon dioxide (see Chapter 6) (i.e., brain stem and diencephalon). However, in the piglet, extreme hypocarbia (<15 mm Hg) is necessary to produce statistically significant decreases in blood flow, and in this animal, the cerebrum and not the brain stem or diencephalon is affected.[922] Perhaps the most consistent observation in the several animal models is that the linear relationship between $PaCO_2$ and CBF becomes curvilinear at tensions lower than 20 to 25 mm Hg[915,920,922]; the decrease in CBF for a given decrease in $PaCO_2$ becomes *considerably less* than it is above this lower range of $PaCO_2$. Additionally, adaptation occurs such that in the newborn lamb, CBF after 6 hours of $PaCO_2$ of 15 mm Hg is not statistically different from that in control animals.[926] Perhaps of greatest importance despite the decreases in CBF in newborn animals, no change in cerebral metabolic rate for oxygen occurs, primarily because of an increase in oxygen extraction.[924,926] Thus, mild hypocarbia may be of little or no danger, although data in the human newborn concerning hypocarbia are of concern (see later).

Perhaps relevant in this context is the demonstration that mild hypocarbia ($PaCO_2$ of 26 mm Hg) interacted adversely with hypoxic-ischemic insults in the immature rat.[929-931] Thus, animals exposed to hypoxia-ischemia during mild hypocarbia sustained a larger decline in CBF, a greater degree of cerebral glucose and energy depletion, and more neuropathological evidence of brain injury than did animals exposed to the same insult but with normocarbia ($PaCO_2$ of 39 mm Hg) or mild hypercarbia ($PaCO_2$ of 54 mm Hg). The latter two groups had better preserved CBF, less severe cerebral biochemical deficits, and less severe brain injury. The mildly hypercarbic animals had the most favorable hemodynamic, biochemical, and neuropathological outcomes.

TABLE 9-43 **Deleterious Consequences of Disturbed Carbon Dioxide Levels**

Hypercarbia (Marked)
Metabolic
  Cerebral acidosis
Vascular
  Pressure-passive cerebral circulation
  Cerebral vasodilation with hemorrhagic complications (e.g., intraventricular hemorrhage, hemorrhagic infarction)
  Intracranial "steal"

Hypocarbia
Vascular
  Diminished cerebral blood flow: ischemic injury

CBF in the human infant is responsive to changes in $Paco_2$, except under conditions of maximal vasodilation in the mechanically ventilated preterm infant (in the first days of life) and in the asphyxiated term infant.[877,914,932-937] *Concern for impaired CBF with vasoconstriction caused by hypocarbia seems warranted.* Thus, in one careful study of 32 ventilated premature infants on the first day of life, values of $Paco_2$ lower than 25 mm Hg were associated with slowing of the EEG tracing and increased cerebral fractional oxygen extraction, likely to be related to decreased cerebral oxygen delivery induced by hypocarbia.[937] Moreover, an increased risk for cystic PVL was shown after cumulative time periods of $Paco_2$ lower than 25 mm Hg.[938-940] An earlier study also suggested a threshold value of 25 mm Hg.[941] Moreover, in another report, 21 of 56 ventilated preterm infants (37%) who were exposed to a maximally low $Paco_2$ value of less than 20 mm Hg at least once during the first 3 days of life developed large periventricular cysts or cerebral palsy, or both.[851] Although the potency of the relationship between hypocarbia and PVL or cerebral palsy, or both, varied somewhat among earlier studies, the relationship has received considerable support.[941-948] One study of 217 term infants with hypoxic-ischemic encephalopathy showed, on multivariate analysis, an association between adverse neurological outcome and $Paco_2$ lower than 20 mm Hg in the first hours of life (odds ratio, 2.34; 95% confidence limits, 1.02 to 5.37; $P = .04$).[900] The risk was accentuated (odds ratio, 4.56) when severe hyperoxia also was present. Similarly, a report of 905 premature infants (birth weight, 501 to 1249 g) measured a *cumulative* index of hypocarbia ($Paco_2 \leq 35$ mm Hg) over the first 7 days of life and found a strong association with the occurrence of cystic PVL, identified as echolucencies on cranial ultrasonography (see Fig. 8-30).[948]

Maintenance of Adequate Perfusion

The maintenance of adequate perfusion to brain is a critical aspect of supportive care. Prevention of additional ischemic injury is important. The basic elements of maintenance of adequate perfusion are summarized in Table 9-44 and in the following discussion.

Recognition of Pressure-Passive Cerebral Circulation

As discussed in Chapter 8 (concerning pathogenesis) and Chapter 6, the cerebral circulation of the infant with hypoxic-ischemic encephalopathy appears to be pressure passive. This occurrence may relate to a disturbance of autoregulation by complicating hypoxemia

TABLE 9-44 Maintenance of Adequate Perfusion
Recognition of pressure-passive cerebral circulation
Recognition of ''normal'' arterial blood pressure level
Avoidance of systemic hypotension (may cause ischemic injury)
Avoidance of systemic hypertension (may cause hemorrhagic complications)
Avoidance of hyperviscosity

or hypercarbia, or both, a postasphyxial impairment of vascular reactivity as observed in experimental models of perinatal asphyxia, an "immature" autoregulatory system with blunted capacity for reactivity because of the deficient arterial muscularis of penetrating cerebral vessels in the third trimester, an intact or partially intact autoregulatory mechanism but with "normal" neonatal blood pressure dangerously close to the downslope of the autoregulatory curve, or a combination of these factors (see Chapters 6 and 8). The important point is that the physician must be aware of the pressure-passive state, must monitor blood pressure continuously and diligently, and must maintain blood pressure at adequate levels to avoid cerebral ischemia or overperfusion. Studies of CBF in human infants with xenon-clearance techniques have documented a *pressure-passive state of the cerebral circulation* in seriously *asphyxiated term infants* (see Chapter 6 and earlier discussion).

The problem of impaired cerebrovascular autoregulation and a *pressure-passive cerebral circulation is particularly frequent in the sick premature infant.* Unlike in term infants, prior asphyxial events are uncommon in premature infants. Numerous studies using invasive and noninvasive methods have shown the pressure-passive state.[932,949-957] In one series (N = 32) of ventilated premature infants studied by near-infrared spectroscopy from the first hours of life, fully 53% were found to have extended periods of a pressure-passive state (Fig. 9-47) (see Chapter 6).[952] *Moreover, the nadirs of blood pressure were often not markedly low* and thus could be readily overlooked. A later study of 90 premature infants used a more sophisticated frequency-based assessment by near-infrared spectroscopy and found that fully 95% of the infants had pressure-passive epochs in the first days of life.[955] The overall mean proportion of pressure-passive time was 20%, although some of the smallest infants were in a pressure-passive state more than 50% of the time. Hypotension (see later) also was a common finding, and the likelihood of a pressure-passive state increased with both decreasing gestational age and hypotension. However, the pressure-passive state fluctuated over time and occurred commonly without low blood pressures. Thus, continuous monitoring of cerebral hemodynamics by a methodology such as near-infrared spectroscopy is necessary to determine whether an infant is in a pressure-passive state at any given blood pressure. Further insights into the causes of the cerebrovascular regulatory abnormality could lead to correction of the abnormality and perhaps prevention of ischemic brain injury in these infants.

The lower limit of the autoregulatory curve in newborns, especially preterm newborns, obviously is of great importance for management purposes. The precise lower limit is unknown and likely fluctuates for a given infant. Critical determining factors, in addition to gestational age, likely include such vasoactive factors as blood gases, seizures, hypoxia-ischemia, and cytokines. Several reports provide insight into the lower limit of the autoregulatory curve.[953,956,957] Thus, in a study of infants of 24 to 30 weeks of gestation on the first day of life, mean blood pressure values lower than

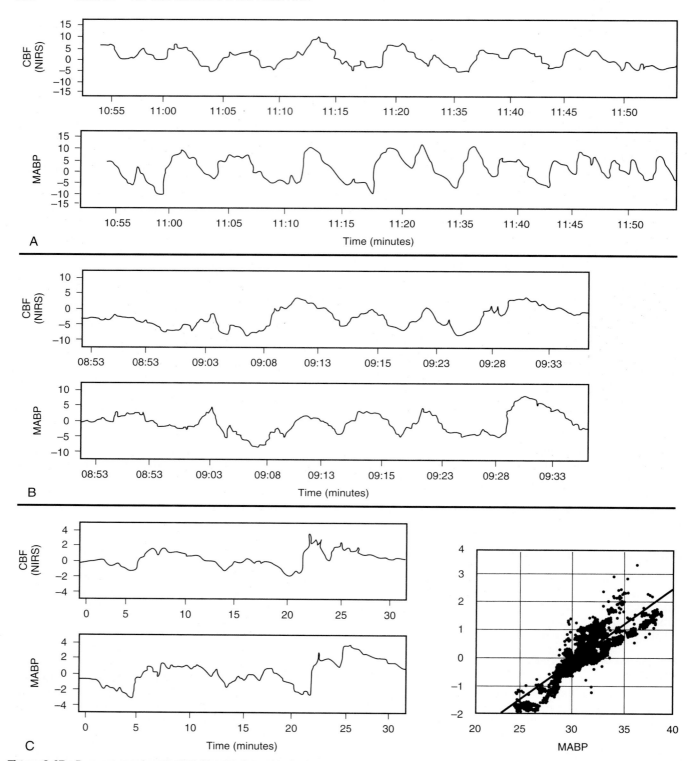

Figure 9-47   **Pressure-passive relationship of cerebral blood flow (CDF), estimated by near-infrared spectroscopy (NIRS; see Chapter 6), and mean arterial blood pressure (MABP), in ventilated premature infants.** Note the parallel changes in arterial blood pressure and cerebral perfusion (**A** to **C**). Note also that the changes in blood pressure are not marked. In **C**, all data points are plotted; the linear relationship between blood pressure and cerebral perfusion is apparent. *(From Tsuji M, Saul JP, du Plessis A, Eichenwald E, et al: Cerebral intravascular oxygenation correlates with mean arterial pressure in critically ill premature infants,* Pediatrics *106:625–632, 2000.)*

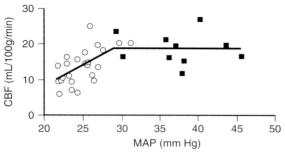

Figure 9-48 **Analysis of cerebral autoregulation in extremely-low-birth-weight infants (mean, 772 g).** Infants studied were either clinically normotensive *(closed squares)* or were clinically hypotensive and studied just before treatment with dopamine *(open circles)*. A break-point in the autoregulation curve relating cerebral blood flow (CBF), determined by near-infrared spectroscopy, to mean arterial blood pressure (MAP) was identified at MAP = 29 mm Hg. *(From Munro MJ, Barfield CP, Walker AM: Hypotensive extremely low birth weight infants have reduced cerebral blood flow, Pediatrics 114:1591–1596, 2004.)*

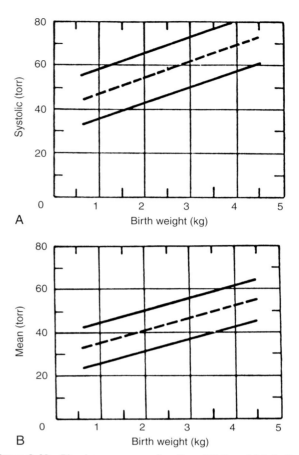

Figure 9-49 **Blood pressure as a function of birth weight. A,** Systolic and, **B,** mean arterial blood pressure (in the first 12 hours of life) as a function of birth weight. *(From Versmold HT, Kitterman JA, Phibbs RH, Gregory GA, et al: Aortic blood pressure during the first 12 hours of life in infants with birth weight 610 to 4,220 grams, Pediatrics 67:607–613, 1981.)*

31 mm Hg were associated with impaired EEG continuity, perhaps related to decreased CBF at such values.[956] Similarly in a study of extremely-low-birth-weight infants (mean birth weight, 772 g; mean gestational age, 26 weeks) by near-infrared spectroscopy, a pressure-passive cerebral circulation resulted when mean arterial blood pressures were less than 30 mm Hg.[953] (Fig. 9-48). However, to what extent, if any, arterial blood pressures lower than 30 mm Hg are clearly dangerous is unclear. Thus, a careful study of cerebral electrical activity and cerebral fractional oxygen extraction, presumably a reflection in part of the adequacy of CBF, in 35 23- to 30-week premature infants showed no electrical abnormality at mean blood pressures higher than 23 mm Hg.[957] Clearly, more data combining cerebral hemodynamic and functional parameters are needed.

Recognition of Normal Arterial Blood Pressure Levels in the Newborn

A series of studies has investigated normal values for arterial blood pressure in the newborn.[958-973a] In the first 12 hours of life, an inverse relationship between birth weight and blood pressure was shown (Table 9-45 and Fig. 9-49). Although this relationship continued over the next 2 days, a postnatal increase in mean blood pressure also was apparent. In a study of 131 premature infants in a neonatal intensive care unit, mean blood pressure over the first 96 hours was described by a linear function (mean blood pressure = 31.6 + (0.1 hours age) + (0.0057

birth weight).[971] It is clear that awareness of these dynamically changing normal values is important for management. In the study depicted in Table 9-45 (n = 131), 43% of the group had mean blood pressures lower than the 10th percentile for weight and postnatal age for 2 consecutive hours at some time during the first 96 hours of life.[971] In a recent study of 90 infants who weighed less than 1500 g at birth, hypotension, defined in this way, was particularly common in the smallest infants, with periods of hypotension exceeding 80% of the epochs studied on days 3 to 5.[955]

TABLE 9-45	Mean Arterial Blood Pressure as a Function of Birth Weight and Postnatal Age					
	HOURS POSTNATAL AGE					
Birth Weight (g)	**3**	**12**	**24**	**48**	**72**	**96**
500	35 (23)*	36 (24)	37 (25)	39 (28)	42 (30)	44 (33)
1000	38 (26)	39 (27)	40 (28)	42 (31)	45 (33)	47 (35)
1500	40 (29)	43 (30)	43 (31)	45 (33)	48 (36)	50 (38)

*Values are for mean blood pressure and, *in parentheses, the 10th percentile for the birth weight and postnatal age.*
Data from Watkins AM, West CR, Cooke RW: Blood pressure and cerebral haemorrhage and ischaemia in very low birthweight infants, *Early Hum Dev* 19:103–110, 1989.

Avoidance of Systemic Hypotension

In view of the aforementioned considerations concerning pressure-passive cerebral circulation and neonatal blood pressure data, it is clear that systemic hypotension must be avoided because of the danger of cerebral hypoperfusion (see Table 9-44). Moreover, because "normal" arterial blood pressure values in the newborn are relatively low and may be dangerously close to the downslope of even an intact autoregulatory curve, the *margin of safety* for arterial blood pressure sufficient to maintain adequate cerebral perfusion is likely to be small. As noted in Chapter 8 concerning pathogenesis, brain regions that are particularly vulnerable include the parasagittal cerebral areas in the term newborn and the periventricular white matter in the premature (and to a lesser extent in the term) newborn. The particular importance of *duration* as well as severity of hypotension in the genesis of brain injury in the premature newborn was shown clearly by a study of 98 infants.[974] Thus, the cumulative effects of hypotension should be watched for and avoided. As noted earlier, the unresolved question, especially in the premature infant, is the definition of hypotension. Common definitions include values of mean arterial blood pressure lower than the 10th percentile for birth weight and postnatal age (see Table 9-45), lower than the infant's gestational age, or less than 30 mm Hg. The most important definition of hypotension, of course, is the blood pressure below which functional or structural injury is likely. This value is generally unknown and likely varies according to multiple associated clinical factors in a given infant.

The principal *causes* of serious systemic hypotension in the asphyxiated infant are *cardiogenic*. Evidence of ischemia to papillary muscle, subendocardial region, and myocardium more diffusely has been demonstrated in asphyxiated infants.[975-983] In a study of 20 asphyxiated term infants, 8 exhibited myocardial dysfunction in the first 2 postnatal days, and this dysfunction was associated with both reduced cardiac output and lower mean CBF velocity than observed on recovery at 3 days.[983] In one study of 86 premature infants (<2000 g) with some evidence of asphyxia (i.e., Apgar scores <3 at 1 minute and <6 at 5 minutes), minimum systolic and diastolic blood pressures were significantly lower postnatally than in infants with normal Apgar scores, and infants with the low Apgar scores who died had lower pressures than those who survived.[970] Cardiogenic shock associated with perinatal asphyxia in the preterm infant was shown to respond to inotropic agents, and in a controlled study of term asphyxiated infants, dopamine was shown to increase cardiac performance and systolic blood pressure.[984,985] However, the mode and the timing of interventions for low blood pressures are controversial.[973,986-988b] The relative roles of volume expansion, dopamine, dobutamine, phosphodiesterase III inhibitors (e.g., milrinone), and corticosteroids are currently under active study.[986-991] Detailed discussion is beyond the scope of this book.

Other important causes of systemic hypotension and apparent impairment of CBF with implications for management include, particularly, patent ductus arteriosus and recurrent apneic spells. In *patent ductus arteriosus*, use of the transcutaneous Doppler ultrasound technique at the anterior fontanelle has shown a marked decrease in CBF velocity during patency of the ductus and an increase after spontaneous, medical (indomethacin), or surgical closure.[992-1000] In many infants, retrograde flow can be documented during diastole. The changes in the cerebral circulation are apparently caused by diminutions in systemic blood pressure, diastolic more than systolic, and by diastolic "runoff" through the ductus. The findings led us to postulate the possibility of "ductal steal" in the premature infant.[992] The demonstration of a markedly higher incidence of PVL (ultrasonographic criteria) among infants with patent ductus arteriosus when retrograde flow in diastole is present supports this notion.[997] It is reasonable to consider whether patent ductus arteriosus, under certain circumstances, may *contribute* to the occurrence of ischemic brain injury in the infant. Whether the apparent value of indomethacin in prevention of intraventricular hemorrhage and improvement of cognitive outcome in male infants[1001,1002] is relevant in this context is possible but not established (see Chapter 11). Indomethacin appears to have a beneficial effect in decreasing cerebral white matter injury, even in the absence of patent ductus arteriosus (see later).[1003] More data are needed on these issues.

Of additional implications for management are data suggesting that serious impairments in cerebral perfusion occur during *apneic spells* and may result from the impaired cardiac function with these spells. In a study of 101 apneic episodes in preterm infants, we observed a striking relationship between decreases in CBF velocity and severity of bradycardia during the apneic episodes (Fig. 9-50).[1004] With bradycardia of 100 beats/minute or less, a prominent decrease in CBF velocity became obvious, and with bradycardia of 80 beats/minute or

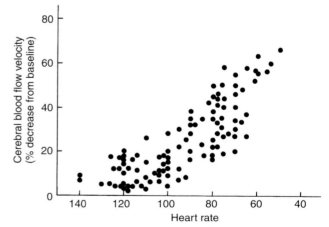

Figure 9-50 **Effect of apnea and bradycardia on cerebral blood flow velocity**. Cerebral blood flow velocity, quantitated as area under the velocity curve, is shown as a function of heart rate with apnea in 15 premature infants. Individual values for 101 separate episodes of apnea and bradycardia are shown. *(From Perlman JM, Volpe JJ: Episodes of apnea and bradycardia in the preterm newborn: Impact on cerebral circulation, Pediatrics 76:333–338, 1985.)*

less, the decrease was marked. The decreases in heart rate were accompanied by decreases in blood pressure, and the latter appeared to cause the changes in the cerebral circulation. Several studies of preterm infants during apnea and bradycardia by near-infrared spectroscopy confirmed the decrease in apparent CBF.[898,1005-1007] When the disturbance in CBF is coupled with the hypoxemia that has been shown to accompany the spells, the dangers to the brain are obvious. Additionally, earlier clinical data showed that the incidence of spastic diplegia is increased in infants with apnea and severe bradycardia.[548] In view of the observations reviewed earlier that correlate spastic diplegia with PVL, the major ischemic lesion of the preterm infant (see "Clinicopathological Correlation" section), the possibility that apneic episodes with severe bradycardia contribute to ischemic brain injury becomes strong. The implication for therapy is obvious: intervention appears to be needed urgently for episodes with bradycardia of 80 beats/minute or less, and in view of the data recorded in Figure 9-50, urgent intervention may be indicated for episodes with bradycardia of 80 to 100 beats/minute.

Avoidance of Systemic Hypertension

The other side of the coin regarding the issue of cerebral ischemia just discussed is cerebral overperfusion. Because of the pressure-passive cerebral circulation, increases in systemic blood pressure, especially abrupt increases, could lead to rupture of certain vulnerable capillaries and thereby to hemorrhagic complications (see Table 9-44). The causes of such elevations in blood pressure, discussed in more detail in Chapter 11, range from apparently innocuous events such as simple handling of the infant to more obvious events such as overly exuberant administration of volume expanders or pressor agents, seizures, pneumothorax, or abrupt closure of patent ductus arteriosus. In the full-term infant, vulnerable capillaries include those at the margins of cerebral infarcts, and thus hemorrhagic infarction could occur. In the premature infant, vulnerable capillaries in the germinal matrix could rupture and result in intraventricular hemorrhage, or those in the region of PVL could burst and produce massive hemorrhagic lesions in cerebral white matter (see Chapter 11). The essential point is that arterial blood pressure must be monitored carefully, and events that lead to abrupt increases in arterial blood pressure must be prevented or corrected promptly.

An additional problem of systemic hypertension in this context is the possibility of occurrence of *ischemic* injury in association with treatment of *chronic* hypertension. The latter is not uncommon in premature infants with bronchopulmonary dysplasia.[1004,1008] In one series of nine infants with chronic hypertension, when previously effective antihypertensive therapy unexpectedly decreased blood pressure markedly and for a mean duration of 17 hours in four patients, oliguria and neurological abnormalities, particularly seizures but also infarction in one case, developed.[1009] The blood pressure, although sharply decreased with the episodes, was not outside the normal range. The data suggest that the cerebrovascular autoregulatory curve was shifted to the right with chronic hypertension, as described in experimental models and in human adults with hypertension,[1010-1013] and rendered the infant vulnerable to decreases in blood pressure not necessarily out of the normal range. Thus, caution is necessary in the treatment of chronic hypertension in the newborn to avoid ischemic complications.

Avoidance of Hyperviscosity

Hyperviscosity, secondary to polycythemia, may occur in the asphyxiated infant[1014,1015] and can compromise cerebral perfusion (see Table 9-44). Hyperviscosity is a recognized cause of impaired CBF in adults.[1016] That this phenomenon can occur in the human newborn is supported by the demonstration of the following: (1) increased cerebrovascular resistance and diminished CBF velocity, determined by Doppler studies in polycythemic infants with hyperviscosity[1017-1020]; and (2) an inverse relationship between blood hemoglobin concentration and CBF, determined by xenon clearance techniques.[933,936,1021,1022] Moreover, improvement in CBF velocity has been shown after partial plasma exchange transfusion.[1017,1019] Additionally, decreased CBF was shown in neonatal piglets with hyperviscosity produced by infusion of cryoprecipitate.[1023] Finally, ischemic lesions, often complicated by hemorrhage, neurological clinical features (jitteriness, lethargy, apnea, and, uncommonly, seizures),[829,830,1024] and impaired cognitive outcome, possibly related to ischemic lesions, have been documented in infants with polycythemia and hyperviscosity.[1020,1025,1026]

Treatment of symptomatic polycythemic infants with partial exchange transfusion is indicated and is beneficial in reducing neurological sequelae. Whether exchange transfusion is beneficial for asymptomatic infants with polycythemia (venous hematocrit >65%) and hyperviscosity (viscosity measurements >2 SD above the mean) is less clear. Each case must be considered separately, but partial exchange transfusion often is recommended if venous hematocrit exceeds 65%, even if the infant is asymptomatic. The critical point is that polycythemia and hyperviscosity must be considered and detected so that therapy can be carried out promptly.

Maintenance of Adequate Glucose Levels

The roles for endogenous glucose stores, particularly *at the time* of the asphyxial insult, and for the addition of exogenous glucose after the insult, remain to be established clearly for the human infant. In Chapter 6, I review the available information based on experiments in immature and mature animals. The former experiments suggest, although not uniformly, a generally beneficial effect of glucose, and the latter experiments suggest a deleterious effect. These experiments are relevant particularly to the treatment of the asphyxiated human *fetus* and, thus, the management of labor and delivery, detailed consideration of which is not within the province of this book.

TABLE 9-46	Maintenance of Adequate Blood Glucose Levels

Maintain a blood glucose concentration of approximately 75 to 100 mg/dL.
Avoid hypoglycemia because it may cause neuronal injury.
Avoid marked hyperglycemia because it may provoke hemorrhage (through a hyperosmolar effect) or may worsen cerebral lactic acidosis.

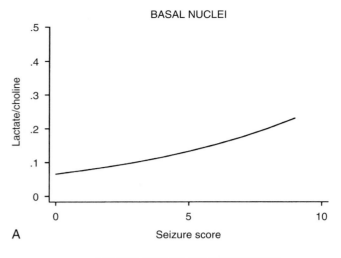

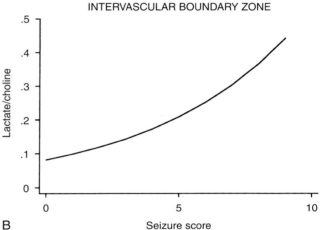

Figure 9-51 **Effect of severity of seizures on regional abnormalities of cerebral metabolites.** Ninety term newborns were studied by proton magnetic resonance spectroscopy on median day of life 6. Seizure severity was scored based on seizure frequency and duration, electroencephalographic findings, and number of anticonvulsant medications. Both graphs show a linear relationship between seizure score and lactate/choline ratio in basal nuclei (lentiform nucleus and thalamus) and in the intervascular boundary zones. *(From Miller SP, Weiss J, Barnwell A, Ferriero DM, et al: Seizure-associated brain injury in term newborns with perinatal asphyxia, Neurology 58:542–548, 2002.)*

The precise role of glucose in the management of the infant who *already has experienced an asphyxial insult* needs to be defined further. As described in detail in Chapter 6, studies in perinatal models of hypoxic-ischemic insults indicate that the effects of glucose administration vary considerably, perhaps because of species and other methodological differences. Neuropathological injury has been reported to be prevented, ameliorated, or accentuated in different models. Improved survival with glucose administration is generally consistent and may relate at least partially to improvement in cardiorespiratory function. Determinations of cerebral lactate and high-energy phosphates by MR spectroscopy as a function of blood glucose in asphyxiated human newborns would aid formulation of recommendations concerning glucose supplementation. On balance, I believe that the available data warrant the recommendation that glucose supplementation be adjusted to maintain a blood glucose level between approximately 75 and 100 mg/dL (Table 9-46).

Control of Seizures

Therapy for seizures begins with careful serial observations to detect clinical seizure activity (Table 9-47; see Chapter 5). Seizures, an accompaniment of the majority of cases of serious hypoxic-ischemic encephalopathy, may cause further injury to brain. For example, in one detailed study of 90 term infants with perinatal asphyxia, each increase in seizure severity score was independently associated with an increase in lactate and a decrease in NAA, assessed by MR spectroscopy (see Chapter 5) (Fig. 9-51).[476] Seizures are associated with a *markedly accelerated cerebral metabolic rate*, and if, as indicated earlier, cerebral metabolism is not operating at optimal aerobic capacity (e.g., because of mitochondrial injury), this acceleration may lead to a rapid fall in brain glucose, an increase in lactate, and a decrease in high-energy phosphate compounds. Moreover, the excessive synaptic release of certain excitotoxic amino acids (e.g., glutamate) also may lead to cellular injury.

TABLE 9-47	Control of Seizures

Recognition of seizure phenomena
Urgency of treatment related to potentially deleterious effects of seizures
Phenobarbital preferred drug as first agent
Potential future therapies: phenobarbital and bumetanide, topiramate

In addition, seizures are associated frequently with hypoventilation and apnea with consequent *hypoxemia and hypercarbia*, the dangers of which have been discussed. Studies with transcutaneous tissue electrodes suggest that these latter changes may occur with seizures that are so subtle that they are readily missed clinically. In addition, neonatal seizures are associated with *abrupt elevations in arterial blood pressure* (see Chapter 5), and hence the possibility of inducing hemorrhage, within either areas of infarction or the germinal matrix (see Chapter 11). Moreover, studies of ischemia in the term fetal lamb indicate that epileptiform activity is a prominent feature in the hours following the insult (maximum at 10 hours, duration of 72 hours) and that cortical neuronal necrosis occurs in the same cortical areas and to a degree that correlates with the extent of epileptiform activity.[1027] Moreover, our own experience and that of others indicate that infants with poorly controlled seizures have more frequent and severe neurological sequelae than infants whose seizures are well controlled.[11,476,1028,1029] Obviously, this difference may relate to the severity of the initial injury rather than to additional injury from repetitive seizures. Indeed, studies in neonatal rats subjected to hypoxia-ischemia and subsequent chemically induced seizures at 2, 6, and 12 hours of recovery showed no accentuation of brain damage compared with histopathological findings in rats subjected to hypoxia-ischemia without induced seizures.[1030-1032] However, the convulsing animals developed hypoglycemia and a mortality rate of 53%, both of which could be improved by glucose supplementation.[1030] Nevertheless, on balance, the data do raise the possibility of a deleterious effect of multiple seizures in the infant with hypoxic-ischemic encephalopathy and demand prospective and controlled study of this issue. Careful attention to glucose homeostasis clearly is critical in this context.

Phenobarbital remains the preferred drug for the treatment of seizures in neonatal hypoxic-ischemic encephalopathy; details of the administration of this drug are described in Chapter 5. The *timing* of treatment has been somewhat controversial. *Pretreatment* with barbiturates (i.e., before the onset of seizures) has been considered because of studies in adult animals that barbiturates in high doses are beneficial in ischemia (by causing reduction of cerebral metabolic rate, cerebral vasoconstriction, reduction of brain edema, or removal of harmful free radicals)[1033-1038] and studies in *perinatal animals* that suggest a beneficial effect in several nonprimate species and in term fetal monkeys.[931,1039-1046] In the study of the fetal monkey by Cockburn and co-workers,[1045] anesthetic doses of pentobarbital that were administered to the mothers produced *anesthesia* in the fetuses, which were then delivered and asphyxiated experimentally. When compared with animals delivered under local anesthesia before asphyxia, the barbiturate-treated animals had prolongation of time to last gasp, accelerated establishment of rhythmic breathing after resuscitation, and less histological evidence of neuronal injury. In the only study of *neonatal monkeys* treated with barbiturates *after birth* but before asphyxia, no beneficial effect on time to last gasp, survival, or CBF could be detected.[1047] In this study, a 20-mg/kg dose of phenobarbital was administered in the 18 hours before asphyxia, and animals were *sedated but not anesthetized*, a potentially important difference from the study of Cockburn and co-workers.[1045] No experimental studies have been reported in which barbiturates have been administered *after* a perinatal asphyxial insult.

Studies of pretreatment of asphyxiated term infants with barbiturates (i.e., before the occurrence of seizures) have shown interesting but not entirely consistent results.[1048,1049] In one randomized controlled trial of 32 severely asphyxiated term infants, thiopental was administered initially at a mean age of 2.3 hours and then by constant infusion over 24 hours.[1049] Seizures occurred in approximately 75% of both treated and control infants. Moreover, mortality rate and

neurological outcome were similar in the two groups. Of concern is that hypotension occurred in nearly 90% of the treated group and required pressor agents in 30%.

An earlier study, which employed a slightly smaller number of severely asphyxiated infants, suggested benefit for relatively high doses of phenobarbital administered shortly after birth.[1050] Fourteen infants were treated within 60 minutes of delivery with phenobarbital (10 mg/kg, followed in 4 hours by 10 mg/kg/day), in addition to assisted ventilation, glucocorticoid, and fresh frozen plasma. (Another group of 16 infants did not receive glucocorticoid or fresh frozen plasma therapy and were given phenobarbital only if seizures did not respond to diazepam.) Plasma levels of phenobarbital in the early-treated infants were approximately 25 µg/mL on the first day and rose to a peak of 40 to 70 µg/mL on the second and third days. Respiratory "insufficiency" was noted at levels higher than approximately 40 µg/mL, and phenobarbital administration "may have prolonged ventilator treatment in some infants."[1050] When compared with infants not treated early with phenobarbital, the early phenobarbital-treated infants had lower mortality rates (14% vs. 50%) and a more frequent normal outcome in survivors (83% vs. 50%). Obviously, the numbers are small, the groups were not comparably treated with respect to factors other than phenobarbital, and the side effects are disturbing.

A later study evaluated the effect of administration of 40 mg/kg of phenobarbital to term infants with "severe asphyxia" (initial arterial pH $\leq$ 7.0 and base deficit of 15 mEq/L or more, Apgar score $\leq$3 at 5 minutes of age, or failure to initiate spontaneous respirations by 10 minutes of age) at a mean age of 6 hours and before the onset of clinical seizures.[1051] Seizures occurred in 9 of 15 treated infants versus 14 of 16 "control" infants (P = .11). At 3 years of age, normal outcome was noted in 11 of 15 treated infants versus only 3 of 16 control infants (P = .003). Thus, although early onset of high-dose phenobarbital therapy was not associated with a statistically significant reduction in the occurrence of seizures, a beneficial effect on neurological outcome was suggested. Further data would be of interest.

Currently, I do not administer phenobarbital routinely before the onset of clinical or electrographic seizures. However, I recommend close observation of the infant and liberal use of the EEG tracing to identify seizures. When available, use of continuous EEG is optimal for management of the asphyxiated infant. When frequent or prolonged electrical seizures are present, I recommend onset of therapy with phenobarbital. Although doses are described in Chapter 5, phenobarbital generally is administered intravenously, with a loading dose of 20 mg/kg, and if seizures are controlled, a maintenance dose of 3 to 4 mg/kg/day is begun 12 hours later. Additional or persistent seizures, as commonly occur, are treated with additional phenobarbital to a maximum loading dose of 40 mg/kg. However, if there is clear indication of hepatic dysfunction, instead of additional phenobarbital, I have used phenytoin and, if necessary, lorazepam, as described in Chapter 5.

Phenobarbital frequently is not optimally effective in the severely asphyxiated infant. This situation results most probably because (1) phenobarbital is a gamma-aminobutyric acid (GABA) agonist, (2) GABA receptors tend to be excitatory in the newborn brain because of high intracellular chloride levels, and (3) the expression of the NKCC1 transporter for chloride influx is activated after hypoxia-ischemia (see Chapter 5).[1052] However, because the agent most often is at least partially effective, I continue to recommend it as first-line agent. It is interesting to speculate that the addition of bumetanide, a diuretic and inhibitor of NKCC1, could render phenobarbital more effective by leading to a decrease in intracellular chloride. More data are needed. Additionally, because another anticonvulsant drug, topiramate, is effective in blocking both neuronal and oligodendroglial injury in neonatal hypoxic-ischemic animal models, this drug could prove especially beneficial. Unfortunately, currently an intravenous preparation of topiramate is not available.

Control of Brain Swelling

The treatment of brain swelling in neonatal hypoxic-ischemic encephalopathy generally is *not* a major concern. As discussed in Chapter 8, neuropathological data indicate that brain swelling is not an early primary event in either the premature or term infant with hypoxic-ischemic encephalopathy, may occur after the first day of life in the term infant in proportion to the degree of tissue necrosis, but is not associated with evidence of transtentorial or transmagnal herniation. Clinical studies, based on serial ICP monitoring by either noninvasive transfontanellar or invasive subarachnoid transducers, indicate that although increased ICP may occur, it develops on the second and third postnatal days in association with tissue necrosis.[87,88,1049,1053-1056] Presumably, this ICP reflects brain swelling secondary to the necrosis, but a contribution of increased intravascular volume from the increased CBF that correlates with poor outcome and occurs with a similar time course is possible (see earlier discussion). The frequency of raised ICP is relatively low; in one study of 32 asphyxiated term newborns, ICP higher than 10 mm Hg occurred in only 22%.[87] Moreover, cerebral perfusion pressure rarely is compromised, and when low cerebral perfusion pressure does occur, it is related to arterial hypotension.[87,88,1049,1054] Thus, although the problem of brain swelling and increased ICP is uncommon, several aspects of management should be considered briefly. These include principally prevention of fluid overload and consideration of more specific therapies for brain swelling (Table 9-48).

Prevention of Fluid Overload

The cornerstone of prevention of serious brain swelling in the asphyxiated newborn infant is *avoidance of fluid overload* (see Table 9-48). Even in the infant with modest tissue injury and secondary brain swelling, a serious increase in brain water content and neurological deterioration may result if excessive fluids are

---

TABLE 9-48 **Control of Brain Swelling**

Prevention of fluid overload: Recognize inappropriate antidiuretic hormone secretion.

Consider therapies for brain swelling if cerebral perfusion is threatened by increased ICP (CPP ≈ MABP − ICP) or if signs of impending transtentorial or transmagnal herniation are present.

CPP, cerebral perfusion pressure; ICP, intracranial pressure; MABP, mean arterial blood pressure.

---

administered. This is particularly the case because the asphyxiated infant may experience *inappropriate ADH secretion* in the first 3 days after an asphyxial insult.[1057-1059] This syndrome has been manifested by hyponatremia (e.g., 110 to 120 mEq/L) and corresponding hypo-osmolality, inappropriately elevated urine osmolality, and continued renal excretion of sodium in the absence of dehydration and in the presence of elevated levels of ADH. Seizures and a bulging anterior fontanelle are the prominent clinical signs, apparently related to the water intoxication. The propensity of the asphyxiated infant for fluid retention *without* the complete syndrome just described is illustrated by a systematic study of 13 asphyxiated term infants; plasma levels of arginine vasopressin were increased over controls by approximately 75-fold on postnatal day 1 and by approximately 15-fold on day 2.[1060] Additionally, the syndrome of inappropriate ADH secretion may be followed by central diabetes insipidus (or the latter may occur alone).[1058] The cause of these disturbances of neurohypophyseal function is unknown, but the hypothalamus is a site of predilection for selective neuronal injury with neonatal hypoxic-ischemic encephalopathy (see Chapter 8). Therefore, careful management of fluids, with avoidance of fluid overload, is important to prevent major degrees of brain swelling and the metabolic derangements associated with water intoxication.

Consideration of Therapies for Brain Swelling

Therapy for brain swelling is reasonable to consider if ICP is shown to be elevated and *if this elevation is likely to impair cerebral perfusion pressure* (see Table 9-48). The latter determination (i.e., imminent impairment of cerebral perfusion pressure) requires knowledge of the level of cerebral perfusion pressure necessary to maintain structural integrity. This level currently is not known definitively. In one study, asphyxiated term infants exhibited a normal outcome with a value for lowest neonatal cerebral perfusion pressure of 33 mm Hg, neurological sequelae with a value of 18 mm Hg, and death with a value of 8 mm Hg.[1061] These investigators suggested that a cerebral perfusion pressure of 25 mm Hg or lower (lower than the third percentile for age) in a term infant "must be viewed with great concern." A subsequent study of asphyxiated infants noted lower scores on the Bayley Scales of Infant Development on follow-up in infants whose mean cerebral perfusion pressure was less than 25 mm Hg.[1049] However, other reports have not observed a close relationship between cerebral perfusion pressure and neurological injury.[87,88,1054] Clearly, more data are needed on the issue of a critical threshold of cerebral perfusion pressure and the duration of time below that threshold required to produce neurological injury. *On balance, available data suggest that arterial hypotension is a much more important factor in producing serious compromises in cerebral perfusion than is elevated ICP.*

Therapies usually considered for brain swelling include principally glucocorticoids (e.g., dexamethasone) or osmotic agents (e.g., mannitol). Currently, no good evidence warrants recommendation for the use of glucocorticoids for this purpose. A role for osmotic agents such as *mannitol* may be suggested because the edema with hypoxic-ischemic injury is primarily cytotoxic, and because osmotic agents are largely confined to the vascular space, benefit may be possible. Indeed, administration of mannitol to term infants with moderate or severe hypoxic-ischemic encephalopathy and increased ICP leads to a decrease in pressure (of ≈ 35%), which is sustained for several hours.[1053,1054] However, no controlled data indicate that such treatment alters outcome. In one controlled study, administration of mannitol in a single dose to asphyxiated infants had no beneficial clinical effect.[1056] An earlier, uncontrolled study also did not provide definitive data for a beneficial effect of mannitol. A careful experimental investigation of hypoxic-ischemic brain injury in the immature rat also showed that mannitol administration could cause a decrease in brain edema (brain water content) but did not alter severity of brain injury.[1062] Thus, I do not currently recommend the routine use of mannitol in the management of neonatal hypoxic-ischemic encephalopathy, even when severe. When measurements of cerebral perfusion pressure indicate declining values, careful attention should be paid to systemic blood pressure, because arterial hypotension is a common cause, perhaps the most common cause, of decreases in cerebral perfusion pressure after asphyxia (see earlier discussion). I would consider therapy with mannitol if cerebral perfusion pressure is threatened markedly because of clearly elevated ICP and if clinical deterioration is not related to marked preexisting cerebral necrosis (see Table 9-48). For more than 25 years, I have not recommended the use of mannitol in any infant with hypoxic-ischemic encephalopathy.

Neuroprotective Interventions

As described in detail in Chapters 6 and 8, the principal mechanisms of neuronal death in hypoxic-ischemic encephalopathy operate after termination of the insult, are initiated by activation of glutamate receptors, occur over hours, and involve accumulation of cytosolic calcium and activation of a variety of calcium-mediated deleterious events, including especially generation of free radicals, such as superoxide anion, hydroxyl radical, and nitric oxide derivatives. Free radical–mediated cell death also appears to be the final common pathway for oligodendroglial death (see Chapters 6 and 8). *The exciting implication concerning management is that interruption of this deleterious cascade,*

TABLE 9-49	Neuroprotective Interventions Implemented in the Human Fetus and Newborn*
Phenobarbital	
Calcium channel blocker	
Magnesium	
Free radical scavenger	
Indomethacin	
Mild hypothermia	

*See text for details.

even after termination of the insult, could prevent or ameliorate the brain injury in perinatal hypoxic-ischemic disease. In Chapter 6, potential neuroprotective interventions shown to be of value in a variety of experimental models of hypoxia-ischemia are discussed and are listed in Table 6-19. Moreover, potential protective interventions for oligodendroglial injury are considered and reviewed in Figure 6-43. In this section, I discuss only those agents studied in human newborns (Table 9-49). One of these agents (phenobarbital) is reviewed earlier concerning treatment of seizures. The other modalities studied in human infants and considered here are calcium channel blockers, magnesium sulfate, free radical scavengers, indomethacin, and mild hypothermia.

Calcium Channel Blockers

Because a central mediator of the cascade to neuronal death is elevated cytosolic calcium, caused in part by enhanced calcium influx, the possibility of a protective effect of calcium channel blockers has been investigated (see Table 9-49). Experimental studies show some benefit. However, a single small study of a calcium channel blocker in treatment of severely asphyxiated infants indicated that further understanding of the toxicity of these agents is necessary before a beneficial effect can be expected.[1063] I am unaware of any current studies of the use of calcium channel blockers in asphyxiated human infants.

Magnesium

Magnesium sulfate has been used for many years in obstetrics as a tocolytic agent for preterm labor and as therapy for preeclampsia. The evidence of its effectiveness for the latter purpose is stronger than that concerning its role as a tocolytic (see Chapter 11). Particular interest for the maternal use of magnesium sulfate in the prevention of neurological deficits in infants born prematurely began with a report that only 7.1% of very-low-birth-weight infants with later cerebral palsy were exposed to maternal magnesium sulfate versus 36% of a control group.[1064] In a subsequent study of approximately 1000 premature infants, those whose mothers received magnesium sulfate had a lower prevalence of cerebral palsy (0.9%) than those whose mothers did not receive this agent (7.7%).[1065] However, subsequent evidence regarding benefit for magnesium sulfate for prevention of cerebral palsy or associated brain lesions or both has not been consistently positive.[1066-1079b]

Study of asphyxiated term infants administered magnesium sulfate postnatally is limited. One report of 22 such infants showed no benefit on aEEG patterns in the neonatal period.[1080]

Experimental studies concerning a beneficial role for magnesium in prevention or amelioration of hypoxic-ischemic death also have yielded conflicting results. Thus, in perinatal hypoxic-ischemic models in the rat, piglet, and fetal lamb, magnesium sulfate treatment either during or immediately following the insult did not ameliorate adverse biochemical (secondary, delayed energy failure), neurophysiological (EEG suppression, seizures), or neuropathological (neuronal necrosis) effects.[1081-1083] Nevertheless, other experimental work supported the potential value of magnesium by several mechanisms (i.e., antiexcitotoxic amino acid [impairs release, blocks the NMDA receptor], antioxidant [essential for glutathione biosynthesis], anticytokine [decreases levels of inflammatory cytokines], and antiplatelet [decreases platelet aggregation] effects).[1084-1090] Perhaps the most likely beneficial effect of magnesium relates to its strong vasodilatory properties, which can lead to an increase in uteroplacental blood flow and perhaps also to improved fetal perfusion.[1091-1095] Such effects also could decrease the likelihood that the infant postnatally would experience a pressure-passive cerebral circulation and thereby cerebral ischemia and periventricular white matter injury (see Chapters 6 and 8).

In summary, at the time of this writing, the potential value of maternal receipt of magnesium sulfate in prevention of the brain injury that results in neurological deficits in premature infants is unresolved. A similar conclusion is warranted concerning postnatal treatment of term asphyxiated infants.

Indomethacin

The possibility that the use of indomethacin for a prolonged course of treatment (≥ 4 days) versus a short course (≤ 3 days) leads to prevention of cerebral white matter injury in premature newborns of 24 to 28 weeks of gestation was suggested by a recent study.[1003] Thus, in a prospective study of 57 infants who were treated with indomethacin to prevent the development of a hemodynamically significant, symptomatic patent ductus arteriosus, a prolonged course of treatment was used when the short course was not effective in closure of the ductus. White matter injury was identified by MRI and was classified as moderate to severe when T1 signal abnormalities were larger than 2 mm or more than three areas of T1 abnormality were noted. Infants who received a short course of indomethacin had a 38% incidence of moderate to severe white matter injury versus only 4% in those who received a prolonged course (Table 9-50).

The basis for the beneficial effect of indomethacin is not known. Patent ductus arteriosus closure did not appear to account for the effect because benefit for prolonged indomethacin course was noted even in the absence of patent ductus.[1003] Possible relevant effects of indomethacin include widening of the range of cerebral vascular autoregulation, prevention of

TABLE 9-50 Preventative Effect of Indomethacin on Cerebral White Matter Injury in Premature Infants*

Indomethacin Treatment	Moderate to Severe White Matter Injury No./Total (Percentage)
Short course (≤ 3 days)	11/29 (38%)
Prolonged course (≥ 4 days)	1/24 (4%)

*White matter injury was determined by magnetic resonance imaging (see text). Infants were born after 24 to 28 weeks of gestation.
Data from Miller SP, Mayer EE, Clyman RI, Glidden DV, et al: Prolonged indomethacin exposure is associated with decreased white matter injury detected with magnetic resonance imaging in premature newborns at 24 to 28 weeks' gestation at birth, *Pediatrics* 117:1626–1631, 2006.

generation of free radicals at the cyclooxygenase step, or anti-inflammatory effects (see Chapter 6). Further data will be of great interest.

Free Radical Scavengers

Central to both hypoxic-ischemic neuronal and oligodendroglial cell death is attack by free radicals (see Chapter 6). Following promising findings in experimental hypoxic-ischemic models of free radical scavengers, a study of the effect of high-dose allopurinol, a xanthine oxidase inhibitor and free radical scavenger, on 11 asphyxiated term infants was performed.[1096] The data suggested a beneficial effect of allopurinol therapy on free radical formation (measured by assay of markers in plasma), cerebral hemodynamics (measured by near-infrared spectroscopy), and electrical brain activity (measured by a cerebral function monitor). Short-term outcome (death, neurological abnormalities at discharge) tended to be more favorable in the treated infants, but the difference did not achieve statistical significance. A more recent report also suggested benefit for allopurinol in asphyxiated term infants.[1097] Further data will be of interest.

Hypothermia

Although for many decades deep hypothermia to body temperatures less than 20° C has been shown to be valuable for neuroprotection during cardiac surgery with circulatory bypass or circulatory arrest, in recent years numerous experimental studies in a variety of models of perinatal hypoxia-ischemia showed a pronounced beneficial effect with induced hypothermia of only a few degrees (i.e., "mild" hypothermia; see Chapter 6). The *principal determinants of neuroprotective benefit* for mild hypothermia have related to *timing* (onset of hypothermia before delayed energy failure and excitatory features, such as seizures, i.e., ≈ 6 hours), *degree* (decrease of body temperature by 3° to 4° C), and *duration* (≈ 72 hours). The *mechanisms of benefit* appear to include decrease in energy consumption, decrease in accumulation of extracellular glutamate, decrease in generation of reactive oxygen and nitrogen species, inhibition of inflammatory mechanisms, and interruption of downstream molecular cascades to apoptosis (see Chapter 6). On the background of the promising results of mild

<table>
<tr><td colspan="4">**TABLE 9-51   Effects of Selective Head Cooling in Term Infants with Hypoxic-Ischemic Encephalopathy***</td></tr>
</table>

Outcome	Hypothermia	Control	*P* Value
Death	33%	38%	0.48
Severe neuromotor disability	19%	31%	0.12
Death or severe disability at 18 months			
Intermediate aEEG	48%	66%	0.02
Severe aEEG	68%	79%	0.51

*Total group included 218 infants with moderate to severe neonatal encephalopathy and abnormal aEEG. Other characteristics included the following: cord pH, 6.9; seizures, 60%; severe aEEG abnormality, 21%; intermediate aEEG abnormality, 79%. Onset of hypothermia, <5.5 hours, rectal temperature, 34° to 35° C, and duration of cooling, 72 hours.

aEEG, amplitude-integrated electroencephalography.

Data from Gluckman PD, Wyatt JS, Azzopardi D, Ballard R, et al: Selective head cooling with mild systemic hypothermia after neonatal encephalopathy: Multicentre randomised trial, *Lancet* 365:663–670, 2005.

<table>
<tr><td colspan="4">**TABLE 9-52   Effects of Whole Body Cooling in Term Infants with Hypoxic-Ischemic Encephalopathy***</td></tr>
</table>

Outcome	Hypothermia	Control	*P* Value
Death	24%	37%	0.08
Disabling cerebral palsy	19%	30%	0.20
Death or moderate or severe disability	44%	62%	0.01

*Total group included 208 infants with moderate or severe neonatal encephalopathy. Other characteristics included the following: cord pH, 6.8 to 6.9; seizures, 45%; severe encephalopathy, 35%; and moderate encephalopathy, 65%. Onset of hypothermia, 4.3 hours, esophageal temperature, 33.5° C; and duration of cooling, 72 hours.

Data from Shankaran S, Laptook AR, Ehrenkranz RA, Tyson JE, et al: Whole-body hypothermia for neonates with hypoxic-ischemic encephalopathy, *N Engl J Med* 353:1574–1584, 2005.

hypothermia in experimental models, multicenter randomized clinical trials in term infants with hypoxic-ischemic encephalopathy have reduced promising findings.[1098-1107a]

Two principal approaches have been used: selective head cooling (by a water-circulating cap, "Cool Cap") or whole body cooling (by water-circulating blankets). The first large-scale multicenter study reported involved *selective head cooling* (Table 9-51).[1102] The total group included 218 infants with moderate to severe encephalopathy and abnormal aEEG. Cooling was begun before 5.5 hours of age and continued for 72 hours. In the minority of infants (n = 46) who had *severe* aEEG abnormalities, no effect on death or severe disability at 18 months was observed. However, in the majority of infants who had *moderate* aEEG abnormalities (n = 172), a significantly lower rate of this unfavorable outcome was observed in the hypothermic group versus the control group (48% vs. 66%, *P* = .02).

Similarly promising results were obtained from the multicenter trial of *whole body cooling* (Table 9-52).[1105] The total group included 208 infants with moderate or severe encephalopathy; aEEG was not used in this study. Cooling was begun at a mean age of 4.3 hours to an esophageal temperature of 33.5° C and was continued for 72 hours. Death or moderate or severe disability occurred in 44% of the hypothermic infants versus 62% of the control infants (*P* = .01).

A third smaller multicenter trial, using whole body hypothermia, also showed benefit.[1103] Cooling was begun within 6 hours and was carried out with ice bags, followed by a cooling blanket, servocontrolled at a rectal temperature of 33° C, for 48 hours. Death or severe disability occurred in 52% of the hypothermic infants versus 84% of the control infants (*P* = .019).

In a meta-analysis of the three trials (N = 478), the relative risk of death or disability for hypothermia versus normothermia was 0.76 with a 95% confidence interval of 0.65 to 0.89.[1107] Further insights into the

magnitude of the benefit of hypothermia should be gained by three other multicenter trials currently in progress in Great Britain, Europe, and Australia.

Many critical issues remain to be resolved. These include the optimal selection criteria, particularly whether the use of aEEG is needed and whether infants who have the most severe disease should be subjected to hypothermia. Whether selective head cooling or whole body cooling is preferable is important, in part because experimental data suggest that optimal protection of cortex may occur at a lower temperature than for deep nuclear structures.[1108] A large MRI study of cooled infants was consistent with this finding,[1109] although a smaller study was not.[1110] Perhaps the most critical issue is whether a *combination* of hypothermia with a pharmacological agent would be synergistic. As discussed in Chapter 6, experimental studies suggest that topiramate, xenon, *N*-acetylcysteine, and a caspase inhibitor may be synergistic with partial hypothermia. More data are need.

Conclusions

The prospective studies of the *individual* agents and interventions discussed in the preceding sections and those likely to be evaluated in the future based on experimental data (see Table 6-19) are necessary and appropriate. However, it seems likely that *combinations* of agents, including those that affect different levels of the cascade to cell death described in Chapter 6, will prove optimal. Moreover, such combinations may include *sequential* administration, beginning intrapartum and continuing postnatally. App-roaches that are likely to affect common initiating mechanisms (e.g., cerebrovascular autoregulation, cerebral ischemia), as well as common downstream mechanisms (e.g., excitotoxicity, free radical attack, especially at multiple sites), will have particular value because both neuronal and oligodendroglial injury could be ameliorated. *Mild hypothermia, glutamate receptor blockers, and free radical scavengers are excellent examples of approaches that affect common downstream mechanisms at multiple sites.* Safety is of prime concern, and currently these approaches appear most promising to be safe as well as effective in the short-term future.

REFERENCES

1. Pierrat V, Haouari N, Liska A, Thomas D, et al: Prevalence, causes, and outcome at 2 years of age of newborn encephalopathy: Population based study, *Arch Dis Child Fetal Neonatal Ed* 90:F257-F261, 2005.
2. Brown JK, Purvis RJ, Forfar JO, Cockburn F: Neurological aspects of perinatal asphyxia, *Dev Med Child Neurol* 16:567-580, 1974.
3. Brown JK: Infants damaged during birth: Perinatal asphyxia. In Hull D, editor: *Recent Advances in Paediatrics*, London: 1976, Churchill Livingstone.
4. MacDonald HM, Mulligan JC, Allen AC, Taylor PM: Neonatal asphyxia. I. Relationship of obstetric and neonatal complications to neonatal mortality in 38,405 consecutive deliveries, *J Pediatr* 96:898-902, 1980.
5. Mulligan JC, Painter MJ, O'Donoghue PA, MacDonald HM, et al: Neonatal asphyxia. II. Neonatal mortality and long-term sequelae, *J Pediatr* 96:903-907, 1980.
6. Finer NN, Robertson CM, Richards RT, Pinnell LE, et al: Hypoxic-ischemic encephalopathy in term neonates: Perinatal factors and outcome, *J Pediatr* 98:112-117, 1981.
7. Low JA, Galbraith RS, Muir DW, Broekhoven LH, et al: The contribution of fetal-newborn complications to motor and cognitive deficits, *Dev Med Child Neurol* 27:578-587, 1985.
8. Low JA, Galbraith RS, Muir DW, Killen HL, et al: The relationship between perinatal hypoxia and newborn encephalopathy, *Am J Obstet Gynecol* 152:256-260, 1985.
9. Low JA, Robertson DM, Simpson LL: Temporal relationships of neuropathologic conditions caused by perinatal asphyxia, *Am J Obstet Gynecol* 160:608-614, 1989.
10. Patterson CA, Graves WL, Bugg G, Sasso SC, et al: Antenatal and intrapartum factors associated with the occurrence of seizures in term infant, *Obstet Gynecol* 74:361-365, 1989.
11. Robertson C, Finer N: Term infants with hypoxic-ischemic encephalopathy: Outcome at 3.5 years, *Dev Med Child Neurol* 27:473-484, 1985.
12. Barabas RE, Barmada MA, Scher MS: Timing of brain insults in severe neonatal encephalopathies with isoelectric EEG, *Pediatr Neurol* 9:39-44, 1993.
13. Stanley FJ, Blair E, Hockey A, Petterson B, et al: Spastic quadriplegia in western Australia: A genetic epidemiological study. I. Case population and perinatal risk factors, *Dev Med Child Neurol* 35:191-201, 1993.
14. Perlman JM, Risser R: Severe fetal acidemia: Neonatal neurologic features and short-term outcome, *Pediatr Neurol* 9:277-282, 1993.
15. Perlman JM, Risser R: Can asphyxiated infants at risk for neonatal seizures be rapidly identified by current high-risk markers? *Pediatrics* 97:456-462, 1996.
16. Gaffney G, Flavell V, Johnson A, Squier M, et al: Cerebral palsy and neonatal encephalopathy, *Arch Dis Child Fetal Neonatal Ed* 70:F195-F200, 1994.
17. Badawi N, Kurinczuk JJ, Keogh JM, Alessandri LM, et al: Antepartum risk factors for newborn encephalopathy: The Western Australian case-control study, *BMJ* 317:1549-1553, 1998.
18. Badawi N, Kurinczuk JJ, Keogh JM, Alessandri LM, et al: Intrapartum risk factors for newborn encephalopathy: The Western Australian case-control study, *BMJ* 317:1554-1558, 1998.
19. Cowan F, Rutherford M, Groenendaal F, Eken P, et al: Origin and timing of brain lesions in term infants with neonatal encephalopathy, *Lancet* 361:736-742, 2003.
20. Miller SP, Ramaswamy V, Michelson D, Barkovich AJ, et al: Patterns of brain injury in term neonatal encephalopathy, *J Pediatr* 146:453-460, 2005.
21. Hagberg B, Hagberg G, Beckung E, Uvebrant P: Changing panorama of cerebral palsy in Sweden. VIII. Prevalence and origin in the birth year period 1991-94, *Acta Paediatr* 90:271-277, 2001.
22. Foley ME, Alarab M, Daly L, Keane D, et al: Term neonatal asphyxial seizures and peripartum deaths: Lack of correlation with a rising cesarean delivery rate, *Am J Obstet Gynecol* 192:102-108, 2005.
23. Stelmach T, Pisarev H, Talvik T: Ante- and perinatal factors for cerebral palsy: Case-control study in Estonia, *J Child Neurol* 20:654-661, 2005.
24. Mimouni F, Miodovnik M, Siddiqi TA, Khoury J, et al: Perinatal asphyxia in infants of insulin-dependent diabetic mothers, *J Pediatr* 113:345-353, 1988.
25. Berg AT: Indices of fetal growth-retardation, perinatal hypoxia-related factors and childhood neurological morbidity, *Early Hum Dev* 19:271-283, 1989.
26. Ounsted M, Moar VA, Scott A: Small-for-dates babies, gestational age, and developmental ability at 7 years, *Early Hum Dev* 19:77-86, 1989.
27. Harel S, Tal-Posener E, Kutai M, Tomer A, et al: Intrauterine growth retardation and brain development. I. Pre and perinatal diagnosis, *Int Pediatr* 6:109-113, 1991.
28. Harel S, Tal-Posener E, Kutai M, Tomer A, et al: Intrauterine growth retardation and brain development. II. Neurodevelopmental outcome, *Int Pediatr* 6:114-120, 1991.
29. Uvebrant P, Hagberg G: Intrauterine growth in children with cerebral palsy, *Acta Paediatr* 81:407-412, 1992.
30. Burke CJ, Tannenberg AE, Payton DJ: Ischemic cerebral injury, intrauterine growth retardation, and placental infarction, *Dev Med Child Neurol* 39:726-730, 1997.
31. Jarvis S, Glinianaia SV, Torrioli MG, Platt MJ, et al: Cerebral palsy and intrauterine growth in single births: European collaborative study, *Lancet* 362:1106-1111, 2003.
32. Tolsa CB, Zimine S, Warfield SK, Freschi M, et al: Early alteration of structural and functional brain development in premature infants born with intrauterine growth restriction, *Pediatr Res* 56:132-138, 2004.
33. Hadders-Algra M, Touwen BC: Body measurements, neurological and behavioural development in six- year-old children born preterm and/or small-for-gestational-age, *Early Hum Dev* 22:1-13, 1990.
34. Blair E, Stanley F: Intrauterine growth and spastic cerebral palsy. I. Association with birth weight for gestational age, *Am J Obstet Gynecol* 162:229-237, 1990.
35. Villar J, de Onis M, Kestler E, Bolaños F, et al: The differential neonatal morbidity of the intrauterine growth retardation syndrome, *Am J Obstet Gynecol* 163:151-157, 1990.
36. Blair E, Stanley F: Intrauterine growth and spastic cerebral palsy. II. The association with morphology at birth, *Early Hum Dev* 28:91-103, 1992.
37. Martikainen MA: Effects of intrauterine growth retardation and its subtypes on the development of the preterm infant, *Early Hum Dev* 28:7-17, 1992.
38. Thordstein M, Kjellmer I: Cerebral tolerance of hypoxia in growth-retarded and appropriately grown newborn guinea pigs, *Pediatr Res* 24:633-638, 1988.
39. Detmer A, Gu W, Carter AM: The blood supply to the heart and brain in the growth retarded guinea pig fetus, *J Dev Physiol* 15:153-160, 1991.
40. Low JA, Galbraith RS, Muir DW, Killen HL, et al: Factors associated with motor and cognitive deficits in children after intrapartum fetal hypoxia, *Am J Obstet Gynecol* 148:533-539, 1984.
41. Nelson KB, Ellenberg JH: Obstetric complications as risk factors for cerebral palsy or seizure disorders, *JAMA* 251:1843-1848, 1984.
42. Niswander K, Henson G, Elbourne D, Chalmers I, et al: Adverse outcome of pregnancy and the quality of obstetric care, *Lancet* 2:827-831, 1984.
43. Nelson KB, Leviton A: How much of neonatal encephalopathy is due to birth asphyxia?, *Am J Dis Child* 145:1325-1331, 1991.
44. Goodwin TM, Belai I, Hernandez P, Durand M, et al: Asphyxial complications in the term newborn with severe umbilical acidemia, *Am J Obstet Gynecol* 167:1506-1512, 1992.
45. Martin-Ancel A, Garcia-Alix A, Gaya F, Cabanas F, et al: Multiple organ involvement in perinatal asphyxia, *J Pediatr* 127:786-793, 1995.
46. Thornberg E, Thiringer K, Odeback A, Milsom I: Birth asphyxia: Incidence, clinical course and outcome in a Swedish population, *Acta Paediatr* 84:927-932, 1995.
47. Hull J, Dodd KL: Falling incidence of hypoxic-ischaemic encephalopathy in term infants, *Br J Obstet Gynaecol* 99:386-391, 1992.
48. Wu YW, Backstrand KH, Zhao S, Fullerton HJ, et al: Declining diagnosis of birth asphyxia in California: 1991-2000, *Pediatrics* 114:1584-1590, 2004.
49. Perlman JM, Tack ED, Martin T, Shackelford G, et al: Acute systemic organ injury in term infants after asphyxia, *Am J Dis Child* 143:617-620, 1989.
50. Pasternak JF, Gorey MT: The syndrome of acute near-total intrauterine asphyxia in the term infant, *Pediatr Neurol* 18:391-398, 1998.
51. Hankins GDV, Koen S, Gei AF, Lopez SM, et al: Neonatal organ system injury in acute birth asphyxia sufficient to result in neonatal encephalopathy, *Obstet Gynecol* 99:688-691, 2002.
52. Shah P, Riphagen S, Beyene J, Perlman M: Multiorgan dysfunction in infants with post-asphyxial hypoxic-ischaemic encephalopathy, *Arch Dis Child* 89:152-155, 2004.
53. Barnett CP, Perlman M, Ekert PG: Clinicopathological correlations in postasphyxial organ damage: A donor organ perspective, *Pediatrics* 99:797-799, 1997.
54. Barberi I, Calabro MP, Cordaro S, Gitto E, et al: Myocardial ischaemia in neonates with perinatal asphyxia: Electrocardiographic, echocardiographic and enzymatic correlations, *Eur J Pediatr* 158:742-747, 1999.
55. Sarnat HB, Sarnat MS: Neonatal encephalopathy following fetal distress: A clinical and electroencephalographic study, *Arch Neurol* 33:696-705, 1976.
56. Levene ML, Kornberg J, Williams TH: The incidence and severity of post-asphyxial encephalopathy in full-term infants, *Early Hum Dev* 11:21-26, 1985.
57. Amiel-Tison C, Ellison P: Birth asphyxia in the full-term newborn: Early assessment and outcome, *Dev Med Child Neurol* 28:671-682, 1986.
58. Volpe JJ: Observing the infant in the early hours after asphyxia. In Gluck L, editor: *Intrauterine Asphyxia and The Developing Fetal Brain*, Chicago: 1977, Year Book.
59. Volpe JJ: Perinatal hypoxic-ischemic brain injury, *Pediatr Clin North Am* 23:383-397, 1976.
60. Sasidharan P: Breathing pattern abnormalities in full term asphyxiated newborn infants, *Arch Dis Child* 67:440-442, 1992.
61. Lien JM, Towers CV, Quilligan EJ, de Veciana M, et al: Term early-onset neonatal seizures: Obstetric characteristics, etiologic classifications, and perinatal care, *Obstet Gynecol* 85:163-169, 1995.
62. Jensen FE, Applegate CD, Holtzman D, Belin TR, et al: Epilep-togenic effect of hypoxia in the immature rodent brain, *Ann Neurol* 29:629-637, 1991.
63. Mannino FL, Trauner DA: Stroke in neonates, *J Pediatr* 102:605-610, 1983.
64. Allan WC, Philip AG: Neonatal cerebral pathology diagnosed by ultrasound, *Clin Perinatol* 12:195-218, 1985.
65. Clancy R, Malin S, Laraque D, Baumgart S, et al: Focal motor seizures heralding stroke in full-term neonates, *Am J Dis Child* 139:601-606, 1985.
66. Levy SR, Abroms IF, Marshall PC, Rosquete EE: Seizures and cerebral infarction in the full-term newborn, *Ann Neurol* 17:366-370, 1985.
67. Fujimoto S, Yokochi K, Togari H, Nishimura Y, et al: Neonatal cerebral infarction: Symptoms, CT findings and prognosis, *Brain Dev* 14:48-52, 1992.
68. Ment LR, Duncan CC, Ehrenkranz RA: Perinatal cerebral infarction, *Ann Neurol* 16:559-568, 1984.

69. Trauner DA, Mannino FL: Neurodevelopmental outcome after neonatal cerebrovascular accident, *J Pediatr* 108:459-461, 1986.

70. Bode H, Strassburg HM, Pringsheim W, Kunzer W: Cerebral infarction in term neonates: Diagnosis by cerebral ultrasound, *Childs Nerv Syst* 2:195-199, 1986.

71. Filipek PA, Krishnamoorthy KS, Davis KR, Kuehnle K: Focal cerebral infarction in the newborn: A distinct entity, *Pediatr Neurol* 3:141-147, 1987.

72. Coker SB, Beltran RS, Myers TF, Hmura L: Neonatal stroke: Description of patients and investigation into pathogenesis, *Pediatr Neurol* 4:219-223, 1988.

73. Hernanz-Schulman M, Cohen W, Genieser NB: Sonography of cerebral infarction in infancy, *AJR Am J Roentgenol* 150:897-902, 1988.

74. Olson DM, Shewmon DA: Electroencephalographic abnormalities in infants with hypoplastic left heart syndrome, *Pediatr Neurol* 5:93-98, 1989.

75. Scher MS, Klesh KW, Murphy TF, Guthrie RD: Seizures and infarction in neonates with persistent pulmonary hypertension, *Pediatr Neurol* 2: 332-339, 1986.

76. Roodhooft AM, Parizel PM, Van Acker KJ, Deprettere AJ, et al: Idiopathic cerebral arterial infarction with paucity of symptoms in the full-term neonate, *Pediatrics* 80:381-385, 1987.

77. Sran SK, Baumann RJ: Outcome of neonatal strokes, *Am J Dis Child* 142:1086-1088, 1988.

78. Voorhies TM, Lipper EG, Lee BC, Vannucci RC, et al: Occlusive vascular disease in asphyxiated newborn infants, *J Pediatr* 105:92-96, 1984.

79. Estan J, Hope P: Unilateral neonatal cerebral infarction in full term infants, *Arch Dis Child Fetal Neonatal Ed* 76:F88-F93, 1997.

80. Koelfen W, Freund M, Varnholt V: Neonatal stroke involving the middle cerebral artery in term infants: Clinical presentation, EEG and imaging studies, and outcome, *Dev Med Child Neurol* 37:204-212, 1995.

81. Rollins NK, Morriss MC, Evans D, Perlman JM: The Role of early MR in the evaluation of the term infant with seizures, *AJNR Am J Neuroradiol* 15:239-248, 1994.

82. de Vries LS, Groenendaal F, Eken P, van Haastert IC, et al: Infarcts in the vascular distribution of the middle cerebral artery in preterm and full-term infants, *Neuropediatrics* 28:88-96, 1997.

83. Mercuri E, Cowan F, Rutherford M, Acolet D, et al: Ischaemic and haemorrhagic brain lesions in newborns with seizures and normal Apgar scores, *Arch Dis Child Fetal Neonatal Ed* 73:F67-F74, 1995.

84. Lee J, Croen LA, Backstrand KH, Yoshida CK, et al: Maternal and infant characteristics associated with perinatal arterial stroke in the infant, *JAMA* 293:723-729, 2005.

85. Ramaswamy V, Miller SP, Barkovich AJ, Partridge JC, et al: Perinatal stroke in term infants with neonatal encephalopathy, *Neurology* 62:2088-2091, 2004.

86. Volpe JJ: Brain death determination in the newborn, *Pediatrics* 80:293-297, 1987.

87. Lupton BA, Hill A, Roland EH, Whitfield MF, et al: Brain swelling in the asphyxiated term newborn: Pathogenesis and outcome, *Pediatrics* 82:139-146, 1988.

88. Clancy R, Legido A, Newell R, Bruce D, et al: Continuous intracranial pressure monitoring and serial electroencephalographic recordings in severely asphyxiated term neonates, *Am J Dis Child* 142:740-747, 1988.

89. Natsume J, Watanabe K, Kuno F, Hayakawa F, et al: Clinical, neurophysiologic, and neuropathological features of an infant with brain damage of total asphyxia type (Myers), *Pediatr Neurol* 13:61-64, 1995.

90. Roland EH, Poskitt K, Rodriguez E, Lupton BA, et al: Perinatal hypoxic-ischemic thalamic injury: Clinical features and neuroimaging, *Ann Neurol* 44:161-166, 1998.

91. Scott H: Outcome of very severe birth asphyxia, *Arch Dis Child* 51:712-716, 1976.

92. Salhab WA, Wyckoff MH, Laptook AR, Perlman JM: Initial hypoglycemia and neonatal brain injury in term infants with severe fetal acidemia, *Pediatrics* 114:361-366, 2004.

93. Goldberg RN, Cabal LA, Sinatra FR, Plajstek CE, et al: Hyperammonemia associated with perinatal asphyxia, *Pediatrics* 64:336-341, 1979.

94. James LS, Meyers RE, Gaull GE: Brain damage in the fetus and newborn from hypoxia or asphyxia. In *Fifty-Seventh Ross Conference on Pediatric Research, 1967*, Columbus, OH: Ross Laboratories, 1967.

95. Fernández F, Verdu A, Quero J, Ferreiros MC, et al: Cerebrospinal fluid lactate levels in term infants with perinatal hypoxia, *Pediatr Neurol* 2:39-42, 1986.

96. Fernández F, Quero J, Verdu A, Ferreiros MC, et al: LDH isoenzymes in CSF in the diagnosis of neonatal brain damage, *Acta Neurol Scand* 74:30-33, 1986.

97. Huang CC, Wang ST, Chang YC, Lin KP, et al: Measurement of the urinary lactate: Creatinine ratio for the early identification of newborn infants at risk for hypoxic-ischemic encephalopathy, *N Engl J Med* 341:328-335, 1999.

98. da Silva S, Hennebert N, Denis R, Wayenberg JL: Clinical value of a single postnatal lactate measurement after intrapartum asphyxia, *Acta Paediatr* 89:320-323, 2000.

99. Ilves P, Blennow M, Kutt E, Magi ML, et al: Concentrations of magnesium and ionized calcium in umbilical cord blood in distressed term newborn infants with hypoxic-ischemic encephalopathy, *Acta Paediatr* 85:1348-1350, 1996.

100. Harrison V, Peat G: Red blood cell magnesium and hypoxic-ischaemic encephalopathy, *Early Hum Dev* 47:287-296, 1997.

101. Roldan A, Figueras-Aloy J, Deulofeu R, Jimenez R: Glycine and other neurotransmitter amino acids in cerebrospinal fluid in perinatal asphyxia and neonatal hypoxic-ischaemic encephalopathy, *Acta Paediatr* 88:1137-1141, 1999.

102. Khashaba MT, Shouman BO, Shaltout AA, Al-Marsafawy HM, et al: Excitatory amino acids and magnesium sulfate in neonatal asphyxia, *Brain Dev* 28:375-379, 2006.

103. Bratteby LE, Swanstrom S: Hypoxanthine concentration in plasma during the first two hours after birth in normal and asphyxiated infants, *Pediatr Res* 16:152-155, 1982.

104. Harkness RA, Simmonds RJ, Coade SB, Lawrence CR: Ratio of the concentration of hypoxanthine to creatinine in urine from newborn infants: A possible indicator for the metabolic damage due to hypoxia, *Br J Obstet Gynaecol* 90:447-452, 1983.

105. Thiringer K: Cord plasma hypoxanthine as a measure of foetal asphyxia: Comparison with clinical assessment and laboratory measures, *Acta Paediatr Scand* 72:231-237, 1983.

106. Saugstad OD: Hypoxanthine as an indicator of hypoxia: Its role in health and disease through free radical production, *Pediatr Res* 23:143-150, 1988.

107. Pietz J, Guttenberg N, Gluck L: Hypoxanthine: A marker for asphyxia, *Obstet Gynecol* 72:762-766, 1988.

108. Russell GA, Jeffers G, Cooke RW: Plasma hypoxanthine: A marker for hypoxic-ischaemic induced periventricular leucomalacia? *Arch Dis Child* 67:388-392, 1992.

109. Oriot D, Betremieux P, Baumann N, Lefrancois C, et al: CSF ascorbic acid and lactate levels after neonatal asphyxia: Preliminary results, *Acta Paediatr* 81:845-846, 1992.

110. Dorrepaal CA, Berger HM, Benders MJ, van Zoeren-Grobben D, et al: Nonprotein-bound iron in postasphyxial reperfusion injury of the newborn, *Pediatrics* 98:883-889, 1996.

111. Bader D, Gozal D, Weingerabend M, Berger A, et al: Neonatal urinary uric acid/creatinine ratio as an additional marker of perinatal asphyxia, *Eur J Pediatr* 154:747-749, 1995.

112. Perlman JM, Risser R: Relationship of uric acid concentrations and severe intraventricular hemorrhage/leukomalacia in the premature infant, *J Pediatr* 132:436-439, 1998.

113. Vilanova JM, Figueras-Aloy J, Rosello J, Gomez G, et al: Arachidonic acid metabolites in CSF in hypoxic-ischaemic encephalopathy of newborn infants, *Acta Paediatr* 87:588-592, 1998.

114. Shi Y, Pan F, Li H, Pan J, et al: Role of carbon monoxide and nitric oxide in newborn infants with postasphyxial hypoxic-ischemic encephalopathy, *Pediatrics* 106:1447-1451, 2000.

115. Yu T, Kui LQ, Ming QZ: Effect of asphyxia on non–protein-bound iron and lipid peroxidation in newborn infants, *Dev Med Child Neurol* 45:24-27, 2003.

116. Ahola T, Fellman V, Kjellmer I, Raivio KO, et al: Plasma 8-isoprostane is increased in preterm infants who develop bronchopulmonary dysplasia or periventricular leukomalacia, *Pediatr Res* 56:88-93, 2004.

117. Inder TE, Mocatta T, Darlow B, Spencer C, et al: Elevated free radical products in the cerebrospinal fluid of VLBW infants with cerebral white matter injury, *Pediatr Res* 52:213-218, 2002.

118. Ogihara T, Hirano K, Ogihara H, Misaki K, et al: Non–protein-bound transition metals and hydroxyl radical generation in cerebrospinal fluid of newborn infants with hypoxic ischemic encephalopathy, *Pediatr Res* 53:594-599, 2003.

119. Ergenekon E, Gucuyener K, Erbas D, Aral S, et al: Cerebrospinal fluid and serum vascular endothelial growth factor and nitric oxide levels in newborns with hypoxic ischemic encephalopathy, *Brain Dev* 26:283-286, 2004.

120. Gulcan H, Ozturk IC, Arslan S: Alterations in antioxidant enzyme activities in cerebrospinal fluid related with severity of hypoxic ischemic encephalopathy in newborns, *Biol Neonate* 88:87-91, 2005.

121. Savman K, Blennow M, Gustafson K, Tarkowski E, et al: Cytokine response in cerebrospinal fluid after birth asphyxia, *Pediatr Res* 41:746-751, 1998.

122. Martin-Ancel A, Carcia-Alix A, Pascual-Salcedo D, Cabanas F, et al: Interleukin-6 in the cerebrospinal fluid after perinatal asphyxia is related to early and late neurological manifestations, *Pediatrics* 100:789-794, 1997.

123. Xanthou M, Fotopoulos S, Mouchtouri A, Lipsou N, et al: Inflammatory mediators in perinatal asphyxia and infection, *Acta Paediatr* 91:92-97, 2002.

124. Chiesa C, Pellegrini G, Panero A, DeLuca T, et al: Umbilical cord interleukin-6 levels are elevated in term neonates with perinatal asphyxia, *Eur J Clin Invest* 33:352-358, 2003.

125. Silveira RC, Procianoy RS: Interleukin-6 and tumor necrosis factor-α levels in plasma and cerebrospinal fluid of term newborn infants with hypoxic-ischemic encephalopathy, *J Pediatr* 143:625-629, 2003.

126. Tekgul H, Yalaz M, Kutukculer N, Ozbek S, et al: Value of biochemical markers for outcome in term infants with asphyxia, *Pediatr Neurol* 31:326-332, 2004.

127. Swanstrom S, Bratteby LE: Hypoxanthine as a test of perinatal hypoxia as compared to lactate, base deficit, and pH, *Pediatr Res* 16:156-160, 1982.

128. Hoo JJ, Goedde HW: Determination of brain type creatine kinase for diagnosis of perinatal asphyxia: Choice of method [letter], *Pediatr Res* 16:806, 1982.

129. Kumpel B, Wood SM, Anthony PP, Brimblecombe FS: Umbilical cord serum creatine kinase BB in the diagnosis of brain damage in the newborn: Problems in interpretation, *Arch Dis Child* 58:382-383, 1983.

130. Walsh P, Jedeikin R, Ellis G, Primhak R, et al: Assessment of neurologic outcome in asphyxiated term infants by use of serial CK-BB isoenzyme measurement, *J Pediatr* 101:988-992, 1982.

131. Worley G, Lipman B, Gewolb IH, Green JA, et al: Creatine kinase brain isoenzyme: Relationship of cerebrospinal fluid concentration to the neurologic condition of newborns and cellular localization in the human brain, *Pediatrics* 76:15-21, 1985.

132. Cuestas RA Jr: Creatine kinase isoenzymes in high-risk infants, *Pediatr Res* 14:935-938, 1980.

133. Amato M, Gambon R, von Muralt G: Prognostic value of serum creatine kinase brain isoenzyme in term babies with perinatal hypoxic injuries, *Helv Paediatr Acta* 40:435-440, 1985.

134. Ezitis J, Finnström O, Hedman G, Rabow L: CK_{BB}-enzyme activity in serum in neonates born after vaginal delivery and cesarean section, *Neuropediatrics* 18:146-148, 1987.

135. Fernéndez F, Verdu A, Quero J, Perez-Higueras A: Serum CPK-BB isoenzyme in the assessment of brain damage in asphyctic term infants, *Acta Paediatr Scand* 76:914-918, 1987.

136. Ruth VJ: Prognostic value of creatine kinase BB-isoenzyme in high risk newborn infants, *Arch Dis Child* 64:563-568, 1989.

137. den Ouden L, van de Bor M, van Bel F, Janssen H, et al: Serum CK-BB activity in the preterm infant and outcome at two and four years of age, *Dev Med Child Neurol* 32:509-514, 1990.

138. De Praeter C, Vanhaesebrouck P, Govaert P, Delanghe J, et al: Creatine kinase isoenzyme BB concentrations in the cerebrospinal fluid of newborns: Relationship to short-term outcome, *Pediatrics* 88:1204-1210, 1991.

139. Sobajima H, Togari H: Cerebrospinal fluid neuron-specific enolase as the prognostic marker for long term neurological sequela in the asphyxiated infants: A multicenter prospective study, *Nagoya Med J* 37:169-178, 1993.

140. Blennow M, Hagberg H, Rosengren L: Glial fibrillary acidic protein in the cerebrospinal fluid: A possible indicator of prognosis in full-term asphyxiated newborn infants? *Pediatr Res* 37:260-264, 1995.

141. Blennow M, Rosengren L, Jonsson S, Forssberg H, et al: Glial fibrillary acidic protein is increased in the cerebrospinal fluid of preterm infants with abnormal neurological findings, *Acta Paediatr* 85:485-489, 1996.

142. Thornberg E, Thiringer K, Hagberg H, Kjellmer I: Neuron specific enolase in asphyxiated newborns: Association with encephalopathy and cerebral function monitor trace, *Arch Dis Child Fetal Neonatal Ed* 72:F39-F42, 1995.

143. Talvik T, Haldre S, Soot A, Hamarik M, et al: Creatine kinase isoenzyme BB concentrations in cerebrospinal fluid in asphyxiated preterm neonates, *Acta Paediatr* 84:1183-1187, 1995.

144. Blennow M, Savman K, Ilves P, Thoresen M, et al: Brain-specific proteins in the cerebrospinal fluid of severely asphyxiated newborn infants, *Acta Paediatr* 90:1171-1175, 2001.

145. Ezgu FS, Atalay Y, Gucuyener K, Tunc S, et al: Neuron-specific enolase levels and neuroimaging in asphyxiated term newborns, *J Child Neurol* 17:842-829, 2002.

146. Wijnberger LDE, Nikkels PGJ, van Dongen AJCM, Noorlander CW, et al: Expression in the placenta of neuronal markers for perinatal brain damage, *Pediatr Res* 51:492-496, 2002.

147. Distefano G, Curreri R, Betta P, Isaja MT, et al: Serial protein S-100 serum levels in preterm babies with perinatal asphyxia and periventricular white matter lesions, *Am J Perinatol* 19:317-322, 2002.

148. Nagdyman N, Komen W, Ko H-K, Muller C, et al: Early biochemical indicators of hypoxic-ischemic encephalopathy after birth asphyxia, *Pediatr Res* 49:502-506, 2001.

149. Nagdyman N, Grimmer I, Scholz T, Muller C, et al: Predictive value of brain-specific proteins in serum for neurodevelopmental outcome after birth asphyxia, *Pediatr Res* 54:270-275, 2003.

150. Gazzolo D, Marinoni E, Di Iorio R, Bruschettini M, et al: Measurement of urinary S100B protein concentrations for the early identification of brain damage in asphyxiated full-term infants, *Arch Pediatr Adolesc Med* 157:1163-1168, 2003.

151. Thorngren-Jerneck K, Alling C, Herbst A, Amer-Wahlin I, et al: S100 protein in serum as a prognostic marker for cerebral injury in term newborn infants with hypoxic ischemic encephalopathy, *Pediatr Res* 55:406-412, 2004.

152. Gazzolo D, Florio P, Ciotti S, Marinoni E, et al: S100B protein in urine of preterm newborns with ominous outcome, *Pediatr Res* 58:1170-1174, 2005.

153. Ruth V, Pohjavuori M, Rovamo L, Salminen K, et al: Plasma beta-endorphin in perinatal asphyxia and respiratory difficulties in newborn infants, *Pediatr Res* 20:577-580, 1986.

154. Ruth V, Autti-Ramo I, Granstrom ML, Korkman M, et al: Prediction of perinatal brain damage by cord plasma vasopressin, erythropoietin, and hypoxanthine values, *J Pediatr* 113:880-885, 1988.

155. Ruth V, Widness JA, Clemons G, Raivio KO: Postnatal changes in serum immunoreactive erythropoietin in relation to hypoxia before and after birth, *J Pediatr* 116:950-954, 1990.

156. Riikonen RS, Korhonen LT, Lindholm DB: Cerebrospinal nerve growth factor: A marker of asphyxia? *Pediatr Neurol* 20:137-141, 1999.

157. Holmes G, Rowe J, Hafford J, Schmidt R, et al: Prognostic value of the electroencephalogram in neonatal asphyxia, *Electroencephalogr Clin Neurophysiol* 53:60-72, 1982.

158. McCutchen CB, Coen R, Iragui VJ: Periodic lateralized epileptiform discharges in asphyxiated neonates, *Electroencephalogr Clin Neurophysiol* 61:210-217, 1985.

159. Scher MS: Midline electrographic abnormalities and cerebral lesions in the newborn brain, *J Child Neurol* 3:135-146, 1988.

160. Scher MS, Dobson V, Carpenter NA, Guthrie RD: Visual and neurological outcome of infants with periventricular leukomalacia, *Dev Med Child Neurol* 31:353-365, 1989.

161. Tharp BR, Scher MS, Clancy RR: Serial EEGs in normal and abnormal infants with birth weights less than 1200 grams: A prospective study with long term follow-up, *Neuropediatrics* 20:64-72, 1989.

162. Novotny EJ Jr, Tharp BR, Coen RW, Bejar R, et al: Positive rolandic sharp waves in the EEG of the premature infant, *Neurology* 37:1481-1486, 1987.

163. Bejar R, Coen RW, Merritt TA, Vaucher Y, et al: Focal necrosis of the white matter (periventricular leukomalacia): Sonographic, pathologic, and electroencephalographic features, *AJNR Am J Neuroradiol* 7:1073-1079, 1986.

164. Marret S, Parain D, Samson-Dollfus D, Jeannot E, et al: Positive rolandic sharp waves and periventricular leukomalacia in the newborn, *Neuropediatrics* 17:199-202, 1986.

165. Scavone C, Radvanyi-Bouvet MF, Morel-Kahn F, Dreyfus-Brisac C: [Coma in full-term newborn infants following acute fetal distress: Electro-clinical evolution], *Rev Electroencephalogr Neurophysiol Clin* 15:279-288, 1985.

166. Pezzani C, Radvanyi-Bouvet MF, Relier JP, Monod N: Neonatal electroencephalography during the first twenty-four hours of life in full-term newborn infants, *Neuropediatrics* 17:11-18, 1986.

167. Grigg-Damberger MM, Coker SB, Halsey CL, Anderson CL: Neonatal burst suppression: Its developmental significance, *Pediatr Neurol* 5:84-92, 1989.

168. Hrachovy RA, Mizrahi EM, Kellaway P: Electroencephalography of the newborn. In Daly DD, Pedley TA, editors: *Current Practice of Clinical Electroencephalography*, 2nd ed, New York: 1990, Raven Press.

169. Bell AH, McClure BG, Hicks EM: Power spectral analysis of the EEG of term infants following birth asphyxia, *Dev Med Child Neurol* 32:990-998, 1990.

170. Takeuchi T, Watanabe K: The EEG evolution and neurological prognosis of neonates with perinatal hypoxia, *Brain Dev* 11:115-120, 1989.

171. Marret S, Parain D, Jeannot E, Eurin D, et al: Positive rolandic sharp waves in the EEG of the premature newborn: A five-year prospective study, *Arch Dis Child* 67:948-951, 1992.

172. Van Lieshout HBM, Jacobs JWFM, Rotteveel JJ, Geven W, et al: The prognostic value of the EEG in asphyxiated newborns, *Acta Neurol Scand* 91:203-207, 1995.

173. Marret S, Parain D, Menard J-F, Blanc T, et al: Prognostic value of neonatal electroencephalography in premature newborns less than 33 weeks of gestational age, *Electroencephalogr Clin Neurophysiol* 102:178-185, 1997.

174. Hayakawa F, Okumura A, Kato T, Kuno K: Disorganized patterns: Chronic-stage EEG abnormality of the late neonatal period following severely depressed EEG activities in early preterm infants, *Neuropediatrics* 28:272-275, 1997.

175. Selton D, Andre M: Prognosis of hypoxic-ischaemic encephalopathy in full-term newborns: Value of neonatal electroencephalography, *Neuropediatrics* 28:276-280, 1997.

176. Baud O, D'Allest A-M, Lacaze-Masmonteil T, Zupan V, et al: The early diagnosis of periventricular leukomalacia in premature infants with positive rolandic sharp waves on serial electroencephalography, *J Pediatr* 132:813-817, 1998.

177. Biagioni E, Bartalena L, Boldrini A, Pieri R, et al: Constantly discontinuous EEG patterns in full-term neonates with hypoxic-ischaemic encephalopathy, *Clin Neurophysiol* 110:1510-1515, 1999.

178. Biagioni E, Mercuri E, Rutherford MA, Cowan F, et al: Combined use of electroencephalogram and magnetic resonance imaging in full-term neonates with acute encephalopathy, *Pediatrics* 107:461-468, 2001.

179. Zeinstra E, Fock JM, Begeer JH, Van Weerden T, et al: The prognostic value of serial EEG recordings following acute neonatal asphyxia in full-term infants, *Eur J Paediatr Neurol* 5:155-160, 2001.

180. Maruyama K, Okumura A, Hayakawa F, Kato T, et al: Prognostic value of EEG depression in preterm infants for later development of cerebral palsy, *Neuropediatrics* 33:133-137, 2002.

181. Vermeulen EJ, Sie LTL, Jonkman EJ, Strijers RLM, et al: Predictive value of EEG in neonates with periventricular leukomalacia, *Dev Med Child Neurol* 45:586-590, 2003.

182. Okumura A, Hayakawa F, Kato T, Kuno K, et al: Developmental outcome and types of chronic-stage EEG abnormalities in preterm infants, *Dev Med Child Neurol* 44:729-734, 2002.

183. Kubota T, Okumura A, Hayakawa F, Kato T, et al: Combination of neonatal electroencephalography and ultrasonography: Sensitive means of early diagnosis of periventricular leukomalacia, *Brain Dev* 24:698-702, 2002.

184. Okumura A, Hayakawa F, Kato T, Maruyama K, et al: Abnormal sharp transients on electroencephalograms in preterm infants with periventricular leukomalacia, *J Biomed Optics* 143:26-30, 2003.

185. Sofue A, Okumura A, Hayakawa F, Watanabe K: Sharp waves in preterm infants with periventricular leukomalacia, *Pediatr Neurol* 29:214-217, 2003.

186. Murray DM, Boylan GB, Ryan CA, Connolly S: Early continuous video-EEG in acute near-total intrauterine asphyxia, *Pediatr Neurol* 35:52-56, 2006.

187. Menache CC, Bourgeois BFD, Volpe JJ: Prognostic value of neonatal discontinuous EEG, *Pediatr Neurol* 27:93-101, 2002.

188. van Rooij LGM, Toet MC, Osredkar D, van Huffelen AC, et al: Recovery of amplitude integrated electroencephalographic background patterns within 24 hours of perinatal asphyxia, *Arch Dis Child Fetal Neonatal Ed* 90:F245-F251, 2005.

189. de Vries LS, HellstromWestas L: Role of cerebral function monitoring in the newborn, *Arch Dis Child Fetal Neonatal Ed* 90:F201-F207, 2005.

190. Thorngren-Jerneck K, Hellstrom-Westas L, Ryding E, Rosen I: Cerebral glucose metabolism and early EEG/aEEG in term newborn infants with hypoxic-ischemic encephalopathy, *Pediatr Res* 54:854-860, 2003.

191. Shalak LF, Laptook AR, Velaphi SC, Perlman JM: Amplitude-integrated electroencephalography coupled with an early neurologic examination enhances prediction of term infants at risk for persistent encephalopathy, *Pediatrics* 111:351-357, 2003.

192. Ter Horst HJ, Sommer C, Bergman KA, Fock JM, et al: Prognostic significance of amplitude-integrated EEG during the first 72 hours after birth in severely asphyxiated neonates, *Pediatr Res* 55:1026-1033, 2004.

193. Shany E, Goldstein E, Khvatskin S, Friger MD, et al: Predictive value of amplitude-integrated electroencephalography pattern and voltage in asphyxiated term infants, *Pediatr Neurol* 35:335-342, 2006.

194. Shany E, Khvatskin S, Golan A, Karplus M: Amplitude-integrated electroencephalography: A tool for monitoring silent seizures in neonates, *Pediatr Neurol* 34:194-199, 2006.

195. Coen RW, McCutchen CB, Wermer D, Snyder J, et al: Continuous monitoring of the electroencephalogram following perinatal asphyxia, *J Pediatr* 100:628-630, 1982.

196. Scher MS: Neonatal encephalopathies as classified by EEG-sleep criteria: Severity and timing based on clinical/pathologic correlations, *Pediatr Neurol* 11:189-200, 1994.

197. Scher MS, Beggarly M: Clinical significance of focal periodic discharges in neonates, *J Child Neurol* 4:175-185, 1989.

198. Rando T, Ricci D, Mercuri E, Frisone F, et al: Periodic lateralized epileptiform discharges (PLEDs) as early indicator of stroke in full-term newborns, *Neuropediatrics* 31:202-205, 2000.

199. Alvarez LA, Lipton RB, Moshé SL: Normal cerebral radionuclide angiogram and electrocerebral silence in the presence of severe cerebral atrophy, *Neuropediatrics* 18:112, 1987.

200. Alvarez LA, Moshé SL, Belman AL, Maytal J, et al: EEG and brain death determination in children, *Neurology* 38:227-230, 1988.

201. Moshé SL, Alvarez LA: Diagnosis of brain death in children, *J Clin Neurophysiol* 3:239-249, 1986.

202. Mizrahi EM, Pollack MA, Kellaway P: Neocortical death in infants: Behavioral, neurologic, and electroencephalographic characteristics, *Pediatr Neurol* 1:302-305, 1985.

203. Moshé SL: Usefulness of EEG in the evaluation of brain death in children: The pros, *Electroencephalogr Clin Neurophysiol* 73:272-275, 1989.

204. Ashwal S, Schneider S: Brain death in the newborn, *Pediatrics* 84:429-437, 1989.

205. Ashwal S: Brain death in the newborn, *Clin Perinatol* 16:501-518, 1989.

206. Medlock MD, Hanigan WC, Cruse RP: Dissociation of cerebral blood flow, glucose metabolism, and electrical activity in pediatric brain death: Case report, *J Neurosurg* 79:752-755, 1993.

207. Okamoto K, Sugimoto T: Return of spontaneous respiration in an infant who fulfilled current criteria to determine brain death, *Pediatrics* 96:518-520, 1995.

208. Fishman MA: Validity of brain death criteria in infants, *Pediatrics* 96: 513-515, 1995.

209. Shewmon DA, Holmes GL, Byrne PA: Consciousness in congenitally decorticate children: Developmental vegetative state as self-fulfilling prophecy, *Dev Med Child Neurol* 41:364-374, 1999.

210. Ashwal S, Schneider S: Failure of electroencephalography to diagnose brain death in comatose children, *Ann Neurol* 6:512-517, 1979.

211. American Academy of Pediatrics Task Force on Brain Death in Children: Report of special Task Force: Guidelines for the determination of brain death in children, *Pediatrics* 80:298-300, 1987.

212. Flodmark O, Becker LE, Harwood-Nash DC, Fitzhardinge PM, et al: Correlation between computed tomography and autopsy in premature and full-term neonates that have suffered perinatal asphyxia, *Radiology* 137:93-103, 1980.

213. Magilner AD, Wertheimer IS: Preliminary results of a computed tomography study of neonatal brain hypoxia: Ischemia, *J Comput Assist Tomogr* 4:457-463, 1980.

214. Fitzhardinge PM, Flodmark O, Fitz CR, Ashby S: The prognostic value of computed tomography as an adjunct to assessment of the term infant with postasphyxial encephalopathy, *J Pediatr* 99:777-781, 1981.

215. Adsett DB, Fitz CR, Hill A: Hypoxic-ischaemic cerebral injury in the term newborn: Correlation of CT findings with neurological outcome, *Dev Med Child Neurol* 27:155-160, 1985.

216. Lipp-Zwahlen AE, Deonna T, Chrzanowski R, Micheli JL, et al: Temporal evolution of hypoxic-ischaemic brain lesions in asphyxiated full-term newborns as assessed by computerized tomography, *Neuroradiology* 27:138-144, 1985.

217. Lipp-Zwahlen AE, Deonna T, Micheli JL, Calame A, et al: Prognostic value of neonatal CT scans in asphyxiated term babies: Low density score compared with neonatal neurological signs, *Neuropediatrics* 16:209-217, 1985.

218. Lipper EG, Voorhies TM, Ross G, Vannucci RC, et al: Early predictors of one-year outcome for infants asphyxiated at birth, *Dev Med Child Neurol* 28:303-309, 1986.

219. Han BK, Towbin RB, De Courten-Myers G, McLaurin RL, et al: Reversal sign on CT: Effect of anoxic/ischemic cerebral injury in children, *AJNR Am J Neuroradiol* 10:1191-1198, 1989.

220. Barkovich AJ: *Pediatric Neuroimaging*, 2nd ed, New York: 1995, Raven Press 1995.

221. Shewmon DA, Fine M, Masdeu JC, Palacios E: Postischemic hypervascularity of infancy: A stage in the evolution of ischemic brain damage with characteristic CT scan, *Ann Neurol* 9:358-365, 1981.

222. Kotagal S, Toce SS, Kotagal P, Archer CR: Symmetric bithalamic and striatal hemorrhage following perinatal hypoxia in a term infant, *J Comput Assist Tomogr* 7:353-355, 1983.

223. Kanarek KS, Gieron MA: Computed tomography demonstration of cerebral calcification in postasphyxial encephalopathy, *J Child Neurol* 1:56-60, 1986.

224. Ansari MQ, Chincanchan CA, Armstrong DL: Brain calcification in hypoxicischemic lesions: An autopsy review, *Pediatr Neurol* 6:94-101, 1990.

225. Pasternak JF: Parasagittal infarction in neonatal asphyxia, *Ann Neurol* 21:202-204, 1987.

226. Naidich TP, Chakera TM: Multicystic encephalomalacia: CT appearance and pathological correlation, *J Comput Assist Tomogr* 8:631-636, 1984.

227. Fitzhardinge PM, Fitz CR, Harwood-Nash DC: Follow-up studies of infants with abnormal neonatal computed tomography (CT) resulting from asphyxia, *Pediatr Res* 12:551, 1978.

228. Barkovich AJ: *Pediatric Neuroimaging*, New York: 1990, Raven Press 1990.

229. Di Chiro G, Arimitsu T, Pellock JM, Landes RD: Periventricular leukomalacia related to neonatal anoxia: Recognition by computed tomography, *J Comput Assist Tomogr* 2:352-355, 1978.

230. Estrada M, El Gammal T, Dyken PR: Periventricular low attenuations: A normal finding in computerized tomographic scans of neonates? *Arch Neurol* 37:754-756, 1980.

231. Penn RD, Trinko B, Baldwin L: Brain maturation followed by computed tomography, *J Comput Assist Tomogr* 4:614-616, 1980.

232. Picard L, Claudon M, Roland J, Jeanjean E, et al: Cerebral computed tomography in premature infants, with an attempt at staging developmental features, *J Comput Assist Tomogr* 4:435-444, 1980.

233. Brant-Zawadzki M, Enzmann DR: Using computed tomography of the brain to correlate low white-matter attenuation with early gestational age in neonates, *Radiology* 139:105-108, 1981.

234. Murakami R, Nakamura H, Mizojiri T, Aida M, et al: A study of brain development in low-birth-weight infants by computerized tomography, *Neuropediatrics* 12:132-142, 1981.

235. Flodmark O, Roland EH, Hill A, Whitfield MF: Periventricular leukomalacia: Radiologic diagnosis, *Radiology* 162:119-124, 1987.

236. Barkovich AJ: *Pediatric Neuroimaging*, 4th ed, Philadelphia: 2005, Lippincott Williams & Wilkins 2005.

237. Siegel MJ, Shackelford GD, Perlman JM, Fulling KH: Hypoxic-ischemic encephalopathy in term infants: Diagnosis and prognosis evaluated by ultrasound, *Radiology* 152:395-399, 1984.

238. Donn SM, Bowerman RA, DiPietro MA, Gebarski SS: Sonographic appearance of neonatal thalamic-striatal hemorrhage, *J Ultrasound Med* 3:231-233, 1984.

239. Kreusser KL, Schmidt RE, Shackelford GD, Volpe JJ: Value of ultrasound for identification of acute hemorrhagic necrosis of thalamus and basal ganglia in an asphyxiated term infant, *Ann Neurol* 16:361-363, 1984.

240. Shen EY, Huang CC, Chyou SC, Hung HY, et al: Sonographic finding of the bright thalamus, *Arch Dis Child* 61:1096-1099, 1986.

241. Cabañas F, Pellicer A, Pérez-Higueras A, Garcia-Alix A, et al: Ultrasonographic findings in thalamus and basal ganglia in term asphyxiated infants, *Pediatr Neurol* 7:211-215, 1991.

242. Eken P, Jansen GH, Groenendaal F, Rademaker KJ, et al: Intracranial lesions in the full-term infant with hypoxic ischaemic encephalopathy: Ultrasound and autopsy correlation, *Neuropediatrics* 25:301-307, 1994.

243. Rutherford MA, Pennock JM, Dubowitz L: Cranial ultrasound and magnetic resonance imaging in hypoxic-ischaemic encephalopathy: A comparison with outcome, *Dev Med Child Neurol* 36:813-825, 1994.

244. Blankenberg FG, Loh NN, Bracci P, DArceuil HE, et al: Sonography, CT, and MR imaging: A prospective comparison of neonates with suspected intracranial ischemia and hemorrhage, *AJNR Am J Neuroradiol* 21:213-218, 2000.

245. Leijser LM, Klein RH, Veen S, Liauw L, et al: Hyperechogenicity of the thalamus and basal ganglia in very preterm infants: Radiological findings and short-term neurological outcome, *Neuropediatrics* 35:283-289, 2004.

246. Hill A, Melson GL, Clark HB, Volpe JJ: Hemorrhagic periventricular leukomalacia: Diagnosis by real time ultrasound and correlation with autopsy findings, *Pediatrics* 69:282-284, 1982.

247. Babcock DS, Ball W Jr: Postasphyxial encephalopathy in full-term infants: Ultrasound diagnosis, *Radiology* 148:417-423, 1983.

248. Slovis TL, Shankaran S, Bedard MP, Poland RL: Intracranial hemorrhage in the hypoxic-ischemic infant: Ultrasound demonstration of unusual complications, *Radiology* 151:163-169, 1984.

249. Levene MI, Williams JL, Fawer CL: *Ultrasound of the Infant Brain*, London: 1985, Blackwell Scientific 1985.

250. Wilson-Davis SL, Lo W, Filly RA: Limitations of ultrasound in detecting cerebral ischemic lesions in the neonate, *Ann Neurol* 14:249-251, 1983.

251. Fischer AQ, Anderson JC, Shuman RM: The evolution of ischemic cerebral infarction in infancy: A sonographic evaluation, *J Child Neurol* 3:105-109, 1988.

252. Adcock LM, Moore PJ, Schlesinger AE, Armstrong DL: Correlation of ultrasound with postmortem neuropathologic studies in neonates, *Pediatr Neurol* 19:263-271, 1998.

253. Golomb MR, Dick PT, MacGregor DL, Armstrong DC, et al: Cranial ultrasonography has a low sensitivity for detecting arterial ischemic stroke in term neonates, *J Child Neurol* 18:98-103, 2003.

254. Cowan F, Mercuri E, Groenendaal F, Bassi L, et al: Does cranial ultrasound imaging identify arterial cerebral infarction in term neonates? *Arch Dis Child Fetal Neonatal Ed* 90:252-256, 2005.

255. Messer J, Haddad J, Casanova R: Transcranial Doppler evaluation of cerebral infarction in the neonate, *Neuropediatrics* 22:147-151, 1991.

256. Levene MI, Wigglesworth JS, Dubowitz V: Hemorrhagic periventricular leukomalacia in the neonate: A real-time ultrasound study, *Pediatrics* 71:794-797, 1983.

257. Bowerman RA, Donn SM, DiPietro MA, D'Amato CJ, et al: Periventricular leukomalacia in the pre-term newborn infant: Sonographic and clinical features, *Radiology* 151:383-388, 1984.

258. Dolfin T, Skidmore MB, Fong KW, Hoskins EM, et al: Diagnosis and evolution of periventricular leukomalacia: A study with real-time ultrasound, *Early Hum Dev* 9:105-109, 1984.

259. Fawer CL, Calame A, Perentes E, Anderegg A: Periventricular leukomalacia: A correlation study between real-time ultrasound and autopsy findings. Periventricular leukomalacia in the neonate, *Neuroradiology* 27:292-300, 1985.

260. McMenamin JB, Shackelford GD, Volpe JJ: Outcome of neonatal intraventricular hemorrhage with periventricular echodense lesions, *Ann Neurol* 15:285-290, 1984.

261. Nwaesei CG, Pape KE, Martin DJ, Becker LE, et al: Periventricular infarction diagnosed by ultrasound: A postmortem correlation, *J Pediatr* 105:106-110, 1984.

262. Dubowitz LM, Bydder GM, Mushin J: Developmental sequence of periventricular leukomalacia: Correlation of ultrasound, clinical, and nuclear magnetic resonance functions, *Arch Dis Child* 60:349-355, 1985.

263. Chow PP, Horgan JG, Taylor KJ: Neonatal periventricular leukomalacia: Real-time sonographic diagnosis with CT correlation, *AJR Am J Roentgenol* 145:155-160, 1985.

264. Weindling AM, Rochefort MJ, Calvert SA, Fok TF, et al: Development of cerebral palsy after ultrasonographic detection of periventricular cysts in the newborn, *Dev Med Child Neurol* 27:800-806, 1985.

265. Bozynski ME, Nelson MN, Matalon TA, Genaze DR, et al: Cavitary periventricular leukomalacia: Incidence and short-term outcome in infants weighing less than or equal to 1200 grams at birth, *Dev Med Child Neurol* 27:572-577, 1985.

266. Calvert SA, Hoskins EM, Fong KW, Forsyth SC: Periventricular leukomalacia: Ultrasonic diagnosis and neurological outcome, *Acta Paediatr Scand* 75:489-496, 1986.

267. Tamisari L, Vigi V, Fortini C, Scarpa P: Neonatal periventricular leukomalacia: Diagnosis and evolution evaluated by real-time ultrasound, *Helv Paediatr Acta* 41:399-407, 1986.

268. Graziani LJ, Pasto M, Stanley C, Pidcock F, et al: Neonatal neurosonographic correlates of cerebral palsy in preterm infants, *Pediatrics* 78:88-95, 1986.

269. Weisglas-Kuperus N, Uleman-Vleeschdrager M, Baerts W: Ventricular haemorrhages and hypoxic-ischaemic lesions in preterm infants: Neurodevelopmental outcome at 3 1/2 years, *Dev Med Child Neurol* 29:623-629, 1987.

270. Graham M, Levene MI, Trounce JQ, Rutter N: Prediction of cerebral palsy in very low birthweight infants: Prospective ultrasound study, *Lancet* 2:593-596, 1987.

271. Fawer CL, Diebold P, Calame A: Periventricular leukomalacia and neurodevelopmental outcome in preterm infants, *Arch Dis Child* 62:30-36, 1987.

272. Stewart A, Hope PL, Hamilton P, Costello AM, et al: Prediction in very preterm infants of satisfactory neurodevelopmental progress at 12 months, *Dev Med Child Neurol* 30:53-63, 1988.

273. Monset-Couchard M, de Bethmann O, Radvanyi-Bouvet MF, Papin C, et al: Neurodevelopmental outcome in cystic periventricular leukomalacia (CPVL) (30 cases), *Neuropediatrics* 19:124-131, 1988.

274. Monset-Couchard M, de Bethmann O, Iritz N, Relier JP: Leucomalacies kystiques neonatals: Anamnèse périnatale chez 30 survivants, *J Gynecol Obstet Biol Reprod* 17:183-189, 1988.

275. Bozynski ME, Nelson MN, Genaze D, Rosati-Skertich C, et al: Cranial ultrasonography and the prediction of cerebral palsy in infants weighing less than or equal to 1200 grams at birth, *Dev Med Child Neurol* 30:342-348, 1988.

276. Nwaesei CG, Allen AC, Vincer MJ, Brown SJ, et al: Effect of timing of cerebral ultrasonography on the prediction of later neuro- developmental outcome in high-risk preterm infants, *J Pediatr* 112:970-975, 1988.

277. Costello AM, Hamilton PA, Baudin J, Townsend J, et al: Prediction of neurodevelopmental impairment at four years from brain ultrasound appearance of very preterm infants, *Dev Med Child Neurol* 30:711-722, 1988.

278. Volpe JJ: Current concepts of brain injury in the premature infant, *AJR Am J Roentgenol* 153:243-251, 1989.

279. de Vries LS, Wigglesworth JS, Regev R, Dubowitz LM: Evolution of periventricular leukomalacia during the neonatal period and infancy: Correlation of imaging and postmortem findings, *Early Hum Dev* 17:205-219, 1988.

280. Hope PL, Gould SJ, Howard S, Hamilton PA, et al: Precision of ultrasound diagnosis of pathologically verified lesions in the brains of very preterm infants, *Dev Med Child Neurol* 30:457-471, 1988.

281. Rodriguez J, Claus D, Verellen G, Lyon G: Periventricular leukomalacia: Ultrasonic and neuropathological correlations, *Dev Med Child Neurol* 32:347-352, 1990.

282. Leviton A, Paneth N: White matter damage in preterm newborns: An epidemiologic perspective, *Early Hum Dev* 24:1-22, 1990.

283. Paneth N, Rudelli R, Monte W, Rodriguez E, et al: White matter necrosis in very low birth weight infants: Neuropathologic and ultrasonographic findings in infants surviving six days or longer, *J Pediatr* 116:975-984, 1990.

284. Pidcock FS, Graziani LJ, Stanley C, Mitchell DG, et al: Neurosonographic features of periventricular echodensities associated with cerebral palsy in preterm infants, *J Pediatr* 116:417-422, 1990.

285. Carson SC, Hertzberg BS, Bowie JD, Burger PC: Value of sonography in the diagnosis of intracranial hemorrhage and periventricular leukomalacia: A postmortem study of 35 cases, *AJNR Am J Neuroradiol* 155:595-601, 1990.

286. Cioni G, Bartalena L, Biagioni E, Boldrini A, et al: Neuroimaging and functional outcome of neonatal leukomalacia, *Behav Brain Res* 49:7-19, 1992.

287. Pellicer A, Cabanas F, Garcia-Alix A, Rodriguez JP, et al: Natural history of ventricular dilatation in preterm infants: Prognostic significance, *Pediatr Neurol* 9:108-114, 1993.

288. Roth SC, Baudin J, McCormick DC, Edwards AD, et al: Relation between ultrasound appearance of the brain of very preterm infants and neurodevelopmental impairment at eight years, *Dev Med Child Neurol* 35:755-768, 1993.

289. Fujimoto S, Yamaguchi N, Togari H, Wada Y, et al: Cerebral palsy of cystic periventricular leukomalacia in low-birth-weight infants, *Acta Paediatr* 83:397-401, 1994.

290. Rogers B, Msall M, Owens T, Guernsey K, et al: Cystic periventricular leukomalacia and type of cerebral palsy in preterm infants, *J Pediatr* 125:S1-S8, 1994.

291. Fazzi E, Orcesi S, Caffi L, Ometto A, et al: Neurodevelopmental outcome at 5-7 years in preterm infants with periventricular leukomalacia, *Neuropediatrics* 25:134-139, 1994.

292. Aziz K, Vickar DB, Sauve RS, Etches PC, et al: Province-based study of neurologic disability of children weighing 500 through 1249 grams at britth in relation to neonatal cerebral ultrasound findings, *Pediatrics* 95:837-844, 1995.

293. Pinto-Martin JA, Riolo S, Cnaan A, Holzman C, et al: Cranial ultrasound prediction of disabling and nondisabling cerebral palsy at age two in a low birth weight population, *Pediatrics* 95:249-254, 1995.

294. Leviton A, Gilles F: Ventriculomegaly, delayed myelination, white matter hypoplasia, and "periventricular" leukomalacia: How are they related? *Pediatr Neurol* 15:127-136, 1996.

295. Whitaker AH, Feldman JF, Van Rossem R, Schonfeld IS, et al: Neonatal cranial ultrasound abnormalities in low birth weight infants: Relation to cognitive outcomes at six years of age, *Pediatrics* 98:719-729, 1996.

296. Allan WC, Vohr B, Makuch RW, Katz KH, et al: Antecedents of cerebral palsy in a multicenter trial of indomethacin for intraventricular hemorrhage, *Arch Pediatr Adolesc Med* 151:580-585, 1997.

297. Bos AF, Martijn A, Okken A, Prechtl HFR: Quality of general movements in preterm infants with transient periventricular echodensities, *Acta Paediatr* 87:328-335, 1998.

298. Dammann O, Leviton A: Duration of transient hyperechoic images of white matter in very-low-birthweight infants: A proposed classification, *Dev Med Child Neurol* 39:2-5, 1997.

299. Kuban K, Sanocka U, Leviton A, Allred EN, et al: White matter disorders of prematurity: Association with intraventricular hemorrhage and ventriculomegaly, *J Pediatr* 134:539-546, 1999.

300. Holling EE, Leviton A: Characteristics of cranial ultrasound white matter echolucencies that predict disability: A review, *Dev Med Child Neurol* 41:136-139, 1998.

301. Kubota T, Okumura A, Hayakawa F, Kato T, et al: Relation between the date of cyst formation observable on ultrasonography and the timing of injury determined by serial electroencephalography in preterm infants with periventricular leukomalacia, *Brain Dev* 23:390-394, 2001.

302. Maalouf EF, Duggan PJ, Rutherford MA, Counsell SJ, et al: Magnetic resonance imaging of the brain in a cohort of extremely preterm infants, *J Pediatr* 135:351-357, 1999.

303. Laub MC, Ingrisch H: Increased periventricular echogenicity (periventricular halos) in neonatal brain: A sonographic study, *Neuropediatrics* 17:39-43, 1986.

304. Di Pietro MA: The periventricular echogenic "blush" on cranial ultrasonography, *AJR Am J Roentgenol* 141:851, 1983.

305. van Wezel-Meijler G, van der Knaap MS, Oosting J, Sie LTL, et al: Predictive value of neonatal MRI as compared to ultrasound in premature infants with mild periventricular white matter changes, *Neuropediatrics* 30:231-238, 1999.

306. Ancel PY, Livinec F, Larroque B, Marret S, et al: Cerebral palsy among very preterm children in relation to gestational age and neonatal ultrasound abnormalities: The EPIPAGE cohort study, *Pediatrics* 117:828-835, 2006.

307. Fedrizzi E, Inverno M, Bruzzone MG, Botteon G, et al: MRI features of cerebral lesions and cognitive functions in preterm spastic diplegic children, *Pediatr Neurol* 15:207-212, 1996.

308. Olsen P, Paakko E, Vainionpaa L, Pyhtinen J, et al: Magnetic resonance imaging of periventricular leukomalacia and its clinical correlation in children, *Ann Neurol* 41:754-761, 1997.

309. Skranes JS, Vik T, Nilsen G, Smevik O, et al: Cerebral magnetic resonance imaging and mental and motor function of very low birth weight children at six years of age, *Neuropediatrics* 28:149-154, 1997.

310. Weisglas-Kuperus N, Baerts W, Fetter W, Sauer P: Neonatal cerebral ultrasound, neonatal neurology and perinatal conditions as predictors of neurodevelopmental outcome in very low birthweight infants, *Early Hum Dev* 31:131-148, 1992.

311. Inder TE, Huppi PS, Warfield S, Kikinis R, et al: Periventricular white matter injury in the premature infant is associated with a reduction in cerebral cortical gray matter volume at term, *Ann Neurol* 46:755-760, 1999.

312. Miller SP, Cozzio CC, Goldstein RB, Ferriero DM, et al: Comparing the diagnosis of white matter injury in premature newborns with serial MR imaging and transfontanel ultrasonography findings, *AJNR Am J Neuroradiol* 24:1661-1669, 2003.

313. Inder TE, Anderson NJ, Spencer C, Wells SJ, et al: White matter injury in the premature infant: A comparison between serial cranial ultrasound and MRI at term, *AJNR Am J Neuroradiol* 24:805-809, 2003.

314. Debillon T, Guyen SN, Muet A, Quere MP, et al: Limitations of ultrasonography for diagnosing white matter damage in preterm infants, *Arch Dis Child Fetal Neonatal Ed* 88:F275-F279, 2003.

315. Vollmer B, Roth SC, Baudin J, Stewart AL, et al: Predictors of long-term outcome in very preterm infants: Gestational age versus neonatal cranial ultrasound, *Pediatrics* 112:1108-1114, 2003.

316. Larroque B, Marret S, Ancel PY, Arnaud C, et al: White matter damage and intraventricular hemorrhage in very preterm infants: The EPIPAGE study, *J Pediatr* 143:477-483, 2003.

317. Vergani P, Locatelli A, Doria V, Assi F, et al: Intraventricular hemorrhage and periventricular leukomalacia in preterm infants, *Obstet Gynecol* 104:225-231, 2004.

318. de Vries LS, Van, Haastert IL, Rademaker KJ, Koopman C, et al: Ultrasound abnormalities preceding cerebral palsy in high-risk preterm infants, *J Pediatr* 144:815-820, 2004.

319. Hamrick SE, Miller SP, Leonard C, Glidden DV, et al: Trends in severe brain injury and neurodevelopmental outcome in premature newborn infants: The role of cystic periventricular leukomalacia, *J Pediatr* 145:593-599, 2004.

320. Wilson-Costello D, Friedman H, Minich N, Fanaroff AA, et al: Improved survival rates with increased neurodevelopmental disability for extremely low birth weight infants in the 1990s, *Pediatrics* 115:997-1003, 2005.

321. Roelants-Van Rijn AM, Groenendaal F, Beek FJA, Eken P, et al: Parenchymal brain injury in the preterm infant: Comparison of cranial ultrasound, MRI and neurodevelopmental outcome, *Neuropediatrics* 32:80-89, 2001.

322. de Vries LS, Connell JA, Dubowitz LM, Oozeer RC, et al: Neurological, electrophysiological and MRI abnormalities in infants with extensive cystic leukomalacia, *Neuropediatrics* 18:61-66, 1987.

323. Byrne P, Welch R, Johnson MA, Darrah J, et al: Serial magnetic resonance imaging in neonatal hypoxic-ischemic encephalopathy, *J Pediatr* 117:694-700, 1990.

324. Keeney SE, Adcock EW, McArdle CB: Prospective observations of 100 high-risk neonates by high-field (1.5 Tesla) magnetic resonance imaging of the central nervous system. II. Lesions associated with hypoxic-ischemic encephalopathy, *Pediatrics* 87:431-438, 1991.

325. Grossman R, Novak G, Patel M, Maytal J, et al: MRI in neonatal dural sinus thrombosis, *Pediatr Neurol* 9:235-238, 1993.

326. Kuenzle C, Baenziger O, Martin E, Thun-Hohenstein L, et al: Prognostic value of early MR imaging in term infants with severe perinatal asphyxia, *Neuropediatrics* 25:191-200, 1994.

327. Martin E, Barkovich AJ: Magnetic resonance imaging in perinatal asphyxia, *Arch Dis Child Fetal Neonatal Ed* 72:62-70, 1995.

328. Rutherford MA, Pennock JM, Schwieso JE, Cowan FM, et al: Hypoxic ischaemic encephalopathy: Early magnetic resonance imaging findings and their evolution, *Neuropediatrics* 26:183-191, 1995.

329. Rutherford M, Pennock J, Schwieso J, Cowan F, et al: Hypoxic-ischaemic encephalopathy: Early and late magnetic resonance imaging findings in relation to outcome, *Arch Dis Child Fetal Neonatal Ed* 75:F145-F151, 1996.

330. Cowan FM, Pennock JM, Hanrahan JD, Manji KP, et al: Early detection of cerebral infarction and hypoxic ischemic encephalopathy in neonates using diffusion-weighted magnetic resonance imaging, *Neuropediatrics* 25:172-175, 1994.

331. Barkovich AJ, Hallam D: Neuroimaging in perinatal hypoxic-ischemic injury, *Ment Retard Dev Disabil Res Rev* 3:1-14, 1997.

332. Aida N, Nishimura G, Hachiya Y, Matsui K, et al: MR imaging of perinatal brain damage: Comparison of clinical outcome with initial and follow-up MR findings, *AJNR Am J Neuroradiol* 19:1909-1921, 1998.

333. Yoshiura T, Iwanaga S, Yamada K, Shrier DA, et al: Perirolandic cortex in infants: Signal intensity on MR images as a landmark of the sensorimotor cortex, *Radiology* 207:385-388, 1998.

334. Rutherford MA, Pennock JM, Counsell SJ, Mercuri E, et al: Abnormal magnetic resonance signal in the internal capsule predicts poor neurodevelopmental outcome in infants with hypoxic-ischemic encephalopathy, *Pediatrics* 102:323-328, 1998.

335. Mercuri E, Rutherford M, Cowan F, Pennock J, et al: Early prognostic indicators of outcome in infants with neonatal cerebral infraction: A clinical, electroencephalogram, and magnetic resonance imaging study, *Pediatrics* 103:103-139, 1999.

336. Mercuri E, Guzzetta A, Haataja L, Cowan F, et al: Neonatal neurological examination in infants with hypoxic ischaemic encephalopathy: Correlation with MRI findings, *Neuropediatrics* 30:83-89, 1999.

337. Rutherford M: *MRI of the Neonatal Brain*, Philadelphia: 2002, WB Saunders 2002.

338. Jouvet P, Cowan FM, Cox P, Lazda E, et al: Reproducibility and accuracy of MR imaging of the brain after severe birth asphyxia, *AJNR Am J Neuroradiol* 20:1343-1348, 1999.

339. Johnson AJ, Lee BCP, Lin WL: Echoplanar diffusion-weighted imaging in neonates and infants with suspected hypoxic-ischemic injury: Correlation with patient outcome, *AJR Am J Roentgenol* 172:219-226, 1999.

340. Robertson RL, Ben-Sira L, Barnes PD, Mulkern RV, et al: MR line scan diffusion imaging of term neonates with perinatal brain ischemia, *AJNR Am J Neuroradiol* 20:1658-1670, 1999.

341. Sie LTL, van der Knaap MS, Oosting J, de Vries LS, et al: MR patterns of hypoxic-ischemic brain damage after prenatal, perinatal or postnatal asphyxia, *Neuropediatrics* 31:128-136, 2000.

342. Mercuri E, Ricci D, Cowan FM, Lessing D, et al: Head growth in infants with hypoxic-isehmic encephalopathy: Correlation with neonatal magnetic resonance imaging, *Pediatrics* 106:235-243, 2000.

343. Tekgul H, Serdaroglu G, Yalman O, Tutuncuoglu S: Prognostic correlative values of the late-infancy MRI pattern in term infants with perinatal asphyxia, *Pediatr Neurol* 31:35-41, 2004.

344. Belet N, Belet U, Incesu LU, Uysal S, et al: Hypoxic-ischemic encephalopathy: Correlation of serial MRI and outcome, *Pediatr Neurol* 31:267-274, 2004.

344a. Liauw L, Palm-Meinders IH, Van der Grond J, Leijser LM, et al: Differentiating normal myelination from hypoxic-ischemic encephalopathy on T1-weighted MR Images: A new approach, *AJNR Am J Neuroradiol* 28:660-665, 2007.

344b. Connolly DJ, Widjaja E, Griffiths PD: Involvement of the anterior lobe of the cerebellar vermis in perinatal profound hypoxia, *AJNR Am J Neuroradiol* 28:16-19, 2007.

344c. Eichler F, Krishnamoorthy K, Grant PE: Magnetic resonance imaging evaluation of possible neonatal sinovenous thrombosis, *Pediatr Neurol* 37:317-323, 2007.

345. Vrenken H, Barkhof F, Uitdehaag BMJ, Castelijns JA, et al: MR spectroscopic evidence for glial increase but not for neuro-axonal damage in MS normal-appearing white matter, *Magn Reson Med* 53:256-266, 2005.

346. Moseley ME, Cohen Y, Mintorovitch J: Early detection of regional cerebral ischemia in cats: Comparison of diffusion- and T2-weighted MRI and spectroscopy, *Magn Reson Med* 14:330-346, 1990.

347. Lutsep HL, Albers GW, DeCrespigny A, Kamar GN, et al: Clinical utility of diffusion-weighted magnetic resonance imaging in the assessment of ischemic stroke, *Ann Neurol* 41:574-580, 1997.

348. Lovblad KO, Laubach HJ, Baird AE, Curtin F, et al: Clinical experience with diffusion-weighted MR in patients with acute stroke, *AJNR Am J Neuroradiol* 19:1061-1066, 1998.

349. Burdette JH, Ricci PE, Petitti N, Elster AD: Cerebral infarction: Time course of signal intensity changes on diffusion-weighted MR images, *AJR Am J Roentgenol* 171:791-795, 1998.

350. Schwamm LH, Koroshetz WJ, Sorensen AG, Wang B, et al: Time course of lesion development in patients with acute stroke: Serial diffusion- and hemodynamic-weighted magnetic resonance imaging, *Stroke* 29:2268-2276, 1998.

351. Baird AE, Warach S: Magnetic resonance imaging of acute stroke, *J Cereb Blood Flow Metab* 18:583-609, 1998.

352. Yoneda Y, Tokui K, Hamihara T, Kitagaki H, et al: Diffusion-weighted magnetic resonance imaging: Detection of ischemic injury 39 minutes after onset in a stroke patient, *Ann Neurol* 45:794-797, 1999.

353. Takeoka M, Soman TB, Yoshii A, Caviness VS, et al: Diffusion-weighted images in neonatal cerebral hypoxic-ischemic injury, *Pediatr Neurol* 26:274-281, 2002.

354. Wolf RL, Zimmerman RA, Clancy R, Haselgrove JH: Quantitative apparent diffusion coefficient measurements in term neonates for early detection of hypoxic-ischemic brain injury: Initial experience, *Radiology* 218:825-833, 2001.

355. Soul JS, Robertson RL, Tzika AA, du Plessis AJ, et al: Time course of changes in diffusion-weighted magnetic resonance imaging in a case of neonatal encephalopathy with defined onset and duration of hypoxic-ischemic insult, *Pediatrics* 108:1211-1214, 2001.

356. Hunt RW, Neil JJ, Coleman LT, Kean MJ, et al: Apparent diffusion coefficient in the posterior limb of the internal capsule predicts outcome after perinatal asphyxia, *Pediatrics* 114:999-1003, 2004.

357. Roelants-Van Rijn AM, Nikkels PGJ, Groenendaal F, van der Grond J, et al: Neonatal diffusion-weighted MR imaging: Relation with histopathology or follow-up MR examination, *Neuropediatrics* 32:286-294, 2001.

358. McKinstry RC, Miller JH, Snyder AZ, Mathur A, et al: A prospective, longitudinal diffusion tensor imaging study of brain injury in newborns, *Neurology* 59:824-833, 2002.

359. Rutherford M, Counsell S, Allsop J, Boardman J, et al: Diffusion-weighted magnetic resonance imaging in term perinatal brain injury: A comparison with site of lesion and time from birth, *Pediatrics* 114:1004-1014, 2004.

360. de Vries LS, Van der Grond J, Van Haastert IC, Groenendaal F: Prediction of outcome in new-born infants with arterial ischaemic stroke using diffusion-weighted magnetic resonance imaging, *Neuropediatrics* 36:12-20, 2005.

360a. Miller SP: Newborn brain injury: Looking back to the fetus, *Ann Neurol* 61:285-287, 2007.

360b. Malik GK, Trivedi R, Gupta RK, Hasan KM, et al: Serial quantitation tensor MRI of the term neonates with hypoxic-ischemic encephalopathy (HIE), *Neuropediatrics* 37:337-343, 2006.

360c. Winter JD, Lee DS, Hung RM, Levin SD, et al: Apparent diffusion coefficient pseudonormalization time in neonatal hypoxic-ischemic encephalopathy, *Pediatr Neurol* 37:255-262, 2007.

361. Copen WA, Schwamm LH, Gonzalez G, Wu O, et al: Ischemic stroke: Effects of etiology and patient age on the time course of the core apparent diffusion coefficient, *Neuroradiology* 221:27-34, 2001.

362. Meng S, Qiao M, Scobie K, Tomanek B, et al: Evolution of magnetic resonance imaging changes associated with cerebral hypoxia-ischemia and a relatively selective white matter injury in neonatal rats, *Pediatr Res* 59:554-559, 2006.

363. Maalouf EF, Duggan PJ, Rutherford MA, Counsell SJ, et al: Magnetic resonance imaging of the brain in a cohort of extremely preterm infants, *J Pediatr* 135:351-357, 1999.

364. Inder TE, Wells SJ, Mogridge N, Spencer C, et al: Defining the nature of the cerebral abnormalities in the premature infant: A qualitative magnetic resonance imaging study, *J Pediatr* 143:171-179, 2003.

365. Counsell SJ, Allsop JM, Harrison MC, Larkman DJ, et al: Diffusion weighted imaging of the brain in preterm infants with focal and diffuse white matter abnormality, *Pediatrics* 112:1-7, 2003.

366. Volpe JJ: Cerebral white matter injury of the premature infant: More common than you think, *Pediatrics* 112:176-179, 2003.

367. Woodward LJ, Edgin JO, Thompson D, Inder TE: Object working memory deficits predicted by early brain injury and development in the preterm infant, *Brain* 128:2578-2587, 2005.

368. Woodward LJ, Anderson PJ, Austin NC, Howard K, et al: Neonatal MRI to predict neurodevelopmental outcomes in preterm infants, *N Engl J Med* 355:685-694, 2006.

369. Dyet LE, Kennea NL, Counsell SJ, Mallouf EF, et al: Natural history of brain lesions in extremely preterm infants studied with serial magnetic resonance imaging from birth and neurodevelopmental assessment, *Pediatrics* 118:536-548, 2006.

370. Miller SP, Ferriero DM, Leonard C, Piecuch R, et al: Early brain injury in premature newborns detected with magnetic resonance imaging is associated with adverse early neurodevelopmental outcome, *J Pediatr* 147:609-616, 2005.

371. Inder T, Huppi PS, Zientara GP, Maier SE, et al: Early detection of periventricular leukomalacia by diffusion-weighted magnetic resonance imaging techniques, *J Pediatr* 134:631-634, 1999.

372. Huppi PS, Maier SE, Peled S, Zientara GP, et al: Microstructural development of human newborn cerebral white matter assessed *in vivo* by diffusion tensor magnetic resonance imaging, *Pediatr Res* 44:584-590, 1998.

373. Miller SP, Vigneron DB, Henry RG, Bohland MA, et al: Serial quantitative diffusion tensor MRI of the premature brain: Development in newborns with and without injury, *J Magn Reson Imag* 16:621-632, 2002.

374. Neil JJ, Shiran SI, McKinstry RC, Schefft GL, et al: Normal brain in human newborns: Apparent diffusion coefficient and diffusion anisotropy measured by using diffusion tensor MR imaging, *Radiology* 209:57-66, 1998.

375. Back SA, Luo NL, Borenstein NS, Levine JM, et al: Late oligodendrocyte progenitors coincide with the developmental window of vulnerability for human perinatal white matter injury, *J Neurosci* 21:1302-1312, 2001.

376. Back SA, Luo NL, Borenstein NS, Volpe JJ, et al: Arrested oligodendrocyte lineage progression during human cerebral white matter development: Dissociation between the timing of progenitor differentiation and myelinogenesis, *J Neuropathol Exp Neurol* 61:197-211, 2002.

377. Kinney HC, Brody BA, Kloman AS, Gilles FH: Sequence of central nervous system myelination in human infancy. II. Patterns of myelination in autopsied infants, *J Neuropathol Exp Neurol* 47:217-234, 1988.

378. Black JA, Waxman SG, Ransom BR, Feliciano MD: A quantitative study of developing axons and glia following altered gliogenesis in rat optic nerve, *Brain Res* 380:122-135, 1986.

379. Fields RD, Waxman SG: Regional membrane heterogeneity in premyelinated CNS axons: Factors influencing the binding of sterol-specific probes, *Brain Res* 443:231-242, 1988.

380. Hildebrand C, Waxman SG: Postnatal differentiation of rat optic nerve fibers: Electron microscopic observations on the development of nodes of Ranvier and axoglial relations, *J Comp Neurol* 224:25-37, 1984.

381. Waxman SG, Black JA, Kocsis JD, Ritchie JM: Low density of sodium channels supports action potential conduction in axons of neonatal rat optic nerve, *Proc Natl Acad Sci U S A* 86:1406-1410, 1989.

382. Wimberger DM, Roberts TP, Barkovich AJ, Prayer LM, et al: Identification of "premyelination" by diffusion-weighted MRI, *J Comput Assist Tomogr* 19:28-33, 1995.

383. Flodmark O, Lupton B, Li D, Stimac GK, et al: MR imaging of periventricular leukomalacia in childhood, *AJNR Am J Neuroradiol* 10:111-118, 1989.

384. Baker LL, Stevenson DK, Enzmann DR: End-stage periventricular leukomalacia: MR evaluation, *Radiology* 168:809-815, 1988.

385. Lipper EG, Ross GS, Heier L, Nass R: Magnetic resonance imaging in children of very low birth weight with suspected brain abnormalities, *J Pediatr* 113:1046-1049, 1988.

386. Sugita K, Takeuchi A, Iai M, Tanabe Y: Neurologic sequelae and MRI in low-birth weight patients, *Pediatr Neurol* 5:365-369, 1989.

387. Konishi Y, Kuriyama M, Hayakawa K, Konishi K, et al: Periventricular hyperintensity detected by magnetic resonance imaging in infancy, *Pediatr Neurol* 6:229-232, 1990.

388. van de Bor M, Guit GL, Schreuder AM, Wondergem J, et al: Early detection of delayed myelination in preterm infants, *Pediatrics* 84:407-411, 1989.

389. Guit GL, van de Bor M, den Ouden L, Wondergem JH: Prediction of neurodevelopmental outcome in the preterm infant: MR-staged myelination compared with cranial US, *Radiology* 175:107-109, 1990.

390. Koeda T, Suganuma I, Kohno Y, Takamatsu T, et al: MR imaging of spastic diplegia: Comparative study between preterm and term infants, *Neuroradiology* 32:187-190, 1990.

391. Feldman HM, Scher MS, Kemp SS: Neurodevelopmental outcome of children with evidence of periventricular leukomalacia on late MRI, *Pediatr Neurol* 6:296-302, 1990.

392. Yokochi K, Aiba K, Kodama M, Fujimoto S: Magnetic resonance imaging in athetotic cerebral palsied children, *Acta Paediatr Scand* 80:818-823, 1991.

393. Yokochi K, Aiba K, Horie M, Inukai K, et al: Magnetic resonance imaging in children with spastic diplegia: Correlation with the severity of their motor and mental abnormality, *Dev Med Child Neurol* 33:18-25, 1991.

394. Truwit CL, Barkovich AJ, Koch TK, Ferriero DM: Cerebral palsy: MR findings in 40 patients, *AJNR Am J Neuroradiol* 13:67-78, 1992.

395. Fujii Y, Konishi Y, Kuriyama M, Maeda M, et al: MRI assessment of myelination patterns in high-risk infants, *Pediatr Neurol* 9:194-197, 1993.

396. Panigrahy A, Barnes PD, Robertson RL, Back SA, et al: Volumetric brain differences in children with periventricular T2-signal hyperintensities: A grouping by gestational age at birth, *AJR Am J Roentgenol* 177:695-702, 2001.

397. Davatzikos C, Barzl A, Lawrie T, Hoon AH, et al: Correlation of corpus callosal morphometry with cognitive and motor function in periventricular leukomalacia, *Neuropediatrics* 34:247-252, 2003.

398. Abernethy LJ, Klafkowski G, Foulder-Hughes LA, Cooke WI: Magnetic resonance imaging and T2 relaxometry of cerebral white matter and hippocampus in children born preterm, *Pediatr Res* 54:868-874, 2003.

399. Carmody DP, Dunn SM, Boddie-Willis AS, DeMarco JK, et al: A quantitative measure of myelination development in infants, using MR images, *Neuroradiology* 46:781-786, 2004.

400. Serdaroglu G, Tekgul H, Kitis O, Serdaroglu E, et al: Correlative value of magnetic resonance imaging for neurodevelopmental outcome in periventricular leukomalacia, *Dev Med Child Neurol* 46:733-739, 2004.

401. Indredavik MS, Skranes JS, Vik T, Heyerdahl S, et al: Low-birth-weight adolescents: Psychiatric symptoms and cerebral MRI abnormalities, *Pediatr Neurol* 33:259-266, 2005.

402. Anderson NG, Laurent I, Woodward LJ, Inder TE: Detection of impaired growth of the corpus callosum in premature infants, *Pediatrics* 118:951-960, 2006.

403. Inder TE, Warfield SK, Wang H, Huppi PS, et al: Abnormal cerebral structure is present at term in premature infants, *Pediatrics* 115:286-294, 2005.

404. Murphy BP, Inder TE, Huppi PS, Warfield S, et al: Impaired cerebral cortical gray matter growth after treatment with dexamethasone for neonatal chronic lung disease, *Pediatrics* 107:217-221, 2001.

405. Thompson DK, Warfield SK, Carlin JB, Pavlovic M, et al: Perinatal risk factors altering regional brain structure in the preterm infant, *Brain* 130:667-677, 2007.

406. Huppi PS, Murphy B, Maier SE, Zientara GP, et al: Microstructural brain development after perinatal cerebral white matter injury assessed by diffusion tensor magnetic resonance imaging, *Pediatrics* 107:455-460, 2001.

407. Arzoumanian Y, Mirmiran M, Barnes PD, Woolley K, et al: Diffusion tensor brain imaging findings at term-equivalent age may predict neurologic abnormalities in low birth weight preterm infants, *AJNR Am J Neuroradiol* 24:1646-1653, 2003.

408. Counsell S, Shen Y, Boardman JP, Larkman D, et al: Axial and radial diffusivity in preterm infants who have diffuse white matter changes on MRI at term equivalent age, *Pediatrics* 117:376-386, 2006.

408a. Rose J, Mirmiran M, Butler EE, Lin CY, et al: Neonatal microstructural development of the internal capsule on diffusion tensor imaging correlates with severity of gait and deficits, *Dev Med Child Neurol* 49:745-750, 2007.

409. Peterson BS, Vohr B, Staib LH, Cannistraci CJ, et al: Regional brain volume abnormalities and long-term cognitive outcome in preterm infants, *JAMA* 284:1939-1947, 2000.

410. Nosarti C, Al-Asady MHS, Frangou S, Stewart AL, et al: Adolescents who were born very preterm have decreased brain volumes, *Brain* 125:1616-1623, 2002.

411. Reiss AL, Kesler SR, Vohr B, Duncan CC, et al: Sex differences in cerebral volumes of 8-year-olds born preterm, *J Pediatr* 145:242-249, 2004.

412. Kesler SR, Ment LR, Vohr B, Pajot SK, et al: Volumetric analysis of regional cerebral development in preterm children, *Pediatr Neurol* 31:318-325, 2004.

413. Allin M, Henderson M, Suckling J, Nosarti C, et al: Effects of very low birthweight on brain structure in adulthood, *Dev Med Child Neurol* 46:46-53, 2004.

414. Fearon P, O'Connell P, Frangou S, Aquino P, et al: Brain volumes in adult survivors of very low birth weight: A sibling-controlled study, *Pediatrics* 114:367-371, 2004.

415. Lodygensky GA, Rademaker KJ, Zimine S, Gex-Fabry M, et al: Structural and functional brain developmental after hydrocortisone treatment for neonatal chronic lung disease, *Pediatrics* 116:1-7, 2005.

416. Vangberg TR, Skranes J, Dale AM, Martinussen M, et al: Changes in white matter diffusion anisotropy in adolescents born prematurely, *Neuroimage* 32:1538-1548, 2006.

417. Nagy Z, Westerberg H, Skare S, Andersson JL, et al: Preterm children have disturbances of white matter at 11 years of age as shown by diffusion tensor imaging, *Pediatr Res* 54:672-679, 2003.

418. Hoon AH, Lawrie WT, Melhem ER, Reinhardt EM, et al: Diffusion tensor imaging of periventricular leukomalacia shows affected sensory cortex white matter pathways, *Neurology* 59:752-756, 2002.

419. Thomas B, Eyssen M, Peeters R, Molenaers G, et al: Quantitative diffusion tensor imaging in cerebral palsy due to periventricular white matter injury, *Brain* 128:2562-2577, 2005.

420. Ajayi-Obe M, Saeed N, Cowan FM, Rutherford MA, et al: Reduced development of cerebral cortex in extremely preterm infants, *Lancet* 356:1162-1163, 2000.

421. Peterson BS, Anderson AW, Ehrenkranz RA, Staib LH, et al: Regional brain volumes and their later neurodevelopmental correlates in term and preterm infants, *Pediatrics* 111:939-948, 2003.

422. Boardman JP, Counsell SJ, Rueckert D, Kapellou O, et al: Abnormal deep grey matter development following preterm birth detected using deformation based morphometry, *Neuroimage* 32:70-78, 2006.

423. Parikh N, Lasky RE, Kennedy KA, Moya FR, et al: Postnatal dexamethasone therapy and cerebral tissue volumes in extremely low birth weight infants, *Pediatrics* 119:265-272, 2007.

423a. Nosarti C, Giouroukou E, Healy E, Rifkin L, et al: Grey and white matter distribution in very preterm adolescents mediates neurodevelopmental outcome, *Brain* 131:205-217, 2008.

424. Isaacs E, Lucas A, Chong WK, Wood SJ, et al: Hippocampal volume and everyday memory in children of very low birth weight, *Pediatr Res* 47:713-720, 2000.

425. Abernethy LJ, Cooke RW, Foulder-Hughes L: Caudate and hippocampal volumes, intelligence, and motor impairment in 7-year-old children who were born preterm, *Pediatr Res* 55:884-893, 2004.

426. Martinussen M, Fischl B, Larsson HB, Skranes J, et al: Cerebral cortex thickness in 15-year-old adolescents with low birth weight measured by an automated MRI-based method, *Brain* 128:2588-2596, 2005.

426a. Counsell SJ, Dyet LE, Larkman DJ, Nunes RG, et al: Thalamo-cortical connectivity in children born preterm mapped using probabilistic magnetic resonance tractography, *Neuroimage* 34:896-904, 2007.

427. Lin Y, Okumura A, Hayakawa F, Kato T, et al: Quantitative evaluation of thalami and basal ganglia in infants with periventricular leukomalacia, *Dev Med Child Neurol* 43:481-485, 2001.

428. Allin M, Matsumoto H, Santhouse AM, Nosarti C, et al: Cognitive and motor function and the size of the cerebellum in adolescents born very pre-term, *Brain* 124:60-66, 2001.

429. Johnsen SD, Tarby TJ, Lewis KS, Bird R, et al: Cerebellar infraction: An unrecognized complication of very low birthweight, *J Child Neurol* 17:320-324, 2002.

430. Peterson BS, Vohr B, Staib LH, Cannistraci CJ, et al: Regional brain volume abnormalities and long-term cognitive outcome in preterm infants, *JAMA* 284:1939-1947, 2000.

431. Mercuri E, Atkinson J, Braddick O, Anker S, et al: Visual function in full-term infants with hypoxic-ischaemic encephalopathy, *Neuropediatrics* 28:155-161, 1997.

432. Argyropoulou MI, Xydis V, Drougia A, Argyropoulou PI, et al: MRI measurements of the pons and cerebellum in children born preterm: Associations with the severity of periventricular leukomalacia and perinatal risk factors, *Neuroradiology* 45:730-734, 2003.

433. Miall LS, Cornette LG, Tanner SF, Arthur RJ, et al: Posterior fossa abnormalities seen on magnetic resonance brain imaging in a cohort of newborn infants, *J Perinatol* 23:396-403, 2003.

434. Srinivasan L, Allsop J, Counsell SJ, Boardman JP, et al: Smaller cerebellar volumes in very preterm infants at term-equivalent age are associated with the presence of supratentorial lesions, *AJNR Am J Neuroradiol* 27:573-579, 2006.

435. Bodensteiner JB, Johnsen SD: Cerebellar injury in the extremely premature infant: Newly recognized but relatively common outcome, *J Child Neurol* 20:139-142, 2005.

436. Johnsen SD, Bodensteiner JB, Lotze TE: Frequency and nature of cerebellar injury in the extremely premature survivor with cerebral palsy, *J Child Neurol* 20:60-64, 2005.

437. Limperopoulos C, Soul JS, Gauvreau K, Huppi PS, et al: Late gestation cerebellar growth is rapid and impeded by premature birth, *Pediatrics* 115:688-695, 2005.

438. Limperopoulos C, Soul JS, Haidar H, Huppi PS, et al: Impaired trophic interactions between the cerebellum and the cerebrum among preterm infants, *Pediatrics* 116:844-850, 2005.

439. Shah DK, Anderson PJ, Carlin JB, Pavlovic M, et al: Reduction in cerebellar volumes in preterm infants: Relationship to white matter injury and neurodevelopment at two years of age, *Pediatr Res* 60:97-102, 2006.

440. Haddad J, Constantinesco A, Brunot B: Single photon emission computed tomography of the brain perfusion in neonates. In Haddad J, Christmann D, Messer J, editors: *Imaging Techniques of the CNS of the Neonates*, New York: 1991, Springer-Verlag.

441. Denays R, Van Pachterbeke T, Tondeur M, Spehl M, et al: Brain single photon emission computed tomography in neonates, *J Nucl Med* 30:1337-1341, 1989.

442. Uvebrant P, Bjure J, Hedstrom A, Ekholm S: Brain single photon emission computed tomography (SPECT) in neuropediatrics, *Neuropediatrics* 22:3-9, 1991.

443. Konishi Y, Kuriyama M, Mori I, Fujii Y, et al: Assessment of local cerebral blood flow in neonates with N-isopropyl-P-[^{123}I] iodoamphetamine

and single photo emission computed tomography, *Brain Dev* 16:450-453, 1995.

444. Volpe JJ, Pasternak JF: Parasagittal cerebral injury in neonatal hypoxic-ischemic encephalopathy: Clinical and neuroradiologic features, *J Pediatr* 91:472-476, 1977.

445. O'Brien MJ, Ash JM, Gilday DL: Radionuclide brain-scanning in perinatal hypoxia/ischemia, *Dev Med Child Neurol* 21:161-170, 1979.

446. Hope PL, Costello AM, Cady EB, Delpy DT, et al: Cerebral energy metabolism studied with phosphorus NMR spectroscopy in normal and birth-asphyxiated infants, *Lancet* 2:366-370, 1984.

447. Wyatt JS, Edwards AD, Azzopardi D, Reynolds EO: Magnetic resonance and near infrared spectroscopy for investigation of perinatal hypoxic-ischaemic brain injury, *Arch Dis Child* 64:953-963, 1989.

448. Roth SC, Azzopardi D, Aldridge R, Cady E, et al: Progression of changes in cerebral energy metabolism in newborn infants studied by ^{31}P magnetic resonance spectroscopy (MRS) following birth asphyxia, *Neuropediatrics* 22:169-170, 1991.

449. Roth SC, Edwards AD, Cady EB, Delpy DT, et al: Relation between cerebral oxidative metabolism following birth asphyxia, and neurodevelopmental outcome and brain growth at one year, *Dev Med Child Neurol* 34:285-295, 1992.

450. Azzopardi D, Wyatt JS, Cady EB, Delpy DT, et al: Prognosis of newborn infants with hypoxic-ischemic brain injury assessed by phosphorus magnetic resonance spectroscopy, *Pediatr Res* 25:445-451, 1989.

451. Cady EB: Phosphorus and proton magnetic resonance spectroscopy of the brain of the newborn human infant. In Bachelard H, editor: *Magnetic Resonance Spectroscopy and Imaging in Neurochemistry*, New York: 1997, Plenum Publishing.

452. Martin E, Buchli R, Ritter S, Schmid R, et al: Diagnostic and prognostic value of cerebral ^{31}P magnetic resonance spectroscopy in neonates with perinatal asphyxia, *Pediatr Res* 40:749-758, 1996.

453. Roth SC, Baudin J, Cady E, Johal K, et al: Relation of deranged neonatal cerebral oxidative metabolism with neurodevelopmental outcome and head circumference at 4 years, *Dev Med Child Neurol* 39:718-725, 1997.

454. Robertson NJ, Cox IJ, Cowan FM, Counsell SJ, et al: Cerebral intracellular lactic alkalosis persisting months after neonatal encephalopathy measured by magnetic resonance spectroscopy, *Pediatr Res* 46:287-296, 1999.

455. Robertson NJ, Cowan FM, Cox IJ, Edwards AD: Brain alkaline intracellular pH after neonatal encephalopathy, *Ann Neurol* 52:732-742, 2002.

456. Pi RB, Li WM, Lee NTK, Chan HHN, et al: Minocycline prevents glutamate-induced apoptosis of cerebellar granule neurons by differential regulation of p38 and Akt pathways, *J Neurochem* 91:1219-1230, 2004.

457. Peden CJ, Rutherford MA, Sargentoni J, Cox IJ, et al: Proton spectroscopy of the neonatal brain following hypoxic-ischaemic injury, *Dev Med Child Neurol* 35:502-510, 1993.

458. Groenendaal F, Veenhoven RH, Van Der Grond J, Jansen GH, et al: Cerebral lactate and N-acetyl-aspartate/choline ratios in asphyxiated full-term neonates demonstrated in vivo using proton magnetic resonance spectroscopy, *Pediatr Res* 35:148-151, 1994.

459. Hanrahan JD, Sargentoni J, Azzopardi D, Manji K, et al: Cerebral metabolism within 18 hours of birth asphyxia: A proton magnetic resonance spectroscopy study, *Pediatr Res* 39:584-590, 1996.

460. Leth H, Toft PB, Peitersen B, Lou HC, et al: Use of brain lactate levels to predict outcome after perinatal asphyxia, *Acta Paediatr* 85:859-864, 1996.

461. Penrice J, Cady EB, Lorek A, Wylezinska M, et al: Proton magnetic resonance spectroscopy of the brain in normal preterm and term infants, and early changes after perinatal hypoxia-ischemia, *Pediatr Res* 40:6-14, 1996.

462. Shu SK, Ashwal S, Holshouser BA, Nystrom G, et al: Prognostic value of ^{1}H-MRS in perinatal CNS insults, *Pediatr Neurol* 17:309-318, 1997.

463. Holshouser BA, Ashwal S, Luh GY, Shu S, et al: Proton MR spectroscopy after acute central nervous system injury: Outcome prediction in neonates, infants, and children, *Radiology* 202:487-496, 1997.

464. Ashwal S, Holshouser BA, Tomasi LG, Shu S, et al: ^{1}H-magnetic resonance spectroscopy determined cerebral lactate and poor neurological outcomes in children with central nervous system disease, *Ann Neurol* 41:470-481, 1997.

465. Hanrahan JD, Cox IJ, Edwards AD, Cowan FM, et al: Persistent increases in cerebral lactate concentration after birth asphyxia, *Pediatr Res* 44:304-311, 1998.

466. Novotny E, Ashwal S, Shevell M: Proton magnetic resonance spectroscopy: An emerging technology in pediatric neurology research, *Pediatr Res* 44:1-10, 1998.

467. Hanrahan JD, Cox IJ, Azzopardi D, Cowan FM, et al: Relation between proton magnetic resonance spectroscopy within 18 hours of birth asphyxia and neurodevelopment at 1 year of age, *Dev Med Child Neurol* 41:76-82, 1999.

468. Amess PN, Penrice J, Wylezinska M, Lorek A, et al: Early brain proton magnetic resonance spectroscopy and neonatal neurology related to neurodevelopmental outcome at 1 year in term infants after presumed hypoxic-ischaemic brain injury, *Dev Med Child Neurol* 41:436-445, 1999.

469. Barkovich AJ, Baranski K, Vigneron D, Partridge JC, et al: Proton MR spectroscopy for the evaluation of brain injury in asphyxiated, term neonates, *AJNR Am J Neuroradiol* 20:1399-1405, 1999.

470. Groenendaal F, RoelantsvanRijn AM, van der Grond J, Toet MC, et al: Glutamate in cerebral tissue of asphyxiated neonates during the first week of life demonstrated in vivo using proton magnetic resonance spectroscopy, *Biol Neonate* 79:254-257, 2001.

471. Barkovich AJ, Westmark KD, Bedi HS, Partridge JC, et al: Proton spectroscopy and diffusion imaging on the first day of life after perinatal asphyxia: Preliminary report, *AJNR Am J Neuroradiol* 22:1786-1794, 2001.

472. Zarifi MK, Astrakas LG, Young Poussaint T, du Plessis AJ, et al: Prediction of adverse outcome with cerebral lactate level and apparent diffusion coefficient in infants with perinatal asphyxia, *Radiology* 225:859-870, 2002.

473. Roelants-van Rijn AM, van der Grond J, de Vries LS, Groenendaal F: Value of ¹H-MRS using different echo times in neonates with cerebral hypoxia-ischemia, *Pediatr Res* 49:356-362, 2001.

474. Miller SP, Newton N, Ferriero DM, Partridge C, et al: Predictors of 30-month outcome after perinatal depression: Role of proton MRS and socioeconomic factors, *Pediatr Res* 52:71-77, 2002.

475. Bartha AI, Foster-Barber A, Miller SP, Vigneron DB, et al: Neonatal encephalopathy: Association of cytokines with MR spectroscopy and outcome, *Pediatr Res* 56:960-966, 2004.

476. Miller SP, Weiss J, Barnwell A, Ferriero DM, et al: Seizure-associated brain injury in term newborns with perinatal asphyxia, *Neurology* 58:542-548, 2002.

477. Khong PL, Tse C, Wong IYC, Lam BCC, et al: Diffusion-weighted imaging and proton magnetic resonance spectroscopy in perinatal hypoxic-ischemic encephalopathy: Association with neuromotor outcome at 18 months of age, *J Child Neurol* 19:872-881, 2004.

478. L'Abee C, de Vries LS, van der Grond J, Groenendaal F: Early diffusion-weighted MRI and 1H-magnetic resonance spectroscopy in asphyxiated full-term neonates, *Biol Neonate* 88:306-312, 2005.

479. da Silva LF, Filho JR, Anes M, Nunes ML: Prognostic value of (1)H-MRS in neonatal encephalopathy, *Pediatr Neurol* 34:360-366, 2006.

480. Shanmugalingam S, Thornton JS, Iwata O, Bainbridge A, et al: Comparative prognostic utilities of early quantitative magnetic resonance imaging spin-spin relaxometry and proton magnetic resonance spectroscopy in neonatal encephalopathy, *Pediatrics* 118:1467-1477, 2006.

481. Volpe JJ, Herscovitch P, Perlman JM, Kreusser KL, et al: Positron emission tomography in the asphyxiated term newborn: Parasagittal impairment of cerebral blood flow, *Ann Neurol* 17:287-296, 1985.

482. Kaufman SA, Miller SP, Ferriero DM, Glidden DH, et al: Encephalopathy as a predictor of magnetic resonance imaging abnormalities in asphyxiated newborns, *Pediatr Neurol* 28:342-346, 2003.

483. Sladky JT, Rorke LB: Perinatal hypoxic-ischemic spinal cord injury, *Pediatr Pathol* 6:87-101, 1986.

484. Clancy RR, Sladky JT, Rorke LB: Hypoxic-ischemic spinal cord injury following perinatal asphyxia, *Ann Neurol* 25:185-189, 1989.

485. Graybiel AM: The basal ganglia: Learning new tricks and loving it, *Curr Opin Neurobiol* 15:638-644, 2005.

486. Monchi O, Petrides M, Strafella AP, Worsley KJ, et al: Functional role of the basal ganglia in the planning and execution of actions, *Ann Neurol* 59:257-264, 2006.

487. Yoshioka H, Mino M, Morikawa Y, Kasubuchi Y, et al: Changes in cell proliferation kinetics in the mouse cerebellum after total asphyxia, *Pediatrics* 76:965-969, 1985.

488. Yoshioka H, Yoshida A, Ochi M, Iino S, et al: Dendritic development of cortical neurons of mice subjected to total asphyxia: A Golgi-Cox study, *Acta Neuropathol* 70:185-189, 1986.

489. Roland EH, Jan JE, Hill A, Wong PK: Cortical visual impairment following birth asphyxia, *Pediatr Neurol* 2:133-137, 1986.

490. Groenendaal F, van Hof-van Duin J: Partial visual recovery in two full-term infants after perinatal hypoxia, *Neuropediatrics* 21:76-78, 1990.

491. Muttitt SC, Taylor MJ, Kobayashi JS, MacMillan L, et al: Serial visual evoked potentials and outcome in term birth asphyxia, *Pediatr Neurol* 7:86-90, 1991.

492. Schenk-Rootlieb AJ, van Nieuwenhuizen O, van der Graaf Y, Wittebol-Post D, et al: The prevalence of cerebral visual disturbance in children with cerebral palsy, *Dev Med Child Neurol* 34:473-480, 1992.

493. Mercuri E, Atkinson J, Braddick O, Anker S, et al: The aetiology of delayed visual maturation: Short review and personal findings in relation to magnetic resonance imaging, *Eur J Paediatr Neurol* 1:31-34, 1997.

494. Mercuri E, Anker S, Guzzetta A, Barnett AL, et al: Visual function at school age in children with neonatal encephalopathy and low Apgar scores, *Arch Dis Child Fetal Neonatal Ed* 89:F258-F262, 2004.

495. Ricci D, Guzzetta A, Cowan F, Haataja L, et al: Sequential neurological examinations in infants with neonatal encephalopathy and low apgar scores: Relationship with brain MRI, *Neuropediatrics* 37:148-153, 2006.

496. Robertson CM, Morrish DW, Wheler GH, Grace MG: Neonatal encephalopathy: An indicator of early sexual maturation in girls, *Pediatr Neurol* 6:102-108, 1990.

497. Maller AI, Hankins LL, Yeakley JW, Butler IJ: Rolandic type cerebral palsy in children as a pattern of hypoxic-ischemic injury in the full-term neonate, *J Child Neurol* 13:313-321, 1998.

498. Koeda T, Takeshita K, Kisa T: Bilateral opercular syndrome: An unusual complication of perinatal difficulties, *Brain Dev* 17:193-195, 1995.

499. Lou HC: Etiology and pathogenesis of attention-deficit hyperactivity disorder (ADHD): Significance of prematurity and perinatal hypoxic-haemodynamic encephalopathy, *Acta Paediatr* 85:1266-1271, 1996.

500. Toft PB: Prenatal and perinatal striatal injury: A hypothetical cause of attention-deficit-hyperactivity disorder? *Pediatr Neurol* 21:602-610, 1999.

501. Lou HC, Rosa P, Pryds O, Karrebaek H, et al: ADHD: Increased dopamine receptor availability linked to attention deficit and low neonatal cerebral blood flow, *Dev Med Child Neurol* 46:179-183, 2004.

502. Sugama S, Ariga M, Hoashi E, Eto Y: Brainstem cranial-nerve lesions in an infant with hypoxic cerebral injury, *Pediatr Neurol* 29:256-259, 2003.

503. Sarnat HB: Watershed infarcts in the fetal and neonatal brainstem: An aetiology of central hypoventilation, dysphagia, Mobius syndrome and micrognathia, *Eur J Pediatr Neurol* 8:71-87, 2004.

504. Krageloh-Mann I, Helber A, Mader I, Staudt M, et al: Bilateral lesions of thalamus and basal ganglia: Origin and outcome, *Dev Med Child Neurol* 44:477-484, 2002.

505. Yokochi K: Clinical profiles of children with cerebral palsy having lesions of the thalamus, putamen and/or peri-rolandic area, *Brain Dev* 26:227-232, 2004.

506. Malamud N: Status marmoratus: A form of cerebral palsy following either birth injury or inflammation of the central nervous system, *J Pediatr* 37:610-619, 1950.

506a. Himmelmann K, Hagberg G, Wiklund LM, Eek MN, et al: Dyskinetic cerebral palsy: A population-based study of children born between 1991 and 1998, *Dev Med Child Neurol* 49:246-251, 2007.

507. Polani PE: The natural history of choreoathetoid cerebral palsy, *Guys Hosp Rep* 108:32-45, 1959.

508. Paine RS: The evolution of infantile postural reflexes in the presence of chronic brain syndromes, *Dev Med Child Neurol* 5:345-361, 1964.

509. Colamaria V, Curatolo P, Cusmai R, Dalla Bernardina B: Symmetrical bithalamic hyperdensities in asphyxiated full-term newborns: An early indicator of status marmoratus, *Brain Dev* 10:57-59, 1988.

510. Burke RE, Fahn S, Gold AP: Delayed-onset dystonia in patients with "static" encephalopathy, *J Neurol Neurosurg Psychiatry* 43:789-797, 1980.

511. Hanson RA, Berenberg W, Byers RK: Changing motor patterns in cerebral palsy, *Dev Med Child Neurol* 12:309-314, 1970.

512. Arvidsson J, Hagberg B: Delayed-onset dyskinetic "cerebral palsy": A late effect of perinatal asphyxia? *Acta Paediatr Scand* 79:1121-1123, 1990.

513. Saint-Hilaire MH, Burke RE, Bressman SB, Brin MF, et al: Delayed-onset dystonia due to perinatal or early childhood asphyxia, *Neurology* 41:216-222, 1991.

514. Crothers B, Paine RS: *The Natural History of Cerebral Palsy*, Cambridge, MA: 1959, Harvard University Press 1959.

515. Hagberg B, Hagberg G, Olow I: The changing panorama of cerebral palsy in Sweden 1954-1970. I. Analysis of the general changes, *Acta Paediatr Scand* 64:187-192, 1975.

516. Kyllerman M, Bager B, Bensch J, Bille B, et al: Dyskinetic cerebral palsy. I. Clinical categories, associated neurological abnormalities and incidences, *Acta Paediatr Scand* 71:543-550, 1982.

517. Rosenbloom L: Dyskinetic cerebral palsy and birth asphyxia, *Dev Med Child Neurol* 36:285-289, 1994.

518. Barnett A, Mercuri E, Rutherford M, Haataja L, et al: Neurological and perceptual-motor outcome at 5-6 years of age in children with neonatal encephalopathy: Relationship with neonatal brain MRI, *Neuropediatrics* 33:242-248, 2002.

519. de Vries LS, Pierrat V, Eken P, Minami T, et al: Prognostic value of early somatosensory evoked potentials for adverse outcome in full-term infants with birth asphyxia, *Brain Dev* 13:320-325, 1991.

520. Lou HC, Henriksen L, Bruhn P: Focal cerebral hypoperfusion in children with dysphasia and/or attention deficit disorder, *Arch Neurol* 41:825-829, 1984.

521. Lou HC, Henriksen L, Bruhn P, Borner H, et al: Striatal dysfunction in attention deficit and hyperkinetic disorder, *Arch Neurol* 46:48-52, 1989.

522. Lou HC, Henriksen L, Bruhn P: Focal cerebral dysfunction in developmental learning disabilities, *Lancet* 335:8-11, 1990.

523. Yokochi K: Clinical profiles of subjects with subcortical leukomalacia and border-zone infarction revealed by MR, *Acta Paediatr* 87:879-883, 1998.

523a. Gonzalez FF, Miller SP: Does perinatal asphyxia impair cognitive function without cerebral palsy? *Arch Dis Child Fetal Neonatal Ed* 91:F454-459, 2006.

524. Larroche JC: *Developmental Pathology of the Neonate*, New York: 1977, Excerpta Medica 1977.

525. Dambska M, Laure-Kamionowska M, Schmidt-Sidor B: Early and late neuropathological changes in perinatal white matter damage, *J Child Neurol* 4:291-298, 1989.

526. Cioni G, Bertuccelli B, Boldrini A, Canapicchi R, et al: Correlation between visual function, neurodevelopmental outcome, and magnetic resonance imaging findings in infants with periventricular leucomalacia, *Arch Dis Child Fetal Neonatal Ed* 82:F134-F140, 2000.

527. Koeda T, Takeshita K: Visuoperceptual impairment and cerebral lesions in spastic diplegia with preterm birth, *Brain Dev* 14:239-244, 1992.

528. Weisglas-Kuperus N, Heersema DJ, Baerts W, Fetter WPF, et al: Visual functions in relation with neonatal cerebral ultrasound, neurology and cognitive development in very-low-birthweight children, *Neuropediatrics* 24:149-154, 1993.

529. Eken P, van Nieuwenhuizen O, van der Graaf Y, Schalij-Delfos NE, et al: Relation between neonatal cranial ultrasound abnormalities and cerebral visual impairment in infancy, *Dev Med Child Neurol* 36:3-15, 1994.

530. Eken P, de Vries LS, van Nieuwenhuizen O, Schalif-Delfos NE, et al: Early predictors of cerebral visual impairment in infants with cystic leukomalacia, *Neuropediatrics* 27:16-25, 1996.

531. Pike MG, Holmstrom G, de Vries LS, Pennock JM, et al: Patterns of visual impairment associated with lesions of the preterm infant brain, *Dev Med Child Neurol* 36:849-862, 1994.

532. Luna B, Dobson V, Scher MS, Guthrie RD: Grating acuity and visual field development in infants following perinatal asphyxia, *Dev Med Child Neurol* 37:330-344, 1995.

533. Cioni G, Fazzi B, Ipata AE, Canapicchi R, et al: Correlation between cerebral visual impairment and magnetic resonance imaging in children with neonatal encephalopathy, *Dev Med Child Neurol* 38:120-132, 1996.

534. Jacobson L, Ek U, Fernell E, Flodmark O, et al: Visual impairment in preterm children with periventricular leukomalacia: Visual, cognitive and neuropaediatric characteristics related to cerebral imaging, *Dev Med Child Neurol* 38:724-735, 1996.

535. Ito J-I, Saijo H, Araki A, Tanaka H, et al: Assessment of visuoperceptual disturbance in children with spastic diplegia using measurements of the lateral ventricles on cerebral MRI, *Dev Med Child Neurol* 38:496-502, 1996.

536. Jongmans M, Mercuri E, Henderson S, de Vries L, et al: Visual function of prematurely born children with and without perceptual-motor difficulties, *Early Hum Dev* 45:73-82, 1996.

537. Cioni G, Fazzi B, Coluccini M, Bartalena L, et al: Cerebral visual impairment in preterm infants with periventricular leukomalacia, *Pediatr Neurol* 17:331-338, 1997.

538. van Holf-van Duin J, Cioni G, Bertuccelli B, Fazzi B, et al: Visual outcome at 5 years of newborn infants at risk of cerebral visual impairment, *Dev Med Child Neurol* 40:302-309, 1998.

539. Powls A, Botting N, Cooke RWI, Stephenson G, et al: Visual impairment in very low birthweight children, *Arch Dis Child Fetal Neonatal Ed* 76:F82-F87, 1997.

540. Singer L, Yamashita T, Lilien L, Collin M, et al: A longitudinal study of developmental outcome of infants with bronchopulmonary dysplasia and very low birth weight, *Pediatrics* 100:987-993, 1997.

541. Harvey E,V, Luna B: Long-term grating acuity and visual-field development in preterm children who experienced bronchopulmonary dysplasia, *Dev Med Child Neurol* 39:167-173, 1997.

542. Lanzi G, Fazzi E, Uggetti C, Cavallini A, et al: Cerebral visual impairment in periventricular leukomalacia, *Neuropediatrics* 29:145-150, 1998.

543. Fedrizzi E, Anderloni A, Bono R, Bova S, et al: Eye-movement disorders and visual-perceptual impairment in diplegic children born preterm: A clinical evaluation, *Dev Med Child Neurol* 40:682-688, 1998.

544. Luoma L, Herrgard E, Martikainen A: Neuropsychological analysis of the visuomotor problems in children born preterm at ≤32 weeks of gestation: A 5-year prospective follow-up, *Dev Med Child Neurol* 40:21-30, 1998.

545. Goyen T-A, Lui K, Woods R: Visual-motor, visual-perceptual, and fine motor outcomes in very-low-birthweight children at 5 years, *Dev Med Child Neurol* 40:76-81, 1998.

546. Hard A-L, Niklasson A, Svensson E, Hellstrom A: Visual function in school-aged children born before 29 weeks of gestation: A population-based study, *Dev Med Child Neurol* 42:100-105, 2000.

547. Guzzetta A, Mazzotti S, Tinelli F, Bancale A, et al: Early assessment of visual information processing and neurological outcome in preterm infants, *Neuropediatrics* 37:278-285, 2006.

548. McDonald A: *Children of Very Low Birthweight: M.E.I.U. Research Monograph No. 1.* London: 1967, Spastics Society and Heineman 1967.

549. Pharoah PO, Cooke T, Rosenbloom L, Cooke RW: Effects of birth weight, gestational age, and maternal obstetric history on birth prevalence of cerebral palsy, *Arch Dis Child* 62:1035-1040, 1987.

550. Fazzi E, Lanzi G, Gerardo A, Ometto A, et al: Neurodevelopmental outcome in very low-birth-weight infants with or without periventricular haemorrhage and/or leucomalacia, *Acta Paediatr* 81:808-811, 1992.

551. Volpe JJ: Value of MR in definition of the neuropathology of cerebral palsy in vivo, *AJNR Am J Neuroradiol* 13:79-83, 1992.

552. Yokochi K, Horie M, Inukai K, Kito H, et al: Computed tomographic findings in children with spastic diplegia: Correlation with the severity of their motor abnormality, *Brain Dev* 11:236-240, 1989.

553. Valkama AM, Paakko ELE, Vainionpaa LK, Lanning FP, et al: Magnetic resonance imaging at term and neuromotor outcome in preterm infants, *Acta Paediatr* 89:348-355, 2000.

554. Staudt M, Pavlova M, Bohm S, Grodd W, et al: Pyramidal tract damage correlates with motor dysfunction in bilateral periventricular leukomalacia (PVL), *Neuropediatrics* 34:182-188, 2003.

555. Ohgi S, Akiyama T, Fukuda M: Neurobehavioural profile of low-birth-weight infants with cystic periventricular leukomalacia, *Dev Med Child Neurol* 47:221-228, 2005.

556. Tang-Wai R, Webster RI, Shevell MI: A clinical and etiologic profile of spastic diplegia, *Pediatr Neurol* 34:212-218, 2006.

557. Krägeloh-Mann I, Hagberg B, Petersen D, Riethmuller J, et al: Bilateral spastic cerebral palsy: Pathogenetic aspects from MRI, *Neuropediatrics* 23:46-48, 1992.

558. Krageloh-Mann I, Petersen D, Hagberg G, Vollmer B, et al: Bilateral spastic cerebral palsy: MRI pathology and origin, analysis from a representative series of 56 cases, *Dev Med Child Neurol* 37:379-397, 1995.

559. Miller SP, Shevell MI, Patenaude Y, O'Gorman AM: Neuromotor spectrum of periventricular leukomalacia in children born at term, *Pediatr Neurol* 23:155-159, 2000.

560. Shevell MJ, Majnemer A, Morin I: Etiologic yield of cerebral palsy: A contemporary case series, *Pediatr Neurol* 28:352-359, 2003.

561. Wu YW, Croen LA, Shah SJ, Newman TB, et al: Cerebral palsy in a term population: Risk factors and neuroimaging findings, *Pediatrics* 118:690-697, 2006.

562. Bax M, Tydeman C, Flodmark O: Clinical and MRI correlates of cerebral palsy: The European Cerebral Palsy Study, *JAMA* 296:1602-1608, 2006.

563. Judas M, Rados M, Jovanov-Milosevic N, Hrabac P, et al: Structural, immunocytochemical, and MR imaging properties of periventricular crossroads of growing cortical pathways in preterm infants, *AJNR Am J Neuroradiol* 26:2671-2684, 2005.

564. Kostovic I, Judas M: Prolonged coexistence of transient and permanent circuitry elements in the developing cerebral cortex of fetuses and preterm infants, *Dev Med Child Neurol* 48:388-393, 2006.

565. Sie LT, Hart AA, van Hof J, de Groot L, et al: Predictive value of neonatal MRI with respect to late MRI findings and clinical outcome. A study in infants with periventricular densities on neonatal ultrasound, *Neuropediatrics* 36:78-89, 2005.

566. Dyet LE, Kennea N, Counsell SJ, Maalouf EF, et al: Natural history of brain lesions in extremely preterm infants studied with serial magnetic resonance imaging from birth and neurodevelopmental assessment, *Pediatrics* 118:536-548, 2006.

567. San Giovanni JP, Allred EN, Mayer DL, Stewart JE, et al: Reduced visual resolution acuity and cerebral white matter damage in very-low-birth-weight infants, *Dev Med Child Neurol* 42:809-815, 2000.

568. Fazzi E, Bova SM, Uggetti C, Signorini SG, et al: Visual-perceptual impairment in children with periventricular leukomalacia, *Brain Dev* 26:506-512, 2004.

569. van den Hout BM, de Vries LS, Meiners LC, Stiers P, et al: Visual perceptual impairment in children at 5 years of age with perinatal haemorrhagic or ischaemic brain damage in relation to cerebral magnetic resonance imaging, *Brain Dev* 26:251-261, 2004.

570. Kapellou O, Counsell SJ, Kennea NL, Dyet L, et al: Abnormal cortical development after premature birth shown by altered allometric scaling of brain growth, *PLOS Med* 3:265, 2006.

571. Saigal S, Stoskopf BL, Streiner DL, Burrows E: Physical growth and current health status of infants who were of extremely low birth weight and controls at adolescence, *Pediatrics* 108:407-415, 2001.

572. Okumura A, Watanabe K, Hayakawa F, Katio T: The timing of brain insults in preterm infants who later developed West syndrome, *Neuropediatrics* 32:245-249, 2001.

573. Ravizza SM, McCormick CA, Schlerf JE, Justus T, et al: Cerebellar damage produces selective deficits in verbal working memory, *Brain* 129:306-320, 2006.

574. Schmahmann JD: Disorders of the cerebellum: Ataxia, dysmetria of thought, and the cerebellar cognitive affective syndrome, *J Neuropsychiatry Clin Neurosci* 16:367-378, 2004.

575. Exner C, Weniger G, Irle E: Cerebellar lesions in the PICA but not SCA territory impair cognition, *Neurology* 63:2132-2135, 2004.

576. Hermann B, Seidenberg M, Sears L, Hansen R, et al: Cerebellar atrophy in temporal lobe epilepsy affects procedural memory, *Neurology* 63:2129-2131, 2004.

576a. Limperopoulos C, Bassan H, Sullivan N, Soul J, et al: Positive screening for autism in ex-preterm infants: Prevalence and risk factors, *Pediatrics* 2008: in press.

577. Klesh KW, Murphy TF, Scher MS, Buchanan DE, et al: Cerebral infarction in persistent pulmonary hypertension of the newborn, *Am J Dis Child* 141:852-857, 1987.

578. Aso K, Scher MS, Barmada MA: Cerebral infarcts and seizures in the neonate, *J Child Neurol* 5:224-228, 1990.

579. Lanska MJ, Lanska DJ, Horwitz SJ, Aram DM: Presentation, clinical course, and outcome of childhood stroke, *Pediatr Neurol* 7:333-341, 1991.

580. Bouza H, Rutherford M, Acolet D, Pennock JM, et al: Evolution of early hemiplegic signs in full-term infants with unilateral brain lesions in the neonatal period: A prospective study, *Neuropediatrics* 25:201-207, 1994.

581. Govaert P, Matthys E, Zecic A, Roelens F, et al: Perinatal cortical infarction within middle cerebral artery trunks, *Arch Dis Child Fetal Neonatal Ed* 82:F59-F63, 2000.

582. Sreenan C, Bhargava R, Robertson CM: Cerebral infarction in the term newborn: Clinical presentation and long-term outcome, *J Pediatr* 137:351-355, 2000.

583. Gunther G, Junker R, Strater R, Schobess R, et al: Symptomatic ischemic stroke in full-term neonates role of acquired and genetic prothombotic risk factors, *Stroke* 31:2437-2441, 2003.

584. Wu YW, March WM, Croen LA, Grether JK, et al: Perinatal stroke in children with motor impairment: A population-based study, *Pediatrics* 114:612-619, 2004.

585. Hanigan WC, Rossi LJ, McLean JM, Wright RM: MRI of cerebral vein thrombosis in infancy: A case report, *Neurology* 36:1354-1356, 1986.

586. Konishi Y, Kuriyama M, Sudo M, Konishi K, et al: Superior sagittal sinus thrombosis in neonates, *Pediatr Neurol* 3:222-225, 1987.

587. Wong VK, LeMesurier J, Franceschini R, Heikali M, et al: Cerebral venous thrombosis as a cause of neonatal seizures, *Pediatr Neurol* 3:235-237, 1987.

588. Baram TZ, Butler IJ, Nelson MD Jr, McArdle CB: Transverse sinus thrombosis in newborns: Clinical and magnetic resonance imaging findings, *Ann Neurol* 24:792-794, 1988.

589. Shevell MI, Silver K, O'Gorman AM, Watters GV, et al: Neonatal dural sinus thrombosis, *Pediatr Neurol* 5:161-165, 1989.

590. Rivkin MJ, Anderson ML, Kaye EM: Neonatal idiopathic cerebral venous thrombosis: An unrecognized cause of transient seizures or lethargy, *Ann Neurol* 32:51-56, 1992.
591. Khurana DS, Buonanno F, Ebb D, Krishnamoorthy KS: The role of anticoagulation in idipathic cerebral venous thrombosis, *J Child Neurol* 11:248-249, 1996.
592. Pohl M, Zimmerbackl LB, Heinen F, Sutor AH, et al: Bilateral renal vein thrombosis and venous sinus thrombosis in a neonate with factor V mutation (FV Leiden), *J Pediatr* 132:159-161, 1998.
593. de Veber G, Andrew M, Adams C, Bjornson B, et al: Cerebral sinovenous thrombosis in children, *N Engl J Med* 345:417-423, 2001.
594. Hunt RW, Badawi N, Laing S, Lam A: Pre-eclampsia: A predisposing factor for neonatal venous sinus thrombosis? *Pediatr Neurol* 25:242-246, 2001.
595. Wu TW, Miller SP, Chin K, Collins AE, et al: Multiple risk factors in neonatal sinovenous thrombosis, *Neurology* 59:438-440, 2002.
596. Fitzgerald KC, Williams LS, Garg BP, Carvalho KS, et al: Cerebral sinovenous thrombosis in the neonate, *Arch Neurol* 63:405-409, 2006.
597. Wulfeck BB, Trauner DA, Tallal PA: Neurologic, cognitive, and linguistic features of infants after early stroke, *Pediatr Neurol* 7:266-269, 1991.
598. Mercuri E, Spano M, Bruccini G, Frisone MF, et al: Visual outcome in children with congenital hemiplegia: Correlation with MRI findings, *Neuropediatrics* 27:184-188, 1996.
599. Mercuri E, Atkinson J, Braddick O, Anker S, et al: Visual function and perinatal focal cerebral infarction, *Arch Dis Child Fetal Neonatal Ed* 75:F76-F81, 1996.
600. Dall'Oglio AM, Bates E, Volterra V, Di Capua M, et al: Early cognition, communication and language in children with focal brain injury, *Dev Med Child Neurol* 36:1076-1098, 1994.
601. Goodman R, Yude C: IQ and its predictors in childhood hemiplegia, *Dev Med Child Neurol* 38:881-890, 1996.
602. Trauner DA, Ballantyne A, Friedland S, Chase C: Disorders of affective and linguistic prosody in children after early unilateral brain damage, *Ann Neurol* 39:361-367, 1996.
603. Bouza H, Dubowitz LM, Rutherford M, Cowan F, et al: Late magnetic resonance imaging and clinical findings in neonates with unilateral lesions on cranial ultrasound, *Dev Med Child Neurol* 36:951-964, 1994.
604. Bouza H, Dubowitz LMS, Rutherford M, Pennock JM: Prediction of outcome in children with congenital hemiplegia: A magnetic resonance imaging study, *Neuropediatrics* 25:60-66, 1994.
605. Mercuri E, Jongmans M, Bouza H, Haataja L, et al: Congenital hemiplegia in children at school age: Assessment of hand function in the non-hemiplegic hand and correlation with MRI, *Neuropediatrics* 30:8-13, 1999.
606. Mercuri E, Cowan F, Gupte G, Manning R, et al: Prothrombotic disorders and abnormal neurodevelopmental outcome in infants with neonatal cerebral infarction, *Pediatrics* 107:1400-1404, 2001.
607. Golomb MR, MacGregor DL, Domi T, Armstrong DC, et al: Presumed pre- or perinatal arterial ischemic stroke: Risk factors and outcomes, *Ann Neurol* 50:163-168, 2001.
608. Mercuri E, Barnett A, Rutherford M, Guzzetta A, et al: Neonatal cerebral infarction and neuromotor outcome at school age, *Pediatrics* 113:95-100, 2004.
609. Nelson KB, Lynch JK: Stroke in newborn infants, *Lancet* 3:150-158, 2004.
610. Lee J, Croen LA, Lindan C, Nash KB, et al: Predictors of outcome in perinatal arterial stroke: A population-based study, *Ann Neurol* 58:303-308, 2005.
611. Boardman JP, Ganesan V, Rutherford M, Saunders DE, et al: Magnetic resonance image correlates of hemiparesis after neonatal and childhood middle cerebral artery stroke, *Pediatrics* 115:321-326, 2005.
612. Cao Y, Vikingstad EM, Huttenlocher PR, Towle VL, et al: Functional magnetic resonance studies of the reorganization of the human hand sensorimotor area after unilateral brain injury in the perinatal period, *Proc Natl Acad Sci U S A* 91:9612-9616, 1994.
613. Lewine JD, Astur RS, Davis LE, Knight JE, et al: Cortical organization in adulthood is modified by neonatal infarct: A case study, *Radiology* 190:93-96, 1994.
614. Maegaki Y, Maeoka Y, Ishii S, Shiota M, et al: Mechanisms of center motor reorganization in pediatric hemiplegic patients, *Neuropediatrics* 28:168-174, 1997.
615. Feldman HM, Holland AL, Kemp SS, Janosky JE: Language development after unilateral brain injury, *Brain Lang* 42:89-102, 1992.
616. Kolk A, Talvik T: Cerebral lateralization and cognitive deficits after congenital hemiparesis, *Pediatr Neurol* 27:356-362, 2002.
617. Bolanos AA, Bleck EE, Firestone P, Young L: Comparison of stereognosis and two-point discrimination testing of the hands of children with cerebral palsy, *Dev Med Child Neurol* 31:371-376, 1989.
618. Wiklund LM, Uvebrant P: Hemiplegic cerebral palsy: Correlation between CT morphology and clinical findings, *Dev Med Child Neurol* 33:512-523, 1991.
619. Guzzetta A, Fazzi B, Mercuri E, Bertuccelli B, et al: Visual function in children with hemiplegia in the first years of life, *Dev Med Child Neurol* 43:321-329, 2001.
620. Lorber J: Hydranencephaly with normal development, *Dev Med Child Neurol* 7:628-631, 1965.
621. Crome L, Sylvester PE: Hydranencephaly (hydrencephaly), *Arch Dis Child* 33:235-245, 1958.
622. Wariyar U, Richmond S, Hey E: Pregnancy outcome at 24-31 weeks' gestation: Neonatal survivors, *Arch Dis Child* 64:678-686, 1989.
623. McCormick MC, Gortmaker SL, Sobol AM: Very low birth weight children: Behavior problems and school difficulty in a national sample, *J Pediatr* 117:687-693, 1990.
624. Msall ME, Buck GM, Rogers BT, Merke D, et al: Risk factors for major neurodevelopmental impairments and need for special education resources in extremely premature infants, *J Pediatr* 119:606-614, 1991.
625. Veelken N, Stollhoff K, Claussen M: Development and perinatal risk factors of very low-birth-weight infants: Small versus appropriate for gestational age, *Neuropediatrics* 23:102-107, 1992.
626. Majnemer A, Rosenblatt B, Riley PS: Influence of gestational age, birth weight, and asphyxia on neonatal neurobehavioral performance, *Pediatr Neurol* 9:181-186, 1993.
627. Thompson CM, Buccimazza SS, Webster J, Malan AF, et al: Infants of less than 1250 grams birth weight at Groote Schuur Hospital: Outcome at 1 and 2 years of age, *Pediatrics* 91:961-968, 1993.
628. Veelken N, Schopf M, Dammann O, Schulte FJ: Etiological classification of cerebral palsy in very low birthweight infants, *Neuropediatrics* 24:74-76, 1993.
629. Project TIotV-OTND: The Vermont-Oxford Trials Network: Very low birth weight outcomes for 1990. Investigators of the Vermont-Oxford Trials Network Database Project, *Pediatrics* 91:540-545, 1993.
630. Halsey CL, Collin MF, Anderson CL: Extremely low birth weight children and their peers: A comparison of preschool performance, *Pediatrics* 91:807-811, 1993.
631. Weisglas-Kuperus N, Koot HM, Baerts W, Fetter WP, et al: Behaviour problems of very low-birthweight children, *Dev Med Child Neurol* 35:406-416, 1993.
632. Stjernqvist K, Svenningsen NW: Extremely-low-birth-weight infants less than 901-g growth and development after one year of life, *Acta Paediatr* 82:40-44, 1993.
633. Msall ME, Rogers BT, Buck GM, Mallen S, et al: Functional status of extremely preterm infants at kindergarten entry, *Dev Med Child Neurol* 35:312-320, 1993.
634. Cooper RL, Goldenberg RL, Creasy RK, Dubard MB, et al: A multicenter study of preterm birth weight and gestational age specific neonatal mortality, *Am J Obstet Gynecol* 168:78-84, 1993.
635. Bhushan V, Paneth N, Kiely JL: Impact of improved survival of very low birth weight infants on recent secular trends in the prevalence of cerebral palsy, *Pediatrics* 91:1094-1100, 1993.
636. Johnson A, Townshend P, Yudkin P, Bull D, et al: Functional abilities at age four years of children born before 29 weeks' of gestation, *Br Med J* 306:1715-1718, 1993.
637. Sung I-K, Vohr B, Oh W: Growth and neurodevelopmental outcome of very low birth weight infants with intrauterine growth retardation: Comparison with control subjects matched by birth weight and gestational age, *J Pediatr* 123:618-624, 1993.
638. McCormick MC, McCarton C, Tonascia J, Brooks-Gunn J: Early educational intervention for very low birth weight infants: Results from the infant health and development program, *J Pediatr* 123:527-533, 1993.
639. Robertson C, Sauve RS, Christianson HE: Province-based study of neurologic disability among survivors weighing 500 through 1249 grams at birth, *Pediatrics* 93:636-640, 1994.
640. Leonard CH, Piecuch RE, Ballard RA, Cooper BA: Outcome of very low birth weight infants: Multiple gestation versus singletons, *Pediatrics* 93:611-615, 1994.
641. Saigal S, Szatmari P, Rosenbaum P, Campbell D, et al: Cognitive abilities and school performance of extremely low birth weight children and matched term control children at age 8 years: A regional study, *J Pediatr* 118:751-760, 1991.
642. Teplin SW, Burchinal M, Johnson-Martin N, Humphry RA, et al: Neurodevelopmental, health, and growth status at age 6 years of children with birth weights less than 1001 grams, *J Pediatr* 118:768-777, 1991.
643. Holtrop PC, Ertzbischoff LM, Roberts CL, Batton DG, et al: Survival and short-term outcome in newborns of 23 to 25 weeks' gestation, *Am J Obstet Gynecol* 170:1266-1270, 1994.
644. Blaymore-Bier J, Pezzullo J, Kim E, Oh W, et al: Outcome of extremely low-birth-weight infants: 1980-1990, *Acta Paediatr* 83:1244-1248, 1994.
645. Saigal S, Feeny D, Furlong W, Rosenbaum P, et al: Comparison of the health-related quality of life of extremely low birth weight children and a reference group of children at age eight years, *J Pediatr* 125:418-425, 1994.
646. Roth SC, Baudin J, Pezzani-Goldsmith M, Townsend J, et al: Relation between neurodevelopmental status of very preterm infants at one and eight years, *Dev Med Child Neurol* 36:1049-1062, 1994.
647. Cooke RWI: Factors affecting survival and outcome at 3 years in extremely preterm infants, *Arch Dis Child Fetal Neonatal Ed* 71:F28-F31, 1994.
648. Brooks-Gunn J, McCarton CM, Casey PH, McCormick M, et al: Early intervention in low-birth-weight premature infants, *JAMA* 272:1257-1262, 1994.
649. Saigal S, Rosenbaum P, Stoskopf B, Hoult L, et al: Comprehensive assessment of the health status of extremely low birth weight children at eight years of age: Comparison with a reference group, *J Pediatr* 125:411-417, 1994.
650. Hack M, Taylor HG, Klein N, Eiben R, et al: School-age outcomes in children with birth weights under 750 g, *N Engl J Med* 331:753-759, 1994.
651. Klebanov PK, Brooks-Gunn J, McCormick MC: Classroom behavior of very low birth weight elementary school children, *Pediatrics* 94:700-708, 1994.
652. Pharoah P, Stevenson CJ, Cooke R, Stevenson RC: Prevalence of behaviour disorders in low birthweight infants, *Arch Dis Child* 70:271-274, 1994.
653. Hille E, Denouden AL, Bauer L, Vandenoudenrijn C, et al: School performance at nine years of age in very premature and very low birth weight infants: Perinatal risk factors and predictors at five years of age, *J Pediatr* 125:426-434, 1994.

654. Goldstein RF, Thompson RJ, Oehler JM, Brazy JE: Influence of acidosis, hypoxemia, and hypotension on neurodevelopmental outcome in very low birth weight infants, *Pediatrics* 95:238-243, 1995.

655. Fanaroff AA, Wright LL, Stevenson DK, Shankaran S, et al: Very-low-birth-weight outcomes of the National Institute of Child Health and Human Development Neonatal Research Network, May 1991 through December 1992, *Am J Obstet Gynecol* 173:1423-1441, 1995.

656. Fawer CL, Besnier S, Forcada M, Buclin T, et al: Influence of perinatal, developmental and environmental factors on cognitive abilities of preterm children without major impairments at 5 years, *Early Hum Dev* 43:151-164, 1995.

657. Roth J, Resnick MB, Ariet M, Carter RL, et al: Changes in survival patterns of very low-birth-weight infants from 1980 to 1993, *Arch Pediatr Adolesc Med* 149:1311-1317, 1995.

658. Philip A: Neonatal mortality rate: Is further improvement possible? *J Pediatr* 126:427-433, 1995.

659. Powls A, Botting N, Cooke R, Marlow N: Motor impairment in children 12 to 13 years old with a birthweight of less than 1250 g, *Arch Dis Child Fetal Neonatal Ed* 73:F62-F66, 1995.

660. Rosenbaum P, Saigal S, Szatmari P, Hoult L: Vineland adaptive behavior scales as a summary of functional outcome of extremely low-birthweight children, *Dev Med Child Neurol* 37:577-586, 1995.

661. Buehler DM, Als H, Duffy FH, McAnulty GB, et al: Effectiveness of individualized developmental care for low-risk preterm infants: Behavioral and electrophysiologic evidence, *Pediatrics* 96:923-932, 1995.

662. Stjernqvist K, Svenningsen NW: Extremely low-birth-weight infants less than 901 g: Development and behaviour after 4 years of life, *Acta Paediatr* 84:500-506, 1995.

663. Lee K, Kim BI, Khoshnood B, Hsieh H, et al: Outcome of very low birth weight infants in industrialized countries: 1947-1987, *Am J Epidemiol* 141:1188-1193, 1995.

664. Wilcox A, Skjaerven R, Buekens P, Kiely J: Birth weight and perinatal mortality, *JAMA* 273:709-711, 1995.

665. LaPine TR, Jackson JC, Bennett FC: Outcome of infants weighing less than 800 grams at birth: 15 years' experience, *Pediatrics* 96:479-483, 1995.

666. Perlman M, Claris O, Hao Y, Pandit P, et al: Secular changes in the outcomes to eighteen to twenty-four months of age of extremely low birth weight infants, with adjustment for changes in risk factors and severity of illness, *J Pediatr* 126:75-87, 1995.

667. O'Callaghan MJ, Burns Y, Gray P, Harvey JM, et al: Extremely low birth weight and control infants at 2 years corrected age: A comparison of intellectual abilities, motor performance, growth and health, *Early Hum Dev* 40:115-125, 1995.

668. Hall A, McLeod A, Counsell C, Thomson L, et al: School attainment, cognitive ability and motor function in a total Scottish very-low-birthweight population at eight years: A controlled study, *Dev Med Child Neurol* 37:1037-1050, 1995.

669. Damman O, Walther H, Allers B, Schjroder M, et al: Development of a regional cohort of very-low-birthweight children at six years: Cognitive abilities are associated with neurological disability and social background, *Dev Med Child Neurol* 38:97-108, 1996.

670. Pinto-Martin JA, Dobson V, Cnaan A, Zhao H, et al: Vision outcome at age 2 years in a low birth weight population, *Pediatr Neurol* 14:281-287, 1996.

671. Hack M, Friedman H, Avroy A, Fanaroff MB: Outcomes of extremely low birth weight infants, *Pediatrics* 98:931-937, 1996.

672. Meadow W, Reimshisel T, Lantos J: Birth weight–specific mortality for extremely low birth weight infants vanishes by four days of life: Epidemiology and ethics in the neonatal intensive care unit, *Pediatrics* 97:636-643, 1996.

673. Sommerfelt K, Troland K, Ellertsen B, Markestad T: Behavioral problems in low-birthweight preschoolers, *Dev Med Child Neurol* 38:927-940, 1996.

674. McCarton CM, Wallace IF, Divon M, Vaughan HG: Cognitive and neurologic development of the premature, small for gestational age infant through age 6: Comparison by birth weight and gestational age, *Pediatrics* 98:1167-1178, 1996.

675. Zupan V, Gonzalez P, Lacaze-Masmonteil T, Boithias C, et al: Periventricular leukomalacia: Risk factors revisited, *Dev Med Child Neurol* 38:1061-1067, 1996.

676. Tyson JE, Younes N, Verter J, Wright LL: Viability, morbidity, and resource use among newborns of 501- to 800-g birth weight, *JAMA* 276:1645-1651, 1996.

677. O'Callaghan MJ, Burns YR, Gray PH, Harvey JM, et al: School performance of ELBW children: A controlled study, *Dev Med Child Neurol* 38:917-926, 1996.

678. McCormick MC, Workman-Daniels D, Brooks-Gunn J: The behavioral and emotional well-being of school-age children with different birth weights, *Pediatrics* 97:18-25, 1996.

679. Saigal S, Feeny D, Rosenbaum P, Furlong W, et al: Self-perceived health status and health-related quality of life of extremely low-birth-weight infants at adolescence, *JAMA* 276:453-459, 1996.

680. Anderson AE, Wildin SR, Woodside M, Swank PR, et al: Severity of medical and neurologic complications as a determinant of neurodevelopmental outcome at 6 and 12 months in very low birth weight infants, *J Child Neurol* 11:215-219, 1996.

681. Monset-Couchard M, de Bethmann O, Kastler B: Mid- and long-term outcome of 89 premature infants weighing less than 1,000 g at birth, all appropriate at gestational age, *Biol Neonate* 70:328-338, 1996.

682. Halsey CL, Collin MF, Anderson CL: Extremely low-birth-weight children and their peers, *Arch Pediatr Adolesc Med* 150:790-794, 1996.

683. Gosch A, Brambring M, Gennat H, Rohlmann A: Longitudinal study of neuropsychological outcome in blind extremely-low-birthweight children, *Dev Med Child Neurol* 39:295-304, 1997.

684. McCarton CM, Brooks-Gunn J, Wallace IF, Bauer CR, et al: Results at age 8 years of early intervention for low-birth-weight premature infants, *JAMA* 277:126-132, 1996.

685. Horbar JD, Badger GJ, Lewit EM, Rogowski J, et al: Hospital and patient characteristics associated with variation in 28-day mortality rates for very low birth weight infants, *Pediatrics* 99:149-156, 1997.

686. Schendel DE, Stockbauer JW, Hoffman HJ, Herman AA, et al: Relation between very low birth weight and developmental delay among preschool children without disabilities, *Am J Epidemiol* 146:740-749, 1997.

687. Piecuch RE, Leonard CH, Cooper BA, Sehring SA: Outcome of extremely low birth weight infants (500 to 999 grams) over a 12-year period, *Pediatrics* 100:633-639, 1997.

688. Koller H, Lawon K, Rose SA, Wallace I, et al: Patterns of cognitive development in very low birth weight children during the first six years of life, *Pediatrics* 99:383-389, 1997.

689. Luoma L, Herrgard E, Martikainen A, Ahonen T: Speech and language development of children born < 32 weeks' gestation: A 5-year prospective follow-up study, *Dev Med Child Neurol* 40:380-387, 1998.

690. Resnick MB, Gomatam SV, Carter RL, Ariet M, et al: Educational disabilities of neonatal intensive care graduates, *Pediatrics* 102:308-314, 1998.

691. Lorenz JM, Wooliever DE, Jetton JR, Paneth N: A quantitative review of mortality and developmental disability in extremely premature newborns, *Arch Pediatr Adolesc Med* 152:425-435, 1998.

692. Pasman JW, Rotteveel JJ, Maassen B: Neurodevelopmental profile in low-risk preterm infants at 5 years of age, *Eur J Paediatr Neurol* 1:7-17, 1998.

693. Sommerfelt K: Long-term outcome for non-handicapped low birth weight infants: Is the fog clearing? *Eur J Pediatr* 157:1-3, 1998.

694. Emsley HCA, Wardle SP, Sims DG, Chiswick ML, et al: Increased survival and deteriorating developmental outcome in 23 to 25 week old gestation infants, 1990–4 compared with 1998–9, *Arch Dis Child Fetal Neonatal Ed* 78:F99-F104, 1998.

695. Pinto-Martin JA, Cnaan A, Zhao H: Short interpregnancy interval and the risk of disabling cerebral palsy in a low birth weight population, *J Pediatr* 132:818-821, 1998.

696. Cooper TR, Berseth CL, Adams JM, Weisman LE: Actuarial survival in the premature infant less than 30 weeks' gestation, *Pediatrics* 101:975-978, 1998.

697. Kramer MS, Platt R, Yang H, Joseph KS, et al: Secular trends in preterm birth: A hospital-based cohort study, *JAMA* 280:1849-1854, 1998.

698. Keller H, Ayub BV, Saigal S, Bar-Or O: Neuromotor ability in 5- to 7-year-old children with very low or extremely low birthweight, *Dev Med Child Neurol* 40:661-666, 1998.

699. Jacobson L, Fernell E, Broberger U, Elk U, et al: Children with blindness due to retinopathy of prematurity: A population-based study. Perinatal data, neurological and ophthalmological outcome, *Dev Med Child Neurol* 40:155-159, 1998.

700. Wilson-Costello D, Borawski E, Friedman H, Redline R, et al: Perinatal correlates of cerebral palsy and other neurologic impairment among very low birth weight children, *Pediatrics* 102:315-322, 1998.

701. Botting N, Powls A, Cooke RWI, Marlow N: Cognitive and educational outcome of very-low-birthweight children in early adolescence, *Dev Med Child Neurol* 40:652-660, 1998.

702. Barton L, Hodgman JE, Pavlova Z: Causes of death in the extremely low birth weight infant, *Pediatrics* 103:446-451, 1999.

703. Hack M, Fanaroff AA: Outcomes of children of extremely low birthweight and gestational age in the 1990's, *Early Hum Dev* 53:193-218, 1999.

704. Wolke D, Meyer R: Cognitive status, language attainment, and prereading skills of 6-year-old very preterm children and their peers: The Bavarian longitudinal study, *Dev Med Child Neurol* 41:94-109, 1999.

705. Paneth N: Classifying brain damage in preterm infants, *J Pediatr* 134:527-529, 1999.

706. McIntire DD, Bloom SL, Casey BM, Leveno KJ: Birth weight in relation to morbidity and mortality among newborn infants, *N Engl J Med* 340:1234-1238, 1999.

707. Palta M, SadehBadawi M, Evans M, Weinstein MR, et al: Functional assessment of a multicenter very-low-birth-weight cohort at age 5 years, *Arch Pediatr Adolesc Med* 154:23-30, 2000.

708. Saigal S, Hoult LA, Streiner DL, Stoskopf BL, et al: School difficulties at adolescence in a regional cohort of children who were extremely low birth weight, *Pediatrics* 105:325-331, 2000.

709. Hack M, Wilson-Costello D, Friedman H, Taylor GH, et al: Neurodevelopment and predictors of outcomes of children with birth weights of less than 1000 g: 1992-1995, *Arch Pediatr Adolesc Med* 154:725-731, 2000.

710. Hille ETM, Lya den Ouden A, Saigal S, Wolke D, et al: Behavioural problems in children who weight 1000 g or less at birth in four countries, *Lancet* 357:1641-1643, 2001.

711. Doyle LW for the Victorian Infant Collaborative Study Group: Outcome at 5 years of age of children 23 to 27 weeks' gestation refining the prognosis, *Pediatrics* 108:134-141, 2001.

712. Salokorpi T, Rautio T, Sajaniemi N, Serenius-Sirve S, et al: Neurological development up to the age of four years of extremely low birthweight infants born in Southern Finland in 1991-94, *Acta Paediatr* 90:218-221, 2001.

713. Pinto-Martin JA, Whitaker AH, Feldman JF, Van Rossem R, et al: Relation of cranial ultrasound abnormalities in low-birthweight infants to motor or cognitive performance at ages 2, 6, and 9 years, *Dev Med Child Neurol* 41:826-833, 1999.

714. Perlman JM: Neurobehavioral deficits in premature graduates of intensive care: Potential medical and neonatal environmental risk factors, *Pediatrics* 108:1339-1348, 2001.

715. Hack M, Taylor HG: Perinatal brain injury in preterm infants and later neurobehavioral function, *JAMA* 284:1973-1974, 2000.

716. Gross SJ, Mettelman BB, Dye TD, Slagle TA: Impact of family structure and stability on academic outcome in preterm children at 10 years of age, *J Pediatr* 138:169-175, 2001.

717. Lee SK, McMillan DD, Ohlsson A, Pendray M, et al: Variations in practice and outcomes in the Canadian NICU network: 1996-1997, *Pediatrics* 106:1070-1079, 2000.

718. Rushe TM, Rifkin L, Stewart AL, Townsend JP, et al: Neuropsychological outcome at adolescence of very preterm birth and its relation to brain structure, *Dev Med Child Neurol* 43:226-233, 2001.

719. Collaborating Centres in SCPE (Surveillance of Cerebral Palsy in Europe): Prevalence and characteristics of children with cerebral palsy in Europe, *Dev Med Child Neurol* 44:633-640, 2002.

720. Hack M, Flannery DJ, Schluchter M, Cartar L, et al: Outcomes in young adulthood for very-low-birth-weight infants, *N Engl J Med* 346:149-157, 2002.

721. Aylward GP: Cognitive and neuropsychological outcomes: More than IQ scores, *Ment Retard Dev Disabil Res Rev* 8:234-240, 2002.

722. Bracewell M, Marlow N: Patterns of motor disability in very preterm children, *Ment Retard Dev Disabil Res Rev* 8:241-248, 2002.

723. Bhutta AT, Cleves MA, Casey PH, Cradock MM, et al: Cognitive and behavioral outcomes of school-aged children who were born preterm, *JAMA* 288:728-737, 2002.

724. Horbar JD, Badger GJ, Carpenter JH, Fanaroff AA, et al: Trends in mortality and morbidity for very low birth weight infants 1991-1999, *Pediatrics* 110:143-151, 2002.

725. Samsom JF, de Groot L, Cranendonk, Bezemer D, et al: Neuromotor function and school performance in 7-year-old children born as high-risk preterm infants, *J Child Neurol* 17:325-332, 2002.

726. Saigal S, den Ouden L, Wolke D, Hoult L, et al: School-age outcomes in children who were extremely low birth weight from four international population-based cohorts, *Pediatrics* 112:943-950, 2003.

727. Tommiska V, Heinonen K, Kero P, Pokela ML, et al: A national two year follow up study of extremely low birthweight infants born in 1996-1997, *Arch Dis Child* 88:29-34, 2003.

728. Ment LR, Vohr B, Allan W, Katz KH, et al: Change in cognitive function over time in very low-birth-weight infants, *JAMA* 289:705-711, 2003.

729. Latal-Hajnal B, Von Siebenthal K, Kovari H, Bucher HU, et al: Postnatal growth in VLBW infants: Significant association with neurodevelopmental outcome, *J Pediatr* 143:163-170, 2003.

730. Rijken M, Stoelhorst GM, Martens SE, van Zwieten PHT, et al: Mortality and neurologic, mental, and psychomotor development at 2 years in infants born less than 27 weeks' gestation: The Leiden follow-up project on prematurity, *Pediatrics* 112:351-358, 2003.

731. Cust AE, Darlow BA, Donoghue DA: Outcomes for high risk New Zealand newborn infants in 1998-1999: A population based, national study, *Arch Dis Child* 88:15-22, 2003.

732. Foulder-Hughes LA, Cooke RWI: Motor, cognitive, and behavioural disorders in children born very preterm, *Dev Med Child Neurol* 45:97-103, 2003.

733. Surman G, Newdick H, Johnson A: Cerebral palsy rates among low-birth-weight infants fell in the 1990s, *Dev Med Child Neurol* 45:456-462, 2003.

734. Johnson A, Bowler U, Yudkin P, Hockley C, et al: Health and school performance of teenagers born before 29 weeks gestation, *Arch Dis Child* 88:190-198, 2003.

735. Larroque B, Breart G, Kaminski M, Dehan M, et al: Survival of very preterm infants: EPIPAGE, a population based cohort study, *Arch Dis Child* 89:139-144, 2004.

736. Mirmiran M, Barnes PD, Keller K, Constantinou JC, et al: Neonatal brain magnetic resonance imaging before discharge is better than serial cranial ultrasound in predicting cerebral palsy in very low birth weight preterm infants, *Pediatrics* 114:992-998, 2004.

737. Breslau N, Paneth NS, Lucia VC: The lingering academic deficits of low birth weight children, *Pediatrics* 114:1035-1040, 2004.

738. Hansen BM, Greisen G: Is improved survival of very-low-birthweight infants in the 1980s and 1990s associated with increasing intellectual deficit in surviving children? *Dev Med Child Neurol* 46:812-815, 2004.

739. Anderson PJ, Doyle LW: Executive functioning in school-aged children who were born very preterm or with extremely low birth weight in the 1990s, *Pediatrics* 114:50-57, 2004.

740. Doyle LW, Victorian Infant Collaborative Study Group: Evaluation of neonatal intensive care for extremely low birth weight infants in Victoria over two decades. I. Effectiveness, *Pediatrics* 113:505-510, 2004.

741. Vohr BR, Wright LL, Dusick AM, Perritt R, et al: Center differences and outcomes of extremely low birth weight infants, *Pediatrics* 145:723-724, 2004.

742. Edwards D: Brain protection for girls and boys, *J Pediatr* 145:723-724, 2004.

743. Therien JM, Worwa CT, Mattia FR, de Regnier R-A: Altered pathways for auditory discrimination and recognition memory in preterm infants, *Dev Med Child Neurol* 46:816-824, 2004.

744. Gray RF, Indurkhya A, McCormick MC: Prevalence, stability, and predictors of clinically significant behavior problems in low birth weight children at 3, 5, and 8 years of age, *Pediatrics* 114:736-743, 2004.

745. Walsh MC, Morris BH, Wrage LA, Vohr BR, et al: Extremely low birth-weight neonates with protracted ventilation: Mortality and 18-month neurodevelopmental outcomes, *J Pediatr* 146:798-804, 2005.

746. Mikkola K, Ritari N, Tommiska V, Salokorpi T, et al: Neurodevelopmental outcome at 5 years of age of a national cohort of extremely low birth weight infants who were born in 1996-1997, *Pediatrics* 116:1391-1400, 2005.

747. Hack M, Taylor HG, Drotar D, Schluchter M, et al: Chronic conditions, functional limitations, and special health care needs of school-aged children born with extremely low-birth-weight in the 1990s, *JAMA* 294:318-325, 2005.

748. Hack M, Taylor HG, Drotar D, Schluchter M, et al: Poor predictive validity of the Bayley Scales of Infant Development for cognitive function of extremely low birth weight children at school age, *Pediatrics* 116:333-341, 2005.

749. Indredavik MS, Skranes JS, Vik T, Heyerdahl S, et al: Low-birth-weight adolescents: Psychiatric symptoms and cerebral MRI abnormalities, *Pediatr Neurol* 33:259-266, 2005.

750. Cooke RWI: Perinatal and postnatal factors in very preterm infants and subsequent cognitive and motor abilities, *Arch Dis Child Fetal Neonatal Ed* 90:F60-F63, 2005.

751. Rose SA, Feldman JF, Jankowski JJ: Recall memory in the first three years of life: A longitudinal study of preterm and term children, *Dev Med Child Neurol* 47:653-659, 2005.

752. Vohr BR, Wright LL, Poole K, McDonald SA: Neurodevelopmental outcomes of extremely low birth weight infants <32 weeks' gestation between 1993 and 1998, *Pediatrics* 116:635-643, 2005.

753. Hajnal BL, Braun-Fahrlander C, von Siebenthal K, Bucher HU, et al: Improved outcome for very low birth weight multiple births, *Pediatr Neurol* 32:87-93, 2005.

754. Fily A, Pierrat V, Delporte V, Breart G, et al: Factors associated with neurodevelopmental outcome at 2 years after very preterm birth: The population-based Nord-Pas-de-Calais EPIPAGE cohort, *Pediatrics* 117:357-366, 2006.

755. Khan NZ, Muslima H, Parveen M, Bhattacharya M, et al: Neurodevelopmental outcomes of preterm infants in Bangladesh, *Pediatrics* 118:280-289, 2006.

756. McCormick MC, Brooks-Gunn J, Buka SL, Goldman J, et al: Early intervention in low birth weight premature infants: Results at 18 years of age for the Infant Health and Development Program, *Pediatrics* 117:771-780, 2006.

757. Saavalainen P, Luoma L, Bowler D, Timonen T, et al: Naming skills of children born preterm in comparison with their term peers at the ages of 9 and 16 years, *Dev Med Child Neurol* 48:28-32, 2006.

758. Delobel-Ayoub M, Kaminski M, Marret S, Burguet A, et al: Behavioral outcome at 3 years of age in very preterm infants: The EPIPAGE study, *Pediatrics* 117:1996-2005, 2006.

759. Power C, Jefferis BJ, Manor O, Hertzman C: The influence of birth weight and socioeconomic position on cognitive development: Does the early home and learning environment modify their effects? *J Pediatr* 148:54-61, 2006.

760. Schmidhauser J, Caflisch J, Rousson V, Bucher HU, et al: Impaired motor performance and movement quality in very-low-birthweight children at 6 years of age, *Dev Med Child Neurol* 48:718-722, 2006.

761. Hintz SR, Kendrick DE, Vohr BR, Kenneth Poole W, et al: Gender differences in neurodevelopmental outcomes among extremely preterm, extremely-low-birthweight infants, *Acta Paediatr* 95:1239-1248, 2006.

762. Tommiska V, Heinonen K, Lehtonen L, Renlund M, et al: No improvement in outcome of nationwide extremely low birth weight infant populations between 1996-1997 and 1999-2000, *Pediatrics* 119:29-36, 2007.

763. Wilson-Costello D, Friedman H, Minich N, Siner B, et al: Improved neurodevelopmental outcomes for extremely low birth weight infants in 2000-2002, *Pediatrics* 119:37-45, 2007.

763a. Farooqi A, Hagglof B, Sedin G, Gothefors L, et al: Mental health and social competencies of 10- to 12-year-old children born at 23 to 25 weeks of gestation in the 1990s: A Swedish national prospective follow-up study, *Pediatrics* 120:118-133, 2007.

763b. Marlow N, Hennessy EM, Bracewell MA, Wolke D: Motor and executive function at 6 years of age extremely preterm birth, *Pediatrics* 120:793-804, 2007.

764. Hoyert DL, Mathews TJ, Menacker F, Strobino DM, et al: Annual summary of vital statistics: 2004, *Pediatrics* 117:168-183, 2006.

765. Martin JA, Hamilton BE, Sutton PD, Ventura SJ, et al: Births: Final data for 2004, *Natl Vital Stat Rep* 55:1-101, 2006.

766. Hamilton BE, Minina AM, Martin JA, Kockanek K, et al: Annual summary of vital statistics: 2005, *Pediatrics* 119:345-360, 2007.

767. El-Metwally D, Vohr B, Tucker R: Survival and neonatal morbidity at the limits of viability in the mid 1990s: 22 to 25 weeks, *J Pediatr* 137:616-622, 2000.

768. Hack M, Taylor G, Klein N, Mercuri-Minich N: Functional limitations and special health care needs of 10- to 14-year old children weighing less than 750 grams at birth, *Pediatrics* 106:554-560, 2000.

769. Lorenz JM, Paneth N: Treatment decisions for the extremely premature infant, *J Pediatr* 137:593-595, 2000.

770. Wood NS, Markow N, Costeloe K, Gibson AT, et al: Neurologic and developmental disability after extremely preterm birth, *N Engl J Med* 343:378-384, 2000.

771. Kilbride HW, Thorstad K, Daily DK: Preschool outcome of less than 801-gram preterm infants compared with full-term siblings, *Pediatrics* 113:742-747, 2004.

772. Sweet MP, Hodgman JE, Pena I, Barton L, et al: Two-year outcome of infants weighing 600 grams or less at birth and born 1994 through 1998, *Obstet Gynecol* 101:18-23, 2003.

773. Wood NS, Costeloe K, Gibson AT, Hennessy EM, et al: The EPICure study: Growth and associated problems in children born at 25 weeks of gestational age or less, *Arch Dis Child Fetal Neonatal Ed* 88:F492-F500, 2003.

774. Lucey JF, Rowan CA, Shiono P, Wilkinson AR, et al: Fetal infants: The fate of 4172 infants with birth weights of 401 to 500 grams—the Vermont Oxford Network experience (1996-2000), *Pediatrics* 113:1559-1566, 2004.

775. Wood NS, Costeloe K, Gibson AT, Hennessy EM, et al: The EPICure study: Associations and antecedents of neurological and developmental disability at 30 months of age following extremely preterm birth, *Arch Dis Child Fetal Neonatal Ed* 90:F134-F140, 2005.

776. Marlow N: Neurocognitive outcome after very preterm birth, *Arch Dis Child Fetal Neonatal Ed* 89:F224-F228, 2004.

777. Shankaran S, Johnson Y, Langer JC, Vohr BR, et al: Outcome of extremely-low-birth-weight infants at highest risk: Gestational age ≤24 weeks, birth weight ≤750 g, and 1-minute Apgar ≤3, *Am J Obstet Gynecol* 191:1084-1091, 2004.

778. Rieger-Fackeldey E, Schulze A, Pohlandt F, Schwarze R, et al: Short-term outcome in infants with a birthweight less than 501 grams, *Acta Paediatr* 94:211-216, 2005.

779. Serenius F, Ewald U, Farooqi A, Holmgren PA, et al: Short-term outcome after active perinatal management at 23-25 weeks of gestation: A study from two Swedish tertiary care centres. II. Infant survival, *Acta Paediatr* 93:1081-1089, 2004.

780. Serenius F, Ewald U, Farooqi A, Holmgren PA, et al: Short-term outcome after active perinatal management at 23-25 weeks. III. Neonatal morbidity, *Acta Paediatr* 93:1090-1097, 2004.

781. Hintz SR, Poole WK, Wright LL, Fanaroff AA, et al: Changes in mortality and morbidities among infants born at less than 25 weeks during the post-surfactant era, *Arch Dis Child Fetal Neonatal Ed* 90:F128-F133, 2005.

782. Louis JM, Ehrenberg HM, Collin MF, Mercer BM: Perinatal intervention and neonatal outcomes near the limit of viability, *Am J Obstet Gynecol* 191:1398-1402, 2004.

783. Marlow N, Wolke D, Bracewell MA, Samara M: Neurologic and developmental disability at six years of age after extremely preterm birth, *N Engl J Med* 352:9-19, 2005.

784. Saigal S, Stoskopf B, Streiner D, Boyle M, et al: Transition of extremely low-birth-weight infants from adolescence to young adulthood: Comparison with normal birth-weight controls, *JAMA* 295:667-675, 2006.

785. Cordero L Jr, Hon EH: Neonatal bradycardia following nasopharyngeal stimulation, *J Pediatr* 78:441-447, 1971.

786. Crawford J: Apgar score and neonatal asphyxia [letter], *Lancet* 1:684-685, 1982.

787. Catlin EA, Carpenter MW, Brann BS 4th, Mayfield SR, et al: The Apgar score revisited: Influence of gestational age, *J Pediatr* 109:865-868, 1986.

788. Marlow N: Do we need an Apgar score? *Arch Dis Child* 67:765-767, 1992.

789. Hegyi T, Carbone T, Anwar M, Ostfeld B, et al: The Apgar score and its components in the preterm infant, *Pediatrics* 101:77-81, 1998.

790. Carter BS, McNabb F, Merenstein GB: Prospective validation of a scoring system for predicting neonatal morbidity after acute perinatal asphyxia, *J Pediatr* 132:619-623, 1998.

791. Leuthner SR, Das UG: Low Apgar scores and the definition of birth asphyxia, *Pediatr Clin North Am* 51:737-745, 2004.

792. Stark AR, Adamkin DH, Batton DG, Bell EF, et al: The Apgar score, *Pediatrics* 117:1444-1447, 2006.

793. Master D, Lie RT, Irgens LM, Bjerkedal T, et al: The association of Apgar score with subsequent death and cerebral palsy: A population-based study in term infants, *J Pediatr* 138:798-803, 2001.

794. Sykes GS, Molloy PM, Johnson P, Gu W, et al: Do Apgar scores indicate asphyxia? *Lancet* 1:494-496, 1982.

795. Silverman F, Suidan J, Wasserman J, Antoine C, et al: The Apgar score: Is it enough? *Obstet Gynecol* 66:331-336, 1985.

796. Dijxhoorn MJ, Visser GH, Touwen BC, Huisjes HJ: Apgar score, meconium and acidaemia at birth in small-for-gestational age infants born at term, and their relation to neonatal neurological morbidity, *Br J Obstet Gynaecol* 94:873-879, 1987.

797. Marrin M, Paes BA: Birth asphyxia: Does the Apgar score have diagnostic value? *Obstet Gynecol* 72:120-123, 1988.

798. Ruth VJ, Raivio KO: Perinatal brain damage: Predictive value of metabolic acidosis and the Apgar score, *BMJ* 297:24-27, 1988.

799. King TA, Jackson GL, Josepy AS, Vedro DA, et al: The effect of profound umbilical artery acidemia in term neonates admitted to a newborn nursery, *J Pediatr* 132:624-629, 1998.

800. Lavrijsen SW, Uiterwaal CS, Stigter RH, de Vries LS, et al: Severe umbilical cord acidemia and neurological outcome in preterm and full-term neonates, *Biol Neonate* 88:27-34, 2005.

801. Nelson KB, Ellenberg JH: Apgar scores as predictors of chronic neurologic disability, *Pediatrics* 68:36-44, 1981.

802. Thomson AJ, Searle M, Russell G: Quality of survival after severe birth asphyxia, *Arch Dis Child* 52:620-626, 1977.

803. Jain L, Ferre C, Vidyasagar D, Nath S, et al: Cardiopulmonary resuscitation of apparently stillborn infants: Survival and long-term outcome, *J Pediatr* 118:778-782, 1991.

804. Perlman JM: Intrapartum hypoxic-ischemic cerebral injury and subsequent cerebral issues: Medicolegal issues, *Pediatrics* 99:851-857, 1997.

805. Ekert P, MacLusky N, Luo XP, Lehotay DC, et al: Dexamethasone prevents apoptosis in a neonatal rat model of hypoxic-ischemic encephalopathy (HIE) by a reactive oxygen species-independent mechanism, *Brain Res* 747:9-17, 1997.

806. Shah PS, Beyene J, To T, Ohlsson A, et al: Postasphyxial hypoxic-ischemic encephalopathy in neonates: Outcome prediction rule within 4 hours of birth, *Arch Pediatr Adolesc Med* 160:729-736, 2006.

807. Ambalavanan N, Carlo WA, Shankaran S, Bann CM, et al: Predicting outcomes of neonates diagnosed with hypoxemic-ischemic encephalopathy, *Pediatrics* 118:2084-2093, 2006.

808. Levene MI, Sands C, Grindulis H, Moore JR: Comparison of two methods of predicting outcome in perinatal asphyxia, *Lancet* 1:67-69, 1986.

809. Shankaran S, Woldt E, Koepke T, Bedard MP, et al: Acute neonatal morbidity and long-term central nervous system sequelae of perinatal asphyxia in term infants, *Early Hum Dev* 25:135-148, 1991.

810. Perlman JM, Tack ED: Renal injury in the asphyxiated newborn infant: Relationship to neurologic outcome, *J Pediatr* 113:875-879, 1988.

811. Lanzi G, Fazzi E, Gerardo A, Ometto A, et al: Early predictors of neurodevelopmental outcome at 12-36 months in very low-birthweight infants, *Brain Dev* 12:482-487, 1990.

812. Nelson KB, Ellenberg JH: The asymptomatic newborn and risk of cerebral palsy, *Am J Dis Child* 141:1333-1335, 1987.

813. Ellenberg JH, Nelson KB: Cluster of perinatal events identifying infants at high risk for death or disability, *J Pediatr* 113:546-552, 1988.

814. Robertson CM, Finer NN: Educational readiness of survivors of neonatal encephalopathy associated with birth asphyxia at term, *J Dev Behav Pediatr* 9:298-306, 1988.

815. Robertson CM, Finer NN, Grace MG: School performance of survivors of neonatal encephalopathy associated with birth asphyxia at term, *J Pediatr* 114:753-760, 1989.

816. Ishikawa T, Ogawa Y, Kanayama M, Wada Y: Long-term prognosis of asphyxiated full-term neonates with CNS complications, *Brain Dev* 9:48-53, 1987.

817. De Souza SW, Richards B: Neurological sequelae in newborn babies after perinatal asphyxia, *Arch Dis Child* 53:564-569, 1978.

818. Fitzhardinge PM, Flodmark O, Ashby S: The prognostic value of computed tomography of the brain in asphyxiated premature infants, *J Pediatr* 100:476-481, 1982.

819. Finer NN, Robertson CM, Peters KL, Coward JH: Factors affecting outcome in hypoxic-ischemic encephalopathy in term infants, *Am J Dis Child* 137:21-25, 1983.

820. Yudkin PL, Johnson A, Clover LM, Murphy KW: Clustering of perinatal markers of birth asphyxia and outcome at age five years, *Br J Obstet Gynaecol* 101:774-781, 1994.

821. Wolf MJ, Wolf B, Bijleveld C, Beunen G, et al: Neurodevelopmental outcome in babies with a low Apgar score from Zimbabwe, *Dev Med Child Neurol* 39:821-826, 1997.

822. Wayenberg J-L, Dramaix M, Vermeylen D, Bormans J, et al: Neonatal outcome after birth asphyxia: Early indicators of prognosis, *Prenat Neonat Med* 3:482-489, 1998.

823. Caravale B, Allemand F, Libenson MH: Factors predictive of seizures and neurologic outcome in perinatal depression, *Pediatr Neurol* 29:18-25, 2003.

824. Dixon G, Badawi N, Kurinczuk JJ, Keogh JM, et al: Early developmental outcomes after newborn encephalopathy, *Pediatrics* 109:26-33, 2002.

825. Badawi N, Felix JF, Kurinezuk JF, Dixon G, et al: Cerebral palsy following term newborn encephalopathy: A population-based study, *Dev Med Child Neurol* 47:293-298, 2005.

826. Miller SP, Latal B, Clark H, Barnwell A, et al: Clinical signs predict 30-month neurodevelopmental outcome after neonatal encephalopathy, *Am J Obstet Gynecol* 190:93-99, 2004.

827. Lindstrom K, Lagerroos P, Gillberg C, Fernell E: Teenage outcome after being born at term with moderate neonatal encephalopathy, *Pediatr Neurol* 35:268-274, 2006.

827a. van Handel M, Swaab H, de Vries LS, Jongmans MJ: Long-term cognitive and behavioral consequences of neonatal encephalopathy following perinatal asphyxia: A review, *Eur J Pediatr* 166:645-654, 2007.

828. Ellis M, Manandhar N, Shrestha PS, Shrestha L, et al: Outcome at 1 year of neonatal encephalopathy in Kathmandu Nepal, *Dev Med Child Neurol* 41:689-695, 1999.

829. Nelson KB, Ellenberg JH: Neonatal signs as predictors of cerebral palsy, *Pediatrics* 64:225-232, 1979.

830. Nelson KB, Broman SH: Perinatal risk factors in children with serious motor and mental handicaps, *Ann Neurol* 2:371-377, 1977.

831. Curtis PD, Matthews TG, Clarke TA, Darling M, et al: Neonatal seizures: The Dublin Collaborative Study, *Arch Dis Child* 63:1065-1068, 1988.

832. Minchom P, Niswander K, Chalmers I, Dauncey M, et al: Antecedents and outcome of very early neonatal seizures in infants born at or after term, *Br J Obstet Gynaecol* 94:431-439, 1987.

833. Tekgul H, Gauvreau K, Soul J, Murphy L, et al: The current etiologic profile and neurodevelopmental outcome of seizures in term newborn infants, *Pediatrics* 117:1270-1280, 2006.

834. al Naqeeb N, Edwards AD, Cowan FM, Azzopardi D: Assessment of neonatal encephalopathy by amplitude-integrated electroencephalography, *Pediatrics* 103:1263-1271, 1999.

835. Douglass LM, Wu JY, Rosman NP, Stafstrom CE: Burst suppression electroencephalogram pattern in the newborn: Predicting the outcome, *J Child Neurol* 17:403-408, 2002.

836. Hellstrom-Westas L, Rosen I, Svenningsen NW: Predictive value of early continuous amplitude integrated EEG recordings on outcome after severe birth asphyxia in full term infants, *Arch Dis Child Fetal Neonatal Ed* 72:F34-F38, 1995.

837. Eken P, Toet MC, Groenendaal F, de Vries LS: Predictive value of early neuroimaging, pulsed Doppler and neurophysiology in full term infants with hypoxic-ischaemic encephalopathy, *Arch Dis Child Fetal Neonatal Ed* 73:F75-F80, 1995.

838. Hellstrom-Westas L, Rosen I: Continuous brain-function monitoring: State of the art in clinical practice, *Semin Fetal Neonatal Med* 11:503-511, 2006.

839. Shepherd AJ, Saunders KJ, McCulloch DL, Dutton GN: Prognostic value of flash visual evoked potentials in preterm infants, *Dev Med Child Neurol* 41:9-15, 1999.

840. Kato T, Watanabe K: Visual evoked potential in the newborn: Does it have predictive value? *Semin Fetal Neonatal Med* 11:459-463, 2006.

841. Hrbek A, Karlberg P, Kjellmer I, Olsson T, et al: Clinical application of evoked electroencephalographic responses in newborn infants. I. Perinatal asphyxia, *Dev Med Child Neurol* 19:34-44, 1977.

842. Willis J, Duncan C, Bell R: Short-latency somatosensory evoked potentials in perinatal asphyxia, *Pediatr Neurol* 3:203-207, 1987.

843. Gibson NA, Graham M, Levene MI: Somatosensory evoked potentials and outcome in perinatal asphyxia, *Arch Dis Child* 67:393-398, 1992.

844. de Vries LS, Eken P, Pierrat V, Daniels H, et al: Prediction of neurodevelopmental outcome in the preterm infant: Short latency cortical somatosensory evoked potentials compared with cranial ultrasound, *Arch Dis Child* 67:1177-1181, 1992.

845. Majnemer A, Rosenblatt B: Prediction of outcome at school entry in neonatal intensive care unit survivors, with use of clinical and electrophysiologic techniques, *J Pediatr* 127:823-830, 1995.

846. Vanhatalo S, Lauronen L: Neonatal SEP: Back to bedside with basic science, *Semin Fetal Neonatal Med* 11:464-470, 2006.

847. Pierrat V, Eken P, Duquennoy C, Sousseau S, et al: Prognostic value of early somatosensory evoked potentials in neonates with cystic leukomalacia, *Dev Med Child Neurol* 35:683-690, 1993.

848. Ishida A, Nakajima W, Arai H, Takahashi Y, et al: Cranial computed tomography scans of premature babies predict their eventual learning disabilities, *Pediatr Neurol* 16:319-322, 1997.

849. de Vries LS, Eken P, Dubowitz LMS: The spectrum of leukomalacia using cranial ultrasound, *Behav Brain Res* 49:1-6, 1992.

850. Saliba E, Bertrand P, Gold F, Marchand S, et al: Area of lateral ventricles measured on cranial ultrasonography in preterm infants: Association with outcome, *Arch Dis Child* 65:1033-1037, 1990.

851. Graziani IJ, Spitzer AR, Mitchell DG: Mechanical ventilation in preterm infants: Neurosonographic and developmental studies, *Pediatrics* 90:515-522, 1993.

852. Fowlie PW, Tarnow-Mordi WO, Gould CR, Strang D: Predicting outcome in very low birthweight infants using an objective measure of illness severity and cranial ultrasound scanning, *Arch Dis Child Fetal Neonatal Ed* 78:F175-F178, 1998.

853. van den Hout BM, Stiers P, Haers M, van der Schouw YT, et al: Relation between visual perceptual impairment and neonatal ultrasound diagnosis of haemorrhagic-ischaemic brain lesions in 5-year old children, *Dev Med Child Neurol* 42:376-386, 2000.

854. Lai FF, Tsou KY: Transient periventricular echodensities and developmental outcome in preterm infants, *Pediatr Neurol* 21:797-801, 1999.

855. Horsch S, Muentjes C, Franz A, Roll C: Ultrasound diagnosis of brain atrophy is related to neurodevelopmental outcome in preterm infants, *Acta Paediatr* 94:1815-1821, 2005.

856. Haataja L, Mercuri E, Guzzetta A, Rutherford MA, et al: Neurologic examination in infants with hypoxic-ischemic encephalopathy at age 9 to 14 months: Use of optimality scores and correlation with magnetic resonance imaging findings, *J Pediatr* 138:332-337, 2001.

857. Eken P, de Vries LS, van der Graaf Y, Meiners LC, et al: Haemorrhagic-ischaemic lesions of the neonatal brain: Correlation between cerebral visual impairment, neurodevelopmental outcome and MRI in infancy, *Dev Med Child Neurol* 37:41-55, 1995.

858. Olsen P, Vainionpaa L, Paakko E, Korkman M, et al: Psychological findings in preterm children related to neurologic status and magnetic resonance imaging, *Pediatrics* 102:329-336, 1998.

859. Skranes J, Vike T, Nilsen G, Smevik O, et al: Can cerebral MRI at age 1 year predict motor and intellectual outcomes in very-low-birthweight children? *Dev Med Child Neurol* 40:256-262, 1998.

860. Kato T, Nishina M, Matsushita K, Hori E, et al: Neuronal maturation and N-acetyl-L-aspartic acid development in human fetal and child brains, *Brain Dev* 19:131-133, 1997.

861. Urenjak J, Williams SR, Gadian DG, Noble M: Specific expression of N-acetylaspartate in neurons, oligodendrocyte-type-2 astrocyte progenitors, and immature oligodendrocytes in vitro, *J Neurochem* 59:55-61, 1992.

862. Groenendaal F, van der Grond J, Witkamp TD, de Vries LS: Proton magnetic resonance spectroscopic imaging in neonatal stroke, *Neuropediatrics* 26:243-248, 1995.

863. Bada HS, Hajjar W, Chua C, Sumner DS: Noninvasive diagnosis of neonatal asphyxia and intraventricular hemorrhage by Doppler ultrasound, *J Pediatr* 95:775-779, 1979.

864. Ando Y, Takashima S, Takeshita K: Cerebral blood flow velocities in postasphyxial term neonates, *Brain Dev* 5:529-532, 1983.

865. van Bel F, van de Bor M, Stijnen T, Baan J, et al: Cerebral blood flow velocity pattern in healthy and asphyxiated newborns: A controlled study, *Eur J Pediatr* 146:461-467, 1987.

866. Archer LN, Levene MI, Evans DH: Cerebral artery Doppler ultrasonography for prediction of outcome after perinatal asphyxia, *Lancet* 2:1116-1118, 1986.

867. Ramaekers VT, Casaer P: Defective regulation of cerebral oxygen transport after severe birth asphyxia, *Dev Med Child Neurol* 32:56-62, 1990.

868. Levene MI, Fenton AC, Evans DH, Archer LN, et al: Severe birth asphyxia and abnormal cerebral blood-flow velocity, *Dev Med Child Neurol* 31:427-434, 1989.

869. Morrison FK, Patel NB, Howie PW, Mires GJ, et al: Neonatal cerebral arterial flow velocity waveforms in term infants with and without metabolic acidosis at delivery1, *Early Hum Dev* 42:155-168, 1995.

870. Ilves P, Talvik R, Talvik T: Changes in Doppler ultrasonography in asphyxiated term infants with hypoxic-ischaemic encephalopathy, *Acta Paediatr* 87:680-684, 1998.

871. Jongeling BR, Badawi N, Kurinczuk JJ, Thonell S, et al: Cranial ultrasound as a predictor of outcome in term newborn encephalopathy, *Pediatr Neurol* 26:37-42, 2002.

872. Ilves P, Lintrop M, Metsvaht T, Vaher U, et al: Cerebral blood-flow velocities in predicting outcome of asphyxiated newborn infants, *Acta Paediatr* 93:523-528, 2004.

873. Marks KA, Mallard EC, Roberts I, Williams CE, et al: Delayed vasodilation and altered oxygenation after cerebral ischemia in fetal sheep, *Pediatr Res* 39:48-54, 1995.

874. Wyatt JS: Near infrared spectroscopy in asphyxiated brain injury, *Clin Perinatol* 20:369-378, 1993.

875. Meek JH, Elwell CE, McCormick DC, Edwards AD, et al: Abnormal cerebral haemodynamics in perinatally asphyxiated neonates related to outcome, *Arch Dis Child Fetal Neonatal Ed* 81:F110-F115, 1999.

876. Skov I, Pryds O, Greisen G, Lou H: Estimation of cerebral venous saturation in newborn infants by near infrared spectroscopy, *Pediatric Res* 33:52-55, 1993.

877. Pryds O, Greisen G, Lou H, Friis-Hansen B: Vasoparalysis associated with brain damage in asphyxiated term infants, *J Pediatr* 117:119-125, 1990.

878. Rosenbaum JL, Almli CR, Yundt KD, Altman DI, et al: Higher neonatal cerebral blood flow correlates with worse childhood neurologic outcome, *Neurology* 49:1035-1041, 1997.

879. Thorngren-Jerneck K, Ohlsson T, Sandell A, Erlandsson K, et al: Cerebral glucose metabolism measured by positron emission tomography in term newborn infants with hypoxic ischemic encephalopathy, *Pediatr Res* 49:495-501, 2001.

880. Shankaran S, Szego E, Eizert D, Siegel P: Severe bronchopulmonary dysplasia: Predictors of survival and outcome, *Chest* 86:607-610, 1984.

881. Huch R, Lucey JF, Huch A: Oxygen: Noninvasive monitoring, *Perinat Care* 2:18-29, 1978.

882. Stark AR, Thach BT: Mechanisms of airway obstruction leading to apnea in newborn infants, *J Pediatr* 89:982-985, 1976.

883. Lucey J, Peabody J, Phillip A: Recurrent undetected hypoxemia and hyperoxia, *Pediatr Res* 11:537-544, 1977.

884. Peabody JL, Gregory GA, Willis MM, Philip AG, et al: Failure of conventional monitoring to detect apnea resulting in hypoxemia, *Birth Defects* 15:274-284, 1979.

885. Peabody J, Phillip A, Lucey J: Disorganized breathing: An important form of apnea and cause of hypoxia, *Pediatr Res* 11:540, 1977.

886. Long JG, Lucey JF, Philip AG: Noise and hypoxemia in the intensive care nursery, *Pediatrics* 65:143-145, 1980.

887. Hiatt IM, Hegyi T, Indyk L, Dangman BC, et al: Continuous monitoring of Po2 during apnea of prematurity, *J Pediatr* 98:288-291, 1981.

888. Cassady G: Transcutaneous monitoring in the newborn infant, *J Pediatr* 103:837-848, 1983.

889. Danford DA, Miske S, Headley J, Nelson RM: Effects of routine care procedures on transcutaneous oxygen in neonates: A quantitative approach, *Arch Dis Child* 58:20-23, 1983.

890. Rosen CL, Glaze DG, Frost JD Jr: Hypoxemia associated with feeding in the preterm infant and full-term neonate, *Am J Dis Child* 138:623-628, 1984.

891. Peabody JL, Emery JR: Noninvasive monitoring of blood gases in the newborn, *Clin Perinatol* 12:147-160, 1985.

892. Hay WW Jr, Thilo E, Curlander JB: Pulse oximetry in neonatal medicine, *Clin Perinatol* 18:441-472, 1991.

893. Poets CF, Samuels MP, Southall DP: Potential role of intrapulmonary shunting in the genesis of hypoxemic episodes in infants and young children, *Pediatrics* 90:385-391, 1992.

894. Singer L, Martin RJ, Hawkins SW, Benson-Szekely LJ, et al: Oxygen desaturation complicates feeding in infants with bronchopulmonary dysplasia after discharge, *Pediatrics* 90:380-384, 1992.

895. Pokela M-L: Pain relief can reduce hypoxemia in distressed neonates during routine treatment procedures, *Pediatrics* 93:379-383, 1994.

896. Poets CF, Stebbens VA, Richard D, Southall DP: Prolonged episodes of hypoxemia in preterm infants undetectable by cardiorespiratory monitors, *Pediatrics* 95:860-863, 1995.

897. Adams JA, Zabaleta IA, Sackner MA: Hypoxemic events in spontaneously breathing premature infants: Etiologic basis, *Pediatr Res* 42:463-471, 1997.

898. Urlesberger B, Kaspirek A, Pichler G, Muller W: Apnea of prematurity and changes in cerebral oxygenation and cerebral blood volume, *Neuropediatrics* 30:29-33, 1999.

899. Kennedy C, Grave GD, Jehle JW: Effect of hyperoxia on the cerebral circulation of the newborn puppy, *Pediatr Res* 5:659, 1971.

900. Klinger G, Beyene J, Shah P, Perlman M: Do hyperoxaemia and hypocapnia add to the risk of brain injury after intrapartum asphyxia? *Arch Dis Child Fetal Neonatal Ed* 90:F49-F52, 2005.

901. Saugstad OD, Ramji S, Irani SF, El-Meneza S, et al: Resuscitation of newborn infants with 21% or 100% oxygen: Follow-up at 18 to 24 months, *Pediatrics* 112:296-300, 2003.

902. Vento M, Asensi M, Sastre J, Garcia-Sala F, et al: Resuscitation with room air instead of 100% oxygen prevents oxidative stress in moderately asphyxiated term neonates, *Pediatrics* 107:642-647, 2001.

903. Vento M, Asensi M, Sastre J, Lloret A, et al: Oxidative stress in asphyxiated term infants resuscitated with 100% oxygen, *J Pediatr* 142:240-246, 2003.

904. Saugstad OD, Ramji S, Rootwelt T, Vento M: Response to resuscitation of the newborn: Early prognostic variables, *Acta Paediatr* 94:890-895, 2005.

905. Saugstad OD, Ramji S, Vento M: Oxygen for newborn resuscitation: How much is enough? *Pediatrics* 118:789-792, 2006.

905a. Higgins RD, Bancalari E, Willinger M, Raju TN: Executive summary of the workshop on oxygen in neonatal therapies: Controversies and opportunities for research, *Pediatrics* 119:790-769, 2007.

906. Lundstrom KE, Pryds O, Greisen G: Oxygen at birth and prolonged cerebral vasoconstriction in preterm infants, *Arch Dis Child Fetal Neonatal Ed* 73:F81-F84, 1995.

907. Lucey JF, Dangman B: A reexamination of the role of oxygen in retrolental fibroplasia, *Pediatrics* 73:82-96, 1984.

908. Nelson LB, Calhoun JH, Harley RD, editors: *Pediatric Ophthalmology*, 3rd ed, Philadelphia: 1991, WB Saunders 1991.

909. Emond D, Lachance C, Gagnon J, Bard H: Arterial partial pressure of oxygen required to achieve 90% saturation of hemoglobin in very low birth weight newborns, *Pediatrics* 91:602-604, 1993.

910. Hannah RS, Hannah KJ: Hyperoxia: Effects on the vascularization of the developing central nervous system, *Acta Neuropathol (Berl)* 51:141-144, 1980.

911. Hansen TN, Tooley WH: Skin surface carbon dioxide tension in sick infants, *Pediatrics* 64:942-945, 1979.

912. Merritt TA, Liyamasawad S, Boettrich C, Brooks JG: Skin-surface CO_2 measurement in sick preterm and term infants, *J Pediatr* 99:782-786, 1981.

913. Hunt CE: Cardiorespiratory monitoring, *Clin Perinatol* 18:473-495, 1991.

914. Kaiser JR, Gauss CH, Williams DK: The effects of hypercapnia on cerebral autoregulation in ventilated very low birth weight infants, *Pediatr Res* 58:931-935, 2005.

915. Reivich M: Arterial pCO_2 and cerebral hemodynamics, *Am J Physiol* 206:25-35, 1964.

916. Haggendal E, Johansson B: Effects of arterial carbon dioxide tension and oxygen saturation on cerebral blood flow autoregulation in dogs, *Acta Physiol Scand Suppl* 258:27-53, 1965.

917. Davis SM, Ackerman RH, Correia JA, Alpert NM, et al: Cerebral blood flow and cerebrovascular CO_2 reactivity in stroke-age normal controls, *Neurology* 33:391-399, 1983.

918. Purves MJ, James IM: Observations on the control of cerebral blood flow in the sheep fetus and newborn lamb, *Circ Res* 25:651-667, 1969.

919. Reivich M, Brann AW Jr, Shapiro H, Rawson J, et al: Reactivity of cerebral vessels to CO_2 in the newborn rhesus monkey, *Eur Neurol* 6:132-136, 1971.

920. Shapiro HM, Greenberg JH, Naughton KV, Reivich M: Heterogeneity of local cerebral blood flow-P_aCO_2 sensitivity in neonatal dogs, *J Appl Physiol* 49:113-118, 1980.

921. Batton DG, Hellmann J, Hernandez MJ, Maisels MJ: Regional cerebral blood flow, cerebral blood velocity, and pulsatility index in newborn dogs, *Pediatr Res* 17:908-912, 1983.

922. Hansen NB, Brubakk AM, Bratlid D, Oh W, et al: The effects of variations in $Paco_2$ on brain blood flow and cardiac output in the newborn piglet, *Pediatr Res* 18:1132-1136, 1984.

923. Young RS, Yagel SK: Cerebral physiological and metabolic effects of hyperventilation in the neonatal dog, *Ann Neurol* 16:337-342, 1984.

924. Reuter JH: Cerebral blood flow and cerebral metabolic rate during hyperventilation in the newborn dog, *Pediatr Res* 19:360-374, 1985.

925. Gleason CA, Hamm C, Jones MD Jr: Cerebral blood flow, oxygenation, and carbohydrate metabolism in immature fetal sheep in utero, *Am J Physiol* 256:R1264-R1268, 1989.

926. Gleason CA, Short BL, Jones MD Jr: Cerebral blood flow and metabolism during and after prolonged hypocapnia in newborn lambs, *J Pediatr* 115:309-314, 1989.

927. Rosenberg AA, Jones MD Jr, Traystman RJ, Simmons MA, et al: Response of cerebral blood flow to changes in Pco_2 in fetal, newborn, and adult sheep, *Am J Physiol* 242:H862-H866, 1982.

928. Kamei A, Ozaki T, Takashima S: Monitoring of the intracranial hemodynamics and oxygenation during and after hyperventilation in newborn rabbits with near-infrared spectroscopy, *Pediatr Res* 35:334-338, 1994.

929. Vannucci RC, Towfighi J, Heitjan DF, Brucklacher RM: Carbon dioxide protects the perinatal brain from hypoxic-ischemic damage: An experimental study in the immature rat, *Pediatrics* 95:868-874, 1995.

930. Vannucci RC, Brucklacher RM, Vannucci SJ: Effect of carbon dioxide on cerebral metabolism during hypoxia-ischemia in the immature rat, *Pediatr Res* 42:24-29, 1997.

931. Vannucci RC: Interventions for perinatal hypoxic-ischemic encephalopathy, *Pediatrics* 100:1004-1014, 1997.

932. Pryds O, Greisen G, Lou H, Friis-Hansen B: Heterogeneity of cerebral vasoreactivity in preterm infants supported by mechanical ventilation, *J Pediatr* 115:638-645, 1989.

933. Pryds O, Greisen G: Effect of P_aCO_2 and haemoglobin concentration on day to day variation of CBF in preterm neonates, *Acta Paediatr Scand Suppl* 360:33-36, 1989.

934. Wyatt JS, Edwards AD, Cope M, Delpy DT, et al: Response of cerebral blood volume to changes in arterial carbon dioxide tension in preterm and term infants, *Pediatr Res* 29:553-557, 1991.

935. Muller AM, Morales C, Briner J, Baenziger O, et al: Loss of CO_2 reactivity of cerebral blood flow is associated with severe brain damage in mechanically ventilated very low birth weight infants, *Eur J Paediatr Neurol* 5:157-163, 1997.

936. Pryds O, Edwards AD: Cerebral blood flow in the newborn infant, *Arch Dis Child Fetal Neonatal Ed* 74:F63-F69, 1996.

937. Victor S, Appleton RE, Beirne M, Marson AG, et al: Effect of carbon dioxide on background cerebral electrical activity and fractional oxygen extraction in very low birth weight infants just after birth, *Pediatr Res* 58:579-585, 2005.

938. Okumura A, Hayakawa F, Kato T, Itomi K, et al: Hypocarbia in preterm infants with periventricular leukomalacia: The relation between hypocarbia and mechanical ventilation, *Pediatrics* 107:469-475, 2001.

939. Kubota H, Ohsone Y, Oka F, Sueyoshi T, et al: Significance of clinical risk factors of cystic periventricular leukomalacia in infants with different birthweights, *Acta Paediatr* 90:302-308, 2001.

940. Murase M, Ishida A: Early hypocarbia of preterm infants: Its relationship to periventricular leukomalacia and cerebral palsy, and its perinatal risk factors, *Acta Paediatr* 94:85-91, 2005.

941. Wiswell TE, Graziani LJ, Kornhauser MS, Stanley C, et al: Effects of hypocarbia on the development of cystic periventricular leukomalacia in premature infants treated with high-frequency jet ventilation, *Pediatrics* 98:918-924, 1996.

942. Calvert SA, Hoskins EM, Fong KW, Forsyth SC: Etiologic factors associated with the development of periventricular leukomalacia, *Acta Paediatr Scand* 76:254-259, 1987.

943. Greisen G, Munck H, Lou H: May hypocarbia cause ischaemic brain damage in the preterm infant? *Lancet* 2:460, 1986.

944. Greisen G, Munck H, Lou H: Severe hypocarbia in preterm infants and neurodevelopmental deficit, *Acta Paediatr Scand* 76:401-404, 1987.

945. Ikonen RS, Janas MO, Koivikko MJ, Laippala P, et al: Hyperbilirubinemia, hypocarbia and periventricular leukomalacia in preterm infants: Relationship to cerebral palsy, *Acta Paediatr* 81:802-807, 1992.

946. Fujimoto S, Togari H, Yamaguchi N, Mizutani F, et al: Hypocarbia and cystic periventricular leukomalacia in premature infants, *Arch Dis Child Fetal Neonatal Ed* 71:F107-F110, 1994.

947. Keszler M, Modanlou HD, Brudno DS, Clark FI, et al: Multicenter controlled clinical trail of high-frequency jet ventilation in preterm infants with uncomplicated respiratory distress syndrome, *Pediatrics* 100:593-599, 1997.

948. Shankaran S, Langer JC, Kazzi SN, Laptook AR, et al: Cumulative index of exposure to hypocarbia and hyperoxia as risk factors for periventricular leukomalacia in low birth weight infants, *Pediatrics* 118:1654-1659, 2006.

949. Lou HC, Lassen NA, Tweed WA, Johnson G, et al: Pressure passive cerebral blood flow and breakdown of the blood-brain barrier in experimental fetal asphyxia, *Acta Paediatr Scand* 68:57-63, 1979.

950. Boylan GB, Young K, Panerai RB, Rennie JM, et al: Dynamic cerebral autoregulation in sick newborn infants, *Pediatr Res* 48:12-17, 2000.

951. von Siebenthal K, Beran J, Wolf M, Keel M, et al: Cyclical fluctuations in blood pressure, heart rate and cerebral blood volume in preterm infants, *Brain Dev* 21:529-534, 1999.

952. Tsuji M, Saul JP, du Plessis A, Eichenwald E, et al: Cerebral intravascular oxygenation correlates with mean arterial pressure in critically ill premature infants, *Pediatrics* 106:625-632, 2000.

953. Munro MJ, Barfield CP, Walker AM: Hypotensive extremely low birth weight infants have reduced cerebral blood flow, *Pediatrics* 114:1591-1596, 2004.

954. Lemmers PM, Toet M, van Schelven LJ, van Bel F: Cerebral oxygenation and cerebral oxygen extraction in the preterm infant: The impact of respiratory distress syndrome, *Exp Brain Res* 173:458-467, 2006.

955. Soul JS, Hammer PE, Tsuji M, Saul JP, et al: Fluctuating pressure-passivity is common in the cerebral circulation of sick premature infants, *Pediatr Res* 61:467-473, 2007.

956. West CR, Groves AM, Williams CE, Harding JE, et al: Early low cardiac output is associated with compromised electroencephalographic activity in very preterm infants, *Pediatr Res* 59:610-615, 2006.

957. Victor S, Marson AG, Appleton RE, Beirne M, et al: Relationship between blood pressure, cerebral electrical activity, cerebral fractional oxygen extraction, and peripheral blood flow in very low birth weight newborn infants, *Pediatr Res* 59:314-319, 2006.

958. Kitterman JA, Phibbs RH, Tooley WH: Aortic blood pressure in normal newborn infants during the first 12 hours of life, *Pediatrics* 44:959-968, 1969.

959. Hall RT, Oliver TK Jr: Aortic blood pressure in infants admitted to a neonatal intensive care unit, *Am J Dis Child* 121:145-147, 1971.

960. Modanlou H, Yeh SY, Siassi B, Hon EH: Direct monitoring of arterial blood pressure in depressed and normal newborn infants during the first hour of life, *J Pediatr* 85:553-559, 1974.

961. Bucci G, Scalamandre A, Savignoni PG, Mendicini M, et al: The systemic systolic blood pressure of newborns with low weight: A multiple regression analysis, *Acta Paediatr Scand Suppl* 229:1-26, 1972.

962. Versmold HT, Kitterman JA, Phibbs RH, Gregory GA, et al: Aortic blood pressure during the first 12 hours of life in infants with birth weight 610 to 4,220 grams, *Pediatrics* 67:607-613, 1981.

963. Adams JH, Brierley JB, Connor RC, Treip CS: The effects of systemic hypotension upon the human brain: Clinical and neuropathological observations in 11 cases, *Brain* 89:235-268, 1966.

964. Sonesson SE, Broberger U: Arterial blood pressure in the very low birth-weight neonate: Evaluation of an automatic oscillometric technique, *Acta Paediatr Scand* 76:338-341, 1987.

965. van Ravenswaaij-Arts CM, Hopman JC, Kollée LA: Influence of behavioural state on blood pressure in preterm infants during the first 5 days of life, *Acta Paediatr Scand* 78:358-363, 1989.

966. Guignard JP, Gouyon JB, Adelman RD: Arterial hypertension in the newborn infant, *Biol Neonate* 55:77-83, 1989.

967. Shortland DB, Evans DH, Levene MI: Blood pressure measurements in very low birth weight infants over the first week of life, *J Perinat Med* 16:93-97, 1988.

968. Weindling AM: Blood pressure monitoring in the newborn, *Arch Dis Child* 64:444-447, 1989.

969. Emery EF, Greenough A, Yuksel B: Effect of gender on blood pressure levels of very low birthweight infants in the first 48 hours of life, *Early Hum Dev* 31:209-216, 1993.

970. Hegyi T, Anwar M, Carbone MT, Ostfeld A, et al: Blood pressure ranges in premature infants. II. The first week of life, *Pediatrics* 97:336-342, 1996.

971. Watkins AM, West CR, Cooke RW: Blood pressure and cerebral haemorrhage and ischaemia in very low birthweight infants, *Early Hum Dev* 19:103-110, 1989.

972. Laughon M, Bose C, Allred E, O'Shjea M, et al: Factors associated with treatment for hypotension in extremely low gestational age newborns during the first postnatal week, *Pediatrics* 119:273-280, 2007.

973. Barrington K: Time for pressure tactics, *Pediatrics* 119:396-397, 2007.

973a. Limperopoulos C, Bassan H, Kalish LA, Ringer SA, et al: Current definitions of hypotension do not predict abnormal cranial ultrasound finding in preterm infants, *Pediatrics* 120:966-977, 2007.

974. Low JA, Froese AB, Galbraith RS, Smith JT, et al: The association between preterm newborn hypotension and hypoxemia and outcome during the first year, *Acta Paediatr* 82:433-437, 1993.

975. Rowe RD, Hoffman T: Transient myocardial ischemia of the newborn infant: A form of severe cardiorespiratory distress in full-term infants, *J Pediatr* 81:243-250, 1972.

976. Bucciarelli RL, Nelson RM, Egan EA, Eitzman DV, et al: Transient tricuspid insufficiency of the newborn: A form of myocardial dysfunction in stressed newborns, *Pediatrics* 59:330-337, 1977.

977. Nelson RM, Bucciarelli RL, Eitzman DV, Egan EA 2d, et al: Serum creatine phosphokinase MB fraction in newborns with transient tricuspid insufficiency, *N Engl J Med* 298:146-149, 1978.

978. Finley JP, Howman-Giles RB, Gilday DL, Bloom KR, et al: Transient myocardial ischemia of the newborn infant demonstrated by thallium myocardial imaging, *J Pediatr* 94:263-270, 1979.

979. Donnelly WH, Bucciarelli RL, Nelson RM: Ischemic papillary muscle necrosis in stressed newborn infants, *J Pediatr* 96:295-300, 1980.

980. Lees MH: Perinatal asphyxia and the myocardium, *J Pediatr* 96:675-678, 1980.

981. Setzer E, Ermocilla R, Tonkin I, John E, et al: Papillary muscle necrosis in a neonatal autopsy population: Incidence and associated clinical manifestations, *J Pediatr* 96:289-294, 1980.

982. Primhak RA, Jedeikin R, Ellis G, Makela SK, et al: Myocardial ischaemia in asphyxia neonatorum: Electrocardiographic, enzymatic and histological correlations, *Acta Paediatr Scand* 74:595-600, 1985.

983. Van Bel F, Walther FJ: Myocardial dysfunction and cerebral blood flow velocity following birth asphyxia, *Acta Paediatr Scand* 79:756-762, 1990.

984. Di Sessa TG, Leitner M, Ti CC, Gluck L, et al: The cardiovascular effects of dopamine in the severely asphyxiated neonate, *J Pediatr* 99:772-776, 1981.

985. Cabal LA, Devaskar U, Siassi B, Hodgman JE, et al: Cardiogenic shock associated with perinatal asphyxia in preterm infants, *J Pediatr* 96:705-710, 1980.

986. Weindling AM, Bentham J: Commentary on "blood pressure in the neonate", *Acta Paediatr* 94:138-140, 2005.

987. Dasgupta SJ, Gill AB: Hypotension in the very low birthweight infant: The old, the new, and the uncertain, *Arch Dis Child Fetal Neonatal Ed* 88:F450-F454, 2003.

988. Barrington KJ, Dempsey EM: Cardiovascular support in the preterm: Treatments in search of indications, *J Pediatr* 148:289-291, 2006.

988a. Osborn DA, Evans N, Kluckow M: Left ventricular contractility in extremely premature infants in the first day and response to inotropes, *Pediatr Res* 61:335-340, 2007.

988b. Osborn DA, Evans N, Kluckow M, Bowen JR, Rieger I: Low superior vena cava flow and effect of inotropes on neurodevelopment to 3 years in preterm infants, *Pediatrics* 120:372-380, 2007.

989. Paradisis M, Evans N, Kuckow M, Osborn D, et al: Pilot study of milrinone for low systemic blood flow in very preterm infants, *J Pediatr* 148:306-313, 2006.

990. Munro MJ, Walker AM, Barfield CP: Hypotensive extremely low birth weight infants have reduced cerebral blood flow, *Pediatrics* 114:1591-1596, 2004.

991. Noori S, Friedlich P, Wong P, Ebrahimi M, et al: Hemodynamic changes after low-dosage hydrocortisone administration in vasopressor-treated preterm and term neonates, *Pediatrics* 118:1456-1466, 2006.

992. Perlman JM, Hill A, Volpe JJ: The effect of patent ductus arteriosus on flow velocity in the anterior cerebral arteries: Ductal steal in the premature newborn infant, *J Pediatr* 99:767-771, 1981.

993. Lipman B, Serwer GA, Brazy JE: Abnormal cerebral hemodynamics in preterm infants with patent ductus arteriosus, *Pediatrics* 69:778-781, 1982.

994. Martin CG, Snider AR, Katz SM, Peabody JL, et al: Abnormal cerebral blood flow patterns in preterm infants with a large patent ductus arteriosus, *J Pediatr* 101:587-593, 1982.

995. Serwer GA, Armstrong BE, Anderson PA: Continuous wave Doppler ultrasonographic quantitation of patent ductus arteriosus flow, *J Pediatr* 100:297-299, 1982.

996. Sonesson SE, Lundell BP, Herin P: Changes in intracranial arterial blood flow velocities during surgical ligation of the patent ductus arteriosus, *Acta Paediatr Scand* 75:36-42, 1986.

997. Shortland DB, Gibson NA, Levene MI, Archer LN, et al: Patent ductus arteriosus and cerebral circulation in preterm infants, *Dev Med Child Neurol* 32:386-393, 1990.

998. Mellander M, Larsson LE: Effects of left-to-right ductus shunting on left ventricular output and cerebral blood flow velocity in 3-day-old preterm infants with and without severe lung disease, *J Pediatr* 113:101-109, 1988.

999. Kurtis PS, Rosendrantz TS, Zalneraitis EL: Cerebral blood flow and EEG changes in preterm infants with patent ductus arteriosus, *Pediatr Neurol* 12:114-119, 1995.

1000. Pladys P, Beuchee A, Wodey E, Treguier C, et al: Patent ductus arteriosus and cystic periventricular leucomalacia in preterm infants, *Acta Paediatr* 90:309-315, 2001.

1001. Ment LR, Vohr BR, Makuch RW, Westerveld M, et al: Prevention of intraventricular hemorrhage by indomethacin in male preterm infants, *J Pediatr* 145:832-834, 2004.

1002. Ment LR, Peterson BS, Meltzer JA, Vohr B, et al: A functional magnetic resonance imaging study of the long-term influences of early indomethacin exposure on language processing in the brains of prematurely born children, *Pediatrics* 118:961-970, 2006.

1003. Miller SP, Mayer EE, Clyman RI, Glidden DV, et al: Prolonged indomethacin exposure is associated with decreased white matter injury detected with magnetic resonance imaging in premature newborns at 24 to 28 weeks' gestation at birth, *Pediatrics* 117:1626-1631, 2006.

1004. Perlman JM, Volpe JJ: Episodes of apnea and bradycardia in the preterm newborn: Impact on cerebral circulation, *Pediatrics* 76:333-338, 1985.

1005. Livera LN, Spencer SA, Thorniley MS, Wickramasinghe YA, et al: Effects of hypoxaemia and bradycardia on neonatal cerebral haemodynamics, *Arch Dis Child* 66:376-380, 1991.

1006. Payer C, Urlesberger B, Pauger M, Muller W: Apnea associated with hypoxia in preterm infants: Impact on cerebral blood volume, *Brain Dev* 25:25-31, 2003.

1007. Pichler G, Urlesberger B, Muller W: Impact of bradycardia on cerebral oxygenation and cerebral blood volume during apnoea in preterm infants, *Physiological Measurement* 24:671-680, 2003.

1008. Abman SH, Warady BA, Lum GM, Koops BL: Systemic hypertension in infants with bronchopulmonary dysplasia, *J Pediatr* 104:928-931, 1984.

1009. Perlman JM, Volpe JJ: Neurologic complications of captopril treatment of neonatal hypertension, *Pediatrics* 83:47-52, 1989.

1010. Barry DI, Strandgaard S, Graham DI, Braendstrup O, et al: Cerebral blood flow in rats with renal and spontaneous hypertension: Resetting of the lower limit of autoregulation, *J Cereb Blood Flow Metab* 2:347-353, 1982.

1011. Strandgaard S: Autoregulation of cerebral circulation in hypertension, *Acta Neurol Scand Suppl* 66:1-82, 1978.

1012. Hankey GJ, Gubbay SS: Focal cerebral ischaemia and infarction due to antihypertensive therapy, *Med J Aust* 146:412-414, 1987.

1013. Fujishima M, Omae T: Lower limit of cerebral autoregulation in normotensive and spontaneously hypertensive rats, *Experientia* 32:1019-1021, 1976.

1014. Black VD, Lubchenco LO: Neonatal polycythemia and hyperviscosity, *Pediatr Clin North Am* 29:1137-1148, 1982.

1015. Hathaway WE: Neonatal hyperviscosity, *Pediatrics* 72:567-569, 1983.

1016. Grotta J, Ackerman R, Correia J, Fallick G, et al: Whole blood viscosity parameters and cerebral blood flow, *Stroke* 13:296-301, 1982.

1017. Rosenkrantz TS, Oh W: Cerebral blood flow velocity in infants with polycythemia and hyperviscosity: Effects of partial exchange transfusion with Plasmanate, *J Pediatr* 101:94-98, 1982.

1018. Bada HS, Korones SB, Kolni HW, Fitch CW, et al: Partial plasma exchange transfusion improves cerebral hemodynamics in symptomatic neonatal polycythemia, *Am J Med Sci* 291:157-163, 1986.

1019. Maertzdorf WJ, Tangelder GJ, Slaaf DW, Blanco CE: Effects of partial plasma exchange transfusion on cerebral blood flow velocity in polycythaemic preterm, term and small for date newborn infants, *Eur J Pediatr* 148:774-778, 1989.

1020. Bada HS, Korones SB, Pourcyrous M, Wong SP, et al: Asymptomatic syndrome of polycythemic hyperviscosity: Effect of partial plasma exchange transfusion, *J Pediatr* 120:579-585, 1992.

1021. Younkin DP, Reivich M, Jaggi JL, Obrist WD, et al: The effect of hematocrit and systolic blood pressure on cerebral blood flow in newborn infants, *J Cereb Blood Flow Metab* 7:295-299, 1987.

1022. Pryds O: Control of cerebral circulation in the high-risk neonate, *Ann Neurol* 30:321-329, 1991.

1023. Goldstein M, Stonestreet BS, Brann BS 4th, Oh W: Cerebral cortical blood flow and oxygen metabolism in normocythemic hyperviscous newborn piglets, *Pediatr Res* 24:486-489, 1988.

1024. Wiswell TE, Cornish JD, Northam RS: Neonatal polycythemia: Frequency of clinical manifestations and other associated findings, *Pediatrics* 78:26-30, 1986.

1025. Black VD, Lubchenco LO, Koops BL, Poland RL, et al: Neonatal hyperviscosity: Randomized study of effect of partial plasma exchange transfusion on long-term outcome, *Pediatrics* 75:1048-1053, 1985.

1026. Delaney-Black V, Camp BW, Lubchenco LO, Swanson C, et al: Neonatal hyperviscosity association with lower achievement and IQ scores at school age, *Pediatrics* 83:662-667, 1989.

1027. Williams CE, Gunn AJ, Mallard C, Gluckman PD: Outcome after ischemia in the developing sheep brain: An electroencephalographic and histological study, *Ann Neurol* 31:14-21, 1992.

1028. Painter MJ, Pippenger C, MacDonald H, Pitlick W: Phenobarbital and diphenylhydantoin levels in neonates with seizures, *J Pediatr* 92:315-319, 1978.

1029. McBride MC, Laroia N, Guillet R: Electrographic seizures in neonates correlate with poor neurodevelopmental outcome, *Neurology* 55:506-513, 2000.

1030. Cataltepe O, Vannucci RC, Heitjan DF, Towfighi J: Effect of status epilepticus on hypoxic-ischemic brain damage in the immature rat, *Pediatr Res* 38:251-257, 1995.

1031. Vannucci RC, Connor JR, Mauger DT, Palmer C, et al: Rat model of perinatal hypoxic-ischemic brain damage, *J Neurosci Res* 55:158-163, 1999.

1032. Towfighi J, Housman C, Mauger D, Vannucci RC: Effect of seizures on cerebral hypoxic-ischemic lesions in immature rats, *Dev Brain Res* 113:83-95, 1999.

1033. Myers RE, Williams MV: Lost opportunities for the prevention of fetal asphyxia: Sedation, analgesia, and general anaesthesia, *Clin Obstet Gynecol* 9:369-414, 1982.

1034. Richter JA, Holtman JR Jr: Barbiturates: Their in vivo effects and potential biochemical mechanisms, *Prog Neurobiol* 18:275-319, 1982.

1035. Steer CR: Barbiturate therapy in the management of cerebral ischaemia, *Dev Med Child Neurol* 24:219-231, 1982.

1036. Smith AL: Barbiturate protection in cerebral hypoxia, *Anesthesiology* 47:285-293, 1977.

1037. Crane PD, Braun LD, Cornford EM, Cremer JE, et al: Dose dependent reduction of glucose utilization by pentobarbital in rat brain, *Stroke* 9:12-18, 1978.

1038. Nilsson L: The influence of barbiturate anaesthesia upon the energy state and upon acid-base parameters of the brain in arterial hypotension and in asphyxia, *Acta Neurol Scand* 47:233-253, 1971.

1039. Snyder FF: The effect of pentobarbital sodium upon the resistance to asphyxia in the newborn, *Fed Proc* 5:97, 1946.

1040. Arnfred I, Secher O: Anoxia and barbiturates, *Arch Int Pharmacodyn Ther* 139:67, 1962.

1041. Miller JA Jr, Miller FS: Factors in neonatal resistance to anoxia. III. Potentiation by narcosis of the effects of hypothermia in the newborn guinea pig, *Am J Obstet Gynecol* 84:44-56, 1962.

1042. Goodlin RC: Drug protection for fetal anoxia, *Obstet Gynecol* 26:9, 1965.

1043. Campbell AG, Milligan JE, Talner NS: The effect of pretreatment with pentobarbital, meperidine, or hyperbaric oxygen on the response to anoxia and resuscitation in newborn rabbits, *J Pediatr* 72:518-527, 1968.

1044. Myers RE: Maternal psychological stress and fetal asphyxia: A study in the monkey, *Am J Obstet Gynecol* 122:47-59, 1975.

1045. Cockburn F, Daniel SS, Dawes GS, James LS, et al: The effect of pentobarbital anesthesia on resuscitation and brain damage in fetal rhesus monkeys asphyxiated on delivery, *J Pediatr* 75:281-291, 1969.

1046. Morishima HO, Yeh MN, James LS: Reduced uterine blood flow and fetal hypoxemia with acute maternal stress: Experimental observation in the pregnant baboon, *Am J Obstet Gynecol* 134:270-275, 1979.

1047. Fisher DE, Paton JB, Behrman RE: The effect of phenobarbital on asphyxia in the newborn monkey, *Pediatr Res* 9:181-184, 1975.

1048. Eyre JA, Wilkinson AR: Thiopentone induced coma after severe birth asphyxia, *Arch Dis Child* 61:1084-1089, 1986.

1049. Goldberg RN, Moscoso P, Bauer CR, Bloom FL, et al: Use of barbiturate therapy in severe perinatal asphyxia: A randomized controlled trial, *J Pediatr* 109:851-856, 1986.

1050. Svenningsen NW, Blennow G, Lindroth M, Gaddlin PO, et al: Brain-oriented intensive care treatment in severe neonatal asphyxia: Effects of phenobarbitone protection, *Arch Dis Child* 57:176-183, 1982.

1051. Hall RT, Hall FK, Daily DK: High-dose phenobarbital therapy in term newborn infants with severe perinatal asphyxia: A randomized, prospective study with three-year follow-up, *J Pediatr* 132:345-348, 1998.

1052. Dai Y, Tang J, Zhang JH: Role of Cl⁻ in cerebral vascular tone and expression of Na^+-K^+-$2Cl^-$ co-transporter after neonatal hypoxia-ischemia, *Can J Physiol Pharmacol* 83:767-773, 2005.

1053. Levene MI, Evans DH: Medical management of raised intracranial pressure after birth asphyxia, *Arch Dis Child* 60:12-16, 1985.

1054. Levene MI, Evans DH, Forde A, Archer LN: Value of intracranial pressure monitoring of asphyxiated newborn infants, *Dev Med Child Neurol* 29:311-319, 1987.

1055. Rochefort MJ, Rolfe P, Wilkinson AR: New fontanometer for continuous estimation of intracranial pressure in the newborn, *Arch Dis Child* 62:152-155, 1987.

1056. Adhikari M, Moodley M, Desai PK: Mannitol in neonatal cerebral oedema, *Brain Dev* 12:349-351, 1990.

1057. Feldman W, Drummond KN, Klein M: Hyponatremia following asphyxia neonatorum, *Acta Paediatr Scand* 59:52-57, 1970.

1058. Khare SK: Neurohypophyseal dysfunction following perinatal asphyxia, *J Pediatr* 90:628-629, 1977.

1059. Kaplan SL, Feigin RD: Inappropriate secretion of antidiuretic hormone complicating neonatal hypoxic-ischemic encephalopathy, *J Pediatr* 92:431-433, 1978.

1060. Speer ME, Gorman WA, Kaplan SL, Rudolph AJ: Elevation of plasma concentrations of arginine vasopressin following perinatal asphyxia, *Acta Paediatr Scand* 73:610-614, 1984.

1061. Raju TN, Doshi U, Vidyasagar D: Low cerebral perfusion pressure: An indicator of poor prognosis in asphyxiated term infants, *Brain Dev* 5:478-482, 1983.

1062. Vannucci RC: Current and potentially new management strategies for perinatal hypoxic-ischemic encephalopathy, *Pediatrics* 85:961-968, 1990.

1063. Levene MI, Gibson NA, Fenton AC, Papathoma E, et al: The use of a calcium-channel blocker, nicardipine, for severely asphyxiated newborn infants, *Dev Med Child Neurol* 32:567-574, 1990.

1064. Nelson KB, Grether JK: Can magnesium sulfate reduce the risk of cerebral palsy in very low birthweight infants? *Pediatrics* 95:263-269, 1995.

1065. Schendel DE, Berg CJ, Yeargin-Allsopp M, Boyle CA, et al: Prenatal magnesium sulfate exposure and the risk for cerebral palsy or mental retardation among very low-birth-weight children aged 3 to 5 years, *JAMA* 276:1805-1810, 1996.

1066. Hauth JC, Goldenberg RL, Nelson KG, duBard MB, et al: Reduction of cerebral palsy with maternal MgSO₄ treatment in newborns weighing 500-1000 g., *Am J Obstet Gynecol* 172:419, 1995.

1067. Paneth N, Jetton J, Pinto-Martin J, Susser M: Magnesium sulfate in labor and risk of neonatal brain lesions and cerebral palsy in low birth weight infants, *Pediatrics* 99:1-10, 1997.

1068. Fine-Smith RB, Roche K, Yelin PB, Walsh KK, et al: Effect of magnesium sulfate on the development of cystic periventricular leukomalacia in preterm infants, *Am J Perinatal* 14:303-307, 1997.

1069. Stigson L, Kjellmer I: Serum levels of magnesium at birth related to complications of immaturity, *Acta Paediatr* 86:991-994, 1997.

1070. Leviton A, Paneth N, Susser M, Reuss ML, et al: Maternal receipt of magnesium sulfate does not seem to reduce the risk of neonatal white matter damage, *Pediatrics* 99:1-5, 1997.

1071. Perlman JM, Riser RC, Gee JB: Pregnancy-induced hypertension and reduced intraventricular hemorrhage in preterm infants, *Pediatr Neurol* 17:29-33, 1997.

1072. Perlman JM: Antenatal glucocorticoid, magnesium exposure, and the prevention of brain injury of prematurity, *Semin Pediatr Neurol* 5:202-210, 1998.

1073. Grether JK, Hoogstrate J, Walsh-Greene E, Nelson KB: Magnesium sulfate for tocolysis and risk of spastic cerebral palsy in premature children born to women without preeclampsia, *Am J Obstet Gynecol* 183:717-725, 2000.

1074. Rantonen T, Ekblad U, Gronlund J, Rikalainen H, et al: Influence of maternal magnesium sulphate and ritodrine treatment on the neonate: A study with six-month follow-up, *Acta Paediatr* 88:1142-1146, 1999.

1075. Mittendorf R, Dambrosia J, Dammann O, Pryde PG, et al: Association between maternal serum ionized magnesium levels at delivery and neonatal intraventricular hemorrhage, *J Pediatr* 140:540-546, 2002.

1076. Crowther CA, Hiller JE, Doyle LW, Haslam RR: Effect of magnesium sulfate given for neuroprotection before preterm birth: A randomized controlled trial, *JAMA* 290:2669-2676, 2003.

1077. Crowther CA, Hiller JE, Doyle LW: Magnesium sulphate for preventing preterm birth in threatened preterm labour, *Cochrane Database Syst Rev* 4:CD001060, 2004.

1078. DiRenzo GC, Mignosa M, Gerli S, Burnelli L, et al: The combined maternal administration of magnesium sulfate and aminophylline reduces intraventricular hemorrhage in very preterm neonates, *Am J Obstet Gynecol* 192:433-438, 2005.

1079. Mittendorf R, Dammann O, Lee KS: Brain lesions in newborns exposed to high-dose magnesium sulfate during preterm labor, *J Perinatol* 26:57-63, 2006.

1079a. Marret S, Marpeau L, Zupan-Simunek V, Eurin D, et al: Magnesium sulphate given before very-preterm birth to protect infant brain: The randomised controlled PREMAG trial, *BJOG* 114:310-318, 2007.

1079b. Harrison V, Fawcus S, Jordaan E: Magnesium supplementation and perinatal hypoxia: Outcome of a parallel group randomised trial in pregnancy, *BJOG* 114:994-1002, 2007.

1080. Groenendaal F, Rademaker CMA, Toet MC, de Vries LS: Effects of magnesium sulphate on amplitude-integrated continuous EEG in asphyxiated term neonates, *Acta Paediatr* 91:1073-1077, 2002.

1081. deHaan HH, Gunn AJ, Williams CE, Heymann MA, et al: Magnesium sulfate therapy during asphyxia in near-term fetal lambs does not compromise the fetus but does not reduce cerebral injury, *Am J Obstet Gynecol* 176:18-27, 1997.

1082. Penrice J, Amess PN, Punwani S, Wylezinska M, et al: Magnesium sulfate after transient hypoxia-ischemia fails to prevent delayed cerebral energy failure in the newborn piglet, *Pediatr Res* 41:443-447, 1997.

1083. Galvin KA, Oorschot DE: Postinjury magnesium sulfate treatment is not markedly neuroprotective for striatal medium spiny neurons after perinatal hypoxia/ischemia in the rat, *Pediatr Res* 44:740-745, 1998.

1084. Hallak M, Irtenkauf SM, Cotton DB: Effect of magnesium sulfate on excitatory amino acid receptors in the rat brain. I. *N*-Methyl-D-aspartate receptor channel complex, *Am J Obstet Gynecol* 175:575-581, 1996.

1085. McDonald JW, Silverstein FS, Johnston MV: Magnesium reduces *N*-methyl-D-aspartate (NMDA)-mediated brain injury in perinatal rats, *Neurosci Lett* 109:234-238, 1990.

1086. Hoffman DJ, Marro PJ, McGowan JE, Mishra OP, et al: Protective effect of MgSO$_4$ infusion on NMDA receptor binding characteristics during cerebral cortical hypoxia in the newborn piglet, *Brain Res* 644:144-149, 1994.

1087. Puza S, Goel R, Hoffman D, Mishra OP, et al: Pretreatment with magnesium protects NMDA receptor in fetal guinea pig brain during hypoxia, *Prenat Neonat Med* 1:349-354, 1996.

1088. Marret S, Gressens P, Gadisseux J-F, Evrard P: Prevention by magnesium of excitotoxic neuronal death in the developing brain: An animal model for clinical intervention studies, *Dev Med Child Neurol* 37:473-484, 1995.

1089. Nakajima W, Ishida A, Takada G: Magnesium attenuates a striatal dopamine increase induced by anoxia in the neonatal rat brain: An in vivo microdialysis study, *Pediatr Res* 41:809-814, 1997.

1090. Regan RF, Jasper E, Guo YP, Panter SS: The effect of magnesium on oxidative neuronal injury in vitro, *J Neurochem* 70:77-85, 1998.

1091. Altura BM, Altura BT, Carella A, Gebrewold A, et al: Mg^{2+}-Ca^{2+} interaction in contractility of vascular smooth muscle: Mg^{2+} versus organic calcium channel blockers on myogenic tone and agonist-induced responsiveness of blood vessels, *Can J Physiol Pharmacol* 65:729-745, 1987.

1092. Scardo JA, Hogg BB, Newman RB: Favorable hemodynamic effects of magnesium sulfate in preeclampsia, *Am J Obstet Gynecol* 173:1249-1253, 1995.

1093. Walsh SW, Romney AD, Wang Y, Walsh MD: Magnesium sulfate attenuates peroxide-induced vasoconstriction in the human placenta, *Am J Obstet Gynecol* 178:7-12, 1998.

1094. Skajaa K, Forman A, Anderson KE: Effects of magnesium on isolated human fetal and maternal uteroplacental vessels, *Acta Physiol Scand* 139:551-559, 1990.

1095. Kim CR, Oh W, Stonestreet BS: Magnesium is a cerebrovasodilator in newborn piglets, *Am J Physiol* 41:511-516, 1997.

1096. Van Bel F, Shadid M, Moison RMW, Dorrepaal CA, et al: Effect of allopurinol on postasphyxial free radical formation, cerebral hemodynamics, and electrical brain activity, *Pediatrics* 101:184-193, 1998.

1097. Gunes T, Ozturk MA, Koklu E, Kose K, et al: Effect of allopurinol supplementation on nitric oxide levels in asphyxiated newborns, *Pediatr Neurol* 36:17-24, 2006.

1098. Gunn AJ, Gluckman PD, Gunn TR: Selective head cooling in newborn infants after perinatal asphyxia: A safety study, *Pediatrics* 102:885-892, 1998.

1099. Azzopardi D, Robertson NJ, Cowan FM, Rutherford MA, et al: Pilot study of treatment with whole body hypothermia for neonatal encephalopathy, *Pediatrics* 106:684-894, 2000.

1100. Battin MR, Dezoete A, Gunn TR, Gluckman PD, et al: Neurodevelopmental outcome of infants treated with head cooling and mild hypothermia after perinatal asphyxia, *Pediatrics* 107:480-484, 2001.

1101. Battin MR, Penrice J, Gunn TR, Gunn AJ: Treatment of term infants with head cooling and mild systemic hypothermia (34.5°C) after perinatal asphyxia, *Pediatrics* 111:244-251, 2003.

1102. Gluckman PD, Wyatt JS, Azzopardi D, Ballard R, et al: Selective head cooling with mild systemic hypothermia after neonatal encephalopathy: Multicentre randomised trial, *Lancet* 365:663-670, 2005.

1103. Eicher DJ, Wagner CL, Katikaneni LP, Hulsey TC, et al: Moderate hypothermia in neonatal encephalopathy: Efficacy outcomes, *Pediatr Neurol* 32:11-17, 2005.

1104. Eicher DJ, Wagner CL, Katikaneni LP, Hulsey TC, et al: Moderate hypothermia in neonatal encephalopathy: Safety outcomes, *Pediatr Neurol* 32:18-24, 2005.

1105. Shankaran S, Laptook AR, Ehrenkranz RA, Tyson JE, et al: Whole-body hypothermia for neonates with hypoxic-ischemic encephalopathy, *N Engl J Med* 353:1574-1584, 2005.

1106. Higgins RD, Raju TN, Perlman J, Azzopardi DV, et al: Hypothermia and perinatal asphyxia: Executive summary of the National Institute of Child Health and Human Development workshop, *J Pediatr* 148:170-175, 2006.

1107. Edwards AD, Azzopardi DV: Therapeutic hypothermia following perinatal asphyxia, *Arch Dis Child Fetal Neonatal Ed* 91:F127-F131, 2006.

1107a. Wyatt JS, Gluckman PD, Liu PY, Azzopardi D, et al: Determinants of outcomes after head cooling for neonatal encephalopathy, *Pediatrics* 119:912-921, 2007.

1108. Iwata O, Thornton JS, Sellwood MW, Iwata S, et al: Depth of delayed cooling alters neuroprotection pattern after hypoxia-ischemia, *Ann Neurol* 58:75-87, 2005.

1109. Rutherford MA, Azzopardi D, Whitelaw A, Cowan F, et al: Mild hypothermia and the distribution of cerebral lesions in neonates with hypoxic-ischemic encephalopathy, *Pediatrics* 116:1001-1006, 2005.

1110. Inder TE, Hunt RW, Morley CJ, Coleman L, et al: Randomized trial of systemic hypothermia selectively protects the cortex on MRI in term hypoxic-ischemic encephalopathy, *J Pediatr* 145:835-837, 2004.

INTRACRANIAL HEMORRHAGE

Intracranial Hemorrhage: Subdural, Primary Subarachnoid, Cerebellar, Intraventricular (Term Infant), and Miscellaneous

Intracranial hemorrhage in the neonatal period is an important clinical problem. Its importance relates to a relatively high frequency of occurrence, accompanied often by serious neurological sequelae or even death. In addition to this high frequency, distinct changes in the spectrum of neonatal intracranial hemorrhage have occurred in the past several decades. These changes have consisted of a marked reduction in traumatic lesions, such as subdural hemorrhage, and a marked increase in lesions characteristic of the premature infant, particularly germinal matrix–intraventricular hemorrhage. The first change is a result of improvements in obstetrical practice. The increased number of hemorrhages characteristic of the premature infant is the result principally of the markedly improved survival rates for such infants, and this, in turn, is related primarily to the advances of modern neonatal intensive care.

In this chapter, I present an overview of neonatal intracranial hemorrhage and the basic elements of recognition. Detailed discussion is devoted to subdural hemorrhage, primary subarachnoid hemorrhage, cerebellar hemorrhage, intraventricular hemorrhage of the *full-term infant*, and certain unusual, miscellaneous examples of neonatal intracranial hemorrhage. The critical problem of germinal matrix–intraventricular hemorrhage of *the premature infant* is discussed separately in Chapter 11, and various traumatic extracranial and intracranial hemorrhages, now generally unusual, are considered in Chapter 22.

OVERVIEW

Classification

The five major, clinically important types of neonatal intracranial hemorrhage (Table 10-1) are (1) subdural hemorrhage, (2) primary subarachnoid hemorrhage, (3) cerebellar hemorrhage, (4) intraventricular hemorrhage, and (5) miscellaneous intraparenchymal hemorrhages (other than cerebellar). Certain general conclusions can be made about each of these types of hemorrhage in terms of the maturation of the affected infant, the relative frequency of the specific type, and

the usual clinical gravity (see Table 10-1). Thus, *subdural hemorrhage*, more frequent in the full-term infant than in the premature infant, is in general uncommon but is usually clinically serious. *Primary subarachnoid hemorrhage*, more frequent in the premature infant than in the full-term infant, is, in general, common but is almost always clinically benign. *Cerebellar hemorrhage*, more frequent in the premature infant than in the full-term infant, is, in general, uncommon but is usually serious. *Intraventricular hemorrhage, almost* exclusively a lesion of the premature infant, is, in contrast to the other three types of hemorrhage, both common and usually serious. *Miscellaneous intraparenchymal hemorrhages*, more frequent in the full-term infant than in the premature infant, are uncommon and are of variable clinical gravity.

Recognition of Hemorrhage

Three Major Steps

Three major steps need to be taken to ensure recognition of neonatal intracranial hemorrhage. First, *predisposing factors* should be identified. As outlined in more detail in subsequent sections, these factors include the gestational history, the details of labor and delivery, the maturation of the baby, the occurrence of "hypoxic" events, the modes of resuscitation, and so forth. Second, definition of *abnormal clinical features* must be made early in the neonatal course. Particular attention should be given to subtle neurological signs, as outlined later. Third, visualization of the site and extent of the hemorrhage should be made by an *imaging technique*, often initially by ultrasound scan and then more definitively by computed tomography (CT) or magnetic resonance imaging (MRI), as illustrated later. Intracranial hemorrhage is often first suspected because a lumbar puncture, often carried out to rule out sepsis, reveals *cerebrospinal fluid* (*CSF*) consistent with hemorrhage. In view of this role of CSF examination, I discuss interpretation of the CSF findings first. (Performance of lumbar puncture can be dangerous in the presence of a major unilateral supratentorial hemorrhage or a large posterior fossa

TABLE 10-1 Major Types of Neonatal Intracranial Hemorrhage

Type of Hemorrhage	Maturation of Infant	Relative Frequency	Usual Clinical Gravity
Subdural	Full term > premature	Uncommon	Serious
Primary subarachnoid	Premature > full term	Common	Benign
Cerebellar	Premature > full term	Uncommon	Serious
Intraventricular	Premature > full term	Common	Serious
Miscellaneous: intraparenchymal, multiple sites	Full term > premature	Uncommon	Variable

hemorrhage (see later). Thus, I do not recommend lumbar puncture as a routine diagnostic procedure for hemorrhage.

Cerebrospinal Fluid in the Recognition of Intracranial Hemorrhage

"Traumatic" Lumbar Puncture. The finding of bloody CSF in a newborn often is attributed to "traumatic" lumbar puncture. This conclusion primarily relates to the relative difficulty of performing the puncture in the newborn but also to the relative frequency of finding bloody CSF in infants without overt neurological signs. I believe that traumatic lumbar puncture in the newborn is much less common than is generally thought. For example, in a study in which we performed lumbar punctures on the third postnatal day in all infants of less than 2000 g in our neonatal intensive care unit, the 76 infants who had *grossly* bloody CSF with elevated protein content were evaluated by CT scan (Table 10-2). Only 6 (8%) had no increased attenuation consistent with blood observable. Subarachnoid blood was detectable in 22 (29%), and intraventricular hemorrhage was noted in 48 (63%).

Although I believe that the finding of bloody CSF in an infant is an indication for a definitive search for a locus of intracranial hemorrhage (see subsequent discussion), certain indirect techniques have been used to determine whether the finding is "real" or related to a "traumatic" lumbar puncture. These approaches include determination of the ratio of fetal to adult hemoglobin in both circulating blood and the blood in CSF, determination of the penetration into CSF of systemically administered fluorescein dye during the collection of CSF, high-intensity transillumination of the frontal subarachnoid space by a fiberoptic device applied to the overlying scalp, determination of CSF glutamine levels, and detection of D-dimers of fibrinogen.[1-5] None of these approaches is in wide use.

TABLE 10-2 Computed Tomography Scan Correlates of Bloody Cerebrospinal Fluid in 76 Infants Weighing Less than 2000 g

Blood on Scan	No. of Patients	Percentage of Total Group
None	6	8%
Subarachnoid	22	29%
Germinal matrix– intraventricular	48	63%

Cerebrospinal Fluid Findings of Intracranial Hemorrhage. CSF findings that indicate intracranial hemorrhage are, primarily, xanthochromia of the centrifuged fluid and elevations of the number of red blood cells (RBCs) and the protein content. Particular emphasis should be placed on the occurrence of *combinations* of findings rather than on a single, isolated abnormality.

Xanthochromia of the CSF develops within several hours after hemorrhage in older children and adults. (In one particularly large study of adults with subarachnoid hemorrhage, nearly 90% exhibited xanthochromia within 12 hours of the ictus.[6]) The evolution of xanthochromia in newborns has not been studied systematically, although I have the impression that it occurs more slowly than in older patients. This slower evolution may relate to a delay in the induction of the enzyme, heme oxygenase, which is located in the arachnoid and is responsible for the conversion of heme to bilirubin, the major pigment accounting for xanthochromia of the CSF.[7] In adult rats, the activity of heme oxygenase reaches peak values 6 to 12 hours after injection of heme into the subarachnoid space.[7] These data are closely comparable to the clinical observations with adult patients cited. Determination of the significance of xanthochromia in newborns is occasionally difficult in the presence of elevated serum bilirubin levels. Although this difficulty is rarely a major consideration, demonstration of spectrophotometric differences between CSF bilirubin pigments derived from the systemic circulation and those derived from the hemorrhage could be used in the evaluation.[8] When xanthochromia is evaluated in the context of the *total CSF profile*, difficulties in assessing significance are very unusual.

The number of *RBCs* that should be considered significant is difficult to state conclusively, in part because of the remarkably wide range of values considered normal (see Chapter 4).[9-16] For example, some observers consider as normal a few hundred RBCs/mm³. In studies of infants in neonatal intensive care facilities, median values of 100 to 200 RBCs/mm³ have been observed. In the only report with ultrasonographic correlates, among 43 infants of less than 1500 g birth weight, the median value was 112, but the mean value was 785, and 20% of CSF samples had more than 1000 RBCs/mm³.[16] These infants did not exhibit ultrasonographic evidence of intracranial hemorrhage. However, exclusion of minor subarachnoid hemorrhage by cranial ultrasonography is not reliable. Thus, the data indicate that findings of more than 100 RBCs/mm³ in the newborn are common, and in the very-low-birth-weight infants, values greater than 1000 occur in a substantial minority in the absence of apparently clinically significant intracranial hemorrhage. Again, the *combination* of findings is important in the evaluation.

Values for CSF *protein* are higher in newborns in an intensive care nursery than in older children. In the series of Sarff and co-workers,[15] an average protein content in CSF of 90 mg/dL was observed for term infants, and a content of 115 mg/dL was observed for preterm infants. We obtained similar data.[14] In general, values for CSF protein are higher in the most premature infants; in one series, the mean value at 26 to 28 weeks of postconceptional age was 177 mg/dL, and at 35 to 37 weeks, it was 109 mg/dL.[16] Values in intracranial hemorrhage are usually severalfold or higher than these.

Finally, determination of the CSF *glucose* level may be helpful in the diagnosis. In term and preterm infants evaluated in a neonatal intensive care unit and free of intracranial infection, the ratios of CSF to blood glucose levels are relatively high (i.e., 0.81 and 0.74, respectively).[15] As with CSF protein levels, values for CSF glucose tend to be higher in the most premature infants; in one series, the mean value at 26 to 28 weeks was 85 mg/dL, and at 38 to 40 weeks, it was 44 mg/dL.[16] After neonatal intracranial hemorrhage, the CSF glucose level is frequently low (Table 10-3).[17-21] Indeed, in one study in which serial lumbar punctures were performed (for therapeutic purposes) on 13 infants with intraventricular hemorrhage, the CSF glucose concentration decreased on subsequent measurements in *all* the infants.[21] Eleven of the 13 infants had CSF glucose values lower than 30 mg/dL at some point subsequent to the hemorrhage, and values of 10 mg/dL or less were common. The low values occurred as early as 1 day after the hemorrhage but usually became apparent between approximately 5 and 15 days after the hemorrhage. (The hypoglycorrhachia observed after subarachnoid hemorrhage in adults reaches lowest values after a similar time interval.[22,23]) The depressed CSF glucose values persist for weeks and have been noted as long as 3 months after the hemorrhage.[18,19]

The basis of hypoglycorrhachia is probably related to an impairment of the mechanisms of glucose transport into CSF. This impairment may occur at the level of the plasma membrane glucose transporter.[23] Other proposed pathogeneses have included glucose use by RBCs or by contiguous brain. The former is ruled out by the lack of correlation between RBC number and CSF glucose level and by the negligible rates of glucose consumption observed when the cellular CSF is incubated in vitro. The possibility of excessive anaerobic use of glucose by contiguous brain rendered hypoxic-ischemic by hemorrhage, ventricular dilation, or other insult[24] appears unlikely in view of simultaneous, serial determinations of CSF glucose and lactate.[21] Thus, in 13 infants described with CSF hypoglycorrhachia, CSF glucose and lactate concentrations decreased pari passu; if anaerobic use of glucose had been operative, a concomitant increase in CSF lactate would have been expected. These observations favor the notion of a defect in glucose transport mechanisms.

An important practical problem arises when the low CSF glucose level is accompanied by pleocytosis and elevated protein content. This not uncommon occurrence is related presumably to meningeal inflammation from blood products and raises the question of bacterial meningitis. Although appropriate cultures are always indicated, and even initiation of antimicrobial therapy may be necessary (until results of cultures are known), the CSF formula of pleocytosis, depressed glucose, and elevated protein content is not infrequent after neonatal intracranial hemorrhage.

The *optimal imaging procedure for diagnosis* becomes apparent in the following discussions of the respective lesions, and the relative value of cranial ultrasonography, CT, and MRI in diagnosis is reviewed in Chapter 4. Suffice it to say here that cranial ultrasonography is often used as a screening procedure, CT is a more definitive approach, and MRI is the most effective methodology. The sometimes confusing features of MRI signal change after neonatal parenchymal hemorrhage are reviewed in Table 10-4. (On the first day after the hemorrhage, CT is perhaps more sensitive for detection of hemorrhage than is MRI.) The MRI changes relate primarily to changes in hemoglobin state, which proceed from predominately intracellular deoxyhemoglobin, to intracellular methemoglobin, to extracellular methemoglobin, and finally hemosiderin.

SUBDURAL HEMORRHAGE

Subdural hemorrhage is the least common of the major varieties of neonatal intracranial hemorrhage. Recognition of the disorder is important because in

---

TABLE 10-3   **Major Features of Hypoglycorrhachia after Neonatal Intracranial Hemorrhage**

Nearly uniform occurrence after major hemorrhage
Onset usually 5 to 15 days after hemorrhage
Duration of weeks to months
Accompanied by concomitant decrease in cerebrospinal fluid lactate level
Mechanism not proved but probably related to impaired glucose transport

---

TABLE 10-4   **Predominant Magnetic Resonance Imaging Signal Changes after Parenchymal Hemorrhage**

Age of Hemorrhage	SIGNAL CHANGES	
	T1 Weighted	T2 Weighted
1–3 days	Isointense	Low
3–10 days	High	Low
10–21 days	High	High
3–6 wk	High	High
6 wk–10 mo	Isointense	Low

Adapted from Rutherford M: *MRI of the Neonatal brain*, Philadelphia: 2002, WB Saunders, and from personal experience.

patients with large hemorrhages, therapeutic intervention can be lifesaving.

Neuropathology

Anatomy of Major Veins and Sinuses

The neuropathology of neonatal subdural hemorrhage is readily understood after a brief review of the major anatomical features of the veins and sinuses involved in the production of such hemorrhage (Fig. 10-1). The deep venous drainage of the cerebrum empties into the great cerebral vein of Galen at the junction of the tentorium and falx. The confluence of the vein of Galen and the inferior sagittal sinus, the latter located in the inferior margin of the falx, forms the straight sinus. This sinus proceeds directly posteriorly and joins the superior sagittal sinus, located in the superior margin of the falx, to form the transverse sinus. Blood in the transverse sinuses, located in the lateral margins of the tentorium, proceeds eventually to the jugular vein. Blood in the posterior fossa in part drains into the occipital sinus, which empties into the torcular. The superficial portion of the cerebrum is drained by the superficial, bridging cerebral veins, which empty into the superior sagittal sinus. Tears of these several veins or venous sinuses, occurring secondary to forces to be described and often accompanying laceration of the dura, result in subdural hemorrhage.

Major Varieties of Subdural Hemorrhage

The major varieties of neonatal subdural hemorrhage include the following (Table 10-5): tentorial laceration with rupture principally of the straight sinus, transverse sinus, vein of Galen, or smaller infratentorial veins;

TABLE 10-5	Neuropathology of Subdural Hemorrhage	
Source of Bleeding	**Location of Hematoma**
Tentorial Laceration Straight sinus, vein of Galen, transverse sinus, and infratentorial veins	Infratentorial (posterior fossa), supratentorial
Occipital Osteodiastasis Occipital sinus	Infratentorial (posterior fossa)
Falx Laceration Inferior sagittal sinus	Longitudinal cerebral fissure
Superficial Cerebral Veins	Surface of cerebral convexity

occipital osteodiastasis with rupture of the occipital sinus; falx laceration with rupture of the inferior sagittal sinus; and rupture of bridging, superficial cerebral veins.

Tentorial Laceration. With *major, lethal tears* of the tentorium, hemorrhage is most often infratentorial.[25-31] This finding is the case particularly with rupture of the vein of Galen or straight sinus or with severe involvement of the transverse sinus. The clots extend into the posterior fossa and, when large, very rapidly result in lethal compression of the brain stem.[25,26,28,32-35] (Massive infratentorial hemorrhage from a rupture of the vein of Galen also may occur without visible tear of the tentorium.)

Lesser degrees of tentorial injury, with the advent of modern brain imaging techniques, are recognized

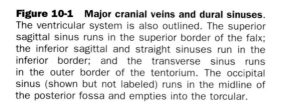

Figure 10-1 **Major cranial veins and dural sinuses.** The ventricular system is also outlined. The superior sagittal sinus runs in the superior border of the falx; the inferior sagittal and straight sinuses run in the inferior border; and the transverse sinus runs in the outer border of the tentorium. The occipital sinus (shown but not labeled) runs in the midline of the posterior fossa and empties into the torcular.

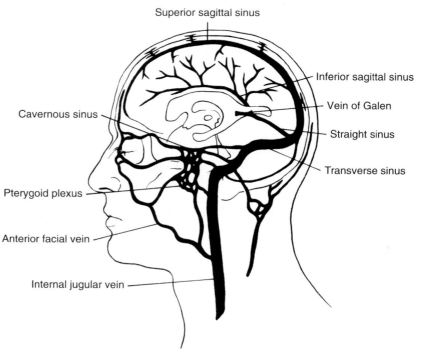

TABLE 10-6   **Spectrum of Tentorial Hemorrhage***
Anterior Extension Excrescence (on free edge of tentorium) Velum interpositum Intraventricular Subarachnoid
Superior Extension Supratentorial subdural Cerebral parenchymal hemorrhage[†]
Inferior Extension Infratentorial (posterior fossa) subdural Cerebellar parenchymal hemorrhage[†]

*See text for references.
[†]Often associated hemorrhage rather than true extension.

now to be more common than the major lethal lacerations just described and probably are much more common than previously suspected. Thus, several series (with a cumulative total of >200 newborns) documented a spectrum of intracranial hemorrhage, primarily subdural, associated with apparent or presumed tentorial injury.[25,27-31,36-44a] This spectrum, summarized in Table 10-6, includes both *infratentorial* (usually retrocerebellar) subdural hemorrhage, secondary to inferior extension, and *supratentorial* subdural hemorrhage, secondary to superior extension (Fig. 10-2). (The infratentorial, posterior fossa subdural hemorrhages may relate also to tear of cerebellar bridging veins, with or without accompanying overt tears of the tentorium.) In addition to infratentorial or supratentorial extension, the hemorrhage of a tentorial tear may remain *confined to the free edge of the tentorium*, most often near the junction of the tentorium and falx, or it may extend *anteriorly* further into the subarachnoid space, velum interpositum, or ventricular system (see Table 10-6). Very minor varieties of this spectrum may account for the relatively high RBC counts in CSF in "normal" newborns (see earlier discussion).

Occipital Osteodiastasis. A prominent traumatic lesion in some infants who die after breech delivery is occipital diastasis with posterior fossa subdural hemorrhage and laceration of the cerebellum (see Table 10-5 and Chapter 22).[41,45,46] The diastasis lesion consists of traumatic separation of the cartilaginous joint between

the squamous and lateral portions of the occipital bone.[45,47] In its most severe form, the dura and occipital sinuses are torn, resulting in massive subdural hemorrhage in the posterior fossa and cerebellar laceration. The bony lesion may be more common than has generally been recognized because it is missed easily at postmortem examination.

Falx Laceration. Laceration of the falx alone is distinctly less common than laceration of the tentorium and usually occurs at a point near the junction of the falx with the tentorium. The source of bleeding is usually the inferior sagittal sinus, and the clot is located in the longitudinal cerebral fissure over the corpus callosum (see Table 10-5).

Superficial Cerebral Vein Rupture. Rupture of the bridging, superficial cerebral veins results in hemorrhage over the cerebral convexity, the well-known convexity subdural hematoma (see Table 10-5). The hematoma is usually more extensive over the lateral aspect of the convexity than near the superior sagittal sinus. Although convexity subdural hemorrhage is usually unilateral, bilateral lesions are not uncommon.[39,40,43,48-50] Subarachnoid blood is a typical accompaniment. Convexity subdural hemorrhage is not a rare event, and, indeed, in small amounts, it is a frequent incidental finding at autopsy of the term infant.[35] The trauma that leads to the hemorrhage may result also in *cerebral contusion*, which, in fact, may dominate the clinical picture.

Pathogenesis

Subdural hemorrhage in the neonatal period is most commonly a traumatic lesion, *when the lesion is large*.[25-31,33,38-41,49,51] Most cases have involved full-term infants. However, as the incidence of grossly traumatic deliveries and of subdural hemorrhages has decreased, the relative proportion of premature infants with subdural hemorrhage has increased. Indeed, in some surveys, the proportion of cases in premature and full-term infants has been approximately similar.[45,52] However, most modern reports still indicate a predominance of full-term infants, especially with cerebral convexity subdural hemorrhages.[27-31,38,40,41,53,54]

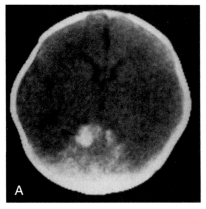 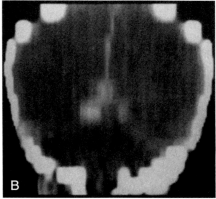

Figure 10-2   Tentorial subdural hemorrhage at the junction of the falx and tentorium. A, Computed tomography (CT) scan along the free margin of tentorium, demonstrating blood accumulated in the quadrigeminal areas and at the free edge of the tentorium (*arrowhead*). **B,** Coronal CT scan, reconstruction view, disclosing the hemorrhage located at the falcotentorial junction. *(From Huang CC, Shen EY: Tentorial subdural hemorrhage in term newborns: Ultrasonographic diagnosis and clinical correlates, Pediatr Neurol 7:171-177, 1991.)*

TABLE 10-7	Pathogenesis of Neonatal Subdural Hemorrhage
At Risk	**Predisposing Factors**
Mother	Primiparous
	Older multiparous
	Small birth canal
Infant	Large full term
	Premature
Labor	Precipitous
	Prolonged
Delivery	Breech extraction
	Foot, face, brow presentation
	Difficult forceps or vacuum extraction
	Difficult rotation

The pathogenesis of *major* neonatal subdural hemorrhage is best considered in terms of predisposing factors referable to the mother, the infant, the duration and progression of labor, and the manner of delivery (Table 10-7). Thus, large subdural hemorrhage is most likely to occur under the following circumstances (1) when the infant is relatively large and the birth canal is relatively small; (2) when the skull is unusually compliant, as in a premature infant; (3) when the pelvic structures are unusually rigid, as in a primiparous or an older multiparous mother; (4) when the duration of labor is either unusually brief, not allowing enough time for dilation of the pelvic structures, or unusually long, subjecting the head to prolonged compression and molding; (5) when the head must pass through a birth canal not gradually adapted to it, as in foot or breech presentation; (6) when the head is subjected to unusual deforming stresses, such as in face or brow presentation; or (7) when the delivery requires difficult vacuum extraction or challenging forceps or rotational maneuvers.

Under the circumstances just described, excessive vertical molding and frontal-occipital elongation or oblique expansion of the head occur (Fig. 10-3). These effects result in stretching of both the falx and one or both leaves of the tentorium, with a tendency for tearing of the tentorium, particularly near its junction with the falx, or, less commonly, tearing of the falx itself. Even if a laceration does not occur, the sinuses into which the vein of Galen drains are stretched, and the result may be a tear of the vein of Galen or its immediate tributaries. Similarly, rupture of cerebellar bridging veins may occur in this context. Tear of the falx occurs particularly with *extreme* frontal-occipital elongation, especially that associated with face or brow presentation. Extreme vertical molding appears to underlie many tears of superficial cerebral veins and the formation of convexity subdural hematoma. In the special case of occipital osteodiastasis with breech delivery, the injury results from suboccipital pressure, which most commonly occurs if the fetus is forcibly hyperextended with the head trapped beneath the symphysis.[41,45] The lower edge of the squamous portion of the occipital bone is displaced in a forward direction, thus lacerating dura, occipital sinus, or cerebellum. (A roughly analogous situation in the supratentorial compartment probably occurs with difficult forceps extractions, which may result in skull fracture, convexity subdural hemorrhage, and cerebral contusion by direct compressive effects.)

Fortunately, many of the aforementioned pathogenetic factors have been eliminated by vastly improved obstetrical practices in most medical centers. Indeed, subdural hemorrhage is by no means invariably a traumatic lesion. For example, coagulation disturbances (e.g., maternal aspirin ingestion, early vitamin K deficiency secondary to maternal phenobarbital administration) may play at least a contributing role in some infants.[40,41,55,56] Moreover, with the advent of intrauterine brain imaging, subdural hematoma has been identified in the fetus before intrapartum events could be responsible.[56-60] In one report, maternal abuse

Figure 10-3 The likely mechanism of tentorial hemorrhage after vacuum extraction. A, The vein of Galen joins the straight sinus and tributaries from the deep venous system at the tentorial notch. **B,** Traction in the occipital-frontal direction produces stress on the vertical axis of the falx and tentorium with kinking of the deep venous system. Engorgement and venous rupture lead to hemorrhage into the surrounding subdural space. *(From Hanigan WC, Morgan AM, Stahlberg LK, Hiller JL: Tentorial hemorrhage associated with vacuum extraction, Pediatrics 85:534-539, 1990.)*

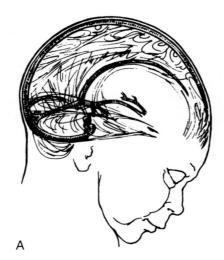

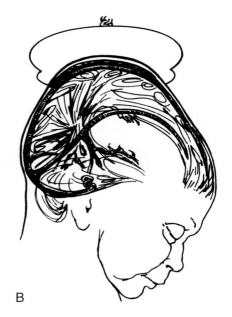

A   B

with blunt abdominal trauma was documented in an infant with bilateral subdural hematomas identified in the first day of life.[49] In other intrauterine cases, other forms of external abdominal pressure or coagulopathy have been important.[56] Moreover, in the largest single series of neonatal subdural hemorrhage (n = 48), 31% of cases had "simple spontaneous" vaginal delivery.[29] Indeed, in one prospective MRI study of 111 asymptomatic term infants, 9 (8%) infants had subdural hemorrhage, and only 5 of these had a complicated vaginal delivery (failed vacuum extraction followed by forceps delivery).[44] In a later study, utilizing 3.0 T-MRI, 15 of 65 (23%) vaginally delivered asymptomatic term infants exhibited small posterior fossa subdural hemorrhages.[44a] At any rate, on modern obstetrical services, subdural hemorrhage of any sort is a very uncommon occurrence. Indeed, considered together, subdural hemorrhages are by far the least common of the major varieties of neonatal intracranial hemorrhages.

Clinical Features

In contrast to the considerable amount of medical writings relative to the neuropathological and radiological aspects of subdural hemorrhage, surprisingly few clinical neurological data are available. However, some important conclusions can be drawn from our own observations and from those recorded by other investigators.[25-32,37,39-41,43,46,54,61-74]

Tentorial Laceration, Occipital Diastasis, and Syndromes Associated with Posterior Fossa Subdural Hematoma

Rapidly Lethal Syndromes. Tentorial laceration with *massive* infratentorial hemorrhage is associated with neurological disturbance from the time of birth. The majority of the most severely affected infants weigh more than 4000 g at birth.[27,33] Initially, the baby demonstrates signs of midbrain-upper pons compression (i.e., stupor or coma, skew deviation of eyes with lateral deviation that is not altered by doll's eyes maneuver, and unequal pupils, with some disturbance of response to light). With such infratentorial hemorrhage, nuchal rigidity with retrocollis or opisthotonos may also be a helpful early sign.[28,61] When these features are associated with bradycardia,[25] a large infratentorial clot with brain stem compression should be suspected. Over minutes to hours, as the clot becomes larger, stupor progresses to coma, pupils may become fixed and dilated, and signs of lower brain stem compression appear. Ocular bobbing and ataxic respirations may occur, and finally, respiratory arrest ensues.

The severe clinical syndrome associated with *occipital osteodiastasis* resembles that described for major tentorial laceration. With occipital osteodiastasis, delivery is characteristically breech. A depressed Apgar score at 1 minute is common, and the course is one of rapid deterioration. In the six infants described by Wigglesworth and Husemeyer,[45] the age at the time of death ranged from 7 to 45 hours.

Less Malignant Syndromes Associated with Posterior Fossa Subdural Hematoma. Less severe clinical syndromes accompany most examples of *posterior fossa subdural hematoma* currently encountered on obstetrical and neonatal services.[27-30,37,40,41,43,54,74] These syndromes appear to result from smaller tears of the tentorium than those just noted, from rupture of bridging veins from superior cerebellum without tentorial tear, or, perhaps, from lesser degrees of occipital diastasis. The clinical syndrome consists of three phases. First, no neurological signs are apparent for a period that varies from several hours after birth (usually a difficult vacuum, forceps, or breech extraction or both) to as much as 3 or 4 days of age. Most commonly, the interval is less than 24 hours. Presumably, this period is associated with slow enlargement of the hematoma. Second, various signs develop referable to increased intracranial pressure (e.g., full fontanelle, irritability, "lethargy"). Most of these signs appear to relate to the evolution of hydrocephalus secondary to a block of CSF flow in the posterior fossa. Third, signs referable to disturbance of brain stem develop, including respiratory abnormalities, apnea, bradycardia, oculomotor abnormalities, skew deviation of eyes, and facial paresis. These deficits relate to direct compressive effects of the posterior fossa hematoma. In addition to brain stem signs, seizures occur in the majority of infants, perhaps because of accompanying subarachnoid blood. In infants who clearly worsen over hours or a day or more, as do approximately one half, lethal brain stem compression may develop.

In more recent years, *particularly small* posterior fossa subdural hemorrhages have been identified by CT or MRI. In one carefully studied series of 26 small subdural hemorrhages detected by CT, 19 were infratentorial, and the leading clinical features were respiratory abnormalities (apnea, "dusky episodes") in approximately 60% and neurological features (subtle seizures, hypotonia) in approximately 40%.[43] None of the infants developed progressive neurological signs.

Falx Laceration

No careful description of the clinical course of falx tears with major subdural hemorrhage is available. However, it is likely that initially bilateral cerebral signs will appear, in view of the locus of the hematoma. However, striking neurological findings probably do not develop until the clot has extended infratentorially, and the resulting syndrome is then similar to that described for tentorial laceration and posterior fossa subdural hematoma.

Cerebral Convexity Subdural Hemorrhage

Subdural hemorrhage over the cerebral convexities is associated with at least three neurological syndromes (Table 10-8). First, and probably most commonly, minor degrees of hemorrhage occur, and *minimal or no clinical signs* are apparent. Irritability, a "hyperalert" appearance, unexplained apneic episodes, or no signs have been noted.[25,43,44]

Second, *signs of focal cerebral disturbance* may occur, with the most common time of onset being the

TABLE 10-8	Neurological Syndromes Associated with Cerebral Convexity Subdural Hemorrhage

Minimal or no clinical signs
Focal cerebral syndrome: hemiparesis, deviation of eyes to side of lesion, focal seizures, homolateral pupillary abnormality
Chronic subdural effusion

second or third day of life. With this syndrome, seizures, often focal, are common and are frequently accompanied by other focal cerebral signs (e.g., hemiparesis, deviation of eyes to the side contralateral to the hemiparesis, although the eyes move by doll's eyes maneuver, because this is a cerebral lesion). These focal cerebral signs are definite, *although usually not striking*. The most distinctive neurological sign with major convexity subdural hemorrhage is dysfunction of the third cranial nerve on the side of the hematoma; this dysfunction is usually manifested by a nonreactive or poorly reactive, dilated pupil.[25,69-72] The latter occurs secondary to compression of the third nerve by herniation of the temporal lobe through the tentorial notch. An excellent example of such a neurological syndrome associated with subdural hematoma was a newborn with hemophilia whom we studied.[72]

A third clinical presentation may be the occurrence of subdural hemorrhage in the neonatal period with few clinical signs and then the development over the next several months of a *chronic subdural effusion*. It is certainly well known that many infants presenting in the first 6 months of life with an enlarging head, increased transillumination, and chronic subdural effusions have no known cause for the lesion and that subdural hemorrhage can evolve into subdural effusion.[75-77]

Diagnosis

The diagnosis of major neonatal subdural hemorrhage depends principally on recognition of the clinical syndrome, with subsequent definitive demonstration by a brain imaging study.

Clinical Syndromes

The clinical syndromes previously reviewed are often sufficiently distinctive to raise the suspicion of subdural hemorrhage, as well as the specific variety thereof. Neurological signs primarily referable to the brain stem should suggest infratentorial hematoma. Neurological signs primarily referable to the cerebrum should suggest convexity subdural hematoma. These signs should provoke more definitive and prompt diagnostic studies because the clinical course may deteriorate very rapidly. Lumbar puncture is *not* a good choice for diagnostic study in this setting because of the possibility of provoking herniation, either of cerebellar tonsils into the foramen magnum in the presence of a posterior fossa subdural hematoma or of temporal lobe into the tentorial notch in the presence of a large unilateral convexity subdural hematoma.

Computed Tomography, Magnetic Resonance Imaging, and Ultrasound Scans

CT is a safe, definitive means of demonstrating the site and extent of neonatal subdural hemorrhage. Examples of the CT demonstration of the varieties of subdural hemorrhage just discussed are shown in Figures 10-2, 10-4, and 10-5.

MRI is more effective than CT in the delineation of posterior fossa subdural hemorrhage (Fig. 10-6).[31, 40,78-80] This particular superiority of MRI in evaluation of posterior fossa hemorrhage applies to other types of lesions in this location (see Chapter 4).

Detection of subdural hematoma by *ultrasound scanning* (Fig. 10-7), although reported, generally is difficult.[28,49,81] Moreover, even when these hematomas

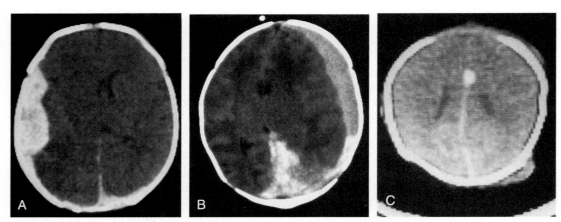

Figure 10-4   Subdural hemorrhage, computed tomography scans. **A**, Convexity subdural hematoma in a newborn with severe hemophilia A. Note the area of increased attenuation on the right, representing the hematoma, and the shift of ventricles to the left. **B**, Convexity subdural hematoma on the left in a 1-day-old infant delivered by forceps for head entrapment. The pupil was dilated on the side of the lesion. Note also deviation of midline structures to the right, and probable tentorial tear, with associated hemorrhage. **C**, Probable falx tear in a newborn of 4780 g delivered by a difficult breech extraction. Note the small circular area of increased attenuation in the midline, representing hemorrhage in the inferior margin of the falx.

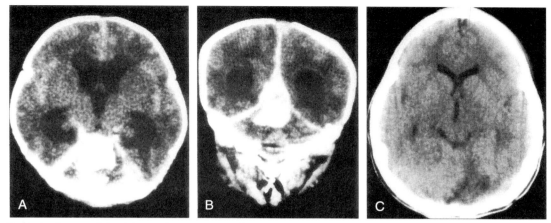

Figure 10-5 **Posterior fossa subdural hemorrhage, computed tomography scans**. In the first 24 hours of life, the infant exhibited apnea, bradycardia, and quadriplegia. **A**, Axial and, **B**, coronal scans show the hemorrhage and obstructive hydrocephalus. **C**, The scan performed 1 year after surgery in the neonatal period shows a small defect in the left cerebellum and normal supratentorial structures. *(From Perrin RG, Rutka JT, Drake JM, Meltzer H, et al: Management and outcomes of posterior fossa subdural hematomas in neonates, Neurosurgery 40:1190-1199, 1997.)*

are detected, the extent and distribution of supratentorial lesions are usually demonstrated far better by CT or MRI and of infratentorial lesions by MRI. The major difficulty of ultrasound scanning in this setting relates to acoustical interference by bone at the margins of the anterior fontanelle and to near-field transducer artifacts.

Skull Radiographs

Occipital osteodiastasis may be demonstrated by skull radiographs. The lateral view shows the lesion (Fig. 10-8).

Prognosis

Infants with major *lacerations of the tentorium and falx* and massive degrees of subdural hemorrhage have a very poor prognosis. Nearly all die; the rare survivor is left with hydrocephalus secondary to obstruction of CSF flow at the tentorial notch or over the convexities. Similarly, severe *occipital diastasis* and its complications have been associated with a poor outcome. Nevertheless, it is possible that early diagnosis could lead to beneficial intervention.

Although they are often serious lesions, *moderate posterior fossa subdural hematomas*, recognized frequently in recent years, primarily by CT and MRI, are

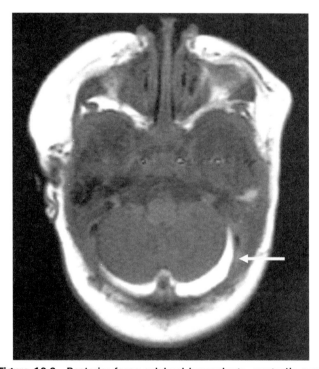

Figure 10-6 **Posterior fossa subdural hemorrhage, magnetic resonance imaging (MRI) scan**. MRI was performed on the tenth postnatal day of an infant born after a complicated breech delivery. Note the increased signal indicative of blood over the cerebellar hemisphere (*arrow*). *(Courtesy of Dr. Omar Khwaja.)*

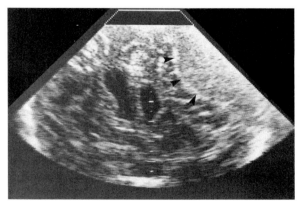

Figure 10-7 **Subdural hemorrhage**. Ultrasound scan of a full-term infant transferred 10 days after traumatic delivery. The coronal scan shows the subdural hemorrhage on the left (margin outlined by *arrowheads*), displacing the ventricles to the right. The subdural lesion was isodense with brain on a computed tomography scan. *(Courtesy of Dr. Gary D. Shackelford.)*

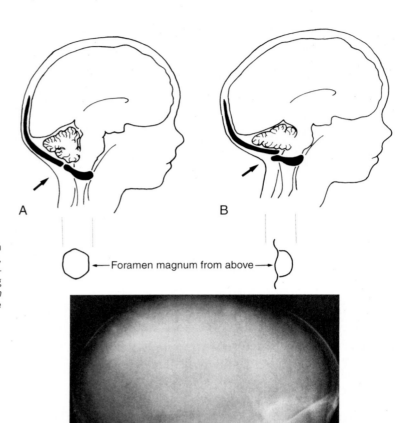

Figure 10-8 Occipital osteodiastasis. Schematic diagram of the cranium, illustrating, **A**, the normal state *(arrow)* and, **B**, occipital osteodiastasis, with posterior fossa encroachment *(arrow)*. **C**, Lateral radiograph of the skull demonstrating occipital osteodiastasis in an autopsy case *(arrow). (From Pape KE, Wigglesworth JS:* Hemorrhage, Ischemia, and the Perinatal Brain. *Philadelphia: 1979, JB Lippincott.)*

associated with an outcome that is variable but dependent on size, rapidity of diagnosis and, when necessary, intervention (Table 10-9).[28-30,37,40,41,54,74] Thus, of 30 surgically treated infants, 80% either were normal or exhibited minor neurological deficits on follow-up. Approximately 15% of surgically treated patients developed communicating hydrocephalus that required shunt placement. Of 40 nonsurgically treated infants, nearly 90% had a favorable outcome (see Table 10-9). In earlier reports, as many as 40% to 50% of infants who did not undergo operations died, probably because of rapidly progressive lesions, the gravity of which escaped prompt detection. The *small* posterior fossa subdural hemorrhages described in hospital-based series are associated with no major sequelae or death.[44,82]

The prognosis of patients with moderate or large *convexity subdural hemorrhage* is relatively good; from 50% to 90% of affected infants are well on follow-up.[29,39-41,71,83] The remainder are left with focal cerebral signs and, occasionally, hydrocephalus. The deficits appear to relate to associated parenchymal lesions. The small convexity subdural hemorrhages detected by widespread imaging in recent years have a generally favorable outcome.[44,82]

Management

Tentorial and Falx Lacerations, Occipital Osteodiastasis, and Posterior Fossa Subdural Hematoma

The severity of the initial trauma and the rapid progression to brain stem compromise have rendered effective treatment nearly impossible in *major* tears of the

TABLE 10-9	Outcome with Posterior Fossa Subdural Hemorrhage*		
	OUTCOME		
Surgical Evacuation (n = 70)	Good to Excellent	Major Sequelae	Deaths
Yes (30)	80%	13%	7%
No (40)	88%	7%	5%

*See text for references; also includes personal cases. Lesions have been of moderate or large size.

tentorium and falx and in overt occipital osteodiastasis with *severe* subdural hemorrhage. Theoretically, rapid surgical evacuation may provide some hope for salvage of the affected baby. Some support for this suggestion is obtained by the experience just reviewed with less severe posterior fossa subdural hematomas (see Table 10-9). Rapid detection and prompt surgical evacuation in the presence of progression of neurological signs have been of value in management of these lesions. However, a normal outcome has been documented in posterior fossa subdural hematoma *without* surgical intervention (see Table 10-9); I have observed several such cases. Thus, *close surveillance alone* is appropriate *in the absence of* major neurological signs, particularly brain stem signs, or worsening neurological status. Surgery should not be delayed if clear neurological deterioration becomes apparent. With small lesions, close surveillance is almost always followed by a favorable outcome.

Cerebral Convexity Subdural Hematoma

Effective management of the infant with an acute convexity subdural hematoma requires careful sequential clinical observation. Surgery is not mandatory if the infant is stable neurologically.[29] The need for surgery is based on large size of the lesion, signs of increased intracranial pressure, and neurological deficits, particularly if findings suggest incipient transtentorial herniation. If a stable subdural hemorrhage evolves to subdural effusion, subdural taps can be used to reduce signs of increased intracranial pressure and to prevent the development of craniocerebral disproportion, the latter serving only to perpetuate subdural bleeding.[76] Repeated subdural taps should not be performed if the infant is asymptomatic and if the head is not growing rapidly. The development of constricting "subdural membranes" was overestimated in the past. Surgery is necessary if subdural taps are not effective in controlling the two complications just discussed. The smaller convexity subdural hemorrhages detected by imaging in recent years rarely require intervention.

PRIMARY SUBARACHNOID HEMORRHAGE

Primary subarachnoid hemorrhage refers to hemorrhage within the subarachnoid space that is not secondary to extension from subdural, intraventricular, or cerebellar hemorrhage. Moreover, also excluded from this category are cases in which subarachnoid blood is secondary to extension from intracerebral hematoma, a structural vascular lesion (e.g., aneurysm or arteriovenous malformation), tumor, hemorrhagic infarction, or major coagulation disturbance (see later discussion of miscellaneous causes of intracranial hemorrhage). Primary subarachnoid hemorrhage, defined in this way, is a very frequent variety of neonatal intracranial hemorrhage, mostly because the category includes the many newborn infants, particularly premature infants, with a few hundred RBCs per cubic millimeter in the CSF. The frequency of *clinically significant* primary subarachnoid hemorrhage was overestimated in the past, particularly in the premature infant but also in

the full-term infant, mostly because of the lack of brain imaging data to identify intraventricular hemorrhage. As reviewed in Table 10-2, in our own series of infants weighing less than 2000 g with grossly bloody CSF, only 29% exhibited subarachnoid hemorrhage alone, and 63% exhibited intraventricular hemorrhage (although with blood also in the subarachnoid space). Moreover, even many term infants with bloody CSF who, in the past, would have been considered to have primary subarachnoid hemorrhage on clinical grounds, have been shown by ultrasound, CT, or MRI scans to have intraventricular hemorrhage (see later section). Finally, a localized variant of subarachnoid hemorrhage, involving the subpial space and superficial cerebral cortex, should also be recognized in this context; this lesion often occurs with subarachnoid hemorrhage and on brain imaging may be difficult to distinguish from typical primary subarachnoid hemorrhage (see later).

Neuropathology

Blood is usually located most prominently in the pia-arachnoid space over the cerebral convexities, especially posteriorly, and in the posterior fossa.[52,84] Small amounts of subarachnoid blood are found not infrequently at postmortem examinations of newborns not suspected clinically of having sustained intracranial hemorrhage.[35] Less commonly, large amounts of blood are observed. The source of the bleeding in primary subarachnoid hemorrhage is presumed to be small vascular channels derived from the involuting anastomoses between leptomeningeal arteries present during brain development.[85] Origin from bridging veins within the subarachnoid space is also possible.[46] At any rate, primary subarachnoid hemorrhage in newborn patients is unlike the dramatic large vessel, arterial hemorrhage in older patients.

Neuropathological complications of neonatal primary subarachnoid hemorrhage are very unusual. Even in major degrees of hemorrhage, significantly increased intracranial pressure with brain stem compression is rare. The only significant, albeit very uncommon, sequela clearly related to the hemorrhage is hydrocephalus. The latter is secondary either to adhesions around the outflow of the fourth ventricle or around the tentorial notch, which result in obstruction to CSF flow, or to adhesions over the cerebral convexities, which result in impaired CSF flow or absorption.

The *variant of subarachnoid hemorrhage* noted earlier involves localized bleeding in the *subpial* region, with involvement of the most superficial aspect of cerebral cortex.[74,86,87] Although this hemorrhage often occurs together with subarachnoid hemorrhage, in subpial hemorrhage, the blood is found beneath the pia and is contiguous with bleeding in the most superficial, largely glial-populated region of cerebral cortex. The usual location for this type of hemorrhage is in the region of the anterior temporal lobe, near the pterion, (a point at the junction of the coronal, squamous, sphenosquamous, and sphenofrontal sutures) or in localized cerebral regions beneath cranial sutures.

Pathogenesis

The pathogenesis of neonatal primary subarachnoid hemorrhage is not entirely understood, but most of the *major* hemorrhages appear to relate, on clinical grounds, to trauma or to circulatory events related to prematurity. The relationships of trauma to the genesis of major subarachnoid hemorrhage are similar in many respects to those described earlier for subdural hemorrhage. The relationships to prematurity are similar to those described in Chapter 11 for germinal matrix–intraventricular hemorrhage of the premature infant. Common to both pathogenetic themes is the substrate of maturation-dependent involution of leptomeningeal anastomotic channels.[85] The pathogenesis of the common smaller subarachnoid hemorrhages is unclear, because most of these hemorrhages occur without any apparent traumatic or circulatory abnormality.

The interesting *subpial hemorrhages* may relate to local trauma with resulting disruption of small veins because the lesions occur at sites in proximity to cranial sutures and to likely movement of bone during normal delivery.[87] Thus, in one series of seven cases, four occurred in proximity to the pterion, and the remainder occurred beneath the coronal or squamosal sutures.[87]

Clinical Features

Three major syndromes with primary subarachnoid hemorrhage can be distinguished (Table 10-10). First, and *undoubtedly most commonly*, minor degrees of hemorrhage occur, and minimal or no signs develop. Second, primary subarachnoid hemorrhage can result in *seizures*, especially in full-term infants (see Chapter 5). The seizures usually have their onset on the second postnatal day. In the interictal period, these babies usually appear remarkably well, and the description "well baby with seizures" often seems appropriate. In the subpial variant, the seizures often are focal, reflecting the localized nature of these lesions.

A third and quite rare syndrome is massive subarachnoid hemorrhage with *catastrophic deterioration* and a rapidly fatal course. The infants usually have sustained severe perinatal asphyxia, sometimes with an element of trauma at the time of birth.[25,33] The neurological syndrome is similar to the catastrophic deterioration described in Chapter 11 for some patients with intraventricular hemorrhage.

Diagnosis

The diagnosis of primary subarachnoid hemorrhage is made usually by CT or MRI. On CT, distinction from

TABLE 10-10	**Neurological Syndromes Associated with Primary Subarachnoid Hemorrhage**

Minimal or no clinical signs
Seizures in full-term infant; considered "well" during interictal period
Catastrophic deterioration

the normal, slightly increased attenuation in the region of the falx and major venous sinuses in the newborn may be difficult. Sometimes, the possibility of primary subarachnoid hemorrhage is raised initially by the findings of an elevated number of RBCs and an elevated protein content in the CSF, usually obtained for another purpose (e.g., to rule out meningitis). Exclusion of another cause of blood in the subarachnoid space (e.g., extension from subdural, cerebellar, or intraventricular hemorrhage) or from certain unusual sources (e.g., tumor, vascular lesions) is made best by CT or MRI. The localized subpial hemorrhages, often with superficial cortical hemorrhage, are observable both by CT or MRI (Fig. 10-9).

Ultrasonography is relatively insensitive in detecting subarachnoid hemorrhage per se because of the normal increase in echogenicity around the periphery of the brain.[88] A large subarachnoid hemorrhage occasionally distends the sylvian fissure and thus becomes detectable, but care must be taken not to confuse a sylvian fissure distended with blood from the wide fissure seen consistently in premature infants and resulting from the normal separation of the frontal operculum and superior temporal region until late in gestation.

Prognosis

In general, the prognosis for infants with primary subarachnoid hemorrhage without serious traumatic or hypoxic injury is good. The specific outcome correlates reliably with the neonatal clinical syndrome. Thus, the many infants with minimal signs in the neonatal period and documentation of subarachnoid blood do well virtually uniformly. Those few full-term infants with seizures as the primary manifestation of the hemorrhage are normal on follow-up in at least 90% of cases (see Chapter 5). The rare patient with a catastrophic course with massive subarachnoid hemorrhage of unknown origin either suffers serious neurological residua or dies. The principal sequela, albeit unusual, after major subarachnoid hemorrhage is hydrocephalus.

Management

The management is essentially that of posthemorrhagic hydrocephalus and is discussed in detail in Chapter 11 in relation to intraventricular hemorrhage of the premature infant.

CEREBELLAR HEMORRHAGE

Cerebellar hemorrhage has been observed in approximately 5% to 10% of autopsy cases in series of neonatal intensive care unit populations.[84,89] The hemorrhage is more common among premature than term infants; in four neuropathological series, the incidence among premature infants less than 32 weeks of gestation or less than 1500 g birth weight, or both, ranged from 15% to 25%.[90-94] In contrast to these neuropathological reports, some large studies of living premature infants by CT did not demonstrate cerebellar hemorrhage.[95,96]

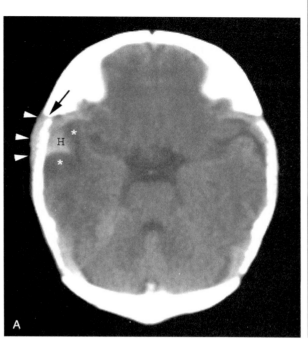 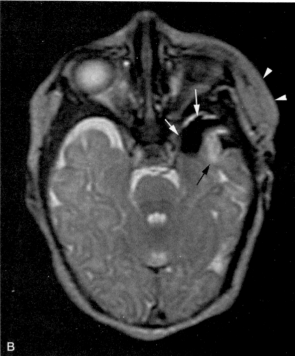

Figure 10-9   Subpial hemorrhage. A, Computed tomography scan performed on the first postnatal day in a term infant with apnea at 8 hours of life; note the hemorrhage (H), which tracks the subpial space and adjacent low-attenuation edema *(asterisks)*. Note also the pterion *(arrow)* and associated soft-tissue swelling *(arrowheads)*. **B,** T2-weighted magnetic resonance imaging scan, performed on the second postnatal day in an infant with apnea and seizures at 24 hours of life, shows subpial hemorrhage *(white arrows)*, which is of low signal in the acute period, in the region of the anterior temporal lobe, near the pterion (see text), a site of predilection for this type of hemorrhage. Parenchymal edema *(black arrow)* and soft tissue swelling *(white arrowheads)* are also apparent. *(From Huang AH, Robertson RL: Spontaneous superficial parenchymal and leptomeningeal hemorrhage in term neonates, AJNR Am J Neuroradiol 25:469-475, 2004.)*

The reason for the discrepancy may not relate simply to differences between dead and living populations. Flodmark and co-workers[94] observed 15 cases of cerebellar hemorrhage at autopsy, all in premature infants, from 79 infants studied by CT for perinatal asphyxia. Among these 15 autopsy-proven cases the hemorrhage was identified by CT in only one. (Ten of the lesions were considered to be "probably below the resolving power of the CT scanner.") Similarly, in infants evaluated by ultrasonography through the anterior fontanelle, the identification of cerebellar hemorrhage is very unusual.[97,98] The advent of imaging through the mastoid fontanelle, the thinnest region of the temporal bone at the junction of the squamosal, lambdoidal, and occipital sutures, has greatly facilitated accurate imaging of the posterior fossa in the newborn.[79,97,99,100] A recent report, based on use of this "mastoid window" in evaluation of 1242 infants weighing less than 1500 g, showed an overall incidence of cerebellar hemorrhage of approximately 3% (Table 10-11).[100] However, the incidence varied markedly as a function of birth weight. *Infants of less than 750 g of birth weight had the highest incidence (i.e., 8.7% overall, and notably, 17% in the last 2 years of the 5-year study).* Infants between 750 and 1499 g exhibited incidences of approximately 2.7%. Indeed, in this large cohort, nearly 60% of all cerebellar hemorrhages were in the infants who weighed less

than 750 g. Thus, cerebellar hemorrhage is particularly a lesion of the most immature infants.

Neuropathology

Four major categories of lesions have been described in infants with cerebellar hemorrhage (Table 10-12). Three categories (primary cerebellar hemorrhage, venous infarction, and extension of intraventricular or subarachnoid hemorrhage *into* cerebellum) probably account for most cases of cerebellar hemorrhage of the *premature* infant. Distinction of hemorrhagic venous infarction from primary cerebellar hemorrhage is very

TABLE 10-11   Incidence of Cerebellar Hemorrhage in Premature Infants

Birthweight	Incidence*
<750 g	20/230 (8.7%)†
750–999 g	4/602 (0.7%)
1000–1499 g	11/410 (2.7%)
Total	35/1242 (2.8%)

*Incidence is expressed as n/N (%).
†Incidence in the last 2 years of the 5-year study period was 17%.
Data from Limperopoulos C, Benson CB, Bassan H, Di Salvo DN, et al: Cerebellar hemorrhage in the preterm infant: Ultrasonographic findings and risk factors, *Pediatrics* 116:717-724, 2005.

TABLE 10-12	Neuropathology of Neonatal "Cerebellar Hemorrhage"

Primary cerebellar hemorrhage
Venous (hemorrhagic) infarction
Extension into cerebellum of intraventricular or subarachnoid blood or both
Traumatic laceration of cerebellum or rupture of major veins or occipital sinus (with or without occipital diastasis)

difficult, even at microscopic examination, and is not considered further in this context. The notion that extension of blood into the cerebellum is important was raised particularly by the studies of Donat and coworkers.[101] In 10 of their 20 cases of cerebellar hemorrhage, secondary dissection of blood into the cerebellum appeared to occur either from the fourth ventricle into the vermis or, less frequently, from the subarachnoid space into the cerebellar hemispheres. In these cases, massive hemorrhage into the lateral ventricles was the original source of the blood. This notion is supported by previous observations of a strong association of cerebellar hemorrhage with cerebral intraventricular hemorrhage.[92,93] Indeed, in the aforementioned study of 1242 premature infants who were less than 1500 g of birth weight, fully 77% of cases were associated with intraventricular hemorrhage.[100] The fourth category of cerebellar hemorrhage, traumatic injury with laceration of cerebellum or with rupture of cerebellar bridging veins or occipital sinus, often occurring with occipital osteodiastasis, is reviewed earlier (see "Subdural Hemorrhage"). This category is more common among the *term* infants with hemorrhage than among the small premature infants.[40,41]

The loci of the hemorrhages within the cerebellum in the *small premature infant* include both the hemisphere and the vermis. The lesions tend to be focal and localized. Approximately 70% of the lesions are localized to one cerebellar hemisphere, and 20% are localized to the vermis (Table 10-13).[100] Smaller lesions have included both subpial and subependymal locations, which are the sites of the germinal matrices in the external granule cell layer and subependymal zones, respectively. In large lesions, the cerebellar cortex and underlying white matter are destroyed (Fig. 10-10). By contrast with the hemispheric predominance in preterm infants, the cerebellar vermis is the initial site of the lesion in the majority of the *term* infants with cerebellar hemorrhage.

TABLE 10-13	Loci of Cerebellar Hemorrhage by Ultrasonography	
Locus		**Occurrence**
Unilateral hemisphere		71%
Vermis		20%
Both hemispheres and vermis		9%
Isolated*		23%

*No supratentorial hemorrhage.
Data from Limperopoulos C, Benson CB, Bassan H, Di Salvo DN, et al: Cerebellar hemorrhage in the preterm infant: Ultrasonographic findings and risk factors, *Pediatrics* 116:717-724, 2005.

Pathogenesis

The pathogenesis of cerebellar hemorrhage is undoubtedly multifactorial, but particular importance can be attributed to traumatic delivery (breech or forceps extractions, or both) and circulatory events related to prematurity.[54,90-93,100,102-104] In the premature infant, the pathogenesis bears similarities to that of intraventricular hemorrhage (see Chapter 11). In the term infant, the pathogenesis appears to relate principally to traumatic events. The pathogenesis of cerebellar hemorrhage is best considered in terms of intravascular, vascular, and extravascular factors (Table 10-14).

Intravascular Factors

Increased Venous Pressure, Compliant Skull. A potentially important factor, in the premature newborn only somewhat more than the term infant, is the *compliant skull*. External pressure, which causes occipital compression, results in forward movement of the upper part of the squamous portion of the occipital bone under the parietal bones, thus distorting the venous sinuses at the torcular and increasing venous pressure. This phenomenon has been demonstrated radiographically and at postmortem examination.[41,46,105] Moreover, forward movement of the lower portion of the squamous bone, as discussed with occipital diastasis, could distort the occipital sinus and its tributaries with a similar effect on venous pressure. These bony distortions would be expected with breech extractions and difficult forceps extractions. In one series of term infants with cerebellar hemorrhage, such intrapartum events were present in the majority of cases.[104]

The possibility that such phenomena could occur *postnatally* was emphasized in a series of patients with cerebellar hemorrhage who had received positive-pressure ventilation by means of a face mask attached by a band across the occiput.[92] The band caused occipital molding and compression of the type just described to result in distortion and obstruction of major venous sinuses. However, use of the face mask is by no means an essential factor because in most other large series of pathologically proven cerebellar hemorrhage in the premature infant, the lesion did not occur in such a clinical setting.[90,91,93,98,100,101] Nevertheless, occipital

TABLE 10-14	Pathogenesis of Cerebellar Hemorrhage

Intravascular Factors
Increased venous pressure (compliant skull)
Pressure-passive cerebellar circulation/ischemia
Disturbed coagulation

Vascular Factors
Vascular integrity tenuous
Involuting vessels: subependymal and subpial germinal matrices

Extravascular Factors
Direct external effects on cerebellar parenchyma and vessels (compliant skull)
Poor vascular support: subependymal and subpial germinal matrices
Extension from intraventricular hemorrhage

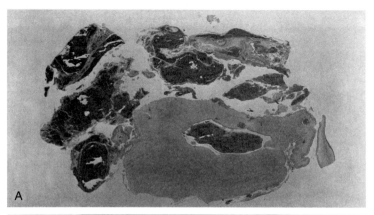

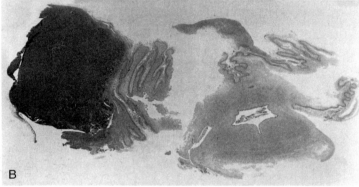

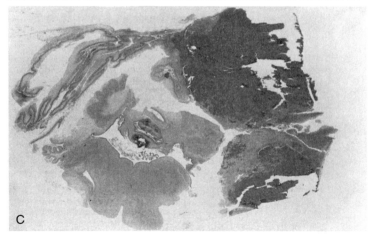

Figure 10-10 Cerebellar hemorrhage in the premature infant; horizontal sections through brain stem and cerebellum. **A**, Hemorrhage involves midline cerebellum and one cerebellar hemisphere. Note also the large amount of blood in the fourth ventricle. **B**, Hemorrhage involves one cerebellar hemisphere, especially the peripheral portion. **C**, Hemorrhage involves the whole cerebellar hemisphere. Note also periventricular hemorrhage in the vermis. (*A, Courtesy of Dr. Margaret L. Grunnet. B and C, From Grunnet ML, Shields WD: Cerebellar hemorrhage in the premature infant, J Pediatr 88:605-608, 1976.*)

compression can occur readily in the small infant by such maneuvers as fixation of the head in the supine position for nursing, bag and mask resuscitation, placement of endotracheal tube, and puncture of scalp vein.[46]

Pressure-Passive Cerebellar Circulation. As discussed in Chapters 6 and 8, the cerebral circulation of the newborn, especially the sick preterm newborn, is pressure passive. If the pressure-passive state of the cerebral circulation also affects the cerebellar circulation, which is likely, then vulnerable capillaries (see vascular factors later) can be exposed to bursts of arterial pressure flow, caused by hypertensive spikes, infusions of colloid, and so forth (see also Chapter 11). Rupture is a potential result. In the most recent large series, several pathogenetic factors potentially

consistent with the occurrence of ischemia included a relation to fetal distress, need for emergency cesarean section, requirement for pressor support, patent ductus arteriosus, and low pH in the early neonatal period (relative to matched controls without cerebellar hemorrhage).[100]

Disturbed Coagulation. Although not common, disturbed coagulation may contribute to pathogenesis. Cerebellar hemorrhage has been described in association with vitamin K deficiency[106] and thrombocytopenia. The latter was present in single cases of cerebellar hemorrhage with methylmalonic acidemia and with propionic acidemia.[107] An infant with cerebellar hemorrhage associated with isovaleric acidemia, a metabolic disorder frequently complicated by thrombocytopenia, had a blood dyscrasia that was not characterized in detail.[108] (Other pathogenetic factors also were present in these patients with organic acidopathies, e.g., infusion of hypertonic solutions, cardiac failure, and cerebellar edema with upward herniation.)

Vascular Factors

Tenuous Vascular Integrity. An intrinsic vulnerability of certain cerebellar capillaries was suggested by Wigglesworth and Husemeyer.[45] Thus, the rich capillary beds of the subpial region and the core of the cerebellar folia are in "a continual process of remodeling," especially in the premature infant. These vessels may be expected to be vulnerable to rupture.

Subependymal and Subpial Germinal Matrix Vessels. Germinal matrices, richly vascularized structures, are present in the cerebellum. In the premature infant, they occur in the subependymal region around the fourth ventricle, and in both the premature and term infant, they are present in the subpial, external granule layer. The latter layer is especially prominent in the premature infant. In the perinatal period, the subependymal region provides glial precursors for migration to cerebellar white matter, and the external granule layer provides neuronal precursors for migration to the internal granule cell layer. These structures and their capillaries are in various stages of involution and, presumably, may be more vulnerable to rupture.

Extravascular Factors

Tear of Cerebellar Parenchyma and Vessels: Compliant Skull. The distortion of vessels discussed earlier concerning the infant's compliant skull could result in rupture by direct effects, rather than or in addition to the effects on venous pressure. Similarly, these compressive forces could cause upward cerebellar herniation, particularly of superior vermis into the tentorial notch, with resulting contusion or laceration. The cerebellar vermis is the usual site of origin of cerebellar hemorrhage in the *term* infant.

Poor Vascular Support: Subependymal and Subpial Germinal Matrix Regions. The subependymal and subpial germinal matrices described earlier are gelatinous regions that provide poor support for the small vessels that course through them. Presumably, this deficiency of extravascular support encourages rupture.

Extension from Intraventricular Hemorrhage. The reasons for the apparent capacity of blood within the fourth ventricle and subarachnoid space of the posterior fossa to dissect into the cerebellum in certain cases are unclear. Moreover, the precise frequency of this cause of "cerebellar" hemorrhage is not known; the 50% frequency suggested by Donat and co-workers[101] is probably too high. In a large recent series, although 77% of cerebellar hemorrhages in premature infants were associated with intraventricular hemorrhage, the hemorrhages were relatively small in about one half of these.[100] Nevertheless, the three factors probably of considerable importance in permitting extension

of blood into the cerebellum in many cases relate to (1) the state of development of the cerebellum (e.g., incomplete myelination of cerebellar white matter and presence of the external granule cell layer), (2) a large quantity of blood associated with the intraventricular hemorrhage, and (3) increased intracranial pressure, especially within the fourth ventricle and subarachnoid space of the posterior fossa.

Clinical Features

The clinical syndrome varies considerably according to the size of the lesion and the gestational age of the infant.* In *term infants*, onset in the first 24 hours has been most common. The neurological syndrome is composed most consistently of signs of brain stem compression, especially apnea or respiratory irregularities, sometimes with bradycardia, and of obstruction to CSF flow, especially full fontanelle, separated sutures, and moderately dilated ventricles on CT or ultrasound scan. Careful examination has also revealed specific additional signs of brain stem disturbance (e.g., skew deviation of eyes, facial paresis, intermittent tonic extension of limbs, opisthotonos, and degrees of quadriparesis).[102-104,110]

The fastest progression of signs has occurred *with large lesions in small premature infants* who soon died, most within 36 hours of onset of deterioration.[90-93] However, in recent years, with detection of the many *smaller lesions in premature infants*, clinical signs referable to the brain stem are subtle or nonexistent.

Diagnosis

The essential issue in recognition of cerebellar hemorrhage is a high index of suspicion. Clinical signs referable to brain stem dysfunction or increased intracranial pressure or both (see "Clinical Features") should provoke careful *ultrasound scan* through the mastoid window. With this approach, the lesions are readily detected (Figs. 10-11 to 10-15).[79,97,100,109,110,112] The cerebellum, especially the vermis, is normally quite echogenic; careful attention to any lack of symmetry in echogenicity is important in diagnosis of the hemorrhage. (Posterior fossa subdural hemorrhage may be difficult to distinguish from intrinsic cerebellar hemorrhage by ultrasound scan,[113] although multiple parasagittal views or imaging through the posterior fontanelle is useful.)

CT and MRI scans are necessary to define the extent and distribution of the lesion most decisively (Fig. 10-16). MRI is especially valuable for assessment of the anatomy of both the posterior fossa and the supratentorial structures.

---

*See references 40,41,54,90,93,98,100,102,103,109-111.

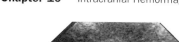

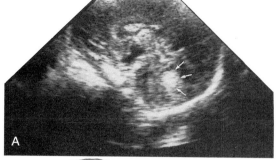

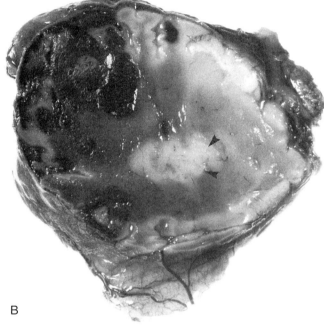

Figure 10-11 **Cerebellar hemorrhage. A,** Ultrasound scan of cerebellar hemorrhage from an infant weighing 1040 g who exhibited clinical deterioration on day 12. Parasagittal scan shows echodense, circular lesion in cerebellar hemisphere *(arrows).* **B,** At postmortem examination, a large cerebellar hemorrhage was observed. *Arrowheads* mark the dentate nucleus.

Prognosis

The outcome in *premature infants* with the largest lesions has been poor. The initial series of cases reported were identified at postmortem examination.[90-93] Subsequently, six premature infants with cerebellar hemorrhage were identified during life, either by CT[54] or by ultrasound scan,[109,110] and all died, often with complicating systemic illness. However, with the detection of the more typical smaller hemorrhages by ultrasonography through the mastoid window in the small premature infant, it has become clear that the outcome is not dire. In a recent series of 35 cases, mortality rate was 14%, although survivors had much longer requirements for supplemental oxygen, mechanical ventilation, and days in the neonatal intensive care unit.[100] In studies of premature infants with longer follow-up and probably somewhat larger lesions, neurological deficits were observed in approximately one-half.[98] In view of the growing awareness of cerebellum in cognitive and behavioral functions, it is of great interest that initial data show that the small premature infants exhibit cognitive deficits in 40% and autism spectrum disorders in 37%.[114]

The outcome in *term infants* in general has been characterized by a high likelihood of subsequent neurological deficits. In two earlier series, of the 10 infants identified during life by CT,[54,102-104] all survived. All 4 infants were treated surgically in one series,[54] and none of 6 was treated surgically in the other series.[102-104] Of the 10 infants, all have subsequent neurological deficits, especially motor, with consistent but variable involvement of intellect. Approximately one half of both surgically treated and nontreated infants developed hydrocephalus that required ventriculoperitoneal shunts. In a later series of 10 infants, neurological deficits were present in the majority of survivors.[98] In one carefully studied group of 6 term infants evaluated at a mean age of 32 months, 5 had prominent deficits relative to cerebellar disturbance, including intention tremor, dysmetria, truncal ataxia, and hypotonia.[104] Such deficits were confirmed in

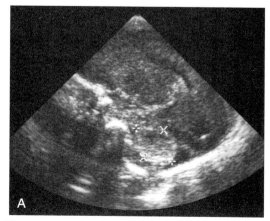

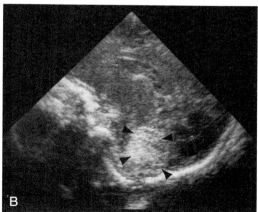

Figure 10-12 **Ultrasound scan of cerebellar hemorrhage.** Sagittal scans from an infant of 650 g birth weight on, **A,** day 1 and, **B,** day 3. The evolving echodense cerebellar hemorrhage is marked by *white crosses* in **A** and *black arrowheads* in **B.**

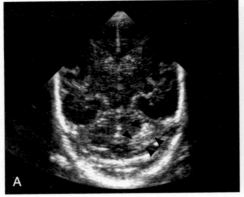
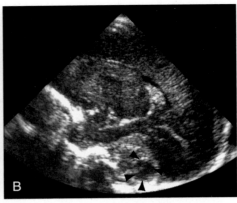

Figure 10-13 Ultrasound scan of cerebellar hemorrhage. **A,** Coronal scan from an infant of 1050 g birth weight on day 7 and, **B,** parasagittal scan from the same infant on day 37. Note echodense cerebellar hemispheral hemorrhage *(arrowheads)* in **A** that evolves to an echolucent area of tissue loss 1 month later in **B.**

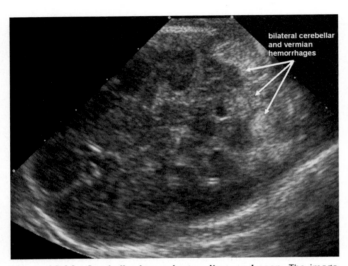

Figure 10-14 Cerebellar hemorrhage, ultrasound scan. The image was obtained through the mastoid fontanelle in a premature infant and shows a bilateral cerebellar hemispheric and vermian hemorrhage. *(From Limperopoulos C, Benson CB, Bassan H, Di Salvo DN, et al: Cerebellar hemorrhage in the preterm infant: Ultrasonographic findings and risk factors, Pediatrics 116:717-724, 2005.)*

later series.[41] Undoubtedly, these clinical phenomena relate to the destruction of cerebellar tissue and perhaps also to subsequent aberrations of cerebellar development. Recall that inward migration of external granule cells to the internal granule cell layer is active in the neonatal period and subsequently in early infancy. Other deficits observed (e.g., cerebral palsy) may relate to the frequently associated supratentorial lesions (see earlier discussion).

Management

Early detection by ultrasound scan, CT, or MRI scan is critical. A high index of suspicion is important. The most difficult issue relates to the decision concerning surgical intervention. Important determining factors include size and location of the hemorrhage, rapidity of neurological deterioration, and seriousness of pulmonary or other systemic disorders that could preclude anesthesia and major surgery. Numerous reports document survival after surgical evacuation by posterior fossa craniotomy in *full-term infants.*[41,54,115-117] However, Fishman and co-workers[102-104] documented survival with no worse neurological sequelae in six full-term infants who were treated with medical support alone. Thus, surgery is not obligatory and, in fact, is probably not indicated unless the infant's neurological status fails to stabilize. Placement of a ventriculoperitoneal shunt is necessary in nearly one half of affected infants, with or without surgical evacuation, and even

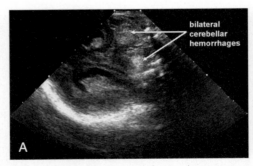
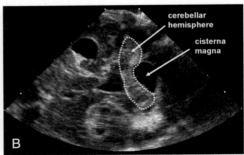

Figure 10-15 Cerebellar hemorrhage, ultrasound scan. Images were obtained through the mastoid fontanelle in a premature infant. In **A,** note the bilateral cerebellar hemispheric hemorrhage, and in **B,** performed 2 months later, note the cerebellar atrophy with enlarged cisterna magna. *(From Limperopoulos C, Benson CB, Bassan H, Di Salvo DN, et al: Cerebellar hemorrhage in the preterm infant: Ultrasonographic findings and risk factors, Pediatrics 116:717-724, 2005.)*

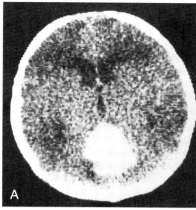

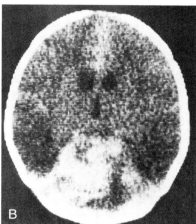

Figure 10-16 **Cerebellar hemorrhage.** Computed tomography scans from two full-term infants, both of whom were delivered by breech extraction and both of whom exhibited rapid neurological deterioration on the first day of life. **A,** Note midline cerebellar hemorrhage, associated with slight dilation of the lateral and third ventricles. **B,** Note bilateral cerebellar hemorrhages, greater on the right, associated with slight dilation of the lateral and third ventricles. *(From Rom S, Serfontein GL, Humphreys RP: Intracerebellar hematoma in the neonate,* J Pediatr *93:486-488, 1978.)*

during the neonatal period, temporary ventriculostomy may be necessary for infants with acute hydrocephalus that occurs before resolution of the obstructing cerebellar hematoma.[102-104]

The appropriate therapeutic approach to the *premature infant* is unclear. Infants with large lesions should be followed for progression as noted for term infants. However, surgery is particularly problematic in very small infants, who unfortunately, are also the most likely to exhibit cerebellar hemorrhage. Most lesions currently identified in premature infants, in my experience, have not required surgical intervention.

INTRAVENTRICULAR HEMORRHAGE OF THE TERM INFANT

Although intraventricular hemorrhage is predominantly a lesion of the premature infant, this variety of hemorrhage has been documented repeatedly by ultrasound, CT, and MRI scans as well as by postmortem study of term infants.[40,52,61,118-143] A few of these hemorrhages are caused by intraventricular extension of blood from large

hemorrhagic infarctions, ruptured vascular lesions (e.g., arteriovenous malformations, aneurysms), or tumors, which are discussed separately (see "Miscellaneous Examples of Neonatal Intracranial Hemorrhage" later). In this section, I consider those cases in which intraventricular hemorrhage per se is the dominant lesion in a *term infant.* Moreover, I emphasize here intraventricular hemorrhages of appreciable size, because minor degrees of intraventricular hemorrhage with or without subependymal or choroid plexus hemorrhage are not rare in asymptomatic full-term infants.[44a,133,139] For example, in one ultrasonographic study of 1000 consecutive healthy term newborns, intracranial hemorrhage was detected in 3.5%, with a subependymal locus in 2.0%, a choroid plexus locus in 1.1%, and a parenchymal locus in 0.4%.[139]

Neuropathology

The neuropathology of major intraventricular hemorrhage of the term infant differs from that of the premature infant (see Chapter 11), primarily in relation to the principal sites of origin of the hemorrhage (Table 10-15). In term infants, *neuropathological studies* indicated that most intraventricular hemorrhages encountered in the early neonatal period emanate from bleeding in the choroid plexus.[46,52,127,132,143] Particularly common sites within the choroid are the posterior tufts in the region of the atrium of the lateral ventricle.[52] In somewhat fewer term infants with intraventricular hemorrhage studied neuropathologically, the site of origin was the subependymal germinal matrix, particularly the region of the thalamocaudate groove (slightly posterior to the region overlying the head of the caudate nucleus as in the premature newborn), which is the last area of matrix to dissipate in the human newborn. Large-scale *ultrasonographic studies* of healthy term newborns examined in the first days of life suggest, however, that the subependymal germinal matrix may be a more common site of intraventricular hemorrhage in the term infant than previously suspected.[133,139] For example, in the study of 1000 term newborns of Heibel and co-workers,[139] of 20 infants with intraventricular blood (albeit generally small amounts in these *asymptomatic* infants), 9 had choroid plexus hemorrhage, and 11 had subependymal germinal matrix hemorrhage.

TABLE 10-15	Sites of Origin of Intraventricular Hemorrhage of the Term Infant*
Choroid plexus (35%)	
Thalamus (24%)	
Subependymal germinal matrix, caudate (17%)	
Periventricular cerebral parenchyma (14%)	
Source unclear (10%)	

*Data derived from brain imaging of 29 full-term infants with intraventricular hemorrhage.
Data from Wu YW, Hamrick SEG, Miller SP, Haward MF, et al: Intraventricular hemorrhage in term neonates caused by sinovenous thrombosis, *Ann Neurol* 54:123-126, 2003.

The conclusions just mentioned concerning site of origin must be interpreted in the context of the two largest studies of *major* intraventricular hemorrhages in *living term infants*, identified by CT scan (n = 19), [136] or by CT and MRI scan (n = 29).[143] In the larger of these two studies (see Table 10-15), the choroid plexus (35%) and thalamus (24%) were the sites of origin in the majority of cases (see Table 10-15).[143] The thalamus was a more common site than the choroid plexus in the earlier study based entirely on CT.[136] Thalamic origin of hemorrhage is associated more prominently than is choroid plexus origin with moderate to severe intraventricular hemorrhage and with venous thrombosis (see later). Subependymal germinal matrix, overlying the caudate, often difficult to distinguish from an apparent caudate origin, accounts for nearly 20% of cases. Intraventricular extension from periventricular hemorrhagic infarction accounts for a small minority of cases (see Table 10-15). With imaging that includes MRI scan, in only approximately 10% is a site of origin of hemorrhage obscure.[143] The neuropathological sequelae of intraventricular hemorrhage (e.g., posthemorrhagic hydrocephalus) are similar in the term and premature infant (see Chapter 11).

Pathogenesis

The principal pathogenetic themes are often multiple, but *apparent disturbances in cerebral blood flow, venous pressure, coagulation, and vascular integrity*, as well as mechanical *trauma*, are prominent.* Many of the pathogenetic factors relative to these themes, discussed in relation to intraventricular hemorrhage of the premature infant, are relevant here (see Chapter 11). However, two aspects of pathogenesis are somewhat different in the term infant compared with the premature infant. First, the role of *trauma* may be somewhat more important in the term infant. Among those cases with adequate perinatal data, an appreciable minority experienced difficult deliveries because of forceps rotations, vacuum-assisted delivery, and breech extractions. The specific relationships between the trauma and the occurrence of intraventricular hemorrhage are not entirely clear, but presumably some of the factors described earlier for cerebellar hemorrhage (see "Pathogenesis") that lead to increases in cerebral venous pressure are important. A second aspect of pathogenesis in the term infant that appears different from that in the preterm infant is the *more prominent role of coagulation disturbance*. Thus, in the largest reported series, 40% of infants tested had coagulation factor abnormalities consistent with a hypercoagulable state, had disseminated intravascular coagulation, or were receiving ECMO.[143]

Recent data strongly indicate an important role for *cerebral sinovenous thrombosis* in the final cascade to intraventricular hemorrhage in the term infant. An earlier report based on CT scanning suggested that thalamic venous hemorrhagic infarction was important in pathogenesis.[136] A later study using MRI demonstrated thrombosis in the vein of Galen or major venous sinuses in approximately 30% of cases of intraventricular hemorrhage and showed parenchymal findings (hemorrhagic infarct) consistent with thrombosis in an additional 25%.[143] Venous thrombosis was associated with nearly all the thalamic infarcts.[143]

Clinical Features

The onset of the neurological syndrome varies with the cause. Infants with perinatal complications usually exhibit distinct abnormalities from the first day or two of life, whereas infants with no clear cause of the syndrome often present later, sometimes as late as the second to fourth *weeks* of life. The neurological syndrome is characterized by irritability, stupor, apnea, and, particularly, seizures.* The seizures are usually focal or multifocal and occur in approximately 50% to 65% of cases. Other features include fever, jitteriness, and signs of increased intracranial pressure (e.g., full fontanelle, vomiting). Approximately 50% of infants with large hemorrhages develop hydrocephalus that requires placement of a ventriculoperitoneal shunt. An additional 20% of infants develop ventricular dilation that ceases progression without therapy. Approximately one half of the infants recover totally within 2 to 3 weeks, and the remainder improve but continue to exhibit neurological abnormalities and subsequently neurological deficits (see "Prognosis").

Diagnosis

The diagnosis of the intraventricular hemorrhage is made readily by ultrasound scan or CT scan, as outlined in more detail in Chapter 11 concerning intraventricular hemorrhage of the premature infant. The thalamic source of origin and any associated venous thrombosis are determined best by MRI scan (Fig. 10-17). MRI also demonstrates parenchymal involvement better than ultrasound or CT and clearly is the preferred imaging modality. MR venography and color Doppler ultrasonography are often useful, in my experience, especially the former. Because of the unusual occurrence of choroid plexus arteriovenous malformation, a lesion that raises serious therapeutic questions, some investigators have suggested angiography in infants with apparent choroid plexus origin of hemorrhage and no apparent causative factors.[142]

Prognosis

At first glance, the overall outcome of intraventricular hemorrhage for the term infant appears to be somewhat worse than that for the premature infant (Table 10-16).[61,119,120,123,129,131,136,138] This apparent difference relates in part to the finding that smaller lesions,

---

*See references 40,61,119,120,123,129,131,134,136-138,143.

*See references 40,61,119,120,123,129,131,134,136,138,141,143.

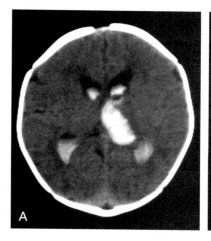
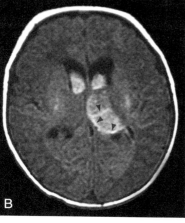

Figure 10-17 Computed tomography (CT) and magnetic resonance imaging (MRI) scans of intraventricular hemorrhage (IVH) originating in the thalamus. A 9-day-old term infant presented with acute onset of vomiting and seizures. **A**, The CT scan shows the IVH and contiguous increased attenuation in the left thalamus. **B**, The MRI scan shows, in addition, a prominent, possibly thrombosed, thalamic vein (*arrowheads*) and likely thalamic infarction.

without parenchymal involvement, make up a greater proportion of the hemorrhages identified in premature infants. For example, in one series of 15 term infants, 67% of hemorrhages were classified as "grade III or IV."[138] In a later series of 9 infants, all 4 of the infants with an unfavorable outcome had "grade III or IV" hemorrhage.[40] In the largest reported series (n = 29), 45% of lesions were "moderate" or "severe."[143] The specific outcome in term infants relates in part to the cause. Those infants with major perinatal complications in the background or on ECMO exhibit neurological deficits in most instances, whereas infants with no etiological factors recognized are usually normal on follow-up examinations. [61,119,120,123,129,131,136,138] The relative frequency of accompanying parenchymal injury appears to underlie the differences in outcome. Infants who develop intraventricular hemorrhage as a consequence of thalamic hemorrhagic infarction have a less favorable outlook than those who do not have thalamic involvement.[120,123,136,144] In the large series of infants with thalamic hemorrhagic lesions with intraventricular hemorrhage (n = 12) reported by Roland and co-workers,[136] 83% had cerebral palsy (usually hemiparesis), whereas only 29% of the term infants with intraventricular hemorrhage without thalamic involvement had cerebral palsy.

Management

Management of intraventricular hemorrhage for term infants is similar to that described in detail in Chapter 11 for premature infants. In addition, the timing and choices of intervention for any posthemorrhagic hydrocephalus that develops are also similar.

TABLE 10-16	Outcome of Intraventricular Hemorrhage of the Term Infant*	
Outcome		**Total**
Normal		55%
Neurological deficits (major)		40%
Hydrocephalus (shunted)		50%
Dead		5%

*Derived from data on 84 infants reported in references listed in text and unpublished personal cases.

MISCELLANEOUS EXAMPLES OF NEONATAL INTRACRANIAL HEMORRHAGE

The major unusual and miscellaneous examples of intracranial hemorrhage are associated with trauma, hemorrhagic infarction, coagulation disturbance, vascular defect, cerebral tumor, and unknown factors (Table 10-17). These examples are reviewed briefly in the following subsections.

Trauma

Although trauma usually results in subdural hemorrhage or primary subarachnoid hemorrhage (see previous sections), epidural, intraventricular, or intracerebral hemorrhage also may be observed. Epidural hemorrhage is discussed in Chapter 22. Intraventricular hemorrhage of the traumatic variety is discussed previously. Traumatic intracerebral hemorrhage is rare, but when it occurs, it is almost always an accompaniment of major extracerebral hemorrhage. Trauma severe enough to produce major hemorrhage most

TABLE 10-17	Miscellaneous Examples of Neonatal Intracranial Hemorrhage
Trauma	
Epidural hemorrhage	
Intracerebral hemorrhage	
Hemorrhagic Infarction	
Embolus	
Venous thrombosis	
Arterial thrombosis	
Coagulation Disturbance	
Thrombocytopenia	
Deficiency of coagulation factors	
Vascular Defect	
Aneurysm	
Arteriovenous malformation	
Coarctation of the aorta	
Cerebral Tumor	
Unknown Cause	
Extracorporeal Membrane Oxygenation	

often results in injury to scalp and skull (see Chapter 22). The precise site and extent of intracranial involvement are best determined by CT or MRI scan.

Hemorrhagic Infarction

Hemorrhagic infarction results when the injured, although functional, capillaries in an ischemic infarct are ruptured by release of an arterial obstruction (e.g., embolus) or by an increase in venous pressure, or when small amounts of bleeding from injured capillaries are not controlled by an intact clotting system. Thus, hemorrhagic infarction is observed in the newborn primarily with (1) embolic arterial occlusion because of distal movement of the embolus, (2) venous thrombosis because of the increase in venous pressure proximally, and (3) arterial thrombosis (or perhaps vasospasm) that is partial (or intermittent) or accompanied by a disturbance of coagulation (see Table 10-17). The specific causes, including sources of emboli, disseminated intravascular coagulation, polycythemia, hypercoagulable states, and so forth, are discussed in Chapter 8. The occurrence of hemorrhagic infarction has been documented frequently in the newborn (see Chapters 8 and 9), and, indeed, most examples of "intracerebral hemorrhage" or "grade IV" intraventricular hemorrhage in the term newborn probably represent hemorrhagic venous infarction (see Chapter 11).[61,120,129,131,138] The clinical accompaniments, diagnosis, and outcome are described in Chapters 9 and 11.

Unilateral thalamic hemorrhagic lesions may represent a specific variety of hemorrhagic infarction.[144-146] This lesion has been observed in both premature and term infants, particularly after perinatal asphyxia or persistent fetal circulation with hypotension. Identification is readily made by cranial ultrasonography (Fig. 10-18). Distinction of hemorrhagic infarction from a primary hemorrhage has not been possible, and no neuropathological data are available. I favor the likelihood of hemorrhagic infarction in view of the nearly constant relationship with prior hypotension. The relationship

of this unilateral hemorrhagic lesion with the bilateral hemorrhagic necrosis observed in thalamus and basal ganglia of asphyxiated term infants (see Chapters 8 and 9) and with the syndrome of intraventricular hemorrhage with apparent thalamic hemorrhagic infarction[136,143] (see the previous section) is not clear. The outcome has been favorable in nearly all infants with unilateral thalamic "hemorrhage," unlike the unfavorable outcome in the thalamic hemorrhagic lesion associated with intraventricular hemorrhage (see earlier discussion). The difference in outcome, of course, could relate to the size of the hemorrhage.

Coagulation Defect

The most common coagulation disturbances *primarily* responsible for neonatal intracranial hemorrhage are thrombocytopenia and defects of a coagulation factor or factors (see Table 10-17).

Thrombocytopenia

Thrombocytopenia of a severe degree may lead to neonatal intracranial hemorrhage. However, the major causes of neonatal thrombocytopenia (i.e., immune disorders, congenital and neonatal infections, maternal drugs, organic acidopathies, and congenital bone marrow hypoplasias) often dominate the clinical picture through extraneural manifestations, including bleeding at various sites. Indeed, except for isoimmune thrombocytopenia, thrombocytopenia is only very uncommonly associated with serious neonatal intracranial hemorrhage.[147]

Neonatal Isoimmune Thrombocytopenia. *Neonatal isoimmune thrombocytopenia* is an unusual but important cause of intrauterine hemorrhagic lesions.[40,138,148-157] This fetal hematological disorder occurs in 0.2 per 1000 live births and is related to passive transfer from mother to fetus of antibodies against a fetal platelet antigen inherited from the father and absent in the mother. In approximately 85% of all cases in white infants, the antigen is the so-called HPA-1a antigen (human platelet antigen 1a). In Japanese infants, the antigen usually is HPA-4a.[154] Other platelet antigens,

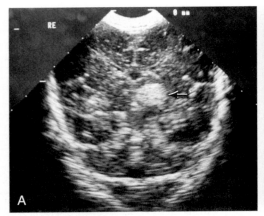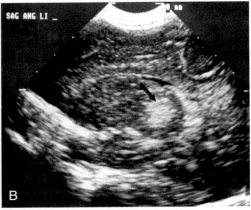

Figure 10-18 Ultrasound scan of unilateral thalamic "hemorrhage." **A,** Coronal and, **B,** sagittal scans obtained on day 3 in an infant of 2120 g with persistent fetal circulation. Note the circular area of echodensity in the region of the thalamus *(arrow in each). (From de Vries LS, Smet M, Goemans N, Wilms G, et al: Unilateral thalamic haemorrhage in the pre-term and full-term newborn, Neuropediatrics 23:153-156, 1992.)*

implicated in the minority of cases, are HPA-3a and HPA-5b.[156,157] Major intrauterine intracranial lesions have been described as a consequence of neonatal isoimmune thrombocytopenia.[40,138,148-153,155-157] Although the lesions are usually characterized as "intracerebral hemorrhage," their frequent location in an apparent vascular distribution, evolution to porencephalic cyst, and reported association with vascular thrombi suggest that at least some are fundamentally ischemic, perhaps with hemorrhage as a secondary event (see also Chapter 8). Moreover, the finding that antibodies to HPA-1a react also with an endothelial cell surface antigen further supports the notion of an ischemic basis for at least a portion of the intrauterine cystic lesions. Optic nerve atrophy or hypoplasia is a common accompaniment of the severe porencephalic lesions.[152,153] Prevention of the intrauterine lesions is difficult because of their frequently early intrauterine occurrence (possible in the second trimester, although usually in the third trimester). Because the risk of recurrence of intracranial hemorrhage in subsequent pregnancies is 80% to 90%, fetal management is critical.

Current management is somewhat controversial. Fetal genotyping by amniocentesis coupled with genotyping of the father will indicate whether the fetus contains the offending antigen and thus is at risk. If the previous affected pregnancy involved fetal intracranial hemorrhage, intravenous immunoglobulin G is administered weekly, beginning in the second trimester, preferably several weeks before the occurrence of hemorrhage in the previous pregnancy.[157-159] This approach leads to elevations of the fetal platelet count and sharp reduction of the risk of fetal intracranial hemorrhage.[160] Although weekly fetal platelet transfusions have been advocated by some investigators, the risk per pregnancy of fetal loss for this procedure is 6%.[161] Thus, cordocentesis, fetal blood sampling, and transfusions have been omitted by some clinicians, with continuation of the weekly immunoglobulin until elective cesarean section at 34 to 38 weeks of gestation.[157] If the previous affected pregnancy was *not* complicated by fetal intracranial hemorrhage, the risk of hemorrhage is only about 7%; in this setting, weekly administration of intravenous immunoglobulin G need not be commenced until 28 to 32 weeks of gestation, with induction of labor at 38 weeks.[157] Intracranial hemorrhage with isoimmune thrombocytopenia also may occur in apparent relation to labor and delivery and consist of subdural hemorrhage, subarachnoid hemorrhage, and intracerebral hemorrhage, often in combination. Management postnatally consists of transfusion of compatible antigen-negative platelets and administration of intravenous immunoglobulin.[154,162,163]

Deficiency of Coagulation Factors

Deficits of coagulation factors also may result in neonatal intracranial hemorrhage (see Table 10-17). The deficits may occur secondary to a congenital deficiency (e.g., hemophilia A), severe liver disease, disseminated intravascular coagulation, or vitamin K deficiency. Except for the first of these examples, evidence of

extraneural bleeding is almost always present. Moreover, with severe liver disease, the clinical picture is usually dominated by systemic disturbances related to hepatic failure. Disseminated intravascular coagulation, also discussed in relation to pathogenesis of cerebral infarction in Chapter 8, can lead to all varieties of intracranial hemorrhage and to extramedullary hematoma of the spinal cord as well.[164] In this context, I briefly review congenital deficiency of coagulation factors, especially hemophilia, and vitamin K deficiency.

Congenital Deficiency of Coagulation Factors. The most common congenital deficiency of a coagulation factor that results in neonatal intracranial hemorrhage is hemophilia. Thus, deficiencies of factor VIII (hemophilia A) or of factor IX (hemophilia B) have been associated with neonatal intracranial hemorrhage.[72,165-168] In one retrospective review of patients with hemophilia, 7 of 119 with hemophilia A and 1 of 31 with hemophilia B developed neonatal intracranial hemorrhage, and all but a single patient had no signs of bleeding at other sites. The hemorrhages occurred during the first 24 hours of life in 4 of the 8 patients, and in the first month in 6 patients. The lesions described have been predominately subdural (see Fig. 10-4A), although intracerebral, cerebellar, and epidural hemorrhages have been observed, often also in association with subdural hemorrhage. Neurological sequelae have occurred in the majority of patients. It is crucial to consider such a coagulation disturbance in unexplained neonatal intracranial hemorrhage, especially subdural hemorrhage in a term infant, to institute appropriate replacement therapy promptly.

Other coagulation defects rarely associated with neonatal intracranial hemorrhage include acquired deficiency of factor VIII (secondary transplacental transfer of an inhibitory antibody),[169] congenital factor X deficiency,[170-172] and congenital fibrinogen deficiency (Fig. 10-19). Fatal intracerebral hemorrhage secondary to bleeding from a hemorrhagic infarct caused by venous thrombosis in the setting of a defect in the antithrombin gene is a rare example of

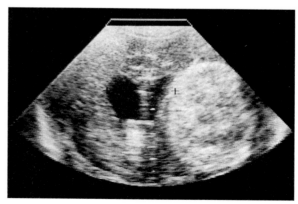

Figure 10-19 Ultrasound scan of hemorrhage into basal ganglia from an infant with congenital fibrinogen deficiency. Note the large circular echodense lesion in the region of the left putamen. *(Courtesy of Dr. Gary Shackelford.)*

lethal hemorrhage resulting from a defect in a procoagulant factor.[173]

Vitamin K Deficiency. Three neonatal syndromes of vitamin K deficiency are recognized: early hemorrhagic disease, with onset in the first 24 hours; classic hemorrhagic disease, with onset between 1 and 7 days; and late hemorrhagic disease, with onset usually in the second month of life. *Early hemorrhagic disease* may be accompanied by intracranial as well as systemic hemorrhage and is usually associated with maternal anticonvulsant therapy, which increases degradation of vitamin K (see Chapter 24). *Classic hemorrhagic disease* is characterized by systemic and, only rarely, intracranial bleeding and is associated with lack of neonatal administration of vitamin K and unknown additional factors.[174]

Late hemorrhagic disease, the major subject of this section, is characterized *particularly by intracranial bleeding*, and the principal cause for the vitamin K deficiency appears to be a combination of low vitamin K content of breast milk (lower than cow's milk and conventional formula) and lack of administration of vitamin K at birth (to augment the "physiologically" lower levels of vitamin K that occur in the newborn).[50,174-187] (Contributing causes may include malabsorption of the fat-soluble vitamin because of diarrhea or cholestatic liver disease, impaired production because of gut sterilization by antibiotic therapy, and maternal drugs.)

The effect on the clotting system is the failure of vitamin K to carboxylate and thereby render functional the clotting factors II (prothrombin), VII, IX, and X, with a resulting prolongation of both the prothrombin time and the partial thromboplastin time.[188] The disorder is especially common in Asia but has been observed in the United States, Great Britain, and many other countries.[50,106,177-187]

The onset usually is not apparent for several weeks, although easy bruising is recorded frequently in the first weeks. In one series, the median age of onset of intracranial hemorrhage was 56 days.[50] The major presenting features are seizures, depressed level of consciousness, and signs of increased intracranial pressure (e.g., tense fontanelle, vomiting). The varieties of hemorrhage have included primarily intracerebral hemorrhage and accompanying subarachnoid hemorrhage, although subdural and intraventricular hemorrhages also have been reported in a substantial minority.[50,106] The diagnosis of the site and extent of hemorrhage is readily made by CT scan (Fig. 10-20). Most affected infants with major intracranial hemorrhage involving cerebral parenchyma and not solely the subarachnoid space have been left with serious neurological deficits. Only 10% to 30% of infants with late hemorrhagic disease and intracranial hemorrhage have been normal on follow-up. The clotting defects are correctable in a matter of hours by vitamin K administration, and the disorder is preventable by prophylactic administration of vitamin K at birth, either intramuscular or oral.[50,181,182,184-187] Using a sensitive assay of vitamin K deficiency (i.e., detection

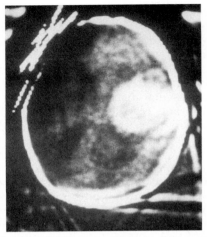

Figure 10-20 Computed tomography scan of intracerebral hemorrhage secondary to vitamin K deficiency. Note the large hematoma in the left cerebral hemisphere.

of protein induced by vitamin K absence [PIVKA-II]), Hathaway and co-workers[182] showed, in a study in Thailand, that a single oral dose at birth reduced the incidence at 1 month of vitamin K deficiency in breast-fed infants to 18% compared with 60% in untreated infants; the incidence was reduced to 6% in infants who were administered vitamin K intramuscularly.[182]

Vascular Defect

The two major intracranial vascular defects that may cause neonatal intracranial hemorrhage are congenital arterial aneurysm and arteriovenous malformation (see Table 10-17). The former is more likely to result in presentation with intracranial hemorrhage than the latter, although both are rare occurrences. A systemic vascular lesion, coarctation of the aorta, is also associated with neonatal intracranial hemorrhage.

Aneurysm

Congenital arterial aneurysm with rupture has been recorded in more than 20 infants in the first 3 months of life.[189-208] The onset of the neurological deterioration is generally abrupt and occurs as early as the first days of life.

The *clinical presentation* is dominated by acute major subarachnoid hemorrhage with signs of increased intracranial pressure (full or bulging anterior fontanelle) and rapid neurological deterioration (Table 10-18). Seizures, often focal, also occur in approximately one half of cases. Focal neurological signs are present in a similar proportion, and their nature relates to the site of the aneurysm (e.g., hemiparesis with middle cerebral artery aneurysm and brain stem signs with aneurysms of the vertebrobasilar circulation). *Sites of the lesions* have consisted of the middle cerebral artery (10 cases), anterior cerebral artery (5 cases), internal carotid artery near its bifurcation into anterior and middle cerebral arteries (2 cases), circle of Willis near the junction of the posterior communicating and posterior cerebral arteries (2 cases), and vertebrobasilar circulation (5 cases). The lesions are usually large. The *anatomical defect* involves the internal elastic lamina

TABLE 10-18	**Aneurysms with Presentation in the First 3 Months of Life***

Clinical Presentation

Subarachnoid hemorrhage, massive, with full or bulging anterior fontanelle and catastrophic neurological deterioration

Seizures, usually focal

Focal neurological signs, nature depending on location of aneurysm or associated intracerebral hematoma

Diagnosis

Computed tomography demonstrates large subarachnoid hemorrhage or intraparenchymal hematoma or both

Magnetic resonance imaging may demonstrate the aneurysm

Cerebral angiography, computed tomography angiography, or magnetic resonance angiography is needed to demonstrate exact site of lesion in vasculature

Outcome

Rapid diagnosis and surgical therapy associated with good outcome

*See text for references.

TABLE 10-19	**Arteriovenous Malformations (Not Involving Vein of Galen) with Presentation in the First 3 Months of Life***

Location

Cerebral hemisphere (15), thalamus–third ventricle (5), choroid plexus (3), posterior fossa (8), spinal cord (2)

Common Presentations

Intracranial hemorrhage (with signs of increased intracranial pressure): intracerebral hemorrhage with or without IVH (6), IVH alone (6), IVH with subdural hemorrhage (1), IVH with massive subarachnoid hemorrhage (1), posterior fossa hemorrhage (4)

Seizures, often focal

Congestive heart failure with cranial bruit

Hydrocephalus

Opisthotonos, brain stem signs (especially posterior fossa lesions)

Paraplegia (spinal cord lesions)

*See text for references. Numbers in parentheses indicate number of reported cases.

IVH, Intraventricular hemorrhage.

and muscularis, which are thinned, fragmented, or absent. The *diagnosis* usually begins with CT, which shows subarachnoid hemorrhage or parenchymal hemorrhage, or both. MRI may demonstrate the aneurysm (Fig. 10-21). Cerebral angiography usually is required to define the anatomical features of the vascular lesion, especially concerning the presence of features (e.g., neck) important for surgical intervention. MR angiography or CT angiography may provide similar information in a less invasive manner. The *outcome* relates in considerable part to the size and location of the lesion. Surgical clipping and cure are often possible, except for so-called *giant aneurysms* or lesions located in vessels that are inaccessible or that cannot be clipped, as with basilar aneurysms. In one report, coil embolization was effective.[207]

Arteriovenous Malformation

Arteriovenous malformation is a rare cause of neonatal intracranial hemorrhage but an important one to recognize and treat appropriately.[142,209-225] Of all neonatal arteriovenous malformations, those that involve the vein of Galen are most common. However, vein of Galen malformations rarely manifest clinically as intracranial hemorrhage and are discussed with brain tumors in Chapter 23. Arteriovenous malformations not involving the vein of Galen but manifesting clinically in the first 3 months of life, the subject of this section, commonly herald their presence by *intracranial hemorrhage* (Table 10-19). (Notably, however, approximately one half of cases in the neonatal period manifest with cardiac manifestations, especially congestive heart failure.) Most commonly, the intracranial hemorrhage is intracerebral or intraventricular, or both. This propensity to produce hemorrhage at these loci relates to the most common sites for the vascular malformations (i.e., cerebral hemispheres, thalamus-third ventricle, and choroid plexus, which together account for 70% of all reported lesions; see Table 10-19). *Other clinical*

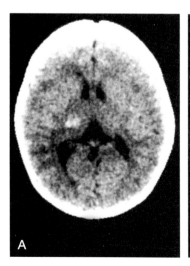
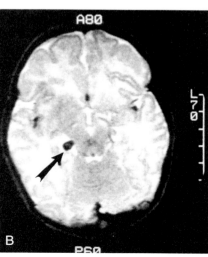

Figure 10-21 **Congenital aneurysm in a 7-week-old infant with a 2-week history of left focal seizures**. **A**, Computed tomography (CT) scan shows only a small hemorrhagic lesion in the right posterior thalamus. **B**, Magnetic resonance imaging scan obtained shortly after the CT scan demonstrated flow void in the perimesencephalic cistern *(arrow)*, consistent with an aneurysm (later proven by cerebral angiography). *(From Putty TK, Luerssen TG, Campbell RL, Boaz JC, et al: Magnetic resonance imaging diagnosis of a cerebral aneurysm in an infant: Case report and review of the literature, Pediatr Neurosurg 16:48-51, 1990-1991.)*

presentations, sometimes occurring with hemorrhage, include seizures, congestive heart failure (secondary to high cardiac output), hydrocephalus (secondary to increased venous pressure or obstruction of CSF pathways), opisthotonos with other brain stem signs (posterior fossa lesions), or paraplegia, either congenital or of abrupt onset in the neonatal period (spinal cord lesions). The *diagnosis* is suspected by the occurrence of unexplained intracranial hemorrhage or one or more of the other clinical features noted in Table 10-19. Color Doppler ultrasonography is an effective means of assessing the site of the lesion.[215,224] Angiography (conventional or MR, or both) is required to identify the anatomical details of the malformation and its vascular feeders. Treatment consists of surgical extirpation and has been curative except in very large lesions or those in loci that preclude surgical attack. Embolic therapy, as in management of vein of Galen malformations (see Chapter 23), is an alternative therapeutic modality.

Coarctation of the Aorta

A major *systemic* vascular defect, coarctation of the aorta, has been associated rarely with the occurrence of intracranial hemorrhage in the newborn (see Table 10-17).[226-228] The hemorrhages documented in the six patients have included subarachnoid, intraventricular, and intracerebral lesions.[227,228] The cause of the hemorrhage in newborns was thought to be systemic hypertension, which, in four of the five infants reported, was only moderate (90 to 110 mm Hg systolic).[227] Cerebral hemorrhage complicates coarctation of the aorta in older patients in as many as 10% of cases and has been attributed in some cases not only to brachiocephalic hypertension but also to frequently associated cerebral aneurysms. In neonatal patients, no cerebral aneurysms have been found on angiography or on postmortem examination, but small aneurysms cannot be excluded. The important points are that infants with coarctation of the aorta must be considered at risk for the occurrence of serious intracranial hemorrhage and that systemic hypertension perhaps need not be dramatic to provoke this complication. Perhaps related to this association is the demonstration of multiple cerebral arteriovenous malformations (although without hemorrhage) in an infant with coarctation of the aorta.[220]

Cerebral Tumor

Hemorrhage associated with brain tumor has been observed in the newborn period. More commonly, the clinical presentation is that of signs of increased intracranial pressure, hydrocephalus, macrocephaly, and focal neurological signs (see Chapter 23).

Unknown Cause

Infants, almost exclusively full term, occasionally exhibit focal parenchymal hemorrhage, usually into cerebral white matter but also into thalamus, basal ganglia, brain stem, or spinal cord without definable cause.[40,61,119,120,123,129,131,155,229-232] The cerebral lesions become manifest most often in the first day or so of life with seizures, frequently focal. Motor deficits are common and are generally predictable by the topography of the lesion. Cerebral lesions may be accompanied by hemiparesis. An infant with a medullary hemorrhage exhibited bilateral diaphragmatic paralysis, impaired sucking and swallowing, and tongue fasciculations.[231] Another infant with a spinal cord hemorrhage exhibited abrupt onset of quadriplegia.[232] Subsequent motor deficits may occur, but full recovery is not unusual. Hydrocephalus has appeared secondary to extension of parenchymal hemorrhage to the lateral ventricles or subarachnoid space. One potential cause for this group of lesions is arteriovenous malformation that is too small to be detected by conventional imaging techniques or is obliterated by the hemorrhage. Some may represent hemorrhagic infarctions not clearly demonstrated by ultrasonography, CT, or MRI.

Extracorporeal Membrane Oxygenation

Extracorporeal membrane oxygenation (ECMO) is a technique of cardiopulmonary bypass used for term and near-term infants with pulmonary failure that is potentially reversible but has not been responsive to trials of conventional or high-frequency ventilation or inhaled nitric oxide. Infants subjected to ECMO have exhibited a variety of intracranial hemorrhagic and ischemic phenomena. The ischemic lesions are reviewed briefly in Chapter 8. The hemorrhagic phenomena are discussed in this context.

Patient Selection and Technique

Infants chosen for ECMO therapy have had intractable respiratory failure secondary to a variety of disorders that have in common a high intrinsic mortality rate (>80%) and a potential for reversibility, either spontaneously or by surgery. The disease states that have led to ECMO therapy in major series have been, in general order of frequency, meconium aspiration syndrome, congenital diaphragmatic hernia, persistent pulmonary hypertension, sepsis, and respiratory distress syndrome.[233-250] The short-term benefit of ECMO is apparent from data collected from 65 centers in North America and elsewhere on more than 3500 newborns; these data show an overall survival rate of 83% in infants with a predicted mortality rate in excess of 80%.[251] The success in recent years of other modalities (e.g., high-frequency oscillatory ventilation, inhaled nitric oxide) has changed the composition of populations treated with ECMO to a somewhat more severe spectrum of disease.

ECMO is carried out by the venoarterial or venovenous technique. The largest reported experience is with the former. In venoarterial ECMO, the right internal jugular vein is cannulated, the catheter is passed into the right atrium, the cranial opening of the jugular vein is permanently ligated, and venous blood from the atrium is drained to the extracorporeal membrane oxygenator. After addition of oxygen and removal of carbon dioxide by the membrane oxygenator, the

TABLE 10-20	Hemorrhagic Lesions in Infants Treated with Extracorporeal Membrane Oxygenation	
Location		**No. of Infants**
Cerebral		
Frontal		12
Parietal		3
Temporal		4
Occipital		6
Periventricular white matter		4
Germinal matrix		17
Intraventricular		6
Basal ganglia		2
Posterior fossa		
Cerebellar		9
Mesencephalon		1
Subarachnoid		4
Total		68

Data from Taylor GA, Fitz CR, Kapur S, Short BL: Cerebrovascular accidents in neonates treated with extracorporeal membrane oxygenation: Sonographic-pathologic correlation, *AJR Am J Roentgenol* 153:355-361, 1989.

blood is warmed and pumped by nonpulsatile flow to the infant through a catheter placed in the right common carotid artery and is directed into the right aortic arch. As with the jugular vein, the cranial opening of the common carotid artery is ligated. (In recent years, reconstruction of the right common carotid artery following termination of ECMO has been carried out commonly.) Anticoagulation therapy with heparin is administered systemically for the duration of the bypass procedure to prevent clotting in the ECMO circuit. With venovenous ECMO, the right common carotid artery is not cannulated, and blood is returned to the central venous circulation.

Intracranial Hemorrhage

Intracranial hemorrhage and ischemic lesions of brain have been documented in infants treated with ECMO.[143,233,234,236-239,244,245,248,250,252-266] In most series, with findings based on brain imaging studies, 20% to 50% of infants exhibit intracranial abnormalities. Approximately 40% of these abnormalities (i.e., those in 10% to 20% of infants) are of major severity. Approximately 40% of the intracranial abnormalities are purely hemorrhagic lesions, approximately 20% are hemorrhagic complicating apparent ischemic lesions, and approximately 40% are nonhemorrhagic ischemic lesions. Ischemic lesions, which consist primarily of periventricular leukomalacia, cerebral infarction (hemorrhagic in ≈50% of cases), and selective neuronal necrosis, are described in Chapter 8.

Hemorrhagic lesions observed in infants treated with ECMO are varied (Table 10-20). In one large series (n = 68), although 34% of lesions were relatively minor germinal matrix or intraventricular hemorrhages, particularly the former, 37% were cerebral parenchymal hemorrhages. Of the cerebral hemorrhages, 40% or more have been observed in unusual locations (i.e., beyond the confines of the anterior circulation and

in the temporal or occipital lobes).[233,254] Additionally, 15% of the hemorrhages, usually serious, have been in the posterior fossa, primarily involving cerebellum (see Table 10-20).[234,238]

The *laterality* of hemorrhagic and ischemic lesions in infants treated with ECMO has been the subject of controversy. In one study, major hemorrhagic cerebral lesions occurred predominantly on the left (seven of nine cases), whereas major ischemic cerebral lesions occurred predominantly on the right (five of six cases).[233] Other reports have not described the left-sided preponderance of hemorrhagic cerebral lesions.[234,238,253,254,266]

The right hemispheric predominance of ischemic lesions has been observed by others.[238,261] For example, in a separate study, 8 of 36 infants exhibited evidence of ischemic lesions, with 5 of the 8 in the right hemisphere, 1 in the left, and 2 bilateral.[238] Moreover, although some reports described a nearly equal distribution of ischemic lesions, the distributions did *not* conform to the left hemisphere predominance characteristic of strokes of other causes in newborns (see Chapter 8). Thus, on balance, the data suggest that focal cerebral infarcts in infants treated with ECMO preferentially affect the right hemisphere.

The hemorrhagic lesions in infants treated with ECMO are identified most readily by ultrasonography during ECMO and by CT or MRI when the infant is not receiving ECMO. Because some of the hemorrhages may be slow to clot as a result of systemic heparinization, some variability in echogenicity on ultrasound scan or in attenuation on CT may be observed, especially acutely (Fig. 10-22). For similar reasons, blood-fluid levels and rapidly expanding hematomas may be observed in affected infants.

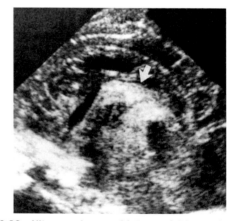

Figure 10-22 **Ultrasound scan of intracranial hemorrhage in association with extracorporeal membrane oxygenation (ECMO).** Sagittal scan from an infant of 35 weeks of gestation with congenital diaphragmatic hernia, treated with ECMO; the ultrasound scan was normal before ECMO. The scan shows a large posterior fossa hemorrhage with characteristically heterogeneous echogenicity. Blood is present also in the third ventricle *(arrow)*. Hemorrhage in the cerebellar parenchyma and in the subarachnoid space cannot be distinguished readily. *(From Taylor GA, Fitz CR, Kapur S, Short BL: Cerebrovascular accidents in neonates treated with extracorporeal membrane oxygenation: Sonographic-pathologic correlation, AJR Am J Roentgenol 153:355-361, 1989.)*

Mechanisms of Hemorrhagic and Ischemic Brain Injury with Extracorporeal Membrane Oxygenation

The mechanisms underlying the hemorrhagic and ischemic brain injury in infants subjected to ECMO are undoubtedly multifactorial. Before discussing the likely mechanisms, I briefly review the cerebral hemodynamic effects as defined primarily by Doppler ultrasonic studies of cerebral blood flow velocity.

Cerebral Hemodynamics in Infants Treated with Extracorporeal Membrane Oxygenation. The *cerebral hemodynamic effects* of ligation of common carotid artery and jugular vein in infants subjected to ECMO have been evaluated by Doppler ultrasonic measurements of cerebral blood flow velocity and by near-infrared spectroscopy.[246,267-275] The principal findings shortly after common carotid ligation are (1) an abrupt initial 50% decrease in systolic flow velocity in the right middle cerebral artery at the time of ligation with a return to 70% of baseline within 5 minutes and (2) a corresponding decline in resistance index and an increase in diastolic flow velocity. Taken together, these data suggest as an initial important hemodynamic effect of ECMO a decline in right cerebral perfusion, followed by vasodilation with a compensatory increase in perfusion. However, measurements of volemic blood flow are not available, and the difficulties of drawing conclusions concerning volemic flow based solely on measurements of blood flow velocity are described in Chapter 4. Nevertheless, the possibility of ischemic injury to the right hemisphere acutely must be considered. However, an acute decline in perfusion to *both* cerebral hemispheres is supported by the findings with near-infrared spectroscopy of an acute decline in oxyhemoglobin concentration and a corresponding increase in deoxyhemoglobin concentration.[246] A decline in perfusion to the left as well as right hemisphere may reflect an inability of the left internal carotid to supply *both* hemispheres acutely. Despite the decrease in flow velocity and oxyhemoglobin concentrations, prompt relative compensation for the common carotid ligation by collateral vessels occurs. Collateral circulation to the right cerebral hemisphere has been shown in the Doppler studies to emanate from (1) the left anterior circulation (i.e., from the anterior communicating artery), (2) the left posterior circulation (i.e., from the posterior communicating artery through the circle of Willis), and (3) from the right external carotid artery to the right internal carotid artery. The action of the collaterals emanating from the left anterior circulation may account for the approximately 50% increase in mean flow velocity in the left internal carotid artery during ECMO and the increase in oxyhemoglobin and decline in deoxyhemoglobin within 60 minutes of onset of ECMO.[246,273]

A second notable hemodynamic effect of ECMO involves the posterior circulation. Thus, *in addition to* potential compromise of the arterial supply to the right anterior circulation, a disturbance of arterial supply to the *posterior circulation* is suggested by Doppler studies.

In one study of 40 infants during ECMO, retrograde flow in the right vertebral artery, consistent with vertebral steal, was observed in 30%.[274] The demonstrations of impaired brachial flow velocity after cannulation and both improvement of brachial flow velocity and reinstitution of anterograde vertebral flow after removal of the arterial cannula suggested that the vertebral artery flow abnormality was related to partial obstruction of the origin of the right subclavian artery by the cannula (from the common carotid artery) in the innominate artery.[274] Whether ischemia in the distribution of the posterior circulation may occur consequent to vertebral steal remains unclear (see later discussion).

A third notable hemodynamic effect of ECMO relates to the effects of ligation of the jugular vein. In a study of 23 consecutive infants subjected to ECMO, Taylor and Walker demonstrated reduction in blood flow velocity in the superior sagittal sinus in 10 (43%).[276] In 9 of these 10 infants, the disturbance in venous flow persisted for over 48 hours and, notably, was followed by the occurrence of a variety of hemorrhagic or ischemic lesions. These observations raise the possibility that jugular venous occlusion may be an important pathogenetic factor for the occurrence of brain injury with ECMO (see later discussion). This finding may be relevant to the frequent occurrence of venous thrombosis in infants on ECMO.[250]

Studies of cerebral blood flow by positron emission tomography and of cerebral vessels by MR angiography suggest that in the weeks *following* ECMO, no major hemodynamic effects are apparent.[277,278] Moreover, the symmetry of cerebral blood flow shown by positron emission tomography was present whether the previously ligated common carotid artery was reanastomosed or not.[277]

Pathogenesis of Intracranial Hemorrhage with Extracorporeal Membrane Oxygenation. The pathogenesis of intracranial hemorrhage with ECMO may relate to one or more of four major factors (Table 10-21). Infants subjected to ECMO have intractable pulmonary failure, commonly complicated by cardiac insufficiency and hypotension. Indeed, in one series of infants with persistent pulmonary hypertension, a common cause for the need for ECMO, approximately 50% of the infants (not treated with ECMO) sustained

---

TABLE 10-21   **Pathogenesis of Hemorrhagic Brain Lesions in Infants Treated with Extracorporeal Membrane Oxygenation**

Prior infarction
Secondary hemorrhage during extracorporeal membrane oxygenation
Heparinization
Increase in cerebral blood flow
Increase in arterial carbon dioxide tension after hypocarbia
Increase in blood pressure with impaired cerebrovascular autoregulation
Collateral circulation: left greater than right hemisphere
Increased central venous pressure
Jugular vein ligation

cerebral infarction.[279] Such infarcts, with their injured microvasculature, would have a high likelihood to become hemorrhagic with reperfusion with ECMO, especially when coupled with other factors that encourage hemorrhage. Venous infarction has been well documented in infants who received ECMO, and extension of hemorrhage into the lateral ventricles is an important cause of intraventricular hemorrhage in these infants.[143,250] The possibility that ischemia predisposes to the occurrence of intracranial hemorrhage with ECMO is also supported by the demonstration of elevated blood lactate levels before ECMO in infants who later developed intracranial hemorrhage relative to lactate levels in infants who did not develop hemorrhage.[280] Other factors of potential importance include heparinization and an abrupt increase in cerebral blood flow with the institution of ECMO. The increase in cerebral blood flow could be related to one or more of three factors. The first of these is the correction of the hypocarbia induced by the hyperventilation used as therapy before institution of ECMO. The hyperemic effect of correction of hypocarbia was clearly shown in an animal model.[281] The second factor is the restoration of the circulation by ECMO in infants who typically are hypotensive before onset of ECMO; the occurrence of impaired cerebrovascular autoregulation, shown in newborn lambs subjected to ECMO,[282] accentuates this factor. Third, cerebral blood flow may increase, particularly in the left hemisphere, as suggested by Doppler studies of the internal carotid artery (see earlier discussion), because the right hemisphere becomes perfused by collaterals (anterior and posterior communicating arteries) emanating from the left hemisphere. (Studies in neonatal animals are inconsistent concerning cerebral hyperperfusion after institution of ECMO.[283,284]) Left hemisphere hyperperfusion would be consistent with the suggestion from studies in human infants of left hemisphere predominance for hemorrhagic cerebral lesions in infants with ECMO (see earlier discussion).

Increased venous pressure, suggested by Doppler studies of venous blood flow velocity in the superior sagittal sinus,[276] may also contribute to the pathogenesis of intracranial hemorrhage (see Table 10-21). Moreover, the venous factor may be particularly important in the pathogenesis of the posterior fossa hemorrhages, which occur with unusually high frequency in infants treated with ECMO (see earlier discussion).

Outcome in Infants Treated with Extracorporeal Membrane Oxygenation. Conclusions concerning outcome in infants treated with ECMO are based on data obtained from a large number of informative studies.[236-238,240-245,247-249,285-301] Data are best evaluated as a function of the birth weight of the infants (Table 10-22). In general, premature infants do less well than heavier and more mature infants.[235,244,248] Thus, overall mortality rates are markedly higher in smaller versus larger infants (see Table 10-22). In one large study of 1524 premature infants treated with ECMO, mortality rate was 39%.[248] Of this cohort, the 185 infants with intracranial hemorrhage had a 57% mortality rate. Similarly, major neuroimaging abnormalities, particularly hemorrhagic, are twice as common in smaller infants. Indeed, major intracranial hemorrhage is a major cause of the higher mortality in smaller infants,[235,244] an observation made first in the earliest years of ECMO therapy.[295] Major developmental delay (developmental quotient <70) is present in 10% to 20% of all infants treated with ECMO, but, again, the rate is considerably higher in smaller (38%) versus larger (8%) infants (see Table 10-22). Major neurological defects occur in approximately 10% to 20% of infants treated with ECMO. Sensorineural hearing loss was observed in 12% and 15% of two well-studied series of infants,[290,297] but the rate was 4% in other series.[289,293] Not unexpectedly, adverse neurological and cognitive outcomes are approximately twice as common in infants who exhibit major hemorrhagic and nonhemorrhagic neuroimaging abnormalities or seizures (or both) in the neonatal period than in infants who do not exhibit such evidence of parenchymal injury.[234,236-238,243,249,266,292,300,301] The number of infants followed to school age has been relatively small. Further data will be of major interest.

TABLE 10-22	Outcome in Infants Treated with Extracorporeal Membrane Oxygenation*		
	PERCENTAGE OF INFANTS		
Outcome	**2000–2500 g**	**>2500 g**	**Total**
Mortality rate	34%	11%	14%
Neuroimaging abnormality (major)	41%	21%	27%
Major intracranial hemorrhage	28%	11%	13%
Developmental quotient <70	38%	8%	12%

*n = 29 for infants with birth weight 2000–2500 g; n = 235 for infants with birth weight >2500 g.
Data from Revenis ME, Glass P, Short BL: Mortality and morbidity rates among lower birth weight infants (2000 to 2500 grams) treated with extracorporeal membrane oxygenation, *J Pediatr* 121:452-458, 1992.

REFERENCES

1. Chaplin ER, Schlueter NA, Phibbs RH, Kitterman JA, et al: Fetal hemoglobin in the diagnosis of neonatal subarachnoid hemorrhage, *Pediatrics* 58:751-754, 1976.
2. Barnhart BJ, Lace JK, Yount JE: Diagnosis of intracranial hemorrhage: Technique using fluorescein, *J Pediatr* 95:289-292, 1979.
3. Donn SM, Sharp MJ, Kuhns LR, Uy JO, et al: Rapid detection of neonatal intracranial hemorrhage by transillumination, *Pediatrics* 64:843-847, 1979.
4. Andersen EA, Bucher D: Cerebrospinal fluid glutamine in intracranial hemorrhage in the newborn, *Acta Paediatr Scand* 75:899-904, 1986.
5. Hill A: Personal communication, 1994.
6. Walton JN: *Subarachnoid haemorrhage*, London: 1956, Churchill Livingstone.
7. Roost KT, Pimstone NR, Diamond I, Schmid R: The formation of cerebrospinal fluid xanthochromia after subarachnoid hemorrhage: Enzymatic conversion of hemoglobin to bilirubin by the arachnoid and choroid plexus, *Neurology* 22:973-977, 1972.
8. Hellstrom B, Kjellin KG: The diagnostic value of spectrophotometry of the CSF in the newborn period, *Dev Med Child Neurol* 12:789-797, 1971.
9. Arnold RG, Zetterstrom R: Proteins in the cerebrospinal fluid in the newborn, *Pediatrics* 27:279-289, 1958.

10. Bauer CH, New MI, Miller JM: Cerebrospinal fluid protein values of premature infants, *J Pediatr* 66:1017-1022, 1965.
11. Gyllensward A, Malmstrom S: The cerebrospinal fluid in mature infants, *Acta Paediatr* 51:933, 1962.
12. Naidoo BT: The cerebrospinal fluid in the healthy newborn infant, *S Afr Med J* 42:933-935, 1968.
13. Otila E: Studies on the cerebrospinal fluid in premature infants, *Acta Paediatr* 35:8, 1948.
14. Escobedo M, Barton L, Volpe J: Cerebrospinal fluid studies in an intensive care nursery, *J Perinat Med* 3:204-210, 1975.
15. Sarff LD, Platt LH, McCracken GH Jr: Cerebrospinal fluid evaluation in neonates: Comparison of high-risk infants with and without meningitis, *J Pediatr* 88:473-477, 1976.
16. Rodriguez AF, Kaplan SL, Mason EO Jr: Cerebrospinal fluid values in the very low birth weight infant, *J Pediatr* 116:971-974, 1990.
17. Mathew OP, Bland HE, Pickens JM, James EJ: Hypoglycorrhachia in the survivors of neonatal intracranial hemorrhage, *Pediatrics* 63:851-854, 1979.
18. Diebler C, Aicardi J: Hemorragie meningée du nourrison et hypoglycorrachie, *Pediatr* 30:1031-1036, 1973.
19. Deonna T, Oberson R: Acute subdural hematoma in the newborn: A case report and review of the literature, *Neuropadiatrie* 5:181-190, 1974.
20. Nelson RM, Bucciarelli RL, Nagel JW: Hypoglycorrhachia associated with intracranial hemorrhage in newborn infants, *J Pediatr* 94:800-803, 1979.
21. Mathew OP, Volpe JJ: Neonatal intraventricular hemorrhage: Hypoglycorrhachia and its relationship to CSF lactate levels, *J Pediatr* 97:292-295, 1980.
22. Troost BT, Walker JE, Cherington M: Hypoglycorrhachia associated with subarachnoid hemorrhage, *Arch Neurol* 19:438-442, 1968.
23. Fishman RA: *Cerebrospinal Fluid in Diseases of the Nervous System*, 2nd ed, Philadelphia: 1992, WB Saunders.
24. Dubynsky O, Vannucci R, Maisels MJ: Post-hemorrhagic encephalopathy in premature infants, *Pediatr Res* 12:551-560, 1978.
25. Craig WS: Intracranial haemorrhage in the newborn, *Arch Dis Child* 13:89, 1938.
26. Haller ES, Nesbitt RE Jr, Anderson GW: Clinical and pathologic concepts of gross intracranial hemorrhage in perinatal mortality, *Obstet Gynecol* 11:179-204, 1956.
27. Welch K, Strand R: Traumatic parturitional intracranial hemorrhage, *Dev Med Child Neurol* 28:156-164, 1986.
28. Huang CC, Shen EY: Tentorial subdural hemorrhage in term newborns: Ultrasonographic diagnosis and clinical correlates, *Pediatr Neurol* 7:171-177, 1991.
29. Hayashi T, Hashimoto T, Fukuda S, Ohshima Y, et al: Neonatal subdural hematoma secondary to birth injury: Clinical analysis of 48 survivors, *Child Nerv Syst* 3:23-29, 1987.
30. Tanaka Y, Sakamoto K, Kobayashi S, Kobayashi N, et al: Biphasic ventricular dilatation following posterior fossa subdural hematoma in the full-term neonate, *J Neurosurg* 68:211-216, 1988.
31. Hanigan WC, Morgan AM, Stahlberg LK, Hiller JL: Tentorial hemorrhage associated with vacuum extraction, *Pediatrics* 85:534-539, 1990.
32. Fleming GB, Morton ED: Meningeal haemorrhage in the newborn, *Arch Dis Child* 5:361, 1930.
33. Grontoft O: Intracranial haemorrhage and blood-brain barrier problems in the newborn, *Acta Path Microbiol Scand* 1:1, 1954.
34. Schwartz P: *Birth injuries of the Newborn: Morphology, Pathogenesis, Clinical Pathology and Prevention*, New York: 1961, Hafner.
35. Towbin A: Central nervous system damage in the premature related to the occurrence of mental retardation. In Angle CR, Bering EA, editors: *Physical Trauma as an Etiologic Agent in Mental Retardation*, Washington, DC: 1979, U.S. Government Printing Office.
36. Blank NK, Strand R, Gilles FH, Palakshappa A: Posterior fossa subdural hematomas in neonates, *Arch Neurol* 35:108-111, 1978.
37. Koch TK, Jahnke SE, Edwards MS, Davis SL: Posterior fossa hemorrhage in term newborns, *Pediatr Neurol* 1:96-99, 1985.
38. Pierre-Kahn A, Renier D, Sainte-Rose C, Hirsch JF: Acute intracranial hematomas in term neonates, *Child Nerv Syst* 2:191-194, 1986.
39. Castillo M, Fordham LA: MR of neurologically symptomatic newborns after vacuum extraction delivery, *AJNR Am J Neuroradiol* 16:816-818, 1995.
40. Hanigan WC, Powell FC, Miller TC, Wright RM: Symptomatic intracranial hemorrhage in full-term infants, *Childs Nerv Syst* 11:698-707, 1995.
41. Perrin RG, Rutka JT, Drake JM, Meltzer H, et al: Management and outcomes of posterior fossa subdural hematomas in neonates, *Neurosurgery* 40:1190-1199, 1997.
42. Holden KR, Titus MO, Van Tassel P: Cranial magnetic resonance imaging examination of normal term neonates: A pilot study, *J Child Neurol* 14:708-710, 1999.
43. Chammanvanakij S, Rollins N, Perlman JM: Subdural hematoma in term infants, *Pediatr Neurol* 26:301-304, 2002.
44. Whitby EH, Griffiths PD, Rutter S, Smith MF, et al: Frequency and natural history of subdural haemorrhages in babies and relation to obstetric factors, *Lancet* 363:846-851, 2004.
44a. Looney CB, Smith JK, Merck LH, Wolfe HM, et al: Intracranial hemorrhage in asymptomatic neonates: Prevalence on MR images and relationship to obstetric and neonatal risk factors, *Radiology* 242:535-541, 2007.
45. Wigglesworth JS, Husemeyer RP: Intracranial birth trauma in vaginal breech delivery: The continued importance of injury to the occipital bone, *Br J Obstet Gynaecol* 84:684-691, 1977.
46. Pape KE, Wigglesworth JS: *Hemorrhage, Ischemia, and the Perinatal Brain*, Philadelphia: 1979, JB Lippincott.
47. Hemsath FA: Birth injury of the occipital bone with a report of thirty-two cases, *Am J Obstet Gynecol* 27:194-201, 1933.
48. Schreiber MS: Some observations on certain head injuries of infants and children, *Med J Aust* 2:930-933, 1957.
49. Stephens RP, Richardson AC, Lewin JS: Bilateral subdural hematomas in a newborn infant, *Pediatrics* 99:619-621, 1997.
50. Aydinli N, Citak A, Caliskan M, Karabocuoglu M, et al: Vitamin K deficiency: Late onset intracranial haemorrhage, *Eur J Paediatr Neurol* 2:199-203, 1998.
51. O'Driscoll K, Meagher D, MacDonald D, Geoghegan F: Traumatic intracranial haemorrhage in firstborn infants and delivery with obstetric forceps, *Br J Obstet Gynaecol* 8:577, 1981.
52. Larroche JC: *Developmental Pathology of the Neonate*, New York: 1977, Excerpta Medica.
53. Flodmark O, Fitz CR, Harwood-Nash DC: CT diagnosis and short-term prognosis of intracranial hemorrhage and hypoxic/ischemic brain damage in neonates, *J Comput Assist Tomogr* 4:775-787, 1980.
54. Scotti G, Flodmark O, Hardwood-Nash DC, Humphreys RP: Posterior fossa hemorrhages in the newborn, *J Comput Assist Tomogr* 5:68-72, 1981.
55. Renzulli P, Tuchschmid P, Eich G, Fanconi S, et al: Early vitamin K deficiency bleeding after maternal phenobarbital intake: Management of massive intracranial haemorrhage by minimal surgical intervention, *Eur J Pediatr* 157:663-665, 1998.
56. Akman CI, Cracco J: Intrauterine subdural hemorrhage, *Dev Med Child Neurol* 42:843-846, 2000.
57. Hanigan WC, Ali MB, Cusack TJ, Miller TC, et al: Diagnosis of subdural hemorrhage in utero: Case report, *J Neurosurg* 63:977-979, 1985.
58. Atluru VL, Kumar IR: Intrauterine chronic subdural hematoma with postoperative tension pneumocephalus, *Pediatr Neurol* 3:306-309, 1987.
59. Mateos F, Esteban J, Martin-Puerto MJ, Miralles M, et al: Fetal subdural hematoma: Diagnosis in utero, *Pediatr Neurosci* 13:125-128, 1987.
60. Rotmensch S, Grannum PA, Nores JA, Hall C, et al: In utero diagnosis and management of fetal subdural hematoma, *Am J Obstet Gynecol* 164:1246-1248, 1991.
61. Scher MS, Wright FS, Lockman LA, Thompson T: Intraventricular hemorrhage in the full-term neonate, *Arch Neurol* 39:769-772, 1982.
62. Von Reuss A: *Diseases of the Newborn*, London: 1920, M.G.
63. Coblentz RG: Cerebellar subdural hematoma in an infant two weeks old with secondary hydrocephalus, *Surgery* 8:771, 1940.
64. Reigh EE, Nelson M: Posterior-fossa subdural hematoma with secondary hydrocephalus, *J Neurosurg* 19:346-348, 1962.
65. Pitlyk PJ, Miller RH, Stayura LA: Subdural hematoma of the posterior fossa: Report of a case, *Pediatrics* 40:436-439, 1967.
66. Carter LP, Pittman HW: Posterior fossa subdural hematoma of the newborn, *J Neurosurg* 34:423-426, 1971.
67. Gilles FH, Shillito J: Infantile hydrocephalus: Retrocerebellar subdural hematoma, *J Pediatr* 76:529-537, 1970.
68. Serfontein GL, Rom S, Stein S: Posterior fossa subdural hemorrhage in the newborn, *Pediatrics* 65:40-43, 1980.
69. Abroms IF, McLennan JE, Mandell F: Acute neonatal subdural hematoma following breech delivery, *Am J Dis Child* 131:192-194, 1977.
70. Deonna T, Calame A, van Melle G, Prod'Hom LS: Hypoglycorrhachia in neonatal intracranial hemorrhage, *Helv Paediatr Acta* 32:351-361, 1977.
71. Schipke R, Riege D, Scoville W: Acute subdural hemorrhage at birth, *Pediatrics* 14:468-474, 1954.
72. Volpe JJ, Manica JP, Land VJ, Coxe WS: Neonatal subdural hematoma associated with severe hemophilia A, *J Pediatr* 88:1023-1025, 1976.
73. Ravenel SD: Posterior fossa hemorrhage in the term newborn: Report of two cases, *Pediatrics* 64:39-42, 1979.
74. Hernansanz J, Munoz F, Rodriquez F: Subdural hematomas of the posterior fossa in normal-weight newborns, *J Neurosurg* 61:972-979, 1984.
75. Matson D: *Neurosurgery of Infancy and Childhood*, Springfield, IL: 1969, Charles C Thomas.
76. Rabe EF, Flynn RE, Dodge PR: Subdural collections of fluid in infants and children: A study of 62 patients with special reference to factors influencing prognosis and the efficacy of various forms of therapy, *Neurology* 18:559-570, 1968.
77. Ney JP, Joseph KR, Mitchell MH: Late subdural hygromas from birth trauma, *Neurology* 65:517, 2005.
78. Keeney SE, Adcock EW, McArdle CB: Prospective observations of 100 high-risk neonates by high-field (1.5 tesla) magnetic resonance imaging of the central nervous system. I. Intraventricular and extracerebral lesions, *Pediatrics* 87:421-429, 1991.
79. Barkovich AJ: *Pediatric Neuroimaging*, 4th ed, Philadelphia: 2005, Lippincott Williams & Wilkins.
80. Rutherford M: *MRI of the Neonatal Brain*, Philadelphia: 2002, WB Saunders.
81. Levene MI, Williams JL, Fawer CL: *Ultrasound of the Infant Brain*, London: 1985, Blackwell Scientific.
82. Chamnanvanakij S, Rollins N, Perlman JM: Subdural hematoma in term infants, *Pediatr Neurol* 26:301-304, 2002.

83. Roberts HM: Intracranial hemorrhage in the newborn, *JAMA* 113:280, 1939.
84. Gilles FH, Leviton A, Dooling EC: *The Developing Human Brain: Growth and Epidemiologic Neuropathology*, Boston: 1983, John Wright.
85. De Reuck JL: Cerebral angioarchitecture and perinatal brain lesions in premature and full-term infants, *Acta Neurol Scand* 70:391-395, 1984.
86. Friede RL: Subpial hemorrhage in infants, *J Neuropathol Exp Neurol* 31:548-556, 1972.
87. Huang AH, Robertson RL: Spontaneous superficial parenchymal and leptomeningeal hemorrhage in term neonates, *AJNR Am J Neuroradiol* 25:469-475, 2004.
88. Shackelford GD, Volpe JJ: Cranial ultrasonography in the evaluation of neonatal intracranial hemorrhage and its complications, *J Perinat Med* 13:293-304, 1985.
89. Rorke LB: *Pathology of Perinatal Brain Injury*, New York: 1982, Raven Press.
90. Grunnet ML, Shields WD: Cerebellar hemorrhage in the premature infant, *J Pediatr* 88:605-608, 1976.
91. Martin R, Roessmann U, Fanaroff A: Massive intracerebellar hemorrhage in low-birthweight infants, *J Pediatr* 89:290-293, 1976.
92. Pape KE, Armstrong DL, Fitzhardinge PM: Central nervous system pathology associated with mask ventilation in the very low birthweight infant: A new etiology for intracerebellar hemorrhages, *Pediatrics* 58:473-483, 1976.
93. Shuman RM, Oliver TK: Face masks defended, *Pediatrics* 58:621-623, 1976.
94. Flodmark O, Becker LE, Harwood-Nash DC, Fitzhardinge PM, et al: Correlation between computed tomography and autopsy in premature and full-term neonates that have suffered perinatal asphyxia, *Radiology* 137:93-103, 1980.
95. Papile LA, Burstein J, Burstein R, Koffler H: Incidence and evolution of subependymal and intraventricular hemorrhage: A study of infants with birth weights less than 1,500 gm, *J Pediatr* 92:529-534, 1978.
96. Ahmann PA, Lazzara A, Dykes FD, Brann AW Jr, et al: Intraventricular hemorrhage in the high-risk preterm infant: Incidence and outcome, *Ann Neurol* 7:118-124, 1980.
97. Merrill JD, Piecuch RE, Fell SC, Barkovich AJ, et al: A new pattern of cerebellar hemorrhages in preterm infants, *Pediatrics* 102:62, 1998.
98. Miall LS, Cornette LG, Tanner SF, Arthur RJ, et al: Posterior fossa abnormalities seen on magnetic resonance brain imaging in a cohort of newborn infants, *J Perinatol* 23:396-403, 2003.
99. Correa F, Enriquez G, Rossello J, Lucaya J, et al: Posterior fontanelle sonography: An acoustic window into the neonatal brain, *AJNR Am J Neuroradiol* 25:1274-1282, 2004.
100. Limperopoulos C, Benson CB, Bassan H, Di Salvo DN, et al: Cerebellar hemorrhage in the preterm infant: Ultrasonographic findings and risk factors, *Pediatrics* 116:717-724, 2005.
101. Donat JF, Okazaki H, Kleinberg F: Cerebellar hemorrhages in newborn infants, *Am J Dis Child* 133:441, 1979.
102. Fishman MA, Percy AK, Cheek WR, Speer ME: Successful conservative management of cerebellar hematomas in term neonates, *J Pediatr* 98:466-468, 1981.
103. Cheek WR, Fishman MA, Speer ME: Cerebellar hemorrhage in the term neonate, *Pediatr Neurosurg* 5:48-58, 1985.
104. Williamson WD, Percy AK, Fishman MA: Cerebellar hemorrhage in the term neonate: Developmental and neurologic outcome, *Pediatr Neurol* 1:356-360, 1985.
105. Newton TH, Gooding CA: Compression of superior sagittal sinus by neonatal calvarial molding, *Radiology* 115:635-640, 1975.
106. Chaou WT, Chou ML, Eitzman DV: Intracranial hemorrhage and vitamin K deficiency in early infancy, *J Pediatr* 105:880-884, 1984.
107. Dave P, Curless RG, Steinman L: Cerebellar hemorrhage complicating methylmalonic and propionic acidemia, *Arch Neurol* 41:1293-1296, 1984.
108. Fischer AQ, Challa VR, Burton BK, McLean W: Cerebellar hemorrhage complicating isovaleric acidemia: A case report, *Neurology* 31:746-748, 1981.
109. Reeder JD, Setzer ES, Kaude JV: Ultrasonographic detection of perinatal intracerebellar hemorrhage, *Pediatrics* 70:385-386, 1982.
110. Perlman JM, Nelson JS, McAlister WH, Volpe JJ: Intracerebellar hemorrhage in a premature newborn: Diagnosis by real-time ultrasound and correlation with autopsy findings, *Pediatrics* 71:159-162, 1983.
111. Fishman M: Personal communication, 1993.
112. Foy P, Dubbins PA, Waldrup L: Ultrasound demonstration of cerebellar hemorrhage in a neonate, *J Clin Ultrasound* 10:196-198, 1982.
113. Grant EG, Schellinger D, Richardson JD: Real-time ultrasonography of the posterior fossa, *J Ultrasound Med* 2:73-87, 1983.
114. Limperopoulos C, Bassan H, Gauvreau K, Robertson RL, et al: Does cerebellar injury in premature infants contribute to the high prevalence of long-term cognitive, learning, and behavioral disability in survivors? *Pediatrics* 120:584-593, 2007.
115. Odeku EL, Adcock KJ: Neonatal hydrocephalus due to intracerebellar hematoma, *Int Surg* 51:302-307, 1969.
116. Schreiber MS: Posterior fossa (cerebellar) haematoma in the newborn, *Med J Aust* 2:713-715, 1963.
117. Rom S, Serfontein GL, Humphreys RP: Intracerebellar hematoma in the neonate, *J Pediatr* 93:486-488, 1978.
118. Donat JF, Okazaki H, Kleinberg F, Reagan TJ: Intraventricular hemorrhage in full-term and premature infants, *Mayo Clin Proc* 53:437-441, 1978.
119. Cartwright GW, Culbertson K, Schreiner RL, Garg BP: Changes in clinical presentation of term infants with intracranial hemorrhage, *Dev Med Child Neurol* 21:730-737, 1979.
120. Palma PA, Miner ME, Morriss FH: Intraventricular hemorrhage in the neonate born at term, *Am J Dis Child* 133:941-944, 1979.
121. Leblanc R, O'Gorman AM: Neonatal intracranial hemorrhage: A clinical and serial computerized tomographic study, *J Neurosurg* 53:642-651, 1980.
122. Ludwig B, Brand M, Brockerhoff P: Post-partum CT examination of the heads of full-term infants, *Neuroradiology* 20:145-154, 1980.
123. Mitchell W, O'Tuama L: Cerebral intraventricular hemorrhage in infants: A widening age spectrum, *Pediatrics* 65:35-39, 1980.
124. Dubowitz LM, Levene MI, Morante A, Palmer P, et al: Neurologic signs in neonatal intraventricular hemorrhage: A correlation with real-time ultrasound, *J Pediatr* 99:127-133, 1981.
125. Flodmark O, Scotti G, Harwood-Nash DC: Clinical significance of ventriculomegaly in children who suffered perinatal asphyxia with or without intracranial hemorrhage: An 18 month follow-up study, *J Comput Assist Tomogr* 5:663-673, 1981.
126. Levene MI, Wigglesworth JS, Dubowitz V: Cerebral structure and intraventricular haemorrhage in the neonate: A real-time ultrasound study, *Arch Dis Child* 56:416-424, 1981.
127. Lacey DJ, Terplan K: Intraventricular hemorrhage in full-term neonates, *Dev Med Child Neurol* 24:332-337, 1982.
128. MacKay RJ, De Crespigny LC, Murton LJ, Roy RN: Intraventricular hemorrhage in term neonates: Diagnosis by ultrasound, *Aust Paediatr J* 18:205-207, 1982.
129. Fenichel GM, Webster DL, Wong WK: Intracranial hemorrhage in the term newborn, *Arch Neurol* 41:30-34, 1984.
130. Nanba E, Eda I, Takashima S: Intracranial hemorrhage in the full-term neonate and young infant: Correlation of the location and outcome, *Brain Dev* 6:435-443, 1984.
131. Bergman I, Bauer RE, Barmada MA: Intracerebellar hemorrhage in the full-term neonatal infant, *Pediatrics* 75:488-496, 1985.
132. Friede RL: *Developmental Neuropathology*, 2nd ed, New York: 1989, Springer-Verlag.
133. Hayden CK, Shattuck KE, Richardson CJ: Subependymal germinal matrix hemorrhage in full-term neonates, *Pediatrics* 75:714-718, 1985.
134. Hill A, Volpe JJ: Pathogenesis and management of hypoxic-ischemic encephalopathy in the term newborn, *Neurol Clin* 3:31-46, 1985.
135. Zorzi C, Angonese I, Nardelli GB, Cantarutti F: Spontaneous intraventricular haemorrhage in utero, *Eur J Pediatr* 148:83-85, 1988.
136. Roland EH, Flodmark O, Hill A: Thalamic hemorrhage with intraventricular hemorrhage in the full-term newborn, *Pediatrics* 85:737-741, 1990.
137. Wehberg K, Vincent M, Garrison B, Dilustro JF, et al: Intraventricular hemorrhage in the full-term neonate associated with abdominal compression, *Pediatrics* 89:327-329, 1992.
138. Jocelyn LJ, Casiro OG: Neurodevelopmental outcome of term infants with intraventricular hemorrhage, *Am J Dis Child* 146:194-197, 1992.
139. Heibel M, Heber R, Bechinger D, Kornhuber HH: Early diagnosis of perinatal cerebral lesions in apparently normal full-term newborns by ultrasound of the brain, *Neuroradiology* 35:85-91, 1993.
140. Weissman BM, Foster D, Baley JE: Primary thalamic hemorrhage in a preterm infant, *Pediatr Neurol* 3:121-122, 1987.
141. Monteiro JP, Roulet-Perez E, Davidoff V, Deonna T: Primary neonatal thalamic haemorrhage and epilepsy with continuous spike-wave during sleep: A longitudinal follow-up of a possible significant relation, *Eur J Paediatr Neurol* 5:41-47, 2001.
142. Heck DV, Gailloud P, Cohen HL, Clatterbuck RE, et al: Choroid plexus arteriovenous malformation presenting with intraventricular hemorrhage, *J Pediatr* 141:710-711, 2002.
143. Wu YW, Hamrick SEG, Miller SP, Haward MF, et al: Intraventricular hemorrhage in term neonates caused by sinovenous thrombosis, *Ann Neurol* 54:123-126, 2003.
144. Trounce JQ, Dodd KL, Fawer CL: Primary thalamic haemorrhage in the newborn: A new clinical entity, *Lancet* 1:190, 1985.
145. Adams C, Hochhauser L, Logan WJ: Primary thalamic and caudate hemorrhage in term neonates presenting with seizures, *Pediatr Neurol* 4:175-177, 1988.
146. de Vries LS, Smet M, Goemans N, Wilms G, et al: Unilateral thalamic haemorrhage in the pre-term and full-term newborn, *Neuropediatrics* 23:153-156, 1992.
147. Burrows RF, Kelton JG: Low fetal risks in pregnancies associated with idiopathic thrombocytopenic purpura, *Am J Obstet Gynecol* 163:1147-1150, 1990.
148. Zalneraitis EL, Young RS, Krishnamoorthy KS: Intracranial hemorrhage in utero as a complication of isoimmune thrombocytopenia, *J Pediatr* 95:611-614, 1979.
149. Palchak AE, Aster RH, Gottschall J, Opitz JM: Effect of maternal-fetal platelet incompatibility on fetal development, *Pediatrics* 74:570, 1984.
150. Naidu S, Messmore H, Caserta V, Fine M: CNS lesions in neonatal isoimmune thrombocytopenia, *Arch Neurol* 40:552-554, 1983.

151. Herman JH, Jumbelic MI, Ancona RJ, Kickler TS: In utero cerebral hemorrhage in alloimmune thrombocytopenia, *J Pediatr Hematol Oncol* 8:312-317, 1986.

152. Manson J, Speed I, Abbott K, Crompton J: Congenital blindness, porencephaly, and neonatal thrombocytopenia: A report of four cases, *J Child Neurol* 3:120-124, 1988.

153. Davidson JE, McWilliam RC, Evans TJ, Stephenson JB: Porencephaly and optic hypoplasia in neonatal isoimmune thrombocytopenia, *Arch Dis Child* 64:858-860, 1989.

154. Matsui K, Ohsaki E, Goto A, Koresawa M, et al: Perinatal intracranial hemorrhage due to severe neonatal alloimmune thrombocytopenic purpura (NAITP) associated with anti-Yuk^b (HPA-4a) antibodies, *Brain Dev* 17:352-355, 1995.

155. Hanigan WC, Powell FC, Palagallo G, Miller TC: Lobar hemorrhages in full-term neonates, *Child Nerv Syst* 11:276-280, 1995.

156. Glade-Bender J, McFarland JG, Kaplan C, Porcelijn L, et al: Anti-HPA-3A induces severe neonatal alloimmune thrombocytopenia, *J Pediatr* 138:862-867, 2001.

157. Kanbai HH, Brand A: Fetal thrombocytopenia. In James DK, Steer PJ, Weiner CP, et al, editors: *High-Risk Pregnancy Management Options*, 3rd ed, Philadelphia: 2006, Elsevier.

158. Radder CM, Brand A, Kanhai HH: A less invasive treatment strategy to prevent intracranial hemorrhage in fetal and neonatal alloimmune thrombocytopenia, *Am J Obstet Gynecol* 185:683-688, 2001.

159. Radder CM, Roelen DL, van de Meer-Prins EMW, Claas FHJ, et al: The immunologic profile of infants born after maternal immunoglobulin treatment and intrauterine platelet transfusions for fetal/neonatal alloimmune thrombocytopenia, *Am J Obstet Gynecol* 191:815-820, 2004.

160. Bussel J, Berkowitz R, McFarland J, Lynch L, et al: Antenatal treatment of neonatal alloimmune thrombocytopenia, *N Engl J Med* 319:1374-1378, 1988.

161. Overton TG, Duncan KR, Jolly M, Letsky E, et al: Serial aggressive platelet transfusion for fetal alloimmune thrombocytopenia: Platelet dynamics and perinatal outcome, *Am J Obstet Gynecol* 186:826-831, 2002.

162. Skacel PO, Contreras M: Neonatal alloimmune thrombocytopenia, *Blood Rev* 3:174-179, 1989.

163. Mueller-Eckhardt C, Kiefel V, Grubert A: High-dose IgG treatment for neonatal alloimmune thrombocytopenia, *Blut* 59:145-146, 1989.

164. Hershenson MB, Hageman JR, Brouillette RT: Neonatal spinal cord dysfunction associated with disseminated intravascular coagulation, *Dev Med Child Neurol* 24:686-691, 1982.

165. Silverstein A: Intracranial bleeding in hemophilia, *Arch Neurol* 3:141-149, 1960.

166. Baehner RL, Strauss HS: Hemophilia in the first year of life, *N Engl J Med* 275:524-528, 1966.

167. Bray GL, Luban NL: Hemophilia presenting with intracranial hemorrhage: An approach to the infant with intracranial bleeding and coagulopathy, *Am J Dis Child* 141:1215-1217, 1987.

168. Yoffe G, Buchanan GR: Intracranial hemorrhage in newborn and young infants with hemophilia, *J Pediatr* 113:333-336, 1988.

169. Ries M, Wolfel D, Maierbrandt B: Severe intracranial hemorrhage in a newborn infant with transplacental transfer of an acquired factor VIII:C inhibitor, *J Pediatr* 127:649-650, 1995.

170. Sumer T, Ahmad M, Sumer NK, Al-Mouzan MI: Severe congenital factor X deficiency with intracranial haemorrhage, *Eur J Pediatr* 145:119-120, 1986.

171. Ermis B, Ors R, Tastekin A, Orhan F: Severe congenital factor X deficiency with intracranial bleeding in two siblings, *Brain Dev* 26:137-138, 2004.

172. Herrmann FH, Navarette M, Salazar-Sanchez L, Carillo JM, et al: Homozygous factor X gene mutations Gly380Arg and Tyr163delAT are associated with perinatal intracranial hemorrhage, *J Pediatr* 146:128-130, 2005.

173. Baud O, Picard V, Durand P, Duchemin J, et al: Intracerebral hemorrhage associated with a novel antithrombin gene mutation in a neonate, *J Pediatr* 139:741-743, 2001.

174. Lane PA, Hathaway WE: Vitamin K in infancy, *J Pediatr* 106:351-359, 1985.

175. Cooper NA, Lynch MA: Delayed hemorrhagic disease of the newborn with extradural hematoma, *BMJ* 1:164-165, 1979.

176. Lorber J, Lilleyman JS, Peile EB: Acute infantile thrombocytosis and vitamin K deficiency associated with intracranial hemorrhage, *Arch Dis Child* 54:471-472, 1979.

177. Lane PA, Hathaway WE, Githens JH: Fatal intracranial hemorrhage in a normal infant secondary to vitamin K deficiency, *Pediatrics* 72:562-564, 1983.

178. McNinch AW, Orme RL, Tripp JH: Haemorrhagic disease of the newborn returns, *Lancet* 1:1089-1090, 1983.

179. Motohara K, Matsukura M, Matsuda I, Iribe K, et al: Severe vitamin K deficiency in breast-fed infants, *J Pediatr* 105:943-945, 1984.

180. Shapiro AD, Jacobson LJ, Arman ME, Manco-Johnson MJ, et al: Vitamin K deficiency in the newborn infant: Prevalence and perinatal risk factors, *J Pediatr* 109:675-680, 1986.

181. Matsuzaka T, Yoshinaga M, Tsuji Y, Yasunaga A, et al: Incidence and causes of intracranial hemorrhage in infancy: A prospective surveillance study after vitamin K prophylaxis, *Brain Dev* 11:384-388, 1989.

182. Hathaway WE, Isarangkura PB, Mahasandana C, Jacobson L, et al: Comparison of oral and parenteral vitamin K prophylaxis for prevention of late hemorrhagic disease of the newborn, *J Pediatr* 119:461-464, 1991.

183. Greer FR, Marshall S, Cherry J, Suttie JW: Vitamin K status of lactating mothers, human milk, and breast feeding infants, *Pediatrics* 88:751-756, 1991.

184. von Kries R, Gobel U: Vitamin K prophylaxis and vitamin K deficiency bleeding (VKDB) in early infancy, *Acta Paediatr* 81:655-657, 1992.

185. American Academy of Pediatrics Vitamin K Ad Hoc Task Force: Controversies concerning vitamin K and the newborn, *Pediatrics* 91:1001-1003, 1993.

186. Matsuzaka T, Tanaka H, Fukuda M, Aoki M, et al: Relationship between vitamin K dependent coagulation factors and anticoagulants (protein-C and protein-S) in neonatal vitamin K deficiency, *Arch Dis Child* 68:297-302, 1993.

187. von Kries R, Hachmeister A, Gobel U: Oral mixed micellar vitamin K for prevention of late vitamin K deficiency bleeding, *Arch Dis Child Fetal Neonatal Ed* 88:F109-F112, 2003.

188. Payne NR, Hasegawa DK: Vitamin K deficiency in newborns: A case report with alpha-1-antitrypsin deficiency and a review of factors predisposing to hemorrhage, *Pediatrics* 73:712-716, 1984.

189. Newcomb AL, Munns GF: Rupture of aneurysm of the circle of Willis in the newborn, *Pediatrics* 3:769-778, 1949.

190. Jones RK, Shearburn EW: Intracranial aneurysm in a four-week-old infant, *J Neurosurg* 18:122-124, 1961.

191. Garcia-Chavez C, Moosy J: Cerebral artery aneurysm in infants: Association with agenesis of the corpus callosum, *J Neuropathol* 24:492-497, 1965.

192. Thompson RA, Pribram HF: Infantile cerebral aneurysm associated with ophthalmoplegia and quadriparesis, *Neurology* 19:785-789, 1969.

193. Pickering LK, Hogan GR, Gilbert EF: Aneurysm of the posterior inferior cerebellar artery, *Am J Dis Child* 119:155-158, 1970.

194. Grode ML, Saunders M, Carton CA: Subarachnoid hemorrhage secondary to ruptured aneurysms in infants, *J Neurosurg* 49:898-902, 1978.

195. Lee YJ, Kandall SR, Ghali VS: Intracerebral arterial aneurysm in a newborn, *Arch Neurol* 35:171-172, 1978.

196. Hungerford GD, Marzluff JM, Kempe LG, Powers JM: Cerebral arterial aneurysm in a neonate, *Neuroradiology* 21:107-110, 1981.

197. Zee C-S, Segall HD, McComb G, Stanley P, et al: Intracranial arterial aneurysms in childhood: More recent considerations, *J Child Neurol* 1:99-114, 1986.

198. Afifi AK, Godersky JC, Menezes A, Smoker WR, et al: Cerebral hemiatrophy, hypoplasia of internal carotid artery and intracranial aneurysm, *Arch Neurol* 44:232-235, 1987.

199. Putty TK, Luerssen TG, Campbell RL, Boaz JC, et al: Magnetic resonance imaging diagnosis of a cerebral aneurysm in an infant, *Pediatr Neurosurg* 91:48-51, 1990.

200. Ferrante L, Fortuna A, Celli P, Santoro A, et al: Intracranial arterial aneurysms in early childhood, *Neurosurgery* 70:420-425, 1988.

201. Frank E, Zusman E: Aneurysms of the distal anterior cerebral artery in infants, *Pediatr Neurosurg* 16:179-182, 1990.

202. Boop FA, Chadduck WM, Sawyer J, Husain M: Congenital aneurysmal hemorrhage and astrocytoma in an infant, *Pediatr Neurosurg* 17:44-47, 1991.

203. Piatt JH, Clunie DA: Intracranial arterial aneurysm due to birth trauma, *J Neurosurg* 77:799-803, 1992.

204. Kuchelmeister K, Schulz R, Bergmann M, Schwuchow R, et al: A probably familial saccular aneurysm of the anterior communicating artery in a neonate, *Childs Nerv Syst* 9:302-305, 1993.

205. Musaynski CA, Carpenter RJ, Armstrong DL: Prenatal sonographic detection of basilar aneurysm, *Pediatr Neurol* 10:70-72, 1994.

206. Pollo C, Meagher-Villmure K, Bernath MA, Vernet O, et al: Ruptured cerebral aneurysm in the early stage of life: A congenital origin? *Neuropediatrics* 35:230-233, 2004.

207. Song JK, Nimi Y, Brisman JL, Fernandez PM, et al: Multiple cerebral aneurysms in a neonate: Occlusion and rupture, *J Neurosurg* 102:81-85, 2005.

208. Kourtopoulos H: Neonatal aneurysms, *J Neurosurg* 103(Suppl):472, 2005.

209. Baird WF, Stitt DG: Arteriovenous aneurysm of the cerebellum in a premature infant, *Pediatrics* 24:455-457, 1959.

210. Ross DA, Walker J, Edwards MS: Unusual posterior fossa dural arteriovenous malformation in a neonate: Case report, *Neurosurgery* 19:1021-1024, 1986.

211. Park TS, Cail WS, Delashaw JB, Kattwinkel J: Spinal cord arteriovenous malformation in a neonate: Case report, *J Neurosurg* 64:322-324, 1986.

212. Esparza J, Perez-Higueras A, Perez-Diaz C, Ramo C: Arteriovenous malformation of the spinal cord in the neonate, *Child Nerv Syst* 3:301-303, 1987.

213. Haase J, Hobolth N, Ringsted J: Growing intracranial arteriovenous malformation in a newborn, *Child Nerv Sys* 2:270-272, 1986.

214. Godersky JC, Menezes AH: Intracranial arteriovenous anomalies of infancy: Modern concepts, *Pediatr Neurosci* 13:242-250, 1987.

215. Tessler FN, Dion J, Vinuela F, Perrella RR, et al: Cranial arteriovenous malformations in neonates: Color Doppler imaging with angiographic correlation, *AJR Am J Roentgenol* 153:1027-1030, 1989.

216. Heafner MD, Duncan CC, Kier EL: Intraventricular hemorrhage in a term neonate secondary to a third ventricular AVM, *J Neurosurg* 63:640-643, 1985.

217. Singman R, Asaikar S, Hotson G, Prose NS: Aplasia cutis congenita and arteriovenous fistula: Case report and review, *Arch Neurol* 47:1255-1258, 1990.

218. Wakai S, Andohl Y, Nagai M, Teramoto C, et al: Choroid plexus arteriovenous malformation in a full-term neonate, *J Neurosurg* 72:127-129, 1990.

219. Malik GM, Sadasivan B, Knighton RS, Ausman JI: The management of arteriovenous malformations in children, *Childs Nerv Syst* 7:43-47, 1991.

220. Tomlinson FH, Piepgras DG, Nichols DA, Rufenacht DA, et al: Remote congenital cerebral arteriovenous fistulae associated with aortic coarctation, *J Neurosurg* 76:137-142, 1992.

221. Hayashi N, Endo S, Oka N, Takeda S, et al: Intracranial hemorrhage due to rupture of an arteriovenous malformation in a full-term neonate, *Child Nerv Syst* 10:344-346, 1994.

222. Rodesch G, Malherbe V, Alvarez H, Zerah M, et al: Nongalenic cerebral arteriovenous malformations in neonates and infants, *Child Nerv Syst* 11:231-241, 1995.

223. Ozek E, Ozek M, Bilgen H, Kilic T, et al: Neonatal intracranial hemorrhage due to rupture of arteriovenous malformation, *Pediatr Neurol* 15:53-56, 1996.

224. Hayashi T, Ichiyama T, Nishikawa M, Furukawa S, et al: A case of a large neonatal arteriovenous malformation with heart failure: Color Doppler sonography, MRI and MR angiography as early non-invasive diagnostic procedures, *Brain Dev* 18:236-238, 1996.

225. Nakayama H, Suzuki S, Hikino S, Tezuka J, et al: Multiple cerebral arteriovenous fistulas and malformations in the neonate, *Pediatr Neurol* 25:236-238, 2001.

226. Keith JD: Coarctation of the aorta. In Keith JD, Rowe RD, Vlad P, editors: *Heart Disease in Infancy and Childhood*, New York: 1978, Macmillan.

227. Young RS, Liberthson RR, Zalneraitis EL: Cerebral hemorrhage in neonates with coarctation of the aorta, *Stroke* 13:491-494, 1982.

228. Mehwald PS, Dittrich S, Grohmann J, Bley T, et al: Coarctation of the aorta presenting as cerebral hemorrhage, *J Pediatr* 146:293, 2005.

229. Aggett PJ, Till K: Intracerebral haematoma with communicating hydrocephalus in a neonate, *Proc R Soc Med* 69:877-879, 1976.

230. Chaplin ER, Goldstein GW, Norman D: Neonatal seizures, intracerebral hematoma, and subarachnoid hemorrhage in full-term infants, *Pediatrics* 63:812-815, 1979.

231. Blazer S, Hemli JA, Sujov PO, Braun J: Neonatal bilateral diaphragmatic paralysis caused by brain stem haemorrhage, *Arch Dis Child* 64:50-52, 1989.

232. Mutoh K, Ito M, Okuno T, Mikawa H, et al: Nontraumatic spinal intramedullary hemorrhage in an infant, *Pediatr Neurol* 5:53-56, 1989.

233. Mendoza JC, Shearer LL, Cook LN: Lateralization of brain lesions following extracorporeal membrane oxygenation, *Pediatrics* 88:1004-1009, 1991.

234. Taylor GA, Fitz CR, Miller MK, Garin DB, et al: Intracranial abnormalities in infants treated with extracorporeal membrane oxygenation: Imaging with US and CT, *Radiology* 165:675-678, 1987.

235. Revenis ME, Glass P, Short BL: Mortality and morbidity rates among lower birth weight infants (2000 to 2500 grams) treated with extracorporeal membrane oxygenation, *J Pediatr* 121:452-458, 1992.

236. Streletz LJ, Bej MD, Graziani LJ, Desai HJ, et al: Utility of serial EEGs in neonates during extracorporeal membrane oxygenation, *Pediatr Neurol* 8:190-196, 1992.

237. Korinthenberg R, Kachel W, Koelfen W, Schultze C, et al: Neurological findings in newborn infants after extracorporeal membrane oxygenation, with special reference to the EEG, *Dev Med Child Neurol* 35:249-257, 1993.

238. Hahn JS, Vaucher Y, Bejar R, Coen RW: Electroencephalographic and neuroimaging findings in neonates undergoing extracorporeal membrane oxygenation, *Neuropediatrics* 24:19-24, 1993.

239. Brunberg JA, Kewitz G, Schumacher RE: Venovenous extracorporeal membrane oxygenation: Early CT alterations following use in management of severe respiratory failure in neonates, *AJNR Am J Neuroradiol* 14:595-603, 1993.

240. Cornish JD, Heiss KF, Clark RH, Strieper MJ, et al: Efficacy of venovenous extracorporeal membrane oxygenation for neonates with respiratory and circulatory compromise, *J Pediatr* 122:105-109, 1993.

241. Robertson C, Finer NN, Sauve RS, Whitfield MF, et al: Neurodevelopmental outcome after neonatal extracorporeal membrane oxygenation, *CMAJ* 152:1981-1988, 1995.

242. Bernbaum J, Schwartz JP, Gerdes M, D'Agostino JA, et al: Survivors of extracorporeal membrane oxygenation at 1 year of age: The relationship of primary diagnosis with health and neurodevelopmental sequelae, *Pediatrics* 96:907-913, 1995.

243. Vaucher YE, Dudell GG, Bejar R, Gist K: Predictors of early childhood outcome in candidates for extracorporeal membrane oxygenation, *J Pediatr* 128:109-117, 1996.

244. Hardart GE, Fackler JC: Predictors of intracranial hemorrhage during neonatal extracorporeal membrane oxygenation, *J Pediatr* 134:156-159, 1999.

245. Desai SA, Stanley C, Gringlas M, Merton DA, et al: Five-year followup of neonates with reconstructed right common carotid arteries after extracorporeal membrane oxygenation, *J Pediatr* 134:428-433, 1999.

246. Van Heist A, Liem D, Hopman J, Van Der Staak F, et al: Oxygenation and hemodynamics in left and right cerebral hemispheres during induction of veno-arterial extracorporeal membrane oxygenation, *J Pediatr* 144:223-228, 2004.

247. Davis PJ, Firmin RK, Manktelow B, Goldman AP, et al: Long-term outcome following extracorporeal membrane oxygenation for congenital diaphragmatic hernia: The UK experience, *J Pediatr* 144:309-315, 2004.

248. Hardart GE, Hardart MK, Arnold JH: Intracranial hemorrhage in premature neonates treated with extracorporeal membrane oxygenation correlates with conceptional age, *J Pediatr* 145:184-189, 2004.

249. Parish AP, Bunyapen C, Cohen MJ, Garrison T, et al: Seizures as a predictor of long-term neurodevelopmental outcome in survivors of neonatal extracorporeal membrane oxygenation (ECMO), *J Child Neurol* 19:930-934, 2004.

250. Wu TW, Miller SP, Chin K, Collins AE, et al: Multiple risk factors in neonatal sinovenous thrombosis, *Neurology* 59:438-440, 2002.

251. Stolar CJ, Snedecor SM, Bartlett RH: Extracorporeal membrane oxygenation and neonatal respiratory failure: Experience from the extracorporeal life support organization, *J Pediatr Surg* 26:563-571, 1991.

252. Kupsky W. Personal communication, 1992.

253. Taylor GA, Fitz CR, Kapur S, Short BL: Cerebrovascular accidents in neonates treated with extracorporeal membrane oxygenation: Sonographic-pathologic correlation, *AJR Am J Roentgenol* 153:355-361, 1989.

254. Taylor GA, Short BL, Fitz CR: Clinical and laboratory observations: Imaging of cerebrovascular injury in infants treated with extracorporeal membrane oxygenation, *J Pediatr* 114:635-639, 1989.

255. Bulas DI, Taylor GA, Fitz CR, Revenis ME, et al: Posterior fossa intracranial hemorrhage in infants treated with extracorporeal membrane oxygenation: Sonographic findings, *AJR Am J Roentgenol* 156:571-575, 1991.

256. Wiznitzer M, Masaryk TJ, Lewin J, Walsh M, et al: Parenchymal and vascular magnetic resonance imaging of the brain after extracorporeal membrane oxygenation, *Am J Dis Ch* 144:1323-1326, 1990.

257. Babcock DS, Han BK, Weiss RG, Ryckman FC: Brain abnormalities in infants on extracorporeal membrane oxygenation: Sonographic and CT findings, *AJR Am J Roentgenol* 153:571-576, 1989.

258. Cilley RE, Zwischenberger JB, Andrews AF, Bowerman RA, et al: Intracranial hemorrhage during extracorporeal membrane oxygenation in neonates, *Pediatrics* 78:699-704, 1986.

259. Bowerman RA, Zwischenberger JB, Andrews AF, Bartlett RH: Cranial sonography of the infant treated with extracorporeal membrane oxygenation, *AJNR Am J Neuroradiol* 6:377-382, 1985.

260. Campbell RL, Bunyapen C, Holmes GL, Howell CG, et al: Right common carotid artery ligation in extracorporeal membrane oxygenation, *J Pediatr* 113:110-113, 1988.

261. Schumacher RE, Barks JDE, Johnston MV, Donn SM, et al: Right-sided brain lesions in infants following extracorporeal membrane oxygenation, *Pediatrics* 82:115-161, 1988.

262. Jarjour IT, Ahdab-Barmada A: Cerebrovascular lesions in infants and children dying after extracorporeal membrane oxygenation, *Pediatr Neurol* 10:13-19, 1994.

263. Graziani LJ, Streletz LJ, Mitchell DG, Merton DA, et al: Electroencephalographic, neuroradiologic, and neurodevelopmental studies in infants with subclavian steal during ECMO, *Pediatr Neurol* 10:97-103, 1994.

264. Evans MJ, Mckeever PA, Pearson GA, Field D, et al: Pathological complications of non-survivors of newborn extracorporeal membrane oxygenation, *Arch Dis Child Fetal Neonatal Ed* 71:F88-F92, 1994.

265. Van Meurs KP, Nguyen HT, Rhine WD, Marks MP, et al: Intracranial abnormalities and neurodevelopmental status after venovenous extracorporeal membrane oxygenation, *J Pediatr* 125:304-307, 1994.

266. Lago P, Rebsamen S, Clancy RR, Pinto-Martin J, et al: MRI, MRA and neurodevelopmental outcome following neonatal ECMO, *Pediatr Neurol* 12:294-305, 1995.

267. Mitchell DG, Merton D, Desai H, Needleman L, et al: Neonatal brain: Color Doppler imaging. II. Altered flow patterns from extracorporeal membrane oxygenation, *Radiology* 167:307-310, 1988.

268. Raju TNK, Kim SY, Meller JL, Srinivasan G, et al: Circle of Willis blood velocity and flow direction after common carotid artery ligation for neonatal extracorporeal membrane oxygenation, *Pediatrics* 83:343-347, 1989.

269. Taylor GA, Catena LM, Garin DB, Miller MK, et al: Intracranial flow patterns in infants undergoing extracorporeal membrane oxygenation: Preliminary observations with Doppler US, *Radiology* 165:671-674, 1987.

270. Taylor GA, Short BL, Glass P, Ichord R: Cerebral hemodynamics in infants undergoing extracorporeal membrane oxygenation: Further observations, *Radiology* 168:163-167, 1988.

271. Mitchell DG, Merton DA, Graziani LJ, Desai HJ, et al: Right carotid artery ligation in neonates: Classification of collateral flow with color Doppler imaging, *Radiology* 175:117-123, 1990.

272. Matsumoto JS, Babcock DS, Brody AS, Weiss RG, et al: Right common carotid artery ligation for extracorporeal membrane oxygenation: Cerebral blood flow velocity measurement with Doppler duplex US, *Radiology* 175:757-760, 1990.

273. Lohrer RM, Bejar RF, Simko AJ, Moulton SL, et al: Internal carotid artery blood flow velocities before, during, and after extracorporeal membrane oxygenation, *Am J Dis Child* 146:201-207, 1992.

274. Alexander AA, Mitchell DG, Merton DA, Desai HJ, et al: Cannula-induced vertebral steal in neonates during extracorporeal membrane oxygenation: Detection with color Doppler US, *Radiology* 182:527-530, 1992.

275. Liem KD, Hopman JCW, Osenburg B, de Haan AFJ, et al: Cerebral oxygenation and hemodynamics during induction of extracorporeal membrane oxygenation as investigated by near infrared spectrophotometry, *Pediatrics* 95:555-561, 1995.

276. Taylor GA, Walker LK: Intracranial venous system in newborns treated with extracorporeal membrane oxygenation: Doppler US evaluation after ligation of the right jugular vein, *Radiology* 183:453-456, 1992.

277. Perlman JM, Altman DI: Symmetric cerebral blood flow in newborns who have undergone successful extracorporeal membrane oxygenation, *Pediatrics* 89:235-239, 1992.

278. Lewin JS, Masaryk TJ, Modic MT, Rose JS, et al: Extracorporeal membrane oxygenation in infants: Angiographic and parenchymal evaluation of the brain with MR imaging, *Radiology* 173:361-365, 1989.

279. Klesh KW, Murphy TF, Scher MS, Buchanan DE, et al: Cerebral infarction in persistent pulmonary hypertension of the newborn, *Am J Dis Child* 141:852-857, 1987.

280. Grayck EN, Meliones JN, Kern FH, Hansell DR, et al: Elevated serum lactate correlates with intracranial hemorrhage in neonates treated with extracorporeal life support, *Pediatrics* 96:914-917, 1995.

281. Gleason CA, Short BL, Jones MD Jr: Cerebral blood flow and metabolism during and after prolonged hypocapnia in newborn lambs, *J Pediatr* 115:309-314, 1989.

282. Short BL, Walker K, Bender KS, Traystman RJ: Impairment of cerebral autoregulation during extracorporeal membrane oxygenation in newborn lambs, *Pediatr Res* 33:289-294, 1993.

283. Short BL, Walker LK, Gleason CA, Jones MD, et al: Effect of extracorporeal membrane oxygenation on cerebral blood flow and cerebral oxygen metabolism in newborn sheep, *Pediatr Res* 28:50-53, 1990.

284. Liem KD, Kollee LAA, Klaessens JHG, de Haan AFJ, et al: The influence of extracorporeal membrane oxygenation on cerebral oxygenation and hemodynamics in normoxemic and hypoxemic piglets, *Pediatr Res* 39:209-215, 1996.

285. Taylor GA, Glass P, Fitz CR, Miller MK: Neurologic status in infants treated with extracorporeal membrane oxygenation: Correlation of imaging findings with developmental outcome, *Radiology* 165:679-682, 1987.

286. Glass P, Miller M, Short B: Morbidity for survivors of extracorporeal membrane oxygenation: Neurodevelopmental outcome at 1 year of age, *Pediatrics* 83:72-78, 1989.

287. Dworetz AR, Moya FR, Sabo B, Gladstone I, et al: Survival of infants with persistent pulmonary hypertension without extracorporeal membrane oxygenation, *Pediatrics* 84:1-6, 1989.

288. O'Rourke PP, Crone RK, Vacanti JP, Ware JH, et al: Extracorporeal membrane oxygenation and conventional medical therapy in neonates with persistent pulmonary hypertension of the newborn: A prospective randomized study, *Pediatrics* 84:957-963, 1989.

289. Schumacher RE, Palmer TW, Roloff DW, La Claire PA, et al: Follow-up of infants treated with extracorporeal membrane oxygenation for newborn respiratory failure, *Pediatrics* 87:451-457, 1991.

290. Hofkosh D, Thompson AE, Nozza RJ, Kemp SS, et al: Ten years of extracorporeal membrane oxygenation: Neurodevelopmental outcome, *Pediatrics* 87:549-555, 1991.

291. Lott IT, McPherson D, Towne B, Johnson D, et al: Long-term neurophysiologic outcome after neonatal extracorporeal membrane oxygenation, *J Pediatr* 116:343-349, 1990.

292. Campbell LR, Bunyapen C, Gangarosa ME, Cohen M, et al: Significance of seizures associated with extracorporeal membrane oxygenation, *J Pediatr* 119:789-792, 1991.

293. Paccioretti DC, Haluschak MM, Finer NN, Robertson C, et al: Auditory brain-stem responses in neonates receiving extracorporeal membrane oxygenation, *J Pediatr* 120:464-467, 1992.

294. Beck R, Anderson KD, Pearson GD, Cronin J, et al: Criteria for extracorporeal membrane oxygenation in a population of infants with persistent pulmonary hypertension of the newborn, *J Pediatr Surg* 21:297-302, 1986.

295. Bartlett RH, Roloff DW, Cornell RG, Andrews AF, et al: Extracorporeal circulation in neonatal respiratory failure: A prospective randomized study, *Pediatrics* 76:479-487, 1985.

296. Glass P, Wagner AE, Papero PH, Rajasingham SR, et al: Neurodevelopmental status at age five years of neonates treated with extracorporeal membrane oxygenation, *J Pediatr* 127:447-457, 1995.

297. Desai S, Kollros PR, Graziani LJ, Streletz LJ, et al: Sensitivity and specificity of the neonatal brain-stem auditory evoked potential for hearing and language deficits in survivors of extracorporeal membrane oxygenation, *J Pediatr* 131:233-239, 1997.

298. Kornhauser MS, Baumgart S, Desai SA, Stanley CW, et al: Adverse neurodevelopmental outcome after extracorporeal membrane oxygenation among neonates with bronchopulmonary dysplasia, *J Pediatr* 132:307-311, 1998.

299. Nield TA, Langenbacher D, Poulsen MK, Platzker ACG: Neurodevelopmental outcome at 3.5 years of age in children treated with extracorporeal life support: Relationship to primary diagnosis, *J Pediatr* 136:338-344, 2000.

300. Goodman M, Gringlas M, Baumgart S, Stanley C, et al: Neonatal electroencephalogram does not predict cognitive and academic achievement scores at early school age in survivors of neonatal extracorporeal membrane oxygenation, *J Child Neurol* 16:745-750, 2001.

301. Amigoni A, Pettenazzo A, Biban P, Suppiej A, et al: Neurologic outcome in children after extracorporeal membrane oxygenation: Prognostic value of diagnostic tests, *Pediatr Neurol* 32:173-179, 2005.

Chapter 11

Intracranial Hemorrhage: Germinal Matrix–Intraventricular Hemorrhage of the Premature Infant

Germinal matrix–intraventricular hemorrhage (IVH) is the most common variety of neonatal intracranial hemorrhage and is characteristic of the premature infant.[1] The importance of the lesion relates not only to its high incidence but also to the essential gravity of the larger examples of IVH and their attendant complications. Moreover, the major forms of brain injury of the premature infant occur most commonly in the context of IVH, either as an apparent consequence of the IVH or as an associated finding.

The *magnitude of the problem* of IVH in the premature infant relates to the relatively high and unchanging incidence of prematurity, the relatively high survival rates of premature infants, and the relatively high incidence of IVH. Thus, in the 4 decades from the 1970s to the present in the United States, the proportion of live births weighing less than 1500 g increased from 1.17% to 1.45%.[2-5] In view of the approximately 4 million live births each year in the United States, approximately 55,000 infants of such very low birth weight will be born yearly in this country alone. In parallel with the large number of premature births has been a continual decline in mortality rates,[6-16] such that approximately 85% to 90% of infants between 500 and 1500 g birth weight survive the neonatal period. Indeed, even among infants of birth weights 500 to 1000 g, current survival rates are approximately 70%.[17-19] Thus, although the incidence of IVH has declined in recent years, large absolute numbers of infants are affected yearly.

The *incidence* of IVH in premature infants, although lower than it was 2 decades ago, is high (Table 11-1). In six well-studied series of premature infants (total of ≈1200) subjected to routine computed tomography (CT) or ultrasound scans and studied in the late 1970s and early 1980s, the incidence generally ranged from 40% to 50%.[20-25] Among this group, our series of 460 infants (birth weight < 2250 g) had an incidence of IVH of 39%.[24] However, subsequently, the incidence of IVH in the mid-1980s in the same unit for infants less than 2000 g birth weight was 29%.[26] Incidences derived from infants studied in the late 1980s were approximately 20%.[27-31] In the mid-1990s, values generally were less than 20% and often approximately 15%.[1,32-35] This historical decrease in incidence, however, does not indicate that IVH is a lessening problem, for two reasons. First, the incidence is directly correlated with the degree of prematurity (Fig. 11-1),[26,32,35-37] and second, survival rates for the smallest premature infants continue to increase. More recently, perhaps reflecting the increased survival of the smallest and sickest infants, overall rates of IVH are generally in the 20% to 25% range.[12,14,16,38,39] Indeed, the incidence of IVH in infants of 500 to 749 g birth weight is approximately 45%.[19] Additionally, the proportion of *severe* IVH is greatest among the most premature infants (see later). Thus, IVH will continue to be a major problem in the modern neonatal intensive care unit.

In this chapter, I review the neuropathology, pathogenesis, clinical features, diagnosis, prognosis, and management of IVH and its complications. The prominent position of this lesion in neonatal medicine has been accompanied by a large increase in work from several disciplines. This chapter attempts to integrate this information in a meaningful way without oversimplifying a clearly complex problem.

NEUROPATHOLOGY

The neuropathology of IVH is best considered in terms of the site of origin (primarily the germinal matrix), the spread of the hemorrhage throughout the ventricular system, the neuropathological consequences of the hemorrhage, and the neuropathological accompaniments not necessarily related directly to the IVH.

The basic lesion in germinal matrix hemorrhage–IVH is bleeding into the subependymal germinal matrix. This region is represented by the ventricular-subventricular zone described in Chapter 2. Over the final 12 to 16 weeks of gestation, this matrix becomes less and less prominent and is essentially exhausted by term (see later discussion). This region is highly cellular, gelatinous in texture, and as would be expected for a structure with active cellular proliferation, richly vascularized. To understand the nature of IVH, it is useful to review first the arterial and venous supply to the germinal matrix.

Arterial Supply to Subependymal Germinal Matrix

The arterial supply to the subependymal germinal matrix is derived particularly from the anterior cerebral

TABLE 11-1	High Incidence of Intraventricular Hemorrhage in Premature Infants*	
Years of Study	**Criteria for Inclusion**	**Incidence**
Late 1970s–1980s	Premature: several different birth weights and gestational ages	40%–50%
Late 1980s	<1500 g	20%
Late 1990s	<1500 g	15%–20%
Present	<1500 g	20%–25%

*See text for references; values for incidence are rounded off.

artery (through Heubner's artery), the middle cerebral artery (primarily through the deep lateral striate branches but also through penetrating branches from surface meningeal branches), and the internal carotid artery (through the anterior choroidal artery) (Fig. 11-2).[40,41] The relative importance of these arteries in the vascular supply to the capillaries of the matrix is not entirely clear; different studies have attributed particular importance to Heubner's artery[40,42] and to the lateral striate arteries.[43] However, it is likely that the terminal branches of this arterial supply constitute a vascular end zone and thus a vulnerability to ischemic injury (see later discussion).

Capillary Network

The rich arterial supply just described feeds an elaborate *capillary bed* in the germinal matrix.[40,42-47] This bed generally is composed of relatively large, irregular endothelial-lined vessels that do not exhibit the characteristics of arterioles or venules and are classified as capillaries or channels, or both. Pape and Wigglesworth[42] characterized the anatomical appearance as "a persisting immature vascular rete in the subependymal matrix which is only remodeled into a definite capillary bed when the germinal matrix disappears." As term approaches, some of the larger endothelial-lined

vessels acquire a collagenous adventitial sheath[43] and can be categorized appropriately as veins,[46] as also described in the matrix of the monkey.[48] The nature of the endothelial-lined vessels in this microvascular bed may be of pathogenetic importance concerning germinal matrix hemorrhage (see later section).

Venous Drainage of Subependymal Germinal Matrix

The rich microvascular network just described is continuous with a well-developed deep venous system. This venous drainage eventually terminates in the great cerebral vein of Galen (Fig. 11-3).[49] In addition

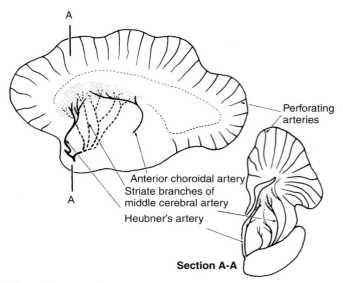

Figure 11-2   Arterial supply. Arterial supply to the subependymal germinal matrix at 29 weeks of gestation. *(From Hambleton G, Wigglesworth JS: Origin of intraventricular haemorrhage in the preterm infant,* Arch Dis Child *51:651–659, 1976.)*

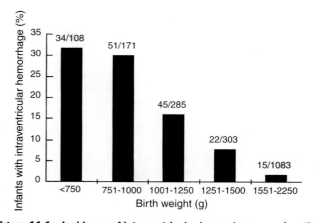

Figure 11-1   Incidence of intraventricular hemorrhage as a function of birth weight of 1950 infants weighing 2250 g or less. The bars represent the percentage of total infants in the range of birth weight, and the numbers at the top of the bars are absolute numbers of infants. *(From Sheth RD: Trends in incidence and severity of intraventricular hemorrhage,* J Child Neurol *13:261–264, 1998.)*

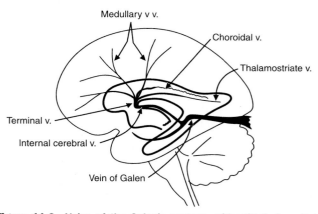

Figure 11-3   Veins of the Galenic system, midsagittal view. Note that the medullary, choroidal, and thalamostriate veins come to a point of confluence to form the terminal vein. The terminal vein, which courses through the germinal matrix, empties into the internal cerebral vein, and the major flow of blood changes direction sharply at that junction.

to the matrix region, this venous system drains blood from the cerebral white matter, choroid plexus, striatum, and thalamus through the medullary, choroidal, thalamostriate, and terminal veins. Indeed, the terminal vein, which runs essentially within the germinal matrix, is the principal terminus of the medullary, choroidal, and thalamostriate veins. The latter three vessels course primarily *anteriorly* to a point of confluence at the level of the head of the caudate nucleus to form the terminal veins, which empty into the internal cerebral vein that courses directly *posteriorly* to join the vein of Galen. Thus, at the usual site of germinal matrix hemorrhage, the direction of blood flow changes in a peculiar U-turn. This feature may have pathogenetic implications (see later section). This venous anatomy is also relevant to the occurrence of periventricular hemorrhagic infarction (see later discussion).

Site of Origin and Spread of Intraventricular Hemorrhage

Site of Origin

The site of origin of IVH characteristically is the *subependymal germinal matrix* (Fig. 11-4). This cellular region immediately ventrolateral to the lateral ventricle serves as the source of cerebral neuronal precursors between approximately 10 to 20 weeks of gestation and in the third trimester provides glial precursors that become cerebral oligodendroglia and astrocytes (see Chapter 2). For reasons discussed later, the many thin-walled vessels in the matrix are a ready source of bleeding. The matrix undergoes progressive decrease in size, from a width of 2.5 mm at 23 to 24 weeks, to 1.4 mm at 32 weeks, to nearly complete involution by approximately 36 weeks.[36] The matrix from 28 to 32 weeks is most prominent in the thalamostriate groove at the level of the head of the caudate nucleus at the site of or slightly posterior to the foramen of Monro,[40,50-54] and this site is the most common for germinal matrix hemorrhage. Before 28 weeks, hemorrhage in persisting matrix over the body of the caudate nucleus may also be found. Hemorrhage from choroid plexus occurs in nearly 50% of infants with germinal matrix hemorrhage and IVH,[55] and, in more mature infants especially, it may be the major site of origin of IVH (see Chapter 10).

The vascular *site of origin* of germinal matrix hemorrhage within the microcirculation of this region appears most commonly to be the prominent endothelial-lined vessels described earlier, not clearly arterial or venous.[40,46,50,54,56-58] Particular importance for vessels in free communication with the venous circulation (e.g., capillary-venule junction or small venules) is suggested by the emergence of solution into germinal matrix hemorrhage from postmortem injection into the jugular veins but not from injection into the carotid artery.[56] Histochemical studies of germinal matrix vessels at the site of hemorrhage also are consistent with an origin at the capillary-venule or small venule level.[58] Multiple microcirculatory sites involving small vessels lined only by endothelium may be involved, depending on the clinical circumstances.

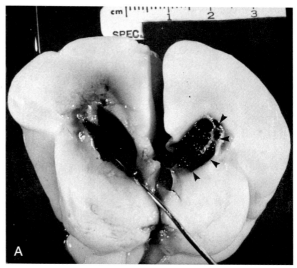

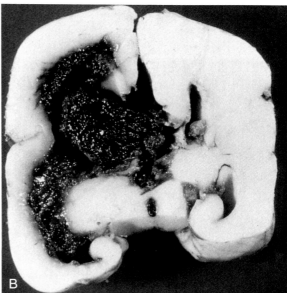

Figure 11-4 **Germinal matrix–intraventricular hemorrhage.** Coronal sections of cerebrum. **A,** Germinal matrix hemorrhage (*arrowheads*) at the level of the head of the caudate nucleus and foramen of Monro (see probe), with rupture into the lateral ventricles. **B,** Massive intraventricular hemorrhage. Obstruction at the foramen of Monro has caused severe, unilateral ventricular dilation.

Spread of Intraventricular Hemorrhage

In the approximately 80% of cases with germinal matrix hemorrhage in which blood enters the lateral ventricles, spread occurs throughout the ventricular system (Fig. 11-5).[40,53,54] Blood proceeds through the foramina of Magendie and Luschka and tends to collect in the basilar cisterns in the posterior fossa; with substantial collections, the blood may incite an obliterative arachnoiditis over days to weeks with obstruction to cerebrospinal fluid (CSF) flow. Other sites at which particulate blood clot may lead to impaired CSF dynamics are the aqueduct of Sylvius and the arachnoid villi (see later discussion of hydrocephalus).

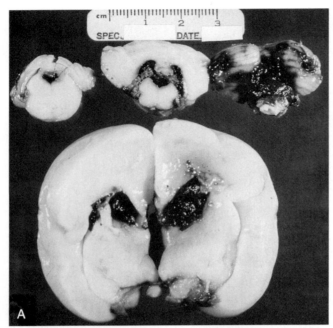

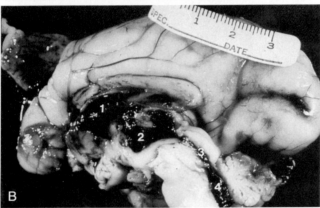

Figure 11-5 Spread of intraventricular hemorrhage. **A**, Coronal and, **B**, sagittal views. In **A**, note blood in the lateral ventricles, aqueduct of Sylvius, the fourth ventricle, and the subarachnoid space around the cerebellum and lower brain stem. In **B**, note blood throughout the ventricular system (the numbers *1* to *4* refer to lateral ventricle, third ventricle, aqueduct, and fourth ventricle, respectively).

Neuropathological Consequences of Intraventricular Hemorrhage

Several neuropathological states occur as apparent consequences of IVH, including, in temporal order of occurrence, germinal matrix destruction, periventricular hemorrhagic infarction, and posthemorrhagic hydrocephalus.

Germinal Matrix Destruction

Destruction of germinal matrix and, perhaps importantly, its glial precursor cells is a consistent and expected feature of germinal matrix hemorrhage.[50,54] The hematoma is frequently replaced by a cyst, the walls of which include hemosiderin-laden macrophages and reactive astrocytes. The destruction of glial precursor cells may have a deleterious influence on subsequent brain development (see later discussion).

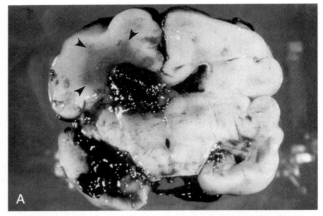

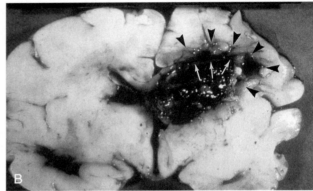

Figure 11-6 **Periventricular hemorrhagic infarction with intraventricular hemorrhage; coronal sections of cerebrum. A**, Early lesion; note evolving hemorrhagic infarction *(arrowheads)* on the same side as larger intraventricular hemorrhage. **B**, More advanced lesion; note hemorrhagic necrosis with liquefaction in periventricular white matter *(arrowheads)* on the same side as larger intraventricular hemorrhage. The ependymal lining is marked by *white arrows*.

Periventricular Hemorrhagic Infarction

Approximately 15% of very-low-birth-weight infants with IVH also exhibit a characteristic parenchymal lesion (i.e., a relatively large region of hemorrhagic necrosis in the periventricular white matter) just dorsal and lateral to the external angle of the lateral ventricle (Fig. 11-6).[13,16,39] The incidence of the lesion increases with decreasing gestational age, such that in infants of less than 1000 g or gestational age less than 28 weeks, periventricular hemorrhagic infarction accounts for approximately 15% to 20% of all cases with IVH (see later).[9,13,16,19,39,59]

Large-scale ultrasonographic studies have defined the *topographic characteristics of periventricular hemorrhagic infarction*. The parenchymal hemorrhagic necrosis is strikingly asymmetrical; in the largest early series reported,[60] 67% of such lesions were exclusively unilateral, and in virtually all the remaining cases, lesions were grossly asymmetrical, although bilateral. Approximately one half of the lesions were extensive and involved the periventricular white matter from frontal to parieto-occipital regions (Fig. 11-7); the remainder were more localized. Approximately 80% of cases were associated with large IVH. Commonly (and mistakenly),

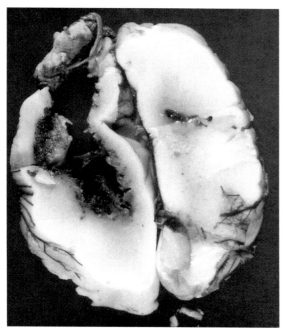

Figure 11-7 **Periventricular hemorrhagic infarction, neuropathology**. Horizontal section of cerebrum above the level of lateral ventricles from a premature infant who died on the sixth postnatal day, 3 days after severe intraventricular hemorrhage. Hemorrhagic necrosis in left cerebral white matter separated from the brain section during fixation and revealed a shaggy margin of the hemorrhagic infarction. See text for details.

the parenchymal hemorrhagic lesion is described as an "extension" of IVH. Several neuropathological studies have shown that simple extension of blood into cerebral white matter from germinal matrix or lateral ventricle does *not* account for the periventricular hemorrhagic necrosis.[24,55,59-65] In a later ultrasonographic report of 58 infants, findings were similar: the lesion was unilateral in 74%, extensive (involving two or more lobar territories) in 67%, and associated with large IVH in 88%.[66] The lobar distribution indicates that the majority of lesions involved the frontal and parietal regions. Approximately 50% of the cases exhibited a midline

shift of cerebral structures, consistent with the severity of the lesions.

Microscopic study of the periventricular hemorrhagic necrosis just described indicates that the lesion is a *hemorrhagic infarction*.[24,60-65,67] The careful studies of Gould and co-workers[62] and Takashima and co-workers[67] emphasized that (1) the hemorrhagic component consists usually of perivascular hemorrhages that follow closely the fan-shaped distribution of the medullary veins in periventricular cerebral white matter (Fig. 11-8) and (2) the hemorrhagic component tends to be most concentrated near the ventricular angle where these veins become confluent and ultimately join the terminal vein in the subependymal region. Thus, the periventricular hemorrhagic necrosis occurring in association with large IVH is, in fact, a *venous infarction*. The *most common neuropathological sequela* of periventricular hemorrhagic infarction is a large *porencephalic cyst* at the site of the lesion, either alone (66%) or in combination with smaller cysts (23%).[66] The large cyst communicates often, although not invariably, with the lateral ventricle.

Periventricular hemorrhagic infarction is distinguishable neuropathologically from secondary hemorrhage into periventricular leukomalacia, which is the ischemic, usually nonhemorrhagic, and symmetrical lesion of periventricular white matter of the premature infant (see later discussion). Distinction of these two lesions in vivo, however, is difficult. Indeed, because the pathogeneses of periventricular hemorrhagic infarction and periventricular leukomalacia overlap (see later discussion), it is to be expected that the lesions often coexist, thereby sometimes causing confusion in interpretation of cranial ultrasound scans.[1] In Table 11-2, I compare the basic features of these two periventricular white matter lesions of the premature infant.

The *pathogenesis* of periventricular hemorrhagic infarction appears to be related causally to the germinal matrix hemorrhage–IVH. A direct relation to the latter lesion seems likely on the basis of three fundamental findings.[60,66] First, 80% to 90% of the reported

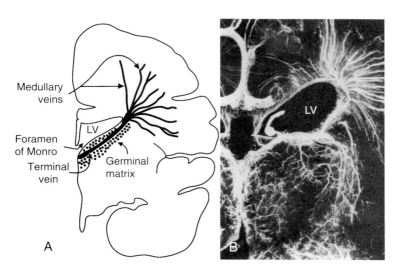

Figure 11-8 **Venous drainage of cerebral white matter in schematic and actual appearances**. **A**, Schematic diagram shows that the medullary veins, arranged in a fan-shaped distribution, drain blood from the cerebral white matter into the terminal vein, which courses through the germinal matrix. **B**, Postmortem venogram obtained from a human newborn shows the actual appearance of the vessels. LV, lateral ventricle. (**B**, From Takashima S, Mito T, Ando Y: Pathogenesis of periventricular white matter hemorrhages in preterm infants, Brain Dev 8:25–30, 1986.)

TABLE 11-2   **Periventricular White Matter Lesions in the Premature Infant with Intraventricular Hemorrhage**

	LESION	
	Periventricular Hemorrhagic Infarction	**Periventricular Leukomalacia**
Likely site of circulatory disturbance	Venous	Arterial
Grossly hemorrhagic	Invariable	Uncommon
Markedly asymmetrical	Nearly invariable	Uncommon
Evolution	Single large cyst	Multiple small cysts

parenchymal lesions are observed in association with large (and almost invariably) asymmetrical germinal matrix hemorrhage–IVH. Second, the parenchymal lesions invariably occurred *on the same side* as the larger amount of germinal matrix and intraventricular blood (Table 11-3). Third, in some cases, the lesions were shown to develop and progress after the occurrence of the germinal matrix hemorrhage–IVH. More than one-half of the lesions were detected after the second postnatal day, when approximately 75% of cases of IVH have already occurred (see "Diagnosis"). The association of large asymmetrical germinal matrix hemorrhage–IVH with progression to ipsilateral periventricular hemorrhagic infarction has been confirmed.[66,68-71] These data suggest that the IVH or its associated germinal matrix hemorrhage leads to obstruction of the terminal veins and thus impaired blood flow in the medullary veins with the occurrence of hemorrhagic venous infarction. A similar conclusion was suggested from a neuropathological study.[62] The timing of this progression to infarction is often very rapid because, in most cases, the severe IVH and the periventricular hemorrhagic infarction are detected simultaneously.

This pathogenetic formulation received strong support from Doppler determinations of blood flow velocity in the terminal vein during the evolution of the infarction in the living premature infant; obstruction of flow in the terminal vein by the ipsilateral germinal matrix hemorrhage–IVH was shown clearly.[72,73] Moreover, the finding of elevated lactate in structures adjacent to the germinal matrix hemorrhage, in the distribution of tributaries of the terminal vein, further supports the occurrence of ischemia secondary to venous obstruction by the matrix hemorrhage.[74]

Finally, a magnetic resonance imaging (MRI) study of acute periventricular hemorrhagic infarction has shown an appearance consistent with a combination of intravascular thrombi and perivascular hemorrhage along the course of the medullary veins within the area of infarction (Fig. 11-9).[75]

The pathogenetic scheme that I consider to account for most examples of periventricular hemorrhagic infarction is shown in Figure 11-10. This scheme should be distinguished from that operative for hemorrhagic periventricular leukomalacia (Fig. 11-11), although the lesions could coexist. The frequency of coexistence of the two lesions is not known. Additionally, the two pathogenetic schemes could operate in sequence; that is, periventricular leukomalacia could become secondarily hemorrhagic (and perhaps a larger area of injury) when germinal matrix hemorrhage or IVH subsequently causes venous obstruction.

Hydrocephalus

A third neuropathological consequence of IVH is progressive posthemorrhagic ventricular dilation (i.e.,

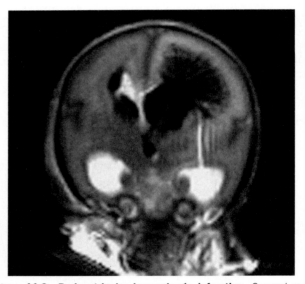

Figure 11-9   **Periventricular hemorrhagic infarction.** Coronal magnetic resonance imaging scan (fast spin-echo image) demonstrating bilateral germinal matrix–intraventricular hemorrhages, with an apparent periventricular hemorrhagic infarction on the side of the larger amount of germinal matrix and intraventricular blood (reader's right). Note the fan-shaped linear distribution of increased signal in the parenchymal lesion (reader's right), consistent with a combination of intravascular thrombi and perivascular hemorrhage along the course of the medullary veins. *(From Counsell SJ, Maalouf EF, Rutherford MA, Edwards AD: Periventricular haemorrhagic infarct in a preterm neonate, Eur J Paediatr Neurol 3:25–28, 1999.)*

TABLE 11-3   **Laterality of Apparent Periventricular Hemorrhagic Infarction and Concurrent Asymmetrical Intraventricular Hemorrhage**

Severity of Intraventricular Hemorrhage	Periventricular Hemorrhagic Infarction Homolateral	Periventricular Hemorrhagic Infarction Contralateral
Grade III	47	0
Grades I–II	5	4

Data from Guzzetta F, Shackelford GD, Volpe S, Perlman JM, et al: Periventricular intraparenchymal echodensities in the premature newborn: Critical determinant of neurologic outcome, *Pediatrics* 78:995–1006, 1986.

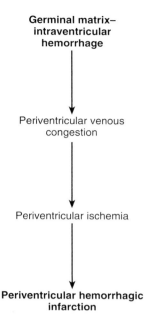

Figure 11-10 **Pathogenesis of periventricular hemorrhagic infarction.** The formulation indicates a central role for germinal matrix–intraventricular hemorrhage in causation of the periventricular venous infarction.

hydrocephalus). The likelihood and the rapidity of evolution of hydrocephalus after IVH are related directly to the quantity of intraventricular blood. Thus, with large IVH, hydrocephalus may evolve over days (*acute* hydrocephalus), and with smaller IVH, the process evolves usually over weeks (*subacute-chronic* hydrocephalus) (see later discussion).

Acute hydrocephalus is accompanied by particulate blood clot, readily demonstrated in life by ultrasound scan (see later discussion). The particulate clot may impair CSF absorption by obstruction of the arachnoid villi. This mechanism may be particularly likely in the newborn, in whom only microscopic arachnoid villi (and not larger, later-appearing arachnoid granulations) are present.[76-78] The possibility that endogenous fibrinolytic mechanisms mediated by plasminogen activation are deficient in the CSF of the premature infant

is suggested by the findings that plasminogen levels are extremely low in CSF of such infants,[79] whereas in infants with recent IVH, the levels of plasminogen activator inhibitor are relatively high.[80,81] This combination of findings may limit the infant's capacity to mediate clot lysis after IVH.

Subacute-chronic hydrocephalus relates most commonly either to an obliterative arachnoiditis in the posterior fossa (which results in either obstruction of fourth ventricular outflow or flow through the tentorial notch) or to aqueductal obstruction by blood clot, disrupted ependyma, and reactive gliosis.[42,50,82-84] The obliterative arachnoiditis is probably most important. Two molecules important in fibroproliferative responses have been shown to be up-regulated in infants with posthemorrhagic hydrocephalus.[85-88] Transforming growth factor-beta1, derived in this setting from platelets, is a cytokine chemotactic for fibroblasts and important in the up-regulation of genes encoding collagen, fibronectin, and other extracellular matrix proteins.[85,87,88] Procollagen 1C-peptide, involved in collagen fiber formation and tissue deposition, also has been shown to be elevated in CSF of infants with posthemorrhagic hydrocephalus.[86]

Neuropathological Accompaniments of Intraventricular Hemorrhage

Several neuropathological states are common accompaniments of IVH, but, in contrast to the states just described, these are apparently not caused by the IVH. The two most common accompaniments are periventricular leukomalacia and selective neuronal necrosis.

Periventricular Leukomalacia

Periventricular leukomalacia, the generally symmetrical, nonhemorrhagic, and apparently ischemic white matter injury of the premature infant (see Chapters 8 and 9), was observed to some degree in 75% of one series of infants who died with IVH.[55] The frequent association of classic necrotic/cystic periventricular leukomalacia and IVH also was emphasized in three other neuropathological reports,[63,67,89] as well as in two large ultrasonographic studies.[16,39] Although it has been reported that approximately 25% of examples of periventricular leukomalacia become hemorrhagic,[55,90] especially when associated coagulopathy is present, this figure includes examples that have been accompanied by large IVH and that probably represent the venous infarction discussed earlier as periventricular hemorrhagic infarction. Takashima and co-workers[67] suggested that the two lesions (i.e., periventricular hemorrhagic infarction and hemorrhagic periventricular leukomalacia) may be distinguishable in part on the basis of topography. Thus, hemorrhagic periventricular leukomalacia has a predilection for periventricular arterial border zones, particularly in the region near the trigone of the lateral ventricles. Venous infarction, especially its most hemorrhagic component, is particularly prominent more anteriorly; that is, the lesion radiates from the periventricular region at the site of confluence of the medullary and terminal veins and

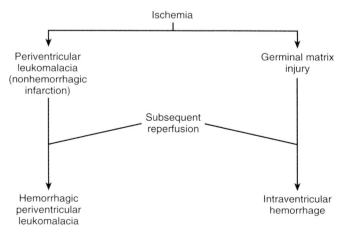

Figure 11-11 **Pathogenesis of hemorrhagic periventricular leukomalacia.**

assumes a roughly triangular, fan-shaped appearance in periventricular white matter. The potential role of IVH in contributing to the occurrence of periventricular leukomalacia is discussed later (see "Mechanisms of Brain Injury").

Selective Neuronal Necrosis

Selective neuronal necrosis, secondary to hypoxia-ischemia in the premature infant, particularly involves the pons, deep nuclear structures, especially, thalamus and basal ganglia, and hippocampus (see Chapter 8). Although each of these lesions is more commonly encountered in association with IVH, the relationship is particularly notable for pontine neuronal necrosis. In two carefully studied neuropathological series,[55,89] 46% and 71% of infants with IVH exhibited pontine neuronal necrosis. Accompanying neuronal necrosis in the subiculum of the hippocampus is common but not invariable.[23,42,77,89,91,92] All the infants with IVH accompanied by pontine neuronal necrosis in the series of Armstrong and co-workers[55] died of respiratory failure; previous investigations had suggested that the pontine lesion is related to hypoxic-ischemic insult, hyperoxia, and hypocarbia (see Chapter 8).[77,93] Involvement of the inferior olivary nucleus often accompanies the pontine disturbance, and thus cerebellar afferent systems are often affected. This involvement could be related causally to the decreased volume of cerebellum observed by volumetric MRI in infants after severe IVH.[94]

PATHOGENESIS

The pathogenesis of IVH is considered best in terms of intravascular, vascular, and extravascular factors. Clearly, the pathogenesis of IVH is multifactorial, and to some extent different combinations of these factors are operative in different patients. Nevertheless, several of the factors are important in every patient, as discussed in the following sections.

Intravascular Factors

Intravascular factors are those that relate primarily to the regulation of blood flow, pressure, and volume in the microvascular bed of the germinal matrix (Table 11-4). Factors that relate to platelet-capillary function and to blood clotting capability may play a contributory pathogenetic role in certain patients.

Fluctuating Cerebral Blood Flow

Major importance for fluctuating cerebral blood flow in the pathogenesis of IVH was shown by a study by Perlman and co-workers[95] of ventilated preterm infants with respiratory distress syndrome. Employing the Doppler technique at the anterior fontanelle to insonate the pericallosal branch of the anterior cerebral artery (the latter an important source of blood supply to the germinal matrix), we asked whether alterations in cerebral blood flow velocity in the first hours and days of life could be identified and related to the subsequent development of IVH. The findings were decisive. Two patterns of cerebral blood flow velocity were noted on the

TABLE 11-4   Pathogenesis of Germinal Matrix–Intraventricular Hemorrhage: Intravascular Factors

Fluctuating Cerebral Blood Flow
Ventilated preterm infant with respiratory distress syndrome

Increase in Cerebral Blood Flow
Systemic hypertension: importance of pressure-passive circulation
Rapid volume expansion
Hypercarbia
Decreased hematocrit
Decreased blood glucose

Increase in Cerebral Venous Pressure
Venous anatomy: U-turn in direction of venous flow
Labor and vaginal delivery
Respiratory disturbances

Decrease in Cerebral Blood Flow (Followed by Reperfusion)
Systemic hypotension: importance of pressure-passive circulation

Platelet and Coagulation Disturbance

first day of life: a stable pattern and a fluctuating pattern (Fig. 11-12). The *stable pattern* was characterized by equal peaks and troughs of systolic and diastolic flow velocity

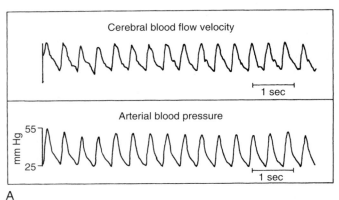

A

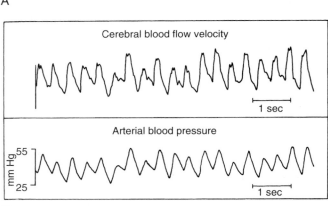

B

Figure 11-12   Cerebral blood flow velocity in ventilated premature infant with respiratory distress syndrome. The *upper trace* of each pair is the cerebral blood flow velocity, obtained at the anterior fontanelle, and the *lower trace* is the simultaneous blood pressure obtained using an umbilical artery catheter. **A**, Stable pattern, and **B**, fluctuating pattern. See text for description.

TABLE 11-5	Relation of Fluctuating Cerebral Blood Flow Velocity to Subsequent Development of Intraventricular Hemorrhage	

Cerebral Blood Flow Velocity Pattern	Subsequent IVH	No IVH
Fluctuating	21	2
Stable	7 *	20

*Other provocative factors (e.g., pneumothorax) present in four patients.
IVH, intraventricular hemorrhage.

(see Fig. 11-12A). In contrast, the *fluctuating pattern* was characterized by marked, *continuous alterations* in both systolic and diastolic flow velocities (see Fig. 11-12B). The cerebral blood flow velocity tracings closely reflected similar patterns of arterial blood pressure, simultaneously obtained from the abdominal aorta through an umbilical artery catheter (see Fig. 11-12). A striking relationship of the fluctuating pattern of cerebral blood flow velocity to the subsequent occurrence of IVH was defined when the infants were studied by serial cranial ultrasound scans (Table 11-5).

The aforementioned observations were important for two reasons. First, they identified a subset of infants with respiratory distress syndrome at extreme risk for the subsequent occurrence of IVH and, therefore, prime candidates for preventive interventions (see later discussion). Second, they suggested a rational pathogenetic mechanism for the development of IVH with the respiratory distress syndrome (i.e., continuous fluctuations of blood flow in the vulnerable matrix microvessels, leading to rupture of these vessels). The relationship between fluctuating cerebral blood flow velocity and occurrence of major IVH was later confirmed.[96] Two studies[97,98] in which fluctuations in flow velocity were less than 10% (coefficient of variation) did not show a correlation of fluctuations with the occurrence of IVH, consistent with the earlier observation of Perlman and co-workers[95] that fluctuations of this small degree do not lead to IVH.

The cause of the fluctuations in both the systemic and cerebral circulations is related primarily to the mechanics of ventilation.[99-103] This notion is supported by the observations that the fluctuations are nearly invariable in infants who breathe out of synchrony with the ventilator and that elimination of the infant's respiratory efforts by muscle paralysis eliminates the fluctuations in the systemic and cerebral circulations (see later discussion). In separate studies, hypercarbia, hypovolemia, hypotension, "restlessness," patent ductus arteriosus, and relatively high inspired oxygen concentrations also have correlated with the occurrence of fluctuations in cerebral blood flow velocity.[96,102-106] The effect of these rapid fluctuations is unrelated to the presence or absence of cerebrovascular autoregulation (see later), because the response time of the latter system ($\approx$5 to 15 seconds) is too slow.

Increases in Cerebral Blood Flow: Importance of Pressure-Passive Circulation

The close temporal correlation between the occurrence of IVH and abrupt increases in arterial blood pressure,

apparent cerebral blood flow (jugular venous occlusion plethysmography), and cerebral blood flow velocity[100,107-112] has supported the earlier suggestion[40] that increases in cerebral blood flow play an important pathogenetic role in IVH. A *particularly likely cause of the premature infant's apparent propensity for dangerous elevations of cerebral blood flow is a pressure-passive state of the cerebral circulation.*[94,113-122] As discussed in Chapter 6, severely impaired cerebrovascular autoregulation was identified in approximately 50% of ventilated very-low-birth-weight infants studied by near-infrared spectroscopy in the first several days of life.[122] Using a more sophisticated approach with the same methodology, Soul and co-workers[117] showed that *fully 87 of 90 infants studied in the first 5 days of life had pressure-passive periods, and for the total group these periods accounted for a mean of 20% of the time.* Indeed, some infants exhibited the pressure-passive state more than 50% of the time. Additionally, hypercarbia and, perhaps, decreased hematocrit or decreased blood glucose may contribute to severe enough elevations in cerebral blood flow in the premature infant to provoke IVH (see later discussion). The developmental aspects of autoregulation and the regulatory factors involved are discussed in detail in Chapter 6.

Elevations of Arterial Blood Pressure and Pressure-Passive Cerebral Circulation. Concerning the role of elevations in arterial blood pressure, the presence of a pressure-passive cerebral circulation would be expected to lead to an increase in cerebral blood flow in association with increases in blood pressure, with the potential consequence being rupture of vulnerable germinal matrix vessels. The striking increase in cerebral blood flow associated with increases in blood pressure can be shown in real time by near-infrared spectroscopy (Fig. 11-13). A decisive demonstration of the relation between pressure-passive cerebral circulation and the occurrence of IVH was obtained from a classic study of 57 preterm infants supported by mechanical ventilation during at least the first 48 hours of life (Fig. 11-14). Infants in whom ultrasonographic signs of severe IVH developed had prior evidence of a pressure-passive cerebral circulation, whereas those with intact cerebrovascular autoregulation developed either no hemorrhage or only mild hemorrhage (see Fig. 11-14).[114,115] The work of Tsuji and co-workers[122] showed that 47% of infants with impaired cerebrovascular autoregulation developed IVH (or periventricular leukomalacia, or both), whereas only 13% of those with intact autoregulation developed these lesions.[122] Consistent with a potential role for arterial hypertension in this setting is the demonstration of a relationship between maximum systolic blood pressure above a threshold value and subsequent occurrence of IVH.[123] The limit for the highest tolerable peak systolic blood pressure was markedly lower for the smaller infants.[123] A particular role for minute-to-minute alterations in blood pressure has also been demonstrated.[124] Moreover, as discussed in Chapter 6, the upper limit of the normal autoregulatory range in the infant is dangerously close to the upper limit of the

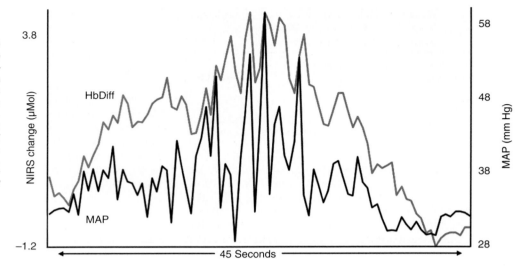

Figure 11-13 Changes in blood pressure (mean arterial pressure [MAP]) and cerebral perfusion (hemoglobin difference [HbDiff]) during a diaper change. Simultaneous tracings were obtained from a premature infant (30 weeks of gestational age). Note the marked, parallel increase in cerebral perfusion, determined by near-infrared spectroscopy (NIRS), and in arterial blood pressure, obtained from an umbilical artery catheter. *(Courtesy of Dr. Adre du Plessis.)*

range of normal blood pressure. Studies in developing animals indicate that the receptor number for specific vasoconstricting prostaglandins, which are important in setting the upper limit of the autoregulatory range in the adult, are low early in maturation and thereby impair protection of the cerebral circulation from increases in blood pressure.[125]

Whether the pressure-passive cerebral circulatory state relates to dysfunctional autoregulation per se, to maximal vasodilation caused by hypercarbia or hypoxemia (or both), to the cranial trauma of even a "normal" vaginal delivery, or to "normal" arterial blood pressures in the premature infant that are dangerously close to the upslope of a normal autoregulatory curve remains unclear. Experimental support for these several possibilities is available (see Chapter 6).[40,100,116,125-132]

Whatever the mechanism, however, the balance of current data imparts particular importance to events that cause elevations in arterial blood pressure, especially abrupt elevations, in the small premature infant.

Causes of Increased Arterial Blood Pressure in the Human Newborn. The causes of abrupt elevations in arterial blood pressure sometimes shown to be accompanied by increased cerebral blood flow velocity by the Doppler technique, or increased cerebral blood volume by near-infrared spectroscopy in the premature infant, are clearly important to detect (and to prevent, whenever possible) (Table 11-6). These causes include the following: such "physiological" events as rapid eye movement (REM) sleep and the first minutes and hours after birth; such "caretaking" concomitants as inadvertent noxious

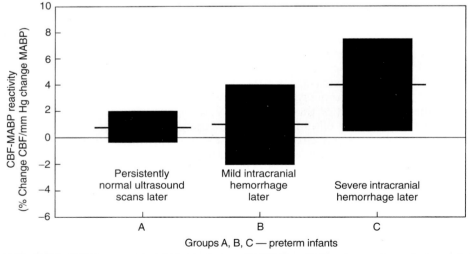

Figure 11-14 Cerebral blood flow (CBF)–mean arterial blood pressure (MABP) reactivities (percentage of change in CBF per millimeter of mercury change in MABP) in premature infants before intracranial hemorrhage. CBF-MABP reactivities were obtained in the first 2 days of life (primarily in the first 24 hours) in 57 mechanically ventilated preterm infants who had normal ultrasound scans at the time of the reactivity measurements and who were followed subsequently by ultrasonography. Groups A, B, and C were determined by the results of the subsequent scans. The average reactivity and 95% confidence limits for each group are shown. Intact autoregulation (i.e., zero value for CBF-MABP reactivity) was present in those infants who had subsequent scans that were normal or showed only mild hemorrhage. Infants who later developed severe hemorrhage had a pressure-passive cerebral circulation. *(Redrawn from Pryds O, Greisen G, Lou H, Friis-Hansen B: Heterogeneity of cerebral vasoreactivity in preterm infants supported by mechanical ventilation, J Pediatr 115:638–645, 1989.)*

TABLE 11-6	Major Causes of Increased Blood Pressure or Cerebral Blood Flow in the Premature Infant*
Related to "Physiological" Events	
Postpartum status	
Rapid eye movement sleep	
Related to Caretaking Procedures	
Noxious stimulation	
Motor activity: spontaneous or with handling	
Tracheal suctioning	
Instillation of mydriatics	
Related to Systemic Complications	
Pneumothorax	
Rapid volume expansion: exchange transfusion, other rapid colloid infusion	
Ligation of patent ductus arteriosus	
Related to Neurological Complications	
Seizure	

*See text for references.

stimulation, abdominal examination, handling (see Fig. 11-13; Fig. 11-15), instillation of mydriatics, and tracheal suctioning (Fig. 11-16); such systemic complications as pneumothorax, exchange transfusion, and rapid infusion of colloid; and such neurological complications as seizures.[107,108,111,133-159]

Although the degree to which these events contribute to the pathogenesis of IVH requires further quantitation and probably depends on concomitant clinical circumstances, particular importance can be attributed to *pneumothorax*.[97,160-165] In one earlier study of nine infants, pneumothorax was accompanied consistently by abrupt elevations of systemic blood pressure and cerebral blood flow velocity, and these circulatory changes were followed within hours by IVH.[161] Studies in newborn dogs documented abrupt increases in arterial blood pressure on rapid evacuation of pneumothorax.[162] Thus, both clinical and experimental data emphasize the potentially deleterious circulatory effects of neonatal pneumothorax.

Relevant Experimental Studies: Role of Hypertension. The particular importance of abrupt increases in systemic blood pressure and cerebral blood flow in pathogenesis has been demonstrated conclusively in elegant *experimental* studies in the newborn beagle puppy[129,166-174] and in the preterm sheep fetus.[175] The newborn puppy, which has been studied most extensively, has a subependymal germinal matrix approximately comparable to that of the human premature infant of 30 to 32 weeks of gestation.[176] Germinal matrix hemorrhage–IVH is produced most readily in this animal by a sequence of hypotension and

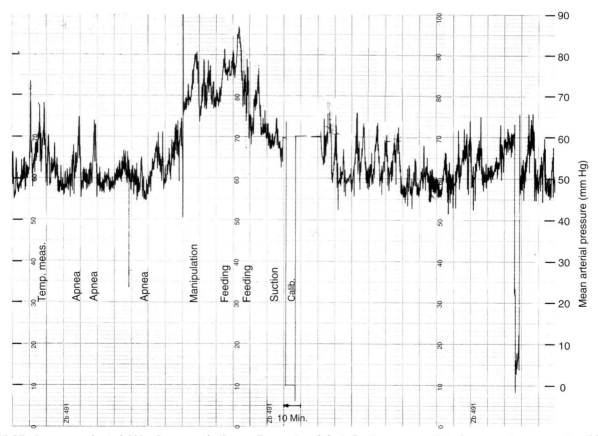

Figure 11-15 **Increases of arterial blood pressure in the small premature infant.** Continuous recording of mean aortic pressure in a 20-hour-old premature infant weighing 880 g. Note the marked and sustained increase with manipulation. The infant subsequently developed an intraventricular hemorrhage. *(From Lou HC, Lassen NA, Friis-Hansen B: Is arterial hypertension crucial for the development of cerebral haemorrhage in premature infants? Lancet 1:1215–1217, 1979.)*

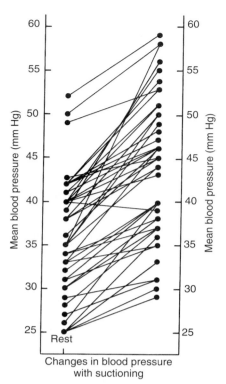

Figure 11-16 **Changes in blood pressure with tracheal suctioning in premature infants**. Note the increase in blood pressure that accompanied suctioning in all but one infant.

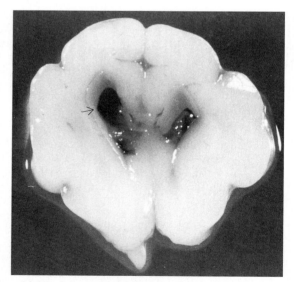

Figure 11-17 **Intraventricular hemorrhage in the newborn beagle puppy**. Gross intraventricular hemorrhage with dilation of the lateral ventricle (*arrow*) in cerebrum of a 24-hour-old puppy subjected to hypertension. *(From Goddard J, Lewis RM, Armstrong DL, Zeller RS: Moderate, rapidly induced hypertension as a cause of intraventricular hemorrhage in the newborn beagle model, J Pediatr 96:1057–1060, 1980.)*

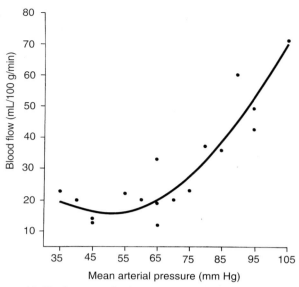

Figure 11-18 **Increase in blood flow to germinal matrix with increase in arterial blood pressure in the newborn dog**. Blood pressure was elevated by infusion of phenylephrine. Blood flow to the germinal matrix was measured by ^{14}C-iodoantipyrine autoradiography. *(From Pasternak JF, Groothuis DR: Autoregulation of cerebral blood flow in the newborn beagle puppy, Biol Neonate 48:100–109, 1985.)*

hypertension produced by blood removal and volume reinfusion (Fig. 11-17). The marked increase in germinal matrix flow provoked by hypertension has been demonstrated strikingly by autoradiography (Fig. 11-18).[129]

Rapid Volume Expansion. The role of *rapid volume expansion* (see Table 11-4) involves not only the administration of blood or other colloid, as described in relation to systemic hypertension, but also the administration of hyperosmolar materials, such as hypertonic sodium bicarbonate. Pressure-passive cerebral circulation may not be the sole or even the principal means by which such infusions may lead to IVH, particularly in the case of *sodium bicarbonate*. Although the dangers of rapid infusion of hyperosmolar solutions had been noted for many years, an association of IVH in the premature infant administered sodium bicarbonate was emphasized initially by Simmons and co-workers[177] from study of an autopsy population. The association was later confirmed in a CT study of premature infants, and the importance of rapidity of infusion was made apparent.[178] Conflicting reports on the pathogenetic role of sodium bicarbonate[163,179-186] relate in part to the failure to take into account such factors as rapidity of administration and also to the problems of extrapolating data to living infants from studies of dead infants, particularly in the case of IVH. At any rate, the mechanism for the effect of rapid infusion of hyperosmolar sodium bicarbonate on intracranial hemorrhage may relate in part to the abrupt elevation of arterial pressure of carbon dioxide ($Paco_2$) that results in the poorly ventilated or nonventilated patient from the buffering effect of the bicarbonate. The elevated $Paco_2$ would then act on cerebral arterioles, by causing an increase in perivascular hydrogen ion (H^+) concentration, to increase cerebral perfusion as outlined next.

Hypercarbia. The role of *hypercarbia* in causing increases in cerebral blood flow of pathogenetic importance for IVH may be appreciable in selected infants.

Hypercarbia, a common accompaniment of respiratory distress syndrome, respiratory complications, apneic episodes, and so forth, has been demonstrated conclusively to be a potent means for increasing cerebral blood flow in experimental studies (see Chapter 6). Indeed, careful studies of mechanically ventilated preterm infants show a pronounced reactivity of cerebral blood flow to changes in $Paco_2$ ($\approx$30% increase in cerebral blood flow per kilopascal [kPa] increase in $Paco_2$) after the first 24 hours of life.[115,116,119,187-190] Notably, in the first 24 hours of life, this normal reactivity was attenuated markedly ($\approx$10% increase in cerebral blood flow per kPa increase in $Paco_2$) in mechanically ventilated infants with normal subsequent ultrasonograms, but it was actually *absent* in infants with subsequent severe IVH.[114] This observation suggested that, in the first day of life at least, hypercarbia of at least a moderate degree may not be a major pathogenetic factor for severe IVH in mechanically ventilated infants. A similar lack of correlation between hypercarbia and IVH is apparent in several other studies.[164,185,191] An increased risk for IVH after hypercarbia, however, is suggested in several other reports,[69,97,192-194] including three that employed multivariate analysis.[165,194,195] In a particularly large study ($n = 463$), hypercarbia (defined as $Paco_2 > 60$ mm Hg) showed a positive relation with IVH.[165,193] In a later study of "permissive hypercapnia" to 45 to 55 mm Hg (versus 35 to 45 mm Hg in the control group) in ventilated premature infants, no statistically significant difference in IVH was noted between the groups, although the incidence of severe IVH was 29% in the permissive hypercapnia group versus 20% in the control group (not statistically significant).[196] Thus, a role for hypercarbia in pathogenesis of IVH may require particularly marked elevations of $Paco_2$. Consistent with this speculation is the demonstration that hypercapnia leads to clearly impaired autoregulation at $Paco_2$ levels above 45 mm Hg (Fig. 11-19).[159] Such levels were shown to be significantly associated with the occurrence of severe IVH and periventricular hemorrhagic infarction in a study of 58 infants.[197]

Decreased Hemoglobin. The role of *decreased hematocrit* in causing increases in cerebral blood flow of pathogenetic importance for IVH may be greater than was previously suspected. Thus, as described in Chapter 6, an inverse correlation exists in the human infant between hemoglobin concentration and cerebral blood flow as well as between the concentration of adult versus fetal hemoglobin (higher hemoglobin oxygen affinity) and cerebral blood flow.[115,116,198-201] In one study of premature infants in the first days of life, cerebral blood flow increased by 12% per 1-mM decrease in hemoglobin.[115,198] The inverse relationship between hematocrit and cerebral blood flow described previously in experimental studies has been suggested to result from changes in arterial oxygen content or blood viscosity. Because alterations in newborn hematocrit to less than 60% have little influence on blood viscosity, the major factor in the studies of human infants is considered to be related to arterial

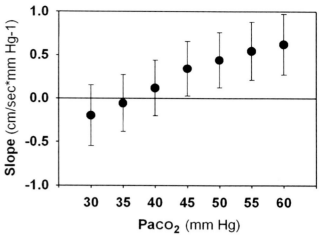

Figure 11-19 **Impaired autoregulation with hypercapnia.** Estimated mean slopes and 95% confidence intervals of the autoregulatory plateau for arterial carbon dioxide tension ($Paco_2$) values 30, 35, 40, 45, 50, 55, and 60 mm Hg for 43 very-low-birth-weight infants. Bars indicate 95% confidence intervals for the mean slopes of the autoregulatory plateaus for $Paco_2$ 30 ($n = 82$), 35 ($n = 94$), 40 ($n = 100$), 45 ($n = 103$), 50 ($n = 100$), 55 ($n = 90$), and 60 mm Hg ($n = 83$). The horizontal line at slope 0 indicates intact autoregulation. The estimated means of the slope of the autoregulatory plateau (cm/sec* mm Hg^{-1}) increased as $Paco_2$ increased ($P = .004$). *(From Kaiser JR, Gauss CH, Williams DK: The effects of hypercapnia on cerebral autoregulation in ventilated very low birth weight infants, Pediatr Res 58:931–935, 2005.)*

oxygen content and thereby cerebral oxygen delivery. Cerebral blood flow presumably increases to maintain cerebral oxygen delivery at a constant level. Consistent with this possibility, apparently "stable" premature infants with low hematocrits (<21%) had clinically unsuspected high cardiac output.[202] The adaptive response of increased cerebral blood flow may become maladaptive if certain vulnerable capillary beds (e.g., in the germinal matrix) are exposed to the elevated cerebral blood flow. When one considers that iatrogenic blood loss, owing to repeated blood sampling, and low initial blood volume are common in sick premature infants, especially during the periods of highest risk for occurrence of IVH, the role of decreased hematocrit as a cause of IVH could be considerable.

Decreased Blood Glucose. *Decreased blood glucose* now should be considered in the evaluation of pathogenetic factors for IVH in view of the observation that cerebral blood flow increases twofold to threefold when blood glucose declines to levels lower than 1.7 mM in the premature infant.[115,188,203] Blood glucose levels lower than 1.7 mM in premature infants are not unusual in the first days of life in many neonatal intensive care units (see Chapter 12). More data are needed on a potential contributory role of low blood glucose in the pathogenesis of IVH.

Increases in Cerebral Venous Pressure

Elevations of cerebral venous pressure may contribute to the occurrence of IVH. Indeed, the potential importance of venous factors is suggested by the demonstration that with postmortem injection of carotid artery or jugular vein in infants with germinal matrix hemorrhage, the injected material entered the hemorrhage only through venous injections.[56] Moreover, careful anatomical studies also are consistent with an origin at the level of the capillary-venule junction or the small venule.[58] The *most important causes* for such increases are labor and delivery, asphyxia, and respiratory complications (see later discussion).

Importance of Venous Anatomy. The particular importance of increased venous pressure in pathogenesis of IVH relates in part to the *venous anatomy* in the region of the germinal matrix (see Fig. 11-3). Thus, the direction of deep venous flow takes a peculiar U-turn in the subependymal region at the level of the foramen of Monro (i.e., the most common site of germinal matrix hemorrhage). At this site also is the point of confluence of the medullary, thalamostriate, and choroidal veins to form, in sequence, the terminal vein and then the internal cerebral vein, which ultimately empties into the vein of Galen.

Labor and Delivery. Concerning labor and delivery, marked increases in cerebral venous pressure must be common accompaniments. Indeed, in one study of 46 infants, when measurement of "fetal head compression pressure" was determined by a compression transducer positioned between the fetal head and the wall of the uterus,[204] the overall mean pressure was 158 mm Hg. *Deformations of the particularly compliant premature skull* are likely to accentuate the increases in venous pressure caused by normal labor. Indeed, the deleterious effects of labor (see later discussion) appear to be most pronounced in the most premature infants.[29,69,186,205,206] The skull deformations can lead to obstruction of major venous sinuses and presumably increased venous pressure.[42,207] Support for this notion has been provided by studies of blood flow velocity in the sagittal sinus, cerebral blood volume, and intracranial pressure during such manipulations as external pressure on the skull or rotation of the neck.[208,209] These effects may be expected to be greater with breech delivery. Available data are somewhat inconsistent concerning a relationship between such factors as presence or absence of labor, duration of labor, mode of delivery, and the occurrence of IVH, although in general the studies were not designed to address these issues specifically.[163,183,210-224] The inconsistency of the data, however, do not rule out a *contributory role* of intrapartum events in causation of IVH in certain infants. Thus, in a study that addressed the role of presence or absence of labor, duration of labor, mode of labor, and potential confounders in a multivariate analysis, Leviton and co-workers[29] showed that infants delivered vaginally were more likely to develop IVH than those delivered abdominally, that labor longer than 12 hours increased risk of IVH regardless of the mode of delivery, and that the occurrence of labor before abdominal delivery increased the incidence of IVH by two to four times, depending on the duration of labor (Table 11-7). In a separate study of 201 very-low-birth-weight infants,

TABLE 11-7	Occurrence of Germinal Matrix Hemorrhage as a Function of Route of Delivery and Duration of Labor	
	ROUTE OF DELIVERY	
Labor	**Vaginal**	**Abdominal**
None	—	6.1% (8/131)
<6 hr	23.2% (19/82)	14.7% (12/129)
6–12 hr	22.5% (9/40)	18.5% (5/27)
>12 hr	32.1% (9/28)	25.0% (3/12)

Data from Leviton A, Fenton T, Kuban KC, Pagano M: Labor and delivery characteristics and the risk of germinal matrix hemorrhage in low birth weight infants, *J Child Neurol* 6:35–40, 1991.

multivariate analysis also indicated an increased risk (2.2-fold) of IVH for infants delivered vaginally, a very low risk (7%) for infants delivered abdominally with no labor, and an increased risk among infants delivered abdominally for labor greater than 10 hours in duration (40%).[225] Subsequent investigations of 229, and 254 infants, respectively, show an increased risk of IVH occurring in the first 3 to 12 hours of life as a function of active labor and vaginal delivery.[69,70,224] Finally, a multicenter study of 4795 infants of less than 1500 g birth weight showed an incidence of "grade III and IV IVH" in 19% of vaginally delivered infants and 11% of those delivered by cesarean section without labor.[206] On balance, these data suggest that labor and delivery influence the risk of IVH in premature infants and have implications concerning a potential role for cesarean section in prevention (see later discussion).

Asphyxia. Concerning *asphyxia*, increased cerebral venous pressure may result from hypoxic-ischemic cardiac failure. The latter is caused by injury of papillary muscle, subendocardial tissue, and myocardium.[226-235] The importance of increased venous pressure in association with asphyxia in the causation of IVH was shown in experimental studies of preterm fetal sheep.[175] It seems likely that increased venous pressure could contribute to the propensity to IVH observed after serious asphyxia. Consistent with this notion are the strong relationships among such factors as severe umbilical cord acidemia, low Apgar scores, the need for neonatal resuscitation, and the occurrence of severe IVH (see later).[197,236] Other factors associated with asphyxia, such as ischemic injury to the germinal matrix and hypercarbia, are also likely important.

Respiratory Disturbances. Concerning *respiratory disturbances*, available data suggest that such factors as positive-pressure ventilation with relatively high peak inflation pressure, tracheal suctioning, abnormalities of the mechanics of respiration, and pneumothorax may be major causes of increased cerebral venous pressure in the premature infant.[235,237-243] Thus, extending earlier observations,[239,242,244] Cowan and Thoresen[237] used Doppler measurements of blood flow velocity in the superior sagittal sinus to demonstrate a striking sensitivity of the venous circulation to the level of peak inflation pressure; the smallest infants exhibited the most marked effects.

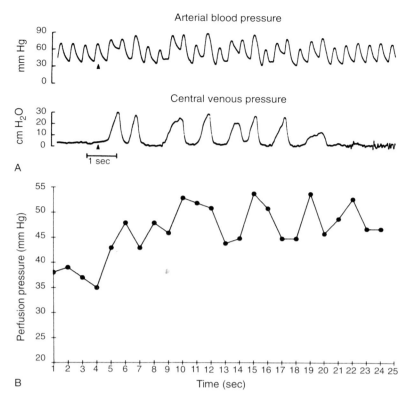

Figure 11-20 Venous pressure response to suctioning. **A,** Simultaneous venous pressure and arterial blood pressure tracings from a premature infant during tracheal suctioning (*arrowhead*). Note the pronounced increases in venous pressure after onset of suctioning. **B,** Graphic plot of calculated changes in perfusion pressure during the same suctioning episode. *(Adapted from Perlman JM, Volpe JJ: Are venous circulatory abnormalities important in the pathogenesis of hemorrhagic and/or ischemic cerebral injury?* Pediatrics *80:705–711, 1987.)*

The possibility of a particular importance for venous abnormalities in causation of IVH was raised by a study of intubated preterm infants with respiratory distress syndrome under conditions in which dangerous alterations in arterial blood pressure occur (i.e., elevations with tracheal suctioning[140] and fluctuations with breathing out of synchrony with the ventilator[99]). The effects on the venous circulation were dramatic.[241] With elevations in arterial blood pressure produced by tracheal suctioning, pronounced changes in venous pressure also occurred (Fig. 11-20A). Moreover, because the magnitude and the direction of the changes in venous pressure often were not similar to those in arterial pressure, striking changes in perfusion pressure resulted (Fig. 11-20B). Similarly, because fluctuations in arterial blood pressure were associated with noncoordinate fluctuations in venous pressure (Fig. 11-21A), pronounced and continuous alterations in perfusion pressure resulted (Fig. 11-21B). Thus, under both circumstances, *decreases* in perfusion pressure by as much as 10 to 20 mm Hg were followed in seconds by abrupt, similar *increases* in perfusion pressure. Because these changes occur essentially on a beat-to-beat basis, it is unlikely that autoregulation, even if functional, could protect critical capillary beds by causing the changes in arteriolar diameter necessary to maintain constant cerebral blood flow under such circumstances. Thus, the previously established role for disturbed mechanics of respiration with fluctuations in arterial blood pressure in the causation of IVH (see Table 11-5)[95] may be mediated as much by alterations on the venous side of the cerebral circulation as by

alterations on the arterial side. A similar conclusion can be drawn for the previously established role[108] in causation of IVH of abruptly increased arterial blood pressure with pneumothorax because this respiratory complication has been shown to cause abruptly increased venous pressure as well.[162,235,245,246] A recent study of 58 cases of severe IVH with periventricular hemorrhagic infarction showed a significant relationship of pneumothorax with the occurrence of the lesion.[197]

Decreases in Cerebral Blood Flow

Importance of Pressure-Passive Cerebral Circulation. Decreases in cerebral blood flow, occurring either prenatally (perhaps primarily intrapartum) or postnatally, may play an important role in pathogenesis of IVH in certain infants. The principal consequence of the decreased cerebral blood flow is injury of germinal matrix vessels, which rupture subsequently on reperfusion. The importance of vascular border zones and end zones in the matrix, as well as the intrinsic vulnerability of the matrix vessels to oxygen deprivation, is emphasized later (see section on vascular factors). As indicated earlier, hemorrhagic hypotension preceding volume reexpansion is the optimal means to produce IVH experimentally in the newborn beagle puppy. In the premature infant, decreases in cerebral blood flow are most likely with perinatal hypoxia-ischemia and with various postnatal events that result in systemic hypotension. Because of the pressure-passive cerebral circulation in sick premature infants, this hypotension can lead to a decrease in cerebral blood flow. Recall that a detailed study of 90 premature

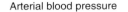
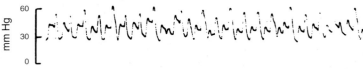

Arterial blood pressure

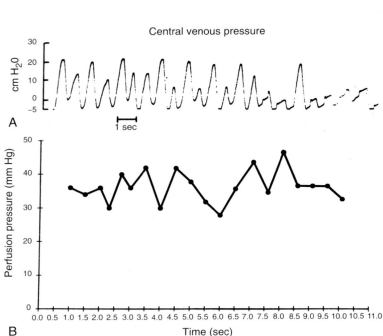

Central venous pressure

1 sec

A

B

Figure 11-21   **Correlation of fluctuations in arterial and venous pressure. A,** Simultaneous venous pressure and arterial blood pressure tracings from an infant with fluctuating blood pressure. Note that the marked fluctuations in arterial pressure are associated with marked fluctuations in venous pressure. **B,** Graphic plot of calculated changes in perfusion pressure in the same infant. *(Adapted from Perlman JM, Volpe JJ: Are venous circulatory abnormalities important in the pathogenesis of hemorrhagic and/or ischemic cerebral injury?* Pediatrics *80:705–711, 1987.)*

infants in the first 5 days of life showed that more than 95% had pressure-passive periods, with a mean total time of pressure-passivity of 20%.[117]

Perinatal Hypoxic-Ischemic Events. Although it is not an obligatory event for development of IVH, the infant with prior perinatal asphyxia clearly has an increased likelihood of developing IVH and, in our experience, the hemorrhage in such infants tends to be relatively large. Indeed, a recent study of 58 infants with periventricular hemorrhagic infarction found a strong association of the lesion with fetal distress and the need for emergency cesarean section, low Apgar scores, and the need for respiratory resuscitation.[197] Perinatal hypoxic-ischemic events presumably explain, at least in part, the relation between low Apgar scores, early acidosis, early use of bicarbonate or pressors, hypocarbia, and the subsequent overall occurrence of IVH, particularly lesions that develop in the first 12 hours.[163,197,224,236,247-249] The mechanism for provocation of IVH with perinatal asphyxia is complex and includes increases in cerebral blood flow associated with impaired vascular autoregulation, increases in cerebral venous pressure, and decreases in cerebral blood flow associated with hypotension, with resulting injury to matrix capillaries. Release of endogenous vasodilators (e.g., adrenomedullin) in the first hours after birth may also play a role in this situation.[250] Studies of the concentrations of brain-specific creatine kinase isoenzymes in cord blood or blood samples

obtained early in the postnatal period or of the hypoxanthine metabolite, uric acid, in blood samples obtained on the first postnatal day, in preterm infants who later developed IVH, support the notion that late intrauterine injury (perhaps asphyxia) may be involved in at least some cases of IVH.[251-253] In one study, those infants who developed IVH had cord blood levels of brain-specific creatine kinase (CK-BB) that were six times greater than those in the infants who did not develop IVH.[251] Moreover, the possibility of a perinatal hypoxic-ischemic insult to brain as a predecessor to IVH is suggested also by the finding of depressed amplitude-integrated electroencephalographic activity before the occurrence of the hemorrhage in 4 of 10 carefully studied preterm infants.[254] In a separate study, early continuous electroencephalographic monitoring detected such abnormalities as excessive discontinuity before the occurrence of IVH.[255] These abnormalities are similar to those produced by hypoxic-ischemic insults (see Chapter 9).

The possibility that increases in intracranial pressure during preterm labor could lead to impaired cerebral blood flow is suggested by studies of preterm fetal sheep.[256] In experiments designed to lead to the increased intracranial pressure associated with fetal cranial deformations during labor, preterm but not near-term fetal sheep were unable to generate a pressor response sufficient to maintain cerebral blood flow, and in fact cerebral blood flow declined by 72% during the 30 minutes of elevated intracranial pressure.

Postnatal Ischemic Events. Importance for *postnatal decreases in cerebral blood flow* in pathogenesis of IVH has been shown by studies using a combination of noninvasive methods to evaluate the cerebral circulation.[224,257-259a] Notably, however, a relationship with decreases in *mean arterial blood pressure*, when infants who developed IVH were compared with infants who did not develop IVH, was not uniformly shown. *Thus, the changes in cerebral hemodynamics could occur without pronounced disturbances of mean arterial blood pressure.* Because impaired autoregulation and fluctuations in blood pressure are both frequent but not necessarily constant in the sick preterm infant,[94] intermittent declines in cerebral blood flow could occur without pronounced changes in mean blood pressure (see Chapter 6). Thus, *continuous measurements of the cerebral circulation are critical in determining changes in cerebral blood flow in the sick, ventilated infant.*

Nevertheless, importance for postnatal decreases in arterial blood pressure in the pathogenesis of IVH is suggested by several studies in which arterial blood pressure was monitored continuously from birth or the first hours of life. In a study of approximately 25,000 very-low-birth-weight infants, severe IVH was three times more common in those infants requiring cardiopulmonary resuscitation (15.3%) at delivery than in those not requiring resuscitation (4.9%).[260] A relationship between arterial hypotension and subsequent occurrence of IVH has been documented frequently.[124,163,261-263] Although the possibility of ischemic insult to germinal matrix in the postnatal period is obvious in association with such occurrences as severe apnea, myocardial failure, sepsis, and so forth, sharp decreases in blood pressure have also been shown to precede the more widely recognized increases provoked by ordinary caretaking procedures.[139] By continuous monitoring of arterial blood pressure during such procedures as auscultation of the chest, taking of temperature, and suctioning, the increases in blood pressure previously noted were shown to be preceded by a decrease in blood pressure. The decreases were most pronounced in the infants requiring the most intensive ventilatory support. The biphasic response of decrease and then increase in blood pressure is qualitatively similar to the sequence required to produce IVH in the beagle puppy (see earlier). The rebound elevation of cerebral blood flow velocity observed after apnea and bradycardia is relevant in this context.[264]

Of particular importance concerning a role for postnatal ischemia is the demonstration by near-infrared spectroscopy in 24 preterm infants in the first 24 hours of life that cerebral blood flow was significantly lower in infants with subsequent demonstration of IVH (median, 7.0 mL/100 g/min) than in those without IVH (median, 12.2 mL/100 g/min).[265] Additionally supportive of a relationship between postnatal ischemic events and the occurrence of IVH is the demonstration of decreased cardiac output in the first 36 hours of life in infants who developed the lesion, especially severe IVH.[266] Similarly, the occurrence of periventricular hemorrhagic infarction with severe IVH was strongly associated with metabolic acidosis in the first days of

life and a need for pressor support and volume expanders.[197] Finally, the beneficial effect of delayed versus immediate clamping of the umbilical cord on the incidence of IVH is considered to be likely caused in considerable part by stabilization of cerebral blood flow and prevention of ischemia.[267]

The contributory role of *maternal intrauterine infection and fetal systemic inflammation* in the pathogenesis of IVH likely is mediated by effects on the cerebral circulation. Although data are not entirely consistent concerning a relationship between chorioamnionitis and the occurrence of IVH, several reports indicate an association with IVH of elevated levels of specific cytokines, especially interleukin-6 (IL-6), in cord or early neonatal blood.[268-275] Infants with chorioamnionitis *and* fetal cord vasculitis had higher IL-6 levels and likelihood of IVH than those with fetal vasculitis alone.[270] The findings suggest that maternal intrauterine infection that leads to a systemic fetal inflammatory response is critical. Indeed, a recent large study of periventricular hemorrhagic infarction ($n = 58$) found no association with maternal fever, maternal infection, or pathologically-confirmed chorioamnionitis.[197] The principal mechanism of the fetal/neonatal cytokine effect is likely circulatory disturbance. Thus, decreased arterial blood pressure, often requiring pressor support, has been shown in the infants with elevated IL-6.[270,273] IL-6, like several other cytokines, has vasodilator properties that likely lead to the decreased blood pressure and presumably cerebral blood flow (Fig. 11-22). Whether IL-6 or related cytokines impair cerebrovascular autoregulation is plausible but not yet shown.

Platelet and Coagulation Disturbances

Disturbances of platelet-capillary function and coagulation may contribute to the pathogenesis of IVH

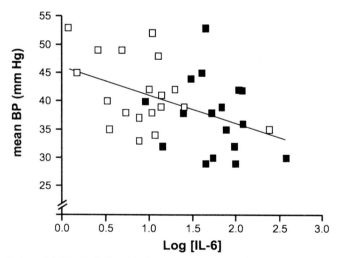

Figure 11-22 Relationship between mean arterial blood pressure (BP) and interleukin-6 (IL-6) concentration. Mean BP was inversely correlated ($R^2 = 0.21$, $P < .01$) with Log IL-6. *Solid square*, chorioamnionitis; *open square*, no chorioamnionitis. *(From Yanowitz TD, Jordan JA, Gilmour CH, Towbin R, et al: Hemodynamic disturbances in premature infants born after chorioamnionitis: Association with cord blood cytokine concentrations, Pediatr Res 51:310–316, 2002.)*

UNIT IV   INTRACRANIAL HEMORRHAGE

(see Table 11-4). The lack of uniformity in results of studies designed to investigate the pathogenetic role of such disturbances, however, emphasizes that the role is likely to be contributory or important only in certain patients.

Platelet-Capillary Function. Regarding platelet-capillary function, an earlier prospective study is of particular interest.[276] Forty percent of infants of less than 1500 g birth weight exhibited platelet counts less than 100,000/mm[3],[251] and most of these thrombocytopenic infants had abnormal bleeding times. The incidences of IVH in thrombocytopenic versus nonthrombocytopenic infants were 78% versus 48% for those weighing less than 1000 g. Additional analysis for other factors potentially important for causation of IVH suggested that the presence of thrombocytopenia was an independent pathogenetic factor. Subsequent work has both confirmed and refuted a role for thrombocytopenia in pathogenesis of IVH.[277-279]

Perhaps relevant to the possibility of disturbed platelet *function* (rather than platelet count) in some infants before occurrence of IVH is the study by Rennie and co-workers[280] of circulating levels of the principal metabolite of prostacyclin in preterm infants. Prostacyclin is a potent perturbant of platelet-capillary function and is produced in elevated amounts, probably by lung, in respiratory distress syndrome and with mechanical ventilation. Evidence was obtained for elevated levels of prostacyclin before the occurrence of IVH. Because prostaglandins additionally have an impact on such factors as cerebral blood flow and free radical production that also may be important in pathogenesis of IVH, it is not clear to what extent effects on platelet-capillary function were independently related to causation of IVH. More data are needed on these issues.

Coagulation. Disagreement exists concerning the role of coagulopathy in causation of IVH. [163,211,277,279,281-291] It could be postulated that prothrombotic disturbances (e.g., factor V Leiden mutation, prothrombin mutation), would increase IVH by provoking deep venous thrombosis or would decrease IVH by preventing extension of small hemorrhages. Because disturbances of coagulation are not uncommon in preterm infants with other provocative factors for IVH (e.g., serious respiratory distress syndrome, asphyxia) or may occur *secondary* to major hemorrhage, an independent pathogenetic role for such disturbances has been difficult to establish. Although administration of fresh frozen plasma was shown in one study to decrease the incidence of IVH,[281] no effect on coagulation measures accompanied the apparent beneficial effect. Moreover, a later investigation failed to show a beneficial effect of prophylactic early fresh frozen plasma in premature infants.[285,292] Administrative of antithrombin III, known to be low in premature infants, did not alter the incidence of IVH in a randomized study.[290]

Potential Role of Drugs. The possibility that *maternal ingestion of certain drugs*, such as aspirin, can result in impaired neonatal hemostasis and provoke IVH was suggested by two earlier reports.[293,294] It is not likely,

TABLE 11-8	Pathogenesis of Germinal Matrix–Intraventricular Hemorrhage: Vascular Factors
Tenuous Capillary Integrity	
Involuting, remodeling capillary bed	
Deficient vascular lining	
Large vascular and luminal area	
Vulnerability of Matrix Capillaries to Hypoxic-Ischemic Injury	
Vascular border zones	
High requirements for oxidative metabolism	

however, that such factors play a major independent role.[283] Similarly, retrospective data suggest that the use of heparin as an intravascular flush to maintain patency of umbilical artery catheters increases the risk of IVH by fourfold.[295] Whether this effect is related to a disturbance of coagulation or to selection bias because of the use of heparin in sick premature infants who develop IVH for other reasons is unclear. A subsequent report also suggested an increasing risk for IVH in premature infants as a function of the daily dose of heparin.[296] More data are needed.

Vascular Factors

Vascular factors are those referable to the blood vessels of the germinal matrix (Table 11-8). As discussed earlier (see "Neuropathology"), the vascular site of origin likely involves the rich microcirculation of the germinal matrix and, specifically, endothelial-lined vessels not readily characterized as arterial or venous. Thus, vascular factors are best grouped in two categories, those suggesting (1) that the integrity of small matrix vessels is tenuous and (2) that these vessels are particularly vulnerable to hypoxic-ischemic injury (see Table 11-8).

Tenuous Vascular Integrity

Three lines of anatomical evidence suggest that the integrity of the microvasculature is tenuous in the germinal matrix (see Table 11-8). First, these vessels, like the germinal matrix itself, are in a process of involution. Pape and Wigglesworth[42] characterized the elaborate capillary bed of the germinal matrix as "a persisting immature vascular rete," an immature microvascular network that is remodeled into a mature capillary bed when the matrix disappears. In keeping with this notion, transmission electron microscopic studies of the matrix reveal many small vessels with absence of a complete basal lamina, a fenestrated lining, and other features characteristic of immature vessels.[297] This involuting remodeling capillary bed may be expected to be more susceptible to rupture than would more mature vessels.

Second, many studies emphasized that the matrix microcirculation is composed of simple endothelial-lined vessels, often of a larger size than capillaries but not readily categorizable as arterioles or venules because of absence of muscle and collagen.[42-45,47,50-53,58,298] Particularly careful studies have documented in detail the absence of muscle[43] and of type VI collagen.[298] Investigators have postulated that such vessels are likely to be more susceptible to rupture. In favor of this postulate is the demonstration in the newborn beagle puppy of matrix vessels that are similar to those just described (i.e., relatively large size and thin walls[299]); these vessels are the sites of hemorrhage in this animal model of germinal matrix hemorrhage–IVH. Recent work emphasized the high vascular density of the germinal matrix and the abundance of small veins, the walls of which are lined only by endothelial cells.[46,300]

Third, an electron microscopic study of cortical and germinal matrix vessels showed a twofold to fourfold-greater diameter of both the vessels and the lumina of the vessels of the germinal matrix versus those of the cortical plate in infants of 25 to 33 weeks of gestation.[301] At 37 weeks of gestation, this difference had disappeared and, notably, the diameters of the matrix vessels and their lumina were twofold to threefold smaller than at 25 to 33 weeks. Thus, in the age range of greatest propensity for occurrence of IVH, the diameters are unusually large, a finding of potential pathogenetic importance because of the Laplace law, which states that the larger the vessel diameter, the greater the total force on the wall at any given pressure.

The possibility should be considered that effects of these maturational deficiencies of germinal matrix vessels underlie the interesting observation that women with a diagnosis of preeclampsia exhibit a lower risk for an infant with IVH (2.5%) than do women without this diagnosis (17%).[30] This lower risk for IVH has been confirmed.[302,303] Infants born to preeclamptic mothers exhibit a variety of features suggestive of accelerated maturation of brain and other organs.[163,304-306]

Vulnerability to Hypoxic-Ischemic Injury

Two features suggest a particular vulnerability of matrix capillaries to hypoxic-ischemic injury (see Table 11-8). First, as shown by Takashima and Tanaka,[41] at the usual site for matrix hemorrhage a vascular border zone exists between the end-fields of the striate and thalamic arteries (Fig. 11-23). The demonstration of heterogeneity of blood flow within the matrix of the beagle puppy may represent the physiological correlate of the anatomical data.[172] Studies of hypotension in the fetal rat also demonstrate a vulnerability of the matrix to ischemia.[307] Thus, it can be postulated that the matrix vessels could be readily injured by ischemia, and, on reperfusion of these injured vessels, hemorrhage could occur. As indicated earlier, this notion is supported by the finding in the

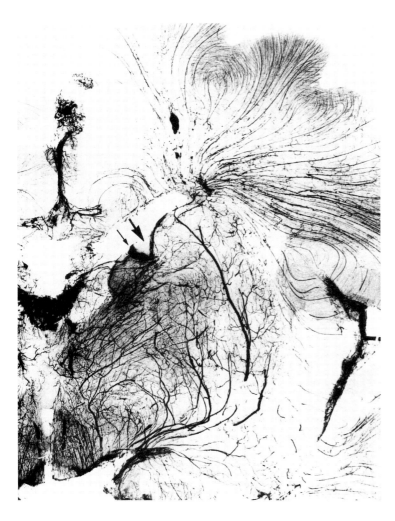

Figure 11-23   Vascular border zone and end zone at the site of germinal matrix hemorrhage. Postmortem arteriography of cerebral hemisphere (coronal section) of a premature infant of 32 weeks of gestational age. Note the triangular avascular area (*large arrow*) at the border zone between the end-fields of the thalamostriate and medullary arteries at the site of a small subependymal hemorrhage (*small arrow*). *(From Takashima S, Tanaka K: Microangiography and vascular permeability of the subependymal matrix in the premature infant, Can J Neurol Sci 5:45–50, 1978.)*

TABLE 11-9	Pathogenesis of Germinal Matrix–Intraventricular Hemorrhage: Extravascular Factors
Deficient vascular support	
Fibrinolytic activity	
Postnatal decrease in extravascular tissue pressure (?)	

beagle puppy model of IVH that the free radical scavenger, superoxide dismutase, prevents hemorrhage caused by the usual hypotension-reperfusion sequence. Similarly, certain studies in human infants (see later discussion) suggest that vitamin E, a free radical scavenger, has a preventive effect on IVH.

Second, matrix capillaries, like other brain capillaries, appear to have a high requirement for oxidative metabolism. Thus, brain endothelial cells have been shown to contain three to five times more mitochondria than do systemic capillary endothelial cells.[308,309] This intense oxidative activity would complement the presence of a vascular border zone in the matrix in enhancing the vulnerability of matrix vessels to ischemic insults.

Extravascular Factors

Extravascular factors are those referable to the space surrounding the germinal matrix capillaries (Table 11-9). These factors are grouped best into the following three categories: deficient vascular support, fibrinolytic activity, and postnatal decrease in extravascular tissue pressure.

Deficient Vascular Support

The germinal matrix can be seen by gross examination to be a gelatinous, friable structure and by microscopic examination to be deficient in supporting mesenchymal and glial elements.[40,50,310] Thus, investigators have suggested that the extravascular space provides poor support for the large, endothelial-lined capillaries that course through it and that are the site of the hemorrhage. This formulation received experimental support from studies of the germinal matrix of the beagle puppy, which showed that large portions of the capillary walls lacked any direct contact with perivascular structures (unlike the capillaries in cerebral cortex or caudate nucleus).[299] Decisive demonstration of the potential importance of deficient vascular support in the human infant is derived from the work of Gould and Howard.[310] Thus, assessing astrocytic fibrillary development by immunocytochemical staining for glial fibrillary acidic protein (GFAP), these investigators showed minimal astrocytic development as late as 27 weeks of gestation and prominent GFAP staining not until 31 weeks (Fig. 11-24). A later detailed study also showed deficient GFAP and astrocytic end-feet overlying the germinal matrix vasculature during the gestational period of 23 to 34 weeks.[311]

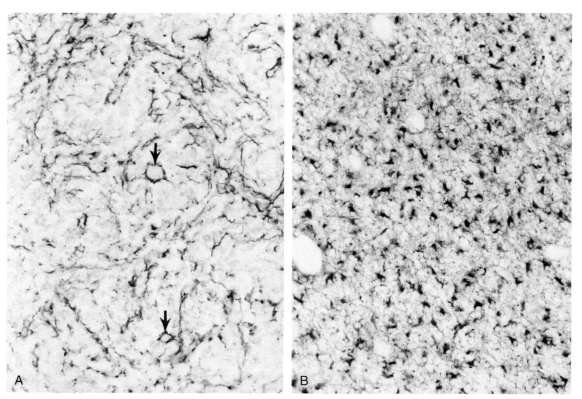

Figure 11-24 **Astrocyte differentiation during gestation**. Glial fibrillary acid protein (GFAP)–stained microscopic sections of germinal matrix at, **A**, 27 weeks and, **B**, 31 weeks of gestation to demonstrate the comparative density of astrocyte differentiation at each gestation. **A**, Capillaries are delineated by the astrocyte fibers terminating on them (*arrows*). **B**, Note the striking increase in GFAP-stained astrocytic fibers at 31 weeks of gestation. *(From Gould SJ, Howard S: An immunohistochemical study of the germinal layer in the late gestation human fetal brain,* Neuropathol Appl Neurobiol *13:421–437, 1987.)*

Because of the role of glial fibers in capillary stabilization, these data suggest an important role for deficient astrocytic development in pathogenesis of IVH in the premature infant.

Fibrinolytic Activity

An excessive amount of fibrinolytic activity has been defined in the periventricular, germinal matrix region of the human premature infant (see Table 11-9).[312,313] Although the source of this activity is not established conclusively, it is likely that the fibrinolytic activity reflects the proteolytic action of the plasmin-generating system. This extracellular proteolytic system is composed of plasminogen activator, plasminogen, and plasmin.[314,315] Plasminogen activator, a protease secreted from cells, activates plasminogen to generate the protease plasmin, which, in turn, can degrade a wide variety of extracellular proteins. This system is involved in many developing, remodeling tissues as a normal maturational process. Fibrinolysis is only one action of this proteolytic system. In developing chick spinal cord, this system is most active during glial proliferation. Moreover, studies in cell culture show that the immature astrocyte (not the mature astrocyte) is the principal source for plasminogen activator and the action of this proteolytic system. Glial proliferation is very active in the germinal matrix at the usual time of occurrence of germinal matrix hemorrhage (see Chapter 2). It is reasonable to suspect that this fibrinolytic activity, an epiphenomenon of the proteolytic system required for remodeling of the germinal matrix, allows the small capillary hemorrhages of the matrix to become the large lesions characteristic of IVH.

Postnatal Decrease in Extravascular Tissue Pressure

The possibility that a postnatal decrease in extravascular tissue pressure causes an increase in the transmural intravascular-extravascular pressure gradient sufficient to provoke hemorrhage was raised by studies of the beagle puppy.[316,317] Administration of prolactin was shown to decrease the incidence and severity of hemorrhage in that animal model. The relevance to hemorrhage in the human premature infant, however, is unclear because the timing of the apparent postnatal decrease in extracellular volume in the premature infant[318-321] (i.e., 2 to 3 days of life) occurs *after* the peak time of occurrence of IVH. A relationship among postnatal weight loss, hypernatremia, and development of IVH could not be demonstrated in a study of 229 infants of less than 1500 g birth weight.[322]

Interaction of Pathogenetic Factors

As indicated throughout the preceding discussion, not *all* the pathogenetic factors operate in every case. *Clinical circumstances dictate which factors are most critical in the individual infant.* Perhaps the best example of the interaction of the most important pathogenetic factors is provided by the clinical situation of the premature infant who is mechanically ventilated for serious respiratory distress syndrome (Fig. 11-25), the clinical setting for the largest proportion of all cases of IVH.

CLINICAL FEATURES

The principal clinical setting for IVH is a premature infant with respiratory distress syndrome severe enough

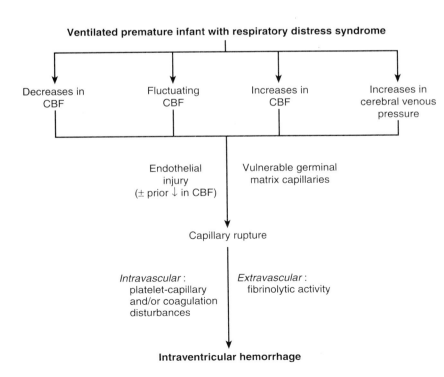

Figure 11-25   Germinal matrix–intraventricular hemorrhage in respiratory distress syndrome. Interaction of major pathogenetic factors for the occurrence of germinal matrix–intraventricular hemorrhage in the ventilated premature infant with respiratory distress syndrome. CBF, cerebral blood flow.

TABLE 11-10	Catastrophic Clinical Syndrome with Germinal Matrix–Intraventricular Hemorrhage

Inexorable evolution in minutes to hours
Neurological features
  Stupor → coma
  Respiratory disturbance → apnea
  Generalized tonic seizures
  ''Decerebrate'' posturing
  Pupils fixed to light
  Eyes fixed to vestibular stimulation
  Flaccid quadriparesis

to require mechanical ventilation. The *time of onset of hemorrhage*, defined most clearly by serial cranial ultrasonography (see ''Diagnosis''), is the first day of life in at least 50% of affected infants, and by 72 hours, approximately 90% of the lesions can be identified. The timing of the initial clinical features, as expected, is similar.

Three Basic Syndromes

Three basic clinical syndromes accompany IVH: (1) a *catastrophic* deterioration (Table 11-10), (2) a *saltatory* deterioration (Table 11-11), and (3) a *''clinically silent''* syndrome. The least common but most dramatic of these is the catastrophic deterioration, which occurs in infants with the most severe hemorrhages. More common is the saltatory deterioration, and *most common of all is the clinically silent syndrome.* The latter two syndromes occur most often, although not exclusively, in infants with smaller lesions.

Catastrophic Syndrome

The catastrophic syndrome is dramatic in presentation (see Table 11-10). The deterioration evolves in minutes to hours and consists of deep stupor or coma, respiratory abnormalities (arrhythmias, hypoventilation, and apnea), generalized tonic seizures, decerebrate posturing, pupils fixed to light, eyes fixed to vestibular stimulation, and flaccid quadriparesis. The clinical distinction between tonic seizures and ''decerebrate'' posturing is very difficult in this setting. Indeed, generalized tonic ''seizures'' in this setting most often do represent posturing rather than an epileptic phenomenon (see Chapter 5). The wide range of frequencies of seizure phenomena recorded with IVH ($\approx$15%

TABLE 11-11	Saltatory Clinical Syndrome with Germinal Matrix–Intraventricular Hemorrhage

Stuttering evolution: hours to days
Neurological features
  Altered level of consciousness
  Altered motility (usually decreased)
  Hypotonia
  Abnormally tight popliteal angle
  Abnormal eye position or movement or both
  Respiratory disturbance

to 35%)[153,323-327] in part reflects this difficulty. In my experience, seizures occurring with IVH early in the neonatal course usually are associated with periventricular hemorrhagic infarction.

This impressive neurological syndrome is associated with numerous other features, for example, falling hematocrit, bulging anterior fontanelle, hypotension, bradycardia, temperature derangements, metabolic acidosis, and abnormalities of glucose and water homeostasis.[325,328-331] The latter include, particularly, inappropriate antidiuretic hormone secretion and, less commonly, diabetes insipidus.[328,331]

I have reasoned that the neurological syndrome reflects the movement of blood through the ventricular system with sequential affection of the diencephalon, midbrain, pons, and medulla. The signs of increased intracranial pressure reflect acute hydrocephalus. The outcome, often poor, reflects the severity of the hemorrhage and, particularly, the extent of complicating parenchymal involvement (see ''Prognosis'').

Saltatory Syndrome

The saltatory syndrome is much more subtle in presentation (see Table 11-11).[332,333] The most common presenting signs are (1) an alteration in the level of consciousness, (2) a change (usually a decrease) in the quantity and quality of spontaneous and elicited motility, (3) hypotonia, and (4) subtle aberrations of eye position and movement (e.g., skew deviation, vertical drift, usually down, and incomplete horizontal movement with doll's eyes maneuver). In some patients, disturbances of respiratory function appear to be concomitants, but more data are needed on this issue. In one careful study of serial clinical evaluations and ultrasonographic examinations, an abnormal popliteal angle was found to be a particularly useful diagnostic sign.[327] Eighty-four percent of premature infants with IVH (versus 10% of infants without hemorrhage) exhibited an abnormally tight angle, perhaps secondary to meningeal irritation. The signs of the saltatory syndrome evolve over many hours, and the deterioration often ceases, only to begin anew after several more hours. This stuttering course may continue for a day or more. The outcome, most often favorable, again relates to the ultimate severity of the hemorrhage and any accompanying parenchymal involvement (see ''Prognosis'').

Clinically Silent Syndrome

The neurological signs of the saltatory syndrome may be so subtle that they are overlooked. Indeed, in a prospective study of infants subjected to clinical assessment and CT scan in the first week of life, only approximately 50% of cases of IVH were correctly predicted to have the lesion on the basis of clinical criteria.[326] The most valuable sign was an unexplained fall in hematocrit or a failure of hematocrit to rise after transfusion. In the serial study of Dubowitz and co-workers,[327] approximately 75% of cases had three or more of the abnormal neurological signs of the saltatory syndrome. Thus, in 25% to 50% of infants with IVH, even careful, serial clinical assessments may fail to reveal a distinct constellation of signs indicative of the lesion.

DIAGNOSIS

Initial Approach

The two essential steps in establishing the diagnosis of IVH are *recognition of the clinical setting* and use of a suitable *screening procedure*. In view of the high incidence of the hemorrhage, I consider the infant at risk to be any premature infant in a neonatal intensive care facility. Thus, such infants should be subjected to a suitable screening procedure.

Although the screening procedure of choice is portable cranial ultrasonography (see "Ultrasound Scan" later), *lumbar puncture*, usually obtained for such purposes as evaluation for sepsis, can provide useful information. The characteristic CSF profile of intracranial hemorrhage consists initially of many red blood cells and elevated protein content, followed shortly by xanthochromia and depressed glucose content (see Chapter 10). The first two of these CSF abnormalities are the most critical in early recognition. The degree of elevation of CSF protein correlates approximately with the severity of the hemorrhage. For example, in one study of 48 cases of CT-proven IVH, the mean CSF protein in the small lesions (subependymal hemorrhage or less than 10% of ventricular area filled with blood) was 254 mg/dL; in the moderate lesions (10% to 50% of the ventricular area filled with blood), it was 746 mg/dL; and in the largest lesions (more than 50% of the ventricular area filled with blood), it was 1668 mg/dL.[334] However, the dispersion of the mean values was so large that the CSF protein content could be used only as an approximation of severity of hemorrhage.

In the following sections, I review the principal means of visualizing germinal matrix hemorrhage–IVH (i.e., ultrasonography) and consider only briefly other brain imaging techniques. Finally, the particular insight into the periventricular hemorrhagic infarction with IVH provided by positron emission tomography (PET), although by no means a conventional diagnostic technique, is demonstrated.

Ultrasound Scan

Ultrasound scan of the neonatal cranium is the procedure of choice in the diagnosis of germinal matrix hemorrhage–IVH. The basic principles of the technique, the features of the instruments used, and the normal anatomical features visualized are described in Chapter 4. Since the initial reports of the value of the technique in diagnosis of IVH,[335-341] a vast experience has demonstrated the reliability and versatility of the procedure in this clinical setting.[15,16,22,33,43,71,195,197,342-366] High-resolution imaging, portable instrumentation, lack of ionizing radiation, and relative affordability have been the major advantages. In the following subsections, I illustrate the value of cranial ultrasound scanning in identification of hemorrhage and in determination of timing, severity, and progression of the lesion.

Identification of the Hemorrhage

Ultrasound scan is effective in identification of all degrees of severity of IVH from isolated germinal matrix hemorrhage to major degrees, with or without periventricular

hemorrhagic infarction. The physical basis of the dense echoes that correlate with the hemorrhage is probably the formation of fibrin mesh within the clot.[360]

The major elemental lesion, of course, is *hemorrhage within the germinal matrix* (Fig. 11-26A). *Intraventricular*

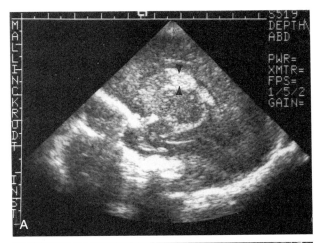

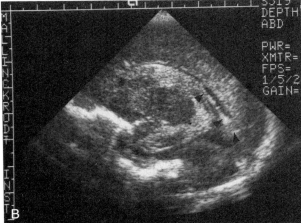

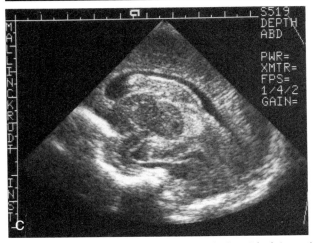

Figure 11-26 Grading the severity of germinal matrix–intraventricular hemorrhage, parasagittal ultrasound scans. A, Grade I. Note echogenic blood in germinal matrix (*arrowheads*) just anterior to anterior tip of choroid plexus, which (normally) also is echogenic. **B,** Grade II. Note echogenic blood (*arrowheads*) filling less than 50% of the ventricular area. **C,** Grade III. Note large blood clot nearly completely filling and distending the entire lateral ventricle.

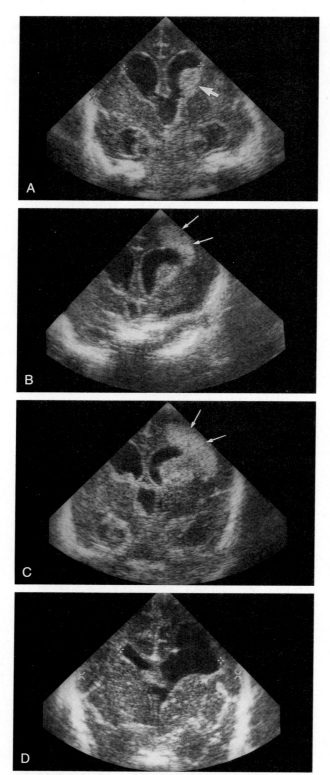

Figure 11-27 Ultrasound scans of evolution of periventricular hemorrhagic infarction. Coronal scans obtained from a premature infant of 30 weeks of gestation on, **A** to **C**, day 7 and, **D**, day 60. The three coronal scans obtained on day 7 were separated by minutes to several hours and show a bulging germinal matrix hemorrhage (*arrow* in **A**) that increases in size (**B** and **C**); with the increasing size, a crescentic periventricular echodensity (*arrows*) consistent with periventricular hemorrhagic infarction develops. Note in **C** the midline shift to the right. **D**, Two months later, a large single porencephalic cyst is observed at the site of the infarction.

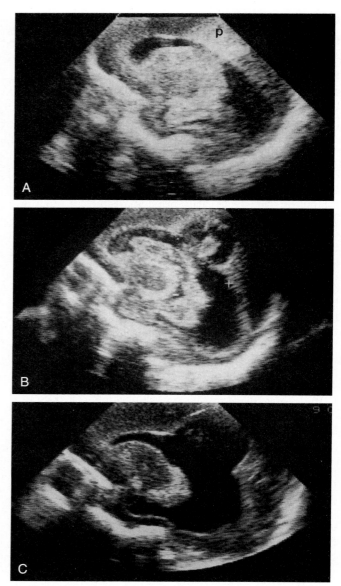

Figure 11-28 Periventricular hemorrhagic infarction with evolution to porencephalic cyst, ultrasound scans. **A**, At 9 days of age, the intraparenchymal lesion (p) and ventricular dilation are visible on parasagittal ultrasound scan. Remaining intraventricular clot is also apparent. **B**, At 3 weeks of age, the cystic cavity becomes apparent, as necrotic tissue and clot retract. **C**, At 2 months of age, a large porencephalic cyst has evolved pari passu with increased ventricular dilation.

bleeding results in echogenic material that fills a portion or all of the lateral ventricular system (see Fig. 11-26B and C). *Periventricular hemorrhagic infarction* complicating major IVH is a striking echogenic lesion, globular, crescentic, or fan shaped in configuration, usually unilateral, and located on the side of the largest amount of germinal matrix or intraventricular blood or both (Fig. 11-27). The echogenic portion of the lesion is located most commonly in the frontal and parietal regions. The subsequent finding of porencephalic cyst at the site of such a hemorrhagic intracerebral lesion (see Fig. 11-27; Fig. 11-28) reflects the essential ischemic nature of the lesion (see "Mechanisms of Brain Injury" later). The *single, large, unilateral* or

TABLE 11-12	Grading of Severity of Germinal Matrix–Intraventricular Hemorrhage by Ultrasound Scan	
Severity	**Description**	
Grade I	Germinal matrix hemorrhage with no or minimal intraventricular hemorrhage (<10% of ventricular area on parasagittal view)	
Grade II	Intraventricular hemorrhage (10%–50% of ventricular area on parasagittal view)	
Grade III	Intraventricular hemorrhage (>50% of ventricular area on parasagittal view; usually distends lateral ventricle)	
Separate notation	Periventricular echodensity (location and extent)	

TABLE 11-13	Approximate Time of Occurrence of Germinal Matrix–Intraventricular Hemorrhage Identified by Ultrasound Scan	
Postnatal Day	**Percentage of Infants with Germinal Matrix–Intraventricular Hemorrhage***	
1	50%	
2	25%	
3	15%	
≥4	10%	

*Approximately 20% to 40% of these infants exhibit progression of hemorrhage over 3 to 5 days.

asymmetrical porencephalic cyst that occurs as a consequence of periventricular hemorrhagic infarction differs from the *multiple, small, symmetrical* cysts observed as a consequence of periventricular leukomalacia (see Chapter 9). The evolution of the typical unilateral or grossly asymmetrical periventricular hemorrhagic infarction after ipsilateral germinal matrix or IVH, or both, has been well documented.[68,197] *Posthemorrhagic ventricular dilation* is demonstrated very well by cranial ultrasound scan. This disorder and its management are discussed in detail later (see "Management").

Grading the Severity of Hemorrhage

The grading system that I have used is based on the presence and amount of blood in the germinal matrix and lateral ventricles (Table 11-12); determination of the presence of blood in the matrix is best made on the coronal scan, and determination of the amount of blood in the lateral ventricles is best made on the parasagittal scan. In this classification, the presence of periventricular hemorrhagic infarction or of other parenchymal lesions is noted separately because these abnormalities generally are not caused simply by "extension" of matrix hemorrhage or IVH into normal brain parenchyma (see earlier discussion and "Mechanisms of Brain Injury" later).

Timing of Hemorrhage

Serial ultrasound scans of premature infants have provided invaluable information concerning the *time of onset of hemorrhage*, and this information, of course, is critical for deciding when to screen for the presence of hemorrhage. In a cumulative series of 105 infants with IVH studied by real-time ultrasonography from the first hours of life, approximately 50% had onset of hemorrhage on the first postnatal day, an additional 25% on the second day, and an additional 15% on the third day (Table 11-13).[37,70,191,247,349,351,354] In a single study of 1105 infants weighing 2000 g or less at birth, approximately 40% of the 265 who developed IVH did so within the first 5 hours of life.[31] The likelihood of onset of hemorrhage on the first postnatal day varies inversely with birth weight; in one series, 62% of hemorrhages in infants between 500 and 700 g birth weight occurred in the first 18 hours.[37] In general, if

screening were to be confined to a single postnatal day in the first days of life, a scan on the fourth postnatal day would be expected to detect approximately 90% of all hemorrhages. However, *progression* of the lesions occurs in approximately 20% to 40% of the affected infants, with maximal extent of the lesion attained usually within 3 to 5 days of the initial diagnosis.[37,343,349,354,356,361] Thus, a second scan after approximately 5 days is necessary to identify maximal extent of hemorrhage in the many infants who exhibit progression. I prefer a regimen of two scans in the first week, with timing of subsequent scans determined by the initial findings and clinical events (see later).

Severity of Hemorrhage

The relative distribution of the severity of IVH has been elucidated more effectively with ultrasound scan than was possible with CT scan because the *single* CT scan usually obtained could not be expected to identify the maximal severity of hemorrhage in many of the cases. With serial ultrasound scans, this problem is obviated. However, large-scale ultrasonographic studies have used different grading systems and inclusion criteria and have often grouped together infants with grade III IVH and periventricular hemorrhagic infarction. The relative distribution of severity of IVH in infants of less than 1500 g birth weight, based on our unpublished data and that in the literature, is shown in Table 11-14.[12-16,19,38,39,367] Approximately 20% of

TABLE 11-14	Severity of Germinal Matrix–Intraventricular Hemorrhage Identified by Ultrasound Scan	
Severity*	**Percentage of Infants with Germinal Matrix–Intraventricular Hemorrhage**	
Grade I	40%	
Grade II	25%	
Grade III	20%	
Intraventricular hemorrhage and apparent periventricular hemorrhagic infarction	15%†	

*See Table 11-13 for grading system.
†In approximately 90%, the accompanying intraventricular hemorrhage was grade III in severity.
From unpublished personal data from approximately 400 premature infants with germinal matrix–intraventricular hemorrhage.

TABLE 11-15 Incidence of Periventricular Hemorrhagic Infarction as a Function of Birth Weight and Year of Delivery*

Year of Delivery	Birth Weight <750 g PHI	Birth Weight 750–1500 g PHI	Birth Weight <1500 g PHI
1997–1999	6%	2%	3%
2000–2002	16%	3%	6%

*The total population was 723 live births for 1997 to 1999 and 616 for 2000 to 2002. Percentages are rounded off.
PHI, periventricular hemorrhagic infarction.
Adapted from Bassan H, Feldman HA, Limperopoulos C, Benson CB, et al: Periventricular hemorrhagic infarction: Risk factors and neonatal outcome, *Pediatr Neurol* 35:85–92, 2006.

the hemorrhages were large (i.e., grade III), with blood usually filling and dilating the lateral ventricles on parasagittal scan (see Table 11-12 for grading system). Approximately 15% of all the infants with hemorrhage had, in addition, large periventricular echodensity consistent with periventricular hemorrhagic infarction. In these infants, the severity of the IVH was grade III in approximately 90%.

Particular emphasis should be placed on large IVH with periventricular hemorrhagic infarction, because this lesion accounts for most of the morbidity attributable to IVH per se. This striking lesion is particularly characteristic of the most immature infants. Thus, in one series of 2667 infants, IVH with periventricular hemorrhagic infarction accounted for 20% to 30% of all IVH in infants born at 24 to 26 weeks of gestation but less than 5% of all IVH at 30 to 32 weeks of gestation.[16] If one considers the *total population* of premature infants who weigh less than 1500 g at birth, the magnitude of the problem of periventricular hemorrhagic infarction is striking. The incidence among 1339 premature infants (<1500 g) is shown as a function of birth weight and two epochs of year of birth in Table 11-15. The *maturation-related effect is shown by highest incidences in the most premature infants (birth weight < 750 g)* such that in the more recent epoch, 2000 to 2002, the incidence among all infants of less than 750 g was approximately 16%.[197] Notably, in these smallest infants, the incidence increased 2.7-fold in the later epoch (see Table 11-15).[197] This increase in incidence in the later years was accompanied by an overall decrease in mortality for infants with birth weight lower than 750 g from 50% in 1997 to 1999 to 36% in 2000 to 2002, and in those infants who died, by a decrease in the incidence of death on the first day of life from 79% to 55%, before the usual occurrence of the periventricular hemorrhagic infarction on the second to fifth days of life (see later). In the same study, of 4435 infants of 1500 to 2550 g birth weight, only 4 (0.1%) exhibited periventricular hemorrhagic infarction.[197]

Computed Tomography Scan

The CT scan demonstrates the site and extent of IVH very effectively.[20,25,325,368-374] Indeed, in the first edition of this book, I stated that "the CT scan is the most definitive means to define the site(s) and extent of periventricular-intraventricular hemorrhage."[100] Ultrasound scan has displaced CT as the principal diagnostic technique, not only because of equivalent resolution

for identification of the hemorrhage but also because CT has the disadvantages of requiring the sick premature infant to be transported and of exposing the brain and eyes to ionizing radiation. CT retains some value, however, for identification of complicating hemorrhagic lesions, such as subdural hemorrhage, hemorrhagic posterior fossa lesions, and certain cerebral parenchymal hemorrhagic abnormalities (see Chapter 4).

Magnetic Resonance Imaging Scan

MRI has been shown to provide excellent images of IVH, especially after the first few days of the hemorrhage.[71,375-380] However, MRI currently cannot supplant ultrasonography in the evaluation of IVH, because the former technique requires transport to the scanner, has a relatively long data acquisition time, precludes the use of metallic materials still often found on neonatal monitoring and support equipment, and is expensive. The effectiveness of MRI in demonstration of the parenchymal details of periventricular hemorrhagic infarction with germinal matrix hemorrhage–IVH was illustrated earlier (see Fig. 11-9).[75]

Positron Emission Tomography

PET, although by no means a routine diagnostic procedure (see Chapter 4), has provided valuable information concerning the basic nature of the critical periventricular hemorrhagic infarction that often accompanies major IVH. Thus, because previous experience with adult patients indicated that measurements of regional cerebral blood flow provided important information concerning the regional structural integrity of brain, we studied a series of six infants who had major IVH complicated by periventricular hemorrhagic involvement with the $H_2^{15}O$ technique to measure regional cerebral blood flow.[64] The infants weighed between 900 and 1200 g at birth and had severe respiratory distress syndrome that required mechanical ventilation. Cranial ultrasonography demonstrated major IVH and the unilateral periventricular echodensity typical of periventricular hemorrhagic infarction in the left frontal white matter. The hemorrhagic lesion did not extend into posterior parietal-occipital white matter.

The PET findings were similar and dramatic in these six patients. First, anteriorly in the region of the periventricular echodensity, cerebral blood flow was reduced markedly (as expected). Second, and unexpectedly, markedly diminished cerebral blood flow was also observed in the posterior cerebral (parietal-occipital)

TABLE 11-16 Short-Term Outcome of Germinal Matrix–Intraventricular Hemorrhage as a Function of Severity of Hemorrhage and Birth Weight*

| Severity of Hemorrhage[†] | DEATHS IN FIRST 14 DAYS[‡] | | PVD (SURVIVORS >14 DAYS)[‡] | |
	<750 g (n = 75)	751–1500 g (n = 173)	<750 g (n = 56)	751–1500 g (n = 165)
Grade I	3/24 (12)	0/80 (0)	1/21 (5)	3/80 (4)
Grade II	5/21 (24)	1/44 (2)	1/16 (6)	6/43 (14)
Grade III	6/19 (32)	2/26 (8)	10/13 (77)	18/24 (75)
Grade III and apparent PHI	5/11 (45)	5/23 (22)	5/6 (83)	12/18 (66)

*Values are n (%).
[†]For grading system, see Table 11-12.
[‡]Deaths occurring later in the neonatal period are not shown; the *total* mortality rates (early and late deaths) are approximately 50% to 100% greater for each grade of hemorrhage and birth weight than those shown in the table for early deaths alone.
PHI, periventricular hemorrhagic infarction; PVD, progressive ventricular dilation.
Data from Murphy BP, Inder TE, Rooks V, Taylor GA, et al: Posthemorrhagic ventricular dilatation in the premature infant: Natural history and predictors of outcome, *Arch Dis Child Fetal Neonatal Ed* 87:F37–F41, 2002.

white matter in the same hemisphere. Indeed, the impairment of cerebral blood flow in the hemisphere containing the parenchymal echodensity was much more extensive in every patient than could be accounted for by the locus of the echodensity.[64] We confirmed this observation in eight subsequent infants studied by PET (unpublished). This larger region of abnormality, delineated by the lower regional cerebral blood flow associated with the periventricular hemorrhagic infarction, presumably contributes importantly to the serious neurological deficits so frequently observed in the survivors of large examples of this lesion (see "Prognosis"). We concluded that the extensive abnormality of cerebral blood flow demonstrated by PET in these patients with periventricular hemorrhagic infarction was indicative primarily of a fixed structural lesion for two reasons. First, the PET lesion was irreversible in two patients studied a second time (after 1 month of age). Second, neuropathological correlation demonstrated extensive infarction in the affected hemisphere in the three infants studied post mortem (see Fig. 11-7 for one of the three cases). Thus, the PET data demonstrated that the periventricular hemorrhagic lesion observed with major IVH and so critical in determining prognosis (see "Prognosis") is indicative of a *larger lesion than was previously suspected by ultrasonography.* The neuropathological data indicate that the lesion is ischemic (i.e., an infarct), presumably venous in origin (see earlier discussion).

PROGNOSIS

Prognosis is best considered in terms of the short-term outcome (mortality rate and development of progressive ventricular dilation) and the long-term outcome (neurological sequelae). I emphasize the relationship of outcome with the severity of hemorrhage and parenchymal abnormalities identifiable on neonatal brain imaging studies, especially the most widely used modality, cranial ultrasonography. In the following discussion, I review our current concepts of short-term and long-term outcomes, and in the major section that follows this one, the mechanisms of brain injury associated with IVH, because these mechanisms obviously are related closely to outcome.

Short-Term Outcome: Mortality Rates and Progressive Ventricular Dilation

The *short-term outcome* relates clearly to the severity of the hemorrhage and to the degree of prematurity. The mortality rates and incidences of progressive posthemorrhagic ventricular dilation (i.e., hydrocephalus) are shown in Table 11-16 as a function of the severity of the hemorrhage, documented primarily by ultrasound scan, and the infant's birth weight.[367] Although the data are derived from a single study of 248 infants, findings of other reports are more or less similar.* Thus, with small lesions, confined to the germinal matrix or accompanied by small amounts of intraventricular blood (grade I), mortality rates are low, comparable to those of small premature infants without hemorrhage, and the frequency of progressive ventricular dilation in survivors is very uncommon. With moderate (grade II) lesions, mortality rates are higher only in the smallest infants (<750 g), and approximately 5% to 15% of survivors develop progressive ventricular dilation. With severe (grade III) lesions (i.e., blood filling the ventricles), mortality rates are approximately 30% in the infants weighing less than 750 g at birth but still less than 10% in the infants with a birth weight of 751 to 1500 g; approximately 75% of survivors exhibit progressive ventricular dilation in both groups. For those infants who, in addition to severe IVH, also exhibit apparent periventricular hemorrhagic infarction, mortality rates approach 50% in the infants weighing less than 750 g at birth and are approximately 20% in those with a birth weight of 751 to 1500 g, and the incidences of subsequent hydrocephalus are still higher. Indeed, for the now prominent population of infants of less than 750 g birth weight, survival without progressive ventricular dilation is very unusual with these severe lesions.

The progressive ventricular dilation that occurs in survivors does not necessarily require a procedure to divert CSF from the lateral ventricles (i.e., ventriculostomy or ventriculoperitoneal shunt). Indeed, many

---

*See references 14,15,19,20,24,33,34,39,161,350,381-399.

TABLE 11-17 Long-Term Outcome: Neurological Sequelae in Survivors with Germinal Matrix–Intraventricular Hemorrhage as a Function of Severity of Hemorrhage*

Severity of Hemorrhage[†]	Incidence of Definite Neurological Sequelae[‡]
Grade I	15%
Grade II	25%
Grade III	50%
Grade III and apparent periventricular hemorrhagic infarction	75%

*See text for references. Data are derived from reports published since 2002 and include personal published and unpublished cases.
[†]For grading system, see Table 11-12.
[‡]Mean values (to nearest 5%); considerable variability among studies was apparent, especially for the severe lesions. Definite neurological sequelae included principally cerebral palsy or mental retardation, or both.

infants, especially with less severe IVH, exhibit cessation of progression, with or without resolution, with no therapy. The natural history of posthemorrhagic ventricular dilation is discussed in more detail under "Management."

Long-Term Outcome: Major Neurological Sequelae

The outcome of the infant with IVH depends in largest part on the degree of associated parenchymal injury. Only an approximate relationship exists between the quantity of intraventricular blood and neurological outcome (Table 11-17).* Thus, although the incidence of major neurological sequelae (spastic motor deficits, major cognitive deficits) after minor degrees of hemorrhage is slightly higher than that in infants without hemorrhage and increases to approximately 50% in infants with severe hemorrhage, a *clearly higher* incidence occurs in infants with IVH complicated by periventricular hemorrhagic infarction or cystic periventricular leukomalacia, or both. *Prognostic estimates* thus are refined considerably by assessment of the presence and the degree of parenchymal injury by detailed imaging. This essential point is discussed in more detail next.

Overall Outcome

Clearly, major determinants of outcome in the premature infant are the presence and severity of associated periventricular hemorrhagic infarction. Although many studies have addressed the outcome in this group, quantitative conclusions are difficult to draw because the selection criteria differ, the numbers of infants are often relatively small, the lesion is not quantitated, and the mortality rates vary, in part because of differences in policies of termination of life support in the severely

*See references 15,24,34-65,68,350,383,385-389,391-392,394-395, 400-441.

affected infant. Nevertheless, more recent studies[15,66,441] provide useful data and complement the largest single study reported earlier ($n = 75$).[60] In the latter study, the *degree* of parenchymal injury was quantitated after identification on ultrasound scan as a large intraparenchymal echodensity (i.e., >1 cm), presumed to represent periventricular hemorrhagic infarction.[60] Among the 75 infants studied, the mortality rate was 59%. This finding should be contrasted with a mortality rate of 8% in the same neonatal unit at the same time for infants with the severest grade of IVH (i.e., grade III, IVH but no associated periventricular hemorrhagic infarction). Among the 22 survivors who could be examined on follow-up, 87% exhibited major motor deficits, and 68% had cognitive function less than 80% of normal. The motor deficits correlated with the topography of the parenchymal lesions and thus consisted of either spastic hemiparesis or asymmetrical spastic quadriparesis. In more recent reports, the incidence of major motor deficits has been lower (i.e., ≈50% in 36 surviving infants <32 weeks of gestational age,[15] and 60% in 30 surviving infants <2500 g birth weight[197]).

Outcome as a Function of Severity of Intraparenchymal Echodensity

Prognostic estimation can be refined by considering the severity of the periventricular hemorrhagic infarction (Table 11-18). Thus, among infants with extensive lesions (i.e., echodensity that included frontoparieto-occipital regions [Fig. 11-29]), 30 of 37 (81%) died, and of the 8 survivors, 7 had subsequent motor deficits.[60] *However, caution is necessary in extrapolating these small numbers to all infants; careful consideration of associated lesions (e.g., periventricular leukomalacia) and other clinical aspects is necessary.* Among infants with *localized* lesions (i.e., echodensity confined to frontal, parietal, or occipital regions [Fig. 11-30]), the outcome was more favorable than after extensive echodensity for both unilateral and bilateral lesions. Thus, major spastic motor deficits occurred in only 50% with unilateral localized lesions, and major cognitive deficits appeared in only 12% of these infants. Even with bilateral localized disease, major cognitive deficits occurred in only 50%. In a recent study,[437,441] only 4 of 12 (33%) infants with unilateral localized lesions had an abnormal motor examination at 2 years of age. Consistent with this *more favorable outcome for localized lesions*, a study of unilateral periventricular echodensities that evolved to porencephalic cyst reported a developmental quotient less than 80 in five of nine localized lesions versus six of seven diffuse lesions; spastic motor deficits occurred in four of nine localized lesions versus seven of seven diffuse lesions.[442] The relationship between the anterior-posterior distribution of periventricular hemorrhagic infarction and outcome is controversial. An earlier report indicated that motor deficits were more likely with posterior than anterior lesions,[442] whereas more recent work found more motor deficits with anterior than posterior lesions.[197,441] Posterior (peritrigonal) lesions have been noted to be especially closely associated with subsequent cognitive deficits[442] and microcephaly.[197,441]

TABLE 11-18   **Outcome of Intraventricular Hemorrhage as a Function of the Severity of Associated Periventricular Intraparenchymal Echodensity**

| Outcome | SEVERITY OF IPE* | | | |
	Unilateral Extensive	Localized	Bilateral Extensive	Localized
Mortality rate	21/27 (78%)	8/23 (35%)	9/11 (82%)	6/14 (43%)
Major motor deficits[†]	5/6 (83%)	4/8 (50%)	2/2 (100%)	5/6 (83%)
Cognitive <75%[‡]	5/6 (83%)	1/8 (12%)	2/2 (100%)	3/6 (50%)

*See text for definitions of "extensive" and "localized."
[†]Includes only overt spastic motor deficits.
[‡]Age range at testing generally 1 to 4 years; tests included varying combinations of Bayley, Stanford-Binet, Vineland, Wechsler, and Verbal Language Development Scales.
IPE, intraparenchymal echodensity.

Clinicopathological Correlation: Periventricular Hemorrhagic Infarction

A particular variety of spastic hemiparesis is characteristic of periventricular hemorrhagic infarction. Involvement of *lower* extremities is as prominent as involvement of upper extremities, in contrast to the greater affection of upper versus lower extremity in the hemiparesis that follows middle cerebral artery infarction in the term infant (see Chapter 9). The reason for this characteristic type of spastic hemiparesis of the premature infant relates to the topography of the neuropathology (Fig. 11-31). Thus, the periventricular locus causes as prominent an affection of descending fibers for lower extremities as for upper extremities. The particular propensity for lesions affecting *posterior* cerebral white matter to result in cognitive deficits may relate to the presence of fibers crucial for associative functions and integration of visual, auditory, and somesthetic input.

MECHANISMS OF BRAIN INJURY

Major Factors

The principal mechanisms of brain injury in the premature infant with IVH can be categorized into those factors of proven importance, those of likely but not yet proven importance, and those of unlikely or rare importance (Table 11-19). Those mechanisms of proven

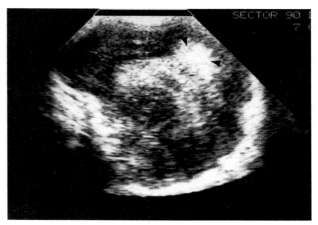

Figure 11-30   **Ultrasound scan of periventricular intraparenchymal echodensity, localized.** Note that the lesion (*arrowheads*) is confined to the posterior parietal region.

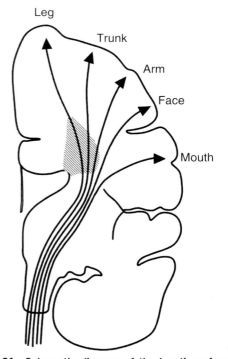

Figure 11-31   **Schematic diagram of the location of periventricular hemorrhagic infarction and descending corticospinal tract motor fibers.** Note that the topography of the lesion accounts for the subsequent spastic hemiparesis with prominent involvement of lower as well as upper extremity.

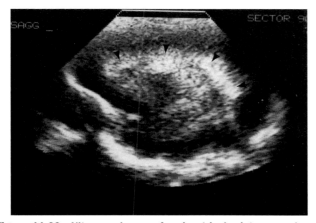

Figure 11-29   **Ultrasound scan of periventricular intraparenchymal echodensity, extensive.** Note that the lesion (*arrowheads*) extends from frontal to occipital regions.

TABLE 11-19   **Mechanisms of Brain Injury with Germinal Matrix–Intraventricular Hemorrhage**

Factors of Proven Importance
Preceding and concomitant ischemic/inflammatory injury, especially periventricular leukomalacia
Destruction of periventricular white matter—periventricular hemorrhagic infarction
Posthemorrhagic hydrocephalus

Factors of Likely but Unproven Importance
Injury to periventricular white matter secondary to intraventricular, parenchymal, or subarachnoid blood products (by generation of free radicals and possibly by vasoconstriction with decreased blood flow)
Destruction of glial precursors in germinal matrix: deleterious effect on myelination
Impairment of subsequent cerebral cortical development

Factors of Unlikely or Rare Importance
Intracranial hypertension and impaired cerebral perfusion (rare)
Arterial vasospasm with focal brain ischemia (?)

importance include the following: (1) preceding and concomitant ischemic/inflammatory injury, especially periventricular leukomalacia; (2) destruction of periventricular white matter–periventricular hemorrhagic infarction; and (3) posthemorrhagic hydrocephalus. Those of likely but unproven importance include the following: (1) injury to periventricular white matter secondary to intraventricular, parenchymal, or subarachnoid blood products (by generation of free radicals and perhaps by vasoconstriction with decreased blood flow); (2) destruction of glial precursors in germinal matrix—deleterious effect on myelination; and (3) impairment of subsequent cerebral cortical development. The factors of rare or unlikely importance include (1) intracranial hypertension and impaired cerebral perfusion and (2) arterial vasospasm with focal brain ischemia.

Factors of Proven Importance

Preceding and Concomitant Ischemic/Inflammatory Injury

Neuropathological studies indicate that infants who die with IVH exhibit principally two lesions related to hypoxic-ischemic and inflammatory insults: periventricular leukomalacia and selective neuronal necrosis, (see earlier "Neuropathology" section). The neuropathological, pathogenetic, and clinical aspects of these lesions are described in Chapter 9.

Destruction of Periventricular White Matter–Periventricular Hemorrhagic Infarction

Numerous follow-up studies that correlated ultrasonographic findings in the neonatal period in patients with IVH with the occurrence of subsequent neurological deficits leave little doubt that ultrasonographic evidence of unilateral or grossly asymmetrical destruction of white matter, the lesion that I referred to previously (see earlier "Neuropathology" and "Prognosis" sections) as periventricular hemorrhagic infarction, is a

highly critical determinant of neurological outcome. Among survivors of severe IVH, this lesion accounts for the largest proportion of the subsequent neurological deficits observed.

The deleterious neurological effects of periventricular hemorrhagic infarction may relate not only to destruction of cerebral white matter per se but also to the effects of the white matter injury on cerebral cortical development. Thus, careful neuropathological study of cerebral cortical organization in infants who died with major hemorrhagic white matter lesions has shown striking alterations in neuronal axonal and dendritic ramifications in areas overlying the white matter destruction.[443] Moreover, in unpublished work from our group, cerebral cortical gray matter volume was shown by three-dimensional MRI to be reduced at term in premature infants with periventricular hemorrhagic infarction.[94] These abnormalities are postulated to be secondary to disturbances of afferent input to and efferent input from the areas of cortex by disruption of the respective white matter axons. Another potential cause of the cortical abnormalities could be destruction of subplate neurons by the white matter infarction.[444] These neurons are critical for cerebral cortical organization and are abundant in subcortical white matter in the human premature infant (see Chapter 2). Whatever the mechanism, these *cerebral cortical* abnormalities with periventricular hemorrhagic infarction could be very important in determining subsequent cognitive deficits and seizure disorders.

Hydrocephalus

Posthemorrhagic hydrocephalus is a major complication of IVH, especially severe lesions, and can contribute importantly to the brain injury associated with IVH. The principal mechanism of brain injury with hydrocephalus is cerebral ischemia. This complication is discussed in detail later under "Management."

Factors of Likely but Unproven Importance

Periventricular White Matter Injury Secondary to Blood Products

The possibility of periventricular white matter injury caused by blood products is raised primarily by experimental studies and by the demonstration that the presence of IVH is associated with a sharply increased risk of ultrasonographic correlates (e.g., echolucencies) of white matter injury.[33,39] In one excellent study, cystic periventricular leukomalacia by ultrasonography was accompanied by IVH in 67% of cases versus only 17% in infants without the cystic injury.[39] A later correlate of white matter injury, nonprogressive ventriculomegaly, is also associated especially with impaired cognitive function in infants with IVH (see Chapter 9).[395,445] Moreover, the neurodevelopmental outcome of preterm infants with later ventricular dilation was worse in those who had associated IVH versus those who did not.[439] Finally, infants with only mild degrees of IVH exhibit a poorer neurodevelopmental outcome than infants with no IVH.[440] The most likely mechanism of white matter injury with intraventricular or parenchymal blood involves *increased free radical formation*, provoked perhaps in part by ischemia-reperfusion but also particularly by local release of iron from the blood.[446-448] Supportive of this suggestion is the demonstration that non–protein-bound iron was found in the CSF of 75% of preterm infants with posthemorrhagic ventriculomegaly for many *weeks* after the IVH.[448] Of particular importance in this context are the recent observations of the crucial role of free radicals in the pathogenesis of cerebral white matter injury in the premature infant (see Chapters 6 and 8).

Destruction of Germinal Matrix and Glial Precursors

As discussed previously (see "Neuropathology" section), one of the consistent neuropathological consequences of IVH is destruction of germinal matrix with its glial precursor cells. These glial precursor cells are destined to give rise to both oligodendroglia and astrocytes (see Chapter 2). The loss of these precursor cells raises two questions. The first is whether the loss of future oligodendroglia results in a subsequent impairment of myelination. The frequent association in infants with IVH of periventricular white matter injury secondary to periventricular hemorrhagic infarction, periventricular leukomalacia, and posthemorrhagic hydrocephalus makes this issue difficult to resolve. Studies of premature infants after the neonatal period by MRI do not suggest that IVH *alone* results in impaired myelination.[449]

The second question raised by the loss of glial precursor cells relates to astrocytic development. Gressens and Evrard and co-workers[450,451] showed that astrocytes destined for supragranular (upper) cortical layers originate and migrate after the occurrence of neuronal migration and are crucial for normal organizational development of the supragranular cerebral cortex. These astrocytic precursors are likely to be destroyed by germinal matrix hemorrhage, thereby raising the possibility of a subsequent disturbance in cortical development.[450,451] Such a disturbance would not be detectable by conventional neuropathological techniques but perhaps could be detected by volumetric MRI (see next section). More data are needed on this important possibility.

Impairment of Subsequent Cerebral Cortical Development

One study of premature infants with IVH uncomplicated by periventricular hemorrhagic infarction or cystic periventricular leukomalacia showed at term reduced cerebral cortical gray matter volume.[452] No difference in subcortical gray matter or white matter volume was noted. Because *noncystic* periventricular leukomalacia may be followed by subsequent impairment of cerebral cortical gray matter development (see Chapters 8 and 9), the possibility that IVH was not the key factor in the volumetric deficit must be considered. Nevertheless, in view of the immediately preceding discussions of the potential deleterious effects of germinal matrix destruction or release of injurious free radicals from subarachnoid blood, these findings are of interest and require confirmation. Recall also in this context the earlier discussion of the deleterious effects of

periventricular hemorrhagic infarction on subsequent cerebral cortical development.

Factors of Unlikely or Rare Importance

Intracranial Hypertension and Impaired Cerebral Perfusion

With massive IVH, intracranial pressure may increase acutely, and, if severe enough, the intracranial hypertension may threaten cerebral perfusion. Cerebral perfusion pressure is related to mean arterial blood pressure minus intracranial pressure. In the presence of severe IVH, I have observed intracranial pressure as high as 250 to 300 mm of CSF with concomitant systemic hypotension. This combination is a *rare* occurrence, however, even with large IVH. Experimental studies of the newborn dog demonstrate that instillation of blood into the lateral ventricles can lead to intracranial hypertension, diminished cerebral perfusion pressure, and impaired cerebral blood flow.[162] However, the levels of intracranial pressure in these animal studies (i.e., 65 mm Hg) were much higher than expected in the clinical situation. Thus, I consider this mechanism of brain injury with IVH to be operative only rarely.

Arterial Vasospasm

In adult patients with subarachnoid hemorrhage secondary to ruptured aneurysm, focal brain ischemia may result from arterial vasospasm. *Disturbances of cerebral blood flow* with parenchymal or subarachnoid blood in experimental models have been demonstrated secondary to local release of vasoconstricting potassium from hemolyzed red blood cells[453,454] or of such vasoconstricting metabolites as prostanoids[455-457] or 5-hydroxytryptamine.[458] The possibility that such a phenomenon occurs in neonatal patients with IVH was suggested by Doppler studies of blood flow velocity in the anterior cerebral artery of 11 infants with IVH studied on the day of occurrence of the hemorrhage.[459] A decrease in diastolic flow velocity, which can be caused by an increase in cerebrovascular resistance (among other factors), was defined.[459] However, a subsequent study of a larger series of infants failed to confirm this finding.[349] Other considerations make it unlikely that arterial vasospasm is an important mechanism of brain injury with IVH. In adults, vasospasm is associated with large amounts of subarachnoid (not intraventricular) blood, and the clinical syndrome caused by the vasospasm appears between 4 and 12 days after the hemorrhage and hardly ever before 48 hours.[460,461] Moreover, the possibility of vasospasm in the newborn, caused by vasoactive products of the blood clot or of damaged tissue, seems unlikely because the walls of cerebral parenchymal vessels do not contain a muscularis, presumably necessary for vasospasm, before 30 weeks of gestation.[43,44]

MANAGEMENT

Management of neonatal germinal matrix hemorrhage–IVH is considered best in terms of (1) prevention,

TABLE 11-20	Prevention of Germinal Matrix–Intraventricular Hemorrhage: Prenatal Interventions

Prevention of premature birth
Transportation in utero
Prenatal pharmacological interventions
  Glucocorticoids
  Phenobarbital
  Vitamin K
  Magnesium sulfate
Optimal management of labor and delivery

(2) initial or acute measures, and (3) treatment of posthemorrhagic ventricular dilation. In the following discussion, I consider these three aspects and conclude with a rational sequence of management.

Prevention

As with many neonatal neurological disorders, the primary goal in management of IVH is prevention. Rational attempts at prevention require an understanding of pathogenesis (see earlier discussion). The relevant prenatal (Table 11-20) and postnatal interventions (see Table 11-22 later) are discussed next in the context of current concepts of pathogenesis discussed earlier.

Prenatal Interventions

Prevention of Premature Birth. The most decisive way to prevent IVH would be to prevent premature birth. Those pathogenetic factors referable to the regulation of cerebral blood flow and the microvascular network of the germinal matrix of the premature brain obviously cannot be altered after birth. Indeed, the magnitude of the problem of IVH relates directly to the fact that annually more than 300,000 premature infants (birth weight <2500 g) are born in the United States (≈7.7% of the 4,000,000 births yearly), and, more important, approximately 60,000 of these infants weigh less than 1500 g at birth.[3-5,462,463] Notably, in the United States, the rate of very low birth weight (i.e., <1500 g) has actually increased from 1.17% to 1.45% in the past 30 years.[2,4,5,462,464-467]

Attempts at prevention of premature birth have been based on three major approaches, operating in sequence: (1) identification of the woman at high *risk* for premature delivery; (2) management of such a woman with a combination of patient education, treatment of infection, comprehensive health care, and early detection of premature labor; and (3) early treatment of premature labor, primarily with tocolytic agents.[2,462,464,465,468-492] Despite comprehensive prevention programs and aggressive use of tocolytic agents, or both, results have not shown consistent benefit.[462,464,465,468-483,485-488,490-492]

Of particular interest has been the beneficial effect of progesterone or 17-alpha-hydroxyprogesterone caproate (17P) in reduction of preterm delivery.[493,494,494a] In one large multicenter, randomized clinical trial of 17P begun at 16 to 20 weeks of gestation in women with a history of previous preterm delivery, the rate of preterm delivery in the 17P-treated group was 36% versus 55% in the placebo group.[493] Notably, the incidence of IVH in these infants who weighed less than 2500 g at birth was 1.3% in the 17P-treated group versus 5.2% in the placebo group. More data are needed.

Transportation in utero. If premature labor and delivery cannot be prevented, then the pregnant woman should be transported to a perinatal center specializing in high-risk deliveries.[495-497] Infants thus transported in utero have a considerably lower incidence of IVH than apparently similar infants transported after delivery.[100] Whether this difference relates to inherently lower risk in pregnant women who are transported compared with those who are not transported, the type of management of labor and delivery, neonatal resuscitation factors, complications during transport, or a combination of these factors is not yet clear.

Prenatal Pharmacological Interventions. Because of the possibility that factors related to labor and delivery or to the immediate postnatal period may play a role in pathogenesis of IVH, a preventive intervention that could be instituted in the presence of impending premature delivery has been sought. Antenatal administration of *glucocorticoids*, usually betamethasone or dexamethasone, currently is the most clearly beneficial antenatal intervention to decrease the incidence of all varieties of IVH (Table 11-21). The beneficial effect was observed initially in studies of the use of antenatal glucocorticoids to promote fetal lung maturation.[498] An early brief report suggested that this therapy resulted in a decreased incidence of IVH postnatally.[499] In a subsequent careful study, the incidence of germinal matrix hemorrhage–IVH was twofold to threefold lower in infants whose mothers received a complete course of steroids antenatally compared with infants whose mothers received no steroids or an incomplete course.[500] A similar beneficial effect of glucocorticoid was observed in a contemporaneous study.[225] Multivariate analysis suggested that the effect was *not* related to a lower incidence of complications of respiratory distress syndrome, although the severity of the respiratory disease was less in the treated infants.[500] A large amount of subsequent work demonstrated the beneficial effect of antenatal glucocorticoids (Fig. 11-32).[206,249,501-514] The beneficial effect has been observed most decisively after a "complete" course of treatment (maternal receipt of two or more doses of

TABLE 11-21	Antenatal Steroids and Prevention of Intraventricular Hemorrhage

Single most effective antenatal pharmacological intervention for prevention of intraventricular hemorrhage
Reduced incidence of both total and severe intraventricular hemorrhage
Reduced incidence of cystic periventricular leukomalacia
Betamethasone preferred over dexamethasone
Mechanism of beneficial effects not established: improved cerebral hemodynamics and maturational benefits most likely

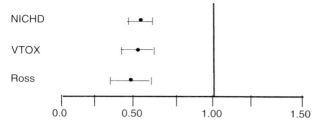

Figure 11-32 Intraventricular hemorrhage and antenatal steroids. Unadjusted odds ratio and 95% confidence intervals for the occurrence of severe intraventricular hemorrhage after antenatal steroid treatment (versus no treatment) in three separate studies of infants of less than 1500 g birth weight (the National Institute of Child Health and Human Development Neonatal Research Network [NICHD], the Vermont-Oxford Trials Network [VTOX], and the database of Ross Laboratories [Ross]). The total number of infants was approximately 18,000. *(Data from Wright LL, Horbar JD, Gunkel H, Verter J, et al: Evidence from multi-center networks on the current use and effectiveness of antenatal corticosteroids in low birth weight infants, Am J Obstet Gynecol 173:263–269, 1995.)*

glucocorticoid within a week of delivery with an interval of 12 hours from the last dose [or 24 hours from the first dose] to delivery) but also has been observed with a "partial" course (less than two doses in the week before delivery.)[206,249,502,504,510] Two issues of importance relate to the benefits and hazards of (1) different corticosteroid preparations and (2) repeated courses of antenatal steroids. Concerning the former, *betamethasone* is preferred over dexamethasone because of more favorable pharmacokinetics, better pulmonary maturation enhancement, and less toxicity.[510,515-519] However, some investigators consider the two agents similar in terms of risks and benefits.[520] *Repeated* antenatal glucocorticoid courses have not been recommended as routine clinical practice because of adverse effects on fetal growth and cerebral cortical maturation, documented in animals[521] and humans.[510,522-527a] However, one randomized clinical trial (*n* = 982) showed benefit of repeat doses for respiratory outcome but no additional benefit concerning incidence of IVH.[528] Another, smaller trial (*n* = 249) of mothers who received a course of betamethasone followed by a single booster dose of betamethasone just before preterm birth showed a trend for worse survival and increased respiratory disease but no effect on incidence of IVH for those receiving the booster dose of betamethasone versus placebo.[529] *The basis for the beneficial effect of antenatal steroids* may relate to the improved cardiovascular stability in the treated infants. Thus, antenatal steroid therapy is associated with less need for blood pressure support and less hypotension postnatally.[502,510,530,531] That this beneficial postnatal hemodynamic effect could be related to improved placental blood flow (and thereby less likelihood of impairment in the infant's cerebrovascular autoregulation) seems possible because antenatal betamethasone has been shown to lead to a decrease in placental vascular resistance.[532] Perhaps relevant in this context is the observation that antenatal steroid administration is associated with a reduced incidence of cystic periventricular leukomalacia postnatally.[509,510,533-535] The possibility also exists that the therapy leads to the beneficial effect on

IVH in part by stimulation of maturation of brain structures (e.g., germinal matrix).[500,502,536]

Antenatal administration of *phenobarbital* led to interesting results in five studies.[537-548] Initial studies raised the possibility that antenatal phenobarbital may have a small protective effect against IVH. However, later work failed to show a significant protective effect. Currently, this approach appears not to be beneficial for prevention of IVH.

Because the function of vitamin K–dependent coagulation factors in preterm infants is approximately 30% to 60% of the function in adults, *vitamin K* was administered intramuscularly to women in premature labor at least 4 hours before delivery in an attempt to prevent IVH.[549] The incidence of IVH in the prenatally treated infants was 5% compared with 33% in the control infants. Although the infants treated prenatally with vitamin K had normal prothrombin activity (compared with 67% of normal in control infants), no statistically significant relationship existed between prothrombin activity and the occurrence of IVH. In a subsequent larger study (*n* = 100), antenatal administration of vitamin K resulted in a lower incidence of total IVH (16% versus 36% in control infants) and of severe IVH (0% versus 11% in control infants).[550] However, uncertainty concerning the role of vitamin K per se persists despite these interesting data. In the two studies, infants in both the control group and the group that received prenatal vitamin K received vitamin K at birth. Other confounding variables make a decisive conclusion about the role of prenatal vitamin K difficult to draw. Moreover, two later studies of antenatal vitamin K administration, combined in one of the studies with antenatal phenobarbital administration, showed no significant beneficial effect on hemostasis or incidence and severity of IVH.[541,551-553] Thus, on balance, it does not appear that antenatal vitamin K is useful for the prevention of IVH.

As described in Chapter 9, some data, although not consistent, indicate that the use of *antenatal magnesium sulfate* (principally for tocolysis) is followed by a lower incidence of cerebral palsy in the premature infants so treated. Although one preliminary report suggested that antenatal magnesium sulfate therapy results in a lower incidence of "grade III or IV IVH," most data do not show a beneficial effect on IVH or cerebral palsy, or both.[302,303,507,554-559a] More concerning, some reports noted an increase in perinatal and postnatal mortality after antenatal magnesium administration.[560,561] Other studies did not show this increased mortality.[558,559a,562] A more recent report showed a decreased incidence of IVH after the combination of antenatal magnesium and aminophylline, but the population was not randomized, and the numbers of infants with IVH were small (1 of 78 in the treated group and 7 of 68 in the control group).[563] A review of the nine best trials concluded that antenatal magnesium sulfate has no beneficial effect on "the risk of neonatal morbidity."[564]

Optimal Management of Labor and Delivery. As discussed earlier concerning pathogenesis, potentially deleterious effects of labor and delivery relate principally to the easily deformed, particularly compliant skull of the premature infant. Such deformations presumably could lead to dangerous elevations of venous pressure and perhaps to an impairment of cerebrovascular autoregulation (analogous to that observed in adult patients with head trauma).[565] Prolonged labor and breech delivery would be considered most likely to lead to such hemodynamic effects, and some, but not all, work supports this contention.* In one large prospective study that employed multivariate analysis (see Table 11-7), abdominal delivery appeared to be protective concerning germinal matrix hemorrhage, and longer duration of labor was deleterious. In a later study, cesarean section before the active phase of labor resulted in a lower frequency of progression to severe IVH but did not affect total incidence of IVH.[567] Another study identified a twofold lower incidence of grade III/IV IVH in infants delivered by cesarean section without labor versus section delivery with labor, but the difference disappeared after logistic regression analysis.[222] Thus, potential value for cesarean section in selected preterm infants for prevention of IVH is suggested by some, but not all, work; more data are needed to define the specific clinical circumstances that should lead to a recommendation for abdominal delivery.

Postnatal Interventions

Newborn Resuscitation. Consideration of the intravascular pathogenetic factors (see "Pathogenesis" earlier) makes it clear that certain practices in newborn resuscitation may increase the likelihood of IVH in the premature infant (Table 11-22). In particular, overly rapid infusion of volume expanders or of hypertonic solutions such as sodium bicarbonate should be avoided.

Concerning cerebrovascular autoregulation, the most important admonition in neonatal resuscitation is to establish adequate ventilation promptly to prevent hypoxemia and hypercarbia, two alterations that result readily in pressure-passive cerebral circulation.[100,115] Because of the latter facts and because hyperventilation in animals[126] and humans[570] sufficient to decrease Pa_{CO_2} to approximately 25 mm Hg restores autoregulation after hypoxia, two retrospective studies of hyperventilation in the first 2 hours of life and the subsequent occurrence of IVH were conducted.[571,572] The data in the initial study suggested that Pa_{CO_2} values less than 35 mm Hg led to a decrease in incidence of subsequent IVH,[572] but a subsequent study failed to confirm this observation.[571] Currently, it seems prudent to recommend that adequate ventilation be established promptly in the resuscitation of the newborn infant and that hypoxemia and hypercarbia be avoided. However, this goal does not require systematic early intubation of all extremely-low-birth-weight infants ($\leq$1000 g) at the slightest signs of respiratory distress.[573] An individualized approach to intubation is important.

---

*See references 22,29,40,44,53,55,69,95,136,142,163,165,183,206, 217-222,225,245,294,299,319,566-569.

TABLE 11-22	Prevention of Germinal Matrix–Intraventricular Hemorrhage: Postnatal Interventions

Newborn resuscitation
Correction of fluctuating cerebral blood flow velocity
  Muscle paralysis
Correction or prevention of other hemodynamic
  disturbances
Correction of abnormalities of coagulation
  Fresh frozen plasma
  Vitamin K
Pharmacological interventions
  Phenobarbital
  Indomethacin
  Ethamsylate
  Vitamin E

Correction of Fluctuating Cerebral Blood Flow Velocity. The nearly invariable relationship between fluctuating cerebral blood flow velocity in the ventilated premature infant with respiratory distress syndrome and the subsequent occurrence of IVH (see Table 11-5) led us to a search for interventions that could prevent this hemodynamic disturbance. Muscle paralysis with pancuronium bromide was found to be highly effective for the rapid conversion of the fluctuating pattern to a stable velocity (Fig. 11-33).[95] Moreover, muscle paralysis eliminated the fluctuations in venous pressure that accompany the cerebral arterial fluctuations (see earlier discussion).[241] Thus, we undertook a prospective, randomized study of muscle paralysis from the first day of life to 72 hours of age in ventilated premature infants with the fluctuating hemodynamic disturbance (Table 11-23).[574] *All* the control infants (i.e., nonparalyzed) developed IVH, consistent with our previous observations.[95] In 7 of the 10 infants, the IVH was severe (i.e., grade III), with or without major periventricular echodensity. In contrast, the paralyzed infants exhibited a sharply reduced incidence of IVH: only 1 of 14 exhibited IVH while paralyzed, and an additional 4 experienced small IVH within 1 to 9 days after cessation of paralysis. In *none* of the paralyzed infants was the

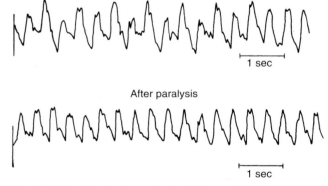

Figure 11-33 **Effect of muscle paralysis on fluctuating cerebral blood flow velocity from a ventilated, preterm infant with respiratory distress syndrome.** Before paralysis, the constantly fluctuating peak systolic and end-diastolic flow velocities are apparent. After paralysis was induced by pancuronium, the fluctuating pattern was eliminated.

TABLE 11-23	Effect of Correction of Fluctuating Cerebral Blood Flow Velocity on Incidence and Severity of Intraventricular Hemorrhage		
		INTRAVENTRICULAR HEMORRHAGE	
Patient Group	No. of Patients	Total	Severe*
Nonparalyzed	10	10 (100%)	7 (70%)
Paralyzed	14	5 (36%)†	0

*Includes grade III intraventricular hemorrhage with or without major periventricular echodensity.

†Four occurred *after cessation* of paralysis.

IVH severe. Thus, the data indicated that correction of fluctuating cerebral blood flow velocity and venous pressure by muscle paralysis in this high-risk patient group resulted in a sharp decrease in overall incidence of IVH, and, more important, in elimination of the clinically important severe hemorrhages.

After completion of the controlled study,[574] we paralyzed 72 ventilated premature infants with the fluctuating circulatory abnormality for the first 72 hours of life. In this group, in which the incidence of IVH was expected to be 90% to 100%, only 5 (7%) infants developed IVH while paralyzed. An additional 7 (10%) developed IVH after muscle paralysis was discontinued. Thus, this continued experience indicated that short-term muscle paralysis of at least this very high-risk patient group leads to a reduction in incidence and severity of IVH.

An important issue for future research is the search for means other than muscle paralysis to correct the fluctuating hemodynamic disturbance and to reduce the incidence and severity of IVH. In one study of 16 ventilated infants, pethidine was shown to be as effective as pancuronium in producing decreases in fluctuations of arterial blood pressure,[575] although the fluctuations before therapy were not as marked as in the studies of Perlman and co-workers.[95,574] Sedative-analgesic agents, such as fentanyl, may have a role in this context,[576,577] although a large, carefully controlled study showed no decrease in major IVH with continuous morphine analgesia.[511] Potentially useful are ventilatory methods, such as the ventilator interaction system capable of automatically modifying ventilator pressures and timing according to an immediately prerecorded interval of the infant's own ventilatory efforts.[578-580]

Correction or Prevention of Other Major Hemodynamic Disturbances. As indicated in the earlier discussion of pathogenesis, increases and decreases in cerebral arterial blood flow and increases in cerebral venous pressure can be involved in the pathogenesis of IVH. Thus, care must be taken to prevent sharp elevations in blood pressure and cerebral blood flow with excessive handling, tracheal suctioning, rapid infusions of blood or other colloid, exchange transfusions, apneic spells, seizures, pneumothorax, and hypercarbia. Fluctuating $Paco_2$ or hypocarbia also should be avoided. Several smaller retrospective studies suggested that

alterations in various monitoring and caretaking procedures, resulting in "minimal stimulation," led to a decrease in incidence of IVH.[581-583] However, the use, of necessity, of historical controls made it difficult to specify the most important alterations. A subsequent prospective study in which infants were randomly assigned to a carefully quantitated "reduced manipulation" protocol (n = 62) or to standard care (n = 94) did not show a significant difference in incidence of IVH (30% in study infants, 37% in control infants).[263]

Muscle paralysis appears to be particularly effective in prevention of pneumothorax[584] and of the abrupt increases in arterial pressure associated with tracheal suctioning, perhaps also an important cause of dangerous hemodynamic disturbances.[139] The value of muscle paralysis in prevention of the venous hemodynamic changes with tracheal suctioning was shown in two studies.[241,585] Similarly, careful control of arterial blood pressure with prevention of hypotension to minimize ischemic injury to the germinal matrix with subsequent hemorrhage on reperfusion is critical (see "Pathogenesis" earlier). Finally, elevations in venous pressure must be avoided by prompt treatment of myocardial impairment (e.g., in the asphyxiated infant) and of factors that may increase intrathoracic pressure and thereby cerebral venous pressure, such as pneumothorax and vigorous tracheal suctioning.

The role of *surfactant* per se in prevention of the hemodynamic disturbances associated with mechanical ventilation of infants with respiratory distress syndrome and thereby IVH is not entirely clear. Thus, a series of earlier studies employing one of at least seven different preparations of surfactant in "prophylactic" or "rescue" trials resulted in findings that were not entirely uniform.[586-605] In general, however, neonatal mortality rates, severity of respiratory distress, and air-block complications (e.g., pneumothorax) were reduced. The incidence and severity of IVH most often were either unchanged or reduced. The occurrence, albeit unusual, of increased incidence of IVH in surfactant-treated infants and the failure of a consistent decrease in incidence of IVH (despite a decrease in respiratory disease) in such infants led to the suspicion that surfactant treatment may have deleterious cerebral hemodynamic effects. Available data suggest that surfactant therapy may cause a transient increase in cerebral blood flow velocity and cerebral blood volume and electroencephalographic depression, but the effects are generally not marked.[606-612] Moreover, no clinical or biochemical evidence of deleterious effects (e.g., serum CK-BB levels) has been demonstrated.[613] In addition, the combined use of antenatal glucocorticoids and postnatal surfactant has added benefits concerning the prevention of IVH.[604,614,615]

Alternative methods of mechanical ventilation (i.e., high-frequency oscillatory ventilation or high-frequency jet ventilation) are not clearly superior to conventional ventilation regarding incidence of IVH.[616-622] Indeed, in initial work, the incidence of severe IVH was higher in infants treated with high-frequency oscillatory ventilation (26%) than in infants treated with conventional mechanical ventilation (18%), and the neurological outcome was poorer in the former group of infants.[619,620] A subsequent multicenter study showed a similarly higher incidence of IVH (36% versus 20%),[621] but four later studies showed no increase in incidence of IVH in infants treated with high-frequency oscillatory ventilation.[622-625] A significantly deleterious effect concerning IVH also was not observed in two studies of high-frequency jet ventilation,[618,626] although an increase in incidence of cystic periventricular leukomalacia was documented in one report.[626] More data are needed on these issues.

The use of *inhaled nitric oxide* for premature infants with severe respiratory failure, related most often to severe respiratory distress syndrome, currently is under active investigation.[627-632d] The gas is used for pulmonary benefits related to its strong pulmonary vasodilator properties. Thus far, no consistent significant differences in the rate of IVH in infants treated with nitric oxide have been reported. One controlled study of 793 infants 34 weeks of gestational age or younger described a decline in "grade 3 or 4" hemorrhage in infants treated with nitric oxide from the first days of life, but only in infants of birth weight 750 to 999 g.[632] Another report described improved neurodevelopmental outcome in infants treated with inhaled nitric oxide, but the neuropathological basis for the improvement was not clear.[627]

Correction of Abnormalities of Coagulation. Although in selected infants abnormalities of coagulation (or of platelet-capillary interactions) may play a role in the pathogenesis of IVH, it is unclear whether interventions to correct or prevent such abnormalities are indicated for all premature infants. Thus, in one controlled study of the administration of fresh frozen plasma (10 mL/kg) to premature infants on admission to the nursery and again at 24 hours of life, treated infants exhibited a decrease in overall incidence of IVH (14% versus 41% in untreated infants).[281] However, no difference in incidence of severe IVH was noted, and no clear effect on coagulation variables could be demonstrated. The possibility was raised that the fresh frozen plasma exerted its benefit by "stabilizing the circulation" rather than by an effect on coagulation. Two later studies of administration of fresh frozen plasma showed no benefit regarding prevention or extension of IVH or on neurological outcome at 2 years.[284,285,292] Thus, at present, no clear indication exists for the routine administration of fresh frozen plasma postnatally to premature infants for prevention of IVH.

Pharmacological Interventions

Phenobarbital. Phenobarbital was evaluated in nine controlled studies as a means to prevent IVH.[163,164,343,633-640] The results were not consistent. Although the studies had small methodological differences, the essential similarities in methods were more prominent; that is, phenobarbital was administered generally from the first hours of life, and phenobarbital levels attained were usually 20 to 25 μg/mL. The first reported series comprised 122 infants[343,635] and indicated that phenobarbital administration led to a decrease in

TABLE 11-24 Effect of Phenobarbital Administration on Incidence and Severity of Intraventricular Hemorrhage

Patient Group	No. of Patients	Total	Severe*
		INTRAVENTRICULAR HEMORRHAGE	
Control	135	26 (19%)	8 (6%)
Phenobarbital	145	51 (35%)	18 (13%)

*Consists of IVH equivalent to our Grade III, with or without major parenchymal echodensity.
Data from Kuban KC, Leviton A, Krishnamoorthy KS, Brown ER, et al: Neonatal intracranial hemorrhage and phenobarbital, *Pediatrics* 77:443–450, 1986.

overall incidence and in severity of IVH. The next five studies did not demonstrate benefit for phenobarbital, although in one the severity but not the overall incidence of IVH was diminished.[634] The largest reported study[164] was composed of 280 intubated premature infants (Table 11-24). The data showed a higher overall incidence of IVH in the phenobarbital-treated infants than in the controls.[164] A meta-analysis of the available trials showed no difference between the phenobarbital-treated group and the control group in occurrence of IVH overall or of severe IVH.[640] The trend was toward increased use of mechanical ventilation in the phenobarbital-treated group. Thus, at present, I do not recommend the use of phenobarbital for prophylaxis for IVH.

The *mechanism of beneficial effect of phenobarbital*, if any, may possibly relate to the dampening of abrupt increases in cerebral blood flow caused perhaps by arterial blood pressure rises associated with motor activity, handling, tracheal suctioning, and related factors.[136,143,641] Phenobarbital administration led to a reduction in occurrence of IVH in the beagle puppy subjected to phenylephrine-induced hypertension, although no effect on the level of rise in blood pressure was observed.[642] Despite the lack of effect of phenobarbital on blood pressure, attenuation of increases in cerebral blood flow produced by hypertension in neonatal animal models has been documented.[174,643-646] However, phenobarbital prevented the cerebral vasodilation associated with hypoxia following hypertension, thus raising the possibility that the agent could be harmful under such clinical circumstances.[645] Notably, phenobarbital was shown to have no significant effect on cerebral blood flow in seven asphyxiated infants when flow was measured 60 minutes after a 20 mg/kg loading dose of the drug.[647] Other potential beneficial effects of phenobarbital include the ability to protect against free radical–mediated ischemia-reperfusion injury, and in experimental studies free radicals have been implicated both in pathogenesis of IVH and in postasphyxial impairment of cerebrovascular autoregulation (see earlier discussion and Chapter 6).[648,649]

Indomethacin. Indomethacin was evaluated in 19 controlled studies as a means to prevent IVH.[650-664a]

TABLE 11-25	**Effect of Prophylactic Indomethacin Administration on Incidence and Severity of Intraventricular Hemorrhage: Effect of Gender***			
	FEMALE PATIENTS (*n* = 196)		**MALE PATIENTS (*n* = 235)**	
	Saline	Indomethacin	Saline	Indomethacin
No IVH	89 (86%)	78 (84%)	93 (78%)	106 (91%)
IVH	14 (14%)	15 (16%)	26 (22%)	10 (9%)
Grade I			5	4
Grade II			12	6
Grade III			1	0
Grade IV			8	0

*Breslow-Day test for homogeneity (female vs. male), *P* = .013 for IVH/no IVH.
IVH, intraventricular hemorrhage.
Data from Ment LR, Vohr BR, Makuch RW, Westerveld M, et al: Prevention of intraventricular hemorrhage by indomethacin in male preterm infants, *J Pediatr* 145:832–834, 2004.

The drug was studied particularly for prophylaxis, rather than treatment, of patent ductus arteriosus, and it was generally administered initially before 12 hours of age. A summary of the pooled results showed that indomethacin administration led to a decrease in incidence of overall IVH (relative risk [RR], 0.88; 95% confidence limits [CI], 0.80 to 0.96) and of severe IVH (RR, 0.66; 95% CI, 0.53 to 0.82).[661,665] In the largest early series (*n* = 431) Ment and co-workers[666] observed a decrease in incidence of total IVH (18% to 12%) and "grade IV" IVH (4.5% to 0.5%). However, in this study, early-onset IVH was excluded, and the marked preponderance of "grade IV" IVH relative to "grade III" IVH (10:1) in the control population was unusual and raised the possibility of an undefined unusual characteristic of the control population.[667] Indeed, in centers where the incidence of grades III and IV IVH in the control population was greater than 10%, indomethacin administration was shown to lead to a significant reduction in these severe hemorrhages (odds ratio [OR], 0.54; 95% CI, 0.36 to 0.82; *P* <.005), whereas in centers where the incidence was less than 10%, indomethacin did not lead to a significant reduction (OR, 0.72; 95% CI, 0.39 to 1.33; *P* <.3).[658] Moreover, the beneficial effects of the agent appeared to be more prominent in larger (>1000 g) rather than smaller (<1000 g) infants; thus, in the former group the OR was 0.42 with a 95% CI of 0.24 to 0.76, *P* <.005, whereas in the latter group, the OR was 0.66 with a 95% CI of 0.37 to 1.18, *P* <.02.[658] However, a later multicenter study (*n* = 1202) of infants of less than 1000 g birth weight confirmed a reduction in severe IVH in the indomethacin-treated group (9%) versus the control group (13%).[663]

An interesting development in this area was the repeat analysis of the data from the earlier study of Ment and co-workers (*n* = 431) (Table 11-25).[662] Thus, the beneficial effect of indomethacin on IVH was shown in *male* but not female patients. A repeat analysis of the later larger study of prophylactic indomethacin (*n* = 1202) showed a weak differential effect of indomethacin by sex; for severe IVH, the incidences in indomethacin-treated versus placebo groups were 9.8% versus 11.7% (OR, 0.46 to 1.44) for female patients but 8.6% versus 14.7% (OR, 0.31 to 0.94) for male patients.[663] The findings are consistent with

previous observations of more neurological and developmental disability in small preterm male versus female infants,[668] and greater disturbance of cerebral cortical volumes on MRI follow-up of male versus female preterm infants.[669] *Thus, on balance, in the total experience with indomethacin, a generally favorable preventive effect of the drug on IVH seems apparent, particularly or exclusively in male patients.* Follow-up of the large series of infants studied by Ment and co-workers showed no difference in development of ultrasonographically demonstrated cystic periventricular leukomalacia or in incidences of cerebral palsy or of cognitive impairment at 36 months of age.[34,670] Other investigators also have shown no beneficial long-term neurodevelopmental effects.[661,664a,665] However, again, when male and female patients are analyzed separately, a clear cognitive benefit is apparent in male but not female patients (Table 11-26). On balance, although the overall data are interesting and provocative, the findings do not appear sufficiently conclusive to recommend routine indomethacin prophylaxis for IVH. This tentative conclusion, however, will need reassessment in the context of the more recent finding that prolonged indomethacin prophylactic exposure in premature newborns of 24 to 28 weeks of gestation is associated with decreased white matter injury detected by MRI (see Chapter 9).[671]

TABLE 11-26	**Effect of Prophylactic Indomethacin Administration on Neurodevelopment: Effect of Gender***		
	AGE AT FOLLOW-UP		
	3 yr	6 yr	8 yr
Female Patients			
Saline	88.5 ± 17.3	92.0 ± 21.7	92.6 ± 22.3
Indomethacin	83.5 ± 22.0	93.2 ± 25.2	90.8 ± 24.8
Male Patients			
Saline	77.8 ± 25.1	86.8 ± 29.8	89.9 ± 30.0
Indomethacin	87.4 ± 20.6	96.6 ± 19.6	95.4 ± 23.4

*Scores are based on the Peabody Picture Vocabulary Test-R. For male patients, saline versus indomethacin, *P* = .017.
Data from Ment LR, Vohr BR, Makuch RW, Westerveld M, et al: Prevention of intraventricular hemorrhage by indomethacin in male preterm infants, *J Pediatr* 145:832–834, 2004.

The mechanisms of a beneficial effect of indomethacin may relate to the circulatory and metabolic consequences of the drug. First, indomethacin was shown in the beagle puppy model of IVH to decrease baseline cerebral blood flow and to diminish the occurrence of IVH after hemorrhagic hypotension and volume reexpansion.[672] The decrease in cerebral blood flow after indomethacin was replicated in several animal models.[673-681] The circulatory effects are presumed to be secondary to the drug's inhibition of prostaglandin biosynthesis. Indeed, studies in newborn piglets showed that indomethacin not only decreased baseline cerebral blood flow by approximately 20% to 30% but also, perhaps more important, attenuated the cerebral hyperemia induced by asphyxia (combined hypoxia-hypercarbia).[682,683] Similarly, and of some concern, Leffler and co-workers[684] showed in the piglet that degrees of hemorrhagic hypotension not severe enough alone to alter cerebral blood flow or cerebral oxygen consumption produced, in the presence of indomethacin treatment, a 40% decrease in cerebral blood flow, 40% to 60% decreases in cerebral oxygen consumption, and coma in 75% of the animals.[674,684] The deleterious effect of indomethacin was associated with a marked decrease in cerebral prostaglandin production and an increase in cerebrovascular resistance. However, a later study of the neonatal piglet with lower doses of indomethacin, comparable to those employed in human infants, did not show blunting of the cerebrovascular dilation provoked by hypercarbia.[685] Moreover, in experiments with the preterm lamb, indomethacin did not accentuate the decline in cerebral oxygen consumption produced by hypotension below the lower limit of the autoregulatory range.[678] More recently, in the newborn piglet the decline in cerebral blood flow induced by indomethacin was compensated by an increase in oxygen extraction fraction and no change in cerebral metabolic rate of oxygen.[680] The decline in cerebral blood flow produced by indomethacin in the several models is consistent with the notion that the drug produces its circulatory effects by inhibition of synthesis of vasodilating prostanoids and thereby stimulation of cerebral vasoconstriction (see Chapter 6).

Studies of human preterm infants suggested that the increase in cerebrovascular resistance and decline in cerebral blood flow observed in perinatal animals also occur in the infant. Thus, a decrease in cerebral blood flow velocity and an increase in resistance indices were documented by the Doppler technique after administration of indomethacin to human infants.[686-692] Indeed, a *decrease in cerebral blood flow after administration of indomethacin* was shown clearly by Pryds and co-workers,[693] who used the xenon clearance method to define in six premature infants a mean decrease in cerebral blood flow of 24%. The effect of indomethacin began within minutes and continued for at least an hour. Studies with near-infrared spectroscopy also clearly documented a decline in cerebral blood volume, flow, and oxygen delivery after administration of indomethacin to human infants.[694-698] An additional manifestation of the vasoconstrictive effect of

indomethacin was a marked attenuation of the cerebrovascular reactivity to carbon dioxide observed after administration of the drug. Perhaps of greatest concern, the decrease in cerebral blood flow and oxygen delivery was accompanied by a prominent decrease in the brain level of oxidized cytochrome oxidase, a finding suggesting that the hemodynamic disturbance was marked enough to decrease cerebral intracellular oxygenation.[695-697] Thus, although the apparent cerebral vasoconstriction produced by indomethacin may be useful for prevention of IVH, under such adverse conditions as hypoxemia, hypercarbia, or hypotension, it seems possible that the normal compensatory circulatory effects, in part mediated by prostanoids, may be blunted. Whether this blunting could lead to ischemic brain injury is unknown, although the studies of human infants with xenon clearance and near-infrared spectroscopy are of concern. Nevertheless, recall that prolonged indomethacin exposure is associated with a *decrease* in white matter injury in premature newborns of 24 to 28 weeks of gestation.[671] Finally, *ibuprofen*, shown to be effective in prophylaxis for patent ductus arteriosus, is not associated with the unfavorable cerebral hemodynamic effects of indomethacin.[699-703] However, prophylactic ibuprofen does not have a preventive effect for IVH.[701,702]

A second aspect of the indomethacin action that may be of benefit in prevention of IVH relates to the inhibition of the formation of free radicals generated by the cyclooxygenase portion of the pathway of prostaglandin biosynthesis (the portion affected by indomethacin).[704] Thus, under circumstances in which this pathway is active, such as ischemia with calcium-activated phospholipase activity leading to formation of arachidonic acid (the lipid precursor of prostaglandins), free radicals could be generated and cause injury to endothelial cells in germinal matrix and thereby IVH. *This mechanism may be of relevance concerning the male versus female effects noted earlier.* Thus, male cells have been shown to be more susceptible to free radical–mediated cell death because of a deficiency in antioxidant defenses at the glutathione peroxidase step.[705]

A third potentially beneficial effect of indomethacin is an acceleration of maturation of microvessels in the germinal matrix. Thus, indomethacin administration to the newborn beagle puppy led to increased laminin deposition in basement membranes of matrix microvessels.[706] This effect was apparent on the second postnatal day, 1 day after the first injection of the drug.

Etamsylate. Etamsylate (formerly ethamsylate) was evaluated in five studies as a means to prevent IVH. In the initial randomized, controlled study of 70 premature infants, etamsylate resulted in a lower overall incidence of IVH (26% versus 51% in untreated infants).[686] However, no decrease in incidence of severe IVH was observed. In a second larger study, not only was a similar decrease in overall incidence of IVH observed, but also the incidence of severe IVH was lower in the etamsylate-treated infants (1 of 10, or 10%) than in the control infants (9 of 28, or 32%).[707] In the third study, a multicenter, randomized, controlled study of 330 premature

TABLE 11-27 Effect of Etamsylate Administration on Incidence and Severity of Intraventricular Hemorrhage

Patient Group	No. of Patients	INTRAVENTRICULAR HEMORRHAGE	
		Total	Severe*
Control	168	60 (36%)	17 (10%)
Etamsylate	162	39 (24%)	8 (5%)

*Consists of intraventricular hemorrhage with "parenchymal hemorrhage."

Data from Benson JW, Drayton MR, Hayward C, Murphy JF, et al: Multicentre trial of ethamsylate for prevention of periventricular haemorrhage in very low birthweight infants, *Lancet* 2:1297–1300, 1986.

infants, etamsylate administration was associated with a lower overall incidence of IVH (24% vs. 36% in untreated infants) and a lower incidence of severe IVH (i.e., IVH with "parenchymal hemorrhage," 5% vs. 10% in untreated infants) (Table 11-27).[708] Similar results were obtained in a randomized controlled study of 171 premature infants in a single center; that is, incidences in treated versus untreated infants were 28% versus 46% for all IVH and 10% versus 24% for severe IVH.[709] Enthusiasm for etamsylate was dampened by the results of an international, multicenter randomized trial that involved 334 infants of less than 32 weeks of gestation.[710] Thus, no difference was seen between the treated and control groups in incidence of all IVH (35% vs. 37%) or of severe IVH or "major" ultrasonographic lesions (13% vs. 12%). Etamsylate in this trial was administered "within 4 hours of birth" (i.e., later than the "1 hour" in two large trials that demonstrated a protective effect of etamsylate).[708,709] However, still more discouraging, long-term follow-up of the cohort shown in Table 11-27 showed no decrease in rates of cerebral palsy in the etamsylate-treated group.[711] Severe cognitive deficit was reduced somewhat, but the results are not conclusive. A systematic review of more than 500 infants enrolled in randomized controlled trials of etamsylate showed a reduction in total IVH but a nonsignificant reduction in "grade 3 or 4" IVH and no overall reduction in mortality or longer-term neurodevelopmental impairment.[712]

The *mechanism of any beneficial effect of etamsylate* is likely to be severalfold. First, the drug has been shown to inhibit prostaglandin synthesis, probably at a site distal to the cyclooxygenase pathway that is affected by indomethacin. Prostacyclin production appears to be particularly strongly affected by etamsylate in the newborn.[713] As discussed in the previous section on pathogenesis, prostacyclin is both a potent vasodilator and a promoter of platelet disaggregation, and it is present at high levels in newborns who subsequently develop IVH. Thus, inhibition of the prostacyclin actions may be involved in the etamsylate prevention of IVH. Of note in this regard, etamsylate was shown in the beagle puppy model to reduce the incidence of IVH, perhaps by an effect on cerebral blood flow.[169] However, in human infants, it may be less likely that the beneficial effect of etamsylate is

related to hemodynamic effects, because no change in cerebral blood flow velocity or resistance index was apparent by Doppler study of 19 very-low-birth-weight infants administered the drug.[714] A second potential beneficial effect of etamsylate may relate to actions at the capillary level. Etamsylate causes a polymerization of hyaluronic acid of capillary basement membrane and promotes platelet adhesiveness, both of which properties would inhibit bleeding from capillaries, a microvascular site of germinal matrix hemorrhage. Finally, because the drug crosses the placenta during labor,[715] prenatal administration to prevent early onset of IVH is a potential consideration.

Vitamin E. Vitamin E was evaluated in several studies as a means to prevent IVH.[163,716-721] In an initial small study ($n = 44$), Chiswick and colleagues[716] demonstrated that intramuscular vitamin E administered to premature infants within 12 hours of birth had no effect on overall incidence of IVH but a threefold lower incidence of severe IVH. A later study in the United States of 134 premature infants also demonstrated a lower overall incidence of IVH in vitamin E–treated infants (16%) than in control infants (34%).[719] In follow-up of the earlier initial observations, Sinha and co-workers[718] then studied 210 premature infants in a randomized, controlled trial. The data showed in vitamin E–treated infants a lower overall incidence of all hemorrhages (54% vs. 30%) and "severe" hemorrhages (41% vs. 11%). However, "severe" hemorrhages in this series included *all* IVH, exclusive only of isolated germinal matrix hemorrhage.

Nevertheless, enthusiasm for the use of vitamin E for prevention of IVH was tempered by the fourth of these studies, that of Phelps and co-workers.[717] This investigation of 287 premature infants was designed to evaluate the efficacy of vitamin E in prevention of retinopathy of prematurity. Vitamin E was administered *intravenously* initially and later by the oral route. The data showed not only that vitamin E did not prevent retinopathy of prematurity, but also that the treated infants exhibited a *higher* incidence of severe IVH (25% in treated infants, 15% in control infants). This effect was most marked in infants less than 1000 g (36% in treated infants, 11% in control infants). The conclusion that vitamin E administration increased the risk of IVH, however, had to be qualified by the recognition that, in the study by Phelps and colleagues, ultrasound scans or other imaging studies were not carried out before the onset of treatment, and the plasma levels of vitamin E were higher than in the study of Sinha and co-workers.[718]

A later report concerning vitamin E focused on the smallest infants (<1000 g), those with the highest risk of the most severe hemorrhages (Table 11-28).[720] Infants were administered intramuscular vitamin E (alpha-tocopherol) from the first day of life, although most were administered the agent after the first hours. A beneficial effect of vitamin E was apparent in the smaller group of infants (501 to 750 g), with a 50% decrease in incidence of total IVH (60% vs. 32%, $P = .045$) and an even more marked decrease in incidence

TABLE 11-28   **Effect of Vitamin E Administration on Incidence and Severity of Intraventricular Hemorrhage**

| Patient Group | No. of Patients | INTRAVENTRICULAR HEMORRHAGE | |
		Total	Severe*
501–750 g			
Control	25	15 (60%)	8 (32%)
Vitamin E	24	7 (29%)	1 (4%)
751–1000 g			
Control	44	20 (45%)	11 (25%)
Vitamin E	44	17 (39%)	10 (23%)

*Comparable to our Grade III with or without parenchymal echodensity.
Data from Fish WH, Cohen M, Franzek D, Williams JM, et al: Effect of intramuscular vitamin E on mortality and intracranial hemorrhage in neonates of 1000 grams or less, *Pediatrics* 85:578–584, 1990.

of IVH of severe variety (29% vs. 4%, P = .023). No increase in mortality rate, sepsis, or necrotizing enterocolitis (previously suggested, potential deleterious effects of vitamin E[722]) was observed in the vitamin E–treated infants. Coupled particularly with the earlier work of Chiswick and colleagues and Sinha and co-workers,[716,718] the observations suggested that vitamin E administration leads to a decrease in incidence *and* severity of IVH, particularly in the smallest infants, who sustain most of the clinically important hemorrhages. A review of 26 randomized clinical trials of relevance to the role of vitamin E concluded that, in preterm infants, vitamin E supplementation reduced the risk of IVH when administered by routes other than intravenous and at serum tocopherol levels that did not exceed 3.5 mg/dL.[721] More data are needed before a recommendation is made for routine clinical use for prevention of IVH.

The *mechanism of any beneficial effect of vitamin E* likely relates to the potent antioxidant properties of the vitamin.[723] Presumably, vitamin E operates as a free radical scavenger to protect matrix capillary endothelial cells from hypoxic-ischemic injury. An important role in prevention of IVH for compounds that either prevent formation of free radicals (e.g., indomethacin) or scavenge these injurious compounds (e.g., vitamin E) is suggested not only by at least some of the clinical studies but also by the experimental observation that administration of superoxide dismutase, the critical metalloenzyme involved in dismutation of the harmful superoxide anion to hydrogen peroxide (see Chapter 6), prevents IVH in the beagle puppy model.[649] Experimental support for a role for vitamin E specifically in prevention of IVH was provided by two animal models (chick and fetal hamsters).[724-726] In both models, vitamin E was shown to reverse an encephalopathy characterized by damaged endothelial cells; indeed, in the fetal hamster model, a particular predilection for vessels of the germinal matrix with the development of matrix hemorrhage and IVH was shown.[724,726] Finally, plasma levels of vitamin E are lower in premature infants than in older infants, and intramuscular vitamin E administration causes a twofold to threefold increase in plasma vitamin E levels within a day.[718]

Conclusions

The advances in understanding the pathogenesis of germinal matrix hemorrhage–IVH, as discussed earlier, led to the formulation of rational interventions to prevent hemorrhages. Both prenatal and postnatal interventions show considerable promise. Prenatal interventions include prevention of premature birth (currently a very elusive goal in the United States), transportation of the premature infant to a tertiary facility in utero rather than after birth (an approach of proven value), *prenatal administration especially of glucocorticoid*, and optimal management of labor and delivery. Postnatal interventions include careful newborn resuscitation, correction of fluctuating cerebral blood flow velocity, correction or prevention of other major hemodynamic disturbances, and correction of abnormalities of coagulation. Of these, the use of muscle paralysis to correct fluctuating cerebral blood flow velocity has shown striking benefit in prevention of IVH in this particular subset of premature infants at high risk for the clinically important severe lesions. Postnatal pharmacological interventions that have been studied in detail include phenobarbital, indomethacin, etamsylate, and vitamin E. No single agent among this group has been shown consistently to lead to a decrease in incidence *and* severity of IVH. Promising current data relate to the postnatal administration particularly of indomethacin. A potential role for vitamin E in the smallest infants deserves further cautious study.

Acute Management

Most often, the physician has been unable to prevent IVH and is faced with the task of managing the infant who has sustained this potentially serious intracranial event. The basic elements of acute management are shown in Table 11-29.

Maintenance of Cerebral Perfusion

The critical initial task is to maintain cerebral perfusion. As discussed previously, cerebral perfusion pressure is related to the mean arterial blood pressure minus the intracranial pressure. With *major* IVH, because of the sometimes decreased arterial blood pressure and occasionally elevated intracranial pressure, cerebral perfusion may be threatened.

TABLE 11-29   **Acute Management of Germinal Matrix–Intraventricular Hemorrhage**

Maintenance of cerebral perfusion
  Cautious control of blood pressure
  Lowering of increased intracranial pressure: rarely indicated
Prevention of cerebral hemodynamic disturbances
  Avoidance of fluctuating or increased arterial blood pressure, hypercarbia, hypoxemia, acidosis, hyperosmolar solutions, rapid volume expansion, pneumothorax, and seizures
Other supportive care
Serial ultrasound scans
Management of posthemorrhagic hydrocephalus

Arterial blood pressure must be maintained at adequate levels (see Chapter 9), although this control of blood pressure must be carried out cautiously because of the likely presence of pressure-passive cerebral circulation. Overly exuberant therapeutic responses may contribute to conversion of a moderate lesion to a severe one.

Intracranial pressure should not be allowed to remain excessive. Optimally, to address this issue best, intracranial pressure should be measured, either at the time of diagnostic lumbar puncture or by anterior fontanelle sensor (see Chapter 4). Intracranial pressure may be elevated with severe hemorrhage; values of approximately 15 mm Hg by anterior fontanelle sensor have been reported.[727] I have documented such elevations *only rarely*. The lower limit of safe cerebral perfusion pressure is discussed in Chapter 9. However, direct measurements of intracranial pressure in all cases of IVH are *not practical*. Selection of those patients with large lesions and clinical signs of increased intracranial pressure (e.g., full anterior fontanelle) is important. I consider the need for active lowering of intracranial pressure (e.g., by ventricular drainage) in acute management of IVH to be *rare*.

Prevention of Cerebral Hemodynamic Disturbances

The other side of the coin concerning cerebral perfusion is avoidance of abrupt increases in cerebral blood flow and the other hemodynamic disturbances important in the pathogenesis of hemorrhage. Such disturbances may lead to progression of hemorrhage. Thus, the factors previously discussed concerning prevention of hemorrhage must be considered: avoidance of fluctuating or increased arterial blood pressure, hypercarbia, hypoxemia, acidosis, hyperosmolar solutions, rapid volume expansion, and pneumothorax. Because seizures may provoke cerebral hyperfusion by an effect on arterial blood pressure as well as by local factors in brain (see Chapter 5), overt seizures should be treated vigorously in the setting of major IVH.

Other Supportive Care

Under this imprecise rubric, I include many therapies, some implied earlier, related to ventilation, circulation, temperature, and metabolic status that are discussed in standard writings on neonatal medicine.

Serial Ultrasound Scans

If the infant survives the acute period, serial assessments of ventricular size by ultrasound scan should be conducted. The interval for the initial assessments should be approximately 4 to 7 days, with the shorter time used for the larger lesions. Serial assessment is necessary because, as discussed later, the classic signs of evolving hydrocephalus (i.e., rapid head growth, full anterior fontanelle, and separated cranial sutures) do not appear for days to weeks *after* ventricular dilation has already commenced.

Prevention and Management of Posthemorrhagic Hydrocephalus

These topics are discussed in the following section.

TABLE 11-30   **Progressive Ventricular Dilation after Intraventricular Hemorrhage**
Etiology: acute, particulate blood clot; chronic, obliterative arachnoiditis in posterior fossa; aqueductal obstruction less commonly
Temporal features: usual onset of progression 1 to 3 weeks after hemorrhage; rapidity of evolution directly related to severity of hemorrhage
Rapid head growth or signs of increased intracranial pressure or both **following** ventricular dilation by days to weeks
Posterior horns of lateral ventricles dilating before, and more severely than, anterior horns

Posthemorrhagic Hydrocephalus

Incidence and Definition

Hydrocephalus, which is progressive ventricular dilation secondary to a disturbance in CSF dynamics, is a not uncommon sequela of IVH (Table 11-30).* As might be expected, the incidence of posthemorrhagic progressive ventricular dilation is related closely to the severity of the initial hemorrhage (see later). However, because ventricular dilation may occur after IVH as a result of periventricular leukomalacia or periventricular hemorrhagic infarction, or both, posthemorrhagic ventriculomegaly should not be equated with hydrocephalus. Indeed, clinical distinction between ventriculomegaly secondary to periventricular cerebral atrophy and ventriculomegaly secondary to hydrocephalus with attendant impairment of CSF dynamics is difficult but critical for formulation of appropriate management decisions. Close surveillance and neuroimaging usually provide the necessary information to make the distinction (see "Management" section later). In general, the development of ventriculomegaly, secondary to atrophy, occurs slowly over several weeks, is not associated with the development of increased intracranial pressure or rapid head growth, and evolves to a state of stable ventricular size; that is, ventricular size neither decreases, as in transient hydrocephalus, nor continues to increase, as in persistently progressive hydrocephalus.

Pathogenesis

The pathogenesis of posthemorrhagic hydrocephalus (see "Neuropathology" earlier) can be considered in terms of either the acute process, apparent within days (particularly after severe IVH), or the subacute-chronic process, apparent within weeks. *Acute* hydrocephalus appears to be secondary to an impairment of CSF absorption caused by particulate blood clot and demonstrable by ultrasound scan (Fig. 11-34).[742] *Subacute-chronic* hydrocephalus presumably is related to the obliterative arachnoiditis in the posterior fossa where the blood tends to collect.[50] The important role of *the combination of deficient fibrinolytic properties and enhanced*

---

*See references 20,22,87,88,161,195,350,354,359,367,383-386,389, 390,392-394,407,408,728-741.

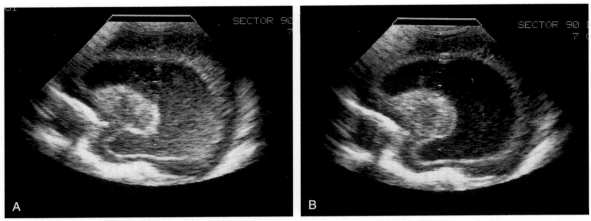

Figure 11-34   Acute hydrocephalus with intraventricular hemorrhage: pathogenesis. Parasagittal ultrasound scans were performed, **A**, immediately after the examiner turned the patient's head from right to left, and, **B**, after 10 minutes. In moderately to markedly dilated lateral ventricles, echogenic particulate matter is prominent immediately after, **A**, turning of head and disappears, **B**, over the next 10 minutes.

fibroproliferative characteristics of the CSF of infants with posthemorrhagic hydrocephalus was discussed earlier (see "Neuropathology"). The deficient fibrinolytic properties may relate to low plasminogen and high plasminogen activator inhibitor levels in CSF of premature infants after IVH.[79-81] The enhanced fibroproliferative properties appear to relate to the up-regulation after IVH of CSF levels of transforming growth factor-beta1 and procollagen 1C-peptide.[85-88] The impairment of CSF flow is usually distal to the outflow of the fourth ventricle because most examples of posthemorrhagic hydrocephalus are of the communicating type. The latter has been demonstrated by radionuclide lumbar cisternography and by ultrasonographic demonstration of a decrease in ventricular size immediately after removal of CSF from the lumbar space.[389,407,738,743,744] Obstruction at the level of the aqueduct by blood clot, debris, and subependymal scarring occurs less commonly.

Evolution

The ventricular dilation may begin essentially with the hemorrhage, especially with marked IVH. More often, definite ventricular dilation and, particularly, the progression thereof begin within 1 to 3 weeks of the hemorrhage. Unfortunately, the traditional clinical criteria of evolving hydrocephalus (i.e., rapid head growth, full anterior fontanelle, and separated cranial sutures) do not appear for days to weeks *after* ventricular dilation has already been present. This phenomenon was surmised on the basis of neuropathological[330,745] and clinical data and then later proved by serial CT studies.[746] The availability of serial ultrasound studies has allowed repeated observation of this occurrence. As discussed in more detail in the "Management" section, the rapidity of progression of posthemorrhagic ventricular dilation relates principally to the severity of the hemorrhage.

Reasons for Ventricular Dilation Before Rapid Head Growth

The reasons for the impressive ventricular dilation before the development of rapid head growth and signs of increased intracranial pressure must relate to

the developmental state of the cerebrum in the premature infant. The three most relevant features are (1) the paucity of cerebral myelin, (2) the relative excess of water in the centrum semiovale, and (3) the relatively large subarachnoid space. In experimental and human hydrocephalus, the cerebral white matter is encroached on, and central gray structures are relatively spared (see later discussion).[747] The paucity of myelin and the relative excess of water in the cerebral white matter of the premature infant would serve to accentuate this general feature of hydrocephalus. It can be postulated that less force is required to compress this immature cerebral white matter than to overcome the restrictions of the dura and skull. This notion is supported by the disproportionate dilation of the occipital versus frontal horns with posthemorrhagic hydrocephalus. The third factor (i.e., the relatively large subarachnoid space in the premature infant, reflected by the enhanced cranial transillumination in the normal premature infant) may have an important contributory effect because this space could be encroached on even after ventricular dilation but before separation of sutures (Figs. 11-35 and 11-36).

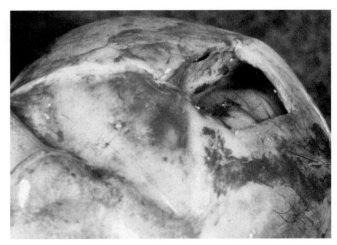

Figure 11-35   Prominent subarachnoid space in the premature infant. Bone has been removed from the left parietal region of an infant of 29 weeks of gestation. Note the large subarachnoid space. *(Courtesy of Dr. James Rohrbaugh.)*

Extracerebral cerebrospinal fluid

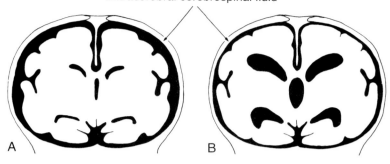

A

B

Figure 11-36 Postulated contributory mechanism for development of posthemorrhagic ventricular dilation before rapid head growth. A, Normal premature brain. **B,** Evolving posthemorrhagic hydrocephalus encroaching on subarachnoid space. *(From Pape KE, Wigglesworth JS:* Haemorrhage, Ischaemia, and the Perinatal Brain, *Philadelphia: 1979, JB Lippincott.)*

Relation of Ventricular Dilation to Brain Injury

The precise relation of progressive posthemorrhagic ventricular dilation to brain injury is unclear. This issue is considered best in terms of experimental and clinical studies.

Experimental Studies. Deleterious effects of hydrocephalus on brain include disturbances of cerebral white matter, cerebral blood vessels, and cerebral cortex.[748] Concerning cerebral white matter, the earliest changes (1 week after induction of experimental hydrocephalus) involve oligodendrocytes and myelin, with a decrease in myelin-associated enzymes (e.g., ceramide galactosyltransferase) and structural proteins (e.g., myelin basic protein). Later, after several weeks, axonal loss and impaired myelination are apparent. Investigators reported that shunting at 1 week, but not at 4 weeks, when axonal loss had occurred, allowed recovery of myelination.[749,750] The late occurrence of axonal loss with hydrocephalus was noted in earlier studies.[751-758] Thus, if this stage is not reached, therapy appears to be beneficial in preventing permanent structural deficits.

A role for *cerebral vascular changes and ischemia* in the genesis of the white matter injury in experimental hydrocephalus is demonstrated by morphological studies that show an attenuation of the caliber of major cerebral vessels and a decrease in the secondary and tertiary vessels in cerebral white matter.[748,755,759] These changes may underlie, at least in part, the decrease in volemic cerebral blood flow and alterations in energy metabolism in hydrocephalic animal models.[748,760-762] Further supportive of cerebral ischemia are the findings in cerebral white matter of increased cerebral rates of glucose metabolism (presumably anaerobic glycolysis), elevated lactate, decreased high-energy phosphates, and elevated free radicals.[763-766] These mechanisms, leading to free radical production, are particularly relevant in view of the data demonstrating the particular vulnerability of differentiating oligodendroglia to free radical attack (see Chapter 6).[767] These biochemical changes and neurochemical signs of axonal loss could be prevented by early shunting in the various experimental models.[748,762,764,768] Moreover, the vascular attenuation may represent the anatomical substrate for the increase in cerebrovascular resistance and decrease in volemic cerebral blood flow and flow velocity in human infants with hydrocephalus (see later discussion).

Of particular additional interest are alterations in *cerebral cortical neurons* in hydrocephalic animal models. Thus, disturbances in catecholaminergic and serotonergic neurotransmitter development and in synaptogenesis and evidence for neuronal degeneration have been delineated.[748,769-779] These effects could reflect, in part, disturbance to ascending and descending axons in cerebral white matter with secondary anterograde and retrograde effects on organizational development of cerebral cortex. When specifically addressed in the various experimental studies, the deleterious effects were shown to be reversible when the hydrocephalic state was corrected early. The specific roles of duration of dilation, severity thereof, and presence and degree of intracranial hypertension in determining reversibility remain to be defined clearly.

Human Studies. Data from studies of infants concerning the deleterious effect of progressive posthemorrhagic ventricular dilation relate to cerebral hemodynamics, neurophysiological function, morphological disturbances, biochemical indicators of hypoxia, and clinical outcome (Table 11-31). The data are sometimes difficult to interpret conclusively because such details as rate of progression, degree and duration of ventriculomegaly, intracranial pressure, preceding parenchymal injury, and neurological outcome are often not provided. Nevertheless, the findings suggest at least transient disturbances.

Concerning *cerebral hemodynamics*, a systematic study of nine infants with posthemorrhagic hydrocephalus initially demonstrated *impaired blood flow velocity* in the anterior cerebral arteries that was reversed with therapy to correct the hydrocephalic state.[108] The disturbance of cerebral blood flow velocity appeared to correlate more closely with ventriculomegaly than with increased intracranial pressure. Subsequent studies of cerebral blood flow velocity confirmed the fundamental observation.[780-796] The principal finding with posthemorrhagic hydrocephalus is evidence for increased cerebrovascular resistance, by means of resistance indices, and for diminished mean cerebral blood flow velocity. Removal of CSF by lumbar puncture or ventricular drainage led to improvement in both parameters, except in infants with ventriculomegaly secondary to periventricular white matter atrophy.

With gradual increases in intracranial pressure and volume, cerebral compliance is sufficient to prevent alterations in cerebral hemodynamics, perhaps in part

TABLE 11-31	**Cerebral Hemodynamic, Neurophysiological, and Biochemical Evidence of at Least Transient Disturbance with Posthemorrhagic Ventricular Dilation in Human Infants***

Cerebral Hemodynamics
Decreased cerebral blood flow velocity–increased cerebrovascular resistance–decreased cerebral compliance (Doppler)
Decreased cerebral blood flow (positron emission tomography)
Decreased cerebral oxygenated hemoglobin, blood volume, and indicator of cerebral blood flow (near-infrared spectroscopy)

Neurophysiological Function
Abnormal visual evoked responses
Abnormal brain stem auditory evoked responses
Abnormal somatosensory evoked responses

Biochemical Parameters
Increased cerebrospinal fluid hypoxanthine
Increased cerebrospinal fluid nonprotein-bound iron
Decreased oxidized cytochrome aa_3 in brain (near-infrared spectroscopy)

*See text for references.

by obliteration of the subarachnoid space and encroachment of the infant's cerebral white matter (see earlier discussion). However, available data suggest that (1) a critical point of altered cerebral compliance is reached when further increases will elevate cerebrovascular resistance, and (2) this critical point can be detected by Doppler measurements of the resistive index (RI) before and after a small increase in intracranial pressure induced by external compression of the anterior fontanelle by the ultrasonic transducer.[794,795] Thus, Taylor and co-workers[741,794,795] showed the following: (1) a close correlation between the (percentage) change in resistive index (ΔRI) before and after compression ([RI after compression − RI before compression]/RI before compression) (Fig. 11-37A) and the intracranial pressure; and, importantly, (2) a clear distinction between ΔRI in infants with posthemorrhagic hydrocephalus who required a shunt versus the ΔRI in infants who had arrest of their posthemorrhagic hydrocephalus (see Fig. 11-37B). All infants who required ventricular drainage had a maximum ΔRI of 45% (or greater), compared with a maximum of 18% in infants who did not require surgical intervention.[795] In this investigation, the compression consisted of depression of the fontanelle "such that any additional pressure results in no further depression of the fontanelle." In my experience, the difficulty with utilization of the ΔRI is the variability of the extent of compression used from measurement to measurement. Moreover, it seems likely that as the progression of the hydrocephalus continues and the baseline diastolic flow declines, the baseline RI will increase, and thus the *percentage* ΔRI will decrease. *Therefore I consider it most important to follow baseline RI and the RI after compression, (according to a consistent mode of compression) as well as the calculated percentage ΔRI, serially, in making therapeutic decisions (see later).* Indeed, *the data show that studies of cerebral blood flow velocity and resistance before therapy may aid in the decision of whether CSF removal is indicated, and studies after therapy may aid in the decision of whether a given therapy (e.g., ventriculoperitoneal shunt) is malfunctioning.* Overall, the findings are consistent with experimental studies that show attenuation of cerebral vessels in models of hydrocephalus (see earlier discussion).

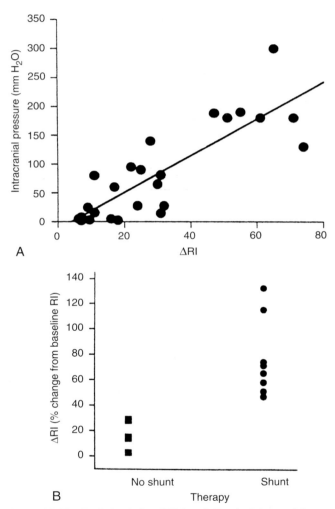

Figure 11-37   **Resistive index (RI) in relation to intracranial pressure or shunt indication**. Relationship of the RI, obtained by Doppler from the pericallosal artery in a series of infants with posthemorrhagic hydrocephalus, as a function of, **A**, intracranial pressure or, **B**, subsequent need for shunt placement. ΔRI is the percentage of change in RI before and after compression of the fontanelle ([RI after compression − RI before compression]/RI before compression). See text for details. *(From Taylor GA, Madsen JR: Neonatal hydrocephalus: Hemodynamic response to fontanelle compression: Correlation with intracranial pressure and need for shunt placement,* Radiology *201:685–689, 1996.)*

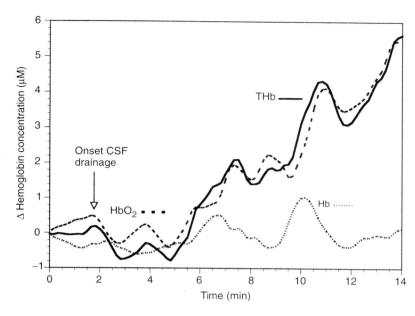

Figure 11-38 Near-infrared spectroscopic measurements of changes in cerebral hemodynamics in posthemorrhagic hydrocephalus, treated by lumbar puncture. Near-infrared spectroscopy was carried out as described in Chapter 4 in a premature infant with posthemorrhagic hydrocephalus, previously untreated. Note the marked increase in cerebral blood volume (total hemoglobin, or THb) on removal of cerebrospinal fluid (CSF) (10 mL/kg). The increase is composed predominantly of oxygenated hemoglobin (HbO₂) and thus appears to be a result primarily of an increase in arterial blood (i.e., cerebral blood flow). Hb, deoxygenated hemoglobin.

Additional studies suggest that the changes in cerebral blood flow velocity parameters just described do reflect lower volemic cerebral blood flow.[797,797a] Thus, we used PET scanning (H₂¹⁵O technique) to show an increase in regional cerebral blood flow in five infants with posthemorrhagic hydrocephalus immediately after removal of CSF by lumbar puncture (unpublished). Moreover, we showed, by near-infrared spectroscopy, evidence for an increase in cerebral blood flow after CSF removal in 16 infants with posthemorrhagic hydrocephalus (Figs. 11-38 and 11-39).[797] The findings included an increase in oxygenated hemoglobin, total hemoglobin (i.e., cerebral blood volume), and the hemoglobin difference (HbO₂ – Hb), an established marker of cerebral blood flow (see Chapter 4).

Concerning *neurophysiological function, visual evoked potentials* have been shown to be altered by posthemorrhagic ventricular dilation. The measurement may be expected to be a sensitive indicator of neurological dysfunction with posthemorrhagic hydrocephalus, because, as noted earlier, the ventricular dilation characteristically affects posterior horns disproportionately. Two studies initially demonstrated prolonged latencies of visual evoked potentials with posthemorrhagic hydrocephalus in the premature infant.[798,799] Improvement in latencies was demonstrated 1 to 2 weeks after placement of a ventriculoperitoneal shunt and within minutes after direct removal of ventricular fluid.[798,799] These data suggest that an axonal disturbance is caused by distention of occipital horns and that this disturbance can be reversed by effective therapy. A second parameter of neurophysiological function, *brain stem auditory evoked potentials*, also has been shown to be altered by posthemorrhagic ventricular dilation and corrected by CSF removal.[800] A similar phenomenon was shown in the hydrocephalic rabbit, in which increased intracranial pressure markedly increased the likelihood of disturbances of brain stem auditory evoked responses with hydrocephalus.[801] The mechanism for the effect is unknown, although the possibility that the auditory system is particularly sensitive to

pressure or traction effects has been raised. A third parameter of neurophysiological function, *somatosensory evoked responses*, also has been shown to be altered by posthemorrhagic ventricular dilation and to be corrected by either spontaneous arrest of ventricular growth or shunt placement.[802] The effect on latency was most marked in infants with increased intracranial pressure. The mechanism of the effect could relate in part to affection of ascending thalamocortical fibers that course around the dilated body of the lateral ventricle.

Concerning *morphological evidence for brain injury* with posthemorrhagic ventricular dilation, data from

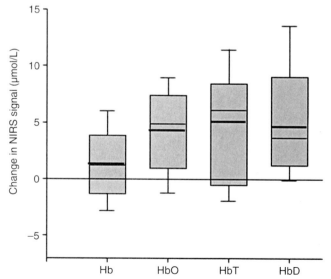

Figure 11-39 Box plot showing the change in signals obtained by near-infrared spectroscopy (NIRS) accompanying cerebrospinal fluid removal. The *box edges* represent the 25th and 75th percentiles, the *thick line* within the box is the mean, and the *error bars* are the fifth and 95th percentiles. Hb, deoxygenated hemoglobin; HbD, the hemoglobin difference; HbO, oxygenated hemoglobin; HbT, total hemoglobin (see text). *(From Soul J, Eichewald E, Walter G, Volpe JJ, et al: CSF removal in infantile posthemorrhagic hydrocephalus results in significant improvement in cerebral hemodynamics, Pediatr Res 55:872–876, 2004.)*

autopsy studies of human infants who did not have markedly advanced disease are few. Studies of biopsies taken at the time of shunt placement have shown four major findings: (1) disruption of ependyma, (2) direct evidence for axonal injury ("axonal ballooning"), (3) lipid-laden microglia, and (4) diminished number of myelinated axons.[748,750,752,803-807] A potential biochemical correlate of this injury is the elevation of CSF levels of such brain-specific proteins as GFAP, neurofilament protein, and S-100 protein in CSF of infants with posthemorrhagic ventricular dilation.[808] These findings are reminiscent of the more carefully controlled observations made in experimental models of hydrocephalus. However, the relation of these changes to the rate of progression and severity of ventriculomegaly, intracranial hypertension, and neurological outcome is unclear.

Biochemical evidence of free radical–mediated injury is suggested by several lines of evidence. Thus, a study of 12 infants with posthemorrhagic hydrocephalus demonstrated *markedly elevated CSF levels of hypoxanthine*, a marker for hypoxic tissue and free radical generation, before treatment.[809] Successful treatment of the ventriculomegaly by lumbar puncture or ventriculoperitoneal shunt led to marked decreases of CSF hypoxanthine levels in all but one infant.[809] Although the morphological effects of hydrocephalus on cerebral vessels and the resulting deleterious cerebral hemodynamic effects (see earlier discussion) appear to be the most probable explanation for tissue hypoxia, the possibility that elevated levels of vasoconstricting eicosanoids (e.g., thromboxanes) or edema-producing eicosanoids (e.g., leukotrienes) are important should be considered. Such eicosanoids have been shown to be elevated in CSF of infants with posthemorrhagic hydrocephalus.[810] Although the source of these compounds remains unclear, and their specific relation to the posthemorrhagic ventricular dilation (effect or association) remains to be established, eicosanoid metabolism by oxygenases results in generation of reactive oxygen species (see Chapter 6). Additionally, elevated levels of non–protein-bound iron have been observed in CSF of premature infants for weeks after IVH.[448] Free iron can lead to generation of the highly injurious hydroxyl radical (see Chapter 6). Additional biochemical evidence for oxygen deficiency at the mitochondrial level is the demonstration by near-infrared spectroscopy of an increase in *brain levels of oxidized cytochrome aa$_3$* after lumbar puncture in infants with posthemorrhagic hydrocephalus accompanied by increased intracranial pressure.[738,811] This observation is consistent with the demonstration by PET of increases in cerebral metabolic rate for oxygen in several infants (one newborn) after treatment of hydrocephalus.[812] More data are needed on these issues.

Finally, several studies concerned with *clinical follow-up* of premature infants with IVH, with and without subsequent hydrocephalus, led investigators to conclude that ventricular dilation contributed to subsequent neurological deficits or that early therapy improved outcome (or both). This issue is addressed in relation to management (see later discussion). In general, it is unclear from the available data how many infants with ventricular dilation had the dilation *because of* brain injury and how many would have had resolution of ventricular dilation and a favorable outcome without intervention. Indeed, the most decisive determinant of outcome in infants with ventricular dilation has appeared to be the extent of prior cerebral parenchymal injury, particularly periventricular hemorrhagic infarction.

Prevention

Because blood products and protein in the CSF presumably lead to the impaired fibrinolysis and the arachnoiditis that causes subsequent hydrocephalus in infants with IVH (see earlier), serial lumbar punctures to remove blood products and administration of fibrinolytic agents to dissolve blood clot have been used to attempt to prevent the development of posthemorrhagic hydrocephalus. Initially, we instituted a prospective controlled study of *serial lumbar punctures* from the *time of diagnosis* of the hemorrhage for *prevention* of hydrocephalus.[334] The rationale for the study was that repeated lumbar punctures would accelerate removal of blood and protein from the CSF and would thereby lessen the chance for the development of hydrocephalus. Thirty-eight infants with moderate or severe IVH identified by CT were randomized to receive serial lumbar punctures or no punctures from the time of diagnosis of the hemorrhage. The data showed no difference in development of hydrocephalus despite punctures performed until CSF was clear and colorless, with protein content less than 180 mg/dL. Although it seemed possible that the relatively small volumes of bloody fluid that could be removed by the punctures accounted for the failure of prophylaxis for hydrocephalus, the observations suggested no benefit for very early serial lumbar punctures for this purpose. A later study of 47 infants with grade III or IV IVH, in whom lumbar punctures were commenced at mean postnatal age of 11 days and continued for 20 days, also failed to show a difference in incidence of subsequent hydrocephalus requiring placement of a ventriculoperitoneal shunt (39% in control group, 42% in treated group).[813] In this study, a mean total of 67 ± 101 mL of CSF was removed with 16 ± 12 lumbar punctures. These data do not bear on the potential of lumbar puncture for *treatment* of posthemorrhagic hydrocephalus after it is established (see later section).

A second approach to prevention of severe posthemorrhagic hydrocephalus involves the use of intraventricular *fibrinolytic* therapy. The approach was stimulated by the observation of successful dissolution of intraventricular blood clots and improved outcome in adults with IVH treated with intraventricular infusion of urokinase.[814,815] Moreover, endogenous fibrinolytic activity was shown to be absent in the CSF of premature infants until at least 17 days after the occurrence of IVH.[816] The impaired endogenous fibrinolytic activity may relate to a combination of low levels of plasminogen in CSF after IVH and of high levels of plasminogen activator inhibitor in the posthemorrhagic CSF (see earlier).[79,80] In an initial encouraging report, Whitelaw and co-workers[817] treated nine infants with evolving posthemorrhagic hydrocephalus at 8 to 27 days of age with intraventricular infusion of streptokinase for 12 to 72 hours. This approach led to detectable fibrinolysis in the infant's CSF, as reflected by an increase in fibrin degradation products in the streptokinase-treated infants.[818] Only one of the nine infants in the initial report ultimately required ventriculoperitoneal shunt, and based on parallel studies in a multicenter trial,[389] approximately 60% of this group would have been expected to develop hydrocephalus requiring shunt placement. A subsequent study of four infants with urokinase resulted in favorable results (i.e., none required a ventriculoperitoneal shunt).[819] A later investigation of 22 preterm infants with progressive posthemorrhagic ventricular dilation treated with intraventricular instillation of recombinant tissue plasminogen activator resulted in the need for shunt placement in 45%, versus 71% in historical controls.[820] This equivocally favorable result was followed by two later studies that recorded no benefit from intraventricular urokinase or streptokinase.[821,822] A Cochrane review "found no good evidence" that streptokinase is useful in this context.[823] It is possible that the usual timing of the onset of therapy, generally after the first week of life, is too late to prevent the progressive changes provoked by the initial blood clots. Early therapy, however, carries the theoretical risk that hemorrhage could be precipitated by the fibrinolytic therapy. An additional possibility for the lack of striking benefit of therapy appears to relate to the finding that *certain infants generate unusually high levels of plasminogen activator inhibitor in their posthemorrhagic CSF* (Fig. 11-40).[80]

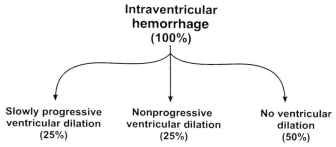

Figure 11-41   Likelihood of progressive ventricular dilation after intraventricular hemorrhage. The schema begins with all infants with intraventricular hemorrhage (*not* germinal matrix hemorrhage alone). Data are derived from 221 infants studied by Murphy and colleagues; numbers are rounded off. *(Data from Murphy BP, Inder TE, Rooks V, Taylor GA, et al: Posthemorrhagic ventricular dilatation in the premature infant: Natural history and predictors of outcome, Arch Dis Child Fetal Neonatal Ed 87:F37–F41, 2002.)*

Currently, it does not appear that *early* intraventricular fibrinolytic therapy has an important role in *prevention* of posthemorrhagic hydrocephalus.

Management of Progressive Posthemorrhagic Ventricular Dilation

Natural History. Management of progressive posthemorrhagic ventricular dilation must begin with recognition of the natural history of the disorder (Figs. 11-41 and 11-42). Although definitions of progressive ventricular dilation and descriptions of evolution,

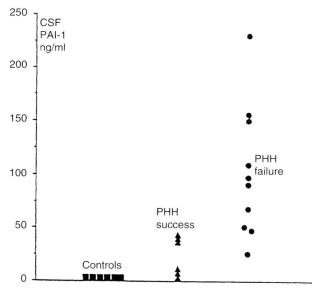

Figure 11-40   Relationship of cerebrospinal fluid (CSF) concentrations of plasminogen activator inhibitor-1 (PAI-1) to success or failure of intraventricular fibrinolytic therapy in premature infants with posthemorrhagic hydrocephalus (PHH). CSF concentrations of PAI-1 are shown for control infants and for those with PHH who responded to intraventricular fibrinolytic therapy (or lumbar puncture) (PHH success) and for those with PHH who did not respond to the fibrinolytic therapy (PHH failure). *(From Hansen A, Whitelaw A, Lapp C, Brugnara C: Cerebrospinal fluid plasminogen activator inhibitor-1: A prognostic factor in posthaemorrhagic hydrocephalus, Acta Paediatr 86:995–998, 1997.)*

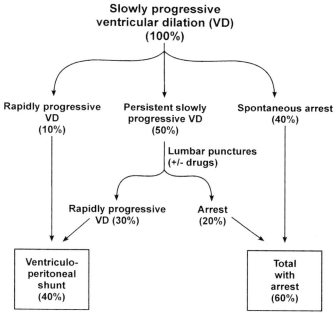

Figure 11-42   Outcome of infants with slowly progressive ventricular dilation (VD). The starting population of infants (100%) is the 25% of infants with intraventricular hemorrhage, shown in Figure 11-41, who developed slowly progressive ventricular dilation. The starting population of slowly progressive ventricular dilation includes only infants of less than 1500 g birth weight, 31% of whom had birth weights lower than 750 g and 81% of whom had grade III or grade IV intraventricular hemorrhage; the population does not include 15% of infants who died (principally of systemic complications of prematurity). *(Data from Murphy BP, Inder TE, Rooks V, Taylor GA, et al: Posthemorrhagic ventricular dilatation in the premature infant: Natural history and predictors of outcome, Arch Dis Child Fetal Neonatal Ed 87:F37–F41, 2002.)*

management, and outcome vary considerably among studies, the data shown in Figures 11-41 and 11-42, based on our personal published and unpublished observations, bear similarities to those reported by others for all infants with IVH (not germinal matrix hemorrhage only) who survive the acute period.* However, readers of previous editions of this book will note a somewhat more aggressive course for progressive posthemorrhagic ventricular dilation, as shown in Figures 11-41 and 11-42, when compared with the course observed in previous years. This change relates to a larger number of extremely-low-birth-weight infants and more severe IVH (see later).[197,367,396,397] Currently, approximately 50% of infants with IVH exhibit no progressive ventricular dilation. This includes the large majority of infants with slight to moderate IVH and the minority of infants with severe IVH (see Table 11-16). Approximately 25% of infants exhibit ventricular dilation that is not progressive and, at least in part, may reflect cerebral white matter injury, such as periventricular leukomalacia (see Chapters 8 and 9). The remaining 25% of infants with IVH develop slowly progressive ventricular dilation (see Fig. 11-41). These infants usually have moderate degrees of ventricular dilation and intracranial pressure measurements that are generally stable and normal or nearly normal. In our experience, mean values for intracranial pressure (anterior fontanelle sensor) in this group are approximately 50 to 80 mm H_2O, near or just above the upper limit of normal (see Chapter 4), and the rate of head growth is appropriate for gestational and postnatal age and nutritional status (see Chapter 3). The term *normal-pressure hydrocephalus* has been used for this group of infants.[161] More refined grouping of infants with posthemorrhagic ventricular dilation have been made with measurements of ventricular width on coronal and sagittal ultrasound scans, of ventricular area by multiple ultrasound scans, and of ventricular volume by ultrasonographic and MRI techniques.[389,731,732,827-830]

Currently, I use serial measurements of (1) rate and severity of progression of ventricular dilation (ultrasonography), (2) rate of head growth, (3) clinical signs of increased intracranial pressure, and (4) resistance index (RI) and ΔRI (see earlier discussion) to follow infants with posthemorrhagic ventricular dilation. (Although I do not perform serial measurements of intracranial pressure, close attention to such measurement is made at any lumbar puncture performed.) On the basis of this experience, summarized in Figure 11-42, four groups of infants can be categorized for management: group I, those with the onset of slowly progressive ventricular dilation (<2 weeks); group II, those with *persistent* slowly progressive ventricular dilation (>2 weeks); group III, those with rapidly progressive ventricular dilation; and group IV, those with apparent arrest of progression, either spontaneous or induced by serial lumbar punctures (see later discussion).

Virtually all infants with progressive posthemorrhagic ventricular dilation begin with the slowly progressive form, and of these infants, approximately 40% exhibit spontaneous arrest, usually with partial or total resolution of the ventricular dilation (see Fig. 11-42). The arrest occurs and resolution commences generally *within 4 weeks* of the development of progressive ventricular dilation. Of the remaining 60% of infants with slowly progressive ventricular dilation, most continue to progress for more than 4 weeks and, if not treated, develop a rapidly progressive process, ultimately with severe ventricular dilation. A smaller proportion of the starting group ($\approx$10%) develop this rapid progression even before 4 weeks (see Fig. 11-42). In these infants, intracranial pressure increases rapidly, usually within days of onset of rapid progression, and is followed closely and consistently by rapid head growth and often by such clinical signs as full anterior fontanelle and separated cranial sutures. Rates of head growth greater than 2 cm/week usually signal the rapid progression,[732,733] although rates greater than 1.5 cm/week are considered indicative of this phase by others.[827] In our experience, values for intracranial pressure in this group may increase rapidly to greater than 150 mm H_2O. The baseline RI and the ΔRI also increase appreciably at this stage (see Fig. 11-37 and earlier discussion).

The severity of the initial IVH is the most critical determinant of not only the likelihood of progressive ventricular dilation (see Table 11-16) but also the temporal evolution and course. Thus, with moderate hemorrhages, the onset of the slowly progressive ventricular dilation is usually after 10 to 14 days, and the likelihood of spontaneous resolution is high. *With severe hemorrhages, the onset of the ventricular dilation may be within several days, the phase of slow progression may be very brief, and the likelihood of spontaneous resolution may be relatively low.* Indeed, in most series, the vast majority of infants who develop rapidly progressive hydrocephalus, either initially or later, experienced severe IVH, with or without periventricular hemorrhagic infarction. In our study of 221 infants with IVH and survival after the acute neonatal period (>14 days), only 7% of infants with grades I/II IVH developed progressive ventricular dilation, whereas approximately 75% and 70% of infants with grades III and IV IVH, respectively, did so (Table 11-32).[367] Additionally, among the group with grade I/II IVH, less than 1% eventually required a ventriculoperitoneal shunt, whereas the incidences were 27% and 33% after grades III and IV IVH. Still more strikingly, among the infants with progressive ventricular dilation, approximately 40% or more of those who had grade III or IV IVH eventually required a ventriculoperitoneal shunt, whereas only 9% (1 of 11) of those who had a grade I/II IVH eventually required shunting. *Thus, progressive ventricular dilation after grade I/II IVH rarely becomes rapidly progressive and requires ventricular drainage, whereas the course of progressive ventricular dilation after grade III/IV IVH is likely to lead to ventricular drainage.*

Four Basic Groups for Management

For the purposes of formulating management, as noted in the previous section, four basic groups can be

---

*See references 20,22,161,195,350,354,359,367,384-386,389,390,392-394,407,408,728,730,732,734,740,824-826.

TABLE 11-32	Progressive Ventricular Dilation, Ventriculoperitoneal Shunt and Mortality as a Function of Severity of IVH				
		VPS IN SURVIVORS[†]			
Severity of IVH*	PVD in Survivors >14 Days Old	PVD	Total		Late Mortality[‡]
Grade I/II	11/160 (7%)	1/11 (9%)	1/160 (0.6%)		14/160 (9%)
Grade III	28/37 (76%)	10/28 (36%)	10/37 (27%)		6/37 (16%)
Grade IV	17/24 (71%)	8/17 (47%)	8/24 (33%)		7/24 (29%)

*Grading as described in Table 11-12, except the combination of intraventricular hemorrhage (IVH) and apparent periventricular hemorrhagic infarction is termed grade IV.
[†]Ventriculoperitoneal shunt (VPS) in infants with progressive ventricular dilation (PVD) and in the total group of infants surviving >14 days.
[‡]Late mortality is death after 14 days; most deaths are related to systemic complications of prematurity.
Data from Murphy BP, Inder TE, Rooks V, Taylor GA, et al: Posthemorrhagic ventricular dilatation in the premature infant: Natural history and predictors of outcome, *Arch Dis Child Fetal Neonatal Ed* 87:F37-F41, 2002.

gleaned from the data. These are summarized in Table 11-33. In the following sections, I discuss the approach to management of these four basic groups of infants with progressive ventricular dilation.

Slowly Progressive Ventricular Dilation (<2 Weeks)

The major therapeutic choices for slowly progressive ventricular dilation of less than 2 weeks in duration (group I) are outlined in Table 11-34.

Close Surveillance. I consider the most appropriate initial step to be close surveillance of changes in ventricular size, rate of head growth, clinical condition, and baseline RI and ΔRI (see Table 11-34). This approach is reasonable because of the relatively high incidence of spontaneous arrest, followed by partial or total resolution of ventriculomegaly in cases of slowly progressive ventricular dilation (Fig. 11-43; see also Fig. 11-42). A crucial question is whether this delay in onset of intervention, while waiting for the occurrence of spontaneous arrest, is deleterious to the developing brain. Although evidence of cerebral hemodynamic and neurophysiological dysfunction with posthemorrhagic hydrocephalus may be obtained (see earlier discussion), available experimental and clinical data suggest, on balance, that any dysfunction is readily reversible and that fixed deficits, structural or functional, do not develop until the process is protracted for many weeks *or* evolves to rapid progression. In a careful, multicenter, randomized controlled trial of

157 infants with posthemorrhagic ventricular dilation, "early lumbar puncture" (mean age at onset, 19 days) did not alter neurological or cognitive outcome in infants managed without lumbar puncture.[389] A marginal beneficial effect of early intervention was suggested for infants with parenchymal lesions at the onset of randomization but only for the combination of cognitive and motor disturbance (*P* = .05) and not for motor disturbance alone.

Persistent Slowly Progressive Ventricular Dilation (>2 Weeks)

Infants who exhibit persistent slowly progressive ventricular dilation beyond 2 weeks (Table 11-35) have been the subject of controversy regarding management. Because spontaneous arrest, if it will occur, does so within 4 weeks, close surveillance for 2 more weeks (to a total of 4 weeks) is reasonable if the patient has no rapid head growth, clinical signs of increased intracranial pressure, or clearly abnormal resistive indices (baseline RI/ΔRI) and if the likelihood of evolution to rapid progression is low (i.e., initiating IVH grade I or II). If progression continues to 4 weeks or if any of the signs of rapid progression just noted appear, intervention is appropriate. I believe currently that serial lumbar punctures are the appropriate choice at this point.

Serial Lumbar Punctures. Cessation of posthemorrhagic ventricular dilation in association with serial lumbar punctures has been well documented.* However, no consensus exists on whether this therapeutic modality is consistently beneficial in arresting progression or improving outcome.[836] Nevertheless, I consider

TABLE 11-33	Management Groups for Posthemorrhagic Hydrocephalus
I.	**Slowly progressive ventricular dilation:** moderate dilation, appropriate rate of head growth, stable RI/ΔRI; <2 wk
II.	**Persistent slowly progressive ventricular dilation:** similar to I, except that duration is >2 wk and rate of head growth and RI/ΔRI may begin to increase
III.	**Rapidly progressive ventricular dilation:** moderate to severe dilation, clearly excessive rate of head growth, RI/ΔRI clearly increased
IV.	**Arrested progression:** spontaneous arrest of ventricular dilation or arrest following lumbar puncture

ΔRI, change in resistive index; RI, resistive index.

TABLE 11-34	Management of Posthemorrhagic Hydrocephalus: Group I
Slowly Progressive Ventricular Dilation: Moderate Dilation, Appropriate Rate of Head Growth (and RI and ΔRI), Duration <2 Wk	
1. Close surveillance	

ΔRI, change in resistive index; RI, resistive index.

*See references 20,350,367,389,390,397,407,734,740,744,831-835.

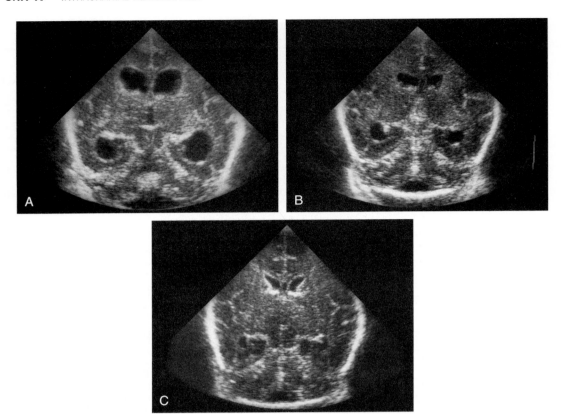

Figure 11-43 **Spontaneous arrest and resolution of slowly progressive posthemorrhagic ventricular dilation**. The coronal ultrasound scans show, **A**, prominent ventricular dilation, which developed slowly over 19 days after intraventricular hemorrhage. The subsequent scans were obtained at, **B**, 26 days and, **C**, 33 days after the hemorrhage. The infant received no therapy for the dilation.

the technique to be useful for at least temporary improvement (i.e., arrest of progression and intermittent decrease in ventricular size) if two criteria are met. The first criterion is to establish the presence of communication between the lateral ventricles and lumbar subarachnoid space, and the second is to remove an adequate quantity (usually a relatively large volume) of CSF.[744] Regarding the first criterion, we have shown that communication is best established by demonstration that removal of CSF causes an immediate decrease in ventricular size that can be documented by ultrasound scan performed immediately after the CSF removal (Fig. 11-44). Alternatively, communication can be shown by demonstrating a decrease in intracranial pressure measured simultaneously at both the anterior fontanelle (anterior fontanelle sensor) and the lumbar subarachnoid space (manometer) with CSF removal.

Concerning the second criterion for ensuring at least temporary benefit from lumbar punctures, it is clear that a substantial volume of CSF must be removed to effect arrest of progression of the hydrocephalic process and intermittent decreases in ventricular size.[350,367,389,390,397,407,744,824] This requirement is not unexpected, because the volume of CSF in the dilated ventricular system may be considerable. Although quantitative data for premature newborns with hydrocephalus are lacking, our observations indicate that, on average, volumes of approximately 10 to 15 mL/kg are most often necessary. The critical volume must be determined for each infant, and cranial ultrasonography before and after CSF removal is important in this regard.

The *timing of onset of therapy* appears to be important. Thus, in a study of 95 infants in the Netherlands with hydrocephalus after grade III IVH, de Vries and coworkers showed that intervention with serial lumbar puncture after the ventricular index[835] exceeded the 97th percentile but before the ventricular size had increased 4 mm higher than that percentile (i.e., "early intervention"), ventriculoperitoneal shunt was required in only 16%.[397,835] Those not treated with lumbar punctures until after the ventricular index had increased to more than 4 mm above the 97th percentile line ultimately required shunt placement in 62%.

Duration of therapy with lumbar punctures is determined according to the response. If daily lumbar punctures lead to cessation of progression, the punctures can be performed at longer intervals, as necessary, to

TABLE 11-35	Management of Posthemorrhagic Hydrocephalus: Group II

Persistent Slowly Progressive Ventricular Dilation: Similar to Group I, except Duration >2 Wk and RI/ΔRI May Begin to Increase
1. Close surveillance for 2 more weeks, especially if initiating intraventricular hemorrhage was grade I or II (see text)
2. Serial lumbar punctures

ΔRI, change in resistive index; RI, resistive index.

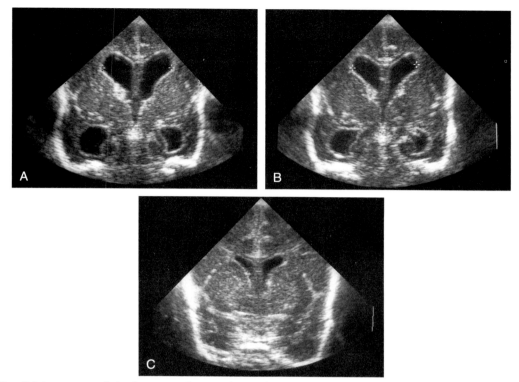

Figure 11-44   **Beneficial response of slowly progressive ventricular dilation to lumbar puncture and removal of cerebrospinal fluid (CSF).** Coronal ultrasound scans were obtained, **A**, immediately before lumbar puncture and, **B**, immediately after removal of 10 mL/kg (body weight) of CSF in a 5-week-old premature infant with progressive posthemorrhagic ventricular dilation. Note the decrease in size of the lateral ventricles after the tap. **C**, Obtained 2 weeks after a 3-week course of serial lumbar punctures. No further therapy was required.

prevent recurrence. In our earlier reported series of 12 infants, a duration of approximately 2 to 3 weeks was necessary in the eight infants who had permanent arrest and partial or total resolution of the dilation.[744] In the remaining four infants, a similar duration did not prevent development of rapidly progressive hydrocephalus, and ventriculoperitoneal shunt was necessary. In our experience the majority of infants with posthemorrhagic hydrocephalus after grade I or II IVH and treated with lumbar punctures undergo arrest with partial or total resolution. However, only the minority respond when the initiating IVH is grade III or IV (see Fig. 11-42).[367]

Complications of lumbar puncture therapy are minimized if the punctures are performed with the infant in the lateral recumbent position with partial neck extension rather than flexion.[744,838] Rare complications reported include meningitis, epidural abscess, vertebral osteomyelitis, and late occurrence of intraspinal epidermoid tumor.[839,840] When large volumes of CSF are removed, attention to fluid status is important to avoid hyponatremia. The risk of complicating meningitis has been unusually high in some small series (e.g., 27%).[841] However, meningitis may be more common in infants with progressive posthemorrhagic ventricular dilation even without intervention. For example, in the large multicenter British trial, infection of CSF occurred in 9% of infants subjected to serial lumbar puncture and in 5% of those managed without puncture.[389] In my experience, the risk of meningitis is on the order of 1%. The use of unstyletted needles has

been associated with the rare examples of late epidermoid tumors.[840] Such needles should be avoided.

The *goal* of lumbar punctures, of course, is to lead to permanent arrest and resolution of persistent slowly progressive ventricular dilation, by intermittently decreasing ventricular size, removing blood products and other toxic compounds (see earlier), and allowing time for reparative processes to result in renewed balance of CSF production and absorption. The value of the decreases in ventricular size may relate in part to the improvements in cerebral blood flow, blood flow velocity, and neurophysiological function (visual, somatosensory, and auditory evoked potentials) described earlier.

Drugs that Decrease Cerebrospinal Fluid Production. As an alternative to serial lumbar punctures, or perhaps as an *additional* therapeutic modality, medications that lead to a decrease in CSF production have been used in treatment of slowly progressive posthemorrhagic hydrocephalus. Two groups of drugs, osmotic agents and carbonic anhydrase inhibitors, have been used in this regard. (A third class of drugs, adenosine triphosphatase inhibitors, such as digoxin, cause a decrease in CSF production that is too brief to be useful clinically.[842,843]) I discuss these agents next because it is likely that they are still used by some neonatologists. *However, I do not believe that the available evidence supports sufficient benefit for this approach.*

Carbonic Anhydrase Inhibitors. The *rationale* for the use of carbonic anhydrase inhibitors in the control of hydrocephalus relates to a reduction in CSF production caused by such agents. Acetazolamide causes a 50% reduction in CSF production, and essentially complete cessation of CSF production can be achieved when acetazolamide and furosemide are used in combination.[844] The effect of acetazolamide on CSF production has been shown in human infants.[845]

The first substantial reported experience with the use of carbonic anhydrase inhibitors in treatment of posthemorrhagic hydrocephalus included 16 infants.[846] Treatment with high dosages of acetazolamide (100 mg/kg/day) and furosemide (1 mg/kg/day) was accompanied by arrest and resolution of ventriculomegaly in 7 infants; the remaining 9 infants required shunt placement. The infants with favorable responses were treated for approximately 6 months. However, no control group was studied, and thus the exact role of the therapy in the improvement is not clear. Complications of therapy included metabolic acidosis that was managed by prophylactic base therapy. In a later study of the efficacy of acetazolamide and furosemide compared with serial lumbar punctures, of 10 infants treated with the two drugs (with supplementation of sodium citrate), only a single infant ultimately required a ventriculoperitoneal shunt.[740] (Three of the 6 infants treated with serial lumbar punctures ultimately required shunts, a proportion not significantly different from that for the drug-treated infants.) Before therapy, these infants had rising intracranial pressure as well as progressive posthemorrhagic ventricular dilation, and thus they may have been more nearly comparable to our group III, with rapidly progressive ventricular dilation, than to infants with persistent, slowly progressive ventricular dilation. Nevertheless, some value for the carbonic anhydrase inhibitors was suggested. Notably, however, 31% of the infants ultimately treated with the two agents ($n = 12$) developed nephrocalcinosis by renal ultrasonography. An earlier report had raised concerns about the possibility that the combination of furosemide and acetazolamide could lead to hypercalciuria and nephrocalcinosis.[847] Furosemide predisposes infants to hypercalciuria by inhibition of renal tubular calcium reabsorption, and acetazolamide encourages precipitation of calcium salts by leading to alkalinization of urine.

Two large studies of the use of acetazolamide and furosemide in the treatment of posthemorrhagic hydrocephalus resulted in the conclusion that the combination "cannot be recommended."[396,739,848] Thus, an international multicenter controlled trial of acetazolamide (100 mg/kg/day) and furosemide (1 mg/kg/day) (with supplements of sodium bicarbonate and potassium chloride, adjusted according to plasma concentrations of sodium, potassium, and bicarbonate) was carried out with 89 infants randomly assigned to "standard therapy" (including 50% with multiple lumbar punctures) and 88 infants to "standard therapy" and the two drugs.[739] Of the drug-treated versus non–drug-treated infants, 51% versus 38% required shunt placement, 19% versus 13% died, and 23% versus 11% (of survivors) exhibited moderate or severe neuromotor impairment. Thus, the drugs were not effective in treating the hydrocephalus. Moreover, 24% of the drug-treated infants developed nephrocalcinosis. A similar lack of benefit and trend toward unfavorable outcome

with acetazolamide and furosemide was shown in a later randomized controlled trial[396] The basis for the apparent worsening of neurological outcome in the drug-treated infants was not established. However, carbonic anhydrase is important in glial differentiation and myelination.[849-852] Perhaps severe inhibition of the enzyme is toxic to developing myelin.

In *conclusion*, the combined and long-term use of acetazolamide (100 mg/kg/day) and furosemide (1 mg/kg/day) does not appear to have clear benefit in therapy and may be associated with risk. Although the use of acetazolamide *alone* has not been studied in a controlled fashion as a complement to lumbar punctures, currently I do not recommend the use of either of these agents in the management of posthemorrhagic hydrocephalus.

Osmotic Agents. The *rationale* for the use of osmotic agents in the control of hydrocephalus is based on observations in cats that indicate an inverse relation between serum osmolarity and CSF formation.[853,854] A 1% change in serum osmolarity resulted in a 15% change in CSF production. Thus, CSF formation could be abolished essentially by a 6.7% increase in serum osmolarity.[854] Glycerol leads to a decrease in CSF production in this manner.[855]

Isosorbide and *glycerol* have been used for treatment of infantile hydrocephalus,[370,856-860] including posthemorrhagic hydrocephalus. Moreover, *glycerol* was used earlier in our unit because of the inconsistent availability of isosorbide.[370,859] Neither agent has been studied in a controlled fashion. Moreover, because of the dangers of hyperosmolality in small preterm infants, I do not recommend this approach to management of posthemorrhagic hydrocephalus.

Rapidly Progressive Ventricular Dilation

The major treatment choices for the third treatment group (group III, i.e., rapidly progressive ventricular dilation) are outlined in Table 11-36. In this clinical setting, close surveillance alone certainly is no longer appropriate because an infant with rapidly progressive ventricular dilation can develop severe ventricular dilation with markedly increased intracranial pressure within days. The specific criteria to be used to define this stage are based on progression of dilation that is measured in days, rising intracranial pressure, rate of head growth in excess of 2.0 cm/week, ventricular size (superior to inferior borders) on a sagittal ultrasound scan of more than 1.5 cm at

TABLE 11-36	Management of Posthemorrhagic Hydrocephalus: Group III

Rapidly Progressive Ventricular Dilation: Moderate to Severe Dilation, Excessive Rate of Head Growth, and RI/ΔRI Clearly Increased
1. Serial lumbar punctures (consider for temporization)
2. Ventricular drainage
   a. Direct external ventricular drain
   b. Tunneled external ventricular drain
   c. Subcutaneous ventricular catheter to reservoir or to subgaleal or supraclavicular spaces
3. Ventriculoperitoneal shunt

ΔRI, change in resistive index; RI, resistive index.

the level of the body of the lateral ventricle just anterior to the trigone, and elevated baseline RI and ΔRI.[389,407,732,734,827] In practice, I place greatest emphasis on the rapidity of progression of dilation, rate of head growth, status of anterior fontanelle and cranial sutures, and serial measurements of Doppler measurements of RI (see earlier discussion and Fig. 11-37).

Serial Lumbar Punctures. Serial lumbar punctures represent the least invasive of the three therapeutic modalities noted in Table 11-36 and may lead to temporary or even permanent arrest of the hydrocephalic process (see Fig. 11-44).[367,397,407,734,740,831,832,835] Cranial ultrasonography before and after the punctures is necessary to ensure that CSF removal leads to a decrease in ventricular size and that the ventricles do not return to the same or larger size too quickly, that is, within a few hours. Considerations concerning management of serial lumbar punctures with rapidly progressive ventricular dilation are similar to those recorded earlier concerning the slowly progressive process, but the essential need to be sure that the effect of CSF removal truly arrests progression deserves reemphasis. *In general, I have not found serial lumbar punctures to provide consistent benefit, either in the short term or the long term, when the hydrocephalic process has reached this stage.* This inconsistency relates either to rapid reaccumulation of CSF after the tap or to obstruction of CSF flow with resulting inability to remove an adequate amount of CSF.

Ventricular Drainage. More often, in my experience, ventricular drainage is necessary for adequate control of rapidly progressive posthemorrhagic hydrocephalus (see Table 11-36).[367,861] This therapy is indicated for infants who have not responded adequately to lumbar puncture and who are not good candidates for placement of ventriculoperitoneal shunt. Reasons for the latter situation are, first, an infant who is too small or too ill to tolerate the surgical procedure and, second, an infant who has bloody or highly proteinaceous CSF that may lead to shunt obstruction. Essentially, the goal of ventricular drainage is temporization, although in a minority of infants, the time gained also allows reopening of pathways of CSF flow and absorption (see later discussion). The *value* of external ventricular drainage in treatment of rapidly progressive ventricular dilation in premature infants has been documented in several studies.[367,384,394,732,737,861-871] Four basic approaches have been used: (1) a novel procedure of ventricular drainage, irrigation, and fibrinolytic therapy ("DRIFT"); (2) a direct external ventricular drain; (3) an external ventricular drain tunneled subcutaneously to an external drip chamber; and (4) a completely internal ventricular drain tunneled to a subcutaneous reservoir, to a surgically established subcutaneous supraclavicular pouch or to the subgaleal space.

Drift. A novel approach of ventricular *drainage, irrigation and fibrinolytic therapy* was shown in a pilot study to be of benefit in the management of rapidly progressive posthemorrhagic hydrocephalus.[88,872] The goals of the procedure are to remove deleterious blood products, antifibrinolytic and fibroproliferative molecules (see earlier), and toxic compounds (free radicals, non–protein-bound iron), to provide the antifibrinolytic agent tissue-type plasminogen activator, and to control intracranial pressure. Two ventricular catheters are placed, one in the frontal horn and one in the occipital horn, tissue-type plasminogen activator is administered intraventricularly, and after 8 hours, irrigation with artificial CSF is commenced and is carried out for 72 hours. In the initial study of 24 infants (median birth weight, 1150 g) with grade III IVH, 16 with parenchymal lesions, only 26% required a ventriculoperitoneal shunt.[872] Outcome was better than in historical controls; in infants with parenchymal lesions, 70% were free of major cognitive deficits and 40% had no major motor deficits, and in infants without parenchymal lesions, all were normal. Subsequently, a multicenter randomized trial ($n=70$) comparing DRIFT with conventional therapy found no difference in the primary outcomes of death or need for shunt.[873] Moreover, 35% of the infants in the DRIFT group developed secondary IVH, usually in the 24 hours after onset of therapy, whereas only 8% of the conventionally treated infants developed such hemorrhage. Thus, currently DRIFT is not indicated for routine clinical practice.

Direct External Ventricular Drains. Direct external ventricular drains have been in use for many years, although less so in recent years (see Table 11-36). The *technique* that we employed initially involved placement of a soft Silastic 21-gauge feeding catheter into the lateral ventricle. The catheter was threaded into the lateral ventricle through a 16-gauge needle-catheter assembly, which was used to enter the lateral ventricle and then removed after the feeding catheter was in place. To facilitate entry of the needle-catheter assembly into the lateral ventricle, an ultrasound scan was obtained just before the ventricular tap. Some investigators have suggested performance of the tap under ultrasonic guidance,[874,875] but we did not find this necessary. The catheter was maintained in a closed system with a reservoir, the height of which can be adjusted to determine intracranial pressure and to regulate rate of drainage. In general, the rate of CSF drainage that I have used is approximately 10 to 15 mL/kg body weight per day. This fluid should be calculated in determining daily fluid requirements. Duration of drainage is generally approximately 5 to 7 days. The use of tunneled catheters (see later discussion) increases the possible duration of drainage, and currently I favor the use of tunneled catheters. Nevertheless, this direct technique is easily applied and remains a useful approach.[876]

In my experience, the *short-term outcome* of direct external ventricular drainage concerning the ventriculomegaly is uniformly favorable; for example, in our initial series, all 19 infants had a striking decrease in ventricular size within 48 hours of placement of the ventriculostomy (Fig. 11-45).[861] Moreover, ventricular decompression was demonstrated also by reduction in intracranial pressures from as high as 150 to 200 mm H_2O to less than 100 mm H_2O in all cases. Subsequent to removal of the ventricular catheter, three infants (16%) required no

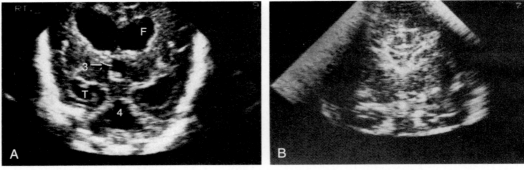

Figure 11-45   **Coronal ultrasound scan in a 13-day-old infant with rapidly progressive posthemorrhagic ventricular dilation. A,** Before ventriculostomy, the scan shows severe dilation of frontal (F) and temporal (T) horns of lateral ventricles as well as of third (3) and fourth (4) ventricles. **B,** The scan obtained after 5 days of external ventricular drainage demonstrates a striking decrease in size of the ventricles.

further therapy. The other 16 infants eventually required placement of a ventriculoperitoneal shunt, some after one or more additional ventriculostomies. After that report, we studied an additional 40 infants with direct external ventricular drainage, and a total of 15% ultimately did not require a ventriculoperitoneal shunt. Thus, although the likelihood of permanent arrest after ventriculostomy was relatively low, the principal benefit was temporization, such that the infant became larger and healthier and the CSF was no longer bloody. These occurrences allowed placement of a ventriculoperitoneal shunt under more favorable conditions.

The other major reported experience with direct external ventricular drainage is that described by Marro and Allan and their co-workers[732] with 24 infants. In this group, mean age at placement of the first drain was 23 days (i.e., generally ≈1 week or so earlier than in our work). Thus, the severity of the process in the patients of Allan and co-workers may have been less. Of the survivors, 57% ultimately required shunt placement, although 80% had more than one ventricular drain placed, and 33% had four or more.[732]

The major *complication* of ventriculostomy is infection. The incidence of infection in our series was 5% of ventriculostomies, somewhat lower than the 9% reported in adults.[877] In the series of Marro and co-workers,[732] 1 of 70 drains was complicated by infection.

Tunneled External Ventricular Drains. The second major approach to external ventricular drainage for neonatal posthemorrhagic hydrocephalus involves not a direct route from the skin surface to the ventricle but rather a *tunneled ventricular catheter* (see Table 11-36). With this approach, a subcutaneous tunnel is established from the point of entry at the skin surface to the point of penetration of the skull and, ultimately, the cerebral wall. The use of a subcutaneous tunnel decreases the risk of infection and thereby allows a longer duration for the drainage (i.e., several weeks versus 5 to 7 days with direct external ventricular drainage). As with direct external ventricular drains, the rate of CSF removal can be modulated by alteration of the height of the external drip chamber. The ultimate need for shunt placement, approximately 70%, is similar to that reported for direct external ventricular drainage.[737,863,866,868] The reported infection rates, approximately 5%, are similar to those reported for direct drains, although clearly the number of

procedures to which the infant is subjected is less with tunneled catheters. Long-term outcome, as with the direct external ventricular drainage, depends principally on the degree of initial parenchymal injury. In one report, 41% of infants with hydrocephalus after "grade III IVH" who were treated with a tunneled drain were normal on follow-up, whereas none of the six similarly treated infants with "grade IV IVH" were normal.[868]

Subcutaneous Ventricular Catheter with a Reservoir. A third major approach to temporizing ventricular drainage, now perhaps the most commonly used, involves a tunneled ventricular catheter that is connected to a subcutaneous reservoir, which can be tapped several times daily for CSF removal (see Table 11-36).[394,397,864,869-871,878] Variations on the connection of a tunneled ventricular catheter to a subcutaneous reservoir are connections either to a surgically prepared subcutaneous pouch in the supraclavicular region or to the subgaleal space.[865,867]

Early experience with the use of ventricular drainage to a subcutaneous reservoir for treatment of rapidly progressive hydrocephalus after "grade III or IV IVH" involved 72 severely affected preterm infants (see Table 11-37).[394] Of this group, 31 (41%) died, and 30 of these 31 had experienced "grade IV IVH." In the entire series, *of the 24 infants with hydrocephalus after "grade III IVH,"* 1 (4%) died, 78% ultimately required shunt placement, 54% had motor deficits, and 8% had a developmental quotient more than 2 SD below the mean on follow-up. *By contrast, of the 48 infants with hydrocephalus after grade IV IVH,* the outcome was much poorer; that is, 30 (62%) died, 94% of the survivors ultimately required shunt placement, all had motor deficits, and fully 78% had a developmental quotient more than 2 SD below the mean. Only 2 of the 71 infants had infection of their reservoir.

In a more recent experience, de Vries and co-workers studied the use of a subcutaneous reservoir after either early or late lumber punctures for hydrocephalus after grade III IVH (see earlier).[397,835] Approximately one third of those infants who continued to progress after early lumbar punctures and were treated with a subcutaneous reservoir required a ventriculoperitoneal shunt. By contrast, approximately 80% of infants who had *more severe* hydrocephalus and were treated with a reservoir immediately or

TABLE 11-37 Outcome of Premature Infants Referred to a Neurosurgical Service with Rapidly Progressive Posthemorrhagic Hydrocephalus Treated Initially with Ventricular Drainage*

Severity of Hemorrhage[†]	OUTCOME				
	No.	Death	Required Shunt	Motor Deficits	Abnormal DQ[‡]
Grade III	24	4%	78%	54%	8%
Grade IV	48	62%	94%	100%	78%

*Rapidly progressive posthemorrhagic hydrocephalus was identified by "progressive and marked ventriculomegaly despite serial lumbar punctures." The ventricular catheter was tunneled to a subcutaneous reservoir, from which "5–20 mL of CSF" was removed daily. Outcome data are rounded off. Note that this selected population of infants was particularly severely affected.
[†]Severity of hemorrhage: grade III is equivalent to grade III in Table 11-13; grade IV includes parenchymal hemorrhagic lesions.
[‡]Abnormal development quotient (DQ): more than 2 SD below the mean.
Data from Levy ML, Masri LS, McComb JG: Outcome for preterm infants with germinal matrix hemorrhage and progressive hydrocephalus, *Neurosurgery* 41:1111–1117, 1997.

after lumbar punctures required ventriculoperitoneal shunts. Overall, 66% of infants treated with a reservoir required a ventriculoperitoneal shunt. *Thus, the possibility that a ventricular drain to a subcutaneous reservoir will be curative and not merely temporization decreases with more severe hydrocephalus.*

In conclusion, the essential point is that ventricular catheterization, which drains CSF externally, either directly or after subcutaneous tunneling, *or preferably, which drains CSF into a subcutaneous reservoir that can be tapped percutaneously,* is *effective temporization* for treatment of rapidly progressive posthemorrhagic hydrocephalus. A minority of infants so treated will escape ultimate ventriculoperitoneal shunt placement, but, more important, the majority who ultimately will require a shunt will be better able to tolerate the procedure and more likely to have CSF free enough of blood products to avoid frequent shunt obstruction.

Ventriculoperitoneal Shunt. Placement of a shunt system that diverts CSF from the lateral ventricles to the peritoneal cavity (definitive therapy for hydrocephalus) (see Table 11-36) has been associated with variable success in reports from many medical centers.[392,394,397,408,734,831,861,879-894] Shunt placement in small premature infants carries a considerable morbidity, secondary to various shunt-related complications, such as ulceration of scalp, ventriculitis, sepsis, and need for frequent revisions. Indeed, poor outcome is related in part to the occurrence of shunt infection. Thus, the value of procedures for temporization (i.e., external ventricular drain and serial lumbar punctures) is considerable. Systematic data for brain injury caused by posthemorrhagic hydrocephalus *alone* are difficult to obtain because major parenchymal lesions play a dominant role in causing subsequent neurological deficits in these infants.[392,394,408,734,831,861,883,885-891,893-895] This fact is demonstrated clearly by the data recorded in Table 11-37. This series of infants, studied more than a decade ago, is not representative of *all* infants with grade III or IV IVH but rather those *selected after referral to a neurosurgical service.* The findings are presented to illustrate a poorer outcome in infants with hydrocephalus after grade III versus grade IV IVH. The principal determinant of unfavorable outcome

appears to relate to the occurrence of parenchymal injury consequent to the IVH (periventricular hemorrhagic infarction) or to preceding ischemic insults (periventricular leukomalacia). However, the brain already injured by hemorrhage or ischemia may be more vulnerable to additional injury from progressive ventricular dilation or elevated intracranial pressure, or both. More data clearly are needed on this issue to design optimal timing of shunt placement. Nevertheless, I believe that undue delay in placement of a ventriculoperitoneal shunt in the infant with rapidly progressive hydrocephalus recalcitrant to other therapies may enhance the likelihood of subsequent neurological deficits.

Arrested Progression: Spontaneous Arrest of Ventricular Dilation or Arrest Following Lumbar Puncture or Drugs That Decrease Cerebrospinal Fluid Production

In previous years, the discussion of management of posthemorrhagic ventricular dilation would be completed after consideration of the patient group just discussed. However, it is now clear that a fourth group (group IV) for management must be recognized (Table 11-38). Thus, of the approximately 60% of infants with slowly progressive ventricular dilation who have exhibited arrest with partial or total resolution of the dilation, either spontaneously or after treatment with serial lumbar punctures or drugs to decrease CSF production (see Fig. 11-42), approximately 5% develop late progressive ventricular dilation (Fig. 11-46). This occurrence is manifested primarily by rapid head growth and a usual age at diagnosis of 3 to 6 months (Fig. 11-47).[367,390] Nearly all infants with this late onset of progressive hydrocephalus have

TABLE 11-38 Management of Posthemorrhagic Hydrocephalus: Group IV

Arrested Progression: Spontaneous Arrest of Ventricular Dilation or Arrest following Lumbar Puncture or Drugs That Decrease Cerebrospinal Fluid Production
Close surveillance for 1 year

Spontaneous or
treatment-associated arrest
60%

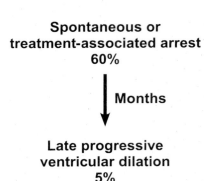

↓ **Months**

Late progressive
ventricular dilation
5%

Figure 11-46 Evolution of late progressive ventricular dilation after arrest of posthemorrhagic hydrocephalus. Arrest occurred either spontaneously or with treatment by serial lumbar punctures and drugs to decrease cerebrospinal fluid production. The starting population is the 60% of the total with progressive ventricular dilation who underwent arrest of progression, as described in Figure 11-42.

required placement of a ventriculoperitoneal shunt. A similar phenomenon has been observed by others.[730,896] The essential clinical point is that even infants with apparent arrest of progressive ventricular dilation, whether spontaneous or induced by interventions, must be followed carefully through the first year, at least with careful attention to head growth, neurological development, and clinical signs of increased intracranial pressure (see Table 11-38).

Rational Sequence for Management of Survivors of Intraventricular Hemorrhage

A rational sequence for management of survivors of IVH can be derived from the considerations reviewed in the preceding sections (Fig. 11-48). Serial ultrasound scans (coupled with determinations of head growth, clinical course, and resistive indices) define the presence, severity, and rapidity of progression of the ventricular dilation. As described earlier, infants with slowly progressive ventricular dilation exhibit moderate dilation, no rapid head growth, and generally stable

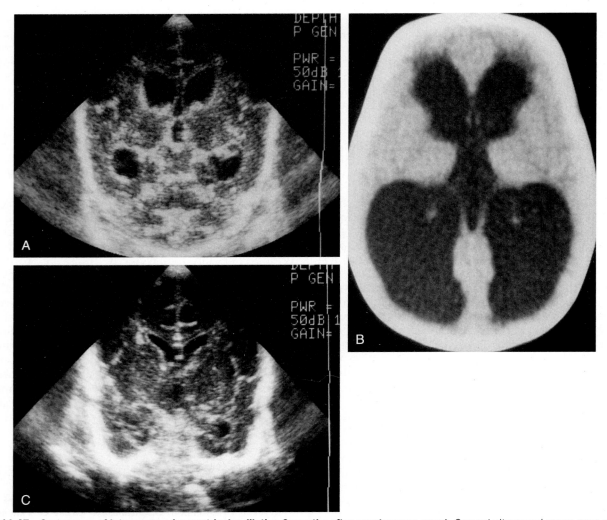

Figure 11-47 Occurrence of late progressive ventricular dilation 6 months after spontaneous arrest. Coronal ultrasound scans were obtained from a premature infant who developed, **A**, posthemorrhagic hydrocephalus, which, **B**, resolved spontaneously. Six months later, the infant developed, over several weeks, irritability, a full fontanelle, and a rapid increase in head circumference. **C**, The computed tomography scan demonstrated marked hydrocephalus, which responded well to placement of a ventriculoperitoneal shunt.

Management of intraventricular hemorrhage
(Serial ultrasound scans, etc. - see text)

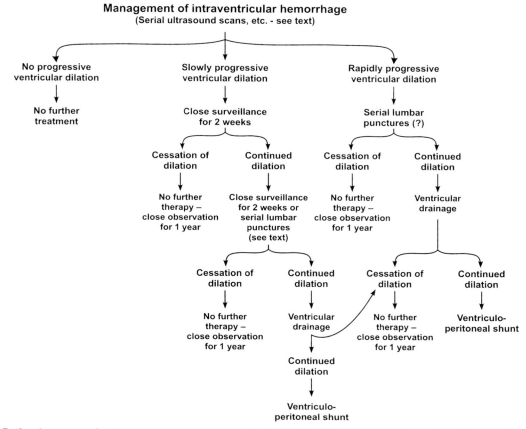

Figure 11-48 Rational sequence for the management of the infant who survives intraventricular hemorrhage. See text for details.

intracranial pressure and resistive indices. In contrast, infants with rapidly progressive ventricular dilation exhibit moderate to severe dilation, rapid head growth, and rapidly rising intracranial pressure and resistive indices. Evolution of persistent, slowly progressive to rapidly progressive cases occurs, as discussed earlier. *Cases with overlapping features are not rare*, but careful consideration of all aspects of the individual case usually allows appropriate categorization and management decisions (see Fig. 11-48).

REFERENCES

1. Volpe JJ: Brain injury in the premature infant: Overview of clinical aspects, neuropathology, and pathogenesis, *Semin Pediatr Neurol* 5:135-151, 1998.
2. Kiely JL, Susser M: Preterm birth, intrauterine growth retardation, and perinatal mortality, *Am J Public Health* 82:343-344, 1992.
3. Guyer B, MacDorman MF, Martin JA, Peters KD, et al: Annual summary of vital statistics: 1997, *Pediatrics* 102:1333-1349, 1998.
4. Guyer B, Hoyert DL, Martin JA, Ventura SJ, et al: Annual summary of vital statistics: 1998, *Pediatrics* 104:1229-1246, 1999.
5. Martin JA, Kochanek KD, Strobino DM, Guyer B, et al: Annual summary of vital statistics: 2003, *Pediatrics* 115:619-634, 2005.
6. Wilcox AJ, Skjoerven R: Birth weight and perinatal mortality: The effect of gestational age, *Am J Public Health* 82:378-382, 1992.
7. Horbar JD, McAuliffe TL, Adler SM, Albersheim S, et al: Variability in 28-day outcomes for very low birth weight infants: An analysis of 11 neonatal intensive care units, *Pediatrics* 82:554-559, 1988.
8. Horbar JD, Badger GJ, Lewit EM, Rogowski J, et al: Hospital and patient characteristics associated with variation in 28-day mortality rates for very low birth weight infants, *Pediatrics* 99:149-156, 1997.
9. Fanaroff AA, Wright LL, Stevenson DK, Shankaran S, et al: Very-low-birth-weight outcomes of the National Institute of Child Health and Human Development Neonatal Research Network, May 1991 through December 1992, *Am J Obstet Gynecol* 173:1423-1141, 1995.
10. McIntire DD, Bloom SL, Casey BM, Leveno KJ: Birth weight in relation to morbidity and mortality among newborn infants, *N Engl J Med* 340:1234-1238, 1999.
11. Lee SK, McMillan DD, Ohlsson A, Pendray M, et al: Variations in practice and outcomes in the Canadian NICU network: 1996–1997, *Pediatrics* 106:1070-1079, 2000.
12. Davis JM, Parad RB, Michele T, Allred E, et al: Pulmonary outcome at 1 year corrected age in premature infants treated at birth with recombinant human CuZn superoxide dismutase, *Pediatrics* 111:469-476, 2003.
13. Darlow BA, Cust AE, Donoghue DA: Improved outcomes for very low birthweight infants: Evidence from New Zealand national population based data, *Arch Dis Child* 88:23-28, 2003.
14. Cust AE, Darlow BA, Donoghue DA: Outcomes for high risk New Zealand newborn infants in 1998–1999: A population based, national study, *Arch Dis Child* 88:15-22, 2003.
15. De Vries LS, Van Haastert IL, Rademaker KJ, Koopman C, et al: Ultrasound abnormalities preceding cerebral palsy in high-risk preterm infants, *J Pediatr* 144:815-820, 2004.
16. Larroque B, Marret S, Ancel PY, Arnaud C, et al: White matter damage and intraventricular hemorrhage in very preterm infants: The EPIPAGE study, *J Pediatr* 143:477-483, 2003.
17. MacDonald H, Committee on Fetus and Newborn: Perinatal care at the threshold of viability, *Pediatrics* 110:1024-1027, 2002.
18. Vohr BR, Wright LL, Dusick AM, Perritt R, et al: Center differences and outcomes of extremely low birth weight infants, *Pediatrics* 113:781-789, 2004.
19. Wilson-Costello D, Friedman H, Minich N, Fanaroff AA, et al: Improved survival rates with increased neurodevelopmental disability for extremely low birth weight infants in the 1990s, *Pediatrics* 115:997-1003, 2005.
20. Ahmann PA, Lazzara A, Dykes FD, Brann AW Jr, et al: Intraventricular hemorrhage in the high-risk preterm infant: Incidence and outcome, *Ann Neurol* 7:118-124, 1980.
21. Holt PJ, Allan WF: The natural history of ventricular dilatation in neonatal intraventricular hemorrhage and its therapeutic implication, *Ann Neurol* 10:293, 1981.
22. Levene MI, Wigglesworth JS, Dubowitz V: Cerebral structure and intraventricular haemorrhage in the neonate: A real-time ultrasound study, *Arch Dis Child* 56:416-424, 1981.
23. Lipscomb AP, Thorburn RJ, Reynolds EO, Stewart AL, et al: Pneumothorax and cerebral haemorrhage in preterm infants, *Lancet* 1:414-416, 1981.

24. McMenamin JB, Shackelford GD, Volpe JJ: Outcome of neonatal intraventricular hemorrhage with periventricular echodense lesions, *Ann Neurol* 15:285-290, 1984.
25. Papile LA, Burstein J, Burstein R, Koffler H: Incidence and evolution of subependymal and intraventricular hemorrhage: A study of infants with birth weights less than 1,500 gm, *J Pediatr* 92:529-534, 1978.
26. Perlman JM, Volpe JJ: Prevention of neonatal intraventricular hemorrhage, *Clin Neuropharmacol* 10:126-142, 1987.
27. Philip AG, Allan WC, Tito AM, Wheeler LR: Intraventricular hemorrhage in preterm infants: Declining incidence in the 1980's, *Pediatrics* 84:797-801, 1989.
28. Allan WC: Intraventricular hemorrhage, *J Child Neurol* 4:512-522, 1989.
29. Leviton A, Fenton T, Kuban KC, Pagano M: Labor and delivery characteristics and the risk of germinal matrix hemorrhage in low birth weight infants, *J Child Neurol* 6:35-40, 1991.
30. Kuban KC, Leviton A, Pagano M, Fenton T, et al: Maternal toxemia is associated with reduced incidence of germinal matrix hemorrhage in premature babies, *J Child Neurol* 7:70-76, 1992.
31. Paneth N, Pinto-Martin J, Gardiner J, Wallenstein S, et al: Incidence and timing of germinal matrix/intraventricular hemorrhage in low birth weight infants, *Am J Epidemiol* 137:1167-1176, 1993.
32. Sheth RD: Trends in incidence and severity of intraventricular hemorrhage, *J Child Neurol* 13:261-264, 1998.
33. Kuban K, Sanocka U, Leviton A, Allred EN, et al: White matter disorders of prematurity: Association with intraventricular hemorrhage and ventriculomegaly, *J Pediatr* 134:539-546, 1999.
34. Ment LR, Vohr B, Oh W, Scott DT, et al: Neurodevelopmental outcome at 36 months' corrected age of preterm infants in the multicenter indomethacin intraventricular hemorrhage prevention trail, *Pediatrics* 98:714-718, 1996.
35. Vohr BR, Wright LL, Dusick AM, Mele L, et al: Neurodevelopmental and functional outcomes of extremely low birth weight infants in the National Institute of Child Health and Human Development Neonatal Research Network, 1993–1994, *Pediatrics* 105:1216-1226, 2000.
36. Szymonowicz W, Schafler K, Cussen LJ, Yu VY: Ultrasound and necropsy study of periventricular haemorrhage in preterm infants, *Arch Dis Child* 59:637-642, 1984.
37. Perlman JM, Volpe JJ: Intraventricular hemorrhage in extremely small premature infants, *Am J Dis Child* 140:1122-1124, 1986.
38. Horbar JD, Badger GJ, Carpenter JH, Fanaroff AA, et al: Trends in mortality and morbidity for very low birth weight infants, 1991–1999, *Pediatrics* 110:143-151, 2002.
39. Hamrick SE, Miller SP, Leonard C, Glidden DV, et al: Trends in severe brain injury and neurodevelopmental outcome in premature newborn infants: The role of cystic periventricular leukomalacia, *J Pediatr* 145:593-599, 2004.
40. Hambleton G, Wigglesworth JS: Origin of intraventricular haemorrhage in the preterm infant, *Arch Dis Child* 51:651-659, 1976.
41. Takashima S, Tanaka K: Microangiography and vascular permeability of the subependymal matrix in the premature infant, *Can J Neurol Sci* 5:45-50, 1978.
42. Pape KE, Wigglesworth JS: *Haemorrhage, Ischaemia, and the Perinatal Brain*, Philadelphia: 1979, JB Lippincott.
43. Kuban KC, Gilles FH: Human telencephalic angiogenesis, *Ann Neurol* 17:539-548, 1985.
44. Haruda F, Blanc WA: The structure of small intracerebral arteries in premature infants and autoregulation of cerebral blood flow, *Ann Neurol* 10:303-304, 1981.
45. Anstrom JA, Brown WR, Moody DM, Thore CR, et al: Anatomical analysis of the developing cerebral vasculature in premature neonates: Absence of precapillary arteriole-to-venous shunts, *Pediatr Res* 52:554-560, 2002.
46. Anstrom JA, Brown WR, Moody DM, Thore CR, et al: Subependymal veins in premature neonates: Implications for hemorrhage, *Pediatr Neurol* 30:46-53, 2004.
47. Ballabh P, Hu FB, Kumarasiri M, Braun A, et al: Development of tight junction molecules in blood vessels of germinal matrix, cerebral cortex, and white matter, *Pediatr Res* 58:791-798, 2005.
48. Lenn NJ, Whitmore L: Gestational changes in the germinal matrix of the normal rhesus monkey fetus, *Pediatr Res* 19:130-135, 1985.
49. Larroche JC: *Developmental Pathology of the Neonate*, New York: 1977, Excerpta Medica.
50. Larroche JC: Intraventricular hemorrhage in the premature neonate. In Korobkin R, Guilleminault C, editors: *Advances in Perinatal Neurology*, vol 1, New York: 1979, SP Medical and Scientific Books.
51. Yakovlev PI: Distribution of the terminal hemorrhages in the brain wall in stillborn premature and nonviable neonates. In Angle CR, Bering EA Jr, editors: *Physical Trauma as an Etiologic Agent in Mental Retardation*, Washington, DC: 1970, U.S. Government Printing Office.
52. Gruenwald P: Subependymal cerebral hemorrhage in premature infants, and its relation to various injurious influences at birth, *Am J Obstet Gynecol* 61:1285-1292, 1951.
53. Leech RW, Kohnen P: Subependymal and intraventricular hemorrhages in the newborn, *Am J Pathol* 77:465-475, 1974.
54. Rorke LB: *Pathology of Perinatal Brain Injury*, New York: 1982, Raven Press.
55. Armstrong DL, Sauls CD, Goddard-Finegold J: Neuropathologic findings in short-term survivors of intraventricular hemorrhage, *Am J Dis Child* 141:617-621, 1987.
56. Nakamura Y, Okudera T, Fukuda S, Hashimoto T: Germinal matrix hemorrhage of venous origin in preterm neonates, *Hum Pathol* 21:1059-1062, 1990.
57. Moody DM, Brown WR, Challa VR, Block SM: Alkaline phosphatase histochemical staining in the study of germinal matrix hemorrhage and brain vascular morphology in a very-low-birth-weight neonate, *Pediatr Res* 35:424-430, 1994.
58. Ghazi-Birry HS, Brown WR, Moody DM, Challa VR, et al: Human germinal matrix: Venous origin of hemorrhage and vascular characteristics, *AJNR Am J Neuroradiol* 18:219-229, 1997.
59. Golden JA, Gilles FH, Rudewlli R, Leviton A: Frequency of neuropathological abnormalities in very low birth weight infants, *J Neuropathol Exp Neurol* 56:472-478, 1997.
60. Guzzetta F, Shackelford GD, Volpe S, Perlman JM, et al: Periventricular intraparenchymal echodensities in the premature newborn: Critical determinant of neurologic outcome, *Pediatrics* 78:995-1006, 1986.
61. Flodmark O, Becker LE, Harwood-Nash DC, Fitzhardinge PM, et al: Correlation between computed tomography and autopsy in premature and full-term neonates that have suffered perinatal asphyxia, *Radiology* 137:93-103, 1980.
62. Gould SJ, Howard S, Hope PL, Reynolds EO: Periventricular intraparenchymal cerebral haemorrhage in preterm infants: The role of venous infarction, *J Pathol* 151:197-202, 1987.
63. Rushton DI, Preston PR, Durbin GM: Structure and evolution of echodense lesions in the neonatal brain: A combined ultrasound and necropsy study, *Arch Dis Child* 60:798-808, 1985.
64. Volpe JJ, Herscovitch P, Perlman JM, Raichle ME: Positron emission tomography in the newborn: Extensive impairment of regional cerebral blood flow with intraventricular hemorrhage and hemorrhagic intracerebral involvement, *Pediatrics* 72:589-601, 1983.
65. Rademaker KJ, Groenendaal F, Jansen GH, Eken P, et al: Unilateral haemorrhagic parenchymal lesions in the preterm infant: Shape, site and prognosis, *Acta Paediatr* 83:602-608, 1994.
66. Bassan H, Benson CB, Limperopoulos C, Feldman HA, et al: Ultrasonographic features and severity scoring of periventricular hemorrhagic infarction in relation to risk factors and outcome, *Pediatrics* 117:2111-2118, 2006.
67. Takashima S, Mito T, Ando Y: Pathogenesis of periventricular white matter hemorrhages in preterm infants, *Brain Dev* 8:25-30, 1986.
68. Perlman JM, Rollins N, Burns D, Risser R: Relationship between periventricular intraparenchymal echodensities and germinal matrix–intraventricular hemorrhage in the very low birth weight neonate, *Pediatrics* 91:474-480, 1993.
69. Ment LR, Oh W, Phillip AGS, Ehrenkranz R, et al: Risk factors for early intraventricular hemorrhage in low birth weight infants, *J Pediatr* 121:776-783, 1992.
70. Shaver DC, Bada HS, Korones SB, Anderson GD, et al: Early and late intraventricular hemorrhage: The role of obstetric factors, *Obstet Gynecol* 80:831-837, 1992.
71. de Vries LS, Roelants-Van Rijn AM, Rademaker KJ, van Haastert IC, et al: Unilateral parenchymal haemorrhagic infarction in the preterm infant, *Eur J Paediatr Neurol* 5:139-149, 2001.
72. Taylor GA: Effect of germinal matrix hemorrhage on terminal vein position and patency, *Pediatr Radiol* 25:S37-S40, 1995.
73. Dean LM, Taylor GA: The intracranial venous system in infants: Normal and abnormal findings on duplex and color Doppler sonography, *AJR Am J Roentgenol* 164:151-156, 1995.
74. Toft PB, Leth H, Peitersen B, Lou HC: Metabolic changes in the striatum after germinal matrix hemorrhage in the preterm infant, *Pediatr Res* 41:309-316, 1997.
75. Counsell SJ, Maalouf EF, Rutherford MA, Edwards AD: Periventricular haemorrhagic infarct in a preterm neonate, *Eur J Paediatr Neurol* 3:25-28, 1999.
76. Clark WEL: On the pachionian bodies, *J Anat* 55:40, 1920.
77. Friede RL: *Developmental Neuropathology*, 2nd ed, New York: 1989, Springer-Verlag.
78. Fawer CL, Levene MI: Elusive blood clots and fluctuating ventricular dilatation after neonatal intraventricular haemorrhage, *Arch Dis Child* 57:158-160, 1982.
79. Whitelaw A, Mowinckel MC, Abildgaard U: Low levels of plasminogen in cerebrospinal fluid after intraventricular haemorrhage: A limiting factor for clot lysis? *Acta Paediatr* 84:933-936, 1995.
80. Hansen A, Whitelaw A, Lapp C, Brugnara C: Cerebrospinal fluid plasminogen activator inhibitor-1: A prognostic factor in posthaemorrhagic hydrocephalus, *Acta Paediatr* 86:995-998, 1997.
81. Hansen AR, Lapp C, Brugnara C: Plasminogen activator inhibitor-1: Defining characteristics in the cerebrospinal fluid of newborns, *J Pediatr* 137:132-134, 2000.
82. Larroche JC: Post-haemorrhagic hydrocephalus in infancy: Anatomical study, *Biol Neonate* 20:287-299, 1972.
83. Fukumizu M, Takashima S, Becker LE: Neonatal posthemorrhagic hydrocephalus: Neuropathologic and immunohistochemical studies, *Pediatr Neurol* 13:230-234, 1995.

84. Fukumizu M, Takashima S, Becker LE: Glial reaction in periventricular areas of the brainstem in fetal and neonatal posthemorraghic hydrocephalus and congenital hydrocephalus, *Brain Dev* 18:40-45, 1996.

85. Whitelaw A, Christie S, Pople I: Transforming growth factor-b1: A possible signal molecule for posthemorrhagic hydrocephalus? *Pediatr Res* 46:576-580, 1999.

86. Heep A, Stoffel-Wagner B, Soditt V, Aring C, et al: Procollagen IC-propeptide in the cerebrospinal fluid of neonates with posthaemorrhagic hydrocephalus, *Arch Dis Child Fetal Neonatal Ed* 87:F34-F36, 2002.

87. Whitelaw A, Thoresen M, Pople I: Posthaemorrhagic ventricular dilatation, *Arch Dis Child Fetal Neonatal Ed* 86:F72-F74, 2002.

88. Whitelaw A, Cherian S, Thoresen M, Pople I: Posthaemorrhagic ventricular dilatation: New mechanisms and new treatment, *Acta Paediatr* 93:11-14, 2004.

89. Skullerud K, Westre B: Frequency and prognostic significance of germinal matrix hemorrhage, periventricular leukomalacia, and pontosubicular necrosis in preterm neonates, *Acta Neuropathol (Berl)* 70:257-261, 1986.

90. Armstrong D, Norman MG: Periventricular leucomalacia in neonates: Complications and sequelae, *Arch Dis Child* 49:367-375, 1974.

91. Torvik A, Skullerud K, Andersen SN, Hurum J, et al: Affection of the hippocampal granule cells in pontosubicular neuron necrosis, *Acta Neuropathol (Berl)* 83:535-537, 1992.

92. Bruck Y, Bruck W, Kretzschmar HA, Lassmann H: Evidence for neuronal apoptosis in pontosubicular neuron necrosis, *Neuropathol Appl Neurobiol* 22:23-29, 1996.

93. Ahdab-Barmada M, Moossy J, Painter M: Pontosubicular necrosis and hyperoxemia, *Pediatrics* 66:840-847, 1980.

94. Soul JS, Limperopoulos C, Bassan H, Zientara G, et al: Reduced gray matter volume in preterm infants with complicated intraventricular hemorrhage measured by three-dimensional magnetic resonance imaging at term, *Ann Neurol* 52:5133-5134, 2002.

95. Perlman JM, McMenamin JB, Volpe JJ: Fluctuating cerebral blood-flow velocity in respiratory-distress syndrome: Relation to the development of intraventricular hemorrhage, *N Engl J Med* 309:204-209, 1983.

96. van Bel F, Van de Bor M, Stijnen T, Baan J, et al: Aetiological role of cerebral blood-flow alterations in development and extension of periintraventricular haemorrhage, *Dev Med Child Neurol* 29:601-614, 1987.

97. Miall-Allen VM, de Vries LS, Dubowitz LM, Whitelaw AG: Blood pressure fluctuation and intraventricular hemorrhage in the preterm infant of less than 31 weeks' gestation, *Pediatrics* 83:657-661, 1989.

98. Kuban KC, Skouteli H, Cherer A, Brown E, et al: Hemorrhage, phenobarbital, and fluctuating cerebral blood flow velocity in the neonate, *Pediatrics* 82:548-553, 1988.

99. Perlman J, Thach B: Respiratory origin of fluctuations in arterial blood pressure in premature infants with respiratory distress syndrome, *Pediatrics* 81:399-403, 1988.

100. Volpe JJ: *Neurology of the Newborn*, 2nd ed, Philadelphia: 1987, Saunders.

101. Jenni OG, Bucher HU, Vonsiebenthal K, Wolf M, et al: Cyclical variations in cerebral blood volume during periodic breathing, *Acta Paediatr* 83:1095-1096, 1994.

102. Mullaart RA, Hopman JC, Rotteveel JJ, Daniels O, et al: Cerebral bood flow fluctuation in neonatal respiratory distress and periventricular haemorrhage, *Early Hum Dev* 37:179-185, 1994.

103. Coughtrey H, Rennie JM, Evans DH: Variability in cerebral blood flow velocity: Observations over one minute in preterm babies, *Early Hum Dev* 47:63-70, 1997.

104. Rennie JM: Cerebral blood flow velocity variability after cardiovascular support in premature babies, *Arch Dis Child* 64:897-901, 1989.

105. Coughtrey H, Rennie JM, Evans DH, Cole TJ: Factors associated with respiration induced variability in cerebral blood flow velocity, *Arch Dis Child* 68:312-316, 1993.

106. Mullaart RA, Hopman JCW, Dehaan AFJ, Rotteveel JJ, et al: Cerebral blood flow fluctuation in low-risk preterm newborns, *Early Hum Dev* 30:41-48, 1992.

107. Goldberg RN, Chung D, Goldman SL, Bancalari E: The association of rapid volume expansion and intraventricular hemorrhage in the preterm infant, *J Pediatr* 96:1060-1063, 1980.

108. Hill A, Perlman JM, Volpe JJ: Relationship of pneumothorax to occurrence of intraventricular hemorrhage in the premature newborn, *Pediatrics* 69:144-149, 1982.

109. Marshall TA, Marshall F 2nd, Reddy PP: Physiologic changes associated with ligation of the ductus arteriosus in preterm infants, *J Pediatr* 101:749-753, 1982.

110. Milligan DW: Failure of autoregulation and intraventricular haemorrhage in preterm infants, *Lancet* 1:896-898, 1980.

111. Funato M, Tamai H, Noma K, Kurita T, et al: Clinical events in association with timing of intraventricular hemorrhage in preterm infants, *J Pediatr* 121:614-619, 1992.

112. Gronlund JU, Kero P, Korvenranta H, Aarimaa T, et al: Cerebral circulation assessed by transcephalic electrical impedance during the first day of life: A potential predictor of outcome? *Early Hum Dev* 41:129-145, 1995.

113. Lou HC, Lassen NA, Friis-Hansen B: Impaired autoregulation of cerebral blood flow in the distressed newborn infant, *J Pediatr* 94:118-121, 1979.

114. Pryds O, Greisen G, Lou H, Friis-Hansen B: Heterogeneity of cerebral vasoreactivity in preterm infants supported by mechanical ventilation, *J Pediatr* 115:638-645, 1989.

115. Pryds O: Control of cerebral circulation in the high-risk neonate, *Ann Neurol* 30:321-329, 1991.

116. Pryds O, Edwards AD: Cerebral blood flow in the newborn infant, *Arch Dis Child Fetal Neonatal Ed* 74:F63-F69, 1996.

117. Soul JS, Hammer PE, Tsuji M, Saul P, et al: Fluctuating pressure-passivity is common in the cerebral circulation of sick premature infants, *Pediatr Res* 61:467-473, 2007.

118. Menke J, Michel E, Hillebrand S, Von Twickel J, et al: Cross-spectral analysis of cerebral autoregulation dynamics in high risk preterm infants during the perinatal period, *Pediatr Res* 42:690-699, 1997.

119. Muller AM, Morales C, Briner J, Baenziger O, et al: Loss of CO_2 reactivity of cerebral blood flow is associated with severe brain damage in mechanically ventilated very low birth weight infants, *Eur J Paediatr Neurol* 5:157-163, 1997.

120. Boylan GB, Young K, Panerai RB, Rennie JM, et al: Dynamic cerebral autoregulation in sick newborn infants, *Pediatr Res* 48:12-17, 2000.

121. von Siebenthal K, Beran J, Wolf M, Keel M, et al: Cyclical fluctuations in blood pressure, heart rate and cerebral blood volume in preterm infants, *Brain Dev* 21:529-534, 1999.

122. Tsuji M, Saul JP, du Plessis A, Eichenwald E, et al: Cerebral intravascular oxygenation correlates with mean arterial pressure in critically ill premature infants, *Pediatrics* 106:625-632, 2000.

123. Perry EH, Bada HS, Ray JD, Korones SB, et al: Blood pressure increases, birth weight-dependent stability boundary, and intraventricular hemorrhage, *Pediatrics* 85:727-732, 1990.

124. Bada HS, Korones SB, Perry EH, Arheart KL, et al: Mean arterial blood pressure changes in premature infants and those at risk for intraventricular hemorrhage, *J Pediatr* 117:607-614, 1990.

125. Chemtob S, Li DY, Abran D, Hardy P, et al: The role of prostaglandin receptors in regulating cerebral blood flow in the perinatal period, *Acta Paediatr* 85:517-524, 1996.

126. Haggendal E, Johansson B: Effects of arterial carbon dioxide tension and oxygen saturation on cerebral blood flow autoregulation in dogs, *Acta Physiol Scand Suppl* 258:27-53, 1965.

127. Laptook A, Stonestreet BS, Oh W: Autoregulation of brain blood flow in the newborn piglet: Regional differences in flow reduction during hypotension, *Early Hum Dev* 6:99-107, 1982.

128. Papile LA, Rudolph AM, Heymann MA: Autoregulation of cerebral blood flow in the preterm fetal lamb, *Pediatr Res* 19:159-161, 1985.

129. Pasternak JF, Groothuis DR: Autoregulation of cerebral blood flow in the newborn beagle puppy, *Biol Neonate* 48:100-109, 1985.

130. Tweed A, Cote J, Lou H, Gregory G, et al: Impairment of cerebral blood flow autoregulation in the newborn lamb by hypoxia, *Pediatr Res* 20:516-519, 1986.

131. Tweed WA, Cote J, Pash M, Lou H: Arterial oxygenation determines autoregulation of cerebral blood flow in the fetal lamb, *Pediatr Res* 17:246-249, 1983.

132. Young RS, Hernandez MJ, Yagel SK: Selective reduction of blood flow to white matter during hypotension in newborn dogs: A possible mechanism of periventricular leukomalacia, *Ann Neurol* 12:445-448, 1982.

133. Goldberg RN: Sustained arterial blood pressure elevation associated with pneumothoraces: Early detection via continuous monitoring, *Pediatrics* 68:775-777, 1981.

134. Isenberg S, Everett S: Cardiovascular effects of mydriatics in low-birth-weight infants, *J Pediatr* 105:111-112, 1984.

135. Lees BJ, Cabal LA: Increased blood pressure following pupillary dilation with 2.5% phenylephrine hydrochloride in preterm infants, *Pediatrics* 68:231-234, 1981.

136. Lou HC, Lassen NA, Friis-Hansen B: Is arterial hypertension crucial for the development of cerebral haemorrhage in premature infants? *Lancet* 1:1215-1217, 1979.

137. Lou HC, Friis-Hansen B: Arterial blood pressure elevations during motor activity and epileptic seizures in the newborn, *Acta Paediatr Scand* 68:803-806, 1979.

138. Moscoso P, Goldberg RN, Jamieson J, Bancalari E: Spontaneous elevation in arterial blood pressure during the first hours of life in the very-low-birth-weight infant, *J Pediatr* 103:114-117, 1983.

139. Omar SY, Greisen G, Ibrahim MM, Youssef AM, et al: Blood pressure responses to care procedures in ventilated preterm infants, *Acta Paediatr Scand* 74:920-924, 1985.

140. Perlman JM, Volpe JJ: Suctioning in the preterm infant: Effects on cerebral blood flow velocity, intracranial pressure, and arterial blood pressure, *Pediatrics* 72:329-334, 1983.

141. Perlman JM, Volpe JJ: Seizures in the preterm infant: Effects on cerebral blood flow velocity, intracranial pressure, and arterial blood pressure, *J Pediatr* 102:288-293, 1983.

142. Sinkin RA, Phillips BL, Adelman RD: Elevation in systemic blood pressure in the neonate during abdominal examination, *Pediatrics* 76:970-972, 1985.

143. Wimberley PD, Lou HC, Pedersen H, Hejl M, et al: Hypertensive peaks in the pathogenesis of intraventricular hemorrhage in the newborn: Abolition by phenobarbitone sedation, *Acta Paediatr Scand* 71:537-542, 1982.

144. Cooke R, Rolfe P, Howat P: Apparent cerebral blood-flow in newborns with respiratory disease, *Dev Med Child Neurol* 21:154-159, 1979.

145. Adams MA, Pasternak JF, Kupfer BM, Gardner TH: A computerized system for continuous physiologic data collection and analysis: Initial report on mean arterial blood pressure in very low-birth-weight infants, *Pediatrics* 71:23-30, 1983.

146. Milligan DW: Cerebral blood flow and sleep state in the normal newborn infant, *Early Hum Dev* 3:321-328, 1979.

147. Rahilly PM: Effects of sleep state and feeding on cranial blood flow of the human neonate, *Arch Dis Child* 55:265-270, 1980.

148. Mukhtar AI, Cowan FM, Stothers JK: Cranial blood flow and blood pressure changes during sleep in the human neonate, *Early Hum Dev* 6:59-64, 1982.

149. Sonesson SE, Lundell BP, Herin P: Changes in intracranial arterial blood flow velocities during surgical ligation of the patent ductus arteriosus, *Acta Paediatr Scand* 75:36-42, 1986.

150. van Ravenswaaij-Arts CM, Hopman JC, Kollée LA: Influence of behavioural state on blood pressure in preterm infants during the first 5 days of life, *Acta Paediatr Scand* 78:358-363, 1989.

151. Blair E, Stanley F: Intrauterine growth and spastic cerebral palsy. I. Association with birth weight for gestational age, *Am J Obstet Gynecol* 162:229-237, 1990.

152. Porter FL, Miller JP, Cole FS, Marshall RE: A controlled clinical trial of local anesthesia for lumbar punctures in newborns, *Pediatrics* 88:663-669, 1991.

153. Hellström-Westas L, Rosen I, Svenningsen NW: Cerebral function monitoring during the first week of life in extremely small low birthweight (ESLBW) infants, *Neuropediatrics* 22:27-32, 1991.

154. Shah AR, Kurth CD, Gwiazdowski SG, Chance B, et al: Fluctuations in cerebral oxygenation and blood volume during endotracheal suctioning in premature infants, *J Pediatr* 120:769-774, 1992.

155. Craig KD, Whitfield MF, Grunau RVE, Linton J, et al: Pain in the preterm neonate: Behavioural and physiological indices, *Pain* 52:287-299, 1993.

156. Porter FL, Wolf CM, Miller JP: The effect of handling and immobilization on the response to acute pain in newborn infants, *Pediatrics* 102:1383-1389, 1998.

157. Anand KJS, McIntosh N, Lagercrantz H, Pelausa E, et al: Analgesia and sedation in preterm neonates who require ventilatory support: Results from the NOPAIN trial, *Arch Pediatr Adolesc Med* 153:331-338, 1999.

158. Greenough A, Cheeseman P, Kavvadia V, Dimitrion G, et al: Colloid infusion in the perinatal period and abnormal neurodevelopmental outcome in very low birth weight infants, *Eur J Pediatr* 161:319-323, 2002.

159. Kaiser JR, Gauss CH, Williams DK: The effects of hypercapnia on cerebral autoregulation in ventilated very low birth weight infants, *Pediatr Res* 58:931-935, 2005.

160. Dykes FD, Lazzara A, Ahmann P, Blumenstein B, et al: Intraventricular hemorrhage: A prospective evaluation of etiopathogenesis, *Pediatrics* 66:42-49, 1980.

161. Hill A, Volpe JJ: Normal pressure hydrocephalus in the newborn, *Pediatrics* 68:623-629, 1981.

162. Batton DG, Hellmann J, Nardis EE: Effect of pneumothorax-induced systemic blood pressure alterations on the cerebral circulation in newborn dogs, *Pediatrics* 74:350-353, 1984.

163. Kuban K, Volpe JJ: Intraventricular hemorrhage: An update, *J Intensive Care Med* 8:157-176, 1993.

164. Kuban KC, Leviton A, Krishnamoorthy KS, Brown ER, et al: Neonatal intracranial hemorrhage and phenobarbital, *Pediatrics* 77:443-450, 1986.

165. Wallin LA, Rosenfeld CR, Laptook AR, Maravilla AM, et al: Neonatal intracranial hemorrhage. II. Risk factor analysis in an inborn population, *Early Hum Dev* 23:129-137, 1990.

166. Goddard-Finegold J, Michael LH: Cerebral blood flow and experimental intraventricular hemorrhage, *Pediatr Res* 18:7-11, 1984.

167. Goddard J, Lewis RM, Armstrong DL, Zeller RS: Moderate, rapidly induced hypertension as a cause of intraventricular hemorrhage in the newborn beagle model, *J Pediatr* 96:1057-1060, 1980.

168. Goddard-Finegold J, Armstrong D, Zeller RS: Intraventricular hemorrhage following volume expansion after hypovolemic hypotension in the newborn beagle, *J Pediatr* 100:796-799, 1982.

169. Ment LR, Stewart WB, Duncan CC: Beagle puppy model of intraventricular hemorrhage: Ethamsylate studies, *Prostaglandins* 27:245-256, 1984.

170. Pasternak JF, Groothuis DR, Fischer JM, Fischer DP: Regional cerebral blood flow in the newborn beagle pup: The germinal matrix is a "low-flow" structure, *Pediatr Res* 16:499-503, 1982.

171. Pasternak JF, Groothuis DR, Fischer JM, Fischer DP: Regional cerebral blood flow in the beagle puppy model of neonatal intraventricular hemorrhage: Studies during systemic hypertension, *Neurology* 33:559-566, 1983.

172. Pasternak JF, Groothuis DR: Regional variability of blood flow and glucose utilization within the subependymal germinal matrix, *Brain Res* 299:281-288, 1984.

173. Ment LR, Stewart WB, Petroff OA, Duncan CC: Thromboxane synthesis inhibitor in a beagle pup model of perinatal asphyxia, *Stroke* 20:809-814, 1989.

174. Goddard-Finegold J, Donley DK, Adham BI, Michael LH: Phenobarbital and cerebral blood flow during hypertension in the newborn beagle, *Pediatrics* 86:501-508, 1990.

175. Reynolds ML, Evans CA, Reynolds EO, Saunders NR, et al: Intracranial haemorrhage in the preterm sheep fetus, *Early Hum Dev* 3:163-186, 1979.

176. Goddard J, Lewis RM, Alcala H, Zeller RS: Intraventricular hemorrhage: An animal model, *Biol Neonate* 37:39-52, 1980.

177. Simmons MA, Adcock EW 3rd, Bard H, Battaglia FC: Hypernatremia and intracranial hemorrhage in neonates, *N Engl J Med* 291:6-10, 1974.

178. Papile LA, Burstein J, Burstein R, Koffler H, et al: Relationship of intravenous sodium bicarbonate infusions and cerebral intraventricular hemorrhage, *J Pediatr* 93:834-836, 1978.

179. Wigglesworth JS, Keith IH, Girling DJ, Slade SA: Hyaline membrane disease, alkali, and intraventricular haemorrhage, *Arch Dis Child* 51:755-762, 1976.

180. Roberton NR, Howat P: Hypernatraemia as a cause of intracranial haemorrhage, *Arch Dis Child* 50:938-942, 1975.

181. Anderson JM, Bain AD, Brown JK, Cockburn F, et al: Hyaline-membrane disease, alkaline buffer treatment, and cerebral intraventricular halphaemorrhage, *Lancet* 1:117-119, 1976.

182. Corbet AJ, Adams JM, Kenny JD, Kennedy J, et al: Controlled trial of bicarbonate therapy in high-risk premature newborn infants, *J Pediatr* 91:771-776, 1977.

183. Murton LJ, Butt WW, Mackay JR: Perinatal factors, periventricular hemorrhage and mortality in very low birthweight infants, *Aust Pediatr J* 21:39-43, 1985.

184. van de, Bor M, Verloove-Vanhorick SP, Brand R: Incidence and prediction of periventricular-intraventricular hemorrhage in very preterm infants, *J Perinat Med* 15:333-339, 1987.

185. Skouteli H, Kuban KC, Leviton A: Arterial blood gas derangements associated with death and intracranial hemorrhage in premature babies, *J Perinatol* 8:336-341, 1988.

186. Pagano M, Leviton A, Kuban K: Early and late germinal matrix hemorrhage may have different antecedents, *Eur J Obstet Gynecol Reprod Biol* 37:47-54, 1990.

187. Greisen G, Trojaborg W: Cerebral blood flow, $Paco_2$ changes, and visual evoked potentials in mechanically ventilated, preterm infants, *Acta Paediatr Scand* 76:394-400, 1987.

188. Pryds O, Greisen G, Friis-Hansen B: Compensatory increase of CBF in preterm infants during hypoglycaemia, *Acta Paediatr Scand* 77:632-637, 1988.

189. Pryds O, Greisen G, Skov LL, Friis-Hansen B: Carbon dioxide-related changes in cerebral blood volume and cerebral blood flow in mechanically ventilated preterm neonates: Comparison of near infrared spectrophotometry and ^{133}xenon clearance, *Pediatr Res* 27:445-449, 1990.

190. Wyatt JS, Edwards AD, Cope M, Delpy DT, et al: Response of cerebral blood volume to changes in arterial carbon dioxide tension in preterm and term infants, *Pediatr Res* 29:553-557, 1991.

191. Levene MI, Fawer CL, Lamont RF: Risk factors in the development of intraventricular haemorrhage in the preterm neonate, *Arch Dis Child* 57:410-417, 1982.

192. van de Bor M, Van Bel F, Lineman R, Ruys JH: Perinatal factors and periventricular-intraventricular hemorrhage in preterm infants, *Am J Dis Child* 140:1125-1130, 1986.

193. Luyt K, Baumer JH, Dunn PM: Hypercarbia during the first 3 days of life is associated with intraventricular haemorrhage, *Pediatr Res* 58:582, 2006.

194. Fabres J, Carlo WA, Phillips V, Howard G, et al: Both extremes of arterial carbon dioxide pressure and the magnitude of fluctuations in arterial carbon dioxide pressure are associated with severe intraventricular hemorrhage in preterm infants, *Pediatrics* 119:299-305, 2007.

195. Szymonowicz W, Yu VY, Wilson FE: Antecedents of periventricular haemorrhage in infants weighing 1250 g or less at birth, *Arch Dis Child* 59:13-17, 1984.

196. Mariani G, Cifuentes J, Carlo WA: Randomized trial of permissive hypercapnia in preterm infants, *Pediatrics* 104:1082-1088, 1999.

197. Bassan H, Feldman HA, Limperopoulos C, Benson CB, et al: Periventricular hemorrhagic infarction: Risk factors and neonatal outcome, *Pediatr Neurol* 35:85-92, 2006.

198. Pryds O, Greisen G: Effect of $Paco_2$ and haemoglobin concentration on day to day variation of CBF in preterm neonates, *Acta Paediatr Scand Suppl* 360:33-36, 1989.

199. Lipp-Zwahlen AE, Müller A, Tuchschmid P, Duc G: Oxygen affinity of haemoglobin modulates cerebral blood flow in premature infants: A study with the non-invasive xenon-133 method, *Acta Paediatr Scand Suppl* 360:26-32, 1989.

200. Ramaekers VT, Casaer P, Marchal G, Smet M, et al: The effect of blood transfusion on cerebral blood-flow in preterm infants: A Doppler study, *Dev Med Child Neurol* 30:334-341, 1988.

201. Younkin DP, Reivich M, Jaggi JL, Obrist WD, et al: The effect of hematocrit and systolic blood pressure on cerebral blood flow in newborn infants, *J Cereb Blood Flow Metab* 7:295-299, 1987.

202. Alkalay AL, Galvis S, Ferry DA, Simmons CF, et al: Hemodynamic changes in anemic premature infants: Are we allowing the hematocrits to fall too low? *Pediatrics* 112:838-845, 2003.

203. Pryds O, Christensen NJ, Friis HB: Increased cerebral blood flow and plasma epinephrine in hypoglycemic, preterm neonates, *Pediatrics* 85:172-176, 1990.

204. Svenningsen L, Lindemann R, Eidal K: Measurements of fetal head compression pressure during bearing down and their relationship to the condition of the newborn, *Acta Obstet Gynecol Scand* 67:129-133, 1988.

205. Leviton A, Pagano M, Kuban KC: Etiologic heterogeneity of intracranial hemorrhages in preterm newborns, *Pediatr Neurol* 4:274-278, 1988.

206. Shankaran S, Bauer CR, Bain R, Wright LL, et al: Prenatal and perinatal risk and protective factors for neonatal intracranial hemorrhage, *Arch Pediatr Adolesc Med* 150:491-497, 1996.

207. Newton TH, Gooding CA: Compression of superior sagittal sinus by neonatal calvarial molding, *Radiology* 115:635-640, 1975.

208. Cowan F, Thoresen M: Changes in superior sagittal sinus blood velocities due to postural alterations and pressure on the head of the newborn infant, *Pediatrics* 75:1038-1047, 1985.

209. Pellicer A, Gaya F, Madero R, Quero J, et al: Noninvasive continuous monitoring of the effects of head position on brain hemodynamics in ventilated infants, *Pediatrics* 109:434-440, 2002.

210. Barrett JM, Boehm FH, Vaughn WK: The effect of type of delivery on neonatal outcome in singleton infants of birth weight of 1,000 g or less, *JAMA* 250:625-629, 1983.

211. Beverley DW, Chance GW, Inwood MJ, Schaus M, et al: Intraventricular haemorrhage and haemostasis defects, *Arch Dis Child* 59:444-448, 1984.

212. Horbar JD, Pasnick M, McAuliffe TL, Lucey JF: Obstetric events and risk of periventricular hemorrhage in premature infants, *Am J Dis Child* 137:678-681, 1983.

213. Kauppila O, Gronroos M, Aro P, Aittoniemi P, et al: Management of low birth weight breech delivery: Should cesarean section be routine? *Obstet Gynecol* 57:289-294, 1981.

214. Low JA, Galbraith RS, Sauerbrei EE, Muir DW, et al: Maternal, fetal, and newborn complications associated with newborn intracranial hemorrhage, *Am J Obstet Gynecol* 154:345-351, 1986.

215. Tejani N, Rebold B, Tuck S, Ditroia D, et al: Obstetric factors in the causation of early periventricular-intraventricular hemorrhage, *Obstet Gynecol* 64:510-515, 1984.

216. Welch RA, Bottoms SF: Reconsideration of head compression and intraventricular hemorrhage in the vertex very-low-birth-weight fetus, *Obstet Gynecol* 68:29-34, 1986.

217. Meidell R, Marinelli P, Pettett G: Perinatal factors associated with early-onset intracranial hemorrhage in premature infants: A prospective study, *Am J Dis Child* 139:160-163, 1985.

218. Bada HS, Korones SB, Anderson GD, Magill HL, et al: Obstetric factors and relative risk of neonatal germinal layer/intraventricular hemorrhage, *Am J Obstet Gynecol* 148:798-804, 1984.

219. Tejani N, Verma U, Hameed C, Chayen B: Method and route of delivery in the low birth weight vertex presentation correlated with early periventricular/intraventricular hemorrhage, *Obstet Gynecol* 69:1-4, 1987.

220. Tejani N, Verma U, Shiffman R, Chayen B: Effect of route of delivery on periventricular/intraventricular hemorrhage in the low birth weight fetus with a breech presentation, *J Reprod Med* 32:911-914, 1987.

221. Hansen A, Leviton A: Labor and delivery characteristics and risks of cranial ultrasonographic abnormalities among very-low-birth-weight infants, *Am J Obstet Gynecol* 181:997-1006, 1999.

222. Wadhawan R, Vohr BR, Fanaroff AA, Perritt RL, et al: Does labor influence neonatal and neurodevelopmental outcomes of extremely-low-birth-weight infants who are born by cesarean delivery? *Am J Obstet Gynecol* 189:501-506, 2003.

223. Synnes AR, Chien L-Y, Peliowski A, Baboolal R, et al: Variations in intraventricular hemorrhage incidence rates among Canadian neonatal intensive care units, *J Pediatr* 138:525-531, 2001.

224. Osborn DA, Evans N, Kluckow M: Hemodynamic and antecedent risk factors of early and late periventricular/intraventricular hemorrhage in premature infants, *Pediatrics* 112:33-39, 2003.

225. O'Shea M, Savitz DA, Hage ML, Feinstein KA: Prenatal events and the risk of subependymal/intraventricular haemorrhage in very low birth-weight neonates, *Paediatr Perinat Epidemiol* 6:352-362, 1992.

226. Bucciarelli RL, Nelson RM, Egan EA, Eitzman DV, et al: Transient tricuspid insufficiency of the newborn: A form of myocardial dysfunction in stressed newborns, *Pediatrics* 59:330-337, 1977.

227. Cabal LA, Devaskar U, Siassi B, Hodgman JE, et al: Cardiogenic shock associated with perinatal asphyxia in preterm infants, *J Pediatr* 96:705-710, 1980.

228. DiSessa TG, Leitner M, Ti CC, Gluck L, et al: The cardiovascular effects of dopamine in the severely asphyxiated neonate, *J Pediatr* 99:772-776, 1981.

229. Donnelly WH, Bucciarelli RL, Nelson RM: Ischemic papillary muscle necrosis in stressed newborn infants, *J Pediatr* 96:295-300, 1980.

230. Finley JP, Howman-Giles RB, Gilday DL, Bloom KR, et al: Transient myocardial ischemia of the newborn infant demonstrated by thallium myocardial imaging, *J Pediatr* 94:263-270, 1979.

231. Lees MH: Perinatal asphyxia and the myocardium, *J Pediatr* 96:675-678, 1980.

232. Nelson RM, Bucciarelli RL, Eitzman DV, Egan EA 2nd, et al: Serum creatine phosphokinase MB fraction in newborns with transient tricuspid insufficiency, *N Engl J Med* 298:146-149, 1978.

233. Rowe RD, Hoffman T: Transient myocardial ischemia of the newborn infant: A form of severe cardiorespiratory distress in full-term infants, *J Pediatr* 81:243-250, 1972.

234. Setzer E, Ermocilla R, Tonkin I, John E, et al: Papillary muscle necrosis in a neonatal autopsy population: Incidence and associated clinical manifestations, *J Pediatr* 96:289-294, 1980.

235. Skinner JR, Milligan DWA, Hunter S, Hey EN: Central venous pressure in the ventilated neonate, *Arch Dis Child* 67:374-377, 1992.

236. Lavrijsen SW, Uiterwaal CSPM, Stigter RH, de Vries LS, et al: Severe umbilical cord acidemia and neurological outcome in preterm and full-term neonates, *Biol Neonate* 88:27-34, 2005.

237. Cowan F, Thoresen M: The effects of intermittent positive pressure ventilation on cerebral arterial and venous blood velocities in the newborn infant, *Acta Paediatr Scand* 76:239-247, 1987.

238. de Lemos RA, Tomasovic JJ: Effects of positive pressure ventilation on cerebral blood flow in the newborn infant, *Clin Perinatol* 5:395-409, 1978.

239. Leahy FA, Durand M, Cates D, Chernick V: Cranial blood volume changes during mechanical ventilation and spontaneous breathing in newborn infants, *J Pediatr* 101:984-987, 1982.

240. Milligan DW: Positive pressure ventilation and cranial volume in newborn infants, *Arch Dis Child* 56:331-335, 1981.

241. Perlman JM, Volpe JJ: Are venous circulatory abnormalities important in the pathogenesis of hemorrhagic and/or ischemic cerebral injury? *Pediatrics* 80:705-711, 1987.

242. Vert P, Nomin P, Sibout M: Intracranial venous pressure in newborns: Variation in physiologic state and in neurologic and respiratory disorders. In Stern L, Friis-Hansen B, Kildeberg P, editors: *Intensive Care in the Newborn*, New York: 1976, Masson.

243. Bucher HU, Vonsiebenthal K, Duc G: Increased cerebral blood volume associated with pneumothorax in preterm infant, *Lancet* 341:1599-1600, 1993.

244. Vert P, Andre M, Sibout M: Continuous positive airway pressure and hydrocephalus, *Lancet* 2:319, 1973.

245. Monin P, Crance JP, Bougie D: Hemodynamics and ventilatory effects of tension on pneumothorax in rabbits. In Stern L, Oh W, Friis-Hansen B, editors: *Intensive Care of the Newborn* vol 2, New York: 1978, Masson.

246. Simmons DH, Hemingway A, Ricchiuti N: Acute circulatory effects of pneumothorax in dogs, *J Appl Physiol* 12:255, 1958.

247. Leviton A, Pagano M, Kuban KC, Krishnamoorthy KS, et al: The epidemiology of germinal matrix hemorrhage during the first half-day of life, *Dev Med Child Neurol* 33:138-145, 1991.

248. Tejani N, Verma UL: Correlation of Apgar scores and umbilical artery acid-base status to mortality and morbidity in the low birth weight neonate, *Obstet Gynecol* 73:597-600, 1989.

249. Heuchan AM, Evans N, Smart DJH, Simpson JM: Perinatal risk factors for major intraventricular haemorrhage in the Australian and New Zealand Neonatal Network, 1995–97, *Arch Dis Child Fetal Neonatal Ed* 86:F86-F90, 2002.

250. Gazzolo D, Marinoni E, Giovannini LG, Letizia C, et al: Circulating adrenomedullin is increased in preterm newborns developing intraventricular hemorrhage, *Pediatr Res* 50:544-547, 2001.

251. Amato M, Gambon R, Howald H, von Muralt G: Correlation of raised cord-blood CK-BB and the development of peri-intraventricular hemorrhage in preterm infants, *Neuropediatrics* 17:173-174, 1986.

252. van de Bor M, Janssen JW, Van Bel F, Ruys JH: Serum creatine kinase BB as predictor of periventricular haemorrhage in preterm infants, *Early Hum Dev* 17:165-174, 1988.

253. Perlman JM, Risser R: Relationship of uric acid concentrations and severe intraventricular hemorrhage/leukomalacia in the premature infant, *J Pediatr* 132:436-439, 1998.

254. Greisen G, Hellström-Westas L, Lou H, Rosen I, et al: EEG depression and germinal layer haemorrhage in the newborn, *Acta Paediatr Scand* 76:519-525, 1987.

255. Connell J, de Vries L, Oozeer R, Regev R, et al: Predictive value of early continuous electroencephalogram monitoring in ventilated preterm infants with intraventricular hemorrhage, *Pediatrics* 82:337-343, 1988.

256. Harris AP, Helou S, Traystman RJ, Jones MD, et al: Efficacy of the Cushing response in maintaining cerebral blood flow in premature and near-term fetal sheep, *Pediatr Res* 43:50-56, 1998.

257. Kluckow M, Evans N: Low superior vena cava flow and intraventricular haemorrhage in preterm infants, *Arch Dis Child Fetal Neonatal Ed* 82:F188-194, 2000.

258. Evans N, Kluckow M, Simmons M, Osborn D: Which to measure, systemic or organ blood flow? Middle cerebral artery and superior vena cava flow in very preterm infants, *Arch Dis Child* 87:181-184, 2002.

259. Kissack CM, Garr R, Wardle SP, Weindling AM: Postnatal changes in cerebral oxygen extraction in the preterm infant are associated with intraventricular hemorrhage and hemorrhagic parenchymal infarction but not periventricular leukomalacia, *Pediatr Res* 56:111-116, 2004.

259a. Osborn DA, Evans N, Kluckow M, Bowen JR, et al: Low superior vena cava flow and effect of inotropes on neurodevelopment to 3 years in preterm infants, *Pediatrics* 120:372-380, 2007.

260. Finer NN, Horbar JD, Carpenter JH: Cardiopulmonary resuscitation in the very low birth weight infant: The Vermont Oxford Network Experience, *Pediatrics* 104:428-434, 1999.

261. Miall-Allen VM, de Vries LS, Whitelaw AG: Mean arterial blood pressure and neonatal cerebral lesions, *Arch Dis Child* 62:1068-1069, 1987.

262. Watkins AM, West CR, Cooke RW: Blood pressure and cerebral hae-morrhage and ischaemia in very low birthweight infants, *Early Hum Dev* 19:103-110, 1989.

263. Bada HS, Korones SB, Perry EH, Arheart KL, et al: Frequent handling in the neonatal intensive care unit and intraventricular hemorrhage, *J Pediatr* 117:126-131, 1990.

264. Ramaekers VT, Casaer P, Daniels H: Cerebral hyperperfusion following episodes of bradycardia in the preterm infant, *Early Hum Dev* 34:199-208, 1993.

265. Meek JH, Tyszczuk L, Elwell CE, Wyatt JS: Low cerebral blood flow is a risk factor for severe intraventricular haemorrhage, *Arch Dis Child Fetal Neonatal Ed* 81:F15-F18, 1999.

266. Evans N, Kluckow M: Early ductal shunting and intraventricular hae-morrhage in ventilated preterm infants, *Arch Dis Child Fetal Neonatal Ed* 75:F183-F186, 1996.

267. Mercer JS, Vohr BR, McGrath MM, Padbury JF, et al: Delayed cord clamping in very preterm infants reduces the incidence of intraventric-ular hemorrhage and late-onset sepsis: A randomized, controlled trial, *Pediatrics* 117:1235-1242, 2006.

267a. Baenziger O, Stolkin F, Keel M, von Siebenthal K, et al: The influence of the timing of cord clamping on postnatal cerebral oxygenation in preterm neonates: A randomized, controlled trial, *Pediatrics* 119:455-459, 2007.

268. Heep A, Behrendt D, Nitsch P, Fimmers R, et al: Increased serum levels of interleukin 6 are associated with severe intraventricular haemorrhage in extremely premature infants, *Arch Dis Child Fetal Neonatal Ed* 88:F501-F504, 2003.

269. Weeks JW, Reynolds L, Taylor D, Lewis J, et al: Umbilical cord blood interleukin-6 levels and neonatal morbidity, *Obstet Gynecol* 90:815-818, 1997.

270. Yanowitz TD, Jordan JA, Gilmour CH, Towbin R, et al: Hemodynamic disturbances in premature infants born after chorioamnionitis: Association with cord blood cytokine concentrations, *Pediatr Res* 51:310-316, 2002.

271. Tauscher MK, Berg D, Brockmann M, Seidenspinner S, et al: Association of histologic chorioamnionitis, increased levels of cord blood cytokines, and intracerebral hemorrhage in preterm neonates, *Biol Neonate* 83:166-170, 2003.

272. Kassal R, Anwar M, Kashlan F, Smulian J, et al: Umbilical vein inter-leukin-6 levels in very low birth weight infants developing intraventric-ular hemorrhage, *Brain Dev* 27:483-487, 2005.

273. Hansen-Pupp I, Harling S, Berg AC, Cilio C, et al: Circulating inter-feron-gamma and white matter brain damage in preterm infants, *Pediatr Res* 58:946-952, 2005.

274. Krediet TG, Kavelaars A, Vreman HJ, Heijnen CJ, et al: Respiratory distress syndrome–associated inflammation is related to early but not late peri/intraventricular hemorrhage in preterm infants, *J Pediatr* 148:740-746, 2006.

275. Babnik J, Stucin-Gantar I, Kornhauser-Cerar L, Sinkovec J, et al: Intrauterine inflammation and the onset of peri-intraventricular hemor-rhage in premature infants, *Biol Neonate* 90:113-121, 2006.

276. Andrew M, Castle V, Saigal S, Carter C, et al: Clinical impact of neonatal thrombocytopenia, *J Pediatr* 110:457-464, 1987.

277. Amato M, Fauchere JC, Hermann U Jr: Coagulation abnormalities in low birth weight infants with peri-intraventricular hemorrhage, *Neuropediatrics* 19:154-157, 1988.

278. Lupton BA, Hill A, Whitfield MF, Carter CJ, et al: Reduced platelet count as a risk factor for intraventricular hemorrhage, *Am J Dis Child* 142:1222-1224, 1988.

279. Shirahata A, Nakamura T, Shimono M, Kaneko M, et al: Blood coagu-lation findings and the efficacy of factor XIII concentrate in premature infants with intracranial, *Thromb Res* 57:755-763, 1990.

280. Rennie JM, Doyle J, Cooke RW: Elevated levels of immunoreactive pros-tacyclin metabolite in babies who develop intraventricular haemorrhage, *Acta Paediatr Scand* 76:19-23, 1987.

281. Beverley DW, Pitts-Tucker TJ, Congdon PJ, Arthur RJ, et al: Prevention of intraventricular haemorrhage by fresh frozen plasma, *Arch Dis Child* 60:710-713, 1985.

282. McDonald MM, Johnson ML, Rumack CM, Koops BL, et al: Role of coagulopathy in newborn intracranial hemorrhage, *Pediatrics* 74:26-31, 1984.

283. Setzer ES, Webb IB, Wassenaar JW, Reeder JD, et al: Platelet dysfunc-tion and coagulopathy in intraventricular hemorrhage in the premature infant, *J Pediatr* 100:599-605, 1982.

284. van de Bor M, Briet E, Van Bel F, Ruys JH: Hemostasis and periventri-cular-intraventricular hemorrhage of the newborn, *Am J Dis Child* 140:1131-1134, 1986.

285. Northern Neonatal Nursing Initiative Trial Group: Randomised trial of prophylactic early fresh-frozen plasma or gelatin or glucose in preterm babies: Outcome at 2 years, *Lancet* 348:229-232, 1996.

286. Ramenghi LA, Gill BJ, Tanner SF, Martinez D, et al: Cerebral venous throm-bosis, intraventricular haemorrhage and white matter lesions in a preterm newborn with factor V (Leiden) mutation, *Neuropediatrics* 33:97-99, 2002.

287. Gopel W, Kattner E, Seidenberg J, Kohlmann t, et al: The effect of Val34Leu polymorphism in the factor XIII gene in infants with a birth weight below 1500 g, *J Pediatr* 140:688-692, 2002.

288. Petaja J, Hiltunen L, Fellman V: Increased risk of intraventricular hemorrhage in preterm infants with thrombophilia, *Pediatr Neurol* 49:643-646, 2001.

289. Gopel W, Gortner L, Kohlmann T, Schultz C, et al: Low prevalence of large intraventricular haemorrhage in very low birthweight infants carry-ing the factor V Leiden or prothrombin G20210A mutation, *Acta Paediatr* 90:1021-1024, 2001.

290. Fulia F, Cordaro S, Meo P, Gitto P, et al: Can the administration of an-tithrombin III decrease the risk of cerebral hemorrhage in premature infants? *Biol Neonate* 83:1-5, 2003.

291. Aronis S, Bouza H, Pergantou H, Kapsimalis Z, et al: Prothrombotic factors in neonates with cerebral thrombosis and intraventricular hemor-rhage, *Acta Paediatr* 91:87-91, 2002.

292. Northern Neonatal Nursing Initiative Trial Group: A randomized trial comparing the effect of prophylactic intravenous fresh frozen plasma, gelatin or glucose on early mortality and morbidity in preterm babies, *Eur J Pediatr* 155:580-588, 1996.

293. Rumack CM, Guggenheim MA, Rumack BH, Peterson RG, et al: Neonatal intracranial hemorrhage and maternal use of aspirin, *Obstet Gynecol* 58:52S-56S, 1981.

294. Stuart MJ, Gross SJ, Elrad H, Graeber JE: Effects of acetylsalicylic-acid ingestion on maternal and neonatal hemostasis, *N Engl J Med* 307:909-912, 1982.

295. Lesko SM, Mitchell AA, Epstein MF, Louik C, et al: Heparin use as a risk factor for intraventricular hemorrhage in low-birth-weight infants, *N Engl J Med* 314:1156-1160, 1986.

296. Malloy MH, Cutter GR: The association of heparin exposure with intra-ventricular hemorrhage among very low birth weight infants, *J Perinatol* 15:185-191, 1995.

297. Pinar MH, Edwards WH, Fratkin J: A transmission electron microscopy study of hyman cerebral cortical and germinal matrix (GM) blood vessels in premature neonate [abstract], *Pediatr Res* 19:394, 1985.

298. Kamei A, Houdou S, Mito T, Konomi H, et al: Developmental change in type VI collagen in human cerebral vessels, *Pediatr Neurol* 8:183-186, 1992.

299. Trommer BL, Groothuis DR, Pasternak JF: Quantitative analysis of cere-bral vessels in the newborn puppy: The structure of germinal matrix vessels may predispose to hemorrhage, *Pediatr Res* 22:23-28, 1987.

300. Ballabh P, Braun A, Nedergaard M: Anatomic analysis of blood vessels in germinal matrix, cerebral cortex, and white matter in developing infants, *Pediatr Res* 56:117-124, 2004.

301. Grunnet ML: Morphometry of blood vessels in the cortex and germinal plate of premature neonates, *Pediatr Neurol* 5:12-16, 1989.

302. Perlman JM, Riser RC, Gee JB: Pregnancy-induced hypertension and re-duced intraventricular hemorrhage in preterm infants, *Pediatr Neurol* 17:29-33, 1997.

303. Leviton A, Paneth N, Susser M, Reuss ML, et al: Maternal receipt of magnesium sulfate does not seem to reduce the risk of neonatal white matter damage, *Pediatrics* 99:1-5, 1997.

304. Hadi HA: Fetal cerebral maturation in hypertensive disorders of preg-nancy, *Obstet Gynecol* 63:214-219, 1984.

305. Gluck L, Kulovich MV: The evaluation of functional maturity. In Gluck L, editor: *Modern Prenatal Medicine*, Chicago: 1974, Year Book.

306. Amiel-Tison C, Pettigrew AG: Adaptive changes in the developing brain during intrauterine stress, *Brain Dev* 13:67-76, 1991.

307. Apak RA, Anlar B, Atilla P, Cakar N: Transient intrauterine hypotension: Effect on newborn rat brain, *Pediatr Res* 49:45-49, 2001.

308. Goldstein GW: Pathogenesis of brain edema and hemorrhage: Role of the brain capillary, *Pediatrics* 64:357-360, 1979.

309. Oldendorf WH, Cornford ME, Brown WJ: The large apparent work capa-bility of the blood-brain barrier: A study of the mitochondrial content of capillary endothelial cells in brain and other tissues of the rat, *Ann Neurol* 1:409-417, 1977.

310. Gould SJ, Howard S: An immunohistochemical study of the germinal layer in the late gestation human fetal brain, *Neuropathol Appl Neurobiol* 13:421-437, 1987.

311. El-Khoury N, Braun A, Hu F, Pandey M, et al: Astrocyte end-feet in germinal matrix, cerebral cortex, and white matter in developing infants, *Pediatr Res* 59:673-679, 2006.

312. Gilles FH, Price RA, Kevy SV, Berenberg W: Fibrinolytic activity in the ganglionic eminence of the premature human brain, *Biol Neonate* 18:426-432, 1971.

313. Takashima S, Tanaka K: Microangiography and fibrinolytic activity in subependymal matrix of the premature brain, *Brain Dev* 4:222-229, 1972.

314. Kalderon N, Williams CA: Extracellular proteolysis: Developmentally regulated activity during chick spinal cord histogenesis, *Brain Res* 390:1-9, 1986.

315. Kalderon N, Ahonen K, Juhasz A, Kirk JP, et al: Astroglia and plasmin-ogen activator activity: Differential activity level in the immature, mature and "reactive" astrocytes. In *Current Issues in Neural Regeneration*, New York: 1988, Alan R. Liss.

316. Coulter DM, LaPine TR, Gooch WM 3rd: Treatment to prevent postna-tal loss of brain water reduces the risk of intracranial hemorrhage in the beagle puppy, *Pediatr Res* 19:1322-1326, 1985.

317. Coulter DM, Gooch WM: Falling intracranial pressure: An important element in the genesis of intracranial hemorrhage in the beagle puppy, *Biol Neonate* 63:316-326, 1993.

318. de Courten GM, Rabinowicz T: Intraventricular hemorrhage in premature infants: Reappraisal and new hypothesis, *Dev Med Child Neurol* 23:389-403, 1981.

319. Donn SM, Philip AG: Early increase in intracranial pressure in preterm infants, *Pediatrics* 61:904-907, 1978.

320. Williams J, Hirsch NJ, Corbet AJ, Rudolph AJ: Postnatal head shrinkage in small infants, *Pediatrics* 59:619-622, 1977.

321. Heimler R, Doumas BT, Jendrzejczak BM, Nemeth PB, et al: Relationship between nutrition, weight change, and fluid compartments in preterm infants during the first week of life, *J Pediatr* 122:110-114, 1992.

322. Lupton BA, Roland EH, Whitfield MF, Hill A: Serum sodium concentration and intraventricular hemorrhage in premature infants, *Am J Dis Child* 144:1019-1021, 1990.

323. Tsiantos A, Victorin L, Relier JP, Dyer N, et al: Intracranial hemorrhage in the prematurely born infant: Timing of clots and evaluation of clinical signs and symptoms, *J Pediatr* 85:854-859, 1974.

324. Amiel C: Intraventricular haemorrhages in the premature infant. II. Clinical diagnosis, *Biol Neonate* 7:57, 1964.

325. Krishnamoorthy KS, Fernandez RA, Momose KJ, DeLong GR, et al: Evaluation of neonatal intracranial hemorrhage by computerized tomography, *Pediatrics* 59:165-172, 1977.

326. Lazzara A, Ahmann P, Dykes F, Brann AW Jr, et al: Clinical predictability of intraventricular hemorrhage in preterm infants, *Pediatrics* 65:30-34, 1980.

327. Dubowitz LM, Levene MI, Morante A, Palmer P, et al: Neurologic signs in neonatal intraventricular hemorrhage: A correlation with real-time ultrasound, *J Pediatr* 99:127-133, 1981.

328. Adams JM, Kenny JD, Rudolph AJ: Central diabetes insipidus following intraventricular hemorrhage, *J Pediatr* 88:292-294, 1976.

329. Cepeda EE, Heilbronner DM, Poland RL: Glucose intolerance in premature infants with massive intracranial hemorrhage (ICH), *Pediatr Res* 12:521-528, 1978.

330. Furzan JA, Rosenfeld CR, Nyson JE: Inappropriate ADH syndrome (IADH) and persistent metabolic acidosis (PMA) in neonatal periventricular hemorrhage (PVH), *Pediatr Res* 12:552, 1978.

331. Moylan FM, Herrin JT, Krishnamoorthy K, Todres ID, et al: Inappropriate antidiuretic hormone secretion in premature infants with cerebral injury, *Am J Dis Child* 132:399-402, 1978.

332. Volpe JJ: Neonatal periventricular hemorrhage: Past, present, and future [editorial], *J Pediatr* 92:693-696, 1978.

333. Volpe JJ: Intracranial hemorrhage in the newborn: Current understanding and dilemmas, *Neurology* 29:632-635, 1979.

334. Mantovani JF, Pasternak JF, Mathew OP, Allan WC, et al: Failure of daily lumbar punctures to prevent the development of hydrocephalus following intraventricular hemorrhage, *J Pediatr* 97:278-281, 1980.

335. Bejar R, Curbelo V, Coen R: Incidence of intraventricular and germinal layer hemorrhage (IVH/GLH) in preterm infants born per vagina and caesarean section, *Pediatr Res* 14:629-630, 1980.

336. Johnson ML, Mack LA, Rumack CM, Frost M, et al: B-mode echoencephalography in the normal and high risk infant, *AJR Am J Roentgenol* 133:375-381, 1979.

337. Pape KE, Blackwell RJ, Cusick G, Sherwood A, et al: Ultrasound detection of brain damage in preterm infants, *Lancet* 1:1261-1264, 1979.

338. Babcock DS, Han BK, LeQuesne GW: B-mode gray scale ultrasound of the head in the newborn and young infant, *AJR Am J Roentgenol* 134:457-468, 1980.

339. Allan WC, Roveto CA, Sawyer LR, Courtney SE: Sector scan ultrasound imaging through the anterior fontanelle: Its use in diagnosing neonatal periventricular-intraventricular hemorrhage, *Am J Dis Child* 134:1028-1031, 1980.

340. London DA, Carroll BA, Enzmann DR: Sonography of ventricular size and germinal matrix hemorrhage in premature infants, *AJR Am J Roentgenol* 135:559-564, 1980.

341. Silverboard G, Horder MH, Ahmann PA, Lazzara A, et al: Reliability of ultrasound in diagnosis of intracerebral hemorrhage and posthemorrhagic hydrocephalus: Comparison with computed tomography, *Pediatrics* 66:507-514, 1980.

342. Babcock DS, Han BK: The accuracy of high resolution, real-time ultrasonography of the head in infancy, *Radiology* 139:665-676, 1981.

343. Donn SM, Roloff DW, Goldstein GW: Prevention of intraventricular haemorrhage in preterm infants by phenobarbitone: A controlled trial, *Lancet* 2:215-217, 1981.

344. Fleischer AC, Hutchison AA, Allen JH, Stahlman MT, et al: The role of sonography and the radiologist-ultrasonologist in the detection and follow-up of intracranial hemorrhage in the preterm neonate, *Radiology* 139:733-736, 1981.

345. Grant EG, Borts FT, Schellinger D, McCullough DC, et al: Real-time ultrasonography of neonatal intraventricular hemorrhage and comparison with computed tomography, *Radiology* 139:687-691, 1981.

346. Mack LA, Wright K, Hirsch JH, Alvord EC, et al: Intracranial hemorrhage in premature infants: Accuracy in sonographic evaluation, *AJR Am J Roentgenol* 137:245-250, 1981.

347. Slovis TL, Kuhns LR: Real-time sonography of the brain through the anterior fontanelle, *AJR Am J Roentgenol* 136:277-286, 1981.

348. Lebed MR, Schifrin BS, Waffran F, Hohler CW, et al: Real-time B scanning in the diagnosis of neonatal intracranial hemorrhage, *Am J Obstet Gynecol* 142:851-861, 1982.

349. Perlman JM, Volpe JJ: Cerebral blood flow velocity in relation to intraventricular hemorrhage in the premature newborn infant, *J Pediatr* 100:956-959, 1982.

350. Shankaran S, Slovis TL, Bedard MP, Poland RL: Sonographic classification of intracranial hemorrhage: A prognostic indicator of mortality, morbidity, and short-term neurologic outcome, *J Pediatr* 100:469-475, 1982.

351. Dolfin T, Skidmore MB, Fong KW, Hoskins EM, et al: Incidence, severity, and timing of subependymal and intraventricular hemorrhages in preterm infants born in a perinatal unit as detected by serial real-time ultrasound, *Pediatrics* 71:541-546, 1983.

352. Hecht ST, Filly RA, Callen PW, Wilson-Davis SL: Intracranial hemorrhage: Late onset in the preterm neonate, *Radiology* 149:697-699, 1983.

353. Pape KE, Bennett-Britton S, Szymonowicz W, Martin DJ, et al: Diagnostic accuracy of neonatal brain imaging: A postmortem correlation of computed tomography and ultrasound scans, *J Pediatr* 102:275-280, 1983.

354. Partridge JC, Babcock DS, Steichen JJ, Han BK: Optimal timing for diagnostic cranial ultrasound in low-birth-weight infants: Detection of intracranial hemorrhage and ventricular dilation, *J Pediatr* 102:281-287, 1983.

355. Bowerman RA, Donn SM, Silver TM, Jaffe MH: Natural history of neonatal periventricular/intraventricular hemorrhage and its complications: Sonographic observations, *AJR Am J Roentgenol* 143:1041-1052, 1984.

356. Levene MI, de Vries L: Extension of neonatal intraventricular haemorrhage, *Arch Dis Child* 59:631-636, 1984.

357. Allan WC, Philip AG: Neonatal cerebral pathology diagnosed by ultrasound, *Clin Perinatol* 12:195-218, 1985.

358. Levene MI, Williams JL, Fawer CL: *Ultrasound of the Infant Brain*, London: 1985, Blackwell Scientific.

359. Rumack CM, Manco-Johnson ML, Manco-Johnson MJ, Koops BL, et al: Timing and course of neonatal intracranial hemorrhage using real-time ultrasound, *Radiology* 154:101-105, 1985.

360. Shackelford GD, Volpe JJ: Cranial ultrasonography in the evaluation of neonatal intracranial hemorrhage and its complications, *J Perinat Med* 13:293-304, 1985.

361. Volpe JJ: Intraventricular hemorrhage and brain injury in the premature infant: Diagnosis, prognosis, and prevention, *Clin Perinatol* 16:387-411, 1989.

362. Fawer CL, Calame A: Ultrasound. In Haddad J, Christmann D, Messer J, editors: *Imaging Techniques of the CNS of the Neonates*, New York: 1991, Springer-Verlag.

363. Haddad J, Messer J, Aranda J: Periventricular haemorrhagic infarction associated with subependymal germinal matrix haemorrhage in the premature newborn: Report of two cases, *Eur J Pediatr* 151:63-65, 1992.

364. Schellinger D, Grant EG, Manz HJ, Patronas NJ: Intraparenchymal hemorrhage in preterm neonates: A broadening spectrum, *AJR Am J Roentgenol* 150:1109-1115, 1988.

365. Rennie JM: *Neonatal Cerebral Ultrasound*, Cambridge: 1997, Cambridge University Press.

366. Adcock LM, Moore PJ, Schlesinger AE, Armstrong DL: Correlation of ultrasound with postmortem neuropathologic studies in neonates, *Pediatr Neurol* 19:263-271, 1998.

367. Murphy BP, Inder TE, Rooks V, Taylor GA, et al: Posthemorrhagic ventricular dilatation in the premature infant: Natural history and predictors of outcome, *Arch Dis Child Fetal Neonatal Ed* 87:F37-F41, 2002.

368. Scott WR, New PF, Davis KR, Schnur JA: Computerized axial tomography of intracerebral and intraventricular hemorrhage, *Radiology* 112:73-80, 1974.

369. Pevsner PH, Garcia-Bunuel R, Leeds N, Finkelstein M: Subependymal and intraventricular hemorrhage in neonates: Early diagnosis by computed tomography, *Radiology* 119:111-114, 1976.

370. Volpe JJ: Neonatal intracranial hemorrhage: Pathophysiology, neuropathology, and clinical features, *Clin Perinatol* 4:77-102, 1977.

371. Rumack CM, McDonald MM, O'Meara OP, Sanders BB, et al: CT detection and course of intracranial hemorrhage in premature infants, *AJR Am J Roentgenol* 131:493-497, 1978.

372. Lee BC, Grassi AE, Schechner S, Auld PA: Neonatal intraventricular hemorrhage: A serial computed tomography study, *J Comput Assist Tomogr* 3:483-490, 1979.

373. Albright L, Fellows R: Sequential CT scanning after neonatal intracerebral hemorrhage, *AJR Am J Roentgenol* 136:949-953, 1981.

374. Siegel MJ, Patel J, Gado MH, Shackelford GD: Cranial computed tomography and real-time sonography in full-term neonates and infants, *Radiology* 149:111-116, 1983.

375. McArdle CB, Richardson CJ, Hayden CK, Nicholas DA, et al: Abnormalities of the neonatal brain: MR imaging. I. Intracranial hemorrhage, *Radiology* 163:387-394, 1987.

376. Haddad J, Constantinesco A, Brunot B: Single photon emission computed tomography of the brain perfusion in neonates. In Haddad J, Christmann D, Messer J, editors: *Imaging Techniques of the CNS of the Neonates*, New York: 1991, Springer-Verlag.

377. Zuerrer M, Martin E, Boltshauser E: MR imaging of intracranial hemorrhage in neonates and infants at 2.35 tesla, *Neuroradiology* 33:223-229, 1991.

378. Barkovich AJ: *Pediatric Neuroimaging*, 3rd ed, New York: 2000, Raven Press.
379. Rutherford M: *MRI of the Neonatal Brain*, Philadelphia: 2002, Saunders.
380. Barkovich AJ: *Pediatric Neuroimaging*, 4th ed, Philadelphia: 2005, Lippincott Williams & Wilkins.
381. Kosmetatos N, Dinter C, Williams ML, Lourie H, et al: Intracranial hemorrhage in the premature: Its predictive features and outcome, *Am J Dis Child* 134:855-859, 1980.
382. Robinson RO, Desai NS: Factors influencing mortality and morbidity after clinically apparent intraventricular haemorrhage, *Arch Dis Child* 56:478-481, 1981.
383. Thorburn RJ, Lipscomb AP, Stewart AL, Reynolds EO, et al: Prediction of death and major handicap in very preterm infants by brain ultrasound, *Lancet* 1:1119-1121, 1981.
384. Allan WC, Holt PJ, Sawyer LR, Tito AM, et al: Ventricular dilation after neonatal periventricular-intraventricular hemorrhage: Natural history and therapeutic implications, *Am J Dis Child* 136:589-593, 1982.
385. Papile LA, Munsick-Bruno G, Schaefer A: Relationship of cerebral intraventricular hemorrhage and early childhood neurologic handicaps, *J Pediatr* 103:273-277, 1983.
386. Stewart AL, Thorburn RJ, Hope PL, Goldsmith M, et al: Ultrasound appearance of the brain in very preterm infants and neurodevelopmental outcome at 18 months of age, *Arch Dis Child* 58:598-604, 1983.
387. Catto-Smith AG, Yu VY, Bajuk B, Orgill AA, et al: Effect of neonatal periventricular haemorrhage on neurodevelopmental outcome, *Arch Dis Child* 60:8-11, 1985.
388. van de Bor M, Verloove-Vanhorick SP, Baerts W, Brand R, et al: Outcome of periventricular-intraventricular hemorrhage at 2 years of age in 484 very preterm infants admitted to 6 neonatal intensive care units in the Netherlands, *Neuropediatrics* 19:183-185, 1988.
389. Ventriculomegaly Trial Group: Randomised trial of early tapping in neonatal posthaemorrhagic ventricular dilatation, *Arch Dis Child* 65:3-10, 1990.
390. Perlman JM, Lynch B, Volpe JJ: Late hydrocephalus after arrest and resolution of neonatal post-hemorrhagic hydrocephalus, *Dev Med Child Neurol* 32:725-729, 1990.
391. Roth SC, Baudin J, McCormick DC, Edwards AD, et al: Relation between ultrasound appearance of the brain of very preterm infants and neurodevelopmental impairment at eight years, *Dev Med Child Neurol* 35:755-768, 1993.
392. Resch B, Gedermann A, Maurer U, Ritschl E, et al: Neurodevelopmental outcome of hydrocephalus following intra-periventricular hemorrhage in preterm infants: Short- and long term results, *Childs Nerv Syst* 12:27-33, 1996.
393. Hansen AR, Allred EN, Leviton A: Predictors of ventriculoperitoneal shunt among babies with intraventricular hemorrhage, *J Child Neurol* 12:381-386, 1997.
394. Levy ML, Masri LS, McComb JG: Outcome for preterm infants with germinal matrix hemorrhage and progressive hydrocephalus, *Neurosurgery* 41:1111-1117, 1997.
395. Ment LR, Vohr B, Allan W, Westerveld M, et al: The etiology and outcome of cerebral ventriculomegaly at term in very low birth weight preterm infants, *Pediatrics* 104:243-248, 1999.
396. Kennedy CR, Ayers S, Campbell MJ, Elbourne D, etal: Randomized, controlled trial of acetazolamide and furosemide in posthemorrhagic ventricular dilation in infancy: Follow-up at 1 year, *Pediatrics* 597-607:597-607, 2001.
397. de Vries LS, Liem KD, van Dijk K, Smit BJ, et al: Early versus late treatment of posthaemorrhagic ventricular dilatation: Results of a retrospective study from five neonatal intensive care units in the Netherlands, *Acta Paediatr* 91:212-217, 2002.
398. Futagi Y, Suzuki Y, Toribe Y, Nakano H, et al: Neurodevelopmental outcome in children with posthemorrhagic hydrocephalus, *Pediatr Neurol* 33:26-32, 2005.
399. Ment LR, Allan WC, Makuch RW, Vohr B: Grade 3 to 4 intraventricular hemorrhage and Bayley scores predict outcome, *Pediatrics* 116:1597-1598(author reply 1598), 2005.
400. Krishnamoorthy KS, Shannon DC, DeLong GR, Todres ID, et al: Neurologic sequelae in the survivors of neonatal intraventricular hemorrhage, *Pediatrics* 64:233-237, 1979.
401. Krishnamoorthy KS, Kuehnle KJ, Todres ID, DeLong GR: Neurodevelopmental outcome of survivors with posthemorrhagic hydrocephalus following grade II neonatal intraventricular hemorrhage, *Ann Neurol* 15:201-204, 1984.
402. Williamson WD, Desmond MM, Wilson GS, Andrew L, et al: Early neurodevelopmental outcome of low birth weight infants surviving neonatal intraventricular hemorrhage, *J Perinat Med* 10:34-41, 1982.
403. de Vries LS, Dubowitz LM, Dubowitz V, Kaiser A, et al: Predictive value of cranial ultrasound in the newborn baby: A reappraisal, *Lancet* 2:137-140, 1985.
404. Fawer CL, Calame A, Furrer MT: Neurodevelopmental outcome at 12 months of age related to cerebral ultrasound appearances of high risk preterm infants, *Early Hum Dev* 11:123-132, 1985.
405. Ment LR, Scott DT, Ehrenkranz RA, Duncan CC: Neurodevelopmental assessment of very low birth weight neonates: Effect of

406. germinal matrix and intraventricular hemorrhage, *Pediatr Neurol* 1:164-168, 1985.
406. TeKolste KA, Bennett FC, Mack LA: Follow-up of infants receiving cranial ultrasound for intracranial hemorrhage, *Am J Dis Child* 139:299-303, 1985.
407. Dykes FD, Dunbar B, Lazarra A, Ahmann PA: Posthemorrhagic hydrocephalus in high-risk preterm infants: Natural history, management, and long-term outcome, *J Pediatr* 114:611-618, 1989.
408. Hanigan WC, Morgan AM, Anderson RJ, Bradle P, et al: Incidence and neurodevelopmental outcome of periventricular hemorrhage and hydrocephalus in a regional population of very low birth weight infants, *Neurosurgery* 29:701-706, 1991.
409. van de Bor M, Ensdokkum M, Schreuder AM, Veen S, et al: Outcome of periventricular-intraventricular haemorrhage at five years of age, *Dev Med Child Neurol* 35:33-41, 1993.
410. van Zeben-van der Aa TM, Verloove-Vanhorick SP, Brand R: Morbidity of very-low-birthweight infants [letter], *Lancet* 1:729-730, 1989.
411. Costello AM, Hamilton PA, Baudin J, Townsend J, et al: Prediction of neurodevelopmental impairment at four years from brain ultrasound appearance of very preterm infants, *Dev Med Child Neurol* 30:711-722, 1988.
412. Lewis M, Bendersky M: Cognitive and motor differences among low birth weight infants: Impact of intraventricular hemorrhage, medical risk, and social class, *Pediatrics* 83:187-192, 1989.
413. Anderson LT, Garcia-Coll C, Vohr BR, Emmons L, et al: Behavioral characteristics and early temperament of premature infants with intracranial hemorrhage, *Early Hum Dev* 18:273-283, 1989.
414. Vohr BR, Garcia-Coll C, Mayfield S, Brann B, et al: Neurologic and developmental status related to the evolution of visual-motor abnormalities from birth to 2 years of age in preterm infants with intraventricular hemorrhage, *J Pediatr* 115:296-302, 1989.
415. Ford LM, Steichen J, Steichen-Asch PA, Babcock D, et al: Neurologic status and intracranial hemorrhage in very-low-birth-weight preterm infants: Outcome at 1 year and 5 years, *Am J Dis Child* 143:1186-1190, 1989.
416. Low JA, Galbraith RS, Sauerbrei EE, Muir DW, et al: Motor and cognitive development of infants with intraventricular hemorrhage, ventriculomegaly, or periventricular parenchymal lesions, *Am J Obstet Gynecol* 155:750-756, 1986.
417. Greisen G, Petersen MB, Pedersen SA, Baekgaard P: Status at two years in 121 very low birth weight survivors related to neonatal intraventricular haemorrhage and mode of delivery, *Acta Paediatr Scand* 75:24-30, 1986.
418. Amato M, Howald H, von Muralt G: Neurological prognosis of high-risk preterm infants with peri-intraventricular hemorrhage and ventricular dilatation, *Eur Neurol* 25:241-247, 1986.
419. Lowe J, Papile L: Neurodevelopmental performance of very-low-birth-weight infants with mild periventricular, intraventricular hemorrhage: Outcome at 5 to 6 years of age, *Am J Dis Child* 144:1242-1245, 1990.
420. Leonard CH, Clyman RI, Piecuch RE, Juster RP, et al: Effect of medical and social risk factors on outcome of prematurity and very low birth weight, *J Pediatr* 116:620-626, 1990.
421. Krishnamoorthy KS, Kuban KC, Leviton A, Brown ER, et al: Periventricular-intraventricular hemorrhage, sonographic localization, phenobarbital, and motor abnormalities in low birth weight infants, *Pediatrics* 85:1027-1033, 1990.
422. Brazy JE, Eckerman CO, Oehler JM, Goldstein RF, et al: Nursery Neurobiologic Risk Score: Important factor in predicting outcome in very low birth weight infants, *J Pediatr* 118:783-792, 1991.
423. Vohr B, Garcia-Coll C, Flanagan P, Oh W: Effects of intraventricular hemorrhage and socioeconomic status on perceptual, cognitive, and neurologic status of low birth weight infants at 5 years of age, *J Pediatr* 121:280-285, 1992.
424. Cooke RW: Early and late cranial ultrasonographic appearances and outcome in very low birthweight infants, *Arch Dis Child* 62:931-937, 1987.
425. Sinha SK, Davies JM, Sims DG, Chiswick ML: Relation between periventricular haemorrhage and ischaemic brain lesions diagnosed by ultrasound in very pre-term infants, *Lancet* 2:1154-1156, 1985.
426. Stewart AL, Reynolds EO, Hope PL, Hamilton PA, et al: Probability of neurodevelopmental disorders estimated from ultrasound appearance of brains of very preterm infants, *Dev Med Child Neurol* 29:3-11, 1987.
427. Weindling AM, Rochefort MJ, Calvert SA, Fok TF, et al: Development of cerebral palsy after ultrasonographic detection of periventricular cysts in the newborn, *Dev Med Child Neurol* 27:800-806, 1985.
428. Graziani LJ, Mitchell DG, Kornhauser M, Pidcock FS, et al: Neurodevelopment of preterm infants: Neonatal neurosonographic and serum bilirubin studies, *Pediatrics* 89:229-234, 1992.
429. Weisglas-Kuperus N, Baerts W, Fetter W, Sauer P: Neonatal cerebral ultrasound, neonatal neurology and perinatal conditions as predictors of neurodevelopmental outcome in very low birthweight infants, *Early Hum Dev* 31:131-148, 1992.
430. Fazzi E, Lanzi G, Gerardo A, Ometto A, et al: Neurodevelopmental outcome in very low-birth-weight infants with or without periventricular haemorrhage and/or leucomalacia, *Acta Paediatr* 81:808-811, 1992.

431. Gibson JY, Masingale TW, Graves GR, LeBlanc MH, et al: Relationship of cranial midline shift to outcome of very-low-birth-weight infants with periventricular hemorrhagic infarction, *J Neuroimaging* 4:212-217, 1994.
432. Aziz K, Vickar DB, Sauve RS, Etches PC, et al: Province-based study of neurologic disability of children weighing 500 through 1249 grams at brith in relation to neonatal cerebral ultrasound findings, *Pediatrics* 95:837-844, 1995.
433. Bouza H, Dubowitz LM, Rutherford M, Cowan F, et al: Late magnetic resonance imaging and clinical findings in neonates with unilateral lesions on cranial ultrasound, *Dev Med Child Neurol* 36:951-964, 1994.
434. de Vries LS, Radenmaker KJ, Groenendaal F, Eken P, et al: Correlation between neonatal cranial ultrasound, MRI in infancy and neurodevelopmental outcome in infants with a large intraventricular haemorrhage with or without unilateral parenchymal involvement, *Neuropediatrics* 29:180-188, 1998.
435. Ames PN, Baudin J, Townsend J, Meek J, et al: Epilepsy in very preterm infants: Neonatal cranial ultrasound reveals a high-risk subcategory, *Dev Med Child Neurol* 40:724-730, 1998.
436. de Vries LS, Groenendaal F, van Haastert IC, Eken P, et al: Asymmetrical myelination of the posterior limb of the internal capsule in infants with periventricular haemorrhagic infarction: An early predictor of hemiplegia, *Neuropediatrics* 30:314-319, 1999.
437. Bassan H, Benson CB, Limperopoulos C, Feldman HA, et al: Ultrasonographic features and severity scoring of periventricular hemorrhagic infarction in relation to risk factors and outcome, *Pediatrics* 117:2111-2118, 2006.
438. Futagi Y, Toribe Y, Ogawa K, Suzuki Y: Neurodevelopmental outcome in children with intraventricular hemorrhage, *Pediatr Neurol* 34:219-224, 2006.
439. Vollmer B, Roth S, Riley K, Sellwood MW, et al: Neurodevelopmental outcome of preterm infants with ventricular dilatation with and without associated haemorrhage, *Dev Med Child Neurol* 48:348-352, 2006.
440. Patra K, Wilson-Costello D, Taylor HG, Mercuri-Minich N, et al: Grades I-II intraventricular hemorrhage in extremely low birth weight infants: Effects on neurodevelopment, *J Pediatr* 149:169-173, 2006.
441. Bassan H, Limperopoulos C, Visconti K, Mayer DL, et al: Neurodevelopmental outcome in survivors of periventricular hemorrhagic infarction, *Pediatrics* 120:785-792, 2007.
442. Blackman JA, McGuinness GA, Bale JF Jr, Smith WL Jr: Large postnatally acquired porencephalic cysts: Unexpected developmental outcomes, *J Child Neurol* 6:58-64, 1991.
443. Marin-Padilla M: Developmental neuropathology and impact of perinatal brain damage. II. White matter lesions of the neocortex, *J Neuropathol Exp Neurol* 56:219-235, 1997.
444. Volpe JJ: Subplate neurons: Missing link in brain injury of the premature infant? *Pediatrics* 97:112-113, 1996.
445. Miller SP, Ferriero DM, Leonard C, Piecuch R, et al: Early brain injury in premature newborns detected with magnetic resonance imaging is associated with adverse early neurodevelopmental outcome, *J Pediatr* 147:609-616, 2005.
446. Rehncrona S, Nielsen Hauge H, Siesjö BK: Enhancement of iron-catalyzed free radical formation by acidosis in brain homogenates: Difference in effect by lactic acid and CO_2, *J Cereb Blood Flow Metab* 9:65-70, 1989.
447. Lackmann GM, Hesse L, Tollner U: Reduced iron-associated antioxidants in premature newborns suffering intracerebral hemorrhage, *Free Radic Biol Med* 20:407-409, 1996.
448. Savman K, Nilsson UA, Blennow M, Kjellmer I, et al: Non-protein-bound iron is elevated in cerebrospinal fluid from preterm infants with posthemorrhagic ventricular dilation, *Pediatr Res* 49:208-212, 2001.
449. van de Bor M, Guit GL, Schreuder AM, Wondergem J, et al: Early detection of delayed myelination in preterm infants, *Pediatrics* 84:407-411, 1989.
450. Gressens P, Richelme C, Kadhim HJ, Gadisseux JF, et al: The germinative zone produces the most cortical astrocytes after neuronal migration in the developing mammalian brain, *Biol Neonate* 61:4-24, 1992.
451. Evrard P, Gressens P, Volpe JJ: New concepts to understand the neurological consequences of subcortical lesions in the premature brain [editorial], *Biol Neonate* 61:1-3, 1992.
452. Vasileiadis GT, Gelman N, Han VK, Williams LA, et al: Uncomplicated intraventricular hemorrhage is followed by reduced cortical volume at near-term age, *Pediatrics* 114:e367-e372, 2004.
453. Edvinsson L, Lou HC, Tvede K: On the pathogenesis of regional cerebral ischemia in intracranial hemorrhage: A causal influence of potassium? *Pediatr Res* 20:478-480, 1986.
454. Stutchfield PR, Cooke RW: Electrolytes and glucose in cerebrospinal fluid of premature infants with intraventricular haemorrhage: Role of potassium in cerebral infarction, *Arch Dis Child* 64:470-475, 1989.
455. Busija DW, Leffler CW: Perivascular blood attenuates noradrenergic but not cholinergic effects on piglet pial arterioles, *Stroke* 21:441-446, 1990.
456. Yakubu MA, Shibata M, Leffler CW: Subarachnoid hematoma attenuates vasodilation and potentiates vasoconstriction induced by vasoactive agents in newborn pigs, *Pediatr Res* 36:589-594, 1994.
457. Yakubu MA, Shibata M, Leffler CW: Hematoma-induced enhanced cerebral vasoconstrictions to leukotriene C_4 and endothelin-1 in piglets: Role of prostanoids, *Pediatr Res* 38:119-123, 1995.
458. Yakubu MA, Leffler CW: 5-Hydroxtryptamine-induced vasoconstriction after cerebral hematoma in piglets, *Pediatr Res* 41:317-320, 1997.
459. Bada HS, Hajjar W, Chua C, Sumner DS: Noninvasive diagnosis of neonatal asphyxia and intraventricular hemorrhage by Doppler ultrasound, *J Pediatr* 95:775-779, 1979.
460. Heros RC, Zervas NT, Varsos V: Cerebral vasospasm after subarachnoid hemorrhage: An update, *Ann Neurol* 14:599-608, 1983.
461. Kistler JP, Crowell RM, Davis KR, Heros R, et al: The relation of cerebral vasospasm to the extent and location of subarachnoid blood visualized by CT scan: A prospective study, *Neurology* 33:424-436, 1983.
462. Goldenberg RL, Rouse DJ: Medical progress: Prevention of premature birth, *N Engl J Med* 339:313-320, 1998.
463. Mattison DR, Damus K, Fiore E, Petrini J, et al: Preterm delivery: A public health perspective, *Paediatr Perinat Epidemiol* 15(Suppl 2):7-16, 2001.
464. Creasy RK: Preterm birth prevention: Where are we? *Am J Obstet Gynecol* 168:1223-1230, 1993.
465. Iams JD, Creasy RK: Preterm labor and delivery. In Creasy RK, Resnik R, Iams JD, editors: *Maternal-Fetal Medicine Principles and Practice*, 5th ed, Philadelphia: 2004, Saunders.
466. Martin JA, Hamilton BE, Sutton PD, Ventura SJ, et al: Births: Final data for 2004, *Natl Vital Stat Rep* 55:1-101, 2006.
467. Hamilton BE, Minina AM, Martin JA, Kockanek K, et al: Annual summary of vital statistics: 2005, *Pediatrics* 119:345-360, 2007.
468. Creasy RK: Preventing preterm birth [editorial], *N Engl J Med* 325:727-729, 1991.
469. Kliegman RM, Rottman CJ, Behrman RE: Strategies for the prevention of low birth weight, *Am J Obstet Gynecol* 162:1073-1083, 1990.
470. Canadian Preterm Labor Investigators Group: Treatment of preterm labor with the beta-adrenergic agonist ritodrine, *N Engl J Med* 327:308-312, 1992.
471. Laros RK Jr, Kitterman JA, Heilbron DC, Cowan RM, et al: Outcome of very-low-birth-weight infants exposed to beta-sympathomimetics in utero, *Am J Obstet Gynecol* 164:1657-1664, 1991.
472. Ferguson JE 2nd, Dyson DC, Schutz T, Stevenson DK: A comparison of tocolysis with nifedipine or ritodrine: Analysis of efficacy and maternal, fetal, and neonatal outcome, *Am J Obstet Gynecol* 163:105-111, 1990.
473. Tucker JM, Goldenberg RL, Davis RO, Copper RL, et al: Etiologies of preterm birth in an indigent population: Is prevention a logical expectation? *Obstet Gynecol* 77:343-347, 1991.
474. Mueller-Heubach E, Reddick D, Barnett B, Bente R: Preterm birth prevention: Evaluation of a prospective controlled randomized trial, *Am J Obstet Gynecol* 160:1172-1178, 1989.
475. Morrison JC: Preterm birth: A puzzle worth solving, *Obstet Gynecol* 76:S5-S12, 1990.
476. Goldenberg RL, Davis RO, Copper RL, Corliss DK, et al: The Alabama preterm birth prevention project, *Obstet Gynecol* 75:933-939, 1990.
477. McLaughlin FJ, Altemeier WA, Christensen MJ, Sherrod KB, et al: Randomized trial of comprehensive prenatal care for low-income women: Effect on infant birth weight, *Pediatrics* 89:128-132, 1992.
478. Roberts WE, Morrison JC, Hamer C, Wiser WL: The incidence of preterm labor and specific risk factors, *Obstet Gynecol* 76:S85-S89, 1990.
479. Hill WC, Fleming AD, Martin RW, Hamer C, et al: Home uterine activity monitoring is associated with a reduction in preterm birth, *Obstet Gynecol* 76:S13-S18, 1990.
480. Main DM, Richardson DK, Hadley CB, Gabbe SG: Controlled trial of a preterm labor detection program: Efficacy and costs, *Obstet Gynecol* 74:873-877, 1989.
481. Konte JM, Creasy RK, Laros RK Jr: California North Coast Preterm Birth Prevention project, *Obstet Gynecol* 71:727-730, 1988.
482. Groome LJ, Goldenberg RL, Cliver SP, Davis RO, et al: Neonatal periventricular-intraventricular hemorrhage after maternal beta-sympathomimetic tocolysis, *Am J Obstet Gynecol* 167:873-879, 1992.
483. Higby K, Xenakis E, Pauerstein CJ, Harbert GM, et al: Do tocolytic agents stop preterm labor? A critical and comprehensive review of efficacy and safety, *Am J Obstet Gynecol* 168:1247-1259, 1993.
484. Hobel CJ, Ross MG, Bemis RL, Bragonier JR, et al: The West Los Angeles preterm birth prevention project. I. Program impact on high-risk women, *Am J Obstet Gynecol* 170:54-62, 1994.
485. Iams J: Prevention of preterm birth, *N Engl J Med* 338:54-56, 1998.
486. Holzman C, Paneth N: Preterm birth: From prediction to prevention, *Am J Public Health* 88:183-184, 1998.
487. Goldenberg RL, Iams JD, Mercer BM, Meis PJ, et al: The preterm prediction study: The value of new vs standard risk factors in predicting early and all spontaneous preterm births, *Am J Public Health* 88:233-238, 1998.
488. Dyson DC, Danbe KH, Bamber JA, Crites YM, et al: Monitoring women at risk for preterm labor, *N Engl J Med* 338:15-19, 1998.
489. Hall RT: Prevention of premature birth: Do pediatricians have a role? *Pediatrics* 105:1137-1140, 2000.
490. Weintraub Z, Solovechick M, Reichman B, Rotschild A, et al: Effect of maternal tocolysis on the incidence of severe periventricular/intraventricular haemorrhage in very low birthweight infants, *Arch Dis Child Fetal Neonatal Ed* 85:F13-F17, 2001.

491. Hack M, Shah D: Periventricular haemorrhage and tocolytic therapies, *Lancet* 359:185-186, 2002.
492. Abbasi S, Gerdes JS, Sehdev HM, Samimi SS, et al: Neonatal outcome after exposure to indomethacin in utero: A retrospective case cohort study, *Am J Obstet Gynecol* 189:782-785, 2003.
493. Meis PJ, Klebanoff M, Thom E, Dombrowski MP, et al: Prevention of recurrent preterm delivery by 17 alpha-hydroxyprogesterone caproate, *N Engl J Med* 348:2379-2385, 2003.
494. Sanchez-Ramos L, Kaunitz AM, Delke I: Progestational agents to prevent preterm birth: A meta-analysis of randomized controlled trials, *Obstet Gynecol* 105:273-279, 2005.
495. Delaney-Black V, Lubchenco LO, Butterfield LJ, Goldson E, et al: Outcome of very-low-birth-weight infants: Are populations of neonates inherently different after antenatal versus neonatal referral? *Am J Obstet Gynecol* 160:545-552, 1989.
496. Kollee LA, Verloove-Vanhorick PP, Verwey RA, Brand R, et al: Maternal and neonatal transport: Results of a national collaborative survey of preterm and very low birth weight infants in the Netherlands, *Obstet Gynecol* 72:729-732, 1988.
497. Kollee LAA, Brand R, Schreuder AM, Ensdokkum MH, et al: 5-year outcome of preterm and very low birth weight infants: A comparison between maternal and neonatal transport, *Obstet Gynecol* 80:635-638, 1992.
498. Roberts WE, Morrison JC: Pharmacologic induction of fetal lung maturity, *Clin Obstet Gynecol* 34:319-327, 1991.
499. Clark CE, Clyman RI, Roth RS, Sniderman SH, et al: Risk factor analysis of intraventricular hemorrhage in low-birth-weight infants, *J Pediatr* 99:625-628, 1981.
500. Leviton A, Kuban K, Pagano M, Allred E, et al: Antenatal corticosteroids appear to reduce the risk of postnatal germinal matrix hemorrhage in intubated low birthweight newborn, *Pediatrics* 81:1083-1088, 1993.
501. Wright LL, Horbar JD, Gunkel H, Verter J, et al: Evidence from multicenter networks on the current use and effectiveness of antenatal corticosteroids in low birth weight infants, *Am J Obstet Gynecol* 173:263-269, 1995.
502. Garland JS, Buck R, Leviton A: Effect of maternal glucocorticoid exposure on risk of severe intraventricular hemorrhage in surfactant-treated preterm infants, *J Pediatr* 126:272-279, 1995.
503. Spinillo A, Capuzzo E, Ometto A, Stronati M, et al: Value of antenatal corticosteroid therapy in preterm birth, *Early Hum Dev* 42:37-47, 1995.
504. Wright LL, Verter J, Younes N, Stevenson D, et al: Antenatal corticosteroid administration and neonatal outcome in very low birth weight infants: The NICHD Neonatal Research Network, *Am J Obstet Gynecol* 173:269-274, 1995.
505. Shankaran S, Bauer CR, Bain R, Wright LL, et al: Relationship between antenatal steroid administration and grades III and IV intracranial hemorrhage in low birth weight infants, *Am J Obstet Gynecol* 173:305-312, 1995.
506. Horbar JD: Antenatal corticosteroid treatment and neonatal outcomes for infants 501 to 1500 gm in the Vermont-Oxford Trials Network, *Am J Obstet Gynecol* 173:275-281, 1995.
507. Perlman JM: Antenatal glucocorticoid, magnesium exposure, and the prevention of brain injury of prematurity, *Semin Pediatr Neurol* 5:202-210, 1998.
508. Arad H, Durkin MS, Hinton VJ, Kuhn L, et al: Long-term cognitive benefits of antenatal corticosteroids for prematurely born children with cranial ultrasound abnormalities, *Am J Obstet Gynecol* 186:818-825, 2002.
509. Agarwal R, Chiswick ML, Rimmer S, Taylor GM, et al: Antenatal steroids are associated with a reduction in the incidence of cerebral white matter lesions in very low birthweight infants, *Arch Dis Child Fetal Neonatal Ed* 86:F96-F101, 2002.
510. Baud O: Antenatal corticosteroid therapy: Benefits and risks, *Acta Paediatr* 93:6-10, 2004.
511. Anand KJS, Hall RW, Desai N, Shephard B, et al: Effects of morphine analgesia in ventilated preterm neonates: Primary outcomes from the NEOPAIN randomised trial, *Lancet* 363:1673-1682, 2004.
512. Foix-Helias L, Baud O, Lenclen R, Kaminski M, et al: Benefit of antenatal glucocorticoids according to the cause of very premature birth, *Arch Dis Child Fetal Neonatal Ed* 90:F46-F48, 2005.
513. Crowley P: Prophylactic corticosteroids for preterm birth, *Cochrane Database Syst Rev* 3:CD000065, 2006.
514. Blickstein I, Reichman B, Lusky A, Shinwell ES: Plurality-dependent risk of severe intraventricular hemorrhage among very low birth weight infants and antepartum corticosteroid treatment, *Am J Obstet Gynecol* 194:1329-1333, 2006.
515. Jobe AH, Soll RF: Choice and dose of corticosteroid for antenatal treatments, *Am J Obstet Gynecol* 190:878-881, 2004.
516. Volpe JJ: Encephalopathy of prematurity includes neuronal abnormalities, *Pediatrics* 116:221-225, 2005.
517. Murphy BP, Inder TE, Huppi PS, Warfield S, et al: Impaired cerebral cortical gray matter growth after treatment with dexamethasone for neonatal chronic lung disease, *Pediatrics* 107:217-221, 2001.
518. Karemaker R, Heijnen CJ, Veen S, Baerts W, et al: Differences in behavioral outcome and motor development at school age after neonatal treatment for chronic lung disease with dexamethasone versus hydrocortisone, *Pediatr Res* 60:745-750, 2006.
519. Parikh N, Lasky RE, Kennedy KA, Moya FR, et al: Postnatal dexamethasone therapy and cerebral tissue volumes in extremely low birth weight infants, *Pediatrics* 119:265-272, 2007.

520. Bar-Lev MRR, Maayan-Metzger A, Matok I, Heyman Z, et al: Short-term outcomes in low birth weight infants following antenatal exposure to betamethasone versus dexamethasone, *Obstet Gynecol* 104:484-488, 2004.
521. Aghajafari F, Murphy K, Matthews S, Ohlsson A, et al: Repeated doses of antenatal corticosteroids in animals: A systematic review, *Am J Obstet Gynecol* 186:843-849, 2002.
522. Lawson EE: Antenatal corticosteroids: Too much of a good thing? *JAMA* 286:1628-1630, 2001.
523. Thorp JA, Jones PG, Knox E, Clark RH: Does antenatal corticosteroid therapy affect birth weight and head circumference? *Obstet Gynecol* 99:101-108, 2002.
524. Modi N, Lewis HJ, Al-Naqeeb N, Ajayi-Obe M, et al: The effects of repeated antenatal glucocorticoid therapy on the developing rat, *Pediatr Res* 50:581-585, 2001.
525. Guinn DA: Repeat courses of antenatal corticosteroids: The controversy continues, *Am J Obstet Gynecol* 190:585-587, 2004.
526. Spinillo A, Viazzo F, Colleoni R, Chiara A, et al: Two-year infant neurodevelopmental outcome after single or multiple antenatal courses of corticosteroids to prevent complications of prematurity, *Am J Obstet Gynecol* 191:217-224, 2004.
527. Guinn DA, Atkinson MW, Sullivan L, Lee M, et al: Single vs weekly courses of antenatal corticosteroids for women at risk of preterm delivery: A randomized controlled trial, *JAMA* 286:1581-1587, 2001.
527a. Stiles AD: Prenatal corticosteroids—early gain, long-term questions, *N Engl J Med* 357:1248-1250, 2007.
528. Crowther CA, Haslam RR, Hiller JE, Doyle LW, et al: Neonatal respiratory distress syndrome after repeat exposure to antenatal corticosteroids: A randomised controlled trial, *Lancet* 367:1913-1919, 2006.
529. Peltoniemi OM, Kari MA, Tammela O, Lehtonen L, et al: Randomized trial of a single repeat dose of prenatal betamethasone treatment in imminent preterm birth, *Pediatrics* 119:290-298, 2007.
530. Padbury JF, Ervin MG, Polk DH: Extrapulmonary effects of antenatally administered steroids, *J Pediatr* 128:167-172, 1996.
531. Moise AA, Wearden ME, Kozinetz CA, Gest AL, et al: Antenatal steroids are associated with less need for blood pressure support in extremely premature infants, *Pediatrics* 95:845-850, 1995.
532. Wallace EM, Baker LS: Effect of antenatal betamethasone administration on placental vascular resistance, *Lancet* 353:1404-1407, 1999.
533. Baud O, Foixl-Helias L, Kaminski M, Audibert F, et al: Antenatal glucocorticoid treatment and cystic periventricular leukomalacia in very premature infants, *N Engl J Med* 341:1190-1196, 1999.
534. Leviton A, Dammann O, Allred EN, Kuban K, et al: Antenatal corticosteroids and cranial ultrasonographic abnormalities, *Am J Obstet Gynecol* 181:1007-1017, 1999.
535. Canterino JC, Verma U, Visintainer PF, Elimian A, et al: Antenatal steroids and neonatal periventricular leukomalacia, *Obstet Gynecol* 97:135-139, 2001.
536. de Zegher F, de Vries L, Pierrat V, Daniels H, et al: Effect of prenatal betamethasone/thyrotropin releasing hormone treatment on somatosensory evoked potentials in preterm newborns, *Pediatr Res* 32:212-214, 1992.
537. Morales WJ, Koerten J: Prevention of intraventricular hemorrhage in very low birth weight infants by maternally administered phenobarbital, *Obstet Gynecol* 68:295-299, 1986.
538. Shankaran S, Cepeda EE, Ilagan N, Mariona F, et al: Antenatal phenobarbital for the prevention of neonatal intracerebral hemorrhage, *Am J Obstet Gynecol* 154:53-57, 1986.
539. Shankaran S, Cepeda EE, Ilagan N, Kauffman RE: Pharmacokinetic basis for antenatal dosing of phenobarbital for the prevention of neonatal intracerebral hemorrhage, *Dev Pharmacol Ther* 9:171-177, 1986.
540. Kaempf JW, Porreco R, Molina R, Hale K, et al: Antenatal phenobarbital for the prevention of periventricular and intraventricular hemorrhage: A double-blind, randomized, placebo-controlled, multihospital trial, *J Pediatr* 117:933-938, 1990.
541. Thorp JA, Ferrettesmith D, Gaston LA, Johnson J, et al: Combined antenatal vitamin K and phenobarbital therapy for preventing intracranial hemorrhage in newborns less than 34 weeks' gestation, *Obstet Gynecol* 86:1-8, 1995.
542. Shankaran S, Cepeda E, Muran G, Mariona F, et al: Antenatal phenobarbital therapy and neonatal outcome. I. Effect on intracranial hemorrhage, *Pediatrics* 97:644-648, 1996.
543. Shankaran S, Woldt E, Nelson J, Bedard M, et al: Antenatal phenobarbital therapy and neonatal outcome. II. Neurodevelopmental outcome at 36 months, *Pediatrics* 97:649-652, 1996.
544. Thorp JA, White RD, Westergom KL, OConnor MA: Intracranial haemorrhage in premature neonates: Epidemiology and prevention, *CNS Drugs* 11:421-433, 1999.
545. Shankaran S, Papile LA, Wright LL, Ehrenkranz RA, et al: The effect of antenatal phenobarbital therapy on neonatal intracranial hemorrhage in preterm infants, *N Engl J Med* 337:466-471, 1997.
546. Crowther C, Henderson-Smart D: Prenatal phenobarbital before very-preterm birth and neurodevelopmental outcome, *Lancet* 360:1529-1530, 2002.
547. Shankaran S, Papile LA, Wright LL, Ehrenkranz RA, et al: Neurodevelopmental outcome of premature infants after antenatal phenobarbital exposure, *Am J Obstet Gynecol* 187:171-177, 2002.

548. Crowther CA, Henderson-Smart DJ: Phenobarbital prior to preterm birth for preventing neonatal periventricular haemorrhage, *Cochrane Database Syst Rev* 3:CD000164, 2002.

549. Pomerance JJ, Teal JG, Gogolok JF, Brown S, et al: Maternally administered antenatal vitamin K1: Effect on neonatal prothrombin activity, partial thromboplastin time, and intraventricular hemorrhage, *Obstet Gynecol* 70:235-241, 1987.

550. Morales WJ, Angel JL, O'Brien WF, Knuppel RA, et al: The use of antenatal vitamin K in the prevention of early neonatal intraventricular hemorrhage, *Am J Obstet Gynecol* 159:774-779, 1988.

551. Kazzi NJ, Ilagan NB, Liang KC, Kazzi GM, et al: Maternal administration of vitamin K does not improve the coagulation profile of preterm infants, *Pediatrics* 84:1045-1050, 1989.

552. Thorp JA, Parriott J, Ferrettesmith D, Meyer BA, et al: Antepartum vitamin K and phenobarbital for preventing intraventricular hemorrhage in the premature newborn: A randomized, double-blind, placebo-controlled trial, *Obstet Gynecol* 83:70-76, 1994.

553. Crowther CA, Henderson-Smart DJ: Vitamin K prior to preterm birth for preventing neonatal periventricular haemorrhage, *Cochrane Database Syst Rev* 1:CD000229, 2001.

554. Hirtz DG, Nelson K: Magnesium sulfate and cerebral palsy in premature infants, *Curr Opin Pediatr* 10:131-137, 1998.

555. Grether JK, Hoogstrate J, Walsh-Greene E, Nelson KB: Magnesium sulfate for tocolysis and risk of spastic cerebral palsy in premature children born to women without preeclampsia, *Am J Obstet Gynecol* 183:717-725, 2000.

556. Rantonen T, Ekblad U, Gronlund J, Rikalainen H, et al: Influence of maternal magnesium sulphate and ritodrine treatment on the neonate: A study with six-month follow-up, *Acta Paediatr* 88:1142-1146, 1999.

557. Mittendorf R, Dambrosia J, Dammann O, Pryde PG, et al: Association between maternal serum ionized magnesium levels at delivery and neonatal intraventricular hemorrhage, *J Pediatr* 140:540-546, 2002.

558. Crowther CA, Hiller JE, Doyle LW, Haslam RR: Effect of magnesium sulfate given for neuroprotection before preterm birth: A randomized controlled trial, *JAMA* 290:2669-2676, 2003.

559. Mittendorf R, Dammann O, Lee KS: Brain lesions in newborns exposed to high-dose magnesium sulfate during preterm labor, *J Perinatol* 26:57-63, 2006.

559a. Marret S, Marpeau L, Zupan-Simunek V, Eurin D, et al: Magnesium sulphate given before very preterm birth to protect infant brain: The randomised controlled PREMAG trial, *BJOG* 114:310-318, 2007.

560. Scudiero R, Khoshnood B, Pryde PG, Lee K-S, et al: Perinatal death and tocolytic magnesium sulfate, *Obstet Gynecol* 96:178-182, 2000.

561. Mittendorf R, Dambrosia J, Pryde PG, Lee K-S, et al: Association between the use of antenatal magnesium sulfate in preterm labor and adverse health outcomes in infants, *Am J Obstet Gynecol* 186:1111-1118, 2002.

562. Farkouh LJ, Thorp JA, Jones PG, Clark RH, et al: Antenatal magnesium exposure and neonatal demise, *Am J Obstet Gynecol* 185:869-872, 2001.

563. DiRenzo GC, Mignosa M, Gerli S, Burnelli L, et al: The combined maternal administration of magnesium sulfate and aminophylline reduces intraventricular hemorrhage in very preterm neonates, *Am J Obstet Gynecol* 192:433-438, 2005.

564. Crowther CA, Hiller JE, Doyle LW: Magnesium sulphate for preventing preterm birth in threatened preterm labour, *Cochrane Database Syst Rev* 2005.

565. Enevoldsen EM, Jensen FT: Autoregulation and CO_2 responses of cerebral blood flow in patients with acute severe head injury, *J Neurosurg* 48:689-703, 1978.

566. Batton DG, Nardis EE: The effect of intraventricular blood on cerebral blood flow in newborn dogs, *Pediatr Res* 21:511-515, 1987.

567. Anderson GD, Bada HS, Shaver DC, Harvey CJ, et al: The effect of cesarean section on intraventricular hemorrhage in the preterm infant, *Am J Obstet Gynecol* 166:1091-1101, 1992.

568. Malloy MH, Onstad L, Wright E: The effect of cesarean delivery on birth outcome in very low birth weight infants: National Institute of Child Health and Human Development Neonatal Research Network, *Obstet Gynecol* 77:498-503, 1991.

569. Grant A, Glazener CM: Elective caesarean section versus expectant management for delivery of the small baby, *Cochrane Database Syst Rev* 4:CD001060, 2002.

570. Paulson OB, Olesen J, Christensen MS: Restoration of autoregulation of cerebral blood flow by hypocapnia, *Neurology* 22:286-293, 1972.

571. Cooke RW, Morgan ME: Hyperventilation at birth and periventricular hemorrhage [letter], *Lancet* 2:450, 1982.

572. Lou HC, Phibbs RH, Wilson SL, Gregory GA: Hyperventilation at birth may prevent early periventricular haemorrhage [letter], *Lancet* 1:1407, 1982.

573. Lindner W, Vobbeck S, Hummler H, Pohlandt F: Delivery room management of extremely low birth weight infants: Spontaneous breathing or intubation? *Pediatrics Aaa* 103:961-967, 1999.

574. Perlman JM, Goodman S, Kreusser KL, Volpe JJ: Reduction in intraventricular hemorrhage by elimination of fluctuating cerebral blood-flow velocity in preterm infants with respiratory distress syndrome, *N Engl J Med* 312:1353-1357, 1985.

575. Miall-Allen VM, Whitelaw AG: Effect of pancuronium and pethidine on heart rate and blood pressure in ventilated infants, *Arch Dis Child* 62:1179-1180, 1987.

576. Hamon I, Hascoet JM, Debbiche A, Vert P: Effects of fentanyl administration on general and cerebral haemodynamics in sick newborn infants, *Acta Paediatr* 85:361-365, 1996.

577. Saarenmaa E, Hultunen P, Leppaluoto J, Meretoja O, et al: Advantages of fentanyl over morphine in analgesia for ventilated newborn infants after birth: A randomized trial, *J Pediatr* 134:144-150, 1999.

578. Rennie JM, South M, Morley CJ: Cerebral blood flow velocity variability in infants receiving assisted ventilation, *Arch Dis Child* 62:1247-1251, 1987.

579. South M, Morley CJ: Synchronous mechanical ventilation of the neonate, *Arch Dis Child* 61:1190-1195, 1986.

580. Shaw NJ, Cooke R, Gill AB, Shaw NJ, et al: Randomised trial of routine versus selective paralysis during ventilation for neonatal respiratory distress syndrome, *Arch Dis Child* 69:479-482, 1993.

581. Adams JM: The controlled nursery environment and neonatal intraventricular hemorrhage, *Focus* 3:3-4, 1985.

582. Bada HS, Korones SB, Green RS: Association between minimum manipulation (MM) and intraventricular hemorrhage (IVH) [abstract], *Pediatr Res* 21:351, 1987.

583. Szymonowicz W, Yu VY, Walker A, Wilson F: Reduction in periventricular haemorrhage in preterm infants, *Arch Dis Child* 61:661-665, 1986.

584. Greenough A, Wood S, Morley CJ, Davis JA: Pancuronium prevents pneumothoraces in ventilated premature babies who actively expire against positive pressure inflation, *Lancet* 1:1-3, 1984.

585. Fanconi S, Duc G: Intratracheal suctioning in sick preterm infants: Prevention of intracranial hypertension and cerebral hypoperfusion by muscle paralysis, *Pediatrics* 79:538-543, 1987.

586. Morley CJ: Surfactant treatment for premature babies: A review of clinical trials, *Arch Dis Child* 66:445-450, 1991.

587. Martin RJ: Neonatal surfactant therapy: Where do we go from here? [editorial], *J Pediatr* 118:555-556, 1991.

588. Corbet A, Bucciarelli R, Goldman S, Mammel M, et al: Decreased mortality rate among small premature infants treated at birth with a single dose of synthetic surfactant: A multicenter controlled trial. American Exosurf Pediatric Study Group 1, *J Pediatr* 118:277-284, 1991.

589. Speer CP, Robertson B, Curstedt T, Halliday HL, et al: Randomized European multicenter trial of surfactant replacement therapy for severe neonatal respiratory distress syndrome: Single versus multiple doses of Curosurf, *Pediatrics* 89:13-20, 1992.

590. Hoekstra RE, Jackson JC, Myers TF, Frantz ID 3rd, et al: Improved neonatal survival following multiple doses of bovine surfactant in very premature neonates at risk for respiratory distress syndrome, *Pediatrics* 88:10-18, 1991.

591. Phibbs RH, Ballard RA, Clements JA, Heilbron DC, et al: Initial clinical trial of EXOSURF, a protein-free synthetic surfactant, for the prophylaxis and early treatment of hyaline membrane disease, *Pediatrics* 88:1-9, 1991.

592. Long W, Thompson T, Sundell H, Schumacher R, et al: Effects of two rescue doses of a synthetic surfactant on mortality rate and survival without bronchopulmonary dysplasia in 700- to 1350-gram infants with respiratory distress syndrome: The American Exosurf Neonatal Study Group I, *J Pediatr* 118:595-605, 1991.

593. Dunn MS, Shennan AT, Zayack D, Possmayer F: Bovine surfactant replacement therapy in neonates of less than 30 weeks' gestation: A randomized controlled trial of prophylaxis versus treatment, *Pediatrics* 87:377-386, 1991.

594. Ware J, Taeusch HW, Soll RF, McCormick MC: Health and developmental outcomes of a surfactant controlled trial: Follow-up at 2 years, *Pediatrics* 85:1103-1107, 1990.

595. Morley CJ, Morley R: Follow up of premature babies treated with artificial surfactant (ALEC), *Arch Dis Child* 65:667-669, 1990.

596. Horbar JD, Soll RF, Sutherland JM, Kotagal U, et al: A multicenter randomized, placebo-controlled trial of surfactant therapy for respiratory distress syndrome, *N Engl J Med* 320:959-965, 1989.

597. Morley CJ, Greenough A, Miller NG, Bangham AD, et al: Randomized trial of artificial surfactant (ALEC) given at birth to babies from 23 to 34 weeks gestation, *Early Hum Dev* 17:41-54, 1988.

598. McCord FB, Curstedt T, Halliday HL, McClure G, et al: Surfactant treatment and incidence of intraventricular haemorrhage in severe respiratory distress syndrome, *Arch Dis Child* 63:10-16, 1988.

599. Merritt TA, Hallman M, Bloom BT, Berry C, et al: Prophylactic treatment of very premature infants with human surfactant, *N Engl J Med* 315:785-790, 1986.

600. Vaucher YE, Harker L, Merritt TA, Hallman M, et al: Outcome at twelve months of adjusted age in very low birth weight infants with lung immaturity: A randomized placebo-controlled trial of human surfactant, *J Pediatr* 122:126-132, 1993.

601. Hallman M, Merritt A, Bry K, Berry C: Association between neonatal care practices and efficacy of exogenous human surfactant: Results of a bicenter randomized trial, *Pediatrics* 91:552-559, 1993.

602. Horbar JD, Wright EC, Onstad L: Decreasing mortality associated with the introduction of surfactant therapy: An observational study of neonates weighing 601 to 1300 grams at birth, *Pediatrics* 92:191-196, 1993.

603. Ferrara TB, Hoekstra RE, Couser RJ, Gaziano EP, et al: Survival and follow-up of infants born at 23 to 26 weeks of gestational age: Effects of surfactant therapy, *J Pediatr* 124:119-124, 1994.

604. Wells JT, Ment LR: Prevention of intraventricular hemorrhage in preterm infants, *Early Hum Dev* 42:209-233, 1995.

605. Vermont-Oxford Neonatan Network: A multicenter, randomized trial comparing synthetic surfactant with modified bovine surfactant extract in the treatment of neonatal respiratory distress syndrome, *Pediatrics* 97:1-6, 1996.

606. van Bel F, de Winter PJ, Wijnands HBG, van de Bor M, et al: Cerebral and aortic blood flow velocity patterns in preterm infants receiving prophylactic surfactant treatment, *Acta Paediatr* 81:504-510, 1992.

607. van de, Bor M, Ma EJ, Walther FJ: Cerebral blood flow velocity after surfactant instillation in preterm infants, *J Pediatr* 118:285-287, 1991.

608. Skov L, Hellström-Westas L, Jacobsen T, Greisen G, et al: Acute changes in cerebral oxygenation and cerebral blood volume in preterm infants during surfactant treatment, *Neuropediatrics* 23:126-130, 1992.

609. Hellström-Westas L, Bell AH, Skov L, Greisen G, et al: Cerebroelectrical depression following surfactant treatment in preterm neonates, *Pediatrics* 89:643-647, 1992.

610. Edwards AD, McCormick DC, Roth SC, Elwell CE, et al: Cerebral hemodynamic effects of treatment with modified natural surfactant investigated by near infrared spectroscopy, *Pediatr Res* 32:532-536, 1992.

611. Bell AH, Skov L, Lundstrom KE, Saugstad OD, et al: Cerebral blood flow and plasma hypoxanthine in relation to surfactant treatment, *Acta Paediatr* 83:910-914, 1994.

612. Roll C, Knief J, Horsch S, Hanssler L: Effect of surfactant administration on cerebral haemodynamics and oxygenation in premature infants: A near infrared spectroscopy study, *Neuropediatrics* 31:16-23, 2000.

613. Amato M, Huppi P, Markus D, Herschkowitz N: Neurological function of immature babies after surfactant replacement therapy, *Neuropediatrics* 22:43-44, 1991.

614. Kari MA, Hallman M, Eronen M, Teramo K, et al: Prenatal dexamethasone treatment in conjunction with rescue therapy of human surfactant: A randomized placebo-controlled multicenter study, *Pediatrics* 93:730-736, 1994.

615. Jobe AH, Mitchell BR, Gunkel JH: Beneficial effects of the combined use or prenatal corticosteroids and postnatal surfactant on preterm infants, *Am J Obstet Gynecol* 168:508-513, 1993.

616. Clark RH, Gerstmann DR, Null DM Jr, deLemos RA: Prospective randomized comparison of high-frequency oscillatory and conventional ventilation in respiratory distress syndrome, *Pediatrics* 89:5-12, 1992.

617. Bryan AC, Froese AB: Reflections on the HIFI trial, *Pediatrics* 87:565-567, 1991.

618. Keszler M, Donn SM, Bucciarelli RL, Alverson DC, et al: Multicenter controlled trial comparing high-frequency jet ventilation and conventional mechanical ventilation in newborn infants with pulmonary interstitial emphysema, *J Pediatr* 119:85-93, 1991.

619. HIFO Study Group: High-frequency oscillatory ventilation compared with conventional mechanical ventilation in the treatment of respiratory failure in preterm infants, *N Engl J Med* 320:88-93, 1989.

620. HIFO Study Group: High-frequency oscillatory ventilation compared with conventional intermittent mechanical ventilation in the treatment of respiratory failure in preterm infants: Neurodevelopmental status at 16 to 24 months of postterm age, *J Pediatr* 117:939-946, 1990.

621. HIFO Study Group: Randomized study of high-frequency oscillatory ventilation in infants with severe respiratory distress syndrome, *J Pediatr* 122:609-619, 1993.

622. Ogawa Y, Miyasaka K, Kawano T, Imura S, et al: A multicenter randomized trial of high frequency oscillatory ventilation as compared with conventional mechanical ventilation in preterm infants with respiratory failure, *Early Hum Dev* 32:1-10, 1993.

623. Clark RH, Yoder BA, Sell MS: Prospective, randomized comparison of high-frequency oscillation and conventional ventilation in candidates for extracorporeal membrane oxygenation, *J Pediatr* 124:447-454, 1994.

624. Gerstmann DR, Minton SD, Stoddard RA, Meredith KS, et al: The Provo multicenter early high frequency oscillatory ventilation trial: Improved pulmonary and clinical outcome in respiratory distress syndrome, *Pediatrics* 98:1044-1057, 1996.

625. Thome U, Kossel H, Lipowsky G, Porz F, et al: Randomized comparison of high frequency ventilation with high-rate intermittent positive pressure ventilation in preterm infants with respiratory failure, *J Pediatr* 135:39-46, 1999.

626. Wiswell TE, Graziani LJ, Kornhauser MS, Cullen J, et al: High-frequency jet ventilation in the early management of respiratory distress syndrome is associated with a greater risk for adverse outcomes, *Pediatrics* 98:1035-1043, 1996.

627. Mestan KKL, Marks JD, Hecox K, Huo D, et al: Neurodevelopmental outcomes of premature infants treated with inhaled nitric oxide, *N Engl J Med* 353:23-32, 2005.

628. Van Meurs KP, Wright LL, Ehrenkranz RA, Lemons JA, et al: Inhaled nitric oxide for premature infants with severe respiratory failure, *N Engl J Med* 353:13-22, 2005.

629. Hascoet JM, Fresson J, Claris O, Hamon I, et al: The safety and efficacy of nitric oxide therapy in premature infants, *J Pediatr* 146:318-323, 2005.

630. Barrington KJ, Finer NN: Inhaled nitric oxide for respiratory failure in preterm infants, *Cochrane Database Syst Rev* 1:CD000509, 2005.

631. Ballard RA, Truog WE, Cnaan A, Martin RJ, et al: Inhaled nitric oxide in preterm infants undergoing mechanical ventilation, *N Engl J Med* 355:343-353, 2006.

632. Kinsella JP, Cutter GR, Walsh WF, Gerstmann DR, et al: Early inhaled nitric oxide therapy in premature newborns with respiratory failure, *N Engl J Med* 355:354-364, 2006.

632a. Tanaka Y, Hayashi T, Kitajima H, Sumi K, et al: Inhaled nitric oxide therapy decreases the risk of cerebral palsy in preterm infants with persistent pulmonary hypertension of the newborn, *Pediatrics* 119:1159-1164, 2007.

632b. Kinsella JP, Abman SH: Inhaled nitric oxide in the premature newborn, *J Pediatr* 151:10-15, 2007.

632c. Hintz SR, Van Meurs KP, Perritt R, Poole WK, et al: Neurodevelopmental outcomes of premature infants with severe respiratory failure enrolled in a randomized controlled trial of inhaled nitric oxide, *J Pediatr* 151:16-22, 2007.

632d. Barrington KJ, Finer NN: Inhaled nitric oxide for preterm infants: A systematic review, *Pediatrics* 120:1088-1099, 2007.

633. Anwar M, Kadam S, Hiatt IM, Hegyi T: Phenobarbitone prophylaxis of intraventricular haemorrhage, *Arch Dis Child* 61:196-197, 1986.

634. Bedard MP, Shankaran S, Slovis TL, Pantoja A, et al: Effect of prophylactic phenobarbital on intraventricular hemorrhage in high-risk infants, *Pediatrics* 73:435-439, 1984.

635. Goldstein GW, Donn SM: Periventricular and intraventricular hemorrhages. In Sarnat HB, editor: *Topics In Neonatal Neurology*, Orlando, FL: 1984, Grune & Stratton.

636. Morgan ME, Massey RF, Cooke RW: Does phenobarbitone prevent periventricular hemorrhage in very low-birth-weight babies? A controlled trial, *Pediatrics* 70:186-189, 1982.

637. Whitelaw A, Placzek M, Dubowitz L, Lary S, et al: Phenobarbitone for prevention of periventricular haemorrhage in very low birth-weight infants: A randomised double-blind trial, *Lancet* 2:1168-1170, 1983.

638. Ruth V, Virkola K, Paetau R, Raivio KO: Early high-dose phenobarbital treatment for prevention of hypoxic-ischemic brain damage in very low birth weight infants, *J Pediatr* 112:81-86, 1988.

639. Chen H-J, Roloff DW: Routine administration of phenobarbital for the prevention of intraventricular hemorrhage in premature infants: Five years' experience, *J Perinatol* 14:15-22, 1994.

640. Whitelaw A: Postnatal phenobarbitone for the prevention of intraventricular hemorrhage in preterm infants, *Cochrane Database Syst Rev* 1:CD001691, 2001.

641. Burgess GH, Oh W, Brann BS, Brubakk AM, et al: Effects of phenobarbital on cerebral blood flow velocity after endotracheal suctioning in premature neonates, *Arch Pediatr Adolesc Med* 155:723-727, 2001.

642. Goddard-Finegold J, Armstrong DL: Reduction in incidence of periventricular, intraventricular hemorrhages in hypertensive newborn beagles pretreated with phenobarbital, *Pediatrics* 79:901-906, 1987.

643. Monin P, Hascoet JM, Vert P: Autoregulation of cerebral blood flow, *Dev Pharmacol Ther* 13:120-128, 1989.

644. Laudignon N, Chemtob S, Beharry K, Rex J, et al: Effect of phenobarbital on cerebral blood flow in the newborn piglet under stress, *Biol Neonate* 50:288-296, 1986.

645. Goddard-Finegold J, Michael LH: Brain vasoactive effects of phenobarbital during hypertension and hypoxia in newborn pigs, *Pediatr Res* 32:103-106, 1992.

646. Yamashita Y, Goddard-Finegold J, Contant CF, Martin CG, et al: Phenobarbital and cerebral blood flow during hypotension in newborn pigs, *Pediatr Res* 33:598-602, 1993.

647. Andersen K, Jensen KA, Ebbesen F: The effect of phenobarbital on cerebral blood flow in newborn infants with foetal distress, *Eur J Pediatr* 153:584-587, 1994.

648. Rosenberg AA, Murdaugh E, White CW: The role of oxygen free radicals in postasphyxia cerebral hypoperfusion in newborn lambs, *Pediatr Res* 26:215-219, 1989.

649. Ment LR, Stewart WB, Duncan CC: Beagle puppy model of intraventricular hemorrhage. Effect of superoxide dismutase on cerebral blood flow and prostaglandins, *J Neurosurg* 62:563-569, 1985.

650. Ment LR, Duncan CC, Ehrenkranz RA, Kleinman CS, et al: Randomized indomethacin trial for prevention of intraventricular hemorrhage in very low birth weight infants, *J Pediatr* 107:937-943, 1985.

651. Ment LR, Duncan CC, Ehrenkranz RA, Kleinman CS, et al: Randomized low-dose indomethacin trial for prevention of intraventricular hemorrhage in very low birth weight neonates, *J Pediatr* 112:948-955, 1988.

652. Rennie JM, Doyle J, Cooke RW: Early administration of indomethacin to preterm infants, *Arch Dis Child* 61:233-238, 1986.

653. Bandstra ES, Montalvo BM, Goldberg RN, Pacheco I, et al: Prophylactic indomethacin for prevention of intraventricular hemorrhage in premature infants, *Pediatrics* 82:533-542, 1988.

654. Hanigan WC, Kennedy G, Roemisch F, Anderson R, et al: Administration of indomethacin for the prevention of periventricular-intraventricular hemorrhage in high-risk neonates, *J Pediatr* 112:941-947, 1988.

655. Bada HS, Green RS, Pourcyrous M, Leffler CW, et al: Indomethacin reduces the risks of severe intraventricular hemorrhage, *J Pediatr* 115:631-637, 1989.

656. Fowlie PW: Prophylactic indomethacin: Systematic review and meta-analysis, *Arch Dis Ch* 74:F81-F87, 1996.

657. Vohr B, Ment LR: Intraventricular hemorrhage in the preterm infant, *Early Hum Dev* 44:1-16, 1996.

658. Clyman RI: Recommendations for the postnatal use of indomethacin: An analysis of four separate treatment strategies, *J Pediatr* 128:601-607, 1996.

659. Schmidt B, Davis P, Moddemann D, Ohlsson A, et al: Long-term effects of indomethacin prophylaxis in extremely-low-birth-weight infants, *N Engl J Med* 344:1966-1972, 2001.

660. Tyson JE: Does indomethacin prophylaxis benefit extremely low birth weight infants? Results of a placebo-controlled multicenter trial: A review of Schmidt B, Davis P, Moddemann D, Ohlsson A, et al: 2001 Long-term effects of indomethacin prophylaxis in extremely low-birth-weight infants, *N Engl J Med* 334:1966-1972, *Pediatr Res* 51:1, 2000.

661. Fowlie PW, Davis PG: Prophylactic indomethacin for preterm infants: A systematic review and meta-analysis, *Arch Dis Child Fetal Neonatal Ed* 88:F464-F466, 2003.

662. Ment LR, Vohr BR, Makuch RW, Westerveld M, et al: Prevention of intraventricular hemorrhage by indomethacin in male preterm infants, *J Pediatr* 145:832-834, 2004.

663. Ohlsson A, Roberts RS, Schmidt B, Davis P, et al: Male/female differences in indomethacin effects in preterm infants, *J Pediatr* 147:860-862, 2005.

664. Clyman RI, Saha S, Jobe A, Oh W: Indomethacin prophylaxis for preterm infants: The impact of 2 multicentered randomized controlled trials on clinical practice, *J Pediatr* 150:46-50, 2007.

664a. Clyman RI, Chorne N: Patent ductus arteriosus: Evidence for and against treatment, *J Pediatr* 150:216-219, 2007.

665. Fowlie PW, Davis PG: Prophylactic intravenous indomethacin for preventing mortality and morbidity in preterm infants, *Cochrane Database Syst Rev* 3:CD000174, 2002.

666. Ment LR, Oh W, Ehrenkranz RA, Philip AG, et al: Low dose indomethacin and prevention of intraventricular hemorrhage: A multicenter randomized trial, *J Pediatr* 124:951-955, 1994.

667. Volpe JJ: Brain injury caused by intraventricular hemorrhage: Is indomethacin the silver bullet for prevention? *Pediatrics* 46:22-31, 1994.

668. Marlow N, Wolke D, Bracewell MA, Samara M: Neurologic and developmental disability at six years of age after extremely preterm birth, *N Engl J Med* 352:9-19, 2005.

669. Reiss AL, Kesler SR, Vohr B, Duncan CC, et al: Sex differences in cerebral volumes of 8-year-olds born preterm, *J Pediatr* 145:242-249, 2004.

670. Allan WC, Vohr B, Makuch RW, Katz KH, et al: Antecedents of cerebral palsy in a multicenter trial of indomethacin for intraventricular hemorrhage, *Arch Pediatr Adolesc Med* 151:580-585, 1997.

671. Miller SP, Mayer EE, Clyman RI, Glidden DV, et al: Prolonged indomethacin exposure is associated with decreased white matter injury detected with magnetic resonance imaging in premature newborns at 24 to 28 weeks' gestation at birth, *Pediatrics* 117:1626-1631, 2006.

672. Ment LR, Stewart WB, Scott DT, Duncan CC: Beagle puppy model of intraventricular hemorrhage: Randomized indomethacin prevention trial, *Neurology* 33:179-184, 1983.

673. Mirro R, Leffler CW, Armstead W, Beasley DG, et al: Indomethacin restricts cerebral blood flow during pressure ventilation of newborn pigs, *Pediatr Res* 24:59-62, 1988.

674. Leffler CW, Busija DW, Beasley DG: Effect of therapeutic dose of indomethacin on the cerebral circulation of newborn pigs, *Pediatr Res* 21:188-192, 1987.

675. Chemtob S, Laudignon N, Beharry K, Rex J, et al: Effects of prostaglandins and indomethacin on cerebral blood flow and cerebral oxygen consumption of conscious newborn piglets, *Dev Pharmacol Ther* 14:1-14, 1990.

676. van Bel F, Klautz JM, Steenduk P, Schipper IB, et al: The influence of indomethacin on the autoregulatory ability of the cerebral vascular bed in the newborn lamb, *Pediatr Res* 34:278-281, 1993.

677. Pourcyrous M, Leffler CW, Bada HS, Korones SB, et al: Cerebral blood flow responses to indomethacin in awake newborn pigs, *Pediatr Res* 35:565-570, 1994.

678. Van Bel F, Bartelds B, Teitel DF, Rudolph AM: Effect of indomethacin on cerebral blood flow and oxygenation in the normal and ventilated fetal lamb, *Pediatr Res* 38:243-250, 1995.

679. Louis PT, Yamashita Y, Del Toro J, Michael LH, et al: Brain blood flow responses to indomethacin during hemorrhagic hypotension in newborn piglets, *Biol Neonate* 66:359-366, 1995.

680. Brown DW, Hadway J, Lee T-Y: Near-infrared spectroscopy measurement of oxygen extraction fraction and cerebral metabolic rate of oxygen in newborn piglets, *Pediatr Res* 54:861-867, 2003.

681. Brown DW, Lee D, Kumaran VS, Lee T-y: Age-dependent cerebral hemodynamic effects of indomethacin in the newborn piglet, *J Appl Physiol* 97:1880-1887, 2004.

682. Leffler CW, Busija DW, Fletcher AM, Beasley DG: Effects of indomethacin upon cerebral hemodynamics of newborn pigs, *Pediatr Res* 19:1160-1164, 1985.

683. Leffler CW, Busija DW, Beasley DG, Fletcher AM, et al: Effects of indomethacin on cardiac output distribution in normal and asphyxiated piglets, *Prostaglandins* 31:183-190, 1986.

684. Leffler CW, Busija DW, Beasley DG, Fletcher AM: Maintenance of cerebral circulation during hemorrhagic hypotension in newborn pigs: Role of prostanoids, *Circ Res* 59:562-567, 1986.

685. Pourcyrous M, Busija DW, Shibata M, Bada HS, et al: Cerebrovascular responses to therapeutic dose of indomethacin in newborn pigs, *Pediatr Res* 45:582-587, 1999.

686. Cowan F: Indomethacin, patent ductus arteriosus, and cerebral blood flow, *J Pediatr* 109:341-344, 1986.

687. van Bel F, Van de Bor M, Stijnen T, Baan J, et al: Cerebral blood flow velocity changes in preterm infants after a single dose of indomethacin: Duration of its effect, *Pediatrics* 84:802-807, 1989.

688. Laudignon N, Chemtob S, Bard H, Aranda JV: Effect of indomethacin on cerebral blood flow velocity of premature newborns, *Biol Neonate* 54:254-262, 1988.

689. Saliba E, Chantepie A, Autret E, Gold F, et al: Effects of indomethacin on cerebral hemodynamics at rest and during endotracheal suctioning in preterm neonates, *Acta Paediatr Scand* 80:611-615, 1991.

690. Mardoum R, Bejar R, Merritt TA, Berry C: Controlled study of the effects of indomethacin on cerebral blood flow velocities in newborn infants, *J Pediatr* 118:112-115, 1991.

691. Hammerman C, Glaser J, Schimmel MS, Ferber B, et al: Continuous versus multiple rapid infusions of indomethacin: Effects on cerebral blood flow velocity, *Pediatrics* 95:244-248, 1995.

692. Yanowitz TD, Yao AC, Werner JC, Pettigrew KD, et al: Effects of prophylactic low-dose indomethacin on hemodynamics in very low birth weight infants, *J Pediatr* 132:28-34, 1998.

693. Pryds O, Greisen G, Johansen KH: Indomethacin and cerebral blood flow in premature infants treated for patent ductus arteriosus, *Eur J Pediatr* 147:315-316, 1988.

694. Edwards AD, Wyatt JS, Richardson C, Potter A, et al: Effects of indomethacin on cerebral haemodynamics in very preterm infants, *Lancet* 335:1491-1495, 1990.

695. McCormick DC, Edwards AD, Brown GC, Wyatt JS, et al: Effects of indomethacin on cerebral oxidized cytochrome oxidase in preterm infants, *Pediatr Res* 33:603-608, 1993.

696. Benders M, Dorrepaul CA, Vandebor M, Vanbel F: Acute effects of indomethacin on cerebral hemodynamics and oxygenation, *Biol Neonate* 68:91-99, 1995.

697. Liem KD, Hopman JC, Kollee LA, Oeseburg B: Effects of repeated indomethacin administration on cerebral oxygenation and haemodynamics in preterm infants: Combined near infrared spectrophotometry and Doppler ultrasound study, *Eur J Pediatr* 153:504-509, 1994.

698. Patel J, Roberts I, Azzopardi D, Hamilton P, et al: Randomized double-blind controlled trial comparing the effects of ibuprofen with indomethacin on cerebral hemodynamics in preterm infants with patent ductus arteriosus, *Pediatr Res* 47:36-42, 2000.

699. Dani C, Bertini G, Reali MF, Murru P, et al: Prophylaxis of patent ductus arteriosus with ibuprofen in preterm infants, *Acta Paediatr* 89:1369-1374, 2000.

700. Mosca F, Bray M, Colnagbi MR, Fumagalli M, et al: Cerebral vasoreactivity to arterial carbon dioxide tension in preterm infants: The effect of ibuprofen, *J Pediatr* 135:644-646, 1999.

701. Gournay V, Roze JC, Kuster A, Daoud P, et al: Prophylactic ibuprofen versus placebo in very premature infants: A randomised, double-blind, placebo-controlled trial, *Lancet* 364:1939-1944, 2004.

702. Van Overmeire B, Allegaert K, Casaer A, Debauche C, et al: Prophylactic ibuprofen in premature infants: A multicentre, randomised, double-blind, placebo-controlled trial, *Lancet* 364:1945-1949, 2004.

703. Naulaers G, Delanghe G, Allegaert K, Debeer A, et al: Ibuprofen and cerebral oxygenation and circulation, *Arch Dis Child Fetal Neonatal Ed* 90:F75-F76, 2005.

704. Pourcyrous M, Leffler CW, Bada HS, Korones SB, et al: Brain superoxide anion generation in asphyxiated piglets and the effect of indomethacin at therapeutic dose, *Pediatr Res* 34:366-369, 1993.

705. Du L, Bayir H, Lai Y, Zhang X, et al: Innate gender-based proclivity in response to cytotoxicity and programmed cell death pathway, *J Biol Chem* 279:38563-38570, 2004.

706. Ment LR, Stewart WB, Ardito TA, Huang E, et al: Indomethacin promotes germinal matrix microvessel maturation in the newborn beagle pup, *Stroke* 23:1132-1137, 1992.

707. Cooke RW, Morgan ME: Prophylactic ethamsylate for periventricular haemorrhage, *Arch Dis Child* 59:82-83, 1984.

708. Benson JW, Drayton MR, Hayward C, Murphy JF, et al: Multicentre trial of ethamsylate for prevention of periventricular haemorrhage in very low birthweight infants, *Lancet* 2:1297-1300, 1986.

709. Chen JY: Ethamsylate in the prevention of periventricular-intraventricular hemorrhage in premature infants, *J Formos Med Assoc* 92:889-893, 1993.

710. The EC Ethamsylate Trial Group: The EC randomised controlled trial of prophylactic ethamsylate for very preterm neonates: Early mortality and morbidity, *Arch Dis Child Fetal Neonatal Ed* 70:F201-F205, 1994.

711. Schulte J, Osborne J, Benson JW, Cooke R, et al: Developmental outcome of the use of etamsylate for prevention of periventricular haemorrhage in a randomised controlled trial, *Arch Dis Child Fetal Neonatal Ed* 90:F31-35, 2005.

712. Hunt RW: Etamsylate for prevention of periventricular haemorrhage, *Arch Dis Child Fetal Neonatal Ed* 90:F3-5, 2005.

713. Rennie JM, Doyle J, Cooke RW: Ethamsylate reduces immunoreactive prostacyclin metabolite in low birthweight infants with respiratory distress syndrome, *Early Hum Dev* 14:239-244, 1986.

714. Rennie JM, Lam PK: Effects of ethamsylate on cerebral blood flow velocity in premature babies, *Arch Dis Child* 64:46-47, 1989.

715. Harrison RF, Matthews T: Intrapartum ethamsylate [letter], *Lancet* 2:296, 1984.

716. Chiswick ML, Johnson M, Woodhall C, Gowland M, et al: Protective effect of vitamin E (DL-alpha-tocopherol) against intraventricular haemorrhage in premature babies, *Br Med J (Clin Res Ed)* 287:81-84, 1983.

717. Phelps DL, Rosenbaum AL, Isenberg SJ, Leake RD, et al: Tocopherol efficacy and safety for preventing retinopathy of prematurity: A randomized, controlled, double-masked trial, *Pediatrics* 79:489-500, 1987.

718. Sinha S, Davies J, Toner N, Bogle S, et al: Vitamin E supplementation reduces frequency of periventricular haemorrhage in very preterm babies, *Lancet* 1:466-471, 1987.

719. Speer ME, Blifeld C, Rudolph AJ, Chadda P, et al: Intraventricular hemorrhage and vitamin E in the very low-birth-weight infant: Evidence for efficacy of early intramuscular vitamin E administration, *Pediatrics* 74:1107-1112, 1984.

720. Fish WH, Cohen M, Franzek D, Williams JM, et al: Effect of intramuscular vitamin E on mortality and intracranial hemorrhage in neonates of 1000 grams or less, *Pediatrics* 85:578-584, 1990.

721. Brion LP, Bell EF, Raghuveer TS: Vitamin E supplementation for prevention of morbidity and mortality in preterm infants, *Cochrane Database Syst Rev* 3:CD003665, 2003.

722. Law MR, Wijewardene K, Wald NJ: Is routine vitamin E administration justified in very low-birthweight infants? *Dev Med Child Neurol* 32:442-450, 1990.

723. Poland RL: Vitamin E for prevention of perinatal intracranial hemorrhage, *Pediatrics* 85:865-867, 1990.

724. Keeler RF, Young S: Role of vitamin E in the etiology of spontaneous hemorrhagic necrosis of the central nervous system of fetal hamsters, *Teratology* 20:127-132, 1979.

725. Pappenheimer AM, Goettsch M: A cerebellar disorder in chicks apparently of nutritional origin, *J Exp Med* 53:11, 1931.

726. Young S, Keeler RF: Hemorrhagic necrosis of the central nervous system of fetal hamsters: Litter incidence and age-related pathological changes, *Teratology* 17:293-301, 1978.

727. Raju TN, Vidyasagar D, Papazafiratou C: Intracranial pressure monitoring in the neonatal ICU, *Crit Care Med* 8:575-581, 1980.

728. Fleischer AC, Hutchison AA, Bundy AL, Machin JE, et al: Serial sonography of posthemorrhagic ventricular dilatation and porencephaly after intracranial hemorrhage in the preterm neonate, *AJR Am J Roentgenol* 141:451-455, 1983.

729. Allan WC, Dransfield DA, Tito AM: Ventricular dilation following periventricular-intraventricular hemorrhage: Outcome at age 1 year, *Pediatrics* 73:158-162, 1984.

730. Fishman MA, Dutton RV, Okumura S: Progressive ventriculomegaly following minor intracranial hemorrhage in premature infants, *Dev Med Child Neurol* 26:725-731, 1984.

731. Brann BS 4th, Qualls C, Papile L, Wells L, et al: Measurement of progressive cerebral ventriculomegaly in infants after grades III and IV intraventricular hemorrhages, *J Pediatr* 117:615-621, 1990.

732. Marro PJ, Dransfield DA, Mott SH, Allan WC: Posthemorrhagic hydrocephalus: Use of an intravenous-type catheter for cerebrospinal fluid drainage, *Am J Dis Child* 145:1141-1146, 1991.

733. Allan WC: The IVH complex of lesions: Cerebrovascular injury in the preterm infant, *Neurol Clin* 8:529-551, 1990.

734. Shankaran S, Koepke T, Woldt E, Bedard MP, et al: Outcome after posthemorrhagic ventriculomegaly in comparison with mild hemorrhage without ventriculomegaly, *J Pediatr* 114:109-114, 1989.

735. Fernell E, Hagberg G, Hagberg B: Infantile hydrocephalus in preterm, low-birth-weight infants: A nationwide Swedish cohort study 1979–1988, *Acta Paediat* 82:45-48, 1993.

736. Pellicer A, Cabanas F, Garcia-Alix A, Rodriguez JP, et al: Natural history of ventricular dilatation in preterm infants: Prognostic significance, *Pediatr Neurol* 9:108-114, 1993.

737. Cornips E, Van Calenbergh F, Plets C, Devlieger H, et al: Use of external drainage for posthemorrhagic hydrocephalus in very low birth weight premature infants, *Childs Nerv Syst* 13:369-374, 1997.

738. du Plessis AJ: Posthemorrhagic hydrocephalus and brain injury in the preterm infant: Dilemmas in diagnosis and management, *Semin Pediatr Neurol* 5:161-179, 1998.

739. International PHVD Drug Trial Group: International randomised controlled trial of acetazolamide and furosemide in posthaemorrhagic ventricular dilatation in infancy, *Lancet* 352:433-440, 1998.

740. Libenson MH, Kaye EM, Rosman NP, Gilmore HE: Acetazolamide and furosemide for posthemorrhagic hydrocephalus of the newborn, *Pediatr Neurol* 20:185-191, 1999.

741. Taylor GA: Sonographic assessment of posthemorrhagic ventricular dilatation, *Radiol Clin North Am* 39:541-551, 2001.

742. Hill AH, Shackelford GD, Volpe JJ: A potential mechanism for pathogenesis for early posthemorrhagic hydrocephalus in the premature newborn, *Pediatrics* 73:19-21, 1985.

743. Donn SM, Roloff DW, Keyes JW Jr: Lumbar cisternography in evaluation of hydrocephalus in the preterm infant, *Pediatrics* 72:670-676, 1983.

744. Kreusser KL, Tarby TJ, Kovnar E, Taylor DA, et al: Serial lumbar punctures for at least temporary amelioration of neonatal posthemorrhagic hydrocephalus, *Pediatrics* 75:719-724, 1985.

745. Korobkin R: The relationship between head circumference and the development of communicating hydrocephalus in infants following intraventricular hemorrhage, *Pediatrics* 56:74-77, 1975.

746. Volpe JJ, Pasternak JF, Allan WC: Ventricular dilation preceding rapid head growth following neonatal intracranial hemorrhage, *Am J Dis Child* 131:1212-1215, 1977.

747. Naidich TP, Epstein F, Lin JP, Kricheff II, et al: Evaluation of pediatric hydrocephalus by computed tomography, *Radiology* 119:337-345, 1976.

748. Del Bigio MR: Cellular damage and prevention in childhood hydrocephalus, *Brain Pathol* 14:317-324, 2004.

749. Del Bigio MR, Kanfer JN, Zhang YW: Myelination delay in the cerebral white matter of immature rats with kaolin-induced hydrocephalus is reversible, *J Neuropathol Exp Neurol* 56:1053-1066, 1997.

750. Del Bigio MR, Wilson MJ, Enno T: Chronic hydrocephalus in rats and humans: White matter loss and behavior changes, *Ann Neurol* 53:337-346, 2003.

751. Milhorat TH, Clark RG, Hammock MK, McGrath PP: Structural, ultrastructural, and permeability changes in the ependyma and surrounding brain favoring equilibration in progressive hydrocephalus, *Arch Neurol* 22:397-407, 1970.

752. Weller RO, Shulman K: Infantile hydrocephalus: Clinical, histological, and ultrastructural study of brain damage, *J Neurosurg* 36:255-265, 1972.

753. Rubin RC, Hochwald GM, Tiell M, Mizutani H, et al: Hydrocephalus. I. Histological and ultrastructural changes in the pre-shunted cortical mantle, *Surg Neurol* 5:109-114, 1976.

754. Hochwald GM: Animal models of hydrocephalus: Recent developments, *Proc Soc Exp Biol Med* 178:1-10, 1985.

755. Del Bigio MR, Bruni JE: Periventricular pathology in hydrocephalic rabbits before and after shunting, *Acta Neuropathol (Berl)* 77:186-195, 1988.

756. McAllister JP 2nd, Cohen MI, O'Mara KA, Johnson MH: Progression of experimental infantile hydrocephalus and effects of ventriculoperitoneal shunts: An analysis correlating magnetic resonance imaging with gross morphology, *Neurosurgery* 29:329-340, 1991.

757. Hale PM, Mcallister JP, Katz SD, Wright LC, et al: Improvement of cortical morphology in infantile hydrocephalic animals after ventriculoperitoneal shunt placement, *Neurosurgery* 31:1085-1096, 1992.

758. Del Bigio MR: Neuropathological changes caused by hydrocephalus, *Acta Neuropathol (Berl)* 85:573-585, 1993.

759. Wozniak M, McLone DG, Raimondi AJ: Micro- and macrovascular changes as the direct cause of parenchymal destruction in congenital murine hydrocephalus, *J Neurosurg* 43:535-545, 1975.

760. Jones HC, Richards HK, Bucknall RM, Pickard JD: Local cerebral blood flow in rats with congenital hydrocephalus, *J Cereb Blood Flow Metab* 13:531-534, 1993.

761. Matsumae M, Sogabe T, Miura I, Sato O: Energy metabolism in kaolin-induced hydrocephalic rat brain, *Childs Nerv Syst* 6:392-396, 1990.

762. Da Silva MC, Michowicz S, Drake JM, Chumas PD, et al: Reduced local cerebral blood flow in periventricular white matter in experimental neonatal hydrocephalus: Restoration with CSF shunting, *J Cereb Blood Flow Metab* 15:1057-1065, 1995.

763. Chumas PD, Drake JM, Del Bigio MR, Da Silva M, et al: Anaerobic glycolysis preceding white matter destruction in experimental neonatal hydrocephalus, *J Neurosurg* 80:491-501, 1994.

764. Da Silva MC, Drake JM, Lemaire C, Cross A, et al: High-energy phosphate metabolism in a neonatal model of hydrocephalus before and after shunting, *J Neurosurg* 81:544-553, 1994.

765. Braun KPJ, Dijkhuizen RM, deGraaf RA, Nicolay K, et al: Cerebral ischemia and white matter edema in experimental hydrocephalus: A combined in vivo MRI and MRS study, *Brain Res* 757:295-298, 1997.

766. Braun KPJ, Vandertop WP, Gooskens RHJM, Tulleken KAF, et al: NMR spectroscopic evaluation of cerebral metabolism in hydrocephalus: A review, *Neurol Res* 22:51-64, 2000.

767. Socci DJ, Bjugstad KB, Jones HC, Pattisapu JV, et al: Evidence that oxidative stress is associated with the pathophysiology of inherited hydrocephalus in the H-Tx rat model, *Exp Neurol* 155:109-117, 1999.

768. Harris NG, Plant HD, Inglis BA, Briggs RW, et al: Neurochemical changes in the cerebral cortex of treated and untreated hydrocephalic rat pups quantified with in vitro H-1-NMR spectroscopy, *J Neurochem* 68:305-312, 1997.

769. Lovely TJ, McAllister J 2nd, Miller DW, Lamperti AA, et al: Effects of hydrocephalus and surgical decompression on cortical norepinephrine levels in neonatal cats, *Neurosurgery* 24:43-52, 1989.

770. Wright LC, McAllister JP 2nd, Katz SD, Miller DW, et al: Cytological and cytoarchitectural changes in the feline cerebral cortex during experimental infantile hydrocephalus, *Pediatr Neurosurg* 16:139-155, 1990.

771. Miyazawa T, Sato K: Learning disability and impairment of synaptogenesis in HTX-rats with arrested shunt-dependent hydrocephalus, *Childs Nerv Syst* 7:121-128, 1991.

772. Miyazawa T, Nishiye H, Sato K, Kobayashi R, et al: Cortical synaptogenesis in congenitally hydrocephalic HTX-rats using monoclonal anti-synaptic vesicle protein antibody, *Brain Dev* 14:75-79, 1992.

773. Suzuki F, Handa J, Maeda T: Effects of congenital hydrocephalus on serotonergic input and barrel cytoarchitecture in the developing somatosensory cortex of rats, *Childs Nerv Syst* 8:18-24, 1992.

774. Suda K, Sato K, Miyazawa T, Arai H: Changes of synapse-related proteins (SVP-38 and Drebrins) during development of brain in congenitally hydrocephalic HTX rats with and without early placement of ventriculoperitoneal shunt, *Pediatr Neurosurg* 20:50-56, 1994.

775. Suda K, Sato K, Takeda N, Miyazawa T, et al: Early ventriculoperitoneal shunt: Effects on learning ability and synaptogenesis of the brain in congenitally hydrocephalic HTX rats, *Child Nerv Syst* 10:19-23, 1994.

776. Miyazawa T, Sato K: Hippocampal synaptogenesis in hydrocephalic HTX-rats using a monoclonal anti-synaptic vesicle protein antibody, *Brain Dev* 16:432-436, 1995.

777. Harris NG, Jones HC, Patel S: Ventricle shunting in young H-Tx rats with inherited congenital hydrocephalus: A quantitative histological study of cortical grey matter, *Child Nerv Syst* 10:293-301, 1994.

778. Zhang YW, DelBigio MR: Growth-associated protein-43 is increased in cerebrum of immature rats following induction of hydrocephalus, *Neuroscience* 86:847-854, 1998.

779. Boillat CA, Jones HC, Kaiser GL, Harris NG: Ultrastructural changes in the deep cortical pyramidal cells of infant rats with inherited hydrocephalus and the effect of shunt treatment, *Exp Neurol* 147:377-388, 1997.

780. Alvisi C, Cerisoli M, Giulioni M, et al: Evaluation of cerebral blood flow changes by transfontanelle Doppler ultrasound in infantile hydrocephalus, *Childs Nerv Syst* 1:244-247, 1985.

781. van den Wijngaard JA, Reuss A, Wladimiroff JW: The blood flow velocity waveform in the fetal internal carotid artery in the presence of hydrocephaly, *Early Hum Dev* 18:95-99, 1988.

782. Norelle A, Fischer AQ, Flannery AM: Transcranial Doppler: A noninvasive method to monitor hydrocephalus, *J Child Neurol* 4:S87-S90, 1989.

783. Fischer AQ, Shuman RM, Anderson JC, Stinson W: *Pediatric Neurosonography: Clinical, Tomographic, and Neuropathologic Correlates*, New York: 1985, John Wiley & Sons.

784. Chadduck WM, Seibert JJ: Intracranial duplex Doppler: Practical uses in pediatric neurology and neurosurgery, *J Child Neurol* 4:S77-S86, 1989.

785. Chadduck WM, Seibert JJ, Adametz J, Glasier CM, et al: Cranial Doppler ultrasonography correlates with criteria for ventriculoperitoneal shunting, *Surg Neurol* 31:122-128, 1989.

786. Seibert JJ, McCowan TC, Chadduck WM, Adametz JR, et al: Duplex pulsed Doppler US versus intracranial pressure in the neonate: Clinical and experimental studies, *Radiology* 171:155-159, 1989.

787. Lui K, Hellmann J, Sprigg A, Daneman A: Cerebral blood-flow velocity patterns in post-hemorrhagic ventricular dilation, *Childs Nerv Syst* 6:250-253, 1990.

788. Goh D, Minns RA, Pye SD, Steers AJ: Cerebral blood flow velocity changes after ventricular taps and ventriculoperitoneal shunting, *Childs Nerv Syst* 7:452-457, 1991.

789. Goh D, Minns RA, Pye SD: Transcranial Doppler (TCD) ultrasound as a noninvasive means of monitoring cerebrohaemodynamic change in hydrocephalus, *Eur J Pediatr Surg* 1:14-17, 1991.

790. Huang C-C, Chio C-C: Duplex color ultrasound study of infantile progressive ventriculomegaly, *Childs Nerv Syst* 7:251-256, 1991.

791. Goh D, Minns RA, Pye SD, Steers AJ: Cerebral blood-flow velocity and intermittent intracranial pressure elevation during sleep in hydrocephalic children, *Dev Med Child Neurol* 34:676-689, 1992.

792. Quinn MW, Ando Y, Levene MI: Cerebral arterial and venous flow-velocity measurements in post-haemorrhagic ventricular dilatation and hydrocephalus, *Dev Med Child Neurol* 34:863-869, 1992.

793. Kempley ST, Gamsu HR: Changes in cerebral artery blood flow velocity after intermittent cerebrospinal fluid drainage, *Arch Dis Child* 69:74-76, 1993.

794. Taylor GA, Phillips MD, Ichord RN, Carson BS, et al: Intracranial compliance in infants: Evaluation with Doppler US, *Radiology* 191:787-791, 1994.

795. Taylor GA, Madsen JR: Neonatal hydrocephalus: Hemodynamic response to fontanelle compression: Correlation with intracranial pressure and need for shunt placement, *Radiology* 201:685-689, 1996.

796. Maertzdorf WJ, Vles JSH, Beuls E, Mulder ALM, et al: Intracranial pressure and cerebral blood flow velocity in preterm infants with posthaemorrhagic ventricular dilatation, *Arch Dis Child* 87:185-188, 2002.

797. Soul J, Eichewald E, Walter G, Volpe JJ, et al: CSF removal in infantile posthemorrhagic hydrocephalus results in significant improvement in cerebral hemodynamics, *Pediatr Res* 55:872-876, 2004.

797a. van Alfen-van der Velden AA, Hopman JC, Klaessens JH, Feuth T, et al: Cerebral hemodynamics and oxygenation after serial CSF drainage in infants with PHVD, *Brain Dev* 29:623-629, 2007.

798. Ehle A, Sklar F: Visual evoked potentials in infants with hydrocephalus, *Neurology* 29:1541-1544, 1979.

799. McSherry JW, Walters CL, Horbar JD: Acute visual evoked potential changes in hydrocephalus, *Electroencephalogr Clin Neurophysiol* 53:331-333, 1982.

800. Walker ML, Cevette MJ, Newberg N, Moss SD, et al: Auditory brain stem responses in neonatal hydrocephalus, *Concepts Pediatr Neurosurg* 7:142-152, 1987.

801. Foltz EL, Blanks JP, McPherson DL: Hydrocephalus: Increased intracranial pressure and brain stem auditory evoked responses in the hydrocephalic rabbit, *Neurosurgery* 20:211-218, 1987.

802. de Vries LS, Pierrat V, Minami T, Smet M, et al: The role of short latency somatosensory evoked responses in infants with rapidly progressive ventricular dilatation, *Neuropediatrics* 21:136-139, 1990.

803. Del Bigio MR, Bruni JE: Changes in periventricular vasculature of rabbit brain following induction of hydrocephalus and after shunting, *J Neurosurg* 69:115-120, 1988.

804. Weller RO, Mitchell J: Cerebrospinal fluid edema and its sequelae in hydrocephalus, *Adv Neurol* 28:111-123, 1980.

805. Weller RO, Wisniewski H, Ishii N, Shulman K, et al: Brain tissue damage in hydrocephalus, *Dev Med Child Neurol Suppl* 20:1-7, 1969.

806. Rowlatt U: The microscopic effects of ventricular dilatation without increase in head size, *J Neurosurg* 48:957-961, 1978.

807. Ulfig N, Bohl J, Neudorfer F, Rezaie P: Brain macrophages and microglia in human fetal hydrocephalus, *Brain Dev* 26:307-315, 2004.

808. Whitelaw A, Rosengren L, Blennow M: Brain specific proteins in posthaemorrhagic ventricular dilatation, *Arch Dis Child Fetal Neonatal Ed* 84:F90-F91, 2001.

809. Bejar R, Saugstad OD, James H, Gluck L: Increased hypoxanthine concentrations in cerebrospinal fluid of infants with hydrocephalus, *J Pediatr* 103:44-48, 1983.

810. White RP, Leffler CW, Bada HS: Eicosanoid levels in CSF of premature infants with posthemorrhagic hydrocephalus, *Am J Med Sci* 299:230-235, 1990.

811. Casaer P, von Siebenthal K, van der Vlugt A, Lagae L, et al: Cytochrome aa3 and intracranial pressure in newborn infants; a near infrared spectroscopy study [letter], *Neuropediatrics* 23:111, 1992.

812. Shirane R, Sato S, Sato K, Kameyama M, et al: Cerebral blood flow and oxygen metabolism in infants with hydrocephalus, *Child Nerv Syst* 8:118-123, 1992.

813. Anwar M, Kadam S, Hiatt IM, Hegyi T: Serial lumbar punctures in prevention of post-hemorrhagic hydrocephalus in preterm infants, *J Pediatr* 107:446-450, 1985.

814. Todo T, Usui M, Takakura K: Treatment of severe intraventricular hemorrhage by intraventricular infusion of urokinase, *J Neurosurg* 74:81-86, 1991.

815. Hansen AR: CNS fibrinolysis: A review of the literature with a pediatric emphasis, *Pediatr Neurol* 18:15-21, 1998.

816. Whitelaw A: Endogenous fibrinolysis in neonatal cerebrospinal fluid, *Eur J Pediatr* 152:928-930, 1993.

817. Whitelaw A, Rivers RP, Creighton L, Gaffney P: Low dose intraventricular fibrinolytic treatment to prevent posthaemorrhagic hydrocephalus, *Arch Dis Child* 67:12-14, 1992.

818. Whitelaw A, Mowinckel M-C, Larsen ML, Rokas E, et al: Intraventricular streptokinase increases cerebrospinal fluid D dimer in preterm infants with posthaemorrhagic ventricular dilatation, *Acta Paediatr* 83:270-272, 1994.

819. Hudgins RJ, Boydston WR, Hudgins PA, Adler SR: Treatment of intraventricular hemorrhage in the premature infant with urokinase, *Pediatr Neurosurg* 20:190-197, 1994.

820. Whitelaw A, Saliba E, Fellman V, Mowinckel C, et al: A phase 1 study of intraventricular recombinant tissue plasminogen activator for the treatment of posthemorrhagic hydrocephalus, *Arch Dis Child Fetal Neonatal Ed* 75:F20-F26, 1996.

821. Luciano R, Verlardi F, Romagnoli C, Papacci P, et al: Failure of fibrinolytic endoventricular treatment to prevent neonatal post-haemorrhagic hydrocephalus: A case-control trial, *Child Nerv Syst* 13:73-76, 1997.

822. Hansen AR, Volpe JJ, Goumnerova LC, Madsen JR: Intraventricular urokinase for the treatment of posthemorrhagic hydrocephalus, *Pediatr Neurol* 17:213-217, 1997.

823. Whitelaw A: Intraventricular streptokinase after intraventricular hemorrhage in newborn infants, *Cochrane Database Syst Rev* 1:CD000498, 2001.

824. Papile LA, Burstein J, Burstein R, Koffler H, et al: Posthemorrhagic hydrocephalus in low-birth-weight infants: Treatment by serial lumbar punctures, *J Pediatr* 97:273-277, 1980.

825. Camfield PR, Camfield CS, Allen AC, Rees EP, et al: Progressive hydrocephalus in infants with birth weights less than 1,500 g, *Arch Neurol* 38:653-655, 1981.

826. Levene MI, Starte DR: A longitudinal study of post-haemorrhagic ventricular dilatation in the newborn, *Arch Dis Child* 56:905-910, 1981.

827. Muller WD, Urlesberger B: Correlation of ventricular size and head circumference after severe intraperiventricular haemorrhage in preterm infants, *Child Nerv Syst* 8:33-35, 1992.

828. Saliba E, Bertrand P, Gold F, Vaillant MC, et al: Area of lateral ventricles measured on cranial ultrasonography in preterm infants: Reference range, *Arch Dis Child* 65:1029-1032, 1990.

829. Kohn MI, Tanna NK, Herman GT, Resnick SM, et al: Analysis of brain and cerebrospinal fluid volumes with MR imaging. I. Methods reliability, and validation, *Radiology* 178:115-122, 1991.

830. Brann BS 4th, Qualls C, Wells L, Papile L: Asymmetric growth of the lateral cerebral ventricle in infants with posthemorrhagic ventricular dilation, *J Pediatr* 118:108-112, 1991.

831. Cooke RW: Early prognosis of low birthweight infants treated for progressive posthemorrhagic hydrocephalus, *Arch Dis Child* 58:410-414, 1983.

832. Lipscomb AP, Thorburn RJ, Stewart AL, Reynolds EO, et al: Early treatment for rapidly progressive post-haemorrhagic hydrocephalus [letter], *Lancet* 1:1438-1439, 1983.

833. Goldstein GW, Chaplin ER, Maitland J, Norman D: Transient hydrocephalus in premature infants: Treatment by lumbar punctures, *Lancet* 1:512-514, 1976.

834. Papile LA, Koffler H, Burstein R, Koops B: Non-surgical treatment of acquired hydrocephalus: Evaluation of serial lumbar puncture, *Pediatr Res* 12:445, 1978.

835. de Vries LS, Benders M, Groenendaal F: Improved outcome in preterm infants with a large intraventricular hemorrhage: A relationship with earlier intervention? [abstract 3590], *Pediatr Res* 58:S322, 2006.

836. Whitelaw A: Repeated lumbar or ventricular punctures in newborns with intraventricular hemorrhage, *Cochrane Database Syst Rev* 2005.

837. Levene MI: Measurement of the growth of the lateral ventricles in preterm infants with real-time ultrasound, *Arch Dis Child* 56:900-904, 1981.

838. Gleason CA, Martin RJ, Anderson JV, Carlo WA, et al: Optimal position for a spinal tap in preterm infants, *Pediatrics* 71:31-35, 1983.

839. Bergman I, Wald ER, Meyer JD, Painter MJ: Epidural abscess and vertebral osteomyelitis following serial lumbar punctures, *Pediatrics* 72:476-480, 1983.

840. Potgieter S, Dimin S, Lagae L, Van Calenbergh F, et al: Epidermoid tumours associated with lumbar punctures performed in early neonatal life, *Dev Med Child Neurol* 40:266-269, 1998.

841. Smith KM, Deddish RB, Ogata ES: Meningitis associated with serial lumbar punctures and post-hemorrhagic hydrocephalus, *J Pediatr* 109:1057-1060, 1986.

842. Neblett CR, Waltz TA Jr, McNeel DP, Harrison GM: Effect of cardiac glycosides on human cerebrospinal-fluid production, *Lancet* 2:1008-1009, 1972.

843. Bass NH, Fallstrom SP, Lundborg P: Digoxin-induced arrest of the cerebrospinal fluid circulation in the infant rat: Implications for medical treatment of hydrocephalus during early postnatal life, *Pediatr Res* 13:26-30, 1979.

844. McCarthy KD, Reed DJ: The effect of acetazolamide and furosemide on cerebrospinal fluid production and choroid plexus carbonic anhydrase activity, *J Pharmacol Exp Ther* 189:194-201, 1974.

845. Carrion E, Hertzog JH, Medlock MD, Hauser GJ, et al: Use of acetazolamide to decrease cerebrospinal fluid production in chronically ventilated patients with ventriculopleural shunts, *Arch Dis Child* 83:68-71, 2001.

846. Shinnar S, Gammon K, Bergman EW Jr, Epstein M, et al: Management of hydrocephalus in infancy: Use of acetazolamide and furosemide to avoid cerebrospinal fluid shunts, *J Pediatr* 107:31-37, 1985.

847. Stafstrom CE, Gilmore HE, Kurtin PS: Nephrocalcinosis complicating medical treatment of posthemorrhagic hydrocephalus, *Pediatr Neurol* 8:179-182, 1992.

848. Whitelaw A: Diuretic therapy for newborn infants with posthemorrhagic ventricular dilatation, *Cochrane Database Syst Rev* 2:CD002270, 2005.

849. Sapirstein VS, Lees MB: Purification of myelin carbonic anhydrase, *J Neurochem* 31:505-511, 1978.

850. Kumpulainen T, Korhonen LK: Immunohistochemical localization of carbonic anhydrase isoenzyme C in the central and peripheral nervous system of the mouse, *J Histochem Cytochem* 30:283-292, 1982.

851. Cammer W: Carbonic anhydrase in myelin and glial cells in the mammalian central nervous system. In Dodgson SJ, Tashian RE, Gros G, et al, editors: *The Carbonic Anhydrases*, New York: 1991, Plenum Publishing.

852. Cammer W, Zhang H: Carbonic anhydrase in distinct precursors of astrocytes and oligodendrocytes in the forebrains of neonatal and young rats, *Dev Brain Res* 67:257-263, 1992.

853. Hochwald GM, Wald A, Malhan C: The sink action of cerebrospinal fluid volume flow: Effect on brain water content, *Arch Neurol* 33:339-344, 1976.

854. Hochwald GM, Wald A, DiMattio J, Malhan C: The effects of serum osmolarity on cerebrospinal fluid volume flow, *Life Sci* 15:1309-1316, 1974.

855. Laurent JP, El-Hibri H, Okumura S: Glycerol's effect on cerebrospinal fluid formation, *Concept Pediatr Neurosurg* 5:84, 1985.

856. Shurtleff DB, Hayden PW, Weeks R, Laurence KM: Temporary treatment of hydrocephalus and myelodysplasia with isosorbide: Preliminary report, *J Pediatr* 83:651-657, 1973.

857. Lorber J: Isosorbide in treatment of infantile hydrocephalus, *Arch Dis Child* 50:431-436, 1975.

858. Salfield AW, Lorber J, Lonton T: Isosorbide in the management of infantile hydrocephalus, *Arch Dis Child* 56:806-814, 1981.

859. Taylor DA, Hill A, Fishman MA, Volpe JJ: Treatment of posthemorrhagic hydrocephalus with glycerol, *Ann Neurol* 10:297, 1981.

860. Liptak GS, Gellerstedt ME, Klionsky N: Isosorbide in the medical management of hydrocephalus in children with myelodysplasia, *Dev Med Child Neurol* 34:150-154, 1992.

861. Kreusser KL, Tarby TJ, Taylor D, Kovnar E, et al: Rapidly progressive posthemorrhagic hydrocephalus: Treatment with external ventricular drainage, *Am J Dis Child* 138:633-637, 1984.

862. Marlin AE: Protection of the cortical mantle in premature infants with posthemorrhagic hydrocephalus, *Neurosurgery* 7:464-468, 1980.

863. Harbaugh RE, Saunders RL, Edwards WH: External ventricular drainage for control of posthemorrhagic hydrocephalus in premature infants, *J Neurosurg* 55:766-770, 1981.

864. McComb JG, Ramos AD, Platzker AC, Henderson DJ, et al: Management of hydrocephalus secondary to intraventricular hemorrhage in the preterm infant with a subcutaneous ventricular catheter reservoir, *Neurosurgery* 13:295-300, 1983.

865. Saladino A, Gainsburg D, Zmora E, Ronen Y, et al: Ventriculosubcutaneous shunt for temporary treatment of neonatal post-IVH hydrocephalus: A technical note, *Childs Nerv Syst* 2:206-207, 1986.

866. Rhodes TT, Edwards WH, Saunders RL, Harbaugh RE, et al: External ventricular drainage for initial treatment of neonatal posthemorrhagic hydrocephalus: Surgical and neurodevelopmental outcome, *Pediatr Neurosci* 13:255-262, 1987.

867. Sklar F, Adegbite A, Shapiro K, Miller K: Ventriculosubgaleal shunts: Management of posthemorrhagic hydrocephalus in premature infants, *Pediatr Neurosurg* 18:263-265, 1992.

868. Weninger M, Mclone DG, Rekate HL, Salzer HR, et al: External ventricular drainage for treatment of rapidly progressive posthemorrhagic hydrocephalus, *Neurosurgery* 31:52-58, 1992.

869. Marlin AE, Rivera S, Gaskill SJ: Treatment of posthemorrhagic ventriculomegaly in the preterm infant: Use of the subcutaneous ventricular reservoir. In Marlin AE, editor: *Concepts in Pediatric Neurosurgery*, Vol 8, Basel: 1988, Karger.

870. Leonhardt A, Steiner HH, Linderkamp O: Management of posthaemorrhagic hydrocephalus with a subcutaneous ventricular catheter reservoir in premature infants, *Arch Dis Child* 64:24-28, 1989.

871. Brockmeyer DL, Wright LC, Walker ML, Ward RM: Management of posthemorrhagic hydrocephalus in the low-birth-weight preterm neonate, *Pediatr Neurosci* 15:302-307, 1989.

872. Whitelaw A, Pople I, Cherian S, Evans DA, et al: Phase I trial of prevention of hydrocephalus after intraventricular hemorrhage in newborn infants by drainage, irrigation and fibrinolytic therapy, *Pediatrics* 111:759-765, 2003.

873. Whitelaw A, Evans D, Carter M, Thoresen M, et al: Randomised clinical trial of prevention of hydrocephalus after intraventricular hemorrhage in premature infants: Brain-washing v tapping fluid, *Pediatrics* 119:e1071-e1078, 2007.

874. Levene MI: Ventricular tap under direct ultrasound control, *Arch Dis Child* 57:873-875, 1982.

875. Afschrift M, Jeannin P, de Praeter C, van Egmond H, et al: Ventricular taps in the neonate under ultrasonic guidance. Technical note, *J Neurosurg* 59:1100-1101, 1983.

876. Weissman LT, Marro PJ, Kessler DL, Sobel DB, et al: Progressive ventricular dilatation (PVD) over the past 22 years [comment], *Arch Dis Child Fetal Neonatal Ed* 88:F257, 2003.

877. Mayhall CG, Archer NH, Lamb VA, Spadora AC, et al: Ventriculostomy-related infections: A prospective epidemiologic study, *N Engl J Med* 310:553-559, 1984.

878. Bass JK, Bass WT, Green GA, Gurtner P, et al: Intracranial pressure changes during intermittent CSF drainage, *Pediatr Neurol* 28:173-177, 2003.

879. Deonna T, Payot M, Probst A, Prod'hom LS: Neonatal intracranial hemorrhage in premature infants, *Pediatrics* 56:1056-1064, 1975.

880. Fitzhardinge PM, Pape P, Arstikaitis M, Boyle M, et al: Mechanical ventilation of infants of less than 1,501 gm birth weight: Health, growth, and neurologic sequelae, *J Pediatr* 88:531-541, 1976.

881. Wise BL, Ballard R: Hydrocephalus secondary to intracranial hemorrhage in premature infants, *Childs Brain* 2:234-241, 1976.

882. Bada HS, Salmon JH, Pearson DH: Early surgical intervention in posthemorrhagic hydrocephalus, *Childs Brain* 5:109-115, 1979.

883. Scharff TB, Anderson DE, Anderson CL, Caldwell CC: Complications of ventriculo-peritoneal shunts in premature infants, *Concept Pediatr Neurosurg* 4:81, 1983.

884. Etches PC, Ward TF, Bhui PS, Peters KL, et al: Outcome of shunted posthemorrhagic hydrocephalus in premature infants, *Pediatr Neurol* 3:136-140, 1987.

885. Davis SL, Tooley WH, Hunt JV: Developmental outcome following posthemorrhagic hydrocephalus in preterm infants: Comparison of twins discordant for hydrocephalus, *Am J Dis Child* 141:1170-1174, 1987.

886. Cooke RW: Determinants of major handicap in post-haemorrhagic hydrocephalus, *Arch Dis Child* 62:504-506, 1987.

887. Sasidharan P, Marquez E, Dizon E, Sridhar CV: Developmental outcome of infants with severe intracranial-intraventricular hemorrhage and hydrocephalus with and without ventriculoperitoneal shunt, *Childs Nerv Syst* 2:149-152, 1986.

888. Boynton BR, Boynton CA, Merritt TA, Vaucher YE, et al: Ventriculoperitoneal shunts in low birth weight infants with intracranial hemorrhage: Neurodevelopmental outcome, *Neurosurgery* 18:141-145, 1986.

889. Lin JP, Goh W, Brown JK, Steers AJW: Neurological outcome following neonatal post-haemorrhagic hydrocephalus: The effects of maximum raised intracranial pressure and ventriculo-peritoneal shunting, *Child Nerv Syst* 8:190-197, 1992.

890. Hislop JE, Dubowitz LM, Kaiser AM, Singh MP, et al: Outcome of infants shunted for post-haemorrhagic ventricular dilatation, *Dev Med Child Neurol* 30:451-456, 1988.

891. Gurtner P, Bass T, Gudeman SK, Penix JO, et al: Surgical management of posthemorrhagic hydrocephalus in 22 low-birth-weight infants, *Child Nerv Syst* 8:198-202, 1992.

892. Heinsbergen I, Rotteveel J, Roeleveld N, Grotenhuis A: Outcome in shunted hydrocephalic children, *Eur J Paediatr Neurol* 6:99-107, 2002.

893. Futagi Y, Suzuki Y, Toribe Y, Nakano H, et al: Neurodevelopmental outcome in children with posthemorrhagic hydrocephalus, *Pediatric Neurology* 33:26-32, 2005.

894. Battaglia D, Pasca MG, Cesarini L, Tartaglione T, et al: Epilepsy in shunted posthemorrhagic infantile hydrocephalus owing to pre- or perinatal intra- or periventricular hemorrhage, *J Child Neurol* 20:219-225, 2005.

895. Fletcher JM, Landry SH, Bohan TP, Davidson KC, et al: Effects of intraventricular hemorrhage and hydrocephalus on the long-term neurobehavioral development of preterm very-low-birthweight infants, *Dev Med Ch Neurol* 39:596-606, 1997.

896. James HE, Bejar R, Merritt AT, Mannino F, et al: Insidious hydrocephalus in the preterm newborn following discharge from the nursery, *Pediatr Neurosci* 13:129-134, 1987.

METABOLIC ENCEPHALOPATHIES

Chapter 12

Hypoglycemia and Brain Injury

Glucose, like oxygen, is of essential and fundamental importance for brain metabolism. Indeed, because oxygen consumption is relatively low in neonatal human brain, and minimal in such areas as cerebral white matter (see Chapter 6), glucose supply to brain may be even more important. The major source of brain glucose is the blood supply, and thus it is readily understood that serious encephalopathy should ensue when the glucose content of blood becomes deficient.

In this chapter, the normal aspects of glucose metabolism in brain are discussed before review of the biochemical derangements with hypoglycemia. The neuropathology of hypoglycemia is described next, and, on the background of the biochemical and neuropathological derangements, the clinical aspects are reviewed. To begin the discussion, an attempt to define hypoglycemia is presented with an explanation of why this attempt is so difficult.

DEFINITION

Definition of the level of blood glucose that should be considered too low is difficult, in part because the newborn does not have the neural capacity to demonstrate consistently, by overt symptoms, when the critical lower limit has been passed. In few areas of neonatal neurology, other than hypoglycemia, has the unproven concept persisted so firmly that a serious disturbance of the neonatal central nervous system is unlikely in the absence of overt neurological signs. Thus, the critical lower limit of blood glucose level for maintenance of neonatal neural integrity in various clinical circumstances is unknown. Moreover, and most important, these lower limits probably are higher when concomitant insults that increase cerebral demand for glucose and that are deleterious to the brain (e.g., hypoxemia and ischemia) accompany hypoglycemia. Indeed, the concept of the additive and potentiating role of hypoglycemia in the production of brain injury in the sick newborn infant may now be the most critical neurological aspect of neonatal hypoglycemia.

Definition of a blood glucose level lower than which hypoglycemia should be designated has been based usually on statistical measures (i.e., marked deviation from "normal" blood glucose levels). Previous determinations of such blood glucose levels in the newborn were derived from infants generally not fed in the first hours of life.[1,2] Such determinations led to the definition of "significant hypoglycemia" in the newborn as a whole

blood glucose concentration lower than 30 mg/dL (<35 mg/dL of plasma) in the term infant and lower than 20 mg/dL (<25 mg/dL of plasma) in the preterm infant. Later determinations of normal plasma glucose suggested that these values are too low (Table 12-1).[3-16] Thus, in one large study of the healthy term infant, mean plasma glucose values reached a nadir of 55 to 60 mg/dL at 1 to 2 hours after birth and began to increase even before first feedings at 3 to 4 hours of age (Fig. 12-1).[3] Mean values from 3 to 72 hours were approximately 70 mg/dL, after which they were approximately 80 mg/dL. Thus, on a statistical basis, *hypoglycemia*, defined as a plasma glucose concentration less than approximately the fifth percentile, could be designated as shown in Table 12-1.

Cornblath and co-workers suggested that the term *hypoglycemia* is not readily defined for individual patients and that "operational thresholds" (i.e., "a concentration of blood or plasma glucose at which clinicians should consider intervention") should be established.[11,17] These thresholds were defined as less than 45 mg/dL (2.5 mmol/L) for "the infant with abnormal clinical signs" and less than 36 mg/dL (2.0 mmol/L) for the asymptomatic infant and the infant "at risk for hypoglycemia" (without regard to gestational or postnatal age).

Importantly, however, such statistical or "operational" definitions do not address whether the threshold level of blood glucose represents the threshold level for neuronal injury. Indeed, determinations of brain stem auditory evoked responses in a small series of term infants showed prolonged latencies at levels lower than approximately 47 mg/dL (Fig. 12-2) (see later discussion).[6] A later report did not detect prolongation of latency to wave V until blood glucose fell to 25 mg/dL, in a single infant.[18] Moreover, in a study of visual evoked potentials in nine hypoglycemic infants, well-defined latencies of

TABLE 12-1	Chemical Definitions of Hypoglycemia in Term Infants
"Hypoglycemia"*	
<35 mg/dL, 0–3 hr	
<40 mg/dL, 3–24 hr	
<45 mg/dL, >24 hr	

*Glucose determined in plasma.

Data from Srinivasan G, Pildes RS, Cattamanchi G, Voora S, et al: Clinical and laboratory observations: Plasma glucose values in normal neonates—a new look, *J Pediatr* 109:114–117, 1986.

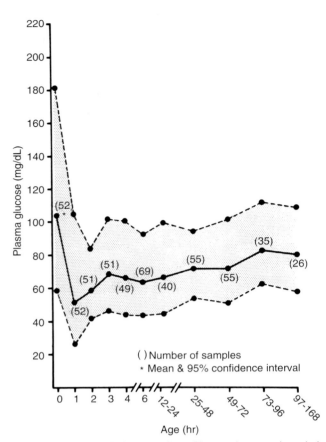

Figure 12-1 **Neonatal glucose values.** Plasma glucose values during the first week of life in healthy term newborns appropriate for gestational age. *(From Srinivasan G, Pildes RS, Cattamanchi G, Voora S, et al: Clinical and laboratory observations: Plasma glucose values in normal neonates—a new look,* J Pediatr *109:114–117, 1986.)*

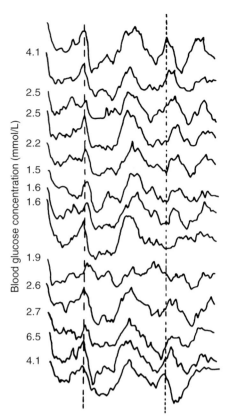

Figure 12-2 **Serial brain stem auditory evoked potentials recorded in a 2-day-old infant in relation to his blood glucose concentration.** The *vertical lines* indicate the latency between wave I and wave V in the initial recording during normoglycemia. Note the prolongation of latency when blood glucose values decreased to 2.5 mmol/L and lower. *(From Koh TH, Aynsley-Green A, Tarbit M, Eyre JA: Neural dysfunction during hypoglycaemia,* Arch Dis Child *63:1353–1358, 1988.)*

visual evoked potentials were observed.[19] The duration of hypoglycemia was not determined but was considered "short."[19] However, careful epidemiological studies suggested a deleterious effect on subsequent cognitive development in infants whose plasma glucose levels were less than approximately 47 mg/dL on at least one occasion on 3 or more separate days (Fig. 12-3).[20] Abnormalities in arithmetic and motor scores persisted at 7.5 to 8 years.[21] In both the neurophysiological and the epidemiological studies that suggest a deleterious effect of hypoglycemia, neonatal neurological signs were minimal or absent. Thus, clearly *duration* and *degree* of depression of blood glucose are crucial. As discussed later, studies of human infants showed an increase in cerebral blood flow (CBF) at glucose values lower than 30 mg/dL and suggested that at a glucose level lower than approximately 54 mg/dL, transport becomes limiting for cerebral glucose use. Additional factors of importance in determination of a critical threshold value of blood glucose are the *rates of CBF and of cerebral utilization of glucose*, as well as the presence of any alternative substrates. Thus, the threshold level of *blood* glucose is different in the infant with *impaired CBF*, as with hypotension, or with *increased cerebral glucose utilization*, as with seizures or with the

anaerobic glycolytic metabolism of hypoxia-ischemia or asphyxia. Currently, I believe that the definition of hypoglycemia must be individualized according to the infant's clinical situation (see "Management" later), and that the normative statistical data shown in Table 12-1 and Figure 12-1 should be considered only starting points.

NORMAL METABOLIC ASPECTS

Brain as the Primary Determinant of Glucose Production

The pathophysiology of neonatal hypoglycemic encephalopathy has as its basis the importance of glucose as the primary metabolic fuel for brain. Glucose for normal brain metabolism is derived from the blood, and glucose production in mammals is primarily a function of the liver. The postnatal induction of hepatic glycogenolysis and gluconeogenesis and the interplay of insulin, glucagon, catecholamines, corticosteroids, and other hormones in the regulation of hepatic glucose metabolism have been reviewed in detail by others.[2,13,15,22-27] It need only be emphasized here that the brain appears to be the major determinant

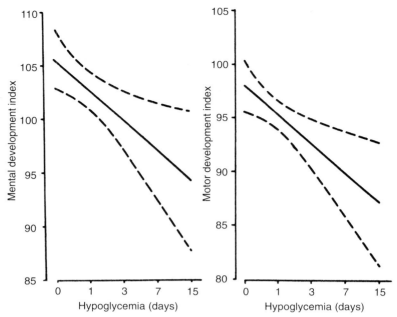

Figure 12-3   Logarithm of days of recorded hypoglycemia lower than 2.6 mmol/L related to Bayley Mental Development Index and Bayley Psychomotor Development Index at 18 months (corrected age) in a series of 433 premature infants. Regression slopes and 95% confidence intervals (*dashed lines*) are shown adjusted for days of ventilation, sex, social class, birth weight, and fetal growth retardation. Data shown are for both sexes and all social classes combined and for no ventilation. For infants ventilated for 1 to 6, 7 to 14, or more than 14 days, subtract 5, 10, or 15 points, respectively, for mental development index and 4.5, 9.0, or 13.5 points, respectively, for psychomotor development index. *(From Lucas A, Morley R, Cole TJ: Adverse neurodevelopment outcome of moderate neonatal hypoglycaemia, BMJ 297:1304–1308, 1988.)*

of (hepatic) glucose production.[28] Thus, glucose production was measured in a series of infants and children from 1 to 25 kg in body weight by a continuous 3- to 4-hour infusion of the nonradioactive tracer, 6,6-dideuteroglucose. Glucose production on a body weight basis was found to be twofold to threefold greater in newborns than in older patients. The infants clearly had disproportionately higher rates of glucose production when compared with adult subjects. This observation becomes understandable when glucose production is plotted as a function of estimated brain weight (Fig. 12-4). The linear relationship suggests that the disproportionately high rates of glucose production in the neonatal period relate to the disproportionately large neonatal brain. Because central nervous system consumption of glucose accounts for 30% or more of total hepatic glucose output, at least in the premature infant, this relationship between glucose production rate and brain weight seems reasonable.[29]

The mechanisms by which utilization of glucose by the brain may regulate hepatic glucose output are unknown. It is possible that the effect is mediated by subtle changes in blood glucose levels, acting directly on pancreatic insulin secretion or on hepatic glucose output. More provocative is the possibility that the brain mediates control over hepatic glucose production by neural or hormonal effectors, originating within the central nervous system.[28] This possibility leads to the interesting logical extension that disturbances of brain may *lead to* disturbances in glucose output by liver and *result in* hypoglycemia or hyperglycemia (see later discussion). Moreover, size of brain

per se may also possibly lead to disturbances in glucose output, secondary to changes in glucose utilization. At any rate, in the normal human, from the newborn period to adulthood, it is now clear a very close relationship exists between brain mass and glucose production.

Glucose Metabolism in Brain

Glucose metabolism in brain is depicted in a simplified fashion in Figure 12-5. Those aspects particularly relevant to this chapter are shown; further review of cerebral glucose and energy metabolism is contained in Chapter 6.[30-37]

Glucose Uptake

Glucose uptake from blood into brain occurs by a process that is not energy dependent but that proceeds faster than expected by simple diffusion (i.e., carrier-mediated, facilitated diffusion). The transport is mediated by a specific protein, a glucose transporter.[34,35,38-42] The brain glucose transporter is concentrated in capillaries, and the concentration of the transporter increases with development. In the rat, the lower apparent blood-brain glucose permeability in the newborn ($\approx$25% of adult values) is related to a lower concentration of the glucose transporter (not to a lower affinity of the transporter for glucose). Studies of human premature infants also suggest that the number of available endothelial transporters is approximately one third to one half the value for human adult brain.[29] The importance of the transporter for brain

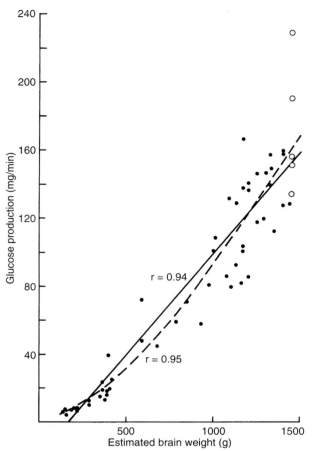

Figure 12-4 **Linear relationship between glucose production and (estimated) brain weight in subjects ranging from premature infants of approximately 1000 g to adults.** Glucose production was measured by continuous infusion of 6,6-dideuteroglucose. The linear and quadratic functions are depicted by *solid* and *dashed lines*, respectively. *(From Bier DM, Leake RD, Haymond MW: Measurement of true glucose production rates in infancy and childhood with 6,6-dideuteroglucose,* Diabetes *26:1016–1023, 1977.)*

function and structure is illustrated by the occurrence of seizures and developmental delay in infants with partial deficiency of the transporter (see Chapters 5 and 16).[39] The glucose concentration normally present in blood in the newborn rat is approximately one fourth that required for glucose uptake to proceed at maximal velocity.[34,43] *Studies of the human premature infant by positron emission tomography indicate that at a plasma glucose level of approximately 3 μmol/mL (i.e., ≈54 mg/dL), transport becomes limiting for cerebral glucose utilization.*[29] *Thus, uptake is one potential site for regulation of glucose metabolism in brain, and this regulation is particularly dependent on changes in blood glucose concentrations.*

Hexokinase

The initial step in glucose utilization in brain is phosphorylation to glucose-6-phosphate by *hexokinase* (see Fig. 12-5). This enzyme is inhibited not only by its product but also by adenosine triphosphate (ATP). Under certain circumstances, hexokinase is an important control point in glycolysis.[37,39,44,45]

Major Fates of Glucose-6-Phosphate

The product of the hexokinase reaction, glucose-6-phosphate, is at an important branch point in glucose metabolism (see Fig. 12-5). From glucose-6-phosphate originate pathways to the formation of glycogen, to the pentose monophosphate shunt, and through glycolysis to pyruvate. *Glycogen* is important as a readily available store of glucose in brain; glycogenolysis is an actively regulated process that is called into play during periods of glucose lack (i.e., hypoglycemia) or accelerated glucose utilization (e.g., oxygen deprivation [with associated anaerobic glycolysis] or seizures). Glycogen is concentrated in astrocytes, and with low brain glucose, astrocytic glycogenolysis is activated to produce glucose-6-phosphate. The latter is converted to lactate, which then enters the neuron for use as an energy source (see later).[45a] The *pentose monophosphate shunt* provides reducing equivalents, important for lipid synthesis, and ribose units, important for nucleic acid synthesis. These two synthetic processes are of particular importance in developing brain. The generation of reducing equivalents also is critical for generation of reduced glutathione, crucial for defense against free radicals and thereby hypoglycemic cellular injury (see later discussion).

The major fate of glucose-6-phosphate in brain is entrance into the *glycolytic pathway*, principally for the ultimate production of *chemical energy* in the form of high-energy phosphate bonds (i.e., ATP and its storage form, phosphocreatine). When oxidized aerobically, each molecule of glucose generates 38 molecules of high-energy phosphate compounds. The next several sections describe the utilization of glucose for energy production.

Phosphofructokinase

The most critical step in the glycolytic pathway is the conversion of fructose-6-phosphate to fructose-1,6-diphosphate; the enzyme involved, phosphofructokinase, is a major regulatory, rate-limiting step in glycolysis (see Fig. 12-5). The enzyme is inhibited by ATP and is activated by adenosine diphosphate (ADP). The ammonium ion (NH_4^+), generated by amino acid transamination, is also a potent activator of this complex.

Pyruvate

The glycolytic pathway ultimately results in the formation of pyruvate, most of which enters the mitochondrion and is converted to acetyl-coenzyme A (acetyl-CoA) (see Fig. 12-5). However, pyruvate also can result in formation of lactate when the cytosolic redox state is shifted toward reduction. Conversely, under the conditions of hypoglycemia (i.e., [1] available lactate and deficient pyruvate, [2] a cytosolic redox state that is normal or shifted toward oxidation, and [3] the action of lactate dehydrogenase), lactate can lead to formation of pyruvate and can become an energy source (see later discussion). Finally, alanine may be converted to pyruvate by transamination and can therefore become a source of glucose or acetyl-CoA.

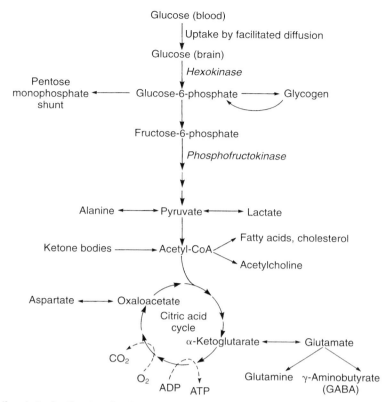

Figure 12-5   Glucose metabolism in brain. See text for details. ADP, adenosine diphosphate; ATP, adenosine triphosphate.

Acetyl-Coenzyme A

The formation of acetyl-CoA by pyruvate dehydrogenase is the major starting point for the citric acid cycle (see Fig. 12-5). This step is an important rate-limiting process in glucose utilization in neonatal brain.[34,35] Acetyl-CoA is also the major starting point for the synthesis of brain lipids and acetylcholine. Moreover, ketone bodies are converted to acetyl-CoA to become an energy source.

Citric Acid Cycle

The citric acid cycle (with the linked electron transport system) ultimately results in the complete oxidation of the carbon of glucose to carbon dioxide and the generation of nearly all the ATP derived from this sugar (see Fig. 12-5). Transamination reactions interface this segment of glucose utilization with certain amino acids, which thereby can be used for energy production.

Glucose as the Primary Metabolic Fuel for Brain

The role of glucose as the primary fuel for the production of chemical energy and the maintenance of normal function in *mature brain* are supported by three main facts.[30,34,35,46] First, the respiratory quotient (i.e., carbon dioxide output/oxygen uptake) of brain is approximately 1, a finding indicating that carbohydrate is the major substrate oxidized by neural tissue.

Glucose is the only carbohydrate extracted by brain in any significant quantity. Second, cerebral glucose uptake is almost completely accounted for by cerebral oxygen uptake. Third, central nervous system function is rapidly and seriously disturbed by hypoglycemia.

Current data support a similar preeminence for glucose in *immature brain*.[30,35,36] Thus, studies in the newborn dog indicated that glucose consumption in brain accounts for 95% of cerebral energy supply.[47] Moreover, studies in term fetal sheep demonstrated that, under aerobic conditions, glucose is the main substrate metabolized for energy production.[48] Glucose/oxygen quotients of approximately 1.1 were obtained in two different laboratories.[48-50] (The glucose/oxygen quotient is equivalent to the arteriovenous difference of glucose [×6] divided by the arteriovenous difference of oxygen and represents the fraction of cerebral oxygen consumption required for the aerobic metabolism of cerebral glucose.) Although the data demonstrated that glucose is the primary substrate metabolized by brain, the finding that the values for glucose/oxygen quotients are slightly but consistently in excess of 1 suggests that a portion of the glucose is used for purposes other than complete oxidation to generate high-energy phosphate bonds. Other data, based on the fate of labeled glucose in brain, indicate that glucose is also used for the synthesis of other materials (e.g., amino acids via transaminations and lipids via appropriate biosynthetic pathways; see Fig. 12-5).[35,46] Syntheses of membrane lipids and proteins, of course, are critical events in developing brain and probably account for a relatively larger proportion of cerebral glucose utilization than in mature brain.

Important *regional* and *developmental* changes in cerebral glucose utilization have been defined, primarily in animals, but also in human infants.[29,30,34-36,51-53] Thus, early in development, regional differences are relatively few, and brain stem structures generally exhibit the highest rates of glucose utilization. With development, increases in cerebral glucose utilization are most prominent, particularly in cerebral cortical regions. In the human infant, the developmental progression in the first year of life occurs first in sensorimotor cortex and thalamus, next in parietal, temporal, and occipital cortices, and last in frontal cortex and association areas.[51,52] Careful studies in animals, focused primarily on electrophysiological maturation of brain stem and diencephalic structures, showed a close correlation between increases in rates of glucose utilization and acquisition of neuronal function.[34]

Alternative Substrates for Glucose in Brain Metabolism

Overview

Although glucose is the primary metabolic fuel for brain, it is apparent that certain other substrates also can be used for energy production and other metabolic purposes. Under normal circumstances, such alternative substrates are probably not of major importance for energy production. However, under conditions in which glucose is limited (e.g., hypoglycemia), alternative substrates may spare brain function and structure. Substances such as lactate, pyruvate, free fatty acids, glycerol, a variety of ketoacids (i.e., ketone bodies), and certain amino acids have been shown to be capable of partially or wholly supporting respiration of *brain tissue slices* and related in vitro systems.[16,33-37,54,55] Certain of these substrates are produced *in brain*

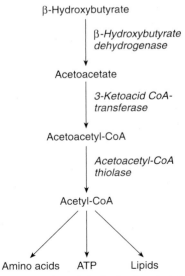

Figure 12-6   Ketone body use in brain. See text for details. ATP, adenosine triphosphate; CoA, coenzyme A.

during hypoglycemia (e.g., amino acids from degradation of protein and fatty acids from degradation of phospholipid) and are potentially utilizable as alternative energy sources (see later discussion). Clearly, however, these latter alternative substrates are not optimal because their sources (i.e., proteins and phospholipids) are largely structural components, and conservation of energy production at the cost of brain structure is not a desirable adaptive response. Moreover, because most of the systemically produced alternative substrates noted either do not appear in appreciable quantities in blood or are not capable of crossing the blood-brain barrier to a major extent, they can contribute relatively little to brain energy levels in hypoglycemia. The two substrates most often considered to be useful as primarily blood-borne, alternative sources of brain energy with hypoglycemia are ketone bodies and lactate, and considerable data show evidence of their value for support of oxidative metabolism in the neonatal brain.[16,30,33-36,56-64]

Ketone Bodies

Appreciable data have accumulated to suggest that ketone bodies may be used as alternative substrates for brain metabolism in the neonatal period. Ketone bodies are taken up by brain by a carrier-mediated transport system and are subsequently used according to the reactions outlined in Figure 12-6.[34,65,66]

Energy Production. Studies of *newborn infants* demonstrated that the cerebral extraction of ketone bodies from blood is markedly greater than in older infants and adults.[34,67] Associated with this finding is an enhanced rate of ketone body utilization in newborn brain. Thus, it was shown that ketone bodies accounted for approximately 12% of total cerebral oxygen consumption in newborns subjected to 6-hour fasts. An enhanced capacity to use ketone bodies was also demonstrated in *human fetal brain*.[68] These data indicate relevance for animal studies that demonstrate relatively high activities for the enzymes involved in ketone body utilization in the immature versus the mature brain.[69-71] These enzymatic activities also have been demonstrated in the human fetal brain.[72]

Thus, the newborn brain, at least under conditions of brief fasting, normally satisfies a small portion of its energy demands by the conversion of ketone bodies to acetyl-CoA, which then proceeds through the citric acid cycle (see Fig. 12-5). Whether ketone bodies satisfy a greater portion of cerebral energy demands when glucose is deficient is a separate issue and not so readily demonstrated (see later). Available data in the newborn dog do not support an important role for ketone bodies in this context (see later discussion).[30,35,47]

Limitations of Hepatic Ketone Synthesis.
Utilization of ketone bodies as alternative substrates for glucose in brain energy production, under conditions of glucose deprivation, depends on the capacity of liver to deliver these compounds to the blood. Data obtained in human newborn infants suggest that hepatic ketone synthesis is restricted during the early

TABLE 12-2 Failure of Ketone Bodies to Increase in Blood with Hypoglycemia

| Infants | KETONE BODIES (mmol/L) | |
	Beta-Hydroxybutyrate	Acetoacetate
Normoglycemic, term, AGA	0.31 ± 0.04	0.06 ± 0.01
Hypoglycemic, term, AGA	0.16 ± 0.03	0.02 ± 0.01
Hypoglycemic, SGA	0.24 ± 0.07	0.03 ± 0.01

AGA, appropriate for gestational age; SGA, small for gestational age.
Data from Stanley CA, Anday EK, Baker L, Delivoria-Papadopoulos M: Metabolic fuel and hormone responses to fasting in newborn infants, *Pediatrics* 64:613–619, 1979.

neonatal period.[73] The findings demonstrate (1) low levels of ketone bodies, (2) failure of ketone bodies to rise with fasting (in contrast to fasting in older children), and (3) failure of ketone bodies to rise with hypoglycemia (Table 12-2). In a subsequent study, relatively low plasma concentrations of ketone bodies were also documented with formula feeding.[74] Because cerebral utilization of ketone bodies linearly depends on plasma concentrations,[68] these data from studies of human infants suggest that *limitations of hepatic ketone synthesis* prevent a major role for these materials as alternative metabolic substrates in brain of human infants with hypoglycemia. *However, these data do not rule out the possibility that exogenous administration of ketone bodies or of exogenous sources of ketone bodies (e.g., fatty acids) could serve as alternative metabolic substrates.* One report demonstrated cerebral uptake of exogenously administered beta-hydroxybutyrate for the management of hypoglycemic infants in the first year of life.[75]

Lactate

Lactate as an important energy source in neonatal hypoglycemia was suggested by elegant experiments in the newborn dog.[30,34,35,47,63,76,77] Thus, determinations of cerebral metabolic rates for oxygen, glucose, lactate, and beta-hydroxybutyrate were accomplished by measurements of CBF and cerebral arteriovenous differences of these compounds.[47] These data then

TABLE 12-3 Lactate as Important Alternative Substrate for Brain Energy Production with Hypoglycemia in the Newborn Dog

| Blood Glucose* | SOURCE OF CEREBRAL ENERGY REQUIREMENTS | | |
	Glucose	Lactate	Beta-Hydroxybutyrate
Normoglycemia	95%	4%	<1%
Hypoglycemia (13 mg/dL)	48%	52%	<1%
Hypoglycemia (5 mg/dL)	42%	56%	2%

*Two hours after injection of insulin (or placebo).
Data from Hernandez MJ, Vannucci RC, Salcedo A, Brennan RW: Cerebral blood flow and metabolism during hypoglycemia in newborn dogs, *J Neurochem* 35:622–628, 1980.

were used to determine the relative proportions of cerebral energy requirements derived from glucose, lactate, and beta-hydroxybutyrate under conditions of normoglycemia and insulin-induced hypoglycemia (Table 12-3). During normoglycemia, the newborn dog obtained 95% of its cerebral energy requirements from glucose and only a small fraction from lactate (4%) and beta-hydroxybutyrate (<1%).[47] With hypoglycemia, in concert with the expected decline in cerebral utilization of glucose, a striking increase in lactate use was observed (see Table 12-3). (No appreciable change in the contribution of ketone body utilization was noted.) In subsequent experiments, no significant decrease in brain high-energy phosphate levels occurred under these conditions.[76] *Thus, the data indicate that increased utilization of lactate spared brain energy levels under conditions of severe hypoglycemia.*

The *mechanisms* by which blood lactate leads to energy production in brain probably include enhanced lactate uptake by the brain from blood and active oxidation to pyruvate by lactate dehydrogenase (see Fig. 12-5). Indeed, available data indicate that lactate uptake in newborn dogs occurs at a rate that exceeds that of adult dogs, even when arterial lactate concentrations are within or near the physiological range.[30,34,35,47,76,78] Concerning conversion of lactate to pyruvate, the activity of lactate dehydrogenase in brain of the perinatal animal has been shown to be relatively high.[34,79-81] Moreover, other data suggest that neonatal brain may have a particular capability to use lactate as a brain energy source as an adaptation to the relative lactic acidemia in the first hours and days after birth.[47,82] Lactic acidemia related to the hypoxic stress of "normal" vaginal delivery has been documented in newborn rats and lambs.[30,34,83,84] These data also bear on the relative resistance of neonatal versus adult brain to hypoglycemic injury (see later). The sparing role of lactate in neonatal hypoglycemia requires further elucidation, but the data from studies of the newborn dog suggest that this role is considerable.

BIOCHEMICAL ASPECTS OF HYPOGLYCEMIA

The *pathophysiological aspects* of the encephalopathy caused by hypoglycemia are best considered in terms of the *initial* biochemical effects on brain metabolism, the *later* effects, and the *combined* effects of hypoglycemia with hypoxemia, ischemia, or seizures. These combined effects may be of major clinical relevance because hypoglycemia uncommonly occurs as an isolated neonatal event and because hypoglycemia not severe enough to cause brain injury alone may attain that capacity when combined with certain other deleterious insults to brain metabolism.

Major Initial Biochemical Effects of Hypoglycemia on Brain Metabolism

Major Biochemical Changes

At the outset, it is crucial to recognize that *no* biochemical effects of hypoglycemia occur as long as the initial

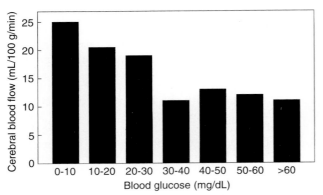

Figure 12-7 **Cerebral blood flow as a function of blood glucose measured 2 hours after birth in 25 premature newborns.** Cerebral blood flow was determined by xenon clearance. Note the increase in cerebral blood flow that begins with blood glucose lower than 30 mg/dL. *(Values are means calculated and redrawn from data from Pryds O, Christensen NJ, Friis HB: Increased cerebral blood flow and plasma epinephrine in hypoglycemic, preterm neonates, Pediatrics 85:172–176, 1990.)*

physiological response of *increased CBF* supplies sufficient glucose to brain. This initial hyperemic response, first described in adult models of hypoglycemia,[33] was documented in neonatal animal models[85,86] and in human infants.[19,87-89] The marked increase in CBF begins in the human infant when blood glucose declines to less than approximately 30 mg/dL (Fig. 12-7). Studies of changes in cerebral blood volume, measured continuously in preterm infants by near-infrared spectroscopy (see Chapter 4), suggested that previously unperfused capillaries are recruited to maintain glucose levels in brain with hypoglycemia.[89] However, clearly with marked decreases in cerebral glucose delivery (e.g., because of marked decreases in blood glucose or impaired CBF, or both) or with marked increases in cerebral glucose utilization (e.g., because of seizure), biochemical derangements begin.

The major *initial* biochemical effects of hypoglycemia on brain metabolism are summarized in Table 12-4.[30,33,35-37,46,47,64,76,90-103] The principal consequences involve cerebral glucose metabolism and the metabolic attempts to preserve cerebral energy status by utilization of alternatives to glucose. Sharp falls

TABLE 12-4	Major Initial Biochemical Effects of Hypoglycemia on Brain Metabolism
↓↓ Brain glucose	
↑ Glycogen → glucose	
↓↓ CMR glucose	
±↓ CMR oxygen	
±↓ ATP, phosphocreatine	
↑ CMR lactate	
↓ Amino acids, ↑ ammonia	
?↑ Ketone body utilization	
↓ Synthesis of acetylcholine	

↓, decreased; ↓↓, moderately decreased; ↑, increased; →, conversion to; ±, with or without; ATP, adenosine triphosphate; CMR, cerebral metabolic rate.

in brain glucose concentrations are expected. Glycogenolysis responds in an attempt to restore some of the brain's supply of glucose. Nevertheless, the result is a sharp decrease in the cerebral metabolic rate for glucose. However, an important feature of hypoglycemia, noted in 1948 in humans,[104] and subsequently studied in more detail in experimental animals,[30,94,99] is a disproportionately smaller disturbance of the cerebral metabolic rate for oxygen. Indeed, in neonatal animals, cerebral metabolic rates of oxygen tend to be unchanged.[30,47] This discrepancy between cerebral utilization of glucose and that of oxygen implies that brain energy needs are being met by alternative substrates to glucose (see next paragraph). Indeed, except in very severe hypoglycemia, significant declines in high-energy phosphate levels in brain are not consistent initial features.

The preservation of oxidative metabolism and high-energy phosphate levels in brain despite the decrease in cerebral glucose metabolic rate presumably relates to the utilization of alternative substrates (see Table 12-4). The major substrates considered are lactate, ketone bodies, and amino acids. As noted previously, *lactate* is the most likely candidate as the *major* alternative substrate for maintenance of brain oxidative metabolism during hypoglycemia, and the increase in its rate of utilization in the newborn dog with hypoglycemia is sufficient to account for the preservation of cerebral metabolic rate for oxygen and of tissue levels of high-energy phosphate compounds (see Table 12-3). The possibility of increased *ketone body* utilization as an additional alternative energy source is suggested by data in adult and young (not newborn) animals.[99,105] However, as described earlier, direct measurements of ketone body utilization in the hypoglycemic newborn dog did not suggest that ketone bodies are important alternative substrates, at least in that insulin-induced model.[30,34,47] Other alternative substrates for glucose or energy production, or both, are *amino acids.* Indeed, a sharp decrease in brain concentrations of most, although not all, amino acids occurs, with a consequent increase in brain ammonia levels (through transamination and deamination reactions; see Table 12-4 and subsequent discussion).

Dissociation of Impaired Brain Function and Energy Metabolism

Changes in brain energy metabolism do not clearly explain the striking changes in clinical signs and electroencephalographic (EEG) activity of brain during the initial phases of hypoglycemia. Thus, although findings differ qualitatively if newborn or adult animals are studied, in general the evolution with hypoglycemia of clinical changes from an alert state to a depressed level of consciousness (and even to seizures) and of EEG changes from normal activity to slowing (and even to burst-suppression patterns and seizure discharges) occurs with no definite change in ATP levels in whole brain or in cerebral cortex and several other brain regions.[30,33,35,46,76,90,98,99] In many respects, this dissociative phenomenon is similar to that observed in the initial phases of hypoxic-ischemic

TABLE 12-5 **Major Later Biochemical Effects of Hypoglycemia on Brain Metabolism**

↓↓↓ Brain glucose
↓↓↓ CMR glucose
↓ CMR oxygen
↓ ATP, phosphocreatine
↑ CMR lactate
↓↓ Amino acids (except glutamate and aspartate),
 ↑ ammonia
↓ Phospholipids, ↑ free fatty acids
↑ Intracellular calcium, ↑ extracellular potassium
↑ Extracellular glutamate
↓ Glutathione, ↑ oxidative stress

↓, decreased; ↓↓, moderately decreased; ↓↓↓, severely decreased; ↑, increased; ATP, adenosine triphosphate; CMR, cerebral metabolic rate.

insults (see Chapter 6). It is unclear whether this occurrence is an adaptive phenomenon (i.e., when faced with an imminent power failure, the brain curtails neuronal activity), perhaps to conserve energy stores.

The *mechanism* by which the dissociation of functional and electrical activity of brain from brain energy levels occurs may relate to certain of the metabolic concomitants of hypoglycemia (see Table 12-4). Such concomitants could include alterations in relative amounts of excitatory and inhibitory amino acids, in tissue levels of ammonia, or in neurotransmitter metabolism. Indeed, the degradation of amino acids described earlier results in an increase in levels of *brain ammonia* that are considered potentially sufficient to produce stupor in adult hypoglycemic animals.[99] Whether such levels are generated in newborn animals is unknown. Data in mature rats rendered hypoglycemic demonstrated that *impaired synthesis of acetylcholine* (see Table 12-4) occurs in the first minutes after onset of hypoglycemia.[93,106] Indeed, only modest decreases in plasma glucose levels caused 20% to 45% decreases in concentrations of acetylcholine and 40% to 60% decreases in synthesis of this neurotransmitter in cortex and striatum.[106] The likely mechanism of this disturbance relates to a decrease in synthesis of acetyl-CoA because of the drastic decrease in brain glucose and, as a consequence, glycolysis. Even with modest hypoglycemia, pyruvate concentrations in brain decrease by 50% in minutes.[99] Data concerning acetylcholine synthesis in hypoglycemic *newborn animals* are lacking, but similar sharp decreases in brain glucose and pyruvate[35,76] levels suggest that the same impairment of acetylcholine synthesis is likely.

Major Later Biochemical Effects of Hypoglycemia on Brain Metabolism

Glucose and Energy Metabolism

The major *later* biochemical effects of hypoglycemia are summarized in Table 12-5. Because the largest amount of available data has been derived from studies of mature animals, and because the limited data in newborn animals suggest some differences (although many similarities) compared with mature animals, in the following discussion I review the major effects on the mature and immature nervous systems separately.

Biochemical Changes in the Mature Animal

Glucose and Energy Metabolism. The biochemical effects of severe or prolonged hypoglycemia include an accentuation of the changes described in the previous section as well as the addition of other effects (Table 12-5). Thus, the decreases in brain glucose level become very marked, the cerebral metabolic rate of glucose falls drastically, and a distinct decrease in cerebral oxidative metabolism and in synthesis of high-energy phosphate compounds becomes apparent.[33,35-37,94,95,97-99,107]

Metabolic Responses to Preserve Brain Energy Levels. To preserve brain energy levels, utilization of endogenous amino acids, derived from protein degradation, glycolytic intermediates, and lactate, continues as described earlier for initial biochemical effects (glycogen is essentially exhausted by this time). Indeed, as a consequence of the utilization of amino acids, ammonia levels in the brain increase markedly (i.e., 10-fold to 15-fold). An additional metabolic response (i.e., phospholipid degradation with the generation of free fatty acids) becomes apparent. The free fatty acids become an energy source in severe hypoglycemia. However, the responses are insufficient in severe and prolonged hypoglycemia to prevent the onset of declines in levels of high-energy phosphate compounds in brain and the occurrences of coma and an isoelectric EEG pattern.[33,99] At this point, an additional series of events develops.

Intracellular Calcium and Cell Injury with Hypoglycemia. At approximately the time of onset of EEG isoelectricity, striking changes in intracellular calcium (Ca^{2+}) and extracellular potassium (K^+) occur and appear to initiate a series of events that result in cell death.[33,35-37,97,107] Thus, at this time, the capacity of the neuron to maintain energy-dependent normal ionic gradients is lost, extracellular Ca^{2+} levels decrease abruptly by approximately sixfold, and extracellular K^+ levels increase by approximately 14-fold. Movements of Ca^{2+} into the cell and of K^+ out of the cell account for these observations. The initiating event is probably failure of the energy-dependent sodium-K^+ (Na^+/K^+) pump, which extrudes Na^+ and retains K^+. With failure of this system, sodium accumulates intracellularly, K^+ is extruded, and sustained membrane depolarization occurs; the intracellular increase of Na^+ then leads to activation of the Na^+/Ca^{2+} exchange system and movement of Ca^{2+} intracellularly in exchange for Na^+. Additional crucial effects of this membrane depolarization are excessive release of excitatory amino acids from synaptic nerve endings and reduced reuptake secondary to failure of glutamate transport; the resulting extracellular accumulation of these excitatory neurotransmitters and consequent activation of glutamate receptors result in a variety of deleterious effects, including influx of Ca^{2+} (see later). Ca^{2+} also may accumulate intracellularly because of

TABLE 12-6   Cerebral Glucose, Pyruvate, Lactate, and High-Energy Phosphates with Hypoglycemia in the Newborn Dog

Blood Glucose (mg/dL)*	CEREBRAL METABOLITE (PERCENTAGE OF CONTROL)[†]				
	Glucose	Pyruvate	Lactate	Phosphocreatine	ATP
20–30	9%	86%	69%	91%	93%
10–20	1%	35%	45%	98%	100%
<10	1%	36%	26%	91%	97%

*Two hours after insulin injection.
[†]All values for glucose, pyruvate, and lactate, but *none* for phosphocreatine and ATP, were statistically significant from control values.
ATP, adenosine triphosphate.
Data from Vannucci RC, Nardis EE, Vannucci SJ, Campbell PA: Cerebral carbohydrate and energy metabolism during hypoglycemia in newborn dogs, *Am J Physiol* 240:R192–R199, 1981.

failure of energy-dependent Ca^{2+} transport mechanisms designed to maintain low cytosolic Ca^{2+} levels (see Chapter 6). The metabolic consequences of these ionic changes appear to be similar to those described in Chapter 6 concerning the mechanisms of cell death with oxygen deprivation. The importance of the cytosolic Ca^{2+}-induced phospholipase activation (see Chapter 6) is emphasized by the observation of an abrupt decline in phospholipid concentration in brain and a further elevation in free fatty acid concentration. The deleterious effects of arachidonate (e.g., generation of free radicals and harmful vasoactive compounds) are summarized in Chapter 6. Thus, the final common pathway to neuronal injury in hypoglycemia may be very similar to that in oxygen deprivation and relates especially to accumulation of cytosolic Ca^{2+}. Moreover, in hypoglycemia, as in hypoxia-ischemia, *massive depletion of high-energy phosphate compounds does not appear to be an obligatory event in producing cell death.*

Role for Excitotoxic Amino Acids in Hypoglycemic Neuronal Death. As discussed in Chapter 6, considerable data indicate that the mechanism of cell death with hypoxia-ischemia is mediated by the extracellular accumulation of excitatory amino acids, which are toxic in high concentrations. *It now appears likely that excitatory amino acids play a major role in mediation of neuronal death with hypoglycemia.* Evidence in support of this conclusion includes the demonstrations of a rise in extracellular concentrations of excitatory amino acids (aspartate and glutamate) in advanced hypoglycemia and an attenuation of neuronal injury by simultaneous administration of antagonists of the *N*-methyl-D-aspartate (NMDA) type of glutamate receptor, both in in vivo models and in cultured neurons.[33,35,36,95,108-119] These observations suggest that the Ca^{2+} accumulation and Ca^{2+}-mediated deleterious events, noted in the previous section and described in detail in Chapter 6, including especially the generation of reactive oxygen and nitrogen species, are intertwined with and provoked in considerable part by activation of the NMDA receptor with resulting influx of Ca^{2+} through the NMDA channel (as well as through voltage-dependent Ca^{2+} channels). The free radicals generated result in DNA damage and, as a consequence, the DNA repair enzyme, poly(ADP-ribose) polymerase-1 (PARP). With excessive activation of PARP and,

as a consequence, adenosine depletion, energy failure and activation of apoptosis occur.[119] PARP inhibitors have been shown to protect neurons from hypoglycemia in in vitro and in vivo experimental models.[119] Thus, the data concerning excitotoxicity and prevention thereof raise interesting new therapeutic possibilities for the prevention or amelioration of hypoglycemic neuronal death, possibilities that exhibit analogies with potential therapies for ischemic neuronal death (see Chapter 6).

Biochemical Changes in the Newborn Animal

Similarities and Differences in Changes in Newborn and Adult Brain. Many of the biochemical effects of hypoglycemia described earlier in adult brain can be documented in neonatal brain, such as sharp decreases in levels of glucose, diminished cerebral utilization of glucose, and diminished concentrations of glycolytic intermediates (Table 12-6).[30,35,36,47,76,96,101,118] However, *certain metabolic differences* from the changes observed in adult brain are prominent (e.g., preservation of phosphocreatine and ATP levels despite severe decreases in glucose levels and markedly greater utilization of lactate as an alternative substrate for energy metabolism). The data contained in Table 12-6 show that hypoglycemia severe enough to deplete brain of glucose almost entirely is accompanied by some preservation of such glycolytic intermediates as pyruvate and lactate and, most strikingly, by complete preservation of phosphocreatine and ATP levels. Indeed, hypoglycemia of comparable severity in the adult animal causes marked reductions in the levels of phosphocreatine and ATP in brain.[98,99]

The relative preservation of the energy status of brain with severe hypoglycemia in the newborn animal is accompanied by a similar *preservation of neurological function and electrical activity.* Thus, in the adult rat, insulin-induced hypoglycemia to plasma glucose values of approximately 35 mg/dL resulted in prominent slowing on the EEG tracing, and plasma glucose values of approximately 30 mg/dL resulted in lethargy and markedly slow activity on the EEG tracing.[98,99] Prolongation of this degree of hypoglycemia for approximately 1 hour resulted in coma and an isoelectric EEG pattern.[98,99] These latter states were attained in less time in the adult animals when plasma glucose levels were reduced to 10 to 15 mg/dL.[98] In contrast, in the newborn rat rendered hypoglycemic to

TABLE 12-7	Major Reasons for the Relative Resistance of the Newborn Animal to Hypoglycemia

Diminished cerebral energy utilization
Increased cerebral blood flow with even moderate hypoglycemia
Increased cerebral uptake and utilization of lactate
Resistance of the heart to hypoglycemia

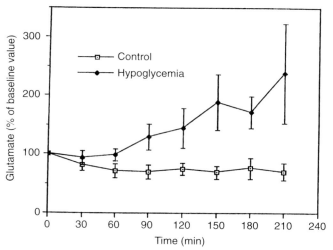

Figure 12-8 Increase in extracellular glutamate with hypoglycemia in the immature rat. The striatal glutamate efflux (i.e., extracellular glutamate) in control ($n=6$) and hypoglycemic ($n=6$) postnatal day 7 rats was determined by microdialysis. Hypoglycemia was produced by insulin injection. In hypoglycemic animals, the striatal glutamate efflux increased gradually and peaked at 240% of control values. *(From Silverstein FS, Simpson J, Gordon KE: Hypoglycemia alters striatal amino acid efflux in perinatal rats: An in vivo microdialysis study, Ann Neurol 28:516–521, 1990.)*

a plasma glucose level of approximately 15 mg/dL, no change in neurological function could be observed over 2 hours.[96] In the newborn dog, prominent slow activity on the EEG tracing was observed only at plasma glucose levels lower than approximately 20 mg/dL. Moreover, at plasma glucose values of approximately 10 to 15 mg/dL (i.e., levels sufficient to cause an isoelectric EEG pattern in the adult dog), considerable electrical activity, albeit slow, was apparent in the newborn dog.[76] Indeed, at this level, seizure discharges often became apparent, and the accompanying respiratory failure and cardiovascular collapse could result in death of the animal.[76]

Reasons for Relative Resistance of Newborn Brain to Hypoglycemia. The data reviewed demonstrate clearly a relative resistance of the newborn versus the adult animal to the deleterious effects of hypoglycemia. The major reasons for this relative resistance are shown in Table 12-7. Of particular importance is the lower cerebral energy requirement in the immature brain with the consequently *lower rate of energy utilization.* This situation, discussed in Chapter 6 concerning the relative resistance of perinatal brain to hypoxic injury, presumably relates first to the less-developed dendritic-axonal ramifications and synaptic connections and, as a consequence, energy-dependent ion pumping and neurotransmitter synthesis. The second reason for the relative resistance of the newborn animal and human to hypoglycemia relates to the *marked increase in CBF*, provoked by even moderate hypoglycemia. As noted earlier, blood glucose levels lower than 30 mg/dL in the human newborn are associated with prominent increases in CBF. In mature animals, severe hypoglycemia is required to lead to increases in CBF. The third reason for the relative resistance to hypoglycemia presumably relates to an *increased capacity for both cerebral uptake and utilization of lactate for brain energy production* (see previous discussion of alternative substrates).[30,34,35,47,120] Fourth, severe hypoglycemia does not have as profound an effect on cardiovascular function in the newborn as in the adult animal.[76] The *relative resistance of the immature heart* relates to its rich endogenous carbohydrate stores (glucose and glycogen), which can be mobilized for energy during hypoglycemia, and the capacity of the immature heart to use fuels other than glucose for energy.[121-123] Thus, although it is clear that more data are needed concerning the impact of hypoglycemia on neonatal brain, current information suggests that cerebral and myocardial metabolic capacities provide remarkable degrees of resistance.

Role for Excitotoxic Amino Acids in Hypoglycemic Neuronal Death. A possible role for excitatory amino acids in the hypoglycemic neuronal death with severe hypoglycemia in neonatal animals, as in mature animals (see earlier discussion), is suggested by studies of severe insulin-induced hypoglycemia in 7-day-old rats.[124] Thus, insulin-induced hypoglycemia caused an increase in striatal extracellular glutamate, measured by microdialysis, with the onset of the increase at blood glucose levels of 20 mg/dL (Fig. 12-8). After 3½ hours of hypoglycemia (terminal glucose level of <5 mg/dL), striatal glutamate was approximately 2.4-fold higher than baseline levels. The increased extracellular glutamate may be caused by failure of high-affinity glutamate uptake mechanisms or by increased release (secondary to synaptic release provoked by membrane depolarization [resulting from Na^+ or Ca^{2+} influx] or by reversal of the Na^+-dependent glutamate transport system [resulting from increased intracellular Na^+], or by both mechanisms). The potential consequence would be excitotoxic neuronal death by the mechanisms described in Chapter 6. Prevention of neuronal death in organotypic hippocampal cultures derived from newborn rat brain and maintained in the absence of glucose by the NMDA receptor antagonist MK-801 also illustrates the importance of excitotoxic mechanisms in hypoglycemic neuronal death.[115] The prevention of neuronal death by addition of the antagonist 30 minutes *after* the insult may have important therapeutic implications. The increase in apparent affinity of the NMDA receptor observed in the hypoglycemic piglet suggests that the excitotoxic potential of glutamate may be enhanced by hypoglycemia.[118]

Glutathione Depletion and Oxidative Stress. A role for oxidative stress in hypoglycemic cell death was suggested by studies of cultured neural cells and a newborn piglet model.[125,126,126a] In cultured cells, glucose deprivation caused a decrease in glutathione levels and then cell death. Glucose is involved in production of reduced glutathione by generating reducing equivalents and by providing a carbon source required for biosynthesis of this critical antioxidant. That the cell death in the studies of cultured glial cells was mediated by oxidative stress and free radical attack was shown by the demonstration of protection by free radical scavengers. Because Ca^{2+} influx and glutamate receptor activation in neurons may lead to generation of free radicals (see Chapter 6), the deleterious effect of reduced glutathione levels could be critical in the final common pathway to cell death with hypoglycemia. Studies of the hypoglycemic newborn piglet showed markedly elevated mitochondrial production of reactive oxygen species.[126] The demonstration that brain-derived neurotrophic factor (BDNF) protected cultured neurons from hypoglycemic injury further suggests a role for oxidative stress because BDNF induces antioxidant systems.[127]

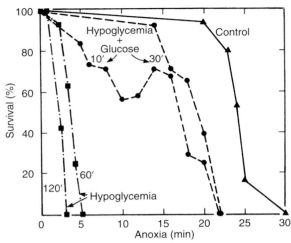

Figure 12-9   **Deleterious effect of hypoglycemia on vulnerability to anoxia (nitrogen breathing).** The percentage of survival of newborn rats was determined as a function of duration of anoxia. Hypoglycemia was produced by insulin injection 1 to 2 hours before the onset of anoxia; some hypoglycemic animals were pretreated with glucose (1.8 g/kg, subcutaneously) either 10 or 30 minutes before anoxia. *(From Vannucci RC, Vannucci SJ: Cerebral carbohydrate metabolism during hypoglycemia and anoxia in newborn rats, Ann Neurol 4:73–79, 1978.)*

Hypoglycemia and Hypoxemia or Asphyxia

Hypoglycemia and Hypoxemia

The vulnerability of immature brain to hypoxemic injury is enhanced by concomitant hypoglycemia, an observation first made in 1942.[128] Studies of cerebral carbohydrate metabolism during hypoxemia and hypoglycemia in newborn rats provided further insight into the mechanism of this effect.[30,96] Thus, newborn rats subjected to hypoxemia by breathing 100% nitrogen exhibited greater mortality rates when they were also subjected to insulin-induced hypoglycemia (Fig. 12-9). Indeed, animals rendered hypoglycemic for 1 hour experienced a fivefold reduction in survival capability, and those hypoglycemic for 2 hours did even worse. Supplementation of hypoglycemic animals with glucose before anoxia improved outcome (see Fig. 12-9). Animals rendered hypoglycemic as well as hypoxemic exhibited less accumulation of lactate in brain and a faster decline in cerebral energy reserves (ATP and phosphocreatine) than those rendered hypoxemic alone. Moreover, glucose supplementation ameliorated the adverse metabolic effects. The mechanism for the enhanced deleterious effect of hypoxemia when hypoglycemia was associated appeared to relate to a diminution in brain glucose reserves and thus retarded glycolytic flux. The improvement with glucose supplementation supports this notion.

Studies of cultured immature glial cells are relevant to the adverse effect of the combination of hypoxemia and hypoglycemia. Thus, not only are immature astrocytes more vulnerable to glucose deprivation than are mature glial cells,[129] but also, of special interest in this context, glucose deprivation markedly accentuates the vulnerability of differentiating glial cells to oxygen deprivation (Fig. 12-10).[130] This effect of glucose deprivation on immature glial cells is apparent in both differentiating astrocytes and oligodendroglia.[130]

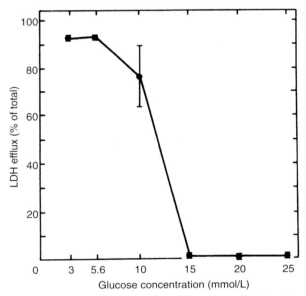

Figure 12-10   **Beneficial effect of glucose on hypoxia-induced cellular injury in differentiating glial cells, primarily astrocytes.** Cellular injury was determined by measurement of efflux of lactate dehydrogenase (LDH) from the damaged cells. Primary glial cell cultures were grown for 18 days, when differentiation was active, and subjected to hypoxia, with the indicated concentrations of glucose in the culture medium. *(From Callahan DJ, Engle MJ, Volpe JJ: Hypoxic injury to developing glial cells: Protective effect of high glucose, Pediatr Res 27:186–190, 1990.)*

Hypoglycemia and Asphyxia

Study of the newborn dog demonstrated the deleterious effect of hypoglycemia when combined with asphyxia.[30,35,120] Thus, to approximate clinical circumstances more closely (than the nitrogen breathing of the experiments just described), neonatal dogs were asphyxiated, with and without prior induction of hypoglycemia to plasma glucose levels of approximately 20 mg/dL. The data showed striking worsening of the cerebral metabolic effects of asphyxia in animals rendered hypoglycemic versus those normoglycemic. Thus, whereas in normoglycemic animals levels of glycolytic substrates subsequent to the phosphofructokinase step increased, secondary to the expected acceleration of anaerobic glycolysis, in hypoglycemic animals no such increase occurred, in keeping with a failure of enhancement of anaerobic glycolysis. Moreover, whereas hypoglycemia alone resulted in little or no alteration in levels of high-energy phosphate compounds, when combined with asphyxia a drastic reduction in these compounds resulted. ATP levels declined with asphyxia by 61% in the hypoglycemic animals compared with only 13% in the normoglycemic animals. Thus, the data extended the findings described earlier with the combination of hypoglycemia and hypoxemia and indicated that hypoglycemia combined with asphyxia leads to greater cerebral metabolic derangements than those observed with asphyxia alone.

A deleterious effect of hypoglycemia in the *postasphyxial* period was shown by studies of newborn lambs.[131] Thus, cerebral fractional oxygen extraction remained depressed relative to values in control or hyperglycemic animals for as long as 4 hours following termination of asphyxia (the last time point studied).

A study of 185 term infants with severe fetal acidemia (umbilical arterial pH <7.00) suggested an important role for postasphyxial postnatal hypoglycemia in the genesis of brain injury.[132] Thus, 27 (14.5%) of the 185 infants had an initial blood glucose level of 40 mg/dL or lower. Of these 27 infants, 56% (15) had an abnormal neurological outcome, whereas only 16% (26) of the 158 infants with a blood glucose level higher than 40 mg/dL had an abnormal outcome. Infants with abnormal outcomes and a blood glucose level of 40 mg/dL or lower did not appear to have sustained a more pronounced asphyxial insult, because they had a higher cord pH (6.86 versus 6.75) and lesser base deficit (−19 versus −23.8). By multivariate logistic analysis, initial blood glucose was significantly associated with abnormal outcome (odds ratio, 18.5; 95% confidence interval, 3.1 to 111.9).

Summary

Taken together, these observations demonstrating that hypoglycemia potentiates the deleterious effects of hypoxemia or asphyxia on newborn mammalian brain and that deleterious effects are potentiated also in the postasphyxial period by hypoglycemia may have major clinical relevance. Indeed, these insults frequently occur together in the clinical arena (see later discussion). The findings raise the possibility that degrees of hypoxemia or asphyxia or both *and* hypoglycemia, which alone would not cause brain injury, may do so when acting in concert.

Hypoglycemia and Ischemia

Enhanced Vulnerability of Hypoglycemic Brain to Ischemic Insult

The vulnerability of brain of *mature animals* to ischemic insult is enhanced by concomitant hypoglycemia.[133] Increases of mortality, acute neurological phenomena (e.g., seizures), and neurological deficits in survivors were apparent in the hypoglycemic versus normoglycemic animals. The mechanism of this effect presumably was similar to that just described; that is, diminished glucose reserves in the hypoglycemic brain were unable to maintain the accelerated glycolytic flux necessary to maintain cerebral energy reserves under anaerobic (ischemic) conditions. (Recall the 19-fold difference in ATP production from glucose metabolism under anaerobic versus aerobic conditions; see Chapter 6.)

The *degree of ischemia* is important in the enhancement of vulnerability of hypoglycemic brain to ischemia. Thus, with only moderate hypotension in the mature rat (blood pressure reduced to 60 mm Hg), although energy failure was enhanced in hypoglycemic brain, neuronal necrosis was not accentuated.[134]

Data relative to *neonatal animals* also suggest a crucial role for blood glucose in determination of ischemic brain injury. Thus, studies of 7-day-old rats subjected to hypoxic-ischemic insult showed an increase in mitochondrial oxidation, in contrast to the decrease observed in the adult brain. This observation indicates a disturbance in the immature brain of glucose influx and utilization, the major source of mitochondrial reducing equivalents.[135] Hypoglycemia presumably would accentuate this disturbance. Direct demonstration of the deleterious additional effect of hypoglycemia in neonatal hypoxia-ischemia was shown in the 7-day-old rat pup.[136] Thus, Yager and coworkers subjected the pups to hypoglycemia by fasting or insulin injection before inducing hypoxia-ischemia. Although the hypoglycemia was relatively mild (i.e., 5.4, 4.3, and 3.4 mmol/L for control, insulin-injected, and fasting animals, respectively), the brain injury was accentuated in the insulin-injected animals. The fasted animals had the least damage, apparently because of enhanced ketogenesis exhibited by this group.

Observations relative to the *neonatal human* that suggest an enhanced vulnerability to ischemic injury with hypoglycemia are derived from studies of infants with hypoplastic left heart syndrome.[137] Thus, periventricular leukomalacia, an ischemic lesion (see Chapter 8), occurred particularly in infants with decreased blood glucose as well as with the presumed ischemia associated with this severe cardiac lesion. In the immature rat with hypoglycemia, of all brain regions, cerebral white matter showed the poorest compensatory increase in blood flow and the greatest reduction in cerebral metabolic rate for glucose.[85]

Impaired Vascular Autoregulation and the Likelihood of Ischemic Insult in Hypoglycemia

The enhanced vulnerability of the hypoglycemic brain to major ischemic insult, as just described, is particularly important because of the likelihood of ischemia to certain brain regions during hypoglycemia with only moderate hypotension. This likelihood relates to the impairment of vascular autoregulation that has been documented with hypoglycemia in experimental studies.[30,33,85,138,139] A tissue autoradiographic technique was used initially to measure regional CBF in 25 brain structures in the hypoglycemic rat. Siesjo and co-workers[139] observed diminutions in CBF with only moderate hypotension (mean arterial blood pressure of 80 mm Hg; i.e., impaired autoregulation) in several brain regions. The latter included the cerebral cortex, hippocampus, and thalamus, each of which exhibits particular vulnerability to hypoglycemic neuronal injury. The regional decreases in blood flow were to values as low as 10% of control values. In separate experiments, diminutions in CBF with hypoglycemia and moderate hypotension were shown to enhance the deterioration of cerebral energy state and, as a consequence, to enhance K+ release from cerebral cortical cells.[140,141] The mechanism of the effect of hypoglycemia on autoregulation remains to be defined. (A disturbance in the synthesis of a neurotransmitter [acetylcholine?] involved in regulation of local cerebrovascular tone seems possible.) The effect of hypoglycemia in the mature animal on cerebrovascular reactivity is not confined to autoregulation and indeed includes reactivity to arterial carbon dioxide pressure and a variety of pharmacological vasodilators and vasoconstrictors.[142,143]

A decisive demonstration of the impairment of cerebrovascular autoregulation with hypoglycemia was made in the *newborn* dog (Fig. 12-11).[85] The mechanism of this effect in the neonate, as in the adult animal, is unclear.[142]

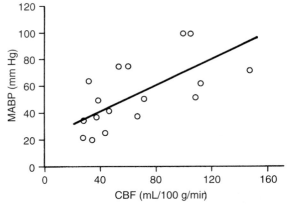

Figure 12-11 **Correlation of cerebral blood flow (CBF) with mean arterial blood pressure (MABP).** A pressure-passive relationship exists between CBF and MABP in the newborn dog during hypoglycemia. *(From Anwar M, Vannucci RC: Autoradiographic determination of regional cerebral blood flow during hypoglycemia in newborn dogs, Pediatr Res 24:41–45, 1988.)*

Summary

The observations reviewed indicate that the cerebral metabolic and vascular derangements caused by hypoglycemia render brain more susceptible to ischemic insults. Thus, major brain ischemia would be expected to result in greater brain injury with hypoglycemia than with normoglycemia. Perhaps more important, the data indicate that ischemia to certain brain regions is particularly likely to occur with even *moderate* hypotension because of the impairment in cerebrovascular autoregulation. The observations emphasize the importance of controlling both circulatory function in hypoglycemic infants and glucose homeostasis in infants experiencing, or at risk for, ischemic insults to brain. Moreover, as with hypoxemia and asphyxia, the data suggest the clinically important possibility that degrees of ischemia and hypoglycemia that alone would not cause brain injury might do so when acting together.

Hypoglycemia and Seizures

Consideration of the effects of seizures on cerebral glucose and energy metabolism (see Chapter 5) leads to the prediction that hypoglycemia would be deleterious in the presence of seizures. Thus, seizures are associated with accelerated energy utilization (secondary to the increased neuronal activity and energy-dependent ion pumping), which leads to a several-fold increase in the rate of glucose utilization. The resulting increased demand for glucose produces a diminution in brain glucose concentrations, despite the maintenance of normal blood glucose concentrations. Therefore, during seizures, if supplies of glucose in brain decrease further because of hypoglycemia, a serious deficit of cerebral energy reserves may be expected to occur particularly rapidly. Earlier studies of paralyzed, ventilated mature rats subjected to bicuculline-induced seizures and concomitant hypoglycemia by starvation demonstrated this deficit.[144] *An additional abnormality* in the hypoglycemic convulsing animals was *a decrease in CBF,* in contrast to an increase in CBF in the convulsing, normoglycemic animals. This decrease in CBF is obviously particularly serious in a situation such as repetitive seizures, in which the supply of exogenous substrate already is limiting for cerebral metabolism. The cause of the decrease in CBF was unclear, although a combination of myocardial dysfunction and impairment of autoregulation could be important (see earlier discussion).

Studies in *newborn monkeys and puppies* also indicated a deleterious effect of the combination of hypoglycemia and seizures.[35,59,145,146] Thus, in the newborn puppy, more severe decreases in cerebral high-energy phosphate compounds occurred with the combination of seizures and hypoglycemia than with hypoglycemia, as just described. Indeed, decreases in blood glucose levels not sufficient to lead to a decrease in phosphocreatine levels resulted in significant decreases when seizures were added.[59] In the newborn monkey, repeated seizures resulted in virtual total depletion of brain glucose and marked depletion of high-energy phosphate levels, and glucose supplementation was required to prevent these changes.[145,146]

The aforementioned data underscore the *importance of controlling seizures in infants with accompanying hypoglycemia.* Moreover, they emphasize the necessity of monitoring glucose homeostasis in any infant exhibiting seizures and again raise the possibility that degrees of hypoglycemia and seizure activity, which alone would not cause brain injury, may do so when acting in concert.

NEUROPATHOLOGY

Definition of the neuropathology of neonatal hypoglycemia has been made particularly difficult by the almost invariable association of other insults, especially hypoxia-ischemia, which also cause brain injury. Nevertheless, data from studies of animals, including subhuman primates, as well as from the few reports of affected human newborns, lead to several conclusions. *First,* hypoglycemia, if severe or prolonged, results in injury to neurons primarily but also to glia. *Second,* the topography of the injury is somewhat different from that observed with hypoxic-ischemic injury. *Third,* when associated with other insults to brain (e.g., hypoxia-ischemia), hypoglycemia of a degree not sufficient to cause brain injury alone probably can play an important contributory role in the genesis of neuronal injury.

Experimental Observations

A distinct correlation between the severity and duration of hypoglycemia and the occurrence of brain injury was demonstrated in studies of monkeys subjected to insulin-induced hypoglycemia with carefully maintained ventilation, perfusion, and temperature.[147,148] Thus, the brain of the adolescent monkey subjected to blood glucose levels of less than 20 mg/dL for more than 2 hours usually exhibited neuropathological aberrations. Of ten such animals, six exhibited cerebral cortical injury, whereas of four animals subjected to this degree of hypoglycemia for less than 2 hours, only one exhibited cerebral cortical injury. The brain injury involved neurons particularly, and the areas especially vulnerable were *cerebral cortex, mainly the parieto-occipital region.* Less commonly involved were neurons of the hippocampus, the caudate nucleus, and the putamen. Detailed studies in the mature rat indicated that the neuronal injury with hypoglycemia is particularly pronounced in regions contiguous to cerebrospinal fluid, such as superficial cerebral cortical layers.[33,134,149-152] This observation suggested that the agent causing the neuronal death is derived from the extracellular space and the evidence, described earlier, that excitotoxic amino acids are involved in the neuronal death is relevant in this context. Moreover, the neuropathological demonstration that the early lesion in hypoglycemic neuronal injury involves dendrites also is consistent with an excitotoxic mechanism.

Limited data are available concerning the potentiating deleterious effects of hypoglycemia and ischemia.

However, a single well-studied monkey that experienced a degree of hypoglycemia (no time when blood glucose level fell to <20 mg/dL) and of moderate hypotension, either of which alone not sufficient to cause brain injury, demonstrated striking neuronal injury in the border zone distribution between the middle cerebral and anterior cerebral arteries.[147,148] This pattern of injury is characteristic of marked falls in cerebral perfusion pressure (see Chapter 8) and demonstrated the potentiating deleterious effect of hypoglycemia with ischemia. This observation corroborates the experimental observations (see earlier discussion) indicating a potentiation of ischemic injury by hypoglycemia.

Human Observations

Neonatal Neuropathology

The limited observations in human newborns suggest that the lessons learned from the animal studies are relevant. Thus, a correlation between the severity and duration of hypoglycemia and the degree of neuronal injury is apparent.[153,154] In one series of 17 largely premature infants, who experienced *transient hypoglycemia* (blood glucose level <20 mg/dL) and "hypoxia" confined to the first day of life, no increase in brain injury could be discerned over and above that expected with the concomitant "hypoxia."[154] In another series, marked and diffuse neuronal injury was apparent in 2- and 3-day-old premature infants whose hypoglycemia was not effectively treated before death.[153] In these *untreated and inadequately treated* patients, the neuronal injury involved essentially every level of the nervous system, including the anterior horn cells of the spinal cord, but with a particular predilection for the *posterior cerebrum,* as in the monkey experiments (see earlier discussion). This posterior cerebral predilection has been demonstrated in the hypoglycemic newborn by computed tomography, magnetic resonance imaging (MRI), and single photon emission computed tomography blood flow scans (Fig. 12-12; see later).[155-165] The lesions in the neuropathological study did not exhibit selective involvement of border zones, or Purkinje cells, as in hypoxic-ischemic injury. Moreover, involvement of upper cortical neuronal layers occurred with neonatal hypoglycemia, a finding, as described earlier, suggestive of an agent (excitatory amino acid?) borne in cerebrospinal fluid. This cortical topography is different from that observed with ischemia (i.e., selective involvement of intermediate and deeper cortical layers).[166-168]

Although neuronal injury dominates the neuropathological picture in neonatal hypoglycemia, concomitant injury to glia is also detectable.[153] Indeed, the classic neuropathological studies of Larroche[167] showed that hypoglycemia is a precedent of periventricular leukomalacia. Moreover, decreased blood glucose was an important pathogenetic factor in careful studies of infants with hypoplastic left heart syndrome, in whom periventricular leukomalacia is a prominent sequela.[137] Studies of oligodendrocyte precursor cells and cerebellar slice cultures showed that hypoglycemia

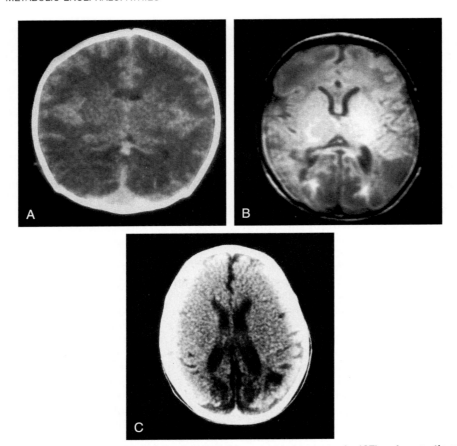

Figure 12-12 **Structural changes with neonatal hypoglycemia, studied by computed tomography (CT) and magnetic resonance imaging (MRI) in a term infant. A**, CT scan at 6 days of age shows a generalized decrease in attenuation, especially posteriorly. **B**, Proton density MRI scan at 19 days of age shows particular involvement of posterior cerebral cortex and subcortical white matter. **C**, CT scan at 78 days of age shows parenchymal loss, especially in the posterior parietal and occipital regions. *(From Spar JA, Lewine JD, Orrison WW: Neonatal hypoglycemia: CT and MR findings, AJNR Am J Neuroradiol 15:1477–1478, 1994.)*

induces apoptotic cell death and inhibits differentiation and myelination.[169] Moreover, the experimental observations of vulnerability of differentiating glial cells to glucose deprivation and to excitatory amino acids (see earlier discussion and Chapter 6) are clearly relevant in this context. These findings may account for the subsequent disturbance of myelination noted in animal studies and in surviving human infants (see later discussion).[167,170]

Neuropathological Sequelae

The neuropathological *sequelae* of severe neonatal hypoglycemic encephalopathy reflect injury particularly to cerebral cortex but also to subcortical white matter, especially posteriorly (see Fig. 12-12C).[155-157,159-164,167,171] These include microcephaly and widened sulci, with atrophic gyri, as well as diminution in myelinated cerebral white matter, with dilated lateral ventricles. The effect on myelination may be a consequence of the glial injury.

Unresolved Issues

Despite the informative aforementioned data, the anatomical correlates of *marginal* hypoglycemia, in combination with other insults (e.g., hypoxemia, ischemia,

and seizures) remain to be defined. Precedent from experimental studies, biochemical and neuropathological in design (see earlier discussions), lead one to expect that these combined insults, which are quite prevalent, may result in brain injury that was not recognized in the past. However, this notion remains to be proven conclusively in the human newborn. Moreover, the impact of these combined insults on *development* of the nervous system, particularly the organizational aspects thereof, is totally unexplored. The application of newer techniques for assessing dendritic and synaptic development (see Chapter 2) in the brains of affected infants is a critical topic for future research.

CLINICAL ASPECTS

The clinical aspects of neonatal hypoglycemia encompass a wide variety of disorders and pathogeneses, with the common denominator being the decrease in blood glucose concentration. Consequently, and not surprisingly, considerable heterogeneities in incidence, occurrence of symptoms, and prognosis are apparent. Nevertheless, certain unifying characteristics can be recognized and are emphasized in the following discussion.

TABLE 12-8 Incidence and Duration of Hypoglycemia in Preterm Infants*

	PLASMA GLUCOSE (MMOL/L)		
	<0.06	<1.6	<2.6
Total Occurrences	10%	28%	66%
Duration (No. of Days Concentration Recorded)			
1	8%	20%	32%
2	1%	4%	18%
≥3	1%	4%	16%

*The population consisted of 661 preterm infants (<1850 g at birth) who survived for more than 48 hours.

Data from Lucas A, Morley R, Cole TJ: Adverse neurodevelopment outcome of moderate neonatal hypoglycaemia, *BMJ* 297:1304–1308, 1988.

Incidence

The incidence of neonatal hypoglycemia in a given population varies considerably, depending on the following: the relative number of preterm and term infants; the time of screening; the time and type of feeding; the control of temperature, ventilation, and circulation; and, above all, the definition of hypoglycemia. In one study of 232 "low-risk" infants in a level 1 nursery, the onset of hypoglycemia occurred at a mean age of 3.4 hours, with incidences of 8% when the definitions were blood glucose level lower than 30 mg/dL in the full-sized term infant and lower than 20 mg/dL in the low-birth-weight infant and 21% when the definition was a blood glucose level lower than 40 mg/dL in all infants.[172] In a large multicenter study of 661 preterm infants with birth weight of less than 1850 g who were subjected to "broadly similar early feeding practices," fully 10% had at least one value of blood glucose less than approximately 10 mg/dL (0.06 mmol/L), 28% at least one value less than approximately 30 mg/dL (1.6 mmol/L), and 66% at least one value less than 45 mg/dL (2.6 mmol/L) (Table 12-8).[20] The proportions were 1%, 4%, and 16% of infants with values less than 10, 30, and 45 mg/dL, respectively, *on 3 or more days* (see later discussion).[20] Among healthy breast-fed term infants, median values were 2.8 to 3.1 mmol/L in two large studies.[12,173] Values did not vary appreciably between 3 and 72 hours of age. Notably, approximately 17% had values of plasma glucose lower than 2.16 mmol/L (<40 mg/dL) at 3 hours of age and 10% had such values at 72 hours.[173] Approximately 5% had values lower than 1.6 mmol/L (<29 mg/dL) at 3 and 72 hours.[173] As outlined later, the incidences of hypoglycemia are highest for certain "high-risk" infants. Thus, although the largest proportion of infants identified as hypoglycemic in the early neonatal period exhibit only transient depressions of blood glucose levels, large absolute numbers of infants do exhibit levels considered low by generally accepted definitions. Thus, we are dealing with a very common disorder.

Clinical Categorization of Neonatal Hypoglycemia

A classification of neonatal hypoglycemia based on the clinical setting, the presence of symptoms, the duration and severity of hypoglycemia, and the time of recognition is depicted in Table 12-9.[1,2,9,11,174-177] *Early transitional-adaptive hypoglycemia* usually occurs in the first 6 to 12 hours after sudden withdrawal of maternally derived substrate at birth. These infants fail to make the appropriate adaptive metabolic adjustments during transition from intrauterine to extrauterine life, hence the term *transitional-adaptive*. *Secondary-associated hypoglycemia* occurs as an associated finding in infants with a variety of disorders, including particularly involvement of the central nervous system. In many respects, this group could be considered a subtype of early transitional-adaptive hypoglycemia. *Classic transient neonatal hypoglycemia* is an extension of an intrauterine disturbance, often undernutrition, that may affect glycogen and lipid stores, gluconeogenic capacity, and endocrine interactions in glucose homeostasis for a brief period of extrauterine life. *Severe recurrent (i.e., not transient) hypoglycemia* is secondary to specific primary enzymatic or metabolic-endocrine abnormalities involving glucose homeostasis.

TABLE 12-9 Clinical Categories of Neonatal Hypoglycemia*

Category	Relative Frequency	WEIGHT AND GESTATION				Proportion Symptomatic	Mean Age at Diagnosis (hr)	Mean Serum Glucose (mg/dL)	Duration of Hypoglycemia
		Term Gestation	LGA	AGA	SGA				
Early transitional-adaptive	+++	+++	++	++	++	+	3	19	Brief
Secondary-associated	++	++	–	+++	++	++	16	16	Brief
Classic transient	+	+++	–	++	+++	++++	17	10	Prolonged
Severe recurrent	–	++++	–	++++	–	++++	18	8	Prolonged

*See text for references.
LGA, large for gestational age; AGA, appropriate for gestational age; SGA, small for gestational age; –, <5%; +, 6% to 25%; ++, 26% to 50%; +++, 51% to 75%; ++++, 76% to 100% of cases.

Early Transitional-Adaptive Hypoglycemia

Early transitional-adaptive hypoglycemia is a relatively common variety of neonatal hypoglycemia (see Table 12-9). The pathophysiology involves one or more of the early adaptive responses to birth (i.e., an up-regulation of glycogenolysis and gluconeogenesis and a blunting of insulin secretion). Thus, included in this somewhat heterogeneous hypoglycemic group are infants whose mothers received excessive glucose intrapartum (resulting in down-regulation of glycogenolysis and gluconeogenesis and increased insulin secretion), large-for-gestational-age infants of diabetic, gestational diabetic, or nondiabetic mothers (resulting in excessive insulin), hypothermic infants (resulting in excessive glucose utilization for heat production and still to be defined factors), or asphyxiated infants (resulting in excessive anaerobic metabolism of glucose, glycogen depletion and hyperinsulinism of unknown causes [see later]). *Preterm* asphyxiated infants are particularly at risk because of diminished glycogen stores (most hepatic glycogen accumulation occurs in the third trimester of pregnancy). *Onset of hypoglycemia* in this category (i.e., early transitional-adaptive) is characteristically *very early*, duration is relatively brief, degree is relatively mild, and response to glucose administration is prompt. Few of these patients exhibit symptoms clearly referable to hypoglycemia.[1,9-11,15,178-181] Prognosis depends to a large extent on any accompanying disorder; the contributory role of the hypoglycemia remains to be clarified. In a study of 185 term infants with severe fetal acidemia and presumed asphyxia, 14% exhibited a blood glucose in the first 30 minutes of 40 mg/dL or lower, and of these infants, 56% had an abnormal short-term neurological outcome.

Secondary-Associated Hypoglycemia

Secondary-associated hypoglycemia also is a relatively common variety of hypoglycemia in patients in neonatal intensive care facilities (see Table 12-9). Included in this group are principally appropriate-for-gestational-age (AGA) term and preterm infants, although small-for-gestational-age (SGA) infants are overrepresented. These infants have been subjected to a variety of *associated illnesses*, which include particularly disorders of the central nervous system, especially asphyxia, intracranial hemorrhage, and congenital anomalies, and such systemic disorders as bacterial sepsis, cold injury, and congenital heart disease (with resulting hypoxia-ischemia). The association of this category with central nervous system disturbances is of particular pathogenetic interest because of the data demonstrating the close relationship between hepatic glucose production and brain mass (see earlier discussion). Thus, the brain disturbance may have an adverse impact on the regulation of hepatic glucose production. Additional pathogenetic factors potentially operative with cerebral disturbance, especially asphyxia, are (1) enhanced cerebral utilization of glucose secondary to anaerobic glycolysis, (2) glycogen depletion secondary to asphyxia-induced catecholamine release, and (3) hypersecretion of insulin.[2,11,15,27,182-184] Secondary hypoglycemia usually has its onset in the first day of life (although usually later than in the early transitional group), duration is relatively brief, degree is relatively mild, and response to glucose therapy is prompt. (In the *severely asphyxiated infant*, onset is earlier, degree is marked, and, if complicated by hyperinsulinism, response to glucose therapy may not be prompt.) Approximately 50% (or more) of the infants in this category exhibit neurological symptoms, although the relation to hypoglycemia is difficult to determine decisively because of the associated disorders. The outlook depends particularly on the associated disorders, but, again, the contributory role of the hypoglycemia remains to be defined.

Classic Transient Neonatal Hypoglycemia

Classic transient neonatal hypoglycemia now accounts for a relatively small proportion of total patients with neonatal hypoglycemia (see Table 12-9). Included in this group are principally SGA term infants, particularly boys, who occasionally have accompanying polycythemia. Intrauterine undernutrition is a dominant feature of the disorder. Pathogenesis includes the following: (1) inadequate production of glucose and energy, because of both diminished glycogen and lipid stores and defective gluconeogenesis; and (2) excessive glucose utilization because of both the relatively large brain (major consumer) compared with the liver (major producer) and, in some infants at least, hyperinsulinism.[2,9,11,15,27,175,178,183] Most infants in this classic category are symptomatic ($\approx$80%)[1]; this group represents the best category for evaluating the relationship between clinical signs and blood glucose levels. The onset of hypoglycemia occurs in the latter part of the first day. The degree of hypoglycemia is moderate to severe, duration can be prolonged, and response to glucose administration requires relatively large amounts. The outlook depends in largest part on the duration and severity of hypoglycemia and, as a corollary, the time before onset of adequate therapy.

Severe Recurrent Hypoglycemia

Severe recurrent hypoglycemia is the least common variety of neonatal hypoglycemia (see Table 12-9). The single feature that distinguishes this group from those just described is the persistence and the recurrence of the hypoglycemia; these disorders are neither transient nor self-limited. Included in this category are principally term AGA infants with primary disorders of glucose homeostasis. The major causes are detailed in Table 12-10.[1,9,11,16,175,178,185-202] The onset of hypoglycemia in these disorders varies with the specific entity, but degree is usually severe, duration is prolonged, and symptoms are almost invariable. The outlook depends primarily on detection of the disorder, institution of specific therapy when possible, and, particularly, rapid and adequate maintenance of blood glucose levels.

The most common causes of persistent hypoglycemia in the newborn are *hyperinsulinemic hypoglycemia of infancy* or *congenital hyperinsulinism*. These disorders relate to abnormalities of the mechanisms of insulin secretion by the pancreatic beta cell. The final stage of insulin secretion is regulated by the action of a

TABLE 12-10	Differential Diagnosis of Severe Recurrent or Persistent Neonatal Hypoglycemia*

Hyperinsulinism
Congenital hyperinsulinism (nesidioblastosis, adenoma spectrum)
Beckwith-Wiedemann syndrome
Macrosomia (without Beckwith-Wiedemann syndrome)

Endocrine Deficiencies
Panhypopituitarism
Isolated growth hormone deficiency
Cortisol deficiency (adrenocorticotropic hormone unresponsiveness, isolated glucocorticoid deficiency, maternal steroid therapy, adrenal hemorrhage, adrenogenital syndrome)
Hypothyroidism
Glucagon deficiency

Hereditary Metabolic Defects
Carbohydrate metabolism (galactosemia, glucose-6-phosphatase deficiency [von Gierke disease], glycogen synthetase deficiency, fructose-1,6-diphosphatase deficiency, phosphoenolpyruvate carboxykinase deficiency)
Amino acid metabolism (maple syrup urine disease, hereditary tyrosinemia)
Organic acid metabolism (pyruvate carboxylase deficiency, propionic acidemia, methylmalonic acidemia), mitochondrial disorders
Fatty acid metabolism (deficiencies of carnitine palmityl transferases I and II and medium and long-chain acyl-coenzyme A dehydrogenases)

*See text for references.

TABLE 12-11	Major Neurological Features in Small-for-Gestational-Age Infants with Hypoglycemia	
Clinical Features		**Symptomatic Infants**
Stupor (usually slight to moderate)		100%(?)
Jitteriness		81%
Seizures		58%
Apnea and other respiratory abnormalities		47%
Irritability		41%
Hypotonia		26%

Data from Cornblath M, Schwartz R: *Disorders of Carbohydrate Metabolism in Infancy*, 2nd ed, Philadelphia: 1976, Saunders.

receptor-channel complex, composed of the sulfonylurea receptor (SUR1) and inwardly rectifying K+ channel (Kir6.2). The channel is closed when the ATP/ADP ratio rises in the beta cell. Closure results in an increase in intracellular K+, membrane depolarization, Ca^{2+} influx, and insulin release.[198,199] Glucose entry through the GLUT2 transporter up-regulates insulin secretion by glucose metabolism, generation of ATP, and closure of the Kir6.2 channel. Another regulator of insulin secretion is the action of glutamate dehydrogenase and generation of ATP from glutamate, with resulting closure of the channel. Glutamate dehydrogenase is allosterically activated by leucine. Of the five major forms of congenital hyperinsulinism, an autosomal recessive defect of SUR1/Kir6.2 and a sporadic form probably also involving the receptor-channel complex, most commonly occur in the newborn period. The sporadic form is associated either with beta-cell microadenomas or diffuse hyperplasia of beta cells.

Neurological Features

The neurological features of neonatal hypoglycemia are best considered in terms of their relative frequency, severity, and nature. These aspects of the clinical syndrome vary as a function of the clinical circumstances (e.g., infant of diabetic mother, infant with asphyxia), as well as of the duration and severity of the hypoglycemia, particularly the length of time before adequate

therapy is instituted (see later section "Seizures: Importance of Duration of Hypoglycemia"). The neurological features that are concomitants of any associated disorders may obscure or accentuate those because of hypoglycemia.

Major Neurological Features

The most representative group of infants to define the neurology of neonatal hypoglycemia is the classic transient group (i.e., SGA infants with classic transient hypoglycemia; Table 12-11).[1,2,9,15,178,203] In my experience, the clinical hallmark of this disorder is the combination of stupor and jitteriness. In standard writings, stupor either is not commented on or is categorized in an imprecise manner (e.g., "lethargy" and "somnolence"). Nevertheless, it is rare to see a symptomatic hypoglycemic SGA infant with a normal level of alertness. Jitteriness occurs in at least 80% of symptomatic infants, and seizures occur in more than 50%. Respiratory disturbances and hypotonia are also relatively common. In my experience, hypotonia is present in the majority of the affected infants, although the precise frequency is difficult to define from reported cases and therefore is probably underestimated in Table 12-11. Further delineation of the relative frequency of the neurological features of neonatal hypoglycemia now is difficult because of close surveillance and prompt treatment of infants at risk.

Seizures: Importance of Duration of Hypoglycemia

The development of seizures exemplifies the importance of temporal factors in determining the occurrence of symptoms in neonatal hypoglycemia (Table 12-12).[204] Late diagnosis, onset of therapy, and control of hypoglycemia were common in the infants who experienced seizures. Infants who remained asymptomatic were identified and were adequately treated earliest. Similar data have been obtained by other investigators.[205] These observations have implications for estimating prognosis, as discussed later.

Brain Imaging in Neonatal Hypoglycemia

A series of reports identified, by brain imaging, a specific pattern of cerebral abnormality involving principally

TABLE 12-12   Seizures and Other Characteristics of the Neurological Syndrome in Neonatal Hypoglycemia as a Function of Duration of Hypoglycemia

Neonatal Clinical Syndrome	Age at Diagnosis (hr)	Therapy Started (hr)	Duration of Hypoglycemia (hr)
Neurological features: seizures	39	43	105
Neurological features: no seizures	10	21	49
No neurological features	9	14	37

Adapted from Koivisto M, Blanco SM, Krause U: Neonatal symptomatic and asymptomatic hypoglycaemia: A follow-up study of 151 children, *Dev Med Child Neurol* 14:603–614, 1972

the parieto-occipital regions.[155-165,206,206a] A total of 55 cases have been reported; I have seen an additional 5 cases (Table 12-13). Consistent with the reported neuropathology (see earlier), the dominant finding has been abnormal signal intensity by MRI in the parieto-occipital region (see Fig. 12-12; Figs. 12-13 and 12-14). The involved areas exhibit restricted diffusion on diffusion-weighted MRI (DWI) (see Figs. 12-13 and 12-14). The topography is seen better in the acute stage by DWI than by conventional MRI. MR spectroscopy shows an elevation of lactate (see Fig.12-14). Although 10% to 15% of the lesions resolve, most are followed in subsequent weeks and months by loss of cerebral cortex and white matter (see Fig. 12-13C), often with ventricular dilation. Occasionally, lesions are apparent in thalamus or basal ganglia, but the involvement of perirolandic and parasagittal cerebral cortex typical of hypoxic-ischemic disease (see Chapter 9) is absent. Although duration of hypoglycemia is difficult to determine from the published reports, the degree of hypoglycemia generally has been marked (see Table 12-13). Thus, 74% of cases had glucose levels of 20 mg/dL or lower, and only 5%

TABLE 12-13   Brain Imaging Abnormalities (and Neurological Outcome) in Severe Neonatal Hypoglycemia*

Neonatal Blood Glucose Levels
≤20 mg/dL: 74%
≤25 mg/dL: 89%
≤30 mg/dL: 95%

Major Imaging Findings
Occipital with or without parietal lesions: 84%
Subsequent atrophy (after lesions): 87%

Neurological Sequelae
Total: 84%
Developmental delay/mental retardation: 84%
Seizures: 66%
Visual impairment: 37%[†]
Microcephaly: 32%

*See text for references.
[†]Testing inconsistent; likely an underestimate.

had levels of 30 mg/dL or higher. Neurological sequelae occurred in most patients (84%) and included developmental deficits or overt mental retardation (84%), seizures (66%), and microcephaly (32%). Visual impairment was described in 37%, but evaluation of visual function was variable. Thus, it is likely that disturbed higher visual function and visual associations are more common, consistent with the locus of the disease. It will be of great interest to determine whether milder degrees of hypoglycemia have milder and transient abnormalities, detectable perhaps by DWI. These observations raise the possibility that neurological features, such as impaired higher visual functions, may have been undetected in previous follow-up studies and indicate that focus on such functions will be important in future work.

Prognosis

Mortality and neurological outcome in neonatal hypoglycemic states relate to the rapidity of onset of adequate therapy and to the associated disorders. Mortality because of untreated hypoglycemia is now rare. Sequelae include, particularly, disturbances of neurological development and intellectual function, visual disturbances, motor deficits, especially spasticity and ataxia, seizure disorders, and microcephaly.* As one may predict from the topography of the neuropathological lesions, disturbances of neurological development and subsequent intellectual function and visual disturbances are the most common deficits, presumably reflecting the cerebral cortical neuronal and white matter (glial) injury.

Relation of Neurological Outcome to Neonatal Neurological Features

A distinct correlation exists between neurological outcome and neonatal clinical features (Table 12-14). This is particularly true when series exclude those infants with secondary associated hypoglycemia, in whom neonatal clinical features and neurological sequelae secondary to the associated disorders are difficult to distinguish from those secondary to the hypoglycemia. In one series of 151 infants with neonatal hypoglycemia followed for 1 to 4 years, the occurrence of seizures as part of the neonatal neurological syndrome was associated with a clearly abnormal outcome in 50% and with transient neurological abnormalities that were no longer apparent in an additional 12%.[204] In contrast, infants with no neonatal neurological features (i.e., asymptomatic) were clearly abnormal on follow-up examination in only 6% of cases. Infants with neurological features, but *not* seizures, did nearly as well as those without any neurological features (see Table 12-14). However, the relatively brief follow-up period in this study is noteworthy.

In a study with a longer follow-up period of 39 hypoglycemic infants, most of whom were SGA,

---

*See references 1,2,9,10,20,175,178,179,203,204,206a,207,208.

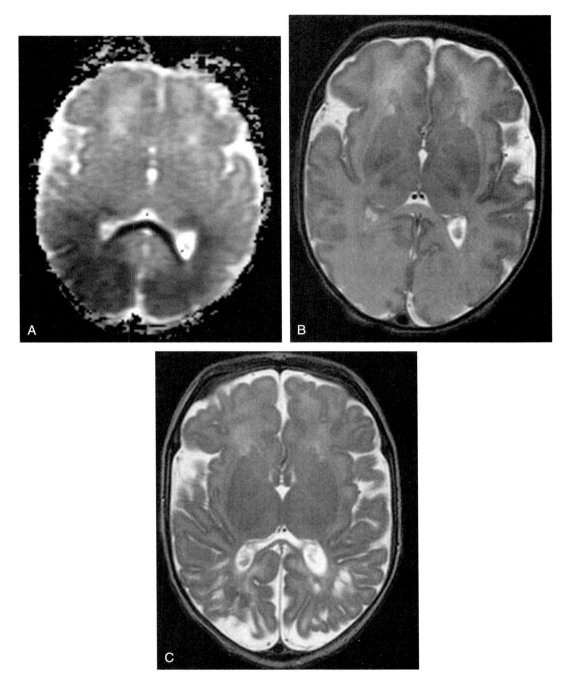

Figure 12-13   **Conventional magnetic resonance imaging (MRI) and diffusion-weighted MRI (DWI) in neonatal hypoglycemia. A,** ADC map (DWI), **B,** T-2 weighted (T2W) MRI on day 6, and **C,** T2W MRI on day 44, from a term infant with a minimum blood glucose of 1.1 mmol/L at 92 hours of age. Note in **A** the area of decreased diffusion (dark in the ADC map) in parieto-occipital cortex, subcortical white matter, and splenium of the corpus callosum, and in **B** the loss of gray-white matter differentiation in the parieto-occipital cortex and white matter on the T2W MRI. In **C,** atrophy of the parieto-occipital region and splenium is apparent on the T2W image at 44 days. *(From Filan PM, Inder TE, Cameron FJ, Kean MJ, et al: Neonatal hypoglycemia and occipital cerebral injury,* J Pediatr *148:552–555, 2006.)*

the prognostic importance of neonatal symptoms was reaffirmed.[1,207] Although mean intelligence quotient (IQ) scores were not significantly different between the total hypoglycemic group and the matched control group, a significantly larger number of the hypoglycemic children (13 of 25) had IQ scores less than 86 than did the control children (6 of 27) at 5 to 7 years of age. Children who did most poorly had *seizures* as part of their neonatal neurological syndrome.

Findings from a multicenter prospective study of preterm infants suggest that even *moderate hypoglycemia* (at least one daily value of plasma glucose <2.6 mmol/L, or ≈47 mg/dL) may be deleterious if it is present for 3 or more days (Table 12-15).[20] The data shown in Table 12-15 indicate an approximately 30% incidence of neurodevelopmental sequelae when moderate hypoglycemia was present for 3 days or more and approximately 40% when it was present for 5 days or more. Notably, relatively

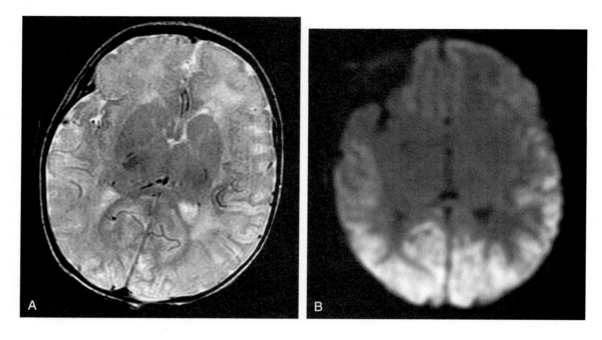

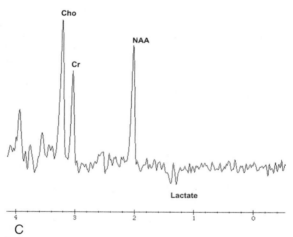

Figure 12-14 **Proton magnetic resonance spectroscopy (MRS) and diffusion-weighted magnetic resonance imaging (DWI) in neonatal hypoglycemia.** Images are from a term infant with minimum blood glucose of 5 mg/dL on day 2. On day 6, **A**, axial T2-weighted magnetic resonance imaging shows subtle loss of gray-white differentiation in parieto-occipital areas. However, in **B**, DWI shows markedly decreased diffusion (high signal) in these regions, and in **C**, MRS demonstrates an elevation of lactate. Cr, creatine; Cho, choline; NAA, *N*-acetylaspartate. *(Courtesy of Dr. Omar Khwaja.)*

TABLE 12-14	Neurological Outcome after Neonatal Hypoglycemia as a Function of Neonatal Neurological Features		
	NEUROLOGICAL OUTCOME*		
Neonatal Clinical Syndrome	**Normal**	**Transient Abnormality**	**Abnormal**
Neurological features: seizures	38%	12%	50%
Neurological features: no seizures	76%	12%	12%
No neurological features	80%	14%	6%

*Follow-up examination was at 1 to 4 years of age.
Adapted from Koivisto M, Blanco SM, Krause U: Neonatal symptomatic and asymptomatic hypoglycaemia: A follow-up study of 151 children, *Dev Med Child Neurol* 14:603–614, 1972.

TABLE 12-15	Neurological Outcome in Preterm Infants with Moderate Hypoglycemia*	
Duration of Hypoglycemia	**Percentage of All Infants Studied**	**Percentage with Neurodevelopmental Impairment***
≥3 days	15%	29%
≥5 days	6%	42%
≥7 days	3%	40%

*Neurodevelopmental impairment consisted of cerebral palsy (≈40%) or developmental delay (i.e., Bayley mental or motor score of ≥70 [≈60%]). The population consisted of 661 preterm infants (<1850 g at birth) who survived for more than 48 hours. Moderate hypoglycemia consisted of at least one daily value of plasma glucose lower than 2.6 mmol/L (≈47 mg/dL).
Data from Lucas A, Morley R, Cole TJ: Adverse neurodevelopment outcome of moderate neonatal hypoglycaemia, *BMJ* 297:1304–1308, 1988.

large proportions of all infants studied were affected (see Table 12-15). These findings emphasize the importance of *duration* of hypoglycemia, even if moderate, in determination of prognosis. Follow-up of this population showed persistence of abnormalities in arithmetic and motor scores at 7.5 to 8 years.[21] One study of 62 SGA preterm infants with neonatal hypoglycemia defined as values lower than 2.6 mmol/L or 47 mg/dL showed a strong correlation with persistent neurodevelopmental deficits and reduced head circumference, *especially in infants with recurrent episodes of moderate hypoglycemia* (compared with infants with a single episode of more pronounced hypoglycemia).[203] The latter point reemphasizes the importance of moderate hypoglycemia.

In recent years, infants at risk for hypoglycemia have been *screened from the first hours of life*, and low glucose levels have been treated promptly. In general, the results have been transient, relatively brief, mild hypoglycemia (<2.2 mmol/L, <40 mg/dL), and a favorable neurological outcome.[181,209] In one small series (*n* = 28) of infants of diabetic mothers, those who had a more clearly low blood glucose level (<1.5 mmol/L, 27 mg/dL) exhibited at the age of 8 years significantly more signs in a validated test of "minimal brain dysfunction," lower Griffiths developmental quotients, and more impulsivity, hyperactivity, and distractibility than infants who had values higher than 1.5 mmol/L.

Unresolved Issues

Of additional importance, and still to be defined, is the outcome in those infants who have neonatal hypoglycemia, marginal in severity, in association with other insults deleterious to the central nervous system. As indicated in the previous sections on biochemical and neuropathological aspects, strong data suggest *additive and potentiating effects of hypoglycemia*.

Of particular importance, in view of the parieto-occipital predominance of the pathology identified in hypoglycemic infants by MRI (see earlier), it is clear that more detailed neurophysiological testing focused on higher visual functions and visual-spatial associations is needed in follow-up studies. Many of these deficits are readily overlooked in conventional follow-up measurements. *Thus, currently the true frequency and full spectrum of neurological sequelae after neonatal hypoglycemia remain to be defined.*

Management

Management of the infant with neonatal hypoglycemia is considered best in terms of *prevention and therapy*. Major advances in both these aspects of management have been made in the past 20 years.

Prevention

Prevention of neonatal hypoglycemia must involve factors related to pregnancy, labor, delivery, and the early neonatal period. These factors are discussed most appropriately in standard texts of perinatology and neonatology. During pregnancy, importance can be attributed to control of maternal diabetes, preeclampsia/eclampsia, nutrition, and factors that cause prematurity. Prevention and control of perinatal asphyxia are clearly of major significance. Of particular relevance *after delivery* are (1) identification of the high-risk infant, (2) minimization of excessive caloric expenditures by maintenance of temperature, (3) implementation of oral feedings within the first 3 or 4 hours of life when possible, (4) careful surveillance for clinical symptoms, and (5) blood glucose level determinations before the first feeding and subsequently according to the clinical setting. Early discharge of preterm infants before firm establishment of oral feedings should be avoided to prevent postdischarge evolution of hypoglycemia.[162,210]

Simple preventive guidelines in *asymptomatic infants* can be summarized as follows.[14,15] In the *healthy appropriately grown term infant*, facilitating normal feeding is sufficient. In *preterm infants* of less than 32 to 34 weeks of gestation or those with respiratory distress, establishment of enteral feedings is relatively slow, and intravenous glucose, generally commencing at 6 mg glucose/kg/minute is needed. For clearly *intrauterine growth-retarded infants*, management depends in part on the initial glucose values but usually includes intravenous glucose infusions and early introduction of enteral feedings. Such infants are likely to require 8 mg/kg/minute of glucose. For *infants of diabetic mothers*, early glucose screening (highest incidence of hypoglycemia is at ≈4 to 6 hours of age), early enteral feeding and regular prefeed glucose monitoring are crucial. Early administration of glucagon to stimulate hepatic glycogenolysis may improve glycemic control. Excessive intravenous glucose should be avoided to prevent overstimulation of the infant's pancreas, already positioned to produce hyperinsulinism.

Therapy

When to Treat. The major issues in therapy relate to when and how to treat. Detection of hypoglycemia at the bedside, previously dependent on Dextrostix determinations, has been facilitated by portable reflectance meters, electrochemical glucose meters, and related instruments.[8,211-213] Confirmation of low values with laboratory determinations is important. Most physicians treat hypoglycemia with glucose infusion even if the infant is asymptomatic. The difficult issue in this context, of course, is the definition of hypoglycemia. This issue was discussed earlier (see "Definition"). At the present time, I consider that several factors support a recommendation to treat both the full-term and premature infant with blood glucose levels of less than 45 to 50 mg/dL. (Thresholds for treatment may be lower in the first 3 hours of life.) These factors include the following: (1) the neurophysiological,[6] epidemiologic,[20,21] and clinical[203] observations that levels less than 50 mg/dL can be associated with evidence for neurophysiological or neurodevelopmental dysfunction; (2) the positron emission tomography observation that cerebral glucose utilization in the premature infant may be limited by glucose transport at levels of plasma glucose less than approximately 54 mg/dL[29]; (3) the likelihood that degrees of hypoglycemia not sufficient to cause brain injury alone may do so when combined with other factors deleterious to the central nervous system; (4) the lack of precise information regarding the level of blood glucose below which neuronal injury is likely to occur; (5) the realization that the parieto-occipital region and higher visual functions are most sensitive to hypoglycemia and that such cortical functions have not been carefully studied in most previous follow-up reports; and (6) the ample experimental evidence that blood glucose levels are not accurate predictors of brain glucose levels, particularly in states such as asphyxia or seizures. It is essential that the physician consider the status of both *cerebral glucose delivery* (i.e., CBF), as well as blood glucose content, and *cerebral glucose utilization*.

How to Treat. If a decision is made to treat an infant, the next issue is the manner of therapy. A small group of infants requires specific therapies for hormonal or enzymatic aberrations; these therapies are discussed in detail elsewhere.[1,2,9,15,190,199] For the large group of infants in whom glucose alone is the mainstay of therapy, a frequent past recommendation was to institute intravenous treatment with a bolus infusion of 0.5 to 1.0 g/kg as 2 to 4 mL/kg of 25% glucose (at a rate of 1 mL/minute),[1] to be followed with a continuous infusion of 8 to 10 mg/kg/minute. However, later data indicated that this bolus infusion of glucose followed by continuous infusion may lead to *hyperglycemia*, especially in small preterm infants who exhibit impaired glucose homeostasis.[2,13,27,214] Hyperglycemia has been shown to cause osmotic diuresis and dehydration, has been associated with increased mortality and, perhaps, intracranial hemorrhage in premature infants, and often is followed by "rebound" hypoglycemia in hyperinsulinemic infants.[2,5,13,27,175,215,216] (Indeed, hyperglycemia can be an important contributory determinant of neurological sequelae even in infants without hypoglycemia.[5,175]) Therefore, it is prudent to avoid the relatively large bolus infusion, particularly in the premature infant. Pildes and co-workers[217] demonstrated particular effectiveness and safety of a *minibolus infusion* of 200 mg/kg (2 mL of 10% glucose injected over 1 minute), immediately

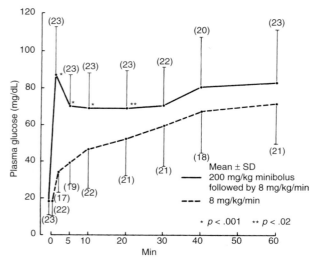

Figure 12-15 Response to minibolus therapy in hypoglycemia. Composite of blood glucose response to 200 mg/kg glucose minibolus followed by 8 mg/kg/minute constant glucose infusion in 23 hypoglycemic newborn infants and composite of blood glucose response to 8 mg/kg/minute constant glucose infusion, without minibolus, in 22 previously studied hypoglycemic infants. *(From Lilien LD, Pildes RS, Srinivasan G: Treatment of neonatal hypoglycemia with minibolus and intravenous glucose infusion,* J Pediatr *97:295–298, 1980.)*

followed by a continuous glucose infusion of 8 mg/kg/minute (Fig. 12-15 and Table 12-16).[217] The minibolus infusion results in rapid correction of blood glucose level (within 1 minute), and a relative stability of values between approximately 70 and 80 mg/dL occurs thereafter with the continuous infusion of 8 mg/kg/minute, approximately the maximum usable dose of glucose in the newborn.[175,218] Thus, for the *symptomatic infant,* I prefer the minibolus infusion. *Careful assessment of the initial clinical response after the minibolus infusion is essential,* especially if the indication for the infusion was seizure, because of variability in the response to blood glucose level; a second minibolus infusion may be necessary. *Continued careful monitoring of clinical response and blood glucose level* also is important because certain infants (e.g., those with hyperinsulinism) may require higher maintenance doses of glucose, whereas some infants require lower maintenance doses to avoid hyperglycemia.[*]

In general, after blood glucose levels are stable at 70 to 100 mg/dL, the dextrose concentration in the infusion is decreased by 2 mg/kg/minute every 6 to 12 hours.[175] Glucose levels are monitored closely and should be maintained at more than 50 mg/dL. For infants whose glucose levels do not increase adequately despite infusion rates of 12 mg/kg/minute or who require infusion rates of more than 12 mg/kg/minute, or if hypoglycemia recurs, the likely cause is hyperinsulinism (see Table 12-16). Treatment for the latter includes diazoxide (suppresses insulin secretion), octreotide (suppresses insulin secretion), or pancreatic surgery.[199] Less likely causes include specific hormonal defects (e.g., hypopituitarism) or a metabolic disorder

TABLE 12-16	Therapy of Neonatal Hypoglycemia*
Symptomatic Infant Glucose: 200 mg/kg as 2 mL/kg of 10% glucose IV	
Following Bolus Infusion, or at Start of Therapy if Infant Is Asymptomatic Glucose: 8 mg/kg/min IV	
If Glucose Rates of 12 mg/kg/min Required for Normoglycemia Treatment depends on disorder: likely hyperinsulinism (diazoxide, octreotide [somatostatin analogue], pancreatic surgery), hormonal defects, metabolic disorder	
Taper and Wean IV Glucose Slowly	

IV, intravenously
*See text for references.

*See references 8,9,13,15,16,27,175,178,217,219,220.

(see earlier), each of which requires specific therapy. Hydrocortisone, previously used in this context at 5 mg/kg every 12 hours, has benefit by increasing gluconeogenesis (from protein sources) and decreasing peripheral glucose utilization. This agent has been used less in recent years, and if administered, should be discontinued as soon as is feasible.[15]

REFERENCES

1. Cornblath M, Schwartz R: *Disorders of Carbohydrate Metabolism in Infancy*, 2nd ed, Philadelphia: 1976, Saunders.
2. Cowett RM: Hypoglycemia and hyperglycemia in the newborn. In Polin RA, Fox WW, editors: *Fetal and Neonatal Physiology*, Philadelphia: 1992, Saunders.
3. Srinivasan G, Pildes RS, Cattamanchi G, Voora S, et al: Clinical and laboratory observations: Plasma glucose values in normal neonates—a new look, *J Pediatr* 109:114-117, 1986.
4. Heck LJ, Erenberg A: Clinical and laboratory observations, *J Pediatr* 110:119-122, 1987.
5. Cornblath M, Schwartz R, Aynsley-Green A, Lloyd JK: Hypoglycemia in infancy: The need for a rational definition, *Pediatrics* 85:834-837, 1990.
6. Koh TH, Aynsley-Green A, Tarbit M, Eyre JA: Neural dysfunction during hypoglycaemia, *Arch Dis Child* 63:1353-1358, 1988.
7. Sann L: Neonatal hypoglycemia, *Biol Neonate* 58:16-21, 1990.
8. Schwartz RP: Neonatal hypoglycemia: How low is too low?, *J Pediatr* 131:171-173, 1997.
9. Polk DH: Disorders of carbohydrate metabolism. In Taeusch HW, Ballard RA, editors: *Avery's Diseases of the Newborn*, 7th ed, Philadelphia: 1998, Saunders.
10. Cowett RM: Hypoglycemia and hyperglycemia in the newborn. In Polin RA, Fox WW, editors: *Fetal and Neonatal Physiology*, 2nd ed, Philadelphia: 1998, Saunders.
11. Cornblath M, Hawdon JM, Williams AF, Aynsley-Green A, et al: Controversies regarding definition of neonatal hypoglycemia: Suggested operational thresholds, *Pediatrics* 105:1141-1145, 2000.
12. Hoseth E, Joergensen A, Ebbesen F, Moeller M: Blood glucose levels in a population of healthy, breast fed, term infants of appropriate size for gestational age, *Arch Dis Child Fetal Neonatal Ed* 83:F117-F119, 2000.
13. Cowett RM, Loughead JL: Neonatal glucose metabolism: differential diagnoses, evaluation, and treatment of hypoglycemia, *Neonatal Netw* 21:9-19, 2002.
14. Deshpande S, Ward Platt M: The investigation and management of neonatal hypoglycaemia, *Semin Fetal Neonatal Med* 10:351-361, 2005.
15. Kalhan SC, Parimi PS: Metabolic and endocrine disorders. In Martin RJ, Fanaroff AA, Walsh MC, editors: *Neonatal-Perinatal Medicine Diseases of the Fetus and Infant*, 8th ed, Philadelphia: 2006, Elsevier.
16. Rozance PJ, Hay WW: Hypoglycemia in newborn infants: Features associated with adverse outcomes, *Biol Neonate* 90:74-86, 2006.
17. Williams AF: Neonatal hypoglycaemia: Clinical and legal aspects, *Semin Fetal Neonatal Med* 10:363-368, 2005.
18. Cowett RM, Howard GM, Johnson J, Vohr B: Brain stem auditory-evoked response in relation to neonatal glucose metabolism, *Biol Neonate* 71:31-36, 1997.
19. Pryds O, Greisen G, Friis-Hansen B: Compensatory increase of CBF in preterm infants during hypoglycaemia, *Acta Paediatr Scand* 77:632-637, 1988.
20. Lucas A, Morley R, Cole TJ: Adverse neurodevelopment outcome of moderate neonatal hypoglycaemia, *BMJ* 297:1304-1308, 1988.
21. Lucas A, Morley R: Outcome of neonatal hypoglycaemia [letter], *BMJ* 318:194, 1999.
22. Hawdon JM, Aynsley-Green A, Alberti KG, Ward Platt MP: The role of pancreatic insulin secretion in neonatal glucoregulation. I. Healthy term and preterm infants, *Arch Dis Child* 68:274-279, 1993.
23. Hawdon JM, Ward Platt MP: Metabolic adaptation in small gestational age infants, *Arch Dis Child* 68:262-268, 1993.
24. Hawdon JM, Weddell A, Aynsley-Green A, Ward Platt MP: Hormonal and metabolic response to hypoglycaemia in small for gestational age infants, *Arch Dis Child* 68:269-273, 1993.
25. Hawdon JM, Aynsley-Green A, Ward Platt MP: Neonatal blood glucose concentrations: Metabolic effects of intravenous glucagon and intragastric medium chain triglyceride, *Arch Dis Child* 68:255-261, 1993.
26. Hawdon JM, Aynsley-Green A, Bartlett K, Ward Platt MP: The role of pancreatic insulin secretion in neonatal glucoregulation. II. Infants with disordered blood glucose homeostasis, *Arch Dis Child* 68:280-285, 1993.
27. Cowett RM, Farrag HM: Selected principles of perinatal-neonatal glucose metabolism, *Semin Neonatol* 9:37-47, 2004.
28. Bier DM, Leake RD, Haymond MW: Measurement of true glucose production rates in infancy and childhood with 6,6-dideuteroglucose, *Diabetes* 26:1016-1023, 1977.
29. Powers WJ, Rosenbaum JL, Dence CS, Markham J, et al: Cerebral glucose transport and metabolism in preterm human infants, *J Cereb Blood Flow Metab* 18:632-638, 1998.
30. Vannucci RC: Perinatal brain metabolism. In Polin RA, Fox WW, editors: *Fetal and Neonatal Physiology*, Philadelphia: 1992, Saunders.
31. Vannucci RC, Yager JY: Glucose, lactic acid, and perinatal hypoxic-ischemic brain damage, *Pediatr Neurol* 8:3-12, 1992.
32. Vannucci RC: Cerebral carbohydrate and energy metabolism in perinatal hypoxic-ischemic brain damage, *Brain Pathol* 2:229-234, 1992.
33. Siesjo BK: Hypoglycemia, brain metabolism and brain damage, *Diabetes Metab Rev* 4:113-144, 1988.
34. Nehlig A, de Vasconcelos AP: Glucose and ketone body utilization by the brain of neonatal rats, *Prog Neurobiol* 40:163-221, 1993.
35. Vannucci RC, Yager JY: Perinatal brain metabolism. In Polin RA, Fox WW, editors: *Fetal and Neonatal Physiology*, 2nd ed, Philadelphia: 1998, Saunders.
36. Yager JY: Hypoglycemic injury to the immature brain, *Clin Perinatol* 29:651-674, 2002.
37. McKenna MC, Gruetter R, Sonnewald U, Waagepetersen HS, et al: Energy metabolism of the brain. In Siegel GJ, Albers RW, Brady ST, et al, editors: *Basic Neurochemistry: Molecular, Cellular and Medical Aspects*, 7th ed, New York: 2006, Elsevier Academic.
38. Lienhard GE, Slot JW, James DE, Mueckler MM: How cells absorb glucose, *Sci Am* 266:86-91, 1992.
39. DeVivo DC, Trifiletti RR, Jacobson RI, Ronen GM, et al: Defective glucose transport across the blood-brain barrier as a cause of persistent hypoglycorrhachia, seizures and developmental delay, *N Engl J Med* 325:703-709, 1991.
40. Fishman RA: The glucose-transporter protein and glucopenic brain injury, *N Engl J Med* 325:731-732, 1991.
41. Vannucci SJ: Developmental expression of GLUT1 and GLUT3 glucose transporters in rat brain, *J Neurochem* 62:240-246, 1994.
42. DiMauro S, DeVivo DC: Diseases of carbohydrate, fatty acid and mitochondrial metabolism. In Siegel JG et al, editors: *Basic Neurochemistry: Molecular, Cellular and Medical Aspects*, 7th ed, New York: 2006, Elsevier.
43. Bachelard HS: Glucose transport and phosphorylation in the control of carbohydrate metabolism in the brain. In Brierley JB, Brown AW, Meldrum BS, editors: *Brain Hypoxia*, Philadelphia: 1971, JB Lippincott.
44. Lowry OH, Passonneau JV: The relationships between substrate and enzymes of glycolysis in the brain, *J Biol Chem* 239:31-42, 1964.
45. Lowry OH, Passonneau JV, Hasselberger FX, Schulz D: Effect of ischemia on known substrates and cofactors of the glycolytic pathway in brain, *J Biol Chem* 239:18-30, 1964.
45a. Brown AM, Ransom BR: Astrocyte glycogen and brain energy metabolism, *Glia* 55:1263-1271, 2007.
46. Ferrendelli JA: Cerebral utilization of nonglucose substrates and their effect in hypoglycemia. In *Brain Dysfunction in Metabolic Disorders*, New York: 1974, Raven Press.
47. Hernandez MJ, Vannucci RC, Salcedo A, Brennan RW: Cerebral blood flow and metabolism during hypoglycemia in newborn dogs, *J Neurochem* 35:622-628, 1980.
48. Mann LI, Duchin S, Halverstram J: The effect of hypoglycemia on fetal brain function and metabolism, *Am J Obstet Gynecol* 117:45-50, 1973.
49. Makowski EL, Schneider JM, Tsoulos NG: Cerebral blood flow, oxygen consumption, and glucose utilization of fetal lambs in utero, *Am J Obstet Gynecol* 114:292-303, 1972.
50. Tsoulos NG, Schneider JM, Colwill JR: Cerebral glucose utilization during aerobic metabolism in fetal sheep, *Pediatr Res* 6:182-186, 1972.
51. Chugani HT, Phelps ME: Maturational changes in cerebral function in infants determined by [18]FDG positron emission tomography, *Science* 231:840-843, 1986.
52. Chugani HT: Positron emission tomography study of human brain functional development, *Ann Neurol* 22:487-497, 1987.
53. Corbett RJT, Laptook AR, Sterett R, Tollefsbol G, et al: The effect of hypercarbia on age-related changes in cerebral glucose transport and glucose-modulated agonal glycolytic rates, *Pediatr Res* 34:370-378, 1993.
54. McIlwain H, Bachelard HS: *Biochemistry and the Central Nervous System*, Edinburgh: 1972, Churchill Livingstone.
55. McDougal DB: Defects in carbohydrate metabolism. In Siegel GJ, Albers RW, Agranoff BW, et al, editors: *Basic Neurochemistry*, Boston: 1981, Little, Brown.
56. Dombrowski GJ Jr, Swiatek KR, Chao KL: Lactate, 3-hydroxybutyrate, and glucose as substrates for the early postnatal rat brain, *Neurochem Res* 14:667-675, 1989.
57. Young RS, Petroff OA, Chen B, Aquila WJ Jr, et al: Preferential utilization of lactate in neonatal dog brain: In vivo and in vitro proton NMR study, *Biol Neonate* 59:46-53, 1991.
58. Bossi E, Kohler E, Herschkowitz N: Utilization of D-β-hydroxybutyrate and oleate as alternate energy fuels in brain cell cultures of newborn mice after hypoxia at different glucose concentrations, *Pediatr Res* 26:478-481, 1989.
59. Young RS, Cowan BE, Petroff OA, Novotny E, et al: In vivo ^{31}P and in vitro ^{1}H nuclear magnetic resonance study of hypoglycemia during neonatal seizure, *Ann Neurol* 22:622-628, 1987.

60. Rosenkrantz TS, Philipps AF, Knox I, Zalneraitis EL, et al: Regulation of cerebral glucose metabolism in normal and polycythemic newborn lambs, *J Cereb Blood Flow Metab* 12:856-865, 1992.
61. Thurston JH, Hauhart RE: Effect of momentary stress on brain energy metabolism in weaning mice: Apparent use of lactate as cerebral metabolic fuel concomitant with a decrease in brain glucose utilization, *Metab Brain Dis* 4:177-186, 1989.
62. Thurston JH, Hauhart RE, Schiro J: β-Hydroxybutyrate reverses insulin-induced hypoglycemic coma in suckling-weaning mice despite low blood and brain glucose levels, *Metab Brain Dis* 1:63-81, 1986.
63. Kliegman RM: Cerebral metabolic response to neonatal hypoglycemia in growth-retarded dogs, *Pediatr Res* 24:649-652, 1988.
64. Lin C-H, Gelardi NL, Cha C-J, Oh W: Cerebral metabolic response to hypoglycemia in severe intrauterine growth-retarded rat pups, *Early Hum Dev* 52:1-11, 1998.
65. Moore TJ, Lione AP, Sugden MC, Regen DM: Beta-hydroxybutyrate transport in rat brain: Developmental and dietary modulations, *Am J Physiol* 230:619-630, 1976.
66. Daniel PM, Love ER, Moorhouse SR, Pratt OE: The transport of ketone bodies into the brain of the rat (in vivo), *J Neurosci* 34:1-13, 1977.
67. Kraus H, Schlenker S, Schwedesky D: Developmental changes of cerebral ketone body utilization in human infants, *Physiol Chem* 355:164-170, 1974.
68. Adam PA, Raiha N, Rahiala E, Kekomaki M: Oxidation of glucose and D-beta-OH-butyrate by the early human fetal brain, *Acta Paediatr Scand* 64:17-24, 1975.
69. Hawkins RA, Williamson DH, Krebs HA: Ketone-body utilization by adult and suckling rat brain in vivo, *Biochem J* 122:13-18, 1971.
70. Page MA, Krebs HA, Williamson DH: Activities of enzymes of ketone-body utilization in brain and other tissues of suckling rats, *Biochem J* 121:49-53, 1971.
71. Spitzer JJ, Weng JT: Removal and utilization of ketone bodies by the brain of newborn puppies, *J Neurochem* 19:2169-2173, 1972.
72. Page MA, Williamson DH: Enzymes of ketone-body utilisation in human brain, *Lancet* 2:66-68, 1971.
73. Stanley CA, Anday EK, Baker L, Delivoria-Papadopoulos M: Metabolic fuel and hormone responses to fasting in newborn infants, *Pediatrics* 64:613-619, 1979.
74. Anday EK, Stanley CA, Baker L, Delivoria-Papadopoulos M: Plasma ketones in newborn infants: Absence of suckling ketosis, *J Pediatr* 98:628-630, 1981.
75. Plecko B, Stoeckler-Ipsiroglu S, Schober E, Harrer G, et al: Oral beta-hydroxybutyrate supplementation in two patients with hyperinsulinemic hypoglycemia: Monitoring of beta-hydroxybutyrate levels in blood and cerebrospinal fluid, and in the brain by in vivo magnetic resonance spectroscopy, *Pediatr Res* 52:301-306, 2002.
76. Vannucci RC, Nardis EE, Vannucci SJ, Campbell PA: Cerebral carbohydrate and energy metabolism during hypoglycemia in newborn dogs, *Am J Physiol* 240:R192-R199, 1981.
77. Young RS, Petroff OA, Chen B, Gore JC, et al: Brain energy state and lactate metabolism during status epilepticus in the neonatal dog: In vivo ^{31}P and $_1$H nuclear magnetic resonance study, *Pediatr Res* 29:191-195, 1991.
78. Cremer JR, Braun LD, Oldendorf WH: Changes during development in transport processes of blood-brain barrier, *Biochim Biophys Acta* 448:633-637, 1976.
79. Kuhlman RE, Lowry OH: Quantitative histochemical changes during the development of the rat cerebral cortex, *J Neurochem* 1:173-180, 1956.
80. Lehrer GM, Bornstein MB, Weiss C, Silides DJ: Enzymatic maturation of mouse cerebral neocortex in vitro and in situ, *Exp Neurol* 26:595-606, 1970.
81. Wilson JE: The relationship between glycolytic and mitochondrial enzymes in the developing rat brain, *J Neurochem* 19:223-227, 1972.
82. Vannucci RC, Duffy TE: Carbohydrate metabolism in fetal and neonatal rat brain during anoxia and recovery, *Am J Physiol* 230:1269-1275, 1976.
83. Comline RS, Silver M: The composition of foetal and maternal blood during parturition in the ewe, *J Physiol* 222:233-256, 1972.
84. Vannucci RC, Duffy TE: Influence of birth on carbohydrate and energy metabolism in rat brain, *Am J Physiol* 226:933-940, 1974.
85. Anwar M, Vannucci RC: Autoradiographic determination of regional cerebral blood flow during hypoglycemia in newborn dogs, *Pediatr Res* 24:41-45, 1988.
86. Mujsce DJ, Christensen MA, Vannucci RC: Regional cerebral blood flow and glucose utilization during hypoglycemia in newborn dogs, *Am J Physiol* 256:H1659-H1666, 1989.
87. Pryds O, Christensen NJ, Friis HB: Increased cerebral blood flow and plasma epinephrine in hypoglycemic, preterm neonates, *Pediatrics* 85:172-176, 1990.
88. Pryds O: Control of cerebral circulation in the high-risk neonate, *Ann Neurol* 30:321-329, 1991.
89. Skov L, Pryds O: Capillary recruitment for preservation of cerebral glucose influx in hypoglycemic, preterm newborns: Evidence for a glucose sensor, *Pediatrics* 90:193-195, 1992.
90. Ferrendelli JA, Chang M: Brain metabolism during hypoglycemia, *Arch Neurol* 28:173-177, 1973.
91. Lewis LD, Ljunggren B, Norberg K, Siesjo BK: Changes in carbohydrate substrates, amino acids and ammonia in the brain during insulin-induced hypoglycemia, *J Neurochem* 23:659-671, 1974.
92. Lewis LD, Ljunggren B, Ratcheson RA, Siesjo BK: Cerebral energy state in insulin-induced hypoglycemia, related to blood glucose and to EEG, *J Neurochem* 23:673-679, 1974.
93. Gibson GE, Blass JP: Impaired synthesis of acetylcholine in brain accompanying mild hypoxia and hypoglycemia, *J Neurochem* 27:37-42, 1976.
94. Norberg K, Siesjo BK: Oxidative metabolism of the cerebral cortex of the rat in severe insulin-induced hypoglycemia, *J Neurochem* 26:345-352, 1976.
95. Behar KL, Hollander JA, Petroff OA: Effect of hypoglycemic encephalopathy upon amino acids, high-energy phosphates, and pHi in the rat brain in vivo: Detection by sequential ^{1}H and ^{31}P NMR spectroscopy, *J Neurochem* 44:1045-1052, 1985.
96. Vannucci RC, Vannucci SJ: Cerebral carbohydrate metabolism during hypoglycemia and anoxia in newborn rats, *Ann Neurol* 4:73-79, 1978.
97. Agardh CD, Chapman AG, Nilsson B, Siesjo BK: Endogenous substrates utilized by rat brain in severe insulin-induced hypoglycemia, *J Neurochem* 36:490-500, 1981.
98. Ratcheson RA, Blank AC, Ferrendelli JA: Regionally selective metabolic effects of hypoglycemia in brain, *J Neurochem* 36:1952-1958, 1981.
99. Ghajar JB, Plum F, Duffy TE: Cerebral oxidative metabolism and blood flow during acute hypoglycemia and recovery in unanesthetized rats, *J Neurochem* 38:397-409, 1982.
100. Kliegman R, Hulman S, Morton S: Altered cerebral substrate utilization by the hypoglycemic dog, *Pediatr Res* 19:314-321, 1985.
101. Petroff OAC, Young RSK, Cowan BE: ^{1}H nuclear magnetic resonance spectroscopy study of neonatal hypoglycemia, *Pediatr Neurol* 4:31-34, 1988.
102. Paschen W, Siesjo BK, Ingvar M, Kossmann KA: Regional differences in brain glucose content in graded hypoglycemia, *Neurochem Pathol* 5:131-142, 1986.
103. Brown AM: Brain glycogen re-awakened, *J Neurochem* 89:537-552, 2004.
104. Kety SS, Woodford RB, Harmel MH: Cerebral blood flow and metabolism in schizophrenia: Effects of barbiturate seminarcosis, insulin coma and electroshock: 1948, *Am J Psychiatry* 151(Suppl):203-209, 1994.
105. Dahlquist G: Cerebral utilization of glucose, ketone bodies, and oxygen in starving infant rats and the effect of intrauterine growth retardation, *Acta Physiol Scand* 98:237-247, 1976.
106. Ghajar JB, Gibson GE, Duffy TE: Regional acetylcholine metabolism in brain during acute hypoglycemia and recovery, *J Neurochem* 44:94-98, 1985.
107. Wieloch T, Harris RJ, Symon L, Siesjo BK: Influence of severe hypoglycemia on brain extracellular calcium and potassium activities, energy, and phospholipid metabolism, *J Neurochem* 43:160-168, 1984.
108. Agardh CD, Folbergrova J, Siesjo BK: Cerebral metabolic changes in profound, insulin-induced hypoglycemia, and in the recovery period following glucose administration, *J Neurochem* 31:1135-1142, 1978.
109. Sandberg M, Butcher SP, Hagberg H: Extracellular overflow of neuroactive amino acids during severe insulin induced hypoglycemia in vivo dialysis of the rat hippocampus, *J Neurochem* 47:178-184, 1986.
110. Butcher SP, Sandberg M, Hagberg H, Hamberger A: Cellular origins of endogenous amino acids released into the extracellular fluid of the rat striatum during severe insulin-induced hypoglycemia, *J Neurochem* 47:722-728, 1987.
111. Wieloch T: Hypoglycemia-induced neuronal damage prevented by an N-methyl-D-aspartate antagonist, *Science* 230:681-683, 1985.
112. Facci L, Leon A, Skaper SD: Hypoglycemic neurotoxicity in vitro: Involvement of excitatory amino acid receptors and attenuation by monosialoganglioside GM1, *Neuroscience* 37:709-716, 1990.
113. Papagapiou MP, Auer RN: Regional neuroprotective effects of the NMDA receptor antagonist MK-801 (dizocilpine) in hypoglycemic brain damage, *J Cereb Blood Flow Metab* 10:270-276, 1990.
114. Monyer H, Goldberg MP, Choi DW: Glucose deprivation neuronal injury in cortical culture, *Brain Res* 483:347-354, 1989.
115. Tasker RC, Coyle JT, Vornov JJ: The regional vulnerability to hypoglycemia-induced neurotoxicity in organotypic hippocampal culture: Protection by early tetrodotoxin or delayed MK-801, *J Neurosci* 12:4298-4308, 1992.
116. Westerberg E, Kehr J, Ungerstedt U, Wieloch T: The NMDA-antagonist MK-801 reduces extracellular amino acid levels during hypoglycemia and prevents striatal damage, *Neurosci Res Com* 3:151-158, 1988.
117. Simon RP, Schmidley JW, Meldrum BS, Swan JH, et al: Excitotoxic mechanisms in hypoglycaemic hippocampal injury, *Neuropathol Appl Neurobiol* 12:567-576, 1986.
118. McGowan JE, Haynesaing AG, Mishra OP, Delivoria-Papadopoulos M: The effect of acute hypoglycemia on the cerebral NMDA receptor in newborn piglets, *Brain Res* 670:283-288, 1995.
119. Suh SW, Aoyama K, Chen YM, Garnier P, et al: Hypoglycemic neuronal death and cognitive impairment are prevented by poly(ADP-ribose) polymerase inhibitors administered after hypoglycemia, *J Neurosci* 23:10681-10690, 2003.
120. Vannucci RC, Nardis EE, Vannucci SJ: Cerebral metabolism during hypoglycemia and asphyxia in newborn dogs, *Biol Neonate* 38:276-286, 1980.

121. Shelley HJ: Glycogen reserves and their changes at birth and in anoxia, *Br Med J* 17:137, 1961.

122. Dawes GS, Mott JC, Shelley HJ: The importance of cardiac glycogen for the maintenance of life in fetal lambs and newborn animals during anoxia, *J Physiol* 152:271-298, 1960.

123. Lee JC, Halloran KH, Taylor JF, Downing SE: Coronary flow and myocardial metabolism in newborn: Effects of hypoxia and acidemia, *Am J Physiol* 224:1381-1387, 1973.

124. Silverstein FS, Simpson J, Gordon KE: Hypoglycemia alters striatal amino acid efflux in perinatal rats: An in vivo microdialysis study, *Ann Neurol* 28:516-521, 1990.

125. Papadopoulos MC, Koumenis IL, Dugan LL, Giffard RG: Vulnerability to glucose deprivation injury correlates with glutathione levels in astrocytes, *Brain Res* 748:151-156, 1997.

126. McGowan JE, Chen L, Gao D, Trush M, et al: Increased mitochondrial reactive oxygen species production in newborn brain during hypoglycemia, *Neurosci Lett* 399:111-114, 2006.

126a. Suh SW, Gum ET, Hamby AM, Chan PH, et al: Hypoglycemic neuronal death is triggered by glucose reperfusion and activation of neuronal NADPH oxidase, *J Clin Invest* 117:910-918, 2007.

127. Kokaia Z, Othberg A, Kokaia M, Lindvall O: BDNF makes cultured dentate granule cells more resistant to hypoglycaemic damage, *Neuroreport* 5:1241-1244, 1994.

128. Himwich HE, Bernstein AO, Herlich H: Mechanisms for the maintenance of life in the newborn during anoxia, *Am J Physiol* 135:387, 1942.

129. Juurlink BHJ, Hertz L, Yager JY: Astrocyte maturation and susceptibility to ischaemia or substrate deprivation, *Dev Neurosci* 3:1135-1137, 1992.

130. Callahan DJ, Engle MJ, Volpe JJ: Hypoxic injury to developing glial cells: Protective effect of high glucose, *Pediatr Res* 27:186-190, 1990.

131. Rosenberg AA, Murdaugh E: The effect of blood glucose concentration on postasphyxia cerebral hemodynamics in newborn lambs, *Pediatr Res* 27:454-459, 1990.

132. Salhab WA, Wyckoff MH, Laptook AR, Perlman JM: Initial hypoglycemia and neonatal brain injury in term infants with severe fetal acidemia, *Pediatrics* 114:361-366, 2004.

133. Siemkowicz E, Hansen AJ: Clinical restitution following cerebral ischemia in hypo-, normo- and hyperglycemic rats, *Acta Neurol Scand* 58:1-8, 1978.

134. Auer RN: Progress review: Hypoglycemic brain damage, *Stroke* 17:699-708, 1986.

135. Yager JY, Brucklacher RM, Vannucci RC: Cerebral oxidative metabolism and redox state during hypoxia-ischemia and early recovery in immature rats, *Am J Physiol* 261:H1102-H1108, 1991.

136. Yager JY, Heitjan DF, Towfighi J, Vannucci RC: Effect of insulin-induced and fasting hypoglycemia on perinatal hypoxic-ischemic brain damage, *Pediatr Res* 31:138-142, 1992.

137. Glauser TA, Rorke LB, Weinberg PM, Clancy RR: Acquired neuropathologic lesions associated with the hypoplastic left heart syndrome, *Pediatrics* 85:991-1000, 1990.

138. Nilsson B, Agardh CD, Ingvar M, Siesjo BK: Cerebrovascular response during and following severe insulin-induced hypoglycemia: CO_2-sensitivity, autoregulation, and influence of prostaglandin synthesis inhibition, *Acta Physiol Scand* 111:455-463, 1981.

139. Siesjo BK, Ingvar M, Pelligrino D: Regional differences in vascular autoregulation in the rat brain in severe insulin-induced hypoglycemia, *J Cereb Blood Flow Metab* 3:478-485, 1983.

140. Pelligrino D, Siesjo BK: Regulation of extra- and intracellular pH in the brain in severe hypoglycemia, *J Cereb Blood Flow Metab* 1:85-96, 1981.

141. Pelligrino D, Yokoyama H, Ingvar M, Siesjo BK: Moderate arterial hypotension reduces cerebral cortical blood flow and enhances cellular release of potassium in severe hypoglycemia, *Acta Physiol Scand* 115:511-513, 1982.

142. Gomez B, García-Villallón AL, Frank A, García JL, et al: Effects of hypoglycemia on the cerebral circulation in awake goats, *Neurology* 42:909-916, 1992.

143. Cipolla MJ, Porter JM, Osol G: High glucose concentrations dilate cerebral arteries and diminish myogenic tone through an endothelial mechanism, *Stroke* 28:405-410, 1997.

144. Blennow G, Folbergrova J, Nilsson B, Siesjo BK: Effects of bicuculline-induced seizures on cerebral metabolism and circulation of rats rendered hypoglycemic by starvation, *Ann Neurol* 5:139-151, 1979.

145. Dwyer BE, Wasterlain CG: Neonatal seizures in monkeys and rabbits: Brain glucose depletion in the face of normoglycemia, prevention by glucose loads, *Pediatr Res* 19:992-995, 1985.

146. Fujikawa DG, Vannucci RC, Dwyer BE, Wasterlain CG: Generalized seizures deplete brain energy reserves in normoxemic newborn monkeys, *Brain Res* 454:51-59, 1988.

147. Meldrum BS, Horton RW, Brierley JB: Insulin-induced hypoglycaemia in the primate: Relationship between physiological changes and neuropathology. In Brierley JB, Meldrum BS, editors: *Brain Hypoxia*, Philadelphia: 1971, JB Lippincott.

148. Brierley JB, Brown AW, Meldrum BS: The neuropathology of insulin induced hypoglycaemia in primate. In Brierley JB, Meldrum BS, editors: *Brain Hypoxia*, Philadelphia: 1971, JB Lippincott.

149. Agardh CD, Kalimo H, Olsson Y, Siesjo BK: Hypoglycemic brain injury. I. Metabolic and light microscopic findings in rat cerebral cortex during profound insulin-induced hypoglycemia and in the recovery period following glucose administration, *Acta Neuropathol (Berl)* 50:31-41, 1980.

150. Auer RN, Kalimo H, Olsson Y, Siesjo BK: The temporal evolution of hypoglycemic brain damage, *Acta Neuropathol (Berl)* 67:13-24, 1985.

151. Auer RN, Wieloch T, Olsson Y, Siesjo BK: The distribution of hypoglycemic brain damage, *Acta Neuropathol (Berl)* 64:177-191, 1984.

152. Kalimo H, Auer RN, Siesjo BK: The temporal evolution of hypoglycemic brain damage, *Acta Neuropathol (Berl)* 67:37-50, 1985.

153. Anderson JM, Milner RD, Strich SJ: Effects of neonatal hypoglycaemia on the nervous system: A pathological study, *J Neurol Neurosurg Psychiatry* 30:295-310, 1967.

154. Griffiths AD, Laurence KM: The effect of hypoxia and hypoglycaemia on the brain of the newborn human infant, *Dev Med Child Neurol* 16:308-319, 1974.

155. Spar JA, Lewine JD, Orrison WW: Neonatal hypoglycemia: CT and MR findings, *AJNR Am J Neuroradiol* 15:1477-1478, 1994.

156. Traill Z, Squier M, Anslow P: Brain imaging in neonatal hypoglycaemia, *Arch Dis Child Fetal Neonatal Ed* 79:F145-F147, 1998.

157. Barkovich AJ, Al Ali F, Rowley HA, Bass N: Imaging patterns of neonatal hypoglycemia, *AJNR Am J Neuroradiol* 19:523-528, 1998.

158. Chiu NT, Huang CC, Chang YC, Lin CH, et al: Technetium-99m-HMPAO brain SPECT in neonates with hypoglycemic encephalopathy, *J Nucl Med* 39:1711-1713, 1998.

159. Kinnala A, Rikalainen H, Lapinleimu H, Parkkola R, et al: Cerebral magnetic resonance imaging and ultrasonography findings after neonatal hypoglycemia, *Pediatrics* 103:724-729, 1999.

160. Caraballo RH, Sakr D, Mozzi M, Guerrero A, et al: Symptomatic occipital lobe epilepsy following neonatal hypoglycemia, *Pediatr Neurol* 31:24-29, 2004.

161. Alkalay AL, Flores-Sarnat L, Sarnat HB, Moser FG, et al: Brain imaging findings in neonatal hypoglycemia: Case report and review of 23 cases, *Clin Pediatr (Phila)* 44:783-790, 2005.

162. Moore AM, Perlman M: Symptomatic hypoglycemia in otherwise healthy, breastfed term newborns, *Pediatrics* 103:837-839, 1999.

163. Murakami Y, Yamashita Y, Matsuishi T, Utsunomiya H, et al: Cranial MRI of neurologically impaired children suffering from neonatal hypoglycaemia, *Pediatr Radiol* 29:23-27, 1999.

164. Cakmakci H, Usal C, Karabay N, Kovanlikaya A: Transient neonatal hypoglycemia: Cranial US and MRI findings, *Eur Radiol* 11:2585-2588, 2001.

165. Filan PM, Inder TE, Cameron FJ, Kean MJ, et al: Neonatal hypoglycemia and occipital cerebral injury, *J Pediatr* 148:552-555, 2006.

166. Friede RL: *Developmental Neuropathology*, 2nd ed, New York: 1989, Springer-Verlag.

167. Larroche JC: *Developmental Pathology of the Neonate*, New York: 1977, Excerpta Medica.

168. Rorke LB: *Pathology of Perinatal Brain Injury*, New York: 1982, Raven Press.

169. Yan H, Rivkees SA: Hypoglycemia influences oligodendrocyte development and myelin formation, *Neuroreport* 17:55-59, 2006.

170. Chase HP, Marlow RA, Dabiere CS, Welch NN: Hypoglycemia and brain development, *Pediatrics* 52:513-520, 1973.

171. Banker BQ: The neuropathological effects of anoxia and hypoglycemia in the newborn, *Dev Med Child Neurol* 9:544-550, 1967.

172. Sexson WR: Incidence of neonatal hypoglycemia: A matter of definition, *J Pediatr* 105:149-150, 1984.

173. Diwakar KK, Sasidhar MV: Plasma glucose levels in term infants who are appropriate size for gestation and exclusively breast fed, *Arch Dis Child Fetal Neonatal Ed* 87:F46-F48, 2002.

174. Gutberlet RL, Cornblath M: Neonatal hypoglycemia revisited, *Pediatrics* 58:10-17, 1976.

175. Pildes RS, Lilien LD: Carbohydrate disorders. In Fanaroff AA, Martin RJ, editors: *Neonatal-Perinatal Medicine, Behrman's Diseases of the Fetus and Infant*, St. Louis, 1987, C.V. Mosby.

176. Mehta A: Prevention and management of neonatal hypoglycaemia, *Arch Dis Child Fetal Neonatal Ed* 70:F54-F65, 1994.

177. Hawdon JM, Platt M, Aynsley-Green A: Prevention and management of neonatal hypoglycaemia [commentary], *Arch Dis Child Fetal Neonatal Ed* 70:F60-F65, 1994.

178. Cowett RM: *Pathophysiology, Diagnosis, and Management of Glucose Homeostasis in the Neonate*, Chicago: 1985, Year Book.

179. Stenninger E, Flink R, Eriksson B, Sahlen C: Long term, neurological dysfunction and neonatal hypoglycaemia after diabetic pregnancy, *Arch Dis Child Fetal Neonatal Ed* 79:F174-F179, 1998.

180. Schaefer-Graf UM, Rossi R, Buhrer C, Siebert G, et al: Rate and risk factors of hypoglycemia in large-for-gestational-age newborn infants of nondiabetic mothers, *Am J Obstet Gynecol* 187:913-917, 2002.

181. Brand PL, Molenaar NL, Kaaijk C, Wierenga WS: Neurodevelopmental outcome of hypoglycaemia in healthy, large for gestational age, term newborns, *Arch Dis Child* 90:78-81, 2005.

182. Lagercrantz H, Bistoletti P: Catecholamine release in the newborn after birth, *Pediatr Res* 11:889-896, 1973.

183. Collins JE, Leonard JV: Hyperinsulinism in asphyxiated and small-for-dates infants with hypoglycemia, *Lancet* 2:311-313, 1984.

184. Klenka HM, Seager J: Hyperinsulinism in asphyxiated and small-for-dates infants with hypoglycemia, *Lancet* 2:975, 1984.
185. Collins J: A practical approach to the diagnosis of metabolic disease in the neonate, *Dev Med Child Neurol* 32:79-86, 1990.
186. Sovik O: Inborn errors of amino acid and fatty acid metabolism with hypoglycemia as a major clinical manifestation, *Acta Paediatr Scand* 78:161-170, 1989.
187. Perelmuter B, Goodman SI, McCabe ER: Galactosaemia with fatal cerebral oedema, *J Inherit Metab Dis* 12:489-490, 1989.
188. Waggoner DD, Buist NRM, Donnell GN: Long-term prognosis in galactosaemia: Results of a survey of 350 cases, *J Inherit Metab Dis* 13:802-818, 1990.
189. Matsuo M, Maeda E, Nakamura H, Koike K, et al: Hepatic phosphoenol-pyruvate carboxykinase deficiency: A neonatal case with reduced activity of pyruvate carboxylase, *J Inherit Metab Dis* 12:336-337, 1989.
190. Zeller J, Bougneres P: Hypoglycemia in infants, *Trends Endocrinol Metab* 3:366-370, 1992.
191. Riudor E: Neonatal onset in fatty acid oxidation disorders: How can we minimize morbidity and mortality, *J Inherit Metab Dis* 21:619-623, 1998.
192. Riudor E, Arranz JA, Anguera R, Salcedo S, et al: Neonatal medium-chain acyl-CoA dehydrogenase deficiency presenting with very high creatine kinase levels, *J Inherit Metab Dis* 21:673-674, 1998.
193. Spiekerkoetter U, Khuchua Z, Yue Z, Strauss AW: The early-onset phenotype of mitochondrial trifunctional protein deficiency: A lethal disorder with multiple tissue involvement, *J Inherit Metab Dis* 27:294-296, 2004.
194. Moore DJ: Medium-chain acyl-CoA dehydrogenase deficiency: A case presentation, *Neonatal Netw* 5:7-13, 2005.
195. Bell JJ, August GP, Blethen SL, Baptista J: Neonatal hypoglycemia in a growth hormone registry: Incidence and pathogenesis, *J Pediatr Endocrinol Metab* 17:629-635, 2004.
196. Cohen MM, Jr: Beckwith-Wiedemann syndrome: Historical, clinico-pathological, and etiopathogenetic perspectives, *Pediatr Dev Pathol* 8:287-304, 2005.
197. Garcia-Cazorla A, Rabier D, Touati G, Chadefaux-Vekemans B, et al: Pyruvate carboxylase deficiency: Metabolic characteristics and new neurological aspects, *Ann Neurol* 59:121-127, 2006.
198. Sperling MA, Menon RK: Differential diagnosis and management of neonatal hypoglycemia, *Pediatr Clin North Am* 51:703-723, 2004.
199. Hussain K: Congenital hyperinsulinism, *Semin Fetal Neonatal Med* 10:369-376, 2005.
200. Hussain K, Aynsley-Green A: Hyperinsulinaemic hypoglycaemia in preterm neonates, *Arch Dis Child Fetal Neonatal Ed* 89:65-67, 2004.
201. Menni F, de Lonlay P, Sevin C, Touati G, et al: Neurologic outcomes of 90 neonates and infants with persistent hyperinsulinemic hypoglycemia, *Pediatrics* 107:476-479, 2001.
202. Raizen DM, Brooks-Kayal A, Steinkrauss L, Tennekoon GI, et al: Central nervous system hyperexcitability associated with glutamate dehydrogenase gain of function mutations, *J Pediatr* 146:388-394, 2005.
203. Duvanel CB, Fawer C-L, Cotting J, Hohlfeld P, et al: Long-term effects of neonatal hypoglycemia on brain growth and psychomotor development in small-for-gestational-age preterm infants, *J Pediatr* 134:492-498, 1999.
204. Koivisto M, Blanco SM, Krause U: Neonatal symptomatic and asymptomatic hypoglycaemia: A follow-up study of 151 children, *Dev Med Child Neurol* 14:603-614, 1972.
205. Fluge G: Clinical aspects of neonatal hypoglycaemia, *Acta Paediatr Scand* 63:826, 1974.
206. Kim SY, Goo HW, Lim KH, Kim ST, et al: Neonatal hypoglycaemic encephalopathy: Diffusion-weighted imaging and proton MR spectroscopy, *Pediatr Radiol* 36:144-148, 2006.
206a. Yalnizoglu D, Haliloglu G, Turanli G, Cila A, et al: Neurologic outcome in patients with MRI pattern of damage typical for neonatal hypoglycemia, *Brain Dev* 29:285-292, 2007.
207. Pildes RS, Cornblath M, Warren I: A prospective controlled study of neonatal hypoglycemia, *Pediatrics* 54:5-14, 1974.
208. Fluge G: Neurological findings at follow-up in neonatal hypoglycaemia, *Acta Paediatr Scand* 64:629-634, 1975.
209. Dalgic N, Ergenekon E, Soysal S, Koc E, et al: Transient neonatal hypoglycemia: Long-term effects on neurodevelopmental outcome, *J Pediatr Endocrinol Metab* 15:319-324, 2002.
210. Hume R, McGeehan A, Burchell A: Failure to detect preterm infants at risk of hypoglycemia before discharge, *J Pediatr* 134:499-502, 1999.
211. Innanen VT, Deland ME, deCampos FM, Dunn MS: Point-of-care glucose testing in the neonatal intensive care unit is facilitated by the use of the Ames glucometer elite electrochemical glucose meter, *J Pediatr* 130:151-155, 1997.
212. Michel A, Kuster H, Krebs A, Kadow I, et al: Evaluation of the Glucometer Elite XL device for screening for neonatal hypoglycaemia, *Eur J Pediatr* 164:660-664, 2005.
213. Ho HT, Yeung WK, Young BW: Evaluation of "point of care" devices in the measurement of low blood glucose in neonatal practice, *Arch Dis Child Fetal Neonatal Ed* 89:F356-F359, 2004.
214. Cowett RM, Andersen GE, Maguire CA, Oh W: Ontogeny of glucose homeostasis in low birth weight infants, *J Pediatr* 112:462-465, 1988.
215. Dweck HS, Cassady G: Glucose intolerance in infants of very low birth weight, *Pediatrics* 53:189-195, 1974.
216. Zarif M, Pildes RS, Vidyasagar D: Insulin and growth hormone responses in neonatal hyperglycemia, *Diabetes* 25:428-433, 1976.
217. Lilien LD, Pildes RS, Srinivasan G: Treatment of neonatal hypoglycemia with minibolus and intravenous glucose infusion, *J Pediatr* 97:295-298, 1980.
218. Bier DM, Leake RD, Arnold KJ: Glucose production rates in infancy and childhood, *Pediatr Res* 10:405-412, 1976.
219. Lilien LD, Grajwer LA, Pildes RS: Treatment of neonatal hypoglycemia with continuous intravenous glucose infusion, *J Pediatr* 91:779-782, 1977.
220. Lilien LD, Rosenfield RL, Baccaro MM, Pildes RS: Hyperglycemia in stressed small premature neonates, *J Pediatr* 94:454-459, 1979.

Chapter 13

Bilirubin and Brain Injury

An important relationship between bilirubin and injury to the neonatal central nervous system has been recognized for many years. The first comprehensive description of the most overt form of bilirubin encephalopathy (i.e., kernicterus) was provided by Schmorl in 1903.[1] The development of therapeutic measures, such as exchange transfusion, and of preventive measures, such as the use of anti-Rh immune globulin to prevent maternal sensitization, has caused a marked decrease in this overt form of bilirubin encephalopathy. However, the evidence for bilirubin neurotoxicity continues to appear. Indeed, in the United States, early discharge of newborns ($\leq$48 hours of age), provoked in considerable part by managed care practices, has resulted in relatively frequent readmission for hyperbilirubinemia in the first 1 to 2 weeks of life.[2-4] A recrudescence in bilirubin brain injury, in part because of this change in practice, is suggested by recent observations.[3-7]

In this chapter, I review normal bilirubin structure and metabolism, the pathophysiology of hyperbilirubinemia and bilirubin neurotoxicity, and the neuropathological and clinical aspects of bilirubin injury to the neonatal central nervous system.

NORMAL BILIRUBIN STRUCTURE AND METABOLISM

Central to an understanding of the relation of bilirubin to neonatal brain injury is an awareness of the normal aspects of bilirubin structure, properties, and metabolism in the newborn. Thus, before the pathophysiology of bilirubin encephalopathies is discussed, certain highly relevant aspects of the chemical structure and solubility of bilirubin, as well as normal bilirubin metabolism, are briefly reviewed.

Bilirubin Structure and Properties

Bilirubin is a catabolic product of the porphyrin ring, derived from heme (see subsequent discussion). This compound can exist in plasma as bilirubin anion (monoanion or dianion form) (Fig. 13-1A) or as bilirubin acid (see Fig. 13-1B). Bilirubin dianion binds actively to albumin. The dianion is not highly soluble in lipid or nonpolar solvents,[8-15] but in view of the two polar carboxyl groups and oxidipyrryl (lactam) groups, it is not surprising that the anionic forms of bilirubin are relatively soluble in polar solvents. Although the

anionic forms were considered previously to be the principal free bilirubin species in plasma, more recent work showed that at physiological pH the acceptance of two hydrogen ions results in bilirubin diacid (see Fig. 13-1B). The diacid has a rigid folded structure, maintained by six internal hydrogen bonds involving all the polar groups, thereby rendering the molecule poorly soluble in aqueous solutions.[16] However, the compound does passively diffuse across plasma membranes of cells (see later). When the concentration of free bilirubin diacid exceeds its limit of aqueous solubility ($\approx$70 nM at physiological pH), the compound exists as soluble oligomers and metastable microaggregates. Moreover, at very high concentrations of the diacid, insoluble precipitates form and may result in major injury to membranes. At *physiological pH*, the species of free bilirubin are approximately 82% diacid, 16% monoanion, and 2% dianion.[16] These chemical properties of bilirubin are important in understanding the neurotoxicity of bilirubin (see later discussion).

Bilirubin Metabolism

Normal bilirubin metabolism is considered best in terms of the following sequential events: (1) production, (2) transport, (3) hepatic uptake, (4) conjugation, (5) excretion, and (6) enterohepatic circulation (Fig. 13-2).[4,15,17-21]

Production

Bilirubin is the end product of the catabolism of heme, the major source of which is circulating hemoglobin (see Fig. 13-2). In the newborn infant, the normal destruction of circulating red blood cells in the reticuloendothelial system accounts for approximately 75% of the daily production of bilirubin. The conversion of the heme moiety to bilirubin requires the sequential action of two enzymes, heme oxygenase (to form biliverdin), and a reduced nicotinamide adenine dinucleotide phosphate (NADPH)–dependent biliverdin reductase (to form bilirubin). Approximately 25% of the daily production of bilirubin in the newborn is derived from sources other than senescent red blood cells. This "other" fraction has two major components: a nonerythropoietic component, resulting from turnover of nonhemoglobin sources of heme (e.g., cytochromes, catalase, peroxidase, and myoglobin), and an erythropoietic component, resulting from destruction of products of ineffective erythropoiesis.

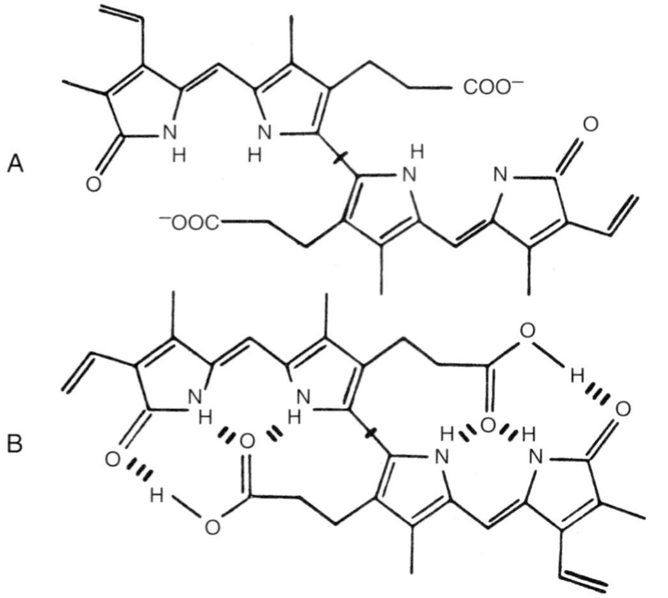

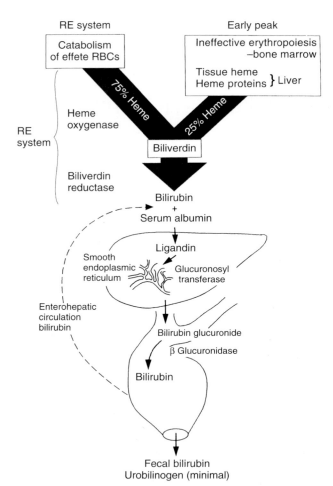

Figure 13-1 **Chemical structures of bilirubin. A,** Bilirubin dianion, with two free carboxyl groups; bilirubin monoanion has one free carboxyl group. **B,** Bilirubin diacid, the predominant form of free bilirubin in plasma at physiological pH. See text for details. *(From Brodersen R: Bilirubin transport in the newborn infant, reviewed in relation to kernicterus, J Pediatr 96:349–356, 1980.)*

Figure 13-2 **Bilirubin metabolism.** See text for details. RBCs, red blood cells; RE system, reticuloendothelial system. *(From Maisels MJ: Jaundice. In Avery G, Fletcher MA, MacDonald MG, editors: Neonatology: Pathophysiology and Management of the Newborn, 5th ed, Philadelphia: 1999, Lippincott Williams & Wilkins.)*

Transport

Bilirubin leaves the site of production in the reticuloendothelial system and is transported in plasma bound to albumin (see Fig. 13-2). Human albumin has a single, tight, high-affinity (or primary) binding site for bilirubin and one or more (probably two) weaker, lower-affinity binding sites.[3,4,15,18,19,22-25] The capacity of serum albumin to bind bilirubin is known as the *binding capacity*, and the strength of the bilirubin-albumin bond is referred to as the *binding affinity*. The amount of *free bilirubin* (i.e., bilirubin not bound to albumin) is very low at physiological pH. These latter three characteristics of a given serum-binding capacity, binding affinity, and amount of free bilirubin can be estimated by in vitro measurements[4,18,26,27] and provide a measure, albeit only approximate, of the amount of bilirubin that may be available to cause neuronal injury (see later discussion).

Hepatic Uptake

Hepatocytes have a selective and highly efficient system for removing unconjugated bilirubin from plasma. This mechanism requires several different organic anion transport proteins.[4,28] Variants of one of these, organic anion transporter 2 (OATP2), may be important in determining the elevated risk of severe hyperbilirubinemia in Asian infants.[29] In the hepatocyte, the transported bilirubin is bound to a cytosolic protein, ligandin, which facilitates transfer to the endoplasmic reticulum, the site of bilirubin conjugation.[4]

Conjugation

Conversion of bilirubin to excretable monoconjugates and diconjugates is carried out primarily by the microsomal enzyme uridine-diphosphate (UDP)–glucuronyl transferase (A1 isoform). The protein is encoded by the *UGT1A1* gene.[4] Variants of the *UGT1A1* gene appear to be important in determining the elevated risk of severe hyperbilirubinemia in Asian infants.[29] The diconjugate accounts for approximately 90% of total bilirubin glucuronide conjugates.[4,15,18,19,30]

Excretion

The conjugated bilirubin is excreted into the bile. Because this event occurs across a concentration gradient, an energy-dependent active transport system is involved.[4,15,30] The conjugated bilirubin is then transported to the small intestine, is primarily further degraded by intestinal bacteria, and is excreted in the stool.

Enterohepatic Circulation

Enterohepatic circulation also occurs. Intestinal beta-glucuronidase hydrolyzes the conjugated bilirubin, thus releasing free bilirubin, which then is reabsorbed and transported by the portal circulation to the liver (see Fig. 13-2).

PATHOPHYSIOLOGY

Hyperbilirubinemia

Although the relationship between serum levels of unconjugated bilirubin and neurotoxicity is not simple (see subsequent sections), a general link can be discerned between neonatal hyperbilirubinemia and the risk of neural injury. Thus, I review briefly here the major causes of neonatal hyperbilirubinemia, including the universal ("physiological") elevation of bilirubin in the newborn.

Major Causes

In the newborn period, numerous disorders may lead to elevated concentrations of unconjugated bilirubin (Table 13-1). These include the following: disorders with *increased production*, principally hemolytic disease, secondary to blood group incompatibility, intrinsic defects of red blood cells or hemoglobin, degradation of extravascular blood (i.e., hemorrhage), polycythemia, sepsis; disorders with disturbed gastrointestinal transit and therefore *increased enterohepatic circulation;* and

TABLE 13-1	**Major Causes of Neonatal Unconjugated Hyperbilirubinemia***

Increased Production
Hemolytic disease
Immune-mediated: Rh or ABO incompatibility
Inherited red blood cell defects: red blood cell membranes (e.g., spherocytosis), hemoglobin (e.g., thalassemias), or red blood cell metabolism (e.g., glucose-6-phosphate dehydrogenase activity[†])
Other
Hematoma, including cerebral, or other extravasation of blood
Polycythemia
Sepsis[†]
Large infants of diabetic mothers

Increased Enterohepatic Circulation
Breast-milk feeding
Pyloric stenosis[†]
Bowel obstruction

Decreased Conjugation
Prematurity
Glucose-6-phosphase dehydrogenase deficiency
Inborn errors (e.g., Crigler-Najjar, Gilbert syndrome)
Hypothyroidism

*Adapted from Maisels MJ: Jaundice. In MacDonald MG, Mullett MD, Seshia MMK, editors: *Avery's Neonatology Pathophysiology and Management of the Newborn*, 6th ed, Philadelphia: 2005, Lippincott Williams & Wilkins.
†Decreased conjugation/clearance also involved.

disorders of bilirubin conjugation, including inherited and acquired defects (e.g., prematurity) and hormonal disturbances (e.g., hypothyroidism).[4,30-33] Central to the frequency of hyperbilirubinemia in the newborn is the development of hyperbilirubinemia that occurs normally and onto which these other causes are grafted. This *physiological jaundice of the newborn* may be better termed *developmental hyperbilirubinemia* because it is very difficult to define precisely when this neonatal process is physiological and when it is pathological.[3,4,20,30,34]

Physiological Hyperbilirubinemia

Definition. *Physiological hyperbilirubinemia* refers to the elevation of serum bilirubin values that occur in essentially every newborn infant in the first week of life. In classic earlier studies of formula-fed white and African American full-term infants, the serum bilirubin level rose gradually to a mean peak of approximately 6 mg/dL by 48 to 72 hours of life and then declined relatively rapidly to a slightly elevated level, approximately 3 mg/dL, at approximately 5 days of life. After the peak bilirubin level was reached, little change then occurred for several days, and then a second, gradual decline occurred, with normal levels reached by approximately 2 weeks.[3,4,35] Thus, two phases could be identified in the human, and the mechanisms underlying these two phases were studied in detail in the neonatal monkey, in which the biphasic course is also apparent.[35] With the current increase in breast-feeding in the United States and elsewhere, peak values for bilirubin clearly are greater than in the earlier studies. Thus, in predominantly breast-fed white and African American term infants, the normal peak value is 8 to 9 mg/dL, and the decline is slower.[4] In Asian newborns (predominantly breast-fed), the peak values, 10 to 14 mg/dL, are still higher than those in white and African American infants.[3,29] In the premature infant, the peak serum bilirubin concentration occurs slightly later than in the full-term infant (i.e., approximately the fourth to fifth day) and is higher (i.e., mean, 10 to 12 mg/dL); normal levels may not be reached until 3 to 4 weeks of age.[36] More importantly, the term *physiological hyperbilirubinemia* in the *premature infant* is misleading because such values are potentially dangerous (see later).[4] Indeed, in infants of very low birth weight, phototherapy is recommended well before values reach 10 to 12 mg/dL (see later).

The *near-term infant* (i.e., 35 to 37 weeks of gestation) presents a situation intermediate between the clearly premature infant and the full-term infant (38 to 42 weeks of gestation). Thus, several studies showed that such infants have a severalfold higher risk of significant hyperbilirubinemia in the first week of life.[37-40] In a careful study through the first 7 days of life, near-term infants exhibited a later and higher peak value of bilirubin than did term infants. Moreover, the higher values declined more slowly in the near-term infants. Overall, 10% of the full-term infants had significant hyperbilirubinemia requiring phototherapy, versus 25% in the near-term group.[40] These data highlight

TABLE 13-2	Probable Mechanisms Involved in Physiological Hyperbilirubinemia

Increased Bilirubin Production
↑ Red blood cell volume
↓ Red blood cell survival
↑ "Other" sources

Increased Enterohepatic Circulation

Decreased Hepatic Uptake of Bilirubin from Plasma
↓ Membrane transport
↓ Ligandin

Defective Bilirubin Conjugation
↓ Uridine-diphosphate–glucuronyl transferase

↑, increased; ↓, decreased.
Data from Maisels MJ: Jaundice. In MacDonald MG, Mullett MD, Seshia MMK, editors: *Avery's Neonatology Pathophysiology and Management of the Newborn*, 6th ed, Philadelphia: 2005, Lippincott Williams & Wilkins.

the importance of particularly close follow-up of near-term infants after hospital discharge (see later).

Mechanisms. The mechanisms considered important in the genesis of physiological hyperbilirubinemia are shown in Table 13-2. Although evidence has been mustered for all these factors, studies of the newborn monkey provided considerable insight into their relative importance.[35] Thus, the *first phase* of hyperbilirubinemia (see previous section) has been shown to relate to the combined effects of (1) increased bilirubin load to the liver and (2) decreased bilirubin-conjugating capacity. The source of the increased bilirubin load to the liver includes both hemoglobin and nonhemoglobin sources, as well as the enterohepatic circulation[41,42]; the latter is increased in the newborn because of deficient bacterial degradation of bilirubin and increased activity of intestinal beta-glucuronidase.[43-45] The defective bilirubin conjugating capacity is related to a diminished activity of hepatic UDP-glucuronyl transferase, which undergoes a rapid developmental change from negligible levels at birth to adult levels after several days.[35] Prematurity results in more severe neonatal hyperbilirubinemia, principally because of a delayed maturation of the hepatic UDP-glucuronyl transferase.[35] More recent studies in human infants refined the earlier observations. Thus, the possibility of impaired transport of bilirubin into the hepatocyte because of genetic variants of organic anion transporters (see earlier) is likely important, perhaps especially in Asian infants.[29] The diminished levels of

ligandin in hepatic cytosol are likely less important. Genetic variants of the *UGT1A1* gene, as well as the long-recognized developmental deficiency of the glucuronyl transferase, may also be important. Increase in the enterohepatic circulation is likely important in *jaundice associated with breast milk feedings* because breast milk contains beta-glucuronidase, which can degrade conjugated bilirubin in the small intestine.[3,4,46] Additionally lipoprotein lipase activity in breast milk has been suggested to lead to increased release of free fatty acids (anions) from triglycerides and thereby to a disturbance of hepatic uptake. Pregnanediol in breast milk also may inhibit bilirubin conjugation. Finally, the common *delay in adequate caloric intake* with breast-feeding is considered of most importance in jaundice associated with breast-feeding; the mechanism of the deleterious effect of caloric deprivation on bilirubin homeostasis remains unclear.[4]

Important Determinants of Neuronal Injury by Bilirubin

The critical event in the genesis of brain injury caused by bilirubin is entrance of bilirubin into brain and exposure to neurons.[4,10,16,18,47-58] Although the essential toxicity of bilirubin occasionally has been questioned,[59-62] the predominance of available data indicates that bilirubin per se is injurious to neurons (see later discussion). Similarly, although the possibility has been considered that bilirubin still bound to albumin may bind to the neuronal plasma membrane and may then be incorporated into the neuronal interior by endocytosis,[62] it now seems clear that bilirubin no longer bound to albumin, i.e., *unbound or "free" bilirubin*, is the form that ultimately leads to neuronal injury.

Interrelationships of Bilirubin, Albumin, and Hydrogen Ion

To derive the important determinants of neuronal injury by bilirubin, it is necessary to recognize the critical reactions shown in Figure 13-3. As noted earlier, at physiological pH the predominant species of unbound bilirubin in plasma is bilirubin acid. Consideration of these equilibria makes it clear that the potential means for increasing exposure of neurons to bilirubin acid would include: increasing the quantity of [bilirubin anion]-albumin (i.e., *unconjugated bilirubin*) and especially thereby unbound or free bilirubin, disturbing the binding of bilirubin anion to albumin, decreasing the quantity of albumin that is free to bind bilirubin, and increasing the quantity of hydrogen ions

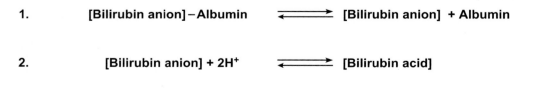

Figure 13-3   Relationships among bilirubin anion, either bound to albumin or "free," hydrogen ion, albumin, and bilirubin acid. See text for details.

TABLE 13-3	Important Determinants of Neuronal Injury by Bilirubin

Concentration of serum unconjugated and free (unbound) bilirubin
Concentration of serum albumin
Bilirubin binding by albumin
Concentration of hydrogen ions (pH)
Blood-brain barrier
Neuronal susceptibility

(i.e., lowering pH) (Table 13-3). Additional factors that interrelate closely with those just enumerated include the status of the blood-brain barrier and the susceptibility of target neurons to bilirubin injury; these factors are considered separately in later sections. In the following discussion of the determinants of bilirubin neurotoxicity, it becomes clear that the importance of each factor must vary with the clinical circumstances (see Table 13-3).

Concentration of Serum Unconjugated and Free Bilirubin

Unconjugated Bilirubin. Although it is generally recognized that serum levels of unconjugated bilirubin must be elevated to cause neurotoxicity, the relationship between such elevations and brain injury is not simple. In the *full-term infant with marked hyperbilirubinemia* secondary to *hemolytic disease*, a clear correlation can be discerned between the occurrence of kernicterus and the maximal recorded level of serum bilirubin (Table 13-4).[4,18,30,36,56,63-65] In a review of 52 infants with hemolytic disease (33 Rh incompatibility, 19 ABO incompatibility), approximately 95% of whom developed kernicterus, the peak total serum bilirubin in both groups was *approximately 32 mg/dL*, with an *approximate range of 18 to 51 mg/dL*.[65]

The neural risk of marked hyperbilirubinemia in *full-term infants without hemolysis* is less clear. Indeed, an earlier analysis of available studies by Newman and Maisels[66] indicated that the risk for neurological

sequelae is distinctly less for hyperbilirubinemic infants without hemolytic disease compared with the risk for infants with hemolytic disease. Subsequent observations supported this contention, including a study by Newman and associates of 140 infants with total serum bilirubin levels of 25 mg/dL.[67] Nevertheless, multiple reports have described the occurrence of kernicterus, identified by neuropathological, neuroradiological, or clinical criteria, after neonatal nonhemolytic hyperbilirubinemia.[5,7,58,65,68-73] In a recent review of 35 selected infants with nonhemolytic, "idiopathic" hyperbilirubinemia and documented acute or chronic bilirubin encephalopathy, all infants had peak total serum bilirubin levels greater than 20 mg/dL (Fig. 13-4).[65] Indeed, more than 90% of the infants with kernicterus had peak levels higher than 25 mg/dL. Notably, however, fully 25% had peak levels lower than 30 mg/dL.

The relationships between neonatal bilirubin values and neurological outcome in *premature infants* are probably different from those in full-term infants. Indeed, kernicterus has been demonstrated repeatedly in the *premature infant without marked hyperbilirubinemia* (see later discussion).[4,30,64,74-83] These infants usually have exhibited a variety of complicating illnesses (e.g., acidosis, hyperbilirubinemia, sepsis, asphyxia, hypothermia, intraventricular hemorrhage, and, rarely, benzyl alcohol exposure). In one often-cited, relatively large collection of premature infants with kernicterus (n = 6), peak total serum bilirubin levels were in excess of 20 mg/dL (range, 22 to 26 mg/dL.[84] However, in this report, the gestational age of the six infants ranged from 34 to 36 weeks. Studies of bilirubin-induced auditory disturbances in smaller premature infants (28 to 32 weeks of gestational age) document neurological dysfunction at much lower bilirubin levels.[85,86] The critical issue of the premature infant is discussed later (see "Clinical Features").

Free Bilirubin. Because of the recognition that the fraction of bilirubin not bound to albumin is the critical component involved in bilirubin entry into the brain and in neurotoxicity (see later) and because of the demonstration of kernicterus in premature infants without markedly elevated levels of unconjugated bilirubin, intensive investigation has been directed toward measurement of the quantity of that fraction of unconjugated serum bilirubin, namely, unbound (i.e., "free") bilirubin.* In general, premature infants with higher levels of free bilirubin exhibit kernicterus at postmortem examination more often than those with lower levels. In a study that did not support this relation, the substantial difference in free bilirubin levels between the seven infants with kernicterus (18.2 nmol/L) and the 23 without kernicterus (11.1 nmol/L) may not have achieved statistical significance in part because of the relatively small numbers.[91] Disturbances of the brain stem auditory-evoked response (BSAER) are observed at lower levels of

TABLE 13-4	Relationship between Maximum Serum Bilirubin Concentration and Kernicterus in Newborns with Hemolytic Disease

Maximum Bilirubin Concentration (mg/dL)	Total No. of Cases	No. with Kernicterus
30–40	11	8 (73%)
25–29	12	4 (33%)
19–24	13	1 (8%)
10–18	24	0

Data from Maisels MJ: Jaundice. In Avery GB, Fletcher MA, MacDonald MG, editors: *Neonatology, Pathophysiology and Management of the Newborn*, 5th ed, Philadelphia: 1999, Lippincott Williams & Wilkins, and Mollison PL, Cutbush M: Haemolytic disease of the newborn. In Gairdner D, editor: *Recent Advances in Pediatrics*, New York: 1954, Blakiston.

---

*See references 3,4,8,18,23,49,55,58,64,85,87-94.

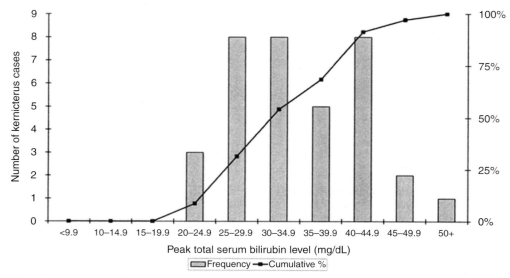

Figure 13-4   **Distribution of peak total serum bilirubin level in term and near-term newborns with idiopathic jaundice who developed kernicterus (n = 35).** The bars refer to frequency, that is, number of cases (left Y-axis) and the line to cumulative percentage (right Y-axis). *(From Ip S, Chung M, Kulig J, O'Brien R, et al: An evidence-based review of important issues concerning neonatal hyperbilirubinemia, Pediatrics 114:e130–e153, 2004.)*

free bilirubin in premature versus full-term infants (see later).[85,86] Nevertheless, it is clear that free bilirubin levels *alone* do not clearly distinguish premature infants who will develop kernicterus from those who will not. Indeed, as concluded in a carefully studied series, although a statistically significant difference in unbound bilirubin concentrations was observed between kernicteric and nonkernicteric infants, the individual values overlapped, so "no clear limits of 'safe' or 'toxic' unbound bilirubin levels can be drawn."[89] The important point is that other determinants (e.g., concerning albumin binding of bilirubin, status of the blood-brain barrier, and neuronal susceptibility; see Table 13-3) also are often present in the sick premature infant and contribute to the likelihood of bilirubin injury (see subsequent sections). Studies in animals support a relationship between free or unbound bilirubin and neuronal injury.[18,54,55,92,95]

Concentration of Serum Albumin

Consideration of the equilibria among albumin-bound bilirubin anion, albumin, hydrogen ion, and bilirubin acid (see Fig. 13-3) makes it apparent that the concentration of serum albumin is important in determining the neurotoxicity of bilirubin (see Table 13-3). At lower concentrations of serum albumin, the overall reaction favors formation of unbound bilirubin anion and, ultimately, bilirubin acid. Indeed, in experimental systems, the toxic effects of bilirubin on enzymatic systems or on cultured cells of neural origin can be reversed by the addition of albumin.[13,51,53-55,95,96,96a] Moreover, evidence indicates that infants at the greatest risk for kernicterus in the absence of marked hyperbilirubinemia (i.e., sick premature infants) usually exhibit concentrations of serum albumin that are lower than in healthy premature and full-term infants.[4,18,74,97] Indeed, in one study of 27 premature infants with kernicterus, serum

albumin levels were statistically significantly lower than in a comparable control group.[98] However, the latter observation has not been entirely consistent, in keeping with the importance of such other factors as the bilirubin binding affinity and binding capacity of albumin (see following discussion).

Bilirubin Binding by Albumin

The capacity of serum albumin to bind bilirubin depends on such factors as the affinity of the albumin for bilirubin and the competition between bilirubin and other endogenous and exogenous anions for albumin binding sites.[3,4,10,13,18,27,52,85,99-111] The clinical importance of the ability of albumin to bind bilirubin is emphasized by the demonstrations that premature infants who develop kernicterus without marked hyperbilirubinemia may have disturbances of the affinity or capacity, or both, of albumin to bind bilirubin.[10,13,27,52,55,89,97,98] Similarly, a relationship between bilirubin-albumin binding and subsequent cognitive outcome of premature infants who required neonatal intensive care further supports the clinical importance of this binding.[112]

Affinity of Newborn Albumin for Bilirubin. The affinity of albumin for bilirubin is less in the newborn than in the older infant.[10,13,18,52,55,109,110,113,113a] Adult levels of binding affinity are not reached until as late as 5 months of age. Moreover, binding affinity is lower in the premature infant than in the term infant and is lower in sick infants than in well infants. The explanation for the lower binding affinity of neonatal albumin is not entirely clear. The search for competing anions or for compositional differences in the protein as the unifying explanation has not been fruitful. The leading possibility is that a difference in *conformation* of the albumin is responsible.[10,52] Moreover, it is likely that the conformational difference relates to the humoral

TABLE 13-5	Factors of Potential Importance in Enhancing Bilirubin Neurotoxicity with Asphyxia*

Impaired bilirubin-albumin binding and increased proportion of free bilirubin (endogenous anions)

Increased proportion of bilirubin as bilirubin acid (acidosis)

Increased blood-brain transport of bilirubin (hypercarbia, increased bilirubin acid, and potentially impaired ATP-dependent transporters)

Enhanced susceptibility of neurons to bilirubin injury (hypoxia-ischemia)

Enhanced susceptibility of neurons to hypoxic-ischemic excitotoxic injury (free bilirubin)

*Probable mechanisms are in parentheses; see text for references.

environment of the neonatal albumin because adult serum albumin infused into newborns loses its superior binding affinity over 24 hours.[114]

Endogenous Anions. Endogenous anions that may compete with bilirubin for albumin binding sites include nonesterified fatty acids and other organic anions.* *Nonesterified fatty acids* are anions at physiological pH and are present in high concentrations with hypothermia, hypoxemia, hypoglycemia, sepsis, starvation, the administration of heparinized blood (through heparin's activation of triglyceride lipase), and intravenous alimentation with lipid. Studies of *asphyxiated infants with metabolic acidosis* demonstrated impaired bilirubin binding to albumin that could not be attributed to the low pH per se.[116] Rather, the data indicated the presence of *organic anions* in the plasma of asphyxiated, acidotic infants that compete with bilirubin for albumin binding sites. This finding may represent one of several mechanisms of potential importance in enhancing bilirubin neurotoxicity with asphyxia (Table 13-5).

Exogenous Anions. Many exogenous anions may compete with bilirubin for albumin binding sites.[†] However, the largest proportion of substances has been shown to displace bilirubin from albumin in vitro and in relatively high concentrations. Agents that appear to be particularly potent competitors for bilirubin binding sites include sulfonamides (especially sulfisoxazole), ibuprofen, various penicillins (especially ceftriaxone, cefotetan, carbenicillin, and moxalactam). Indeed, ceftriaxone is a more potent bilirubin displacer than is sulfisoxazole.[108,121] Although benzoate esters, previously used commonly as antimicrobial preservatives for a variety of injectable preparations (e.g., diazepam), exhibit a bilirubin-displacing effect in vitro, studies of patients treated with such preparations have yielded results that do not suggest that such an effect occurs in vivo.[100]

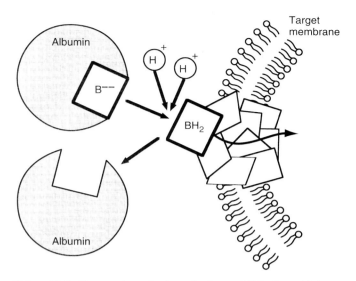

Figure 13-5 **Proposed mechanism of advanced bilirubin acid deposition in the lipid bilayer of cellular membranes.** See text for details. B⁻, Bilirubin anion; BH₂, bilirubin acid. *(Adapted from Brodersen R: Binding of bilirubin to albumin and tissues. In Stern L, editor: Physiological and Biochemical Basis for Perinatal Medicine, Basel: 1981, Karger.)*

Concentration of Hydrogen Ions: Acidosis

Results of experimental and clinical studies indicate that acidosis facilitates the neurotoxicity of bilirubin.[11,13,18,54-56,91,98,122-126] Experimental data suggest that the principal deleterious effect of acidosis occurs at the level of cellular binding or uptake of bilirubin, or both.[11,13,54,55,125,127,128] Thus, enhanced binding and uptake of bilirubin in the presence of acidosis have been demonstrated with cells in tissue culture, liposomes, red blood cell membranes, rat brain slices, and rat brain in vivo.[11,13,54,55,127-131] It is likely that the striking increase in brain bilirubin levels in neonatal rat brain observed during and shortly after nitrogen breathing[132] also relates to acidosis. Moreover, the acidosis associated with asphyxia may be similarly important in enhancing the bilirubin neurotoxicity of that insult (see Table 13-5). The mechanism by which acidosis leads to increased neuronal binding or brain uptake of bilirubin, or both, presumably relates to the conversion of bilirubin anion to bilirubin acid (see Fig. 13-3) on acceptance of two hydrogen ions. Bilirubin anion binds to cellular surface membrane components, primarily phospholipids, but also gangliosides and sphingomyelin, and this binding is increased by decreased pH.[54,133] This electrostatic interaction of the bilirubin anion and the cationic membrane lipid moieties is followed rapidly by formation of bilirubin acid in the membrane, aggregation of bilirubin acid, irreversible binding to the membrane, and membrane injury or uptake, or both (see later discussion) (Fig. 13-5). This effect of acidosis, when exerted at the level of the endothelial cells of the blood-brain barrier, perhaps could lead to increased transport of bilirubin across the barrier into brain, in addition to the effect exerted at the level of the neuron (i.e., bilirubin acid binding, neuronal uptake, and neuronal death; see later sections concerning blood-brain barrier and mechanisms of neurotoxicity).

---

*See references 4,10,13,18,52,55,85,99,100,104,105,107,108, 115-117.

†See references 4,10,13,18,52,55,85,100,104,105,107,108,118-121.

TABLE 13-6	Brain Transport Mechanisms Prevent High Cellular Bilirubin

Bilirubin entry into the CNS potentially can occur across the blood-brain barrier and blood (choroid plexus)-CSF barrier

Prevention of high cellular (and CSF) bilirubin levels depends on the action of two large families of ABC transporters, which function by hydrolysis of ATP

These transporters, the MRPs and MDR/PGPs, are located in neurons, glia, and capillary endothelial cells (blood-brain barrier and blood-CSF barrier)

The function of MRPs and MDR/PGPs is to export bilirubin from brain cells to the extracellular space and then across capillary endothelial cells to blood (similar transport from CSF to blood by the choroid plexus transporters also occurs)

Disturbances in action of these transporters, because of genetic variants or perhaps ATP depletion, could play a major role in determining neuronal susceptibility to bilirubin injury.

ABC, adenosine triphosphate–binding cassettes; ATP, adenosine triphosphate; CNS, central nervous system; CSF, cerebrospinal fluid; MDR/PGP, multidrug-resistance P-glycoprotein; MRP, multidrug-resistant protein.
Data from references 16, 57, and 135.

Blood-Brain Barrier

Bilirubin entry into the central nervous system potentially can occur across the blood-brain or the blood (choroid plexus)–cerebrospinal fluid barrier. It is likely, although not established, that transport across the blood-brain barrier is the more important of these two mechanisms. The blood-brain barrier is composed of the brain capillary endothelial cells with characteristic tight intercellular junctions. The choroid plexus does not contain such tight junctions. Insights into bilirubin transport mechanisms, although incomplete at the time of this writing, have identified key processes that attempt to protect brain cells from accumulation of intracellular bilirubin. These transport mechanisms are summarized in Table 13-6. Two families of ABC (adenosine triphosphate [ATP] binding cassette) transporters, which function by ATP hydrolysis, appear to be involved.[16,57,134,135] The function of these transporters is to export bilirubin from neurons and glia to the extracellular space and thence to the blood by capillary endothelial cells of the blood-brain barrier. A similar process extrudes bilirubin from cerebrospinal fluid to blood through the cells of the choroid plexus. These transporters are up-regulated with hyperbilirubinemia. However, disturbance in their function (e.g., genetic variants and possibly energy depletion) could render the brain in a given infant highly susceptible to bilirubin accumulation within neurons and glia, with resulting neurotoxicity. Further data will be of great interest.

In this context, it is most reasonable to consider bilirubin entry into the brain across either an intact or a disrupted blood-brain barrier (Table 13-7). The clinical circumstances largely determine the status of the blood-brain barrier (see Table 13-7).

Bilirubin Transport across an Intact Blood-Brain Barrier.

The likelihood of passage of bilirubin across an *intact blood-brain barrier* is suggested by the finding

TABLE 13-7	Bilirubin Transport and the Blood-Brain Barrier

Bilirubin Transport across Intact Blood-Brain Barrier
Unbound (free) bilirubin: passive diffusion
Increased cerebral blood flow (hypercarbia, seizure)

Bilirubin Transport across Disrupted Blood-Brain Barrier
Hyperosmolar load (hyperosmolar solutions, exchange transfusion)
Hypercarbia with acidosis
Asphyxia
Acidosis (?),* benzyl alcohol (?)
Vasculitis (meningitis)
Abrupt increase in arterial blood pressure and/or venous pressure (?), pneumothorax (?)

*Question marks indicate experimental data that are suggestive but not yet conclusive.

that free bilirubin binds to phospholipid (e.g., plasma membrane phospholipid of capillary endothelial cells). Such bilirubin-phospholipid complexes are very lipophilic,[8,10,12,14,16,52,54,57] and thus they would be expected to move bilirubin across the blood-brain barrier readily (Fig. 13-6). Therefore, those aforementioned factors that lead to elevations of bilirubin no longer bound to albumin (i.e., "free" bilirubin) would be expected to enhance movement of bilirubin across the blood-brain barrier. Studies in animals demonstrated such movement across the intact blood-brain barrier,[54,136-141] and the occurrence of kernicterus in older children and adults with apparently intact blood-brain barrier further supports this concept.[142,143] As noted earlier, the predominant species of unbound bilirubin in plasma is the diacid with the minority as the monoanion or dianion. These species readily diffuse across cell membranes.[16] When free bilirubin is only moderately higher than its aqueous

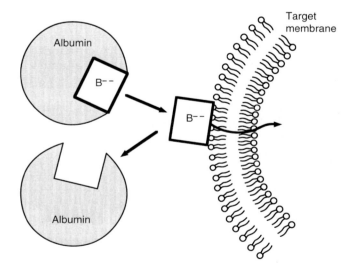

Figure 13-6 Proposed mechanism of bilirubin entry into cells and passage across an intact blood-brain barrier. Bilirubin anion (B⁻ ⁻) [or bilirubin acid (BH₂)] binds to membrane phospholipid of the target plasma membrane (e.g., brain endothelial cell, neuronal or glial cell) and is transported across the membrane as a lipid-soluble, bilirubin-phospholipid complex.

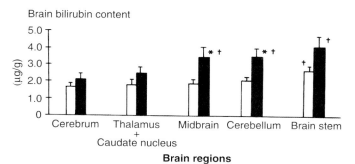

Figure 13-7   **Increase in brain bilirubin content with hypercarbia (arterial carbon dioxide pressure, ≈70 mm Hg) and consequent increased cerebral blood flow in the neonatal piglet.** *Open bars* show regional brain bilirubin content in the control group ($n = 14$); *closed bars* show regional brain bilirubin content in the hypercarbia group ($n = 10$). Note the increase in brain bilirubin in several brain regions with hypercarbia. Mean ± SEM; *, $P < .05$ as compared with control;[†], $P < .05$ as compared with cerebral value within the same group. *(From Burgess GH, Oh W, Bratlid D, Brubakk AM, et al: The effects of brain blood flow on brain bilirubin deposition in newborn piglets, Pediatr Res 19:691–696, 1985.)*

saturation (≈70 nM), soluble oligomers and metabolic microaggregates of the diacid form and bind to the outer leaflet of the plasma membrane. The result is a modest perturbation of membrane structure that may enhance further uptake of bilirubin (see Fig. 13-5). These occurrences merge with the mechanism of bilirubin transport across a disrupted blood-brain barrier (see following section). Conditions such as acidosis that favor formation of bilirubin acid (see Fig. 13-3) may be expected to provoke this series of events. Studies of isolated brain capillary cells support this notion of toxicity of bilirubin to endothelia, with an effect on membrane transport.[144]

A role for *increased cerebral blood flow* in enhanced transport of bilirubin across an intact blood-brain barrier may be predicted if, as just discussed, bilirubin can be transported across an intact blood-brain barrier. Direct demonstration of an increase in bilirubin transport by an increase in cerebral blood flow was made in studies of neonatal piglets subjected to moderate hypercarbia (Fig 13-7).[145] No increase in albumin uptake occurred, and thus the blood-brain barrier remained intact under these conditions. The implications of this observation are considerable, because abrupt increases in cerebral blood flow are not uncommon in the premature infant, particularly the sick infant, with impaired cerebrovascular autoregulation (see Chapters 6, 9, and 11).

Bilirubin Transport across a Disrupted Blood-Brain Barrier. The likelihood of passage of bilirubin, even still bound to albumin, across a *disrupted blood-brain barrier*, caused by exposure to *hyperosmolar materials*, is suggested by results of experimental studies, primarily in the rat (see Table 13-7).[54,55,60,62,146-150] Thus, unilateral kernicterus was produced in the rat by infusion of bilirubin-albumin after reversible opening of the blood-brain barrier was accomplished on the same side by infusion of hypertonic arabinose.[60] The infusion of hyperosmolar materials is a well-established means for disturbing endothelial tight junctions and thereby the blood-brain barrier.[151-153] That it was indeed the bilirubin-albumin complex that entered the brain was shown by demonstration of an increase in brain concentration of albumin as well as bilirubin in

the affected hemisphere.[60] Subsequent studies confirmed the increase in brain bilirubin concentration under these conditions.[54,55,148,150,154,155] An *approximate* similarity of the topography of the bilirubin deposition to that of kernicterus was reported in the initial work, but the critical question concerning whether the brain bilirubin deposition was followed by neuronal injury was not answered.[60] However, subsequent studies demonstrated alterations in electroencephalogram and in brain energy metabolism parallel to the uptake of bilirubin (Fig. 13-8).[148,149] These data raise the possibility that sudden or sustained increases in serum osmolality (e.g., in the sick premature infant administered hypertonic glucose or sodium bicarbonate, or in association with hypothalamic disturbance after asphyxia or intraventricular hemorrhage, or following exchange transfusion) could lead to abrupt increases in brain bilirubin levels, even in the absence of marked hyperbilirubinemia.[54,55,156]

A second potential means of disrupting the blood-brain barrier in the newborn is *hypercarbia* (see Table 13-7). Thus, experimental data suggest that hypercarbia can disturb the blood-brain barrier and can induce kernicterus in puppies.[157,158] A careful study of the rat demonstrated that marked hypercarbia (carbon dioxide pressure [P_{CO_2}], 100 mm Hg), independent of acidosis, caused a more than twofold increase in brain bilirubin concentration as well as in the brain albumin level.[159] The mechanism of the effect of hypercarbia could involve the impact of maximal vasodilation and an abrupt increase in cerebral blood flow on the integrity of the blood-brain barrier. These data raise the possibility that hypercarbia in the sick premature infant could contribute to the transport of bilirubin into the brain of the infant without marked hyperbilirubinemia.

Asphyxia may lead to disruption of the blood-brain barrier, at least in mature animals (see Table 13-7).[146] Moreover, kernicterus has been produced readily in the asphyxiated but not in the nonasphyxiated monkey or rabbit.[160,161] In addition, asphyxia is necessary to produce bilirubin neuronal injury in the adult rat,[162] and in the Gunn rat it leads to hearing impairment at levels of bilirubin otherwise insufficient to lead to injury.[163] It is tempting to suggest that the association of

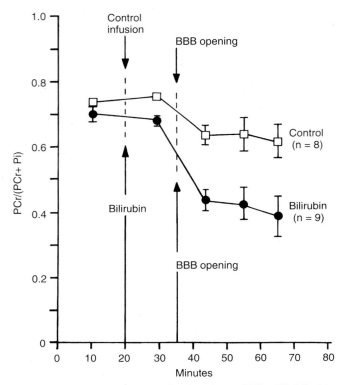

Figure 13-8 **Changes in phosphocreatine (PCr)/(PCr + inorganic phosphorus [Pi]) with bilirubin and control infusions before and after hyperosmolar opening of the blood-brain barrier.** Results expressed as mean ± SD; values were obtained by magnetic resonance spectroscopy. BBB, blood-brain barrier. *(From Ives NK, Bolas NM, Gardiner RM: The effects of bilirubin on brain energy metabolism during hyperosmolar opening of the blood-brain barrier: An in vivo study using 31P nuclear magnetic resonance spectroscopy, Pediatr Res 26:356–361, 1989.)*

kernicterus and asphyxia in the human infant could reside, at least in part, on the basis of a disturbance in the blood-brain barrier. However, the only direct measurement of albumin transport across the blood-brain barrier in an asphyxiated perinatal animal involved the fetal lamb, and no significant increase in transport could be demonstrated.[164] The possibility that asphyxia, by way of the associated acidosis, could lead to enhanced formation of bilirubin acid at the endothelial cell surface, injury to the blood-brain barrier, and the transport of *bilirubin acid* (see previous section) remains to be determined. Moreover, the marked hypercarbia associated with asphyxia could lead to increased brain uptake of bilirubin through both an intact blood-brain barrier, as described earlier, and a disrupted blood-brain barrier, as just described. Finally, the ATP-dependent transporters on brain endothelial cells (see Table 13-6) perhaps could be impaired by the energy depletion of asphyxia. This issue requires further study, but it may add to the mechanisms of potentiation of bilirubin neurotoxicity with asphyxia (see Table 13-5).

The possibility that *severe acidosis per se* may lead to the disruption of the blood-brain barrier through the deposition of bilirubin acid was considered earlier. The relationship of kernicterus with benzyl alcohol exposure (see later discussion) could be based, at least in part, on such a mechanism. More data are needed on this issue.

Intracranial infection, particularly meningitis, is associated with *vasculitis* and a clearly compromised blood-brain barrier (see Chapter 21) (see Table 13-7). A possible role for this mechanism in the genesis of kernicterus is suggested by clinical data.[165] Thus, in two affiliated neonatal facilities, four infants with kernicterus were observed at postmortem examination over 5 years; of these four babies, each exhibited sepsis and two had meningitis. Whether the effect of sepsis-meningitis was at the level of the blood-brain barrier, enhanced neuronal susceptibility to bilirubin injury because of concomitant neuronal injury (see later discussion), or a combination of these factors requires further study. Nevertheless, these and other data[166] indicate that the infant with sepsis-meningitis is at enhanced risk for the development of kernicterus, perhaps secondary to a disturbance in the blood-brain barrier.

Finally, the possibility that the blood-brain barrier can be disrupted transiently by abrupt *increases in blood pressure, especially in the infant with impaired autoregulation, or in venous pressure*, with an associated increase in transport of bilirubin into brain, is suggested by several lines of evidence (see Table 13-7). First, as noted earlier, circumstances that cause an increase in cerebral blood flow, such as hypercarbia, are associated with the increased transport of bilirubin into brain. An *abrupt increase in blood pressure* in the sick infant with a pressure-passive cerebral circulation would be expected to cause an abrupt increase in cerebral blood flow (see Chapters 6 and 11). Seizure, which causes an abrupt increase in blood pressure and cerebral blood flow in the newborn (see Chapter 5), also may lead to transient disruption of the blood-brain barrier. Such a disruption was documented shortly after a seizure in the human adult and was delineated carefully in animal models.[167,168] *Abrupt increases in venous pressure* are common in sick premature infants, particularly in relation to respiratory disturbances (see Chapter 11). Pneumothorax was documented to result in disruption of the blood-brain barrier in piglets.[169,170] More data are needed concerning the possibility that transient disruptions in the blood-brain barrier are an important means for entry of bilirubin into the neonatal brain.

Neuronal Susceptibility

The distinctive regional topography of brain injury with kernicterus (see subsequent discussion) and the predilection for involvement of neurons indicate a selective susceptibility of specific neurons to bilirubin injury. The possibility that the *distinctive regional topography* relates to the topography of bilirubin transport across the blood-brain barrier, particularly the disrupted barrier, was suggested by some experimental data,[60,147] reviewed previously, but not by other findings.[148,150] Moreover, a simple relationship of the topography of injury with patterns of highest regional cerebral blood flow or metabolic rate also is not apparent.

The predilection of bilirubin injury for *neurons* rather than glia (see later discussion of neuropathology) was reproduced in cultured cells.[55,171,172] This predilection may relate to aspects of neuronal surface membranes (e.g., abundance of gangliosides) that lead more readily to binding of bilirubin and to the initial steps leading to membrane injury (see later discussion of mechanisms of neurotoxicity). This speculation is only one of many possible explanations, however.

Perhaps of particular clinical importance, available data suggest that *concomitant injury to neurons* enhances the likelihood of bilirubin encephalopathy. The potentiating role of asphyxia may be a good example of this effect (see Table 13-5). Thus, in this circumstance, concomitant injury to neurons may render the cell more susceptible to uptake of and injury by bilirubin, and as will be discussed regarding mechanisms of neurotoxicity, exposure of neurons to bilirubin may enhance the susceptibility to hypoxic-ischemic excitotoxic neuronal injury. As noted earlier, these factors related to neuronal susceptibility are among several other factors that may underlie the increased likelihood of bilirubin encephalopathy with asphyxia (see Table 13-5). Nevertheless, it also must be considered that other insults to neurons by such factors as hypoglycemia, metabolic aberrations, intracranial hemorrhage, infection, trauma, or exposure to toxic agents may have critical additive effects with bilirubin by producing concomitant injury to neurons. The role of such factors in enhancing neuronal susceptibility to injury could be very important and requires further study. The demonstrations that bilirubin toxicity to cultured cells is enhanced by otherwise nontoxic concentrations

of tumor necrosis factor-alpha and endotoxin (lipopolysaccharide) suggest a mechanism whereby sepsis-meningitis could enhance neuronal susceptibility to bilirubin injury.[173,174] The role of endotoxin and cytokines in bilirubin-induced excitotoxicity (see later) is also relevant to this issue.[174,175] Finally, the observation that immature rat brain is rich in heme oxygenase,[176] which could lead ultimately to the formation of bilirubin from local heme sources, raises the possibility that certain neurons could be exposed to particularly high local concentrations of bilirubin. Further information concerning the factors that could activate heme oxygenase or increase availability of its substrate, or both, would be of interest concerning neuronal susceptibility to bilirubin injury.

Mechanisms of Bilirubin Neurotoxicity
Spectrum of Effects of Bilirubin on Cellular Functions

The mechanism of injury of neurons by bilirubin is not entirely resolved, but recent work has provided important insights (see later). Previous work indicated that bilirubin exerts a deleterious effect on a wide variety of cellular events. Various in vitro and in vivo studies, primarily with animals, including Gunn rats, demonstrated disturbances in glucose utilization, oxidative phosphorylation, glycogen synthesis, citric acid cycle function, cyclic adenosine monophosphate synthesis, amino acid and protein metabolism, DNA synthesis, lipid metabolism, myelination, synthesis and transport of neurotransmitters, ion transport, synaptic transmission, excitatory amino acid homeostasis, cytosolic calcium levels, free radical homeostasis, and apoptotic/survival balance (Table 13-8).[18,50,51,56,96,149,174,177-204] Notably, however, most, although not all, of this earlier work involved exposure to levels of free bilirubin that far exceeded those expected in the clinical setting. However, several earlier observations are consistent with later work and deserve particular attention.

A particular importance for disturbance of mitochondrial function and thereby energy metabolism was suggested by several studies using biochemical

TABLE 13-8	Potential Mechanisms for Bilirubin Neurotoxicity*
Impairment of	
Glucose utilization	
Oxidative phosphorylation, adenosine triphosphate levels	
DNA synthesis	
Protein synthesis	
Activity of many enzymes	
Protein phosphorylation	
Neurotransmitter synthesis	
Ion transport	
Synaptic transmission	
Excitatory amino acid homeostasis	
Cytosolic calcium concentration	
Free radical homeostasis	
Apoptotic/survival balance	

*Based on numerous studies performed in vivo and in vitro (cultured cells, tissue extracts); see text for references.

TABLE 13-9	Brain Energy Metabolites 15 Minutes after Intracarotid Infusion of Osmotic Agent (Arabinose) and Bilirubin in the Rat*		
Metabolite		**Control**	**Bilirubin**
Phosphocreatine		4.93	2.04
Adenosine triphosphate		2.83	1.72
Glycogen		2.82	1.20
Glucose		2.95	1.02
Lactate		2.27	10.55

*Values are mmol/kg brain tissue; all differences are significant at the P < .05 level.

Data from Wennberg RP, Johansson BB, Folbergrova J, Siesjo BK: Bilirubin-induced changes in brain energy metabolism after osmotic opening of the blood-brain barrier, *Pediatr Res* 30:473–478, 1991.

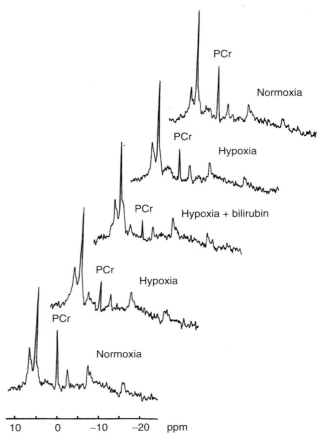

Figure 13-9 **Deleterious effect of bilirubin in the presence of hypoxia in brain slices.** A representative sequence of spectra collected hourly over a 5-hour experimental period is shown. Alterations in the superfusate are as labeled, with progression from *bottom left* to *top right*. Bilirubin at a concentration of 40 μmol/L (bilirubin/albumin molar ratio, 5:1) in combination with hypoxia was associated with a reversible fall in phosphocreatine (PCr) to less than the steady-state reduction observed during hypoxia (tracing immediately above). *(From Ives NK, Cox DWG, Gardiner RM, Bachelard HS: The effects of bilirubin on brain energy metabolism during normoxia and hypoxia: An in vitro study using 31P nuclear magnetic resonance spectroscopy, Pediatr Res 23:569–573, 1988.)*

measurements and magnetic resonance (MR) spectroscopy to analyze energy metabolites, including high-energy phosphate levels. Thus, a rapid decline in high-energy phosphate levels was observed in brain 15 minutes after entrance of bilirubin by disruption of the blood-brain barrier (Table 13-9).[195] The findings were indicative of a disturbance in oxidative phosphorylation, with the depletion of glucose and glycogen and accumulation of lactate indicative of an increase in glycolytic rates in an attempt to restore energy potential. Moreover, similar experiments, using MR spectroscopy, documented in vivo the disturbance in high-energy phosphate levels (see Fig. 13-8).[149] The importance of hypoxia in potentiating the effect of bilirubin on energy metabolism was also shown by MR spectroscopy in a similar model (Fig. 13-9).[196] Consistent with these observations, various earlier primarily morphological studies in the Gunn rat and other experimental models suggested that the mitochondrion is particularly involved in bilirubin toxicity.[190,191,205-207]

Involvement of excitotoxic mechanisms in bilirubin-induced injury emanated initially from the demonstrations in the Gunn rat that (1) bilirubin-induced neuronal injury could be blocked by administration of the *N*-methyl-D-aspartate (NMDA) receptor antagonist, MK-801, and (2) excitotoxic neuronal injury induced by injection of NMDA into striatum is accentuated by bilirubin entry into the region.[204] These observations suggested that excitotoxic mechanisms could contribute to the neuronal injury caused by bilirubin. The sequence of events then could be similar to that described in hypoxia-ischemia (see Chapter 6) and in hypoglycemia (see Chapter 12), whereby a disturbance in high-energy phosphate levels leads to impairment of energy-dependent glutamate uptake mechanisms in both nerve terminals and astrocytes, a resulting accumulation of extracellular glutamate, and neuronal death initiated by activation of glutamate receptors, particularly the NMDA receptor. The demonstration of an impairment of glutamate uptake mechanisms by synaptic vesicles treated with bilirubin[203] suggested that bilirubin itself could cause or accentuate the increase in extracellular glutamate.

These considerations provided an additional reason for a link between hypoxic-ischemic insults and bilirubin neuronal injury (see Table 13-5). Moreover, the finding that the *combination* of lipopolysaccharide and bilirubin exacerbated excitotoxic neuronal injury induced by bilirubin suggests a mechanism whereby sepsis could increase the risk of kernicterus.[174]

Potential Sequence for Bilirubin Neurotoxicity

More recent work placed the initial observations of bilirubin-induced energy depletion and excitotoxicity in the context of a broader cellular and molecular scheme (Fig. 13-10).[16,57,208] Since the early 2000s, studies based on concentrations of free bilirubin more relevant to the clinical setting suggest that the principal subcellular compartments affected are the *plasma membrane* and the *mitochondrion*, and the major cell types involved are the *neuron* and the *astrocyte*.

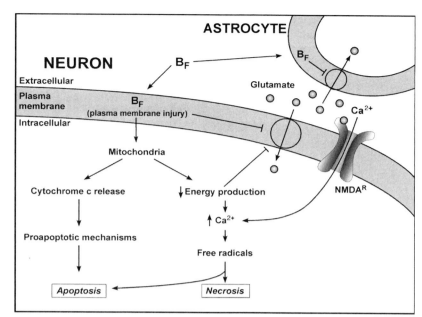

Figure 13-10 **Potential sequence for bilirubin neurotoxicity.** See text for details. Note the particular importance of mitochondrial disturbance and impaired glutamate homeostasis with increased extracellular glutamate and resulting excitotoxicity. B_F, free bilirubin; Ca^{2+}, calcium; NMDA, N-methyl-D-aspartate.

Plasma Membrane and Excitotoxicity. Although bilirubin dianion and its rapidly formed diacid can bind to phospholipids and diffuse passively across the plasma membrane, plasma membrane disturbance also can occur. The results are accentuation of bilirubin uptake and disturbance of certain plasma membrane functions (e.g., glutamate transport). Impairment of glutamate transport in neurons and *especially astrocytes* causes an increase in extracellular glutamate.[172,174,209] The result is excessive activation of neuronal NMDA receptors with an increase in cytosolic calcium, generation of free radicals, and neuronal necrosis or apoptosis, or both, as described for hypoxia-ischemia in Chapter 6. Prevention of bilirubin-induced injury by specific inhibitors of the NMDA receptor (e.g., MK-801) supports this formulation.[204,209-212] Astrocytes also sustain injury from unconjugated bilirubin, although vulnerability to cell death is less than that for neurons.[172,174] However, impairment of *glutamate transport* is greater in astrocytes than in neurons, and thus the accumulation of extracellular glutamate attributable to astrocytic dysfunction is greater than that for neurons (see Fig. 13-10). Additionally, astrocytes exposed to bilirubin release such cytokines as tumor necrosis factor-alpha and interleukin-1beta, which also impair glutamate transport, and therefore the action of these cytokines may add to the accumulation of extracellular glutamate (see Fig. 13-10).[175] Finally, because high-affinity sodium-dependent glutamate transport is impaired secondary to energy depletion and the resulting disturbance of ionic gradients (see Chapter 6), the energy depletion associated with bilirubin mitochondrial toxicity (see next) adds to the transport failure (or even reversal) and accumulation of extracellular glutamate.

Importance of the Mitochondrion. In addition to the plasma membrane and excitotoxic effects, bilirubin exposure in clinically relevant concentrations has important effects on *mitochondria* (see Fig. 13-10).[16,211-213] What results is not only diminished energy production, but also permeabilization of mitochondrial membranes and release of cytochrome c.[57] The latter then leads to apoptotic neuronal death by binding to apoptosis protease activating factor-1, activation of caspases, and execution of the cell death program.

Final Common Pathway to Cell Death. The final common pathway for both the plasma membrane effects with excitotoxicity and the mitochondrial disturbances includes an increase in cytosolic calcium and the generation of free radicals (see Fig. 13-10) (see Chapter 6).[208,214] The result is either apoptotic or necrotic cell death, or both. Both neurons and astrocytes can be affected, although neurons are more vulnerable. (More recent work suggests that bilirubin is also toxic to oligodendrocytes and that generation of reactive nitrogen species are important in this process.[215]) The intensity and duration of the stimulus determine whether neuronal death will be apoptotic or necrotic (see Chapter 6), with high bilirubin concentrations or longer exposures, or both, resulting in necrosis and lower concentrations or shorter exposures resulting in apoptosis.[216] A particular, although not exclusive, importance for apoptotic cell death with bilirubin toxicity was suggested by the observation that inhibition of the proapoptotic enzyme p38 MAP kinase by minocycline prevented cerebellar neuronal cell death with bilirubin exposure.[217] (This effect was likely independent of the antimicroglial effects of

TABLE 13-10 **Potential Novel Interventions versus Bilirubin Neurotoxicity***

TABLE 13-10 **Potential Novel Interventions versus Bilirubin Neurotoxicity***

N-methyl-D-aspartate receptor blockers (e.g., memantine, dextromethorphan, magnesium, MK-801)
Antioxidant therapies (free radical scavengers, antioxidant enzyme mimetics)
Antiapoptotic agents
Combinations of interventions

*Based on experimental studies (see text for references).

TABLE 13-11 **Neuropathological States with Bilirubin Staining of Brain Nuclei**

Acute bilirubin encephalopathy, or kernicterus, of the full-term (or premature) infant *with* marked hyperbilirubinemia
Acute bilirubin encephalopathy, or kernicterus, of the premature infant *without* marked hyperbilirubinemia
Secondary bilirubin staining of brain nuclei of the premature infant (*without* marked hyperbilirubinemia)

minocycline, as discussed in Chapter 6.) Moreover, minocycline administered to the newborn Gunn rat prevented the marked apoptotic cell death that resulted in cerebellar hypoplasia in that animal.[217] *Combination* of *antiapoptotic* (caspase inhibitor) and *antiexcitoxic* (MK-801) agents may exhibit *synergy* in neuronal protection from bilirubin toxicity.[212]

Implications for Therapy

The sequence outlined in Fig. 13-10 and the supporting experimental data suggest several promising sites for therapeutic intervention (Table 13-10). Thus, blockade of NMDA receptors has been shown to be highly effective, depending on the model. MK-801 is the most effective NMDA inhibitor but unfortunately is not clinically safe (see Chapters 6 and 9). However, memantine, magnesium, or dextromethorphan would be potentially more useful. Scavenging of free radicals with such agents as vitamin E or related compounds or enhancing antioxidant defenses with antioxidant enzyme mimetics may be of potential value (see Chapters 6 and 9). Antiapoptotic interventions may also be beneficial (see Chapter 9), and the beneficial effects of minocycline in the Gunn rat are relevant in this context. *Combinations* of interventions may have *synergistic* effects, as noted earlier for antiapoptotic (caspase inhibitor) and antiexcitotoxic (MK-801) agents. At any rate, the recent insights into the mechanisms of bilirubin neurotoxicity raise important new possibilities for prevention of this injury.

NEUROPATHOLOGY

The classic neuropathology of acute bilirubin encephalopathy consists of two essential features: bilirubin staining of specific nuclear groups *and* neuronal necrosis.[166,218-223] The former is the earliest and most dramatic finding of bilirubin encephalopathy, and the latter is a later occurrence (in subsequent days), presumably in large part a consequence of the bilirubin uptake. Although the bilirubin staining of nuclei gives rise to the term *kernicterus*, to avoid later confusion I use this term for encephalopathy that includes *both* the staining *and* evidence for neuronal injury.

Three neuropathological states should be recognized in association with bilirubin staining of brain nuclei in the newborn (Table 13-11). The first two states (acute bilirubin encephalopathy, or kernicterus by my definition) occur in the full-term (or premature) infant with marked hyperbilirubinemia or in the premature infant *without* marked hyperbilirubinemia.

The third variety, bilirubin staining *without* related neuronal injury, also occurs in the premature infant without marked hyperbilirubinemia.[222-225]

In the following discussion, the neuropathology of acute bilirubin encephalopathy or kernicterus is reviewed in detail as the essential variety of bilirubin injury to the central nervous system. Because the pathological features of the disorder in the full-term (or premature) infant with marked hyperbilirubinemia and in the premature infant *without* marked hyperbilirubinemia are similar, these disorders are discussed together. (Indeed, these two neuropathological states appear to differ principally only in pathogenesis.) Finally, briefer note is made of the third variety of bilirubin staining of brain, the apparently secondary staining of brain nuclei by bilirubin (see Table 13-11).

Acute Bilirubin Encephalopathy-Kernicterus

The essential hallmarks of acute bilirubin encephalopathy, or kernicterus, are bilirubin staining of neurons and neuronal necrosis. These characteristics are discussed separately next, although they are inextricably intertwined.

Bilirubin Staining

Bilirubin staining is most apparent in fresh specimens or in frozen sections, especially in infants surviving only several days, and it occurs in a characteristic topography (Table 13-12).[70,166,218-223,226] Those regions most commonly affected are as follows: basal ganglia, particularly the globus pallidus and subthalamic nucleus; hippocampus, specifically, the so-called sectors CA2,3; substantia nigra; various cranial nerve nuclei, particularly the oculomotor, vestibular, auditory (especially cochlear nuclei but also superior olivary complex, nuclei of lateral lemniscus, inferior colliculi) and facial nerve nuclei; various other brain stem nuclei, particularly the reticular formation of pons and the inferior olivary nuclei; certain cerebellar nuclei, particularly the dentate; and anterior horn cells of the spinal cord. Similarities among the topography in full-term (or premature) infants with marked hyperbilirubinemia, premature infants *without* marked hyperbilirubinemia, and the homozygous Gunn rat are striking (see Table 13-12) and support the concept of the essential neurotoxicity of bilirubin. The period of prominent brain pigmentation lasts for only approximately 7 to 10 days, and this phase is accompanied by the commencement of the neuronal changes that result in chronic (postkernicteric) bilirubin encephalopathy.

TABLE 13-12 Comparative Neuropathology of Acute Bilirubin Encephalopathy or Kernicterus

Topography of Injury	Full-Term Infants, Marked Hyperbilirubinemia	Premature Infants, *No* Marked Hyperbilirubinemia	Homozygous Gunn Rats
Globus pallidus	+	+	+
Subthalamic nucleus	+	+	+
Hippocampus	+	+	+
Hypothalamus	+	–	+
Substantia nigra	+	+	+
Cranial nerve nuclei*	+	+	+
Reticular formation (brain stem)	+	+	
Cerebellum			
Dentate nuclei	+	+	–
Purkinje cells	–	+	+
Spinal cord, anterior horn cells	+	+	+

*Includes oculomotor and auditory nuclei; see text for details.
+, present; –, absent.
Data from Ahdab-Barmada M, Moossy J: The neuropathology of kernicterus in the premature neonate: Diagnostic problems, *J Neuropathol Exp Neurol* 43:45–56, 1984.

Neuronal Injury

Topography. The distribution of neuronal injury corresponds closely to the distribution of the bilirubin staining (see Table 13-12). An intimate relationship between bilirubin deposition and the neuronal injury is suggested by this similarity in topography. However, the relationship is not invariable. For example, little or no staining is apparent in Purkinje cells, but impressive neuronal loss is very common in this region, especially in the premature infant. In anticipation of the clinical sequelae of chronic (postkernicteric) bilirubin encephalopathy (see subsequent discussion), I should reemphasize that the major regions of neuronal injury include basal ganglia, brain stem nuclei for oculomotor function, and brain stem auditory (cochlear) nuclei.

Prominent involvement of cerebral cortical neurons is *not* a feature of kernicterus and, when present, appears to be related primarily to concomitant hypoxic-ischemic injury. However, it is possible that a degree of involvement of cerebral cortex would be recognized more commonly if more sophisticated neuropathological techniques than classic light microscopy could be used. Thus, in electron microscopic studies of the Gunn rat, Jew and Sandquist[206] observed qualitatively similar, yet clearly less severe, ultramicroscopic changes in neurons of cerebral cortex as in those of the cochlear nuclei or hippocampus.

Cytopathology. The cytopathology of kernicterus is distinctive and undergoes a characteristic evolution.[70,220,221] Thus, in the first several days, the early neuronal changes consist of swollen granular cytoplasm, often with microvacuolation and disruption of neuronal and nuclear membranes (Fig. 13-11). Yellow pigment often is prominent. By the end of the first week, dissolution of affected neurons becomes apparent, and nuclear and plasma membranes become poorly defined. In subsequent days to weeks, neuronal loss, often with mineralization, and astrocytosis are prominent.

Relation to Hypoxic-Ischemic Injury. The neuropathology of kernicterus is clearly different from that of hypoxic-ischemic injury in terms of the topography of the injury (Table 13-13). Additionally, the early basophilic, swollen neuron of bilirubin injury differs clearly

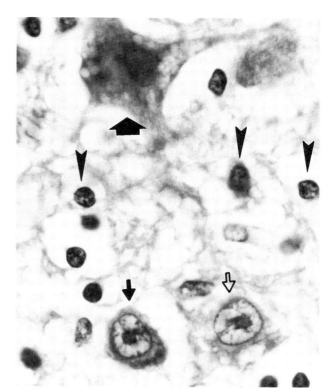

Figure 13-11 Neuronal changes in kernicterus; large neurons, third cranial nerve nucleus. Note early vacuolation of cytoplasm with loss of Nissl substance (*small open arrow*), increased nuclear density with irregular, hazy nuclear membrane (*large dark arrow*), relatively well-preserved neuron (*small dark arrow*), and pyknotic nuclei of necrotic neurons (*arrowheads*). (From Ahdab-Barmada M: Hyperbilirubinemia in the Newborn, *Columbus, OH: 1983, Ross.*)

TABLE 13-13 Major Differences in Topography of Neuropathology between Kernicterus and Hypoxic-Ischemic Encephalopathy

Brain Region	Kernicterus	Hypoxic-Ischemic Encephalopathy
Cerebral cortex and/or periventricular white matter	−	+
Basal ganglia		
Caudate-putamen	−	+
Globus pallidus	+	−
Hippocampus	Sectors CA2,3	Sector CA1
Thalamus	Subthalamic nucleus	Anterior and lateral nuclei
Substantia nigra	Reticulata	Compacta
Cochlear nuclei	+	−
Dentate nuclei	+	−

cytopathologically from the shrunken eosinophilic neuron of hypoxic-ischemic encephalopathy. Although these two encephalopathies may coexist, a hypoxic-ischemic insult sufficient to cause its characteristic encephalopathy is *not* necessary for the resultant neuropathological picture of kernicterus. This observation supports the aforementioned conclusion that *although asphyxial insults may be important in the pathogenesis of kernicterus in certain infants*, insults sufficient to cause major hypoxic-ischemic brain injury are not obligatory.

Secondary Bilirubin Staining of Brain of Premature Infants

Bilirubin may stain brain regions injured by other insults. Striking examples of such secondary bilirubin staining of discrete hypoxic-ischemic lesions (e.g., periventricular leukomalacia) are well known. The demonstration of more diffuse bilirubin staining of the brain of premature infants (i.e., without the characteristic topography of kernicterus just described) probably is of this variety (see Table 13-11).[224,225,227] Thus, although the staining was said to exhibit similarity to that in kernicterus, *no neuronal changes* were observed in the regions observed to have the staining when the fresh brain was examined. Indeed, after fixation, only 2 of 32 brains exhibited any microscopic evidence of bilirubin staining.[224] This lack of retention of bilirubin after brain fixation, and especially the absence of evidence of neuronal injury, indicated that the bilirubin staining of the fresh brain was not that of kernicterus, as I described it earlier. The principal pathological feature in the premature infants with secondary bilirubin staining was a diffuse, spongy change principally of the cerebral cortex and white matter, without associated neuronal injury. Whether this abnormality represented an artifactual change or the effect of concomitant major hypoxic-ischemic or other injury was not clear. At any rate, bilirubin staining did not appear to be related to the structural disturbance and presumably was a secondary phenomenon.

CLINICAL ASPECTS OF ACUTE AND CHRONIC BILIRUBIN ENCEPHALOPATHIES

The clinical features in infants who have sustained bilirubin injury to brain in the neonatal period depend on the topography and intensity of the neuropathological findings and their interrelations with brain maturation. Thus, important determining features are the severity of the hyperbilirubinemia (including associated clinical factors), the duration, and the postconceptional age of the infant. These issues are discussed later. In the following, I consider both the clinical features observed in the newborn period (i.e., acute bilirubin encephalopathy associated with kernicterus) and the principal sequelae to this neonatal injury (i.e., chronic postkernicteric bilirubin encephalopathy). Because the clinical correlates of both the acute and chronic bilirubin encephalopathies of the *full-term (or premature) infant with marked hyperbilirubinemia* are understood most clearly, and because the disorder in this group of infants serves as the prototype for bilirubin injury to the neonatal nervous system, I describe those correlates in detail. However, as described earlier (see "Neuropathology"), similar neuropathological findings are observed in the *premature infant without marked hyperbilirubinemia;* the acute and chronic clinical correlates in this important group of infants *remain to be defined fully*. I discuss the somewhat limited available data relevant to this group in the context of the better-defined information available concerning the infants with marked hyperbilirubinemia.

Clinical Features

Acute Bilirubin Encephalopathy-Kernicterus

The occurrence of neonatal clinical features in full-term infants with marked hyperbilirubinemia who either have died with pathologically proven kernicterus or have survived to develop the clinical syndrome of chronic bilirubin encephalopathy of the postkernicteric type was documented in the older literature relative to erythroblastosis fetalis (Table 13-14).[222,228,229] Most affected infants exhibited a definite neurological syndrome, although 15% of those with proven kernicterus failed to exhibit any definite neurological signs.

The characteristics of the neonatal neurological syndrome in infants with marked hyperbilirubinemia were defined particularly in older writings and have been

TABLE 13-14 Occurrence of Clinical Features in Acute Bilirubin Encephalopathy

Clinical Features	Percentage of Cases
No definite neurological signs	15%
Equivocal neurological signs	20%–30%
Definite neurological signs	55%–65%

Data from Van Praagh R: Diagnosis of kernicterus in the neonatal period, *Pediatrics* 28:870–876, 1961, and Jones MH, Sands R, Hyman CB: Longitudinal study of the incidence of central nervous system damage following erythroblastosis fetalis, *Pediatrics* 14:346–350, 1954.

TABLE 13-15	Major Clinical Features of Acute Bilirubin Encephalopathy

Initial Phase
Slight stupor ("lethargic," "sleepy")
Slight hypotonia, paucity of movement
Poor sucking; slightly high-pitched cry

Intermediate Phase
Moderate stupor: irritability
Tone variable, usually increased; some with
   retrocollis-opisthotonos
Minimal feeding; high-pitched cry

Advanced Phase
Deep stupor to coma
Tone usually increased; pronounced
   retrocollis-opisthotonos
No feeding; shrill cry

supplemented in recent years with experience that included premature infants.[4,5,68,72,83-85,208,230-237] In my experience, the major neurological features involve abnormalities of *(1) level of consciousness, (2) tone and movement, and (3) brain stem function, especially relating to feeding and cry* (Table 13-15). I believe that the aberrations of level of consciousness relate principally to the involvement of neurons of reticular formation, aberrations of tone and movement relate to nuclei of the basal ganglia (globus pallidus and subthalamic nucleus), and disorders of brain stem function pertain to the relevant cranial nerve nuclei. The severity of the abnormalities appears to correlate, at least approximately, with both the severity of the hyperbilirubinemia and duration thereof and the gestational age of the infant. In general, overt neurological features are somewhat less common in small premature infants than in full-term or near-term infants, although an increase in apnea and bradycardia has been documented in hyperbilirubinemic infants of 25 to 32 weeks of gestational age versus those without hyperbilirubinemia.[81,85,86] I find it useful to consider the clinical features of acute bilirubin encephalopathy in three major phases of increasing severity, which, in marked hyperbilirubinemia, evolves generally over several days (see Table 13-15).

Initial Phase. As the syndrome first evolves, stupor, hypotonia, and a paucity of movement are prominent and are usually accompanied by poor sucking (see Table 13-15). These signs clearly are not specific and must raise the question of a variety of primary and secondary disorders of the central nervous system. Recognition of these signs as a signal of acute bilirubin encephalopathy and a need for prompt therapeutic intervention is important because a drastic deterioration in prognosis results if the syndrome progresses markedly.

Intermediate Phase. The cardinal signs of the next phase usually appear within 2 to 3 days and consist of moderate stupor, often with irritability, and a tendency for tone to *increase*, especially with stimulation. The increase in tone involves especially extensor muscle groups, and the infant begins to exhibit backward arching of the neck (retrocollis) or of the back (opisthotonos) (see Table 13-15). In some previous reports, this hypertonia is often referred to as *spasticity*. This term is inaccurate because the increase in tone is probably extrapyramidal rather than corticospinal in origin. (Fever occurred in 80% of the patients studied by Van Praagh,[229] did not relate to any clearly recognized cause, and may have been on a diencephalic basis. Such a high frequency of fever has not been my experience.) If untreated, infants who exhibit the principal features of the intermediate phase, including hypertonia, are highly likely to progress to the ominous next phase. In the series collected by Johnson and colleagues of 81 infants who appeared to be in the late intermediate phase and who were followed through 18 months of age, 75 (93%) developed "classic kernicteric sequelae."[72]

Advanced Phase. In the most severely affected infants, the clinical syndrome evolves, usually after several days, to the advanced phase, characterized by deep stupor or even coma, consistently increased tone, no feeding, and a striking shrill cry (see Table 13-15). Typically, pronounced retrocollis and opisthotonos are easily elicited by stimulation or are observed spontaneously (Fig. 13-12). Seizures occur in the *minority* of infants with acute bilirubin encephalopathy, although a frequency of 50% was recorded in one older series.[238] It appears likely that seizures are most often a manifestation of a concomitant process, such as hypoxic-ischemic injury. When infants reach the advanced phase of the disease, most have irreversible injury and the subsequent development of chronic postkernicteric bilirubin encephalopathy (see later). However, the converse may not be true. In a prospective series of 100 infants with hyperbilirubinemia secondary to erythroblastosis fetalis, approximately 10% of infants with no or minimal signs in the newborn period later developed the clinical features of chronic bilirubin encephalopathy.[228] This occurrence may be more common in premature infants.[80,81,83,84]

Chronic Postkernicteric Bilirubin Encephalopathy following Marked Neonatal Hyperbilirubinemia

Major Features and Temporal Evolution. Chronic bilirubin encephalopathy of the classic postkernicteric type was described particularly well in older studies of infants who experienced marked hyperbilirubinemia secondary to Rh incompatibility (Table 13-16).[222,239,240] However, the more recent literature and my personal experience confirm the essential clinical features.* The temporal evolution of the encephalopathy is particularly interesting. *In the first year of life*, the characteristic features are hypotonia (evolving from the neonatal hypertonia), active deep tendon reflexes,

_____

*See references 5,7,69,72,80,81,83,84,208,230,241-246.

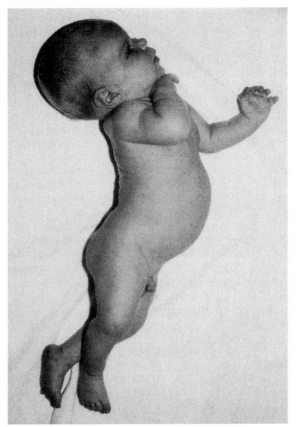

Figure 13-12 **Retrocollis and opisthotonos in a 1-month-old infant with kernicterus.** The kernicterus was secondary to Crigler-Najjar syndrome. *(Courtesy of Dr. M. Jeffrey Maisels.)*

persistent and often obligatory tonic neck reflex (and righting reflex), and delayed acquisition of motor skills.[239] The first three of these features provide an important clue, although not a flagrantly obvious one, of more serious motor disturbances to follow. The constellation of findings particularly characteristic of chronic bilirubin encephalopathy of the postkernicteric type (see Table 13-16) usually does not become apparent until *after the age of 6 months to 1 year*. The extrapyramidal motor disturbances may not be well developed for several years. The major features of the fully developed encephalopathy are extrapyramidal movement abnormalities, gaze disturbances, and auditory deficits. Intellect is relatively spared. Dental dysplasia is a very frequent accompaniment of chronic bilirubin encephalopathy,[4,72] and the term *clinical tetrad of bilirubin injury* often is used to refer to the three neurological features just noted and the dental dysplasia.

TABLE 13-16 **Major Clinical Features of Chronic Postkernicteric Bilirubin Encephalopathy**

Extrapyramidal abnormalities, especially athetosis
Gaze abnormalities, especially of upward gaze
Auditory disturbance, especially sensorineural hearing loss
Intellect relatively spared

Extrapyramidal Movement Abnormalities. The most striking neurological feature of the syndrome is the extrapyramidal disturbance (see Table 13-16). These motor phenomena are present to a variable degree in nearly every case and, in the most severely affected cases, consist principally of athetosis. The slow, writhing movements characteristically involve all limbs, although the upper extremities are usually affected more severely than are the lower extremities. Swallowing, phonation, and facial movement are also involved. Dystonic posturing is also a common extrapyramidal feature, and the associated increased tone is often mistakenly termed *spasticity*. In severely affected children, the limb movements may exhibit features of chorea (rapid, jerky movements), ballismus (wide amplitude, flailing movements), or, least commonly, tremor (small amplitude, distal movements). The abnormal movements, especially athetosis, and the increased tone typical of dystonia tend to fluctuate, a dynamic feature more common in the extrapyramidal syndrome of kernicterus than in the syndrome associated with status marmoratus (see Chapter 9).[226] In a minority of cases, the extrapyramidal abnormalities may be apparent only with attempts at skilled movement. The extrapyramidal syndrome reflects the disturbance of basal ganglia, particularly globus pallidus and subthalamic nucleus, the neuropathological hallmark of the encephalopathy.

Gaze Abnormalities. Gaze abnormalities occur in most patients (see Table 13-16) and usually involve vertical gaze, particularly upward gaze. Occasionally, both horizontal and vertical movements are affected. In most affected cases, vertical eye movements can be elicited by the doll's eyes maneuver,[240] thus indicating that the lesion probably is above the level of the oculomotor nuclei. However, a few patients also exhibit apparent paralytic gaze palsies. The neuropathological correlate for the supranuclear palsies is involvement of neurons of upper midbrain,[247] and the nuclear palsies reflect the neuronal injury in appropriate cranial nerve nuclei in the brain stem. Gaze disturbances require careful examination and are frequently overlooked.

Auditory Abnormalities. Disturbances of hearing have been well documented.[85,208,239-241,246,248-251] In most cases, the auditory disturbance is a high-frequency loss, usually bilateral. The hearing deficit, even when severe, very often escapes clinical detection for months or even longer, and this may be reflected in delayed acquisition of language. Delayed development and progression of sensorineural loss in the first months of life, after normal hearing studies in the neonatal period, have been observed.[241] In one well-studied series of infants with chronic bilirubin encephalopathy, 63% had moderate or severe hearing loss.[252] More subtle forms of auditory imperception also are common.[240,250,253] Studies of BSAERs[85,86,93,106,109,208,251,254-270a] and morphological data in human infants[166,220,221,248] indicate that the pathological substrate for the auditory disturbances resides principally in neurons in the brain stem, particularly the cochlear nuclei, and perhaps, in the auditory nerve. Thus, the hearing disturbance is principally central (brain stem) and, to a lesser extent, peripheral in origin. The crucial role for bilirubin in pathogenesis is apparent from experimental studies that established the relationship between the auditory disturbances and bilirubin uptake and deposition.[85,95,271-274] Studies in human infants showed a relationship not only with serum bilirubin levels but also with impaired bilirubin albumin binding,[106] as well as with the combination of bilirubin level and acidosis.[262] The last observation is particularly suggestive of the formation of injurious bilirubin acid in brain (see earlier discussion of determinants of neuronal injury). Amelioration of abnormal brain stem evoked responses with intervention has been documented.[269]

In recent years, the occurrence of *auditory neuropathy* or *auditory dyssynchrony* has been identified as an important sequela of bilirubin-induced injury.[208,246,275] Recognition of auditory dyssynchrony is important because the clinical characteristics and treatment of this disorder differ from those of more typical hearing loss. This auditory disorder is defined as absent or abnormal BSAERs with normal tests of inner ear function. Thus, tests of the mechanical integrity of the inner ear (otoacoustic emissions) or of the outer hair cells of the inner ear (cochlear microphonics) are normal, in the presence of absent BSAER or of abnormal brain stem latencies. *Children with auditory neuropathy may have little or no hearing loss but exhibit abnormal processing of sound.* It appears that conduction in the large, heavily myelinated afferent auditory pathways is not synchronized.[275] Functional effects include difficulties with sound localization and speech discrimination, and although abnormal BSAERs may resolve, this central auditory processing disorder becomes apparent. Importantly, initial data indicate that children with auditory neuropathy and hearing loss appear to respond favorably to cochlear implantation.[275] More data are needed on these issues.

The possibilities that impairment of auditory function is the most consistent abnormality associated with chronic postkernicteric bilirubin encephalopathy and, as a corollary, that the auditory system is the most sensitive neural system to clinically overt bilirubin injury have not been clarified decisively. In the acute period, detection of abnormalities of the BSAER is a very sensitive indicator of bilirubin-induced neural dysfunction (see later discussion). Documentation has been made of subsequent hearing impairment secondary to neonatal bilirubin injury *without* the development of associated athetosis.[5,85,86,250,252,275] This observation may be relevant to the possibility of bilirubin auditory neurotoxicity in the premature infant without marked hyperbilirubinemia (see later).

Intellectual Deficits. Marked intellectual deficits occur only in the minority of patients in unselected populations.[239] In patients with athetosis secondary to severe kernicterus (secondary to hemolytic disease) studied by Byers and co-workers,[239] only approximately 25% of the group had an intelligence quotient

TABLE 13-17   Intelligence of 19 Patients with Severe Chronic Bilirubin Encephalopathy, Kernicteric Type, Secondary to Hemolytic Disease

Intelligence Quotient	No. (Percentage of Total)
90–100	7 (37%)
70–90	4 (21%)
50–50	3 (16%)
<50	1 (5%)
Testing unsatisfactory	4 (21%)

Data from Byers RK, Paine RS, Crothers B: Extrapyramidal cerebral palsy with hearing loss following erythroblastosis, *Pediatrics* 15:248–254, 1955.

(IQ) of less than 70 (Table 13-17). Unfortunately, these patients often have been considered mistakenly to be mentally retarded because of their contorted countenance and writhing limbs, as well as undetected disturbances in audition. Indeed, most recent studies suggest that intellect is *relatively spared* in chronic bilirubin encephalopathy.[65] In the 81 surviving infants reviewed by Johnson and associates,[72] "intelligence appears to have been spared in almost all infants," although the survivors were not evaluated systematically. The clinician must be alert to the possibilities that the movement disorder may mask spared cognitive function or that auditory deficits may disturb language development and thus must recognize that intellectual function is usually relatively spared in this disorder. The *relative* sparing of cerebral cortex on neuropathological examination is compatible with this observation.

Chronic Bilirubin Encephalopathy without Marked Neonatal Hyperbilirubinemia

The striking syndrome of chronic postkernicteric bilirubin encephalopathy after marked hyperbilirubinemia led to the postulate that neurological involvement may be less severe, caused by less than marked neonatal hyperbilirubinemia, shorter durations of hyperbilirubinemia, prematurity, or a combination of these factors. It is most useful to formulate two questions in this context. *First* do full-term infants without marked hyperbilirubinemia experience subsequent neurological deficits secondary to bilirubin neurotoxicity? *Second*, do premature infants without marked hyperbilirubinemia experience a different spectrum of neurological deficits than do term infants without marked hyperbilirubinemia? As will become apparent, these questions are interrelated but are considered separately in the following discussion.

Neurological Sequelae in Term Infants without Marked Hyperbilirubinemia. The possibility that brain injury may occur secondary to intermediate levels of bilirubin and without a recognizable neonatal neurological syndrome in term infants has been the subject of numerous reports.[4,65,66,208,250,252,268, 276-283] Results of these studies are variable; several documented an early delay in motor development, but most detected no significant ultimate effect on neurological development or cognition at ages

4 to 13 years.[4,66,250,252,268,270,277-282,284] Effects, when present, were greatest in studies that included infants of low birth weight and infants with pathological evidence of amniotic fluid infection (i.e., chorioamnionitis).[278,279] The former observations are relevant to the subsequent discussion of premature infants, and the latter are relevant to the previous discussion of the potentiating effects on bilirubin neurotoxicity of infection through an increase in the transport of bilirubin across the blood-brain barrier, enhanced neuronal susceptibility to bilirubin injury, or both. *Nevertheless, even in these reports, the effects, when present and although statistically significant, are modest.* In view of recent data concerning auditory dyssynchrony (see earlier) in infants with normal or nearly normal hearing,[208] the possibility of previously undetected central auditory processing deficits after moderate hyperbilirubinemia cannot be excluded.

Neurological Sequelae in Premature Infants without Marked Hyperbilirubinemia. Several syndromes of chronic bilirubin encephalopathy appear established in premature infants without marked hyperbilirubinemia (Table 13-18). Thus, autopsy (see earlier) and imaging studies (see later) demonstrated *classic kernicterus* in premature infants with bilirubin levels less than 20 mg/dL. Most commonly the hyperbilirubinemia was nonhemolytic but complicated by such factors as sepsis, acidosis, and other features that increase the risk of bilirubin neurotoxicity.

Of great interest has been the possibility that moderate hyperbilirubinemia in very-low-birth-weight infants can lead to *partial forms* of chronic bilirubin encephalopathy. The most compelling data are available for a *predominantly auditory* partial form. Thus, study of hearing loss in surviving premature infants suggests that auditory impairment may be the principal neurological manifestation of bilirubin neurotoxicity in the premature infant without marked hyperbilirubinemia. In one detailed study of 30 premature infants with documented hearing loss on follow-up, multivariate testing demonstrated peak serum bilirubin concentration (12 mg/dL) to be positively associated and exchange transfusion to be negatively associated with subsequent hearing loss.[261] Only one of the infants exhibited choreoathetosis (and impaired upgaze), and approximately 60% had hearing loss as their only subsequent abnormality. Similarly, moderate hyperbilirubinemia was associated with hearing loss in preterm infants in other reports,[253,261,262,285] and in one of these reports the additional association of duration of

hyperbilirubinemia and associated acidosis with the occurrence of hearing loss lent further credence to bilirubin (perhaps bilirubin acid) as the neurotoxic agent. In a study of 221 surviving infants of less than 1000 g birth weight, peak serum bilirubin levels higher than 10 mg/dL were predictive of deafness (odds ratio, 4.80; 95% confidence interval, 1.46 to 15.73) but not of the motor deficits of "cerebral palsy" or of developmental delay. Other studies attest to abnormalities of the neonatal BSAER in premature infants with only moderate hyperbilirubinemia,[85,86,208,237,286] although often the abnormalities resolve with treatment of the hyperbilirubinemia. *However, the data indicate the particular sensitivity of the auditory nuclei of the brain stem in the premature infant.* Consistent with this conclusion, one report concerning 2575 surviving infants of less than 1000 g birth weight showed a direct correlation of peak serum bilirubin concentrations with hearing impairment (Fig. 13-13).[287] In view of the observations regarding classic postkernicteric encephalopathy that indicate impairment of the auditory system, when carefully evaluated, to be a most sensitive indication of bilirubin injury, these findings suggest similarly that hearing loss may be the principal manifestation of bilirubin neurotoxicity in the premature infant without marked hyperbilirubinemia. Nevertheless, with more aggressive use of phototherapy and exchange transfusion, more recent data suggest that the frequency of such neurotoxicity is relatively low.[253,261,262] Finally, in a still-to-be-defined proportion of premature infants with bilirubin-induced hearing loss, motor abnormalities, often not marked, are present.[208] Thus, it is likely that a related partial form of chronic bilirubin encephalopathy in this context is a *mixed auditory and motor form* (see Table 13-18).

The possibility that a third partial form is *predominantly motor* has been suggested.[208] An earlier report of 831 premature infants followed in the Netherlands indicated that moderate hyperbilirubinemia was associated with later neurological impairment manifested primarily by cerebral palsy.[77] Thus, at the age of 2 years, a significant increase in such neurological impairment was observed after neonatal hyperbilirubinemia in the moderate range. A subsequent study of this large Dutch population at 5 years of age showed a relationship between hyperbilirubinemia only in infants with intracranial hemorrhage.[78] The odds ratio for impairment increased from 1.0 for maximum serum bilirubin concentrations of 8.7 mg/dL to 3.3 for concentrations of 11.7 to 14.6 mg/dL and to 5.6 for concentrations of 14.7 to 17.5 mg/dL. However, ultrasonographic data did not allow the potentially confounding effect of periventricular lesions (e.g., echodensities, cysts) to be evaluated. Two subsequent reports of 249 and 494 preterm infants with moderate hyperbilirubinemia did evaluate the confounding effects of both intracranial hemorrhage and periventricular lesions and found no consistent relation between the subsequent occurrence of "cerebral palsy" or "developmental problems" and maximum serum bilirubin concentration.[282,288] Thus, on balance, a relationship between moderate hyperbilirubinemia in the preterm infant and subsequent major motor deficits is unclear but does not appear likely.

TABLE 13-18 **Chronic Bilirubin Encephalopathy without Marked Hyperbilirubinemia in Premature Infants***

Chronic bilirubin encephalopathy: classic postkernicteric
Chronic bilirubin encephalopathy: partial forms
    Predominantly auditory
    Mixed auditory and motor, often mild
    Predominantly motor (?)

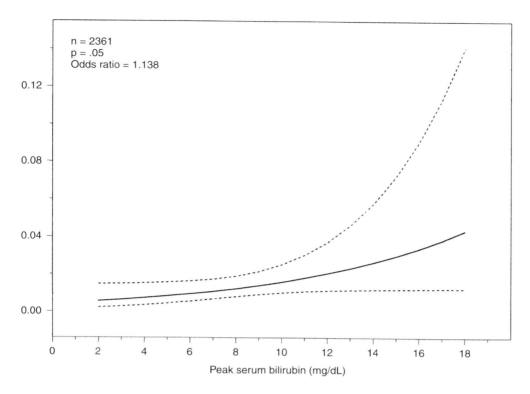

n = 2361
p = .05
Odds ratio = 1.138

Peak serum bilirubin (mg/dL)

Figure 13-13 **Proportion of infants requiring hearing aids as a function of peak serum bilirubin level in the neonatal period.** Population consisted of 2575 infants of 401 to 1000 g birth weight and followed until 18 to 22 months of postconceptional age. The peak serum bilirubin level during the neonatal period is shown on the *X*-axis, and the proportion of infants with hearing aids is shown on the *Y*-axis. The *dotted lines* represent 95% confidence intervals. *(From Oh W, Tyson JE, Fanaroff AA, Vohr BR, et al: Association between peak serum bilirubin and neurodevelopmental outcomes in extremely low birth weight infants, Pediatrics 112:773–779, 2003.)*

Indeed, in view of the apparent sensitivity of the auditory system of the premature infant to bilirubin, I doubt that a predominantly motor partial form of chronic bilirubin encephalopathy is likely in the premature infant (see Table 13-18).

Finally, the possibility that cognitive impairment is a feature of neurotoxicity caused by moderate hyperbilirubinemia in the premature infant was raised. Follow-up of 2575 infants of less than 1000 g birth weight showed a correlation between peak serum bilirubin levels and Psychomotor Developmental Index values lower than 70; however, the effect was modest (odds ratio, 1.057; *P* = .05), and the cerebral white matter was evaluated only by cranial ultrasonography. Thus, confounding could not be excluded. Thus, currently it seems unlikely that moderate hyperbilirubinemia leads to cognitive impairment in the premature infant. Moreover, an analysis of 224 children with a birth weight less than 2000 g who were followed to 6 years of age showed no associations among maximum bilirubin level, duration of exposure to bilirubin, or measures of bilirubin-albumin binding at bilirubin levels lower than 20 mg/dL (Fig. 13-14).[289] A more recent study of 128 infants of less than 800 g birth weight also showed no statistically significant relationship between moderate hyperbilirubinemia and cognitive impairment.[290]

Diagnosis

Serum Bilirubin Measurements

The goal in diagnosis is to identify the infant who is likely to develop brain injury from bilirubin before the

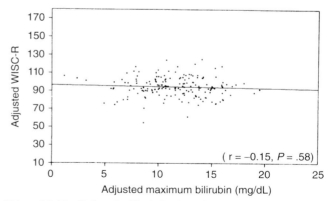

Adjusted maximum bilirubin (mg/dL)

(r = –0.15, P = .58)

Figure 13-14 **Full-scale Wechsler Intelligence Scale for Children-Revised (WISC-R) score at 6 years by maximum bilirubin level for children of less than 2000 g birth weight.** Values were obtained using multiple regression analysis. *(From Scheidt PC, Graubard BI, Nelson KB, Hirtz DG, et al: Intelligence at six years in relation to neonatal bilirubin level: Follow-up of the National Institute of Child Health and Human Development clinical trial of phototherapy, Pediatrics 87:797–806, 1991.)*

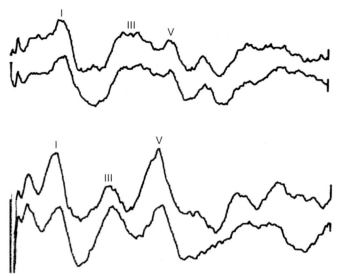

Figure 13-15 Auditory brain stem evoked responses before (*upper tracings*) and after (*lower tracings*) exchange transfusion in an infant with hyperbilirubinemia. The *horizontal axis* represents time, and the *vertical axis* represents amplitude. Waves I, III, and V are indicated in both pairs of tracings. Increased wave amplitude and reduced latencies are apparent after exchange transfusion. (*From Nwaesei CG, Van Aerde J, Boyden M, Perlman M: Changes in auditory brainstem responses in hyperbilirubinemic infants before and after exchange transfusion,* Pediatrics *74:800–803, 1984.*)

occurrence of the neurotoxicity. Toward this goal, certain tests have been devised to determine in an infant's serum the "free" bilirubin, essentially the concentration of unconjugated bilirubin not bound to albumin, the bilirubin binding capacity of albumin, and the bilirubin binding affinity of albumin.[4,18,27,106,268,291] Although these measures have proved to be of some value in predicting which infants develop kernicterus, the most reproducible tests are not easily applied clinically, and the data are not consistent or conclusive enough to state that one or more of the measures accomplish the goal of identifying the infant susceptible to bilirubin injury before neurotoxicity occurs. More detailed discussion of these measures is available elsewhere.[3,4,18,58,268]

Brain Stem Auditory Evoked Responses and Other Electrophysiological Measures

The more refined laboratory techniques just described indicate the clinical setting for bilirubin neurotoxicity but do not indicate whether neuronal injury has occurred or is imminent. Early detection of bilirubin neurotoxicity may be possible by the use of *brain stem evoked response audiometry*. Thus, many studies documented distinct disturbances of the BSAERs with hyperbilirubinemia, and several documented improvement when bilirubin levels decreased over days or promptly after exchange transfusion (Fig. 13-15).*

---

*See references 3,4,85,86,93,106,109,208,237,241,251,255-260, 263-265,267,268,270,270a,286,292,293.

The most consistently observed abnormalities involved the threshold for all waves, latency for wave I, and conduction times between waves I, III, and V. In general, the effects indicated both peripheral and brain stem disturbance, with a predominance of the latter, and correlated with neuropathological findings indicative of injury to auditory nerve and cochlear nuclei as well as to superior olivary nuclei and inferior colliculi. The adverse effects were observed at serum bilirubin concentrations in the upper teens (i.e., not marked hyperbilirubinemia) in term and near-term infants, with effects at lower concentrations in premature infants. Reversibility when the level of serum bilirubin is lowered was consistent. In keeping with the clinical observations reviewed previously concerning the vulnerability of the auditory pathway to bilirubin injury, the data indicated that brain stem evoked response audiometry is a sensitive technique for detecting bilirubin neuronal disturbance and, perhaps, imminent neuronal injury. However, the evidence for neuronal *dysfunction* provided by abnormal evoked response audiometry in hyperbilirubinemic infants is not necessarily or even usually followed by evidence of structural *neuronal injury* (i.e., subsequent fixed hearing deficits). Thus, the very sensitivity of the technique presents problems in the diagnosis of true bilirubin neurotoxicity. Nevertheless, the method holds considerable promise for the early identification of the infant at risk for neuronal injury. In my preliminary experience, based on the clinical classification of the phases of acute bilirubin encephalopathy (see earlier), the initial clinical phase is accompanied by marginal increases in latencies, usually not out of the normal ranges for age; the intermediate phase is accompanied by definite prolongation of latencies and a decrease in amplitude of the major waves; and the advanced phase is accompanied by severely prolonged latencies and depressed amplitudes or no definable waves at all.

The possibility that evaluation of *somatosensory evoked responses* may be useful in assessment of bilirubin neurotoxicity was raised by well-established data.[294] Thus, in a study of 59 term infants, the central conduction time (from cervical cord to cerebral cortex) correlated directly with bilirubin levels above approximately 15 mg/dL (250 μmol/L) (Fig. 13-16). This abnormality disappeared by 5 weeks of age. Further data will be of interest.

The possibility that assessment of *visual evoked responses* will be useful in the assessment of bilirubin neurotoxicity was raised by a study of 72 hyperbilirubinemic infants.[295] Earlier reports of 11 hyperbilirubinemic infants and studies of developing Gunn rats suggested that bilirubin may affect the visual system.[237,259,296,297] In the large study of 72 infants, a striking relationship between the major wave latency and maximal serum bilirubin level was observed in the first week of life (Fig. 13-17).[295] The latencies returned to normal by 8 weeks of age in nearly all infants. Thus, this electrophysiological approach, as with the BSAER, may be too sensitive to distinguish the infant with a fixed deficit from one with a transient deficit.

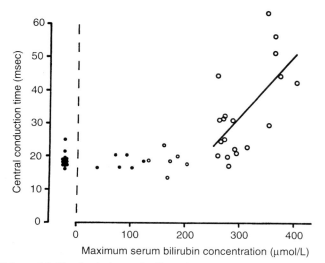

Figure 13-16 Central conduction time of the somatosensory evoked potential as a function of maximum serum bilirubin concentration among term infants. *(From Bongers-Schokking JJ, Colon EJ, Hoogland RA, Van Den Brande JL, et al: Somatosensory evoked potentials in neonatal jaundice,* Acta Paediatr Scand *79:148–155, 1990.)*

Transient abnormalities of the *electroencephalogram* were observed in two detailed studies of hyperbilirubinemic term newborns.[237,298] The disturbances included decreased amplitudes, slowed frequencies, delayed maturation and multifocal spikes. The changes do not appear consistent enough to use for diagnostic

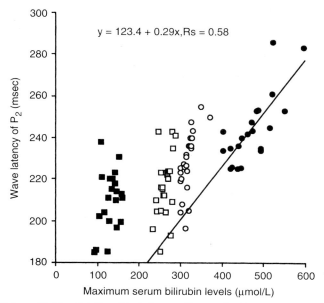

$$y = 123.4 + 0.29x, Rs = 0.58$$

Figure 13-17 Relationship between the maximal neonatal serum bilirubin level and the latency of wave P$_2$ of the visual evoked response, obtained on the same day. The four groups were classified according to maximal serum bilirubin level as: control (*solid squares*) (*n* = 22), low (*open squares*) (*n* = 26), moderate (*open circles*) (*n* = 25), and severe (*closed circles*) (*n* = 21). Regression line for the severe group (*P* <.0001). *(From Chen YJ, Kang WM: Effects of bilirubin on visual evoked potentials in term infants,* Eur J Pediatr *154:662–666, 1995.)*

TABLE 13-19	**Value of Magnetic Resonance Imaging in Identification of Acute and Chronic Bilirubin Encephalopathy**

Approximately 75 reported cases studied by MRI; includes 11 premature infants with only moderate hyperbilirubinemia

Globus pallidus affected bilaterally and symmetrically in approximately 90%, subthalamic nucleus in approximately 40%, and hippocampus in approximately 5%

In first 3 weeks, lesions seen best on T1-weighted images; chronic lesions seen best on T2- weighted images

Acute lesions may disappear and not be replaced by chronic lesions; frequency unclear

Presence of the *chronic* abnormality on MRI consistently associated with the classic clinical features of chronic postkernicterus bilirubin encephalopathy; however, a few cases with the classic clinical syndrome do *not* have detectable MRI abnormality of globus pallidus

MRI, magnetic resonance imaging.

purposes. Moreover, their clinical significance is unclear.

Magnetic Resonance Imaging

In contrast to common structural imaging modalities, ultrasonography and computed tomography, *MR imaging (MRI)* has been of major value in the identification of both acute and chronic bilirubin encephalopathy (Table 13-19).* Most infants reported were term or near-term infants with marked hyperbilirubinemia. However, similar abnormalities were detected in 11 premature infants, most of whom had only moderate hyperbilirubinemia.[80,81,83,301] The principal findings are bilateral and symmetric abnormalities of globus pallidus in approximately 90%, subthalamic nucleus in approximately 40%, and rarely hippocampus. The lesions are seen best in the acute period, first several weeks of life, on T1-weighted images (Fig. 13-18), and later, chronic lesions, on T2-weighted images (Fig. 13-19). The abnormalities of globus pallidus and subthalamic nucleus should be distinguished from the typical involvement in hypoxic-ischemic disease of putamen and thalamus. The acute lesions may be transient and, with clinical recovery, may disappear. Infants who exhibit the chronic abnormality on T2-weighted images consistently exhibit the classic clinical features of chronic postkernicteric bilirubin encephalopathy (see earlier). However, the converse is not true (i.e., occasional children with the classic clinical syndrome have normal MRI findings).

MR spectroscopy provides additional information in the acute period. A decrease in the *N*-acetylaspartate/choline ratio in "basal ganglia," consistent with neuronal injury, was shown in the first 3 weeks in an infant with a bilirubin concentration higher than 25 mg/dL and later development of athetosis; four other infants with similar bilirubin levels but normal ratios did not develop athetosis, although follow-up was relatively

---

*See references 68,69,80,81,83,233,237,243,244,292,299-301.

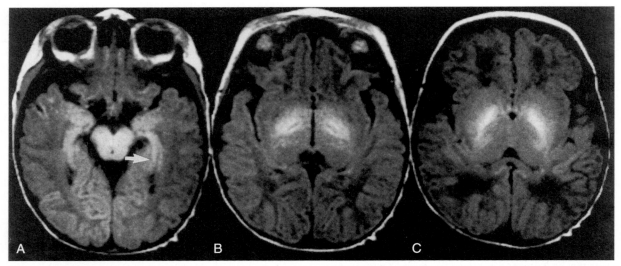

Figure 13-18 Series of three axial T1-weighted magnetic resonance images in a 16-day-old infant with the clinical and biochemical features of acute bilirubin encephalopathy. In **A**, note the abnormal high signal intensity in the hippocampus in the medial temporal lobe (*arrow*). In **B** and **C**, note the abnormal high signal intensity in the globus pallidus but not putamen. Less prominent high signal intensity is present in the ventroposterolateral nucleus of the thalamus **(C)**. All the findings were less prominent on T2-weighted images (not shown). The topography of the findings is typical of kernicterus. *(From Penn AA, Enzmann DR, Hahn JS, Stevenson DK: Kernicterus in a full-term infant, Pediatrics 93:1003–1006, 1994.)*

brief (12 to 24 months).[234] The single infant with sequelae also exhibited opisthotonus and abnormal signal in the globus pallidus on MRI. Thus, it is not clear that the MR spectroscopy results added appreciably to the evaluation of the infant. In another report, six infants with hyperbilirubinemia and MRI findings of kernicterus exhibited on MR spectroscopy elevated ratio of glutamate/glutamine to creatine in "basal ganglia."[245] The authors suggested that the finding reflected an increase in extracellular glutamate, consistent with a role for excitotoxicity in the neuronal injury of kernicterus (see earlier).

Management

The essential aspect of the management of bilirubin encephalopathy is prevention. Although major efforts are directed at prevention and control of neonatal hyperbilirubinemia per se, other factors such as prematurity, acidosis, hypoalbuminemia, hypoxia-ischemia, infection, or other insults to the central nervous system may be as important in the genesis of bilirubin neurotoxicity, at least under certain circumstances (see preceding discussions). These additional deleterious factors must be treated vigorously, when possible, and the search should continue for other such factors that still elude detection.

In this section, I address briefly the prevention and treatment of neonatal hyperbilirubinemia and, in particular, the choice of therapy as a function of the infant's gestational age, postnatal age, and bilirubin level. More detailed discussions are available from excellent sources in neonatology.[84,302-306] Five major aspects of management of neonatal hyperbilirubinemia should be recognized (Table 13-20): (1) prevention,

(2) early detection, (3) phototherapy, (4) exchange transfusion, and (5) other therapies.

Prevention

Prevention of hemolytic disease of the newborn begins with maternal screening for isoimmunization. Prevention of the most serious form of hemolytic disease (i.e., that resulting from Rh incompatibility) has been accomplished to a major extent through the widespread use of anti-Rh immune globulin to prevent maternal sensitization.[307-310] Infants known to be affected in utero have been treated successfully with intrauterine blood transfusion.[311-317]

Surveillance and Early Detection

Careful surveillance and early detection of the infant at risk for brain injury by bilirubin begin with recognition of infants at risk for severe hyperbilirubinemia. Recognition requires a systematic approach to the infant (Table 13-21) and awareness of major risk factors for development of severe hyperbilirubinemia (Table 13-22).[4,304-306] These issues have been reviewed previously in this chapter. Worthy of emphasis is measurement of total serum bilirubin. In recent years, transcutaneous bilirubin measurements of bilirubin have been developed and appear promising, at least for screening.[4,318-321] Most importantly, bilirubin levels should be evaluated in the context of hour-specific nomograms (Fig. 13-20).[4,84,303-305] Those infants in the high-risk zone or with a rapid rate of rise require further evaluation for a cause of their hyperbilirubinemia and a decision concerning therapy (see later).

Identification of the infant experiencing acute bilirubin encephalopathy requires careful clinical assessment, and if possible, evaluation of BSAERs and

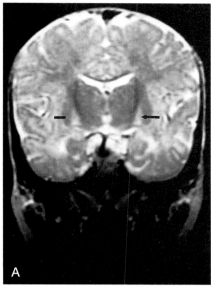

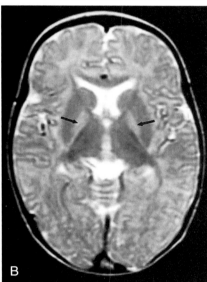

Figure 13-19 **MRI scans (T2-weighted).** Coronal (**A**) and axial (**B**) planes in a 6-month-old infant who had a serum bilirubin concentration of 30 mg/dL at 2 weeks of age. Note the distinct increased signal bilaterally in the globus pallidus (*arrows*), a site of predilection for ker- nicterus. *(Courtesy of Drs. Tina Young-Poissants and Charles Barlow.)*

TABLE 13-20	**Management of Neonatal Hyperbilirubinemia**

Prevention
Maternal screening for isoimmunization
Maternal use of anti-Rh immune globulin
Fetal blood transfusion

Surveillance and Early Detection

Phototherapy

Exchange Transfusion

Other Therapies
Heme oxygenase inhibitors: metalloporphyrins
Phenobarbital
Enterohepatic circulation enhancement (agar/orlistat)

TABLE 13-21	**Selected Key Elements of the American Academy of Pediatrics Guideline on Management of Hyperbilirubinemia in the Newborn 35 Weeks or More of Gestation**

Measure total serum bilirubin (or transcutaneous bilirubin) on infants jaundiced in the first 24 hours.
Interpret all bilirubin levels according to the infant's age in hours.
Recognize that infants less than 38 weeks of gestation, particularly those breast-fed, are at higher risk of devel- oping hyperbilirubinemia and require closer surveillance and monitoring.
Perform a systematic assessment on all infants before dis- charge for the *risk* of severe hyperbilirubinemia.
Provide appropriate follow-up based on risk assessment and time of discharge.
Treat newborns when indicated with phototherapy or exchange transfusion.

Adapted from Maisels MJ, Baltz RD, Bhutani VK, Newman TB, et al: Management of hyperbilirubinemia in the newborn infant 35 or more weeks of gestation, *Pediatrics* 114:297–316, 2004.

MRI, as discussed earlier. Vigorous therapy should be instituted in the presence of overt acute bilirubin encephalopathy because the process is potentially reversible.

Phototherapy

Phototherapy refers to the exposure of the infant to light with high-energy output near the maximum absorption peak of bilirubin (450 to 460 nm). This pro- cedure exposes the bilirubin circulating in superficial capillaries to the light and stimulates photoisomeriza- tion of bilirubin to a form that is water soluble and can be excreted in bile without conjugation.[4,322-330] This approach is effective as a means of preventing or treating moderate hyperbilirubinemia.[4,265,327-329,331-334] It has been particularly effective in the pre- mature infant with nonhemolytic jaundice. With care- ful attention to temperature, fluid balance, and eye

TABLE 13-22	**Major Risk Factors for Development of Severe Hyperbilirubinemia in Infants 35 Weeks or More of Gestation**

Predischarge total serum bilirubin (or transcutaneous biliru- bin) in the high-risk zone (see Fig. 13-20)
Jaundice in the first 24 hours of life
Blood group incompatibility with positive direct antiglobulin test or other hemolytic disease (e.g., glucose-6-phos- phate dehydrogenase deficiency)
Gestational age 35 to 36 weeks
Exclusive breast-feeding (especially if feeding not going well or weight loss excessive)
Cephalhematoma or significant bruising
Sibling with history of phototherapy
East Asian race

Adapted from Maisels MJ, Baltz RD, Bhutani VK, Newman TB, et al: Management of hyperbilirubinemia in the newborn infant 35 or more weeks of gestation, *Pediatrics* 114:297–316, 2004.

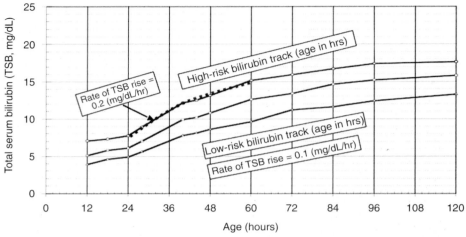

Figure 13-20 **Hour-specific bilirubin nomogram for term and near-term healthy infants.** The nomogram illustrates the rate of rise in total serum bilirubin (TSB) between 24 to 60 hours of age for the high-risk track (95th percentile) at 0.2 mg/dL/hr, the intermediate-risk track (75th percentile) at 0.15 mg/dL/hr, and the low-risk track (40th percentile) at 0.10 mg/dL/hr. See text for details. *(From Bhutani VK, Johnson LH, Keren R: Diagnosis and management of hyperbilirubinemia in the term neonate: For a safer first week, Pediatr Clin North Am 51:843–861, 2004.)*

occlusion, this procedure is safe and yet effective.[4,325,327-329,331,335] Currently recommended guidelines for the use of phototherapy are shown in Table 13-23 for low-birth-weight infants and in Figure 13-21 for near-term and term infants.[4] The importance of associated risk factors (e.g., hemolytic disease, asphyxia, sepsis, acidosis, low albumin, immaturity) are demonstrated.

Exchange Transfusion

Exchange transfusion is the treatment of choice for hyperbilirubinemia when the most aggressive intervention is necessary.[4,268,328,331,336] Albumin is a useful adjunct to exchange transfusion and increases the amount of bilirubin removed by the procedure; however, care must be taken to prevent volume overload. Exchange transfusion lowers the blood

bilirubin concentration rapidly, and when performed by experienced personnel, the procedure is relatively harmless. In one review of 66 exchange transfusions, although 74% were associated with an adverse event (primarily thrombocytopenia [44%], hypocalcemia [29%], metabolic acidosis [24%]), most of these events were asymptomatic and were readily treated.[337] Some data, however, indicate appreciable changes in cerebral blood volume and intracranial pressure coincident with the infusion and removal of blood during exchange transfusion, even when relatively small aliquots are used.[338,339] This occurrence presumably relates to the pressure-passive cerebral circulation demonstrated in the newborn by more direct techniques (see Chapter 6), and it presumably reflects an increase in cerebral blood flow with infusion and a decrease in cerebral blood flow with removal of blood. These observations raise the possibility of precipitating hemorrhagic or ischemic injury to the cerebrum during exchange transfusion, especially if a degree of asphyxia has occurred to disturb cerebrovascular autoregulation and to enhance the pressure-passive state of the cerebral circulation (see Chapter 6).

A crucial issue is which hyperbilirubinemic infant to treat with exchange transfusion. Current recommendations are shown in Table 13-23 for low-birth-weight infants and in Figure 13-22 for term and near-term infants.[304] The guidelines are categorized according to level of "risk," based on such factors as isoimmune hemolytic disease, glucose-6-phosphate dehydrogenase deficiency, asphyxia, sepsis, acidosis, low albumin, or relative immaturity.

Other Therapies

Other therapies for neonatal hyperbilirubinemia have been used or are under development.[4,268,317,328,340-356] These interventions have been directed at several steps

TABLE 13-23	Guidelines for the Use of Phototherapy and Exchange Transfusion in Low-Birth-Weight Infants*	
	TOTAL BILIRUBIN LEVEL (mg/dL [μmol/L])	
Birth Weights (g)	**Phototherapy**	**Exchange Transfusion**
≤1500	5–8 (85–140)	13–16 (220–275)
1500–1999	8–12 (140–200)	16–18 (275–300)
2000–2499	11–14 (190–240)	18–20 (300–340)

*Lower bilirubin concentrations should be used for infants who are sick (e.g., sepsis, acidosis, hypoalbuminemia) or who have hemolytic disease.

From Maisels MJ: Jaundice. In MacDonald MG, Mullett MD, Seshia MMK, editors: *Avery's Neonatology: Pathophysiology and Management of the Newborn*, 6th ed, Philadelphia: 2005, Lippincott Williams & Wilkins

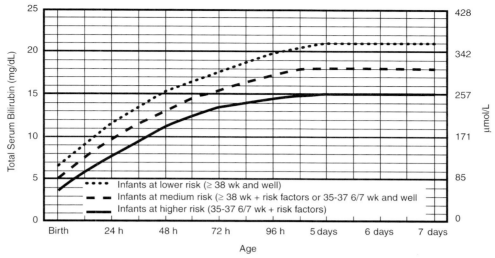

Figure 13-21 **Guidelines for phototherapy in hospitalized infants 35 weeks of gestation or more.** The guidelines are based on limited evidence and the levels shown are approximations. The following points are important. Use total serum bilirubin (TSB); do not subtract direct reacting or conjugated bilirubin. Risk factors are isoimmune hemolytic disease, glucose-6-phosphate dehydrogenase deficiency, asphyxia, significant lethargy, temperature instability, sepsis, acidosis, and albumin lower than 3.0 g/dL (if measured). For well infants 35 to 37 6/7 weeks of gestation, TSB levels for intervention can be adjusted around the medium risk line. It is an option to intervene at lower TSB levels for infants closer to 35 weeks and at higher TSB levels for those closer to 37 6/7 weeks. It is an option to provide conventional phototherapy in the hospital or at home at TSB levels of 2 or 3 mg/dL (35 to 50 mmol/L) lower than those shown, but home phototherapy should not be used in any infant with risk factors. *(From Maisels MJ, Baltz RD, Bhutani VK, Newman TB, et al: Management of hyperbilirubinemia in the newborn infant 35 or more weeks of gestation,* Pediatrics *114:297–316, 2004.)*

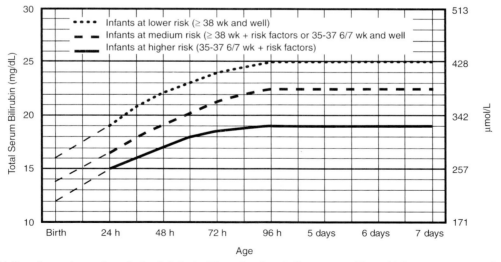

Figure 13-22 **Guidelines for exchange transfusion in infants 35 weeks of gestation or more.** The guidelines are based on limited evidence, and the levels shown are approximations. The following points are important. The *dashed lines* for the first 24 hours indicate uncertainty owing to a wide range of clinical circumstances and a range of responses to phototherapy. Immediate exchange transfusion is recommended if infant shows signs of acute bilirubin encephalopathy (hypertonia, arching, retrocollis, opisthotonos, fever, high-pitched cry) or if total serum bilirubin (TSB) is 5 mg/dL (85 μmol/L) or more above these lines. Risk factors are isoimmune hemolytic disease, glucose-6-phosphate dehydrogenase deficiency, asphyxia, significant lethargy, temperature instability, sepsis, and acidosis. Measure serum albumin and calculate the bilirubin/albumin ratio, which can be used as an additional factor in determining for exchange transfusion. Use TSB; do not subtract direct reacting or conjugated bilirubin. If the infant is well and 35 to 37 6/7 weeks of gestation (median risk), one can individualize TSB levels for exchange based on actual gestational age. *(From Maisels MJ, Baltz RD, Bhutani VK, Newman TB, et al: Management of hyperbilirubinemia in the newborn infant 35 or more weeks of gestation,* Pediatrics *114:297–316, 2004.)*

in bilirubin metabolism. Thus, bilirubin production has been inhibited at the rate-limiting heme oxygenase step by treatment with metalloporphyrins. The hepatic conjugation of bilirubin has been induced by phenobarbital, administered both antenatally and postnatally. The enterohepatic circulation has been enhanced by administration of agar, which binds to bilirubin in the intestine, inhibits reabsorption, and thereby promotes excretion, or orlistat, an intestinal lipase inhibitor, which enhances bilirubin excretion by still-to-be-defined mechanisms. Currently, none of these therapies is in wide clinical use.

REFERENCES

1. Schmorl G: Zur kenntie des icterus neonatorum, *Verh Dtsch Ges Pathol* 6:109, 1903.
2. Wiley CC, Lai N, Hill C, Burke G: Nursery practices and detection of jaundice after newborn discharge, *Arch Pediatr Adolesc Med* 152:972-975, 1998.
3. Wong RJ: Neonatal jaundice and liver disease. In Martin RJ, Fanaroff AA, Walsh MC, editors: *Neonatal-Perinatal Medicine Diseases of the Fetus and Infant*, 8th ed, Philadelphia: 2006, Elsevier.
4. Maisels MJ: Jaundice. In MacDonald MG, Mullett MD, Seshia MMK, editors: *Avery's Neonatology: Pathophysiology and Management of the Newborn*, 6th ed, Philadelphia: 2005, Lippincott Williams & Wilkins.
5. Maisels MJ, Newman TB: Kernicterus in otherwise healthy, breast-fed term newborns, *Pediatrics* 96:730-733, 1995.
6. Brown AK, Johnson L: Loss of concern about jaundice and the emergence of kernicterus in full term infants in the era of managed care. In Fanaroff AA, Klaus MH, editors: *Yearbook of Neonatal-Perinatal Medicine*, St. Louis: 1996, Mosby.
7. Johnson LH, Brown AK: A pilot registry for acute and chronic kernicterus in term and near-term infants [abstract], *Pediatrics* 104:736, 1999.
8. Brodersen R: Bilirubin solubility and interaction with albumin and phospholipid, *J Biol Chem* 254:2364-2369, 1979.
9. Brodersen R: Bilirubin transport in the newborn infant, reviewed in relation to kernicterus, *J Pediatr* 96:349-356, 1980.
10. Brodersen R, Robertson A: Chemistry of bilirubin and its interaction with albumin. In Levine RL, Maisel MJ, editors: *Hyperbilirubinemia in the Newborn: Report of the Eighty-fifth Ross Conference on Pediatric Research*, Columbus, OH: 1983, Ross.
11. Brodersen R, Stern L: Aggregation of bilirubin in injectates and incubation media: Its significance in experimental studies of CNS toxicity, *Neuropediatrics* 18:34-36, 1987.
12. Leonard M, Noy N, Zakim D: The interactions of bilirubin with model and biological membranes, *J Biol Chem* 264:5648-5652, 1989.
13. Brodersen R, Stern L: Deposition of bilirubin acid in the central nervous system: A hypothesis for the development of kernicterus, *Acta Paediatr Scand* 79:12-19, 1990.
14. Hayward D, Fedunec S, Chan G, Davis PJ, et al: Bilirubin diffusion through lipid membranes, *Biochim Biophys Acta* 8600:149-153, 1986.
15. Rosenthal P: Bilirubin metabolism in the fetus and neonate. In Polin RA, Fox WW, editors: *Fetal and Neonatal Physiology*, Philadelphia: 1992, Saunders.
16. Ostrow JD, Pascolo L, Shapiro SM, Tiribelli C: New concepts in bilirubin encephalopathy, *Eur J Clin Invest* 33:988-997, 2003.
17. Rubaltelli FF: Bilirubin metabolism in the newborn, *Biol Neonate* 63:133-138, 1993.
18. Cashore WJ: Bilirubin metabolism and toxicity in the newborn. In Polin RA, Fox WW, editors: *Fetal and Neonatal Physiology*, 2nd ed, Philadelphia: 1998, Saunders.
19. MacMahon JR: Bilirubin metabolism. In Taeusch H, Ballard RA, editors: *Avery's Diseases of the Newborn*, 7th ed, Philadelphia: 1998, Saunders.
20. Maisels MJ: What's in a name? Physiologic and pathologic jaundice: The conundrum of defining normal bilirubin levels in the newborn, *Pediatrics* 118:805-807, 2006.
21. Maisels MJ, Kring E: The contribution of hemolysis to early jaundice in normal newborns, *Pediatrics* 118:276-279, 2006.
22. Jacobsen J: Binding of bilirubin to human serum albumin: Determination of the dissociation constants, *FEBS Lett* 5:112-114, 1969.
23. Jacobsen J, Wennberg RP: Determination of unbound bilirubin in the serum of newborns, *Clin Chem* 20:783, 1974.
24. Lee K, Gartner LM, Zarafu I: Fluorescent dye method for determination of the bilirubin binding capacity of serum albumin, *J Pediatr* 86:280-285, 1975.
25. Levine RL: Fluorescence-quenching studies of the binding of bilirubin to albumin, *Clin Chem* 23:2292-2301, 1977.
26. Cashore WJ, Gartner LM, Oh W, Stern L: Clinical application of neonatal bilirubin-binding determinations: Current status, *J Pediatr* 83:827-833, 1978.
27. Cashore WJ: Bilirubin binding tests. In Levine RL, Maisels MJ, editors: *Hyperbilirubinemia in the Newborn: Report of the Eighty-fifth Ross Conference on Pediatric Research*, Columbus, OH: 1983, Ross.
28. Watchko JF: Genetics and the risk of neonatal hyperbilirubinemia, *Pediatr Res* 56:677-678, 2004.
29. Huang MJ, Kua KE, Teng HC, Tang KS, et al: Risk factors for severe hyperbilirubinemia in neonates, *Pediatr Res* 56:682-689, 2004.
30. Maisels MJ: Jaundice in the newborn, *Pediatr Rev* 3:305-313, 1982.
31. MacMahon JR, Stevenson DK, Oski FA: Unconjugated hyperbilirubinemias. In Taeusch H, Ballard RA, editors: *Avery's Diseases of the Newborn*, 7th ed, Philadelphia: 1998, Saunders.
32. Kaplan M, Algur N, Hammerman C: Onset of jaundice in glucose-6-phosphate dehydrogenase-deficient neonates, *Pediatrics* 108:956-959, 2001.
33. Kaplan M, Muraca M, Vreman HJ, Hammerman C, et al: Neonatal bilirubin production-conjugation imbalance: Effect of glucose-6-phosphate dehydrogenase deficiency and borderline prematurity, *Arch Dis Child Fetal Neotal Ed* 90:F123-F127, 2005.
34. MacMahon JR: Physiologic jaundice. In Taeusch H, Ballard RA, editors: *Avery's Diseases of the Newborn*, 7th ed, Philadelphia: 1998, Saunders.
35. Gartner LM, Lee K, Vaisman S: Development of bilirubin transport and metabolism in the newborn rhesus monkey, *J Pediatr* 90:513, 1977.
36. Maisels MJ: Jaundice. In Avery GB, Fletcher MA, MacDonald MG, editors: *Neonatology, Pathophysiology and Management of the Newborn*, 5th ed, Philadelphia: 1999, Lippincott Williams & Wilkins.
37. Newman TB, Xiong B, Gonzales VM, Escobar GJ: Prediction and prevention of extreme neonatal hyperbilirubinemia in a mature health maintenance organization, *Arch Pediatr Adolesc Med* 154:1140-1147, 2000.
38. Gale R, Seidman DS, Dollberg S, Stevenson DK: Epidemiology of neonatal jaundice in the Jerusalem population, *J Pediatr Gastroenterol Nutr* 10:82-86, 1990.
39. Maisels MJ, Kring E: Length of stay, jaundice, and hospital readmission, *Pediatrics* 101:995-998, 1998.
40. Sarici SU, Serdar MA, Korkmaz A, Erdem G, et al: Incidence, course, and prediction of hyperbilirubinemia in near-term and term newborns, *Pediatrics* 113:775-780, 2004.
41. Yamamoto T, Skanderbeg J, Zipursky A, Israels LG: The early appearing bilirubin: Evidence for two components, *J Clin Invest* 44:31-41, 1965.
42. Pearson HA: Life-span of the fetal red blood cell, *J Pediatr* 70:166-171, 1967.
43. Brodersen R, Hermann LS: Intestinal reabsorption of unconjugated bilirubin: A possible contributing factor in neonatal jaundice, *Lancet* 1:1242, 1963.
44. Ulstrom RA, Eisenklam E: The enterohepatic shunting of bilirubin in the newborn infant. I. Use of oral activated charcoal to reduce normal serum bilirubin values, *J Pediatr* 65:27, 1964.
45. Poland RL, Odell GB: Physiological jaundice: The enterohepatic circulation of bilirubin, *N Engl J Med* 284:2, 1971.
46. Watchko JF: Vigintiphobia revisited, *Pediatrics* 115:1747-1753, 2005.
47. Diamond I: Bilirubin binding and kernicterus. In Schulman I, editor: *Advances in Pediatrics*, Chicago: 1969, Year Book.
48. Odell GB, Seungdamrong S, Odell JL: The displacement of bilirubin from albumin, *Birth Defects Orig Artic Ser* 13:192-204, 1976.
49. Brodersen R: Prevention of kernicterus, based on recent progress in bilirubin chemistry, *Acta Paediatr Scand* 66:625, 1977.
50. Karp WB: Biochemical alterations in neonatal hyperbilirubinemia and bilirubin encephalopathy: A review, *Pediatrics* 64:361, 1979.
51. Cowger ML: Bilirubin encephalopathy. In Gaull GE, editor: *Biology of Brain Dysfunction*, New York: 1975, Plenum.
52. Brodersen R: Binding of bilirubin to albumin and tissues. In Stern L, editor: *Physiological and Biochemical Basis for Perinatal Medicine*, Basel: 1981, Karger.
53. Cashore WJ: The neurotoxicity of bilirubin, *Clin Perinatol* 17:437-447, 1990.
54. Bratlid D: How bilirubin gets into the brain, *Clin Perinatol* 17:449-465, 1990.
55. Cashore WJ: Bilirubin metabolism and toxicity in the newborn. In Polin RA, Fox WW, editors: *Fetal and Neonatal Physiology*, Philadelphia: 1992, Saunders.
56. MacMahon JE: Bilirubin toxicity, encephalopathy, and kernicterus. In Taeusch H, Ballard RA, editors: *Avery's Diseases of the Newborn*, 7th ed, Philadelphia: 1998, Saunders.
57. Ostrow JD, Pascolo L, Brites D, Tiribelli C: Molecular basis of bilirubin-induced neurotoxicity, *Trends Mol Med* 10:65-70, 2004.
58. Wennberg RP, Ahlfors CE, Bhutani VK, Johnson LH, et al: Toward understanding kernicterus: A challenge to improve the management of jaundiced newborns, *Pediatrics* 117:474-485, 2006.
59. Levine RL: Bilirubin: Worked out years ago?, *Pediatrics* 64:380-385, 1979.
60. Levine RL, Fredericks WR, Rapoport SI: Entry of bilirubin into the brain due to opening of the blood-brain barrier, *Pediatrics* 69:255-259, 1982.
61. Levine RL: The toxicology of bilirubin. In Levine RL, Maisels MJ, editors: *Hyperbilirubinemia in the Newborn: Report of the Eighty-fifth Ross Conference on Pediatric Research*, Columbus, OH: 1983, Ross.

62. Levine RL: Bilirubin and the blood-brain barrier. In Levine RL, Maisels MJ, editors: *Hyperbilirubinemia in the Newborn: Report of the Eighty-fifth Ross Conference on Pediatric Research*, Columbus, OH: 1983, Ross.

63. Mollison PL: Haemolytic disease of the newborn. In Gairdner D, editor: *Recent Advances in Pediatrics*, New York: 1954, Blakiston.

64. Maisels MJ: Clinical studies of the sequelae of hyperbilirubinemia. In Levine RL, Maisels MJ, editors: *Hyperbilirubinemia in the Newborn: Report of the Eighty-fifth Ross Conference on Pediatric Research*, Columbus, OH: 1983, Ross.

65. Ip S, Chung M, Kulig J, O'Brien R, et al: An evidence-based review of important issues concerning neonatal hyperbilirubinemia, *Pediatrics* 114:e130-e153, 2004.

66. Newman TB, Maisels MJ: Evaluation and treatment of jaundice in the term newborn: A kinder, gentle approach, *Pediatrics* 89:809-818, 1992.

67. Newman TB, Liljestrand P, Jeremy RJ, Ferriero DM, et al: Outcomes among newborns with total serum bilirubin levels of 25 mg per deciliter or more, *N Engl J Med* 354:1889-1900, 2006.

68. Penn AA, Enzmann DR, Hahn JS, Stevenson DK: Kernicterus in a full-term infant, *Pediatrics* 93:1003-1006, 1994.

69. Yokochi K: Magnetic resonance imaging in children with kernicterus, *Acta Paediatr* 84:937-939, 1995.

70. Perlman JM, Rogers BB: Kernicteric findings at autopsy in two sick near term infants, *Pediatrics* 99:612-615, 1998.

71. Hanko E, Lindemann R, Hansen TWR: Spectrum of outcome in infants with extreme neonatal jaundice, *Acta Paediatr* 90:782-785, 2001.

72. Johnson LH, Bkutani V, Brown AK: System-based approach to management of neonatal jaundice and prevention of kernicterus, *J Pediatr* 140:396-403, 2002.

73. Ebbesen F, Andersson C, Verder H, Grytter C, et al: Extreme hyperbilirubinaemia in term and near-term infants in Denmark, *Acta Paediatr* 94:59-64, 2005.

74. Stern L, Denton RL: Kernicterus in small premature infants, *Pediatrics* 35:483-485, 1965.

75. Gartner LM, Snyder RN, Chabon RS, Bernstein J: Kernicterus: High incidence in premature infants with low serum bilirubin concentrations, *Pediatrics* 45:906-917, 1970.

76. Jardine DS, Rogers K: Relationship of benzyl alcohol to kernicterus, intraventricular hemorrhage, and mortality in preterm infants, *Pediatrics* 83:153-160, 1989.

77. van de Bor M, van Zeben-van der Aa TM, Verloove-Vanhorick SP, Brand R, et al: Hyperbilirubinemia in preterm infants and neurodevelopmental outcome at 2 years of age: Results of a national collaborative survey, *Pediatrics* 83:915-920, 1989.

78. van de Bor M, Ens-Dokkum M, Schreuder AM, Veen S, et al: Hyperbilirubinemia in low birth weight infants and outcome at 5 years of age, *Pediatrics* 89:359-364, 1992.

79. Watchko JF, Claassen D: Kernicterus in premature infants: Current prevalence and relationship to NICHD phototherapy study exchange criteria, *Pediatrics* 93:996-999, 1994.

80. Okumura A, Hayakawa F, Kato T, Itomi K, et al: Preterm infants with athetoid cerebral palsy: Kernicterus? *Arch Dis Child Fetal Neonatal Ed* 84:F136-F137 2001.

81. Govaert P, Lequin M, Swarte R, Robben S, et al: Changes in globus pallidus with (Pre)term kernicterus, *Pediatrics* 112:1256-1263, 2003.

82. Merhar SL, Gilbert DL: Clinical (video) findings and cerebrospinal fluid neurotransmitters in 2 children with severe chronic bilirubin encephalopathy, including a former preterm infant without marked hyperbilirubinemia VIDEO, *Pediatrics* 116:1226-1230, 2005.

83. Sugama S, Soeda A, Eto Y: Magnetic resonance imaging in three children with kernicterus, *Pediatr Neurol* 25:328-331, 2001.

84. Bhutani VK, Johnson LH, Shapiro SM: Kernicterus in sick and preterm infants (1999–2002): A need for an effective preventive approach, *Semin Perinatol* 28:319-325, 2004.

85. Amin SB: Clinical assessment of bilirubin-induced neurotoxicity in premature infants, *Semin Perinatol* 28:340-347, 2004.

86. Amin SB, Charafeddine L, Guillet R: Transient bilirubin encephalopathy and apnea of prematurity in 28 to 32 weeks gestational age infants, *J Perinatol* 25:386-390, 2005.

87. Valaes T, Kapitlnik J, Kauffmann NA: Experience with Sephadex gel filtration in assessing the risk of bilirubin encephalopathy in neonatal jaundice. In Bergsma D, Blondheim SH, editors: *Bilirubin Metabolism in the Newborn*, New York: 1976, Elsevier.

88. Wennberg RP, Lau M, Rasmussen LF: Clinical significance of unbound bilirubin, *Pediatr Res* 10:434-444, 1976.

89. Cashore WJ, Oh W: Unbound bilirubin and kernicterus in low-birth-weight infants, *Pediatrics* 69:481-485, 1982.

90. Pledger DR, Scott JM, Belfield A: Kernicterus at low levels of serum bilirubin: The impact of bilirubin albumin-binding capacity, *Biol Neonate* 41:38-44, 1982.

91. Ritter DA, Kenny JD, Norton HJ, Rudolph AJ: A prospective study of free bilirubin and other risk factors on the development of kernicterus in premature infants, *Pediatrics* 69:260-266, 1982.

92. Hansen TWR, Bartlid D: Bilirubin and brain toxicity, *Acta Paediatr Scand* 75:513-522, 1986.

93. Funato M, Tamai H, Shimada S, Nakamura H: Vigintiphobia, unbound bilirubin, and auditory brainstem responses, *Pediatrics* 93:50-53, 1994.

94. Ahlfors CE: Criteria for exchange transfusion in jaundiced newborns, *Pediatrics* 93:488-494, 1994.

95. Kuriyama M, Konishi Y, Sudo M: Auditory brainstem response in hyperbilirubinemic rats: Part II, *Pediatr Neurol* 7:375-379, 1991.

96. Schiff D, Shan G, Pozansky M: Bilirubin toxicity in neural cell lines N115 and NBR10A, *Pediatr Res* 19:908-911, 1985.

96a. Calligaris SD, Bellarosa C, Giraudi P, Wennberg RP, et al: Cytotoxicity is predicted by unbound and not total bilirubin concentration, *Pediatr Res* 62:576-580, 2007.

97. Cashore WJ, Oh W, Brodersen R: Reserve albumin and bilirubin toxicity index in infant serum, *Acta Paediatr Scand* 72:415-419, 1983.

98. Kim MH, Yoon JJ, Sher J, Brown AK: Lack of predictive indices in kernicterus: A comparison of clinical and pathologic factors in infants with or without kernicterus, *Pediatrics* 66:852-858, 1980.

99. Bratlid D: The effect of free fatty acids, bile acids and hematin on bilirubin binding by human erythrocytes, *Scand J Clin Lab Invest* 30:107-112, 1972.

100. Brodersen R, Friis-Hansen B, Stern L: Drug-induced displacement of bilirubin from albumin in the newborn, *Dev Pharmacol Ther* 6:217-229, 1983.

101. Freeman J, Lesko SM, Mitchell AA, Epstein MF, et al: Hyperbilirubinemia following exposure to pancuronium bromide in newborns, *Dev Pharmacol Ther* 14:209-215, 1990.

102. Lam BC, Wong HN, Yeung CY: Effect of indomethacin on binding of bilirubin to albumin, *Arch Dis Child* 65:690-691, 1990.

103. Meisel P, Jahrig D, Beyersdorff E, Jahrig K: Bilirubin binding and acid-base equilibrium in newborn infants with low birthweight, *Acta Paediatr Scand* 77:496-501, 1988.

104. Brodersen R, Robertson A: Ceftriaxone binding to human serum albumin: Competition with bilirubin, *Mol Pharmacol* 36:478-483, 1989.

105. Fink S, Karp W, Robertson A: Effect of penicillins on bilirubin-albumin binding, *J Pediatr* 113:566-568, 1988.

106. Esbjorner E, Larsson P, Leissner P, Wranne L: The serum reserve albumin concentration for monoacetyldiaminodiphenyl sulphone and auditory evoked responses during neonatal hyperbilirubinaemia, *Acta Paediatr Scand* 80:406-412, 1991.

107. Robertson A, Brodersen R: Effect of drug combinations on bilirubin-albumin binding, *Dev Pharmacol Ther* 17:95-99, 1991.

108. Robertson A, Karp W, Brodersen R: Bilirubin displacing effect of drugs used in neonatology, *Acta Paediatr Scand* 80:1119-1127, 1991.

109. Ahlfors CE, DiBasio-Erwin D: Rate constants for dissociation of bilirubin from its binding sites in neonatal (cord) and adult sera, *J Pediatr* 108:295-298, 1986.

110. Ritter DA, Kenny JD: Bilirubin binding in premature infants from birth to 3 months, *Arch Dis Child* 61:352-356, 1986.

111. Maisels MJ: Jaundice. In Winters R, Cox K, Dickmeyer ME, editors: *Neonatology: Pathophysiology and Management of the Newborn*, Philadelphia: 1994, JB Lippincott.

112. Hansen RL: Neurodevelopment and serum bilirubin in preterm infants, *J Dev Behav Pediatr* 12:287-293, 1991.

113. Kapitulnik J, Horner-Mibashan R, Blondheim S: Increase in bilirubin-binding affinity of serum with age of infant, *J Pediatr* 86:442-445, 1975.

113a. Bender GJ, Cashore WJ, Oh W: Ontogeny of bilirubin-binding capacity and the effect of clinical status in premature infants born at less than 1300 grams, *Pediatrics* 120:1067-1073, 2007.

114. Ebbesen F, Brodersen R: Albumin administration combined with phototherapy in treatment of hyperbilirubinemia in low birth weight infants, *Acta Paediatr Scand* 70:649-653, 1981.

115. Odell GB, Cukier JO, Ostrea EM: The influence of fatty acids on the binding of bilirubin to albumin, *J Lab Clin Med* 89:295-307, 1977.

116. Perlman M, Kapitulnik J, Blondheim SH: Bilirubin binding and neonatal acidosis, *Clin Chem* 27:1872-1874, 1981.

117. Ostrea EM Jr, Bassel M, Fleury CA, Bartos A, et al: Influence of free fatty acids and glucose infusion on serum bilirubin binding to albumin: Clinical implications, *J Pediatr* 102:426-432, 1983.

118. Robertson A, Karp W: Effect of pancuronium on bilirubin-albumin binding, *J Pediatr* 101:463-465, 1982.

119. Shankaran S, Pantoja A, Poland RL: Indomethacin and bilirubin-albumin binding, *Dev Pharmacol Ther* 4:124-131, 1982.

120. Stutman HR, Parker KM, Marks MI: Potential of moxalactam and other new antimicrobial agents for bilirubin-albumin displacement in neonates, *Pediatrics* 75:294-398, 1985.

121. Martin E, Fanconi S, Kalin P, Zwingelstein C, et al: Ceftriaxone-bilirubin-albumin interactions in the neonate: An in vivo study, *Eur J Pediatr* 152:530-534, 1993.

122. Diamond I, Schmid R: Experimental bilirubin encephalopathy: The mode of entry of bilirubin-^{14}C into the nervous system, *J Clin Invest* 45:678-689, 1966.

123. Silberberg DH, Johnson L, Ritter L: Factors influencing toxicity of bilirubin in cerebellum tissue culture, *J Pediatr* 77:386-396, 1970.

124. Cowger ML: Mechanism of bilirubin toxicity on tissue culture cells: Factors that affect toxicity, reversibility by albumin, and comparisons with other respiratory poisons and surfactants, *Biochem Med* 5:1-16, 1971.

125. Sugita K, Sata T, Nakajima H: Effects of pH and hypoglycemia on bilirubin cytotoxicity in vitro, *Biol Neonate* 52:22-25, 1987.

126. Wennberg RP, Gospe SM, Rhine WD, Seyal M, et al: Brainstem bilirubin toxicity in the newborn primate may be promoted and reversed by modulating P_{CO_2}, Pediatr Res 34:6-9, 1993.

127. Nelson T, Jacobsen J, Wennberg RP: Effect of pH on the interaction of bilirubin with albumin and tissue culture cells, Pediatr Res 8:963-967, 1974.

128. Cashore WJ, Oh W: Effect of acidosis on bilirubin uptake by rat brain in vivo, Pediatr Res 13:523-534, 1979.

129. Eriksen EF, Danielsen H, Brodersen R: Bilirubin-liposome interaction, J Biol Chem 254:4269-4274, 1981.

130. Sato M, Kashiwamata S: Interaction of bilirubin with human erythrocyte membranes, Biochem J 210:489-496, 1983.

131. Kashiwamata S, Suzuki F, Semba RK: Affinity of young rat cerebral slices for bilirubin and some factors influencing its transfer to the slices, Jpn J Exp Med 50:303-311, 1980.

132. Mayor F, Pages M, Diez-Guerra J: Effect of postnatal anoxia on bilirubin levels in rat brain, Pediatr Res 19:231-236, 1985.

133. Vasquez J, Garcia-Calvo M, Valdivieso F: Interaction of bilirubin with the synaptosomal plasma membrane, J Biol Chem 263:1255-1262, 1988.

134. Watchko JF, Daood MJ, Hanse TW: Brain bilirubin content is increased in P-glycoprotein–deficient transgenic null mutant mice, Pediatr Res 44:763-766, 1998.

135. Hanko E, Topmmarello S, Watchko JF, Hanse TWR: Administration of drugs known to inhibit P-glycoprotein increases brain bilirubin and alters the regional distribution of bilirubin in rat brain, Pediatr Res 54:441-445, 2003.

136. Ohsugi M, Sato H, Yamamura H: Transfer of bilirubin covalently bound to I-125 albumin from blood to brain in the Gunn rat newborn, Biol Neonate 62:416-423, 1992.

137. Hansen TWR, Oyasaeter S, Stiris T, Bratlid D: Effects of sulfisoxazole, hypercarbia, and hyperosmolality on entry of bilirubin and albumin into brain regions in young rats, Biol Neonate 56:22-30, 1989.

138. Ives NK, Gardiner RM: Blood-brain barrier permeability to bilirubin in the rat studied using intracarotid bolus injection and in situ brain perfusion techniques, Pediatr Res 27:436-441, 1990.

139. Hansen TW: Acute entry of bilirubin (B) into rat brain regions [abstract], Pediatr Res 33:214A, 1993.

140. Lee C, Oh W, Stonestree BS, Cashore WJ: Permeability of the blood brain barrier for ^{125}I-albumin–bound bilirubin in newborn piglets, Pediatr Res 25:452-456, 1989.

141. Roger C, Koziel V, Vert P, Nehlig A: Autoradiographic mapping of local cerebral permeability to bilirubin in immature rats: Effects of hyperbilirubinemia, Pediatr Res 39:64-71, 1995.

142. Waser M, Kleihues P, Frick P: Kernicterus in an adult, Ann Neurol 19:595-598, 1986.

143. Labrune PH, Myara A, Francoual J, Trivin F, et al: Cerebellar symptoms as the presenting manifestations of bilirubin encephalopathy in children with Crigler-Najjar type I disease, Pediatrics 89:768-770, 1992.

144. Katoh-Semba R, Kashiwamata S: Interaction of bilirubin with brain capillaries and its toxicity, Biochim Biophys Acta 632:290, 1980.

145. Burgess GH, Oh W, Bratlid D, Brubakk AM, et al: The effects of brain blood flow on brain bilirubin deposition in newborn piglets, Pediatr Res 19:691-696, 1985.

146. Rapoport SI: Reversible osmotic opening of the blood-brain barrier for experimental and therapeutic purposes. In Levine RL, Maisels MJ, editors: Hyperbilirubinemia in the Newborn: Report of the Eighty-fifth Ross Conference on Pediatric Research, Columbus, OH: 1983, Ross.

147. Levine RL: Neonatal jaundice, Acta Paediatr Scand 77:177-182, 1988.

148. Wennberg RP, Hance AJ: Experimental bilirubin encephalopathy: Importance of total bilirubin, protein binding, and blood-brain barrier, Pediatr Res 20:789-792, 1986.

149. Ives NK, Bolas NM, Gardiner RM: The effects of bilirubin on brain energy metabolism during hyperosmolar opening of the blood-brain barrier: An in vivo study using ^{31}P nuclear magnetic resonance spectroscopy, Pediatr Res 26:356-361, 1989.

150. Hansen TWR: Bilirubin entry into and clearance from rat brain during hypercarbia and hyperosmolality, Pediatr Res 39:72-76, 1995.

151. Chiueh CC, Sun CL, Kopin IJ: Entry of [^{3}H]norepinephrine, [^{125}I] albumin and Evans blue from blood into brain following unilateral osmotic opening of the blood-brain barrier, Brain Res 145:291-301, 1978.

152. Rapoport SI, Hori M, Klatzo I: Reversible osmotic opening of the blood-brain barrier, Science 173:1026-1028, 1971.

153. Barranger JA, Rapoport SI, Fredericks WR: Modification of the blood-brain barrier: Increased concentration and fate of enzymes entering the brain, Proc Natl Acad Sci U S A 76:481-485, 1979.

154. Bratlid D, Cashore WJ, Oh W: Effect of serum hyperosmolality on opening of blood-brain barrier for bilirubin in rat brain, Pediatrics 71:909-912, 1983.

155. Burgess GH, Stonestreet BS, Cashore WJ, Oh W: Brain bilirubin deposition and brain blood flow during acute urea-induced hyperosmolality in newborn piglets, Pediatr Res 19:537-542, 1985.

156. Blazer S, Linn S, Hocherman I, Alon U, et al: Acute increase in serum tonicity following exchange transfusion: Increased risk for the very low birthweight infant during the first 48 hours of life, Acta Paediatr Scand 79:1182-1185, 1990.

157. Johansson B, Nilsson B: The pathophysiology of blood brain barrier dysfunction induced by severe hypercapnia and by epileptic brain activity, Acta Neuropathol 38:153-158, 1977.

158. Lending M, Slobody LB, Mestern J: The relationship of hypercapnoea to the production of kernicterus, Dev Med Child Neurol 9:145-151, 1967.

159. Bratlid D, Cashore WJ, Oh W: Effect of acidosis on bilirubin deposition in rat brain, Pediatrics 73:431-434, 1984.

160. Lucey JF, Hibbard E, Behrman RE: Kernicterus in asphyxiated newborn rhesus monkeys, Exp Neurol 9:43, 1964.

161. Chen HC, Lien IN, Lu TC: Kernicterus in newborn rabbits, Am J Pathol 46:331-343, 1965.

162. Jirka JH, Duckrow B, Kendig JW, Maisels MJ: Effect of bilirubin on brainstem auditory evoked potentials in the asphyxiated rat, Pediatr Res 19:556-560, 1985.

163. Silver S, Kapitulnik J, Sohmer H: Contribution of asphyxia to the induction of hearing impairment in jaundiced Gunn rats, Pediatrics 95:579-583, 1995.

164. Tweed WA, Cote J, Pash M, Lou H: Arterial oxygenation determines autoregulation of cerebral blood flow in the fetal lamb, Pediatr Res 17:246-249, 1983.

165. Pearlman MA, Gartner LM, Lee K: The association of kernicterus with bacterial infection in the newborn, Pediatrics 65:26-29, 1980.

166. Larroche JC: Developmental Pathology of the Neonate, New York: 1977, Excerpta Medica.

167. Plum F, Posner JB, Troy B: Cerebral metabolic and circulatory responses to induced convulsions in animals, Arch Neurol 18:1-13, 1968.

168. Lorenzo AV, Chirahige L, Liang M, Barlow CF: Temporary alteration of cerebrovascular permeability to plasma protein during drug-induced seizures, Am J Physiol 223:268-277, 1972.

169. Joo F: A unifying concept on the pathogenesis of brain oedemas, Neuropathol Appl Neurobiol 13:161-176, 1987.

170. Temesvari P, Kovacs J: Selective opening of the blood-brain barrier in newborn piglets with experimental pneumothorax, Neurosci Lett 93:38-43, 1988.

171. Notter MF, Kendig JW: Differential sensitivity of neural cells to bilirubin toxicity, Pediatr Res 19:393, 1985.

172. Silva RFM, Rodrigues CMP, Brites D: Rat cultured neuronal and glial cells respond differently to toxicity of unconjugated bilirubin, Pediatr Res 51:535-541, 2002.

173. Ngai KC, Yeung CY: Additive effect of tumor necrosis factor-α and endotoxin on bilirubin cytotoxicity, Pediatr Res 45:526-530, 1999.

174. Falcao AS, Fernandes A, Brito MA, Silva RFM, et al: Bilirubin-induced inflammatory response, glutamate release, and cell death in rat cortical astrocytes are enhanced in younger cells, Neurobiol Dis 20:199-206, 2005.

175. Fernandes A, Silva RF, Falcao AS, Brito MA, et al: Cytokine production, glutamate release and cell death in rat cultured astrocytes treated with unconjugated bilirubin and LPS, J Neuroimmunol 153:64-75, 2004.

176. Bergeron M, Ferriero DM, Sharp FR: Developmental expression of heme oxygenase-1 (HSP32) in rat brain: An immunocytochemical study, Dev Brain Res 105:181-194, 1998.

177. Cowger ML, Igo RP, Labbe RF: The mechanism of bilirubin toxicity studies with purified respiratory enzyme and tissue culture systems, Biochemistry 4:2763-2770, 1965.

178. Ogasawara N, Watanabe T, Goto H: A potent inhibitor of NAD;pl-linked isocitrate dehydrogenase by bilirubin, J Biochem 68:441-448, 1970.

179. Yamaguchi T: Inhibition of glutamate dehydrogenase by bilirubin, J Biochem 68:441-449, 1970.

180. Noir BA, Boveris A, Garaza Pereira AM, Stoppani AO: Bilirubin: A multisite inhibitor of mitochondrial respiration, FEBS Lett 27:270-274, 1972.

181. Kashiwamata S, Niwa F, Katch R, Higashida H: Malate dehydrogenase of bovine cerebellum: Inhibition of bilirubin, J Neurochem 24:189-191, 1975.

182. Weil ML, Menkes JH: Bilirubin interaction with ganglioside: Possible mechanism in kernicterus, Pediatr Res 9:791-793, 1975.

183. Girotti AW: Glyceraldehyde-3-phosphate dehydrogenase in the isolated human erythrocyte membrane: Selective displacement by bilirubin, Arch Biochem Biophys 173:210-218, 1976.

184. Shepard RE, Moreno FJ, Cashore WJ, Fain JN: Effect of bilirubin on fat cell metabolism and lipolysis, Am J Physiol 237:E504-509, 1979.

185. Brann BS, Cashore WJ, Patrick R, Oh W: In vitro effect of bilirubin on dopamine synthesis in adult rat brain synaptosomes, Pediatr Res 19:335-341, 1985.

186. Brann BS, Stonestreet BS, Oh W, Cashore WJ: The effect of bilirubin (BR) on cerebral cortex (CC) O2 and glucose metabolism in piglets (P), Pediatr Res 19:335-342, 1985.

187. Hansen TW, Tydal T, Jorgensen H, Bratlid D: The effect of bilirubin on the uptake of 5-HT and dopamine in rat brain synaptosomes, Pediatr Res 19:390-397, 1985.

188. Nakamura H, Uetani Y, Takada S: Inhibitory action of bilirubin on O2 production by polymorphonuclear leucocytes (PMN), Pediatr Res 29:355-364, 1985.

189. Schiff D, Shan G, Pozansky M: Bilirubin toxicity of neural cells in culture, Pediatr Res 19:362-368, 1985.

190. Amit Y, Chan G, Fedunec S, Poznansky MJ, et al: Bilirubin toxicity in a neuroblastoma cell line N-115. I. Effects on Na$^+$K$^+$ ATPase, [^{3}H] thymidine uptake, L-[^{35}S] methionine incorporation, and mitochondrial function, *Pediatr Res* 25:364-368, 1989.

191. Amit Y, Poznansky MJ, Schiff D: Bilirubin toxicity in a neuroblastoma cell line N-115. II. Delayed effects and recovery, *Pediatr Res* 25: 369-372, 1989.

192. Hansen TWR, Bratlid D, Walaas I: Bilirubin decreases phosphorylation of synapsin I, a synaptic vesicle-associated neuronal phosphoprotein, in intact synaptosomes from rat cerebral cortex, *Pediatr Res* 23:219-223, 1988.

193. Hansen TWR, Paulsen O, Gjerstad L, Bratlid D: Short-term exposure to bilirubin reduces synaptic activation in rat transverse hippocampal slices, *Pediatr Res* 23:453-456, 1988.

194. Shapiro SM, Churn SB, DeLorenzo RJ, Conlee JW: Bilirubin toxicity selectively decreases neuronal CaM kinase II enzyme activity [abstract], *Pediatr Res* 33:236, 1993.

195. Wennberg RP, Johansson BB, Folbergrova J, Siesjo BK: Bilirubin-induced changes in brain energy metabolism after osmotic opening of the blood-brain barrier, *Pediatr Res* 30:473-478, 1991.

196. Ives NK, Cox DWG, Gardiner RM, Bachelard HS: The effects of bilirubin on brain energy metabolism during normoxia and hypoxia: An in vitro study using ^{31}P nuclear magnetic resonance spectroscopy, *Pediatr Res* 23:569-573, 1988.

197. Brann BS, Stonestreet BS, Oh W, Cashore WJ: The in vivo effect of bilirubin and sulfisoxazole on cerebral oxygen, glucose, and lactate metabolism in newborn piglets, *Pediatr Res* 25:135-141, 1987.

198. Cashore WJ, Kilguss NV: Bilirubin decreases dopamine release in striatal synaptosomes [abstract], *Pediatr Res* 33:206A, 1993.

199. Amato MM, Kilguss NV, Gelardi NL, Cashore WJ: Dose-effect relationship of bilirubin on striatal synaptosomes in rats, *Biol Neonate* 66:288-293, 1994.

200. Roger C, Koziel V, Vert P, Nehlig A: Regional cerebral metabolic consequences of bilirubin in rat depend upon post-gestational age at the time of hyperbilirubinemia, *Dev Brain Res* 87:194-202, 1995.

201. Roger C, Koziel V, Vert P, Nehlig A: Mapping of the consequences of bilirubin exposure in the immature rat: Local cerebral metabolic rates for glucose during moderate and severe hyperbilirubinemia, *Early Hum Dev* 43:133-144, 1995.

202. Hansen TWR, Mathiesen SBW, Walaas SI: Bilirubin has widespread inhibitory effects on protein phosphorylation, *Pediatr Res* 39:1072-1077, 1996.

203. Roseth S, Hansen TWR, Fonnum F, Walaas SI: Bilirubin inhibits transport of neurotransmitters in synaptic vesicles, *Pediatr Res* 44:312-316, 1998.

204. McDonald JW, Shapiro SM, Silverstein FS, Johnston MV: Role of glutamate receptor-mediated excitotoxicity in bilirubin-induced brain injury in the Gunn rat model, *Exp Neurol* 150:21-29, 1998.

205. Mustafa MG, King TE: Binding of bilirubin with lipid: A possible mechanism of its toxic reactions in mitochondria, *J Biol Chem* 245:1084, 1970.

206. Jew JY, Sandquist D: CNS changes in hyperbilirubinemia, *Arch Neurol* 36:149-154, 1979.

207. Jew JY, Williams TH: Ultrastructural aspects of bilirubin encephalopathy in cochlear nuclei of the Gunn rat, *J Anat* 124:599-614, 1977.

208. Shapiro SM: Definition of the clinical spectrum of kernicterus and bilirubin-induced neurologic dysfunction (BIND), *J Perinatol* 25:54-59, 2005.

209. Ostrow JD, Pascolo L, Tieibelli C: Reassessment of the unbound concentrations of unconjugated bilirubin in relation to neurotoxicity in vitro, *Pediatr Res* 54:98-104, 2003.

210. Grojean S, Lievre V, Koziel V, Vert P, et al: Bilirubin exerts additional toxic effects in hypoxic cultured neurons from the developing rat brain by the recruitment of glutamate neurotoxicity, *Pediatr Res* 49:507-513, 2001.

211. Hansen TW, Tommarello S, Allen JW: Subcellular localization of bilirubin in rat brain after in vivo i.v. administration of [^{3}H] bilirubin, *Pediatr Res* 49:203-207, 2001.

212. Hanko E, Hansen TW, Almaas R, Paulsen R, et al: Synergistic protection of a general caspase inhibitor and MK-801 in bilirubin-induced cell death in human NT2-N neurons, *Pediatr Res* 59:72-77, 2006.

213. Watchko JF: Bilirubin induced apoptosis in vitro: Insights for kernicterus: Commentary on the article by Hanko et al. on page 179, *Pediatr Res* 57:177-178, 2005.

214. Brito MA, Brites D, Butterfield DA: A link between hyperbilirubinemia, oxidative stress and injury to neocortical synaptosomes, *Brain Res* 1026:33-43, 2004.

215. Genc S, Genc K, Kumral A, Baskin H, et al: Bilirubin is cytotoxic to rat oligodendrocytes in vitro, *Brain Res* 985:135-141, 2003.

216. Hanko E, Hansen TW, Almaas R, Lindstad J, et al: Bilirubin induces apoptosis and necrosis in human NT2-N neurons, *Pediatr Res* 57:179-184, 2005.

217. Lin S, Wei X, Bales KR, Paul AB, et al: Minocycline blocks bilirubin neurotoxicity and prevents hyperbilirubinemia-induced cerebellar hypoplasia in the Gunn rat, *Eur J Neurosci* 22:21-27, 2005.

218. Friede RL: *Developmental Neuropathology*, 2nd ed, New York: 1989, Springer-Verlag.

219. Norman MG: Perinatal brain damage, *Perspect Pediatr Pathol* 4:41-92, 1978.

220. Ahdab-Barmada M, Moossy J: Kernicterus reexamined, *Pediatrics* 71:463-464, 1983.

221. Ahdab-Barmada M, Moossy J: The neuropathology of kernicterus in the premature neonate: Diagnostic problems, *J Neuropathol Exp Neurol* 43: 45-56, 1984.

222. Connolly AM, Volpe JJ: Clinical features of bilirubin encephalopathy, *Clin Perinatol* 17:371-379, 1990.

223. Turkel SB: Autopsy findings associated with neonatal hyperbilirubinemia, *Clin Perinatol* 17:381-396, 1990.

224. Turkel SB, Miller CA, Guttenberg ME: A clinical pathologic reappraisal of kernicterus, *Pediatrics* 69:267-272, 1982.

225. Turkel SB: Clinical and pathologic correlations with kernicterus and yellow pulmonary hyaline membranes. In Leveine RL, Maisels MJ, editors: *Hyperbilirubinemia in the Newborn: Report of the Eighty-fifth Ross Conference on Pediatric Research*, Columbus, OH: 1983, Ross.

226. Hayashi M, Satoh J, Sakamoto K, Morimatsu Y: Clinical and neuropathological findings in severe athetoid cerebral palsy: A comparative study of globo-Luysian and thalamo-putaminal groups, *Brain Dev* 13:47-51, 1991.

227. Turkel SB, Guttenberg ME, Moynes DR, Hodgman JE: Lack of identifiable risk factors for kernicterus, *Pediatrics* 66:502-506, 1980.

228. Jones MH, Sands R, Hyman CB: Longitudinal study of the incidence of central nervous system damage following erythroblastosis fetalis, *Pediatrics* 14:346-350, 1954.

229. Van Praagh R: Diagnosis of kernicterus in the neonatal period, *Pediatrics* 28:870-876, 1961.

230. Wolf MJ, Wolf B, Bijleveld C, Beunen G, et al: The predictive value of developmental testing of extremely jaundiced African infants, *Dev Med Child Neurol* 40:405-410, 1998.

231. Johnson L, Brown AK, Bhutani VK: BIND: A clinical score for bilirubin induced neurologic dysfunction in newborns [abstract], *Pediatrics* 104:746, 1999.

232. Dennery PA, Seidman DS, Stevenson DK: Drug therapy: Neonatal hyperbilirubinemia, *N Engl J Med* 344:581-590, 2001.

233. Shah Z, Chawla A, Patkar D, Pungaonkar S: MRI in kernicterus, *Australas Radiol* 47:55-57, 2003.

234. Groenendaal F, van der Grond J, de Vries LS: Cerebral metabolism in severe neonatal hyperbilirubinemia, *Pediatrics* 114:291-294, 2004.

235. Coskun A, Yikilmaz A, Kumandas S, Karahan OI, et al: Hyperintense globus pallidus on T1-weighted MR imaging in acute kernicterus: Is it common or rare? *Eur Radiol* 15:1263-1267, 2005.

236. Mansi G, DeMaio C, Araimo G, Rotta I, et al: "Safe" hyperbilirubinemia is associated with altered neonatal behavior, *Biol Neonate* 83:19-21, 2003.

237. AlOtaibi SF, Blaser S, MacGregor DL: Neurological complications of kernicterus, *Can J Neurol Sci* 32:311-315, 2005.

238. Craig WB: Convulsive movements in the first ten days of life, *Arch Dis Child* 35:336-345, 1960.

239. Byers RK, Paine RS, Crothers B: Extrapyramidal cerebral palsy with hearing loss following erythroblastosis, *Pediatrics* 15:248-254, 1955.

240. Perlstein MA: The late clinical syndrome of posticteric encephalopathy, *Pediatr Clin North Am* 7:665-674, 1960.

241. Worley G, Erwin CW, Goldstein RF, Provenzale JM, et al: Delayed development of sensorineural hearing loss after neonatal hyperbilirubinemia: A case report with brain magnetic resonance imaging, *Dev Med Child Neurol* 38:271-278, 1996.

242. Wolf MJ, Beunen G, Casaer P, Wolf B: Extreme hyperbilirubinaemia in Zimbabwean neonates: Neurodevelopmental outcome at 4 months, *Eur J Pediatr* 156:803-807, 1997.

243. Yilmaz Y, Alper G, Kilicoglu G, Celik L, et al: Magnetic resonance imaging findings in patients with severe neonatal hyperbilirubinemia, *J Child Neurol* 16:452-455, 2001.

244. Paksoy Y, Koc H, Genc BO: Bilateral mesial temporal sclerosis and kernicterus, *J Comput Assist Tomogr* 28:269-272, 2004.

245. Oakden WK, Moore AM, Blaser S, Noseworthy MD: 1H MR spectroscopic characteristics of kernicterus: A possible metabolic signature, *AJNR Am J Neuroradiol* 26:1571-1574, 2005.

246. Shapiro SM: Bilirubin toxicity in the developing nervous system, *Pediatr Res* 29:410-421, 2003.

247. Hoyt CS, Billson FA, Alpins N: The supranuclear disturbances of gaze in kernicterus, *Ann Ophthalmol* 10:1487-1492, 1978.

248. Gerrard J: Nuclear jaundice and deafness, *J Laryngol Otol* 66:39-46, 1952.

249. Keaster J, Hyman CB, Harris I: Hearing problems subsequent to neonatal hemolytic disease or hyperbilirubinemia, *Am J Dis Child* 117:406-410, 1969.

250. Johnston WH, Angara V, Baumal R: Erythroblastosis fetalis and hyperbilirubinemia: A five-year followup with neurological, psychological and audiological evaluation, *Pediatrics* 39:88-92, 1967.

251. Hung KL: Auditory brainstem responses in patients with neonatal hyperbilirubinemia and bilirubin encephalopathy, *Brain Dev* 11:297-301, 1989.

252. Hyman CB, Keaster J, Hanson V: CNS abnormalities after neonatal hemolytic disease or hyperbilirubinemia, *Am J Dis Child* 117:395-405, 1969.

253. Doyle LW, Keir E, Kitchen WH, Ford GW, et al: Audiologic assessment of extremely low birth weight infants: A preliminary report, *Pediatrics* 90:744-749, 1992.

254. Chisin R, Perlman M, Sohmer H: Cochlear and brain stem responses in hearing loss following neonatal hyperbilirubinemia, *Ann Otolaryngol Rhinol Laryngol* 88:352-357, 1979.

255. Wennberg RP, Ahlfors CE, Bickers R, McMurtry CA, et al: Abnormal auditory brainstem response in a newborn infant with hyperbilirubinemia: Improvement with exchange transfusion, *J Pediatr* 100:624-626, 1982.

256. Perlman M, Fainmesser P, Sohmer H: Auditory nerve-brainstem evoked responses in hyperbilirubinemic neonates, *Pediatrics* 72:658-664, 1983.

257. Lenhardt ML, McArtor R, Bryant B: Effects of neonatal hyperbilirubinemia on the brainstem electric response, *J Pediatr* 104:281-284, 1984.

258. Nwaesei CG, Van Aerde J, Boyden M, Perlman M: Changes in auditory brainstem responses in hyperbilirubinemic infants before and after exchange transfusion, *Pediatrics* 74:800-803, 1984.

259. Chin KC, Taylor MJ, Perlman M: Improvement in auditory and visual evoked potential in jaundiced preterm infants after exchange transfusion, *Arch Dis Child* 60:714-717, 1985.

260. Deliac PH, Demarquez JL, Barberot JP, Sandler B, et al: Brainstem auditory evoked potentials in icteric full-term newborns: Alterations after exchange transfusion, *Neuropediatrics* 21:115-118, 1990.

261. Bergman I, Hirsch RP, Fria TJ, Shapiro SM, et al: Cause of hearing loss in the high-risk premature infant, *J Pediatr* 106:95-101, 1985.

262. de Vries LS, Lary S, Dubowitz LMS: Relationship of serum bilirubin levels to ototoxicity and deafness in high-risk low-birth-weight infants, *Pediatrics* 76:351-354, 1985.

263. Kuriyama M, Konishi Y, Mikawa H: The effect of neonatal hyperbilirubinemia on the auditory brainstem response, *Brain Dev* 8:240-245, 1986.

264. Kuriyama M, Tomiwa K, Konishi Y, Mikawa H: Improvement in auditory brainstem response of hyperbilirubinemic infants after exchange transfusions, *Pediatr Neurol* 2:127-132, 1986.

265. Tan KL, Skurr BA, Yip YY: Phototherapy and the brain-stem auditory evoked response in neonatal hyperbilirubinemia, *J Pediatr* 120:306-308, 1992.

266. Vohr BR: New approaches to assessing the risks of hyperbilirubinemia, *Clin Perinatol* 17:293-306, 1990.

267. Streletz LJ, Graziani LJ, Branca PA, Desai HJ, et al: Brainstem auditory evoked potentials in full-term and preterm newborns with hyperbilirubinemia and hypoxemia, *Neuropediatrics* 17:66-71, 1986.

268. Maisels MJ: Jaundice. In Avery GB, Fletcher MA, MacDonald MG, editors: *Neonatology, Pathophysiology and Management of the Newborn*, 4th ed, Philadelphia: 1994, JB Lippincott.

269. Wong V, Chen WX, Wong KY: Short- and long-term outcome of severe neonatal nonhemolytic hyperbilirubinemia, *J Child Neurol* 21:309-315, 2006.

270. Chen WX, Wong VC, Wong KY: Neurodevelopmental outcome of severe neonatal hemolytic hyperbilirubinemia, *J Child Neurol* 21:474-479, 2006.

270a. Jiang ZD, Chen C, Liu TT, Wilkinson AR: Changes in brainstem auditory evoked response latencies in term neonates with hyperbilirubinemia, *Pediatr Neurol* 37:35-41, 2007.

271. Karplus M, Lee C, Cashore WJ, Oh W: The effects of brain bilirubin deposition on auditory brain stem evoked responses in rats, *Early Hum Dev* 16:185-194, 1988.

272. Hansen TW, Cashore WJ, Oh W: Changes in piglet auditory brainstem response amplitudes without increases in serum or cerebrospinal fluid neuron-specific enolase, *Pediatr Res* 32:524-529, 1992.

273. Shapiro SM: Reversible brainstem auditory evoked potential abnormalities in jaundiced Gunn rats given sulfonamide, *Pediatr Res* 34:629-633, 1993.

274. Shapiro SM: Somatosensory and brainstem auditory evoked potentials in the Gunn rat model of acute bilirubin neurotoxicity, *Pediatr Res* 52:844-849, 2002.

275. Shaia WT, Shapiro SM, Spencer RF: The jaundiced Gunn rat model of auditory neuropathy/dyssynchrony, *Laryngoscope* 115:2167-2173, 2005.

276. Odell GB, Storey GNB, Rosenberg LA: Studies in kernicterus. III. The saturation of serum proteins with bilirubin during neonatal life and its relationship to brain damage at five years, *J Pediatr* 76:12-21, 1970.

277. Bengtsson B, Verneholt J: A followup study of hyperbilirubinemia in healthy, full-term infants without isoimmunization, *Acta Paediatr Scand* 63:70-80, 1974.

278. Scheidt PC, Mellits D, Hardy JB, Drage JS, et al: Toxicity to bilirubin in neonates: Infant development during first year in relation to maximum neonatal serum bilirubin concentration, *J Pediatr* 91:292-297, 1977.

279. Naeye RL: Amniotic fluid infections, neonatal hyperbilirubinemia and psychomotor impairment, *Pediatrics* 62:497-503, 1978.

280. Rubin RA, Balow B, Fisch RO: Neonatal serum bilirubin levels related to cognitive development at ages 4 through 7 years, *J Pediatr* 94:601-604, 1979.

281. Newman TB, Klebanoff MA: Neonatal hyperbilirubinemia and long-term outcome: Another look at the collaborative perinatal project, *Pediatrics* 92:651-657, 1993.

282. O'Shea TM, Dillard RG, Klinepeter KL, Goldstein DJ: Serum bilirubin levels, intracranial hemorrhage, and the risk of developmental problems in very low birth weight neonates, *Pediatrics* 90:888-892, 1992.

283. Ross G: Hyperbilirubinemia in the 2000s: What should we do next, *Am J Perinatol* 20:415-424, 2003.

284. Soorani-Lunsing I, Wolth HA, Hadders-Algra M: Are moderate degrees of hyperbilirubinemia in health term neonates really safe for the brain?, *Pediatr Res* 50:701-705, 2001.

285. Hack M, Wilson-Costello D, Friedman H, Taylor GH, et al: Neurodevelopment and predictors of outcomes of children with birth weights of less than 1000 g: 1992-1995, *Arch Pediatr Adolesc Med* 154:725-731, 2000.

286. Smith CM, Barnes GP, Jacobson CA, Oelberg DG: Auditory brainstem response detects early bilirubin neurotoxicity at low indirect bilirubin values, *J Perinatol* 24:730-732, 2004.

287. Oh W, Tyson JE, Fanaroff AA, Vohr BR, et al: Association between peak serum bilirubin and neurodevelopmental outcomes in extremely low birth weight infants, *Pediatrics* 112:773-779, 2003.

288. Graziani LJ, Mitchell DG, Kornhauser M, Pidcock FS, et al: Neurodevelopment of preterm infants: Neonatal neurosonographic and serum bilirubin studies, *Pediatrics* 89:229-234, 1992.

289. Scheidt PC, Graubard BI, Nelson KB, Hirtz DG, et al: Intelligence at six years in relation to neonatal bilirubin level: Follow-up of the National Institute of Child Health and Human Development clinical trial of phototherapy, *Pediatrics* 87:797-806, 1991.

290. Yeo KL, Perlman M, Hao Y, Mullaney P: Outcomes of extremely premature infants related to their peak serum bilirubin concentrations and exposure to phototherapy, *Pediatrics* 102:1426-1431, 1998.

291. Sykes E, Epstein E: Laboratory measurement of bilirubin, *Clin Perinatol* 17:397-416, 1990.

292. Harris MC, Bernbaum JC, Polin JR, Zimmerman R, et al: Developmental follow-up of breastfed term and near-term infants with marked hyperbilirubinemia, *Pediatrics* 107:1075-1080, 2001.

293. Amin SB, Ahlfors CE, Orlando MS, Dalzell LE, et al: Bilirubin and serial auditory brainstem responses in premature infants, *Pediatrics* 107:664-670, 2001.

294. Bongers-Schokking JJ, Colon EJ, Hoogland RA, Van Den Brande JL, et al: Somatosensory evoked potentials in neonatal jaundice, *Acta Paediatr Scand* 79:148-155, 1990.

295. Chen YJ, Kang WM: Effects of bilirubin on visual evoked potentials in term infants, *Eur J Pediatr* 154:662-666, 1995.

296. Silver S, Kapitulnik J, Sohmer H: Postnatal development of flash visual evoked potentials in the jaundiced Gunn rat, *Pediatr Res* 30:469-472, 1991.

297. Silver S, Sohmer H, Kapitulinik J: Visual evoked potential abnormalities in jaundiced Gunn rats treated with sulfadimethoxine, *Pediatr Res* 38:258-261, 1995.

298. Gurses D, Kilic I, Sahiner T: Effects of hyperbilirubinemia on cerebrocortical electrical activity in newborns, *Pediatr Res* 52:125-130, 2002.

299. Harris MC, Bernbaum JC, Polin JR, Polin RA: Developmental follow-up of breast fed term infants with bilirubin brain injury: Resolution of clinical signs [abstract], *Pediatr Res* 43:217A, 1998.

300. Shapiro SM, Geiger AS, O'Tuama L, Baron MS: Abnormalities on magnetic resonance imaging (MRI) in children with kernicterus [abstract], *Pediatr Res* 60:1261, 2005.

301. Okumura A, Hayakawa F, Maruyama K, Kubota T, et al: Single photon emission computed tomography and serial MRI in preterm infants with kernicterus, *Brain Dev* 28:348-352, 2006.

302. Maisels MJ, Watchko JF: Treatment of jaundice in low birthweight infants, *Arch Dis Child Fetal Neonatal Ed* 88:F459-F463, 2003.

303. Bhutani VK, Johnson LH, Keren R: Diagnosis and management of hyperbilirubinemia in the term neonate: For a safer first week, *Pediatr Clin North Am* 51:843-861, 2004.

304. Maisels MJ, Baltz RD, Bhutani VK, Newman TB, et al: Management of hyperbilirubinemia in the newborn infant 35 or more weeks of gestation, *Pediatrics* 114:297-316, 2004.

305. Keren R, Bhutani VK, Luan X, Nihtianova S, et al: Identifying newborns at risk of significant hyperbilirubinaemia: A comparison of two recommended approaches, *Arch Dis Child* 90:415-421, 2005.

306. Newman TB, Liljestrand P, Escobar GJ: Combining clinical risk factors with serum bilirubin levels to predict hyperbilirubinemia in newborns, *Arch Pediatr Adolesc Med* 159:113-119, 2005.

307. Pollack W, Freda VJ, Gorman JG: 10 years of disease prevention, *Perinat Care* 2:8, 1978.

308. Clarke CA, 1989: Preventing Rhesus babies: The Liverpool research and follow up, *Arch Dis Child* 64:1734-1740, 1989.

309. Howard H, Martlew V, McFadyen I, Clarke C, et al: Consequences for fetus and neonate of maternal red cell allo-immunization, *Arch Dis Child Fetal Neonatal Ed* 78:F62-F66, 1998.

310. MacKenzie IZ, Bowell P, Gregory H, Pratt G, et al: Routine antenatal Rhesus D immunoglobulin prophylaxis: The results of a prospective 10 year study, *Br J Obstet Gynaecol* 106:492-497, 1999.

311. Bowe ET: Management of Rh disease, *Perinat Care* 2:16, 1978.

312. Greene MF, Frigdetto FD: Intrauterine transfusion. In Nelson NM, editor: *Current Therapy in Neonatal-Perinatal Medicine*, St. Louis: 1985, Mosby.

313. Liley HG: Rescue in inner space: Management of Rh hemolytic disease, *J Pediatr* 131:340-342, 1997.

314. Janssens HM, de Haan MJJ, van Kamp IL, Brand R, et al: Outcome for children treated with fetal intravascular transfusions because of severe blood group antagonism, *J Pediatr* 131:373-380, 1997.

315. Hudon L, Moise KJ, Hegemier SE, Hill RM, et al: Long-term neurodevelopmental outcome after intrauterine transfusion for the treatment of fetal hemolytic disease, *Am J Obstet Gynecol* 179:858-863, 1998.

316. Grab D, Paulus WE, Bommer A, Buck G, et al: Treatment of fetal erythroblastosis by intravascular transfusions: Outcome at 6 years, *Obstet Gynecol* 93:165-168, 1999.

317. Trevett TN, Dorman K, Lamvu G, Moise KJ: Antenatal maternal administration of phenobarbital for the prevention of exchange transfusion in neonates with hemolytic disease of the fetus and newborn, *Am J Obstet Gynecol* 192:478-482, 2005.

318. Maisels MJ, Ostrea EM Jr, Touch S, Clune SE, et al: Evaluation of a new transcutaneous bilirubinometer, *Pediatrics* 113:1628-1635, 2004.

319. Szabo P, Wolf M, Bucher HU, Haensse D, et al: Assessment of jaundice in preterm neonates: Comparison between clinical assessment, two transcutaneous bilirubinometers and serum bilirubin values, *Acta Paediatr* 93:1491-1495, 2004.

320. Karolyi L, Pohlandt F, Muche R, Franz AR, et al: Transcutaneous bilirubinometry in very low birthweight infants, *Acta Paediatr* 93:941-944, 2004.

321. Grohmann K, Roser M, Rolinski B, Kadow I, et al: Bilirubin measurement for neonates: Comparison of 9 frequently used methods, *Pediatrics* 117:1174-1183, 2006.

322. McDonagh AF, Lightner DA: "Like a shrivelled blood orange": Bilirubin, jaundice, and phototherapy, *Pediatrics* 75:443-455, 1985.

323. Lightner DA, McDonagh AF: Molecular mechanisms of phototherapy for neonatal jaundice, *Acc Chem Res* 17:417-421, 1984.

324. Ennever JF, Costarino AT, Knox T: Where does the bilirubin go when you turn on the lights? *Pediatr Res* 19:218-220, 1985.

325. Ennever JF: Blue light, green light, white light, more light: Treatment of neonatal jaundice, *Clin Perinatol* 17:467-481, 1990.

326. Ennever JF: Phototherapy for neonatal jaundice. In Polin RA, Fox WW, editors: *Fetal and Neonatal Physiology*, Philadelphia: 1992, Saunders.

327. Maisels MJ: Why use homeopathic doses of phototherapy? *Pediatrics* 98:283-287, 1996.

328. MacMahon JR, Stevenson DK, Oski FA: Management of neonatal hyperbilirubinemia. In Taeusch H, Ballard RA, editors: *Avery's Diseases of the Newborn*, 7th ed, Philadelphia: 1998, Saunders.

329. Ennever JF: Phototherapy for neonatal jaundice. In Polin RA, Fox WW, editors: *Fetal and Neonatal Physiology*, 2nd ed, Philadelphia: 1998, Saunders.

330. Yetman RJ, Parks DK, Huseby V, Mistry K, et al: Rebound bilirubin levels in infants receiving phototherapy, *J Pediatr* 133:705-707, 1998.

331. Maisels MJ: Hyperbilirubinemia. In Nelson NM, editor: *Current Therapy in Neonatal-Perinatal Medicine*, St. Louis: 1985, Mosby.

332. Brown AK, Kim MH, Wu PY, Bryla DA: Efficacy of phototherapy in prevention and management of neonatal hyperbilirubinemia, *Pediatrics* 75:393-400, 1985.

333. Scheidt PC, Bryla DA, Nelson KB, Hirtz DG, et al: Phototherapy for neonatal hyperbilirubinemia: Six-year follow-up of the National Institute of Child Health and Human Development clinical trial, *Pediatrics* 85:455-463, 1990.

334. Martinez JC, Maisels MJ, Otheguy L, Garcia H, et al: Hyperbilirubinemia in the breast-fed newborn: A controlled trial of four interventions, *Pediatrics* 91:470-473, 1993.

335. Lipsitz PJ, Gartner LM, Bryla DA: Neonatal and infant mortality in relation to phototherapy, *Pediatrics* 75:422-426, 1985.

336. Linderkamp O, Riegel KP: Exchange transfusion. In Nelson NM, editor: *Current Therapy in Neonatal-Perinatal Medicine*, St. Louis: 1985, Mosby.

337. Patra K, Storfer-Isser A, Siner B, Moore J, et al: Adverse events associated with neonatal exchange transfusion in the 1990s, *J Pediatr* 144:626-631, 2004.

338. Bada HS, Chua C, Salmon JH, Hajjar W: Changes in intracranial pressure during exchange transfusion, *J Pediatr* 94:129-132, 1979.

339. van de Bor M, Benders MJ, Dorrepaal CA, van Bel F, et al: Cerebral blood volume changes during exchange transfusions in infants born at or near term, *J Pediatr* 125:617-621, 1994.

340. Valaes TN, Harvey-Wilkes K: Pharmacologic approaches to the prevention and treatment of neonatal hyperbilirubinemia, *Clin Perinatol* 17:245-273, 1990.

341. Rodgers PA, Stevenson DK: Developmental biology of heme oxygenase, *Clin Perinatol* 17:275-391, 1990.

342. Vreman H, Rodgers P, Stevenson DK: Zinc protoporphyrin administration for suppression of increased bilirubin production by iatrogenic hemolysis in Rhesus neonates, *J Pediatr* 117:292-297, 1990.

343. Landaw SA, Drummond GS, Kappas A: Targeting of heme oxygenase inhibitors to the spleen markedly increases their ability to diminish bilirubin production, *Pediatrics* 84:1091-1096, 1989.

344. Mullon CJ, Tosone CM, Langer R: Simulation of bilirubin detoxification in the newborn using an extracorporeal bilirubin oxidase reactor, *Pediatr Res* 26:452-457, 1989.

345. McDonagh A: Purple versus yellow: Preventing neonatal jaundice with tin-porphyrins, *J Pediatr* 113:777-781, 1988.

346. Kappas A, Drummond GS, Manola T, Petmezaki S, et al: Sn-protoporphyrin use in the management of hyperbilirubinemia in term newborns with direct Coombs-positive ABO incompatibility, *Pediatrics* 81:485-497, 1988.

347. Delaney JK, Mauzerall D, Drummond GS, Kappas A: Photophysical properties of Sn-porphyrins: Potential clinical implications, *Pediatrics* 81:498-504, 1988.

348. Fort FL, Gold J: Phototoxicity of tin protoporphyrin, tin mesoporphyrin, and tin diiododeuteroporphyrin under neonatal phototherapy conditions, *Pediatrics* 84:1031-1037, 1989.

349. Galbraith RA, Drummond GS, Kappas A: Suppression of bilirubin production in the Crigler-Najjar type I syndrome: Studies with the heme oxygenase inhibitor tin-mesoporphyrin, *Pediatrics* 89:175-182, 1992.

350. Dennery PA, Vreman HJ, Rodgers PA, Stevenson DK: Role of lipid peroxidation in metalloporphyrin-mediated phototoxic reactions in neonatal rats, *Pediatr Res* 33:87-91, 1993.

351. Caglayan S, Candemir H, Aksit S, Kansoy S, et al: Superiority of oral agar and phototherapy combination in the treatment of neonatal hyperbilirubinemia, *Pediatrics* 92:86-89, 1993.

352. Valaes T, Petmezaki S, Henschke C, Drummond GS, et al: Control of jaundice in preterm newborns by an inhibitor of bilirubin production: Studies with tin-mesoporphyrin, *Pediatrics* 93:1-11, 1994.

353. Kappas A, Drummond GS, Henschke C, Valaes T: Direct comparison of Sn-mesoporphyrin, an inhibitor of bilirubin production, and phototherapy in controlling hyperbilirubinemia in term and near-term newborns, *Pediatrics* 95:468-474, 1995.

354. Kappas A: A method for interdicting the development of severe jaundice in newborns by inhibiting the production of bilirubin, *Pediatrics* 113:119-123, 2004.

355. Suresh GK, Martin CL, Soll RF: Metalloporphyrins for treatment of unconjugated hyperbilirubinemia in neonates, *Cochrane Database Syst Rev* 2:CD004207, 2003.

356. Hafkamp AM, Havinga R, Ostrow JD, Tiribelli C, et al: Novel kinetic insights into treatment of unconjugated hyperbilirubinemia: Phototherapy and orlistat treatment in Gunn rats, *Pediatr Res* 59:506-512, 2006.

Chapter 14

Hyperammonemia and Other Disorders of Amino Acid Metabolism

Since the late 1950s, numerous disorders of amino acid metabolism have been described with major implications for the developing nervous system. Although each of the disorders is rare, collectively they are important for two major reasons. First, they represent causes of devastating disturbances of neurological development that are potentially treatable, and second, they provide insight into normal and abnormal brain metabolism.

Disorders of amino acid metabolism are defined, in this context, as those in which the major accumulating metabolite is an amino acid and the enzymatic defect involves the initial step (or, in one case, the second step) in the metabolism of the amino acid. In this chapter, I discuss in most detail those disorders of amino acid metabolism of especial importance in the neonatal period (e.g., maple syrup urine disease, nonketotic hyperglycinemia, and the urea cycle defects). Because urea cycle defects are characterized particularly by hyperammonemia, they are discussed in the larger context of neonatal hyperammonemia.

OVERVIEW OF AMINOACIDOPATHIES WITH NEONATAL NEUROLOGICAL MANIFESTATIONS

Disorders of amino acid metabolism associated with neurological manifestations in the first month of life are shown in Table 14-1. Many other disorders manifest later in infancy and childhood, including variants of most of those conditions listed in the table. The major clinical features include altered level of consciousness, seizures, vomiting (and impaired feeding), and delayed neurological development. In the following sections, I emphasize maple syrup urine disease, nonketotic hyperglycinemia, and hyperammonemia, including the urea cycle defects, because these are the most common disorders. The other disorders in Table 14-1 are very rare and are noted only briefly (see "Miscellaneous Amino Acid Disorders" later). Pyridoxine dependency is discussed in Chapter 5.

MAPLE SYRUP URINE DISEASE

Maple syrup urine disease, in its classic form, is a fulminating neonatal neurological disorder caused by a disturbance in the metabolism of the branched-chain, essential amino acids, leucine, isoleucine, and valine. The disturbance involves the second step in the degradation of these compounds (i.e., oxidative decarboxylation).[1]

Normal Metabolic Aspects

Transamination

The first two steps in the degradation of the branched-chain amino acids (BCAAs) are shown in Figure 14-1. The initial transamination is thought to occur through a single transaminase.[1] The usual amino acceptor for the transamination is alpha-ketoglutarate, which is converted to glutamate.

Oxidative Decarboxylation

The transaminations result in the formation of the three branched-chain ketoacids (BCKAs), which then undergo oxidative decarboxylation through a dehydrogenase complex to the corresponding short-chain fatty acids (see Fig. 14-1).[1,2] Oxidative decarboxylation of the three alpha-ketoacids is particularly active in liver, kidney, heart, and brain. This reaction is a multistep sequence that requires thiamine pyrophosphate and lipoic acid. The former is of clinical importance because of the occurrence of thiamine-responsive varieties of maple syrup urine disease.[1]

Biochemical Aspects of Disordered Metabolism

Enzymatic Defect and Essential Consequences

The enzymatic defect in maple syrup urine disease involves the oxidative decarboxylation of the BCKAs. The obvious consequence is a marked elevation in body fluid levels of the BCKAs and the BCAAs. The importance of these accumulated materials in the genesis of the short-term and long-term neurological abnormalities associated with maple syrup urine disease is indicated by the favorable response to diets low in the BCAAs.[1,3] Available data suggest that both the BCAAs and the BCKAs have deleterious effects on brain, and the precise effect depends in considerable part on the nature of the experimental system examined.

TABLE 14-1   Disorders of Amino Acid Metabolism Associated with Neurological Manifestations in the First Month of Life

Disorder	Major Clinical Features	Enzymatic Defect
Urea cycle defects*	Vomiting, stupor, seizures	Carbamyl phosphate synthase, ornithine transcarbamylase, argininosuccinic acid synthetase, argininosuccinase
Maple syrup urine disease*	Stupor, seizures, dystonia, odor of maple syrup	Branched-chain ketoacid decarboxylase
Nonketotic hyperglycinemia*	Stupor, seizures, hiccups	Glycine decarboxylase
Hypervalinemia	Stupor, delayed development	Valine transaminase
Phenylketonuria	Vomiting, musty order	Phenylalanine hydroxylase
Lysinuric protein intolerance	Vomiting, hypotonia	Transport of cationic amino acids (lysine, arginine, ornithine)
Pyridoxine dependency[†]	Seizures	Glutamic acid decarboxylase (pyridoxal phosphate action), decreased gamma-aminobutyric acid synthesis

*Most common disorders and discussed in this chapter.
[†]See Chapter 5.

Biochemical Effects of Excess Branched-Chain Amino Acids or Ketoacids, or Both

Neurochemical effects associated with excessive quantities of BCAAs, BCKAs, or both, appear to be caused primarily by *alterations of brain amino acids* and by *energy failure* (Table 14-2). The alterations of amino acids include a marked increase in BCAAs and a depletion of non-BCAAs. The latter depletion results in part because of impaired amino acid transport across the blood-brain barrier caused by the large quantities of competing BCAAs. However, *cellular* depletion occurs also secondary to the large influx of leucine, which enters brain from blood more readily than any other amino acid.[4] Leucine first enters astrocytes, which surround brain capillaries, and is metabolized by the BCAA transaminase to the alpha-ketoacid, alpha-ketoisocaproate (KIC; see Fig. 14-1). KIC enters neurons and a BCAA transaminase, which uses an amino group of glutamate, reaminates KIC to leucine, forming alpha-ketoglutarate, thereby consuming glutamate. The alpha-ketoglutarate becomes available for the aminotransferase of aspartate and thus consumes aspartate. The result of the latter process is a diminution in the malate-aspartate shuttle for providing reducing equivalents to the mitochondrion. The result is diminished function of the election transport chain, coupled with a direct effect of BCAAs on the chain and on creatine kinase.[4-6] The disturbance in mitochondrial metabolism results not only in

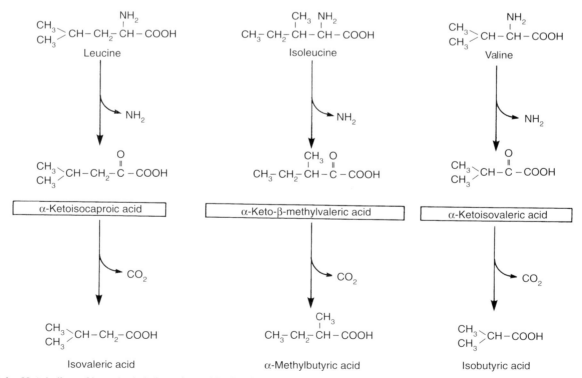

Figure 14-1   **Metabolism of branched-chain amino acids.** The first step is a transamination, and the second step is an oxidative decarboxylation. The latter is defective in maple syrup urine disease; the ketoacids (*enclosed in boxes*) accumulate in body fluids.

TABLE 14-2 Neurochemical Consequences of Excessive Branched-Chain Amino Acids and Ketoacids

Principal Causes
Alterations of Amino Acids
Accumulation of BCAAs, especially leucine
Impaired transport of non-BCAAs
Excessive consumption of amino acids, especially glutamate
Energy Failure
Impaired electron transport
Impaired creatine kinase

Principal Consequences
Alteration of Neurotransmitters
Reduced gamma-aminobutyric acid
Reduced glutamate
Reduced serotonin
Impaired Protein Synthesis
Decreased myelin synthesis
Increased Cytosolic Calcium
Cytoskeletal disturbance
Free radical generation
Cell Edema
Osmotic effects of BCAAs, especially leucine, and of BCKAs, especially KIC.
Altered membrane properties
Cell Death

BCAAs, branched-chain amino acids; BCKAs, branched-chain keto-acids; KIC, alpha-ketoisocaproate.

energy failure but also in impaired pyruvate metabolism and increased lactate (see later).

The principal consequences of the altered amino acids and the energy failure are multiple (see Table 14-2). Consequences of the amino acid abnormalities include *alterations of neurotransmitters* derived from amino acids (i.e., reduced gamma-aminobutyric acid [GABA], glutamate, and serotonin).[7,8] A second effect of the amino acid abnormalities is disturbed protein synthesis, with multiple effects, including myelin synthesis (see later).[9,10] The *energy failure* likely initiates a cascade to cell death that begins with increase in cytosolic calcium.[11] The deleterious effects of cytosolic calcium are reviewed in Chapter 6 and include generation of free radicals, shown to be involved in cell death produced by experimental models of maple syrup urine disease.[12-15] A deleterious calcium-mediated effect on cytoskeleton also has been shown.[16-18] The cell edema that is a prominent feature of classic maple syrup urine disease (see later) appears to relate in part to the osmotic effect of the large accumulation of BCAAs, especially leucine, and BCKAs, especially KIC. Additionally, it is likely that the energy failure results in altered ionic balance, because of failure of adenosine triphosphate (ATP)–dependent ion pump, and as a consequence, cell edema. Cell death is the final result.

Importance of Branched-Chain Ketoacids

Many of the demonstrated deleterious effects in maple syrup urine disease in animal models in vivo and in

other systems in vitro have been associated with the branched-chain *keto*acids. Of these, the ketoacid of leucine (i.e., KIC) is the most critical (see Fig. 14-1). Thus, clinical neurological deficits in human infants are correlated best with leucine administration or with blood leucine levels (KIC not measured directly),[1,19-21] and of the branched-chain ketoacids, only KIC inhibits myelination in cultures of cerebellum. Indeed, other adverse effects described in Table 14-2 involving energy failure, free radical generation, cytosolic calcium accumulation, cytoskeletal disturbance, and cell death have been shown in experimental models particularly or exclusively with KIC. If the ketoacids and especially KIC are critical endogenous toxins, this will have major implications for brain because the transaminations of the BCAAs are particularly active in brain (unlike the decarboxylation of the alpha-ketoacids) and would facilitate formation of the ketoacids at the site of greatest sensitivity.

Clinical Features

Of the five types of maple syrup urine disease (classic, intermediate, intermittent, thiamine-responsive, and lipoamide dehydrogenase deficiency), the classic variety consistently manifests in the newborn period. The onset is in the latter part of the first week and is characterized by poor feeding, vomiting, and stupor (Table 14-3).[1,20-27] Abnormalities of tone appear; initial fluctuations between hypotonia and hypertonia are followed quickly by dystonic posturing. Opisthotonos, jaw rigidity, and dysphagia become apparent. Seizures occur in approximately one half of symptomatic infants. The characteristic odor of maple syrup may not be present in the early neonatal period. Cerumen is the best source of the odor. Approximately one half of infants exhibit a bulging anterior fontanelle and signs of increased intracranial pressure. If the disease is not recognized and treated appropriately, death in the first weeks of life is common. The disorder is more fulminating and malignant than phenylketonuria. In phenylketonuria, the clinical presentation is usually delayed for several weeks and is insidious in onset,

TABLE 14-3 Common Features of Maple Syrup Urine Disease

Clinical Features
Vomiting
Stupor, coma
Dystonia
Seizures
Odor of maple syrup (burnt sugar)
Full fontanelle

Metabolic Features
Acidosis
Branched-chain amino acidemia (or aciduria)
Branched-chain ketoacidemia (or aciduria)
Hypoglycemia

Neuropathological Features
Myelin disturbance
Dendritic abnormalities

perhaps because the ketoacids of phenylalanine metabolism are derived from a minor pathway, whereas the ketoacids of BCAA metabolism are derived from the major metabolic pathway.

Interesting and helpful clinical signs in acute maple syrup urine disease are ocular abnormalities.[20,22,23] These abnormalities have consisted of fluctuating ophthalmoplegias, including internuclear ophthalmoplegia. Ophthalmoplegia may be total, and oculocephalic and oculovestibular reflexes may be absent. In addition, I have seen two infants with maple syrup urine disease who had opsoclonus. Fluctuating ophthalmoplegias and related eye signs should always raise the possibility of serious metabolic encephalopathy in the newborn period. These findings are not confined to maple syrup urine disease; similar observations have been made in nonketotic hyperglycinemia (see later section). The ocular abnormalities may be associated with signs of lower cranial nerve dysfunction, including facial diplegia, absent gag reflex, and weak cry. The frequent impairment of feeding may also partly result from such dysfunction. This constellation of ocular and other cranial nerve signs is often initially mistaken for hypoxic-ischemic encephalopathy or a myopathic disorder.

Neurodiagnostic Studies

The diagnosis of maple syrup urine disease is made on the basis of clinical and metabolic features, but neurodiagnostic studies of value include the electroencephalogram (EEG) and brain imaging. The EEG during the first 2 weeks demonstrates a characteristic "comblike" rhythm, consisting of bursts and runs of 5 to 7 Hz, primarily monophasic negative activity in the central and central-parasagittal regions during both wakefulness and sleep, especially quiet sleep (Fig. 14-2).[28] The abnormality disappears by 40 days after the initiation of dietary therapy. This rhythm may be present on a background of burst suppression, which also disappears after the onset of therapy. This rhythm on the EEG differs from the alpha and theta bursts of normal infants (see Chapter 4) in their presence during both wakefulness and sleep; in neurologically normal infants, the bursts are present only in quiet and transitional sleep.[28] Because of the prominent involvement of brain stem (see later), brain stem auditory evoked responses show impaired brain stem latencies (between waves 1 and 5) with a normal wave 1.[29]

Brain imaging techniques of value in evaluation of the infant with maple syrup urine disease include cranial ultrasonography, computed tomography (CT), and, especially, magnetic resonance imaging (MRI). Cranial ultrasonography, often of minimal value in acute neonatal metabolic disorders, shows increased echogenicity in periventricular white matter, basal ganglia, and thalami, and by imaging through the squamosal "temporal window," in brain stem.[30,31] CT shows decreased attenuation, especially in cerebral white matter and deep nuclear structures (Fig. 14-3).[32] MRI and, especially, diffusion-weighted MRI are most valuable. The consistent abnormality on T2-weighted images is symmetrical hyperintensity in cerebellar white matter,

dorsal brain stem, cerebral peduncles, thalamus, posterior limb of the internal capsule, globus pallidus, and perirolandic cerebral white matter.[32-39] Still more striking than findings on T2-weighted images, diffusion-weighted MRI shows a striking increased signal (decreased diffusion) in the same areas (see Fig. 14-3). The diffusion values are reduced by 70% to 80%. The abnormality is reversible with prompt treatment of the metabolic disorder. However, a subsequent abnormal signal indicative of abnormal myelin is a common sequela,[40] and overt volume loss is noted in infants who are not effectively or promptly treated. The diffusion-weighted MRI findings are consistent with *cytotoxic edema* particularly affecting myelinated regions. The findings are consistent with the neuropathology (see later). Principal abnormalities on MR spectroscopy include elevated lactate as well as elevated BCAAs and BCKAs, consistent with the adverse effects of the latter on energy metabolism (see earlier and Fig. 14-3).

Genetics

Genetic data indicate autosomal recessive inheritance. Thus, familial occurrence, affected male and female infants who are products of consanguineous marriages, and biochemical investigations indicating heterozygosity in parents have been documented.[1] The molecular genetic data thus far do not show a straightforward correlation between genotype and phenotype. Most neonatal onset cases have involvement of the E1 catalytic component (i.e., the thiamine pyrophosphate–dependent decarboxylase).[41] An exception to the variation in molecular defects in general populations, in which the incidence of the disease is 1 in 185,000 newborns, is the single mutation in nearly all Mennonite cases in the United States, in which the incidence is 1 in 176 newborns.[1,27]

Metabolic Features

The major metabolic correlates of maple syrup urine disease are metabolic acidosis, branched-chain aminoacidemia and aminoaciduria, branched-chain ketoacidemia and ketoaciduria, and hypoglycemia (see Table 14-3). Hypoglycemia appears in approximately 50% of the affected infants.

As indicated earlier, the enzymatic defect involves the oxidative decarboxylation of the BCKAs (see Fig. 14-1), which causes the accumulation of the BCAAs and BCKAs. This enzymatic defect can be identified in fresh leukocytes and cultured skin fibroblasts or lymphocytes for diagnosis.[1]

The genesis of the secondary metabolic defects appears to be related principally to the massive accumulation of BCAAs and BCKAs, especially leucine and its alpha-ketoacid, KIC. The ketoacids result in ketoacidosis, and hypoglycemia is thought to relate principally to the accumulation of leucine.[21] The precise mechanism for the hypoglycemia seen in this disorder is probably multifactorial; a deficiency in gluconeogenic substrates, especially alanine, may be most important.[42] A contributory role of leucine in increasing insulin secretion seems possible but is unproven (see Chapter 12).

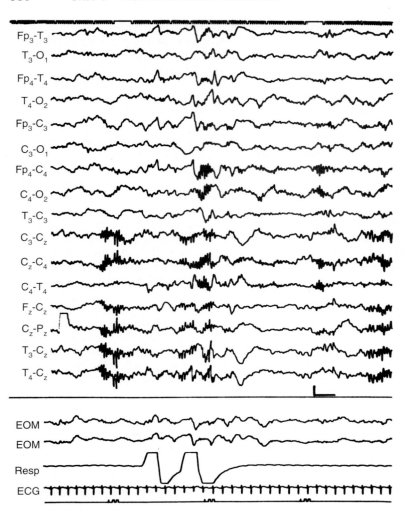

Figure 14-2 Unique electroencephalographic (EEG) pattern in maple syrup urine disease depicting bursts of 4- to 5-Hz comblike activity in active sleep at 13 days of age. Bursts are abundant in the central parasagittal region (C_z), with occasional spread to the right central region (C_4), and they also appear independently in C_4. Note also the abnormal respirations (Resp). Calibration: 50 μV, 1 second. EOM, extraocular muscles. *(From Tharp BR: Unique EEG pattern (comb-like rhythm) in neonatal maple syrup urine disease,* Pediatr Neurol 8:65–68, 1992.)

Neuropathology

The neuropathological features vary with the onset and severity of disease, the type of therapy, and the age at death. Several general conclusions seem warranted.[1,21,42-49] The *younger infant* may exhibit a slightly enlarged and edematous brain. Neuronal changes are minimal and nonspecific. The most prominent parenchymal disturbance involves myelin and consists of vacuolation ("spongy state"). This latter abnormality is most marked in the youngest patients, especially in regions of white matter that myelinate rapidly and near the time of active disease. *Older patients* show a diminution of myelin. A reduction of oligodendrocytes parallels the extent of myelin deficiency. Signs of myelin breakdown are minimal or absent. Because a similar progression from myelin vacuolation to disturbed myelin deposition is seen in several mutant mice with metabolic defects in myelin formation,[50-52] it has been considered that the major brain defect observed in maple syrup urine disease and related states (e.g., non-ketotic hyperglycinemia, phenylketonuria, and ketotic hyperglycinemia) involves myelin formation. It is likely that such a myelin defect in metabolic disorders could be caused by disturbances of the synthesis of myelin lipids (e.g., certain fatty acids, as in ketotic

hyperglycinemia) or of myelin proteins (as in the amino acid disorders).

The *chemical correlates* of the neuropathological findings are diminutions in the levels of myelin lipids as well as myelin proteolipid protein (Table 14-4). The neuropathological and chemical findings of disturbed myelination and the later evidence of such disturbance on MRI scans are less apparent or absent in patients treated from early infancy (see Table 14-4).[47,53-55]

An additional neuropathological feature involves *neuronal development* and consists primarily of deficiencies in dendritic development and in quantities of dendritic spines, sites of synaptic contacts (Fig. 14-4).[49] Additional abnormalities include aberrant orientation of cerebral cortical neurons. Neuronal loss, although not a prominent feature of this disease, is usually apparent in cerebellar granule cells.

Management

Prevention

Prenatal diagnosis and prevention of maple syrup urine disease by therapeutic abortion are well-established approaches.[1,21,26] Fibroblasts grown from cultured amniotic cells have been shown to decarboxylate the BCAAs,[3,56] and this approach can be used for prenatal diagnosis.[1,3,21,26] Cultured cells derived from chorionic villus biopsy have allowed diagnosis in the first trimester of gestation.[1]

Early Detection

After birth of an affected child, early detection is critical.[1,3,57,57a] Institution of therapy at 5 days of age or less has been followed by normal intellectual outcome (see earlier discussion). Moreover, institution of therapy after 14 days of age is very uncommonly followed by normal intellect. Distinction from other causes of metabolic acidosis in the neonatal period is important (see Chapter 15). The early clinical features and the odor of maple syrup, especially in cerumen, are most helpful in making the clinical diagnosis. Neonatal blood screening by the Guthrie test generally provides key information only after several days. The use of tandem mass spectrometry to quantify amino acids in whole blood filter paper specimens is highly sensitive, is accurate, and is faster than the Guthrie bacterial inhibition assay.[27]

Acute Therapy

Acute episodes are managed by lowering toxic levels of BCAAs and BCKAs and by limiting protein catabolism and promoting protein anabolism.[1,27] Although peritoneal dialysis is effective and has been lifesaving,[3] hemodialysis is still more effective.[58,59] Continuous hemofiltration by a pump-assisted, high-flow venovenous system may be as effective and more convenient,

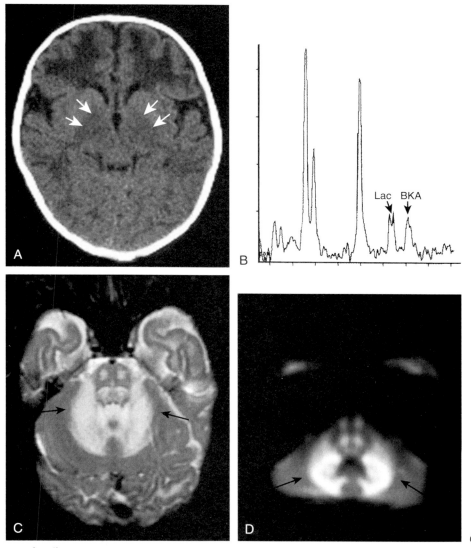

Continued

Figure 14-3 **Maple syrup urine disease, acute neonatal phase. A,** Axial computed tomography image shows low attenuation (*arrows*) in the globi pallidi and posterior limbs of the internal capsules. **B,** Proton magnetic resonance imaging with TE = 288 milliseconds shows abnormal peak at 0.9 ppm (BKA) representing branched-chain amino acids and branched-chain alpha-ketoacids and an abnormal peak at 1.33 ppm (Lac) representing lactate. **C, E,** and **G,** Axial T2-weighted images show abnormal T2 prolongation (*arrows*) in the brain stem, cerebellar white matter, posterior limb of the internal capsule, and centrum semiovale. **D, F,** and **H,** Axial diffusion-weighted images show hyperintensity representing reduced diffusion in the area of T2 prolongation (*arrows*). The diffusion abnormality is more conspicuous than the T2 change in the centrum semiovale. *(From Barkovich AJ: Pediatric Neuroimaging, 4th ed, Philadelphia: 2005, Lippincott Williams & Wilkins.)*

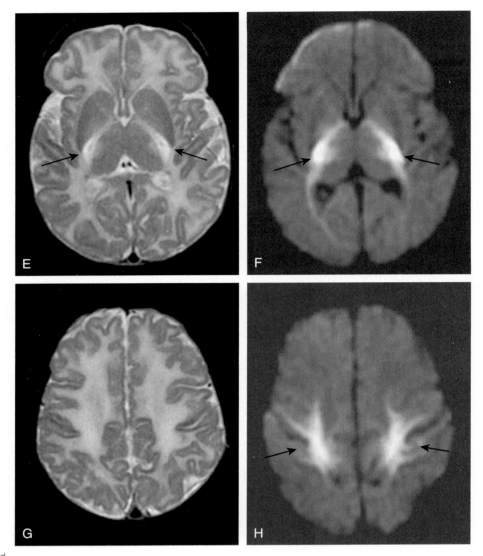

Figure 14-3, *cont'd*

TABLE 14-4 **Alterations of White Matter Lipids and Proteolipid Protein in Maple Syrup Urine Disease**

Age of Infant	Total Lipid	Cerebrosides	Proteolipid Protein
	(PERCENTAGE OF CONTROL)		
16 days	90%	50%	67%
25 days	66%	–	64%
20 months	82%	66%	57%
36 months*	81%	93%	79%

*Treated with diet low in branched-chain amino acids from 35 days of age.
Data from Prensky AL, Carr S, Moser HW: Development of myelin in inherited disorders of amino acid metabolism, *Arch Neurol* 19:552–558, 1968.

albeit somewhat slower than conventional intermittent hemodialysis.[1,60] Enteral and parenteral feeding is instituted with the goal to lower plasma leucine levels promptly.[27] Signs of brain edema are managed with mannitol, furosemide, and intravenous sodium supplementation to replace urinary sodium losses and to maintain a serum sodium level greater than 140 mg/L.[27]

Long-Term Therapy

Subsequent therapy includes a diet that initially contains no BCAAs.[1,3,21] Control of plasma leucine levels is especially crucial, and the adequacy of this control correlates with intellectual outcome in infants with classic maple syrup urine disease.[61] When plasma levels of BCAAs have become normal, these amino acids are added to maintain blood levels at slightly above normal values. With further clinical improvement, milk and certain other natural foods are added

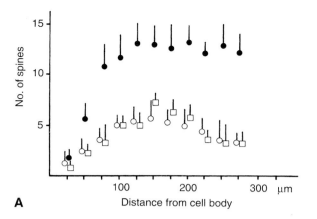

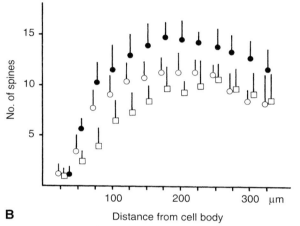

Figure 14-4 Diminished number of synaptic spines in maple syrup urine disease (MSUD). Distribution of synaptic spines on basal dendrites of pyramidal neurons in the, **A**, visual and, **B**, motor cortex of a patient with MSUD and age-matched control. A marked reduction of spine density in MSUD is noted compared with the control. *Open circles*, layer 5 of MSUD; *open squares*, layer 3 of MSUD; *closed circles*, layer 5 of control. *(From Kamei A, Takashima S, Chan F, Becker LE: Abnormal dendritic development in maple syrup urine disease, Pediatr Neurol 8:145–147, 1992.)*

in an amount that does not exceed the requirements for BCAAs. Close supervision is mandatory because relapses may occur with minor infections or for no apparent reason. A more favorable outcome is related particularly to early onset of therapy, careful biochemical monitoring, and early introduction of natural foods

to provide adequate nutrition, especially protein anabolism.[19,55,57,62]

When dietary therapy is instituted before the onset of symptoms (detection because of an earlier affected sibling), a normal neurological outcome can be achieved.[27,57] In infants who develop symptoms, the time of detection and institution of therapy are very important. In one earlier study, those detected and treated at 5 days of age or less had a mean intelligence quotient (IQ) of 97 ± 13 versus 65 ± 20 in those detected and treated at 6 or more days of age.[57] In a more recent study, with particularly vigorous metabolic care, most infants with onset of therapy in the second week had favorable neurological outcomes.[27]

NONKETOTIC HYPERGLYCINEMIA (GLYCINE ENCEPHALOPATHY)

Nonketotic hyperglycinemia is an inborn error of metabolism in which large amounts of glycine accumulate in body fluids and in which a serious neonatal neurological disorder occurs. The disturbance involves the cleavage of glycine to carbon dioxide and a one-carbon fragment. This disorder is approximately twice as common as ketotic hyperglycinemia (see Chapter 15), from which it should be distinguished. Because nonketotic hyperglycinemia involves the central nervous system directly, the term *glycine encephalopathy* may be more appropriate.

Normal Metabolic Aspects

Glycine, the simplest of amino acids, is nonessential, because it can be synthesized in numerous ways in humans.[63,64] It is abundant in most proteins, and, indeed, approximately 50% of ingested glycine is involved in the *synthesis of protein* (Fig. 14-5).[63] In addition, however, a large portion of glycine is *converted to serine*, which, in turn, is involved in the synthesis of phospholipids, as well as oxidation to carbon dioxide through the citric acid cycle (see Fig. 14-5). Glycine is also cleaved to a one-carbon fragment that then is used in a wide variety of synthetic reactions. Additionally, glycine is the precursor for such other critical compounds as purines, glutathione, and porphyrins.

The major roles of glycine as a *neurotransmitter* are almost certainly crucial for the neurological features of nonketotic hyperglycinemia. It is now clear that glycine has *two* neurotransmitter roles in the central

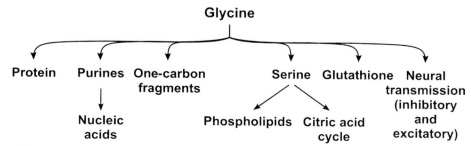

Figure 14-5 Major metabolic fates of glycine.

TABLE 14-5 **Glycine Receptors Involved in Neurotransmission and Their Relation to Nonketotic Hyperglycinemia**

	GLYCINE RECEPTORS	
	Classic	**NMDA**
Major sites in central nervous system	Spinal cord, brain stem	Diffuse, including cerebral cortex, basal ganglia, cerebellum
Primary action	Inhibitory	Excitatory
Mechanism of action	Opens chloride channel	Potentiates activation of NMDA receptor by glutamate
Developmental feature	Excitatory early in brain development (?)	Most abundant early in development
Antagonist	Strychnine	NMDA antagonist (MK-801), glycine site antagonist (HA-966)
Potential clinical correlates	Respiratory failure, weakness, hypotonia	Seizures, myoclonus, neuronal toxicity

NMDA, N-methyl-D-aspartate.

nervous system, one inhibitory and one excitatory, and these roles are influenced by maturation (Table 14-5).[64-71] The "classic" glycine receptor is inhibitory and is located primarily in spinal cord and brain stem. This receptor is inhibited by strychnine. However, this receptor, like the $GABA_A$ receptor, appears to be excitatory during early brain development in animal models.[64,72] The basis of such early excitatory characteristics may be similar to that for the early excitatory $GABA_A$ receptors (see Chapter 5); thus, the immature brain appears to have increased intracellular chloride because of delayed maturation of the chloride exporter.[73] The result would be chloride efflux and depolarization (excitation), rather than chloride influx and hyperpolarization (inhibition) when glycine activation of its receptor opens the chloride channel. Whether all or a portion of these classic glycine receptors are also excitatory in the human newborn brain is unknown. The possibility that both inhibitory and excitatory receptors are present in the brain stem is suggested by the frequency of both apnea and hiccups in newborns with nonketotic hyperglycinemia. Additionally, glycine acts at a second receptor site, associated with the N-methyl-D-aspartate (NMDA) receptor-channel complex, and potentiates the action of glutamate at this receptor. This receptor is located throughout the central nervous system, including cerebrum and cerebellum. Thus, glycine acting at this second receptor is excitatory and indeed can lead to glutamate-induced excitotoxic neuronal death (see later discussion). The excitation may be reflected clinically in the recalcitrant seizures in newborns with nonketotic hyperglycinemia. Because the neonatal nervous system is particularly sensitive to NMDA receptor-mediated neuronal death (see Chapter 6), it is clear

that characteristics of the immature central nervous system cause glycine to be both excitatory and neurotoxic.[68] In addition, the binding of glycine to the NMDA receptor increases postnatally in human cerebral cortical neurons by 100% from term to 6 months.[74] These issues are directly relevant to the clinical, neuropathological, and therapeutic aspects of nonketotic hyperglycinemia (see later discussions).

Biochemical Aspects of Disordered Metabolism

Enzymatic Defect and Essential Consequences

The enzymatic defect in nonketotic hyperglycinemia involves the glycine cleavage enzyme system, which converts the C_1 of glycine to carbon dioxide and results in the formation of a hydroxymethyl derivative of tetrahydrofolate, the key one-carbon donor (Fig. 14-6).[63,64,75-77] A potential particular importance of the glycine cleavage system in early brain development is suggested by the finding of threefold to fivefold higher activities in brain of the first trimester fetus than in brain of the adult.[78] The enzyme is expressed early in development in neural stem/progenitor cells in the germinative zones and then later in radial glial cells.[79] Moreover, glycine receptors in developing cerebrum are important in early neuronal development and differentiation.[80] These considerations could explain, in part, the disturbances in axonal and later myelin development that likely underlie the defects in corpus callosum observed in nonketotic hyperglycinemia (see later).

Abnormalities of two of the four component proteins (i.e., P-protein [the pyridoxal-dependent decarboxylase] and T-protein [a tetrahydrofolate-requiring component]) of the cleavage enzyme system have been identified as the molecular abnormality in the severe

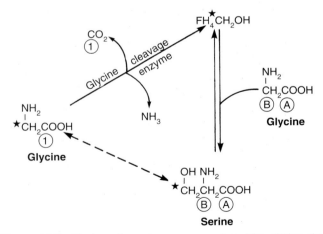

Figure 14-6 **Glycine cleavage enzyme system.** The glycine that serves as substrate for the cleavage enzyme is shown on the *left* of the figure; the C_1 is marked with the *circled numeral* and the C_2 with a *star*. A defect in the glycine cleavage enzyme is accompanied by a defect in the formation of *(1)* carbon dioxide from the C_1 of glycine and *(2)* the C_3 of serine from the C_2 of glycine. (*Adapted from Nyhan WL: Nonketotic hyperglycinemia. In Scriver CR, Beaudet AL, Sly WS, et al, editors: The Metabolic Basis of Inherited Disease, 6th ed, New York: 1989, McGraw-Hill.*)

neonatal cases.[63,64,71,81,82] In one study of 30 cases, 87% exhibited a defect of the P-protein, and the remainder had a defect of the T-protein.[71] The data clarified the earlier in vivo observations in affected infants of defects in the formation of carbon dioxide from the C_1 of glycine and in the formation of the C_3 of serine from the C_2 of glycine (see Fig. 14-6).[63,83-85]

This aminoacidopathy is distinctive in that the enzymatic defect has been shown to occur in *brain*,[63-66,71,75,76,86,87] and, indeed, this fact is probably critical in the pathogenesis of the functional and structural features of the disorder. The immediate result is markedly elevated brain concentrations of glycine. Hyperglycinemia from other causes, including *ketotic* hyperglycinemia, is *not* associated with elevated levels of glycine in brain or with disturbance of glycine cleavage in brain.[76,88] Several lines of evidence suggest that the presence of the defect in *brain* and the resulting accumulation of *glycine in brain* are critical in the neurotoxicity. First, a deficiency of the product of the glycine cleavage reaction (i.e., the one-carbon tetrahydrofolate derivative) is not likely to be highly important because this compound can be generated by other pathways. Second, administration to very young patients with nonketotic hyperglycinemia of sodium benzoate, which is effective in lowering the *plasma* glycine level (through the formation of a water-soluble excretable conjugate) but not the cerebrospinal fluid (CSF) glycine level, does not have consistently beneficial neurological effects (see later discussion). Third, strychnine, a centrally acting antagonist of glycine, is effective in improving certain aspects of the neurological status of at least some affected patients (see later discussion).

Biochemical Effects of Excessive Brain Glycine

The mechanism of the deleterious effect of glycine on neurological *function* may relate to glycine's neurotransmitter roles. Both inhibitory and excitatory actions likely occur. Concerning *inhibition*, the classic inhibitory glycine receptor may account, in part, for the apparent suppression of ventilation through action on the brain stem neurons crucial for respiratory drive, as well as for the hypotonia and weakness through action on spinal cord neurons. Concerning *excitation*, three factors may be relevant. Thus, first, as noted earlier, early in brain development some classic inhibitory glycine receptors may be excitatory. Hiccups, which likely represent a brain stem excitatory effect, may relate to paradoxically excitatory glycine receptors (see earlier). Second, any existing inhibitory glycine receptors could exhibit desensitization with persistent exposure to high concentrations of glycine. Indeed, evidence indicates that excess glycine may result in a desensitization of glycine receptors at the postsynaptic membrane, which would result in diminished inhibition of certain pathways.[89] Third, probably the most potent excitatory influence of glycine is exerted at the NMDA receptor, as described earlier. The result of these excitatory influences could include seizures, hyperexcitability, and myoclonus.

The mechanism of the deleterious effect of glycine on neural *structure* may relate to a disturbance in myelin proteins and to excitotoxic neuronal effects. Neuropathological observations demonstrate a striking *myelin disturbance* in nonketotic hyperglycinemia, similar to that observed with maple syrup urine disease and other aminoacidopathies. Because protein synthesis is disturbed when one amino acid is present in markedly abnormal quantities, one possibility is that excessive brain glycine leads to the myelin disturbance by causing a defect in the synthesis of one or more myelin proteins. In addition, *neuronal loss* in cerebrum and cerebellum may be excitotoxic (see later discussion). Disturbances in cerebral development, of prenatal origin (see later), may relate to both the deficient action of the glycine cleavage enzyme and the excessive action of glycine on glycine and NMDA receptors. Thus, as noted earlier, the glycine cleavage system is important in developing neuroepithelium in stem/progenitor cells and in radial glial cells. The action of glycine on both the glycine and NMDA receptors is important in brain development; in excess, these actions could be deleterious. One such deleterious effect could be excitotoxicity mediated by the NMDA receptor.

Clinical Features

The onset of nonketotic hyperglycinemia in the typical case is in the first days of life, most commonly the first 2 days of life, with ineffective suck, impaired ventilatory effort (or apnea), stupor, hypotonia, seizures, multifocal myoclonus, and hiccups (Table 14-6).[19,63-65,71,87,90-103] Approximately two thirds of infants exhibit the onset before 48 hours of life; onset in the first hours of life is not unusual, and abnormal fetal movements suggestive of myoclonus or hiccups have been observed.[64,100,104-109] Seizures occur on the first postnatal day in approximately 15%, by day 3 in nearly 50%, and by day 30 in approximately 70% of patients.[102] Hiccups are a particularly helpful (although not constant) clinical sign. A mother of one of my affected newborn patients volunteered before the diagnosis was suspected that she felt that her fetus experienced frequent hiccups. As with maple syrup urine disease, interesting and useful neurological signs

TABLE 14-6	Common Features of Nonketotic Hyperglycinemia (Glycine Encephalopathy)
Clinical Features	
Seizures	
Stupor, coma	
Myoclonus	
Hiccups	
Ventilatory failure	
Metabolic Features	
Hyperglycinemia (hyperglycinuria)	
Neuropathological Features	
Myelin disturbance	
Neuronal excitotoxicity	

include a variety of ophthalmoplegias, which may be fluctuating in character. Of particular importance is the need for mechanical ventilation in approximately two thirds of patients. Rapid evolution of intractable seizures, stimulus-sensitive myoclonus, and coma are common.

The *neonatal EEG* is abnormal in at least 90% of infants. The most common finding is the burst-suppression pattern, and nonketotic hyperglycinemia is the most common metabolic cause of the syndrome of early myoclonic encephalopathy (myoclonic seizures, burst-suppression EEG; see Chapter 5). Brain stem auditory evoked responses are characterized by delayed brain stem conduction times (e.g., wave I to V latency).[97,110]

Brain imaging is notable in the neonatal period for the relatively frequent findings of agenesis or hypoplasia of the corpus callosum and abnormalities of cerebral white matter, with subsequent evidence of hypomyelination and to a lesser extent, cerebral cortical atrophy. The CT scan may demonstrate decreased attenuation of the cerebral white matter (Fig. 14-7A) and partial or complete agenesis of the corpus callosum.[111-114] MRI is superior to CT in demonstrating these features (Figs. 14-7B and 14-8). Thus, decreased attenuation of cerebral white matter may be observed, but more strikingly, on diffusion-weighted MRI, one sees increased signal (decreased diffusion) in dorsal brain stem, cerebral peduncles, and posterior limbs of the internal capsule (see Fig. 14-8).[37,115-121] These features are consistent with the vacuolating myelinopathy observed at neuropathological examination (see later), as is also seen in maple syrup urine disease (see earlier) The abnormalities of corpus callosum are best visualized in vivo by MRI and occur in at least 20% of cases.[32,98,114,117,119] Progression of findings to abnormal signal and then atrophy of cerebral white matter and, to a lesser extent, cerebral cortex is common.[98,118,119] MR spectroscopy shows a striking increase in brain glycine levels, consistent with the locus of the enzymatic defect (see earlier) (Fig. 14-9).[32,117,119,122,123] In conventional short-echo spectra, glycine cannot be distinguished from the normal myoinositol peak; with long-echo spectra, the elevation of glycine is seen clearly (see Fig. 14-9).[123]

A syndrome of *transient neonatal nonketotic hyperglycinemia*, which clinically can be indistinguishable from the better-known classic neonatal form first described, has been elucidated.[64,85,124-129] The clinical presentation has been characterized by the onset of seizures in the first days of life with hypotonia and depressed level of consciousness; one infant exhibited coma and respiratory failure. All infants survived, and six of eight were normal neurologically on follow-up. The diagnosis was made by finding increased concentrations of glycine in the CSF, urine, and plasma, with the most consistent elevation in the CSF. The metabolic abnormalities disappeared within 2 to 8 weeks. A transient defect in the glycine cleavage enzyme is presumed but has not been documented. The existence of this syndrome with a markedly better outcome than that associated with the more typical persistent form raises difficult ethical issues in management of classic nonketotic

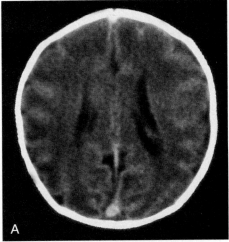

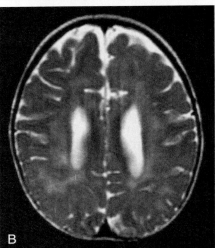

Figure 14-7 **Computed tomography (CT) and magnetic resonance imaging (MRI) features of nonketotic hyperglycinemia. A,** CT scan obtained at 4 days of age in an affected infant with refractory seizures. Note the marked and diffuse decrease in attenuation in cerebral white matter. **B,** T2-weighted MRI scan obtained at 2 years of age, when the child exhibited severe seizures and mental retardation. Note the increased signal in cerebral white matter, the enlarged ventricles, and the marked paucity of myelin. Atrophy of cerebral cortex is manifested by enlarged subarachnoid spaces.

hyperglycinemia. In the latter disorder, cessation of life support often is considered in the severely ill infant early in the clinical course because of the very poor prognosis, despite the typical occurrence of recovery of ventilatory function later in the neonatal period.

Clinical distinction of transient nonketotic hyperglycinemia from *atypical variants of nonketotic hyperglycinemia* is also difficult.[130-133] These infants also present clinically like those with classic nonketotic hyperglycinemia, and the outcome has ranged from normal neurological status to death early in infancy. The distinction of this milder variant from transient neonatal nonketotic hyperglycinemia is based on resolution of the metabolic defects in the latter but not fully in the former. Moreover, the milder forms have been shown to be associated with considerable (20% to 30%) residual glycine cleavage enzyme activity. Decisive distinction from true transient disease requires determination

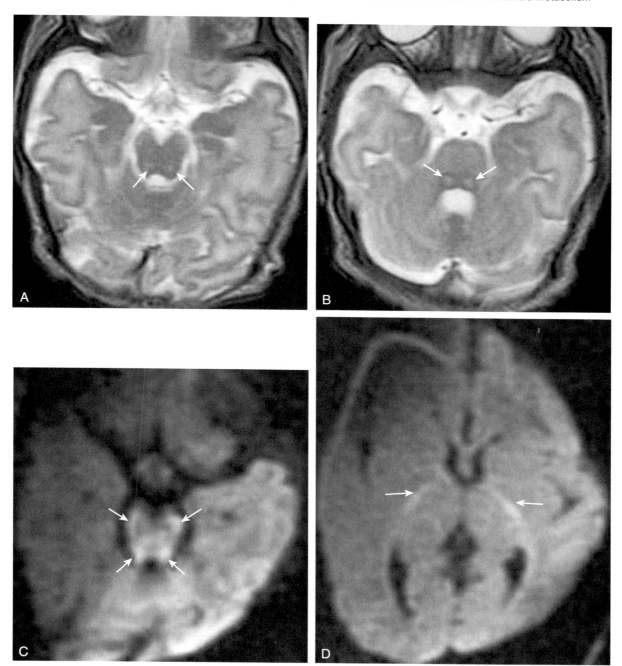

Figure 14-8 **Nonketotic hyperglycinemia, conventional and diffusion-weighted (DWI) magnetic resonance imaging (MRI).** The infant was 15 days old and had nonketotic hyperglycinemia. Note in **A** and **B**, T2-weighted MRI scans, hyperintense lesions in the dorsal midbrain and pons (*arrows*). DWI of the middle-to-upper brain stem, **C**, shows more conspicuous and additional hyperintense (restricted diffusion) lesions (*arrows*). DWI at the level of the cerebral hemispheres, **D**, shows prominent hyperintensity in the posterior limbs of the internal capsules (*arrows*). *(From Khong PL, Tse C, Wong IY, Lam BC, et al: Diffusion-weighted imaging and proton magnetic resonance spectroscopy in perinatal hypoxic-ischemic encephalopathy: Association with neuromotor outcome at 18 months of age, J Child Neurol 19:872–881, 2004.)*

of glycine cleavage activity, which generally requires liver biopsy. It is hoped that molecular genetic analyses will become available in the near future.

The *outcome* of nonketotic hyperglycinemia has been generally poor.[64] Overall, approximately 35% of infants die, often in the neonatal period, and most survivors have serious neurological disturbances, including mental retardation, recurrent seizures, and severe abnormalities (e.g., hypsarrhythmia) on the EEG. Recent data suggest

notable gender differences in outcome (Table 4-7).[102] Thus, in one series of 65 infants, although overall 12% died in the neonatal period, the gender-specific mortality rates were 28% for female patients and 0% for male patients. Indeed, the overall median age at death was 2.6 years for male patients versus less than 1 month for female patients. The male advantage was noted also for outcome. Of survivors 3 years or older, although severe deficits occurred overall in 60%, gender-specific rates of

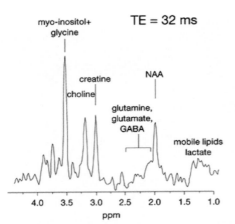
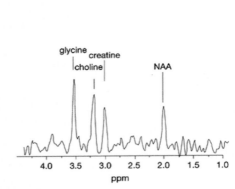

Figure 14-9   **Nonketotic hyperglycinemia, magnetic resonance (MR) spectroscopy.** On postnatal day 7, proton MR spectroscopy from parieto-occipital white matter of an infant with nonketotic hyperglycinemia shows the high intensity of glycine at 3.55 ppm. With conventional short echo times (TE = 32 milliseconds) glycine and myoinositol cannot be separated, whereas with long echo times (TE = 136 milliseconds), the elevation of glycine is readily distinguished. GABA, gamma-aminobutyric acid; NAA, N-acetylaspartate. *(From Huisman TA, Thiel T, Steinmann B, Zeilinger G, et al: Proton magnetic resonance spectroscopy of the brain of a neonate with nonketotic hyperglycinemia: In vivo–in vitro (ex vivo) correlation, Eur Radiol 12:858–861, 2002.)*

poor outcome were 100% for female patients and 29% for male patients. Of the original 65 infants, 10 infants (15%) could walk and say or sign words, and these infants were all male. None of these 10 infants were neurologically normal, however. Therapeutic intervention may modify the unfavorable outcome in nonketotic hyperglycinemia (see later).

Distinction from Ketotic Hyperglycinemia

It is important to distinguish nonketotic hyperglycinemia from ketotic hyperglycinemia, particularly in view of the observation that not all patients with ketotic hyperglycinemia exhibit consistent ketosis.[63,134] Early therapeutic intervention may be particularly beneficial in ketotic hyperglycinemia. Although this is not yet clearly the case with severe nonketotic hyperglycinemia, some observations raise the hope that specific therapy will become available (see later section). Features helpful in the distinction of nonketotic and ketotic hyperglycinemia are included in Table 14-8.

Genetics

Genetic data indicate autosomal recessive inheritance.[64,71] Thus, familial occurrence, parental consanguinity, and intermediate molecular defects in heterozygotes have been recorded.

Metabolic Features

The major biochemical correlate of nonketotic hyperglycinemia is marked accumulation of glycine in blood, urine, and CSF.[64,96] Particularly characteristic is the accumulation of glycine in the CSF. Values range generally between 85 and 280 μmol/L, with control subjects generally having values less than 10 μmol/L.[63,64,71,76,84,135] The ratio of the concentration of glycine in CSF to that in plasma, an important diagnostic measure, generally ranges from 0.09 to 0.25 μmol/L, with control values approximately 0.02 μmol/L.[63,64] This pronounced elevation of CSF glycine level is not observed in other varieties of hyperglycinemia,[75] and it presumably relates to the presence of the enzymatic defect in brain in the patients with nonketotic hyperglycinemia. A distinct correlation exists between the degree of elevation of the ratio of CSF glycine to plasma glycine and the severity of the clinical phenotype. The defect in the glycine cleavage reaction

TABLE 14-7	Outcome of Neonatal Nonketotic Hyperglycinemia: Notable Gender Differences*

Mortality

Neonatal mortality: 12% overall, *0% in male patients*, 28% in female patients

Median age of death: *2–6 yr in male patients*, <1 mo in female patients

Overall mortality (neonatal and later): 34% (similar for male and female patients)

Outcome (Survivors ≥ 3 Years)

"Walk and say/sign words": 40% overall, *71% of male patients, 0% of female patients*

Severe deficits: 60% overall, *29% of male patients, 100% of female patients*

*Starting population: n=65, 36 males, 29 females.
Data from Hoover-Fong JE, Shah S, Van Hove JL, Applegarth D, et al: Natural history of nonketotic hyperglycinemia in 65 patients, *Neurology* 63:1847–1853, 2004.

TABLE 14-8	Nonketotic versus Ketotic Hyperglycinemia	
	Nonketotic	**Ketotic**
Severe neonatal illness	+	+
Seizures	+	+
Hiccups	+	−
Ketoacidosis	−	+
Neutropenia-thrombocytopenia	−	+
Primary defect in glycine metabolism	+	−
Dietary therapy effective	−	+

+, present; −, absent.

(see Fig. 14-6) in brain, liver, and probably other tissues adequately explains the accumulation of glycine in all body fluids. As noted earlier, elevated levels of glycine in the brain of living infants with the disease have been demonstrated by MR spectroscopy.

Neuropathology

Neuropathological findings from studies of more than 20 infants have been described.[63-65,84,87,90,92,97,135-141] The dominant abnormality has involved myelin, and the nature of the disturbance is similar to that noted for ketotic hyperglycinemia, maple syrup urine disease, and various other aminoacidopathies.[64,87] The essential features are vacuolation of and diminution in myelin (Fig. 14-10). No striking involvement of neurons or sign of myelin breakdown is noted. Vacuolation is more common in younger patients, and myelin

diminution is more common in older patients, findings suggesting that myelin formation is deranged and the early sign of this derangement is vacuolation. Ultrastructural studies support the notion of origin of the vacuoles from newly formed myelin sheaths (Fig. 14-11).[90,97,139] Involvement is greatest in those systems that myelinate around the time of birth. A prenatal onset of the process is supported by the finding of partial or total agenesis of the corpus callosum (see earlier discussion). MRI studies have also shown abnormalities of gyral development in occasional cases.[32,117] Whether such abnormalities could be related to the expression during development of the glycine cleavage system in radial glial cells (see earlier) is an intriguing possibility. More detailed MRI studies will be of interest.

Neuronal injury in cerebrum has not been described consistently at autopsy. Severe *cerebellar* neuronal

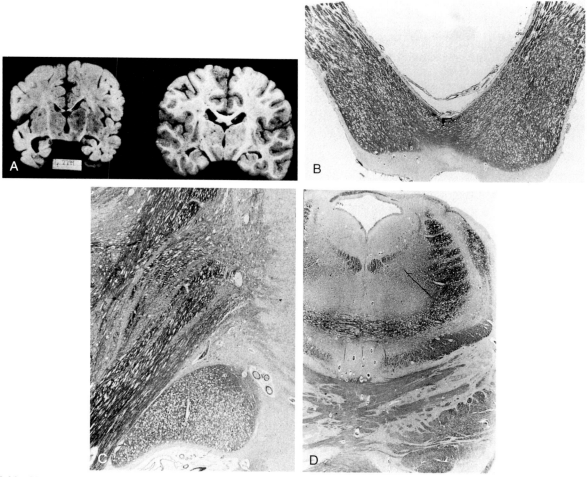

Figure 14-10 Myelin disturbance in nonketotic hyperglycinemia. These sections were obtained from a 24-month-old infant who exhibited lethargy and poor feeding from the first day of life, onset of seizures in the second week, and subsequent failure of neurological development. **A,** Coronal section of cerebrum from the patient *(left)* and from an age-matched control *(right).* Note the differences in bulk of cerebral white matter, corpus callosum, and internal capsules. **B,** Optic nerves and chiasm; note the vacuolated myelin. **C,** Coronal section of the internal capsule. Note vacuolation in the fibers of the capsule *(upper portion* of the figure) and also of the optic tract *(lower portion* of the figure). **D,** Horizontal section of the midbrain. Note vacuolation of the medial longitudinal fasciculus, the superior cerebellar peduncle, and the lateral lemniscus. *(From Shuman RM, Leech RW, Scott CR: The neuropathology of the nonketotic and ketotic hyperglycinemias: Three cases, Neurology 28:139–146, 1978.)*

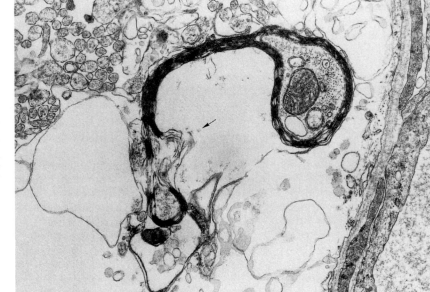

Figure 14-11 **Myelin vacuolation in nonketotic hyperglycinemia.** This electron micrograph of the pontine tegmentum demonstrates that the microvacuolation is splitting the myelin lamellae *(arrow)*. (Epon-embedded lead citrate and uranyl acetate–stained ultrathin section, × 20,650.) *(From Scher MS, Bergman I, Ahdab-Barmada M, Fria T: Neurophysiological and anatomical correlations in neonatal nonketotic hyperglycinemia, Neuropediatrics 17:137–143, 1986.)*

necrosis has been documented.[65] Thus, the possibility of excitotoxic neuronal injury initiated at the NMDA receptor (see earlier discussion) has not been defined clearly, although this occurrence seems likely. As noted earlier, apparent cerebral cortical atrophy is a common feature on brain imaging studies in infants who survive beyond the neonatal period.

Management

Prevention

Demonstration of very low or no activity of the glycine cleavage system in biopsy samples of chorionic villus has allowed diagnosis in the first trimester.[64,71,78] On the basis of such prenatal identification, prevention by therapeutic abortion has been performed.

Early Detection

Early detection is important because institution of therapy in the neonatal period provides the best opportunity to ameliorate, albeit partially, the very unfavorable neurological outcome (see later discussion). A serious ethical issue arises with the severely affected infant who requires ventilatory support. With the unfavorable prognosis characteristic of this disease, the decision to discontinue life support measures frequently arises. Because the severe respiratory failure often resolves later in the neonatal period (see earlier discussion), the continuation of early life support measures may result in recovery of ventilatory function but with a very poor neurological outcome. With the recognition of *transient* nonketotic hyperglycinemia, however, the decision to discontinue ventilatory support early in the neonatal period in infants with nonketotic hyperglycinemia has become especially difficult. Moreover, recent therapeutic

attempts provide some reason for hope in this disorder (see next section).

Therapeutic Attempts

Sodium Benzoate. The major therapeutic challenges are to reduce glycine at the site of injury (i.e., the central nervous system) and to reduce the deleterious effects of glycine at the NMDA receptor and other neural sites. Sodium benzoate has been used to lower glycine in *blood* because an amide bond between glycine and benzoate is formed, and the resulting hippuric acid is excreted. The plasma glycine levels are reduced to near normal but, unfortunately, *CSF* glycine levels often are not similarly affected.[63,64,84,108,142-144] However, with doses as high as 750 mg/kg/day, a substantial decline in CSF glycine levels has been effected, and a decrease in seizures has been reported.[63,64] Moreover, with doses nearly as high, a decrease in brain (as well as CSF) glycine levels has been shown by MR spectroscopy.[145] Unfortunately, however, thus far no beneficial effect on cognitive development has been reported with benzoate therapy.

Strychnine. The initial therapeutic approach directed at the effects of glycine in the central nervous system was the use of strychnine.[91,93,94,110,141,146] The rationale for administration of this drug is its role as a specific antagonist of the inhibitory glycine receptor at the postsynaptic membrane.[147,148] In general, severely affected neonatal patients have not had apparent benefit, despite onset of therapy from the first hours or days of life.[93,110,141] The principal reason for the lack of benefit from strychnine presumably relates to the finding that the drug has no effect on glycine's allosteric activation of the NMDA receptor and thereby excitotoxicity.

Benzodiazepines. A class of agents that acts principally by enhancing GABA receptor inhibitory function, the benzodiazepines, has been used in infants with nonketotic hyperglycinemia.[63,107,149] A beneficial response on seizure frequency, often at relatively high doses, has been observed in some patients. However, antiepileptic effects have been inconstant, and no beneficial effect on neurological development has been observed. The latter failure probably relates, in part, to a lack of effect of benzodiazepines at the NMDA receptor and the concept that GABA$_A$ receptors in the newborn may be largely excitatory (see Chapter 5).

Excitatory Amino Acid Antagonists. A theoretically promising therapy in nonketotic hyperglycinemia involves agents that are excitatory amino acid antagonists.[64,71,82,85,104,105,107-109,144,150-152] In general, the most commonly used agents have been dextromethorphan (or ketamine), in combination with sodium benzoate. Tryptophan, which is metabolized to kynurenic acid, an antagonist of glycine's action at the NMDA receptor, also has been used. The most commonly employed agent has been dextromethorphan, at a dose of 5 to 40 mg/kg/day. Considerable interpatient variability in metabolism requires careful surveillance of dose and effects.[108] However, a beneficial effect on seizures has been documented, although such effects have not been consistently uniform or persistent. Moreover, amelioration of cognitive deficits has generally not been achieved. Further improvements in development of NMDA antagonists, with specific action at the glycine site on the NMDA receptor, may lead to more favorable effects on outcome. Antenatal therapy with such an agent may be necessary for optimal benefit. The findings of hypoplastic corpus callosum, elevated levels of CSF glycine at *birth*, the absence of glycine cleavage activity in *fetal brain*, and the occurrence of severe neurological signs in the first hour of life all support this contention (see earlier).

Conclusions. The data just reviewed are disappointing concerning effective therapy of nonketotic hyperglycinemia. Use of sodium benzoate and an NMDA antagonist theoretically is the best current combination. Additional anticonvulsant therapy may be required. Nevertheless, it does not appear that this approach, even if improved with newer agents, will correct all the deficits in this disorder. The reasons for this prediction relate to several factors. First, it is likely that brain injury or maldevelopment, or both, occur in utero because of the locus of the enzymatic defect in brain (i.e., a locus unavailable to the benefits of placental function). Second, the role of the disturbance of myelination in the genesis of the intellectual failure and some of the other neurological disturbances in nonketotic hyperglycinemia presumably is largely separate from the neurotransmitter effects of glycine.

HYPERAMMONEMIA

Hyperammonemia in the neonatal period may result in serious derangements of neurological function and structure. The Krebs-Henseleit urea cycle is the major pathway of ammonia elimination in mammals, and thus defects in the enzymes catalyzing the five steps of this pathway are important causes of hyperammonemia. Neonatal hyperammonemia results from defects of the first four of these five steps. Elevations of blood ammonia levels occur in certain other inborn errors of metabolism and also have been demonstrated in a significant proportion of premature infants and asphyxiated infants (Table 14-9). In the latter two instances, the hyperammonemia is not secondary to an inborn error of ammonia metabolism. (Not listed in Table 14-9 is hyperammonemia with hepatic failure or with total parenteral nutrition, because the severity of the hyperammonemia is rarely marked and clinical phenomena referable to the hyperammonemia are most unusual in these settings.) In the following discussion, I review the normal aspects of ammonia metabolism, the biochemical aspects of disordered metabolism, and the principal clinical syndromes associated with neonatal hyperammonemia. Emphasis is placed not only on the deficits in the urea cycle enzymes but also on the disturbance observed in premature infants. Hyperammonemia associated with perinatal asphyxia is discussed in Chapter 9.

Normal Metabolic Aspects

Major Sources and Fates of Ammonia

The major sources of ammonia in mammals are amino acids and purine nucleotides (amino groups of adenine, guanine, and their derivatives).[153] Although small amounts of ammonia are used for the synthesis of certain amino acids (primarily by transamination) and pyrimidines, the principal fate of ammonia is biosynthesis of urea through the urea cycle for waste nitrogen disposal (Fig. 14-12).

TABLE 14-9	Major Causes of Hyperammonemia in the Neonatal Period

Urea Cycle Defects
Carbamyl phosphate synthetase
Ornithine transcarbamylase
Argininosuccinic acid synthetase
Argininosuccinase

Organic Acid Disorders
Propionic acidemia
Methylmalonic acidemia
Isovaleric acidemia
beta-Ketothiolase deficiency
Pyruvate dehydrogenase deficiency
Mitochondrial (electron transport) disorders
Glutaric aciduria, type II
Multiple carboxylase deficiency
Fatty acid oxidation defect

Lysine Protein Intolerance

Hyperornithinemia, Hyperammonemia, and Homocitrullinemia

Transient Hyperammonemia of Prematurity

Perinatal Asphyxia

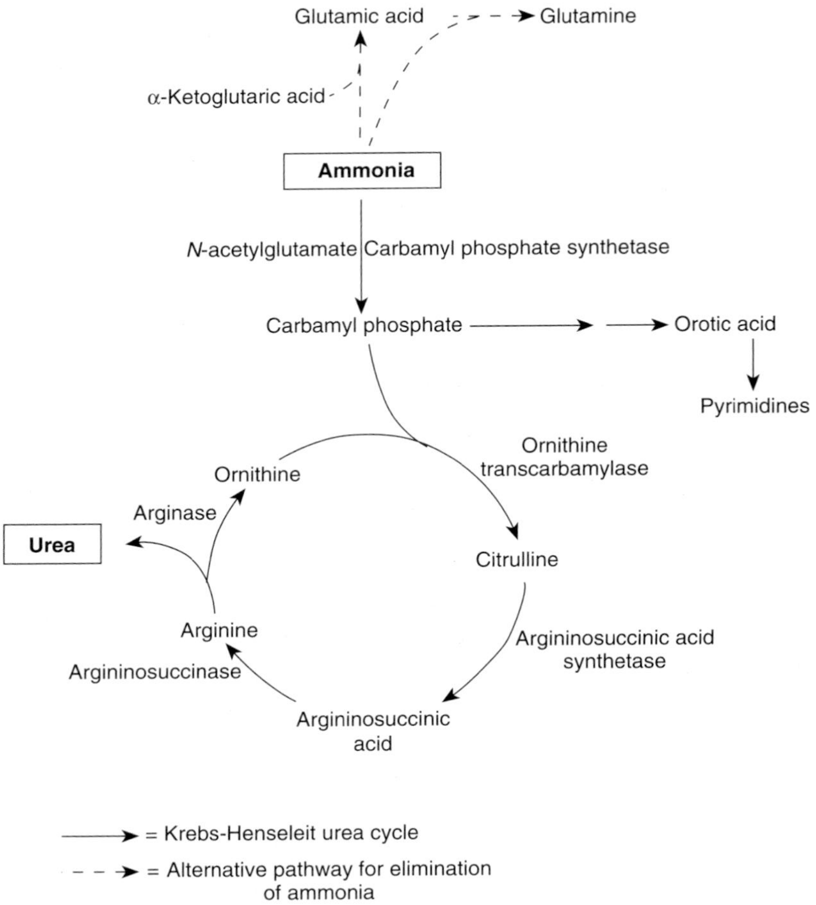

Figure 14-12 Major aspects of ammonia metabolism, particularly in *liver*. See text for details. The upper portion, depicted by *dotted arrows*, indicates ammonia metabolism in *brain*, that is, utilization of two molecules of ammonia for the sequential transamination of alpha-ketoglutarate to form glutamic acid and of the latter, by glutamine synthetase, to form glutamine.

Urea Cycle

The urea cycle consists of five steps, the first two of which are catalyzed by the mitochondrial enzymes carbamyl phosphate synthetase and ornithine transcarbamylase and the latter three of which are catalyzed by the cytosolic enzymes argininosuccinic acid synthetase, argininosuccinase, and arginase (see Fig. 14-12).[153,154] An important obligatory positive effector of carbamyl phosphate synthetase is *N*-acetylglutamate, which is synthesized in the mitochondrion from acetyl-coenzyme A and glutamate. The liver is the only organ that is quantitatively important in urea synthesis.[153,155] In human neonatal brain, only argininosuccinic acid synthetase is present in significant quantities (i.e., 155% of the hepatic activity), whereas activities of carbamyl phosphate synthetase, ornithine transcarbamylase, argininosuccinase, and arginase are present in relatively small quantities (3%, 0.2%, 14%, and 2% of the respective hepatic activities).[156]

Ammonia Disposal in Brain

Ammonia is formed constantly in brain, and, indeed, ammonia concentrations in brain in adult animals are 60% to 100% higher than in blood.[157-159] Ammonia in brain is eliminated by diffusion and by conversion to glutamate and, particularly, to glutamine (see Fig. 14-10). Glutamine also may diffuse from brain. At least one mode of glutamine transport from brain involves a transporter shared with tryptophan, so glutamine efflux from brain is accompanied by tryptophan influx into brain (see later discussion).[154,160]

Biochemical Aspects of Disordered Metabolism

Enzymatic Defects and Essential Consequences

Of the major causes of hyperammonemia in the perinatal period (see Table 14-9), those studied in most detail involve the enzymes catalyzing the reactions of the urea cycle. These disorders affect the hepatic enzymes and, to a variable extent, the enzymes in other tissues. Hyperammonemia is a prominent consequence and, depending on the site of the enzymatic block, so are aberrations of amino acids in blood or urine. The causes of the striking disturbances in function and structure of the central nervous system observed with these hyperammonemic states are not entirely understood. Mechanisms that are supported by some experimental and clinical evidence are displayed in Figure 14-13 and are discussed in the next sections.

Biochemical Effects of Excessive Ammonia

Ammonia may have a variety of toxic effects on brain (see Fig. 14-13). These effects involve several

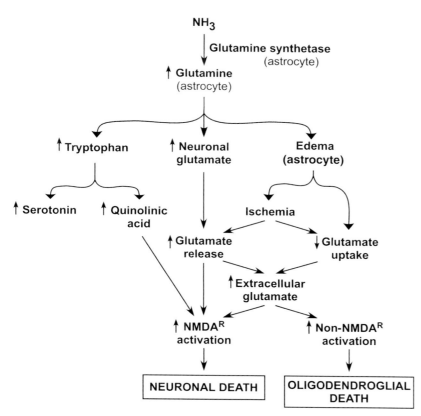

Figure 14-13   **Principal mechanisms by which ammonia (NH$_3$) is toxic to developing brain**. NMDA[R], receptor for *N*-methyl-D-aspartate. See text for details.

neurotransmitter molecules and thereby result in major perturbations of neural function.[160-163] Moreover, because such excitatory neurotransmitter molecules as glutamate and quinolinic acid can lead to neuronal and perhaps oligodendroglial death, these effects result in serious structural lesions as well.

The metabolism of ammonia to glutamine appears to be of particular importance in the acute toxicity of hyperammonemia (see Fig. 14-13).[153,154,160,161,163-170] Thus, with hyperammonemia, the brain glutamine level increases because of glutamine synthesis from glutamate through the glutamine synthetase reaction with ammonia (see Figs. 14-12 and 14-13). In one animal model, when glutamine synthesis is blocked by inhibition of the synthetase, hyperammonemia is no longer toxic.[165] Marked increases in brain glutamine levels were documented by MR spectroscopy during acute hyperammonemia in two infants with ornithine transcarbamylase deficiency.[32,168] Moreover, a newborn with arginase deficiency and only a slightly elevated blood ammonia level but a markedly elevated CSF glutamine level was severely symptomatic (including coma) and died.[171] The functional effects of increased brain glutamine may be marked. A major functional effect, induction of stupor or coma, is a well-documented result of elevated brain glutamine.

Of still greater importance are the *likely structural consequences* of increased glutamine synthesis (see Fig. 14-13). Perhaps most critically, increased glutamine efflux from brain is accompanied by increased tryptophan influx, because these two amino acids share a common transporter.[154,160,161] This increased tryptophan is metabolized to *serotonin* and to *quinolinic acid.*

Serotonin may contribute to the genesis of the stupor and coma. Quinolinic acid is a neurotoxin that activates the NMDA type of glutamate receptor to lead to excitotoxic neuronal death. Batshaw and co-workers[160,172] documented twofold to tenfold elevations of quinolinic acid in newborns with hyperammonemic coma.[160,172] Moreover, the peak toxicity of quinolinic acid in developing rat brain was shown to be at 7 postnatal days, a maturational age comparable to the human newborn infant.[173] Quinolinic acid administered to late gestation fetal sheep resulted in widespread lipid peroxidation in brain;[174] this result could relate, in part, to NMDA excitotoxicity, calcium influx, and generation of reactive oxygen species (see Chapter 6). Related additional deleterious effects of increased brain glutamine include an increase in neuronal levels of glutamate because of the action of the astrocytic-neuronal glutamine-glutamate cycle, in which glutamine diffuses from astrocytes to neurons and is converted to glutamate. The elevated neuronal glutamate then leads to increased glutamate release and the potential for excitotoxic neuronal death (see Fig. 14-13). Another related deleterious effect of the elevated glutamine levels in astrocytes is the induction of astrocytic swelling (see Fig. 14-13) and thereby impaired microcirculatory blood flow with resulting ischemia. The result would be excitotoxic neuronal death because of excessive glutamate release and decreased glutamate uptake as described in Chapter 6 regarding ischemia. Reports of a sharp decline in mortality and in ATP depletion resulting from acute ammonia toxicity by administration of MK-801 before the infusion of ammonium acetate in animal models support the possibility of excitotoxicity mediated by NMDA receptors.[160,161,175,176] Thus, neuronal injury in hyperammonemia may relate to excitotoxic effects at the NMDA receptor provoked by quinolinic acid and by glutamate. In view of the receptor-mediated toxicity of glutamate to oligodendroglia (see Chapter 6), glutamate-induced injury also may be relevant to the deficit in oligodendroglia (see Fig. 14-13) and myelin observed in hyperammonemic brain injury (see "Neuropathology" later).

A disturbance in energy metabolism may help to initiate some of the excitotoxic effects just described and may be important in contributing to additional later effects of hyperammonemia. Thus, with prolonged hyperammonemia, *impairment in brain energy* reserves becomes apparent, especially in brain stem and cerebellum.[157,158,176-178] The cause of the disturbance in brain energy production is unknown. A disturbance in pyruvate utilization (see earlier discussion) may be important in this context and may account in part for the small increases in brain lactate documented in animal models and on proton MR spectroscopy in some affected infants.[32,179-181] Of additional importance is an apparent *disturbance in transport of reducing equivalents (reduced nicotinamide adenine dinucleotide [NADH]) from cytosol to mitochondria.*[180] This disturbance could result in a deficit of NADH for the mitochondrial electron transport chain, inhibit oxidative energy coupling, and lead to a fall in ATP levels.[180] Moreover, in one animal model of hyperammonemia, the NMDA antagonist, MK-801, blocked the decline in ATP levels, a finding thereby suggesting that the energy impairment was *caused* by the excitotoxic effects.[176] Nevertheless, only very marked hyperammonemia, prolonged hyperammonemia, or both, will cause appreciable changes in brain energy levels.[181,182] *On balance, therefore, the deleterious effects on neurotransmitter molecules just discussed seem more crucial than do primary alterations in energy metabolism in the genesis of the functional and structural effects of hyperammonemia.*

Urea Cycle Defects

The best-documented causes of severe neonatal hyperammonemia are deficiencies in the urea cycle enzymes. The overall incidence of these disorders is approximately 1 in 30,000 live births.[154,183,184] Although certain differences in clinical and metabolic features occur, the neonatal forms of these defects of the urea cycle exhibit distinct similarities in clinical, metabolic, and neuropathological features (Table 14-10). The *clinical syndrome* consists almost invariably of onset most commonly between 24 and 72 hours of life, poor feeding (sometimes with vomiting), disturbed level of consciousness (i.e., stupor or coma), hyperventilation, and seizures. Highly distinctive is tachypnea (and occasionally respiratory alkalosis), presumably a central effect of hyperammonemia and reminiscent of the central hyperventilation noted in hepatic coma.[185,186] This finding may lead to suspicion of respiratory illness. In one large series of newborn male infants with ornithine transcarbamylase deficiency (n = 74), at the time of

TABLE 14-10 Common Features of Neonatal Hyperammonemic States

Clinical Features
Vomiting, poor feeding
Stupor, coma
Hyperventilation
Seizures

Metabolic Features
Marked hyperammonemia
Aminoacidemia (aminoaciduria)
Respiratory alkalosis

Neuropathological Features
Acute
Brain swelling
Alzheimer type II astrocytes
Variable neuronal injury
Spongy change in white matter
Chronic
Neuronal loss
Myelin deficiency

onset of symptoms at approximately 60 hours of age, mean pH was 7.5 and mean carbon dioxide pressure was 24 mm Hg.[187] Hyperammonemia in the neonatal disorders is marked, the course is fulminating, and mortality is high. Approximately 70% of these infants die, and at least 60% to 80% of survivors are mentally retarded, despite neonatal diagnosis and intervention.[153,163,187-191a] Infants treated from birth (detected because of affected siblings) and *before development of hyperammonemic coma* have had IQs within the low normal range.[163] Neuropathological features have included, acutely, brain swelling, swollen astrocytes with the appearance of Alzheimer type II protoplasmic glia (the hallmark of hyperammonemic encephalopathy),[192-194] variable overt neuronal injury, and mild spongy change in white matter. The chronic neuropathology consists of marked cerebral neuronal loss and myelin deficiency. Management of the affected infants is similar in most respects and is considered separately after discussion of the individual entities. The diagnostic flow chart for neonatal hyperammonemia shown in Figure 14-14 is cited in the discussion of the separate disorders.

Carbamyl Phosphate Synthetase Deficiency (Congenital Hyperammonemia Type I)

Clinical Features. Carbamyl phosphate synthetase deficiency results in hyperammonemia in the first days of life.[153,154,188,191,191a,194-209] The onset has been as early as 24 hours of life and consists principally of vomiting, stupor or coma, and seizures. Infants usually exhibit hypotonia, although hypertonia and opisthotonos have been observed as well. The "respiratory distress" frequently reported may represent the tachypnea of hyperammonemia.

The *clinical course* is fulminating. Approximately 65% to 75% of reported patients have died, usually in the neonatal period. Of the survivors, only a few have been free of mental retardation on follow-up.[188,189,191,202,206,207] Early detection and treatment

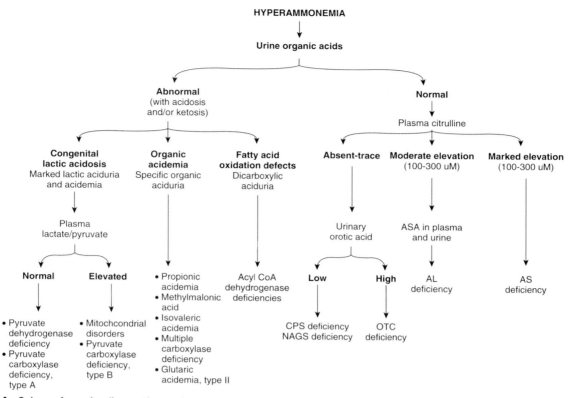

Figure 14-14 **Scheme for major diagnostic considerations in hyperammonemia in the newborn.** Plasma levels of amino acids and lactate and urinary levels of organic acids and orotic acid are important in the diagnostic scheme. AL, argininosuccinate lyase; AS, argininosuccinate synthetase; ASA, argininosuccinic acid; CoA, coenzyme A; CPS, carbamyl phosphate synthetase; CSF, cerebrospinal fluid; NAGS, *N*-acetylglutamate synthetase; OTC, ornithine transcarbamylase.

by dietary and other means are mandatory to preserve significant brain function.

Brain imaging has shown, on CT, findings consistent with severe diffuse cerebral edema. MRI shows particularly bilateral injury to lentiform nuclei (globus pallidus more than putamen), insular and perirolandic cerebral cortex, and subjacent white matter.[32,194,209] Thalamus is relatively spared, a finding helpful in distinction from hypoxic-ischemic encephalopathy.

The *enzymatic defect* is inherited as an autosomal recessive trait. In several large series of cases of urea cycle disorders with neonatal onset, 10% to 20% had carbamyl phosphate synthetase deficiency.[153,184,189,191,191a]

Metabolic Features. Hyperammonemia is moderate to marked in most patients, although levels only two to three times normal have been reported. Other biochemical characteristics include elevated blood glutamine level, absent or trace plasma citrulline level, and normal or diminished urine orotic acid level (see Fig. 14-14). These abnormalities are understandable in view of the pathways of ammonia metabolism (see Fig. 14-12). The occurrence of absent or trace quantities of plasma citrulline is helpful in distinguishing carbamyl phosphate synthetase deficiency from the more distal deficits of the urea cycle.[153,154] However, citrulline levels may be very low in the first days of life in unaffected infants with very low protein intakes.[154,210]

The lack of elevated urinary orotic acid also is useful in distinction from more distal defects (see Fig. 14-14).

Carbamyl phosphate synthetase activity is severely depressed in liver (i.e., none to ≈20% of control values).[153] The enzymatic defect is also detectable in biopsy specimens of duodenal and rectal tissue.[202,211] The deficiency in enzymatic activity is related to a disturbance of enzyme quantity with neither immunoreactive enzyme protein nor mRNA for the enzyme detectable.[212,213] The gene is located on the distal long arm of chromosome 2 (2q35), and mutations have been identified.[153,214]

Rare infants with a *defect in synthesis of N-acetylglutamate*, the allosteric activator of carbamyl phosphate synthetase, and thereby with deficient activity of the enzyme have been reported.[215-220] This disorder at later ages appears to be amenable to treatment with *N*-carbamyl-L-glutamate.[220] The latter substance is a structural analogue of *N*-acetylglutamate that activates carbamyl phosphate synthetase in vitro and is resistant to hepatic degradation. The analogue leads to improvement in hyperammonemia in hours and has been used as a diagnostic test.[221]

Neuropathology. Neuropathological data are few.[194,222] The most consistent findings are the presence acutely of swollen astrocytes with the characteristics of Alzheimer type II glia and brain swelling.

The findings of brain swelling and swollen astrocytes were reproduced by acute hyperammonemia in the young monkey.[223] Neuronal injury can be severe acutely and may reflect excitotoxic injury secondary to hyperammonemia (see earlier discussion). Subsequent brain imaging findings suggest both cortical neuronal and cerebral white matter atrophy.[153,194,197,199,209] Among deep nuclear structures a predilection for putamen and globus pallidus, with relative sparing of thalamus, was noted earlier. The possibility that the oligodendroglial-myelin disturbance also could be related, at least in part, to excitatory amino acids, was discussed earlier.

Ornithine Transcarbamylase Deficiency (Congenital Hyperammonemia Type II)

Clinical Features. Ornithine transcarbamylase deficiency, the most common of the urea cycle defects, results in a severe neonatal syndrome in male infants.[153,154,187-189,191,191a,208,224-234] The disease in female patients is later in onset and is less severe. However, neonatal onset has been reported in approximately 2% of affected female patients, and approximately 50% of male patients with ornithine transcarbamylase deficiency present after the neonatal period.[189,191,231,235,236] Among neonatal-onset urea cycle disorders, ornithine transcarbamylase deficiency accounts for 55% to 60% of cases.[153,184,190,191,191a] As with carbamyl phosphate synthetase deficiency, the affected infant, a boy in nearly all cases, is normal at birth and appears well for the first day or so after birth. The characteristic syndrome of feeding difficulty, stupor, seizures, hypotonia (more often than hypertonia), and tachypnea then appears and evolves rapidly. If not detected promptly and treated, infants progress to coma and death in the first week of life.[153,187,189] In one large series, 46% of infants died in the neonatal period.[187] However, with very early detection and therapy (see following sections), most infants survive the neonatal period, and of long-term survivors, 30% to 60% are not overtly mentally retarded on follow-up.[187,188] However, normal cognitive outcome is rare.

Brain imaging shows findings, on CT, consistent with diffuse cerebral edema during the acute period. MRI shows injury in cerebral cortex, especially depths of sulci, basal ganglia, especially globus pallidus and putamen, and subcortical white matter (Fig. 14-15).[32]

The *enzymatic defect* is inherited as an X-linked trait.[153,233,237] In general, severe neonatal disease occurs in hemizygous male infants, and heterozygous female infants exhibit later onset and generally milder disease. In affected families, ornithine transcarbamylase deficiency was complete in the male patients and partial in the female patients. Fathers were normal, and mothers exhibited partial enzymatic deficiency. The gene is located on the short arm of the X-chromosome (Xp21.1), and approximately 140 mutations have been identified.[153,232]

Metabolic Features. Hyperammonemia and elevated blood glutamine levels occur, as with carbamyl phosphate synthetase deficiency; however, in addition, orotic acid (and related pyrimidine metabolites) appears in the blood and is excreted in large amounts in the urine.[153,154,187,228] This feature reflects overproduction because of the excessive amounts of carbamyl phosphate available (see Fig. 14-12), and it is helpful in distinguishing ornithine transcarbamylase deficiency from carbamyl phosphate synthetase deficiency (see Fig. 14-14). The prominent respiratory alkalosis was noted earlier.

Most male infants affected with the malignant neonatal form of ornithine transcarbamylase deficiency have less than 2% of normal hepatic enzymatic activity.[153] The enzymatic defect is also demonstrable in leukocytes and in duodenal or rectal tissue.[202,211,232,238]

Neuropathology. The relatively scant neuropathological data provide evidence of brain swelling and Alzheimer type II astrocytes with acute encephalopathy. The occurrence of symmetrical infarcts, with cavitation, particularly at the base of sulci and located at the junction of gray and white matter, is of particular interest (Fig. 14-16) because this lesion is considered characteristic of diminished cerebral perfusion in the context of brain swelling and increased intracranial pressure.[239,240] In severe cases, the neuropathological features evolve promptly to neuronal necrosis in cerebral cortex and basal ganglia and to spongiform change of cerebral white matter.[241-243] The chronic neuropathological sequelae are cortical neuronal and cerebral white matter atrophy. The earlier cysts subsequently may evolve to areas of cortical ulegyria.[243]

Two detailed neuropathological studies of infants who died 1 and 6 years after severe neonatal disease demonstrated almost total destruction of cerebral cortex and subjacent cerebral white matter, with numerous Alzheimer type II astrocytes throughout.[243,244] Because the patients died long after the neonatal period and had numerous seizures, it is difficult to determine how much of the brain injury related solely to the metabolic defect. In another case, "mild sponginess" of the cerebral white matter with numerous Alzheimer type II astrocytes was observed.[230] As noted earlier, the astrocytic change is a characteristic abnormality of the hyperammonemic encephalopathy observed in older patients with hepatic disease and in experimental animals.[192,193] Neuronal abnormalities of the type observable after hypoxic-ischemic insult have been reported,[230] and these findings raise the possibility of excitotoxic neuronal death (see earlier discussion).

Argininosuccinic Acid Synthetase Deficiency (Citrullinemia)

Clinical Features. Argininosuccinic acid synthetase deficiency occurs in several clinical forms, including a severe neonatal variety. In several large series, argininosuccinic acid synthetase deficiency accounted for approximately 15% to 20% of cases of urea cycle disorders with neonatal onset, and approximately 80% of cases of argininosuccinic acid synthetase deficiency were of neonatal onset.[153,184,189-191] In neonatal-onset

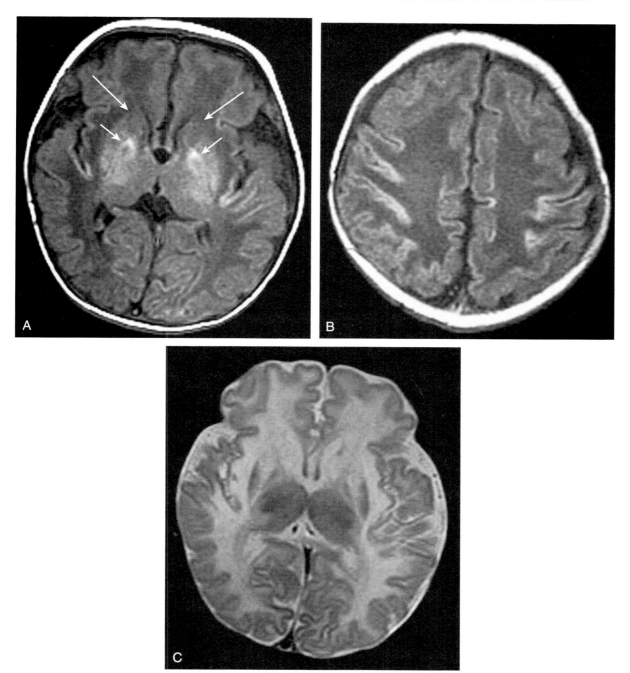

Figure 14-15   Ornithine transcarbamylase deficiency, magnetic resonance imaging scans. A and **B,** Short-echo 550/16 images show hyperintensity in the lentiform nuclei, particularly the globi pallidi *(small white arrows),* insular cortex, and perirolandic cortex, in addition to hypointensity of the caudate heads *(large white arrows).* **C,** Axial T2-weighted image shows diffusely abnormal hyperintensity of the white matter (which is isointense to cerebrospinal fluid and the basal ganglia, indicating diffuse edema). *(From Barkovich AJ:* Pediatric Neuroimaging, *4th ed, Philadelphia: 2005, Lippincott Williams & Wilkins.)*

cases, following a brief symptom-free period after birth, the clinical syndrome begins in the first few days of life. Onset on the first postnatal day, before the institution of feeding, has been reported.[154,212] Most commonly, however, the onset is between 24 and 72 hours of age. Poor feeding, vomiting, tachypnea, alteration of muscle tone, and seizures are the most common features.[63,153,188,245-257] A careful study of the EEG in three affected infants showed the burst-suppression pattern typical of neonatal hyperammonemia and a

close correlation of the severity of the pattern (i.e., the length of the interburst interval) on the EEG with both the degree of hyperammonemia and depression of level of consciousness (Figs. 14-17 and 14-18).[253] Brain imaging shows findings similar to those described for carbamyl phosphate synthetase deficiency and ornithine transcarbamylase deficiency (see earlier). In the initial series of reported cases, nearly all infants died in the neonatal period. In two relatively large later series, only 1 of 23 infants died, but 16 of the 18 survivors were

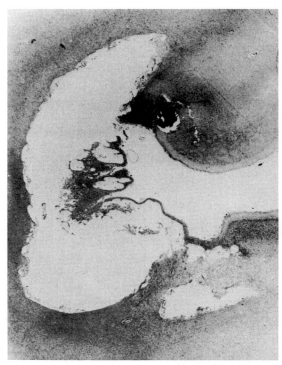

Figure 14-16 **Cystic necrosis of cerebral cortex and immediately subjacent subcortical white matter in ornithine transcarbamylase deficiency.** The infant died at 17 days of age. *(From Filloux F, Townsend JJ, Leonard C: Ornithine transcarbamylase deficiency: Neuropathologic changes acquired in utero, J Pediatr 108:942–945, 1986.)*

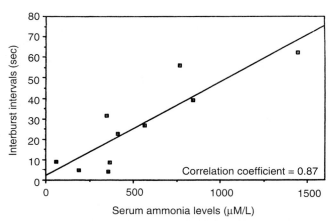

Figure 14-18 **Correlation of serum ammonia levels and interburst intervals in three newborns with citrullinemia.** Note the significant linear relationship between the serum ammonia levels and the interburst durations in three newborns with citrullinemia. *(From Clancy RR, Chung HJ: EEG changes during recovery from acute severe neonatal citrullinemia, Electroencephalogr Clin Neurophysiol 78:222–227, 1991.)*

mentally retarded on follow-up.[188,189] The mode of inheritance is autosomal recessive.[153]

Metabolic Features. Hyperammonemia with citrullinemia often is not as marked as in carbamyl phosphate synthetase and ornithine transcarbamylase deficiencies.[246-248] A massive increase in plasma concentration of citrulline is characteristic (see Fig. 14-14). Orotic aciduria may also occur (see Fig. 14-12).

Affected newborns have exhibited hepatic activities of argininosuccinic acid synthetase that are less than 20%

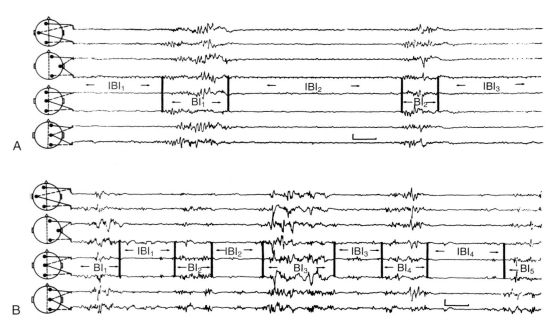

Figure 14-17 **Burst-suppression electroencephalogram (EEG) in hyperammonemia caused by severe neonatal citrullinemia.** **A,** Segment of burst-suppression EEG recorded in an infant when the serum ammonia level was 1445 μmol/L. A 10-minute continuous epoch was chosen for quantitative analysis of the burst (e.g., BI_1, BI_2) and interburst (e.g., IBI_1, IBI_2) intervals. **B,** The same patient recorded during recovery after the serum ammonia level fell to 355 μmol/L. Note the markedly decreased duration of the interburst intervals. Calibration: 50 μV, 2 seconds. *(From Clancy RR, Chung HJ: EEG changes during recovery from acute severe neonatal citrullinemia, Electroencephalogr Clin Neurophysiol 78:222–227, 1991.)*

of normal values. The enzymatic defect can be demonstrated readily in cultured skin fibroblasts and in lymphocytes.[258,259] Many different mutations of the gene, located on chromosome 9q, have been identified.[153]

Neuropathology. Infants who have died with the fulminating neonatal disorder have exhibited signs of brain edema. Indeed, in one report, marked elevations of intracranial pressure were documented and were shown to correlate with the severity of the neurological features.[255] Moreover, the characteristic cortical-subcortical cystic infarcts observed with severe neonatal ornithine transcarbamylase deficiency and considered pathognomonic of diminished cerebral perfusion secondary to elevated intracranial pressure have been documented in neonatal citrullinemia.[260] Patients with survival beyond the acute period exhibit features of neuronal loss, impaired myelin formation, and Alzheimer type II glial cells.[245,246,248,251]

Argininosuccinase Deficiency (Argininosuccinic Aciduria)

Clinical Features. One of the several clinical forms of argininosuccinase (argininosuccinic acid lyase) deficiency is a severe neonatal type.[153,154,189] In several series, approximately 10% to 15% of patients with urea cycle disorders of neonatal onset exhibited this enzyme deficiency, and approximately 80% of patients with argininosuccinic deficiency had a neonatal onset.[153,184,189,191,191a] As in the other neonatal forms of urea cycle defects, apparently normal newborn infants develop symptoms after approximately 24 hours of life. Poor feeding, stupor, and tachypnea, progressing to vomiting, seizures, and coma, constitute the clinical syndrome.[153,156,188,189,261-267] Abnormally fragile hair, characterized by dry, brittle strands with microscopically visible nodular swellings of the shafts (trichorrhexis nodosa), has been observed at as early as 2 weeks of age.[267] Although most of the initially reported patients died in the neonatal period, later experience indicated that only the minority of patients whose condition is detected and treated from the neonatal period die.[188,189,191] However, nearly all survivors are mentally retarded on follow-up examinations. The neonatal form of argininosuccinase deficiency is inherited as an autosomal recessive trait.[212]

Metabolic Features. Hyperammonemia and increased levels of argininosuccinic acid and, to a lesser extent, citrulline in blood and urine are present in the neonatal cases (see Fig. 14-14). Elevated blood glutamine levels and prominent orotic aciduria reflect the alternate pathways of ammonia metabolism (see Fig. 14-12).

Argininosuccinase activity is uniformly severely depressed in liver.[153] The enzymatic defect is detectable in cultured skin fibroblasts as well. Enzyme activity in brain is relatively spared.[268] The gene is located on chromosome 7q.

Neuropathology. The acute neuropathology is likely to be similar to that described earlier for the other

defects of the urea cycle but has not been reported, to my knowledge. Impressive disturbances of myelination have been described in chronic cases.[261,269] In the study of Solitare and co-workers,[269] a patient 8 months of age had an extensive deficit in myelin, with the only significant myelin observed in the dorsal columns of the spinal cord. The likelihood that this observation reflected a disturbance in myelin *formation* rather than myelin destruction is indicated by the absence of myelin breakdown products or of gliosis in the affected areas. The earlier discussion of potential glutamate-induced oligodendroglial injury may be relevant in this context. In addition to these deficits, the patient had numerous astrocytes of the Alzheimer type II variety.

Arginase Deficiency (Hyperargininemia)

Arginase deficiency, although identified at birth by measurement of the plasma arginine level in siblings of a previously affected patient, generally is not characterized by distinct clinical abnormalities in the newborn period.[153,270,271] In a series of 92 cases of urea cycle disorders of neonatal onset, only a single case of arginase deficiency was found.[189] In one more recent neonatal case, blood ammonia was only slightly elevated (194 μg/dL [114 μmol/L], with normal <100 μg/dL).[171] However, the infant evolved on the second to third day from tachypnea to multiple seizures to apnea and coma. MRI showed diffuse edema, and CSF *glutamine* was markedly elevated (9587 μmol/L, with the upper limit of normal 771 μmol/L). The infant died despite hemodialysis. A postmortem examination revealed acute neuronal injury throughout cerebral cortex, with Alzheimer type II astrocytes and diffuse gliosis of cerebral white matter. The findings strongly support the role of *glutamine* as the toxic factor in this and other urea cycle disorders.

In the more common later-onset cases of arginase deficiency, the clinical syndrome becomes apparent later in infancy and is characterized by recurrent vomiting, spastic diplegia, epilepsy, and mental retardation, often with distinct progression of neurological deficits.[153,271-274] Dietary therapy begun at 18 hours of age in a sibling of an affected child (plasma arginine level elevated at 3 hours of age) resulted in normal growth and neurological development at 32 months of age.[270]

Other Inherited Metabolic Disorders with Neonatal Hyperammonemia

Various other inherited metabolic disorders may result in hyperammonemia (see Table 14-9). Although metabolic features other than hyperammonemia (particularly acidosis, ketosis, or both) usually predominate, hyperammonemia may dominate the clinical syndrome and may strongly raise the possibility of a primary defect in the urea cycle. These disorders are considered briefly in the following sections.

Organic Acid Disorders

Disorders of organic acid metabolism are discussed in Chapter 15, but it is appropriate here to note that significant hyperammonemia may occur in the neonatal period in several of these disorders, particularly propionic acidemia, methylmalonic acidemias, and beta-ketothiolase deficiency, but also isovaleric acidemia, glutaric aciduria type II, multiple carboxylase deficiency, pyruvate dehydrogenase deficiency, and fatty acid oxidation defects. These disorders are accompanied by acidosis, ketosis, or both (see Fig. 14-14), and are discussed in Chapter 15. The mechanism of the hyperammonemia in the organic acid disorders is unknown, but available data indicate that the coenzyme A derivatives of the accumulated organic acids are potent inhibitors of human liver carbamyl phosphate synthetase (see Chapter 15 for details).[154,275] This observation imparts particular importance to the report of undetectable carbamyl phosphate synthetase activity in liver homogenates from a patient with methylmalonic acidemia.[276]

Lysinuric Protein Intolerance

Lysinuric protein intolerance may have its clinical onset in the neonatal period with poor feeding, vomiting, hypotonia, and hyperammonemia (see Table 14-9).[277] The molecular defect is in the membrane transport of the cationic amino acids lysine, arginine, and ornithine. The mechanism of the hyperammonemia is unknown, although a deficiency of ornithine and perhaps arginine and thereby dysfunction of the urea cycle is possible. Consistent with such a formulation, citrulline, which is transported by a different mechanism in the intestine, abolishes hyperammonemia when it is administered orally. Treatment consists of a low-protein diet and oral citrulline supplementation. Neurological development is generally normal in adequately treated patients.

Hyperornithinemia, Hyperammonemia, and Homocitrullinemia

The clinical features of hyperornithinemia, hyperammonemia, and homocitrullinemia may appear in the first weeks of life with protein intolerance, stupor, and seizures (see Table 14-9).[278-281] Subsequent neurological development may be impaired, but early detection and treatment of hyperammonemia and long-term dietary therapy have been associated with normal neurological development.[279,281] The major biochemical findings include hyperornithinemia and homocitrullinemia, in addition to hyperammonemia and orotic aciduria. The basic defect involves transport of ornithine into the mitochondrion through the ornithine transporter protein,[280,282-284] with ammonia metabolism affected secondarily because of functional impairment at the ornithine transcarbamylase step.

Acquired Disorders with Neonatal Hyperammonemia

Most recognized patients with severe neonatal hyperammonemia have exhibited inherited disorders of the urea cycle or organic acid metabolism. However, other inherited metabolic defects (as just discussed), as well as a variety of acquired disorders, may result in severe neonatal hyperammonemia (see Table 14-9). Hepatic failure and total parenteral nutrition are uncommon examples of the noninherited disorders.[153,285] Worthy of particular attention is *a syndrome of significant hyperammonemia in the preterm infant that appears to be transient and reversible but can be fatal if undetected or inadequately treated.*[286-295] This syndrome is reviewed next. Possibly, a related syndrome is hyperammonemia observed after perinatal asphyxia, as discussed in Chapter 9.

Transient Hyperammonemia of the Preterm Infant

Clinical Features. Transient *symptomatic* hyperammonemia of the preterm infant has been described in more than 100 infants (Table 14-11).[286-289,291,292,295-297] Radiographic and clinical evidence of hyaline membrane disease, albeit often mild, is consistent. Many patients are near-term premature infants. The onset of central nervous system phenomena is the first or second postnatal day in most patients, often before any protein-containing feeding or intravenous solution is provided. This very early onset differs from that seen in urea cycle disorders. Seizures are common presenting signs. Stupor progresses rapidly to coma. Pupils frequently are fixed to light, and eyes are not movable by oculocephalic stimulation. Indeed, the combination of coma with absent pupillary responses and eye movements suggested advanced hypoxic-ischemic injury or severe intracranial hemorrhage before the diagnosis of transient symptomatic hyperammonemia was sought and discovered. A dramatic response to exchange transfusion, peritoneal dialysis, or hemodialysis has been observed repeatedly. As many as 10 exchange transfusions may be required to control the hyperammonemia. Spontaneous recovery occurs over days to a week or so.

The *prognosis* for transient hyperammonemia is not clear, in part because the spectrum of the disorder has not been defined precisely. Thus, in the experience of the group that reported the first series of patients, the disorder was "encountered much more frequently than inherited disorders of the urea cycle."[286] *In more recent years, for unknown reasons, this disorder has been much less common.* In view of the fulminating course and the clinical features of transient hyperammonemia of the preterm infant, it is likely that infants with this disorder in the past died with the diagnosis of severe perinatal

TABLE 14-11	Transient Hyperammonemia of the Preterm Infant

Clinical Features
Stupor, coma
Seizures
Fixed, dilated (>midposition) pupils

Metabolic Features
Marked hyperammonemia

Pathogenesis
Combination of slow development of urea cycle function with disturbance in hepatic blood flow or oxygen supply (?)

asphyxia, intracranial hemorrhage, sepsis, and so forth. Conversely, it is also likely that less severely affected patients recovered before the correct diagnosis was established. In reported cases, mortality rates of approximately 20% to 30% and rates of neurological sequelae in survivors of approximately 35% to 45% were documented.[292,295-297] With early detection and appropriate therapy, survival without sequelae is an appropriate and attainable goal in this disorder.

Metabolic Features. Hyperammonemia has been marked (see Table 14-11); initial values range from 844 to 3400 mg/dL, and peak values are as high as 7640 mg/dL. Elevations of plasma glutamine level and orotic acid excretion have been observed. Analysis of the urea cycle enzymes in liver of several infants revealed normal values.

Pathogenesis. The pathogenesis of transient hyperammonemia is unknown. Possible mechanisms include deficiency in the development of urea cycle function, either because of insufficient levels of urea cycle intermediates or enzymatic activities, inadequate hepatic blood flow, platelet aggregation with impairment of the hepatic microcirculation, and hypoxia-ischemia.[286,291-294,298] The possibility that the normal delay in development of the urea cycle is exacerbated in certain infants because of hypoxic-ischemic insult or other causes of impaired hepatic blood flow is raised by available data.

With regard to the possibility of limiting substrate quantities, investigators have shown that approximately 50% of (asymptomatic) preterm infants have an approximately twofold increase in blood ammonia level, accompanied by a decrease in blood arginine and ornithine levels, and that the hyperammonemia can be lowered by the oral administration of arginine.[290,299] One explanation for this *asymptomatic arginine-responsive hyperammonemia* in the preterm infant is inadequate activation by arginine of the synthesis of *N*-acetylglutamate, which is necessary for carbamyl phosphate synthetase activity (see Fig. 14-12). The cause of the decreased levels of arginine is unclear. Whether this defect in normal preterm infants is exacerbated greatly by illness, such as respiratory disease, and then results in the massive hyperammonemia of the symptomatic syndrome just described remains to be determined. The occurrence of marked hyperammonemia in severely asphyxiated newborn infants (see Chapter 9) suggests further the possibility that transient hyperammonemia of the preterm "may represent the extreme end of the spectrum of disease that occurs in sick or asphyxiated premature infants."[286] A detailed study showed that transient *asymptomatic* hyperammonemia, whether or not treated with arginine in the neonatal period, is followed by normal neurological outcome at 30 months of age.[290]

Management of Neonatal Hyperammonemia

The basic elements in the management of the infant with hyperammonemia are shown in Table 14-12.

Not all aspects of management are applicable to every patient, and these differences are discussed subsequently.

Antenatal Diagnosis and Prevention

Antenatal diagnosis is of particular value with defects of the urea cycle. Each of the four defects of the urea cycle discussed earlier can be identified antenatally.[153] Techniques include measurement of an abnormal metabolite in amniotic fluid (the metabolite proximal to the enzymatic defect), analysis of DNA from chorionic villus samples or cultured amniocytes, and enzyme analysis of cultured amniocytes or liver biopsy samples obtained in utero. Details are provided in standard sources.[153] These data can be used to provide either information with regard to therapeutic abortion or early institution of postnatal therapeutic measures.

Early Detection

Detection of the aforementioned disorders as rapidly as possible cannot be overemphasized. The fulminating course of serious neonatal hyperammonemia is observed in all the disorders discussed previously, including transient hyperammonemia of the preterm infant. Early detection and prompt institution of therapy may make the difference between the onset of irreversible central nervous system injury and recovery.

A striking demonstration of the importance of prompt intervention is derived from a study of two large series, consisting of 116 infants with neonatal hyperammonemic coma secondary to congenital defects of the urea cycle.[188,189] Survival rates were 34% and 92% in the two studies. In the series with the better survival rate, although 92% of infants survived the neonatal period, approximately 80% of the survivors were mentally retarded (mean IQ, 43), and 17% had seizure disorders, despite careful management of diet and the utilization of supplements to increase alternative pathways of waste nitrogen excretion. The most distinct correlate of outcome was *duration of neonatal coma;* four of five infants with coma for less than 3 days had a normal IQ on follow-up versus none of seven with coma for more than 5 days.

TABLE 14-12	**Management of Neonatal Hyperammonemia**
Antenatal Diagnosis and Prevention	
Early Neonatal Detection	
Ammonia Removal	
Hemodialysis, peritoneal dialysis, hemofiltration	
Alternate Pathways	
Benzoate, phenylacetate, phenylbutyrate, citrulline, arginine	
Dietary	
Protein restriction, essential amino acids, nonprotein caloric sources	
Excitatory Amino Acid Antagonists (?)	
Gene Therapy (?)	
Liver transplantation, virally mediated gene transfer	

Subsequent work confirmed the importance of duration of severe hyperammonemia.[163,184,191a,300]

The *initial or peak ammonia level* may contribute prognostic information; in a large series of 88 patients with urea cycle disorders, when plasma ammonia concentrations exceeded 300 µmol/L initially or 480 µmol/L at peak, none of the patients had a normal cognitive outcome.[190] However, these data were obtained by questionnaires, and treatment was carried out to a considerable degree at "local hospitals." Moreover, peak ammonia values were not correlated with neurocognitive outcome in other work.[163] Therefore, the threshold values should be interpreted cautiously. I consider *duration* more important than absolute levels of blood ammonia in determination of outcome.

Careful observations of 15 infants with defects of the urea cycle, *treated prospectively from birth*, indicated a distinctly more favorable prognosis than that observed in infants treated because of hyperammonemic coma.[301] Thus, of the 12 survivors studied, only 1 was mentally retarded, 4 were within the range of normal intelligence, and the remaining 7 had only mild deficits. The only newborns who died were 3 of the 8 with ornithine transcarbamylase deficiency.

Ammonia Removal

The major therapeutic approaches for the rapid removal of ammonia (and glutamine) are hemodialysis, peritoneal dialysis, and hemofiltration techniques (see Table 14-12).[58,60,153,154,187,300,302-306] In the late 1980s, the major choice for therapy was between *peritoneal dialysis* and *exchange transfusion*.[212] A large study showed that peritoneal dialysis is the more effective procedure.[307] The superiority of dialysis over exchange transfusion in the removal of water-soluble metabolites (ammonia and glutamine) versus a metabolite confined to the intravascular space (e.g., bilirubin bound to albumin) is perhaps not surprising. Survival rates were 20% in those newborns treated with exchange transfusion, 50% in those treated with peritoneal dialysis after exchange transfusion, and 100% in those treated only with peritoneal dialysis.

Later work demonstrated the superiority of *hemodialysis* relative to peritoneal dialysis.[58,153,154,187,300,302,305,308,309] Indeed, the ammonia clearance is approximately 10-fold greater by hemodialysis than by peritoneal dialysis. However, hemodialysis is a complicated procedure, requiring expensive equipment and considerably skilled personnel. *Hemofiltration techniques* (continuous arteriovenous or venovenous) are somewhat less complex.[60,306] However, ammonia removal by hemofiltration techniques is generally slower and less effective than with hemodialysis, and the latter currently is the preferred approach.[153,187,300]

Alternate Pathways of Waste Nitrogen Excretion

The value of specific supplements in stimulating alternate pathways of waste nitrogen excretion has been established (see Table 14-12; Fig. 14-19).[153,154,163,184,188,191a,256,302-304,310-314] Thus, (*sodium*) *benzoate* results in acylation of glycine, the latter formed from ammonia and bicarbonate, and the resulting hippuric acid is readily excreted. Similarly, (*sodium*) *phenylacetate* acetylates glutamine, the latter formed from ammonia by the transamination of glutamate, which itself is formed by transamination of alphaketoglutarate. The resulting phenylacetylglutamine is readily excreted. More recently, phenylacetate has been superseded by the congener phenylbutyrate,[313,314] and some data suggest that high-dose monotherapy with phenylbutyrate (without sodium benzoate) may provide the best survival rates.[153] In carbamyl phosphate deficiency and ornithine transcarbamylase deficiency, *citrulline* supplementation promotes the formation of argininosuccinate and provides a source of arginine. *Arginine* supplementation stimulates the synthesis and excretion of citrulline in argininosuccinic acid synthetase deficiency and of argininosuccinate in argininosuccinase deficiency (in addition to correcting the hypoargininemia in these two disorders).

Excitatory Amino Acid Antagonists (?)

The observations described earlier (see "Biochemical Effects of Excessive Ammonia") suggest that deleterious effects of elevated glutamine levels, with increased tryptophan influx and metabolism to the excitotoxin quinolinic acid, and the accumulation of extracellular glutamate, both acting at the NMDA receptor, could be crucial in the induction of neuronal death in congenital hyperammonemia. The potential value of administration of an NMDA antagonist, such as dextromethorphan (see earlier sections "Biochemical Effects of Excessive Ammonia" and "Nonketotic Hyperglycinemia"), is raised by experimental and clinical data. However, such therapy will require careful study in a relevant animal model; in a study of quinolinate-induced brain injury in developing rat brain, *pretreatment* with the NMDA receptor antagonist, MK-801, led to enhanced neuronal injury, although treatment with the antagonist *minutes after* quinolinate exposure blocked the injury.[173] More information is needed concerning the issue of excitatory amino acid antagonists in hyperammonemia.

Gene Therapy

Gene therapy in urea cycle disorders has consisted of adenovirally mediated gene transfer, hepatocyte infusion, or liver transplantation.[153,315-319] *Management of neonatal-onset urea cycle disorders has consisted of isolated hepatocyte infusion and especially liver transplantation.* Infusion of isolated hepatocytes obtained by collagenase treatment of donated liver has provided temporary metabolic stability.[317] However, long-term use of this approach currently does not appear feasible. Orthoptic liver transplantation has been of limited long-term neurological benefit in neonatal onset cases when transplantation is instituted after the first year of life. However, two more recent reports of *transplantation at less than 1 year of age (2 to 11 months) in neonatal onset carbamyl phosphate synthetase deficiency and ornithine transcarbamylase deficiency* showed not only major metabolic benefits but also comparatively improved neurological outcomes.[316,319] Although long-term data are lacking, the surviving infants do exhibit delayed

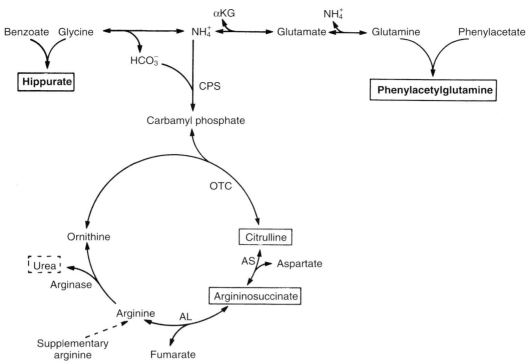

Figure 14-19 Alternate pathways of waste nitrogen excretion in disorders of the urea cycle. Complete deficiencies in carbamyl phosphate synthetase (CPS), ornithine transcarbamylase (OTC), argininosuccinate synthetase (AS), and argininosuccinase (AL) lead to decreased urea synthesis and neonatal hyperammonemic coma. Alternative pathways of nitrogen excretion are as follows. Arginine supplementation stimulates the synthesis and excretion of citrulline in citrullinemia (AS deficiency) and of argininosuccinate in argininosuccinic aciduria (AL deficiency). In all urea cycle disorders, sodium benzoate acylates glycine to form hippurate, and sodium phenylacetate acetylates glutamine to form phenylacetylglutamine. (More recently, sodium phenylbutyrate has been used instead of sodium phenylacetate; see text.) Both waste nitrogen products *(boxed compounds)* are readily excreted in urine. HCO_3^-, bicarbonate; αKG, alpha-ketoglutarate; HCO_4^+, ammonium. *(From Msall M, Batshaw ML, Suss R: Neurologic outcome in children with inborn errors of urea synthesis: Outcome of urea-cycle enzymopathies, N Engl J Med 310:1500, 1984.)*

neurological development. *Nevertheless, aggressive early metabolic management followed by liver transplantation in early infancy may ultimately prove to be the preferred therapy.*

Dietary Therapy

The emergency procedures for ammonia removal described earlier for the newborn with severe hyperammonemia should be followed by appropriate dietary therapy.* The cornerstone of the diet is *low protein content*.[184,204,249,266,267,270,302,303,321] Additionally, abundant *nonprotein calories* and *essential amino acids* are important to prevent protein catabolism. In carbamyl phosphate deficiency and ornithine transcarbamylase deficiency, supplementation with *citrulline*, the important metabolite of the urea cycle just distal to the two enzymatic blocks, is important. Similarly, in argininosuccinic acid synthetase and argininosuccinase deficiencies, *arginine* is the crucial distal amino acid added.

MISCELLANEOUS AMINO ACID DISORDERS

As indicated earlier in this chapter, other disorders of amino acid metabolism have been reported to occur in the newborn period, albeit very rarely (see Table 14-1). Thus, *hypervalinemia*, secondary to a defect in valine

transaminase, has been described in an infant with vomiting, stupor, and delayed development.[21,55,322] *Phenylketonuria* now rarely manifests clinically in the first month of life because of neonatal screening and early intervention[323,324]; vomiting and a peculiar musty odor to the infant's urine, skin, and hair were prominent signs.[325] The enzymatic defect involves phenylalanine hydroxylase. *Lysinuric protein intolerance* is discussed earlier in the section on hyperammonemia, because this rare disorder may have its onset in the newborn period with prominent hyperammonemia. The molecular defect involves transport of cationic amino acids. *Pyridoxine dependency* results in neonatal seizures, sometimes with intrauterine onset, and is discussed in Chapter 5. The defect involves synthesis of GABA. Rare isolated cases of neonatal seizures, other neurological deficits, or both, have been reported with hyperbeta-alaninemia, sarcosinemia, and carnosinemia.[325-334]

REFERENCES

1. Chuang DT, Shih VE: Maple syrup urine disease (branched-chain keto-aciduria). In Schriver CR, Beaudet AL, Sly WS, et al, editors: *The Metabolic and Molecular Bases of Inherited Disease*, 8th ed, New York: 2001, McGraw-Hill.
2. Harris RA, Joshi M, Jeoung NH, Obayashi M: Overview of the molecular and biochemical basis of branched-chain amino acid catabolism, *J Nutr* 135:1527S-1530S, 2005.
3. Dancis J, Snyderman SE: Maple syrup urine disease. In Nelson NM, editor: *Current Therapy in Neonatal-Perinatal Medicine*, Toronto: 1985, Decker.

---

*See references 153,154,184,188,204,302,303,310,311,314,320.

4. Yudkoff M, Daikhin Y, Nissim A, Horyn O, et al: Brain amino acid requirements and toxicity: The example of leucine, *J Nutr* 135:1531S-1538S 2005.

5. Sgaravatti AM, Rosa RB, Schuck PF, Ribeiro CA, et al: Inhibition of brain energy metabolism by the alpha-keto acids accumulating in maple syrup urine disease, *Biochim Biophys Acta* 1639:232-238 2003.

6. Pilla C, Cardozo RF, Dutra-Filho CS, Wyse AT, et al: Creatine kinase activity from rat brain is inhibited by branched-chain amino acids in vitro, *Neurochem Res* 28:675-679 2003.

7. Gortz P, Koller H, Schwahn B, Wendel U, et al: Disturbance of cultured rat neuronal network activity depends on concentration and ratio of leucine and alpha-ketoisocaproate: Implication for acute encephalopathy of maple syrup urine disease, *Pediatr Res* 53:320-324, 2003.

8. Fernstrom JD: Branched-chain amino acids and brain function, *J Nutr* 135:1539S-1546S, 2005.

9. Silberberg DH: Maple syrup urine disease metabolites studied in cerebellum cultures, *J Neurochem* 16:1141-1146, 1969.

10. Dreyfus PM, Prensky AL: Further observations studied on the biochemical lesion in maple syrup urine disease, *Nature* 214:276, 1967.

11. Funchal C, Zamoner A, dos Santos AQ, Moretto MB, et al: Evidence that intracellular Ca^{2+} mediates the effect of alpha-ketoisocaproic acid on the phosphorylating system of cytoskeletal proteins from cerebral cortex of immature rats, *J Neurol Sci* 238:75-82, 2005.

12. Fontella FU, Gassen E, Pulrolnik V, Wannmacher CM, et al: Stimulation of lipid peroxidation in vitro in rat brain by the metabolites accumulating in maple syrup urine disease, *Metab Brain Dis* 17:47-54, 2002.

13. Bridi R, Araldi J, Sgarbi MB, Testa CG, et al: Induction of oxidative stress in rat brain by the metabolites accumulating in maple syrup urine disease, *Int J Dev Neurosci* 21:327-332, 2003.

14. Bridi R, Latini A, Braum CA, Zorzi GK, et al: Evaluation of the mechanisms involved in leucine-induced oxidative damage in cerebral cortex of young rats, *Free Radic Res* 39:71-79, 2005.

15. Bridi R, Braun CA, Zorzi GK, Wannmacher CM, et al: Alpha-keto acids accumulating in maple syrup urine disease stimulate lipid peroxidation and reduce antioxidant defences in cerebral cortex from young rats, *Metab Brain Dis* 20:155-167, 2005.

16. Funchal C, Dos Santos AQ, Jacques-Silva MC, Zamoner A, et al: Branched-chain alpha-keto acids accumulating in maple syrup urine disease induce reorganization of phosphorylated GFAP in C6-glioma cells, *Metab Brain Dis* 20:205-217, 2005.

17. Funchal C, Gottfried C, de Almeida LM, dos Santos AQ, et al: Morphological alterations and cell death provoked by the branched-chain alpha-amino acids accumulating in maple syrup urine disease in astrocytes from rat cerebral cortex, *Cell Mol Neurobiol* 25:851-867, 2005.

18. Funchal C, Gottfried C, De Almeida LM, Wajner M, et al: Evidence that the branched-chain alpha-keto acids accumulating in maple syrup urine disease induce morphological alterations and death in cultured astrocytes from rat cerebral cortex, *Glia* 48:230-240, 2004.

19. Snyderman SE, Norton PM, Roitman E, Holt LE Jr: Maple syrup urine disease with particular reference to dietotherapy, *Pediatrics* 34:454-472, 1964.

20. MacDonald JT, Sher PK: Ophthalmoplegia as a sign of metabolic disease in the newborn, *Neurology* 27:971-973, 1977.

21. Danner DJ, Elsas LJ: Disorders of branched chain amino acid and keto acid metabolism. In Scriver CR, Beaudet AL, Sly WS, et al, editors: *The Metabolic Basis of Inherited Disease*, 6th ed, New York: 1989, McGraw-Hill.

22. Zee DS, Freeman JM, Holtzman NA: Ophthalmoplegia in maple syrup urine disease, *J Pediatr* 84:113-115, 1974.

23. Chhabria S, Tomasi LG, Wong PW: Ophthalmoplegia and bulbar palsy in variant form of maple syrup urine disease, *Ann Neurol* 6:71-72, 1979.

24. Mantovani JF, Naidich TP, Prensky AL, Dodson WE, et al: MSUD: Presentation with pseudotumor cerebri and CT abnormalities, *J Pediatr* 96:279-281, 1980.

25. Mikati MA, Dudin GE, Der Kaloustian VM, Benson PF, et al: Maple syrup urine disease with increased intracranial pressure, *Am J Dis Child* 136:642-643, 1982.

26. Wendel U, Rudiger HW, Passarge E, Mikkelsen M: Maple syrup urine disease: Rapid prenatal diagnosis by enzyme assay, *Humangenetik* 19:127-128, 1973.

27. Morton DH, Strauss KA, Robinson DL, Puffenberger EG, et al: Diagnosis and treatment of maple syrup disease: A study of 36 patients, *Pediatrics* 109:999-1008, 2002.

28. Tharp BR: Unique EEG pattern (comb-like rhythm) in neonatal maple syrup urine disease, *Pediatr Neurol* 8:65-68, 1992.

29. Geal-Dor M, Adelman C, Levi H, Goitein K, et al: Changes in the auditory nerve brainstem evoked responses in a case of maple syrup urine disease, *Dev Med Child Neurol* 46:184-186, 2004.

30. Tu YF, Chen CY, Lin YJ, Chang YC, et al: Neonatal neurological disorders involving the brainstem: Neurosonographic approaches through the squamous suture and the foramen magnum, *Eur Radiol* 15:1927-1933, 2005.

31. Fariello G, Dionisi-Vici C, Orazi C, Malena S, et al: Cranial ultrasonography in maple syrup urine disease, *AJNR Am J Neuroradiol* 17:311-315, 1996.

32. Barkovich AJ: *Pediatric Neuroimaging*, 4th ed, Philadelphia: 2005, Lippincott Williams & Wilkins.

33. Cavalleri F, Berardi A, Burlina AB, Ferrari F, et al: Diffusion-weighted MRI of maple syrup urine disease encephalopathy, *Neuroradiology* 44:499-502, 2002.

34. Ha JS, Kim TK, Eun BL, Lee HS, et al: Maple syrup urine disease encephalopathy: A follow-up study in the acute stage using diffusion-weighted MRI, *Pediatr Radiol* 34:163-166, 2004.

35. Jan W, Zimmerman RA, Wang ZJ, Berry GT, et al: MR diffusion imaging and MR spectroscopy of maple syrup urine disease during acute metabolic decompensation, *Neuroradiology* 45:393-399, 2003.

36. Righini A, Ramenghi LA, Parini R, Triulzi F, et al: Water apparent diffusion coefficient and T2 changes in the acute stage of maple syrup urine disease: Evidence of intramyelinic and vasogenic-interstitial edema, *J Neuroimaging* 13:162-165, 2003.

37. Patay Z: Diffusion-weighted MR imaging in leukodystrophies, *Eur Radiol* 15:2284-2303, 2005.

38. Parmar H, Sitoh YY, Ho L: Maple syrup urine disease: Diffusion-weighted and diffusion-tensor magnetic resonance imaging findings, *J Comput Assist Tomogr* 28:93-97, 2004.

39. Sakai M, Inoue Y, Oba H, Ishiguro A, et al: Age dependence of diffusion-weighted magnetic resonance imaging findings in maple syrup urine disease encephalopathy, *J Comput Assist Tomogr* 29:524-527, 2005.

40. Schonberger S, Schweiger B, Schwahn B, Schwarz M, et al: Dysmyelination in the brain of adolescents and young adults with maple syrup urine disease, *Mol Genet Metab* 82:69-75, 2004.

41. Nellis MM, Kasinski A, Carlson M, Allen R, et al: Relationship of causative genetic mutations in maple syrup urine disease with their clinical expression, *Mol Genet Metab* 80:189-195, 2003.

42. Haymond MW, Karl IE, Feigin RD, DeVivo D, et al: Hypoglycemia and maple syrup urine disease: Defective gluconeogenesis, *Pediatr Res* 7:500-508, 1973.

43. Menkes JH, Hurst PL, Craig JM: A new syndrome: Progressive familial infantile cerebral dysfunction associated with an unusual urinary substance, *Pediatrics* 14:462-467, 1954.

44. Crome L, Dutton G, Ross CF: Maple syrup urine disease, *J Pathol Bacteriol* 81:379-384, 1961.

45. Silberman J, Dancis J, Feigin I: Neuropathological observations in maple syrup urine disease, *Arch Neurol* 5:351-363, 1961.

46. Menkes JH, Philippart M, Fiol RE: Cerebral lipids in maple syrup urine disease, *J Pediatr* 66:584-594, 1965.

47. Menkes JH, Solcher H: Maple syrup urine disease: Effects of diet therapy on cerebral lipids, *Arch Neurol* 16:486-491, 1967.

48. Voyce MA, Montgomery JN, Crome L, Bowman J, et al: Maple syrup urine disease, *J Ment Defic Res* 11:231-238, 1967.

49. Kamei A, Takashima S, Chan F, Becker LE: Abnormal dendritic development in maple syrup urine disease, *Pediatr Neurol* 8:145-147, 1992.

50. Samorajski T, Friede RL, Reimer PR: Hypomyelination in the quaking mouse: Model for the analysis of disturbed myelin formation, *J Neuropathol Exp Neurol* 29:507-523, 1970.

51. Torii J, Adachi M, Volk BW: Histochemical and ultrastructural studies of inherited leukodystrophy in mice, *J Neuropathol Exp Neurol* 30:278-289, 1971.

52. Watanabe I, Bingle GJ: Dysmyelination in "quaking" mouse: An electron microscope study, *J Neuropathol Exp Neurol* 31:352-369, 1972.

53. Prensky AL, Carr S, Moser HW: Development of myelin in inherited disorders of amino acid metabolism, *Arch Neurol* 19:552-558, 1968.

54. Muller K, Kahn T, Wendel U: Is demyelination a feature of maple syrup urine disease? *Neuropediatrics* 9:375-382, 1993.

55. Chuang DT, Shih VE: Disorders of branched chain amino acid and keto acid metabolism. In Scriver CR, Beaudet AL, Sly WS, editors: *The Metabolic and Molecular Bases of Inherited Disease*, 7th ed, New York: 1995, McGraw-Hill.

56. Dancis J: Maple syrup urine disease. In Dorfman A, editor: *Antenatal Diagnosis*, Chicago: 1972, University of Chicago Press.

57. Kaplan P, Mazur A, Field M, Berlin JA, et al: Intellectual outcome in children with maple syrup urine disease, *J Pediatr* 119:46-50, 1991.

57a. Simon E, Fingerhut R, Baumkotter J, Konstantopoulou V, et al: Maple syrup urine disease: favourable effect of early diagnosis by newborn screening on the neonatal course of the disease, *J Inherit Metab Dis* 29:532-537, 2006.

58. Rutledge SL, Havens PL, Haymond MW, McLean RH, et al: Neonatal hemodialysis: Effective therapy for the encephalopathy of inborn errors of metabolism, *J Pediatr* 116:125-128, 1989.

59. Puliyanda DP, Harmon WE, Peterschmitt MJ, Irons M, et al: Utility of hemodialysis in maple syrup urine disease, *Pediatr Nephrol* 17:239-242, 2002.

60. Thompson GN, Butt WW, Shann FA, Kirby DM, et al: Continuous venovenous hemofiltration in the management of acute decompensation in inborn errors of metabolism, *J Pediatr* 118:879-884, 1991.

61. Hoffmann B, Helbling C, Schadewaldt P, Wendel U: Impact of longitudinal plasma leucine levels on the intellectual outcome in patients with classic MSUD, *Pediatr Res* 59:17-20, 2006.

62. Clow CL, Reade TM, Scriver CR: Outcome of early and long-term management of classical maple syrup urine disease, *Pediatrics* 68:856-862, 1981.

63. Nyhan WL: Nonketotic hyperglycinemia. In Scriver CR, Beaudet AL, Sly WS, et al, editors: *The Metabolic Basis of Inherited Disease*, 6th ed, New York: 1989, McGraw-Hill.
64. Hamosh A, Johnston MV: Nonketotic hyperglycinemia. In Schriver CR, Beaudet AL, Sly WS, et al, editors: *The Metabolic and Molecular Bases of Inherited Disease*, 8th ed, New York: 2001, McGraw-Hill.
65. Agamanolis DP, Potter JL, Lundgren DW: Neonatal syndrome associated with subclinical varicella zoster virus and influenza A infection, *Pediatr Neurol* 9:140-143, 1993.
66. Kish SJ, Dixon LM, Burnham WM, Perry TL, et al: Brain neurotransmitters in glycine encephalopathy, *Ann Neurol* 24:458-461, 1988.
67. Patel J, Zinkand WC, Thompson C, Keith R, et al: Role of glycine in the N-methyl-D-aspartate-mediated neuronal cytotoxicity, *J Neurochem* 54:849-854, 1990.
68. McDonald JW, Johnston MV: Physiological and pathophysiological roles of excitatory amino acids during central nervous system development, *Brain Res Brain Res Rev* 15:41-70, 1990.
69. Aprison MH, Davidoff RA, Werman R: Glycine: Its metabolic and possible transmitter roles in nervous tissue, *Handbook Neurochem* 3:381-404, 1970.
70. Krnjevic K: Chemical nature of synaptic transmission in vertebrates, *Physiol Rev* 54:418, 1974.
71. Tada K, Kure S: Nonketotic hyperglycinemia: Molecular lesions and pathophysiology, *Int Pediatr* 8:52-59, 1993.
72. Cherubini E, Gaiarsa JL, Ben-Ari Y: GABA: An excitatory transmitter in early postnatal life, *Trends Neurosci* 14:515-519, 1991.
73. Dzhala VI, Talos DM, Sdrulla DA, Brumback AC, et al: NKCC1 transporter facilitates seizures in the developing brain, *Nat Med* 11:1205-1213, 2005.
74. Slater P, McConnell SE, D'Souza SW, Barson AJ: Postnatal changes in N-methyl-D-aspartate receptor binding and stimulation by glutamate and glycine of [³H]-MK-801 binding in human temporal cortex, *Br J Pharmacol* 108:1143-1149, 1993.
75. Perry TL, Urquhart N, MacLean J: Nonketotic hyperglycinemia, *N Engl J Med* 292:1269-1273, 1975.
76. Perry TL, Urquhart N, Hansen S: Studies of the glycine cleavage enzyme system in brain from infants with glycine encephalopathy, *Pediatr Res* 12:1192-1197, 1977.
77. Motokawa Y, Kikuchi G, Narisawa K, Arakawa T: Reduced level of glycine cleavage system in the liver of hyperglycinemia patients, *Clin Chem Acta* 79:173-181, 1977.
78. Hayasaka K, Tada K, Fueki N, Alkawa J: Prenatal diagnosis of nonketotic hyperglycinemia: Enzymatic analysis of the glycine cleavage system in chorionic villi, *J Pediatr* 116:444-446, 1990.
79. Ichinohe A, Kure S, Mikawa S, Ueki T, et al: Glycine cleavage system in neurogenic regions, *Eur J Neurosci* 19:2365-2370, 2004.
80. Nguyen MD, Julien JP, Rivest S: Innate immunity: The missing link in neuroprotection and neurodegeneration? *Nat Rev Neurosci* 3:216-227, 2002.
81. Tada K, Kure S: Non-ketotic hyperglycinaemia: Molecular lesion, diagnosis and pathophysiology, *J Inherit Metab Dis* 16:691-703, 1993.
82. Applegarth DA, Toone JR: Glycine encephalopathy (nonketotic hyperglycinaemia): Review and update, *J Inherit Metab Dis* 27:417-422, 2004.
83. Ando T, Nyhan WL, Gerritsen T: Metabolism of glycine in the nonketotic form of hyperglycinemia, *Pediatr Res* 2:254-263, 1968.
84. Baumgartner R, Ando T, Nyhan WL: Nonketotic hyperglycinemia, *J Pediatr* 75:1022-1030, 1969.
85. Hamosh A, Johnston MV, Valle D: Nonketotic hyperglycinemia. In Scriver CR, Beaudet AL, Sly WS, et al, editors: *The Metabolic and Molecular Bases of Inherited Disease*, 7th ed, New York: 1995, McGraw-Hill.
86. Hiraga K, Kochi H, Hayasaka K: Defective glycine cleavage system in nonketotic hyperglycinemia: Occurrence of a less active glycine decarboxylase and an abnormal aminomethyl carrier protein, *J Clin Invest* 68:525-534, 1981.
87. Shuman RM, Leech RW, Scott CR: The neuropathology of the nonketotic and ketotic hyperglycinemias: Three cases, *Neurology* 28:139-146, 1978.
88. Bachmann C, Mihatsch MJ, Baumgartner RE: Nicht-ketotische hyperglyzinamie: Perakuter verlauf im neugeborenalter, *Helv Paediatr Acta* 26:228-243, 1971.
89. Ranson BR: Possible pathophysiology of neurologic abnormalities associated with nonketotic hyperglycinemia [letter], *N Engl J Med* 294:1295-1296, 1976.
90. Agamanolis DP, Potter JL, Herrick MK, Sternberger NH: The neuropathology of glycine encephalopathy: A report of five cases with immunohistochemical and ultrastructural observations, *Neurology* 32:975-985, 1982.
91. Arneson D, Ch'ien LT, Chance P, Wilroy RS: Strychnine therapy in nonketotic hyperglycinemia, *Pediatrics* 63:369-373, 1979.
92. Slager UT, Berggren RL, Marubayashi S: Nonketotic hyperglycinemia: Report of a case and review of the clinical, chemical and pathological changes, *Ann Neurol* 1:399-402, 1977.
93. Von Wendt L, Simila S, Saukkonen AL, Koivisto M: Failure of strychnine treatment during the neonatal period in three Finnish children with nonketotic hyperglycinemia, *Pediatrics* 65:1166-1169, 1980.
94. Von Wendt L, Simila S, Saukkonen AL: Prenatal brain damage in nonketotic hyperglycinemia, *Am J Dis Child* 135:1072, 1981.
95. Garcia-Castro JM, Isales-Forsythe CM, Levy HL: Prenatal diagnosis of nonketotic hyperglycinemia, *N Engl J Med* 306:79-81, 1982.
96. Langan TJ, Pueschel SM: Nonketotic hyperglycinemia: Clinical, biochemical and therapeutic considerations, *Curr Probl Pediatr* 13:130, 1983.
97. Scher MS, Bergman I, Ahdab-Barmada M, Fria T: Neurophysiological and anatomical correlations in neonatal nonketotic hyperglycinemia, *Neuropediatrics* 17:137-143, 1986.
98. Press GA, Barshop BA, Haas RH, Nyhan WL, et al: Abnormalities of the brain in nonketotic hyperglycinemia: MR manifestations, *AJNR Am J Neuroradiol* 10:315-321, 1988.
99. Holmqvist P, Polberger S: Neonatal non-ketotic hyperglycinemia (NKH) diagnoses and management in two cases, *Neuropediatrics* 16:191-193, 1985.
100. Lu FL, Wang PJ, Hwu WL, Tsou Yau KI, et al: Neonatal type of nonketotic hyperglycinemia, *Pediatr Neurol* 20:295-300, 1999.
101. Chen PT, Young C, Lee WT, Wang PJ, et al: Early epileptic encephalopathy with suppression burst electroencephalographic pattern: An analysis of eight Taiwanese patients, *Brain Dev* 23:715-720, 2001.
102. Hoover-Fong JE, Shah S, Van Hove JL, Applegarth D, et al: Natural history of nonketotic hyperglycinemia in 65 patients, *Neurology* 63:1847-1853, 2004.
103. Applegarth DA, Toone JR: Glycine encephalopathy (nonketotic hyperglycinemia): Comments and speculations, *Am J Med Genet A* 140:186-188, 2006.
104. Zammarchi E, Donati MA, Ciani F, Pasquini E, et al: Failure of early dextromethorphan and sodium benzoate therapy in an infant with nonketotic hyperglycinemia, *Neuropediatrics* 25:274-276, 1994.
105. Tegtmeyer-Metzdorf H, Roth B, Gunther M, Theisohn M, et al: Ketamine and strychnine treatment of an infant with nonketotic hyperglycinaemia, *Eur J Pediatr* 154:649-653, 1995.
106. Alemzadeh R, Gammeltoft K, Matteson K: Efficacy of low-dose dextromethorphan in the treatment of nonketotic hyperglycinemia, *Pediatrics* 97:924-926, 1996.
107. Boneh A, Degani Y, Harari M: Prognostic clues and outcome of early treatment of nonketotic hyperglycinemia, *Pediatr Neurol* 15:137-141, 1996.
108. Hamosh A, Maher JF, Bellus GA, Rasmussen SA, et al: Long-term use of high-dose benzoate and dextromethorphan for the treatment of nonketotic hyperglycinemia, *J Pediatr* 132:709-713, 1998.
109. Deutsch SI, Rosse RB, Mastropaolo J: Current status of NMDA antagonist interventions in the treatment of nonketotic hyperglycinemia, *Clin Neuropharmacol* 21:71-79, 1998.
110. Markand ON, Garg BP, Brandt IK: Nonketotic hyperglycinemia: Electroencephalographic and evoked potential abnormalities, *Neurology* 32:151-156, 1982.
111. Valavanis A, Schubiger O, Hayek J: Computed tomography in nonketotic hyperglycinemia, *Comput Tomogr* 5:265-270, 1981.
112. Dobyns WB: Agenesis of the corpus callosum and gyral malformations are frequent manifestations of nonketotic hyperglycinemia, *Neurology* 39:817-820, 1989.
113. Kolodny EH: Agenesis of the corpus callosum: A marker for inherited metabolic disease?, *Neurology* 39:847-848, 1989.
114. Nissenkorn A, Michelson M, Ben-Zeev B, Lerman-Sagie T: Inborn errors of metabolism: A cause of abnormal brain development, *Neurology* 56:1265-1272, 2001.
115. Khong PL, Lam BC, Chung BHY, Wong KY, et al: Diffusion-weighted MR imaging in neonatal nonketotic hyperglycinemia, *AJNR Am J Neuroradiol* 24:1181-1183, 2003.
116. Paupe A, Bidat L, Sonigo P, Lenclen R, et al: Prenatal diagnosis of hypoplasia of the corpus callosum in association with non-ketotic hyperglycinemia, *Ultrasound Obstet Gynecol* 20:616-619, 2002.
117. Shah DK, Tingay DG, Fink AM, Hunt RW, et al: Magnetic resonance imaging in neonatal nonketotic hyperglycinemia, *Pediatr Neurol* 33:50-52, 2005.
118. Mourmans J, Majoie CB, Barth PG, Duran M, et al: Sequential MR imaging changes in nonketotic hyperglycinemia, *AJNR Am J Neuroradiol* 27:208-211, 2006.
119. Sener RN: Nonketotic hyperglycinemia: Diffusion magnetic resonance imaging findings, *J Comput Assist Tomogr* 27:538-540, 2003.
120. Sener RN: Diffusion magnetic resonance imaging patterns in metabolic and toxic brain disorders, *Acta Radiol* 45:561-570, 2004.
121. Mourmans J, Majoie CB, Barth PG, Duran M, et al: Sequential MR imaging changes in nonketotic hyperglycinemia, *AJNR Am J Neuroradiol* 27:208-211, 2006.
122. Vila A, Chabrol B, Confort-Gouny FNS, Viout P, et al: Magnetic resonance spectroscopy study of glycine pathways in nonketotic hyperglycinemia, *Pediatr Res* 52:292-300, 2002.
123. Huisman TA, Thiel T, Steinmann B, Zeilinger G, et al: Proton magnetic resonance spectroscopy of the brain of a neonate with nonketotic hyperglycinemia: In vivo–in vitro (ex vivo) correlation, *Eur Radiol* 12:858-861, 2002.
124. Schiffmann R, Kaye EM, Willis JK, Africk D, et al: Transient neonatal hyperglycinemia, *Ann Neurol* 25:201-203, 1989.
125. Luden AS, Davidson A, Goodman SI, Greene CL: Transient nonketotic hyperglycinemia in neonates, *J Pediatr* 114:1013-1015, 1989.
126. Eyskens FJ, Van Doorn JW, Marien P: Neurologic sequelae in transient nonketotic hyperglycinemia of the neonate, *J Pediatr* 121:620-621, 1992.

127. Zammarchi E, Donati MA, Ciani F: Transient neonatal nonketotic hyperglycinemia: A 13-year follow-up, *Neuropediatrics* 36:328-330, 1995.
128. Korman SH, Gutman A: Pitfalls in the diagnosis of glycine encephalopathy (non-ketotic hyperglycinemia), *Dev Med Child Neurol* 44:712-720, 2002.
129. Aliefendioglu D, Aslan AT, Coskun T, Dursun A, et al: Transient nonketotic hyperglycinemia: Two case reports and literature review, *Pediatr Neurol* 28:151-155, 2003.
130. Kure S, Ichinohe A, Kojima K, Sato K, et al: Mild variant of nonketotic hyperglycinemia with typical neonatal presentations: Mutational and in vitro expression analyses in two patients, *J Pediatr* 144:827-829, 2004.
131. Korman SH, Boneh A, Ichinohe A, Kojima K, et al: Persistent NKH with transient or absent symptoms and a homozygous GLDC mutation, *Ann Neurol* 56:139-143, 2004.
132. Flusser H, Korman SH, Sato K, Matsubara Y, et al: Mild glycine encephalopathy (NKH) in a large kindred due to a silent exonic GLDC splice mutation, *Neurology* 64:1426-1430, 2005.
133. Dinopoulos A, Matsubara Y, Kure S: Atypical variants of nonketotic hyperglycinemia, *Mol Genet Metab* 86:61-69, 2005.
134. Wadlington WB, Kilroy A, Ando T: Hyperglycinemia and propionyl CoA carboxylase deficiency and episodic severe illness without consistent ketosis, *J Pediatr* 86:707-712, 1975.
135. Ziter FA, Bray PF, Madsen JA, Nyhan WL: The clinical findings in a patient with nonketotic hyperglycinemia, *Pediatr Res* 2:250-253, 1968.
136. Rushton DI: Spongy degeneration of the white matter of the central nervous system associated with hyperglycinuria, *J Clin Pathol* 21:456-462, 1968.
137. Anderson JM: Spongy degeneration in the white matter of the central nervous system in the newborn: Pathological findings in three infants, one with hyperglycinaemia, *J Neurol Neurosurg Psychiatry* 32:328-337, 1969.
138. Corbeel L, Tada K, Colombo JP: Methylmalonic acidaemia and nonketotic hyperglycinaemia: Clinical and biochemical aspects, *Arch Dis Child* 50:103-109, 1975.
139. Brun A, Borjeson M, Hultberg B: Neonatal non-ketotic hyperglycinemia: A clinical, biochemical and neuropathological study including electron microscopic findings, *Neuropaediatrie* 10:195-205, 1979.
140. Dalla Bernardina B, Aicardi J, Goutieres F, Plouin P: Glycine encephalopathy, *Neuropaediatrie* 10:209-225, 1978.
141. MacDermot KC, Nelson W, Reichert CM, Schulman JD: Attempts at use of strychnine sulfate in the treatment of nonketotic hyperglycinemia, *Pediatrics* 65:61-64, 1980.
142. Scriver CR, White A, Sprague W, Horwood SP: Plasma-CSF glycine ratio in normal and non-ketotic hyperglycinemia subjects, *N Engl J Med* 293:778, 1975.
143. Krieger I, Winbaum ES, Eisenbrey AB: Cerebrospinal fluid glycine in non-ketotic hyperglycinemia: Effect of treatment with sodium benzoate and a ventricular shunt, *Metabolism* 26:517-524, 1977.
144. Hamosh A, McDonald JW, Valle D, Francomano CA, et al: Dextromethorphan and high-dose benzoate therapy for nonketotic hyperglycinemia in an infant, *J Pediatr* 121:131-135, 1992.
145. Heindel W, Kugel H, Roth B: Noninvasive detection of increased glycine content by proton MR spectroscopy in the brains of two infants with nonketotic hyperglycinemia, *AJNR Am J Neuroradiol* 14:629-635, 1993.
146. Gitzelmann R, Steinmann B, Otten A: Nonketotic hyperglycinemia treated with strychnine, a glycine receptor antagonist, *Helv Paediatr Acta* 32:517-525, 1978.
147. Curtis DR, Duggan AW, Johnston GA: The specificity of strychnine as a glycine antagonist in the mammalian spinal cord, *Exp Brain Res* 12:547-565, 1971.
148. Johnson GAR: Amino acid inhibitory transmitters in the central nervous system. In Hockman CH, Bieger D, editors: *Chemical Transmission in the Mammalian Central Nervous System*, Baltimore: 1976, University Park Press.
149. Matalon R, Naidu S, Hughes JR, Michals K: Nonketotic hyperglycinemia: Treatment with diazepam—a competitor for glycine receptors, *Pediatrics* 71:581-584, 1983.
150. Ohya Y, Ochi N, Mizutani N, Hayakawa C, et al: Nonketotic hyperglycinemia: Treatment with NMDA antagonist and consideration of neuropathogenesis, *Pediatr Neurol* 7:65-68, 1991.
151. Schmitt B, Steinmann B, Gitzelmann R, Thun-Hohenstein L, et al: Nonketotic hyperglycinemia: Clinical and electrophysiologic effects of dextromethorphan, an antagonist of the NMDA receptor, *Neurology* 43:421-424, 1993.
152. Chien YH, Hsu CC, Huang A, Chou SP, et al: Poor outcome for neonatal-type nonketotic hyperglycinemia treated with high-dose sodium benzoate and dextromethorphan, *J Child Neurol* 19:39-42, 2004.
153. Brusilow SW, Horwich AL: Urea cycle enzymes. In Schriver CR, Beaudet AL, Sly WS, et al, editors: *The Metabolic and Molecular Bases of Inherited Disease*, 8th ed, New York: 2001, McGraw-Hill.
154. Batshaw ML: Inborn errors of urea synthesis, *Ann Neurol* 35:133-141, 1994.
155. Ratner S: Enzymes of arginine and urea synthesis, *Adv Enzymol Relat Areas Mol Biol* 39:1-90, 1973.
156. Glick NR, Snodgrass PJ, Schafer IA: Neonatal argininosuccinic aciduria with normal brain and kidney but absent liver argininosuccinate lyase activity, *Am J Hum Genet* 28:22-30, 1976.
157. Schenker S, McCandless DW, Brophy E, Lewis M: Studies on the intracerebral toxicity of ammonia, *J Clin Invest* 46:838-848, 1967.
158. Hindfelt B, Siesjo BK: Cerebral effects of acute ammonia intoxication. II. The effect upon energy metabolism, *Scand J Clin Lab Invest* 28:365-374, 1971.
159. Duffy T, Plum F: Seizures and comatose states. In Siegel GJ, Albers RW, Katzman R, et al, editors: *Basic Neurochemistry Boston*, 1976, Little, Brown.
160. Robinson MB, Batshaw ML: Neurotransmitter alterations in congenital hyperammonemia, *Ment Retard Dev Disabil Res Rev* 1:201-207, 1995.
161. Butterworth RF: Effects of hyperammonaemia on brain function, *J Inherit Metab Dis* 21:6-20, 1998.
162. Colombo JP, Bachmann C, Cervantes H, Kokorovic M, et al: Tyrosine uptake and regional brain monoamine metabolites in a rat model resembling congenital hyperammonemia, *Pediatr Res* 39:1036-1040, 1996.
163. Gropman AL, Batshaw ML: Cognitive outcome in urea cycle disorders, *Mol Genet Metab* 81:58-62, 2004.
164. de Graaf AA, Deutz NE, Bosman DK, Chamuleau RA, et al: The use of in vivo proton NMR to study the effects of hyperammonemia in the rat cerebral cortex, *NMR Biomed* 4:31-37, 1991.
165. Hawkins RA, Jessy J: Hyperammonaemia does not impair brain function in the absence of net glutamine synthesis, *Biochem J* 277:697-703, 1991.
166. Jessy J, DeJoseph RM, Hawkins RA: Hyperammonaemia depresses glucose consumption throughout the brain, *Biochem J* 277:693-696, 1991.
167. Chamuleau RA, Boman DK: What the clinician can learn from MR glutamine/glutamate assays, *NMR Biomed* 4:103-108, 1991.
168. Connelly A, Cross JH, Gadian DG, Hunter JV, et al: Magnetic resonance spectroscopy shows increased brain glutamine in ornithine carbamoyl transferase deficiency, *Pediatr Res* 33:77-81, 1993.
169. Rao VLR, Murthy CRK: Hyperammonemic alterations in the metabolism of glutamate and aspartate in rat cerebellar astrocytes, *Neurosci Lett* 138:107-110, 1992.
170. Kanamori K, Ross BD, Chung JC, Kuo EL: Severity of hyperammonemic encephalopathy correlates with brain ammonia level and saturation of glutamine synthetase in vivo, *J Neurochem* 67:1584-1594, 1996.
171. Picker JD, Puga AC, Levy HL, Marsden D, et al: Arginase deficiency with lethal neonatal expression: Evidence for the glutamine hypothesis of cerebral edema, *J Pediatr* 142:349-352, 2003.
172. Batshaw ML, Robinson MB, Hyland K, Djali S, et al: Quinolinic acid in children with congenital hyperammonemia, *Ann Neurol* 34:676-681, 1993.
173. Trescher WH, McDonald JW, Johnston MV: Quinolinate-induced injury is enhanced in developing rat brain, *Dev Brain Res* 83:224-232, 1994.
174. Yan E, Castillo-Melendez M, Smythe G, Walker D: Quinolinic acid promotes albumin deposition in Purkinje cell, astrocytic activation and lipid peroxidation in fetal brain, *Neuroscience* 134:867-875, 2005.
175. Marcaida G, Felipo V, Hermenegildo C, Miñana MD, et al: Acute ammonia toxicity is mediated by the NMDA type of glutamate receptors, *FEBS Lett* 296:67-68, 1992.
176. Kosenko E, Kaminsky Y, Grau E, Miñana MD, et al: Brain ATP depletion induced by acute ammonia intoxication in rats is mediated by activation of the NMDA receptor and Na^+,K^+-ATPase, *J Neurochem* 63:2172-2178, 1994.
177. Schenker S, Breen KJ, Hoyumpa AM: Hepatic encephalopathy: Current status, *Gastroenterology* 66:121-151, 1974.
178. Hindfelt B, Plum F, Duffy TE: Effect of acute ammonia intoxication on cerebral metabolism in rats with portacaval shunts, *J Clin Invest* 59:386-396, 1977.
179. McKhann GM, Tower DB: Ammonia toxicity and cerebral oxidative metabolism, *Am J Physiol* 200:420-424, 1961.
180. Hindfelt B, Siesjo BK: Cerebral effects of acute ammonia intoxication. II. The effect upon energy metabolism, *Scand J Clin Lab Invest* 28:365-374, 1971.
181. Kauppinen RA, Williams SR, Brooks KJ, Bachelard HS: Effects of ammonium on energy metabolism and intracellular pH in guinea pig cerebral cortex studied by ^{31}P and ^1H nuclear magnetic resonance spectroscopy, *Neurochem Int* 19:495-504, 1991.
182. Ratnakumari L, Qureshi IA, Butterworth RF: Effects of congenital hyperammonemia on the cerebral and hepatic levels of the intermediates of energy metabolism in SPF mice, *Biochem Biophys Res Commun* 184:746-751, 1992.
183. Koch R: Introduction to urea cycle symposium, *Pediatrics* 68:271-272, 1981.
184. Wilcken B: Problems in the management of urea cycle disorders, *Mol Genet Metab* 81:S86-S91, 2004.
185. Shannon DC, Wichser J, Kazemi H: Hyperventilation and hyperammonemia, *Pediatr Res* 7:423, 1973.
186. Plum F, Posner JB: *The Diagnosis of Stupor and Coma*, Philadelphia: 1981, FA Davis.
187. Maestri NE, Clissold D, Brusilow SW: Neonatal onset ornithine transcarbamylase deficiency: A retrospective analysis, *J Pediatr* 134:268-272, 1999.
188. Msall M, Batshaw ML, Suss R: Neurologic outcome in children with inborn errors of urea synthesis: Outcome of urea-cycle enzymopathies, *N Engl J Med* 310:1500, 1984.
189. Uchino T, Endo F, Matsuda I: Neurodevelopmental outcome of long-term therapy of urea cycle disorders in Japan, *J Inherit Metab Dis* 21:151-159, 1998.

190. Bachmann C: Outcome and survival of 88 patients with urea cycle disorders: A retrospective evaluation, *Eur J Pediatr* 162:410-416, 2003.
191. Nassogne M, Heron B, Touati G, Rabier D, et al: Urea cycle defects: Management and outcome, *J Inherit Metab Dis* 28:407-414, 2005.
191a. Enns GM, Berry SA, Berry GT, Rhead WJ, et al: Survival after treatment with phenylacetate and benzoate for urea-cycle disorders, *N Engl J Med* 356:2282-2292, 2007.
192. Victor M, Adams RD, Cole M: The acquired (non-Wilsonian) type of chronic hepatocerebral degeneration, *Medicine (Baltimore)* 44:345-396, 1965.
193. Cavanagh JB, Kyu MH: Type II Alzheimer change experimentally produced in astrocytes in the rat, *J Neurol Sci* 12:63-75, 1971.
194. Takeoka M, Soman TB, Shih VE, Caviness VS, et al: Carbamyl phosphate synthetase 1 deficiency: A destructive encephalopathy, *Pediatr Neurol* 24:193-199, 2001.
195. Freeman JM, Nicholson JF, Masland WS: Ammonia intoxication due to a congenital defect in urea synthesis, *J Pediatr* 65:1039-1047, 1964.
196. Hindfelt B, Siesjo BK: Cerebral effects of acute ammonia intoxication. II. The effect upon energy metabolism, *Scand J Clin Lab Invest* 28:365-374, 1971.
197. Arashima S, Matsuda I: A case of carbamyl phosphate synthetase deficiency, *Tohoku J Exp Med* 107:143-147, 1972.
198. Gelehrter TD, Snodgrass PJ: Lethal neonatal deficiency of carbamyl phosphate synthetase, *N Engl J Med* 290:430-433, 1974.
199. Batshaw M, Brusilow S, Walser M: Treatment of carbamyl phosphate synthetase deficiency with keto analogues of essential amino acids, *N Engl J Med* 292:1085-1090, 1975.
200. Oberholzer BB, Palmer T: Increased excretion of N-carbamyl compounds in patients with urea cycle defects, *Clin Chim Acta* 68:73-79, 1976.
201. Hommes FA, de Groot CJ, Wilmink CW, Jonxis JH: Carbamyl-phosphate-synthetase deficiency in an infant with severe cerebral damage, *Arch Dis Child* 44:688-693, 1969.
202. Hoogenraad NJ, Mitchell JD, Don NA: Detection of carbamyl phosphate synthetase I deficiency using duodenal biopsy samples, *Arch Dis Child* 55:292-295, 1980.
203. Jaeken J, Devlieger H, Bachmann C: Carbamyl phosphate synthetase deficiency with lethal neonatal outcome, *Eur J Pediatr* 139:72-75, 1982.
204. Donn SM, Banagale RC: Neonatal hyperammonemia, *Pediatr Rev* 5:203-214, 1984.
205. Kakinuma H, Ohtake A, Ogura N: Two siblings with complete carbamyl phosphate synthetase I deficiency, *Acta Paediatr* 26:16, 1984.
206. Trauner DA, Self TW: Detection of urea cycle enzymopathies in childhood, *Arch Neurol* 41:758-760, 1984.
207. Van de Bor M, Mooy P, van Zoeren D, Berger R, et al: Successful treatment of severe carbamyl phosphate synthetase I deficiency, *Arch Dis Child* 59:1183-1185, 1984.
208. Leonard JV, Morris AA: Urea cycle disorders, *Semin Neonatol* 7:27-35, 2002.
209. Takanashi JI, Barkovich AJ, Cheng SF, Weisiger K, et al: Brain MR imaging in neonatal hyperammonemic encephalopathy resulting from proximal urea cycle disorders, *AJNR Am J Neuroradiol* 24:1184-1187, 2003.
210. Batshaw ML, Berry GT: Use of citrulline as a diagnostic marker in the prospective treatment of urea cycle disorders, *J Pediatr* 118:913-918, 1991.
211. Matsushima A, Orii T: The activity of carbamylphosphate synthetase I (CPS I) and ornithine transcarbamylase (OTC) in the intestine and the screening of OTC deficiency in the rectal mucosa, *J Inherit Metab Dis* 4:83-84, 1981.
212. Brusilow SW, Horwich AL: Urea cycle enzymes. In Schriver CR, Beaudet AL, Sly WS, et al, editors: *The Metabolic and Molecular Bases of Inherited Disease*, 7th ed, New York: 1995, McGraw-Hill.
213. Ohtake A, Miura S, Mori M: A carbamyl phosphate synthetase 1 deficiency with no detectable messenger RNA activity, *Acta Paediatr* 26:262, 1984.
214. Summar ML: Molecular genetic research into carbamoyl-phosphate synthase I: Molecular defects and linkage markers, *J Inherit Metab Dis* 21:30-39, 1998.
215. Bachmann C, Brandis M, Weissenbarth-Riedel E, Burghard R, et al: N-Acetylglutamate synthetase deficiency, a second patient, *J Inherit Metab Dis* 11:191-193, 1988.
216. Schubiger G, Bachmann C, Barben P, Colombo JP, et al: N-Acetylglutamate synthetase deficiency: Diagnosis, management and follow-up of a rare disorder of ammonia detoxication, *Eur J Pediatr* 150:353-356, 1991.
217. Pandya AL, Koch R, Hommes FA, Williams JC: N-Acetylglutamate synthetase deficiency: Clinical and laboratory observations, *J Inherit Metab Dis* 14:685-690, 1991.
218. Guffon N, Vianeysaban C, Bourgeois J, Rabier D, et al: A new neonatal case of N-acetylglutamate synthase deficiency treated by carbamylglutamate, *J Inherit Metab Dis* 18:61-65, 1995.
219. Elpeleg O, Shaag A, Ben-Shalom E, Schmid T, et al: N-acetylglutamate synthase deficiency and the treatment of hyperammonemic encephalopathy, *Ann Neurol* 52:845-849, 2002.
220. Caldovic L, Morizono H, Daikhin Y, Nissim I, et al: Restoration of ureagenesis in N-acetylglutamate synthase deficiency by N-carbamylglutamate, *J Pediatr* 145:552-554, 2004.

221. Guffon N, Schiff M, Cheillan D, Wermuth B, et al: Neonatal hyperammonemia: The N-carbamoyl-L-glutamic acid test, *J Pediatr* 147:260-262, 2005.
222. Friede RL: *Developmental Neuropathology*, 2nd ed, New York: 1989, Springer-Verlag.
223. Voorhies TM, Ehrlich MC, Duffy TE, Petito CK, et al: Acute hyperammonemia in the young primate: Physiologic and neuropathologic correlates, *Pediatr Res* 17:970-975, 1983.
224. Scott CR, Teng CC, Goodman SI: X-linked transmission of ornithine-transcarbamylase deficiency, *Lancet* 2:1148, 1972.
225. Campbell AG, Rosenberg LE, Snodgrass PJ, Nuzum CT: Ornithine transcarbamylase deficiency: A cause of lethal neonatal hyperammonemia in males, *N Engl J Med* 288:1-6, 1973.
226. Kang ES, Snodgrass PJ, Gerald PS: Ornithine transcarbamylase deficiency in the newborn infant, *J Pediatr* 82:642-649, 1973.
227. Goldstein AS, Hoogenraad NJ, Johnson JD: Metabolic and genetic studies of a family with ornithine transcarbamylase deficiency, *Pediatr Res* 8:5-12, 1974.
228. Snyderman SE, Sansaricq C, Phansalkar SV: The therapy of hyperammonemia due to ornithine transcarbamylase deficiency in a male neonate, *Pediatrics* 56:65-73, 1975.
229. Guibaud P, Baxter P, Bourgeois J: Severe ornithine transcarbamylase deficiency: Two and a half years survival with normal development, *Arch Dis Child* 59:477-479, 1984.
230. Kornfeld M, Woodfin BM, Papile L: Neuropathology of ornithine carbamyl transferase deficiency, *Acta Neuropathol (Berl)* 65:261-264, 1985.
231. Pridmore CL, Clarke J, Blaser S: Ornithine transcarbamylase deficiency in females: An often overlooked cause of treatable encephalopathy, *J Child Neurol* 10:369-374, 1995.
232. Tuchman M, Morizono H, Rajagopal BS, Plante RJ, et al: The biochemical and molecular spectrum of ornithine transcarbamylase deficiency, *J Inherit Metab Dis* 21:40-58, 1998.
233. Gordon N: Ornithine transcarbamylase deficiency: A urea cycle defect, *Eur J Paediatr Neurol* 7:115-121, 2003.
234. Valik D, Sedova Z, Starha J, Zeman J, et al: Acute hyperammonaemic encephalopathy in a female newborn caused by a novel, de novo mutation in the ornithine transcarbamylase gene, *Acta Paediatr* 93:710-711, 2004.
235. Lacey DJ, Duffner PK, Cohen ME, Mosovich L: Unusual biochemical and clinical features in a girl with ornithine transcarbamylase deficiency, *Pediatr Neurol* 2:51-53, 1986.
236. Finkelstein JE, Hauser ER, Leonard CO, Brusilow SW: Late-onset ornithine transcarbamylase deficiency in male patients, *J Pediatr* 117:897-902, 1990.
237. Short EM, Conn HO, Snodgrass PJ: Evidence for X-linked dominant inheritance of ornithine transcarbamylase deficiency, *N Engl J Med* 288:7-12, 1973.
238. Wolfe DM, Gatfield PD: Leukocyte urea cycle enzymes in hyperammonemia, *Pediatr Res* 9:531-535, 1975.
239. Filloux F, Townsend JJ, Leonard C: Ornithine transcarbamylase deficiency: Neuropathologic changes acquired in utero, *J Pediatr* 108:942-945, 1986.
240. Janzer RC, Fried RL: Perisulcal infarcts: Lesions caused by hypotension during increased intracranial pressure, *Ann Neurol* 6:399-404, 1979.
241. Harding BN, Leonard JV, Erdohazi M: Ornithine transcarbamylase deficiency: Neuropathological study, *Eur J Pediatr* 141:215-220, 1984.
242. Kendall BE, Kingsley DP, Leonard JV: Neurological features and computed tomography of the brain in children with ornithine transcarbamylase deficiency, *J Neurol Neurosurg Psychiatry* 46:28-34, 1983.
243. Yamanouchi H, Yokoo H, Yuhara Y, Maruyama K, et al: An autopsy case of ornithine transcarbamylase deficiency, *Brain Dev* 24:91-94, 2002.
244. Bruton CJ, Corsellis JA, Russell A: Hereditary hyperammonemia *Brain* 93:423-434, 1970.
245. Van der Zee SP, Trijbels JM, Monnens LA, Hommes FA, et al: Citrullinaemia with rapidly fatal neonatal course, *Arch Dis Child* 46:847-851, 1971.
246. Ghisolfi J, Augier D, Martinez J, Barthe P, et al: Forme neo-natale de citrullinemie a evolution mortelle rapide, *Pediatrie* 28:55-59, 1972.
247. Roerdink FH, Gouw WL, Okken A, van der Blij JF, et al: Citrullinemia: Report of a case, with studies on antenatal diagnosis, *Pediatr Res* 7:863-869, 1973.
248. Wick H, Bachmann C, Baumgartner R, Brechbuhler T, et al: Variants of citrullinaemia, *Arch Dis Child* 48:636-641, 1973.
249. Danks DM, Tippett P, Zentner G: Severe neonatal citrullinaemia, *Arch Dis Child* 49:579-581, 1974.
250. Thoene J, Beach B, Kulovich S: Keto acid treatment of neonatal citrullinemia, *Am J Hum Genet* 27:88, 1975.
251. Martin JJ, Farriaux JP, De Jonghe P: Neuropathology of citrullinaemia, *Acta Neuropathol* 56:303-306, 1982.
252. Donn SM, Thoene JG, Wilson GN: Prevention of neonatal hyperammonemia in citrullinemia, *Pediatr Res* 19:247-253, 1985.
253. Clancy RR, Chung HJ: EEG changes during recovery from acute severe neonatal citrullinemia, *Electroencephalogr Clin Neurophysiol* 78:222-227, 1991.
254. Sanjurjo P, Rodriguez-Soriano J, Vallo A, Arranz A, et al: Neonatal citrullinaemia with satisfactory mental development, *Eur J Pediatr* 150:730-731, 1991.

255. Wayenberg JL, Vermeylen D, Gerlo E, Pardou A: Increased intracranial pressure in a neonate with citrullinaemia, *Eur J Pediatr* 151:132-133, 1992.

256. Melnyk AR, Matalon R, Henry BW, Zeller WP, et al: Prospective management of a child with neonatal citrullinemia, *J Pediatr* 122:96-98, 1993.

257. Majoie CB, Mourmans JM, Akkerman EM, Duran M, et al: Neonatal citrullinemia: Comparison of conventional MR, diffusion-weighted, and diffusion tensor findings, *AJNR Am J Neuroradiol* 25:32-35, 2004.

258. Kennaway NG, Harwood PJ, Ramberg DA, Koler RD, et al: Citrullinemia: Enzymatic evidence for genetic heterogeneity, *Pediatr Res* 9:554-558, 1975.

259. Spector EB, Bloom AD: Citrullinemic lymphocytes in long-term culture, *Pediatr Res* 7:700-705, 1973.

260. Martin JJ, Farriaux JP, De Jonghe PD: Neuropathology of citrullinemia, *Acta Neuropathol (Berl)* 56:303-306, 1982.

261. Baumgartner R, Scheidegger S, Stalder G, Hottinger A: Neonatal death due to argininosuccinic aciduria, *Helv Paediatr Acta* 23:77-106, 1968.

262. Levin B, Dobbs RH: Hereditary metabolic disorders involving the urea cycle, *Proc R Soc Med* 61:773-774, 1968.

263. Carton D, De Schrijver F, Kint J, Van Durme J, et al: Argininosuccinic aciduria: Neonatal variant with rapidly fatal course, *Acta Paediatr Scand* 58:528-534, 1969.

264. Farriaux JP, Pieraert C, Fontaine G: Survival of infant with argininosuccinic aciduria to three months of age [letter], *J Pediatr* 86:639, 1975.

265. Francois B, Cornu G, de Meyer R: Peritoneal dialysis and exchange transfusion in a neonate with argininosuccinic aciduria, *Arch Dis Child* 51:228-231, 1976.

266. Brusilow SW, Batshaw ML: Arginine therapy of argininosuccinase deficiency, *Lancet* 1:124-127, 1979.

267. Collins FS, Summer GK, Schwartz RP, Parke JC: Neonatal argininosuccinic aciduria: Survival after early diagnosis and dietary management, *J Pediatr* 96:429-431, 1980.

268. Perry TL, Wirtz ML, Kennaway NG, Hsia YE: Amino acid and enzyme studies of brain and other tissues in an infant with argininosuccinic aciduria, *Clin Chim Acta* 105:257-267, 1980.

269. Solitare GB, Shih VE, Nelligan DJ, Dolan TF: Argininosuccinic aciduria: Clinical, biochemical, anatomical and neuropathological observations, *J Ment Defic Res* 13:153-170, 1969.

270. Snyderman SE, Sansaricq C, Norton PM, Goldstein F: Argininemia treated from birth, *J Pediatr* 95:61-63, 1979.

271. Prasad AN, Breen JC, Ampola MG, Rosman NP: Argininemia: A treatable genetic cause of progressive spastic diplegia simulating cerebral palsy: Case reports and literature review, *J Child Neurol* 12:301-309, 1997.

272. Cederbaum SD, Shaw KN, Valente M: Hyperargininemia, *J Pediatr* 90:569-573, 1977.

273. Snyderman SE, Sansaricq C, Chen WJ, Norton PM, et al: Argininemia, *J Pediatr* 90:563-568, 1977.

274. Lambert MA, Marescau B, Desjardins M, Laberge M, et al: Hyperargininemia: Intellectual and motor improvement related to changes in biochemical data, *J Pediatr* 118:420-424, 1991.

275. Gruskay JA, Rosenberg LE: Inhibition of hepatic mitochondrial carbamyl phosphate synthetase (CPSI) by acyl CoA esters: Possible mechanism of hyperammonemia in the organic acidemias, *Pediatr Res* 13:475-482, 1979.

276. Shapiro LJ, Bocian ME, Raijman L, Cederbaum SD, et al: Methylmalonyl-CoA mutase deficiency associated with severe neonatal hyperammonemia: Activity of urea cycle enzymes, *J Pediatr* 93:986-988, 1978.

277. Simell O: Lysinuric protein intolerance and other cationic aminoacidurias. In Scriver CR, Beaudet AL, Sly WS, et al, editors: *The Metabolic and Molecular Bases of Inherited Disease,* 8th ed, New York: 2001, McGraw-Hill.

278. Shih VE, Laframboise R, Mandell R, Pichette J: Neonatal form of the hyperornithinaemia, hyperammonaemia, and homocitrullinuria (HHH) syndrome and prenatal diagnosis, *Prenat Diagn* 12:717-723, 1992.

279. Zammarchi E, Ciani F, Pasquini E, Bopnocore G, et al: Neonatal onset of hyperornithinemia-hyperammonemia-homocitrullinuria syndrome with favorable outcome, *J Pediatr* 131:440-443, 1997.

280. Valle D, Simell O: The hyperornithinemias. In Scriver CR, Beaudet AL, Sly WS, et al, editors: *The Metabolic and Molecular Bases of Inherited Disease,* 8th ed, New York: 2001, McGraw-Hill.

281. Salvi S, Santorelli FM, Bertini E, Boldrini R, et al: Clinical and molecular findings in hyperornithinemia-hyperammonemia-homocitrullinuria syndrome, *Neurology* 57:911-914, 2001.

282. Camacho JA, Obie C, Biery B, Goodman BK, et al: Hyperornithinaemia-hyperammonaemia-homocitrullinuria syndrome is caused by mutations in a gene encoding a mitochondrial ornithine transporter, *Nat Genet* 22:151-158, 1999.

283. Tsujino S, Kanazawa N, Ohashi T, Eto Y, et al: Three novel mutations (G27E, insAAC, R179X) in the *ORNT1* gene of Japanese patients with hyperornithinemia, hyperammonemia, and homocitrullinuria syndrome, *Ann Neurol* 47:625-631, 2000.

284. Camacho JA, Mardach R, Rioseco-Camacho N, Ruiz-Pesini E, et al: Clinical and functional characterization of a human ORNT1 mutation (T32R) in the hyperornithinemia-hyperammonemia-homocitrullinuria (HHH) syndrome, *Pediatr Res* 60:423-429, 2006.

285. Glasgow AM, Kapur S, Miller MK, Brudno S: Neonatal hyperammonemia resulting from severe in utero hepatic necrosis, *J Pediatr* 108:136-138, 1986.

286. Ballard RA, Vinocur B, Reynolds JW, Wennberg RP, et al: Transient hyperammonemia of the preterm infant, *N Engl J Med* 299:920-925, 1978.

287. Jaeken J, Devlieger H, Melchior S, Van Paemel G, et al: Transient hyperammonemia in a preterm neonate, *Acta Paediatr Belg* 32:287-288, 1979.

288. Le Guennec JC, Qureshi IA, Bard H, Siriez JY, et al: Transient hyperammonemia in an early preterm infant, *J Pediatr* 96:470-472, 1980.

289. Ellison PH, Cowger ML: Transient hyperammonemia in the preterm infant: Neurologic aspects, *Neurology* 31:767-770, 1981.

290. Batshaw ML, Wachtel RC, Cohen L: Neurologic outcome in premature infants with transient asymptomatic hyperammonemia, *J Pediatr* 108:271-275, 1986.

291. Van Geet C, Vandenbossche L, Eggermont E, Devlieger H, et al: Possible platelet contribution to pathogenesis of transient neonatal hyperammonaemia syndrome, *Lancet* 337:73-75, 1991.

292. Yoshino M, Sakaguchi Y, Kuriya N, Ohtani Y, et al: A nationwide survey on transient hyperammonemia in newborn infants in Japan: Prognosis of life and neurological outcome, *Neuropediatrics* 22:198-202, 1991.

293. Boehm G, Teichmann B, Jung K: Development of urea-synthesizing capacity in preterm infants during the first weeks of life, *Biol Neonate* 59:1-4, 1991.

294. Boehm G, Muller DM, Beyreiss K, Raiha NC: Evidence for functional immaturity of the ornithine-urea cycle in very-low-birth-weight infants, *Biol Neonate* 54:121-125, 1988.

295. Giacoia GP, Padilla-Lugo A: Severe transient neonatal hyperammonemia, *Am J Perinatol* 3:249-254, 1986.

296. Hudak ML, Jones MD, Brusilow SW: Differentiation of transient hyperammonemia of the newborn and urea cycle enzyme defects by clinical presentation, *J Pediatr* 107:712-719, 1985.

297. Chung MY, Chen CC, Huang LT, Ko TY, et al: Transient hyperammonemia in a neonate, *Acta Paediatr Taiwan* 46:94-96, 2005.

298. Eggermont E, Devlieger H, Marchal G, Jaeken J, et al: Angiographic evidence of low portal liver perfusion in transient neonatal hyperammonemia, *Acta Paediatr* 33:163-169, 1980.

299. Batshaw ML, Wachtel RC, Thomas GH, Starrett A, et al: Arginine responsive asymptomatic hyperammonemia in premature infants, *J Pediatr* 105:86-91, 1984.

300. Summar M: Current strategies for the management of neonatal urea cycle disorders, *J Pediatr* 138:S30-S39, 2001.

301. Maestri NE, Hauser ER, Bartholomew D, Brusilow SW: Prospective treatment of urea cycle disorders, *J Pediatr* 119:923-928, 1991.

302. Cederbaum SD: The treatment of urea cycle disorders, *Int Pediatr* 7:61-66, 1992.

303. Batshaw ML, Monahan PS: Treatment of urea cycle disorders, *Enzyme* 38:242-250, 1987.

304. Thoene JG: Treatment of urea cycle disorders, *J Pediatr* 134:255-256, 1999.

305. McBryde KD, Kudelka TL, Kershaw DB, Brophy PD, et al: Clearance of amino acids by hemodialysis in argininosuccinate synthetase deficiency, *J Pediatr* 144:536-540, 2004.

306. Hiroma T, Nakamura T, Tamura M, Kaneko T, et al: Continuous venovenous hemodiafiltration in neonatal onset hyperammonemia, *Am J Perinatol* 19:221-224, 2002.

307. Batshaw ML, Brusilow SW: Acute management of hyperammonemic coma in congenital urea cycle enzymopathies (UCE): Peritoneal dialysis (PD) vs exchange transfusion (ET), *J Pediatr* 97:893-900, 1980.

308. Donn SM, Swartz RD, Thoene JG: Comparison of exchange transfusion, peritoneal dialysis, and hemodialysis for the treatment of hyperammonemia in an anuric newborn infant, *J Pediatr* 95:67-70, 1979.

309. Wiegand C, Thompson T, Bock GH, Mathis RK, et al: The management of life-threatening hyperammonemia: A comparison of several therapeutic modalities, *J Pediatr* 96:142-144, 1980.

310. Walser M: Urea cycle disorders and other hereditary hyperammonemic syndromes. In Stanbury JB, Wyngaarden JB, Frederickson DS, editors: *The Metabolic Basis of Inherited Disease,* New York: 1983, McGraw-Hill.

311. Brusilow SW, Valle DL: Symptomatic inborn errors of metabolism in the neonate. In Nelson NM, editor: *Current Therapy in Neonatal Perinatal Medicine,* Toronto: 1985, Decker.

312. Batshaw ML, Brusilow S, Waber L, Blom W, et al: Treatment of inborn errors of urea synthesis: Activation of alternative pathways of waste nitrogen synthesis and excretion, *N Engl J Med* 306:1387-1392, 1982.

313. Feillet F, Leonard JV: Alternative pathway therapy for urea cycle disorders, *J Inherit Metab Dis* 21:101-111, 1998.

314. Batshaw ML, MacArthur RB, Tuckman M: Alternative pathway therapy for urea cycle disorders: Twenty years later, *J Pediatr* 138:46-55, 2001.

315. Whittington PF, Alonso EM, Boyle JT, Molleston JP, et al: Liver transplantation for the treatment of urea cycle disorders, *J Inherit Metab Dis* 21:112-118, 1998.

316. Ensenauer R, Tuchman M, ElYoussef M, Kotagal S, et al: Management and outcome of neonatal-onset ornithine transcarbamylase deficiency following liver transplantation at 60 days of life, *Mol Genet Metab* 84:363-366, 2005.

317. Horslen SP, McCowan TC, Goertzen TC, Warkentin PI, et al: Isolated hepatocyte transplantation in an infant with a severe urea cycle disorder, *Pediatrics* 111:1262-1267, 2003.

318. Batshaw ML, Robinson MB, Ye X, Pabin C, et al: Correction of ureagenesis after gene transfer in an animal model and after liver transplantation in humans with ornithine transcarbamylase deficiency, *Pediatr Res* 46:588-593, 1999.

319. McBride KL, Miller G, Carter S, Karpen S, et al: Developmental outcomes with early orthotopic liver transplantation for infants with neonatal-onset urea cycle defects and a female patient with late-onset ornithine transcarbamylase deficiency, *Pediatrics* 114:e523-e526, 2004.

320. Tuchman M, Mauer SM, Holzknecht RA, Summar ML, et al: Prospective versus clinical diagnosis and therapy of acute neonatal hyperammonaemia in 2 sisters with carbamyl phosphate synthetase deficiency, *J Inherit Metab Dis* 15:269-277, 1992.

321. Snodgrass PJ: Biochemical aspects of urea cycle disorders, *Pediatrics* 68:273-283, 1981.

322. Wada Y, Tada K, Minagawa A, Yoshida T, et al: Idiopathic valinemia: Probably a new entity of inborn error of valine metabolism, *Tohoku J Exp Med* 81:46-55, 1963.

323. Doherty LB, Rohr FJ, Levy HL: Detection of phenylketonuria in the very early newborn blood specimen, *Pediatrics* 87:240-244, 1991.

324. Platt LD, Koch R, Azen C, Hanley WB, et al: Maternal phenylketonuria collaborative study, obstetric aspects and outcome: The first six years, *Am J Obstet Gynecol* 166:1150-1162, 1992.

325. Scriver CR, Kaufman S: Hyperphenylalaninemia: Phenylalanine hydroxylase deficiency. In Schriver CR, Beaudet AL, Sly WS, et al, editors: *The Metabolic and Molecular Bases of Inherited Disease*, 8th ed, New York: 2001, McGraw-Hill.

326. Scriver CR, Pueschel S, Davies E: Hyperbetaalaninemia associated with beta-aminoaciduria and gamma-aminobutyricaciduria, somnolence, and seizures, *N Engl J Med* 174:635-643, 1966.

327. Scriver CR, Perry TL, Nutzenadel W: Disorders of beta-alanine, carnosine, and homocarnosine metabolism. In Stanbury JB, Wyngaarden JB, Frederickson DS, editors: *The Metabolic Basis of Inherited Disease*, New York: 1983, McGraw-Hill.

328. Gerritsen T, Waisman HA: Hypersarcosinemia: An inborn error of metabolism, *N Engl J Med* 275:66-69, 1966.

329. Scott CR, Clark SH, Teng CC, Swedberg KR: Clinical and cellular studies of sarcosinemia, *J Pediatr* 77:805-811, 1970.

330. Perry TL, Hansen S, Tischler B, Bunting R, et al: Carnosinemia: A new metabolic disorder associated with neurologic disease and mental defect, *N Engl J Med* 277:1219-1227, 1967.

331. Scott CR: Sarcosinemia. In Scriver CR, Beaudet AL, Sly WS, et al, editors: *The Metabolic Basis of Inherited Disease*, 6th ed, New York: 1989, McGraw-Hill.

332. Sweetman L: Branched chain organic acidurias. In Scriver CR, Beaudet AL, Sly WS, et al, editors: *The Metabolic Basis of Inherited Disease*, 6th ed, New York: 1989, McGraw-Hill.

333. Scriver CR, Perry TL: Disorders of ω-amino acids in free and peptide-linked forms. In Schriver CR, Beaudet AL, Sly WS, et al, editors: *The Metabolic Basis of Inherited Disease*, 6th ed, New York: 1989, McGraw Hill.

334. Scott CR: Sarcosinemia. In Scriver CR, Beaudet AL, Sly WS, et al, editors: *The Metabolic and Molecular Bases of Inherited Disease*, 7th ed, New York: 1995, McGraw Hill.

Chapter 15

Disorders of Organic Acid Metabolism

A series of metabolic disorders with prominent neurological accompaniments and serious deleterious effects on the developing central nervous system has been described under the designation *organic acid disorders*. The term *organic acid* is particularly imprecise but, unfortunately, appears to be firmly entrenched in the medical literature. Strictly speaking, organic acids should include amino acids, fatty acids, ketoacids, and a variety of other endogenous and exogenous acids. Disorders of amino acids are discussed in Chapter 14. In this chapter, I discuss the disorders of organic acids that are associated with prominent neurological phenomena in the neonatal period *and* that have been reported in more than a few infants.

OVERVIEW OF MAJOR ORGANIC ACID DISORDERS AND NEONATAL METABOLIC ACIDOSIS

The organic acid disorders enumerated in Table 15-1 are important causes of severe neonatal metabolic acidosis. The major acids that accumulate vary according to the site of the metabolic defect, as outlined subsequently. Lactic acidosis is a very frequent accompaniment. A simplified scheme for the differential diagnosis of neonatal lactic acidosis is shown in Figure 15-1. In the following sections, I discuss principally the disorders of metabolism of propionate and methylmalonate, pyruvate, and branched-chain ketoacids. The rare other organic acid disorders and a fatty acid oxidation disorder (see Table 15-1) are described briefly at the conclusion of the chapter. The mitochondrial disorders are discussed in Chapter 16. The disorders of carbohydrate metabolism listed in Table 15-1 and renal tubular acidosis either manifest clinically only rarely in the neonatal period or exhibit primarily nonneurological syndromes and are not reviewed further.

DISORDERS OF PROPIONATE AND METHYLMALONATE METABOLISM

Disorders of propionate and methylmalonate metabolism are uncommon but serious neonatal neurological disturbances. These disorders are the most common of the so-called organic acid abnormalities. In an earlier large series (105 cases) of patients with organic acidurias with neonatal onset, disorders of propionate and methylmalonate metabolism accounted for 40% of the total.[1] Later reported experiences have been similar.[2-7] These diseases share certain common features (Table 15-2).

Normal Metabolic Aspects

Propionate and methylmalonate are vital intermediates in the catabolism of lipid and protein.[8] The major pathway of the metabolism of propionate and methylmalonate is shown in Figure 15-2. Although propionyl–coenzyme A (CoA) formation from isoleucine catabolism is depicted, this organic acid is also the product of the catabolism of valine, methionine, threonine, cholesterol (side chain), and odd-chain fatty acids.[8] Involved in the propionate and methylmalonate pathway are two vitamins, biotin and vitamin B_{12}. Biotin is the coenzyme for propionyl-CoA carboxylase, and adenosyl cobalamin (a derivative of vitamin B_{12}) is the coenzyme for methylmalonyl-CoA mutase. Indeed, some of the disorders of this pathway are responsive to large doses of these vitamins (see later section). The product of the pathway, succinyl-CoA, enters the tricarboxylic acid cycle, where pyruvate is formed from reaction with oxaloacetate.

Certain alternate and minor metabolic pathways are important in understanding the disorders of this pathway (see Fig. 15-2) Thus, propionyl-CoA also can be metabolized to lactate and can be used in the synthesis of odd-numbered fatty acids. Methylmalonyl-CoA can be used in the synthesis of methyl-branched fatty acids.

Biochemical Aspects of Disordered Metabolism

Enzymatic Defects and Essential Consequences

The enzymes affected in the disorders of propionate and methylmalonate metabolism are shown in Figure 15-2. The resulting metabolic consequences (e.g., acidosis, hyperammonemia, and hyperglycinemia) are diverse, and their pathogeneses are now understood to a considerable degree.

Acidosis

The acidosis in disorders of propionate and methylmalonate metabolism results, at least in part, from the accumulation of the acids proximal to the primary enzymatic blocks. However, the degree of acidosis often is greater than can be accounted for by these compounds. Other sources of acidemia include conversion of

TABLE 15-1	Major Causes of Metabolic Acidosis in the Neonatal Period

Disorders of Propionate-Methylmalonate Metabolism
Propionic acidemia
Methylmalonic acidemia

Disorders of Pyruvate and Mitochondrial Energy Metabolism
Pyruvate dehydrogenase deficiency
Pyruvate carboxylase deficiency
Defects of the electron transport chain (complexes I, IV, V)

Disorders of Branched-Chain Amino Acid–Ketoacid Metabolism
Maple syrup urine disease
Isovaleric acidemia
beta-Methylcrotonyl–CoA carboxylase deficiency
beta-Ketothiolase deficiency
Hydroxymethylglutaryl–CoA lyase deficiency
Mevalonic aciduria

Disorders of Fatty Acid Metabolism
Medium-chain acyl–CoA dehydrogenase deficiency

Other Organic Acid Disorders
Multiple carboxylase deficiency
Glutaric acidemia, type II
Glutathione synthetase deficiency (5-oxoprolinuria)
Sulfite oxidase deficiency (molybdenum cofactor deficiency)

Disorders of Carbohydrate Metabolism
Galactosemia
Glycogen storage disease, type I (von Gierke glucose-6-phosphatase deficiency)
Fructose-1,6-diphosphatase deficiency
Phosphoenolpyruvate carboxykinase deficiency

Renal Tubular Acidosis

TABLE 15-2	Common Features of Disorders of Propionate and Methylmalonate Metabolism

Clinical Features
Vomiting
Tachypnea
Stupor, coma
Seizures

Metabolic Features
Acidosis
Propionic acidemia with or without methylmalonic acidemia (aciduria)
Hyperglycinemia
Hyperammonemia

Other Features
Neutropenia, anemia, thrombocytopenia

Neuropathological Features
Myelin disturbance
Basal ganglia injury (caudate, putamen in propionic acidemia; globus pallidus in methylmalonic acidemia)
Cerebral cortical atrophy (later)

excessive propionate to lactate by a normally minor metabolic pathway (see Fig. 15-2), inhibition of pyruvate dehydrogenase[8] with resulting increased conversion of pyruvate to lactate, and accumulation of ketone bodies by poorly understood mechanisms.

Hyperammonemia

The *hyperammonemia* that is a nearly consistent feature of the neonatal varieties of propionate and

methylmalonate disturbances appears to result from two closely related mechanisms.[8-13] Both relate to an accumulation of the CoA esters of the acids proximal to the enzymatic blocks (particularly propionyl-CoA, tiglyl-CoA [a metabolite of isoleucine], and methylmalonyl-CoA) and to the effects of these derivatives on the activity of carbamyl phosphate synthetase, the first step in the Krebs-Henseleit urea cycle (see Chapter 14). Thus, these CoA esters have been shown to have a direct inhibitory effect on carbamyl phosphate synthetase and an indirect inhibitory effect at this step by inhibition of the synthesis of *N*-acetylglutamate, the important activator of carbamyl phosphate synthetase (see Fig. 14-12). Hyperammonemia and acidosis have major deleterious effects on the brain (see Chapter 14) and are thought to be major determinants of the acute neurological dysfunction and brain injury that result in the neonatal period.

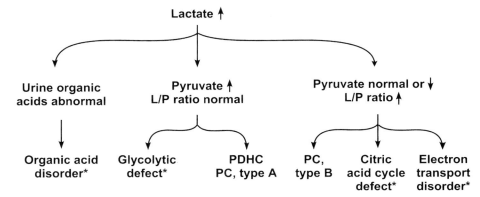

Figure 15-1   Simplified scheme for differential diagnosis of neonatal lactic acidosis. Note the critical initial role of determinations of urine organic acids and blood lactate and pyruvate levels and ratio. L/P ratio, lactate-to-pyruvate ratio; PC, pyruvate carboxylase (deficiency); PDHC, pyruvate dehydrogenase complex (deficiency). *Organic acid disorders: propionic acidemia, methylmalonic acidemia, isovaleric acidemia, multiple carboxylase deficiency, fatty acid oxidation defects, among others. *Glycolytic defects: glucose-6-phosphatase, fructose-1,6-diphosphatase, phosphoenolpyruvate carboxykinase deficiencies. *Citric acid cycle defects: fumarase and succinate dehydrogenase deficiencies. *Electron transport disorders: see mitochondrial disorders in Chapter 16.

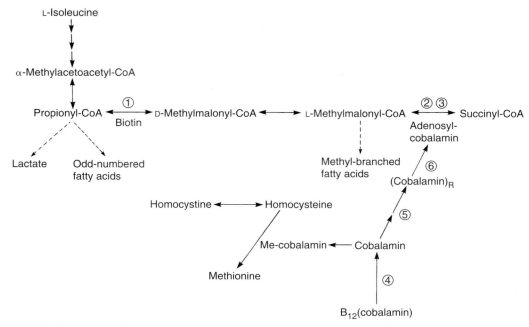

Figure 15-2 **Metabolism of propionate and methylmalonate and sites of defects in their metabolism**. Major pathways are shown by solid arrows, and alternate minor pathways by broken arrows. Sites of defects are numbered and include *(1)* propionyl–coenzyme A (CoA) carboxylase, *(2)* and *(3)* methylmalonyl-CoA mutase (two different structural defects), *(4)* cobalamin binding, internalization, lysosomal release and cytosolic reduction, *(5)* mitochondrial cobalamin reductase, and *(6)* mitochondrial adenosyltransferase. See text for details. *(Adapted from Fenton WA, Gravel RA, Rosenblatt DS: Disorders of propionate and methylmalonate metabolism. In Schriver CR, Beaudet AL, Sly WS, et al, editors:* The Metabolic and Molecular Bases of Inherited Disease, *8th ed, New York: 2001, McGraw-Hill.)*

Hyperglycinemia

A striking aspect of propionate and methylmalonate metabolism is *hyperglycinemia*. This condition is unlike the nonketotic hyperglycinemia described in Chapter 14 because of the association of ketoacidosis (i.e., ketotic versus nonketotic hyperglycinemia) and because the glycine abnormality is a secondary and not a primary metabolic phenomenon. Analogous to the cause of the hyperammonemia in these disorders of the propionate and methylmalonate pathway, the cause of the hyperglycinemia appears related to an inhibition of glycine cleavage by the accumulation of branched-chain alpha-ketoacids and, more specifically, their CoA derivatives.

A disturbance of glycine cleavage was demonstrated indirectly and directly in studies of patients *with ketotic hyperglycinemia* caused by deficiencies of propionyl-CoA carboxylase and methylmalonyl-CoA mutase, as well as of isovaleryl-CoA dehydrogenase and beta-ketothiolase (the latter two disorders of branched-chain amino acid metabolism are discussed later).[3,4,14-18] Analyses of the individual protein components of the glycine cleavage system of patients with propionic acidemia and methylmalonic acidemia have shown that the H-protein, one of the four proteins of the system, is the component initially inactivated.[19]

That *the impairment of glycine metabolism* involves the inhibition of the glycine cleavage system *by CoA derivatives* of accumulated metabolites is suggested by data based on studies of rat liver.[20] In vitro studies of the solubilized hepatic glycine cleavage system show marked inhibition by CoA derivatives found in the catabolic pathway for isoleucine. Such derivatives would be expected to accumulate in the disorders of the propionate and methylmalonate pathway (see Fig. 15-2). Coupled with the data referable to the genesis of the hyperammonemia, these observations suggest that the *CoA derivatives of the accumulated organic acids* are responsible for the major, critical, secondary metabolic effects that accompany the primary enzymatic disorders.

Myelin Disturbance and Fatty Acid Abnormalities

In the disorders associated with the accumulation of propionic and methylmalonic acids, *a disturbance of myelin*, detectable by neuropathological examination (see "Neuropathology"), appears to be important in the genesis of the neurological sequelae.[21-24] Vacuolation of myelin appears in the first months of life and is followed by an apparent disturbance of myelin formation.[21,24] The magnetic resonance imaging (MRI) correlate of the myelin disturbance, present in many reported cases (see later), is, acutely, diffusely swollen, T2-hyperintense cerebral white matter, followed later by white matter atrophy. The genesis of the myelin disturbance is not clear but may be related to changes in the fatty acid composition of oligodendroglial membranes. Distinct changes exist in the composition of fatty acids in the brain of patients with disorders resulting in the accumulation of propionate or methylmalonate,[25-29] and these changes can be reproduced in cultured rat glial cells.[30,31] The major alterations are increases in the amounts of *odd-numbered*

TABLE 15-3 **Fatty Acid Composition of Brain Lipids with Disorder of Propionate-Methylmalonate Metabolism**

Brain Lipid Class	ODD-NUMBERED FATTY ACIDS		METHYL-BRANCHED FATTY ACIDS	
	Control (%)	Patient (%)*	Control (%)	Patient (%)*
Choline phospholipid	Trace	9.8%	—	2.1%
Sphingomyelin	7.5%	18.2%	—	—
Cerebroside	18.9%	29.0%	—	—
Sulfatide	21.7%	31.1%	—	—

*Child with methylmalonic aciduria.
Data from Ramsey RB, Scott T, Banik NL: Fatty acid composition of myelin isolated from the brain of patient with cellular deficiency of co-enzyme forms of vitamin B_{12}, *J Neurol Sci* 34:221-232, 1977.

and methyl-branched fatty acids (see later). These increases have been demonstrated in phospholipids (i.e., components of all cellular membranes) as well as in myelin lipids (e.g., cerebrosides and sulfatides; Table 15-3).[28] Because the fatty acid composition of membrane lipids is important not only for structural integrity but also for the function of a variety of membrane proteins (e.g., enzymes, transport carriers, surface receptors),[32] these alterations may have major implications for the genesis of the neurological dysfunction and the disturbance of myelination.

Disturbances of Fatty Acid Synthesis

The fatty acid abnormalities described in the previous section are caused presumably by disturbances of fatty acid synthesis. The nature of the disturbances observed in disorders of propionate and methylmalonate metabolism is depicted in Figure 15-3. Thus, under normal circumstances, de novo synthesis of fatty acids in brain is catalyzed by the multienzyme complex fatty acid synthetase.[33,34] The first two carbons (i.e., the primer) of the resulting even-numbered fatty acids (primarily the 16-carbon acid, palmitic acid) are derived from

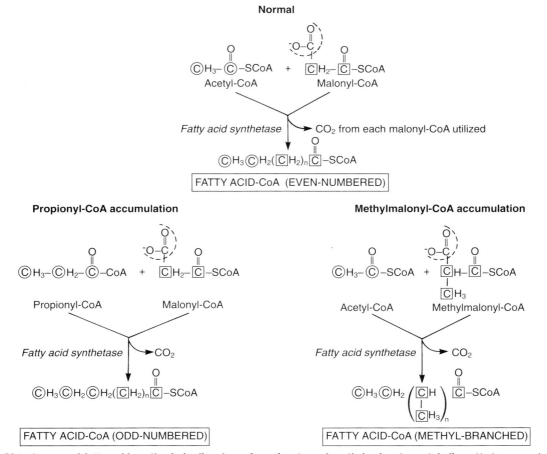

Figure 15-3 **Disturbances of fatty acid synthesis in disorders of propionate and methylmalonate metabolism**. Under *normal conditions*, the enzyme complex, fatty acid synthetase, catalyzes the addition of two-carbon fragments from malonyl–coenzyme A (CoA) to the single primer molecule of acetyl-CoA to form even-numbered fatty acids. With *propionyl-CoA accumulation*, this three-carbon compound replaces acetyl-CoA as primer, and therefore with the addition of the two-carbon fragments from malonyl-CoA, odd-numbered fatty acids result. With *methylmalonyl-CoA accumulation*, this branched compound replaces malonyl-CoA, and therefore methyl-branched fatty acids result.

acetyl-CoA, whereas the remaining carbons for chain elongation are derived from the two-carbon units obtained from malonyl-CoA (see Fig. 15-3). *When propionyl-CoA is present in excessive amounts, it can replace acetyl-CoA with a three-carbon fragment as primer*, and, thus, an odd-numbered fatty acid results after the addition of the two-carbon units from malonyl-CoA (see Fig. 15-3). *When methylmalonyl-CoA is present in excessive amounts, it can replace malonyl-CoA*, and, thus, a methyl-branched unit is derived from malonyl-CoA, resulting in methyl-branched fatty acids (see Fig. 15-3). These unusual fatty acids are incorporated into cellular membranes, including myelin, as discussed in the previous section.

Propionic Acidemia and Propionyl–Coenzyme A Carboxylase Deficiency

Propionic acidemia is caused by a defect in the first step of the pathway from propionyl-CoA to succinyl-CoA, a step catalyzed by the enzyme propionyl-CoA carboxylase.

Clinical Features

Onset is in the first days of life, with a dramatic clinical syndrome consisting primarily of vomiting, stupor, tachypnea, and seizures (see Table 15-2).[7,8,35-37] The usual time of onset is the second to fourth days of life.[38,39] Infants whose condition is not diagnosed and treated properly rapidly lapse into coma and die. Indeed, in earlier studies, approximately 75% of patients died in early infancy.[1] However, even with "early diagnosis and vigorous treatment," median survival in a later series was only 3 years.[38] More recent improvements in management have resulted in improved survival rates.[39] In one series of six infants, all survived the neonatal period.[36] Lethal cerebellar hemorrhage, occurring in association with thrombocytopenia and hyperosmolar bicarbonate therapy, has occasionally been observed in the neonatal period.[40] Survivors of the neonatal period are prone to episodic attacks of vomiting and stupor, with severe ketoacidosis, often precipitated by infection, and to subsequent retardation of neurological development. Of 11 infants reported in one series, no survivor had an intelligence quotient (IQ) higher than 60.[38] Similar cognitive impairment was documented in a later series of six infants.[36] In a recent series of 38 infants, 95% had "cognitive and neurologic" deficits.[39] Chorea or dystonia has been observed in 20% to 40% of surviving children, and this extrapyramidal involvement is common in this disorder (see later discussion of neuropathology).[38,41]

The genetic data for this disorder indicate *autosomal recessive* inheritance. This conclusion is based, in part, on the pattern of familial occurrence, partial disturbance of enzymatic activity in parents, and complementation testing of cells in culture.[7,8,13]

Metabolic Features

Major Findings. The constellation of ketoacidosis, propionic acidemia, hyperglycinemia (and hyperglycinuria), hyperammonemia, neutropenia, anemia, and thrombopenia is characteristic and composes the *"ketotic hyperglycinemia" syndrome.*[8] However, hyperglycinemia with propionic acidemia and propionyl-CoA carboxylase deficiency has occurred in the neonatal period without consistent ketonuria.[42] This finding is important because patients with disorders of propionate and methylmalonate metabolism should be managed differently from those with the more common nonketotic hyperglycinemia described in Chapter 14.

Enzymatic Defect. The enzymatic defect involves propionyl-CoA carboxylase.[8,43] Structural alterations of the two nonidentical subunits (alpha and beta) of the carboxylase molecules account for the enzymatic defect.[8] The enzyme contains four copies each of the alpha and beta subunits, with the gene for the alpha subunit encoded on chromosome 13 and the gene for the beta subunit encoded on chromosome 3.[8] Because this enzyme requires biotin for activity, the possibility of a defect in activation or binding of biotin to the carboxylase apoprotein as the basis of the disturbed activity in certain patients must be considered. The initial observation of a beneficial response of one patient to large amounts of biotin suggested that such an additional defect may occur.[44] The delineation of impaired activity of propionyl-CoA carboxylase (as well as of other carboxylases) in two disorders of biotin metabolism, holocarboxylase synthetase deficiency and biotinidase deficiency, corroborated this suggestion (see later discussion). However, only one of these disorders (holocarboxylase synthetase deficiency) consistently causes prominent clinical phenomena in the newborn, as discussed later.

Pathogenesis of Metabolic Features. The genesis of the various metabolic consequences of this disorder is now understood to a considerable degree. The origins of the *hyperglycinemia* and the *hyperammonemia* relate to the secondary effects of the CoA derivatives of certain of the accumulated metabolites on the pathways of glycine cleavage and ammonia detoxification by the urea cycle (see earlier discussion). The *acidosis* must relate to several factors (i.e., accumulation of the propionic acid proximal to the primary enzymatic block, of lactate produced by the alternate pathway of propionate degradation, and of the various acids that accumulate proximal to propionic acid as a consequence of continuing degradation of branched-chain and other amino acids).

Increased numbers of *odd-numbered fatty acids* have been observed in the tissues of infants with propionic acidemia.[29,45,46] The genesis of the odd-numbered fatty acids relates to the utilization of propionyl-CoA as a primer for the fatty acid synthetase reaction, as described previously (see Fig. 15-3).

Neuropathology

A well-studied *neonatal* case of propionic acidemia involved a 1-month-old patient.[21] The dominant neuropathological findings involved myelin and consisted of marked *vacuolation*, with a less striking *diminution* of the amount of myelin. Similar pathological findings have been described in other affected cases.[22,24]

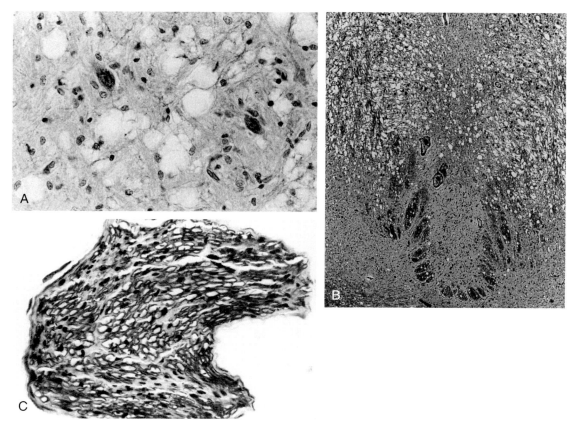

Figure 15-4   Myelin disturbance in propionic acidemia in a 26-day-old infant who exhibited lethargy, poor feeding, tachypnea, profound metabolic acidosis in the first week of life, and generalized seizures in the third week. **A**, Vacuolation of myelinated fibers traversing the globus pallidus. **B**, Vacuolation of the medial longitudinal fasciculus just rostral to the trochlear nucleus. **C**, Demyelination and endoneurial fibrosis of a mixed spinal nerve of the lumbosacral plexus. *(From Shuman RM, Leech RW, Scott CR: The neuropathology of the nonketotic and ketotic hyperglycinemias: Three cases,* Neurology *28:139-146, 1978.)*

The disturbance of myelin is similar to that noted in nonketotic hyperglycinemia and other aminoacidopathies (see Chapter 14). Vacuolation appears to be the early change, occurring principally in systems actively myelinating at the time of the illness (e.g., medial lemniscus, superior cerebellar peduncle, posterior columns, and peripheral nerve in the 1-month-old patient of Shuman and co-workers[21]) (Fig. 15-4). The impaired myelination appears to occur subsequent to the vacuolation.[21] Vacuolation has been observed in oligodendrocytes in areas just before myelination.[24] The cause of this defect in myelination in ketotic hyperglycinemia may relate to the disturbance of fatty acid synthesis and the resultant altered fatty acid composition of myelin (see earlier discussion). Thus, the odd-numbered fatty acids may alter the stability of the oligodendroglial-myelin membrane, thereby impairing oligodendroglial differentiation and rendering the newly formed myelin unstable. Vacuolation and the subsequent deficit of myelin would result. Other possibilities, such as disturbance of synthesis of myelin proteins because of the amino acid imbalance (e.g., the elevated glycine levels), must be considered as well.[21]

An interesting additional feature of the neuropathology of propionic acidemia is the *prominence of involvement of the basal ganglia* in patients who survive for several or more years.[47-49] Thus, neuronal loss and gliosis are prominent, and, in one case, the addition of aberrant myelin bundles caused a "marbled" appearance, reminiscent of status marmoratus of perinatal asphyxia (see Chapter 8). In contrast to methylmalonic acidemia (see later), caudate and putamen, rather than globus pallidus, are preferentially involved.[50] The importance of excitotoxicity in the basal ganglia neuronal injury and the potential role of glycine in the genesis of excitotoxic neuronal injury (see discussion of nonketotic hyperglycinemia in Chapter 4) are of interest in this context. The involvement of basal ganglia in older infants and children has been documented repeatedly by brain imaging.[37,51] Finally, this derangement of basal ganglia may underlie the relative frequency of extrapyramidal movement disorders observed subsequently in infants with propionic acidemia.[38,47] Cerebral cortical atrophy is noted in survivors of several years or more.[50,52]

As with several other metabolic disorders in which the enzymatic defect is present in brain (see later), agenesis or hypoplasia of the corpus callosum may result (Fig. 15-5). Indeed, the presence of callosal abnormalities, without an obvious syndromic or other cause, should raise the possibility of a metabolic disorder.

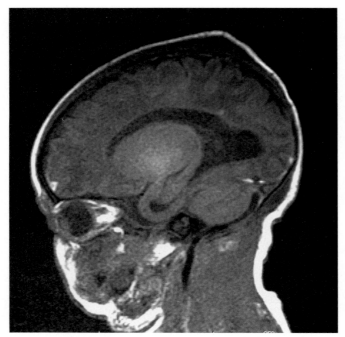

Figure 15-5 Propionic acidemia, magnetic resonance imaging (MRI) scan. An infant with severe lactic acidosis was scanned on the sixth day of life. This T1-weighted MRI scan shows absence of the corpus callosum. (Courtesy of Dr. Omar Khwaja.)

Management

Antenatal Diagnosis. Antenatal diagnosis has been accomplished by measuring propionyl-CoA carboxylase activity in cultured amniotic fluid cells or chorionic villus samples, by analyzing metabolites in amniotic fluid, and by molecular genetic testing of DNA extracted from fetal cells.[7,8,15,53] Thus, the possibility of preventing the disorder is real.

Early Detection. Early diagnosis, particularly in distinguishing this disorder from other causes of severe metabolic acidosis in the neonatal period (see Table 15-1), is critical. Identification of the accompanying metabolic features is particularly valuable in this regard. Organic acid analysis of urine by tandem mass spectrometry is especially useful. Definitive diagnosis is established by measurement of propionyl-CoA carboxylase activity in leukocytes or cultured fibroblasts.

Acute and Long-Term Therapy. Acute episodes should be treated by withdrawing all protein and administering sodium bicarbonate parenterally. Hyperammonemia may be severe enough to require specific measures for ammonia removal, as described in Chapter 14. Subsequently, a low-protein diet (restricted especially in isoleucine, valine, methionine, and threonine) is administered.[8] The use of gastrostomy feeding to guarantee nutritional intake has been valuable.[36] Supplementation with L-carnitine may be indicated, because the excretion of carnitine as propionyl carnitine may lead to decreased plasma levels of free carnitine, and supplementation with carnitine has produced beneficial clinical and metabolic responses in isolated patients.[8] Oral antibiotic therapy to reduce propionate production by bacteria in the gastrointestinal tract may also be useful later.[8]

Biotin. Because some biochemical benefit was observed in one infant treated with biotin, large doses of this vitamin are worthy of a trial in affected patients.[44,45,54] Biotin responsiveness should be assessed by observation of changes in metabolite levels in blood and urine and in enzyme activity in white blood cells. The effect of biotin in vitro on the enzyme in cultured fibroblasts may be useful in determining the likelihood of a beneficial response in vivo.[13] Marked biotin responsiveness is characteristic of multiple carboxylase deficiency (see later discussion).

Gene Therapy. Liver transplantation early in infancy may be of value in the management of neonatal-onset propionic acidemia.[7] Approximately 20 patients so treated have been reported.[55,56] Initial mortality rates after transplantation exceeded 50%, and thus the number of infants followed sufficiently long after transplant is small. However, the most recent survival rates have improved, and prevention of severe acidotic episodes has been noted.[56] A beneficial effect on neurological development remains to be defined.

Methylmalonic Acidemias

Methylmalonic acidemias constitute the single most frequent group of organic disorders.[6,8] The accumulation of large quantities of methylmalonic acid in blood and urine is associated with at least five discrete metabolic defects (see Fig. 15-2): (1 and 2) defects of methylmalonyl-CoA mutase (two different defects of the mutase apoenzyme, one resulting in complete deficiency and the other in partial deficiency of the mutase), (3 and 4) defects in the synthesis of adenosylcobalamin, and (5) defective synthesis of both adenosylcobalamin and methylcobalamin (Table 15-4).[7,8,45,57-59] The latter three defects of vitamin B_{12} metabolism result in diminished activity of

TABLE 15-4	Methylmalonic Acidemias: Biochemical and Metabolic Features*	
METABOLIC ACCUMULATION		
Defective Enzyme	**Methylmalonic Acid**	**Homocysteine**
Methylmalonic acid mutase	+	−
Mitochondrial cobalamin reductase (*cblA*)	+	−
Mitochondrial cobalamin adenosyltransferase (*cblB*)	+	−
Abnormal lysosomal or cytosolic cobalamin metabolism (*cblC, cblD, cblF*)	+	+

*See text for references.

methylmalonyl-CoA mutase, for which adenosylcobalamin is a coenzyme. Additionally, the last of these defects *also* results in diminished activity of the methyltransferase required for methylation of homocysteine; the formation of the methyltransferase requires methylcobalamin. In one series of 45 carefully studied patients with methylmalonic acidemia (without homocystinuria), 15 had complete mutase deficiency, 5 had partial mutase deficiency, 14 had deficient mitochondrial cobalamin reductase, and 11 had deficient cobalamin adenosyltransferase (the latter two defects resulting in defective synthesis of adenosylcobalamin).[45] These disorders are discussed collectively.

Clinical Features

The clinical features are similar to those noted for disorders of propionate metabolism (i.e., vomiting, stupor, tachypnea and seizures; see Table 15-2). Onset of these features in the neonatal period depends on the nature of the enzymatic defect (Table 15-5). Neonatal onset is most likely with complete mutase deficiency, and nearly all neonates with this severe enzymatic lesion present in the first 7 days of life. Fewer than half of all patients with the other three metabolic defects present in the first 7 days. The outcome also is related to the type of metabolic defect (see Table 15-5). The gravity of outcome correlates approximately with the frequency of neonatal onset. Thus, infants with complete mutase deficiency nearly invariably die or exhibit subsequent neurological impairment. In earlier series, mortality rates for such patients were approximately 60%, although in more recent series, approximately 30% of infants have died.[6,8] In a series of 20 infants, the range of subsequent IQ was 65 to 84, with a median of 75.[60] One infant with severe mutase deficiency detected at 3 weeks of age by neonatal screening was reported to be normal at the age of 5 years after treatment with a low-protein diet.[61] Patients with methylmalonic acidemias who survive are subject to episodic decompensation, especially with minor

intercurrent infections. *Brain imaging* reveals the abnormalities of myelin as noted earlier for propionic acidemia. Involvement of basal ganglia, similarly, is very common, but in the case of methylmalonic acidemia, it involves *globus pallidus* rather than the caudate/putamen as in propionic acidemia.[50,51,62-65]

The smaller number of infants, approximately 35, reported with a defect in cobalamin metabolism characterized by impaired synthesis of *both* methylcobalamin *and* adenosylcobalamin (see Table 15-4) (see the next section, "Metabolic Features") and onset in the first month of life also had a generally unfavorable neurological outcome (not shown in Table 15-5).[59,66-70] The clinical and neuroradiological features were similar, albeit milder, than those observed in patients with the mutase deficiencies, and the metabolic features included *homocystinuria* as well as methylmalonic acidemia. At least 80% subsequently exhibited mental retardation, and completely normal intellectual functioning was very unusual. Available genetic data indicate that these disorders all exhibit *autosomal recessive* inheritance.[8]

Metabolic Features

Major Findings. The constellation of severe ketoacidosis, methylmalonic acidemia, hyperglycinemia, hyperammonemia, neutropenia, and thrombopenia is characteristic. Approximately 40% of neonatal patients have also exhibited significant hypoglycemia with their attacks of ketoacidosis.

As noted earlier, approximately 35 infants were observed with a genetic defect that resulted in impaired synthesis of *both* methylcobalamin and adenosylcobalamin and the additional metabolic feature of homocysteinemia/homocystinuria.[8,59,66-68,70] However, unlike the classic homocystinuria resulting from cystathionine synthase deficiency (which is associated with elevated levels of methionine and depressed levels of cystathionine), this type is associated with *hypomethioninemia and cystathioninuria* (the product of homocysteine and serine) (see Fig. 15-2).

Enzymatic Defects. The enzymatic defects in methylmalonic acidemias involve the methylmalonyl-CoA mutase apoenzyme (two major defects) and the metabolism of vitamin B_{12} (three major defects), as noted in the introduction to this section (see Table 15-4). The defects have been demonstrated primarily in liver and in cultured fibroblasts.[7,8,15,45,58,59,71,72]

The two major defects of the mutase apoenzyme result, as noted earlier, in either complete or partial deficiency of enzyme activity. In most reported examples of complete deficiency of mutase activity, little or no immunoreactive enzyme protein was present.[8,58] In the cases with partial deficiency of activity, a presumably altered enzyme with defective catalytic function was present, because the amount of immunologically reactive protein varied from 20% to 100% of control values.[8,58]

The three major sites of the defects in vitamin B_{12} metabolism are shown in Figure 15-2. Under normal circumstances, vitamin B_{12}, bound to a carrier protein,

TABLE 15-5	Time of Onset and Outcome in Methylmalonic Acidemias According to Type of Metabolic Defect			
	METABOLIC DEFECT			
Onset or Outcome	**mut•**	**mut⁻**	**cblA**	**cblB**
Age at Onset				
0–7 days	80%	40%	42%	33%
8–30 days	7%	20%	—	22%
> 30 days	13%	40%	58%	55%
Outcome				
Dead	60%	40%	8%	30%
Impaired	40%	20%	23%	40%
Well	—	40%	69%	30%

cblA, deficiency of mitochondrial cobalamin reductase; cblB, deficiency of cobalamin adenosyltransferase; mut•, complete mutase deficiency; mut⁻, partial mutase deficiency.

Data from Rosenberg LE, Fenton WA: Disorders of propionate and methylmalonate metabolism. In Scriver CR, Beaudet AL, Sly WS, et al, editors: *The Metabolic Basis of Inherited Disease*, 6th ed, New York: 1989, McGraw-Hill.

is internalized by the cell through endocytosis; the endosome is taken up by the lysosome, proteases of which degrade the carrier protein, and the cobalamin is released into the cytosol, where reduction and methylation take place. A portion of the cobalamin released into the cytosol enters the mitochondrion for reduction and adenosylation.[45,73] The defect that results in impaired synthesis of both methylcobalamin and adenosylcobalamin involves an event after binding and internalization (i.e., after cellular uptake).[8] The defects of vitamin B_{12} metabolism have been defined through studies of cultured fibroblasts from affected patients.[8,45,74-76]

Pathogenesis of Metabolic Features. The causes of the various metabolic consequences of the methylmalonic acidemias are similar in many ways to those described for other disorders in the propionate and methylmalonate pathway, especially regarding the *hyperglycinemia* and the *hyperammonemia*. The *ketoacidosis* is not as readily accounted for because it is more severe than would be expected from the accumulation of methylmalonic acid. Methylmalonyl-CoA is an inhibitor of pyruvate carboxylase, and its product, succinyl-CoA, is involved in gluconeogenesis by conversion to pyruvate (see earlier discussion). Together, these effects could lead to an impairment of gluconeogenesis to account for the *hypoglycemia* in nearly one half of the neonatal cases and, secondarily, to increased catabolism of lipid, with resultant ketosis and acidosis.[77]

The accumulation of *odd-numbered and methyl-branched fatty acids* in neural and other tissues of affected patients[26,28] relates, respectively, to

substitution of propionyl-CoA for acetyl-CoA as primer for the fatty acid synthetase reaction and to the substitution of methylmalonyl-CoA for malonyl-CoA for chain elongation in the same reaction (see Fig. 15-3). The genesis of the defects of sulfur amino acid metabolism in the disorder with impaired synthesis of both methylcobalamin and adenosylcobalamin relates to a disturbance of the methylation of homocysteine to form methionine; the enzyme for this reaction, methionine synthase, requires methylcobalamin (see Fig. 15-2). The consequences of the disturbance of homocysteine methylation, as noted earlier, are *homocystinuria, hypomethioninemia,* and *cystathioninuria,* the last resulting because some of the accumulated homocysteine is converted to cystathionine.

Neuropathology

The neuropathological features of the methylmalonic acidemias suggest a derangement of myelination.[27,78,79] An abnormality of myelin with features similar to those described for propionic acidemia has been observed.[27] Particular involvement of spinal nerve roots rather than central myelin was noted in one premature infant studied.[78] Whether the myelin defect relates to the abnormal accumulation of odd-numbered and methyl-branched fatty acids in glial membranes, as discussed earlier, remains to be established.

A carefully studied infant of 36 weeks of gestation (death at 4 days of age) exhibited selective death of immature neurons (i.e., residual neuronal cells in germinal matrix), migrating neuroblasts, and neurons of the external granule cell layer of cerebellum (Fig. 15-6). The cytological characteristics, marked karyorrhexis,

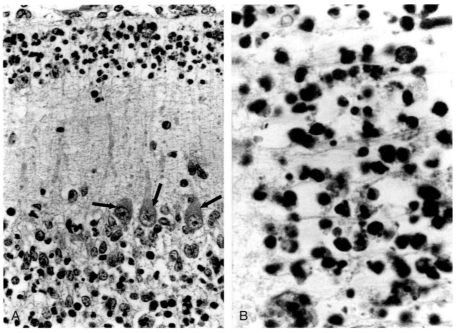

Figure 15-6 **Selective death of immature neurons in a 4-day-old infant with methylmalonic acidemia. A,** Photomicrograph of the cerebellar cortex shows karyorrhectic immature neuroblasts in the external *(top)* and internal granule cell layers *(bottom).* Purkinje cells *(arrows)* are relatively well preserved. **B,** At higher magnification, karyorrhexis in the external granule cell layer is prominent. *(From Sum JM, Twiss JL, Horoupian DS: Selective death of immature neurons in methylmalonic acidemia of the neonate: A case report,* Acta Neuropathol (Berl) *85:217-221, 1993.)*

were compatible with apoptotic cell death (see Chapter 2) and suggested that the toxic effect of the metabolites of methylmalonic acidemia particularly involved provocation of apoptosis of immature neuronal cells. Involvement of the external granule cell layer of cerebellum may be related etiologically to the occasional occurrence of cerebellar hemorrhage with methylmalonic acidemia.[40]

As noted earlier, as with propionic acidemia, evidence for basal ganglia lesions has been obtained by brain imaging later in infancy and childhood. In methylmalonic acidemias, the globus pallidus is preferentially affected. This finding is consistent with the occurrence of dystonia and extrapyramidal features on follow-up in approximately 20% to 25% of cases of methylmalonic acidemia of neonatal onset.[60]

Management

Antenatal Diagnosis. Antenatal detection of the methylmalonic acidemias has been accomplished primarily by detecting elevated methylmalonate content in the amniotic fluid and maternal urine and by enzymatic assay of cultured amniotic fluid cells (mutase activity and adenosylcobalamin synthesis).[8,45,57,80-83] The possibility of prenatal therapy with cobalamin supplements was shown initially by demonstrating a decrease in maternal excretion of methylmalonic acid after administration of such supplements to the mother of an affected fetus.[57,82] A subsequent case, treated similarly in utero and postnatally, had normal growth and development in early infancy.[84] However, because at least 60% of *neonatal* cases are not cobalamin responsive,[6,8,60] this approach may not be highly useful for the majority of affected fetuses.

In the rare infants with the combined defect resulting in both methylmalonic acidemia and homocystinuria, large doses of hydroxycobalamin also are important.[85] Betaine, another methyl donor, also may be beneficial. Follow-up data are too sparse to assess effects on neurological development. It is likely that both prenatal and postnatal therapy will be critical.[70,85]

Early Detection and Acute and Long-Term Therapy. Early detection in the neonatal period and the importance of acute and long-term therapy are essentially as described for propionic acidemia. Therapy consists of a low-protein diet or a diet low in the amino acid precursors of methylmalonate, supplemented with cobalamin (see next section) and L-carnitine.[8] The possible role of antibiotic therapy to reduce production of methylmalonate by bacteria in the gastrointestinal tract may also be relevant in this condition.[8,58]

Vitamin B$_{12}$. Because some patients with isolated methylmalonic acidemias respond to vitamin B$_{12}$ (see earlier discussion), a trial of this vitamin as hydroxycobalamin in high doses is indicated in such patients.[8,45,54,58,86] In a series of 21 infants with neonatal-onset methylmalonic acidemia, of the 11 who responded to vitamin B$_{12}$, 3 were normal on follow-up, whereas of the 10 who did not respond to vitamin B$_{12}$, none was normal.[6]

Gene Therapy. As with propionic acidemia, liver transplantation has been used in infants with methylmalonic acidemia.[55,56] Initial results in transplanted infants were not clearly beneficial. The situation is complicated in methylmalonic acidemia because the defective enzyme is active not only in liver but also in kidney and brain. Later renal failure is a recognized complication of the disease. Whether early liver transplantation or combined liver-kidney transplantation is optimal is currently under study.

DISORDERS OF PYRUVATE AND MITOCHONDRIAL ENERGY METABOLISM

Disorders of pyruvate and mitochondrial energy metabolism have been the topic of active research in the past two decades and constitute uncommon but serious neonatal neurological disorders. Together with disorders of propionate and methylmalonate metabolism and of branched-chain ketoacid metabolism, these disorders are important examples of organic acid disturbances. In large part because of the difficulties in studying the complex enzyme systems involved, the elucidation of abnormalities of pyruvate and mitochondrial energy metabolism has been relatively recent.

Disorders of pyruvate and mitochondrial energy metabolism may lead to striking metabolic acidosis with lactic acidemia in the neonatal period. Disorders related to *pyruvate metabolism* may involve either the Krebs citric acid cycle or the electron transport system. *Disorders of the citric acid cycle* with neonatal onset include deficiencies of alpha-ketoglutarate decarboxylation (dihydrolipoyl dehydrogenase deficiency), succinate dehydrogenase, or fumarase.[87] However, because only a few well-studied neonatal cases have been documented, these disorders are not discussed in detail. Fumarase deficiency with fumaric acidemia is the most common of these conditions with a neonatal presentation. Reports delineate a rare neonatal or early infantile syndrome of hypotonia, seizures, dysmorphic facial features, frontal bossing, microcephaly, neonatal polycythemia, diffuse polymicrogyria, dysgenetic corpus callosum, hypomyelination, and ventriculomegaly.[87-89] *Disorders of the electron transport chain* are more common. In addition to the metabolic abnormalities, the prominent features of these disorders include manifestations of encephalopathy, myopathy, or both, and thus they are discussed in Chapters 16 and 19. In this chapter, I focus on disorders of pyruvate metabolism, because the metabolic manifestations, particularly *lactic acidemia*, tend to dominate the neonatal clinical presentation.

Normal Metabolic Aspects

Pyruvate occupies a central position in intermediary metabolism (Fig. 15-7).[87,90,91] It is formed primarily from glucose through the process of glycolysis, in brain as in other tissues. The major metabolic fates of

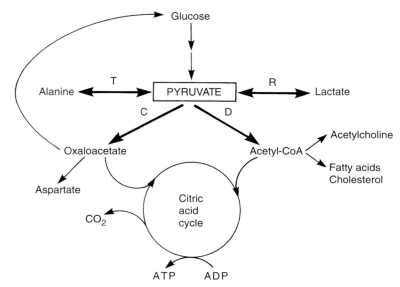

Figure 15-7   Major metabolic fates of pyruvate. See text for details. ADP, adenosine diphosphate; ATP, adenosine triphosphate; C, carboxylation; CoA, coenzyme A; D, decarboxylation; R, reduction; T, transamination.

pyruvate are shown in Figure 15-7 and are summarized in Table 15-6.

Transamination results in the formation of alanine, used, in part, for protein synthesis. The reverse reaction is particularly important in liver for gluconeogenesis from alanine.

Reduction to lactate is catalyzed by lactate dehydrogenase. Lactate can be used for gluconeogenesis through the reversal of this reaction.

Pyruvate *carboxylation*, catalyzed by the biotin-dependent enzyme pyruvate carboxylase, results in the formation of oxaloacetate. This step is critical in gluconeogenesis in liver and in several other tissues (but not to any significant extent in brain).[90] Oxaloacetate also is an important intermediate in the citric acid cycle, and this reaction plays a role in priming the cycle. Oxaloacetate transamination results in the formation of aspartate, an excitatory neurotransmitter in brain, a precursor for protein synthesis, and an important component of the urea cycle.

Pyruvate *decarboxylation*, catalyzed by the thiamine-dependent pyruvate dehydrogenase complex, is an

exceedingly important reaction in all tissues, including brain, in view of the nature of its product, acetyl-CoA. The reaction thereby plays a major role in citric acid cycle function, in adenosine triphosphate synthesis, and in the syntheses of acetylcholine and lipids (i.e., fatty acids and cholesterol).

Biochemical Aspects of Disordered Metabolism

Enzymatic Defects and Essential Consequences

Of the four major fates of pyruvate, impairment of two, decarboxylation and carboxylation, has been described (see later discussion). Defects in the pyruvate dehydrogenase complex and in pyruvate carboxylase have been the enzymatic defects for these disorders. Both defects cause accumulation of pyruvate, lactate, and alanine proximal to the enzymatic block, but obviously the consequences distal to the enzymatic blocks differ to some degree.

Relation to Acute Neurological Dysfunction and to Neuropathology

The mechanisms for brain injury in defects of the pyruvate dehydrogenase complex or of pyruvate carboxylase include acute and more long-lasting effects. The common metabolic feature of these disorders, *lactic acidosis*, may be very important in causing the acute neurological dysfunction. Moreover, an irreversible structural deficit is a likely consequence when the acidosis is severe and prolonged.

A second metabolic feature, important in the genesis of the acute neurological dysfunction associated with disturbances in pyruvate metabolism, is impairment of the synthesis of factors important in *neurotransmission*. Thus, a deficiency of pyruvate dehydrogenase complex activity may be expected to lead to a diminution in the

TABLE 15-6   Major Metabolic Fates of Pyruvate
Transamination
Gluconeogenesis
Alanine synthesis
Reduction
Lactate formation
Carboxylation
Gluconeogenesis
Aspartate synthesis
"Prime" citric acid cycle
Decarboxylation
Energy production
Lipid synthesis
Acetylcholine synthesis

synthesis of acetylcholine (an established and important neurotransmitter).[90,91] A deficiency of pyruvate carboxylase activity, with resulting decreased synthesis of oxaloacetate and function of the citric acid cycle, could lead to a disturbance of the excitatory amino acid transmitters, aspartate (a transamination product of oxaloacetate) and glutamate (a transamination product of the citric acid cycle intermediate alpha-ketoglutarate).

A third metabolic feature, probably important in the genesis of both acute and chronic effects, is impairment of *energy production*.[90] This impairment would be expected with a disturbance of acetyl-CoA synthesis by pyruvate dehydrogenase complex deficiency, but the disturbance of oxaloacetate synthesis by pyruvate carboxylase deficiency may also have a similar consequence.

A fourth metabolic feature, which may be of particular importance in the genesis of the long-term irreversible structural deficits, is a disturbance in the *synthesis of brain lipids and proteins*. Disturbed pyruvate dehydrogenase complex activity would be expected to lead to impairment in the synthesis of fatty acids and cholesterol, critical constituents of neural membranes, including myelin, by impairment of acetyl-CoA formation. Experimental support for this notion is available.[92] Deficits of pyruvate dehydrogenase complex and of pyruvate carboxylase also would lead to an alteration in levels of certain amino acids (e.g., alanine and aspartate) and perhaps thereby to a secondary disturbance of protein synthesis. The relative roles of these several factors remain to be defined in the inborn errors of pyruvate decarboxylation and carboxylation.

Pyruvate Dehydrogenase Complex Deficiency

Clinical Features

In general, pyruvate dehydrogenase complex deficiency is associated with three major categories of clinical phenotype, divisible according to age of onset: (1) neonatal types, (2) infantile form (onset, 3 to 6 months), and (3) later-onset benign forms with episodic ataxia.[87,90,91,93-96] The infantile form is characterized particularly by hypotonia, cranial nerve signs (especially ophthalmoplegia), ataxia, delayed development, ventilatory disturbance, and other features, and it is most often (≈85% of cases) associated with the neuropathological features of Leigh syndrome (see Chapter 16). The later-onset forms may be punctuated by transient episodes of ataxia or paraparesis, but, overall, development is normal or only mildly disturbed.

The *clinical features of the neonatal forms of pyruvate dehydrogenase complex deficiency* consist of two basic syndromes: (1) marked lactic acidosis, often with dysmorphic craniofacial features and brain anomalies; and (2) Leigh syndrome. Newborns with Leigh syndrome overlap with those with the infantile forms of pyruvate dehydrogenase complex deficiency with slightly later onset of Leigh syndrome, noted in the previous

TABLE 15-7	Common Features of Pyruvate Dehydrogenase Complex Deficiency with Neonatal Onset
Clinical Features	
Stupor, coma	
Tachypnea	
Seizures	
Hypotonia	
Dysmorphic facial features	
Metabolic Features	
Acidosis	
Lactic and pyruvic acidemia	
Hyperalaninemia	
Neuropathological Features	
Cerebral cortical and white matter atrophy	
Subcortical white matter cysts	
Cerebral gyral abnormalities (polymicrogyria, pachygyria)	
Impaired myelination	
Agenesis of the corpus callosum	
Dysgenetic brainstem and cerebellum	
Subacute necrotizing encephalopathy (Leigh syndrome)*	

*See Chapter 16.

paragraph and discussed in Chapter 16. In this group, the onset of symptoms generally is in the first week of life and is often within the first 24 hours.[90,93-109]

The major clinical features of the *more common of the two neonatal forms (i.e., marked lactic acidosis)* include stupor, tachypnea, hypotonia, and seizures (Table 15-7). The infant's course may be fulminating, with coma evolving in hours to a day or so. Most of the infants with this severe presentation have died in the first year of life. Newborns with pyruvate dehydrogenase complex deficiency may exhibit prominent craniofacial dysmorphic features (Fig. 15-8) and signs of cerebral dysgenesis.[87,89-91,94,96,110-114] The features of dysgenesis include partial or total agenesis of the corpus callosum, ventricular dilation, gyral

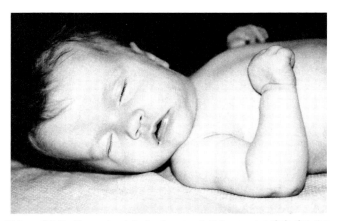

Figure 15-8 **Pyruvate dehydrogenase deficiency: craniofacial dysmorphism.** This affected girl shows frontal bossing, an upturned nose, a thin upper lip, and low-set ears. *(From De Meirleir L, Lissens W, Wayenberg JL, Michotte A, et al: Pyruvate dehydrogenase deficiency: Clinical and biochemical diagnosis, Pediatr Neurol 9:216-220, 1993.)*

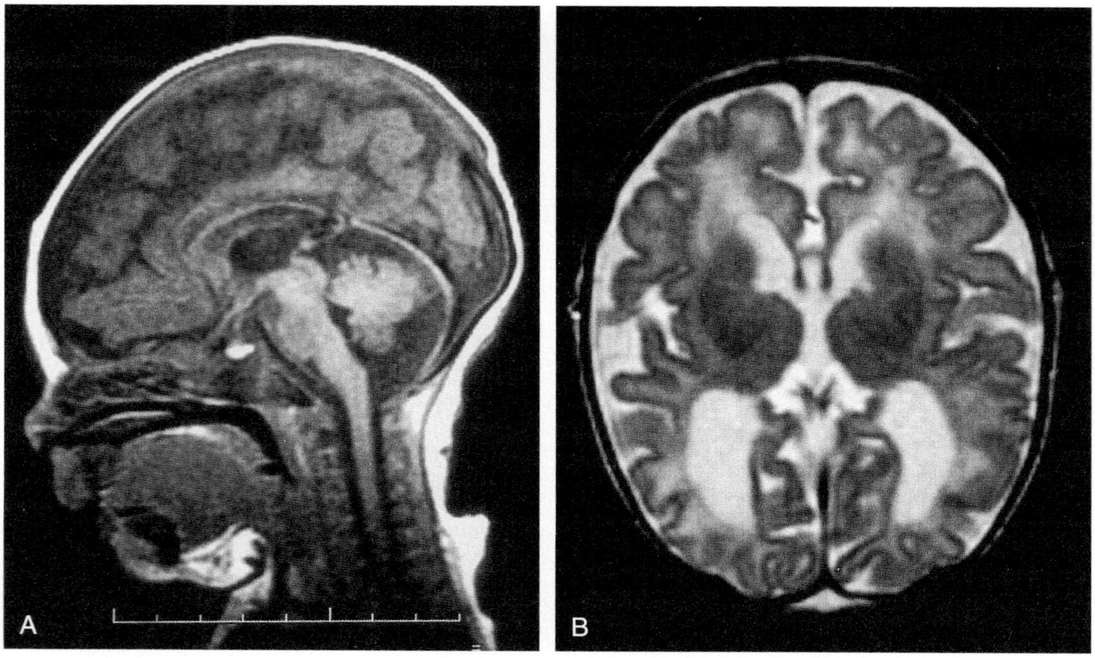

Figure 15-9 **Brain abnormalities in a 2-day-old infant girl with pyruvate dehydrogenase complex deficiency. A,** T1-weighted magnetic resonance imaging (MRI) shows markedly hypoplastic corpus callosum, decreased signal intensity in cerebral white matter, and enlarged subarachnoid spaces. **B,** Axial T2-weighted MRI shows markedly increased signal intensity in cerebral white matter, ventriculomegaly, and enlarged subarachnoid spaces. The infant's MR spectroscopy (not shown) demonstrated markedly elevated lactate resonance.

abnormalities, subependymal heterotopias, hypoplasia of hindbrain structures (brain stem and cerebellum), and ectopic olivary nuclei. Severe impairment of neurological development, often with microcephaly, is the rule in survivors.

Brain imaging, especially MRI, shows the structural features in cerebrum and posterior fossa structures.[89,96,115-117] Prenatal onset is indicated by the frequent finding of abnormal corpus callosum (Fig. 15-9). Moreover, MR spectroscopy has demonstrated an increased pyruvate signal as well as increased lactate.[115]

Genetic data indicate that the disorder most often is inherited in an X-linked dominant fashion. Thus, although nearly equal numbers of male and female patients exhibit defects of the pyruvate dehydrogenase complex, infants with somewhat less severe disease tend to be female. It is likely that severe mutations in hemizygous males are incompatible with life, whereas such severe mutations in females can be tolerated to some extent.[118] Although living male infants tend to exhibit the most severe phenotypes, female infants also may exhibit severe disease. It is now known that most neonatal-onset cases are caused by a defect of the E_{1alpha} subunit of the complex.[87,90,91,94-96,106,109,118-120] The gene for the E_{1alpha} subunit has been localized to the short arms of the X-chromosome (Xp22.1 to 22.2). As noted earlier, hemizygous male infants and heterozygous female infants may exhibit disease. Bias of X-inactivation toward expression of the mutant allele appears to be important in determining the occurrence of the disease and its severity in the heterozygous female infants.[90,109,112,121]

Metabolic Features

Major Findings. The hallmarks of a disturbance of pyruvate utilization (accumulations in blood of pyruvic and lactic acids and of alanine) are present (see Table 15-7). Distinction from other causes of neonatal metabolic acidosis (see Table 15-1) is aided by the accompanying hyperalaninemia and by the lack of accumulation of propionate or methylmalonic acid. The lactate-to-pyruvate ratio is usually normal (see Fig. 15-1). (Certain patients also exhibit elevated concentrations of alpha-ketoglutarate, branched-chain amino acids, and ketone bodies.[93,101,103,104,122]) The systemic acidosis may be relatively mild in the presence of more marked elevations of cerebrospinal fluid pyruvate and lactate or marked elevations in brain lactate, determined by MR spectroscopy.[96,113,123,124] This discrepancy may be more common in female infants and has been attributed to nonrandom X-inactivation with particular affection of brain.[94] The important point concerning the diagnostic evaluation is not to rely exclusively on measurements of lactate in blood.

Enzymatic Defects. The enzymatic defects have included five different components of the pyruvate dehydrogenase complex (Table 15-8). Thus, defects in pyruvate decarboxylase, lipoate acetyltransferase, lipoate dehydrogenase, and the regulatory phosphatase were described in numerous studies.[90,91,93-96,98-100,102-104,109,118,120,125-128] Additionally, a protein important in function of both lipoate components, so-called *protein X,* was shown to be defective in approximately 13 neonatal cases.[129,130] Most neonatal patients have had defects of

TABLE 15-8   **Pyruvate Dehydrogenase Complex**
Pyruvate Decarboxylase (Thiamine Dependent) Pyruvate → two-carbon unit + carbon dioxide
Lipoate Acetyltransferase Two-carbon unit + reduced lipoate → acetyl-CoA + oxidized lipoate
Lipoate Dehydrogenase Oxidized lipoate → reduced lipoate
Regulatory Enzymes Kinase (adenosine triphosphate dependent): inactivates the first reaction Phosphatase (magnesium, calcium dependent): activates the first reaction

the E_{1alpha} subunit, the gene located on the X-chromosome.[90,91,93,96] Defective pyruvate dehydrogenase complex activity was demonstrated in brain as well as liver, skeletal muscle, lymphocytes, and cultured fibroblasts.[90,93,98,122] However, notably, in affected female patients, apparently heterozygous for the E_{1alpha} defect, perhaps because of tissue-specific X-inactivation, pyruvate dehydrogenase complex activity may be *normal* in fibroblasts, lymphocytes, and muscle, with the genetic defect clearly present in brain.[94] Thus, because of such tissue-specific expression, a high index of suspicion for the disorder must exist, and multiple tissues (e.g., liver) may require analysis to detect the enzymatic defect.

Pathogenesis of Metabolic Features. The genesis of the metabolic defects relates to the impairment of the conversion of pyruvate to acetyl-CoA. Thus, the *acidosis* is accounted for particularly by the accumulation of pyruvic and lactic acids. The *hyperalaninemia* is related to the accumulation of pyruvate (see Fig. 15-7). Those rare patients with a defect in the lipoate dehydrogenase exhibit elevations of alpha-ketoglutarate and branched-chain ketoacids because the lipoate dehydrogenase in the three complexes (pyruvate dehydrogenase, alpha-ketoglutarate dehydrogenase, and branched-chain ketoacid dehydrogenase) appears to be the same enzyme.[104]

Neuropathology

The neuropathological findings include evidence both of destructive disease and of disturbance in brain development with onset as early as the first 20 weeks (see Table 15-7). This timing is based on the occurrence of agenesis of the corpus callosum and migrational defects in cerebrum (e.g., gyral abnormalities, heterotopias) and brain stem (e.g., ectopic olivary nuclei, brain stem hypoplasia) (see Fig. 15-9; Fig. 15-10). The gyral and callosal abnormalities have been detected by intrauterine MRI.[115-117] Neuropathological findings overall have included cerebral cortical and white matter atrophy and cystic lesions in subcortical white matter in the majority of cases, and evidence of disturbance of brain development in at least one third (see Fig. 15-10).[89-91,93,110-117,120] In approximately one third, predominantly male patients, neuropathological features of Leigh disease, including bilateral putaminal

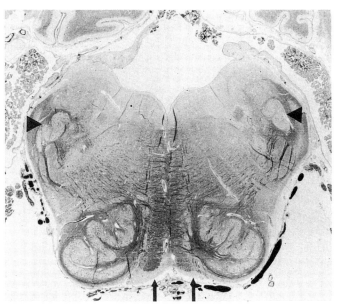

Figure 15-10   **Pyruvate dehydrogenase deficiency: neuropathology.** Transverse section of the medulla shows dorsal ectopic foci *(arrowheads)* of the inferior olives and absent pyramids *(arrows)*. *(From De Meirleir L, Lissens W, Wayenberg JL, Michotte A, et al: Pyruvate dehydrogenase deficiency: Clinical and biochemical diagnosis, Pediatr Neurol 9:216-220, 1993.)*

necrosis (see Chapter 16),[95,106] have been observed, but the full spectrum of Leigh disease is more common in cases with infantile (≈3 to 6 months) onset. The dysgenetic findings tend to be more prominent in female patients[96] and consist of polymicrogyria, pachygyria, cerebral heterotopias, malformed inferior olivary nuclei, and hypoplastic brain stem (including absence of corticospinal tracts), as well as cerebral hypomyelination and absence of hypoplastic corpus callosum. These disturbances suggest abnormalities in neuronal migration, axonal development, and subsequently myelination. Such disturbances have been observed in genetically manipulated mice with pyruvate dehydrogenase deficiency.[131]

Disturbances in myelination have been recognized for many years (Fig. 15-11).[100] Thus, in the initial report, two children from the same family exhibited considerable diminution in myelin in the cerebrum, brain stem, cerebellum, and spinal cord. No sign of myelin destruction or of neuronal injury was observed. Myelin vacuolation, as observed in infants with various disorders of amino acid and organic acid metabolism, was noted in an infant with onset of disease in the second month and death at 18 months.[105] The nearly uniform occurrence of evidence by brain imaging of diminished cerebral white matter with ventriculomegaly is consistent with an impairment in myelination.[90,91,110,111,113-117,132]

Management

Antenatal Diagnosis. Neither antenatal diagnosis nor prevention by therapeutic abortion has been reported. DNA diagnostic techniques hold considerable promise for prenatal diagnosis.[90,94]

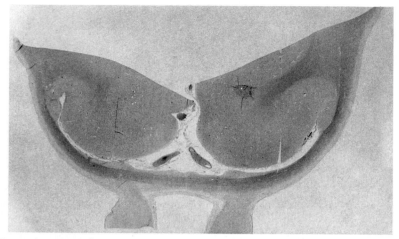

Figure 15-11 **Myelin disturbance in pyruvate dehydrogenase complex deficiency.** In infancy, this 6-year-old child exhibited hypotonia and impaired neurological development and subsequently manifested spastic quadriplegia, choreoathetosis, seizures, and episodes of severe acidosis. This coronal section was stained for myelin, through the cingulate gyri above and the corpus callosum below. The corpus callosum is very thin, and both the corpus and subcortical white matter are very lightly stained because of the paucity of myelin. *(From Cederbaum SD, Blass JP, Minkoff N, Brown WJ, et al: Sensitivity to carbohydrate in a patient with familial intermittent lactic acidosis and pyruvate dehydrogenase deficiency, Pediatr Res 10:713-720, 1976.)*

Early Detection and Acute Therapy. Early detection and acute therapy are critical. The severe acute acidosis requires treatment with intravenous fluids and sodium bicarbonate and may require peritoneal dialysis. Therapy with dichloroacetate causes a decrease in both blood and brain lactate.[91,96,133] This agent inhibits pyruvate dehydrogenase kinase and thereby favors activation of the enzyme. Moreover, the drug also decreases the rate of degradation of the E_{1alpha} subunit and thereby causes an increase in total cellular pyruvate dehydrogenase complex activity.[134,135] The increased conversion of pyruvate to acetyl-CoA decreases the severity of the lactic acidosis.

Long-Term Therapy. Long-term therapy usually includes a diet that is relatively high in fat (e.g., ketogenic diet), because fat, unlike carbohydrate, provides a source of acetyl-CoA (through ketone bodies) that bypasses the pyruvate dehydrogenase step. Particular care must be taken to provide enough calories as fat to make the patient ketonemic but not hypoglycemic or acidotic.[90,93,96,136] Clinical data have shown a beneficial effect of the ketogenic diet on neurological development.[96]

Because thiamine dependence has been reported in some cases of pyruvate dehydrogenase complex deficiency,[90,137,138] a trial of large doses of *thiamine* is appropriate.[93] Similarly, a therapeutic trial of *lipoic acid* may be considered.[54,93] Additionally, because excretion of carnitine derivatives of metabolic acids may lead to secondary carnitine deficiency, L-carnitine supplementation may be useful.[93] Finally, *dichloroacetate* appears to have value in long-term treatment of pyruvate dehydrogenase complex deficiency, especially if the deficiency is not complete.[90,91,93,96,97,139]

Pyruvate Carboxylase Deficiency

Clinical Features

The clinical presentation of pyruvate carboxylase deficiency consists of two major syndromes: (1) a fulminating syndrome of neonatal onset, associated with severe enzyme deficiency caused by absence of the apoenzyme (usually termed the French phenotype or type B); and (2) a syndrome usually of slightly later onset, 2 to 5 months of age, somewhat less severe, associated with partial enzyme activity, and an alteration in catalytic efficiency of the enzyme (type A).[3,4,90,93,96,109,122,140,141] (Onset in the neonatal period, however, can occur in the type A cases.) The neonatal syndrome in the type B disorder has been described in approximately 20 infants and is characterized by the clinical features described in Table 15-9.[10,90,93,140-146] Similarities to the features of pyruvate dehydrogenase complex deficiency are apparent. Macrocephaly may be a distinctive feature of pyruvate carboxylase deficiency, and although the condition is reported commonly, the exact incidence is unclear because of the frequent lack of data on head circumference measurement. A recent report emphasized the high frequency of a movement disorder and unusual ocular behavior.[141] The movement disorder consisted of episodic stimulus-sensitive tremors interspersed with diffuse hypokinesia and lack of facial expression. The ocular findings consisted of fixed gaze, interspersed with pendular nystagmus and episodic conjugate eye movements. Both features are reminiscent of the extrapyramidal features observed with inborn defects of monoamine neurotransmitter biosynthesis (see Chapter 16). Disturbances of neurotransmitter synthesis likely occur in pyruvate carboxylase deficiency (see later). All the infants died by 4 months of life.

TABLE 15-9 Common Features of Pyruvate Carboxylase Deficiency with Neonatal Onset

Clinical Features
Stupor, coma
Tachypnea
Seizures
Hypotonia

Metabolic Features
Acidosis
Lactic and pyruvic acidemia
Hyperalaninemia
Low aspartic acid levels
Hypoglycemia
Hyperammonemia, citrullinemia, hyperlysinemia
Ketosis

Neuropathological Features
Cerebral cortical and white matter atrophy
Periventricular white matter cysts
Impaired myelination

The genetic data available on the neonatal patients indicate *autosomal recessive* inheritance. Intermediate depression of enzymatic activity has been demonstrated in parents of affected patients.[147]

Metabolic Features

Major Findings. The hallmarks of a disorder of pyruvate metabolism, accumulations in blood of pyruvic and lactic acids and alanine, are present. The levels of lactate in the neonatal patients with pyruvate carboxylase deficiency are significantly higher than in the patients with later onsets. The lactate-to-pyruvate ratios in severe (type B) neonatal-onset cases are often normal because of increased cytosolic reduction; in less severely affected type A cases, the ratio is usually normal.[90] Because of the important role of pyruvate carboxylase in hepatic gluconeogenesis (see Fig. 15-7), hypoglycemia is common; median blood glucose was approximately 30 mg/dL in a recent series.[141] Moreover, because of the disturbance in oxaloacetate biosynthesis (see Fig. 15-7), the function of the Krebs cycle is impaired, and aspartate is depleted. Aspartate depletion results in impaired function of the urea cycle, which requires this amino acid; thus, hyperammonemia, citrullinemia, and hyperlysinemia occur.

Enzymatic Defect. The enzymatic defect involves pyruvate carboxylase and has been demonstrated in brain, liver, kidney, and cultured fibroblasts of affected patients.[9,10,90,93,96,122,141-143,146,147] In the neonatal-onset variety, essentially no enzyme activity can be demonstrated, and in most patients, both the pyruvate carboxylase apoenzyme and its mRNA are virtually absent.

Pathogenesis of Metabolic Features. The genesis of the metabolic disturbances relates to the defect in pyruvate carboxylation. As noted earlier, proximal to the enzymatic block, pyruvic and lactic acids accumulate and contribute to the *acidosis*. *Hyperalaninemia* is another proximal consequence of the enzymatic block. *Hyperammonemia*, citrullinemia, and hyperlysinemia occur as a consequence of the disturbance in the urea cycle caused by the depletion of aspartate, in turn caused by the disturbance of oxaloacetate production. An increased conversion of pyruvate to acetyl-CoA occurs as a consequence of the defect in pyruvate carboxylation and, because of the disturbance of the Krebs cycle, acetyl-CoA is converted preferentially to fatty acids and ultimately to ketone bodies, resulting in the ketosis.

In brain, a disturbance in neurotransmitter metabolism is likely, and this disturbance involves the astrocyte and particularly glutamate and gamma-aminobutyric acid. Thus, pyruvate carboxylase in brain is abundant in astrocytes but not in neurons.[90] The resulting deficit in oxaloacetate leads to a defect in citric acid cycle function and thereby alpha-ketoglutarate biosynthesis. The latter is important because, normally, successive transaminations result in formation of glutamate and glutamine. Glutamine then diffuses to neurons, where glutamate is generated and is used as a neurotransmitter and for restoration of the citric acid cycle for energy production and synthetic processes. Failure of this so-called anaplerotic role results in depletion of the neurotransmitters, glutamate and its product gamma-aminobutyric acid. The neurotransmitter defects may underlie some of the unusual neonatal neurological features (see earlier), whereas the disturbances of energy production and synthetic processes could lead to neuronal dysgenesis and death.[90]

Neuropathology

Neuropathological features are indicative of both destructive and developmental disturbances (see Table 15-9).[90,93,96,140,141,146,148] Thus, cerebral cortical neuronal loss, white matter atrophy, and periventricular cysts in cerebral white matter suggest destructive disease. Indeed, the brain imaging picture of apparent periventricular leukomalacia in an infant with lactic acidosis should suggest pyruvate carboxylase deficiency. The white matter lesions have been documented in utero by fetal ultrasonography at 29 weeks of gestation.[140] Vacuolated white matter and subsequent impairment of myelination have been well documented.

Management

Antenatal Diagnosis. Antenatal diagnosis has been accomplished by demonstration of deficient pyruvate carboxylase activity in amniotic fluid cells.[90,147] Prevention by therapeutic abortion thus is possible.

Early Detection and Acute Therapy. Early detection is critical. Treatment of the acute episode with glucose, alkali, and, if necessary, peritoneal dialysis has been lifesaving. However, beneficial effects have been only transient in cases of neonatal onset.

Long-Term Therapy. Dietary therapy is difficult. A relatively high-carbohydrate diet with sufficient amounts of protein for growth is recommended, but

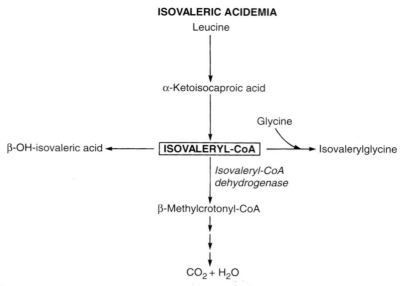

Figure 15-12   **Metabolic defect in isovaleric acidemia.** Isovaleryl–coenzyme A (CoA), a product of leucine catabolism, accumulates because of the impairment of isovaleryl-CoA dehydrogenase.

no systematic demonstrations of efficacy have been reported.[93] A diet relatively high in fat, as used in pyruvate dehydrogenase complex deficiency, is not indicated in this setting, at least in part because ketosis is a prominent feature of this disorder (see earlier discussion). Aspartic acid supplementation is appropriate, as is a trial of biotin, a critical cofactor for pyruvate carboxylase. Recent reports suggest that triheptanoin, an odd-carbon (seven carbons) triglyceride, and citrate may be useful in improving metabolic status by providing an alternative energy source (ketone bodies).[141,149] Further data will be of interest.

Gene Therapy. Orthoptic liver transplantation in a single case produced partial metabolic improvement but no benefit for neurological development.[150]

DISORDERS OF BRANCHED-CHAIN KETOACID METABOLISM

Branched-chain ketoacids, derived from the branched-chain amino acids leucine, isoleucine, and valine, are involved in several disorders with manifestations in the neonatal period (see Table 15-1). These disorders include classic maple syrup urine disease, isovaleric acidemia, beta-methylcrotonyl-CoA carboxylase deficiency, beta-ketothiolase deficiency, and hydroxy-methylglutaryl (HMG)–CoA lyase deficiency.[54,151] Of these disorders, maple syrup urine disease is the most common and is discussed in Chapter 14 as a disorder of amino acid metabolism. Isovaleric acidemia is the next most common, accounting for approximately 15% of all organic acidurias in one large series,[2] and it is reviewed in detail next. Deficiencies of beta-methyl-crotonyl–CoA carboxylase, beta-ketothiolase, and HMG-CoA lyase are very rare in the newborn and are discussed only briefly.

Isovaleric Acidemia

Isovaleric acidemia results from a defect in leucine catabolism at the step immediately distal to that which is the basis for maple syrup urine disease. The defect involves the conversion of isovaleric acid to beta-methylcrotonyl–CoA (Fig. 15-12). The latter compound is metabolized further by beta-methylcrotonyl–CoA carboxylase (see later discussion).

Clinical Features

Two clinical phenotypes are recognized: an acute, severe neonatal form and a chronic intermittent form with onset later in infancy. The neonatal form accounts for approximately half of all cases, and survivors often develop intermittent episodes later in infancy.[151] Onset of the disease is usually in the first days of life (most often 3 to 6 days of age), and the presenting clinical features are similar to those associated with disorders of propionate and methylmalonate metabolism (see Table 15-2).[151-158] Thus, vomiting, tachypnea, and stupor or coma are common (Table 15-10). In addition,

TABLE 15-10	Common Features of Isovaleric Acidemia
Clinical Features	
Vomiting	
Tachypnea	
Stupor, coma	
Odor of sweaty feet	
Metabolic Features	
Acidosis	
Isovaleric acidemia (aciduria)	
Isovaleryl glycinuria, beta-hydroxyisovaleric aciduria	
Hyperammonemia	
Other Features	
Neutropenia or thrombocytopenia	

the accumulation of isovaleric acid in body fluids (e.g., urine and sweat) imparts a characteristic offensive odor of "sweaty feet." The course is fulminating. Thrombocytopenia and neutropenia, or pancytopenia, are common. Overall, in earlier studies, more than half of the infants died in the neonatal period, and most of the survivors exhibited mental retardation and other signs of brain injury. However, more recently, earlier detection and more aggressive short-term and long-term therapy (see later discussion) have improved survival rates markedly, and only a minority of survivors have exhibited prominent neurological sequelae.[151,159] The presence of affected siblings of both sexes and the demonstration of intermediate deficiency of leucine catabolism and levels of dehydrogenase in heterozygotes indicate that inheritance in this disorder is *autosomal recessive.*[151,154,156]

Metabolic Features

Major Findings. The characteristic metabolic features are severe acidosis, isovaleric acidemia and aciduria, isovalerylglycinuria, beta-hydroxyisovaleric acidemia and aciduria, and pancytopenia (see Fig. 15-12). Mild to moderate hyperammonemia is common. Occasionally, patients exhibit hypocalcemia, the basis for which is unclear. Mild hyperglycinemia may occur during the acute episodes, and thus the ketotic hyperglycinemia syndrome can be caused by this defect.[16]

Enzymatic Defect. The enzymatic defect involves isovaleryl-CoA dehydrogenase. This conclusion was based initially on studies of the accumulated metabolites and the metabolism of leucine in cultured fibroblasts.[156,160] The enzymatic defect has been demonstrated directly.[151,156,161,162] A recently developed enzymatic method allows identification of the defect in only a few hours from the time of initial blood sampling.[163]

Pathogenesis of Metabolic Features. The genesis of the metabolic defects is understood to a considerable degree. The *acidosis* relates, in part, to the accumulation of isovaleric acid, which, during periods of decompensation, reaches approximately 1000-fold normal concentrations in plasma.[151] In addition, accumulations of ketone bodies and lactate contribute significantly to the acidosis. These accumulations result from a disturbance of mitochondrial function, including pyruvate dehydrogenase, caused by the isovaleric acid (more specifically, the CoA derivative thereof).[164,165] The mitochondrial disturbance may account for the impairment of brain high-energy phosphates documented in an affected infant by phosphorus MR spectroscopy.[158] *The excessive excretion of isovalerylglycine and of beta-hydroxyisovaleric acid* reflects alternate pathways of isovaleric acid metabolism (see Fig. 15-12). Quantitatively, the more important of these pathways is the conjugation of isovaleric acid with glycine by the enzyme glycine-*N*-acylase to form the water-soluble conjugate, isovalerylglycine. This conjugate is excreted very rapidly, and indeed, during periods of remission, very little free isovaleric acid can be detected in the patient's urine.

Because this process is so active, *hyperglycinemia* is less likely to develop in this disorder than in other disorders causing the ketotic hyperglycinemia syndrome, as demonstrated by the only occasional report of hyperglycinemia. By analogy with disorders of the propionate and methylmalonate pathway, the hyperglycinemia is probably caused by inhibition of glycine cleavage by the CoA derivative of the accumulated alpha-ketoisocaproic acid, the ketoacid that is the immediate precursor of isovaleric acid (see Fig. 15-12). Similarly, the moderate *hyperammonemia* that is observed also relates to the effects of the CoA derivative on the carbamyl phosphate step of the Krebs-Henseleit urea cycle.

Neuropathology

I am unaware of any detailed neuropathological study of isovaleric acidemia of neonatal onset. One infant was reported to have cerebellar hemorrhage at autopsy[157]; the cause may be analogous to that of the cerebellar hemorrhage of propionic and methylmalonic acidemia (hypertonic sodium bicarbonate, thrombocytopenia, involvement of external granule cell layer; see earlier discussion). "White matter edema" and vacuolation have been observed,[157] but whether these findings are analogous to the myelin disturbance typical of other amino acid and organic acid disturbances is not yet clear.

Management

Antenatal Diagnosis. Prenatal diagnosis has been accomplished by demonstration of either undetectable or minimal isovaleryl dehydrogenase activity in cultured amniocytes or elevated levels of isovalerylglycine in amniotic fluid.[151]

Early Detection. Early detection is critical. Distinction from the other causes of severe metabolic acidosis in the neonatal period is necessary (see Table 15-1). The odor of sweaty feet is the most helpful feature in the clinical detection of isovaleric acidemia.

Acute and Long-Term Therapy. Short-term therapy includes glucose and bicarbonate infusion to reduce endogenous protein catabolism and to control acidosis.[151] Later therapy consists of a diet low in protein to decrease the amount of leucine catabolized to isovaleryl-CoA and supplementation with glycine and carnitine.[3,4,151,159,166-169] The use of *glycine* has proved to be highly valuable in the treatment of both the acute episode and subsequently. The principle for administering glycine is based on the finding that the isovalerylglycine conjugate, formed from glycine and isovaleryl-CoA, is rapidly excreted by the kidneys. This excretion provides a means for rapid elimination of the accumulated isovaleric acid. Because the Michaelis constant (K_m) of glycine-*N*-acylase is higher than the intracellular concentration of glycine, the provision of exogenous glycine would be expected to increase conjugation of isovaleric acid.[170] Cohn and coworkers[171] initially treated two very sick infants who had isovaleric acidemia in the first month of life with 250 mg/kg of glycine, with dramatic biochemical benefit within 3 days and normalization of the neurological examination within 2 weeks. On a maintenance dosage of glycine (800 mg daily) and a low-protein diet, these infants experienced normal neurological development by 6 and 13 months of age. Subsequent work supports the value of this approach.[151,159]

Supplementation with *carnitine* is based on the finding that, with the accumulation of isovaleric acid and related organic acids, isovalerylcarnitine and carnitine esters of the other acids are markedly excreted, thus resulting in a secondary carnitine deficiency.[151,166-168] The administration of carnitine corrects the carnitine deficiency and provides a means of removal of toxic isovaleric acid through easily excreted isovalerylcarnitine.

Beta-Methylcrotonyl–Coenzyme A Carboxylase Deficiency

The product of the isovaleryl dehydrogenase reaction, beta-methylcrotonyl–CoA, undergoes carboxylation (see Fig. 15-12) by a specific carboxylase. With widespread use of tandem mass spectroscopy–based neonatal screening programs, deficiency of beta-methylcrotonyl–CoA carboxylase appears to be among the most frequent organic acid abnormalities.[172] However, the phenotype is variable, ranging from severe neonatal onset to asymptomatic adults. Only about 10 cases have presented in the neonatal period.[151,172-176] The clinical syndrome consisted of stupor, difficulty with feeding, vomiting, tachypnea, and acidosis. Hypoglycemia was a common feature. Several infants died, but long-term outcome in most survivors is unknown. High-dose biotin therapy has been beneficial.

Hydroxymethylglutaryl–Coenzyme A Lyase Deficiency

HMG–CoA lyase deficiency is a third defect in the catabolism of the branched-chain amino acid leucine.[151,177] The *clinical course* of this autosomal recessive disorder is characterized by onset in the neonatal period in approximately 50% of cases, with stupor, tachypnea, vomiting, and hypotonia.[3,4,144,151,177-181]

Approximately 10% of infants have had overt seizures. Hepatomegaly is an important finding on physical examination. The course is complicated by severe hypoglycemia, and as a consequence, without prompt intervention, approximately half of the affected infants have died. However, several infants promptly treated have exhibited normal subsequent development, and mortality rates have declined markedly. MRI has shown marked abnormalities of cerebral white matter.[180] Neuropathological data are scant, but one 6½-month-old infant exhibited "diffuse white matter spongiosis" and "gliosis" on a brain biopsy.[182] The *major metabolic features* include metabolic acidosis and severe hypoglycemia. The cause of the hypoglycemia may be related to the enzymatic defect (see next paragraph), which impairs ketone body formation and hence the glucose sparing of these alternative substrates. The combination of severe hypoglycemia and deficient ketone bodies causes the brain to be exquisitely vulnerable to the hypoglycemia, because the organ is deprived of a major alternative substrate. The metabolic acidosis is caused by the accumulated organic acids proximal to the enzymatic block. Hyperammonemia, which may be severe, has been observed in approximately half of infants. A secondary carnitine deficiency, secondary to excessive urinary excretion of acylcarnitines, as in other organic acid disorders, is common. The *enzymatic defect* involves the terminal step in leucine catabolism, the conversion of HMG-CoA to acetoacetate and acetyl-CoA (Fig. 15-13).[151,177-179,181,183]

Management consists of early detection, prompt and vigorous treatment of both acidosis *and* hypoglycemia, and a subsequent dietary regimen with restriction of leucine and carnitine supplementation. Normal outcome has been reported in several infants identified early and treated effectively.

Mevalonic Aciduria

Mevalonic aciduria, a relatively recently recognized disorder of leucine catabolism, is associated with two clinical phenotypes, a severe neonatal variety and

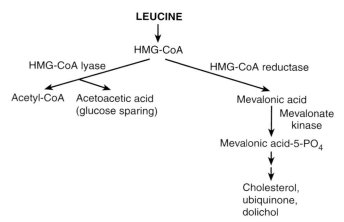

Figure 15-13 Terminal steps in leucine catabolism showing sites of action of hydroxymethylglutaryl (HMG)–coenzyme A (CoA) lyase and mevalonate kinase. PO_4, phosphate.

a more commonly recognized later-onset disorder.[151,184-189] The few reported newborns have exhibited dysplastic facial features, cataracts, hepatosplenomegaly, and anemia. Only one of the three carefully studied newborns had metabolic acidosis in the neonatal period, and acidosis does not appear to be a prominent feature of this disease. Subsequent neurological development has been impaired, hypotonia has been prominent, and neuroimaging has shown development of cerebellar atrophy. The mevalonic acid level is elevated in body fluids. The enzymatic defect involves mevalonate kinase (see Fig. 15-13), which is crucial in the synthesis of cholesterol for cellular membranes, ubiquinone for the electron transport chain, and dolichol for synthesis of the oligosaccharide moieties of glycoproteins. The disorder is autosomal recessive and is classified among disorders of branched-chain organic acid metabolism because the substrate for the reaction, HMG-CoA, is a product of leucine catabolism. Prenatal diagnosis by analysis of mevalonate kinase in a sample of chorionic villus has been accomplished at 12 weeks of gestation.[190] Suitable therapy has not been developed.

Beta-Ketothiolase Deficiency

Beta-ketothiolase deficiency is a defect in the catabolism of the branched-chain amino acid isoleucine.[3,4,151,177] The autosomal recessive disorder is primarily episodic in *clinical course*, and most patients have had onset months *after* the neonatal period. One infant developed vomiting in the neonatal period that became so severe by 4 weeks of age that a pyloromyotomy was performed,[191,192] a mistake in diagnosis and treatment not infrequently made with organic acid disorders.[193] Subsequently, the infant developed stupor and tachypnea before the correct diagnosis was made, and appropriate dietary therapy was instituted.

The *major metabolic features* in the infant reported[191,192] included ketoacidosis, hyperglycinemia, hyperammonemia, and pancytopenia (i.e., the ketotic hyperglycinemia syndrome). The accumulated CoA derivatives of the ketoacids proximal to the enzymatic block presumably caused the secondary metabolic abnormalities, as described for disorders of propionate and methylmalonate metabolism. Notably, hyperglycinemia has not been a feature of the cases of later onset. The *enzymatic defect* involves the terminal beta-ketothiolase in isoleucine catabolism, the product of which is propionate (see Fig. 15-2).[151,177,191,192,194,195]

Management consists of early detection, prompt treatment of acidosis, and subsequent moderate dietary protein restriction. Normal development has been observed in promptly treated infantile cases, except for the one neonatal case.

DISORDERS OF FATTY ACID OXIDATION

Disorders of mitochondrial fatty acid oxidation manifest very uncommonly in the neonatal period. In part, this finding may relate to the relatively high carbohydrate feeding of the newborn and the relatively uncommon need for fatty acid oxidation for energy production (e.g., during fasting). Fatty acid oxidation is particularly active in mitochondria of liver and muscle (both cardiac and skeletal) and consists of 20 individual steps (see Chapter 19). After cellular uptake of the fatty acid and cytosolic generation of the fatty acyl-CoA, the sequence of steps includes transesterification of the acyl-CoA derivative by carnitine palmityltransferase I (CPT I) before mitochondrial translocation by the carnitine acylcarnitine translocase, reesterification of acylcarnitine to acyl-CoA by the mitochondrial CPT II, and then beta-oxidation of the fatty acyl-CoA by the appropriate beta-oxidation series of enzymes.[196]

Because fatty acid oxidation is particularly active in muscle, some fatty acid oxidation disorders manifest in early infancy with prominent hypotonia and weakness, often with signs of cardiomyopathy; these disorders are discussed in Chapter 19. The most common such disorder with neonatal onset, albeit still rare, is carnitine transporter deficiency (primary carnitine deficiency).

Because fatty acid oxidation is particularly active in liver, as well as in muscle, fatty acid oxidation disorders may manifest with striking metabolic disturbances, especially hypoglycemia (without ketones, i.e., hypoketotic hypoglycemia), hyperammonemia, metabolic acidosis (usually mild), and dicarboxylic aciduria (fatty acid intermediates).[196,197] The clinical presentation often includes vomiting, altered level of consciousness, seizures, hypotonia more than hypertonia, and cardiac dysfunction. Sudden death may occur if the diagnosis is not established promptly and therapy instituted. Of all fatty acid oxidation disorders, medium-chain acyl-CoA dehydrogenase deficiency is associated with most cases of neonatal onset (see next paragraph). Rare examples of neonatal onset of the other fatty acid oxidation disorders are included in Table 15-11.[196-212]

Medium-Chain Acyl–Coenzyme A Dehydrogenase Deficiency

Of the inherited defects in the beta-oxidation of fatty acids, impairment of *medium-chain acyl-CoA hydrogenase* has been reported to cause clinical features in the newborn in approximately 10% to 20% of cases.[196,197,211,213-222] The clinical presentation has consisted of stupor, hypotonia, poor feeding, and respiratory difficulties. The onset of the illness has been related to the beginning of breast-feeding, a situation sometimes associated with relative fasting. Metabolic features have included only mild metabolic acidosis, hypoglycemia (without ketones, i.e., hypoketotic hypoglycemia), hyperammonemia, and dicarboxylic aciduria. The ratio of acylcarnitines to free carnitine is markedly elevated. Creatine kinase may be elevated, sometimes markedly. Approximately 45% of infants have died during the acute episode, usually before the correct diagnosis. The diagnosis is established by quantitation of medium-chain fatty acids (C_6 to C_{12}) and demonstration of the enzymatic defect in leukocytes or fibroblasts. The gene for this

TABLE 15-11	Fatty Acid Oxidation Disorders with Neonatal Onset*

Carnitine Transporter Deficiency*
Weakness, hypotonia, cardiomyopathy

Mitochondrial Carnitine-Acylcarnitine Translocase Deficiency
Sudden neonatal death

Carnitine Palmityltransferase I Deficiency
Bradycardia, cardiorespiratory arrest

Carnitine Palmityltransferase II Deficiency
Apnea, seizures, dysmorphic craniofacial features, cardiomyopathy, cystic dysplasia of brain and kidneys, neonatal death

Mitochondrial Trifunctional Protein Deficiency
Hypotonia, cardiomyopathy

Medium-Chain Acyl-CoA Dehydrogenase Deficiency*
Stupor, hypotonia, poor feeding

Medium-Chain 3-Ketoacyl–CoA Thiolase
Vomiting, acidosis, rhabdomyolysis, neonatal death

Short-Chain Acyl–CoA Dehydrogenase Deficiency
Seizures, jitteriness

Long-Chain Hydroxy-Acyl–CoA Dehydrogenase Deficiency
Hypoglycemia, hypotonia, cardiomyopathy, vomiting

Very-Long-Chain Acyl–CoA Dehydrogenase Deficiency
Seizures, stupor, metabolic acidosis, cardiomyopathy

*Most common with neonatal onset; *carnitine transporter deficiency* is discussed in Chapter 19, and *medium-chain acyl–coenzyme A dehydrogenase deficiency* is discussed in this chapter).

autosomal recessive disorder is located on the short arm of chromosome 1, and a single mutation accounts for nearly all cases. Therapy includes aggressive treatment of hypoglycemia and avoidance of fasting. Subsequently, a high-carbohydrate, low-fat diet is appropriate. Most infants also receive carnitine supplementation. Normal development has been documented after prompt diagnosis and institution of therapy.

OTHER ORGANIC ACID DISORDERS

Four additional organic acid disorders with manifestations in the newborn do not correspond to the

TABLE 15-12	Multiple Carboxylase Deficiency

Biotin-Dependent Carboxylases Affected
Propionyl–CoA carboxylase
Pyruvate carboxylase
beta-Methylcrotonyl–CoA carboxylase
Acetyl-CoA carboxylase

Two Basic Types
Holocarboxylase synthetase deficiency: neonatal onset common
Biotinidase deficiency: neonatal onset uncommon, usually later onset (median, 3 months)

categories described in the preceding sections. These are multiple carboxylase deficiency, multiple acyl-CoA dehydrogenase deficiency (glutaric acid, type II), glutathione synthetase deficiency (5-oxoprolinuria), and sulfite oxidase deficiency. These disorders are associated with metabolic acidosis (see Table 15-1).

Multiple Carboxylase Deficiency

Multiple carboxylase deficiency affects four carboxylases and consists of two essential types (Table 15-12).[3,4,223-228] The underlying disturbance involves metabolism of biotin, a vitamin essential for the action of carboxylases. Biotin is attached covalently to the apoenzymes to form the holoenzymes by a holocarboxylase synthetase, and biotin is recovered from the degraded enzyme by biotinidase. A disturbance of the former results in the neonatal form of multiple carboxylase deficiency, and a defect in biotinidase results in a later onset form of multiple carboxylase deficiency.

Holocarboxylase Synthetase Deficiency

The typical neonatal form of multiple carboxylase deficiency is related to holocarboxylase synthetase deficiency and has been reported in approximately 45 infants.[3,4,227-237] The *clinical course* of this autosomal recessive disorder is characterized by onset in the first days of life of stupor, vomiting, tachypnea, hypotonia, and, sometimes, seizures. A nonspecific skin rash, often erythematous and desquamating, is a common feature. Several infants have died before diagnosis and institution of appropriate therapy (see later discussion).

The *major metabolic features* include metabolic ketoacidosis, moderate hyperammonemia, hypoglycemia, and an organic acidemia that includes propionate, lactate, and beta-methylcrotonate. The metabolic features are caused principally by deficiencies of the following three carboxylases: propionyl-CoA carboxylase (propionic acidemia and hyperammonemia; see Fig. 15-2), pyruvate carboxylase (lactic acidemia and hypoglycemia; see Fig. 15-7), and beta-methylcrotonyl–CoA carboxylase (beta-methylcrotonic acidemia and beta-methylcrotonylglycinuria; see Fig. 15-12).

The *enzymatic defect* involves holocarboxylase synthetase, the enzyme that catalyzes the covalent linking of biotin to the three apocarboxylases enumerated. As noted earlier, biotin is essential as the carboxyl carrier for the propionyl-CoA, pyruvate, and beta-methylcrotonyl–CoA carboxylases. The mutation usually involves the biotin-binding domain of the apoenzyme, and the resulting enzyme has a markedly increased K_m (i.e., decreased affinity) for biotin. Partial responsiveness to exogenous biotin is thus explained. In rare instances, the mutation involves a different domain, and the resulting enzyme has a less impaired K_m but greatly reduced maximal velocity (maximal carboxylase activity).[223,228] These infants have a poor response to biotin. The enzymatic defect is demonstrable in cultured fibroblasts and in leukocytes. Prenatal diagnosis is possible by measurement of abnormal organic acids in the amniotic fluid or deficient carboxylase activities in cultured amniocytes.

Therapy of this disorder is principally *biotin* in high doses. This approach has been highly effective, and normal development and growth have been documented in the fetus after therapy commenced in the second or third trimester of pregnancy, as well as in newborns treated early postnatally.

Later-Onset Form: Biotinidase Deficiency

Although the second major form of multiple carboxylase deficiency, biotinidase deficiency, typically results in later onset (median age, 3 months), approximately 10% of patients exhibit onset in the first weeks of life.[6,124,223-226,236,238-245] The clinical features are similar to those observed with holocarboxylase synthetase deficiency, although *seizures* and hypotonia appear to be more common in biotinidase deficiency. Skin rash (dry, squamous appearance) and alopecia are common accompaniments. Subsequent neurological findings include ataxia, hearing loss, optic atrophy, and developmental delay. The diagnosis is suspected by the demonstration of the metabolic features described for holocarboxylase synthetase deficiency, but urinary organic acids occasionally are normal, and cerebrospinal fluid organic acid analysis may be required to show the metabolic defect.[124] Neuropathological features include vacuolation of white matter, defective myelination, and focal necrotizing lesions with vascular proliferation and gliosis, similar to those observed in Leigh disease but more diffuse in distribution.[223,240] The vacuolation of myelin is similar to that observed in many other amino acid and organic acid disorders and probably accounts for the abnormalities of white matter observed on reported computed tomography and MRI scans. The diagnosis is made by detection of low biotinidase in serum, leukocytes, or fibroblasts. Treatment with biotin is effective and should be instituted early in the disease to ensure a favorable outcome. A strikingly favorable response to therapy is illustrated in Figure 15-14.[226]

Multiple Acyl–Coenzyme A Dehydrogenase Deficiency: Glutaric Acidemia Type II

Only in recent years has it become clear that glutaric acidemia type II is not rare (Table 15-13).[3,4,246-249] The molecular defect involves a side chain to the main electron transport chain in the mitochondrion for the coupling of electron transport to the synthesis of adenosine triphosphate. The side chain is composed of electron transfer flavoprotein (ETF) and ETF-ubiquinone oxidoreductase (ETF-QO), which are involved in the transfer of electrons from multiple flavoprotein acyl-CoA and other dehydrogenases to the main respiratory chain. A defect of this side chain thus affects multiple dehydrogenase reactions, including fatty acid oxidation, branched-chain amino acid catabolism, and glutaryl-CoA catabolism, among other processes (see Table 15-13).

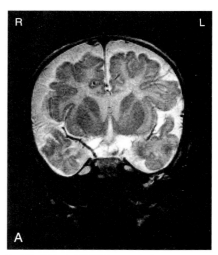

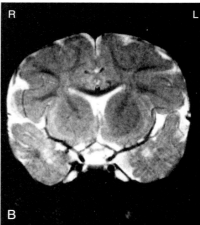

Figure 15-14 Coronal T2-weighted magnetic resonance imaging scans in an infant with biotinidase deficiency. **A,** Scan performed at 6 weeks of age shows high signal intensity in cerebral white matter and markedly enlarged subarachnoid spaces. The infant had developed a skin rash at 3 weeks and generalized seizures at 6 weeks. **B,** Scan performed at 14½ months of age, after 13 months of treatment with oral biotin, is normal. *(From Haagerup A, Andersen JB, Blichfeldt S, Christensen MF: Biotinidase deficiency: Two cases of very early presentation,* Dev Med Child Neurol *39:832-835, 1997.)*

TABLE 15-13	Multiple Acyl–CoA Dehydrogenase Deficiency: Glutaric Acidemia Type II

Major Acyl–CoA Dehydrogenases Affected
Fatty acyl–CoA dehydrogenases (long-chain, medium-chain, short-chain beta-oxidation)
Isovaleryl–CoA dehydrogenase (branched-chain amino acid catabolism)
Methylbutyryl–CoA dehydrogenase (branched-chain amino acid catabolism)
Glutaryl–CoA dehydrogenase (lysine, tryptophan catabolism)

Molecular Defects
Electron transport flavoprotein
Electron transport flavoprotein–ubiquinone oxidoreductase (most common defect in neonatal form with congenital anomalies)

Three basic clinical phenotypes are recognized[3,4,246-257]: (1) a severe neonatal onset form with congenital anomalies; (2) a rarer neonatal onset form without anomalies; and (3) a milder, later-onset variety. The *clinical features* of the classic neonatal syndrome include high frequency of premature birth and onset in the first 24 to 48 hours of stupor, tachypnea, vomiting, hypotonia, and sometimes seizures. Hepatomegaly, enlarged kidneys, facial dysmorphism, rocker-bottom feet, muscular defects of the anterior abdominal wall, abnormal external genitalia, and the odor of sweaty feet (involvement of isovaleryl dehydrogenase) are characteristic. The hypotonia may be so severe as to suggest a neuromuscular disorder. Infants without anomalies are less common but are otherwise similar. Rapid progression and death within a week are characteristic of the neonatal disease with anomalies, and survival for a few months is more common in the neonatal disease without anomalies.

The *pathological features* are interesting and characteristic.[246] Thus, microvesicular fatty change is prominent in liver, kidney, and myocardium. The kidneys are enlarged and cystic, a diagnosis made in life by ultrasonography or computed tomography. The *brain* shows focal cortical dysplasia with changes indicative of impaired neuronal migration. Warty protrusions over cerebral cortex, especially in the temporoparietal regions, have been demonstrated. Additionally dysgenesis of the corpus callosum has been described.[89] MRI has shown hypoplasia of temporal lobes, abnormal signal in the basal ganglia (especially caudate and putamen) and periventricular white matter, and cerebellar vermian hypoplasia.[50,258]

The *major metabolic features* consist of severe metabolic acidosis, severe hypoglycemia (without ketonemia or ketonuria), moderate hyperammonemia, and organic and fatty acidemia. The fatty acids include glutaric, isobutyric, and isovaleric acids. These fatty acids accumulate because of deficiencies of the dehydrogenases responsible for the degradation of the CoA derivatives of these compounds. Acylcarnitines, as a consequence, are usually elevated. The mitochondrial disturbance in brain is reflected by the finding by MR spectroscopy of elevated lactate.[248]

The *enzymatic defect* involves multiple dehydrogenases and is based on a deficiency of either ETF-QO or ETF. Severe disease with anomalies is associated much more commonly with ETF-QO deficiency than with ETF deficiency.[246,247] The defect is demonstrable in cultured fibroblasts. Prenatal diagnosis is accomplished most readily by demonstration of abnormal organic acids, usually glutarate, in amniotic fluid. However, diagnosis in the 17th week of gestation has been accomplished by immunoblot analysis and pulse-chase experiments.[259]

Therapy for this disorder requires vigorous supplementation acutely with glucose and alkali. Despite neonatal onset of therapy, outcome has been generally poor.[246] The demonstration of multiple systemic anomalies (e.g., polycystic kidneys and dysmorphic features) and cerebral dysplasia suggestive of migrational defect in many patients indicates that intrauterine disturbance may occur, and thus fetal therapy may be required. Treatment with a diet restricted in fat and protein and supplemented with riboflavin and L-carnitine has been generally unsuccessful in infants with the common severe disease and variably effective in those with less severe disease, usually of later onset.[246,249,256] A riboflavin-responsive form of glutaric acidemia, type II, manifesting later in infancy with severe white matter disease, has been reported.[260]

Glutaric Acidemia Type I

The syndrome of multiple acyl-CoA dehydrogenase deficiency, glutaric acidemia type II, should be distinguished from glutaric acidemia type I, which is caused by an isolated deficiency of glutaryl-CoA dehydrogenase.[261] This disorder typically has its onset in later infancy or early childhood with an extrapyramidal syndrome, especially with dystonia and dyskinesia, and developmental delay.[3,4,184,185,249,261-274] However, notably, *macrocephaly* is *present at birth* or in very early infancy in nearly all patients. (Macrocephaly and rapid head growth in early infancy may also herald the occurrence of a rarer but related disorder, L-2-hydroxyglutaric aciduria.[275-278] Perhaps similarly related to glutaric acidemia type I is a separate rare disorder, D-2-hydroxyglutaric aciduria, in which macrocephaly occurs, but only in the minority of infants, whereas neonatal seizures and hypotonia occur in the majority.[279,280]) Initially, in glutaric acidemia type I, the macrocephaly may be only relative, but head growth that crosses percentile lines is characteristic. Subtle neurological signs (e.g., hypotonia, irritability, and jitteriness) are present frequently before the onset of the overt disease at approximately 1 year. MRI scan in early infancy shows frontotemporal atrophy and delayed myelination (Fig. 15-15). The overt clinical presentation at approximately 1 year of age is characterized in 75% of cases by an acute encephalopathic syndrome in association with infection and accompanied by vomiting, seizures, and coma. Following the acute event, the infant develops a progressive neurological syndrome characterized especially by dystonia and other extrapyramidal manifestations. MRI at this time shows destruction and atrophy of basal ganglia, decreased attenuation of cerebral white matter, and frontal-temporal atrophy, severe and progressive. Neuropathological findings include striatal necrosis and spongy myelinopathy. The importance of early detection (i.e., in the first months of life before the occurrence of the acute encephalopathy and subsequent neurological deterioration) and of institution of therapy (oral carnitine, dietary therapy, and vigorous supportive therapy with intercurrent infection) is emphasized by the report of normal development in 20 of 21 such managed "presymptomatic" infants with the disease.[273] Early detection may require repeated determinations of urinary organic acids, because single measurements may be normal or nearly normal.[249,261,273] Determination of cerebrospinal fluid organic acids may be a more reliable analysis in such situations.[124]

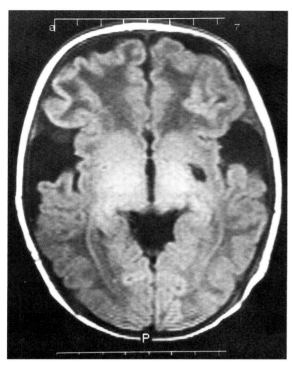

Figure 15-15   Axial T1-weighted magnetic resonance imaging scan performed on a 2-month-old infant with glutaric acidemia, type I. The scan, ordered because of macrocephaly and subtle neurological signs (hypotonia, irritability, jitteriness), shows very prominent sylvian fissures with marked frontotemporal atrophy and decreased signal intensity in cerebral white matter. Small subdural effusions are also apparent in the frontotemporal regions. *(From Hoffman GF, Athanassopoulos S, Burlina AB, Duran M, et al: Clinical course, early diagnosis, treatment and prevention of disease in glutaryl-CoA dehydrogenase deficiency,* Neuropediatrics *27:115-123, 1996.)*

5-Oxoprolinuria

5-Oxoprolinuria has been described in approximately 60 patients, of whom approximately 50% are newborns.[3,4,281-285] This disorder manifests in the *first days of life* with severe metabolic acidosis and evidence of hemolysis. Approximately one half of the reported patients exhibited neurological signs, usually stupor or coma. The *major metabolic features* are 5-oxoprolinemia and 5-oxoprolinuria as well as acidosis. The *enzymatic defect* involves glutathione synthetase, which catalyzes the formation of the tripeptide glutathione from glutamylcysteine and glycine. An increase in glutamylcysteine results, and, as a consequence, excessive amounts of 5-oxoproline, involved in the formation of the former, accumulate in blood and urine. The defect is demonstrable in cultured fibroblasts and erythrocytes. The glutathione deficiency in erythrocytes may account for the hemolysis and jaundice that may occur in the neonatal period. *Therapy* with glucose and sodium bicarbonate is crucial acutely, and subsequently vitamins E and C are administered as free radical scavengers. The latter are used because it is postulated that affected infants have increased sensitivity to oxidative stress. Approximately 25% of affected newborns have died during acute episodes. Infants may remain well between intermittent episodes of acidosis, provoked most often by infection.

Sulfite Oxidase Deficiency/Molybdenum Cofactor Deficiency

Sulfite oxidase deficiency may occur as an isolated enzymatic defect or in combination with xanthine dehydrogenase deficiency as part of molybdenum cofactor (MOCO) deficiency. MOCO is essential for the action of both enzymes (as well as aldehyde oxidase, involved in xanthine biosynthesis). At least 80 cases of sulfite oxidase deficiency have been reported; approximately 75% have been related to MOCO deficiency.[286-298a] Because the neurological features and neuropathology in both forms of sulfite oxidase deficiency are identical, it is assumed that sulfite oxidase deficiency per se is the enzymatic defect responsible for the neural phenomena. Studies with genetically manipulated mice defective in synthesis of MOCO support this conclusion.[299]

The *clinical presentation* is usually in the first days of life, with feeding difficulties, vomiting, and seizures.[286-290,292-296,298,298a,300-303] Seizures are often difficult to control. Approximately 75% of infants exhibit facial dysmorphisms (puffy cheeks, small nose, long philtrum). A course involving progression to spasticity, severe mental retardation, and microcephaly occurs in survivors. Dislocated lenses and a seborrheic rash appear later in infancy, but their presence is a clue to the correct diagnosis. Dislocated lenses have been observed as early as 2 months of age.

Brain imaging studies show progressive destruction of neuronal structures (i.e., cerebral cortex, basal ganglia, thalamus, and cerebellum) and of white matter with widespread diminution of and cystic changes within myelin (Fig. 15-16). *Neuropathological evaluation* confirms a widespread destructive process of neurons and white matter with astrocytic gliosis (Fig. 15-17). The disease has resulted in death in approximately 75% of the neonatal-onset cases, usually in infancy. *Metabolic features* are notable for excretion of sulfite, S-sulfocysteine, taurine, and xanthine (the last of these accumulates in MOCO deficiency but not in isolated sulfite oxidase deficiency). Lactic acidosis is not unusual and may raise the possibility of one of the other disorders noted in Table 15-1. The *diagnosis* should be considered in the newborn with seizures of unknown origin; a sulfite strip test on a *fresh* urine sample is a simple screening procedure.[288,304] However, false-negative and false-positive results can occur. Mass spectrometry is a more sensitive approach for diagnosis. The level of blood uric acid, the product of the xanthine dehydrogenase reaction, is depressed in the MOCO deficiency form of the disease, and detection of hypouricemia thus is a second valuable and simple screening test. A third test is detection of low plasma homocysteine.[298a] The *enzymatic defect* involves sulfite oxidase, either in isolation or more commonly, secondary to MOCO deficiency (when xanthine

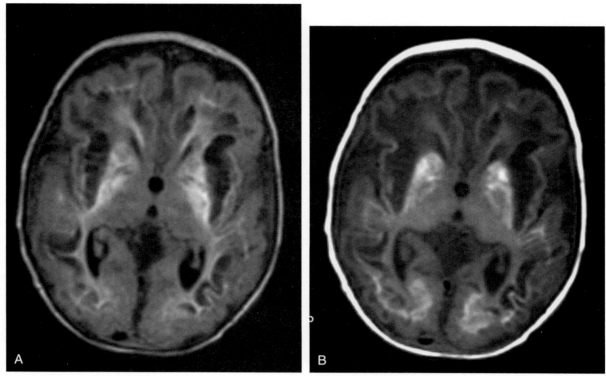

Figure 15-16 **Sulfate oxidase deficiency (isolated), magnetic resonance imaging (MRI) scans. A** and **B**, Axial MRI scans obtained in an affected infant at 31 days show striking cystic lesions diffusely within the white matter, with accompanying abnormal signal and thinning of the cerebral cortex, most marked in the perisylvian regions. Note also the involvement of basal ganglia bilaterally. *(From Dublin AB, Hald JK, Wootton-Gorges SL: Isolated sulfite oxidase deficiency: MR imaging features,* AJNR Am J Neuroradiol *23:484-485, 2002.)*

dehydrogenase is also impaired), and is detectable in cultured fibroblasts, cultured amniocytes, and chorionic villi samples. In general, no clearly effective *therapy* is available. Administration of diets low in sulfur-containing amino acids and supplementation

with sulfate have produced positive biochemical responses but no lasting clinical improvement.[304] A recent experimental report suggested benefit with administration of a precursor of MOCO distal to the most common MOCO synthetic block.[297,299]

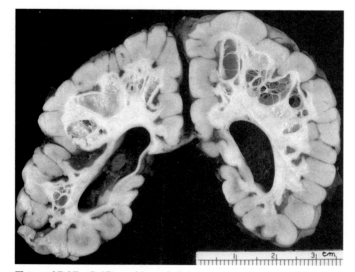

Figure 15-17 **Sulfite oxidase deficiency secondary to molybdenum cofactor deficiency: neuropathology.** This infant died at 9 months of age. Note the striking and diffuse cystic change in white matter, with atrophic cortical gyri and widening of sulci. Compare with Figure 15-16. *(From Salman MS, Ackerley C, Senger C, Becker L: New insights into the neuropathogenesis of molybdenum cofactor deficiency,* Can J Neurol Sci *29:91-96, 2002.)*

REFERENCES

1. Rousson R, Guibaud P: Long-term outcome of organic acidurias: Survey of 105 French cases (1967-1983), *J Inherit Metab Dis*, 7:10-12, 1984.
2. Chaves-Carballo E: Detection of inherited neurometabolic disorders: A practical clinical approach, *Pediatr Clin North Am*, 39:801-820, 1992.
3. Ozand PT, Gascon GG: Organic acidurias: A review. I, *J Child Neurol*, 6:196-219, 1991.
4. Ozand PT, Gascon GG: Organic acidurias: A review. II, *J Child Neurol*, 6:288-303, 1991.
5. Rashed M, Ozand PT, Aqeel AA, Gascon GG: Experience of King Faisal Specialist Hospital and Research Center with Saudi organic acid disorders, *Brain Dev*, 16:1-6, 1994.
6. Hori D, Hasegawa Y, Kimura M, Yang Y, et al: Clinical onset and prognosis of Asian children with organic acidemias, as detected by analysis of urinary organic acids using GC/MS, instead of mass screening, *Brain Dev*, 27:39-45, 2005.
7. Deodato F, Boenzi S, Santorelli FM, Dionisi-Vici C: Methylmalonic and propionic aciduria, *Am J Med Genet C Semin Med Genet*, 142:104-112, 2006.
8. Fenton WA, Gravel RA, Rosenblatt DS: Disorders of propionate and methylmalonate metabolism. In Schriver CR, Beaudet AL, Sly WS, et al, editors: *The Metabolic and Molecular Bases of Inherited Disease*, 8th ed, New York: 2001, McGraw-Hill.
9. Gruskay JA, Rosenberg LE: Inhibition of hepatic mitochondrial carbamyl phosphate synthetase (CPSI) by acyl CoA esters: Possible mechanism of hyperammonemia in the organic acidemias, *Pediatr Res*, 13:475-482, 1979.
10. Coude FX, Sweetman L, Nyhan WL: Inhibition by propionyl coenzyme A of N-acetylglutamate synthetase of rat liver mitochondria: A possible explanation for hyperammonemia in propionic and methylmalonic acidemia, *J Clin Invest*, 64:1544-1551, 1979.
11. Rabier D, Cathelineau L, Briand P, Kamoun P: Propionate and succinate effects on acetylglutamate biosynthesis by rat liver mitochondria, *Biochem Biophys Res Commun*, 91:456-460, 1979.

12. Cathelineau L, Briand P, Ogier H, Charpentier C, et al: Occurrence of hyperammonemia in the course of 17 cases of methylmalonic acidemia, *J Pediatr*, 99:279-280, 1981.
13. Wolf B, Hsia YE, Sweetman L, Gravel R, et al: Propionic acidemia: A clinical update, *J Pediatr*, 99:835-846, 1981.
14. Ando T, Nyhan WL, Connor JD, Rasmussen K, et al: The oxidation of glycine and propionic acid in propionic acidemia with ketotic hyperglycinemia, *Pediatr Res*, 6:576-583, 1972.
15. Morrow G 3rd, Barness LA, Cardinale GJ, Abeles RH, et al: Congenital methylmalonic acidemia: Enzymatic evidence for two forms of the disease, *Proc Natl Acad Sci U S A*, 63:191-197, 1969.
16. Ando T, Klingberg WG, Ward AN: Isovaleric acidemia presenting with altered metabolism of glycine, *Pediatr Res*, 5:478-483, 1971.
17. Hillman RE, Sowers LH, Cohen JL: Inhibition of glycine oxidation in cultured fibroblasts by isoleucine, *Pediatr Res*, 7:945-947, 1973.
18. Hillman RE, Otto EF: Inhibition of glycine-serine interconversion in cultured human fibroblasts by products of isoleucine catabolism, *Pediatr Res*, 8:941-945, 1974.
19. Hayasaka K, Narisawa K, Satoh T, Tateda H, et al: Glycine cleavage system in ketotic hyperglycinemia: A reduction of H-protein activity, *Pediatr Res*, 16:5-7, 1982.
20. Kolvraa S: Inhibition of the glycine cleavage system by branched-chain amino acid metabolites, *Pediatr Res*, 13:889-893, 1979.
21. Shuman RM, Leech RW, Scott CR: The neuropathology of the nonketotic and ketotic hyperglycinemias: Three cases, *Neurology*, 28:139-146, 1978.
22. Friede RL: *Developmental Neuropathology*, 2nd ed, New York: 1989, Springer-Verlag.
23. Steinman L, Clancy RR, Cann H, Urich H: The neuropathology of propionic acidemia, *Dev Med Child Neurol*, 25:87-94, 1983.
24. Prosenc N, Stoltenburg-Didinger G: Spongy encephalopathy in ketotic hyperglycinemia, *Brain Dev*, 16:445-449, 1995.
25. Frenkel EP: Abnormal fatty acid metabolism in peripheral nerves of patients with pernicious anemia, *J Clin Invest*, 52:1237-1245, 1973.
26. Kishimoto Y, Williams M, Moser HW, Hignite C, et al: Branched-chain and odd-numbered fatty acids and aldehydes in the nervous system of a patient with deranged vitamin B_{12} metabolism, *J Lipid Res*, 14:69-77, 1973.
27. Dayan AD, Ramsey RB: An inborn error of vitamin B_{12} metabolism associated with cellular deficiency of coenzyme forms of the vitamin, *J Neurol Sci*, 23:117-128, 1974.
28. Ramsey RB, Scott T, Banik NL: Fatty acid composition of myelin isolated from the brain of patient with cellular deficiency of co-enzyme forms of vitamin B_{12}, *J Neurol Sci*, 34:221-232, 1977.
29. Wendel U: Abnormality of odd-numbered long-chain fatty acids in erythrocyte membrane lipids from patients with disorders of propionate metabolism, *Pediatr Res*, 25:147-150, 1989.
30. Cardinale GJ, Carty TJ, Abeles RH: Effect of methylmalonyl coenzyme A, a metabolite which accumulates in vitamin B_{12} deficiency, on fatty acid synthesis, *J Biol Chem*, 245:3771-3775, 1970.
31. Barley FW, Sato G, Abeles RH: An effect of vitamin B_{12} deficiency in tissue culture, *J Biol Chem*, 247:4270-4276, 1972.
32. Stubbs CD, Smith AD: The modification of mammalian membrane polyunsaturated fatty acid composition in relation to membrane fluidity and function, *Biochim Biophys Acta*, 779:89-137, 1984.
33. Volpe JJ, Kishimoto Y: Fatty acid synthetase of brain: Development, influence of nutritional and hormonal factors and comparison with liver enzyme, *J Neurochem*, 19:737-753, 1972.
34. Volpe JJ, Vagelos PR: Fatty acid synthetase of mammalian brain, liver and adipose tissue: Regulation by prosthetic group turnover, *Biochim Biophys Acta*, 326:293-304, 1973.
35. Childs B, Nyhan WL, Borden M, Bard L, et al: Idiopathic hyperglycinemia and hyperglycinuria: New disorder of amino acid metabolism, *J Pediatr*, 27:522-528, 1961.
36. North KN, Korson MS, Gopal YR, Rohr FJ, et al: Neonatal-onset propionic acidemia: Neurologic and developmental profiles, and implications for management, *J Pediatr*, 126:916-922, 1995.
37. Bergman AJ, Van Der Knaap MS, Smeitink JA, Duran M, et al: Magnetic resonance imaging and spectroscopy of the brain in propionic acidemia: Clinical and biochemical considerations, *Pediatr Res*, 40:404-409, 1996.
38. Surtees R, Matthews EE, Leonard JV: Neurologic outcome of propionic acidemia, *Pediatr Neurol*, 8:333-337, 1992.
39. Sass JO, Hofmann M, Skladal D, Mayatepek E, et al: Propionic acidemia revisited: A workshop report, *Clin Pediatr (Phila)*, 43:837-843, 2004.
40. Dave P, Curless RG, Steinman L: Cerebellar hemorrhage complicating methylmalonic and propionic acidemia, *Arch Neurol*, 41:1293-1296, 1984.
41. Al-Essa M, Bakheet S, Patay Z, Al-Shamsan L, et al: ^{18}Fluoro-2-deoxyglucose (^{18}FDG) PET scan of the brain in propionic acidemia: Clinical and MRI correlations, *Brain Dev*, 21:312-317, 1999.
42. Wadlington WB, Kilroy A, Ando T, Sweetman L, et al: Hyperglycinemia and propionyl CoA carboxylase deficiency and episodic severe illness without consistent ketosis, *J Pediatr*, 86:707-712, 1975.
43. Hsia YE, Scully KJ, Rosenberg LE: Inherited propionyl-CoA carboxylase deficiency in ketotic hyperglycinemia, *J Clin Invest*, 50:127-130, 1971.
44. Barnes ND, Hull D, Balgobin I, Gompertz D: Biotin-responsive propionic acidemia, *Lancet*, 2:244-245, 1970.
45. Rosenberg LE, Fenton WA: Disorders of propionate and methylmalonate metabolism. In Scriver CR, Beaudet AL, Sly WS, et al, editors: *The Metabolic Basis of Inherited Disease*, 6th ed, New York: 1989, McGraw-Hill.
46. Hommes FA, Kuipers JR, Elema JD, Jansen JF, et al: Propionic acidemia, a new inborn error of metabolism, *Pediatr Res*, 2:519-524, 1968.
47. Harding BN, Leonard JV, Erdohazi M: Propionic acidaemia: A neuropathological study of two patients presenting in infancy, *Neuropathol Appl Neurobiol*, 17:133-138, 1991.
48. Hamilton RL, Haas RH, Nyhan WL, Powell HC, et al: Neuropathology of propionic acidemia: A report of two patients with basal ganglia lesions, *J Child Neurol*, 10:25-30, 1995.
49. Haas RH, Marsden DL, Capistranoestrada S, Hamilton R, et al: Acute basal ganglia infarction in propionic acidemia, *J Child Neurol*, 10:18-22, 1995.
50. Barkovich AJ: *Pediatric Neuroimaging*, 4th ed, Philadelphia: 2005, Lippincott Williams & Wilkins.
51. Brismar J, Ozand PT: CT and MR of the brain in disorders of the propionate and methylmalonate metabolism, *AJNR Am J Neuroradiol*, 15:1459-1473, 1994.
52. Feliz B, Witt DR, Harris BT: Propionic acidemia: A neuropathology case report and review of prior cases, *Arch Pathol Lab Med*, 127:e325-e328, 2003.
53. Perez-Cerda C, Perez B, Merinero B, Desviat LR, et al: Prenatal diagnosis of propionic acidemia, *Prenat Diagn*, 24:962-964, 2004.
54. Brusilow SW, Valle DL: Symptomatic inborn errors of metabolism in the neonate. In Nelson NM, editor: *Current Therapy in Neonatal Perinatal Medicine*, Toronto: 1985, Decker.
55. Meyburg J, Hoffmann GF: Liver transplantation for inborn errors of metabolism, *Transplantation*, 80:S135-S137, 2005.
56. Morioka D, Kasahara M, Takada Y, Corrales JP, et al: Living donor liver transplantation for pediatric patients with inheritable metabolic disorders, *Am J Transplant*, 5:2754-2763, 2005.
57. Matsui SM, Mahoney MJ, Rosenberg LE: The natural history of the inherited methylmalonic acidemias, *N Engl J Med*, 308:857, 1983.
58. Tanpaiboon P: Methylmalonic acidemia (MMA), *Mol Genet Metab*, 85:2-6, 2005.
59. Longo D, Fariello G, Dionisi-Vici C, Cannata V, et al: MRI and ^{1}H-MRS findings in early-onset cobalamin C/D defect, *Neuropediatrics*, 36:366-372, 2006.
60. Nicolaides P, Leonard J, Surtees R: Neurological outcome of methylmalonic acidaemia, *Arch Dis Child*, 78:508-512, 1998.
61. Treacy E, Clow C, Mamer OA, Scriver CR: Methylmalonic acidemia with a severe chemical but benign clinical phenotype, *J Pediatr*, 122:428-429, 1993.
62. Burlina AP, Manara R, Calderone M, Catuogno S, et al: Diffusion-weighted imaging in the assessment of neurological damage in patients with methylmalonic aciduria, *J Inherit Metab Dis*, 26:417-422, 2003.
63. Michel SJ, Given CA 2nd, Robertson WC Jr: Imaging of the brain, including diffusion-weighted imaging in methylmalonic acidemia, *Pediatr Radiol*, 34:580-582, 2004.
64. Takeuchi M, Harada M, Matsuzaki K, Hisaoka S, et al: Magnetic resonance imaging and spectroscopy in a patient with treated methylmalonic acidemia, *J Comput Assist Tomogr*, 27:547-551, 2003.
65. Yesildag A, Ayata A, Baykal B, Koroglu M, et al: Magnetic resonance imaging and diffusion-weighted imaging in methylmalonic acidemia, *Acta Radiol*, 46:101-103, 2005.
66. Biancheri R, Cerone R, Schiaffino MC, Caruso U, et al: Cobalamin (Cbl) C/D deficiency: Clinical neurophysiological and neuroradiologic findings in 14 cases, *Neuropediatrics*, 32:14-22, 2001.
67. Rossi A, Cerone R, Biancheri R, Gatti R, et al: Early-onset combined methylmalonic aciduria and homocystinuria: Neuroradiologic findings, *AJNR Am J Neuroradiol*, 22:554-563, 2001.
68. Bodamer OA, Sahoo T, Beaudet AL, O'Brien WE, et al: Creatine metabolism in combined methylmalonic aciduria and homocystinuria, *Ann Neurol*, 57:557-560, 2005.
69. Ricci D, Pane M, Deodato F, Vasco G, et al: Assessment of visual function in children with methylmalonic aciduria and homocystinuria, *Neuropediatrics*, 36:181-185, 2005.
70. Huemer M, Simma B, Fowler B, Suormala T, et al: Prenatal and postnatal treatment in cobalamin C defect, *J Pediatr*, 147:469-472, 2005.
71. Morrow G, Mahoney MJ, Mathews C, Lebowitz J: Studies of methylmalonyl coenzyme A carbonylmutase activity in methylmalonic acidemia. I. Correlation of clinical, hepatic and fibroblast data, *Pediatr Res*, 9:641-644, 1975.
72. Kang ES, Snodgrass PJ, Gerald PS: Methylmalonyl-CoA racemase defect: Another cause of methylmalonic aciduria, *Pediatr Res*, 8:875-879, 1972.
73. Fenton WA, Rosenberg LE: Disorders of propionate and methylmalonate metabolism. In Scriver CR, Beaudet AL, Sly WS, et al, editors: *The Metabolic and Molecular Bases of Inherited Disease*, 7th ed, New York: 1995, McGraw-Hill.
74. Rosenberg LE, Lilljeqvist AC, Hsia YE, Rosenbloom FM: Vitamin B_{12} dependent methylmalonic aciduria: Defective B_{12} metabolism in cultured fibroblasts, *Biochem Biophys Res Commun*, 37:607-614, 1969.
75. Mahoney MJ, Hart AC, Steen VD, Rosenberg LE: Methylmalonic acidemia: Biochemical heterogeneity in defects of 5'deoxy-adenosylcobalamin synthesis, *Proc Natl Acad Sci U S A*, 72:2799-2803, 1975.

76. Mahoney MJ, Rosenberg LE, Mudd SH, Uhlendorf BW: Defective metabolism of vitamin B_{12} in fibroblasts from patients with methylmalonic aciduria, *Biochem Biophys Res Commun*, 44:375-381, 1971.

77. Oberholzer VG, Levin B, Burgess EA, Young WF: Methylmalonic aciduria: An inborn error of metabolism leading to chronic metabolic acidosis, *Arch Dis Child*, 42:492-504, 1967.

78. Sum JM, Twiss JL, Horoupian DS: Selective death of immature neurons in methylmalonic acidemia of the neonate: A case report, *Acta Neuropathol (Berl)*, 85:217-221, 1993.

79. Kanaumi T, Takashima S, Hirose S, Kodama T, et al: Neuropathology of methylmalonic acidemia in a child, *Pediatr Neurol*, 34:156-159, 2006.

80. Marrow G 3rd, Schwartz RH, Hallock JA, Barness LA: Prenatal detection of methylmalonic acidemia, *J Pediatr*, 77:120-123, 1970.

81. Mahoney MJ, Rosenberg LE, Lindblad B, Waldenström J, et al: Prenatal diagnosis of methylmalonic aciduria, *Acta Paediatr Scand*, 64:44-48, 1975.

82. Ampola MG, Mahoney MJ, Nakamura E, Tanaka K: Prenatal therapy of a patient with vitamin B_{12} responsive methylmalonic acidemia, *N Engl J Med*, 293:313-317, 1975.

83. Blass JP: Inborn errors of pyruvate metabolism. In Stanbury JB, Wyngaarden JB, Frederickson DS, editors: *The Metabolic Basis of Inherited Disease*, New York: 1983, McGraw-Hill.

84. van der Meer SB, Spaapen LJ, Fowler B, Jakobs C, et al: Prenatal treatment of a patient with vitamin B_{12}–responsive methylmalonic acidemia, *J Pediatr*, 117:923-926, 1990.

85. Rosenblatt DS, Fenton WA: Inherited disorders of folate and cobalamin transport and metabolism. In Scriver CR, Beaudet AL, Sly WS, et al, editors: *The Metabolic and Molecular Bases of Inherited Disease*, 8th ed, New York: 2001, McGraw-Hill.

86. Chalmers RA, Bain MD, Mistry J, Tracey BM, et al: Enzymologic studies on patients with methylmalonic aciduria: Basis for a clinical trial of deoxyadenosylcobalamin in a hydroxocobalamin-unresponsive patient, *Pediatr Res*, 30:560-563, 1991.

87. Pithukpakorn M: Disorders of pyruvate metabolism and the tricarboxylic acid cycle, *Mol Genet Metab*, 85:243-246, 2005.

88. Kerrigan JF, Aleck KA, Tarby TJ, Bird R, et al: Fumaric aciduria: Clinical and imaging features, *Ann Neurol*, 47:583-588, 2000.

89. Nissenkorn A, Michelson M, Ben-Zeev B, Lerman-Sagie T: Inborn errors of metabolism: A cause of abnormal brain development, *Neurology*, 56:1265-1272, 2001.

90. Robinson BH: Lactic acidemia: Disorders of pyruvate carboxylase and pyruvate dehydrogenase. In Scriver CR, Beaudet MD, Sly WS, et al, editors: *The Metabolic and Molecular Bases of Inherited Disease*, 8th ed, New York: 2001, McGraw-Hill.

91. DeVivo DC: Complexities of the pyruvate dehydrogenase complex, *Neurology*, 51:1247-1249, 1998.

92. Volpe JJ, Marasa JC: A role for thiamine in the regulation of fatty acid and cholesterol biosynthesis in cultured cells of neural origin, *J Neurochem*, 30:975-981, 1978.

93. DeVivo DC: The expanding clinical spectrum of mitochondrial diseases, *Brain Dev*, 15:1-22, 1993.

94. De Meirleir L, Lissens W, Wayenberg JL, Michotte A, et al: Pyruvate dehydrogenase deficiency: Clinical and biochemical diagnosis, *Pediatr Neurol*, 9:216-220, 1993.

95. Matthews PM, Marchington DR, Squier M, Land J, et al: Molecular genetic characterization of an X-linked form of Leigh's syndrome, *Ann Neurol*, 33:652-655, 1993.

96. De Meirleir L: Defects of pyruvate metabolism and the Krebs cycle, *J Child Neurol*, 17(Suppl 3):S26-S33, 2002.

97. Robinson BH: Lactic acidemia. In Scriver CR, Beaudet AL, Sly WS, et al, editors: *The Metabolic Basis of Inherited Disease*, 6th ed, New York: 1989, McGraw-Hill.

98. Farrell DF, Clark AF, Scott CR, Wennberg RP: Absence of pyruvate decarboxylase activity in man: A cause of congenital lactic acidosis, *Science*, 187:1082-1084, 1975.

99. Robinson BH, Sherwood WG: Pyruvate dehydrogenase phosphatase deficiency: A cause of congenital chronic lactic acidosis in infancy, *Pediatr Res*, 9:935-939, 1975.

100. Cederbaum SD, Blass JP, Minkoff N, Brown WJ, et al: Sensitivity to carbohydrate in a patient with familial intermittent lactic acidosis and pyruvate dehydrogenase deficiency, *Pediatr Res*, 10:713-720, 1976.

101. Haworth JC, Perry TL, Blass JP, Hansen S, et al: Lactic acidosis in three sibs due to defects in both pyruvate dehydrogenase and alpha-ketoglutarate dehydrogenase complexes, *Pediatrics*, 58:564-572, 1976.

102. Stromme JH, Borud O, Moe PJ: Fatal lactic acidosis in a newborn attributable to a congenital defect of pyruvate dehydrogenase, *Pediatr Res*, 10:62-66, 1976.

103. Robinson BH, Taylor J, Sherwood WG: Deficiency of dihydrolipoyl dehydrogenase (a component of the pyruvate and alpha-ketoglutarate dehydrogenase complexes): A cause of congenital chronic lactic acidosis in infancy, *Pediatr Res*, 11:1198-1202, 1977.

104. Taylor J, Robinson BH, Sherwood WG: A defect in branched-chain amino acid metabolism in a patient with congenital lactic acidosis due to dihydrolipoyl dehydrogenase deficiency, *Pediatr Res*, 12:60-62, 1978.

105. Prick M, Gabreëls F, Renier W, Trijbels F, et al: Pyruvate dehydrogenase deficiency restricted to brain, *Neurology*, 31:398-404, 1981.

106. Old SE, De Vivo DC: Pyruvate dehydrogenase complex deficiency: Biochemical and immunoblot analysis of cultured skin fibroblasts, *Ann Neurol*, 26:746-751, 1989.

107. Patel MS: Biochemical and molecular aspects of pyruvate dehydrogenase complex deficiency, *Int Pediatr*, 7:16-22, 1992.

108. Byrd SE, Naidich TP: Common congenital brain anomalies, *Radiol Clin North Am*, 26:755-772, 1988.

109. Robinson BH, MacKay N, Chun K, Ling M: Disorders of pyruvate carboxylase and the pyruvate dehydrogenase complex, *J Inherit Metab Dis*, 19:452-462, 1996.

110. Cross JH, Connelly A, Gadian DG, Kendall BE, et al: Clinical diversity of pyruvate dehydrogenase deficiency, *Pediatr Neurol*, 10:276-283, 1994.

111. Otero LJ, Brown GK, Silver K, Arnold DL, et al: Association of cerebral dysgenesis and lactic acidemia with X-linked PDH E1α subunit mutations in females, *Pediatr Neurol*, 13:327-332, 1995.

112. Fujii T, Van Coster RN, Old SE, Medori R, et al: Pyruvate dehydrogenase deficiency: Molecular basis for intrafamilial heterogeneity, *Ann Neurol*, 36:83-89, 1994.

113. Shevell MI, Matthews PM, Scriver CR, Brown RM, et al: Cerebral dysgenesis and lactic acidemia: An MRI/MRS phenotype associated with pyruvate dehydrogenase deficiency, *Pediatr Neurol*, 11:224-229, 1994.

114. Takahashi S, Oki J, Miyamoto A, Tokumitsu A, et al: Autopsy findings in pyruvate dehydrogenase E1α deficiency: Case report, *J Child Neurol*, 12:519-524, 1997.

115. Zand DJ, Simon EM, Pulitzer SB, Wang DJ, et al: In vivo pyruvate detected by MR spectroscopy in neonatal pyruvate dehydrogenase deficiency, *AJNR Am J Neuroradiol*, 24:1471-1474, 2003.

116. Wada N, Matsuishi T, Nonaka M, Naito E, et al: Pyruvate dehydrogenase E1α subunit deficiency in a female patient: Evidence of antenatal origin of brain damage and possible etiology of infantile spasms, *Brain Dev*, 26:57-60, 2004.

117. Robinson JN, Norwitz ER, Mulkern RV, Brown SA, et al: Prenatal diagnosis of pyruvate dehydrogenase deficiency using magnetic resonance imaging, *Prenat Diagn*, 21:1053-1056, 2001.

118. Cameron JM, Levandovskiy V, Mackay N, Tein I, et al: Deficiency of pyruvate dehydrogenase caused by novel and known mutations in the E1alpha subunit, *Am J Med Genet A*, 131:59-66, 2004.

119. DeVivo DC, Van Coster RN: Leigh syndrome: Clinical and biochemical correlates. In Fukuyama Y, Kamoshita S, Ohtsuka C, et al, editors: *Modern Perspectives of Child Neurology*, Tokyo: 1991, Japanese Society of Child Neurology.

120. Fujii T, Alvarez MBG, Sheu K-F, R., Kranz-Eble PJ, et al: Pyruvate dehydrogenase deficiency: The relation of the E1β subunit deficiency, *Pediatr Neurol*, 14:328-334, 1996.

121. Matthews PM, Brown RM, Otero L, Marchington D, et al: Neurodevelopmental abnormalities and lactic acidosis in a girl with a 20-bp deletion in the X-linked pyruvate dehydrogenase E1α subunit gene, *Neurology*, 43:2025-2030, 1993.

122. Breningstall GN: Approach to diagnosis of oxidative metabolism disorders, *Pediatr Neurol*, 9:81-93, 1993.

123. Robinson BH: Lactic acidemia (disorders of pyruvate carboxylase, pyruvate dehydrogenase). In Scriver CR, Beaudet AL, Sly WS, et al, editors: *The Metabolic and Molecular Bases of Inherited Disease*, 7th ed, New York: 1995, McGraw-Hill.

124. Hoffmann GF, Surtees RAH, Wevers RA: Cerebrospinal fluid investigations for neurometabolic disorders, *Neuropediatrics*, 29:59-71, 1998.

125. Kuroda Y, Kline JJ, Sweetman L: Abnormal pyruvate and alpha-ketoglutarate dehydrogenase complexes in a patient with lactic acidemia, *Pediatr Res*, 13:928-931, 1979.

126. Mahbubul-Huq AH, Ito M, Naito E, Saijo T, et al: Demonstration of an unstable variant of pyruvate dehydrogenase protein (E_1) in cultured fibroblasts from a patient with congenital lactic acidemia, *Pediatr Res*, 30:11-14, 1991.

127. Elpeleg ON, Ruitenbeek W, Jakobs C, Barash V, et al: Congenital lactic-acidemia caused by lipoamide dehydrogenase deficiency with favorable outcome, *J Pediatr*, 126:72-74, 1995.

128. Dey R, Mine M, Desguerre I, Slama A, et al: A new case of pyruvate dehydrogenase deficiency due to a novel mutation in the PDX1 gene, *Ann Neurol*, 52:273-277, 2003.

129. Geoffroy V, Fouque F, Benelli C, Poggi F, et al: Defect in the X-lipoyl-containing component of the pyruvate dehydrogenase complex in a patient with neonatal lactic acidemia, *Pediatrics*, 97:267-272, 1996.

130. Brown RM, Head RA, Morris AA, Raiman JA, et al: Pyruvate dehydrogenase E3 binding protein (protein X) deficiency, *Dev Med Child Neurol*, 48:756-760, 2006.

131. Pliss L, Pentney RJ, Johnson MT, Patel MS: Biochemical and structural brain alterations in female mice with cerebral pyruvate dehydrogenase deficiency, *J Neurochem*, 91:1082-1091, 2004.

132. Moroni I, Bugiani M, Bizzi A, Castelli G, et al: Cerebral white matter involvement in children with mitochondrial encephalopathies, *Neuropediatrics*, 33:79-85, 2002.

133. Toth PP, El-Shanti H, Elvins S, Rhead WJ, et al: Transient improvement of congenital lactic acidosis in a male infant with pyruvate decarboxylase deficiency treated with dichloroacetate, *J Pediatr*, 123:427-430, 1993.

134. Morten KJ, Caky M, Matthews PM: Stabilization of the pyruvate dehydrogenase E1α subunit by dichloroacetate, *Neurology*, 51:1331-1335, 1998.

135. Morten KJ, Beattie P, Brown GK, Matthews PM: Dichloroacetate stabilizes the mutant E1α subunit in pyruvate dehydrogenase deficiency, *Neurology*, 53:612-616, 1999.

136. Falk RE, Cederbaum SD, Blass JP, Gibson GE, et al: Ketogenic diet in the management of pyruvate dehydrogenase deficiency, *Pediatrics*, 58:713-721, 1976.

137. Hommes FA, Berger R, Luit-de-Haan G: The effect of thiamine treatment on the activity of pyruvate dehydrogenase: Relation to the treatment of Leigh's encephalomyelopathy, *Pediatr Res*, 7:616-619, 1973.

138. Wick H, Schweizer K, Baumgartner R: Thiamine dependency in a patient with congenital lactic acidemia due to pyruvate dehydrogenase deficiency, *Agents Actions*, 7:405-410, 1978.

139. Stacpoole PW, Moore GW, Kornhauser DM: Metabolic effects of dichloroacetate in patients with diabetes mellitus and hyperproteinemia, *N Engl J Med*, 298:526-530, 1978.

140. Brun N, Robitaille Y, Grignon A, Robinson BH, et al: Pyruvate carboxylase deficiency: Prenatal onset of ischemia-like brain lesions in two sibs with the acute neonatal forum, *Am J Med Genet*, 84:94-101, 1999.

141. Garcia-Cazorla A, Rabier D, Touati G, Chadefaux-Vekemans B, et al: Pyruvate carboxylase deficiency: Metabolic characteristics and new neurological aspects, *Ann Neurol*, 59:121-127, 2006.

142. Brunette MG, Delvin E, Hazel B, Scriver CR: Thiamine-responsive lactic acidosis in a patient with deficiency low-Km pyruvate carboxylase activity in liver, *Pediatrics*, 50:702-711, 1972.

143. Saudubray JM, Marsac C, Charpentier C: Neonatal congenital lactic acidosis with pyruvate carboxylase deficiency in two siblings, *Acta Paediatr Scand*, 65:717-721, 1976.

144. Van Biervliet JP, Bruinvis L, van der Heiden C, Ketting D, et al: Report of a patient with severe, chronic lactic acidaemia and pyruvate carboxylase deficiency, *Dev Med Child Neurol*, 19:392-401, 1977.

145. Vidailhet M, Lefebvre E, Beley G, Marsac C: Neonatal lactic acidosis with pyruvate carboxylase inactivity, *J Inherit Metab Dis*, 4:131-136, 1981.

146. Pineda M, Campistol J, Vilaseca MA, Briones P, et al: An atypical French form of pyruvate carboxylase deficiency, *Brain Dev*, 17:276-279, 1995.

147. Marsac C, Augereau C, Feldman G, Wolf B, et al: Prenatal diagnosis of pyruvate carboxylase deficiency, *Clin Chim Acta*, 119:121-127, 1982.

148. Atkin BM, Buist NR, Utter MF, Leiter AB, et al: Pyruvate carboxylase deficiency and lactic acidosis in a retarded child without Leigh's disease, *Pediatr Res*, 13:109-116, 1979.

149. Mochel F, DeLonlay P, Touati G, Brunengraber H, et al: Pyruvate carboxylase deficiency: Clinical and biochemical response to anaplerotic diet therapy, *Mol Genet Metab*, 84:305-312, 2005.

150. Nyhan WL, Khanna A, Barshop BA, Naviaux RK, et al: Pyruvate carboxylase deficiency: Insights from liver transplantation, *Mol Genet Metab*, 77:143-149, 2002.

151. Sweetman L, Williams JC: Branched chain organic acidurias. In Schriver CR, Beaudet AL, Sly WS, et al, editors: *The Metabolic and Molecular Bases of Inherited Disease*, 8th ed, New York: 2001, McGraw-Hill.

152. Tanaka K, Budd MA, Efron ML, Isselbacher KJ: Isovaleric acidemia: A new genetic defect of leucine metabolism, *Proc Nat Acad Sci U S A*, 56:236-242, 1966.

153. Budd MA, Tanaka K, Holmes LB: Isovaleric acidemia: Clinical features of a new genetic defect of leucine metabolism, *N Engl J Med*, 277:321-327, 1967.

154. Levy HL, Erickson AM: Isovaleric acidemia. In Nyhan WL, editor: *Heritable Disorders of Amino Acid Metabolism: Patterns of Clinical Expression and Genetic Variation*, New York: 1974, John Wiley.

155. Tanaka K: Disorders of organic acid metabolism. In Gaull G, editor: *Biology of Brain Dysfunction*, New York: 1975, Plenum.

156. Tanaka K, Mandell R, Shih VE: Metabolism of (1-14 C) and (2-14 C) leucine in cultured skin fibroblasts from patients with isovaleric acidemia, *J Clin Invest*, 58:164-172, 1976.

157. Fischer AQ, Challa VR, Burton BK, McLean W: Cerebellar hemorrhage complicating isovaleric acidemia: A case report, *Neurology*, 31:746-748, 1981.

158. Lorek AK, Penrice JM, Cady EB, Leonard JV, et al: Cerebral energy metabolism in isovaleric acidaemia, *Arch Dis Child Fetal Neonatal Ed*, 74:F211-F213, 1996.

159. Berry GT, Yudkoff M, Segal S: Isovaleric acidemia: Medical and neurodevelopmental effects of long-term therapy, *J Pediatr*, 113:58-64, 1988.

160. Shih VE, Mandell R, Tanaka K: Diagnosis of isovaleric acidemia in cultured fibroblasts, *Clin Chim Acta*, 48:437-439, 1973.

161. Rhead WJ, Tanaka K: Demonstration of a specific mitochondrial isovaleryl-CoA dehydrogenase deficiency in fibroblasts from patients with isovaleric acidemia, *Proc Natl Acad Sci U S A*, 77:580-583, 1980.

162. Hyman DB, Tanaka K: Isovaleryl-CoA dehydrogenase activity in isovaleric acidemia fibroblasts using an improved tritium release assay, *Pediatr Res*, 20:59-61, 1986.

163. Tajima G, Sakura N, Yofune H, Dwi Bahagia Febriani A, et al: Establishment of a practical enzymatic assay method for determination of isovaleryl-CoA dehydrogenase activity using high-performance liquid chromatography, *Clin Chim Acta*, 353:193-199, 2005.

164. Gregersen N: The specific inhibition of the pyruvate dehydrogenase complex from pig kidney by propionyl-CoA and isovaleryl-CoA, *Biochem Med*, 26:20-27, 1981.

165. Clark JB, Land JM: Phenylketonuria and maple syrup disease and their association with brain mitochondrial substrate utilization. In Hommes FA, Van den Berg CJ, editors: *Normal and Pathological Development of Energy Metabolism*, New York: 1975, Academic Press.

166. Mayatepek E, Kurczynski TW, Hoppel CL: Long-term L-carnitine treatment in isovaleric acidemia, *Pediatr Neurol*, 7:137-140, 1991.

167. Roe CR, Millington DS, Maltby DA, Kahler SG, et al: L-Carnitine therapy in isovaleric acidemia, *J Clin Invest*, 74:2290-2295, 1984.

168. de Sousa C, Chalmers RA, Stacey TE, Tracey BM, et al: The response to L-carnitine and glycine therapy in isovaleric acidemia, *Eur J Pediatr*, 144:451-456, 1978.

169. Naglak M, Salvo R, Madsen K, Dembure P, et al: The treatment of isovaleric acidemia with glycine supplement, *Pediatr Res*, 24:9-13, 1988.

170. Bartlett K, Gompertz D: The specificity of glycine-N-acylase and acylglycine excretion in the organic acidaemias, *Biochem Med*, 10:15-23, 1974.

171. Cohn RM, Yudkoff M, Rothman K, Segal S: Isovaleric acidemia: Use of glycine therapy in neonates, *N Engl J Med*, 299:996-999, 1978.

172. Dantas MF, Suormala T, Randolph A, Coelho D, et al: 3-Methylcrotonyl-CoA carboxylase deficiency: Mutation analysis in 28 probands, 9 symptomatic and 19 detected by newborn screening, *Hum Mutat*, 26:164, 2005.

173. Lehnert W, Niederhoff H, Suormala T, Baumgartner ER: Isolated biotin-resistant 3-methylcrotonyl-CoA carboxylase deficiency: Long-term outcome in a case with neonatal onset, *Eur J Pediatr*, 155:568-572, 1996.

174. Oude Luttikhuis HG, Touati G, Rabier D, Williams M, et al: Severe hypoglycaemia in isolated 3-methylcrotonyl-CoA carboxylase deficiency: A rare, severe clinical presentation, *J Inherit Metab Dis*, 28:1136-1138, 2005.

175. Baykal T, Gokcay GH, Ince Z, Dantas MF, et al: Consanguineous 3-methylcrotonyl-CoA carboxylase deficiency: Early onset necrotizing encephalopathy with lethal outcome, *J Inherit Metab Dis*, 28:229-233, 2005.

176. Baumgartner MR, Dantas MF, Suormala T, Almashanu S, et al: Isolated 3-methylcrotonyl-CoA carboxylase deficiency: Evidence for an allele-specific dominant negative effect and responsiveness to biotin therapy, *Am J Hum Genet*, 75:790-800, 2004.

177. Mitchell GA, Fukao T: Inborn errors of ketone body metabolism. In Scriver CR, Beaudet AL, Sly WS, et al, editors: *The Metabolic and Molecular Bases of Inherited Disease*, 8th ed, New York: 2001, McGraw-Hill.

178. Schutgens RB, Heymans H, Ketel A, Veder HA, et al: Lethal hypoglycemia in a child with a deficiency of 3-hydroxy-3-methylglutaryl coenzyme A lyase, *J Pediatr*, 94:89-91, 1979.

179. Gibson KM, Breuer J, Nyhan WL: 3-Hydroxy-3-methylglutaryl-coenzyme A lyase deficiency: Review of 18 reported patients, *Eur J Pediatr*, 148:180-186, 1988.

180. Yalcinkaya C, Dincer A, Gunduz E, Ficicioglu C, et al: MRI and MRS in HMG-CoA lyase deficiency, *Pediatr Neurol*, 20:375-380, 1999.

181. Muroi J, Yorifuji T, Uematsu A, Shigematsu Y, et al: Molecular and clinical analysis of Japanese patients with 3-hydroxy-3-methylglutaryl CoA lyase (HL) deficiency, *Hum Genet*, 107:320-326, 2000.

182. Zoghbi HQ, Spence JE, Beaudet AL, O'Brien WE, et al: Atypical presentation and neuropathological studies in 3-hydroxy-3-methylglutaryl-CoA lyase deficiency, *Ann Neurol*, 20:367-369, 1986.

183. Barash V, Mandel H, Sella S, Geiger R: 3-hydroxy-3-methylglutaryl-coenzyme A lyase deficiency: Biochemical studies and family investigation of four generations, *J Inherit Metab Dis*, 13:156-164, 1990.

184. Hoffmann GF, Trefz FK, Barth PG, Bohles HJ, et al: Glutaryl-coenzyme A dehydrogenase deficiency: A distinct encephalopathy, *Pediatrics*, 88:1194-1203, 1991.

185. Hoffmann GF, Trefz FK, Barth PG, Böhles HJ, et al: Macrocephaly: An important indication for organic acid analysis, *J Inherit Metab Dis*, 14:329-332, 1991.

186. Hoffmann G, Gibson KM, Brandt IK, Bader PI, et al: Mevalonic aciduria: An inborn error of cholesterol and nonsterol isoprene biosynthesis, *N Engl J Med*, 314:1610-1614, 1986.

187. Hoffmann GF, Charpentier C, Mayatepek E, Mancini J, et al: Clinical and biochemical phenotype in 11 patients with mevalonic aciduria, *Pediatrics*, 91:915-921, 1993.

188. Mancini J, Philip N, Chabrol B, Divry P, et al: Mevalonic aciduria in 3 siblings: A new recognizable metabolic encephalopathy, *Pediatr Neurol*, 9:243-246, 1993.

189. Raupp P, Varady E, Duran M, Wanders RJ, et al: Novel genotype of mevalonic aciduria with fatalities in premature siblings, *Arch Dis Child Fetal Neonatal Ed*, 89:F90-F91, 2004.

190. Rolland MO, Cuisset L, Le Bozec J, Guffon N, et al: First-trimester enzymatic and molecular prenatal diagnosis of mevalonic aciduria, *J Inherit Metab Dis*, 28:1141-1142, 2005.

191. Keating JP, Feigin RD, Tenenbaum SM, Hillman RE: Hyperglycinemia with ketosis due to a defect in isoleucine catabolism, *Pediatrics*, 50:890-895, 1972.

192. Hillman RE, Keating JP: beta-Ketothiolase deficiency as a cause of the ketotic hyperglycinemia syndrome, *Pediatrics*, 53:221-225, 1974.

193. Nyhan WL: Heritable metabolic disease in the differential diagnosis of asphyxia. In Gluck L, editor: *Intrauterine Asphyxia and the Developing Fetal Brain*, Chicago: 1977, Year Book.

194. Gompertz D, Saudubray JM, Charpentier C, Bartlett K, et al: A defect in isoleucine metabolism associated with alpha-methyl-beta-hydroxybutyric and alpha-methylacetoacetic aciduria: Quantitative in vivo and in vitro studies, *Clin Chim Acta*, 57:269-281, 1974.

195. Yamaguchi S, Sakai A, Fukao T, Wakazono A, et al: Biochemical and immunochemical study of seven families with 3-ketothiolase deficiency: Diagnosis of heterozygotes using immunochemical determination of the ratio of mitochondrial acetoacetyl-CoA thiolase and 3-ketoacyl-CoA thiolase proteins, *Pediatr Res*, 33:429-432, 1993.

196. Roe CR, Ding J: Mitochondrial fatty acid oxidation disorders. In Scriver CR, Beaudet MD, Sly WS, et al, editors: *The Metabolic and Molecular Bases of Inherited Disease*, 8th ed, New York: 2001, McGraw-Hill.

197. Riudor E: Neonatal onset in fatty acid oxidation disorders: How can we minimize morbidity and mortality? *J Inherit Metab Dis*, 21:619-623, 1998.

198. Dawson DB, Waber L, Hale DE, Bennett MJ: Transient organic aciduria and persistent lacticacidemia in a patient with short-chain acyl-coenzyme A dehydrogenase deficiency, *J Pediatr*, 126:69-71, 1995.

199. North KN, Hoppel CL, Degirolami U, Kozakewich H, et al: Lethal neonatal deficiency of carnitine palmitoyltransferase II associated with dysgenesis of the brain and kidneys, *J Pediatr*, 127:414-420, 1995.

200. Chalmers RA, Stanley CA, English N, Wigglesworth JS: Mitochondrial carnitine-acylcarnitine translocase deficiency presenting as sudden neonatal death, *J Pediatr*, 131:220-225, 1997.

201. Tyni T, Palotie A, Vinikka L, Valanne L, et al: Long-chain 3-hydroxy-acyl-coenzyme A dehydrogenase deficiency with the G1528C mutation: Clinical presentation of thirteen patients, *J Pediatr*, 130:67-76, 1997.

202. Kamuo T, Indo Y, Souri M, Aoyama T, et al: Medium chain 3-ketoacyl-coenzyme A thiolase deficiency: A new disorder of mitochondrial fatty acid β-oxidation, *Pediatr Res*, 42:569-576, 1997.

203. Sluysmans T, Tuerlinckx D, Hubinont C, Verellen-Dumoulin C, et al: Very long chain acyl-coenzyme A dehydrogenase deficiency in two siblings: Evolution after prenatal diagnosis and prompt management, *J Pediatr*, 131:444-446, 1997.

204. Tyni T, Pihko H: Long-chain 3-hydroxyacyl-CoA dehydrogenase deficiency, *Acta Paediatr*, 88:237-245, 1999.

205. Pons R, Cavadini P, Baratta S, Invernizzi F, et al: Clinical and molecular heterogeneity in very-long-chain acyl-coenzyme A dehydrogenase deficiency, *Pediatr Neurol*, 22:98-105, 2000.

206. Tamaoki Y, Kumura M, Hasegawa Y, Iga M, et al: A survey of Japanese patients with mitochondrial fatty acid β-oxidation and related disorders as detected from 1985 to 2000, *Brain Dev*, 24:675-680, 2002.

207. Invernizzi F, Burlina AB, Donadio A, Giordano G, et al: Lethal neonatal presentation of carnitine palmitoyltransferase I deficiency, *J Inherit Metab Dis*, 24:601-602, 2001.

208. Bok LA, Vreken P, Wijburg FA, Wanders RJA, et al: Short-chain Acyl-CoA dehydrogenase deficiency: Studies in a large family adding to the complexity of the disorder, *Pediatrics*, 112:1152-1155, 2003.

209. Den Boer ME, Dionisi-Vici C, Chakrapani A, Van Thuijl AO, et al: Mitochondrial trifunctional protein deficiency: A severe fatty acid oxidation disorder with cardiac and neurologic involvement, *J Pediatr*, 142:684-689, 2003.

210. Vladutiu GD, Quackenbush EJ, Hainline BE, Albers S, et al: Lethal neonatal and severe late infantile forms of carnitine palmitoyltransferase II deficiency associated with compound heterozygosity for different protein truncation mutations, *J Pediatr*, 141:734-736, 2002.

211. Derks TG, Reingoud DJ, Waterham HR, Gerver WJ, et al: The natural history of medium-chain acyl CoA dehydrogenase deficiency in the Netherlands: Clinical presentation and outcome, *J Pediatr*, 148:665-670, 2006.

212. Mikati MA, Chaaban HR, Karam PE, Krishnamoorthy KS: Brain malformation and infantile spasms in a SCAD deficiency patient, *Pediatr Neurol*, 36:48-50, 2007.

213. Hale DE, Bennett MJ: Fatty acid oxidation disorders: A new class of metabolic diseases, *J Pediatr*, 121:1-11, 1992.

214. Leung KC, Hammond JW, Chabra S, Carpenter KH, et al: A fatal neonatal case of medium-chain acyl-coenzyme A dehydrogenase deficiency with homozygous A->G985 transition, *J Pediatr*, 121:965-968, 1992.

215. Catzeflis C, Bachmann C, Hale DE, Coates PM, et al: Early diagnosis and treatment of neonatal medium-chain acyl-CoA dehydrogenase deficiency: Report of two siblings, *Eur J Pediatr*, 149:577-581, 1990.

216. Nobukuni Y, Yokoo T, Ohtani Y, Endo F, et al: Neonatal onset of medium-chain acyl-CoA dehydrogenase deficiency in two siblings, *Brain Dev*, 10:129-134, 1988.

217. Wilcken B, Carpenter KH, Hammond J: Neonatal symptoms in medium chain acyl coenzyme-A dehydrogenase deficiency, *Arch Dis Child*, 69:292-294, 1993.

218. Iafolla AK, Thompson RJ, Roe CR: Medium-chain acyl-coenzyme A dehydrogenase deficiency: Clinical course in 120 affected children, *J Pediatr*, 124:409-415, 1994.

219. Ziadeh R, Hoffman EP, Fiengold DN, Hoop RC, et al: Medium chain acyl-CoA dehydrogenase deficiency in Pennsylvania: Neonatal screening shows high incidence and unexpected mutation frequencies, *Pediatr Res*, 37:675-678, 1995.

220. Burlina AB, Bennett MJ, Gregersen N, Barba BD, et al: Medium-chain acyl-CoA dehydrogenase deficiency presenting in the neonatal period: The first Italian case, *Eur J Pediatr*, 154:940-941, 1995.

221. Riudor E, Arranz JA, Anguera R, Salcedo S, et al: Neonatal medium-chain acyl-CoA dehydrogenase deficiency presenting with very high creatine kinase levels, *J Inherit Metab Dis*, 21:673-674, 1998.

222. Moore DJ: Medium-chain acyl-CoA dehydrogenase deficiency: A case presentation, *Neonatal Netw*, 5:7-13, 2005.

223. Wolf B: Disorders of biotin metabolism. In Scriver CR, Beaudet MD, Sly WS, et al, editors: *The Metabolic and Molecular Bases of Inherited Disease*, 8th ed, New York: 2001, McGraw-Hill.

224. Bousounis DP, Camfield PR, Wolf B: Reversal of brain atrophy with biotin treatment in biotinidase deficiency, *Neuropediatrics*, 24:214-217, 1993.

225. Kalayci O, Coskun T, Tokatli A, Demir E, et al: Infantile spasms as the initial symptom of biotinidase deficiency, *J Pediatr*, 124:103-104, 1994.

226. Haagerup A, Andersen JB, Blichfeldt S, Christensen MF: Biotinidase deficiency: Two cases of very early presentation, *Dev Med Child Neurol*, 39:832-835, 1997.

227. Morrone A, Malvagia S, Donati MA, Funghini S, et al: Clinical findings and biochemical and molecular analysis of four patients with holocarboxylase synthetase deficiency, *Am J Med Genet*, 111:10-18, 2002.

228. Wilson CJ, Myer M, Darlow BA, Stanley T, et al: Severe holocarboxylase synthetase deficiency with incomplete biotin responsiveness resulting in antenatal insult in Samoan neonates, *J Pediatr*, 147:115-118, 2005.

229. Wolf B: Disorders of biotin metabolism. In Scriver CR, Beaudet AL, Sly WS, et al, editors: *The Metabolic and Molecular Bases of Inherited Disease*, New York: 1995, McGraw-Hill.

230. Burri BJ, Sweetman L, Nyhan WL: Mutant holocarboxylase synthetase: Evidence for the enzyme defect in early infantile biotin-responsive multiple carboxylase deficiency, *J Clin Invest*, 68:1491-1495, 1981.

231. Packman S, Sweetman L, Baker H, Wall S: The neonatal form of biotin-responsive multiple carboxylase deficiency, *J Pediatr*, 99:418-420, 1981.

232. Wolf B, Hsia YE, Sweetman L, Feldman G, et al: Multiple carboxylase deficiency: Clinical and biochemical improvement following neonatal biotin treatment, *Pediatrics*, 68:113-118, 1981.

233. Packman S, Cowan MJ, Golbus MS, Caswell NM, et al: Prenatal treatment of biotin-responsive multiple carboxylase deficiency, *Lancet*, 1:1435-1438, 1982.

234. Roth KS, Yang W, Allan L, Saunders M, et al: Prenatal administration of biotin in biotin responsive multiple carboxylase deficiency, *Pediatr Res*, 16:126-129, 1982.

235. Sweetman L, Nyhan WL, Sakati NA, Ohlsson A, et al: Organic aciduria in neonatal multiple carboxylase deficiency, *J Inherit Metab Dis*, 5:49-53, 1982.

236. Wolf B, Feldman GL: The biotin-dependent carboxylase deficiencies, *Am J Hum Genet*, 34:699-716, 1982.

237. Packman S, Caswell N, Gonzalez-Rios MC, Kadlecek T, et al: Acetyl CoA carboxylase in cultured fibroblasts: Differential biotin dependence in the two types of biotin-responsive multiple carboxylase deficiency, *Am J Hum Genet*, 36:80-92, 1984.

238. Suormala TM, Baumgartner ER, Wick H, Scheibenreiter S, et al: Comparison of patients with complete and partial biotinidase deficiency: Biochemical studies, *J Inherit Metab Dis*, 13:76-92, 1990.

239. Wolf B, Grier RE, McVoy JR, Heard GS: Biotinidase deficiency: A novel vitamin recycling defects, *J Inherit Metab Dis*, 1:53-58, 1985.

240. Honavar M, Janota I, Neville BGR, Chalmers RA: Neuropathology of biotinidase deficiency, *Acta Neuropathol (Berl)*, 84:461-464, 1992.

241. Salbert BA, Pellock JM, Wolf B: Characterization of seizures associated with biotinidase deficiency, *Neurology*, 43:1351-1354, 1993.

242. Collins JE, Nicholson NS, Dalton N, Leonard JV: Biotinidase deficiency: Early neurological presentation, *Dev Med Child Neurol*, 36:263-270, 1994.

243. Moslinger D, Muhl A, Suormala T, Baumgartner R, et al: Molecular characterisation and neuropsychological outcome of 21 patients with profound biotinidase deficiency detected by newborn screening and family studies, *Eur J Pediatr*, 162(Suppl 1):S46-49, 2003.

244. Grunewald S, Champion MP, Leonard JV, Schaper J, et al: Biotinidase deficiency: A treatable leukoencephalopathy, *Neuropediatrics*, 35:211-216, 2004.

245. Weber P, Scholl S, Baumgartner ER: Outcome in patients with profound biotinidase deficiency: Relevance of newborn screening, *Dev Med Child Neurol*, 46:481-484, 2004.

246. Frerman FE, Goodman SI: Defects of electron transfer flavoprotein and electron transfer flavoprotein–ubiquinone oxidoreductase: Glutaric acidemia type II. In Scriver CR, Beaudet MD, Sly WS, et al, editors: *The Metabolic and Molecular Bases of Inherited Disease*, 8th ed, New York: 2001, McGraw-Hill.

247. Loehr JP, Goodman SI, Frerman FE: Glutaric acidemia type II: Heterogeneity of clinical and biochemical phenotypes, *Pediatr Res*, 27:311-315, 1990.

248. Shevell MI, Didomenicantonio G, Sylvain M, Arnold DL, et al: Glutaric acidemia type II: Neuroimaging and spectroscopy evidence for developmental encephalomyopathy, *Pediatr Neurol*, 12:350-353, 1995.

249. Gordon N: Glutaric aciduria types I and II, *Brain Dev*, 28:136-140, 2006.

250. Bohm N, Uy J, Kiessling M, Lehnert W: Multiple acyl-CoA dehydrogenation deficiency (glutaric aciduria type II), congenital polycystic kidneys, and symmetric warty dysplasia of the cerebral cortex in two newborn brothers. II. Morphology and pathogenesis, *Eur J Pediatr*, 139:60-65, 1982.

251. Goodman SI, Stene DO, McCabe ER, Norenberg MD, et al: Glutaric acidemia type II: Clinical, biochemical, and morphologic considerations, *J Pediatr*, 100:946-950, 1982.

252. Lehnert W, Wendel U, Lindenmaier S, Bohm N: Multiple acyl-CoA dehydrogenation deficiency (glutaric aciduria type II), congenital polycystic kidneys, and symmetric warty dysplasia of the cerebral cortex in two brothers. I. Clinical, metabolical, and biochemical findings, *Eur J Pediatr*, 132:56-59, 1982.

253. Goodman SI, Reale M, Berlow S: Glutaric acidemia type II: A form with deleterious intrauterine effects, *J Pediatr*, 102:411-413, 1983.

254. Christensen E, Kolvraa S, Gregersen N: Glutaric aciduria type II: Evidence for a defect related to the electron transfer flavoprotein or its dehydrogenase, *Pediatr Res*, 18:663-667, 1984.

255. Mooy PD, Przyrembel H, Giesberts MA, Scholte HR, et al: Glutaric aciduria type II: Treatment with riboflavine, carnitine and insulin, *Eur J Pediatr*, 143:92-95, 1984.

256. Verjee ZH, Sherwood WG: Multiple acyl-CoA dehydrogenase deficiency: A neonatal onset case responsive to treatment, *J Inherit Metab Dis*, 8:137-138, 1985.

257. Stockler S, Radner H, Karpf EF, Hauer A, et al: Symmetric hypoplasia of the temporal cerebral lobes in an infant with glutaric aciduria type II (multiple acyl-coenzyme A dehydrogenase deficiency), *J Pediatr*, 124:601-604, 1994.

258. Takanashi J-I, Fujii K, Sugita K, Kohno Y: Neuroradiologic findings in glutaric aciduria type II, *Pediatr Neurol*, 20:142-145, 1999.

259. Yamaguchi S, Shimizu N, Orii T, Fukao T, et al: Prenatal diagnosis and neonatal monitoring of a fetus with glutaric aciduria type II due to electron transfer flavoprotein (β-subunit) deficiency, *Pediatr Res*, 30:439-443, 1991.

260. Uziel G, Garavaglia B, Ciceri E, Moroni I, et al: Riboflavin-responsive glutaric aciduria type II presenting as a leukodystrophy, *Pediatr Neurol*, 13:333-335, 1995.

261. Goodman SI, Frerman FE: Organic acidemias due to defects in lysine oxidation: 2-ketoadipic acidemia and glutaric acidemia. In Schriver CR, Beaudet AL, Sly WS, et al, editors: *The Metabolic and Molecular Bases of Inherited Disease*, 8th ed, New York: 2001, McGraw-Hill.

262. Land JM, Goulder P, Johnson A, Hockaday J: Glutaric aciduria type 1: An atypical presentation together with some observations upon treatment and the possible cause of cerebral damage, *Neuropediatrics*, 23:322-326, 1992.

263. Soffer D, Amir N, Elpeleg ON, Gomori JM, et al: Striatal degeneration and spongy myelinopathy in glutaric acidemia, *J Neurol Sci*, 107:199-204, 1992.

264. Mandel H, Braun J, El-Peleg O, Christensen E, et al: Glutaric aciduria type 1: Brain CT features and a diagnostic pitfall, *Neuroradiology*, 33:75-78, 1991.

265. Haworth JC, Booth FA, Chudley AE, deGroot GW, et al: Phenotypic variability in glutaric aciduria type I: Report of fourteen cases in five Canadian Indian kindreds, *J Pediatr*, 118:52-58, 1991.

266. Bergman I, Finegold D, Gartner JC, Zitelli BJ, et al: Acute profound dystonia in infants with glutaric acidemia, *Pediatrics*, 83:228-234, 1989.

267. Yager JY, McClarty BM, Seshia SS: CT-scan findings in an infant with glutaric aciduria type 1, *Dev Med Child Neurol*, 30:808-820, 1988.

268. Chow CW, Haan EA, Goodman SI, Anderson RM, et al: Neuropathology in glutaric acidaemia type 1, *Acta Neuropathol (Berl)*, 76:590-594, 1988.

269. Iafolla AK, Kahler SG: Megalencephaly in the neonatal period as the initial manifestation of glutaric aciduria type I, *J Pediatr*, 114:1004-1006, 1989.

270. Amir N, Elpeleg O, Shalev RS, Christensen E: Glutaric aciduria type I: Enzymatic and neuroradiologic investigations of two kindreds, *J Pediatr*, 114:983-989, 1989.

271. Drigo P, Burlina AB, Battistella PA: Subdural hematoma and glutaric aciduria type I, *Brain Dev*, 15:460-461, 1993.

272. Brismar J, Ozand PT: CT and MR of the brain in glutaric acidemia type I: A review of 59 published cases and a report of 5 new patients, *AJNR Am J Neuroradiol*, 16:675-683, 1995.

273. Hoffman GF, Athanassopoulos S, Burlina AB, Duran M, et al: Clinical course, early diagnosis, treatment and prevention of disease in glutaryl-CoA dehydrogenase deficiency, *Neuropediatrics*, 27:115-123, 1996.

274. Kolker S, Garbade SF, Greenberg CR, Leonard JV, et al: Natural history, outcome, and treatment efficacy in children and adults with glutaryl-CoA dehydrogenase deficiency, *Pediatr Res*, 59:840-847, 2006.

275. Diogo L, Fineza I, Canha J, Borges L, et al: Macrocephaly as the presenting feature of L-2-hydroxyglutaric aciduria in a 5-month-old boy, *J Inherit Metab Dis*, 19:369-370, 1996.

276. Chen E, Nyhan WL, Jakobs C, Greco CM, et al: L-2-Hydroxyglutaric aciduria: Neuropathological correlations and first report of severe neurodegenerative disease and neonatal death, *J Inherit Metab Dis*, 19:335-343, 1996.

277. de Klerk JBC, Huijmans JGM, Stroink H, Robben SGF, et al: L-2-Hydroxyglutaric aciduria: Clinical heterogeneity versus biochemical homogeneity in a sibship, *Neuropediatrics*, 28:314-317, 1997.

278. D'Incerti L, Farina L, Moroni I, Uziel G, et al: L-2-Hydroxyglutaric aciduria: MRI in seven cases, *Neuroradiology*, 40:727-733, 1998.

279. van der Knaap MS, Jakobs C, Hoffmann GF, Nyhan WL, et al: D-2-Hydroxyglutaric aciduria: Biochemical marker or clinical disease entity? *Ann Neurol*, 45:111-119, 1999.

280. Korman SH, Salomons GS, Gutman A, Brooks R, et al: D-2-Hydroxyglutaric aciduria and glutaric aciduria type 1 in siblings: Coincidence, *or linked disorders? Neuropediatrics*, 35:151-156, 2004.

281. Divry P, Roulaud-Parrot F, Dorche C, Zabot MT, et al: 5-Oxoprolinuria (glutathione synthetase deficiency): A case with neonatal presentation and rapid fatal outcome, *J Inherit Metab Dis*, 14:341-344, 1991.

282. Larsson A, Anderson ME: Glutathione synthetase deficiency and other disorders of the γ-glutamyl cycle. In Schriver CR, Beaudet AL, Sly WS, et al, editors: *The Metabolic and Molecular Bases of Inherited Disease*, 8th ed, New York: 2001, McGraw-Hill.

283. Njalsson R, Norgren S: Physiological and pathological aspects of GSH metabolism, *Acta Paediatr*, 94:132-137, 2005.

284. Ristoff E, Mayatepek E, Larsson A: Long-term clinical outcome in patients with glutathione synthetase deficiency, *J Pediatr*, 139:79-87, 2001.

285. Bruggemann LW, Groenendaal F, Ristoff E, Larsson A, et al: Glutathione synthetase deficiency associated with antenatal cerebral bleeding, *J Inherit Metab Dis*, 27:275-276, 2004.

286. Johnson JL, Duran M: Molybdenum cofactor deficiency and isolated sulfite oxidase deficiency. In Schriver CR, Beaudet AL, Sly WS, et al, editors: *The Metabolic and Molecular Bases of Inherited Disease*, 8th ed, New York: 2001, McGraw-Hill.

287. Brown GK, Scholem RD, Croll HB, Wraith JE, et al: Sulfite oxidase deficiency: Clinical, neuroradiologic, and biochemical features in two new patients, *Neurology*, 39:252-256, 1989.

288. Slot HMJ, Overweg-Plandsoen WCG, Bakker HD, Abeling GGM, et al: Molybdenum-cofactor deficiency: An easily missed cause of neonatal convulsions, *Neuropediatrics*, 24:139-142, 1993.

289. Schuierer G, Kurlemann G, Bick U, Stephani U: Molybdenum-cofactor deficiency: CT and MR findings, *Neuropediatrics*, 26:51-54, 1995.

290. Rupar CA, Gillett J, Gordon BA, Ramsey DA, et al: Isolated sulfite oxidase deficiency, *Neuropediatrics*, 27:299-304, 1996.

291. Dublin AB, Hald JK, Wootton-Gorges SL: Isolated sulfite oxidase deficiency: MR imaging features, *AJNR Am J Neuroradiol*, 23:484-485, 2002.

292. Arslanoglu S, Yalaz M, Goksen D, Coker M, et al: Molybdenum cofactor deficiency associated with Dandy-Walker complex, *Brain Dev*, 23:815-818, 2001.

293. Salman MS, Ackerley C, Senger C, Becker L: New insights into the neuropathogenesis of molybdenum cofactor deficiency, *Can J Neurol Sci*, 29:91-96, 2002.

294. Teksam O, Yurdakok M, Coskun T: Molybdenum cofactor deficiency presenting with severe metabolic acidosis and intracranial hemorrhage, *J Child Neurol*, 20:155-157, 2005.

295. Tan WH, Eichler FS, Hoda S, Lee MS, et al: Isolated sulfite oxidase deficiency: A case report with a novel mutation and review of the literature, *Pediatrics*, 116:757-766, 2005.

296. Macaya A, Brunso L, Fernandez-Castillo N, Arranz JA, et al: Molybdenum cofactor deficiency presenting as neonatal hyperekplexia: A clinical, biochemical and genetic study, *Neuropediatrics*, 36:389-394, 2005.

297. Schwarz G: Molybdenum cofactor biosynthesis and deficiency, *Cell Mol Life Sci*, 62:2792-2810, 2005.

298. Hobson EE, Thomas S, Crofton PM, Murray AD, et al: Isolated sulphite oxidase deficiency mimics the features of hypoxic ischaemic encephalopathy, *Eur J Pediatr*, 164:655-659, 2005.

298a. Basheer SN, Waters PJ, Lam CW, Acquaviva-Bourdain C, et al: Isolated sulfite oxidase deficiency in the newborn: Lactic acidaemia and leukoencephalopathy, *Neuropediatrics*, 38:38-41, 2007.

299. Reiss J, Bonin M, Schwegler H, Sass JO, et al: The pathogenesis of molybdenum cofactor deficiency, its delay by maternal clearance, and its expression pattern in microarray analysis, *Mol Genet Metab*, 85:12-20, 2005.

300. Vianey-Liaud C, Desjacques P, Gaulme J, Dorche C, et al: A new case of isolated sulphite oxidase deficiency with rapid fatal outcome, *J Inherit Metab Dis*, 11:425-426, 1988.

301. Arnold GL, Greene CL, Stout JP, Goodman SI: Molybdenum cofactor deficiency, *J Pediatr*, 123:595-598, 1993.

302. Hansen LK, Wulff K, Dorche C, Christensen E: Molybdenum cofactor deficiency in two siblings: Diagnostic difficulties, *Eur J Pediatr*, 152:662-664, 1993.

303. Boles RG, Ment LR, Meyn MS, Horwich AL, et al: Short-term response to dietary therapy in molybdenum cofactor deficiency, *Ann Neurol*, 34:742-744, 1993.

304. Johnson JL: Wadman SK: Molybdenum cofactor deficiency and isolated sulfite oxidase deficiency. In Scriver CR, Beaudet AL, Sly WS, et al, editors: *The Metabolic and Molecular Bases of Inherited Disease*, 7th ed, New York: 1995, McGraw-Hill.

Chapter 16

Degenerative Diseases of the Newborn

Certain degenerative disorders of the developing nervous system may be manifested clinically in the neonatal period. Because most of these disorders are related to a disturbance in the metabolism of a lipid or some other compound, they are discussed most appropriately in this series of chapters concerned with metabolic disorders. Indeed, clinical overlap of some of these degenerative disorders with some of the metabolic disorders discussed in previous chapters will be apparent. Nevertheless, the diseases discussed in this chapter are best considered as a more or less distinct group. Early diagnosis is important for delineation of prognosis, genetic counseling, and, in a few instances, institution of specific therapy. Because these are relatively rare disorders, discussion of each entity is brief.

MAJOR DISORDERS

From the clinical standpoint, I find it useful to separate the degenerative disorders into those that affect primarily gray matter and those that involve primarily white matter (Table 16-1). (At later ages, disorders that affect specific regions of the brain [e.g., basal ganglia in Huntington or Wilson disease or cerebellum in ataxia telangiectasia], so-called "system" degenerations, comprise a third major category.) In general, disorders of gray matter are characterized by the appearance early in the disease of seizures, myoclonus, spikes or sharp activity on the electroencephalogram, failure of cognitive development ("dementia"), and retinal disease, whereas disorders of white matter are characterized by the appearance early in the disease of marked motor deficits and slow activity on the electroencephalogram. Although overlap in the clinical features and even in the topography of the neuropathology between the two broad categories is considerable, I retain the separation. A few disorders, involving specific subcellular organelles (e.g., peroxisomes, mitochondria) or other, still-to-be-defined defects affect both gray and white matter prominently, and these must be considered separately (see Table 16-1). This chapter focuses on only those diseases for which recording of more than an isolated case or two with neonatal manifestations is available. The salient features of the disorders are outlined in Tables 16-2 to 16-5. Many of these disorders are abnormalities of degradation of sphingolipids (Fig. 16-1), as noted in the individual discussions later.

DISORDERS PRIMARILY AFFECTING GRAY MATTER

Disorders primarily affecting gray matter are discussed best according to the presence or absence of accompanying visceral storage. Visceral storage is identified clinically by hepatosplenomegaly and is often accompanied by abnormalities of long bones and by coarse facial features.

No Visceral Storage

Tay-Sachs Disease

Tay-Sachs disease is the prototype of a degenerative disease of gray matter in infancy (see Table 16-2). Onset in the first few weeks of life, although uncommon, may occur. (More commonly, onset is at approximately 3 months.) The principal initial *clinical features* are irritability and hypersensitivity to auditory and often other sensory inputs. A cherry-red spot, caused by ganglioside storage in retinal ganglion cells imparting a yellowish tint around the normally red fovea, is apparent on funduscopic examination. This abnormality has been identified as early as 2 days of age.[1,2] The subsequent course is characterized by myoclonic seizures, motor deterioration, blindness, macrencephaly, and death in the third or fourth year of life. (A clinical variant with organomegaly and bony abnormalities similar to those in generalized GM_1 gangliosidosis [see later discussion] is termed *Sandhoff variant* of Tay-Sachs disease.[1]) The *diagnosis* is established by identification in white blood cells or fibroblasts of the enzymatic defect, which involves hexosaminidase A (see Fig. 16-1). (In Sandhoff variant, both hexosaminidase A and B are deficient.) The disorder is inherited in an autosomal recessive manner and is especially common in Ashkenazi Jews. *Neuropathology* is characterized by generalized neuronal storage of GM_2 ganglioside and by markedly dilated neuronal processes (meganeurites).[2,3] *Neuroimaging (magnetic resonance imaging [MRI])* shows abnormal signal in thalamus and, subsequently, marked atrophy of cerebral cortex and deep nuclear structures; cerebral white matter shows increased T2 signal.[4] Although no known therapy exists, genetically engineered neural progenitor cells have been shown to correct the enzymatic defect in co-cultured human Tay-Sachs fibroblasts and to secrete active enzyme throughout fetal and neonatal mouse brain after

TABLE 16-1 Degenerative Diseases of the Nervous System with Manifestations in the Newborn

Gray Matter
No Visceral Storage
Tay-Sachs disease (GM$_2$ gangliosidosis)
Congenital neuronal ceroid-lipofuscinosis
Alpers disease
Menkes disease
With Visceral Storage
GM$_1$ gangliosidosis
GM$_2$ gangliosidosis (Sandhoff variant)
Niemann-Pick disease
Gaucher disease
Farber disease
Infantile sialic acid storage disease

White Matter
Canavan disease
Alexander disease
Krabbe disease
Pelizaeus-Merzbacher disease
Leukodystrophy with cerebral calcifications and cerebro-
  spinal fluid pleocytosis (Aicardi-Goutieres disease)

Gray and White Matter
Peroxisomal disorders: neonatal adrenoleukodystrophy,
  Zellweger syndrome
Mitochondrial disorder: Leigh syndrome, other
  mitochondrial encephalopathies
Other disorders: congenital disorder of glycosylation,
  pontocerebellar hypoplasia type 2

TABLE 16-3 Neonatal Disorders that Mimic Gray Matter Degenerations at Presentation

Epileptic Syndromes (see Chapter 5)
Early myoclonic epilepsy
Early infantile epileptic encephalopathy (Ohtahara syndrome)
Malignant migrating partial seizures

Metabolic Disorders (see Chapters 14 and 15)
Nonketotic hyperglycinemia
Sulfite oxidase deficiency: molybdenum cofactor deficiency
Multiple carboxylase deficiency: biotinidase deficiency
Multiple acyl–coenzyme A dehydrogenase deficiency
  (glutaric aciduria type II)

Other Disorders
Pyridoxine dependency (see Chapter 5)
Glucose transporter deficiency (see Chapter 5)
Rett syndrome (male patients)

cellular transplantation.[5] *Prenatal diagnosis* can be made readily by enzymatic analysis for hexosaminidase A in cultured amniotic fluid cells or chorionic villus samples.[1] Attempted *therapy* with bone marrow transplantation has not altered the course of the disease.[6]

Congenital Neuronal Ceroid-Lipofuscinosis
Neuronal ceroid-lipofuscinosis consists of a group of neuronal degenerative disorders characterized by accumulation of the lipopigments ceroid and lipofuscin.

TABLE 16-2 Degenerative Diseases Primarily of Gray Matter (No Visceral Storage)

Disease	Clinical Features	Metabolic-Enzymatic Features	Pathology
Tay-Sachs disease (GM$_2$ gangliosidosis)	Stimulus-sensitive myoclonus, irritability, hypotonia, weakness, cherry-red macula (virtually all); later seizures, blindness, and macrocephaly	GM$_2$ ganglioside accumulation in brain; hexosaminidase A deficiency	Neurons distended by GM$_2$ ganglioside throughout the central nervous system
Congenital neuronal ceroid-lipofuscinosis	Neonatal seizures (severe), apnea, microcephaly, developmental arrest, followed by regression and vegetative state	Cathepsin D deficiency	Marked brain atrophy; diffuse neuronal loss with gliosis, autofluorescent granular material in neurons, glia, and macrophages, electron microscopy—osmiophilic granules
Alpers disease	Myoclonus (often stimulus-sensitive), seizures (severe), developmental arrest followed by regression, visual and auditory deficits common, evidence of hepatic dysfunction late	Elevated lactate/pyruvate levels in cerebrospinal fluid (and blood); deficient catalytic subunit of mitochondrial DNA polymerase gamma (mutated gene *POLG*) with mitochondrial DNA depletion and impaired function of electron transport chain at multiple sites	Marked brain atrophy; severe neuronal loss with astrocytosis, spongiosis, and capillary proliferation, especially in cerebral cortex, particularly occipital (striate) cortex
Menkes disease (kinky hair disease)	Hypothermia, hypotonia, poor feeding, poor weight gain, seizures, developmental arrest and then regression; cherubic face; colorless, friable, "steely" hair	Low serum copper and ceruloplasmin levels; cultured fibroblasts: reduced efflux of copper, elevated copper content; deficient activity of many copper-containing enzymes; molecular defect of a cation transporting ATPase	Neuronal loss with gliosis in cerebral cortex and cerebellum, marked proliferation of dendritic tree (especially of Purkinje cells), focal axonal swellings ("torpedoes"); myelin loss with gliosis and arterial changes

TABLE 16-4   Degenerative Diseases Primarily of Gray Matter (with Visceral Storage)

Disease	Clinical Features	Metabolic-Enzymatic Features	Pathology
GM$_1$ gangliosidosis	Sucking and swallowing impairment, hypotonia, decreased movement; edema, coarse facies, hepatosplenomegaly, cherry-red macula (50%)	GM$_1$ ganglioside accumulation in brain, beta-galactosidase deficiency	Neurons distended by GM$_1$ ganglioside throughout CNS
GM$_2$ gangliosidosis (Sandhoff variant)	See Tay-Sachs disease; also hepatosplenomegaly	See Tay-Sachs disease; also globoside accumulates in viscera, hexosaminidase A and B deficiency	See Tay-Sachs disease
Niemann-Pick disease (type 1A, "infantile")	Feeding impairment, failure to thrive, developmental arrest and then regression, cherry-red macula (50%), hepatosplenomegaly	Sphingomyelin (and cholesterol) accumulate in brain; sphingomyelinase deficiency	Neurons distended with sphingomyelin throughout CNS; foam cells in leptomeningeal and perivascular spaces
Gaucher disease (type 2, "acute neuronopathic" or "infantile")	Retrocollis, strabismus, trismus, dysphagia, aspiration, spasticity, hepatosplenomegaly, hydrops fetalis	Glucocerebroside accumulates in brain; glucocerebrosidase (beta-glucosidase) deficiency	Gaucher cells (lipid-laden histiocytes) in perivascular spaces and in parenchyma; neuronal death and neuronophagia throughout CNS, especially in brain stem
Farber disease (lipogranulomatosis) type 1, classic	Painful swelling of joints, (later periarticular nodules), hoarse cry, feeding disturbance, failure to thrive, hypotonia, muscle atrophy, areflexia or hyporeflexia, hepatomegaly (50%)	Ceramide accumulates in tissues; ceramidase deficiency	Neurons distended by glycolipid (ceramide?), especially anterior horn cells, less prominently in brain stem, basal ganglia, and least in cortex
Infantile sialic acid storage disease (also sialidosis type II, and galactosialidosis)	Fetal ascites/hydrops, neonatal hypotonia, impaired feeding, developmental arrest followed by regression; ascites, coarse facies, white hair, hepatosplenomegaly	Sialic acid accumulates in tissues, including brain, and in body fluids; defect of sialic acid transport across lysosomal membrane; similar phenotype with sialidosis secondary to deficiency of alpha-neuraminidase (sialidosis type II) or of alpha-neuraminidase and beta-galactosidase (galactosialidosis)	Neurons distended with sialic acid, especially in diencephalon, brain stem, and spinal cord; prominent axonal spheroids; myelin deficiency

CNS, central nervous system.

At least eight mutant genes and clinical forms are now recognized.[7-11a] The form of most relevance in this context is congenital neuronal ceroid-lipofuscinosis (Norman-Wood disease). This form should be distinguished from the more common and well-known early infantile disorder (Haltia-Santavuori disease). In the latter disorder, the usual age of onset is 6 to 18 months. The rarer congenital form is apparent at birth (see Table 16-2), and approximately 11 cases have been reported.[12-17] The clinical phenotype is dramatic. Postnatal respiratory insufficiency, severe neonatal seizures, and microcephaly are nearly consistent *clinical features*. Failure of neurological development and development of vegetative state, usually with recalcitrant seizures, are followed by death, usually in the first days or weeks of life. The absence of electroretinographic responses and the development of an isoelectric electroencephalogram are characteristic. Neuroimaging (MRI) shows marked and progressive atrophy of cerebral cortex, thalamus, and striatum (Fig. 16-2). The diagnosis should be considered in a newborn with severe seizures and microcephaly of unknown origin. *Diagnosis* is based initially on identification of the autofluorescent lipopigments in lymphocytes, skin, or rectal mucosa, present as granular material on electron microscopic examination. *Neuropathological findings* are characterized by diffuse neuronal loss (Fig. 16-3) with accumulation of the

TABLE 16-5 Degenerative Diseases Primarily of White Matter

Disease	Clinical Features	Metabolic-Enzymatic Features	Pathology
Canavan disease (spongy degeneration of the white matter)	Macrocephaly with rapid head growth, poor visual fixation, hypotonia and later spasticity, developmental arrest, seizures and then regression, spasticity	N-Acetylaspartic acid accumulates in brain and in urine and plasma; N-acetylaspartoacylase deficiency detectable in fibroblasts	Myelin deficiency, spongy vacuolation of white matter, especially subcortical, with involvement of globus pallidus and thalamus
Alexander disease (leukodystrophy with diffuse Rosenthal fiber formation)	Macrocephaly with rapid head growth, developmental arrest, seizures, and then regression, spasticity	De novo, dominant gain-of-function mutation of glial fibrillary acidic protein (GFAP)	Myelin deficiency, Rosenthal fiber formation in fibrillary astrocytes, especially in subpial, perivascular and subependymal loci
Krabbe disease (globoid cell leukodystrophy)	Irritability, poor feeding, stimulus-sensitive tonic spasms, hypertonia, opisthotonos, developmental arrest and later regression, blind, decerebration	Galactosylsphingosine accumulates in brain; galactosylceramidase I deficiency (a beta-galactosidase)	Myelin deficiency, multinucleated globoid cells (macrophages), and diminished oligodendroglia; peripheral neuropathy (segmental demyelination)
Pelizaeus-Merzbacher disease	Abnormal eye movements ("nystagmus"), laryngeal stridor, head titubation, jerky movements, hypotonia (later spasticity), developmental arrest (later deterioration), seizures (2/3); X-linked recessive (Pelizaeus-Merzbacher–like disease [PMLD]; autosomal recessive)	Defect in gene (duplication, mutation or deletion) encoding myelin proteolipid protein (PMLD; defect in gene encoding connexin 47)	Severe myelin deficiency, usually total but occasionally with preserved islands of myelin; decreased number of mature oligodendrocytes; gliosis, occasional sudanophilic material
Leukodystrophy with cerebral calcifications and cerebrospinal fluid pleocytosis (Aicardi-Goutieres syndrome)	Irritability, poor feeding, ocular abnormalities, hypertonia or hypotonia, weakness, jitteriness, dystonia, oral-facial dyskinesias, occasionally seizures, developmental arrest, microcephaly, and spasticity	Defect in TREX1, gene encoding a DNA exonuclease	Severe myelin deficiency, marked fibrillary gliosis, diffuse/focal calcifications, focal collections of inflammatory cells, microangiopathy

lipopigment granules of ceroid-lipofuscin in neurons, glia, and macrophages. Marked infiltration with astrocytes and microglia is apparent. The recently reported *molecular defect* involves the cathepsin D gene, present in homozygous form in patients.[10] The encoded protein, cathepsin D, is a lysosomal protease.

Alpers Disease

The term *Alpers disease*, inappropriately applied in the past to a heterogeneous group of disorders, refers to those relatively uncommon examples, usually familial and consistent with autosomal recessive inheritance, of a progressive degenerative disease of gray matter without neuronal storage or other pathognomonic cytological features and with subsequent hepatic disease.[18-29] Affected infants exhibit the *clinical hallmarks* of gray matter disease, seizures, and myoclonus (often stimulus sensitive) in the first weeks and months of life (see Table 16-2). Hypotonia and vomiting are also prominent features. In one series, 4 of 26 infants had clear onset within the first 2 months of life. Hepatic disease becomes apparent usually after 9 months of age (mean age, 35 months), but more frequent assessment of serum transaminase levels before the appearance of hepatomegaly demonstrates hepatic dysfunction earlier.[23] Most infants die by 3 years of age.

Neuropathological study shows striking cortical neuronal loss with spongy change and gliosis, worse in the deeper cortical layers and especially prominent in the striate cortex (Fig. 16-4). Frequently, capillary proliferation is apparent, and the constellation of pathological change resembles that of Leigh disease, a

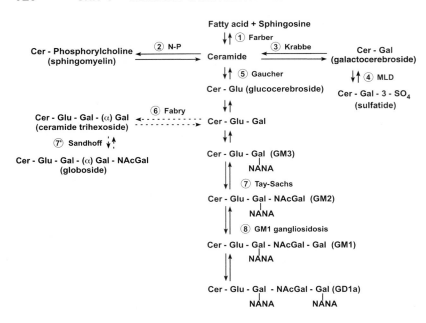

Figure 16-1 **Sphingolipid metabolism and disorders**. The disorders of sphingolipid metabolism involve degradative enzymes: *(1)* Farber disease, ceramidase deficiency; *(2)* Nieman-Pick (N-P) disease, sphingomyelinase deficiency; *(3)* Krabbe disease, galactocerebrosidase deficiency; *(4)* metachromatic leukodystrophy (MLD), arylsulfatase A deficiency; *(5)* Gaucher disease, glucocerebrosidase deficiency; *(6)* Fabry disease, ceramide trihexosidase deficiency; *(7)* Tay-Sachs disease, hexosaminidase A deficiency; *(7′)* Sandhoff disease, hexosaminidase A and B deficiencies; *(8)* GM₁ gangliosidosis, beta-galactosidase deficiency. NANA, *N*-acetylneuraminic acid.

mitochondrial disorder (see later discussion). Earlier data suggested that Alpers disease was a *mitochondrial disorder* because of the finding in several series of patients of elevated blood and cerebrospinal fluid (CSF) lactate and various abnormalities of the electron transport chain.[25-37a] More recently, the disorder was shown to involve mutations in the gene encoding the catalytic subunit of mitochondrial DNA polymerase γ (*POLG*).[26-28] The result is mitochondrial DNA depletion and impaired function of the electron transport chain at multiple sites.

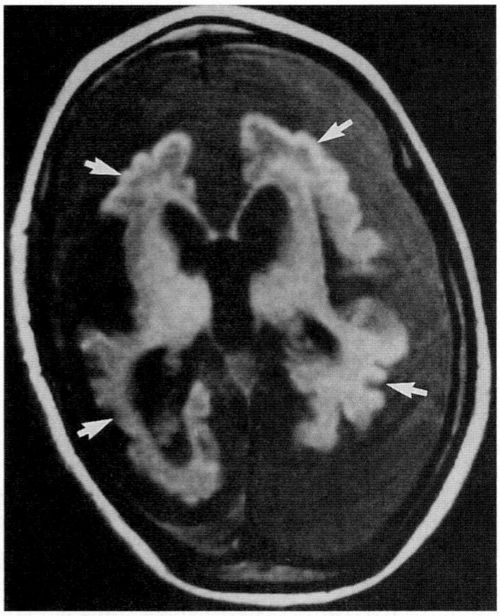

Menkes Disease

Menkes disease (kinky or steely-hair disease, trichopoliodystrophy) is an X-linked disorder of copper metabolism with onset in the severe form of the disease characteristically in the neonatal period.[38-45] Premature delivery, a cherubic face, hypothermia, and hyperbilirubinemia are common neonatal *clinical features* (see Table 16-2). Hypotonia, lethargy, poor feeding, neurological deterioration, and seizures

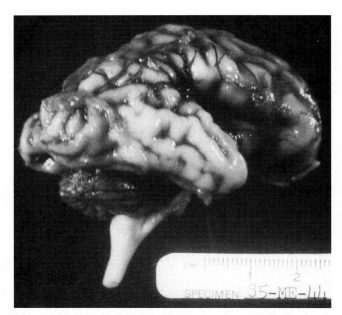

Figure 16-2 **Early infantile neuronal ceroid-lipofuscinosis: magnetic resonance imaging (MRI) scan**. This T1-weighted MRI scan, performed at 4 years of age, shows striking cortical atrophy and markedly dilated lateral ventricles, secondary to atrophy. The shriveled cortical surface is marked by *arrows;* the low signal intensity surrounding the brain is extracerebral fluid. In congenital neuronal ceroid-lipofuscinosis, the atrophy is present in the first weeks and months of life (see Fig. 16-3). *(From Confort-Gouny S, Chabrol B, Vion-Dury J, Mancini J, et al: MRI and localized proton MRS in early infantile form of neuronal ceroid-lipofuscinosis, Pediatr Neurol 9:57-60, 1993.)*

Figure 16-3 **Congenital infantile neuronal ceroid-lipofuscinosis: neuropathology**. This infant was microcephalic at birth, developed status epilepticus, died at 36 hours of age, and exhibited microscopic findings of neuronal ceroid-lipofuscinosis. Note the marked cerebral cortical atrophy with shriveled gyri and marked widening of the sylvian fissure. *(From Barohn RJ, Dowd DC, Kagan-Hallet KS: Congenital ceroid-lipofuscinosis, Pediatr Neurol 8:54-59, 1992.)*

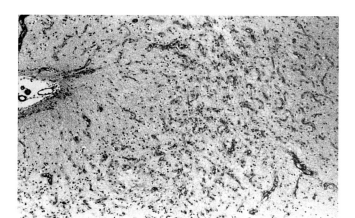

Figure 16-4 Alpers disease: neuropathology. This photomicrograph of the cerebral cortex was obtained at autopsy from a 21-month-old infant with poor feeding and hypotonia in the neonatal period, subsequent development of myoclonic seizures with hypsarrhythmia, minimal neurological development, and, finally, microcephaly, spastic quadriparesis, and an isoelectric electroencephalogram. The cerebral cortex was devoid of neuronal elements and exhibited pronounced spongy changes involving the lower cortical layers and capillary proliferation, shown in extreme form in the figure. *(Courtesy of Dr. Hart Lidov.)*

finding of low serum copper and ceruloplasmin levels; in the early neonatal period, serum values may be normal or elevated but decline over the ensuing weeks, whereas in normal infants, serum values increase postnatally. Studies of cultured fibroblasts show increased retention and reduced efflux of labeled copper, features that can be used for *prenatal diagnosis* by the study of cultured amniotic fluid cells (second trimester) or chorionic villus samples (first trimester).[43,46]

Neuropathological examination shows striking cortical neuronal loss, gliosis, and subcortical myelin loss associated with severe axonal degeneration (see Table 16-2). Axonal changes are especially marked in cerebellum. The evolution of the cerebral parenchymal changes is followed best by MRI scans (Fig. 16-5). Intracranial arterial abnormalities are characteristic. The latter have been identified as striking tortuosities around the circle of Willis by MR angiography as early as 5 weeks of age.[40,41] The essential *biochemical defect* in the disease involves copper transport across specific cellular compartments (i.e., the placenta, gastrointestinal tract, and blood-brain barrier), with a resulting failure of formation of copper-containing enzymes. The latter include tyrosinase (causing depigmentation of hair), lysyl oxidase (causing defective elastin-collagen cross-linking, and arterial intimal defects), superoxide dismutase (causing vulnerability to free radicals), cytochrome oxidase (causing impaired energy production), and dopamine-beta-hydroxylase (causing impaired catecholamine synthesis). The latter three defects perhaps are most important for the neurological phenomena. The responsible gene is located

develop promptly. In the neonatal period, the hair is usually fine and colorless, but shortly thereafter, the more characteristic, friable, kinky appearance (feeling like fine sandpaper) develops. I have noted the sandpaper feel in the neonatal period, however. Recalcitrant seizures and neurological deterioration lead to death, usually in the second year. *Diagnosis* is confirmed by the

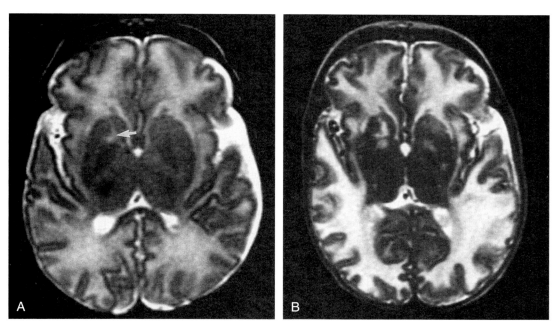

Figure 16-5 Evolution of cerebral parenchymal changes in Menkes disease, as shown by magnetic resonance imaging (MRI). The infant presented with severe refractory seizures at 6 weeks of age, after premature delivery at 30 weeks of gestation. **A,** Axial T2-weighted MRI at 8 weeks of age shows a moderate degree of cerebral cortical atrophy, a focal area of high signal intensity in the right putamen *(arrow),* and moderately high signal intensity in cerebral white matter. **B,** Axial T2-weighted MRI at 14 weeks of age shows marked progression with multiple lesions in basal ganglia and thalami, more cortical atrophy, and markedly higher signal intensity in cerebral white matter. MR spectroscopy at the time of the second MRI showed markedly elevated lactate and markedly depressed *N*-acetylaspartic acid in basal ganglia and cerebral white matter.

on the X-chromosome (Xq13), and the mutant protein is a cation transporting adenosine triphosphatase.[43,47] Attempts to correct the copper deficiency in brain have included parenteral administration of copper histidine, and clinical response, although inconsistent, occasionally has been promising.[41-43,48-50]

Disorders Mimicking Gray Matter Degeneration

Several neonatal disorders in which seizures are a prominent manifestation may mimic onset of a gray matter degeneration (with no visceral storage) (see Table 16-3). It is critical to recognize these disorders, in part because early management may require specific interventions. The group is best divided into recognized epileptic syndromes, certain metabolic disorders, and several other disorders (see Table 16-3). The epileptic syndromes are reviewed in Chapter 5, and the metabolic disorders are discussed in Chapter 14 or 15. Of the other disorders, pyridoxine dependency and glucose transporter deficiency are discussed in Chapter 5.

Rett syndrome, an X-linked disorder caused by a mutation in the gene encoding methyl-CpG-binding protein 2 *(MECP2)*, is a well-known, clinically defined disorder of female patients, with clinical onset in the first year of life, initially with deceleration of head growth. However, in recent years, approximately 30 male patients with the *MECP2* mutation have been recognized, and approximately half of these patients have had a neonatal encephalopathy.[51-60] Although the phenotype is variable, most of the patients with neonatal-onset have had seizures, often with apnea, followed by development of microcephaly, mental retardation, motor deficits, and autonomic dysfunction, including apneic spells. Most of the infants with neonatal onset have died in the first 2 years of life. The diagnosis is made by DNA analysis of the *MECP2* gene.

Gray Matter Degenerations with Visceral Storage

Six neuronal degenerations with infantile onset are accompanied by prominent visceral storage (see Tables 16-1 and 16-4). Although these disorders eventually may exhibit the hallmark of a neuronal process (seizures), this feature often appears later in the course of the disease or even not at all. Thus, in this group of disorders, it often is difficult in the neonatal period or in early infancy to recognize the disease as one affecting primarily neurons. However, other clinical features are usually distinctive enough to lead to a high degree of suspicion of the correct diagnosis (see later discussions).

GM$_1$ Gangliosidosis

Manifestations of the generalized form of *GM$_1$ gangliosidosis* commonly appear in the first weeks of life (see Table 16-4).[2,61-63] *Clinical features* include abnormalities of sucking and swallowing, hypotonia, and a cherry-red spot. Seizures, the hallmark of gray matter disease, are usually not present until after 1 year of age. Generalized edema is a striking early feature.[61,63] Because of systemic storage of mucopolysaccharide, coarse facies, subperiosteal bony abnormalities, and hepatosplenomegaly are present. Progression to death in the second year is characteristic. *Diagnosis* is based on identification in white blood cells or fibroblasts of the enzymatic defect, which involves beta-galactosidase (see Fig. 16-1). The gene is located on chromosome 3. The disorder is inherited in an autosomal recessive manner. *Neuropathology* is characterized by the generalized neuronal storage of GM$_1$ ganglioside and by the meganeurites noted for Tay-Sachs disease. *Neuroimaging (MRI)*, as for Tay-Sachs GM$_2$ gangliosidosis, initially shows abnormal signal in thalamus and subsequently marked cerebral cortical and deep nuclear atrophy; cerebral white matter shows increased T2 signal.[4] Neuronal storage and elevated brain ganglioside content have been observed as early as 22 weeks of gestation.[64,65] This observation has important implications concerning the need for intervention during fetal life with enzyme or gene replacement therapy, when such therapy is further developed. *Prenatal diagnosis* of the enzymatic defect is possible by analysis of cultured amniotic fluid cells.

GM$_2$ Gangliosidosis (Sandhoff Variant)

GM$_2$ gangliosidosis, or the Sandhoff variant of Tay-Sachs disease, is similar clinically to Tay-Sachs disease except for the addition of visceromegaly. The major features were reviewed earlier in relation to Tay-Sachs disease. In this disorder, not only is GM$_2$ ganglioside stored in brain because of the defect in hexosaminidase A, but also globoside is stored in the viscera, because the enzymatic defect involves both hexosaminidase A and B. Both isoforms are required for removal of the terminal *N*-acetylglucosamine from globoside (see Fig.16-1).

Niemann-Pick Disease

The acute infantile form of *Niemann-Pick disease* may be noted in the first weeks of life (see Table 16-4).[2,66] Feeding difficulties are common, and a cherry-red spot is apparent in nearly 50% of cases. Hepatosplenomegaly, caused primarily by storage of sphingomyelin, is prominent. Neurological features are often not pronounced until several weeks or months of age, when developmental arrest and then regression occur. Seizures are not a common feature early in the disease. Death occurs most frequently in the first several years. *Diagnosis* is established by identification in white blood cells or fibroblasts of the enzymatic defect, which involves a diminution of sphingomyelinase activity to less than 10% of normal (see Fig.16-1). The disorder is inherited in an autosomal recessive manner. *Neuropathology* is characterized by neuronal storage of sphingomyelin, most prominent in the cerebellum, brain stem, and spinal cord. Foam cells, laden with lipid and representing macrophages, are prominent in the meninges and perivascular spaces. *Prenatal diagnosis* is possible by identification of the enzymatic defect in cultured amniotic fluid cells or chorionic villus samples. Attempted *therapy* with bone marrow transplantation has not altered the course of the disease.[6]

Gaucher Disease

The infantile neuronopathic form of *Gaucher disease* (type 2) is noted in the neonatal period in 10% of cases.[67–69] The most common presenting *clinical features* are retrocollis (hyperextension of neck), strabismus (or other oculomotor abnormalities), and spasticity (see Table 16-4). Other brain stem signs, dysphagia and trismus, are common. Hepatosplenomegaly secondary to storage of glucocerebroside is present. Dermatological findings, particularly thin, reflective skin characterized as "collodion," "cellophane," or "ichthyosis," are common in the neonatal cases. A particularly severe form with hydrops fetalis and arthrogryposis is recognized.[70] The subsequent course of infants with neonatal Gaucher disease generally is fulminating, with death by 2 or 3 months of age. *Diagnosis* is based on identification in white blood cells, fibroblasts, or liver of the enzymatic defect, which involves beta-glucosidase (see Fig. 16-1). The disorder is inherited in an autosomal recessive manner. *Neuropathology* is characterized by little or no neuronal storage of glucocerebroside, but neuronal loss is present, especially in the brain stem. Basal ganglia and cerebellum also are particularly involved. Gaucher cells, lipid-laden histiocytes, often with the cytoplasmic appearance of wrinkled tissue paper, are present in perivascular spaces and are free in brain parenchyma. Neuronal death with microglial nodules and gliosis appears to occur in proximity to these cells, a finding suggesting the possibility of a toxic effect from the stored lipid or a product thereof (glucosylsphingosine?). *Prenatal diagnosis* is possible by identification of the enzymatic defect in cultured amniotic fluid cells or chorionic villus specimens. The possibility of *therapy* in the less severely affected infants is suggested by successes in patients with the nonneuronopathic forms of Gaucher disease who were treated with recombinant human macrophage-targeted glucocerebrosidase.[6,71,72] Other approaches in nonneuronopathic cases have included drugs that decrease glucocerebroside biosynthesis, bone marrow transplantation, or introduction into bone marrow or other sites of somatic cells (e.g., fibroblasts) into which the normal gene for glucocerebrosidase was introduced by retrovirally mediated gene transfer.[6,67,71,72] Theoretically, the correction or arrest of the neurological disease could be accomplished because this disorder involves the reticuloendothelial system, particularly the bone marrow, and thus entry of the transplanted cells into the central nervous system (i.e., the major limitation of gene therapy of other lysosomal disorders) may not be required.[67] However, currently, no data indicate a benefit for any of these approaches in the *infantile-onset* type 2 neuronopathic disorder.

Farber Disease

In the classic type 1 form of *Farber disease*, as with most other neuronal degenerations with visceral storage, determining that gray matter is primarily involved may be difficult. Thus, the initial *clinical features* are primarily painful swelling of joints, subcutaneous modules, and hoarse cry (see Table 16-4).[73] Subsequently, feeding disturbance leading to failure to thrive is prominent. Perhaps the most pronounced neurological features are hypotonia, weakness, muscle atrophy, and areflexia or hyporeflexia, probably reflecting involvement of anterior horn cells and peripheral nerve roots. Consistent with the latter involvement is the finding of elevated CSF protein levels in nearly all cases and electromyographic findings of denervation. Hepatomegaly is prominent in approximately 75% of cases. Disturbances of swallowing, aspiration, and pulmonary disease lead to death at 1 to 2 years of age. Ceramide accumulates in tissue. *Neuronal storage* occurs, especially in anterior horn cells and brain stem. *Diagnosis* is established by detection of the marked defect in ceramidase in cultured fibroblasts (see Fig. 16-1). *Prenatal diagnosis* is possible by the analysis of cultured amniotic fluid cells. Attempted *therapy* by bone marrow transplantation has provided some benefit for regression of nodules (which contain ceramide-laden macrophages) and associated joint pain but no apparent neurological benefit.[6,7,31]

Infantile Sialic Acid Storage Disease (and Sialidoses)

Sialic acid is a critical component of the oligosaccharide portion of many glycoproteins. Two varieties of disturbance of sialic acid metabolism may result in neonatal disease with neuronal storage. One of these is related to a disorder of sialic acid transport and is sometimes referred to as *infantile sialic acid storage disease* or *sialuria*. The other disturbance is related to a defect in the lysosomal enzyme that degrades the oligosaccharides containing sialic acid (i.e., neuraminidase or sialidase) and is often referred to as *sialidosis*.[2,62,74-81] The prototypical *clinical presentation* of both infantile sialic acid storage disease and sialidosis with onset in utero or the neonatal period includes generalized edema (including fetal ascites/hydrops), feeding disturbance, marked hepatosplenomegaly, hypotonia, coarse dysmorphic facies, and radiographic abnormalities of long bones (Fig. 16-6). In infantile sialic acid storage disease, thin, white hair is a consistent feature (see Fig. 16-6), not noted in the sialidoses. Severe anemia, failure to thrive, developmental arrest, and then regression subsequently develop. *Diagnosis* of the infantile sialic acid storage disorder or sialuria (i.e., the disorder of lysosomal transport of sialic acid) is made by identification of large increases in free sialic acid in plasma and urine and normal activity in fibroblasts of alpha-neuraminidase activity. The diagnosis of sialidosis can be suspected by identification of sialic acid–containing oligosaccharides and glycoproteins in urine, but it is made definitively by the demonstration of deficient alpha-neuraminidase activity. In a subtype of sialidosis, *galactosylsialidosis*, beta-galactosidase activity is also impaired, and the defect involves another lysosomal protein necessary for the activity of both enzymes (cathepsin A). *Neuropathology* of these disorders is characterized by neuronal storage of either free sialic acid in infantile

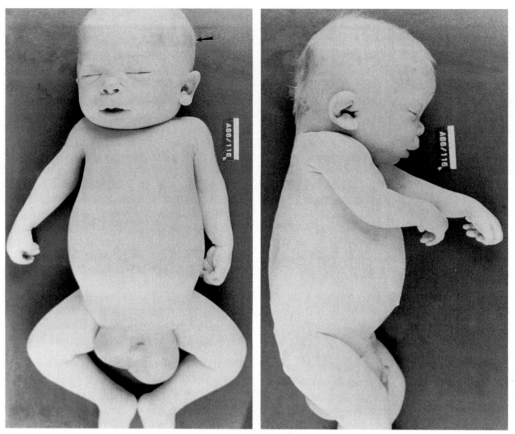

Figure 16-6 **Infantile sialic acid storage disease: postmortem photographs.** Note the coarse dysmorphic facies, generalized edema, abdominal distention, inguinal hernias, bilateral hydroceles, and white hair *(arrow). (From Pueschel SM, O'Shea PA, Alroy J, Ambler MW, et al: Infantile sialic acid storage disease associated with renal disease, Pediatr Neurol 4:207-212, 1988.)*

sialic acid storage disease or sialic acid–containing oligosaccharides and glycoproteins in the sialidoses. *Prenatal diagnosis* is made by identification of elevated free sialic acid levels in cultured amniotic fluid cells in infantile sialic acid storage disorder and of deficient alpha-neuraminidase activity in the sialidoses. (Other disorders of glycoprotein degradation [i.e., mannosidosis and fucosidosis] have their onset beyond the neonatal period.)

DISORDERS PRIMARILY AFFECTING WHITE MATTER

Canavan Disease

Canavan disease, spongy degeneration of the white matter, is an autosomal recessive disorder that commonly begins in the first days and weeks of life; approximately 20% of patients exhibit first signs at birth, an additional 10% in the first month, and a further 10% to 20% by the end of the second month.[24,82-97] *Clinical features* documented in the first days and weeks of life include poor visual fixation, irritability, and poor suck (see Table 16-5). These features are followed over the ensuing weeks by marked hypotonia, weakness, nystagmus, and failure to attain motor milestones. Macrocephaly becomes apparent in the first 6 to 12

months of life in more than 50% of cases and ultimately in 90% of affected infants. As the disease progresses, hypotonia gives way to spasticity, decorticate posture, intellectual failure, optic atrophy, and then death in early to late childhood. Visual evoked responses are abnormal early in the disease, and these neurophysiological abnormalities precede the onset of blindness. *Diagnosis* is suspected by the clinical features. The computed tomography (CT) scan shows decreased attenuation of white matter, and MRI shows strikingly increased signal on T2-weighted images (Fig. 16-7). The particular involvement of subcortical white matter, especially early in the disease, distinguishes Canavan disease from Krabbe disease (see later). Also characteristic is involvement of thalamus and especially globus pallidus with relative sparing of putamen (see Fig. 16-7).[4] Elevation of *N*-acetylaspartate (NAA) levels in brain is detected by proton MR spectroscopy.[4,93,98] *Diagnosis* is established by the demonstration of *increased levels of NAA in urine and of decreased activity of N-acetylaspartoacylase (ASPA) activity in cultured fibroblasts.*[91-93,96,97,99-105] Elevated levels of NAA have been documented in Canavan disease early in infancy, in urine of a mother with an affected 4-month fetus, and in brain of 5- and 8-month-old fetuses.[104] Deficient aspartoacylase activity has been detected in brain postmortem.[91-93,101] NAA is normally

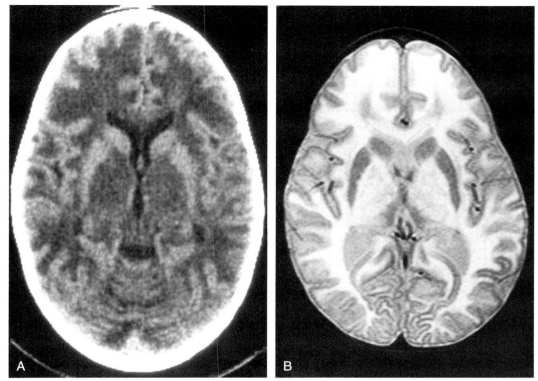

Figure 16-7   Canavan disease. A, Computed tomography (CT) and, **B,** T2-weighted magnetic resonance imaging (MRI) scans. This infant had onset of developmental retardation and macrocephaly noted in early infancy, and scans were carried out at 27 months of age. Note the markedly low attenuation of cerebral white matter on the CT scan **(A)** and the very high signal intensity of the cerebral white matter on the T2-weighted MRI scan **(B).** Note in both scans the involvement of thalamus and globus pallidus, with sparing of putamen, a pattern characteristic of Canavan disease. *(From Marks HG, Caro PA, Wang ZY, Detre JA, et al: Use of computed tomography, magnetic resonance imaging, and localized 1H magnetic resonance spectroscopy in Canavan's disease: A case report,* Ann Neurol *30:106-110, 1991.)*

present in high concentration in neurons, whereas the acylase activity is predominantly localized in the oligodendrocyte. Recent studies in a mouse model of Canavan disease indicated that NAA is synthesized in neurons and is transported to oligodendrocytes, where the action of ASPA generates acetate critical for myelin lipid synthesis (Fig. 16-8).[106] Consistent with this notion is the demonstration that the developmental increase of ASPA in oligodendrocytes parallels cerebral myelination.[107] The possibility has been raised that, in Canavan disease, the accumulated NAA in oligodendrocytes acts as an osmolyte to lead to intramyelinic

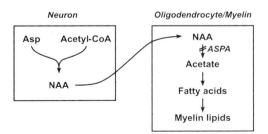

Figure 16-8   Metabolism of *N*-acetylaspartic acid (NAA) in the neuron and oligodendrocyte/myelin. NAA is synthesized in the neuron from aspartate (Asp) and acetyl–coenzyme A (Acetyl-CoA) and is transported to the oligodendrocyte, where NAA is metabolized by *N*-acetylaspartoacylase (ASPA), the enzyme deficient in Canavan disease.

edema. It may be that the deficiency in ASPA leads both to decreased myelin lipid synthesis at the time of active cerebral myelination and to an osmotic disturbance in developing myelin. The major *neuropathological features* are strikingly deficient myelin and widespread vacuolization (spongy degeneration) of white matter, especially in subcortical regions.

More recent attempts at *therapy* have included virally and nonvirally mediated gene transfer methods and lithium (which causes a decrease in elevated brain NAA levels by unknown mechanisms).[97,108,109] Initial findings are encouraging, but more data are needed. A less complex approach may be acetate supplementation, in view of the importance of NAA as an acetate source in the oligodendrocyte/myelin unit.[106] *Prenatal diagnosis* has been made by detection of elevated NAA levels in amniotic fluid and deficient ASPA activity in cultured amniotic fluid cells or chorionic villus samples. However, the most reliable method of diagnosis is DNA analysis.

Alexander Disease

Alexander disease may have its onset in the first weeks of life (≈30% of infantile cases), and the most frequent initial *clinical features* are macrocephaly, failure to attain early motor milestones and, interestingly, seizures (see Table 16-5).[24,110-122] Progressive spastic quadriparesis, seizures, and failure of neurological development later become prominent, and death after a median survival of 3.5 years is most common. *Diagnosis* is suggested by the clinical features and brain imaging findings. CT shows decreased attenuation in frontal white matter especially, and after contrast injection, areas of increased attenuation (most notably subependymal) are noted early in the disease, particularly around the tips of the frontal horns (Fig. 16-9A).[4,112-114,121-124] Cranial ultrasonography has been reported to show increased echogenicity of cerebral white matter early in the disease.[125] MRI findings are characteristic and include increased signal in frontal white matter, with posterior extension, with abnormalities also of basal ganglia, especially caudate heads and anterior putamina, and of brain stem tegmentum and periaqueductal regions (Fig. 16-9B and C). The brain stem changes coupled with the occasional finding of elevated lactate on MR spectroscopy may initially suggest Leigh disease.[115] The major *neuropathological features* are a severe deficiency of myelin and eosinophilic deposits within fibrillary astrocytes (Rosenthal fibers). These deposits have been shown by electron microscopy to be associated with an accumulation of disordered glial filaments.[119,126,127] The Rosenthal fibers in Alexander disease are enriched in a protein, crystallin, that is characteristic of lens but is also synthesized in astrocytes.[112,128-130] The crystallin

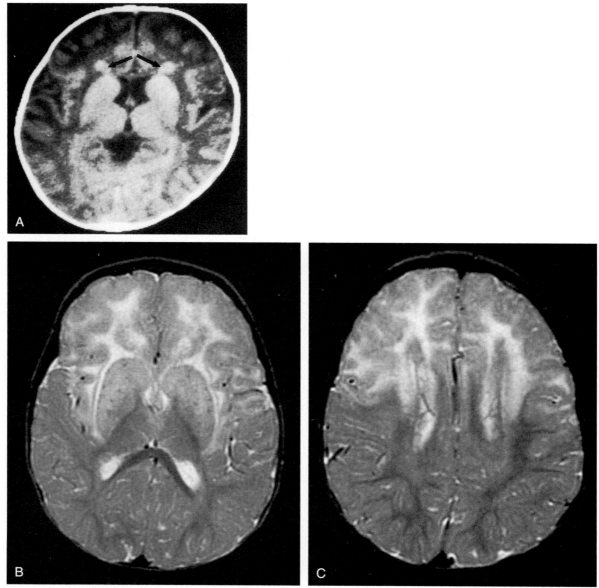

Figure 16-9 **Alexander disease: computed tomography (CT) and magnetic resonance imaging (MRI) scans. A,** The postcontrast CT scan shows low attenuation in the cerebral white matter bilaterally, especially in the frontal regions, but enhancement *(arrows)* in the subependymal region around the tips of the frontal horns of the lateral ventricles. **B** and **C,** MRI scans show T2 prolongation in frontal white matter and basal ganglia bilaterally. *(A, From Pridmore CL, Baraitser M, Harding B, Boyd SG, et al: Alexander's disease: Clues to diagnosis, J Child Neurol 8:134-144, 1993; B and C, from Barkovich AJ: Pediatric Neuroimaging, 4th ed, Philadelphia: 2005, Lippincott Williams & Wilkins.)*

molecules are ubiquitinated, and this modification appears to have altered their biophysical properties to result in insoluble aggregates of abnormally large ubiquitinated crystallin molecules.[112] The fibers represent the intermediate filaments of astrocytes, composed of glial fibrillary acidic protein (GFAP). The molecular defect has been shown to be a de novo, dominant (i.e., heterozygous), missense mutation of the gene for GFAP.[119-122,127,131,132] The latter results in a so-called toxic gain of function. The recent finding of elevated levels of GFAP in the CSF of affected patients is consistent with the molecular defect and suggests potential value for diagnosis.[118]

Krabbe Disease

Krabbe disease, an *autosomal recessive disorder*, has its onset in the first weeks of life, before the median age of onset of 4 months of age, in approximately 25% of cases.[111,133-139] The early *clinical features* are characteristic and consist of irritability, hypersensitivity to stimulation, startle responses, and increased tone (see Table 16-5). Poor feeding and unexplained, recurrent fever are common. Marked spasticity, severe stimulus-sensitive tonic extensor spasms, and decerebration then develop.[133-141] Although macrocephaly has been reported to occur, small head size is more common. The CSF protein level is markedly elevated, compatible with the accompanying peripheral neuropathy. The neuropathy may be detected in the neonatal period by measurement of nerve conduction velocities.[142,143]As a result, deep tendon reflexes may be absent in advanced disease. *Diagnosis* is based on identification in white blood cells or fibroblasts of the enzymatic defect, which involves a beta-galactosidase, galactosylceramidase I (see Fig. 16-1).[134,138,144] *Neuroimaging* findings include relatively early in the disease, by CT, increased attenuation in the thalamus (Fig. 16-10A).[4] MRI is notable for showing particular involvement of cerebellar white matter and periventricular and central cerebral white matter, sparing subcortical myelin (in contrast to Canavan disease) (Fig. 16-10B and C).[4]

Suzuki and co-workers[134,144,145] clarified the *basic biochemical nature* of this disease (Fig. 16-11). Because brain galactosylceramide (galactocerebroside) concentrations were found *not* to be elevated in Krabbe disease, it became apparent that degradation of galactosylceramide is not the essential defect. However, psychosine (galactosylsphingosine) is elevated in the brain in Krabbe disease. Suzuki and co-workers showed that the enzyme missing in infantile Krabbe disease is galactosylceramidase I, which catalyzes the removal of galactose from galactosylsphingosine (psychosine) as well as from galactosylceramide (see Fig. 16-11). Psychosine is highly toxic to oligodendroglia, and injections of psychosine into the brain lead to the neuropathology of Krabbe disease. Galactosylceramidase II, which is not defective in Krabbe disease, can degrade galactosylceramide but not psychosine, thus explaining the failure of galactosylceramide concentrations to increase (see Fig. 16-11). The major *neuropathological features* include severe deficiencies of oligodendroglia and myelin and collections of large, multinucleated globoid cells (Fig. 16-12).[24] These cells are essentially macrophages. The deficiency of galactosylceramidase has been demonstrated in the brain.[134,145,146] *Prenatal diagnosis* is accomplished by assay of the enzyme in cultured amniotic fluid cells or chorionic villus samples. Recent work has suggested a major advance in *therapy* of this disorder. Previous research showed that bone marrow transplantation is beneficial in late-onset disease but not in the early-onset infantile disease.[6,71] Because of the importance of very early initiation of therapy in the infantile disease, transplantation of umbilical cord blood was carried out after myeloablative chemotherapy in asymptomatic newborns ($n = 11$; 12 to 44 days) and symptomatic infants ($n = 14$; 142 to 352 days) with Krabbe disease.[147] Donor cell engraftment and survival were 100% and 100%, respectively, in the asymptomatic newborns, and 100% but only 43% in the symptomatic newborns. The surviving infants had restoration of blood galactocerebrosidase levels. In the *asymptomatic* infants, over a median follow-up of 3 years, progressive cerebral myelination and normal cognitive development occurred; mild to moderate motor disturbances were present. Children who underwent transplantation after the onset of symptoms had minimal neurological improvement. *The findings indicate the importance of transplantation as early as possible and the value of umbilical cord blood.*

Pelizaeus-Merzbacher Disease

One form of the three basic varieties of *Pelizaeus-Merzbacher disease* typically has its onset in utero or during the first weeks of life. This so-called *connatal form* is distinguished from *classic disease* primarily on the basis of rate of progression (faster in the connatal cases), age at death (first decade in connatal cases versus second decade in classic cases), and in severity of the neuropathology (total demyelination in connatal cases versus partial demyelination with a tigroid appearance in the classic cases). *Transitional* cases are intermediate in severity. Because the molecular genetics and the clinical features of these three forms overlap considerably, distinction among them can be difficult, especially in infants with onset in the first weeks of life. At least 50 neonatal-onset, apparent connatal cases have been reported.[148-171] The most consistent initial *clinical features* have been nystagmus, horizontal or rotatory, and inspiratory stridor (see Table 16-5). Head titubation, jerky movements of head or limbs, and hypotonia are prominent. Seizures occur in approximately 75% of patients with neonatal-onset cases, thereby suggesting a gray matter disorder and confusing establishment of diagnosis. Visual evoked responses are usually abnormal, consistent with the disturbance of central myelin. *Diagnosis* is suspected on clinical grounds. *MRI shows a striking absence of myelin*, with increased signal on T2-weighted images (Fig. 16-13). CT may show decreased attenuation of cerebral white matter, but findings are not as consistently abnormal as with MRI. MR spectroscopy is distinctive; notable findings include elevation of

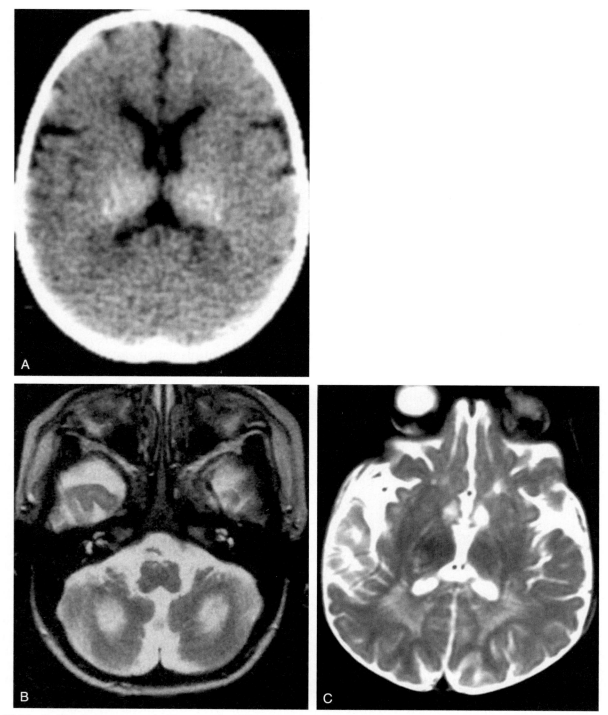

Figure 16-10 **Krabbe disease: computed tomography (CT) and magnetic resonance imaging (MRI) scans.** **A,** The axial CT scan shows prominent increased attenuation in the thalamus bilaterally. **B** and **C,** The T2-weighted MRI scans show abnormal high signal intensity in the cerebellar white matter **(B)** and in the cerebral white matter **(C).** Note in **C** that the high signal intensity spares the subcortical white matter (unlike in Canavan disease). *(From Barkovich AJ: Pediatric Neuroimaging, 4th ed, Philadelphia: 2005, Lippincott Williams & Wilkins.)*

choline-containing compounds, NAA and *N*-acetylaspartyl glutamate, glutamine, and myoinositol.[168-170] The findings are consistent, respectively, with reduced oligodendroglia with dysmyelination, increased axonal packing, and astrogliosis. *Neuropathology* is striking; myelin is virtually absent, with diminished

oligodendroglia and gliosis (Fig. 16-14). Small amounts of sudanophilic material, reflecting myelin breakdown products, may be present. *X-linked recessive* inheritance is consistent. The defect involves the gene on the X-chromosome encoding proteolipid protein *(PLP)*,[161,164-167,171-179] a crucial structural protein of

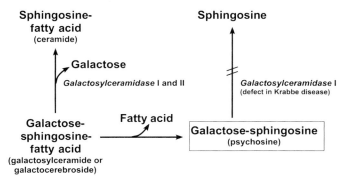

Sphingosine-
fatty acid
(ceramide)

Sphingosine

Galactose

Galactosylceramidase I and II

Galactosylceramidase I
(defect in Krabbe disease)

Galactose-
sphingosine-
fatty acid
(galactosylceramide or
galactocerebroside)

Fatty acid

Galactose-sphingosine
(psychosine)

Figure 16-11   Mechanism for the increase in galactose-sphingosine (psychosine) in Krabbe disease. Galactosylceramidase I, the isoform absent in Krabbe disease, is required for the metabolism of psychosine to sphingosine. Galactosylceramidase II, present in Krabbe disease, provides some activity for conversion of galactosylceramide to ceramide.

myelin accounting for 50% of myelin protein. Pelizaeus-Merzbacher disease in all its forms is caused by mutations in *PLP*, with approximately 60% to 70% of cases related to duplications of the gene, point mutations in 15% to 20%, and the remainder being deletions. The neonatal-onset cases have been associated with duplications and deletions. The result of the former is multiple copies of proteolipid protein, and of the latter, deletion of both proteolipid protein and its post-transcriptional alternatively spliced protein product DM20.[171,180]

A disorder phenotypically closely related to Pelizaeus-Merzbacher disease, with a hypomyelinative leukoencephalopathy but *autosomal recessive inheritance*, has been termed *Pelizaeus-Merzbacher–like disease* (PMLD).[181] Like connatal Pelizaeus-Merzbacher disease, PMLD manifests with nystagmus in the newborn period. However, the subsequent course in PMLD differs from that of connatal, X-linked Pelizaeus-Merzbacher disease (i.e., exhibits slower progression with greater preservation of cognitive functions and development of at least partial myelination of the corticospinal tracts by MRI). The molecular defect in

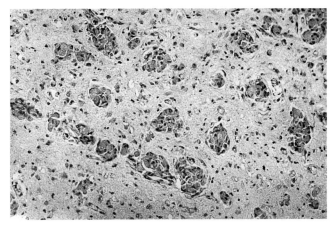

Figure 16-12   Krabbe disease: neuropathology. This photomicrograph of the cerebral white matter in an affected infant shows the large, multinucleated globoid cells. *(Courtesy of Dr. Kunihiko Suzuki.)*

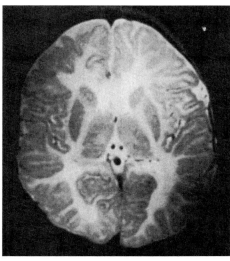

Figure 16-13   Pelizaeus-Merzbacher disease: magnetic resonance imaging (MRI) scan. This T2-weighted MRI scan was obtained from a 13-month-old infant with a history of onset of abnormal eye and head movements at 12 days, hypotonia, and subsequent failure of motor development. The brain biopsy confirmed the diagnosis of Pelizaeus-Merzbacher disease. Note the increased signal in cerebral white matter and the virtual absence of myelin. *(From Scheffer IE, Baraitser M, Wilson J, Harding B, et al: Pelizaeus-Merzbacher disease: Classical or connatal? Neuropediatrics 22:71-78, 1991.)*

PMLD involves the *GJA12* gene, which encodes connexin 47. The connexins are a family of proteins that form intercellular channels of gap junctions, between multiple cell types, including oligodendrocytes.

Other rare sudanophilic hypomyelinative/dysmyelinative leukodystrophies may be related to Pelizaeus-Merzbacher disease and perhaps may be secondary to defects of other structural proteins of myelin.[158,182-185] The best established of these is *Cockayne syndrome*, an autosomal recessive disorder with the neuropathological finding of patchy tigroid demyelination, as in classic Pelizaeus-Merzbacher disease. In the classic form, Cockayne syndrome type I, the development of postnatal growth failure, a "cachectic," "elfin," "progeroid" facial appearance, pigmentary retinopathy, impaired neurological development, sensorineural hearing loss, and cutaneous photosensitivity become apparent *after* the first months of life.[186,187] In the less common severe form, Cockayne syndrome type II, *newborns* have already exhibited growth failure in utero, have markedly impaired postnatal somatic and head growth, and have poor to absent neurological development. Congenital cataracts and more rapid development of auditory and cutaneous complications are features of this severe form. The disturbance of myelination in Cockayne syndrome affects the peripheral as well as the central nervous system and is manifested by elevated CSF protein level, slow nerve conduction velocities, and nerve biopsy specimens showing segmental demyelination. In the central nervous system, imaging studies show, in addition to the myelin disturbance, calcification of basal ganglia, a helpful diagnostic feature. The basic *biochemical disturbance* in the

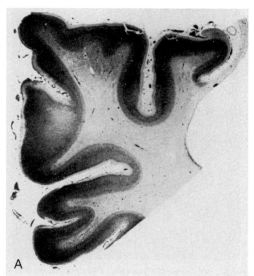

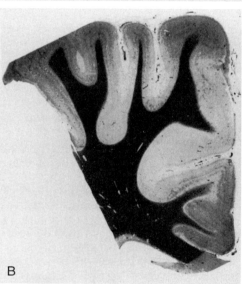

Figure 16-14 Pelizaeus-Merzbacher disease: neuropathology. The infant died at 6 months of age with a history of onset of seizures at 1 month of age, followed by failure of neurological development, hypotonia, hyperreflexia, and clonus. **A,** Frontal white matter is absent. Compare with **B,** an age-matched control infant. *(From Scheffer IE, Baraitser M, Wilson J, Harding B, et al: Pelizaeus-Merzbacher disease: Classical or connatal? Neuropediatrics 22:71-78, 1991.)*

disease involves DNA metabolism and ultrasensitivity to ultraviolet light, with abnormal DNA repair mechanisms detectable in cultured skin fibroblasts. Infants with the severe form of the disease die usually by the age of 6 or 7 years.

Leukodystrophy with Cerebral Calcifications (Aicardi-Goutieres Syndrome)

Leukodystrophy with cerebral calcifications, a rare autosomal recessive disorder, initially described clearly by Aicardi and Goutieres, has been identified in approximately 100 cases.[188-209] Approximately one third of patients have had the onset of the disease within the first postnatal month (see Table 16-5). *Clinical features* include

irritability, poor feeding, ocular abnormalities (especially ocular "jerking"), hypertonia more than hypotonia, weakness, jitteriness, dystonia, oralfacial dyskinesias, and, occasionally, seizures. Developmental arrest, microcephaly, and spastic quadriparesis follow, with death often in the first several years of life. Persistent *CSF pleocytosis* has been consistent. CSF protein levels are slightly elevated in fewer than 50% of patients. *Elevated CSF levels of interferonalpha* also are a consistent finding. *Brain imaging* is distinctive. Ultrasonography shows echogenicity of periventricular white matter, a frequent finding in early infantile white matter degenerations.[193] CT demonstrates decreased attenuation of cerebral white matter and calcifications, which may be diffuse, periventricular, or in basal ganglia (Fig. 16-15). The calcification most characteristically affects putamen and cerebellar dentate nuclei. MRI scan shows diffuse hyperintensity of cerebral white matter on T2-weighted images (see Fig. 16-15). Cerebellar atrophy is a common accompaniment. *Neuropathology* consists of a marked decrease of myelin, striking fibrillary gliosis, and the calcifications, which are located primarily in walls of blood vessels. Perivascular collections of inflammatory cells have been noted, but no viral particles or other evidence of viral infection have been detected. The microangiopathy may be accompanied by thromboses and microinfarction. The elevated CSF levels of interferon-alpha raise the possibility that the cytokine is causally related to the cerebral disorder.[210] Transgenic animals with astrocyte-targeted interferonalpha showed neuropathological features mimicking those found in Aicardi-Goutieres syndrome. Some infants with the syndrome exhibit cutaneous vascular lesions similar to those observed in patients treated with interferon-alpha.[208] Interferon-alpha treatment of young infants with vascular malformations has been associated with the development of spastic diplegia, a finding thus suggesting injury to developing white matter by the cytokine.[211] Recent work shows an immune perturbation caused by mutation of *TREX1*, encoding a DNA exonuclease.[211a,211b]

DISORDERS AFFECTING BOTH GRAY AND WHITE MATTER

Two broad categories of disease affect subcellular structures and thereby result in degenerative disorders with prominent effects on *both* gray and white matter: peroxisomal disorders and mitochondrial disorders (see Table 16-1; Table 16-6). An additional group that involves both gray and white matter, a group that I term *other disorders*, also must be included (see Tables 16-1 and 16-6). These latter disorders have a strong *regional* predilection. The peroxisomal disorders are represented in the newborn by *Zellweger (cerebrohepatorenal) syndrome* and *neonatal adrenoleukodystrophy*, and the mitochondrial disorders in this context are represented by *Leigh syndrome* (and related encephalopathies). (The other mitochondrial disorder with possible neonatal presentation, Alpers disease, manifests as a gray matter

Figure 16-15 Leukodystrophy with cerebral calcifications: computed tomography (CT) and magnetic resonance imaging (MRI) scans. **A,** The CT scan, obtained at 2 months of age, shows bilateral calcifications in the periventricular white matter and in the basal ganglia and decreased attenuation of the frontal and occipital white matter. **B,** The T2-weighted MRI scan, obtained from a separate patient at 9 months of age, shows increased signal intensity in the cerebral white matter and decreased signal intensity in areas of calcification *(arrows). (From Boltshauser E, Steinlin M, Boesch C, Martin E, et al: Magnetic resonance imaging in infantile encephalopathy with cerebral calcification and leukodystrophy,* Neuropediatrics *22:33-35, 1991.)*

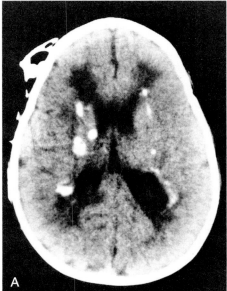
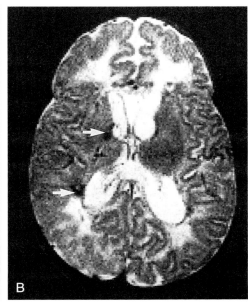

TABLE 16-6	Degenerative Diseases Affecting Both Gray and White Matter		
Disease	**Clinical Features**	**Metabolic-Enzymatic Features**	**Pathology**
Zellweger syndrome (cerebrohepatorenal syndrome)	Craniofacial dysmorphism, hypotonia, weakness, impaired feeding, seizures, optic atrophy, renal cysts, calcific stippling, later blindness, deafness, relative macrocephaly, moderately rapid progression to vegetative state	Evidence of deficiency of multiple peroxisomal functions: elevated very-long-chain fatty acids, pipecolic acid and bile acid intermediate levels, deficient synthesis of plasmalogens; a disorder of peroxisomal biogenesis; molecular defect affecting proteins involved in peroxisomal biogenesis (peroxins), encoded by specific genes *(PEX)*	Severe neuronal migrational defects; major features include pachygyria (especially parasagittal region) and microgyria (especially lateral convexity), with heterotopias also involving cerebellum and inferior olivary nuclei; myelin disturbance as described next for neonatal adrenoleukodystrophy, although less severe
Neonatal adrenoleukodystrophy	Similar to Zellweger syndrome (above), but less severe, course less rapid, and absence of renal cysts and calcific stippling	Similar to Zellweger syndrome (above), except findings generally less severe; molecular defect affects proteins involved in peroxisomal biogenesis (peroxins) encoded by specific genes *(PEX)*	Myelin deficiency and loss, diffuse but especially marked in cerebellum; sudanophilic material, perivascular mononuclear cells, trilamellar inclusions in macrophages; neuronal migrational defects, although less prominent and consistent than in Zellweger syndrome
Leigh syndrome	Hypotonia, weakness, respiratory abnormalities, impaired feeding, oculomotor abnormalities, facial weakness, seizures, developmental arrest with development later of movement disorders and regression.	Elevated lactate-pyruvate in cerebrospinal fluid, variably in serum; deficiency in pyruvate dehydrogenase complex, cytochrome-*c* oxidase (complex IV), reduced nicotinamide adenine dinucleotide–coenzyme Q reductase (complex I), or adenosine triphosphatase subunit 6 (complex V)	Focal, symmetrical, spongiform necrosis especially in diencephalon and brain stem, particularly surrounding third ventricle, aqueduct, and fourth ventricle, characterized by necrosis (relative sparing of neurons), demyelination, vascular proliferation and astrocytosis

Table continued on following page

TABLE 16-6	Degenerative Diseases Affecting Both Gray and White Matter (Continued)		
Disease	**Clinical Features**	**Metabolic-Enzymatic Features**	**Pathology**
Other mitochondrial encephalopathies	Various combinations of the above manifestations	Elevated lactate – pyruvate as for Leigh syndrome; enzymatic defects overlap (see text)	Cellular pathology similar to Leigh syndrome, but regions affected differ; may be principally cerebral white matter and various combinations of the regions involved in Leigh syndrome
Congenital disorder of glycosylation (CDG) type 1a (CDG1a): carbohydrate-deficient glycoprotein syndrome	Facial dysmorphisms, abnormal subcutaneous fat, abnormal eye movements, hypotonia, joint contractures, cardiac-liver-renal abnormalities; subsequent developmental arrest, seizures, ataxia, strokelike episodes	Abnormally glycosylated transferrin, coagulation factors, hormones, lysosomal enzymes, other glycoproteins; phosphomannomutase deficiency (CDG1a)	Cerebellar hypoplasia; often with pontine hypoplasia (i.e., pontocerebellar hypoplasia); neuronal loss and gliosis, especially in cerebellum but also in cerebral cortex, basal ganglia, thalamus, pons, inferior olives, and spinal cord; polyneuropathy
Pontocerebellar hypoplasia type 2	Impaired sucking and swallowing, jitteriness; later progressive microcephaly, extrapyramidal dyskinesias, epilepsy, severe mental retardation	Unknown	Neuronal loss and gliosis, especially in ventral pons and cerebellum, less so in inferior olivary nuclei; moderate cerebral cortical neuronal degeneration and atrophy

degeneration, as discussed earlier.) The other disorders are congenital disorders of glycosylation (CDG) (formerly termed carbohydrate-deficient glycoprotein syndrome) and pontocerebellar hypoplasia (PCH; see Table 16-6).

Peroxisomal Disorders

Peroxisomal functions include both *catabolic activities* (e.g., beta-oxidation of very-long-chain fatty acids, degradation of hydrogen peroxide by catalase, pipecolic acid metabolism, oxidation of phytanic acid) and *anabolic* activities (e.g., biosyntheses of plasmalogens and of bile acids).[212-216] Peroxisomal disorders are divided into two broad groups: disorders of peroxisomal assembly, in which there is a decrease in the number or structure of peroxisomes with multiple peroxisomal enzymes affected (group I); and disorders of single peroxisomal enzymes, with normal peroxisomal number and structure (group II) (Table 16-7).

More than 90% of the cases of peroxisomal disorders with consistent and prominent onset in the neonatal period consist of Zellweger syndrome and neonatal adrenoleukodystrophy. The only single enzyme deficiency with consistent and prominent onset in the newborn period is peroxisomal D-bifunctional protein deficiency, which exhibits many features comparable to those of Zellweger syndrome.[213,214,216,217] The fundamental defect in the disorders of peroxisome biogenesis involves mutations in genes involved in peroxisomal biogenesis.[215,216,218-224] These genes principally encode for integral peroxisome membrane or matrix proteins or receptors involved in targeting cytosolic proteins to the peroxisome.

Zellweger Syndrome

Zellweger syndrome is the prototypical disorder of peroxisome biogenesis that characteristically manifests in the neonatal period.[212,213,215,216,225-239] The *clinical features* include a distinctively dysmorphic craniofacial appearance (Fig. 16-16), cataracts, pigmentary retinopathy, hepatomegaly, glomerulocystic disease of kidneys, and calcific stippling of patellae, hips, and other epiphyses (see Table 16-6; Table 16-8). The neurological syndrome is striking and includes severe visual and auditory impairment and marked hypotonia and weakness. The latter two features are accompanied by areflexia and may be sufficiently severe to raise the possibility

TABLE 16-7	Classification of Peroxisomal Disorders
Group I: Disorders of Peroxisomal Assembly: Activities of Multiple Peroxisomal Enzymes Deficient	
Zellweger cerebrohepatorenal syndrome	
Neonatal adrenoleukodystrophy	
Infantile Refsum disease	
Rhizomelic chondrodysplasia punctata	
Group II: Activity of Only One Peroxisomal Enzyme Deficient: Peroxisomes Normal in Number and Structure	
X-linked adrenoleukodystrophy	
D-bifunctional protein deficiency	
Acyl–coenzyme A oxidase deficiency	
beta-Ketothiolase deficiency	
Other	

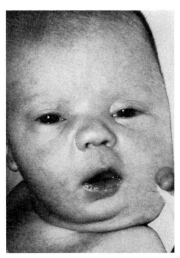

Figure 16-16 **Zellweger syndrome: craniofacial appearance.** This infant, at 2 weeks of age, exhibits a high and wide head (turribrachycephaly), high brow, flat supraorbital ridges, "jowly" cheeks, wide-set eyes, and small mouth.

TABLE 16-8 **Clinical, Morphological, and Biochemical Features of Zellweger Syndrome and Neonatal Adrenoleukodystrophy in the Neonatal Period**

Feature	Zellweger Syndrome	Neonatal Adrenoleuko-dystrophy
Clinical		
Dysmorphic craniofacial appearance	++	+
Hypotonia and weakness	++	+
Seizures	++	+
Cataracts	++	+
Pigmentary retinopathy	++	+
Visual and auditory impairment	++	+
Hepatomegaly	++	+
Renal cysts	+	−
Calcific stippling	+	−
Mean age at death	6 mo	3 yr
Morphological		
Neuronal migrational defect	++	+
Myelin disturbance	+	++
Adrenal atrophy	−	++
Biochemical		
↑ Very-long-chain fatty acids	++	+
↑ Bile acid intermediates	++	+
↓ Plasmalogen synthesis	++	+
↑ Pipecolic acid	++	+
↓ Phytanic acid oxidase	+	+
↑ Phytanic acid	−*	−*

*Develops later in first year.
+, usually present; ++, prominent; −, absent; ↑, increased; ↓, decreased.

of Werdnig-Hoffman disease.[240] Neonatal seizures are characteristic. Neurological deterioration is marked, and death by 6 months of age is common.[215,239] The basic *biochemical defect* involves peroxisome biogenesis; peroxisomal membrane "ghosts" are present, but the organelle's enzymes are absent. Because of the failure of import of enzymes into the peroxisome, the proteins are degraded in the cytosol. Catalase is not degraded but is found in the cytosol, an abnormal site for this enzyme. The total number of peroxisomes is markedly decreased.[215,224]

Diagnosis is based on the clinical features and the finding of deficiency of multiple peroxisomal functions manifested particularly by marked elevations in plasma of very-long-chain fatty acids, pipecolic acid, and bile acid intermediates and by a deficiency of plasmalogens in red blood cells (see Table 16-8). MRI is effective for the demonstration of the neuropathology.[4,241] The *neuropathology* is characterized especially by neuronal migration defects, especially pachygyria and polymicrogyria (see Chapter 2).[215,242,243] In addition to the neuronal migrational defects, the cerebral white matter is abnormal. Accumulation of sudanophilic lipids and deficiency of myelin have suggested sudanophilic leukodystrophy.[212] The molecular basis for the neuronal migrational and the myelin abnormalities may relate principally to the disorder of very-long-chain fatty acid oxidation. Thus, levels of these fatty acids are particularly high in the peroxisomal disorders with migrational abnormalities (i.e., Zellweger syndrome, neonatal adrenoleukodystrophy, and the single enzyme defect, D-bifunctional protein deficiency).[215-217,244,245] The last of these also is accompanied by elevation of bile acid intermediates, probably an unlikely perturbant of neuronal migration. Concerning the potential role of very-long-chain fatty acids in the myelin disturbance, an apparent beneficial effect of dietary supplementation of docosahexanoic acid (22:6n3) on cerebral myelin, as visualized by MRI, is supportive.[246] Thus, levels of this polyunsaturated fatty acid are decreased in brain of patients with disorders of peroxisome biogenesis, because of the defect in oxidation of saturated very-long-chain fatty acids of 26 carbons to those of 22 carbons. The *molecular defect* in Zellweger syndrome involves the genes encoding proteins necessary for peroxisome biogenesis, termed peroxins (*PEX*).[215,216] Peroxisome biogenesis begins with synthesis of peroxisomal matrix and membrane proteins on cytosolic ribosomes, post-translational targeting, docking at the peroxisomal membrane surface, and import into the organelle. In Zellweger syndrome, *PEX1* is the most common affected gene and is involved in import of peroxisomal matrix proteins.

No effective *therapy* has been described for Zellweger syndrome. A report of a beneficial effect of dietary supplementation of docosahexanoic acid on retinal function, myelination, and perhaps clinical features in five patients with disorders of peroxisomal biogenesis requires confirmation.[221,246] Moreover, somewhat promising is the demonstration that treatment of Zellweger syndrome fibroblasts with the peroxisome proliferator, sodium 4-phenylbutyrate, resulted in an increase in peroxisomal number.[224] Nevertheless, the fact that Zellweger syndrome involves a marked disturbance of brain development that occurs before 20 weeks of gestation suggests that postnatal therapies are not likely to be markedly beneficial.

Neonatal Adrenoleukodystrophy

Neonatal leukodystrophy, unlike the X-linked disease of older children, is an autosomal recessive disorder with a characteristic *clinical presentation* (see Tables 16-6 and 16-8).[212,215,216,225-230,238,239,247-251] Infants exhibit a dysmorphic craniofacial appearance, similar to but not as marked as that seen in Zellweger syndrome (see later discussion). Neurological features include hypotonia, weakness, impaired feeding, and optic atrophy, findings probably largely secondary to white matter disease, and seizures, consistent with gray matter disease. Relative macrocephaly, visual and auditory impairment, and neurological deterioration to death at approximately 3 years of age are typical. *Diagnosis* is based on the clinical features and the finding of deficiency of multiple peroxisomal functions, manifested particularly by elevations in plasma of very-long-chain fatty acids, pipecolic acid, and bile acid intermediates and by deficiency of plasmalogens in red blood cells (see Table 16-8). As with the clinical features, the metabolic abnormalities are not as marked as in Zellweger syndrome.[213,215,252] The basic *biochemical defect* involves peroxisome biogenesis, as in Zellweger syndrome; peroxisomal membrane "ghosts" are present, but the organelle's enzymes are absent or are severely deficient.[215,253] The total number of peroxisomes is markedly decreased.[224] As in Zellweger syndrome, the *molecular defect* involves peroxins encoded by specific *PEX* genes. The several defects that lead to the disease have involved targeting of cytosolic proteins, docking, and import into the peroxisome.[216]

Neuropathology is characterized by marked and diffusely decreased myelin, perivascular mononuclear "inflammatory" cells, trilamellar inclusions in macrophages, and sudanophilic lipid in reactive astrocytes. The myelin disturbance is somewhat more severe than in Zellweger syndrome.[212] Peripheral nerve myelin is also involved. In addition to the central white matter disease, evidence of neuronal migration defect is present (see discussion of Zellweger syndrome). The migrational defect in neonatal adrenoleukodystrophy is not as severe as in Zellweger syndrome. MRI identifies both the white matter disease and the neuronal migrational defects.[254] As discussed in relation to Zellweger syndrome, the relation of the biochemical disturbances to the migrational abnormalities is not entirely clear, but evidence suggests that the abnormality of very-long-chain fatty acids is crucial (see also Chapter 2). Consistent with this notion is the finding that plasma levels of very-long-chain fatty acids in neonatal adrenoleukodystrophy, although markedly elevated, are not as high as in Zellweger syndrome.[216,252]

No effective *therapy* has been described in the neonatal form of adrenoleukodystrophy. However, attempts to correct the elevated very-long-chain fatty acid levels in X-linked adrenoleukodystrophy by dietary restriction and by decreasing endogenous synthesis through administration of the monounsaturated fatty acids, oleate and erucate (Lorenzo's oil)[255-259] led to inconsistent evidence of biochemical and neurophysiological improvement. Initiation of treatment *before the onset of symptoms* has clearly been beneficial.[260] Whether such an approach would be beneficial in neonatal adrenoleukodystrophy is less clear because of the prenatal onset of the neuropathology and the wider spectrum of the biochemical disturbance. Perhaps of more relevance is the potential benefit of dietary supplementation with docosahexanoic acid in management of disorders of peroxisomal biogenesis, as described for Zellweger syndrome.[246] When cultured fibroblasts from patients with neonatal adrenoleukodystrophy are treated with sodium 4-phenylbutyrate, an increase in peroxisomal number and an improvement in peroxisomal biochemical functions are observed.[224] Whether similar peroxisomal proliferating agents are effective in vivo will be important to determine.[223,224] *Prenatal diagnosis* is possible by assaying very-long-chain fatty acid levels in cultured amniotic fluid cells or chorionic villus samples.

Mitochondrial Disorders

Five clinical disorders related to mitochondrial disease cause striking encephalopathic syndromes in the pediatric age group: Leigh syndrome, Alpers disease, myoclonic epilepsy with ragged red fibers (MERRF), mitochondrial encephalomyopathy–lactic acidosis-strokelike episodes (MELAS), and Kearns-Sayre syndrome (progressive external ophthalmoplegia plus).[36,261-270] Of these, *Leigh syndrome* and *Alpers disease* (see earlier discussion of gray matter degenerations) are observed relatively frequently in the neonatal period. Moreover, it is now clear that *other mitochondrial encephalopathies* also occur in the newborn period and in early infancy and do not conform to the classic features of Leigh syndrome or Alpers disease. Because overlap among these other mitochondrial encephalopathies seems greater with Leigh syndrome than with Alpers disease, I include these conditions here in the discussion of Leigh syndrome. Among other neonatal-onset mitochondrial disorders, an important mitochondrial myopathy secondary to cytochrome c oxidase deficiency is described in Chapter 19, and defects in pyruvate metabolism with predominant lactic acidosis are described in Chapter 15.

Leigh Syndrome and Other Mitochondrial Encephalopathies

Leigh syndrome is characterized most commonly by clinical onset later in infancy and early childhood, but neonatal onset is well documented.[263,269,271-297a] The principal *clinical features* have been hypotonia, weakness, respiratory abnormalities (including central neurogenic hypoventilation [Ondine's curse]), oculomotor abnormalities, facial weakness, and impaired feeding (see Table 16-6). Seizures, developmental arrest, and then disorders of movement (especially dystonia) and deterioration to death in the first year or so of life have been typical of neonatal-onset cases. Onset later in infancy is associated with slower deterioration, and approximately 50% of cases survive for 5 years.[287] *Diagnosis* is suspected on the basis of the clinical features. Brain imaging is notable for decreased attenuation of the putamen on CT and, on T2-weighted images of MRI, increased signal in putamen, accompanied also by abnormalities in globus pallidus, caudate, periventricular white matter, corpus callosum, midbrain (especially the periaqueductal region), and lower brain stem (Fig. 16-17).[4,287,295,298-302] Cranial ultrasonography may show increased echogenicity in the putamen and caudate.[300] Spatially localized proton MR spectroscopy has detected elevated levels of lactate in areas shown to be involved on T2-weighted images.[4,295,301,303,304] CSF lactate levels are elevated nearly uniformly, whereas ratios of blood lactate to pyruvate may or may not be elevated.[30,31,287,305] Fibroblast cultures or tissue samples (muscle, liver, other tissues) have shown *biochemical defects* most commonly involving the pyruvate dehydrogenase complex, particularly the nuclear-encoded gene for the E_{1alpha} subunit, cytochrome c oxidase (complex IV), reduced nicotinamide adenine dinucleotide–coenzyme Q reductase (complex I), or ATP synthase subunit 6 (complex V) (Table 16-9).[263,266-270,275,279-281,283,286-289,294,297,306-314] The defect of cytochrome oxidase activity, the most common of the four, involves not the oxidase itself but usually a nuclear-encoded protein, SURF-1, involved in the assembly of cytochrome oxidase activity.[268,269,293,302,307,310] A second

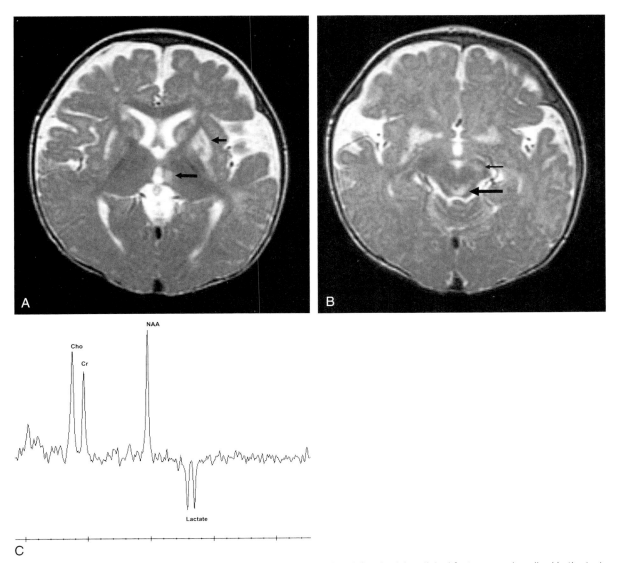

Figure 16-17 **Leigh syndrome: magnetic resonance imaging (MRI) scans.** This infant had the clinical features as described in the text and lactic acidemia. Axial T2-weighted MRI shows abnormal high signal intensity in **(A)** putamen *(short arrow)*, caudate (not marked), and thalamus *(long arrow)*, and in **(B)** the periaqueductal region *(thick arrow)* and cerebral peduncle *(thin arrow)*. **C,** MR spectroscopy shows elevated brain lactate. Cho, choline; Cr, creatine; NAA, *N*-acetylaspartate. (Courtesy of Dr. Omar Khwaja.)

TABLE 16-9 Leigh Syndrome: Major Molecular Defects Identified*

Molecular Defect	Percentage of Total	Usual Inheritance†
Complex I	32%	Autosomal recessive, maternal, or X-linked
Complex IV (cytochrome oxidase)	37%	Autosomal recessive
Complex V (ATP synthase, subunit 6-mtDNA mutation)	17%	Maternal
Pyruvate dehydrogenase complex (E_{1alpha} subunit)	14%	X-linked

*See text for references. Rare cases have been reported secondary to pyruvate carboxylase deficiency, mitochondrial encephalomyopathy–lactic acidosis–strokelike episodes (MELAS) mutation, mitochondrial DNA depletion, mitochondrial DNA deletions, complex II deficiency, and complex III deficiency.

†Many cases are not familial (i.e., they represent new mutations in the affected infant).

ATP, adenosine triphosphate.

assembly gene, *SCO2*, has been implicated, especially in neonatal-onset cases.[269,310] However, in the latter cases, the topography of the abnormalities on brain imaging is not typical for Leigh syndrome, and fulminating hypertrophic cardiomyopathy is distinctive.[269,310] The distribution of the major biochemical defects and their usual mode of inheritance in infants with Leigh syndrome is shown in Table 16-9. Rare cases of Leigh syndrome have been associated with deficiency of pyruvate carboxylase deficiency, MELAS mutation, mitochondrial DNA depletion, mitochondrial DNA deletions, complex II deficiency, and complex III deficiency.[268,291,292,315,316] *Neuropathology* of Leigh syndrome is distinctive and is characterized by symmetrical focal necrotic lesions with demyelination, spongy change, vascular proliferation, and gliosis. The areas especially involved are in the periventricular and periaqueductal regions of brain stem and the diencephalic regions around the third ventricle, especially thalamus, basal ganglia (especially putamen), and subcortical white matter. *Therapy* has included dichloroacetate (to activate the pyruvate dehydrogenase complex), respiratory chain components (e.g., coenzyme Q10), artificial electron acceptors (e.g., ascorbate), free radical scavengers (e.g., vitamin E), and metabolites or cofactors (e.g., L-carnitine).[36,265,268,301,317] Strikingly beneficial responses have not been observed in patients with Leigh syndrome of neonatal onset.

Other mitochondrial encephalopathies with onset in the newborn period or early infancy do not conform to the classic features of Leigh syndrome but sometimes overlap enough to be characterized as "Leigh-like" disorders.[268-270,287,295,296,297a,310] However, these other mitochondrial encephalopathies may exhibit quite different topographic features (e.g., cerebral white matter changes suggestive of leukodystrophy[318-323] or evidence of cerebral or cerebellar atrophy, or both).[324] The clinical features often include fragments of those seen in Leigh syndrome. Mitochondrial disease is established by the findings of elevated lactate in CSF and brain, enzymatic and molecular genetic features indicative of disturbances of mitochondrial proteins (especially in the electron transport chain), and *cellular* pathology comparable to that described for Leigh syndrome. *The principal difference is topography of lesions. The essential clinical point is that newborns and very young infants with evidence for* encephalopathy of diverse topographies and accompanied by elevated CSF or brain lactate should be investigated carefully for a mitochondrial disorder. The presence of systemic phenomena (e.g., cardiomyopathy, nephropathy, hepatopathy) should enhance the suspicion of such a disorder.

Other Disorders

Other degenerative disorders with neonatal onset and involvement of both gray and white matter are linked by the occurrence in both of hypoplasia of hindbrain structures, especially the pontocerebellar regions (see Table 16-6). The two disorders, CDG1a (previously termed carbohydrate-deficient glycoprotein syndrome) and PCH, however, differ considerably in clinical features, genetics, and apparent underlying biochemical disturbance.

Congenital Disorders of Glycosylation Type 1a (Carbohydrate-Deficient Glycoprotein Syndromes)

CDGs, previously termed carbohydrate-deficient glycoprotein syndromes, comprise a family of multisystemic disorders, of which one variety, CDG1a, is by far the most common and best characterized.[325-337a] The following discussion is focused on CDG1a (see Table 16-6). This *autosomal recessive* disorder exhibits a characteristic *clinical presentation*, which includes mild facial dysmorphism (large, dysplastic ears), abnormal subcutaneous fat distribution (fat pads over buttocks, "orange peel" skin), inverted nipples, and joint contractures. Neurological features include "rolling" vertical or horizontal eye movements, alternating internal strabismus, hypotonia, and hyporeflexia. Subsequently, developmental failure, strokelike episodes, ataxia, moderate to severe cognitive defects, epilepsy, and retinal pigmentary degeneration are prominent. Although the neuropathology appears to progress, in a strict sense the lack of a progressively deteriorating course and frequent survival to adulthood, albeit in a disabled state, argue against a relentlessly progressive degenerative disorder of the nervous system. The multisystem involvement includes cardiac (cardiomyopathy, pericardial effusions, hydrops fetalis), hepatic (hepatomegaly, liver dysfunction), renal (nephrotic syndrome), and, later, reproductive (hypogonadism) effects. Approximately 20% of infants die in the first years of life because of systemic failure or status epilepticus.[331] The *biochemical defect* involves glycosylation of proteins (i.e., synthesis of glycoproteins), and the most common defect (i.e., that for CDG1a) involves the phosphomannomutase involved in conversion of mannose-6-phosphate to mannose-1-phosphate, a key early intermediate in dolichol-linked glycoprotein synthesis. Dolichol-linked glycoprotein synthesis is *N*-linked, that is, the glycan is attached to the protein by the amide group of asparagine on the protein. *N*-linked glycoprotein synthesis is involved in CDG, whereas the other major pathway of glycoprotein synthesis in mammals, *O*-linked synthesis, which involves linkage of the glycan to the hydroxyl moiety of serine or threonine, is involved in certain congenital muscular dystrophies (see Chapter 19). *Diagnosis* of CDG1a is established on the basis of the clinical features and the biochemical consequences of the basic defect. These abnormalities include reduction in blood levels of various compounds because of lack of their glycosylated transport proteins (albumin, thyroxine-binding globulin, thyroxine, cholesterol, and coagulation factors, especially factor XI and antithrombin). The diagnosis is usually made by demonstration of deficiently glycosylated transferrin by isoelectrofocusing. *Neuropathology* includes pontocerebellar hypoplasia, with neuronal loss and gliosis especially in cerebellum but also in cerebral cortex, basal ganglia, thalamus, and brain stem. The involvement of neurons in brain stem and cerebellum particularly affects the pons, inferior olives, and Purkinje cells and granule cells of the cerebellum. Pontocerebellar hypoplasia is readily detected by MRI (Fig. 16-18). Polyneuropathy with decreased myelin is also apparent and accounts for

decreased motor nerve conduction velocities and the hyporeflexia. No known *therapy* exists.

Pontocerebellar Hypoplasia Type 2

PCH is a heterogeneous group of disorders with the common feature of hypoplasia of cerebellum and brain stem, especially pons (Table 16-10). (Because the inferior olivary nuclei often also are involved, the term *olivopontocerebellar hypoplasia* is sometimes used.) Thus far, nearly all the disorders have exhibited autosomal recessive inheritance. PCH type 1 is associated with severe degeneration of anterior horn cells and is noted in Chapters 17 and 18 in relation to arthrogryposis multiplex congenita and Werdnig-Hoffman disease. Cerebromuscular dystrophies with prominent cerebellar and, to a lesser extent, brain stem hypoplasia are discussed in Chapter 19. Some examples of mitochondrial disorders, especially involving the electron transport chain, may be associated with pontocerebellar hypoplasia (see earlier).[338,339] Because PCH type 2 has the clinical characteristics of a degenerative disorder of the central nervous system, it is discussed here.

Type 2 PCH exhibits a striking *clinical presentation* apparent from the first days of life.[340-347a] The neonatal neurological syndrome consists particularly of abnormalities of sucking and swallowing and jitteriness. Seizures are less common. Subsequently, head circumference, which is within the normal range at birth, increases at a markedly reduced rate, such that progressive microcephaly develops. A striking extrapyramidal syndrome (chorea, athetosis, dystonia) is characteristic. In addition, epilepsy, severe cognitive deficits, and markedly impaired visual responses ensue. Approximately 40% of patients have died in childhood. Families without dyskinesias have been described and could represent variants or separate genetic disorders.[348,349] One of these has been mapped to 7q11-21.[349] *Diagnosis* of PCH type 2 is suspected from the clinical features. MRI shows the hypoplasia of pons and cerebellum, both vermis and hemispheres, particularly the latter (Fig. 16-19). A moderate degree of cerebral cortical atrophy is also apparent later in the course. *Neuropathology* is striking. Pontine hypoplasia with severe reduction of ventral pontine neurons, cerebellar hypoplasia with marked involvement of internal granule cells and dentate nuclei, and moderate loss of

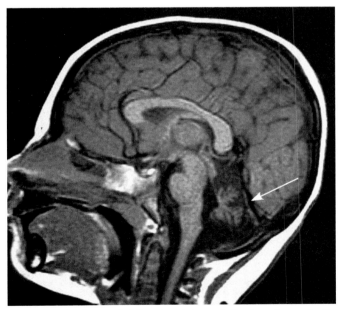

Figure 16-18 **Congenital disorder of glycosylation type 1a: magnetic resonance imaging (MRI) scan.** Sagittal T1-weighted MRI shows very small cerebellar vermis with shrunken folia and enlarged fissures *(arrow)*. Note that the pons is relatively preserved, unlike in pontocerebellar hypoplasia type 2. *(From Barkovich AJ: Pediatric Neuroimaging, 4th ed, Philadelphia: 2005, Lippincott Williams & Wilkins.)*

TABLE 16-10	Major Forms of Pontocerebellar Hypoplasia Encountered in the Neonatal Period*
Pontocerebellar hypoplasia type 1	
Pontocerebellar hypoplasia type 2	
Congenital disorder of glycosylation type 1a	
Cerebromuscular dystrophies	
Walker-Warburg syndrome	
Muscle-eye-brain disease	
Mitochondrial disorder	

*Excludes intrauterine or early postnatal destructive disorders and several other rare syndromic disorders exhibiting pontocerebellar hypoplasia and other distinctive dysmorphic features.

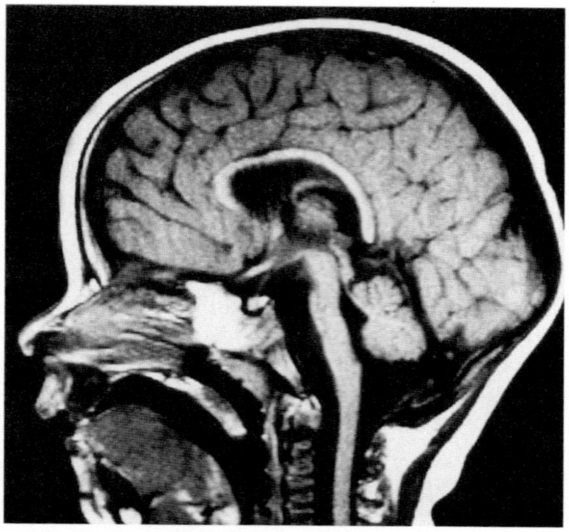

Figure 16-19 Midsagittal T1-weighted magnetic resonance imaging scan of an infant with pontocerebellar hypoplasia type 2. Note the hypoplastic pons and cerebellar vermis. The cerebellar hemispheres, not seen in this image, also were hypoplastic. *(From Barth PG, Blennow G, Lenard HG, Begeer JH, et al: The syndrome of autosomal recessive pontocerebellar hypoplasia, microcephaly, and extrapyramidal dyskinesia [pontocerebellar hypoplasia type 2]: Compiled data from 10 pedigrees, Neurology 45:311-317, 1995.)*

neurons in the inferior olivary nuclei are the prominent features. Gliosis accompanies the neuronal changes. Some degree of cerebral cortical neuronal degeneration also is apparent. No *therapy* is known for this disorder, the biochemical basis (or bases) for which remains to be established.

Several other disorders characterized by autosomal recessively inherited pontocerebellar hypoplasia, with some features resembling PCH type 2, have been reported.[350] Infants with pontocerebellar hypoplasia but, additionally, optic atrophy have been designated as having PCH type 3, those with relative preservation of vermis have PCH type 4, and those with relative preservation of cerebellar hemispheres have PCH type 5. Until the molecular genetic defects are identified, the nosology of these rare forms will remain unclear.

REFERENCES

1. Gravel RA, Kalback MM, Proia RL, Sandhoff K, et al: The G_{M2} gangliosidoses. In Scriver CR, Beaudet MD, Sly WS, et al, editors: *The Metabolic and Molecular Bases of Inherited Disease*, 8th ed, New York: 2001, McGraw-Hill.
2. Suzuki K, Suzuki K: Lysosomal diseases. In Graham DI, Lantos PL, editors: *Greenfield's Neuropathology*, 7 ed, London: 2002, Arnold Publishers.
3. Purpura DP, Suzuki K: Distortion of neuronal geometry and formation of aberrant synapses in neuronal storage disease, *Brain Res*, 116:1-21, 1976.
4. Barkovich AJ: *Pediatric Neuroimaging*, 4th ed, Philadelphia: 2005, Lippincott Williams & Wilkins.
5. Lacorazza HD, Flax JD, Snyder EY, Jendoubi M: Expression of human β-hexosaminidase α-subunit gene (the gene defect of Tay-Sachs disease) in mouse brains upon engraftment of transduced neural progenitor cells, *Nat Med*, 2:424-429, 1996.
6. Malatack JJ, Consolini DM, Bayever E: The status of hematopoietic stem cell transplantation in lysosomal storage disease, *Pediatr Res*, 29:391-403, 2003.
7. Wisniewski KE, Zhong N, Philippart M: Pheno/genotypic correlations of neuronal ceroid lipofuscinoses, *Neurology*, 57:576-581, 2001.
8. Mole SE: The genetic spectrum of human neuronal ceroid-lipofuscinoses, *Brain Pathol*, 14:70-76, 2004.
9. Ezaki J, Kominami E: The intracellular location and function of proteins of neuronal ceroid lipofuscinoses, *Brain Pathol*, 14:77-85, 2004.
10. Siintola E, Partanen S, Stromme P, Haapanen A, et al: Cathepsin D deficiency underlies congenital human neuronal ceroid-lipofuscinosis, *Brain*, 129:1438-1445, 2006.
11. Mole SE: Neuronal ceroid lipofuscinoses (NCL), *Eur J Paediatr Neurol*, 10:255-257, 2006.
11a. Persaud-Sawin DA, Mousallem T, Wang C, Zucker A, et al: Neuronal ceroid lipofuscinoses: A common pathway? *Pediatr Res*, 61:146-152, 2007.
12. Norman R, Wood NW: Congenital form of amaurotic family idiocy, *J Neurol Psychiatry*, 4:175-190, 1941.
13. Brown NJ, Corner BD, Dodgson MC: A second case in the same family of congenital familial cerebral lipoidosis resembling amaurotic family idiocy, *Arch Dis Child*, 29:48-54, 1954.
14. Garborg I, Torvik A, Hals J, Tangsrud SE, et al: Congenital neuronal ceroid-lipofuscinosis, *Acta Pathol Microbiol Immunol Scand*, 95:119-125, 1987.
15. Humphreys S, Lake BD, Scholtz CL: Congenital amaurotic idiocy: A pathological, histochemical, biochemical and ultrastructural study, *Neuropathol Appl Neurobiol*, 11:475-484, 1985.
16. Sandbank U: Congenital amaurotic idiocy, *Pathol Eur*, 3:226-229, 1968.
17. Barohn RJ, Dowd DC, Kagan-Hallet KS: Congenital ceroid-lipofuscinosis, *Pediatr Neurol*, 8:54-59, 1992.
18. Sandbank U, Lerman P: Progressive cerebral poliodystrophy—Alpers' disease: Disorganized giant neuronal mitochondria on electron microscopy, *J Neurol Neurosurg Psychiatry*, 35:749-755, 1972.
19. Alcala H, Kotagal S: Alpers' disease: A distinct clinical-pathological entity, *Ann Neurol*, 16:382, 1984.
20. Harding BN: Progressive neuronal degeneration of childhood with liver disease (Alpers-Huttenlocher syndrome): A personal review, *J Child Neurol*, 5:273-287, 1990.
21. Harding BN, Egger J, Portmann B, Erdohazi M: Progressive neuronal degeneration of childhood with liver disease: A pathological study, *Brain*, 109:181-206, 1986.
22. Egger J, Harding BN, Boyd SG, Wilson J, et al: Progressive neuronal degeneration of childhood (PNDC) with liver disease, *Clin Pediatr (Phila)*, 26:167-173, 1987.
23. Narkewicz MR, Sokol RJ, Beckwith B, Sondheimer J, et al: Liver involvement in Alpers disease, *J Pediatr*, 119:260-267, 1991.
24. Harding BN, Surtees R: Metabolic and neurodegenerative diseases of childhood. In Graham DI, Lantos PL, editors: *Greenfield's Neuropathology*, 7 ed, London: 2002, Arnold Publishers.
25. Tesarova M, Mayr JA, Wenchich L, Hansikova H, et al: Mitochondrial DNA depletion in Alpers syndrome, *Neuropediatrics*, 35:217-223, 2004.
26. Naviaux RK, Nguyen KV: POLG mutations associated with Alpers' syndrome and mitochondrial DNA depletion, *Ann Neurol*, 55:706-712, 2004.
27. Nguyen KV, Ostergaard E, Ravn SH, Balslev T, et al: POLG mutations in Alpers syndrome, *Neurology*, 65:1493-1495, 2005.
28. Ferrari G, Lamantea E, Donati A, Filosto M, et al: Infantile hepatocerebral syndromes associated with mutations in the mitochondrial DNA polymerase-gamma A, *Brain*, 128:723-731, 2005.
29. Davidson G, Mancuso M, Ferraris S, Quinzii C, et al: POLG mutations and Alpers syndrome, *Ann Neurol*, 57:921-923, 2005.
30. Tulinius MH, Holme E, Kristiansson B, Larsson NG, et al: Mitochondrial encephalomyopathies in childhood. I. Biochemical and morphologic investigations, *J Pediatr*, 119:242-250, 1991.
31. Tulinius MH, Holme E, Kristiansson B, Larsson NG, et al: Mitochondrial encephalomyopathies in childhood. II. Clinical manifestations and syndromes, *J Pediatr*, 119:251-259, 1991.
32. Prick M, Gabreëls F, Renier W, Trijbels F, et al: Pyruvate dehydrogenase deficiency restricted to brain, *Neurology*, 31:398-404, 1981.
33. Prick MJ, Gabreëls FJ, Renier WO, Trijbels JM, et al: Progressive infantile poliodystrophy (Alpers' disease) with a defect in citric acid cycle activity in liver and fibroblasts, *Neuropediatrics*, 13:108-111, 1982.
34. Gabreëls F, Prick M, Renier W: Progressive infantile poliodystrophy (Alpers' disease) associated with disturbed NADH oxidation, lipid myopathy and abnormal muscle mitochondria. In Busch H, Jennekens F, Scholte H, editors: *Mitochondria and Muscular Diseases*, Beetsterzwaag: 1981, Mefar.
35. Prick MJ, Gabreëls FJ, Trijbels JM, Janssen AJ, et al: Progressive poliodystrophy (Alpers' disease) with a defect in cytochrome aa₃ in muscle: A report of two unrelated patients, *Clin Neurol Neurosurg*, 85:57-70, 1983.
36. Shoffner JM: Oxidative phosphorylation diseases. In Scriver CR, Beaudet MD, Sly WS, et al, editors: *The Metabolic and Molecular Bases of Inherited Disease*, 8th ed, New York: 2001, McGraw-Hill.
37. Flemming K, Ulmer S, Duisberg B, Hahn A, et al: MR spectroscopic findings in a case of Alpers-Huttenlocher syndrome, *AJNR Am J Neuroradiol*, 23:1421-1423, 2002.
37a. Sarzi E, Bourdon A, Chretien D, Zarhrate M, et al: Mitochondrial DNA depletion is a prevalent cause of multiple respiratory chain deficiency in childhood, *J Pediatr*, 150:531-534, 534 e531-536, 2007.
38. Grover WD, Johnson WC, Henkin RI: Clinical and biochemical aspects of trichopoliodystrophy, *Ann Neurol*, 5:65-71, 1979.
39. Menkes JH: Kinky hair disease: Twenty five years later, *Brain Dev*, 10:77-79, 1988.

40. Leventer RJ, Kornberg AJ, Phelan EM, Kean MJ: Early magnetic resonance imaging findings in Menke's disease, *J Child Neurol*, 12:222-224, 1997.

41. Menkes JH: Menkes disease and Wilson disease: Two sides of the same copper coin. I. Menkes disease, *Eur J Paediatr Neurol*, 3:147-158, 1999.

42. Pedespan JM, Jouaville LS, Cances C, Letellier T, et al: Menkes disease: Study of the mitochondrial respiratory chain in three cases, *Eur J Paediatr Neurol*, 3:167-170, 1999.

43. Culotta VC, Gitlin JD: Disorders of copper transport. In Scriver CR, Beaudet MD, Sly WS, et al, editors: *The Metabolic and Molecular Bases of Inherited Disease*, 8th ed, New York: 2001, McGraw-Hill.

44. Hsich GE, Robertson RL, Irons M, du Plessis AJ: Cerebral infarction in Menkes' disease, *Pediatr Neurol*, 23:425-428, 2000.

45. Borm B, Moller LB, Hausser I, Emeis M, et al: Variable clinical expression of an identical mutation in the *ATP7A* gene for Menkes disease/occipital horn syndrome in three affected males in a single family, *J Pediatr*, 145:119-121, 2004.

46. Tonnesen T, Horn N: Prenatal and postnatal diagnosis of Menkes disease, an inherited disorder of copper metabolism, *J Inherit Metab Dis*, 12:207-214, 1989.

47. Vulpe C, Levinson B, Whitney S: Isolation of a candidate gene for Menkes disease and evidence that it encodes a copper-transporting ATPase, *Nat Genet*, 3:7-13, 1993.

48. Kollros PR, Dick RD, Brewer GJ: Correction of cerebrospinal fluid copper in Menkes kinky hair disease, *Pediatr Neurol*, 7:305-307, 1991.

49. Sherwood G, Sarkar B, Kortsak AS: Copper histidinate therapy in Menkes' disease: Prevention of progressive neurodegeneration, *J Inherit Metab Dis*, 12:393-396, 1989.

50. Danks DM: Disorders of copper transport. In Scriver CR, Beaudet AL, Sly WS, et al, editors: *The Metabolic and Molecular Bases of Inherited Disease*, 7th ed, New York: 1995, McGraw-Hill.

51. Meloni I, Bruttini M, Longo I, Mari F, et al: A mutation in the Rett syndrome gene, *MECP2*, causes X-linked mental retardation and progressive spasticity in males, *Am J Hum Genet*, 67:982-985, 2000.

52. Schanen NC, Kurcznski TW, Brunelle D, Woodcock MM, et al: Neonatal encephalopathy in two boys in families with recurrent Rett syndrome, *J Child Neurol*, 13:229-231, 1998.

53. Villard L, Cardoso AK, Chelly PJ, Tardieu PM, et al: Two affected boys in a Rett syndrome family: Clinical and molecular findings, *Neurology*, 55:1188-1193, 2000.

54. Geerdink N, Rotteveel JJ, Lammens M, Sistermans EA, et al: *MECP2* mutation in a boy with severe neonatal encephalopathy: Clinical, neuropathological and molecular findings, *Neuropediatrics*, 33:33-36, 2002.

55. Ben Zeev B, Yaron Y, Schanen C, Wolf H, et al: Rett syndrome: Clinical manifestations in males with *MECP2* mutations, *J Child Neurol*, 17:20-24, 2002.

56. Moog U, Smeets EE, Van Roozendaal KE, Schoenmakers S, et al: Neurodevelopmental disorders in males related to the gene causing Rett syndrome in females *(MECP2)*, *Eur J Paediatr Neurol*, 7:5-12, 2003.

57. Leuzzi V, Di Sabato ML, Zollino M, Montanaro ML, et al: Early-onset encephalopathy and cortical myoclonus in a boy with *MECP2* gene mutation, *Neurology*, 63:1968-1970, 2004.

58. Lynch SA, Whatley SD, Ramesh V, Sinha S, et al: Sporadic case of fatal encephalopathy with neonatal onset associated with a *T158M* missense mutation in *MECP2*, *Arch Dis Child*, 88:250-252, 2003.

59. Budden SS, Dorsey HC, Steiner RD: Clinical profile of a male with Rett syndrome, *Brain Dev*, 27:S69-S71, 2005.

60. Kankirawatana P, Leonard H, Ellaway C, Scurlock J, et al: Early progressive encephalopathy in boys and *MECP2* mutations, *Neurology*, 67:164-166, 2006.

61. Abu-Dalu KI, Tamary H, Livni N, Rivkind AI, et al: GM1 gangliosidosis presenting as neonatal ascites, *J Pediatr*, 100:940-943, 1982.

62. O'Brien JS: β-Galactosidase deficiency (G$_{M1}$ gangliosidosis, galactosialidosis, and Morquio syndrome type B): Ganglioside sialidase deficiency (mucolipidosis IV). In Scriver CR, Beaudet AL, Sly WS, et al, editors: *The Metabolic Basis of Inherited Disease*, 6th ed, New York: 1989, McGraw-Hill.

63. Suzuki Y, Oshima A, Nanba E: β-Galactosidase deficiency (β-galactosidosis): G$_{M1}$ gangliosidosis and Morquio B disease. In Scriver CR, Beaudet MD, Sly WS, et al, editors: *The Metabolic and Molecular Bases of Inherited Disease*, 8th ed, New York: 2001, McGraw-Hill.

64. Bieber FR, Mortimer G, Kolodny EH, Driscoll SG: Pathologic findings in fetal GM1 gangliosidosis, *Arch Neurol*, 43:736-738, 1986.

65. Yamano T, Shimada M, Okada S, Yutaka T, et al: Ultrastructural study on nervous system of fetus with GM1-gangliosidosis type 1, *Acta Neuropathol (Berl)*, 61:15-20, 1983.

66. Schuchman EH, Desnick RJ: Niemann-Pick disease types A and B: Acid sphingomyelinase deficiencies. In Scriver CR, Beaudet MD, Sly WS, et al, editors: *The Metabolic and Molecular Bases of Inherited Disease*, 8th ed, New York: 2001, McGraw-Hill.

67. Barranger JA, Ginns EI: Glucosylceramide lipidoses: Gaucher disease. In Scriver CR, Beaudet AL, Sly WS, et al, editors: *The Metabolic Bass of Inherited Disease*, 6th ed, New York: 1989, McGraw-Hill.

68. Sidransky E, Sherer DM, Ginns EI: Gaucher disease in the neonate: A distinct Gaucher phenotype is analogous to a mouse model created by targeted disruption of the glucocerebrosidase gene, *Pediatr Res*, 32:494-498, 1992.

69. Beutler E, Grabowski GA: Gaucher disease. In Scriver CR, Beaudet AL, Sly WS, et al, editors: *The Metabolic and Molecular Bases of Inherited Disease*, 7th ed, New York: 1995, McGraw-Hill.

70. Sidransky E, Tayebi N, Stubblefield BK, Eliason W, et al: The clinical, molecular, and pathological characterisation of a family with two cases of lethal perinatal type 2 Gaucher disease, *J Med Genet*, 33:132-136, 1995.

71. Wilcox WR: Lysosomal storage disorders: The need for better pediatric recognition and comprehensive care, *J Pediatr*, 144:S3-S14, 2004.

72. Beutler E, Grabowski G: Gaucher disease. In Scriver CR, Beaudet MD, Sly WS, et al, editors: *The Metabolic and Molecular Bases of Inherited Disease*, 8th ed, New York: 2001, McGraw-Hill.

73. Moser HW, Linke T, Fensom AH, Levade T, et al: Acid ceramidase deficiency: Farber lipogranulomatosis. In Scriver CR, Beaudet MD, Sly WS, et al, editors: *The Metabolic and Molecular Bases of Inherited Disease*, 8th ed, New York: 2001, McGraw-Hill.

74. Pueschel SM, O'Shea PA, Alroy J, Ambler MW, et al: Infantile sialic acid storage disease associated with renal disease, *Pediatr Neurol*, 4:207-212, 1988.

75. Thomas GH: Disorders of glycoprotein degradation: α-Mannosidosis, β-mannosidosis, fucosidosis, and sialidosis. In Scriver CR, Beaudet MD, Sly WS, et al, editors: *The Metabolic and Molecular Bases of Inherited Disease*, 8th ed, New York: 2001, McGraw-Hill.

76. Gahl WA, Renlund M, Thoene JG: Lysosomal transport disorders: Cystinosis and sialic acid storage disorders. In Scriver CR, Beaudet AL, Sly WS, et al, editors: *The Metabolic Basis of Inherited Disease*, 6th ed, New York: 1989, McGraw-Hill.

77. Berra B, Gornati R, Rapelli S, Gatti R, et al: Infantile sialic acid storage disease: Biochemical studies, *Am J Med Genet*, 58:24-31, 1995.

78. d'Azzo A, Andria G, Strisciuglio P, Galjard H: Galactosialidosis. In Scriver CR, Beaudet MD, Sly WS, et al, editors: *The Metabolic and Molecular Bases of Inherited Disease*, 8th ed, New York: 2001, McGraw-Hill.

79. Patel MS, Callahan JW, Zhang SQ, Chan AKJ, et al: Early-infantile galactosialidosis: Prenatal presentation and postnatal follow-up, *Am J Med Genet*, 85:38-47, 1999.

80. Lemyre E, Russo P, Melancon SB, Gagne R, et al: Clinical spectrum of infantile free sialic acid storage disease, *Am J Med Genet*, 82:385-391, 1999.

81. Froissart R, Cheillan D, Bouvier R, Tourret S, et al: Clinical, morphological, and molecular aspects of sialic acid storage disease manifesting in utero, *J Med Genet*, 42:829-836, 2005.

82. Hogan GR, Richardson EP: Spongy degeneration of the nervous system (Canavan's disease): Report of a case in an Irish-American family, *Pediatrics*, 35:284, 1965.

83. Adachi M, Schneck L, Cara J, Volk BW: Spongy degeneration of the central nervous system (van Bogaert and Bertrand type; Canavan's disease): A review, *Hum Pathol*, 4:331-347, 1973.

84. Gascon GG, Ozand PT, Mahdi A, Jamil A, et al: Infantile CNS spongy degeneration—14 cases: Clinical update, *Neurology*, 40:1876-1882, 1990.

85. von Moers A, Sperner J, Michael T, Scheffner D, et al: Variable course of Canavan disease in two boys with early infantile aspartoacylase deficiency, *Dev Med Child Neurol*, 33:824-828, 1991.

86. Michelakakis H, Giouroukos S, Divry P, Katsarou E, et al: Canavan disease: Findings in four new cases, *J Inherit Metab Dis*, 14:267-268, 1991.

87. Echenne B, Divry P, Vianey-Liaud C: Spongy degeneration of the neuraxis (Canavan–van Bogaert disease) and *N*-acetylaspartic aciduria, *Neuropediatrics*, 20:79-81, 1989.

88. Sacks O, Brown WJ, Aguilar MJ: Spongy degeneration of white matter, *Neurology*, 15:165-171, 1965.

89. Anderson JM: Spongy degeneration in the white matter of the central nervous system in the newborn: Pathological findings in three infants, one with hyperglycinaemia, *J Neurol Neurosurg Psychiatry*, 32:328-337, 1969.

90. Zelnik N, Luder AS, Elpeleg ON, Gross-Tsur V, et al: Protracted clinical course for patients with Canavan disease, *Dev Med Child Neurol*, 35:346-358, 1993.

91. Matalon R, Kaul R, Michals K: Canavan disease: Biochemical and molecular studies, *J Inherit Metab Dis*, 16:744-752, 1993.

92. Matalon R, Michals K, Kaul R: Canavan disease: From spongy degeneration to molecular analysis, *J Pediatr*, 127:511-517, 1995.

93. Matalon R, Michaels-Matalon K: Molecular basis of Canavan disease, *Eur J Paediatr Neurol*, 2:69-76, 1998.

94. Traeger EC, Rapin I: The clinical course of Canavan disease, *Pediatr Neurol*, 18:207-212, 1998.

95. Gordon N: Canavan disease: A review of recent developments, *Eur J Paediatr Neurol*, 5:65-69, 2001.

96. Beaudet AL: Aspartoacylase deficiency (Canavan Disease). In Scriver CR, Beaudet MD, Sly WS, et al, editors: *The Metabolic and Molecular Bases of Inherited Disease*, 8th ed, New York: 2001, McGraw-Hill.

97. Kumar S, Mattan NS, de Vellis J: Canavan disease: A white matter disorder, *Ment Retard Dev Disabil Res Rev*, 12:157-165, 2006.

98. Marks HG, Caro PA, Wang ZY, Detre JA, et al: Use of computed tomography, magnetic resonance imaging, and localized 1H magnetic resonance spectroscopy in Canavan's disease: A case report, *Ann Neurol*, 30:106-110, 1991.

99. Divry P, Vianey-Liaud C, Gay C, Macabeo V, et al: *N*-Acetylaspartic aciduria: Report of three new cases in children with a neurological syndrome associating macrocephaly and leukodystrophy, *J Inherit Metab Dis*, 11:307-308, 1988.

100. Matalon R, Michals K, Sebesta D, Deanching M, et al: Aspartoacylase deficiency and N-acetylaspartic aciduria in patients with Canavan disease, *Am J Med Genet*, 29:463-471, 1988.

101. Matalon R, Kaul R, Casanova J, Michals K, et al: SSIEM Award: Aspartoacylase deficiency: The enzyme defect in Canavan disease, *J Inherit Metab Dis*, 12:329-331, 1989.

102. Jakobs C, ten Brink HJ, Langelaar SA, Zee T, et al: Stable isotope dilution analysis of N-acetylaspartic acid in CSF, blood, urine and amniotic fluid: Accurate postnatal diagnosis and the potential for prenatal diagnosis of Canavan disease, *J Inherit Metab Dis*, 14:653-660, 1991.

103. Kelley RI, Stamas JN: Quantification of N-acetyl-L-aspartic acid in urine by isotope dilution gas chromatography mass spectrometry, *J Inherit Metab Dis*, 15:97-104, 1992.

104. Elpeleg ON: N-Acetylaspartic aciduria in young age, *Neuropediatrics*, 23:112, 1992.

105. Burlina AP, Ferrari V, Divry P, Gradowska W, et al: N-Acetylaspartylglutamate in Canavan disease: An adverse effector? *Eur J Pediatr*, 158:406-409, 1999.

106. Madhavarao CN, Arun P, Moffett JR, Szucs S, et al: Defective N-acetylaspartate catabolism reduces brain acetate levels and myelin lipid synthesis in Canavan's disease, *Proc Natl Acad Sci U S A*, 102:5221-5226, 2005.

107. Kirmani BF, Jacobowitz DM, Namboodiri MAA: Developmental increase of aspartoacylase in oligodendrocytes parallels CNS myelination, *Dev Brain Res*, 140:105-115, 2003.

108. Leone P, Janson CG, Bilianuk L, Wang Z, et al: Aspartoacylase gene transfer to the mammalian central nervous system with therapeutic implications for Canavan disease, *Ann Neurol*, 48:27-38, 2000.

109. Janson CG, Assadi M, Francis J, Bilaniuk L, et al: Lithium citrate for Canavan disease, *Pediatr Neurol*, 33:235-243, 2005.

110. Wohlwill FJ, Bernstein J, Yakovlev PI: Dysmyelinogenic leukodystrophy, *J Neuropathol Exp Neurol*, 18:359-383, 1959.

111. Adams RD, Lyon G: *Neurology of Hereditary Metabolic Diseases of Children*, New York: 1982, McGraw-Hill.

112. Neal JW, Cave EM, Singhrao SK, Cole G, et al: Alexander's disease in infancy and childhood: A report of 2 cases, *Acta Neuropathol (Berl)*, 84:322-327, 1992.

113. Pridmore CL, Baraitser M, Harding B, Boyd SG, et al: Alexander's disease: Clues to diagnosis, *J Child Neurol*, 8:134-144, 1993.

114. Springer S, Erlewein R, Naegele E, Becker I, et al: Alexander disease: Classification revisited and isolation of a neonatal form, *Neuropediatrics*, 31:86-92, 2000.

115. Gingold MK, Bodensteiner JB, Schochet SS, Jaynes M: Alexander's disease: Unique presentation, *J Child Neurol*, 14:325-329, 1999.

116. Bassuk AG, Joshi A, Burton BK, Larsen MB, et al: Alexander disease with serial MRS and a new mutation in the glial fibrillary acidic protein gene, *Neurology*, 61:1014-1016, 2003.

117. Gordon N: Alexander disease, *Eur J Paediatr Neurol*, 7:395-399, 2003.

118. Kyllerman M, Rosengren L, Wiklund LM, Holmberg E: Increased levels of GFAP in the cerebrospinal fluid in three subtypes of genetically confirmed Alexander disease, *Neuropediatrics*, 36:319-323, 2005.

119. Messing A, Goldman JE, Johnson AB, Brenner M: Alexander disease: New insights from genetics, *J Neuropathol Exp Neurol*, 60:563-573, 2001.

120. Meins M, Brockmann K, Yadav S, Haupt M, et al: Infantile Alexander disease: A GFAP mutation in monozygotic twins and novel mutations in two other patients, *Neuropediatrics*, 33:194-198, 2002.

121. van der Knaap MS, Salomons GS, Li R, Franzoni E, et al: Unusual variants of Alexander's disease, *Ann Neurol*, 57:327-338, 2005.

122. Li R, Johnson AB, Salomons G, Goldman JE, et al: Glial fibrillary acidic protein mutations in infantile, juvenile, and adult forms of Alexander disease, *Ann Neurol*, 57:310-326, 2005.

123. Trommer BL, Naidich TP, Dal Canto MC, McLone DG, et al: Noninvasive CT diagnosis of infantile Alexander disease: Pathologic correlation, *J Comput Assist Tomogr*, 7:509-516, 1983.

124. Farrell K, Chuang S, Becker LE: Computed tomography in Alexander's disease, *Ann Neurol*, 15:605-607, 1984.

125. Bosnjak V, Besenski N, Della-Marina BM, Polak J: Ultrasonography in hereditary degenerative diseases of the cerebral white matter in infancy, *Neuropediatrics*, 19:208-211, 1988.

126. Schochet SS Jr, Lampert PW, Earle KM: Alexander's disease: A case report with electron microscopic observations, *Neurology*, 18:543-549, 1968.

127. Jaeken J: Alexander disease and intermediate filaments in astrocytes: A fatal gain of function, *Eur J Paediatr Neurol*, 5:151-153, 2001.

128. Goldman JE: Regulation of oligodendrocyte differentiation, *Trends Neurosci*, 15:359-362, 1992.

129. Iwaki T, Kume-Iwaki A, Liem RK, Goldman JE: αβ-crystallin is expressed in non-lenticular tissues and accumulates in Alexander's disease brain, *Cell*, 57:71-78, 1989.

130. Herndon RM: Is Alexander's disease a nosologic entity or a common pathologic pattern of diverse etiology? *J Child Neurol*, 14:275-278, 1999.

131. Graf WD, Sarnat HB: Intermediate filament proteinopathies: From cytoskeletons to genes to functional nosology, *Neurology*, 58:1451-1453, 2002.

132. Gorospe JR, Naidu S, Johnson AB, Puri V, et al: Molecular findings in symptomatic and pre-symptomatic Alexander disease patients, *Neurology*, 58:1494-1500, 2002.

133. Clarke JT, Ozere RL, Krause VW: Early infantile variant of Krabbe globoid cell leucodystrophy with lung involvement, *Arch Dis Child*, 56:640-642, 1981.

134. Suzuki K, Suzuki Y, Suzuki K: Galactosylceramide lipidosis: Globoid-cell leukodystrophy (Krabbe disease). In Scriver CR, Beaudet AL, Sly WS, et al, editors: *The Metabolic and Molecular Bases of Inherited Disease*, 7th ed, New York: 1995, McGraw-Hill.

135. Hagberg B: Krabbe's disease: Clinical presentation of neurological variants, *Neuropediatrics*, 15:11-15, 1984.

136. Ida H, Rennert OM, Watabe K, Eto Y, et al: Pathological and biochemical studies of the fetal Krabbe disease, *Brain Dev*, 16:480-484, 1995.

137. Zafeiriou DI, Anastasiou AL, Michaelakaki EM, Augoustidou-Savvopoulos PA, et al: Early infantile Krabbe disease: Deceptively normal magnetic resonance imaging and serial neurophysiological studies, *Brain Dev*, 19:488-491, 1997.

138. Wenger DA, Suzuki K, Suzuki Y, Suzuki K: Galactosylceramide lipidosis: Globoid cell leukodystrophy (Krabbe disease). In Scriver CR, Beaudet MD, Sly WS, et al, editors: *The Metabolic and Molecular Bases of Inherited Disease*, 8th ed, New York: 2001, McGraw-Hill.

139. Sahai I, Baris H, Kimonis V, Levy HL: Krabbe disease: Severe neonatal presentation with a family history of multiple sclerosis, *J Child Neurol*, 20:826-828, 2005.

140. Hagberg B, Kollberg H, Sourander P, Akesson HO: Infantile globoid cell leukodystrophy (Krabbe's disease): A clinical and genetic study of 32 Swedish cases 1953–1967, *Neuropadiatrie*, 1:74-88, 1969.

141. Martin JJ, Leroy JG, Ceuterick C, Libert J, et al: Fetal Krabbe leukodystrophy: A morphologic study of two cases, *Acta Neuropathol (Berl)*, 53:87-91, 1981.

142. Lieberman JS, Oshtory M, Taylor RG, Dreyfus PM: Perinatal neuropathy as an early manifestation of Krabbe's disease, *Arch Neurol*, 37:446-447, 1980.

143. Husain AM, Altuwaijri M, Aldosari M: Krabbe disease: Neurophysiologic studies and MRI correlations, *Neurology*, 63:617-620, 2004.

144. Kobayashi T, Goto I, Yamanaka T, Suzuki Y, et al: Infantile and fetal globoid cell leukodystrophy: Analysis of galactosylceramide and galactosylsphingosine, *Ann Neurol*, 24:517-522, 1988.

145. Suzuki K: Twenty five years of the "psychosine hypothesis": A personal perspective of its history and present status, *Neurochem Res*, 23: 251-259, 1998.

146. Suzuki K, Suzuki Y: Globoid cell leucodystrophy (Krabbe's disease): Deficiency of galactocerebroside beta-galactosidase, *Proc Natl Acad Sci U S A*, 66:302-309, 1970.

147. Escolar ML, Poe MD, Provenzale JM, Richards KC, et al: Transplantation of umbilical-cord blood in babies with infantile Krabbe's disease, *N Engl J Med*, 352:2069-2081, 2005.

148. Ulrich J, Herschkowitz N: Seitelberger's connatal form of Pelizaeus-Merzbacher disease: Case report, clinical, pathological and biochemical findings, *Acta Neuropathol (Berl)*, 40:129-136, 1977.

149. Seitelberger F: Pelizaeus-Merzbacher disease. In Vonken PJ, Bruyn GW, editors: *Handbook of Clinical Neurology*, Amsterdam: 1970, Elsevier North-Holland.

150. Renier WO, Gabreels FJ, Hustinx TW, Jaspar HH, et al: Connatal Pelizaeus-Merzbacher disease with congenital stridor in two maternal cousins, *Acta Neuropathol (Berl)*, 54:11-17, 1981.

151. Scheffer IE, Baraitser M, Wilson J, Harding B, et al: Pelizaeus-Merzbacher disease: Classical or connatal? *Neuropediatrics*, 22:71-78, 1991.

152. Haenggeli CA, Engel E, Pizzolato GP: Connatal Pelizaeus-Merzbacher disease, *Dev Med Child Neurol*, 31:803-807, 1989.

153. Cassidy SB, Sheehan NC, Farrell DF, Grunnet M, et al: Connatal Pelizaeus-Merzbacher disease: An autosomal recessive form, *Pediatr Neurol*, 3:300-305, 1987.

154. Boulloche J, Aicardi J: Pelizaeus-Merzbacher disease: Clinical and nosological study, *J Child Neurol*, 1:233-239, 1986.

155. Begleiter ML, Harris DJ: Autosomal recessive form of connatal Pelizaeus-Merzbacher disease, *Am J Med Genet*, 33:311-313, 1989.

156. Novotny EJ Jr: Arthrogryposis associated with connatal Pelizaeus-Merzbacher disease: Case report, *Neuropediatrics*, 19:221-223, 1988.

157. Shimomura C, Matsui A, Choh H, Funahashi M, et al: Magnetic resonance imaging in Pelizaeus-Merzbacher disease, *Pediatr Neurol*, 4:124-125, 1988.

158. Baudon JJ, Escourolle R, Polonovski C, Berger B, et al: Leucodystrophie soudanophile congénitale massive: Étude anatomo-clinique d'une observation, *Ann Pediatr (Paris)*, 1973:501-506, 1973.

159. Sugita K, Ishii M, Takanashi J, Suzuki N, et al: Pelizaeus-Merzbacher disease: Cellular hypersensitivity to ultraviolet light, *Brain Dev*, 14:44-47, 1992.

160. Apkarian P, Koetsveldbaart JC, Barth PG: Visual evoked potential characteristics and early diagnosis of Pelizaeus-Merzbacher disease, *Arch Neurol*, 50:981-985, 1993.

161. Carango P, Funanage VL, Quiros RE, Debruyn CS, et al: Overexpression of DM20 messenger RNA in two brothers with Pelizaeus-Merzbacher disease, *Ann Neurol*, 38:610-617, 1995.

162. Nezu A, Kimura S, Uehara S, Osaka H, et al: Pelizaeus-Merzbacher-like disease: Female case report, *Brain Dev*, 18:114-118, 1996.

163. Wang PJ, Young C, Liu HM, Chang YC, et al: Neurophysiologic studies and MRI in Pelizaeus-Merzbacher disease: Comparison of classic and connatal forms, *Pediatr Neurol*, 12:47-53, 1995.

164. Wang PJ, Hwu WL, Lee WT, Wang TR, et al: Duplication of proteolipid protein gene: A possible major cause of Pelizaeus-Merzbacher disease, *Pediatr Neurol*, 17:125-128, 1997.

165. Komaki H, Sasaki M, Yamamoto T, Iai M, et al: Connatal Pelizaeus-Merzbacher disease associated with the Jimpy^{msd} mice mutation, *Pediatr Neurol*, 20:309-311, 1999.

166. Inoue K, Osaka H, Imaizumi K, Nezu A, et al: Proteolipid protein gene duplications causing Pelizaeus-Merzbacher disease: Molecular mechanism and phenotypic manifestations, *Ann Neurol*, 45:624-632, 1999.

167. Golomb MR, Walsh LE, Carvalho KS, Christensen CK, et al: Clinical findings in Pelizaeus-Merzbacher disease, *J Child Neurol*, 19:328-331, 2004.

168. Plecko B, Stockler-Ipsiroglu S, Gruber S, Mlynarik V, et al: Degree of hypomyelination and magnetic resonance spectroscopy findings in patients with Pelizaeus Merzbacher phenotype, *Neuropediatrics*, 34:127-136, 2003.

169. Takanashi J, Inoue K, Tomita M, Kurihara A, et al: Brain *N*-acetylaspartate is elevated in Pelizaeus-Merzbacher disease with *PLP1* duplication, *Neurology*, 58:237-241, 2002.

170. Hanefeld FA, Brockmann K, Pouwels PJ, Wilken B, et al: Quantitative proton MRS of Pelizaeus-Merzbacher disease: Evidence of dys- and hypomyelination, *Neurology*, 65:701-706, 2005.

171. Wolf NI, Sistermans EA, Cundall M, Hobson GM, et al: Three or more copies of the proteolipid protein gene *PLP1* cause severe Pelizaeus-Merzbacher disease, *Brain*, 128:743-751, 2005.

172. Gencic S, Abuelo D, Ambler M, Hudson LD: Pelizaeus-Merzbacher disease: An X-linked neurologic disorder of myelin metabolism with a novel mutation in the gene encoding proteolipid protein, *Am J Hum Genet*, 45:435-442, 1989.

173. Pratt VM, Trofatter JA, Larsen MB, Hodes ME, et al: New variant in exon 3 of the proteolipid protein (PLP) gene in a family with Pelizaeus-Merzbacher disease, *Am J Med Genet*, 43:642-646, 1992.

174. Otterbach B, Stoffel W, Ramaekers V: A novel mutation in the proteolipid protein gene leading to Pelizaeus-Merzbacher disease, *Biol Chem Hoppe-Seyler*, 374:75-83, 1993.

175. Hodes ME, Pratt VM, Dlouhy SR: Genetics of Pelizaeus-Merzbacher disease, *Dev Neurosci*, 15:383-394, 1993.

176. Boespflug-Tanguy O, Mimault C, Melki J, Cavagna A, et al: Genetic homogeneity of Pelizaeus-Merzbacher disease: Tight linkage to the proteoliprotein locus in 16 affected families, *Am J Hum Genet*, 55:461-467, 1994.

177. Gow A, Lazzarini RA: A cellular mechanism governing the severity of Pelizaeus-Merzbacher disease, *Nat Genet*, 13:422-428, 1996.

178. Osaka H, Kawanishi C, Inoue K, Onishi H, et al: Pelizaeus-Merzbacher disease: Three novel mutations and implication for locus heterogeneity, *Ann Neurol*, 45:59-64, 1999.

179. Garbern JY: Pelizaeus-Merzbacher disease: Pathogenic mechanisms and insights into the roles of proteolipid protein 1 in the nervous system, *J Neurol Sci*, 228:201-203, 2005.

180. Percy AK: Pelizaeus-Merzbacher disease: Splice sites are nice sites for disease expression, *Neurology*, 55:1072-1073, 2000.

181. Bugiani M, Al Shahwan S, Lamantea E, Bizzi A, et al: *GJA12* mutations in children with recessive hypomyelinating leukoencephalopathy, *Neurology*, 67:273-279, 2006.

182. Sarnat HB, Adelman LS: Perinatal sudanophilic leukodystrophy, *Am J Dis Child*, 125:281-285, 1973.

183. Ramsey RB, Banik NL, Ramsey PT, Cuzner ML, et al: Neurochemical findings in a perinatal sudanophilic leukodystrophy rich in steryl ester, *J Neurol Sci*, 30:95-111, 1976.

184. Wolf NI, Willemsen MA, Engelke UF, van der Knaap MS, et al: Severe hypomyelination associated with increased levels of *N*-acetylaspartylglutamate in CSF, *Neurology*, 62:1503-1508, 2004.

185. Uhlenberg B, Schuelke M, Ruschendorf F, Ruf N, et al: Mutations in the gene encoding gap junction protein alpha 12 (Connexin 46.6) cause Pelizaeus-Merzbacher–like disease, *Am J Hum Genet*, 75:251-260, 2004.

186. Nance MA, Berry SA: Cocayne syndrome: Review of 140 cases, *Am J Med Genet*, 42:68-84, 1992.

187. Cleaver JE, Kraemer KH: Xeroderma pigmentosum. In Scriver CR, Baudet AL, Sly WS, et al, editors: *The Metabolic Basis of Inherited Disease*, 6th ed, New York: 1989, McGraw-Hill.

188. Razavi-Encha F, Larroche JC, Gaillard D: Infantile familial encephalopathy with cerebral calcifications and leukodystrophy, *Neuropediatrics*, 19:72-79, 1988.

189. Babbitt DP, Tang T, Dobbs J, Berk R: Idiopathic familial cerebrovascular ferrocalcinosis (Fahr's disease) and review of differential diagnosis of intracranial calcification in children, *AJR Am J Roentgenol*, 105:352-358, 1969.

190. Jervis GA: Microcephaly with extensive calcium deposits and demyelination, *J Neuropathol Exp Neurol*, 13:318-329, 1954.

191. Melchior JC, Benda C, Yakovlev P: Familial idiopathic cerebral calcifications in childhood, *Am J Dis Child*, 99:787-803, 1960.

192. Troost D, van Rossum A, Veiga-Pires J, Willemse J: Cerebral calcifications and cerebellar hypoplasia in two children: Clinical, radiologic and neuropathological studies—a separate neurodevelopmental entity, *Neuropediatrics*, 15:102-109, 1984.

193. Boltshauser E, Steinlin M, Boesch C, Martin E, et al: Magnetic resonance imaging in infantile encephalopathy with cerebral calcification and leukodystrophy, *Neuropediatrics*, 22:33-35, 1991.

194. Bonnemann CG, Meinecke P: Encephalopathy of infancy with intracerebral calcification and chronic spinal fluid lymphocytosis: Another case of the Aicardi-Goutieres syndrome, *Neuropediatrics*, 23:157-161, 1992.

195. Tolmie JL, Shillito P, Hughesbenzie R, Stephenson J: The Aicardi-Goutieres syndrome (familial, early onset encephalopathy with calcifications of the basal ganglia and chronic cerebrospinal fluid lymphocytosis), *J Med Genet*, 32:881-884, 1995.

196. Verrips A, Hiel JA, Gabreels FJ, Wesseling P, et al: The Aircardi-Goutieres syndrome: Variable clinical expression in two siblings, *Pediatr Neurol*, 16:323-325, 1997.

197. McEntagart M, Kamel H, Lebon P, King MD: Aicardi-Goutieres syndrome: An expanding phenotype, *Neuropediatrics*, 29:163-167, 1998.

198. Goutieres F, Aicardi J, Barth PG, Lebon P: Aicardi-Goutieres syndrome: An update and results of interferon-α studies, *Ann Neurol*, 44:900-907, 1998.

199. Ostergaard JR, Christensen T, Nehen AM: A distinct difference in clinical expression of two siblings with Aicardi-Goutieres syndrome, *Neuropediatrics*, 30:38-41, 1999.

200. Barth PG: The neuropathology of Aicardi-Goutieres syndrome, *Eur J Paediatr Neurol*, 6:A27-A31, 2002.

201. Rasmussen M, Skullerud K, Bakke SJ, Lebon P, et al: Cerebral thrombotic microangiopathy and antiphospholipid antibodies in Aicardi-Goutieres syndrome: Report of two sisters, *Neuropediatrics*, 36:40-44, 2005.

202. Lanzi G, Fazzi E, D'Arrigo S: Aicardi-Goutieres syndrome: A description of 21 new cases and a comparison with the literature, *Eur J Paediatr Neurol*, 6:A9-A22, 2002.

203. Abdel-Salam GMH, Zaki MS, Lebon P, Meguid NA: Aicardi-Goutieres syndrome: Clinical and neuroradiological findings of 10 new cases, *Acta Paediatr*, 93:929-936, 2004.

204. Lanzi G, Fazzi E, D'Arrigo S, Orcesi S, et al: The natural history of Aicardi-Goutieres syndrome: Follow-up of 11 Italian patients, *Neurology*, 64:1621-1624, 2005.

205. Aicardi J: Aicardi-Goutieres syndrome: Special type early-onset encephalopathy, *Eur J Paediatr Neurol*, 6:A1-A7, 2002.

206. Ostergaard JR, Christensen T: Aicardi-Goutieres syndrome: Neuroradiological findings after nine years of follow-up, *Eur J Paediatr Neurol*, 8:243-246, 2004.

207. Robertson NJ, Stafler P, Battini R, Cheong J, et al: Brain lactic alkalosis in Aicardi-Goutieres syndrome, *Neuropediatrics*, 35:20-26, 2004.

208. Goutieres F: Aicardi-Goutieres syndrome, *Brain Dev*, 27:201-206, 2005.

209. Sanchis A, Cervero L, Bataller A, Tortajada JL, et al: Genetic syndromes mimic congenital infections, *J Pediatr*, 146:701-705, 2005.

210. Lebon P, Meritet JF, Krivine A, Rozenberg F: Interferon and Aicardi-Goutieres syndrome, *Eur J Paediatr Neurol*, 6:A47-A53, 2002.

211. Barlow CF, Priebe CJ, Mulliken JB, Barnes PD, et al: Spastic diplegia as a complication of interferon Alfa-2a treatment of hemangiomas of infancy, *J Pediatr*, 132:527-530, 1998.

211a. Crow YJ, Hayward BE, Parmar R, Robins P, et al: Mutations in the gene encoding the 3'-5' DNA exonuclease TREX1 cause Aicardi-Goutieres syndrome at the AGS1 locus, *Nat Genet*, 38:917-920, 2006.

211b. Rice G, Patrick T, Parmar R, Taylor CF, et al: Clinical and molecular phenotype of Aicardi-Goutieres syndrome, *Am J Hum Genet*, 81:713-725, 2007.

212. Lazarow PB, Moser HW: Disorders of peroxisome biogenesis. In Scriver CR, Beaudet AL, Sly WS, et al, editors: *The Metabolic and Molecular Bases of Inherited Disease*, 7th ed, New York: 1995, McGraw-Hill.

213. Moser HW: Peroxisomal disorders, *Ment Retard Dev Disabil Res Rev*, 2:177-183, 1996.

214. Wanders RJ, Barth PG, Heymans HS: Single peroxisomal enzyme deficiencies. In Scriver CR, Beaudet MD, Sly WS, et al, editors: *The Metabolic and Molecular Bases of Inherited Disease*, 8th ed, New York: 2001, McGraw-Hill.

215. Gould SJ, Raymond GV, Valle D: The peroxisome biogenesis disorders. In Scriver CR, Beaudet MD, Sly WS, et al, editors: *The Metabolic and Molecular Bases of Inherited Disease*, 8th ed, New York: 2001, McGraw-Hill.

216. Moser HW: Lysosomal and peroxisomal disease. In Siegel GJ, Albers RW, Brady ST, et al, editors: *Basic Neurochemistry: Molecular, Cellular and Medical Aspects*, New York: 2006, Elsevier.

217. Ferdinandusse S, Denis S, Mooyer PA, Dekker C, et al: Clinical and biochemical spectrum of D-bifunctional protein deficiency, *Ann Neurol*, 59:92-104, 2006.

218. Reuber BE, Germain-Lee E, Collins CS: Mutations in *PEX1* are the most common cause of peroxisome biogenesis disorders, *Nat Genet*, 17:445-448, 1997.

219. Powers JM, Moser HW: Peroxisomal disorders: Genotype, phenotype, major neuropathologic lesions and pathogenesis, *Brain Pathol*, 8:101-120, 1998.

220. Yahraus T, Braverman N, Dodt G: The peroxisome biogenesis disorder group 4 gene, *PXAAA1*, encodes a cytoplasmic ATPase required for stability of the *PTS1* receptor, *EMBO J*, 15:2914-2923, 1996.

221. Noetzel MJ: Fish oil and myelin: Cautious optimism for treatment of children with disorders of peroxisome biogenesis, *Neurology*, 51:5-7, 1998.

222. Geisbrecht BV, Collins CS, Reuber BE, Gould SJ: Disruption of a *PEX1-PEX6* interaction is the most common cause of the neurologic disorders Zellweger syndrome, neonatal adrenoleukodystrophy, and infantile Refsum disease, *Proc Natl Acad Sci U S A*, 95:8630-8635, 1998.

223. Rizzo WB: Peroxisome 1, 2, 3..., *Ann Neurol*, 47:281-283, 2000.
224. Wei H, Kemp S, McGuinness MC, Moser AB, et al: Pharmacological induction of peroxisomes in peroxisome biogenesis disorders, *Ann Neurol*, 47:286-296, 2000.
225. Percy AK: Metabolic disease with central nervous system involvement, *Curr Opin Pediatr*, 3:950-958, 1991.
226. Moser HW: New approaches in peroxisomal disorders, *Dev Neurosci*, 9:1-18, 1987.
227. Moser HW: The peroxisome: Nervous system role of a previously underrated organelle: The 1987 Robert Wartenberg lecture, *Neurology*, 38:1617-1627, 1988.
228. Naidu S, Moser AE, Moser HW: Phenotypic and genotypic variability of generalized peroxisomal disorders, *Pediatr Neurol*, 4:5-12, 1988.
229. Gordon N: Peroxisomal disorders, *Brain Dev*, 9:571-575, 1987.
230. Wanders RJ, van Roermund CW, Schutgens RB, Barth PG, et al: The inborn errors of peroxisomal β-oxidation: A review, *J Inherit Metab Dis*, 13:4-36, 1990.
231. Gartner J, Chen WW, Kelley RI, Mihalik SJ, et al: The 22-kD peroxisomal integral membrane protein in Zellweger syndrome: Presence, abundance, and association with a peroxisomal thiolase precursor protein, *Pediatr Res*, 29:141-146, 1991.
232. Balfe A, Hoefler G, Chen WW, Watkins PA: Aberrant subcellular localization of peroxisomal 3-ketoacyl-CoA thiolase in the Zellweger syndrome and rhizomelic chondrodysplasia punctata, *Pediatr Res*, 27:304-310, 1990.
233. Shimozawa N, Suzuki Y, Orii T, Yokota S, et al: Biochemical and morphologic aspects of peroxisomes in the human rectal mucosa: Diagnosis of Zellweger syndrome simplified by rectal biopsy, *Pediatr Res*, 24:723-727, 1988.
234. Schram AW, Strijland A, Hashimoto T, Wanders RJ, et al: Biosynthesis and maturation of peroxisomal β-oxidation enzymes in fibroblasts in relation to the Zellweger syndrome and infantile Refsum disease, *Proc Natl Acad Sci U S A*, 83:6156-6158, 1986.
235. Govaerts L, Colon E, Rotteveel J, Monnens L: A neurophysiological study of children with the cerebro-hepato-renal syndrome of Zellweger, *Neuropediatrics*, 16:185-190, 1985.
236. Wilson GN, Holmes RG, Custer J, Lipkowitz JL, et al: Zellweger syndrome: Diagnostic assays, syndrome delineation, and potential therapy, *Am J Med Genet*, 24:69-82, 1986.
237. Aubourg P, Robain O, Rocchiccioli F, Dancea S, et al: The cerebro-hepato-renal (Zellweger) syndrome: Lamellar lipid profiles in adrenocortical, hepatic mesenchymal, astrocyte cells and increased levels of very long chain fatty acids and phytanic acid in the plasma, *J Neurol Sci*, 69:9-25, 1985.
238. Kamei A, Houdou S, Takashima S, Suzuki Y, et al: Peroxisomal disorders in children: Immunohistochemistry and neuropathology, *J Pediatr*, 122:573-579, 1993.
239. Baumgartner MR, Poll-The BT, Verhoeven NM, Jakobs C, et al: Clinical approach to inherited peroxisomal disorders: A series of 27 patients, *Ann Neurol*, 44:720-730, 1998.
240. Baumgartner MR, Verhoeven NM, Jakobs C, Roels F, et al: Defective peroxisome biogenesis with a neuromuscular disorder resembling Werdnig-Hoffman disease, *Neurology*, 51:1427-1432, 1998.
241. Nakai A, Shigematsu Y, Nishida K, Kikawa Y, et al: MRI findings of Zellweger syndrome, *Pediatr Neurol*, 13:346-348, 1995.
242. Volpe JJ, Adams RD: Cerebro-hepato-renal syndrome of Zellweger: An inherited disorder of neuronal migration, *Acta Neuropathol (Berl)*, 20:175-198, 1972.
243. Evrard P, Caviness VS Jr, Prats-Vinas J, Lyon G: The mechanism of arrest of neuronal migration in the Zellweger malformation: An hypothesis bases upon cytoarchitectonic analysis, *Acta Neuropathol (Berl)*, 41:109-117, 1978.
244. Kaufmann WE, Theda C, Naidu S, Watkins PA, et al: Neuronal migration abnormality in peroxisomal bifunctional enzyme defect, *Ann Neurol*, 39:268-271, 1996.
245. Watkins PA, McGuinness MC, Raymond GV, Sisk JM, et al: Distinction between peroxisomal bifunctional enzyme and acyl-CoA oxidase deficiencies, *Ann Neurol*, 38:472-477, 1995.
246. Martinez M, Vazquez E: MRI evidence that docosahexaenoic acid ethyl ester improves myelination in generalized peroxisomal disorders, *Neurology*, 51:26-32, 1998.
247. Kelley RI, Datta NS, Dobyns WB, Hajra AK, et al: Neonatal adrenoleukodystrophy: New cases, biochemical studies, and differentiation from Zellweger and related peroxisomal polydystrophy syndromes, *Am J Med Genet*, 23:869-901, 1986.
248. Mito T, Takada K, Akaboshi S, Takashima S, et al: A pathological study of a peripheral nerve in a case of neonatal adrenoleukodystrophy, *Acta Neuropathol (Berl)*, 77:437-440, 1989.
249. Wolff J, Nyhan WL, Powell H, Takahashi D, et al: Myopathy in an infant with a fatal peroxisomal disorder, *Pediatr Neurol*, 2:141-146, 1986.
250. Aubourg P, Scotto J, Rocchiccioli F, Feldmann-Pautrat D, et al: Neonatal adrenoleukodystrophy, *J Neurol Neurosurg Psychiatry*, 49:77-86, 1986.
251. Brown FR, Voigt R, Singh AK, Singh I: Peroxisomal disorders: Neurodevelopmental and biochemical aspects, *Am J Dis Child*, 147:617-626, 1993.
252. Moser AB, Kreiter N, Bezman L, Lu SE, et al: Plasma very long chain fatty acids in 3,000 peroxisome disease patients and 29,000 controls, *Ann Neurol*, 45:100-110, 1999.
253. Santos MJ, Imanaka T, Shio H, Small GM, et al: Peroxisomal membrane ghosts in Zellweger syndrome: Aberrant organelle assembly, *Science*, 239:1536-1538, 1988.
254. van der Knaap MS, Valk J: The MR spectrum of peroxisomal disorders, *Neuroradiology*, 33:30-37, 1991.
255. Moser AB, Borel J, Odone A, Naidu S, et al: A new dietary therapy for adrenoleukodystrophy: Biochemical and preliminary clinical results in 36 patients, *Ann Neurol*, 21:240-249, 1987.
256. Kaplan PW, Tusa RJ, Shankroff J, Heller JE, et al: Visual evoked potentials in adrenoleukodystrophy: A trial with glycerol trioleate and Lorenzo oil, *Ann Neurol*, 34:169-174, 1993.
257. Moser HW: Lorenzo oil therapy for adrenoleukodystrophy: A prematurely amplified hope, *Ann Neurol*, 34:121-122, 1993.
258. Rizzo WB: Lorenzo oil: Hope and disappointment, *N Engl J Med*, 329:801-802, 1993.
259. Moser HW, Smith KD, Watkins PA, Powers J, et al: X-linked adrenoleukodystrophy. In Scriver CR, Beaudet MD, Sly WS, et al, editors: *The Metabolic and Molecular Bases of Inherited Disease*, 8th ed, New York: 2001, McGraw-Hill.
260. Moser HW, Raymond GV, Lu SE, Muenz LR, et al: Follow-up of 89 asymptomatic patients with adrenoleukodystrophy treated with Lorenzo's oil, *Arch Neurol*, 62:1073-1080, 2005.
261. DiMauro S, Bonilla E, Lombes A, Shanske S, et al: Mitochondrial encephalomyopathies, *Pediatr Neurol*, 8:483-506, 1990.
262. DiMauro S, Moraes CT, Schon EA: Mitochondrial encephalomyopathies: Problems of classification. In Sato T, DiMauro S, editors: *Progress in Neuropathology*, New York: 1991, Raven Press.
263. DeVivo DC: The expanding clinical spectrum of mitochondrial diseases, *Brain Dev*, 15:1-22, 1993.
264. Poulton J: Mitochondrial DNA and genetic disease, *Dev Med Child Neurol*, 35:833-840, 1993.
265. DiMauro S: Mitochondrial encephalomyopathies: What next? *J Inherit Metab Dis*, 19:489-503, 1996.
266. DiMauro S, Schon EA: Mechanisms of disease: Mitochondrial respiratory-chain diseases, *N Engl J Med*, 348:2657-2668, 2003.
267. Zeviani M, Di Donato S: Mitochondrial disorders, *Brain*, 127:2153-2172, 2004.
268. DiMauro S, Hirano M: Mitochondrial encephalomyopathies: An update, *Neuromusc Dis*, 15:276-286, 2005.
269. Bohm M, Pronicka E, Karczmarewicz E, Pronicki M, et al: Retrospective, multicentric study of 180 children with cytochrome c oxidase deficiency, *Pediatr Res*, 59:21-26, 2006.
270. DiMauro S, DeVivo DC: Diseases of carbohydrate, fatty acid and mitochondrial metabolism. In Siegel GJ, Albers RW, Brady ST, et al, editors: *Basic Neurochemistry: Molecular, Cellular and Medical Aspects*, 7th ed, New York: 2006, Elsevier.
271. Tom MI, Rewcastle NB: Infantile subacute necrotizing encephalopathy, *Neurology*, 12:624, 1962.
272. Lewis AJ: Infantile subacute necrotizing encephalopathy, *Can Med Assoc J*, 93:878-881, 1965.
273. Feigin I, Kim HS: Subacute necrotizing encephalomyelopathy in a neonatal infant, *J Neuropathol Exp Neurol*, 36:364-372, 1977.
274. Seitz RJ, Langes K, Frenzel H, Kluitmann G, et al: Congenital Leigh's disease: Panencephalomyelopathy and peripheral neuropathy, *Acta Neuropathol (Berl)*, 64:167-171, 1984.
275. Old SE, De Vivo DC: Pyruvate dehydrogenase complex deficiency: Biochemical and immunoblot analysis of cultured skin fibroblasts, *Ann Neurol*, 26:746-751, 1989.
276. Lombes A, Nakase H, Tritschler HJ, Kadenbach B, et al: Biochemical and molecular analysis of cytochrome c oxidase deficiency in Leigh's syndrome, *Neurology*, 41:491-498, 1991.
277. DiMauro S, Servidei S, Zeviani M, DiRocco M, et al: Cytochrome c oxidase deficiency in Leigh syndrome, *Ann Neurol*, 22:498-506, 1987.
278. Paulus W, Peiffer J: Intracerebral distribution of mitochondrial abnormalities in 21 cases of infantile spongy dystrophy, *J Neurol Sci*, 95:49-62, 1990.
279. Shoffner JM, Fernhoff PM, Krawiecki NS, Caplan DB, et al: Subacute necrotizing encephalopathy: Oxidative phosphorylation defects and the ATPase 6 point mutation, *Neurology*, 42:2168-2174, 1992.
280. Sperl W, Ruitenbeek W, Sengers RC, Trijbels JM, et al: Combined deficiencies of the pyruvate dehydrogenase complex and enzymes of the respiratory chain in mitochondrial myopathies, *Eur J Pediatr*, 151:192-195, 1992.
281. Matthews PM, Marchington DR, Squier M, Land J, et al: Molecular genetic characterization of an X-linked form of Leigh's syndrome, *Ann Neurol*, 33:652-655, 1993.
282. Macaya A, Munell F, Burke RE, De Vivo DC: Disorders of movement in Leigh syndrome, *Neuropediatrics*, 24:60-67, 1993.
283. Yoshinaga H, Ogino T, Ohtahara S, Sakuta R, et al: A T-to-G mutation at nucleotide pair 8993 in mitochondrial DNA in a patient with Leigh's syndrome, *J Child Neurol*, 8:129-133, 1993.
284. Samsom JF, Barth PG, Devries J, Menko FH, et al: Familial mitochondrial encephalopathy with fetal ultrasonographic ventriculomegaly and intracerebral calcifications, *Eur J Pediatr*, 153:510-516, 1994.

285. Dionisi-Vico C, Ruitenbeck W, Fariello G, Bentlage H, et al: New familial mitochondrial encephalopathy with macrocephaly, cardiomyopathy, and complex I deficiency, *Ann Neurol*, 42:661-665, 1997.

286. Morris AA, Leonard JV, Brown GK, Bidouki SK, et al: Deficiency of respiratory chain complex I is a common cause of Leigh disease, *Ann Neurol*, 40:25-30, 1996.

287. Rahman S, Blok RB, Dahl HH, Danks DM, et al: Leigh syndrome: Clinical features and biochemical and DNA abnormalities, *Ann Neurol*, 39:343-351, 1996.

288. DiMauro S, DeVivo DC: Genetic heterogeneity in Leigh syndrome, *Ann Neurol*, 40:5-7, 1996.

289. Kirby DM, Crawford M, Cleary MA, Dahl HH, et al: Respiratory chain complex I deficiency: An underdiagnosed energy generation disorder, *Neurology*, 52:1255-1264, 1999.

290. Feillet F, Mousson B, Grignon Y, Leonard JV, et al: Necrotizing encephalopathy and macrocephaly with mitochondrial complex I deficiency, *Pediatr Neurol*, 20:305-308, 1999.

291. Absolon MJ, Harding CO, Fain DR, Mack KJ: Leigh syndrome in an infant resulting from mitochondrial DNA depletion, *Pediatr Neurol*, 24:60-63, 2001.

292. Sue CM, Bruno C, Andrea AL, Cargan A, et al: Infantile encephalopathy associated with the MELAS *A3243G* mutation, *J Pediatr*, 134:696-700, 1999.

293. Sacconi S, Salviati L, Sue CM, Shanske S, et al: Mutation screening in patients with isolated cytochrome c oxidase deficiency, *Pediatr Res*, 53:224-230, 2003.

294. McFarland R, Kirby DM, Fowler KJ, Ohtake A, et al: De novo mutations in the mitochondrial *ND3* gene as a cause of infantile mitochondrial encephalopathy and complex I deficiency, *Ann Neurol*, 55:58-64, 2004.

295. Dinopoulos A, Cecil KM, Schapiro MB, Papadimitriou A, et al: Brain MRI and proton MRS findings in infants and children with respiratory chain defects, *Neuropediatrics*, 36:290-301, 2005.

296. Esteitie N, Hinttala R, Wibom R, Nilsson H, et al: Secondary metabolic effects in complex I deficiency, *Ann Neurol*, 58:544-552, 2005.

297. Fernandez-Moreira D, Ugalde C, Smeets R, Rodenburg RJ, et al: X-linked *NDUFA1* gene mutations associated with mitochondrial encephalomyopathy, *Ann Neurol*, 61:73-83, 2007.

297a. Debray FG, Lambert M, Chevalier I, Robitaille Y, et al: Long-term outcome and clinical spectrum of 73 pediatric patients with mitochondrial diseases, *Pediatrics*, 119:722-733, 2007.

298. Medina L, Chi TL, DeVivo DC, Hilal SK: MR findings in patients with subacute necrotizing encephalomyelopathy (Leigh syndrome): Correlation with biochemical defect, *AJNR Am J Neuroradiol*, 11:379-384, 1990.

299. Kimura S, Kobayashi T, Amemiya F: Myelin splitting in the spongy lesion in Leigh encephalopathy, *Pediatr Neurol*, 7:56-58, 1991.

300. Yamagata T, Yano S, Okabe I, Miyao M, et al: Ultrasonography and magnetic resonance imaging in Leigh disease, *Pediatr Neurol*, 6:326-329, 1990.

301. Kimura S, Ohtuki N, Nezu A, Tanaka M, et al: Clinical and radiologic improvements in mitochondrial encephalomyelopathy following sodium dichloroacetate therapy, *Brain Dev*, 19:535-540, 1997.

302. Farina L, Chiapparini L, Uziel G, Bugiani M, et al: MR findings in Leigh syndrome with COX deficiency and *SURF-1* mutations, *AJNR Am J Neuroradiol*, 23:1095-1100, 2002.

303. Detre JA, Wang ZY, Bogdan AR, Gusnard DA, et al: Regional variation in brain lactate in Leigh syndrome by localized 1H magnetic resonance spectroscopy, *Ann Neurol*, 29:218-221, 1991.

304. Krägeloh-Mann I, Grodd W, Schoning M, Marquard K, et al: Proton spectroscopy in 5 patients with Leigh's disease and mitochondrial enzyme deficiency, *Dev Med Child Neurol*, 35:769-776, 1993.

305. van Erven PM, Gabreëls FJ, Ruitenbeek W, Renier WO, et al: Familial Leigh's syndrome: Association with a defect in oxidative metabolism probably restricted to brain, *J Neurol*, 234:215-219, 1987.

306. Ciafaloni E, Santorelli FM, Shanske S, Deonna T, et al: Maternally inherited Leigh syndrome, *J Pediatr*, 122:419-422, 1993.

307. Tiranti V, Jaksch M, Hofmann S, Galimberti C, et al: Loss-of-function mutations of *SURF-1* are specifically associated with Leigh syndrome with cytochrome c oxidase deficiency, *Ann Neurol*, 46:161-166, 1999.

308. DiMauro S: Mitochondrial encephalomyopathies: Back to mendelian genetics, *Ann Neurol*, 45:693-694, 1999.

309. DeVivo DC: Solving the COX puzzle, *Ann Neurol*, 45:142-143, 1999.

310. Sue CM, Karadimas C, Checcarelli N, Tanji K, et al: Differential features of patients with mutations in two COX assembly genes, *SURF-1* and *SCO2*, *Ann Neurol*, 47:589-595, 2000.

311. Marin-Garcia J, Goldenthal MJ: Mitochondrial biogenesis defects and neuromuscular disorders, *Pediatr Neurol*, 22:122-129, 2000.

312. Meulemans A, Lissens W, Coster RV, Meirleir LD, et al: Analysis of the mitochondrial encoded subunits of complex I in 20 patients with a complex I deficiency, *Eur J Paediatr Neurol*, 8:299-306, 2004.

313. Coenen MJ, van den Heuvel LP, Ugalde C, Ten Brinke M, et al: Cytochrome c oxidase biogenesis in a patient with a mutation in COX10 gene, *Ann Neurol*, 56:560-564, 2004.

314. Crimi M, Papadimitriou A, Galbiati S, Palamidou P, et al: A new mitochondrial DNA mutation in *ND3* gene causing severe Leigh syndrome with early lethality, *Pediatr Res*, 55:842-846, 2004.

315. Filiano J, Goldenthal M, Mamourian A, Hall C, et al: Mitochondrial DNA depletion in Leigh syndrome, *Pediatr Neurol*, 26:239-242, 2002.

316. Fujii T, Okuno T, Ito M, Mutoh K, et al: MELAS of infantile onset: Mitochondrial angiopathy or cytopathy? *J Neurol Sci*, 103:37-41, 1991.

317. Bindoff L: Treatment of mitochondrial disorders: Practical and theoretical issues, *Eur J Paediatr Neurol*, 3:201-208, 1999.

318. Moroni I, Bugiani M, Bizzi A, Castelli G, et al: Cerebral white matter involvement in children with mitochondrial encephalopathies, *Neuropediatrics*, 33:79-85, 2002.

319. de Lonlay-Debeney P, von Kleist-Retzow JC, Hertz-Pannier L, Peudenier S, et al: Cerebral white matter disease in children may be caused by mitochondrial respiratory chain deficiency, *J Pediatr*, 136:209-214, 2000.

320. Kang PB, Hunter JV, Melvin JJ, Selak MA, et al: Infantile leukoencephalopathy owing to mitochondrial enzyme dysfunction, *J Child Neurol*, 17:421-428, 2002.

321. Brockmann K, Bjornstad A, Dechent P, Korenke G, et al: Succinate in dystrophic white matter: A proton magnetic resonance spectroscopy finding characteristic for complex II deficiency, *Ann Neurol*, 52:38-46, 2002.

322. Bianchi MC, Tosetti M, Battini R, Manca ML, et al: Proton MR spectroscopy of mitochondrial diseases: Analysis of brain metabolic abnormalities and their possible diagnostic relevance, *AJNR Am J Neuroradiol*, 24:1958-1966, 2003.

323. Hung PC, Wang HS: A previously undescribed leukodystrophy in Leigh syndrome associated with *T9176C* mutation of the mitochondrial ATPase 6 gene, *Dev Med Child Neurol*, 49:65-67, 2007.

324. Garcia-Cazorla A, De Lonlay P, Nassogne MC, Rustin P, et al: Long-term follow-up of neonatal mitochondrial cytopathies: A study of 57 patients, *Pediatrics*, 116:1170-1177, 2005.

325. Bawle EV, Kupsky WJ, D'Amato CJ, Becker CJ, et al: Familial infantile olivopontocerebellar atrophy, *Pediatr Neurol*, 13:14-18, 1995.

326. Hagberg BA, Blennow G, Kristiansson B, Stibler H: Carbohydrate-deficient glycoprotein syndromes: Peculiar group of new disorders, *Pediatr Neurol*, 9:255-262, 1993.

327. Jaeken J, Casaer P: Carbohydrate-deficient glycoconjugate (CDG) syndromes: A new chapter of neuropaediatrics, *Eur J Paediatr Neurol*, 2:61-66, 1997.

328. Veneselli E, Biancheri R, DiRocco M, Tortorelli S: Neurophysiological findings in a case of carbohydrate-deficient glycoprotein (CDG) syndrome type 1 with phosphomannomutase deficiency, *Eur J Paediatr Neurol*, 2:239-244, 1998.

329. Grunewald S, Matthijis G: Congenital disorders of glycosylation (CDG): A rapidly expanding group of neurometabolic disorders, *Neuropediatrics*, 31:57-59, 2000.

330. Hanefeld F, Korner C, Holzbach-Eberle U, von Figura K: Congenital disorder of glycosylation-1c: Case report and genetic defect, *Neuropediatrics*, 31:60-62, 2000.

331. Jaeken J, Matthijs G, Carchon H, Van Schaftingen E: Defects of N-glycan synthesis. In Scriver CR, Beaudet MD, Sly WS, et al, editors: *The Metabolic and Molecular Bases of Inherited Disease*, 8th ed, New York: 2001, McGraw-Hill.

332. Miosser-Chauvet E, Mikaeloff Y, Heron D, Merzoug V, et al: Neurological presentation in pediatric patients with congenital disorders of glycosylation type I, *Neuropediatrics*, 34:1-6, 2003.

333. Grunewald S, Matthus G, Jaeken J: Congenital disorders of glycosylation: A review, *Pediatr Res*, 52:618-624, 2002.

334. Aronica E, van Kempen AA, van der Heide M, Poll-The BT, et al: Congenital disorder of glycosylation type Ia: A clinicopathological report of a newborn infant with cerebellar pathology, *Acta Neuropathol (Berl)*, 109:433-442, 2005.

335. Miura Y, Tay SK, Aw MM, Eklund EA, et al: Clinical and biochemical characterization of a patient with congenital disorder of glycosylation (CDG) IIx, *J Pediatr*, 147:851-853, 2005.

336. Eklund EA, Sun L, Westphal V, Northrop JL, et al: Congenital disorder of glycosylation (CDG)-Ih patient with a severe hepato-intestinal phenotype and evolving central nervous system pathology, *J Pediatr*, 147:847-850, 2005.

337. Collins AE, Ferriero DM: The expanding spectrum of congenital disorders of glycosylation, *J Pediatr*, 147:728-730, 2005.

338. de Koning TJ, de Vries LS, Groenendaal F, Ruitenbeek W, et al: Pontocerebellar hypoplasia associated with respiratory-chain defects, *Neuropediatrics*, 30:93-95, 1999.

339. Scaglia F, Wong LJ, Vladutiu GD, Hunter JV: Predominant cerebellar volume loss as a neuroradiologic feature of pediatric respiratory chain defects, *AJNR Am J Neuroradiol*, 26:1675-1680, 2005.

340. Barth PG, Blennow G, Lenard HG, Begeer JH, et al: The syndrome of autosomal recessive pontocerebellar hypoplasia, microcephaly, and extrapyramidal dyskinesia (pontocerebellar hypoplasia type 2): Complied data from 10 pedigrees, *Neurology*, 45:311-317, 1995.

341. Barbot C, Carneiro G, Melo J: Pontocerebellar hypoplasia with microcephaly and dyskinesia: Report of two cases, *Dev Med Child Neurol*, 39:554-557, 1997.

342. Zelnik N, Dobyns WB, Forem SL, Kolodny EH: Congenital pontocerebellar atrophy in three patients: Clinical, radiologic and etiologic considerations, *Neuroradiology*, 38:684-687, 1996.

343. Malandrini A, Palmeri S, Villanova M, Parrotta E, et al: A syndrome of autosomal recessive pontocerebellar hypoplasia with white matter abnormalities and protracted course in two brothers, *Brain Dev*, 19:209-211, 1997.

344. Hashimoto K, Takeuchi Y, Kida Y, Hasegawa H, et al: Three siblings of fatal infantile encephalopathy with olivopontocerebellar hypoplasia and microcephaly, *Brain Dev*, 20:169-174, 1998.
345. Barth PG: Pontocerebella hypoplasia: How many types? *Eur J Paediatr Neurol*, 4:161-162, 2000.
346. Chaves-Vischer V, Pizzolato GP, Hanquinet S, Maret A, et al: Early fatal pontocerebellar hypoplasia in premature twin sisters, *Eur J Paediatr Neurol*, 4:171-176, 2000.
347. Coppola G, Muras I, Pascotto A: Pontocerebellar hypoplasia type 2 (PCH2): Report of two siblings, *Brain Dev*, 22:188-192, 2000.
347a. Steinlin M, Klein A, Haas-Lude K, Zafeiriou D, et al: Pontocerebellar hypoplasia type 2: Variability in clinical and imaging findings, *Eur J Paediatr Neurol*, 11:146-152, 2007.

348. Dilber E, Mujgan F, Ahmetoglu A: Pontocerebellar hypoplasia in two siblings with dysmorphic features, *J Child Neurol*, 17:64-66, 2002.
349. Rajab A, Mochida GH, Hill A, Bodell GA, et al: A novel form of ponto-cerebellar hypoplasia maps to chromosome 7q11-21, *Neurology*, 60: 1664-1667, 2003.
350. Patel MS, Becker LE, Toi A, Armstrong DL, et al: Severe, fetal-onset form of olivopontocerebellar hypoplasia in three sibs: PCH type 5? *Am J Med Genet A*, 140:594-603, 2006.

DISORDERS OF THE MOTOR SYSTEM

Neuromuscular Disorders: Motor System, Evaluation, and Arthrogryposis Multiplex Congenita

Neuromuscular disorders may cause dramatic disability in the neonatal period. The dominant features of these disorders are muscle weakness and hypotonia. In this context, I consider as neuromuscular disorders those that predominantly involve the motor system, from its origins in the cerebral cortex to its termination in the muscle.

This and the next two chapters are concerned with neuromuscular disorders. In this chapter, the motor system is described in terms of its anatomical and physiological organization; special additional emphasis is placed on the development and the biochemical features of muscle. The evaluation of disorders of the motor system in the newborn is reviewed. Finally, arthrogryposis multiplex congenita, a syndrome that represents a common manifestation of many disorders of the neuromuscular apparatus, is discussed as a prelude to the more detailed discussions of the various diseases of the neonatal motor system in the next two chapters.

MOTOR SYSTEM

The control of movement and tone in the human nervous system is highly complex, and major lacunae in knowledge exist in our understanding of this control in the neonatal period. Nevertheless, it is reasonable to expect that the anatomical systems critical for control of movement and tone in the mature nervous system are operative, although undoubtedly to varying extents, in the immature nervous system. In the following discussion, the major components of the central and peripheral nervous systems that are important for the control of movement and tone are briefly reviewed. The discussion is organized in the framework used in the next two chapters for the categorization of diseases that disturb muscle power and tone in the human infant.

Levels above the Lower Motor Neuron

Control of muscle power and tone begins in the central nervous system at levels above the lower motor neuron (Table 17-1). This control is mediated in largest part by the major motor efferent system, the corticospinal and corticobulbar tracts, often termed the *pyramidal system* because a major portion of these tracts originates in the pyramidal cells of the motor cortex of the cerebrum. Also important in control, primarily through effects on cerebral cortical motor centers, are the basal ganglia and cerebellum. Certain other descending tracts that have an impact on the lower motor neuron involved in muscle power and tone are the rubrospinal, reticulospinal, and vestibulospinal tracts, sometimes collectively referred to as the *bulbospinal tracts*.

Corticospinal and Corticobulbar Tracts

The corticospinal tract is the major efferent system concerned with movement of axial and appendicular musculature; the corticobulbar tract is concerned with movement of muscles innervated by the cranial nerves. The origin of this system in the mature subhuman primate is principally from pyramidal cells, with the following distributions: motor cortex, 31%; premotor cortex, 29%; and parietal lobe, 40%.[1] The topographic representation of the homunculus on the contralateral cerebral cortex (see Fig. 9-41) provides an estimate of the somatotopic origin of these fibers. This system descends through the posterior limb of the internal capsule, the cerebral peduncles, and the pontine tegmentum, decussates in the ventral medulla, and then descends in the lateral column of the spinal cord. A small portion of the system does not decussate and descends uncrossed in the anterior column of the spinal cord. The corticospinal tract subserves refined volitional movements, although the precise contribution to movement in the human newborn is not known entirely.

Basal Ganglia

The system of basal ganglia, sometimes categorized by the less precise term *extrapyramidal system*, principally consists of five major nuclear masses: caudate, putamen, globus pallidus, subthalamic nucleus, and substantia nigra.[1] These nuclei do not project to the lower motor neuron directly but rather influence muscle power and tone primarily by effects on the corticospinal system. The major afferent centers are the caudate and putamen (the corpus striatum), and the

TABLE 17-1	Major Components of the Motor System
Levels above the Lower Motor Neuron	
Corticospinal-corticobulbar tracts	
Basal ganglia	
Cerebellum	
Other components ("bulbospinal")	
Rubrospinal tracts	
Reticulospinal tracts	
Vestibulospinal tracts	
Lower Motor Neuron	
Cranial nerve motor nuclei	
Anterior horn cells	
Peripheral Nerve	
Neuromuscular Junction	
Presynaptic	
Postsynaptic	
Muscle	

major efferent center is the globus pallidus. Output from the globus pallidus is relayed to the cortical motor neurons principally by way of the thalamus.

Cerebellum

The cerebellum is a complex system of neurons concerned with coordination of somatic motor activity, regulation of muscle tone, and mechanisms that influence and maintain posture and equilibrium.[1] Afferent connections are derived from muscle and tendon stretch receptors and the visual, auditory, vestibular, and somesthetic sensory systems and are conveyed principally through the inferior and middle cerebellar peduncles in the brain stem. Efferent connections are conveyed principally through the superior cerebellar peduncle to the red nucleus (and then to the rubrospinal tract), the vestibular nuclei (and then to the vestibulospinal tract), and the thalamus (and then to cerebral cortical motor neurons). Thus, the control of movement and tone by the cerebellum ultimately is by way of other motor systems. The hypotonia observed in cerebellar disease may be mediated primarily by decreased muscle fusimotor activity.[2,3]

Other Components

The other major components of the motor system include the rubrospinal, reticulospinal, and vestibulospinal tracts, sometimes collectively known as the bulbospinal tracts. *The nerve fibers of these tracts, unlike most other fibers of the motor system, are myelinated in the third trimester and may play a particularly important role in control of movement and tone in the premature and full-term newborn.*[2,3]

Rubrospinal Tract. The rubrospinal tract originates in the red nucleus in the midbrain, decussates, and then descends in the lateral aspect of the spinal cord. Major afferents are from the cerebellar and cerebral cortices, and the rubrospinal tract projects to nuclei in the brain stem and cerebellum before reaching the spinal cord. The most important function of the rubrospinal tract is the control of muscle tone in *flexor*

muscle groups.[1] It is tempting to speculate that this system is particularly important in the term newborn because of the impressive flexor tone in the limbs (see Chapter 3).

Reticulospinal Tracts. Reticulospinal tracts emanate from neurons of the reticular formation in the pontine and medullary tegmentum and descend in the anterior aspect of the spinal cord. Afferents are derived from all sensory systems and from the cerebral cortex. This system has *major* functional effects on muscle activity and tone, principally through action on the gamma motor neurons in the anterior horn of the spinal cord, which innervate the contractile portions of the muscle spindle.[1] Indeed, the reticulospinal system presumably mediates the impressive changes in tone observed in infants according to the level of alertness.

Vestibulospinal Tract. The vestibulospinal tract arises from the lateral vestibular nucleus and descends in the anterolateral aspect of the spinal cord. Afferents are derived primarily from the labyrinth (and vestibular portion of the eighth nerve) and the cerebellum. An increase in *extensor* muscle tone is observed with stimulation of the lateral vestibular nucleus. This system may play a role in the newborn in the mediation of reflex activity associated with vestibular input and extensor muscle activity (e.g., tonic neck and Moro reflexes).[4]

Lower Motor Neuron

The suprasegmental influences just described play on the final common pathway of the motor system, the motor unit. The term *motor unit* refers to the lower motor neuron (i.e., *anterior horn cell* or *brain stem neuron of the cranial nerve nucleus*), the peripheral nerve (or cranial nerve), the neuromuscular junction, and the innervated muscle.

In the spinal cord, anterior horn cells are arranged such that neurons subserving function of extensor muscles are located ventrally, flexor muscles dorsally, proximal muscles laterally, and distal muscles medially. The two major types of efferent neurons are the predominant large cells that innervate striated muscle and the less abundant small cells that innervate the fibers of the muscle spindle, the stretch receptors. The latter are important in determining the activity of stretch ("tendon") reflexes and receive input from the aforementioned suprasegmental tracts.

Peripheral Nerve

The large anterior horn cells, concerned with innervation of skeletal muscle, exit through the anterior roots to the *peripheral nerve*. The nerve fibers conduct the nerve impulse with a velocity directly proportional to their diameter and the size of their myelin sheath. (In addition to transmission of the nerve impulse, these fibers also transport a variety of compounds, including enzymes, neurotransmitters, organelles, and nutrient materials, to the distal aspect of the fiber.) The terminal aspect of the nerve fiber ramifies into a variable number of smaller fibers that form motor endplates at the neuromuscular junction. The axon of one motor nerve supplies a variable number of skeletal muscle fibers. In the larger muscles involved in postural control, a single anterior horn cell may provide motor endplates to more than 100 muscle fibers.[1] In smaller muscles (e.g., of the thumb) concerned with highly skilled movement, a single anterior horn cell provides endplates for only a few fibers.

Neuromuscular Junction

The neuromuscular junction contains the terminal nerve branch with its specialized *presynaptic ending,* which lies in a specialized trough of the postsynaptic *muscle* plasma membrane (sarcolemma). A synaptic cleft separates the two membranes. When the nerve impulse arrives at the presynaptic site, calcium enters the presynaptic axoplasm and causes the release of vesicles of acetylcholine. The neurotransmitter then diffuses across the synaptic cleft, binds with a specific postsynaptic receptor on the sarcolemma, and alters the permeability of the muscle membrane. Depolarization and a muscle action potential result if enough receptors are activated. This electrical signal is transmitted along the muscle membrane and then internally by a system of invaginations of the sarcolemma to provoke the events leading to muscle contraction. The coupling of excitation and contraction is discussed in more detail subsequently.

Muscle

Development

The chronology and major features of the development of skeletal muscle in the human are summarized in Table 17-2. These features provide information of value in interpreting the pathological significance of specific findings of the muscle biopsy in the newborn and in establishing anatomical correlates for certain developmental changes in muscle function (see subsequent discussion).

Premyoblastic Stage. The premyoblastic stage, occurring in the first 5 weeks of gestation, is characterized principally by the differentiation of primitive mesenchymal cells to myoblasts.

Myoblastic Stage. The myoblastic stage, which follows in the next several weeks, is dominated by active proliferation of myoblasts. Synthesis of the contractile proteins begins.

Myotubular Stage. During the myotubular stage, from approximately 8 to 15 weeks of gestation, myoblasts fuse to form the syncytium characteristic of human skeletal muscle. Nuclei are located centrally, unlike the peripheral location of mature muscle. Myofilaments of the contractile proteins, actin and myosin, develop the longitudinal organization necessary for formation of myofibrils. The sarcotubular system, the invaginations of the sarcolemma so important in excitation-contraction coupling, is formed. Axonal terminals contact muscle by 11 weeks, and motor endplates begin to appear at 14 weeks of gestation.

Myocytic Stage. The myocytic stage, occurring from 15 to 20 weeks, is characterized by migration of nuclei to the periphery of the myotube. Active synthesis of myofibrils continues.

Early Histochemical Differentiation. In the stage of early histochemical differentiation, during the period from 20 to 24 weeks, approximately 5% to 10% of fibers develop prominent quantities of oxidative enzymes and correspond to type I fibers; these are distinctly large fibers.[5] The remaining fibers, designated type II because of their adenosine triphosphatase (ATPase) concentration, predominate (Fig. 17-1).[6] These small fibers are relatively undifferentiated and categorized as type IIc fibers, to be distinguished from

TABLE 17-2 **Human Muscle Development**		
Developmental Stage	**Time (Wk of Gestation)**	**Major Developmental Events**
Premyoblastic	0–5	Differentiation of mesenchymal cells to myoblasts
Myoblastic	5–8	Proliferation of myoblasts
Myotubular	8–15	Formation of syncytium with central nuclei, myofibrils, sarcotubular system, and early endplates
Myocyte	15–20	Movement of nuclei to periphery Continued synthesis of myofibrils
Early histochemical differentiation	20–24	Differentiation of fiber types I and II; type II fibers predominate
Intermediate histochemical differentiation	24–34	Increase in size of type II fibers
Late histochemical differentiation	34–38	Development of equal numbers of fiber types I and II due to marked increase in small type I fibers
Mature myocyte	> 38	Increase in size of all muscle fibers

Data from Sarnat HB: In Korobkin R, Guilleminault C, editors: *Advances in Perinatal Neurology,* New York: 1979, Spectrum Publications; and Schloon H, Schlottmann J, Lenard HG, Goebel HH: The development of skeletal muscles in premature infants, *Eur J Pediatr* 131:49–60, 1979.

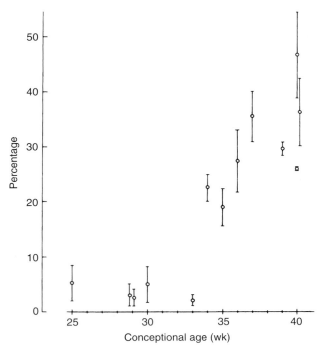

Figure 17-1 **Type I fibers as a percentage of total fiber population from the autopsy specimens of several muscles of infants of the gestational ages shown.** Percentages were calculated from all the muscles studied for each subject and are given as means ± SD. Note the very low percentage of type I fibers before 34 weeks of gestation and the onset of a dramatic increase in percentage at that time. *(From Schloon H, Schlottmann J, Lenard HG, Goebel HH: The development of skeletal muscles in premature infants, Eur J Pediatr 131:49–60, 1979.)*

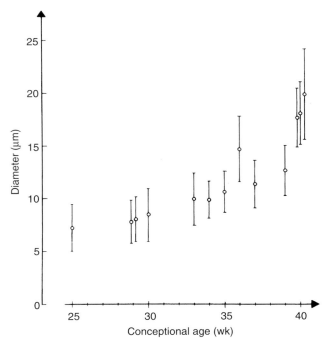

Figure 17-2 **Increase in muscle fiber diameter with maturation, from autopsy specimens of muscle as described in Figure 17-1.** Means ± SD of fiber diameter were calculated from all the muscles studied for each subject. Note the increase in diameter in the last weeks of gestation, especially after 38 weeks. *(From Schloon H, Schlottmann J, Lenard HG, Goebel HH: The development of skeletal muscles in premature infants, Eur J Pediatr 131:49–60, 1979.)*

the differentiated type IIa and IIb fibers that develop in the ensuing weeks and months.[7]

Intermediate Histochemical Differentiation. In the stage of intermediate histochemical differentiation, between 24 and 34 weeks of gestation, the predominant change is a modest increase in size of type II fibers.[6] No significant changes in type I fiber size occur during this period.

Late Histochemical Differentiation. In the stage of late histochemical differentiation, during a relatively brief period from 34 to 38 weeks, a dramatic change occurs.[6] Small type I fibers appear in large numbers (see Fig. 17-1).[6] Near the end of this stage, almost equal numbers of the two muscle fiber types are observed.

Mature Myocytic Stage. Subsequent development (i.e., the mature myocytic stage), after 38 weeks, is characterized particularly by increasing size of individual muscle fibers (Fig. 17-2). Indeed, with continued synthesis of myofibrillar components, the mean diameter of muscle fibers increases approximately fourfold from term to 13 years of age.[8]

Importance of Motor Innervation. The factors governing the developmental sequence of myogenesis are not entirely understood, although motor innervation

likely plays an important role. *Denervation* of the soleus muscle in the newborn rat, when myogenesis is at the myotubular stage, results in a *severe maturational delay*, with persistence of myotubes and failure of histochemical differentiation.[9] The role of the motor neuron in *determination of muscle fiber type* has been demonstrated by cross-innervation and reinnervation after denervation experiments.[10,11] Thus, muscle fiber type can be changed according to the motor innervation. In addition to the roles in differentiation, motor innervation also plays an *important trophic role*, in that disturbances of motor innervation also result in defective growth of affected fibers.

Contractile Elements

The major contractile elements of skeletal muscle are the longitudinally oriented filaments, two sets of which can be recognized: thick and thin. These filaments are arranged in repeating units, imparting the striated appearance to the muscle cell. The two sets of filaments in each repeating unit become cross-linked only on excitation, and contraction of muscle then is effected by a relative sliding motion of the cross-linked filaments.

The major myofibrillar proteins that make up the thin and thick filaments are shown in Table 17-3. The principal protein of the thin filament is actin, and that of the thick filament is myosin. The interaction of these filamentous proteins is regulated by proteins in the thin filaments, the tropomyosin-troponin complex. Troponin itself is a complex of three proteins,

TABLE 17-3	Major Contractile Elements: Myofibrillar Proteins	
Protein	**Location**	**Function**
Myosin	Thick filament	Contraction
Actin	Thin filament	Contraction
Tropomyosin, troponin	Thin filament	Regulation of actin-myosin interaction; provision of calcium requirement

TABLE 17-5	Muscle Fiber Types	
Type	**Major Enzymatic Features**	**Major Physiological Features**
I	Oxidative enzymes (e.g., NADH-tetrazolium reductase)	Slow sustained activity
II	Glycolytic enzymes (e.g., phosphorylase; ATPase [high pH])	Rapid bursts of activity

NADH, nicotinamide adenine dinucleotide.

one of which binds calcium and, in so doing, allows tropomyosin to change its position within the thin filament to permit the combination of myosin with actin that then leads to contraction.

Excitation and Contraction Coupling

Major insight into the coupling of muscle excitation and contraction has been gained.[12] The major events in the fascinating sequence are depicted in Table 17-4. The initial event is the release of the prepackaged vesicles of acetylcholine from the presynaptic nerve ending, provoked by the arrival of the nerve action potential and the subsequent influx of calcium. Acetylcholine traverses the synaptic cleft and binds to a specific postsynaptic receptor on the sarcolemma, thus initiating depolarization of the muscle membrane. Propagation of depolarization occurs along the sarcolemma as well as interiorly. This penetration of depolarization into the interior of the cell occurs by way of the transverse tubules, which are continuous with the outer membrane. In close contact with these tubules is the sarcoplasmic reticulum, membranous sacs rich in calcium. With the inward propagation of depolarization, calcium is released from the sarcoplasmic reticulum and binds with a peptide of the troponin complex. This allows the movement of tropomyosin within the thin filament alluded to previously, the result of which is the interaction of actin and myosin necessary for contraction. Contraction results when actin combines with myosin, thereby causing a stimulation of myosin ATPase activity and hydrolysis of ATP. This occurrence is critical because ATP serves to dissociate actin-myosin cross-links. With a decrease in ATP the cross-links occur, and the relative sliding motion of the

TABLE 17-4	Major Events in Excitation-Contraction Coupling
The motor nerve action potential causes release of acetylcholine at the neuromuscular junction. Acetylcholine initiates depolarization of the muscle cell membrane. Depolarization penetrates into the interior of the muscle cell through the transverse tubules. The adjacent sarcoplasmic reticulum releases calcium. Calcium binds to the troponin component, thus allowing tropomyosin to change position within the thin filament and, in turn, actin to interact with myosin. Interaction of actin and myosin causes sliding movement of the thin and thick filaments and contraction.	

filaments causes contraction. Relaxation is associated with the return of calcium into the sarcoplasmic reticulum, an event mediated by an ATP-dependent calcium pump.

Biochemical Features

Energy is required for the work of muscle contraction, and thus the major task of muscle metabolism is to generate ATP. However, the synthesis of structural, contractile, and other components is obviously also of great importance, particularly during myogenesis. The major metabolic mechanisms for energy production in muscle differ primarily according to the functional requirements of a given fiber.

Two essential fiber types can be recognized by histochemical criteria (Table 17-5). *Type I fibers* are generally concerned with slow, sustained activities and are rich in oxidative enzymes. *Type II fibers* are generally concerned with rapid bursts of activity and are rich in glycogenolytic (phosphorylase) and glycolytic enzymes. Although the metabolic and physiological correlates are complex, it appears that fibers involved in rapid bursts of activity derive their ATP principally from carbohydrate metabolism (i.e., glycogenolysis and glycolysis). When more sustained activity is needed, glycogen stores are not adequate, and another source of ATP is needed; in largest part, this source is lipid (i.e., fatty acid).[13]

Carbohydrate Metabolism. Glucose and glycogen metabolism and the operation of the citric acid cycle are discussed in Chapters 6 and 12 and are similar in muscle. (The disorders of carbohydrate metabolism associated with muscle disease are noted in Chapters 18 and 19.)

Fatty Acid Utilization. The utilization of lipid for energy is particularly characteristic of muscle. The free fatty acid that serves as a source of energy is derived primarily from blood. To be used for production of high-energy phosphate, free fatty acids initially must be activated to their respective coenzyme A (CoA) derivatives (Table 17-6). The enzyme involved is fatty acyl-CoA synthase, located primarily on the outer surface of the mitochondrial membrane.[14] Fatty acyl-CoA derivatives do not cross the mitochondrial membrane. Carnitine, the obligatory carrier of these derivatives across this membrane, is actively transported

TABLE 17-6 **Fatty Acid Utilization in Muscle**

Activation of fatty acid: *fatty acyl-CoA synthase*
Fatty acid + CoA + ATP → fatty acyl-CoA + ADP + P_i
Transfer to carnitine: *carnitine-palmitoyltransferase I*
Fatty acyl-CoA + carnitine → fatty acyl-carnitine + CoA
Transfer to intramitochondrial CoA: *carnitine-palmitoyl transferase II*
Fatty acyl-carnitine + CoA → fatty acyl-CoA + carnitine
Oxidation to acetyl-CoA: *beta-oxidation system*
Fatty acyl-CoA + O_2 + ADP + P_i → acetyl-CoA + ATP (by electron equivalents)
Oxidation of acetyl-CoA: *citric acid cycle*
Acetyl-CoA + O_2 + ADP + P_i → CO_2 + H_2O + ATP
For palmitic acid:
Palmityl-CoA + 23 O_2 + 131 ADP + 131 P_i → CoA + 16 CO_2 + 146 H_2O + 131 ATP

ADP, adenosine diphosphate; ATP, adenosine triphosphate; CoA, coenzyme A; P_i, inorganic phosphate.

into muscle.[15] At the outer surface of the mitochondrial membrane, carnitine-palmitoyl transferase I catalyzes the formation of the carnitine derivative of the long-chain fatty acid (usually palmitic acid). This compound then traverses the mitochondrial barrier, and, on the inner surface, the enzyme carnitine-palmitoyl transferase II regenerates the CoA derivative. The intramitochondrial fatty acyl-CoA then undergoes beta-oxidation to acetyl-CoA, a process during which electron equivalents (in the form of reduced flavin adenine dinucleotide and reduced nicotinamide adenine dinucleotide [NADH]) are produced; the latter are used by the electron transport system in the production of ATP (see Chapter 6). Acetyl-CoA is then oxidized by the citric acid cycle and electron transport system with the formation of additional ATP. As shown in Table 17-6, the complete oxidation of palmityl-CoA through this sequence results in 131 molecules of ATP. Because one molecule of ATP is used for the formation of palmityl-CoA, *a net synthesis of* 130 *molecules of ATP* results from the utilization of one molecule of palmitic acid by the system. The importance of lipids for energy production in muscle is emphasized by the occurrence of certain myopathies associated with derangements in this pathway (see Chapter 19).

EVALUATION OF DISORDERS OF THE MOTOR SYSTEM

History

The importance of acquiring a careful history frequently is overlooked in the evaluation of the infant with a motor disorder. The pertinent historical features will become apparent in the subsequent discussions of the various disorders. However, certain findings that initially may not be considered relevant to a motor abnormality (e.g., polyhydramnios) may prove to be valuable clues to diagnosis (e.g., myotonic dystrophy). Moreover, the family history should be supplemented by examination of the infant's parents. The myotonia and facial weakness of myotonic dystrophy or the pes

cavus and leg weakness of familial polyneuropathy are easily overlooked in many affected adults.

Physical Examination

The physical examination must be performed carefully and completely. As will become apparent later, dysmorphic features, cardiac abnormalities, respiratory insufficiency, hepatomegaly, and the like may be features of certain disorders of the motor system. Congenital hip dislocation and other joint contractures are particularly common features in neonatal motor disorders; these and related joint abnormalities are discussed in more detail later (see "Arthrogryposis Multiplex Congenita").

The neurological evaluation of the motor system is discussed in detail in Chapter 3. As explained later, the anatomical site of the disorder of the motor system is best ascertained by careful determination of muscle bulk, power, tone, tendon reflexes, primary neonatal reflexes, and the presence or absence of myotonia, myasthenia, and fasciculations. Other neurological features, such as abnormalities of cranial nerve function, sensory discrimination, or the occurrence of seizures, provide useful supplementary information in selected instances.

Laboratory Studies

Although the major emphasis of this and the next two chapters is on disorders of the *motor unit* that result in hypotonia and weakness in the neonatal period, disorders of the brain and descending motor tracts in the spinal cord nearly always enter into the differential diagnosis. These disorders and their evaluation are discussed in other chapters, but appropriate diagnostic procedures may include the following: computed tomography, magnetic resonance imaging, and ultrasound brain scanning; computed tomography, magnetic resonance imaging, or conventional radiography of the spine; and myelography. Simple radiographs of the ribs and long bones often show marked thinning, hypomineralization, and, occasionally, diaphyseal fractures, caused most probably by intrauterine immobility.[16-18]

The *major laboratory investigations* for evaluation of disorders of the *motor unit* involve (1) examination of the cerebrospinal fluid (CSF), (2) serum enzyme levels, (3) nerve conduction velocities, (4) electromyogram (EMG), and (5) muscle biopsy. Nerve biopsy is necessary in selected cases. Examinations of the function of cardiac muscle (electrocardiogram, echocardiogram) and even smooth muscle (barium swallow and upper gastrointestinal series) may be helpful adjuncts.

Cerebrospinal Fluid

The major value of the examination of CSF in the evaluation of disorders of the motor unit is determination of the protein concentration. Elevations are common accompaniments of polyneuropathy.

Serum Enzyme Levels

Enzymes most consistently elevated in blood in diseases of muscle are creatine kinase (CK), aldolase, and aspartate aminotransferase (AST, formerly known as serum glutamic-oxaloacetic transaminase [SGOT]).

Creatine Kinase. The most useful of the serum enzymes is CK, specific isozymes of which are found in skeletal (and cardiac) muscle and in brain. Interpretation of serum CK values must be made with the awareness that levels are usually elevated severalfold in the first few days after vaginal delivery. Because such elevations are not observed after elective cesarean section, investigators have suggested that muscle compression during vaginal delivery causes leakage of the enzyme into the bloodstream.[19-21]

CK levels are not elevated in disorders of the anterior horn cell, peripheral nerve, and neuromuscular junction. Indeed, CK values are not elevated in all disorders of muscle. Values within normal limits are observed usually with neonatal myotonic dystrophy and frequently with congenital myopathies. Moreover, CK levels do not correlate necessarily with muscle weakness. CK levels may be exceedingly high in infants with preclinical Duchenne muscular dystrophy or with certain types of congenital muscular dystrophy (see later). Nevertheless, in general, this highly sensitive test is a useful indicator of muscle disease.

Aldolase. Aldolase levels change in a manner similar to CK. In neonatal neurology, evaluation of the quantity of this enzyme generally adds little information and is not necessary.

Aspartate Aminotransferase. Determinations of *AST levels* may add useful information because this enzyme, unlike CK, is not confined to muscle and brain; rather, it is also concentrated in liver. Thus, in the evaluation of a neuromuscular disorder with hepatic involvement (e.g., Pompe glycogen storage disease), the level of AST may be elevated and that of CK may be normal because of minimal muscle disease (although marked disturbance of anterior horn cell) but prominent hepatic disease.

Nerve Conduction Velocity

Estimation of nerve conduction velocity is a valuable and relatively simple technique in determining the presence of a disorder of the peripheral nerve. The median, ulnar, and peroneal nerves are usually studied initially; surface electrodes are sufficient for adequate measurements. Assessment of the distal sensory nerve action potential in the median nerve is important in assessment of peripheral neuropathy because the finding of a normal sensory nerve action potential is sufficient to exclude an abnormality between the dorsal root ganglion and the distal sensory nerve.[22-25] Because the conduction velocity of motor nerves depends on the diameter of the nerve and thickness of the myelin sheath, it is not surprising that motor nerve conduction velocities are lower in the newborn than in the adult (see Chapter 4). Nerve conduction velocity is particularly depressed in disorders associated with demyelination or failure of myelination and is less severely depressed in disorders of the axon (see Chapter 18).

Infants with anterior horn cell disease (e.g., Werdnig-Hoffmann disease) have normal nerve conduction velocities, although a modest decrease in the velocity may occur later in the course of the disease, presumably because of selective loss of anterior horn cells of large, well-myelinated nerve fibers.[24,26] Nerve conduction velocities are normal in disorders of the neuromuscular junction and, of course, muscle.

Electromyography

Basic Features. Examination of the electrical activity of muscle provides useful information about every level of the motor unit. Methodological details concerning performance of the EMG in the newborn have been delineated[22-25]; patience, flexibility, and skill are crucial for obtaining useful data. A concentric needle electrode is used, and potentials are displayed on a monitor. Important information is obtained with the muscle *at rest* and with *spontaneous or elicited* (e.g., movement of needle) *contraction*. No electrical activity occurs in normal muscle at rest. With contraction, electrical activity appears. The normal potential is summated and is derived from individual muscle fiber potentials of a motor unit (i.e., the motor unit potential). The *amplitude, duration, number, and conformation* of the motor unit potential are observed. The normal potential in the newborn is usually biphasic or triphasic, with an amplitude of 100 to 700 µV and a duration of 5 to 9 milliseconds (Fig. 17-3).[22-24,26] The number of potentials increases with vigorous contraction and obscures the baseline (i.e., normal interference pattern; see Fig. 17-3). The *amplitude and duration* of the motor unit potential relate to the number of muscle fibers innervated by the anterior horn cell for that motor unit. The *number* of motor unit potentials observed is determined principally by the number of functioning anterior horn cells.

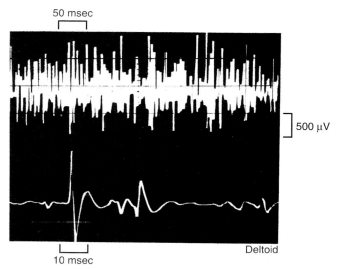

Figure 17-3 Normal electromyogram. The *upper trace* shows a normal "interference pattern" resulting from the summation of motor unit potentials on contraction; the baseline is obliterated. The *lower trace* shows a normal single triphasic motor unit potential (note the faster time scale). *(From Dubowitz V: Muscle Disorders in Childhood, 2nd ed, Philadelphia: 1978, Saunders.)*

TABLE 17-7 Electromyographic Findings in Neuromuscular Disorders

State of Muscle Examined	Observed Activity*	SITE OF LESION		
		Anterior Horn Cell	Peripheral Nerve	Muscle
Rest	Fibrillation	+	+	−†
	Fasciculation	+	−‡	−
Contraction	Amplitude	↑	N−↓	↓
	Duration	↑	N−↓	↓
	Number	↓	N−↓	N (−↓)
	Polyphasics	More and of larger size	More and of variable size	More and of smaller size

*No activity is observed in normal muscle *at rest.* With voluntary or elicited *contraction*, the four listed characteristics of the summated motor unit potential are observed.

†Fibrillations occasionally may be observed in polymyositis, myotonic dystrophy, myotubular myopathy, nemaline myopathy, congenital fiber type disproportion, and glycogen storage myopathies (types II, V, and VII); the other electromyographic features of myopathy aid in the distinction from anterior horn cell or peripheral nerve disease.

‡Fasciculations are observed occasionally in peripheral neuropathies with presumed involvement of the anterior horn cell.

+, present; −, absent; N, normal; ↑, increased; ↓, decreased.

Adapted from sources listed in the text.

Polyphasic potentials, normal in small amounts, occur when the muscle fibers of the motor unit are unusually numerous, are separated by increased distance, or both. Abnormalities of the EMG in neuromuscular disorders are summarized in Table 17-7.[22-24,27]

Anterior Horn Cell Disorders. In disorders of the anterior horn cell, spontaneous fibrillations (i.e., short-duration, low-amplitude potentials) and fasciculations (i.e., high-amplitude, long-duration, often polyphasic potentials) appear at rest (see Table 17-7; Figs. 17-4 and 17-5). Fibrillation potentials are small because they are derived from denervated muscle fibers. Fasciculation potentials, which originate from "irritable" anterior horn cells, are large and are of long duration because the territory of the affected motor neuron is expanded, secondary to reinnervation of adjacent denervated muscle fibers by terminal axonal sprouts.

With contraction, the number of motor unit potentials is decreased because of the reduced number of anterior horn cells (see Table 17-7). The amplitude is large and the duration is long because of the collateral reinnervation noted previously. Polyphasic potentials are abundant and large for the same reason.

Peripheral Nerve Disorders. In disorders of the peripheral nerve, spontaneous fibrillations appear at rest because of the presence of denervated muscle fibers (see Table 17-7). However, fasciculations do not generally occur because the anterior horn cells are not the primary site of the disease.

With contraction, motor unit potentials are not strikingly altered in amplitude and duration until later in the course of the disease. The number of motor unit potentials is decreased because of the loss of enough terminal fibers to denervate whole motor units.

Muscle Disorders. In disorders of muscle, neither fasciculations nor fibrillations should appear at rest because disease of the anterior horn cell and denervation of

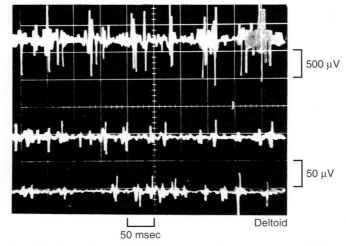

500 μV

50 μV

50 msec   Deltoid

Figure 17-4 Electromyogram showing fibrillation potentials, from an infant with anterior horn cell (Werdnig-Hoffmann) disease. In *the upper trace*, note the reduced interference pattern and visible baseline between potentials. The *lower traces* show spontaneous biphasic, small (≈50 to 100 μV) potentials at rest (i.e., fibrillation potentials), indicative of denervation. *(From Dubowitz V: Muscle Disorders in Childhood, 2nd ed, Philadelphia: 1978, Saunders.)*

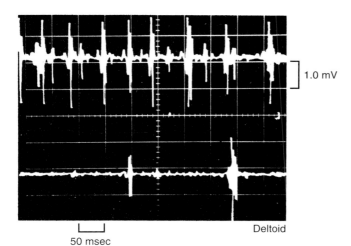

1.0 mV

Deltoid

50 msec

Figure 17-5 **Electromyogram showing fasciculation potentials, from a child with anterior horn cell disease**. The *upper trace* shows a reduced interference pattern and large-amplitude polyphasic potentials (the scale is twice that of the *upper trace* of Figure 17-4). The *lower trace* shows spontaneous, large-amplitude polyphasic potentials at rest (i.e., fasciculation potentials), characteristic of anterior horn cell disease (the scale is 20 times that of the lower trace of Figure 17-4, which shows fibrillation potentials). *(From Dubowitz V: Muscle Disorders in Childhood, 2nd ed, Philadelphia: 1978, Saunders.)*

muscle fibers are not present. However, in some infantile myopathies, fibrillations may be seen (see Table 17-7).

With contraction, motor unit potentials are decreased in amplitude and duration because the size of the motor unit is decreased (see Table 17-7; Fig. 17-6). The number of motor unit potentials, however, is relatively less affected because the anterior horn cells are intact. This relative sparing of the number of motor unit potentials is a helpful point in the identification of

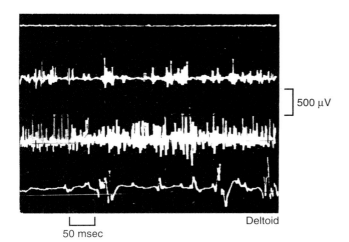

500 μV

Deltoid

50 msec

10 msec for bottom record

Figure 17-6 **Electromyogram showing myopathic changes from a child with Duchenne dystrophy**. The *upper trace*, obtained at rest, shows the normal electrical silence, with no spontaneous potentials. The second and third traces, at moderate and full muscle contraction, show a typical myopathic pattern with full interference pattern but low-amplitude, short-duration, polyphasic potentials. The *bottom trace* (at higher speed) demonstrates individual polyphasic potentials. *(From Dubowitz V: Muscle Disorders in Childhood, 2nd ed, Philadelphia: 1978, Saunders.)*

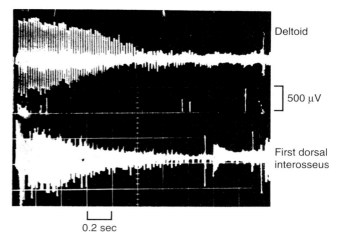

Deltoid

500 μV

First dorsal interosseus

0.2 sec

Figure 17-7 **Electromyograms showing myotonia from a child with congenital myotonic dystrophy (*upper trace*) and his mother (*lower trace*)**. Note the characteristic burst of spontaneous repetitive motor unit potentials with gradual waning. *(From Dubowitz V: Muscle Disorders in Childhood, 2nd ed, Philadelphia: 1978, Saunders.)*

muscle disease. Polyphasic potentials are abundant because of the increased separation of the individual muscle fibers of the motor unit, a result of the random fiber loss.

Myotonia. *Myotonia*, the electrical phenomenon characteristic of myotonic dystrophy, is very difficult to demonstrate in the young infant. The classic myotonic pattern consists of a spontaneous burst of potentials in rapid succession with gradual waning (Fig. 17-7). When the electrical pattern is broadcast, the acoustic pattern is characteristic and resembles the sound of a "dive bomber."

Myasthenia. The *myasthenic phenomenon* is striking and characteristic. This electrical correlate of the clinical fatigability of muscle is demonstrable by repetitive nerve stimulation and observation of the waning in size of the motor unit potential (Fig. 17-8). Improvement after the injection of an anticholinesterase drug (e.g., neostigmine or edrophonium) establishes the diagnosis. However, the converse is not true (i.e., in some types of congenital myasthenic syndromes, no improvement occurs after anticholinesterase treatment; see Chapter 18).

Muscle Biopsy

Value and Indications. Examination of a biopsy specimen of muscle is usually the single most definitive diagnostic procedure in the evaluation of the infant with a disorder of the motor unit. The definition of specific diagnosis provides important information for several reasons: (1) determination of prognosis; (2) genetic counseling; and (3) institution of specific therapy, if available, and appropriate supportive therapy (e.g., physical therapy, occupational therapy, and orthopedic intervention).

The indications for muscle biopsy in the neonatal period must be determined for each individual case. Occasionally, clinical features, family history,

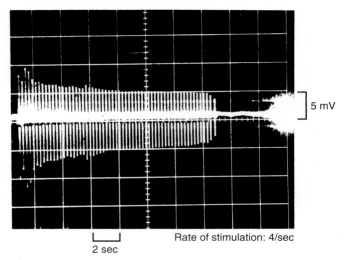

Rate of stimulation: 4/sec

2 sec

Figure 17-8 **Electromyogram in myasthenia gravis.** Note the waning of the size of the motor unit potential on repetitive stimulation of the nerve. *(From Dubowitz V: Muscle Disorders in Childhood, 2nd ed, Philadelphia: 1978, Saunders.)*

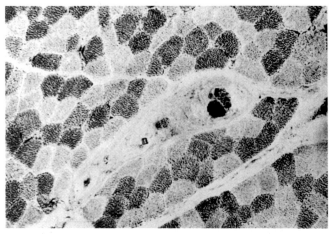

Figure 17-9 **Fiber types of normal muscle in transverse section.** Note the checkerboard appearance of the different fiber types. Type I fibers are dark in this section, stained for oxidative enzyme activity (reduced nicotinamide adenine dinucleotide-tetrazolium reductase stain, × 200). *(From Dubowitz V: Muscle Disorders in Childhood, 2nd ed, Philadelphia: 1978, Saunders.)*

determination of serum enzyme levels, electrophysiological data, or DNA analysis may establish a diagnosis (e.g., myotonic dystrophy, myasthenia gravis, or Werdnig-Hoffman disease). However, often the diagnosis remains uncertain, and the need for examination of muscle is apparent. Although biopsy in the neonatal period is feasible and probably preferable,[28,29] the difficulties of interpreting the muscle biopsy specimen have led others to suggest deferring the procedure for a few months, if possible.[30] My colleagues and I prefer early biopsy, despite the occasional problems in interpretation.

Technique. Two basic techniques have been used in newborn infants: open biopsy and needle biopsy.[26,28,31-33] I prefer open biopsy. Both procedures are performed while the patient is under local anesthesia and have been effective.

Muscle specimens should be prepared for histological, histochemical, electron microscopic, and, perhaps, biochemical studies. Histological and histochemical studies are performed on frozen specimens. A separate sample for electron microscopy must be fixed in glutaraldehyde. Biochemical studies are performed on either fresh or frozen material.

For histological study, hematoxylin and eosin and Gomori trichrome stains are used most often. As the clinical situation dictates, periodic acid–Schiff is used for glycogen, and oil red O is used for lipid. For histochemical studies the most common stains are NADH-tetrazolium reductase (oxidative enzyme), phosphorylase (glycogenolytic enzyme), and myosin ATPase (at high and low pH). Type I fibers are rich in oxidative enzyme activity and low in glycogenolytic and glycolytic activity, and they exhibit low ATPase activity at high pH. Type II fibers are relatively low in oxidative enzyme activity and rich in glycogenolytic and glycolytic activity, and they exhibit high ATPase activity at high pH.

Major Abnormalities. As reviewed previously (see Table 17-2), normal human skeletal muscle is nearly mature from a histological and histochemical standpoint by the latter part of the third trimester. Subsequent development consists principally of an increase in the size of fibers. The full-term newborn has a checkerboard or mosaic distribution of approximately equal numbers of type I and II fibers (Fig. 17-9).[28] Muscle fibers are approximately equal in size and are in close approximation (Fig. 17-10). The major abnormalities observed through histological and histochemical examinations of the muscle biopsy specimen are reviewed in Table 17-8. *No specific abnormalities* of muscle are observed in newborn infants with disorders of the motor system at *levels above the lower motor neuron*

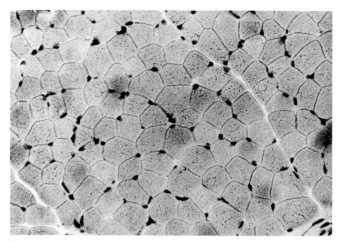

Figure 17-10 **Normal muscle in transverse section.** Note the polygonal fibers, closely approximated to each other, with peripherally placed subsarcolemmal nuclei and only slight variation in fiber size (hematoxylin and eosin stain, ×200). *(From Dubowitz V: Muscle Disorders in Childhood, 2nd ed, Philadelphia: 1978, Saunders.)*

TABLE 17-8	Major Histological-Histochemical Abnormalities in the Muscle Biopsy in Disorders of the Motor System

Levels above the Lower Motor Neuron
None*

Anterior Horn Cell
Loss of checkerboard appearance with type grouping[†]
Grouped atrophy[†]
Panfascicular atrophy[†]

Peripheral Nerve
Grouped atrophy, although grouping often not marked

Neuromuscular Junction
None

Muscle
Nongrouped atrophy
Degenerated fibers
Variations in fiber size
Central nuclei
Increased connective tissue and fat
With or without more distinctive changes (e.g., central cores, rods, storage of glycogen or lipid, absence of enzyme [cytochrome c oxidase])

*Fiber type disproportion may be observed.
[†]Classic early features of anterior horn cell involvement (i.e., loss of checkerboard appearance followed by grouped atrophy) are usually not observed with severe Werdnig-Hoffmann disease; marked *panfascicular atrophy* with involvement of both fiber types is prominent.

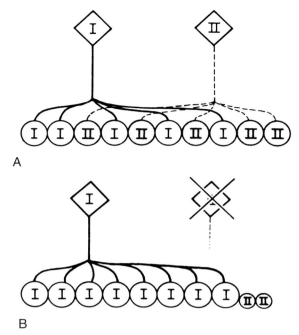

Figure 17-11 Evolution of type grouping with denervation. **A,** Normal. The checkerboard distribution of type I and type II fibers is determined by the corresponding pattern of innervation of the fibers by different anterior horn cells. **B,** Denervation. The anterior horn cell innervating the type II fibers has degenerated, and many of the corresponding fibers have been reinnervated by terminal axonal sprouts of the surviving anterior horn cell. A group of type I fibers results.

(except perhaps for fiber type disproportion discussed in Chapter 19) or at the *neuromuscular junction*.

The pattern of *denervation* is observed with disease of the anterior horn cell. In older infants, this pattern consists initially of a loss of the normal checkerboard appearance with type grouping by histochemical study; the fibers of the motor unit initially denervated by loss of its anterior horn cell are reinnervated by axon terminals from adjacent anterior horn cells (Fig. 17-11). When the anterior horn cells then are lost, atrophy of a *group* of fibers and hence the hallmark of denervation (i.e., *grouped atrophy*) occur (Fig. 17-12). However, in newborns with severe anterior horn cell disease, type grouping and grouped atrophy are observed very uncommonly, and the characteristic finding is severe *panfascicular atrophy* with involvement of both fiber types (see discussion of Werdnig-Hoffmann disease in Chapter 18). This rarity of type grouping and grouped atrophy may relate to the rapidity and severity of the anterior horn cell disorder in the fetus and newborn, with resulting lack of time or capacity for the axonal sprouting and reinnervation required to produce the classic denervation myohistological features of older infants with less severe disease. Similarly, with severe polyneuropathies of fetal onset, diffuse atrophy is more likely than type grouping and grouped atrophy.

The basic denervation pattern is to be contrasted with the *myopathic* pattern. In this latter instance, the involvement of muscle fibers is more or less random, and thus *nongrouped atrophy* is the essential feature (Fig. 17-13). Variations in fiber size, central nuclei, and increased connective tissue and fat are common to most myopathies. In the newborn, degenerative changes in muscle

fibers are less obvious than at later ages, and signs of arrested maturation (e.g., persistent myotubes) may occur (see, especially, discussion of congenital myotonic dystrophy in Chapter 19). Histochemical stains may demonstrate certain very distinctive changes (e.g., central cores, rod bodies) that are discussed in more detail in Chapter 19. Similarly, glycogen and lipid stains may suggest a glycogenosis or lipid storage myopathy, and electron microscopy may be indicative of a mitochondrial or related myopathy.

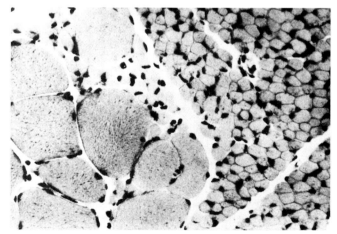

Figure 17-12 Grouped atrophy with denervation from a child with anterior horn cell disease. Note the large group of uniformly atrophic fibers on the right side of the figure (i.e., grouped atrophy). *(From Dubowitz V: Muscle Disorders in Childhood, 2nd ed, Philadelphia: 1978, Saunders.)*

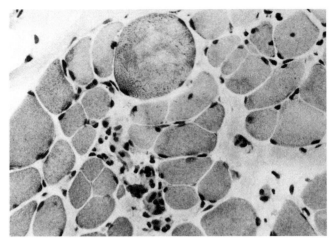

Figure 17-13 Nongrouped atrophy with myopathy from a child with Duchenne dystrophy. Note the nongrouped random abnormalities throughout the section consisting of variation in fiber size, central nuclei, degenerating fibers undergoing phagocytosis (*lower left*), and separation of fibers by increased connective tissue. *(From Dubowitz V: Muscle Disorders in Childhood, 2nd ed, Philadelphia: 1978, Saunders.)*

ARTHROGRYPOSIS MULTIPLEX CONGENITA

Arthrogryposis multiplex congenita refers to a syndrome, apparent at birth, that is characterized by fixed positions of multiple joints and an associated limitation of movement. The term *arthrogryposis* is derived from the Greek and literally means "bent joint." Arthrogryposis multiplex congenita is a *syndrome* and not a disease entity and is discussed here because, to varying degrees, it is a *manifestation of many fetal and neonatal disorders of the motor system*. Indeed, disturbances at each of the major levels of the nervous system listed in Table 17-1 have been associated with arthrogryposis. Overall, arthrogryposis multiplex congenita is not rare; the incidence is generally approximately 1 in 3000 live births.[34]

Clinical Features

The essential clinical features of this syndrome are fixed position and limitation of movement of the affected joints. Distal joints are more frequently and more severely affected than are proximal joints. Most common manifestations are talipes equinovarus and flexion deformities of the wrists (Fig. 17-14), but involvement of more proximal joints is also frequent. Both the upper and lower extremities are most commonly affected; lower extremities only, slightly less commonly; and upper extremities only, least commonly. Webbing of affected joints, especially the knee, may be present, and congenital dislocations of the hips are also common.

Muscles are usually atrophic, thus rendering a fusiform appearance to the joints. Hypotonia and weakness

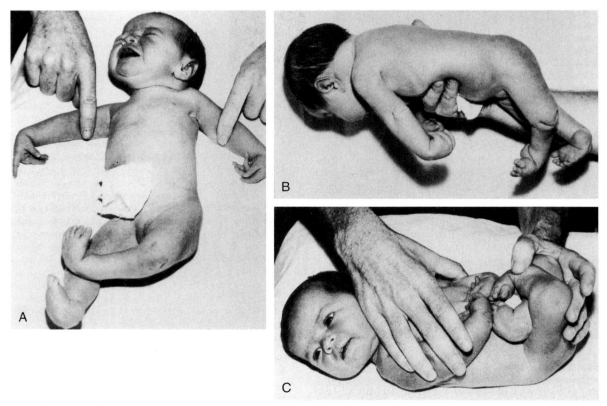

Figure 17-14 Arthrogryposis multiplex congenita in a newborn with congenital fiber type disproportion. A, Deformities of the hands, ankles, and knees. **B,** Good posture of the head and trunk in ventral suspension. **C,** Arms and legs folded into a presumptive intrauterine posture. *(From Dubowitz V: Muscle Disorders in Childhood, 2nd ed, Philadelphia: 1978, Saunders.)*

of the preserved movement occur. Tendon reflexes are depressed and are often absent. Elicitation of tendon reflexes often is hindered by the joint contractures.

At least half of patients with arthrogryposis multiplex congenita exhibit "congenital anomalies" of other organs, craniofacial structures, other parts of the musculoskeletal system, or the central nervous system.[7,34-37] Indeed, more than 150 syndromes are known in which arthrogryposis is a predominant sign.[34,36,37] Some of the associated extraneural anomalies are relatively minor (e.g., clinodactyly and undescended testes), whereas others are lethal (e.g., pulmonary hypoplasia and renal agenesis). Certain of the abnormalities of jaw (micrognathia), tongue, and palate may underlie the approximately 60% incidence of subsequent feeding disturbances.[38] Some of the constellations of anomalies (severe arthrogryposis, camptodactyly, pulmonary hypoplasia) have been designated eponymically (e.g., Pena-Shokeir phenotype).[39-41] However, because the causes of the Pena-Shokeir phenotype are multiple (see later discussion), the designation of such a syndrome appears to serve little clear purpose. Similarly, the "whistling face" Freeman-Sheldon syndrome of arthrogryposis has been associated with both autosomal dominant and autosomal recessive inheritance,[42-44] and it could be considered a variety of arthrogryposis in which involvement of oral-buccal and chin muscles is particularly marked. Banker[7] has emphasized particularly the strong relation among the "congenital anomalies" usually observed with arthrogryposis multiplex congenita and their nearly consistent pathogenetic basis in a disturbance of intrauterine movement rather than a primary disturbance of development (Table 17-9).

TABLE 17-9	"Congenital Anomalies" Commonly Observed in Severe Arthrogryposis Multiplex Congenita and Likely Pathogeneses
Anomaly*	**Likely Pathogenesis**
Micrognathia	Impaired facial and masticatory movements
Retrognathia	Impaired masticatory movements
High arched or cleft palate	Impaired tongue movement and micrognathia
Wide flat nose	Impaired head and facial movements (?)
Low-set ears	Impaired head movements (?)
Short neck	Impaired neck movements
Pulmonary hypoplasia	Impaired breathing movements
Clinodactyly, camptodactyly	Impaired finger movements
Polyhydramnios	Impaired swallowing

*Anomalies present in approximately 10% to 40% cases of arthrogryposis multiplex congenita studied at autopsy by Banker BQ: Arthrogryposis multiplex congenita: spectrum of pathologic changes, *Hum Pathol* 17:656–672, 1986.

Pathogenesis

The development of fixed joints with limitation of movement in most cases is secondary *to impaired intra-uterine motility, almost invariably the result of muscle weakness.*[7,34,45-48] The postural deformities are caused by contractures of muscle with fibrous (not bony) ankylosis of the joints. The time of onset of the paralytic process determines, in part, the severity of the arthrogryposis; onset in the first trimester may be associated with pterygium formation at the neck and elbows.[49] The positions of the deformities are related, in large part, to muscle imbalance around the joints involved; neuropathological data support this notion.[46] The intrauterine position of the fetus may also play a role in determining the configuration of the deformities. The basic concept that impaired motility secondary to muscle weakness is the critical common denominator is supported by experiments with developing chicks and with fetal rats in which infusion of the neuromuscular blocker curare either into incubating eggs or into the fetal animals resulted in fixed postures of neck and limbs that corresponded to intrauterine position.[50,51] Pulmonary hypoplasia, micrognathia, polyhydramnios, short umbilical cord, and fetal growth retardation were documented in the fetal rats as in the human,[51] findings further supporting the notion that intrauterine impairments of movement underlie most of the "congenital anomalies" often observed with arthrogryposis (see Table 17-9). Supporting clinical data include the usual association of arthrogryposis multiplex congenita with neuromuscular diseases with intrauterine onset (see following discussion), as well as the occurrence of the disorder after the administration of drugs to the pregnant woman that cause diminished motor activity.[52] Disturbance of intrauterine movement is also presumed to be the cause of those unusual cases of arthrogryposis multiplex congenita occurring with intrauterine mechanical restrictions, such as amniotic band, small or malformed pelvis or uterus, or oligohydramnios.[47,53,54]

Arthrogryposis multiplex congenita not infrequently is an inherited disorder. In one series of 350 cases, 14% exhibited autosomal dominant inheritance, 7% were autosomal recessive, and 2% were X-linked recessive.[36] Most infants with autosomal recessive inheritance exhibited anomalies (often severe) of other body areas as well as of the central nervous system, whereas infants with autosomal dominant inheritance only uncommonly exhibited severe associated anomalies.[36] A relatively common, autosomal dominant variety of arthrogryposis affects principally hands and feet, is termed *distal arthrogryposis*, and responds particularly well to physical therapy.[37] The sites of involvement of the motor system among familial cases of arthrogryposis are diverse, although the lower motor neuron is most commonly affected.[7,34,36,39,48,49,54-64]

Pathology

The basis for the weakness that leads to arthrogryposis multiplex congenita resides at every major level of the motor system (Table 17-10).

TABLE 17-10 Major Causes of Arthrogryposis Multiplex Congenita

Site of Major Pathological Findings	Disorder
Cerebrum–brain stem	Microcephaly; migrational disorders: lissencephaly-pachygyria (e.g., Zellweger syndrome), schizencephaly, polymicrogyria, agenesis of corpus callosum; fetal alcohol syndrome; cytomegalovirus infection; pontocerebellar hypoplasia (type I); dentato-olivary dysplasia; leptomeningeal angiomatosis; encephaloclastic processes: neuronal destruction, porencephalies, hydranencephaly, multicystic encephalomalacia; hydrocephalus
Anterior horn cell	Developmental agenesis–hypoplasia–dysgenesis (amyoplasia congenita); anterior horn cell destruction; autosomal recessive, X-linked and autosomal dominant anterior horn cell degenerations; severe Werdnig-Hoffmann disease; Möbius syndrome; cervical spinal atrophy; lumbar spinal atrophy; lumbosacral meningomyelocele; sacral agenesis; other
Peripheral nerve or root	Hypomyelinative polyneuropathy; axonal polyneuropathy; neurofibromatosis
Neuromuscular junction	Infant of myasthenic mother; congenital myasthenia; infant of mother with multiple sclerosis (?)
Muscle	Congenital muscular dystrophy (merosin positive and merosin negative); congenital myotonic dystrophy; myotubular myopathy; central core disease; nemaline myopathy; congenital polymyositis; congenital fiber type disproportion; glycogen storage myopathy (muscle phosphorylase deficiency, phosphofructokinase deficiency); mitochondrial myopathy
Primary disorder of joint or connective tissue	Marfan syndrome; other disorders of connective tissue; intrauterine periarticular inflammation
Intrauterine mechanical obstruction	Uterine abnormality; amniotic bands; oligohydramnios; twin pregnancy; extrauterine pregnancy

Cerebrum or Brain Stem

Major intrauterine disorders of the cerebrum or brain stem or both have resulted in arthrogryposis multiplex congenita (see Table 17-10).[7,34,41,42,48,55,65-90] The proportion of cases with *exclusive* involvement of cerebrum or brain stem (and not also of the spinal cord) is approximately 10% to 35%. When spinal cord is evaluated, particularly postmortem but also by EMG in vivo, concomitant involvement of anterior horn cells is often discovered to accompany the more conspicuous central disorders.[7,73-76,78,80,82,83,88] This combination of findings is apparent particularly with pontocerebellar hypoplasia, type I, characterized by atrophy of neurons of the pons, cerebellum, and anterior horn cells (see Chapter 18). Although dysgenetic anomalies account for the majority of this category of cases, encephaloclastic lesions (e.g., ischemic or infectious in origin) and intrauterine hydrocephalus also have been causative. Severity of the disturbance of the motor system has been marked in the infants with central disorders, and thus, not unexpectedly (see earlier discussion), the resulting severe arthrogryposis with pulmonary hypoplasia often has led to the designation of Pena-Shokeir syndrome in this group. In a series of 15 infants with arthrogryposis multiplex congenita *and* ventilator dependence in the neonatal period, 9 had severe disease of cerebrum or brain stem, or both.[74] In a carefully studied series of 68 infants identified retrospectively, 23 (34%) had cerebral lesions.[87]

Anterior Horn Cell

Disease of the anterior horn cell has been demonstrated many times (see Table 17-10), and the anterior horn cell may be the most common single site of disease in arthrogryposis multiplex congenita.[*] This diverse group of disorders appears to account for at least 20% to 25% of cases of arthrogryposis multiplex congenita.[7,87,98,99,112] This proportion increases considerably when anterior horn cell disturbances occurring in association with abnormalities at higher levels of the central nervous system are included. The basic abnormalities of anterior horn cell are dysgenetic, destructive, or degenerative. *Dysgenetic abnormalities*, which are associated with disturbances of number or migration of neurons of the anterior horns, predominate (Fig. 17-15).[7] A likely example of this category is amyoplasia congenita (see later). *Destructive disorders* consist primarily of apparent intrauterine ischemic events. The association of arthrogryposis with maternal misoprostol exposure (oral or vaginal) may relate to ischemic injury to anterior horn cells.[34,118] *Degenerative disorders* include anterior horn cell degenerations with anatomical features often similar to those of Werdnig-Hoffmann disease (see Chapter 18). However, with one exception (see Chapter 18), when involvement of chromosome 5q has been sought specifically, no relationship with the gene locus of spinal muscular atrophy has been found.[109,110,115-117,119] Autosomal recessive and, rarely, X-linked recessive or autosomal dominant syndromes have been delineated.[73,100,101,108-111,113,115-117,120] At least six autosomal recessive phenotypes dominate the severe degenerative syndromes with arthrogryposis. One is a disorder termed *lethal congenital contracture syndrome*, which is associated with

---

*See references 7,46,49,59,61,62,67,73,74,83,87,91-117.

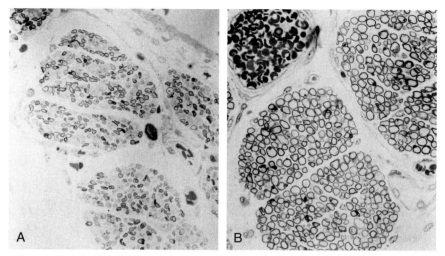

Figure 17-15   Arthrogryposis and dysgenesis of the anterior horns compared with normal findings. Alterations in, **A**, the anterior root of a newborn infant with arthrogryposis and dysgenesis of the anterior horns, compared with, **B**, the anterior root of an age-matched control infant. Note in the root from the arthrogryptic infant **(A)** the large areas devoid of myelinated fibers, without evidence of degeneration. Concordance between the severity of the alteration in the anterior roots and the absence or dysgenesis of the anterior horn cells (not shown) was noted. *(From Banker BQ: Arthrogryposis multiplex congenita: Spectrum of pathologic changes,* Hum Pathol *17:656–672, 1986.)*

intrauterine hydrops, growth retardation, and fetal death; severe neuronal loss in the anterior horns and extreme atrophy of skeletal muscle are present.[73,109,111] The gene has been localized to chromosome 9q34.[111] A related disorder, possibly a less severe form of the first, is associated with slightly less severe anterior horn cell degeneration and severe but not extreme muscle atrophy.[73,108] All the affected infants have died by 20 days of age. A second autosomal recessive disorder, much less common, is pontocerebellar hypoplasia type 1, discussed in the previous section (also see Chapter 16). A third autosomal recessive disorder with severe weakness and hypotonia, as well as mild contractures, is also associated with diaphragmatic paralysis, the need for mechanical ventilation, and a generally lethal course (often designated *SMARD1* for spinal muscular atrophy with respiratory distress); the disorder is genetically distinct from Werdnig-Hoffman disease (see Chapter 18).[115] A fourth disorder, X-linked recessive (Xq11.3-q11.32), is characterized by primarily distal arthrogryposis multiplex congenita, lower facial weakness, and a progressive course.[120] A fifth disorder, variably considered either X-linked or autosomal recessive, is characterized by severe weakness and hypotonia, with arthrogryposis and, notably, *long bone fractures.*[117] Whether this group is homogeneous is unclear. A sixth anterior horn cell disorder, autosomal dominant (localized to chromosome 12q23-q24) or sporadic, is associated with *involvement primarily of lower limbs* and severe, albeit usually nonprogressive disability.[116] The severity of the process and the features on the EMG and myohistological examination suggest that this process is an anterior horn cell degeneration, largely completed by the postnatal period.

The *clinical distinction* of the three major categories of anterior horn cell involvement (dysgenetic, destructive, or degenerative) in an infant with arthrogryposis is difficult. The findings of neurological deterioration,

fasciculations, and grouped atrophy suggest active degenerative disease rather than a dysgenetic or a completed destructive process. *Among probable dysgenetic types,* the relatively common clinical entity termed *amyoplasia* or *amyoplasia congenita* is perhaps the prototype.[34] This disorder has been said to account for as many as one third of all newborns with arthrogryposis.[34] In a large series of infants with arthrogryposis, of 16 with anterior horn cell involvement, 14 had amyoplasia.[87] Clinically, these infants are distinctive and exhibit symmetric involvement of all four limbs, with the upper extremities characteristically in a "waiter's tip" position. The latter relates to internally rotated, adducted shoulders, extended elbows, pronated forearms, and flexed wrists and fingers. Talipes equinovarus is nearly invariable. Common associations are facial hemangioma and digital defects. The EMG shows a reduced number of motor units but no fasciculations. Muscle biopsy (see later) is distinctive, with affected muscles replaced by fatty and fibrous tissue.

Among the degenerative disorders, the clinical features of six principal genetic disorders involving the anterior horn cell (and genetically distinct from Werdnig-Hoffman disease) were described earlier in relation to the pathological features (see "Pathology"). Particular note should be made of the *relative lack of arthrogryposis in typical Werdnig-Hoffman disease.* Thus, only approximately 10% to 20% of infants with typical, chromosome 5q–linked Werdnig-Hoffmann disease exhibit contractures, which are mild and usually restricted to distal limbs.[96] In a series of 68 infants with overt arthrogryposis, only 1 infant had Werdnig-Hoffman disease.[87] The reason for the relatively low incidence of joint deformity in such a severe intrauterine disorder of movement is not known definitely, but it may relate to the uniformity of the disturbance of anterior horn cells, unlike the relative preservation of some anterior horn cells in dysgenetic or destructive

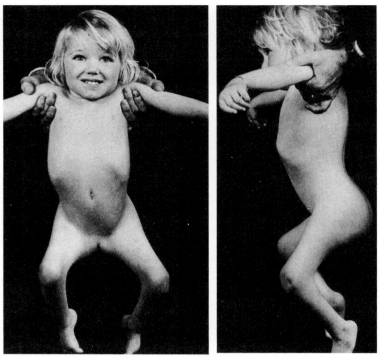

Figure 17-16   **Arthrogryposis multiplex congenita in a child with congenital peripheral neuropathy.** Note the fixed flexion of the hips and knees, equinus of feet, and ulnar deviation of hands. *(From Dubowitz V: Muscle Disorders in Childhood, 2nd ed, Philadelphia: 1978, Saunders.)*

disorders, and hence the possibility of contracture formation.[46] The important clinical point is that severe generalized arthrogryposis multiplex congenita, even related to anterior horn cell degeneration, is extremely unlikely to represent typical, chromosome 5q–linked (survival motor neuron) spinal muscular atrophy (see Chapter 18). *An exception*, as noted earlier, is the small group of very severe chromosomal 5q–linked cases of prenatal onset described in Chapter 18.

As many as one third to one half of infants with Möbius syndrome may exhibit arthrogryposis, a finding reflecting involvement of the lower motor neuron in the spinal cord as well as in the brain stem in this disorder.[34,47,48,67,121] Fixed contractures of the lower limbs are frequent accompaniments of disorders of neural tube development (e.g., lumbosacral meningomyelocele and sacral agenesis).[122,123] Isolated cervical or lumbar arthrogryposis secondary to nonprogressive anterior horn cell involvement, not defined more clearly, also has been reported.[48,102,103,105,106,114]

Peripheral Nerve

Disorder of the peripheral nerve has been shown to result in arthrogryposis multiplex congenita (Fig. 17-16 and Table 17-10).[7,26,48,74,87,93,119,124-132] However, peripheral neuropathy is relatively rare as the basis for arthrogryposis; in the series of Banker,[7] only 2 of 96 patients with arthrogryposis had peripheral nerve disease. In a series of 15 ventilator-dependent newborns with arthrogryposis, 1 infant had congenital (hypomyelinative) neuropathy.[74] In a well-studied retrospective series of 68 infants, only 1 infant had (hypomyelinative)

neuropathy.[87] In virtually all reported cases, the neuropathy was hypomyelinative (see Chapter 18), although I have seen a single patient with combined axonal-hypomyelinative neuropathy.

Neuromuscular Junction

Disorder of the neuromuscular junction is a rare cause of arthrogryposis multiplex congenita (see Table 17-10). One series of infants born to myasthenic mothers exhibited arthrogryposis multiplex congenita and other signs of fetal immobility (e.g., pulmonary hypoplasia).[32,34,48,119,133-141] A relationship of transplacentally transferred antiacetylcholine receptor antibody with fetal immobility was suggested by the correlation of maternal antibody titers with the fetal abnormalities in several patients, as well as by the improvement in fetal motility and the onset of fetal breathing in a woman after treatment with plasmapheresis and prednisone caused a decrease in antibody titers.[138] The woman, who had had two previous pregnancies complicated by arthrogryposis and pulmonary hypoplasia, delivered an infant with no contractures (although transient neonatal myasthenia gravis did occur).[138] In one sibship of six affected infants, the mother's myasthenia gravis was asymptomatic and was previously undetected.[139]

Congenital myasthenia gravis also has been associated with the occurrence of arthrogryposis multiplex congenita.[74,142-147] The most common defect resulting in arthrogryposis is endplate acetylcholine receptor deficiency caused by a mutation of rapsyn (receptor-associated protein at the synapse), which is critical for receptor clustering (see Chapter 18). In a series of

15 ventilator-dependent newborns with arthrogryposis, the only infant with a treatable disorder had congenital myasthenia, an observation emphasizing the importance of an edrophonium test in infants with arthrogryposis of unknown origin, especially before elective cessation of ventilator support.[74]

Arthrogryposis of varying severity was reported in seven infants born to mothers with multiple sclerosis.[148,149] I have seen one such case. The EMG and muscle biopsy were normal. The cause of the fetal immobility is unclear, but a reasonable speculation is that the disturbance was at the level of the neuromuscular junction. This occurrence must be very rare because a more recent review of 649 births to women with multiple sclerosis did not report any cases of arthrogryposis.[150]

Muscle

Disorders of muscle are well-recognized causes of arthrogryposis multiplex congenita (see Table 17-10). Differences in the incidence of myopathic causes are apparent between series of arthrogryposis studied during life and post mortem. Thus, in the series of 96 autopsy cases studied by Banker,[7] only 6 had myopathic disorders. However, in more than 200 well-studied *living* cases evaluated by EMG, muscle biopsy, or both, approximately 20% to 40% of cases of arthrogryposis were related to myopathy.[87,98,119,151] In my experience, the most common myopathic causes of arthrogryposis are congenital muscular dystrophy, congenital myotonic dystrophy, and myotubular myopathy. However, several other myopathies have been reported in association with arthrogryposis (see Fig. 17-14).* These disorders are described in detail in Chapter 19.

Primary Disorder of Joint or Connective Tissue

Approximately 10% of cases of arthrogryposis multiplex congenita appear to relate to a primary disorder of joint or associated connective tissue (see Table 17-10).[34,36,37,47] Such is the case for Marfan syndrome and related congenital contractural arachnodactyly disorders, usually classified among the nine types of distal arthrogryposis.[34,37,48,87,162,163] Experimental and clinical observations suggested a possible role for intrauterine inflammatory disease of muscle or of periarticular tissue as rare causes.[164,165]

Intrauterine Mechanical Obstruction

Mechanical constriction of fetal movement may lead to a variety of joint contractures (see Table 17-10). Important causes include uterine structural abnormalities, amniotic bands, oligohydramnios, and multiple fetuses. Although these contractures may be generalized and may simulate arthrogryposis multiplex congenita, they often are focal and restricted, reflecting the specific nature of the mechanical obstruction.

---

*See references 26,48,60,64,86,87,93,98,99,119,151-161a.

Diagnosis

The occurrence of arthrogryposis multiplex congenita is an indication for a careful evaluation to determine the presence and nature of a disorder of the motor system. Accurate diagnosis is important for definition of prognosis, genetic counseling, and plan of therapy. Careful assessment of central nervous system with clinical examination and brain imaging is critical because of the relatively high frequency of central disorders, especially with severe arthrogryposis multiplex congenita. Evaluation of the neuromuscular apparatus requires serum enzyme analysis, EMG, nerve conduction velocities, and often muscle biopsy. Examinations of the CSF or nerve biopsy may also be appropriate. In certain cases, the muscle is found to be relatively well preserved on biopsy, and in such cases, the prognosis may be good.[26] However, even in some disorders that have a pronounced abnormality of muscle (e.g., amyoplasia), the prognosis for useful function, including walking, is very good.[34] Similarly, certain varieties of congenital myopathy (e.g., congenital fiber-type disproportion) are often associated with a favorable prognosis, whereas others (e.g., congenital myotonic or severe congenital muscular dystrophy) have a less favorable outlook.

Two myopathic patterns commonly observed with arthrogryposis (i.e., *fiber type predominance* and *disproportion* and aplasia of muscle [*amyoplasia*]) should be discussed further. *Fiber type predominance*, which is an increase in the percentage of one fiber type, or *fiber type disproportion*, which is a reduction in diameter of one fiber type (usually type 1 fibers), or both predominance and disproportion may occur. These findings may indicate congenital myopathy (see Chapter 19), but often (20 of 96 cases in the Banker series[7]) they are observed in arthrogrypotic infants with no evidence of myopathy or neurogenic disturbance. Investigators have postulated that such patients have had an intrauterine disturbance in the neural modulation of muscle differentiation, secondary to either undetected central nervous system or anterior horn cell abnormality, as the cause for the fiber type predominance or disproportion.[7,166,167] The pattern of *amyoplasia* also reflects a disturbance of muscle formation related to neural (i.e., anterior horn cell) disturbance. Most probably, amyoplasia represents the severe end of a continuum of disturbance of neural induction of muscle proliferation and growth and is related to severe anterior horn cell maldevelopment with very early onset (Figs. 17-17 and 17-18). Whenever possible, careful quantitative analysis of the number and organization of anterior horn cells in cases of arthrogryposis of unknown causes is needed.

Management

Determination of a diagnosis that is as specific as possible is an important starting point in patient management. The basic elements of management and their usual sequence of progression are (1) passive stretching, (2) serial casting, and (3) surgical release procedures.[26,34,168-175] Passive stretching exercises, often augmented by flexible supports, should be

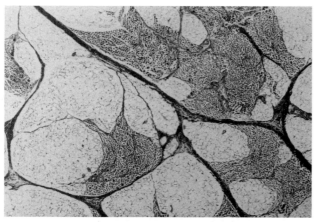

Figure 17-17 **Amyoplasia in an infant with arthrogryposis and dysgenesis of the central nervous system that included the anterior horn cells.** The muscle fibers are very small in cross section. Portions of fasciculi or whole fasciculi have been replaced by adipose tissue (hematoxylin and eosin stain, × 70). *(From Banker BQ: Arthrogryposis multiplex congenita: Spectrum of pathologic changes, Hum Pathol 17:656–672, 1986.)*

instituted first. Because the best responses to physical therapy are usually achieved in the first few months, the onset of such intervention should not be delayed. When needed, these initial procedures are followed by serial casting with lightweight splints. Because the rigidity of joints results from fibrous and not bony ankylosis, these procedures may be particularly beneficial. Marked and persistent deformities can be improved by the surgical release of periarticular tendons and ligaments. Even with major degrees of deformity, a surprising amount of improvement in functional capabilities may be achieved. Infants with progressive disorders or with severe central nervous system involvement, or both (see Table 17-10), respond to therapy in only a limited fashion, if at all.

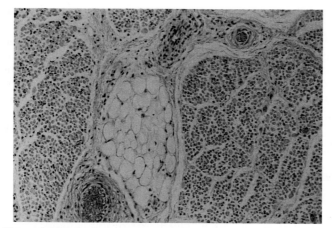

Figure 17-18 **Hypoplasia of muscle in an infant with arthrogryposis and dysgenesis of the anterior horns.** The muscle fibers are small, as is the entire muscle (hematoxylin and eosin stain, × 180). *(From Banker BQ: Arthrogryposis multiplex congenita: Spectrum of pathologic changes, Hum Pathol 17:656–672, 1986.)*

REFERENCES

1. Carpenter MB: *Human Neuroanatomy*, Baltimore: 1983, Williams & Wilkins.
2. Sarnat HB: Cerebral dysgeneses and their influence on fetal muscle development, *Brain Dev* 8:495-499, 1986.
3. Sarnat HB: Do the corticospinal and corticobulbar tracts mediate functions in the human newborn? *Can J Neurol Sci* 16:157-160, 1989.
4. Pasternak JF, Volpe JJ: Neuromuscular problems. In Paxson CL, editor: *Van Leeuwen's Newborn Medicine*, Chicago: 1979, Year Book.
5. Sarnat HB: Neuromuscular disorders in the neonatal period. In Korobkin R, Guilleminault C, editors: *Advances in Perinatal Neurology*, New York: 1979, Spectrum Publications.
6. Schloon H, Schlottmann J, Lenard HG, Goebel HH: The development of skeletal muscles in premature infants, *Eur J Pediatr* 131:49-60, 1979.
7. Banker BQ: Arthrogryposis multiplex congenita: Spectrum of pathologic changes, *Hum Pathol* 17:656-672, 1986.
8. Brooke MH, Engel WK: The histographic analysis of human muscle biopsies with regard to fiber types. IV. Children's biopsies, *Neurology* 19:591-605, 1969.
9. Engel WK, Karpati G: Impaired skeletal muscle maturation following neonatal neurectomy, *Dev Biol* 17:713-723, 1968.
10. Karpati G, Engel WK: "Type grouping" in skeletal muscles after experimental reinnervation, *Neurology* 18:447-455, 1968.
11. Romanul FC, Van der Meulen JP: Slow and fast muscles after cross innervation: Enzymatic and physiologic changes, *Arch Neurol* 17:387-402, 1967.
12. Samaha F, Gergely J: Biochemistry of muscle and muscle disorders. In Siegel GJ, Albers RW, Katzman R, et al, editors: *Basic Neurochemistry*, Boston: 1993, Little, Brown.
13. DiMauro S, Eastwood AB: Disorders of glycogen and lipid metabolism. In Griggs RC, Moxley RT, editors: *Treatment of Neuromuscular Diseases*, New York: 1977, Raven Press.
14. van Tol A: Aspects of long-chain acyl-CoA metabolism, *Mol Cell Biochem* 7:19, 1975.
15. DiMauro S, Bonilla E, Zeviani M: Mitochondrial myopathies, *Ann Neurol* 17:521-538, 1985.
16. Osborne JP, Murphy EG, Hill A: Thin ribs on chest X-ray: A useful sign in the differential diagnosis of the floppy newborn, *Dev Med Child Neurol* 25:343-345, 1983.
17. Rodriguez JI, Palacios J, Garcia-Alix A, Pastor I, et al: Effects of immobilization on fetal bone development: A morphometric study in newborns with congenital neuromuscular diseases with intrauterine onset, *Calcif Tissue Int* 43:335-339, 1988.
18. Rodriguez JI, Garcia-Alix A, Palacios J, Paniagua R: Changes in the long bones due to fetal immobility caused by neuromuscular disease: A radiographic and histological study, *J Bone Joint Surg Am* 70:1052-1060, 1988.
19. Bodensteiner J, Zellweger H: Creatine phosphokinase in normal neonates and young infants, *J Lab Clin Med* 77:853-858, 1971.
20. Drummond LM: Creatine phosphokinase levels in the newborn and their use in screening for Duchenne muscular dystrophy, *Arch Dis Child* 54:362-366, 1979.
21. Sutton TM, O'Brien FJ, Kleinberg F, House RF Jr, et al: Serum levels of creatine phosphokinase and its isoenzymes in normal and stressed neonates, *Mayo Clin Proc* 56:150-154, 1981.
22. Jones HR: EMG evaluation of the floppy infant: Differential diagnosis and technical aspects, *Musc Nerv* 13:338-347, 1990.
23. Jones HR: Pediatric electromyography. In Brown WF, Bolton CF, editors: *Clinical Electromyography*, 2nd ed, Boston: 1993, Butterworth-Heinemann.
24. Jones HR, Bolton CF, Harper C Jr: *Pediatric Clinical Electromyography*, Philadelphia: 1996, Lippincott-Raven.
25. Swoboda KJ, Edelbol-Eeg-Olofsson K, Harmon RL, Bolton CF, et al: Pediatric electromyography. In Jones HR Jr, DeVivo DC, Darras BT, editors: *Neuromuscular Disorders of Infancy, Childhood, and Adolescence: A Clinician's Approach*, Philadelphia: 2003, Butterworth Heinemann.
26. Dubowitz V: *Muscle Disorders in Childhood*, 2nd ed, Philadelphia: 1978, Saunders.
27. Cohen HL, Brumlik J: *Manual of Electroneuromyography*, Hagerstown, MD: 1976, Harper & Row.
28. Sarnat HB: Diagnostic value of the muscle biopsy in the neonatal period, *Am J Dis Child* 132:782-785, 1978.
29. Sarnat HB: Pathology of spinal muscular atrophy. In Gamstorp I, Sarnat HB, editors: *Progressive Spinal Muscular Atrophies*, New York: 1984, Raven Press.
30. Brooke MH, Carroll JE, Ringel SP: Congenital hypotonia revisited, *Muscle Nerve* 2:84-100, 1979.
31. Curless RG, Nelson MB: Needle biopsies of muscles in infants for diagnosis and research, *Dev Med Child Neurol* 17:592-601, 1975.
32. Dubowitz V: *Muscle Disorders in Childhood*, 2nd ed, Philadelphia: 1995, Saunders.
33. Anthony DC, De Girolami U, Shapiro F: Muscle biopsy. In Jones HR Jr, DeVivo DC, Darras BT, editors: *Neuromuscular Disorders of Infancy, Childhood, and Adolescence: A Clinician's Approach*, Philadelphia: 2003, Butterworth Heinemann.
34. Hall J, Vincent A: Arthrogryposis. In Jones HR Jr, DeVivo DC, Darras BT, editors: *Neuromuscular Disorders of Infancy, Childhood, and Adolescence: A Clinician's Approach*, Philadelphia: 2003, Butterworth Heinemann.

35. Beckerman RC, Buchino JJ: Arthrogryposis multiplex congenita as part of an inherited symptom complex: Two case reports and a review of the literature, *Pediatrics* 61:417-422, 1978.
36. Hall JG: Genetic aspects of arthrogryposis, *Clin Orthop Relat Res* 194:44-53, 1985.
37. Hall JC: Overview of arthrogryposis. In Staheli LT, Hall JG, Jaffe KM, et al, editors: *Arthrogryposis*, Cambridge: 1998, Cambridge University Press.
38. Robinson RO: Arthrogryposis multiplex congenita: Feeding, language and other health problems, *Neuropediatrics* 21:177-178, 1990.
39. Pena CE, Miller F, Budzilovich GN, Feigin I: Arthrogryposis multiplex congenita: Report of two cases of radicular type with familial incidence, *Neurology* 18:92-930, 1968.
40. Pena SD, Shokeir MH: Syndrome of camptodactyly, multiple ankyloses, facial anomalies, and pulmonary hypoplasia: A lethal condition, *J Pediatr* 85:373-375, 1974.
41. Lavi E, Montone KT, Rorke LB, Kliman HJ: Fetal akinesia deformation sequence (Pena-Shokeir phenotype) associated with acquired intrauterine brain damage, *Neurology* 41:1467-1468, 1991.
42. Illum N, Reske-Nielsen E, Skovby F, Askjaer SA, et al: Lethal autosomal recessive arthrogryposis multiplex congenita with whistling face and calcifications of the nervous system, *Neuropediatrics* 19:186-192, 1988.
43. Alves AF, Azevedo ES: Recessive form of Freeman-Sheldon's syndrome or "whistling face", *J Med Genet* 14:139-141, 1977.
44. Sauk JJ, Delaney JR, Reaume C, Brandjord R, et al: Electromyography of oral-facial musculature in craniocarpaltarsal dysplasia (Freeman-Sheldon syndrome), *Clin Genet* 6:132-137, 1974.
45. Swinyard CA: Concepts of multiple congenital contractures (arthrogryposis) in man and animals, *Teratology* 25:247-258, 1982.
46. Clarren SK, Hall JG: Neuropathologic findings in the spinal cords of 10 infants with arthrogryposis, *J Neurol Sci* 58:89-102, 1983.
47. Swinyard CA, Bleck EE: The etiology of arthrogryposis (multiple congenital contractures), *Clin Orthop Relat Res* 194:15-29, 1985.
48. Gordon N: Arthrogryposis multiplex congenita, *Brain Dev* 20:507-511, 1998.
49. Herva R, Conradi NG, Kalimo H, Leisti J, et al: A syndrome of multiple congenital contractures: Neuropathological analysis on five fetal cases, *Am J Med Genet* 29:67-76, 1988.
50. Drachman DB, Coulombre AJ: Experimental clubfoot and arthrogryposis multiplex congenita, *Lancet* 2:523-526, 1962.
51. Moessinger AC: Fetal akinesia deformation sequence: An animal model, *Pediatrics* 72:857-863, 1983.
52. Jago RH: Arthrogryposis following treatment of maternal tetanus with muscle relaxants, *Arch Dis Child* 45:277-279, 1970.
53. Kite JH: Arthrogryposis multiplex congenita: Review of fifty-four cases, *South Med J* 48:1141-1146, 1955.
54. Swinyard CA, Mayer V: Multiple congenital contractures, *JAMA* 183:23-27, 1963.
55. Lindhout D, Hageman G, Beemer FA, Ippel PF, et al: The Pena-Shokeir syndrome: Report of nine Dutch cases, *Am J Med Genet* 21:655-668, 1985.
56. Friedlander HL, Westin GW, Wood WL: Arthrogryposis multiplex congenita: A review of forty-five cases, *J Bone Joint Surg* 50:89-105, 1968.
57. Lebenthal E, Shochet SB, Adam A, Seelendfreund M, et al: Arthrogryposis multiplex congenita: Twenty-three cases in an Arab kindred, *Pediatrics* 46:891-899, 1970.
58. Rosemann A, Arad I: Arthrogryposis multiplex congenita: Neurogenic type with autosomal recessive inheritance, *J Med Genet* 11:91-98, 1974.
59. Nezelof C, Dupart MC, Jaubert F, Eliachar E: A lethal familial syndrome associating arthrogryposis multiplex congenita, renal dysfunction, and a cholestatic and pigmentary liver disease, *J Pediatr* 94:258-260, 1979.
60. Kalyanaraman K, Kalyanaraman UP: Myopathic arthrogryposis with seizures and abnormal electroencephalogram, *J Pediatr* 100:247-250, 1982.
61. Sul YC, Mrak RE, Evans OB, Fenichel GM: Neurogenic arthrogryposis in one identical twin, *Arch Neurol* 39:717-718, 1982.
62. Herva R, Leisti J, Kirkinen P, Seppanen U: A lethal autosomal recessive syndrome of multiple congenital contractures, *Am J Med Genet* 20:431-439, 1985.
63. Kawira EL, Bender HA: Brief clinical report: An unusual distal arthrogryposis, *Am J Med Genet* 20:425-429, 1985.
64. Hennekam RC, Barth PG, Van Lookeren CW, De Visser M, et al: A family with severe X-linked arthrogryposis, *J Pediatr* 150:656-660, 1991.
65. Ek JI: Cerebral lesions in arthrogryposis multiplex congenita, *Acta Paediatr* 47:302-316, 1958.
66. Hageman G, Willemse J: Arthrogryposis multiplex congenita: Review with comment, *Neuropediatrics* 14:6-11, 1983.
67. Banker BQ: Neuropathologic aspects of arthrogryposis multiplex congenita, *Clin Orthop Relat Res* 194:30-43, 1985.
68. Davis JE, Katousek DK: Fetal akinesia deformation sequence in previable fetuses, *Am J Med Genet* 29:77-87, 1988.
69. Hageman G, Willemse J, van Ketel BA, Barth PG, et al: The heterogeneity of the Pena-Shokeir syndrome, *Neuropediatrics* 18:45-50, 1987.
70. Bisceglia M, Zelante I, Bosman C, Cera R, et al: Pathologic features in two siblings with the Pena-Shokeir I syndrome, *Eur J Pediatr* 146:283-287, 1987.
71. Massa G, Casaer B, Ceulemans B, Van Eldere S: Arthrogryposis multiplex congenita associated with lissencephaly: A case report, *Neuropediatrics* 19:24-26, 1988.
72. Choi BH, Ruess WR, Kim RC: Disturbances in neuronal migration and laminar cortical organization associated with multicystic encephalopathy in the Pena-Shokeir syndrome, *Acta Neuropathol (Berl)* 69:177-183, 1986.
73. Vuopala K, Leisti J, Herva R: Lethal arthrogryposis in Finland: A clinico-pathological study of 83 cases during thirteen years, *Neuropediatrics* 25:308-315, 1995.
74. Bianchi DW, Van Marter LJ: An approach to ventilator-dependent neonates with arthrogryposis, *Pediatrics* 94:682-686, 1994.
75. Hageman G, Hoogenraad TU, Prevo RL: The association of cortical dysplasia and anterior horn arthrogryposis: A case report, *Brain Dev* 16:463-466, 1995.
76. Brodtkorb E, Torbergsen T, Nakken KO, Andersen K, et al: Epileptic seizures, arthrogryposis, and migrational brain disorders: A syndrome, *Acta Neurol Scand* 90:232-240, 1994.
77. Perlman J, Burns DK, Twickler DM, Weinberg AG: Fetal hypokinesia syndrome in the monochorionic pair of a triplet pregnancy secondary to severe disruptive cerebral injury, *Pediatrics* 96:521-523, 1995.
78. Razavi FE, Larroche JC, Roume J, Gonzales M, et al: Lethal familial fetal akinesia sequence (FAS) with distinct neuropathological pattern: Type III lissencephaly syndrome, *Am J Med Genet* 62:16-22, 1996.
79. Baker EM, Khorasgani MG, Gardner-Medwin D, Gjholkar A, et al: Arthrogryposis multiplex congenita and bilateral parietal polymicrogyria in association with the intrauterine death of a twin, *Neuropediatrics* 27:54-56, 1996.
80. Hevner RF, Horoupian DS: Pena-Shokeir phenotype associated with bilateral opercular polymicrogyria, *Pediatr Neurol* 15:348-351, 1996.
81. Sztriha L, Al-Gazali LI, Varady E, Goebel HH, et al: Autosomal recessive micrencephaly with simplified gyral pattern, abnormal myelination and arthrogryposis, *Neuropediatrics* 30:141-145, 1999.
82. Gorgen-Pauly U, Sperner J, Reiss I, Gehl, et al: Familial pontocerebellar hypoplasia type 1 with anterior horn cell disease, *Eur J Paediatr Neurol* 3:33-38, 1999.
83. Muntoni F, Goodwin F, Sewry C, Cox P, et al: Clinical spectrum and diagnostic difficulties of infantile ponto-cerebellar hypoplasia type 1, *Neuropediatrics* 30:243-248, 1999.
84. Takano T, Aotani H, Takeuchi Y: Asymmetric arthrogryposis multiplex congenita with focal pachygyria, *Pediatr Neurol* 25:247-249, 2001.
85. Charollais A, Lacroix C, Nouyrigat V, Devictor D, et al: Arthrogryposis and multicystic encephalopathy after acute fetal distress in the end stage of gestation, *Neuropediatrics* 32:49-52, 2001.
86. Witters I, Moerman P, Fryne JP: Fetal akinesia deformation sequence: A study of 30 consecutive in utero diagnoses, *Am J Med Genet* 113:23-28, 2002.
87. Darin N, Kimber E, Kroksmark A-K, Tulinius M: Multiple congenital contractures: Birth prevalence, etiology, and outcome, *J Pediatr* 140:61-67, 2002.
88. Rudnik-Schoneborn S, Sztriha L, Aithala GR, Houge G, et al: Extended phenotype of pontocerebellar hypoplasia with infantile spinal muscular atrophy, *Am J Med Genet A* 117:10-17, 2003.
89. Castro-Gago M, Iglesias-Meleiro JM, Blanco-Barca MO, Grande-Seijo M, et al: Neurogenic arthrogryposis multiplex congenita and velopharyngeal incompetence associated with chromosome 22q11.2 deletion, *J Child Neurol* 20:76-78, 2005.
90. Saito Y, Hayashi M, Miyazono Y, Shimogama T, et al: Arthrogryposis multiplex congenita with callosal agenesis and dentato-olivary dysplasia, *Brain Dev* 28:261-264, 2006.
91. Imamura M, Yamanaka N, Nakamura F, Oyanagi K: Arthrogryposis multiplex congenita: An autopsy case of a fatal form, *Hum Pathol* 12:699-704, 1981.
92. Moerman P, Fryns JP, Goddeeris P, Lauweryns JM: Multiple ankylosis, facial anomalies, and pulmonary hypoplasia associated with severe antenatal spinal muscular atrophy, *J Pediatr* 103:238-241, 1983.
93. Hageman G, Jennekens FG, Vette JK, Willemse J: The heterogeneity of distal arthrogryposis, *Brain Dev* 6:273-283, 1984.
94. Brandt SA: A case of arthrogryposis multiplex congenita anatomically appearing as a foetal spinal muscular atrophy, *Acta Paediatr* 34:365-371, 1961.
95. Drachman DB, Banker BQ: Arthrogryposis multiplex congenita: Case due to disease of the anterior horn cells, *Arch Neurol* 5:77-93, 1961.
96. Byers RK, Banker BQ: Infantile muscular atrophy, *Arch Neurol* 5:140-164, 1961.
97. Amick LD, Johnson WW, Smith HL: Electromyographic and histopathologic correlations in arthrogryposis, *Arch Neurol* 16:512-523, 1967.
98. Jones HR: Personal communication, 1993.
99. Strehl E, Vanasse M: EMG and needle muscle biopsy studies in arthrogryposis multiplex congenita, *Neuropediatrics* 16:225-227, 1985.
100. Greenberg F, Fenolio KR, Hejtmancik F, Armstrong D, et al: X-linked infantile spinal muscular atrophy, *Arch J Dis Child* 142:217-219, 1988.
101. Hall JG, Reed SD, Scott CI: Three distinct types of X-linked arthrogryposis seen in six families, *Clin Genet* 21:81-97, 1982.
102. Fleury P, Hageman G: A dominantly inherited lower motor neuron disorder presenting at birth with associated arthrogryposis, *J Neurol Neurosurg Psychiatry* 48:1037-1048, 1985.
103. Darwish H, Sarnat H, Archer C, Brownell K, et al: Congenital cervical spinal atrophy, *Muscle Nerve* 4:106-110, 1981.
104. Robertson WL, Glinski LP, Kirkpatrick SJ, Pauli RM: Further evidence that arthrogryposis multiplex congenita in the human sometimes is caused by an intrauterine vascular accident, *Teratology* 45:345-351, 1992.
105. Tsukamoto H, Inagaki M, Tomita Y, Ohno K: Congenital caudal spinal atrophy: A case report, *Neuropediatrics* 23:260-262, 1992.
106. Hageman G: Congenital brachial arthrogryposis, *J Neurol Neurosurg Psychiatry* 56:365-368, 1993.
107. Frijns C, Vandeutekom J, Frants RR, Jennekens F: Dominant congenital benign spinal muscular atrophy, *Muscle Nerve* 17:192-197, 1994.

108. Vuopala K, Ignatius J, Herva R: Lethal arthrogryposis with anterior horn cell disease, *Hum Pathol* 26:12-19, 1995.
109. Vuopala K, Makela-Bengs P, Suomalainen A, Herva R, et al: Lethal congenital contracture syndrome: A fetal anterior horn cell disease is not linked to the SMA 5q locus, *J Med Genet* 32:36-38, 1995.
110. Rudnik-Schoneborn S, Forkert R, Hahnen E, Wirth B, et al: Clinical spectrum and diagnostic criteria of infantile spinal muscular atrophy: Further delineation on the basis of SMN gene deletion findings, *Neuropediatrics* 27:8-15, 1996.
111. Makela-Bengs P, Jarvinen N, Vuopala K, Suomalainen A, et al: Assignment of the disease locus for lethal congenital contracture syndrome to a restricted region of chromosome 9q34, by genome scan using five affected individuals, *Am J Hum Genet* 63:506-516, 1998.
112. Torres AR, Jones HR, Darras BT: Electromyography and biopsy correlation study of infants with arthrogryposis multiplex congenita, *Ann Neurol* 46:535-541, 1999.
113. Mercuri E, Goodwin F, Sewry C, Dubowitz V, et al: Diaphragmatic spinal muscular atrophy with bulbar weakness, *Eur J Paediatr Neurol* 4:69-72, 2000.
114. Kaiboriboon K, Hayat GR: Congenital cervical spinal atrophy: An intrauterine hypoxic insult, *Neuropediatrics* 32:330-334, 2001.
115. Rudnik-Schoneborn S, Stolz P, Varon R, Grohmann K, et al: Long-term observations of patients with infantile spinal muscular atrophy with respiratory distress type 1 (SMARD1), *Neuropediatrics* 35:174-182, 2004.
116. Mercuri E, Messina S, Kinali M, Cini C, et al: Congenital form of spinal muscular atrophy predominantly affecting the lower limbs: A clinical and muscle MRI study, *Neuromuscul Disord* 14:125-129, 2004.
117. Kizilates SU, Talim B, Sel K, Kose G, et al: Severe lethal spinal muscular atrophy variant with arthrogryposis, *Pediatr Neurol* 32:201-204, 2005.
118. Coelho KE, Sarmento MV, Veiga CM, Speck-Martins CE, et al: Misoprostol embryotoxicity: Clinical evaluation of fifteen patients with arthrogryposis, *Am J Med Genet* 95:297-301, 2000.
119. Kang PB, Lidov HGW, David WS, Torres A, et al: Diagnostic value of electromyography and muscle biopsy in arthrogryposis multiplex congenita, *Ann Neurol* 54:790-795, 2003.
120. Crawford TO: Infantile botulism. In Jones HR Jr, DeVivo DC, Darras BT, editors: *Neuromuscular Disorders of Infancy, Childhood, and Adolescence: A Clinician's Approach*, Philadelphia: 2003, Butterworth Heinemann.
121. Henderson JL: The congenital facial diplegia syndrome: Clinical features, pathology and etiology, *Brain* 62:381-395, 1939.
122. Dodge PR: Congenital neuromuscular disorders, *Proc Assoc Res Nerv Ment Dis* 38:479, 1960.
123. Sarnat HB, Case ME, Graviss R: Sacral agenesis: Neurology and neuropathologic features, *Neurology* 26:1124-1129, 1976.
124. Moore BH: Some orthopedic relationships of neurofibromatosis, *J Bone Joint Surg* 23:109, 1941.
125. Hooshmand H, Martinez AJ, Rosenblum WI: Arthrogryposis multiplex congenita: Simultaneous involvement of peripheral nerve and skeletal muscle, *Arch Neurol* 24:561-572, 1971.
126. Gibson DA, Urs ND: Arthrogryposis multiplex congenita, *J Bone Joint Surg Br* 3:483-493, 1970.
127. Palix C, Coignet J: Un cas de polyneuropathie périphérique néonatale par amyelinisation, *Pediatrie* 23:201-207, 1978.
128. Yuill GM, Lynch PG: Congenital non-progressive peripheral neuropathy with arthrogryposis multiplex, *J Neurol Neurosurg Psych* 37:316-323, 1974.
129. Boylan KB, Ferriero DM, Greco CM, Sheldon RA, et al: Congenital hypomyelination neuropathy with arthrogryposis multiplex congenita, *Ann Neurol* 31:337-340, 1992.
130. Seitz RJ, Wechsler W, Mosny DS, Lenard HG: Hypomyelination neuropathy in a female newborn presenting as arthrogryposis multiplex congenita, *Neuropediatrics* 17:132-136, 1986.
131. Folkerth RD, Guttentag SH, Kupsky WJ, Kinney HC: Arthrogryposis multiplex congenita with posterior column degeneration and peripheral neuropathy: A case report, *Clin Neuropathol* 12:25-33, 1993.
132. Takada E, Koyama N, Ogawa Y, Itoyama S, et al: Neuropathology of infant with Pena-Shokeir I syndrome, *Pediatr Neurol* 10:241-243, 1994.
133. Holmes LB, Driscoll SG, Bradley WG: Contractures in a newborn infant of a mother with myasthenia gravis, *J Pediatr* 96:1067-1069, 1980.
134. Pasternak JF, Hageman J, Adams MA: Exchange transfusion in neonatal myasthenia, *J Pediatr* 99:644-646, 1981.
135. Shepard MK: Arthrogryposis multiplex congenita in sibs, *Birth Defects Orig Artic Ser* 7:127, 1971.
136. Dulitzky F, Sirota L, Landman J, Homburg R: An infant with multiple deformations born to a myasthenic mother, *Helv Paediatr Acta* 42:173-176, 1987.
137. Moutard-Codou ML, Delleur MM, Doulac O, Morel E, et al: Myasthenie néo-natale sévère avec arthrogrypose, *Press Med* 16:615-618, 1987.
138. Carr SR, Gilchrist JM, Abuelo DN, Clark D: Treatment of antenatal myasthenia gravis, *Obstet Gynecol* 78:485-489, 1991.
139. Brueton LA, Huson SM, Cox PM, Shirley I, et al: Asymptomatic maternal myasthenia as a cause of the Pena-Shokeir phenotype, *Am J Med Genet* 92:1-6, 2000.
140. Hoff JM, Daltveit AK, Gilhus NE: Myasthenia gravis: Consequences for pregnancy, delivery, and the newborn, *Neurology* 61:1362-1366, 2003.
141. Dalton P, Clover L, Wallerstein R, Stewart H, et al: Fetal arthrogryposis and maternal serum antibodies, *Neuromuscul Disord* 16:481-491, 2006.
142. Smit LM, Barth PG: Arthrogryposis multiplex congenita due to congenital myasthenia, *Dev Med Child Neurol* 22:371-374, 1980.
143. Eymard B, Morel E, Harpey JP, Teyssier G, et al: Dosage des anticorps antirecepteur de l'acetylcholine dans les syndromes myastheniques de nouveau-né, *Presse Med* 15:1019-1022, 1986.
144. Vajsar J, Sloane A, MacGregor DL, Ronen GM, et al: Arthrogryposis multiplex congenita due to congenital myasthenic syndrome, *Pediatr Neurol* 12:237-241, 1995.
145. Burke G, Cossins J, Maxwell S, Robb S, et al: Distinct phenotypes of congenital acetylcholine receptor deficiency, *Neuromuscul Disord* 14:356-364, 2004.
146. Harper CM: Congenital myasthenic syndromes, *Semin Neurol* 24:111-123, 2004.
147. Barisic N, Muller JS, Paucic-Kirincic E, Gazdik M, et al: Clinical variability of CMS-EA (congenital myasthenic syndrome with episodic apnea) due to identical CHAT mutations in two infants, *Eur J Paediatr Neurol* 9:7-12, 2005.
148. Livingstone IR, Sack GH: Arthrogryposis multiplex congenita occurring with maternal multiple sclerosis, *Arch Neurol* 41:1216-1217, 1984.
149. Hall JG, Reed SD: Teratogens associated with congenital contractures in humans and in animals, *Teratology* 25:173-191, 1982.
150. Dahl J, Myhr KM, Daltveit AK, Hoff JM, et al: Pregnancy, delivery, and birth outcome in women with multiple sclerosis, *Neurology* 65:1961-1963, 2005.
151. Vasta I, Kinali M, Messina S, Guzzetta A, et al: Can clinical signs identify newborns with neuromuscular disorders? *J Pediatr* 146:73-79, 2005.
152. Banker BQ, Victor M, Adams RD: Arthrogryposis multiplex due to congenital muscular dystrophy, *Brain* 80:319-334, 1957.
153. Pearson CM, Fowler WG: Hereditary non-progressive muscular dystrophy inducing arthrogryposis syndrome, *Brain* 86:75-88, 1963.
154. Sarnat HB, Silbert SW: Maturational arrest of fetal muscle in neonatal myotonic dystrophy, *Arch Neurol* 33:466-474, 1976.
155. Brooke MH: A neuromuscular disease characterized by fiber type disproportion. In Kakulas BA, editor: *Clinical Studies in Myology*, New York: 1973, Elsevier.
156. Sells JM, Jaffe KM, Hall JG: Amyoplasia, the most common type of arthrogryposis: The potential for good outcome, *Pediatrics* 97:225-231, 1996.
157. Vuopala K, Pedrosadomellof F, Herva R, Leisti J, et al: Familial fetal akinesia deformation sequence with a skeletal muscle maturation defect, *Acta Neuropathol (Berl)* 90:176-183, 1995.
158. Laubscher B, Janzer RC, Kruhenbuhl S, Hirt L, et al: Ragged-red fibres and complex I deficiency in a neonate with arthrogryposis congenita, *Pediatr Neurol* 17:249-251, 1997.
159. Vielhaber S, Feistner H, Schneider W, Weis J, et al: Mitochondrial complex I deficiency in a female with multiplex arthrogryposis congenita, *Pediatr Neurol* 22:53-56, 2000.
160. Philpot J, Counsell S, Bydder G, Sewry CA, et al: Neonatal arthrogryposis and absent limb muscles: A muscle developmental gene defect? *Neuromuscul Disord* 11:489-493, 2001.
161. Kirschner J, Hausser I, Zou YQ, Schreiber G, et al: Ullrich congenital muscular dystrophy: Connective tissue abnormalities in the skin support overlap with Ehlers-Danlos syndromes, *Am J Med Genet A* 132:296-301, 2005.
161a. Tajsharghi H, Kimber E, Holmgren D, Tulinius M, et al: Distal arthrogryposis and muscle weakness associated with a beta-tropomyosin mutation, *Neurology* 68:772-775, 2007.
162. Hecht F, Beals RK: New syndrome of congenital contractural arachnodactyly originally described by Marfan in 1896, *Pediatrics* 49:574, 1972.
163. McKusick VA: Heritable disorders of connective tissue. VII. The Hurler syndrome, *J Chronic Dis* 3:360-389, 1956.
164. Fitti RM, D'Auria TM: Arthrogryposis multiplex congenita, *J Pediatr* 48:787-789, 1956.
165. Drachman DB, Weiner LP, Price DL, Chase J: Experimental arthrogryposis caused by viral myopathy, *Arch Neurol* 33:362-367, 1976.
166. Adams C, Becker L, Murphy EG: Neurogenic arthrogryposis multiplex congenita: clinical and muscle biopsy findings, *Pediatr Neurosci* 14:97-102, 1988.
167. Uchida T, Nonaka I, Yokochi K, Kodama K: Arthrogryposis multiplex congenita: Histochemical study of biopsied muscles, *Pediatr Neurol* 1:169-173, 1985.
168. Carlson WO, Speck GJ, Vicari V, Wenger DR: Arthrogryposis multiplex congenita: A long-term followup study, *Clin Orthop Relat Res* 194:115-123, 1985.
169. Hahn G: Arthrogryposis: Pediatric review and habilitative aspects, *Clin Orthop Relat Res* 194:104-114, 1985.
170. Palmer PM, MacEwen GD, Bowen JR, Matthews PA: Passive motion therapy for infants with arthrogryposis, *Clin Orthop Relat Res* 194:54-59, 1985.
171. Staheli LT: Orthopedic management principles. In Staheli LT, Hall JG, Jaffe KM, et al, editors: *Arthrogryposis*, Cambridge: 1998, Cambridge University Press.
172. Bach A, Almquist E, LaGrone M: Upper limb and spine. In Staheli LT, Hall JG, Jaffe KM, et al, editors: *Arthrogryposis*, Cambridge: 1998, Cambridge University Press.
173. Staheli LT: Lower extremity management. In Staheli LT, Hall JG, Jaffe KM, et al, editors: *Arthrogryposis*, Cambridge: 1998, Cambridge University Press.
174. Jaffe KM: Rehabilitation: Scope and principles. In Staheli LT, Hall JG, Jaffe KM, et al, editors: *Arthrogryposis*, Cambridge: 1998, Cambridge University Press.
175. Graubert CS, Chaplin DL, Jaffe KM: Physical and occupational therapy. In Staheli LT, Hall JG, Jaffe KM, et al, editors: *Arthrogryposis*, Cambridge: 1998, Cambridge University Press.

Chapter 18

Neuromuscular Disorders: Levels above the Lower Motor Neuron to the Neuromuscular Junction

An effective means of attaining an understanding of the major disorders of the neonatal motor system is to organize the approach to these disorders on the basis of the major affected anatomical site within the motor system. Thus, in this chapter and in Chapter 19, I review disorders of the neonatal motor system according to the following specific anatomical levels: levels above the lower motor neuron and at the lower motor neuron, the peripheral (and cranial) nerve, the neuromuscular junction, and, finally, the muscle.

The major unifying clinical manifestations of the disorders are *hypotonia and weakness*, not necessarily occurring with similar severity, as discussed later. In this chapter, all disorders, except those related to the involvement of muscle (see Chapter 19), are reviewed, principally in terms of clinical features, results of pertinent laboratory studies, pathological features, pathogenesis and etiology, and management.

LEVELS ABOVE THE LOWER MOTOR NEURON

Disorders leading to hypotonia and weakness that are secondary to the involvement of anatomical levels above the lower motor neuron are summarized in Table 18-1. These disorders are best discussed here as a group, because most are reviewed in detail in other sections of this book. Although the group is rather diverse, three features are generally useful in establishing the locus of the hypotonia at an anatomical level above the lower motor neuron. First, in these so-called *central disorders*, hypotonia is usually more severe than weakness, and, indeed, some affected infants, although "floppy," exhibit strong movements when stimulated. Second, tendon reflexes are usually preserved, although it is unusual to observe the hallmark of central hypotonia as seen after the first weeks and months of life: *hyperactive* tendon reflexes. Thus, as with weakness, hypotonia is more marked than is involvement of the tendon reflexes. Third, other signs of central involvement are frequently present; particular note should be made of seizures.

Congenital Encephalopathies

For the purposes of this section, *congenital encephalopathies* are defined as those with onset before or during the perinatal period and affecting principally cerebrum, brain stem, or cerebellum (see Table 18-1). In contrast to degenerative encephalopathies, these disorders are *not progressive*, although worsening may occur if infectious, metabolic, or endocrine disturbance is not corrected.

Hypoxia-Ischemia

Hypoxic-ischemic encephalopathy is by far the most common cause of hypotonia in the newborn period. Other features of this disorder are described in Chapter 9. In patients with minor degrees of this encephalopathy, hypotonia may be the principal neurological abnormality.

Intracranial Hemorrhage and Infection

Intracranial hemorrhage (see Chapters 10 and 11) and *intracranial infection* (bacterial and nonbacterial; see Chapters 20 and 21) are relatively uncommon causes of hypotonia in the absence of other features that distinguish these disorders.

Metabolic Disorders

The *metabolic* disturbances that can result in hypotonia in the newborn period are extremely diverse. Abnormal increases or decreases in electrolyte levels, acidemia, hypoglycemia, increases in divalent cation levels, severe hyperbilirubinemia, aminoacidopathies (including syndromes with hyperammonemia), organic acid disturbances, sepsis, and intoxication of the fetus by administration (usually intrapartum) of analgesics, sedatives, or anesthetics to the mother are the most common of these metabolic disturbances (see Chapters 12 to 15).

Other rarer metabolic disorders should also be considered. An important category encompasses neurotransmitter disturbances, the most common of which is aromatic L-amino acid decarboxylase deficiency.[1] Neonatal onset occurs in more than 50% of cases, and hypotonia and feeding difficulties are prominent early findings.[2-6] Diagnosis is suggested by the finding of reduced catecholamine metabolites in cerebrospinal fluid (CSF), and it is established by the demonstration of markedly reduced plasma aromatic L-amino acid decarboxylase activity. Subsequent findings include hypokinesia, oculogyric crises, movement disorders, and autonomic disturbances.

TABLE 18-1	Hypotonia and Weakness: Levels above the Lower Motor Neuron

Congenital (Nonprogressive) Encephalopathies
Hypoxia-ischemia*
Intracranial hemorrhage
Intracranial infection
Metabolic
 Multiple (see text)
Endocrine
 Hypothyroid
Trauma
Developmental disturbance
 Cerebral* (e.g., Prader-Willi syndrome, neuronal migration
  disorders)
 Cerebellar

Degenerative (Progressive) Encephalopathies
See Chapter 16

Spinal Cord Disorders
Trauma
Developmental

*The two most common causes.

TABLE 18-2	Major Neonatal Features of Prader-Willi Syndrome*

Hypotonia with diminished tendon reflexes
Poor feeding with poor weight gain
Weak cry: often "squeaky," not sustained
Craniofacial characteristics
 Dolichocephaly, narrow bifrontal diameter
 Almond-shaped eyes
 Small mouth with thin upper lip and downturned corners of
  mouth
Hypogonadism (male: undescended testes; scrotal hypopla-
 sia; female: absence or severe hypoplasia of labia
 minora and/or clitoris)
History of fetal inactivity
Normal neuromuscular studies
Neuropathological and molecular genetic studies suggest-
 ing disturbed neuronal and axonal development
Chromosomal disturbance: deletion of the proximal long
 arm of chromosome 15 (15q11-q13 region) in 70%; uniparental (maternal) disomy in 20%–25%; imprinting
 defect in 2%–5%.

*See text for references.

Endocrine Disorders

Hypothyroidism is an important endocrine disorder that may produce neonatal hypotonia. A large tongue, temperature instability, feeding problems, constipation, hoarse cry, dry mottled skin, prolonged jaundice, and delayed skeletal maturation should suggest hypothyroidism.[7,8] Neonatal screening of filter paper blood samples has proved superior to clinical recognition and is of considerable value in early detection of hypothyroidism.[7-12] It is critical to identify and to treat hypothyroidism promptly because of the deleterious effect of the thyroid deficiency on brain development (see Chapter 2).

Trauma

Trauma may result in hemorrhagic and nonhemorrhagic lesions of brain, which are uncommon causes of hypotonia, particularly in the absence of other features that dominate the clinical syndrome. Details are provided in Chapters 10 and 22.

Developmental Disturbance

Aberrations of *brain development* are relatively frequent findings among the neonatal causes of hypotonia referable to anatomical levels above the lower motor neuron. Cerebrum and cerebellum are the principal sites of involvement in these cases. Developmental disturbances of *cerebrum*, which may result in striking hypotonia, are reviewed in Chapter 2. *Disturbances of neuronal migration* are the most prominent cerebral causes. Important examples of cerebral hypotonia are the cerebrohepatorenal syndrome of Zellweger, the oculocerebrorenal syndrome of Lowe, and Prader-Willi syndrome. The *cerebrohepatorenal syndrome of Zellweger* is discussed in Chapter 2 among disorders of neuronal migration.

The *oculocerebrorenal syndrome of Lowe* is an X-linked recessive disorder, characterized by ocular abnormalities (cataracts and congenital glaucoma), marked hypotonia, cryptorchidism, and renal abnormalities (proteinuria and generalized aminoaciduria). Subsequent development is markedly retarded. The cerebral abnormality has not been defined clearly.

Prader-Willi syndrome is characterized by striking neonatal hypotonia, accompanied by diminished deep tendon reflexes, poor feeding, weak cry, and often a history of fetal inactivity.[13-27] Careful attention to the clinical and other features described in Table 18-2 allows diagnosis in the neonatal period before development of the complete syndrome of hyperphagia, obesity, short stature, and cognitive impairment.[13,28-30] The intelligence quotient is less than 70 in 85% of cases, most commonly (75%) in the 40 to 69 range, and is always less than 84.[30] Normal neuromuscular studies and the associated later clinical features (e.g., cognitive impairment) support the conclusion that the hypotonia is on a central basis. The limited neuropathological studies thus far conducted indicate frequent abnormalities of gyral development, hypoplasia of corpus callosum, and minor cerebral, brain stem, and cerebellar migrational anomalies.[26,27] A careful magnetic resonance imaging (MRI) study also showed gyral anomalies reminiscent of polymicrogyria.[31] Two of the proteins deficient in Prader-Willi syndrome (i.e., necdin and Magel 2) are critically involved in neuronal differentiation and axonal outgrowth.[32] More data will be of great interest. The diagnosis is established by detection of the chromosome 15 deletion by fluorescent in situ hybridization (FISH) in the 70% of patients so affected. The approximately 25% of patients with uniparental disomy have normal FISH study results but an abnormal DNA methylation test. The risk of recurrence is less than 1%. The 2% to 5% of cases associated with an imprinting defect are detected by DNA methylation studies; recurrence risk in this small group is 50%. Various other probable disturbances of cerebral development (e.g., eponymic syndromes and chromosomal aberrations), some alluded to in Chapters 1 and 2, may cause neonatal hypotonia, but more distinguishing features usually dominate the clinical syndrome.

Developmental disturbance of *cerebellum* may lead to neonatal hypotonia (see Chapter 1). In one carefully studied series of seven such cases, neonatal hypotonia, occasionally severe, occurred without weakness.[33] Jerky eye movements were prominent, and truncal titubation was apparent within a few weeks. Ataxia and intention tremor appeared later in the first year. Computed tomography scans or pneumoencephalograms demonstrated a strikingly enlarged cisterna magna with symmetrical hypoplasia of the cerebellum. The combination of hypotonia, jerky eye movements, and radiographic findings was diagnostic. Pathological study showed nearly complete absence of internal granule cells, with relatively preserved numbers of Purkinje cells. I have seen several similar cases and have been impressed by the hypotonia present in early infancy with Dandy-Walker malformation and Joubert syndrome and related disorders, all disorders of cerebellar development (see Chapter 1).

Degenerative Encephalopathies

Most degenerative disorders of infancy manifest after the first weeks of life. However, many of these disorders may cause hypotonia in the newborn period (see Chapter 16).

Spinal Cord Disorders

Disorders of the spinal cord are frequently overlooked causes of hypotonia and weakness in newborn (see Table 18-1). *Traumatic injury* is a relatively common cause, and the traumatic event may go undetected in the absence of a careful history (see Chapter 22). *Developmental disorders* (e.g., dysraphic states) are associated usually with signs restricted to lower or, less commonly, upper extremities and are recognized more readily (see Chapter 1).

LEVEL OF THE LOWER MOTOR NEURON

Disorders affecting the lower motor neuron are the most frequent causes of *severe* hypotonia *and* weakness in the neonatal period. The major disorders to be distinguished are listed in Table 18-3. Of these, type 1 spinal muscular atrophy (SMA) or Werdnig-Hoffmann disease is the most common and most important.

TABLE 18-3	Hypotonia and Weakness: Level of the Lower Motor Neuron

Spinal muscular atrophy type 1 (Werdnig-Hoffmann disease; also type 0)
Spinal muscular atrophy variants (anterior horn cell disorders not linked to chromosome 5q)
Neurogenic arthrogryposis multiplex congenita
Glycogen storage disease type II (Pompe disease)
Hypoxic-ischemic injury
Neonatal poliomyelitis (other enteroviruses?)

Spinal Muscular Atrophy Type 1 (Werdnig-Hoffmann Disease)

Type 1 SMA or *Werdnig-Hoffmann disease* refers to the severe, infantile, hereditary form of anterior horn cell degeneration. This disorder is autosomal recessively inherited. The earliest descriptions of hereditary degeneration of anterior horn cell with onset in infancy were by Werdnig in Austria and Hoffmann in Germany from 1891 to 1900.[34-37] Although the original cases described by Werdnig and Hoffmann did not have their onset in the first weeks of life, the severe, early onset form of SMA type 1 is often referred to as Werdnig-Hoffmann disease. This severe form of SMA (i.e., type 1) is defined by onset before 6 months of age, failure to develop the ability to sit, and death usually by less than 2 years of age (see later discussion).[24,24a] (This definition contrasts with that for SMA type. 2, which is defined as onset less than 18 months of age, failure to develop the ability to stand, and death after 2 years of age, and with that for SMA type. 3, which is defined as onset after 18 months of age, ability to stand and usually walk, and death in adulthood.)

More recent recognition of several very severe cases of SMA with clear prenatal onset, multiple joint contractures, ventilatory compromise at birth, early deficits of facial movement, bone fractures, and death by 3 months led to the recognition of an additional type, termed type 0.[38-40] Although these cases occur rarely, it is critical to recognize that the diagnosis of SMA is not excluded by the findings of overt arthrogryposis, respiratory failure at birth, or bone fractures.

Clinical Features

Onset. SMA type 1 is clinically apparent at birth or in the first several months of life.[41-44] In one large series, clinical onset was at birth in 35%, in the first month in 16%, in the second month in 23%, and from the end of the second month to the sixth month in 26%.[45] The finding of onset before 6 months with a median age of onset of 1 to 2 months is consistent.[41,42,45-52] Onset in utero is supported by the observation that in most patients with SMA type 1 *presenting at birth or in the early neonatal period*, decreased and weak fetal movements in the last trimester are reported by the patients' mothers.[42] Neuropathological data (see later) have documented prenatal onset.[53] In particularly severely affected infants, neonatal asphyxia or respiratory distress may occur.[54] As just noted, some particularly severely affected infants (type 0) also may exhibit early deficits of facial movement, arthrogryposis, severe diffuse weakness, and early death.[38-40] In those infants whose disease is not apparent at birth, onset in the first weeks is often acute.[55] Indeed, clinical progression to severe disability characteristically occurs over a time course measured in days to a week or so. These clinical findings have a correlate from electrophysiological studies that show marked deterioration of motor function over a 1- to 2-week period postnatally.[44]

Neurological Features. The neurological features are highly consistent and striking (Table 18-4).[38,39,41,42,45,48-50,52,55-57] *Hypotonia* is severe and generalized.

TABLE 18-4	Type 1 Spinal Muscular Atrophy (Werdnig-Hoffmann Disease): Common Clinical Features

Hypotonia: severe, generalized
Weakness: severe, generalized, or proximal > distal
Areflexia
Characteristic posture
Collapsed chest
Weak cry
Difficulty sucking and swallowing
Relatively preserved facial movement
Normal extraocular movements
Normal sensory function
Normal sphincter function

Unlike the situation with disorders of the cerebrum and other central causes of hypotonia, *weakness* is similarly severe. Most infants exhibit generalized weakness, but when it is possible to make a distinction between proximal and distal muscles, a proximal

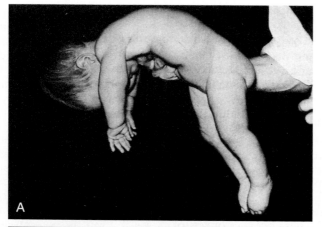

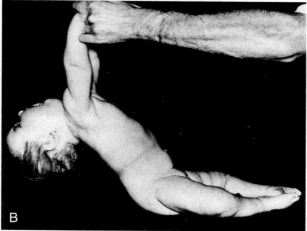

Figure 18-1 **Type 1 spinal muscular atrophy (Werdnig-Hoffmann disease): clinical manifestations of weakness of limb and axial musculature in a 6-week-old infant with severe weakness and hypotonia from birth.** Note the marked weakness of, **A**, the limbs and trunk on ventral suspension and, **B**, the neck on pull to sit. *(From Dubowitz V: Muscle Disorders in Childhood, 2nd ed, Philadelphia: 1978, Saunders.)*

more than distal distribution is discernible. Only minimal movements at hips and shoulders may be elicited in the presence of active movements of hands and feet. The lower extremities are affected more severely than the upper extremities. Involvement of the axial musculature of the trunk and neck is particularly severe, and the resulting deficits are obvious with ventral suspension and pull-to-sit maneuvers (Fig. 18-1). Muscle *atrophy* is also severe and generalized, although the severity may be difficult to appreciate fully in the newborn. Indeed, the replacement of atrophied muscle by connective tissue may further hinder the appreciation of atrophy. *Fasciculations* of limbs are observed rarely, but an analogous phenomenon may be the characteristic fine rhythmic "tremor" of the extended fingers *(polyminimyoclonus)* most commonly observed in less severe cases.[42] Total *areflexia* is the rule, although rarely some reflex response, albeit depressed, can be elicited.

The pattern of weakness of limbs leads to a characteristic posture, characterized particularly by a frog-leg posture with the upper extremities abducted and either externally rotated or internally rotated ("jug handle") at the shoulders (Fig. 18-2). The chest is almost always anteriorly collapsed and bell shaped, with an associated distention of the abdomen and intercostal recession with breathing (see Fig. 18-2). These features relate to weakness of the intercostal muscles and the relatively preserved diaphragmatic function. Contractures of the limbs, usually only at wrists and ankles, are evident in 10% to 20% of infants with onset in utero or in the first month of life.[41,56,58-60]

Involvement of *cranial nerve nuclei* is less striking than of anterior horn cells, at least early in the clinical course. Thus, extraocular movements are normal, and facial motility is relatively well preserved. Indeed, the pathetic picture of a bright-eyed, nearly totally paralyzed infant is characteristic of Werdnig-Hoffmann disease. Sucking and swallowing are affected early in the course in approximately half of cases. Fasciculations and atrophy of the tongue, clinical signs in anterior horn cell disorders of slightly later onset, are apparent in only about one third to one half of patients with the disease occurring at birth or in the first month.[49,56]

Particularly noteworthy differential diagnostic features in the neurological examination include the presence of *normal sphincter and sensory functions*. Both these functions would be expected to be affected with major spinal cord disease, and sensory function with peripheral nerve disease. The patient's alert state with normal visual and auditory responses rules against a central disorder. *Total* areflexia and absence of ptosis, ophthalmoplegia, and facial weakness rule against a variety of primary diseases of muscle. Distinction from type II glycogen storage disease (Pompe disease) can be most difficult, but this much less common disease is usually accompanied by prominent involvement of the heart and enlargement of the tongue.

Several rare genetic variants of infantile SMA should be distinguished from type 1 SMA just described. These *SMA variants* and their mode of inheritance include the association of SMA with (1) primary

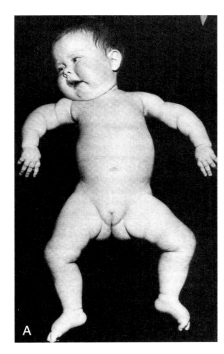
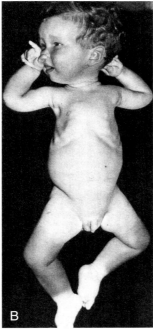

Figure 18-2 Type 1 spinal muscular atrophy (Werdnig-Hoffmann disease): characteristic postures. **A**, 6-week-old and, **B**, 1-year-old infants with severe weakness and hypotonia from birth. Note in **A** the frog-leg posture of the lower limbs and internal rotation ("jug handle") or, **B**, external rotation at shoulders. Note also intercostal recession, especially evident in **B**, and normal facial expressions. *(From Dubowitz V: Muscle Disorders in Childhood, 2nd ed, Philadelphia: 1978, Saunders.)*

respiratory insufficiency secondary to diaphragmatic involvement (autosomal recessive), (2) pontocerebellar atrophy (type 1 pontocerebellar atrophy; see Chapter 17) (autosomal recessive), and (3) congenital arthrogryposis, both with and without bone fractures (autosomal recessive and X-linked, respectively).[24,52,61-64] None of these disorders is linked to the genetic region on chromosome 5 involved in type 1 SMA (see later discussion).

Course. The course of type 1 SMA is a close function of the age of onset (Table 18-5).* Infants with clear *prenatal onset of very severe disease* with respiratory failure at birth, marked diffuse weakness, and early deficits of facial movement (i.e., type 0 SMA) usually die by 3 months of age.[38-40] Those infants with clinical onset in the first 2 months of life have a range of median age at death of 4 to 8 months, with maximum survival rarely exceeding 12 to 18 months. Infants with clinical onsets after 2 months of age have clearly longer median and maximum survival times (see Table 18-5). Recent work suggests even longer survival times.[66a] Moreover, although infants who ultimately prove to have type 2 SMA have a peak age at onset between 8 and 14 months,[50] an occasional infant exhibits onset before 6 months and has a chronic course, including attainment of sitting or even walking, with prolonged survival.[24,42,48,49,55-57,66-69] This portion of the type 2 SMA cases usually can be distinguished from type 1 SMA in the early stages of the disease because of a more insidious onset and slower initial deterioration. Death in type 1 SMA usually relates to intercurrent

respiratory complications. These complications are caused by aspiration because of defective swallowing, hypoventilation because of impaired intercostal muscle function, and impaired clearing of tracheal secretions secondary to weak or absent cough because of weak abdominal muscles.

Laboratory Studies

Serum Enzymes. The creatine kinase (CK) level is normal in type 1 SMA.[24]

Electromyography. The electromyogram (EMG) may be difficult to perform in the young infant, but with patience the major features of anterior horn cell disease are usually observed (see Table 17-7). Thus, at rest, fasciculations and fibrillations are apparent. With muscle contraction, one sees a reduced number of

TABLE 18-5	Survival as a Function of Age of Onset in Type 1 Spinal Muscular Atrophy*	
	AGE AT DEATH (MO)	
Age at Onset (mo)	**Median**	**Maximum**
Birth	4–6	10–12
0–1	6–7	10–18
1–2	7–8	10–12
2–3	14–20	20–25†
3–6	18–20	24–30

*Based on cumulative series of 100 infants from two separate studies: Thomas NH, Dubowitz V: The natural history of type 1 (severe) spinal muscular atrophy, *Neuromuscul Disord* 4:497–502, 1994; and Ignatius J: The natural history of severe spinal muscular atrophy: Further evidence for clinical subtypes, *Neuromuscul Disord* 4:527–528, 1994.

†Excludes 3 of 18 infants with survival to 8, 10, and 18 years.

*See references 24a,38,39,41,42,44,45,48,49,51,52,56,65,66.

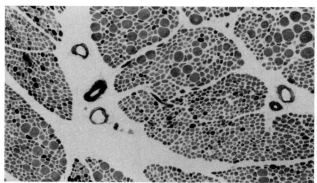

Figure 18-3   Type 1 spinal muscular atrophy (Werdnig-Hoffmann disease): muscle biopsy showing diffuse, panfascicular atrophy in an affected infant. The large muscle fibers are type I. The atrophy is so marked that a grouped pattern cannot be defined readily (adenosine triphosphatase stain, pH 9.4, ×172). *(From Banker BQ: Hum Pathol 17:656, 1986.)*

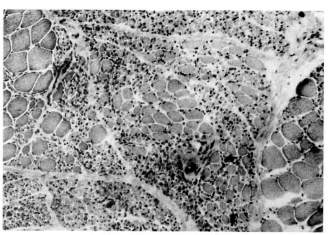

Figure 18-4   Type 1 spinal muscular atrophy (Werdnig-Hoffmann disease): muscle biopsy showing grouped atrophy at the age of 6 months in an infant with later onset and less severe disease than in the infant whose biopsy is illustrated in Figure 18-3. Note the presence of groups of atrophic fibers, interspersed with groups of presumed larger fibers (Verhoeff–van Gieson stain, ×95). *(From Dubowitz V: Muscle Disorders in Childhood, 2nd ed, Philadelphia: 1978, Saunders.)*

motor unit potentials that are of increased amplitude and duration. In general, although no simple relationship exists between features on the EMG and outcome,[24,70,71] one study showed a strong correlation between the degree of depression of the compound muscle action potential and functional outcome.[44]

Nerve Conduction Velocity. Motor nerve conduction velocities are usually normal, although in particularly severe disease, a slight reduction may be observed.[72] This finding suggests a disproportionate loss of anterior horn cells that give rise to the largest, fastest conducting fibers. Some patients with particularly severe cases of type 1 SMA have exhibited signs of severe neuropathy.[73-75]

Muscle Biopsy. The muscle biopsy of a patient with Werdnig-Hoffmann disease with clinically apparent findings at birth or in the first month usually exhibits advanced changes of denervation (see Chapter 17). Characteristically, pronounced atrophy of all fibers of both types within entire fascicles of muscle (i.e., *panfascicular atrophy*) occurs (Fig. 18-3). The early signs of denervation (i.e., loss of checkerboard appearance, type grouping, or even grouped atrophy; see Chapter 17), features of anterior horn cell disease later in infancy (Fig. 18-4), are nearly absent. This virtual absence of signs of terminal axonal sprouting and reinnervation (see Chapter 17) is probably indicative of the severe, fulminating process involving anterior horn cells that causes widespread elimination before such compensatory attempts can occur. A consistent increase in connective tissue is associated with the marked atrophy of muscle (see Fig. 18-4). Hypertrophy of predominantly type I fibers, often in clusters, is an additional characteristic feature. The finding that these hypertrophic fibers often occur in clusters suggests the possibility of reinnervation. The distribution of the histopathological findings parallels the generalized pattern of muscle weakness; the diaphragm is conspicuously less affected.[56] Diagnosis by genetic testing may obviate the need for muscle biopsy in the typical case (see later).

Other Studies. The identification of the q11.2-13.3 region of chromosome 5 as the site of the genetic defect in Werdnig-Hoffmann disease led to the development of molecular diagnostic techniques (see "Pathogenesis and Etiology" later). Radiographs of the chest are useful in demonstrating the chest deformity, the thin ribs characteristic of severe congenital neuromuscular disease,[76-78] and the marked atrophy of muscle. In the rare, very severe type 0 disease, long bone fractures may be observed.[40]

Studies with real-time ultrasonography of limbs have demonstrated several types of changes (i.e., an increase in the intensity of echoes from muscle and the degree of muscle atrophy).[24,79] The echogenicity of muscle correlates well with the severity of histopathological changes observed in biopsy specimens.

Neuropathology

Essential Cellular Changes. The major neuropathological changes are confined to the anterior horn cells of the spinal cord and the motor nuclei of cranial nerves (Table 18-6).[24,53,56,80-83] The essential cellular changes in infantile cases are (1) depletion of the

TABLE 18-6	Type 1 Spinal Muscular Atrophy (Werdnig-Hoffmann Disease): Neuropathology
Anterior Horn Cells	
Decreased number	
Degenerative changes	
Neuronophagia	
Gliosis	
Cranial Nerve Nuclei	
Cellular changes as for anterior horn cells	
Usually affected: V (motor), VII, IX, X, XI, and XII	
Occasionally affected: VI	

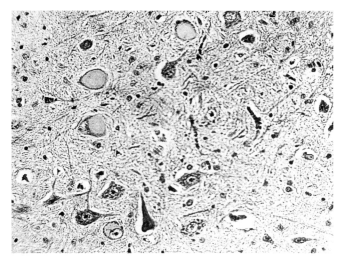

Figure 18-5   Type 1 spinal muscular atrophy (Werdnig-Hoffmann disease): neuronal degeneration in the hypoglossal nucleus. Note the distended neuronal cell bodies, with chromatolytic change as well as pyknotic shrunken cells. Infiltration with pleomorphic microglia and astrocytes is also evident. *(From Dubowitz V:* Muscle Disorders in Childhood, *2nd ed, Philadelphia: 1978, Saunders.)*

number of neurons, (2) degenerative changes of neurons, (3) neuronophagia, and (4) infiltration with microglia and astrocytes (Fig. 18-5). Enhanced apoptosis of anterior horn cell neurons is the most prominent feature during fetal life.[53] Some workers also described cytological findings indicative of immaturity of neurons and suggested impaired development, as well as degeneration, of neurons.[80] The depletion of neurons may be so marked that few, if any, remain in an anterior horn or cranial nerve nucleus. The degenerative changes consist particularly of central chromatolysis, characterized by rounded and distended neuronal cell bodies with eccentric nuclei and Nissl substance displaced to the periphery. Neuronophagia is not prominent, although it is readily demonstrated. The glial response consists of both microglia and astrocytes and is particularly prominent in the ventral aspect of the anterior horns.

Topography. In severe Werdnig-Hoffmann disease, anterior horn cells are affected diffusely, with a particularly prominent affection of the ventromedial group. Cranial nerve nuclei involved invariably and markedly are of cranial nerves VII, IX, X, XI, and XII. The motor nucleus of nerve V is affected in approximately 70% of cases, and the abducens nucleus is involved in fewer than 50% of cases.[56]

Other areas of the motor system are not consistently involved. Hypoxic changes are occasionally observed in hippocampal neurons and Purkinje cells of cerebellum.[56] As noted later, associated degenerative changes in pontocerebellar structures are a feature of an SMA variant that is genetically distinct from type 1 SMA.

The motor nerves exhibit the changes expected from a loss of anterior horn cells (i.e., a decrease in number of myelinated fibers particularly and an increase in connective tissue).[56] Striking atrophy with glial proliferation may be apparent in the proximal anterior roots. Indeed, the glial proliferation may be so conspicuous that some workers have attributed to it a pathogenetic role.[84] The view that the glial infiltration is a secondary event is more widely accepted.[43,80,83,85] Perhaps of greater interest is the demonstration of changes typical of axonal neuropathy in some severe cases.[73-75,83,86] Such changes have led to the suggestion that the anterior horn cell degeneration is a secondary phenomenon, although the most prevalent view is that the neuropathic abnormalities are secondary.

Pathogenesis and Etiology. It is now clear that the acute, early-onset, type 1 form of SMA (Werdnig-Hoffmann disease), as well as the rare, very severe type 0 form and the later-onset, chronic forms (types 2 and 3), are all related to a genetic defect that involves the q13 region of chromosome 5.[24,43,52,65,83,87-97] The SMA region consists of a large inverted duplication containing two copies of the gene deleted (or mutated) in SMA (i.e., the survival motor neuron [*SMN*] gene; Fig. 18-6). Thus, on each chromosome 5 are two copies of SMN: telomeric *(SMN1)* and centromeric *(SMN2)* copies. The deletions involve the telomeric copy. Homozygous deletions of the *SMN1* gene

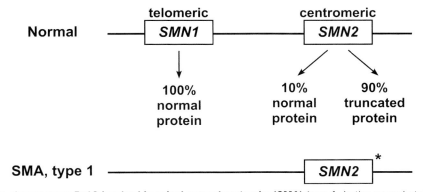

Figure 18-6   The region on chromosome 5q13 involved in spinal muscular atrophy (SMA) type 1. In the normal state, two copies of *SMN1* are present (i.e., a telomeric copy that produces 100% normal protein and a centromeric copy that produces approximately 10% normal protein). With SMA type 1, the telomeric copy contains a deletion (or much less commonly a mutation) and the centromeric copy (*) may increase or decrease in copy number. See text for details.

occur in approximately 95% of cases of SMA, and the remainder are related to mutations in the gene.[43,44,52,98-100b] The nearly identical *SMN2* gene, which contains a single nucleotide change in exon 7 that profoundly influences splicing, produces primarily 90% of a truncated protein lacking exon 7 and having a short half-life and only approximately 10% of the normal protein. Because of the genomic instability of this duplicated region of chromosome 5, *SMN2* copy number may increase or decrease in the presence of the deleted *SMN1* gene. The importance of this phenomenon in this context is that abundant evidence in animal models and now in humans shows that *the copy number of SMN2 is the most critical determinant of the severity of the SMA phenotype*.[38,39,43,44,99-100b] Thus, approximately 90% of SMA type 1 cases have only one (65%) or two (25%) copies of *SMN2*, whereas SMA types 2 and 3 cases have two or more copies in 85% and 100%, respectively.[100]

The biological functions of *SMN1* and its relationship with SMA are beginning to be elucidated.[43,99,101-105a] The SMN protein interacts with other proteins in a multimolecular complex and appears to be involved principally in RNA metabolism. The most critical function of SMN is in the assembly of the ribonucleoproteins of the so-called *spliceosome*, which is critically involved in the removal of introns from pre-RNA and splicing together of exons in mature RNA, for many proteins. The biological functions potentially affected are many, but most recent work suggests that axonal growth and maintenance are key roles. Impairment thereof perhaps could result in the subsequent neuronal apoptosis and degeneration observed in neuropathological studies (see earlier). More data are needed.

Management. Type 1 SMA that is apparent at birth or in the first month of life is usually accompanied by serious disturbances of sucking and swallowing early in infancy. Frequent aspiration of the oropharynx is needed, and usually cessation of oral feedings and institution of tube feeding are required before long to ensure adequate nutrition. Indeed, when dysphagia becomes severe enough to preclude reasonable nutrition and is complicated by frequent aspirations, many clinicians recommend gastrostomy or gastrojejunostomy feeding. This maneuver is carried out not to prolong life but to improve the patient's quality of life and particularly to reduce parental anxiety associated with attempts at oral feeding. Surveillance for respiratory infection must be diligent, because this complication is the usual mode of demise for these unfortunate babies. The intensity of therapy (e.g., antibiotics, chest physical therapy, postural drainage, noninvasive positive pressure ventilation, and even tracheostomy and long-term mechanical ventilation) sometimes is difficult to determine decisively.[106-111b] Tracheostomy and mechanical ventilation have been associated with survival into childhood,[51,66,66a] although longer survival occurs, albeit rarely, without such invasive intervention.[24] The quality of life in such bed-ridden infants and children is a grave concern. More important,

range-of-motion exercises are used to prevent contractures and, I feel, to help the parents "do something" for their infant. In severe Werdnig-Hoffmann disease, my approach is foremost to provide emotional support to the parents and to ensure as much comfort as possible for the infant. I indicate to the family our current understanding of the dire outcome and recommend careful attention to oral-pharyngeal secretions, measures to ensure adequate nutrition, and diligent therapy of respiratory infections. I discuss the complex issues related to *long-term* mechanical ventilation.

Recent insights into the molecular genetic aspects of SMA have led to some potentially promising interventions. Thus, because of the presence of one or more copies of *SMN2*, the possibility of enhancing production by *SMN2* of full-length messenger RNA and SMN protein has been raised. Currently, the most promising approach is the use of histone deacetylase inhibitors.[99,112-114] Histone deacetylases deacetylate and thereby change the conformation of DNA-associated histone proteins, thus altering access of genes to messenger RNA. Histone deacetylase inhibitors have been shown to up-regulate full-length SMN protein from the *SMN2* gene. Studies in cultured cells and animal models and, more recently, in human carriers and patients showed increased production of full-length SMN. Currently, the most promising agents are sodium phenylbutyrate, hydroxyurea, and valproate. Clinical trials in SMA type 1 will be of great interest. The first such trial did not show benefit for phenylbutyrate in children with SMA type 2.[115]

Spinal Muscular Atrophy Variants

At least four disorders with primary involvement of anterior horn cells, clinical presentation at birth, and subsequent course of progressive deterioration (or severe static disability) mimic SMA in the neonatal period. However, these disorders are not linked to chromosome 5q and do not involve *SMN*. Thus, the term *SMA variants* seems most appropriate until the molecular bases are further clarified. At least four disorders should be distinguished (Table 18-7).

SMA with respiratory distress type 1 (SMARD1) is a striking disorder.[64,116-120] From the first days of life, intrauterine growth retardation, mild hypotonia, weak cry, and mild distal contractures are noted. Between 1 and 6 months of age, respiratory distress secondary to diaphragmatic paralysis becomes obvious, and progressive primary distal lower limb weakness ensues. Motor, sensory, and autonomic disturbances develop. Most infants die in infancy or childhood. The responsible gene *(IGHMBP2)* encodes immunoglobulin mu-binding protein 2, the function of which is unclear.

Pontocerebellar hypoplasia type 1 manifests clinically at birth with arthrogryposis, hypotonia, weakness, and bulbar deficits (swallowing difficulty, stridor).[121-124] Subsequent features include progressive bulbar deficits, nystagmus, microcephaly, and cognitive deficits. Brain imaging shows pontocerebellar hypoplasia and cerebral atrophy. Although the disorder is likely autosomal recessive, the molecular defect is unknown.

TABLE 18-7 **Spinal Muscular Atrophy Variants: Progressive or Severe Neonatal Anterior Horn Cell Disease Not Linked to *SMN****

Variant	Major Features
SMA with respiratory distress type 1 (SMARD1)	Mild hypotonia, weak cry, distal contractures initially; respiratory distress from diaphragmatic paralysis 1–6 mo, progressive distal weakness; autosomal recessive, locus 11q13.2, gene: immunoglobulin mu-binding protein 2 (*IGHMBP2*)
Pontocerebellar hypoplasia type 1	Arthrogryposis, hypotonia, weakness, bulbar deficits early; later, microcephaly, extraocular defects, cognitive deficits: pontocerebellar hypoplasia; molecular defect unknown; likely autosomal recessive
X-linked infantile SMA with bone fractures	Arthrogryposis, hypotonia, weakness, congenital bone fractures, respiratory failure, lethal course as in severe type 1 SMA: most cases X-linked (X9/11.3-q11.2); a few cases likely autosomal recessive
Congenital SMA with predominant lower limb involvement	Arthrogryposis, hypotonia, weakness, especially distal lower limbs early; non-progressive but severe disability; autosomal dominant or sporadic; locus 12q23-24

*See text for references.
SMA, spinal muscular atrophy.

X-linked infantile SMA with congenital bone fractures manifests clinically in the neonatal period with arthrogryposis, hypotonia, and weakness.[43,99,125-127] Congenital fractures of long bones and ribs are common. Respiratory failure and progressive weakness lead to death in the first days to weeks in most infants. Anterior horn cell loss is marked. Approximately 80% of cases have been in male infants, and linkage to Xp11.3-q11.2 has been shown. However, some cases likely are autosomal recessive.

Congenital SMA predominantly affecting the lower limbs is the only autosomal dominant disorder of this group.[43,99,128] Presentation at birth is with talipes equinovarus and lower limb hypotonia. EMG and muscle biopsy show signs of anterior horn cell disease. The subsequent course is marked by severe weakness of the lower extremities, although it is generally nonprogressive. The disorder is linked to chromosome 12q23-q24, but the molecular defect is unknown.

Neurogenic Arthrogryposis Multiplex Congenita

Generalized and Localized Types

The term *neurogenic* has been applied to cases of arthrogryposis multiplex congenita secondary to involvement of either anterior horn cell or peripheral nerve (see Chapter 17). Obvious overlap exists with type 0 SMA and with the SMA variants just discussed. I prefer to use the term *neurogenic arthrogryposis multiplex congenita* for the clearly *nonprogressive* forms of arthrogryposis related to anterior horn cell or peripheral nerve disease. By far the most common variety is amyoplasia congenita related to a dysgenetic disturbance of anterior horn cells, described in Chapter 17. Thus, because this generalized form of arthrogryposis multiplex congenita secondary to anterior horn cell has been discussed, I consider in this section only the localized forms.

Cervical Form. A group of infants with a cervical form of anterior horn cell disease and arthrogryposis was described.[129-132] The striking findings in the neonatal period were signs of severe symmetrical lower motor neuron deficit in the upper extremities in the absence of a history suggestive of traumatic injury of spinal cord or brachial plexus. Atrophy and flaccid weakness of upper extremities and the proximal and distal muscle groups were marked, and flexor contractures at the elbow and interphalangeal joints were apparent. Bulbar muscles were not affected. Lower extremities were normal. The course was nonprogressive. Onset in utero was suggested by the presence of flexion contractures, and onset in the first trimester was suggested by the presence of poorly formed palmar creases. The nature of the intrauterine insult to cervical anterior horn cells was not clear. One patient with a clinically similar case had intramedullary telangiectasia.[133]

Caudal Form. A caudal form of anterior horn cell disease with arthrogryposis was described as an apparently sporadic disorder with involvement localized to the lower extremities.[134,135] Weakness, hypotonia, areflexia, and multiple joint contractures were the major features. A few patients later developed signs in the upper extremities and fasciculations of the tongue after several years.[134] Whether these cases represent a different disorder from the SMA variant with predominant lower limb weakness described earlier (see Table 18-7) is unknown.

Laboratory Studies. EMG and muscle biopsy in both the generalized and local forms of neurogenic arthrogryposis multiplex congenita usually demonstrate signs of denervation (see Chapter 17). In the localized forms, the possibility of a correctable structural lesion of the cervical cord or the lumbosacral cord and cauda equina should be ruled out by appropriate studies.

Type II Glycogen Storage Disease (Pompe Disease)

Type II glycogen storage disease, Pompe disease, is an inherited disorder, transmitted in an autosomal recessive manner. The disease is associated with glycogen deposition in anterior horn cells (as well as in skeletal and cardiac muscle, liver, and brain) and with striking weakness and hypotonia in early infancy.

Clinical Features

Onset. Onset of the Pompe disease may be apparent in the first days of life, although the median age at symptom onset in the largest series ($n = 168$) was 2.0 months.[24,136-141]

Neurological Features. Initially, the weakness and hypotonia may be so severe that type 1 SMA is considered the probable diagnosis. The concurrence of fasciculations of tongue and difficulty sucking, crying, and swallowing further mimics this primary anterior horn cell degeneration. However, several clinical features help to distinguish Pompe disease from Werdnig-Hoffmann disease. *First,* cardiac involvement, resulting from accumulation of glycogen, is prominent in Pompe disease; radiographs demonstrate an enlarged globular heart, and electrocardiograms demonstrate evidence of myocardiopathy with shortened PR interval, elevated R waves, and inverted T waves. *Second,* the tongue, although weak and perhaps even fasciculating, is usually *large* in Pompe disease because of the glycogen accumulation, unlike the small, atrophic tongue of Werdnig-Hoffmann disease. *Third,* the skeletal muscles, although weak, are usually prominent in Pompe disease, because of glycogen accumulation (i.e., a true hypertrophy), and they have a characteristic rubbery feel. This finding is unlike the atrophy of Werdnig-Hoffmann disease. *Fourth,* the liver usually is enlarged and readily palpable in Pompe disease. Tendon reflexes are variable in glycogen storage disease. Most patients have preserved tendon reflexes early in the clinical course and later have total areflexia.

A recent report described a delay in myelination, determined by MRI, in five patients with infantile-onset Pompe disease.[142] The clinical correlates of this disturbance remain to be clarified. Deposition of glycogen is a feature of human oligodendroglial development.

Clinical Course. The clinical course is malignant. Infants require ventilatory support at a median age of 6 months, and death in one large series ($n = 168$) occurred at a median age of approximately 9 months.[141] In another series ($n = 153$), the median age at death was 6 months.[140] Survival rates at 12 months of age are approximately 25%, with only 17% ventilator free; at 18 months, the respective values are 12% and 7%.[141] Death is related usually to a combination of cardiac involvement and respiratory complications caused by thoracic muscle weakness and bulbar paralysis.

Laboratory Studies. The serum CK level is elevated because of cardiac and skeletal muscle involvement, and the serum transaminases also are usually elevated because of the combination of muscle and hepatic disease, with the former predominating.[136,140] Muscle biopsy reveals large amounts of periodic acid–Schiff–positive material. Large vacuoles are apparent when standard fixation procedures are used, although some periodic acid–Schiff–positive material usually remains.[143] The EMG reveals fibrillations but often also signs of myopathic disorder because of prominent muscle involvement (see Chapter 19). An additional characteristic feature is "irritability" of muscle with the occurrence of pseudomyotonic bursts of discharges. The large R waves on electrocardiography are particularly helpful signs in diagnosis.

Neuropathology. The neuropathology of Pompe disease is characterized by a striking increase in glycogen throughout the central and peripheral nervous systems (including the myenteric plexus of rectal mucosa). The accumulation of glycogen in the anterior horn cells is the most striking change.[144]

Pathogenesis and Etiology. The biochemical defect involves alpha-glucosidase (acid maltase) activity (Fig. 18-7).[138,145,146] This enzyme catalyzes the *lysosomal* pathway of glycogen degradation, presumably used during normal turnover of cellular constituents. (The major pathway of glycogen degradation, used for glucose-6-phosphate production, occurs in the *cytosol* and is catalyzed by phosphorylase.) Thus, in Pompe disease, the largest accumulation of glycogen is apparent in lysosomal structures. The enzymatic defect is demonstrable in muscle or cultured fibroblasts.[146,147] Moreover, the enzyme is also present in fibroblasts grown from amniotic fluid cells, and this procedure can be used for prenatal diagnosis.[139,148]

Management. Attempts to replenish alpha-glucosidase by bone marrow transplantation have been unsuccessful.[149] However, very promising preliminary results are available for the use of enzyme replacement therapy, involving recombinant human alpha-glucosidase, at least for survival and cardiac and skeletal muscle function.[150-152] Additionally, a recent study of five infants treated from a median age of 6 months showed improvement in myelination by MRI in four of the patients.[142]

Neonatal Poliomyelitis

Neonatal poliomyelitis in this section refers to infection with poliovirus acquired either in utero or in the first 4 weeks of life. Only one case has been reported in the United States in the approximately 40 years since the widespread use of live oral poliovirus vaccine (Sabin vaccine).[153] An additional infantile case with onset at 3 months of age occurred 1 month after administration of live oral polio vaccine.[154] However, poliomyelitis at later ages is still observed, not only in other parts of the world but in the United States among certain religious groups that prohibit vaccination of children. In addition, approximately nine cases per year of poliomyelitis caused by *vaccine-related* poliovirus still occur in the United States. Indeed, the single neonatal case reported in the past 3 decades in this country acquired the infection by contact with a recently vaccinated infant with diarrhea.[153] Moreover, other enteroviruses rarely cause

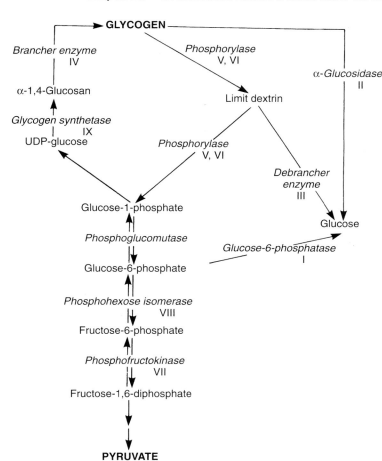

Figure 18-7   Major steps in glycogen metabolism. The enzymatic sites of disease are as follows: I, glucose-6-phosphatase (von Gierke disease); II, alpha-glucosidase or acid maltase (Pompe disease); III, debrancher enzyme; IV, brancher enzyme; V, muscle phosphorylase; VI, liver phosphorylase; VII, phosphofructokinase; VIII, phosphohexose isomerase; IX, glycogen synthetase; and (no numerical designation) phosphoglucomutase. UDP-glucose, uridine diphosphoglucose.

a paralytic syndrome in older patients and, theoretically at least, could cause a neonatal disorder comparable to poliomyelitis. For these reasons, brief attention to neonatal poliomyelitis is warranted here.

Clinical Features

Onset. The disorder may be apparent at birth or may develop in the first weeks of life.[153,155–159] Because the incubation period of the disease is approximately 10 days, infants affected at birth or in the first week presumably were affected in utero.

Neurological Features. Most patients present with diffuse flaccid paralysis that is usually asymmetrical.[56] Apnea may be the initial clinical feature.[153] Not uncommonly, encephalitic involvement results in cerebral signs, including seizures. Respiratory failure may ensue promptly. Moreover, contractures can evolve rapidly, and care must be taken to avoid the postnatal development of arthrogryposis multiplex. Asymmetrical paresis is a common sequel.

Laboratory Studies. The diagnosis is established by viral isolation from the stool. CSF pleocytosis with elevated protein content occurs.

Neuropathology. The neuropathological features in the newborn are often more severe than in the adult. The qualitative features are similar. Neuronal necrosis,

neuronophagia, and perivascular cuffing with inflammatory cells involve neurons of the anterior horns, motor nuclei of the brain stem, roof nuclei of the cerebellum, diencephalon, and motor cortex of the cerebrum.

Pathogenesis and Etiology. Neonatal poliomyelitis is caused by infection of neurons by poliovirus, a classic neurotropic virus. The acquisition of virus may occur prenatally or early postnatally. The demonstration of maternal viremia and placental infection and the recovery of virus from meconium of stillborn infants of diseased mothers support the concept of intrauterine infection by transplacental mechanisms. Because of the incubation period for poliomyelitis, infants affected after approximately 10 days of age presumably were infected during delivery by contamination with infected stool or by postnatal exposure.

Management. Management is entirely supportive.

LEVEL OF THE PERIPHERAL NERVE

Disorders affecting the peripheral nerve are the least defined of those leading to hypotonia and weakness in the neonatal period. However, the more frequent consideration of disorders of peripheral nerve as the cause of motor deficits in neonatal patients, the more frequent use of refined techniques for studying nerve histology, such as electron microscopy, and the

TABLE 18-8	Hypotonia and Weakness: Level of the Peripheral Nerve

Chronic Motor-Sensory Polyneuropathy
Myelin
Hypomyelination*
  Autosomal recessive
  Sporadic
Hypomyelination and demyelination-remyelination (onion bulbs)
  Autosomal recessive*
  Autosomal dominant*
  Sporadic
  Other (associated with axonal disease or focal hypermyelination)
Chronic inflammatory demyelinating polyneuropathy
Neuronal-Axonal (Rare)
Autosomal recessive
Autosomal dominant
Sporadic
Subcellular
Mitochondrial: disorders of electron transport, pyruvate dehydrogenase
Cytoskeletal structures: intermediate filaments (i.e., giant axonal neuropathy), neurofilaments (i.e., infantile neuroaxonal dystrophy)
Lysosomal: Krabbe disease

Congenital Sensory Neuropathies
Familial dysautonomia, congenital sensory neuropathy with or without anhidrosis and mental retardation

Acute Polyneuropathy
Guillain-Barré syndrome

*Each accounts for approximately 25% of all chronic infantile motor-sensory polyneuropathies.

TABLE 18-9	Congenital Polyneuropathy with Hypomyelination and Clinical Onset at Birth*	

Clinical Features	Percentage of Total
Neurological Deficits	
Severe weakness and hypotonia (at birth)	70%
Arthrogryposis multiplex congenita	17%
Age of Walking	
None (most died; see below)	70%
With help (1½–5 yr)	19%
Unassisted (2–6 yr)	11%
Outcome	
Dead (1 hr–4½ yr)	40%
Alive (14 mo–26 yr)	60%
Motor Nerve Conduction Velocity	
≤5 m/sec or unrecordable	96%
Onion Bulbs	
Absent[†]	33%
Present[‡]	67%
Major Genes Involved	
Myelin protein zero (MPZ), peripheral myelin protein 22 (PMP22), early growth response element 2 (EGR2), myotubularin-related protein 2 (MTMR2), ganglioside-induced differentiation-associated protein 1 (GDAP1), periaxin (PRX).	

*See text for references; values shown are percentages of total number of cases for which data are available. All infants had neonatal clinical features and congenital neuropathy with hypomyelination, with or without onion bulbs, on nerve biopsy.
†Approximately 85% died (ages 1 hr–4½ yr).
‡Of these, 81% survived (14 mo–21 yr).

explosion in application of molecular genetics lead to the conclusion that disease at this level is probably considerably more common than was previously suspected. The major disorders to be considered in the neonatal period are shown in Table 18-8. The categorization is somewhat arbitrary because available reports suggest some overlap, as well as the need for more definitive means of study.

Chronic Motor-Sensory Polyneuropathy: Myelin Disease

In chronic motor-sensory polyneuropathies (see Table 18-8) we include several groups of cases, somewhat heterogeneous in basic type but readily identified as affected with a disorder of peripheral nerve myelin. The disorders are categorized best as those that appear to involve a failure of the Schwann cell's role of synthesis and maintenance of myelin (i.e., characterized by *hypomyelination*). In many cases, an additional feature, related to proliferation of Schwann cells and fibroblasts, is *"onion bulb" formation*, with evidence of demyelination-remyelination. In a rare third group, the disturbance of myelin is *inflammatory*. I discuss the two most commonly recognized of these three categories, the hypomyelinative and the hypomyelinative-demyelinating-remyelinating polyneuropathies, together, because their clinical features overlap, and in many respects the disorders are interrelated.

Congenital Polyneuropathies with Hypomyelination, with or without Demyelination and Remyelination

In this group I include those neuropathies associated with hypomyelination alone and those with hypomyelination and evidence of demyelination-remyelination (i.e., onion bulb formation). Those disorders with onion bulb formation were previously termed *Dejerine-Sottas disease* or *hereditary motor sensory neuropathy (HMSN) type III*. The principal overall features of the entire group are summarized in Table 18-9.[160-215]

Clinical Features

In most cases, the disorder has its *onset* in utero and manifests at birth. The dominant *neurological features* in the neonatal period are hypotonia and weakness. Involvement usually is generalized, and the distal more than proximal involvement characteristic of peripheral nerve disease has been difficult to demonstrate in the newborn period. This pattern of weakness, however, usually becomes obvious after several months. Muscle atrophy is usually marked. Tendon reflexes are very hypoactive or, more often, absent. Arthrogryposis multiplex congenita has been a feature in a number of cases and may be very prominent (see Table 18-9).

The involvement of musculature innervated by *cranial nerves* has been variable. Impairment of feeding is common, but the nature of the disturbance is not usually characterized. Clear involvement of facial movement is not common, and extraocular abnormalities have not been reported.

Involvement of the *sensory system* is a valuable feature to elicit for identification of neuropathy. Elicitation of sensory deficits in the neonatal patient requires very careful examination (see Chapter 3). Definitive evaluation of the sensory system usually also requires electrophysiological data (see later discussion). Most patients (70%) never walk, and only 11% eventually do so unassisted (see Table 18-9). Approximately 40% of infants die, and a clear relation to severity of disease, as reflected in the presence or absence of evidence for demyelination-remyelination (i.e., onion bulbs on nerve biopsy), is apparent. Thus, approximately 85% of infants with absence of onion bulbs have died, whereas 81% of those with onion bulbs survive (see Table 18-9).

Three reports of infants with the clinical electrophysiological and pathological features of congenital hypomyelinating polyneuropathy who improved spontaneously after months and were normal or markedly improved at 18 or 19 months and 9 years, respectively, raised the possibility of a transient, reversible form of this disorder.[199,200,203] These observations suggest the need for some caution in rendering a dismal prognosis with the neonatal diagnosis of this form of neuropathy.

Laboratory Studies

Serum Enzymes. The CK level is normal.

Electromyography. The EMG indicates changes of denervation, as outlined in Table 17-7.

Nerve Conduction Velocity. Determination of nerve conduction velocity is critical and is too frequently overlooked in the evaluation of the hypotonic and weak newborn. In most severely affected infants, a drastic reduction in motor nerve conduction velocity has been demonstrated, and values of approximately 5 m/second or less are recorded in nearly all (see Table 18-9). In many infants (including several of my patients), impulse transmission could not be detected. The absence of sensory nerve action potentials is also common.[216]

Muscle Biopsy. Muscle biopsy usually shows evidence of denervation (see Table 17-8), but the muscle histology occasionally may appear remarkably preserved in the presence of severe disease of nerve. The correct diagnosis may be suggested by examination of intramuscular nerves within the biopsy specimen of muscle. Changes seen in full form on nerve biopsy (see later discussion) may be suggested from such examination.

Other Studies. The CSF protein concentration is a valuable adjunct to the diagnosis of infantile polyneuropathy. The CSF protein concentration is almost always elevated, even in the first weeks of life. The elevation usually becomes more marked with age, and occasionally a CSF protein concentration that is only marginally elevated in the first weeks of life becomes markedly elevated later in infancy.

Neuropathology

The diagnosis of peripheral nerve disease is established by examination of a nerve biopsy specimen. The sural nerve, which has a limited distribution over the skin of the foot, is usually chosen for biopsy. The major abnormalities are *hypomyelination* and *onion bulb formation*.

Hypomyelination. In the congenital hypomyelinative neuropathies, the essential feature has been the virtual absence of myelin sheaths (Fig. 18-8). If any myelin is present, large-diameter nerve fibers, which normally

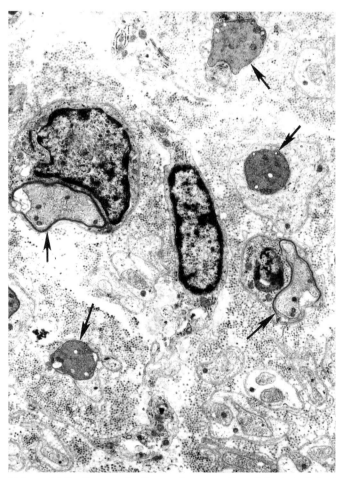

Figure 18-8 Hypomyelination polyneuropathy. This infant had severe, generalized hypotonia and weakness of facial movement, sucking, swallowing, and limb movement from the first days of life. The cerebrospinal fluid protein level was slightly elevated on several occasions, and motor nerve conduction velocities were markedly reduced to 2 to 3 m/second. The infant died at 9½ months of age. The electron micrograph shows several axons *(arrows)*, each surrounded by a Schwann cell, one of which is sectioned through its nucleus (N). Note the marked paucity of myelin lamellae. No onion bulb formation is present. *(Courtesy of Dr. Andrew W. Zimmerman.)*

are heavily myelinated, are conspicuous by the paucity of myelination. The normal proportion between diameter size and thickness of myelin sheath thus is lost. No signs of myelin destruction can be discerned; the lack of a demyelinating process is supported by biochemical studies, which showed no accumulation of cholesterol ester, the chemical hallmark of demyelination. Accompanying these changes may be a modest proliferation of Schwann cells and endoneurial fibroblasts.

Onion Bulb Formation. In many cases, so-called *onion bulb formation* has been detected. This morphological change is associated with the proliferation of Schwann cells and, to a lesser extent, endoneurial fibroblasts. Individual axons become invested by multiple Schwann cells. The multiple concentric lamellae of Schwann cell processes and, to a lesser extent, collagen fibers render the onion bulb appearance (Fig. 18-9). In the youngest and most severely affected patients, the concentric lamellae consist principally of basement membrane of Schwann cells, there remaining little of Schwann cell plasma membrane.[175] In older and usually less severely affected patients, the proliferative changes cause considerable separation of nerve fibers and an increase in the transverse diameter of the nerve, hence the term *interstitial hypertrophy*. In such patients, nerves may be palpable, particularly the posterior auricular in the neck, the ulnar at the elbow, and the peroneal at the fibular head.

Pathogenesis and Etiology

The pathogenesis of congenital hypomyelinative neuropathies is diverse but in general involves a disturbance of myelin formation or maintenance. The major genes involved, myelin protein zero *(MPZ)*, peripheral myelin protein 22 *(PMP22)*, early growth response element 2 *(EGR2)*, myotubularin-related protein 2 *(MTMR2)*, ganglioside-induced differentiation-associated protein 1 *(GADP1)*, and periaxin *(PRX)*, are either structural myelin or Schwann cell proteins or transcription factors.[195,197,201-215,217,218]

Congenital hypomyelinative neuropathies overall have occurred sporadically and by autosomal recessive, autosomal dominant, or X-linked recessive inheritance. The last of these is related to a connexin-32 defect and nearly always presents clinically in childhood. The *purely hypomyelinative* cases have occurred sporadically or by autosomal recessive inheritance. Among the *hypomyelinative group with onion bulb formation* (Dejerine-Sottas disease or HMSN III), autosomal recessive inheritance is most common, but autosomal dominant inheritance has been defined (often categorized as a subtype of HMSN I or Charcot-Marie-Tooth disease).

Autosomal dominant inheritance may be more common than suspected. Thus, when nerve conduction velocity determinations have been performed in apparently unaffected parents of some affected infants, clear evidence of disease has been detected. Indeed, in the series of 20 patients with congenital polyneuropathy described by Hagberg and Lyon,[160,192] 5 had clear evidence of autosomal dominant inheritance and

appeared to represent the HMSN I or Charcot-Marie-Tooth disease. The most common genetic defect for the latter phenotype is a duplication of the chromosomal 17p region that contains *PMP22*.[196,212] Although neonatal electrophysiological abnormalities have been identified in 17p duplication cases, clinical neonatal onset is unusual, but it does occur.[207] Autosomal dominant point mutations of both *PMP22* and *P0* have been shown to lead to congenital hypomyelinating neuropathy and could have accounted for the earlier observations of Hagberg and Lyon.[195,197,198,201-205]

Less commonly, hypomyelinative-demyelinating-remyelinating forms are associated with axonal disease or with focal areas of hypermyelination, in addition to onion bulbs.[212,219] These focal myelin thickenings or *tomacula*, presumably reflect a separate defect in the Schwann cell that differs from those seen in the more typical cases described in Table 18-9.

Management

Supportive measures (see the earlier discussion of Werdnig-Hoffmann disease) are important, particularly because many patients live for years. It is critical to prevent contractures, scoliosis, and recurrent pulmonary infection and to optimize the motor function that is retained.

Chronic Inflammatory Demyelinating Neuropathy

Chronic inflammatory demyelinating neuropathy is a relatively common acquired neuropathy of older children and adults. The disorder is important to recognize because it is treatable. It may be apparent in the neonatal period.[220-224] Decrease in fetal movement and the occurrence of contractures indicate that prenatal onset may occur. The newborn exhibits a poor suck and is hypotonic and weak. Weakness is either in a distal more than proximal or distal equal to proximal distribution. Areflexia is common. The diagnosis is suggested by the finding of elevated CSF protein level, delayed motor nerve conduction velocities (<70% of normal and usually considerably less), and electrophysiological evidence of multifocal disease. Nerve biopsy shows diminution in myelin, evidence of segmental demyelination and remyelination, but especially subperineurial and endoneurial edema with inflammatory cells. Treatment with corticosteroids has been markedly beneficial. Thus, in infants with signs of demyelinating neuropathy and no evidence of a familial disorder, this disorder should be considered seriously, because therapy can lead to major clinical improvement. Notably, one reported patient began to improve *without therapy* by 2 months and fully recovered by age 6 months.[223]

Chronic Motor-Sensory Neuropathy: Neuronal-Axonal Disease

A rare cause of hypotonia and weakness in the newborn period is peripheral nerve disease on the basis of

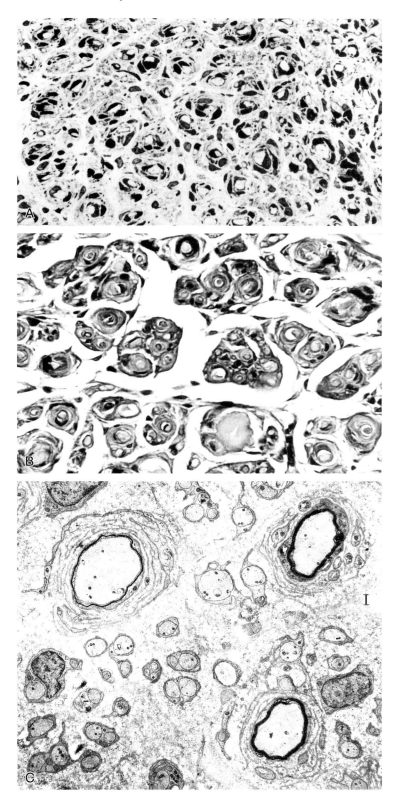

Figure 18-9   Chronic polyneuropathy with onion bulb formation. A, From an infant with hypotonia and weakness from birth, elevated cerebrospinal fluid protein level, and motor nerve conduction velocities markedly reduced to approximately 2 m/second. The sural nerve (which underwent biopsy when the child was 5½ years of age) shows total lack of myelin sheaths and, around individual axons, an increase in the number of Schwann cells arranged concentrically, assuming an onion bulb pattern (toluidine blue–O stain, ×500). **B**, From an infant with severe, generalized hypotonia and weakness from birth. The child died at 22 months of age after a splinting procedure. The anterior nerve root of lumbar cord shows prominent onion bulb formations around poorly myelinated nerve fibers. **C**, From an infant with delayed motor development, areflexia, and distal muscular atrophy. This electron micrograph of the sural nerve, which underwent biopsy in the child at 2½ years of age, shows nerve fibers separated by an increased amount of collagen. Note particularly the three poorly myelinated nerve fibers with onion bulb formations. (**A**, *From Kennedy WR, Sung JH, Berry JF: A case of congenital hypomyelination neuropathy,* Arch Neurol *34:337–345, 1977;* **B** *and* **C**, *from Anderson RM, Dennett X, Hopkins IJ, Shield LK: Hypertrophic interstitial polyneuropathy in infancy,* J Pediatr *82:619–624, 1973.*)

neuronal-axonal involvement. Two groups of patients with neuronal-axonal neuropathy should be distinguished: those with and those without associated Werdnig-Hoffmann disease.

Axonal polyneuropathy unassociated with Werdnig-Hoffmann disease has been reported only rarely.[116,119,] [120,160,192,225-231] In the series of 20 cases of congenital polyneuropathy studied by Hagberg and Lyon,[160] only a single case was of the neuronal-axonal type. Neonatal features have included marked hypotonia and weakness and respiratory distress. Arthrogryposis multiplex congenita may be present. The clinical

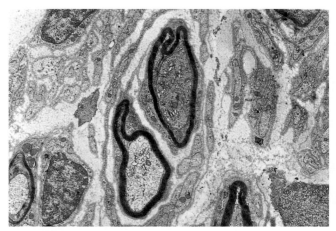

Figure 18-10 **Congenital axonal neuropathy with hypomyelination-demyelination.** Electron micrograph of onion bulb surrounding two fibers with axonal alterations (×6000). *(From Guzzetta F, Ferrière G: Congenital neuropathy with prevailing axonal changes,* Acta Neuropathol (Berl) *68:185–190, 1985.)*

course is usually static or subject to improvement. Results of the EMG and muscle biopsy indicate denervation. Nerve conduction velocities are normal or only modestly depressed, in contrast to the markedly depressed velocities in hypomyelinative neuropathy (see later discussion). Sural nerve biopsy shows axonal degeneration (Fig. 18-10). Secondary changes in myelin surrounding the degenerating axons may occur (see Fig. 18-10). Sporadic cases have been most common, although autosomal dominant inheritance has been recorded.[225] A subset of these cases, with a more severe course, consists of infants with *SMARD1*, discussed earlier, because of accompanying anterior horn cell disease (see "Spinal Muscular Atrophy Variants").[116,119,120,231]

Neuronal-axonal polyneuropathy associated with Werdnig-Hoffmann disease has been described in numerous reports.[73-75,232-242] The infants studied generally have died in the first year of life with the clinical features of Werdnig-Hoffmann disease and with loss of axons noted at postmortem examination, in addition to the characteristic changes of anterior horn cells. Whether the degree of axonal loss is greater than that expected from the involvement of anterior horn cells of Werdnig-Hoffmann disease is difficult to judge from published data. However, of greater interest, disturbance of *sensory* nerve conduction velocity has been demonstrated, and axonal loss and glial infiltration have been reported in *dorsal* as well as ventral roots and in dorsal root ganglia at postmortem examination. Indeed, in one study, impairment of sensory nerve conduction velocities was said to be present in approximately 40% of cases of infantile SMA.[239] In two severely affected sibships, associated with a homozygous deletion of the *SMN* gene, sensory as well as motor nerves were inexcitable on electrophysiological testing.[73,242] The unusually severe nature of the deletion raised the possibility in these cases, and perhaps also in the others reported, that neuronal-axonal polyneuropathy described with Werdnig-Hoffmann disease

represents one end of a continuum of the spectrum of pathology observable with this disease. More data, with accompanying molecular genetic studies, are needed on this issue.

Chronic Motor-Sensory Polyneuropathy: Subcellular

Various other neurological disorders, in which a specific *subcellular structure* or biochemical component thereof is affected, occasionally are recognizable in the first month of life and may have associated disease of peripheral nerve (see Table 18-8), including mitochondrial disease, cytoskeletal disorders (giant axonal neuropathy [intermediate filaments], infantile neuroaxonal dystrophy [neurofilaments]), and certain lysosomal disorders (Krabbe disease). Infantile neuroaxonal dystrophy is not a disorder of the neonatal period; the pathology of peripheral nerve has been defined.[243] For practical purposes, Krabbe disease does not deserve serious consideration here because central nervous system phenomena usually dominate the clinical presentation and course (see Chapter 16). However, impaired motor nerve conduction velocities have been documented in the second month in Krabbe disease.[244] Thus, in this section, I review briefly only the neuropathic aspects of mitochondrial disease, as well as giant axonal neuropathy.

Mitochondrial Disease

Peripheral neuropathy is a common feature of *mitochondrial disease*. As discussed in Chapter 16 in relation to degenerative diseases of the central nervous system, mitochondrial disease, such as Leigh disease, may lead to hypotonia and weakness on the basis of disease above the lower motor neuron. However, in addition, some infants with mitochondrial disease have had electrophysiological and histological evidence of peripheral nerve involvement.[245-249] In a well-studied series of 43 cases of congenital lactic acidosis related primarily to deficiency of pyruvate dehydrogenase activity or various elements of the electron transport chain (complexes I to IV, isolated or in combination), all exhibited neonatal hypotonia.[249] Nerve conduction studies carried out later in infancy provided evidence of neuropathic disease in 42 of the 43. Approximately 70% exhibited signs indicative of both axonal and demyelinative disease. The EMG may reveal fibrillation potentials, findings supporting the concept of a denervating process.[246,247] Nerve conduction velocities generally are reduced by approximately 15%, more consistent with axonal than myelin disease. No such studies of neonatal patients are available. Histological abnormalities of nerve have included evidence for axonal and myelin involvement.[245-247]

Giant Axonal Neuropathy

The unusual disorder of *giant axonal neuropathy* is characterized by onset after the first year of life of chronic, slowly progressive, primarily motor neuropathy.[250-260] However, onset in the neonatal period with marked hypotonia, weakness, and areflexia has been reported.[254,260-262] A nearly constant accompaniment is tightly curled, kinky, poorly pigmented scalp hair that may be apparent in the neonatal period (the hair abnormality is usually more obvious after the first months of life). Nerve histology is striking: axons are greatly enlarged and are filled with disarrayed neurofilaments. Accumulation of filaments in Schwann cells may account for the associated demyelination.[251] Involvement of neurons and oligodendroglia of the central nervous system may cause progressive cognitive and motor deficits and striking abnormality of cerebral white matter, especially on MRI scans.[252,256,257,260] The demonstrations of disordered filaments in astrocytes and fibroblasts[260,263] involving the principal proteins of intermediate filaments (i.e., glial fibrillary acidic protein [astrocytes] and vimentin [fibroblasts]) led to the suggestion that the disease represents a disturbance of organization of intermediate filaments.[254,264] The genetic defect has been localized to chromosome 16q24, and the giant axonal neuropathy gene *(GAN)* encodes the protein gigaxomin.[258,259] Gigaxomin appears to play an important role in the integrity of the cytoskeletal structure through interaction with a microtubule-associated protein.

Congenital Sensory Neuropathies

Currently, *sensory neuropathies* with clinical presentation in the neonatal period include at least three basic disorders: congenital sensory neuropathy, a similar congenital neuropathy with anhidrosis, and familial dysautonomia (Riley-Day syndrome; see Table 18-8). The three disorders are inherited in an autosomal recessive manner and are classified as hereditary sensory neuropathies types II (congenital sensory neuropathy), III (familial dysautonomia), and IV (congenital sensory neuropathy with anhidrosis) in the classic classification system of Dyck and Ohta.[265] (Hereditary sensory neuropathy type I exhibits clinical presentation in late childhood to early adulthood.) Because autonomic phenomena are common in all these disorders, *hereditary sensory autonomic neuropathies* may be a better term.[266,267] These sensory disorders are discussed in this chapter on motor abnormalities because hypotonia and areflexia are very common features.

Congenital Sensory Neuropathy

The designation of *congenital sensory neuropathy* has been applied to a variety of cases of sensory neuropathy with onset in infancy and either slow or no progression of disease. Of these cases, patients with onset in the neonatal period consistently have exhibited the *nonprogressive* course.[267-271] Because evaluation of sensory and autonomic nerve function, the prominent sites of involvement, is difficult in the newborn, the clinical presentation often suggests a motor disturbance because of the presence of *hypotonia, areflexia, feeding disturbance,* and, occasionally, *limb weakness.* These deficits are presumably related to the disturbance of afferent input from muscle and the muscle spindle. With careful examination and with maturation of the infant, marked impairment of pain, touch, and temperature

develops. Less consistently recorded have been disturbances of hearing, smell, and taste, although more careful testing probably would indicate that such disturbances are common. Although less commonly evaluated, such autonomic disturbances as defective lacrimation, impaired axonal flare after stimulation with intradermal histamine, and absence of fungiform papillae have been recorded. However, sweating is normal, and mental retardation is absent. Infants with dysmorphic facies[272,273] and with skeletal dysplasia[274] have been described.

Diagnosis is established by demonstration of a normal EMG and normal motor nerve conduction velocities but grossly impaired or absent sensory nerve conduction responses. *Sural nerve biopsy* demonstrates most characteristically a marked reduction in *myelinated fibers* (Fig. 18-11), but without evidence of myelin degeneration or defective myelin formation around the few remaining observable large fibers, which have normal-appearing myelin sheaths (in contrast to congenital hypomyelinative motor neuropathies, in which the many large fibers have little or no myelin sheaths). The essential pathogenesis is unclear, but a defect in *formation of nerve fibers* destined for myelination seems possible.

Congenital Sensory Neuropathy with Anhidrosis

Congenital sensory neuropathy with anhidrosis is a clinical disorder with many similarities to that just recorded but with lack of sweating and with mental retardation.[275-285] (This disorder is sometimes termed *congenital insensitivity to pain with anhidrosis.*) Both autosomal

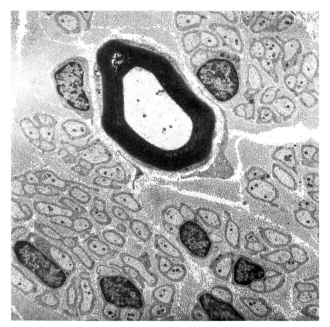

Figure 18-11   Congenital sensory neuropathy from an infant with the clinical features described in the text as characteristic of this disorder. This electron micrograph shows many small unmyelinated fibers but, importantly, only a single myelinated fiber *(upper center)*; the myelin sheath is normal. The unmyelinated small fibers exhibit no signs of axonal disease. Several normal Schwann cell nuclei are visible in the lower portion of the micrograph. *(Courtesy of Drs. Franco Guzzetta and Gerard Ferrière.)*

recessive inheritance and sporadic occurrence have been recorded. Nerve biopsy has shown an almost complete absence of *small* myelinated *and* unmyelinated fibers.[277,279,280,282-287] The particular absence of small fibers accounts for the defect of sweating; the cause of the intellectual impairment is unknown. The molecular genetic defect involves the tyrosine kinase receptor A gene *(TRKA)*. The encoded TRKA protein is a receptor tyrosine kinase that is phosphorylated in response to nerve growth factor.[284,285] Nerve growth factor is critical for the survival of sympathetic ganglion neurons and nociceptive sensory neurons in the dorsal root ganglia.

Familial Dysautonomia (Riley-Day Syndrome)

Familial dysautonomia, a rare, autosomal recessive disorder, usually becomes apparent in the first year of life, although recognition in the neonatal period, albeit very uncommon, is possible.[207,270,287-294] Because of the serious implications for prognosis and genetic counseling, diagnosis early in infancy is important.

The most helpful *clinical features* in the neonatal period include Ashkenazi Jewish parents, feeding difficulty with tracheal aspiration, abnormal "rolling" tongue movements, nasal cry, peculiar jerky limb movements, hypotonia, and episodes of marked irritability with retrocollis and opisthotonos (Table 18-10).[288,292] A recent report described unexplained episodic somnolence (duration, 4 to 15 hours) in a newborn with familial dysautonomia.[294] Corneal reflexes are absent, and tendon reflexes are depressed. Absent fungiform papillae, miosis after dilute methacholine, lack of axonal flare after intradermal histamine, and defective lacrimation complete the syndrome. Clinical progression is common, although variable in severity.

Sural nerve biopsy distinguishes Riley-Day syndrome from those just described. Thus, a drastic reduction in *unmyelinated* fibers is observed; much less disturbance of myelinated fibers is present.[289,293]

The genetic defect is localized to chromosome 9q31-33, and the responsible gene *(IKBKAP)* encodes an I kappa-beta kinase–associated protein.[287] The protein appears critical for development as well as continued survival of the sensory and autonomic neurons involved.

TABLE 18-10   **Most Common Neonatal Abnormalities in Familial Dysautonomia***

Abnormality	Percentage of Total
Poor or no suck reflex	62%
Gavage feeding in nursery	32%
Hypotonia	44%
Hypothermia	26%
Aspiration	20%

*Based on 49 cases with (later) proven familial dysautonomia; in only 5 was the diagnosis made in the neonatal period, and each of these patients had affected siblings.
Adapted from Axelrod FB, Porges RF, Sein ME: Neonatal recognition of familial dysautonomia, *J Pediatr* 110:946–948, 1987.

Acute Polyneuropathy

The evolution of *acute, predominantly motor polyneuropathy* with hypotonia and weakness has been documented in infants in the first weeks of life.[295-302] In four cases, diminished fetal movement was noted. Because of the self-limited course, it seems possible that neonatal cases have been mistaken for other transient causes of hypotonia and weakness. A recognizable infection may be apparent a week or more previously. In two cases, the mother had Guillain-Barré syndrome during her pregnancy. In affected infants, hypotonia and weakness evolve over days. Two other mothers had inflammatory bowel disease and anti-GM1 neuropathy. Areflexia and involvement of cranial nerves (especially VII) are common. Respiratory failure may ensue.

The diagnosis is suggested by an elevated CSF protein concentration in the absence of pleocytosis (i.e., albuminocytological dissociation). Nerve conduction velocities are severely depressed: in five patients, motor nerve conduction velocities were less than 8 m/second.[295,296,299,300,302]

If respiratory support is accomplished, recovery is the rule, often within 1 to 2 months. Recovery in acute infantile polyneuropathy may be more rapid than in the analogous Guillain-Barré syndrome of older patients, but more data are needed on this point. One infant treated with intravenous immunoglobulin began improvement within 48 hours, but complete recovery did not occur for several months.[302]

LEVEL OF THE NEUROMUSCULAR JUNCTION

Disorders of the neuromuscular junction are infrequent causes of neonatal hypotonia and weakness. However, such disorders are critical to recognize because therapeutic intervention is usually beneficial and, indeed, lifesaving. Those disorders that are observed in the neonatal period are listed in Table 18-11. The prototype is myasthenia.

Myasthenia

Myasthenia is characterized principally by muscle weakness provoked by activity and relieved by rest. In an analysis of nearly 500 patients with myasthenia gravis, 11% were observed to have their first symptom in infancy or childhood,[303] 8% were affected after the age of 1 year, and 3% were affected before the age of 1 year. The last group was composed of 2% who were

TABLE 18-11   **Hypotonia and Weakness: Level of the Neuromuscular Junction**

Myasthenia Neonatal transient Congenital (hereditary) myasthenic syndromes (see Table 18-13)
Toxic-Metabolic Conditions Hypermagnesemia Antibiotics, aminoglycosides
Infantile Botulism

born of myasthenic mothers and experienced *transient* neonatal myasthenia gravis and 1% who were born of nonmyasthenic mothers and possibly had a congenital myasthenic syndrome.

Later work demonstrated that congenital myasthenic syndromes are heterogeneous in clinical presentation and course and, in general, are characterized by inherited defects in neuromuscular transmission (see later discussion). Thus, these syndromes are intrinsically different from the typical autoimmune disorder recognized as myasthenia gravis in older infants, children, and adults; indeed, the youngest age at onset of autoimmune myasthenia gravis reported is 6 to 12 months.[304] Interestingly, 55% of reported infants with onset of autoimmune myasthenia gravis before the age of 3 years were born prematurely.[305,306]

Neonatal Transient Myasthenia Gravis

The dramatic myasthenic syndrome of *neonatal transient myasthenia gravis*, described initially in 1942, occurs in approximately 10% to 20% of infants born to myasthenic mothers.[303,307-313] The disorder has important implications for the pathogenesis of myasthenia gravis (see later discussion).

Clinical Features. *Onset* of neonatal transient myasthenia gravis in approximately two thirds of the cases is within the first hours after birth, although this often occurs *after* an apparently normal period immediately following delivery.[24,308,309] In nearly 80% of patients, onset is apparent by 24 hours, and the latest onset is 3 days.[308] Thus, if an infant of a myasthenic mother has an onset of hypotonia and weakness on the fourth postnatal day or beyond, some other condition should be suspected.

The *neurological features* are usually dramatic and may evolve very rapidly (Table 18-12).[24,55,303,308,309,314-320] Disturbance of cranial nerve musculature is prominent. Nearly all patients exhibit feeding difficulties with weakness of sucking and swallowing. Gavage feedings are required in approximately one third of patients. Respiratory difficulties occur in two thirds and result from an inability to handle pharyngeal secretions and from weakness of respiratory muscles. Ventilation is

TABLE 18-12　Clinical Manifestations of Neonatal Transient Myasthenia Gravis

Clinical Manifestation	Percentage of Total
Feeding disturbance	87%
Gavage feeding required	31%
Respiratory disturbance	65%
Weak cry	60%
Facial weakness	54%
Generalized muscle weakness	69%
Hypotonia (marked)*	48%
Ptosis	15%
Oculomotor disturbance	8%

*Hypotonia of some degree is essentially a constant feature.
Data from Namba T, Brown SB, Grob D: Neonatal myasthenia gravis: Report of two cases and review of the literature, *Pediatrics* 45:488–504, 1970.

required in approximately 30% of cases. The cry is weak, and facial diplegia is obvious in approximately 60% of affected infants. Generalized muscle weakness is readily recognized in approximately 70% of cases, and hypotonia is marked in approximately 50%. Hypotonia of some degree is nearly a constant feature. However, tendon reflexes are usually normally active, and no fasciculations can be discerned. In contrast to the most common congenital myasthenic syndrome (see subsequent section), eye signs are *uncommon;* ptosis is apparent in only 15% of patients, and oculomotor disturbance is seen in fewer than 10% of these infants.

A few infants exhibit signs of intrauterine onset of weakness manifested especially by arthrogryposis (see Chapter 17).[24,222,309,313,314,321-325] Polyhydramnios, pulmonary hypoplasia, and neonatal death are common in these more severely affected infants.

Most infants (≈80%) with the typical neonatal onset require anticholinesterase therapy for the disorder, and the mean duration of the illness in survivors is 18 days.[308,309] In previous years, approximately 10% of infants died with the disease, most often because of delayed, inadequate, or absent therapy.[308] Neonatal death now is rare.[309]

Diagnosis at the Bedside. Diagnosis is usually readily apparent in the presence of the clinical syndrome in the infant of a myasthenic mother. Occasionally, the mother's disease is not known to her physician or to her, and the diagnosis may be less obvious. Observation of the infant's response to anticholinesterase medication is the important diagnostic test. The choice of drug for the test is somewhat controversial. Neostigmine methylsulfate, 0.04 mg/kg, administered intramuscularly or subcutaneously, is commonly used. The maximum effect occurs after approximately 15 to 30 minutes. Muscarinic effects (e.g., diarrhea and excessive tracheal secretions) may require atropine. An advantage of neostigmine is the relatively long duration of beneficial effect (1 to 3 hours). If edrophonium is used, a suitable dose is 0.15 mg/kg, administered intramuscularly or subcutaneously, or 0.15 mg/kg administered intravenously in fractional amounts over several minutes, after a test dose of 0.03 mg/kg. A beneficial effect is apparent within 3 to 5 minutes and persists for approximately 10 to 15 minutes. In evaluation of the clinical response to anticholinesterase medication, it is important to choose a quantifiable clinical feature (e.g., sucking or swallowing ability, ventilatory function, facial or limb movement, or crying volume).

Laboratory Studies. The serum CK level, standard EMG (amplitude, duration, and number of motor unit potentials), nerve conduction velocities, and CSF protein concentration are normal. Muscle biopsy, studied by conventional techniques, is also normal.

The diagnosis is confirmed by demonstration of the *myasthenic* phenomenon on electrophysiological testing (see Chapter 17). Thus, in one careful study, repetitive nerve stimulation at a frequency of 10 impulses/second

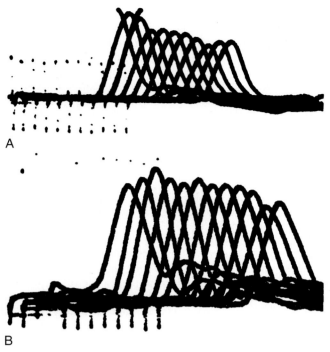

Figure 18-12 **Electromyogram in neonatal transient myasthenia gravis: beneficial effect of edrophonium. A,** Repetitive stimulation of the median motor nerve with supramaximal stimulus intensity at a rate of 3 Hz demonstrated a decremental response of 23% between the first and fifth responses. **B,** A 10-minute rest period followed to eliminate any possibility of postexercise facilitation. Edrophonium was infused intravenously (0.15 mg/kg). Repetitive stimulation within 120 seconds of infusion revealed complete repair of the decremental response. *(From Hays RM, Michaud LJ: Neonatal myasthenia gravis: Specific advantages of repetitive stimulation over edrophonium testing,* Pediatr Neurol *4:245–247, 1988.)*

resulted in a 40% decrement of the amplitude of the motor unit potential within 1 second.[326] With faster frequencies (e.g., 50 impulses/second), a nearly 50% decrement was observed within 100 milliseconds. Measurable improvement in this decrement can be observed after the injection of anticholinesterase medication (Fig. 18-12). Studies of the muscle response to repetitive nerve stimulation must be interpreted with the awareness that newborn infants exhibit less neuromuscular reserve than do older children, and premature infants have less reserve than do full-term infants. Thus, Koenigsberger and co-workers[327] demonstrated an average decrement of 24% in 12 of 17 normal infants at the end of a 15-second train of 20 impulses/second, and an average decrement of 51% in all 17 infants at the end of a similar train of 50 impulses/second.[327] However, with 10 impulses/second, no decrement occurred in these normal infants either during or at the end of the train, in contrast to the observations in neonatal transient myasthenia gravis, as noted earlier. Most commonly used is a 5-second train of 2 to 3 impulses/second with supramaximal stimuli.[309,317]

Pathology. No data in regard to pathology are available for neonatal myasthenia gravis. By conventional techniques, no consistent histological abnormality is observed in myasthenia gravis in older patients.

Pathogenesis and Etiology. The essential defect in autoimmune myasthenia gravis is considered to be a decrease in available acetylcholine receptors at the postsynaptic muscle membrane.[309,328] This decrease is related to a circulating antibody to acetylcholine receptor protein.[329] These antibodies bind to a subunit of the extracellular domain of the acetylcholine receptor and lead to the myasthenic physiological defect in vivo and in vitro.[309,320,329-334] The mechanisms by which the antibodies produce the decrease in available receptors are as follows: (1) acceleration of degradation of receptors; (2) blocking of acetylcholine access to acetylcholine receptors; and (3) induction of local deposition of complement, including the membrane attack complement complex.[24,320,329,331,335,336]

The occurrence of myasthenia in infants of myasthenic mothers for many years stimulated a search for a humoral factor transmitted across the placenta. Antiacetylcholine receptor antibody appears to be the factor. Thus, affected infants nearly invariably exhibit elevated antibody levels, and clinical improvement has been associated with lowering of antibody levels by exchange transfusion.[222,319,337-343] Moreover, fetal breathing movements have become apparent when maternal antibody levels are lowered by plasmapheresis,[321] and transient myasthenia gravis has been documented in an infant with neonatal lupus erythematosus and antiacetylcholine receptor antibodies.[344] Moreover, in one careful study, a relationship between the maternal antibody titer and the occurrence of transient neonatal myasthenia gravis was shown.[314]

The relationship between maternal antibody level and transmission of the transient neonatal disorder level has been refined by determination of ratio of antibody levels to the fetal versus the adult type of acetylcholine receptor. Thus, a high ratio in the pregnant woman is associated with a high likelihood for transmission (Fig. 18-13).[318] This observation may have pathogenetic implications because the newborn may have a relatively high proportion of fetal-type acetylcholine receptors.[318] Nevertheless, several observations indicate that host factors also must play an important role in pathogenesis: (1) only 10% to 20% of all infants of myasthenic mothers develop the transient neonatal syndrome; (2) among mothers who have had an affected infant, the incidence of recurrence rises markedly to approximately 75%[308,309,314]; (3) no invariable correlation exists between occurrence of symptoms and the level of neonatal antibodies[310,342,345]; and (4) asymptomatic myasthenic mothers in either spontaneous remission or remission induced by thymectomy have given birth to infants who had similar antibody titers to those of the mother and who developed typical transient neonatal myasthenia gravis.[341,346] Thus, factors referable to the infant may govern the impact of the antiacetylcholine receptor antibody. The findings of both marked prolongation of elevated antibody levels and immunochemical differences between the antibody of mother and infant in symptomatic versus

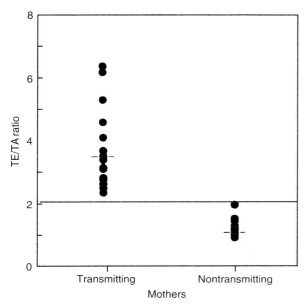

Figure 18-13 Distribution of antifetal (TE) and antiadult (TA) muscle acetylcholine receptor antibody titer ratio (TE/TA) in mothers transmitting or not transmitting neonatal transient myasthenia gravis. *(From Gardnerova M, Eymard B, Morel E, Faltin M, et al: The fetal/adult acetylcholine receptor antibody ratio in mothers with myasthenia gravis as a marker for transfer of the disease to the newborn, Neurology 48:50–54, 1997.)*

asymptomatic infants suggest that symptomatic infants synthesize antiacetylcholine receptor antibodies in addition to receiving passively transferred maternal antibody.[342] Consistent with this notion, antibody levels in affected newborns have been shown to increase after the lowering induced by exchange transfusion.[319] Finally, the possibility of a genetic predisposition to the disorder in certain infants is raised by the observation that infants with the same composition of certain myasthenia-related human leukocyte antigens (HLAs) as exhibited by their mothers develop symptomatic disease, whereas infants with a different HLA composition do not.[309] More data are needed on these issues.

Management. The management of neonatal transient myasthenia gravis is based on careful surveillance of the infant at risk and prompt diagnosis with the early signs of disease. The strong possibility that the infant likely to be affected can be identified prenatally by determination of the ratio of antibody levels to the fetal versus the adult type of acetylcholine receptor is raised by the work described earlier. Therapy is primarily twofold: supportive care and anticholinesterase medication.

Supportive therapy is critical and is addressed principally to the difficulties with feeding and respiration. Frequent feedings of small volumes are helpful to avoid fatigue and the possibility of aspiration. Tube feeding should be provided in patients with severe disease. Pharyngeal secretions should be suctioned and respiratory support provided as needed. The condition of these infants can deteriorate very rapidly. Aminoglycoside antibiotics should be avoided, if possible, because of their deleterious effect on neuromuscular function (see later section).

Anticholinesterase therapy has been used in approximately 80% of patients. In previous years, approximately 50% of those infants who died did not receive therapy. It is better to treat an infant with marginal deficits than to risk serious deterioration. Neostigmine is the drug of choice and is best administered initially intramuscularly or subcutaneously as the methylsulfate derivative in a dose of 0.04 mg/kg, approximately 20 minutes before feedings. Nasogastric administration of 0.4 mg/kg 30 minutes before feedings is an alternative. Pyridostigmine bromide, in a dose of 4 to 10 mg, also could be used by gavage before feeding. Conversion to oral administration can be accomplished when the infant is stable and is swallowing well.

Exchange transfusion may be an adjunct in management. Thus, three reports described clinical improvement in association with decrease in levels of antiacetylcholine receptor antibody caused by exchange transfusion.[222,319,343] Exchange transfusion did not produce clinical benefit in three other reported infants.[342,347] Moreover, when it does produce benefit, the response is transient. Thus, the possible role of exchange transfusion is not yet entirely clear. In two reports, high-dose intravenous immunoglobulin was highly effective in one case and not clearly effective in another.[319,347]

Congenital Myasthenic Syndromes: Overview

Congenital (hereditary) myasthenic syndromes are caused by a variety of defects of the neuromuscular junction and are characterized by weakness and fatigability and by the phenomenon on the EMG of myasthenia from the first days or weeks of life. The disorders differ in a central way from later-onset myasthenia gravis and its transient neonatal counterpart; thus, the congenital syndromes are *not* related to an immune process but are caused by *genetic defects of the neuromuscular junction.* The latter are described subsequently, but the development of new morphological, electrophysiological, biochemical, and molecular genetic techniques for study of the neuromuscular junction is leading to definitions of new disorders. Although at least 16 congenital myasthenic syndromes are recognized,[348-353] relatively few exhibit *overt* neonatal onset. The major congenital myasthenic syndromes, including those with neonatal onset as a common feature, are reviewed in Table 18-13. Although phenotypic variability and some overlap exist, several clinical features are common to these syndromes (Table 18-14).[24,348,351-370] As a group, these disorders are rare, but the following two categories are the most common among the group.

Congenital Myasthenic Syndromes: Acetylcholine Receptor Deficiency (Congenital Myasthenia)

The designation *congenital myasthenia* previously referred to the most common of the congenital myasthenic syndromes. This disorder (or, better, group of disorders) was described initially by Bowman[371] in 1948.

TABLE 18-13   Major Congenital Myasthenic Syndromes*

Basic Abnormality	Usual Inheritance	Neonatal Onset Common	Extraocular Muscle Weakness Common	Response to AChE Inhibitor
Presynaptic Abnormalities				
Defects in ACh synthesis (congenital choline acetyltransferase deficiency or familial infantile myasthenia)	Recessive	+	−	+
Paucity of synaptic vesicles	Recessive	+	−	+
Synaptic Abnormalities				
AChE deficiency	Recessive	+	+	−
Postsynaptic Abnormalities				
ACh receptor deficiency (subunit defect)	Recessive	+	+	+
ACh receptor deficiency (rapsyn mutation)	Recessive	+	−	+
Slow-channel syndrome	Dominant	±	+	−
Fast-channel syndrome	Dominant	±	+	−

*Most common congenital myasthenic syndromes.
ACh, acetylcholine; AChE, acetylcholinesterase; +, present; −, absent; ±, variable.

The disorder is related to deficiency of endplate acetylcholine receptors (see later discussion) and now is most commonly referred to as *endplate acetylcholine receptor deficiency*. Two subtypes should be recognized; the more common is related to a defect of a subunit of the acetylcholine receptor, and the somewhat less common is caused by a defect of a protein involved in clustering of the receptors (see later and Table 18-13).

Clinical Features. Although *onset* of this type of myasthenia is in the first weeks of life, the identification of the disorder is often made after that time. From available data, it seems likely that the correct diagnosis would be established in many cases in the newborn period if the physician's index of suspicion were higher.

The *neurological features* of the form associated with a *subunit deficiency* are characterized by prominent ptosis and ophthalmoplegia (see Table 18-13).* Ptosis is usually the prominent feature in the first weeks of life, and ophthalmoplegia becomes obvious in the ensuing months. Facial weakness and weak sucking and crying are common, but feeding difficulties are not usually marked. Hypotonia and weakness often are not apparent, except after considerable activity. The *clinical course*, with some exceptions, is benign. Anticholinesterase medication is useful for treating the facial weakness, feeding difficulties, and limb weakness but is not particularly effective for treating the ophthalmoplegia, which tends to persist.

The *neurological features* of the form of endplate acetylcholine receptor deficiency related to a *mutation of rapsyn* (receptor-associated protein at the synapse), important for clustering of the receptors, is usually more severe than is the case for subunit deficiency (see Table 18-13).[353,370,376-378] In the early-onset cases of rapsyn deficiency, *arthrogryposis multiplex*

congenita, severe *bulbar symptoms*, and the frequent need for assisted ventilation are prominent. The *clinical course* is more severe with rapsyn deficiency than with a subunit mutation, and frequent, severe exacerbations result in respiratory failure.

Diagnosis at the Bedside. Diagnosis of both forms of endplate acetylcholine receptor deficiency is made best by observation of the response to parenteral anticholinesterase drugs, as described previously for neonatal transient myasthenia gravis.

Laboratory Studies. The initial laboratory evaluation is similar to that described for neonatal transient myasthenia gravis. The decremental response of muscle action potentials with repetitive stimulation has been documented in endplate acetylcholine receptor deficiency or congenital myasthenia.[304,352-356,370,379,380] However, more detailed analysis is required for definitive diagnosis (see Table 18-14).

Pathology. No morphological abnormality at the site of the defect (i.e., the neuromuscular junction) has been described.

TABLE 18-14   Congenital Myasthenic Syndromes: Common Features

Familial occurrence
Autosomal recessive > autosomal dominant
Early ocular involvement: ptosis > ophthalmoparesis
Early facial and bulbar involvement
Response to anticholinesterase drugs*
Diagnosis often requires the following: single-fiber electromyogram; single-nerve stimulation; specific staining for acetylcholine receptors, receptor subunits, acetylcholinesterase; electron microscopy of motor endplate; in vitro electrophysiological studies; molecular genetic analyses

*Except for acetylcholinesterase deficiency syndrome and slow-channel and fast-channel syndromes.

---

*See references 24,303,304,348,352,353,355,356,362,364,370,372-375.

Pathogenesis and Etiology. Two major types of molecular defect underlying endplate acetylcholine receptor deficiency have been described, and both are inherited in an autosomal recessive manner.* Thus, occurrence in siblings in approximately 50% of families and with consanguineous parents has been documented. Earlier studies indicated that the inherited defects at the neuromuscular junction involved the endplate acetylcholine receptor (see Table 18-13).[355,356,380,381] Thus, a deficiency of the number or function of acetylcholine receptors, measured by alpha-bungarotoxin binding studies and electrophysiologically, was defined. The two molecular forms underlying this defect involve a *mutation in a subunit protein* or in *rapsyn*, active in receptor clustering. Of the four subunits of the acetylcholine receptor, the epsilon subunit of the receptor is involved in most cases.[24,348,349,351-353,364,367,370,382,383] The disorder is usually related to a mutation in the gene for the epsilon subunit and less commonly in the promoter for this subunit. Rapsyn deficiency is only slightly less common than the subunit deficiency.

Management. The essential aspects of management involve the use of anticholinesterase medications, as discussed for neonatal transient myasthenia gravis. Anticholinesterase medication is not invariably beneficial.[352,353,355,356,370,384] 3,4-Diaminopyridine, which increases nerve terminal acetylcholine release, may be beneficial alone or in combination with anticholinesterase medication.[385] Steroid therapy and thymectomy have not been useful, in accordance with the nonimmune basis of the disorder. The nonimmune basis is evidenced by the lack of circulating acetylcholine receptor antibodies.[304,380]

Congenital Myasthenic Syndromes: Congenital Choline Acetyltransferase Deficiency (Familial Infantile Myasthenia or Congenital Myasthenic Syndrome with Episodic Apnea)

Congenital choline acetyltransferase deficiency, formerly referred to as *familial infantile myasthenia* or, more recently, *congenital myasthenic syndrome with episodic apnea*, is a presynaptic defect and the second most common type of congenital myasthenic syndrome with onset in the neonatal period (see Table 18-13). In contrast to endplate acetylcholine receptor deficiency, this disorder is based on a *presynaptic defect*. Like endplate acetylcholine receptor deficiency, the disorder is inherited in an autosomal recessive manner and has its onset in the neonatal period.† However, several features, readily delineated at the patient's bedside, help to distinguish this form of myasthenia from the transient form and from acetylcholine receptor deficiency (see later discussion).

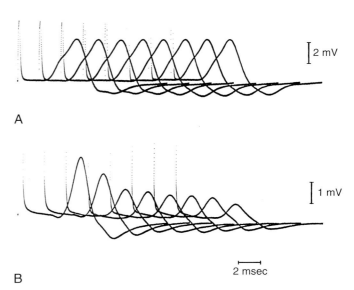

Figure 18-14 Electromyogram in familial infantile myasthenia. In this repetitive nerve stimulation study, recordings were obtained from the left abductor digiti minimi using surface stimulating and recording electrodes. **A**, A 3-Hz stimulation at rest shows no decrement. **B**, At 4 minutes after 2 minutes of continuous stimulation of ulnar nerve at 10 Hz, a decrement of 54% (fifth/first response) occurred. (*From Matthes JW, Kenna AP, Fawcett PRW: Familial infantile myasthenia: A diagnostic problem,* Dev Med Child Neurol *33:912–929, 1991.*)

Clinical Features. *At birth*, infants are hypotonic and cyanotic and require resuscitative efforts. Episodes of apnea occur, and prominent feeding difficulties result from deficits of sucking and swallowing. Facial weakness is prominent, but eye movements are normal and usually remain so. Ptosis may be present but is not striking. Generalized weakness is common. After the serious neonatal course, appropriately treated infants (anticholinesterase medication) improve, and *spontaneous remission* often ensues in the first months of life. However, the disease may *recur* later in infancy and, indeed, develop so abruptly with respiratory infection that apnea and death result. A family history of sudden infant death syndrome in previously born siblings is not uncommon. In general, despite the episodic course, *improvement* with age is the rule.

Diagnosis at the Bedside. Diagnosis is suspected by observation of a beneficial response to parenteral anticholinesterase medication. A decremental response of the muscle to repetitive nerve stimulation requires more prolonged stimulation (several minutes) and more rapid rates (10 Hz) than required for other neonatal myasthenias (Fig. 18-14). This electrophysiological aspect relates to the fundamental *presynaptic* defect, which involves acetylcholine synthesis or release (see later discussion).

Laboratory Studies. Although decremental responses to repetitive stimulation are present in this disorder, as in the other myasthenic disorders, elicitation of the abnormality may require more prolonged stimulation in familial infantile myasthenia.[380,388]

---

*See references 24,304,348,351-353,355,356,364,367,370,373,378,380.

†See references 24,304,352,353,355,356,360,369,372,380,386-392.

Pathology. No morphological abnormality is demonstrable at the neuromuscular junction.

Pathogenesis and Etiology. The inherited defect at the neuromuscular junction is presynaptic in location and in the gene that codes for choline acetyltransferase *(CHAT)*, the rate-limiting enzyme in resynthesis of acetylcholine from acetyl–coenzyme A and choline within the nerve terminal (see Table 18-13).[351-353]

Management. Anticholinesterase drugs form the cornerstone of therapy. Moreover, therapy should be continued despite improvement or apparent remission, to avoid the occurrence of apnea and sudden death. 3,4-Diaminopyridine may produce transient benefit but then may worsen symptoms as acetylcholine stores are depleted and are not replenished sufficiently quickly. Close surveillance is necessary indefinitely, because serious respiratory exacerbations have been reported, even in adults with this disorder.[390]

Toxic-Metabolic Defects of the Neuromuscular Junction

Various exogenous and endogenous toxins and metabolites may disturb the function of the neuromuscular junction. Of these, the most important for neonatal patients are magnesium and certain antibiotics (see Table 18-11).

Hypermagnesemia

Neonatal hypermagnesemia may result in a striking paralytic syndrome. The disorder most often is secondary to administration to the mother of large quantities of intravenous magnesium sulfate for the treatment of eclampsia before delivery.

Clinical Features. The clinical syndrome is usually apparent at birth with hypoventilation or apnea, severe weakness and hypotonia, and hyporeflexia or areflexia.[393-395] In addition to manifestations relating to *skeletal muscular involvement*, evidence of depression of the *central nervous system* (e.g., stupor or coma) and disturbed function of *smooth muscle* (e.g., abdominal distention and absent bowel sounds) may occur. The smooth muscle dysfunction may be so severe that meconium plug syndrome develops.[395] Infants provided supportive therapy recover within approximately 3 days, although serum magnesium levels may remain elevated longer.

Laboratory Studies. The diagnosis is confirmed by the observation of elevated serum magnesium levels (usually >4.5 mEq/L). Electrophysiological studies with repetitive stimulation demonstrate impaired neuromuscular function.[395] Prolonged post-tetanic facilitation and absent post-tetanic exhaustion are characteristic findings.[396]

Pathogenesis and Etiology. The pathogenesis of weakness and hypotonia with hypermagnesemia relates to the effect of magnesium at the presynaptic side of the neuromuscular junction, in contrast to the postsynaptic disturbance in neonatal transient myasthenia or endplate acetylcholine receptor deficiency. Hypermagnesemia results in an impairment of release of acetylcholine from the presynaptic nerve ending. This effect is a result of antagonism of the releasing effect of calcium, and, indeed, calcium counteracts the toxic effects of magnesium to a variable degree.

Management. Management of hypermagnesemia is based on vigorous support. A clearly beneficial role for calcium supplementation was not supported by the few clinical trials available.[394] *Hypocalcemia, however, should be particularly avoided.* Exchange transfusion has been useful in the management of the very severely affected infant who is not responsive to supportive therapy.[397]

Antibiotics

Certain antibiotics, particularly the aminoglycosides, may disturb neuromuscular function. The drugs reported to have toxic effects include kanamycin, gentamicin, neomycin, colimycin, streptomycin, and polymyxin.[398-400] Drug-induced cases have been recorded in the neonatal period.[398,401] Although this disorder has not been recognized in infants with myasthenia, the particular sensitivity of older patients with myasthenia to these drugs[399,402] makes it imperative in infants with myasthenia to avoid their use or, when necessary, to use such drugs under carefully controlled conditions. A similar conclusion applies to infants with botulism (see subsequent discussion).

Clinical Features. The clinical syndrome in otherwise neurologically normal infants has occurred most commonly with the administration of large quantities of drug, such as at the time of abdominal surgery (intraperitoneal lavage) or pulmonary surgery (intrapleural lavage), retrograde pyelography, and intravenous therapy. Postoperative occurrence has been associated with the combined use of a curare-type drug during anesthesia and an aminoglycoside antibiotic following surgery. Evolution to apnea, bulbar paralysis, and generalized flaccid paralysis occurs within 2 hours.[398] Additional diagnostic signs, when present, include pupillary dilation, atonic bladder, and paralytic ileus.

Laboratory Studies. The diagnosis is based usually on clinical evidence, although electrophysiological studies demonstrate impaired neuromuscular transmission.[399]

Pathogenesis and Etiology. The pathogenesis of the neuromuscular disturbance is impairment of presynaptic mobilization of acetylcholine caused by the antibiotic per se.[400]

Management. Management principally consists of recognition of the syndrome and elimination of the source of the excessive amount of drug. Support of respiration is critical. Neostigmine has been used with benefit.[398] Calcium may play an adjunct role, and, at the least, hypocalcemia should be corrected promptly.

Infantile Botulism

Clearly recognized for the first time in 1976,[403] *infantile botulism* is a relatively common disorder. The infantile disease is the result of intestinal infection by *Clostridium botulinum*, rather than ingestion of preformed toxin, as in the more common form of botulism observed in older patients. Previously reported infants with "acute polyneuropathy" probably include those with botulism.[404] More than 1000 cases have been identified in the United States, and currently approximately 70 to 100 cases per year are reported. The disorder has been identified in countries around the world.[43,405-420] Many other infants with transient hypotonia and weakness may represent unidentified cases of infantile botulism.

Clinical Features

Onset. Infantile botulism has a characteristic time of onset, between approximately 2 weeks and 6 months of age, with a median age of 10 weeks.[43,403-407,409,410,416,417,419-428] Thus, although most cases have occurred after the neonatal period, approximately 15% manifest in the first month, and infants as young as 54 hours and 6 days of age have been symptomatic with the disease.[411-415,418,419] The patient's presenting problems are usually constipation, poor feeding, hypotonia, and weakness.

Neurological Features. A striking neurological syndrome evolves over days, usually within a week after initial constipation, floppiness, and feeding problems. Almost invariable features include facial diplegia, weak suck, weak cry ("mewlike" or "sheeplike"), impaired swallowing and gag, peripheral weakness, and hypotonia. The resulting paucity of facial expression and minimal limb movement also gives the appearance of "lethargy." The paralytic process usually progresses in a descending direction (in contrast to the ascending direction in Guillain-Barré syndrome) and is generally symmetrical (in contrast to the asymmetrical flaccid paralysis in poliomyelitis). Ptosis is relatively common, but disturbances of extraocular function occur only in the minority of patients. Particularly helpful in diagnosis are the nearly invariable abnormalities of pupillary function. Pupillary size is most often midposition or dilated, and reaction to light is *absent* or is recognizably *impaired*. The pupillary abnormality is accentuated readily (or made apparent when not clear) by repetitive elicitation of the pupillary light reflex. Thus, an initially nearly normal response fatigues rapidly. Pupillary abnormality is the most helpful clinical feature distinguishing this disorder from congenital myasthenic syndromes (Table 18-15).

Clinical Course. The course of the disorder is variable, and, with increasing recognition of the illness, less severely affected cases have been

TABLE 18-15   Infantile Botulism versus Congenital Myasthenic Syndrome

	Infantile Botulism	Congenital Myasthenic Syndrome
Generalized hypotonia and weakness	+	±
Facial weakness, ptosis	+	+
Pupillary abnormality	+	−
Constipation	+	−
Response to anticholinesterase	−	+
Electromyogram	Incremental response	Decremental response

+, Present; −, absent; ±, variable.

recognized.[43,405,406,408-410,412,419,420] Evolution usually occurs over several or more days, except in rare cases in which evolution to a nadir in hours or a day or so can occur (see botulinum serotype F, later). In most cases, tube feeding is required. Ventilatory support is needed in approximately 70% of cases, from a few days to months.[410,412,421] The duration of the illness has been as long as 4 months, but 1 to 2 months is more common.[43,412,419,421,428] In earlier reports, among approximately 200 confirmed cases, the fatality rate was approximately 2%.[407,410] A later study of 57 infants found no fatalities.[412] Approximately 5% of infants experience a relapse within 1 to 2 weeks,[429,430] but in general the disorder is self-limiting.

A role for this disorder in the genesis of sudden infant death syndrome was suggested by epidemiological and microbiological data. Thus, Arnon and coworkers,[423] in 280 autopsy studies in infants, isolated *C. botulinum* from 10. Of these infants, 9 suffered sudden infant death syndrome and represented 4.3% of all cases of the syndrome in the series. Subsequent observations added support for a relationship between infantile botulism and sudden infant death syndrome,[419,431,432] although the possibility that the relationship does not hold for all regions was suggested by other data.[43,419,433,434] More importantly, these observations emphasize the suddenness and rapidity with which the disease may evolve.[419,423,431,432] The abrupt onset of apnea or need for mechanical ventilation near the onset of this disease, or both, is common in neonatal cases.[43,414-416,419]

Laboratory Studies. With few exceptions, serum enzyme levels, CSF protein concentration, nerve conduction velocities, and muscle biopsy have been normal. The diagnosis is established by observing, *in this clinical setting*, three consistent EMG findings. The first, observed in more than 90% of cases, is an *incremental response* in the muscle action potential produced by high rates (20 and 50 Hz) of repetitive nerve stimulation, a finding characteristic of a presynaptic neuromuscular blockade (Fig. 18-15).[43,396,427] This so-called *tetanic facilitation* results from enhanced acetylcholine release as a consequence of increased intracellular calcium concentration at the presynaptic terminal. The

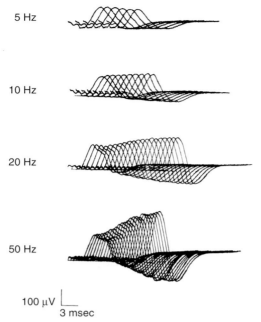

5 Hz

10 Hz

20 Hz

50 Hz

100 µV

3 msec

Figure 18-15 **Electromyogram in infantile botulism: incremental response obtained with repetitive stimulation of the left median nerve from the innervated abductor pollicis brevis at the rates shown.** A striking incremental response is observable at the higher rates of stimulation, especially at 50 Hz. *(From Cornblath DR, Sladky JT, Sumner AJ: Clinical electrophysiology of infantile botulism, Muscle Nerve 6:448, 1983.)*

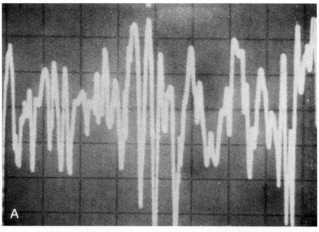

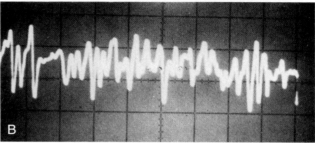

Figure 18-16 **Electromyogram in infantile botulism: brief-duration, small-amplitude, overly abundant motor unit potentials (BSAP). A,** Normal pattern of infant muscle. **B,** Brief-duration, small-amplitude, overly abundant (for the amount of power exerted) motor unit potentials (i.e., BSAP pattern) from an infant with botulism. *(From Johnson RO, Clay SA, Arnon SS: Diagnosis and management of infant botulism, Am J Dis Child 133:586–593, 1979.)*

related post-tetanic facilitation is also a feature of the disorder. The second consistent finding consists of the presence of prolonged post-tetanic facilitation (>120 seconds) and the absence of posttetanic exhaustion.[396] The third consistent finding is *the brief-duration, small-amplitude, overly abundant motor unit potentials (BSAP) pattern* (Fig. 18-16).[43,396,427] This pattern is caused by presynaptic block of many motor units but not of all the axonal terminals in the units.[435] (Additional findings include abnormal spontaneous activity [e.g., fibrillations], observed in approximately 50% of cases and caused by functional denervation of the muscle fibers.[216,427]) The EMG may be normal initially,[412,413] but usually a repeat study shows the characteristic findings. Indeed, if *all three* of the consistent EMG findings are present, and hypermagnesemia is excluded, the diagnosis of infantile botulism is considered the only possibility.[396] Isolation of *C. botulinum* from the stool is an important diagnostic adjunct.

Pathology. Muscle biopsy is normal.[421] This observation is to be expected in view of the nature of the defect (see following discussion).

Pathogenesis and Etiology. The defect at the neuromuscular junction is *presynaptic* in location. The botulinum toxin impairs acetylcholine release from cholinergic nerve terminals.[43,419,436-440] The neurotoxin is composed of a heavy chain (100 kDa) and a light chain (50 kDa). The heavy chain binds to specific gangliosides on the nerve terminal, the toxin then enters the nerve ending, and the light chain separates and carries

out proteolytic attack on specific proteins involved in synaptic vesicle docking and exocytosis. Botulinum neurotoxin types A and B, produced by *C. botulinum*, account for nearly all cases of infantile botulism, whereas neurotoxin types E and F, produced by *Clostridium butyricum* and *Clostridium barati*, respectively, account for isolated cases. The cases caused by types E and F evolve more rapidly and recover more promptly than do the cases caused by types A and B. In the United States, cases caused by type A neurotoxin are most prevalent west of the Mississippi River, and those caused by type B neurotoxin are more common east of the Mississippi River.

As just noted, the source of the toxin is *C. botulinum* (or rarely *C. barati* or *C. butyricum*) infection in the gastrointestinal tract.[43,403,419,421-423,425] Thus, this disorder is a *toxic infection*, in contrast to the more widely recognized type of botulism observed in older patients (i.e., ingestion of preformed toxin, or toxic ingestion). The source of the organism has been difficult to establish, in part because of its wide distribution in soil and dust.

After the initial recognition of infantile botulism, epidemiological and laboratory investigations, particularly of hospitalized patients with infantile botulism in California, led to the conclusion that 35% of the cases were caused by ingestion of honey.[425] *The honey was found to harbor* C. botulinum *spores.* Subsequent data confirmed the initial observation.[405] These findings led to the recommendation that infants less than 1 year of age not be given honey. Later work implicated honey as the source of the organism in only approximately 16% of all cases, and, more important, in infants less than 2 months of age, honey was not a statistically significant factor.[43,411] A more recent study of 122 infants reported honey exposure in only 5% to 7%.[428] Other patients have had similar *Clostridium* strains isolated from both their stool and dust in their immediate environment (vacuum cleaners and soil). Indeed, in careful studies in Pennsylvania, honey was not an important source of the organism, but contact with soil and dust was critical.[410] Residence near an active residential construction site occurred in 87% of cases in a recent series of 34 cases.[420] In two series of infants less than 2 months of age, living in a rural area or on a farm was the only significant predisposing factor, a finding further supporting environmental contact with soil and dust as crucial.[43,411,415,419] My most recent patient was a 2-week old infant whose father was a landscaper. An interesting recent report described an infant presenting at 54 hours of life with *C. barati* infection and type F botulinum neurotoxin who was born to parents in a rural setting.[418]

Remaining to be determined are the host factors (e.g., intestinal flora and immunological status) that allow the infection to become established in the young infant and not in the similarly exposed older child. Early data attributed particular importance to the first few weeks of exposure to food after a diet of only human breast milk.[43,409,410] The combination of loss of immunological factors of a human breast milk diet and the dramatic perturbation of gut flora caused by the change to other food may make the infant particularly vulnerable, for the first several weeks after this change, to colonization by the botulinum organism. Clinical and experimental data support this formulation.[409,410] However, more important in the youngest infants is poorly developed anaerobic fecal flora, which is important in protection from colonization by C. botulinum.[411]

Management. The most critical aspects of management are early recognition of infantile botulism, careful surveillance, particularly of respiratory status, and intervention at the early signs of ventilatory compromise. The disease can evolve exceedingly rapidly. Tube feeding and ventilatory support may be required for many days or weeks. Aminoglycosides should be avoided particularly; these antibiotics have been shown to potentiate muscular weakness and to precipitate respiratory failure in infantile botulism because of their effect on acetylcholine release at the neuromuscular junction.[43,419,441]

A *major advance in therapy has been the use of human botulism immune globulin for use in infant botulism.*[419,420,428,428a] This preparation is derived from pooled plasma of adults immunized with pentavalent botulinum toxoid and selected for high titers of antibodies versus type A and B toxin. When this preparation is administered early in the course of the disease, marked reductions in hospital stay (2.6 weeks versus 5.7 weeks), length of mechanical ventilation (1.8 versus 4.4 weeks), and length of tube feeding (3.6 weeks versus 10 weeks) have been observed.[419,428]

REFERENCES

1. Volpe JJ: Neonatal hypotonia. In Jones HR Jr, DeVivo DC, Darras BT, editors: *Neuromuscular Disorders of Infancy, Childhood, and Adolescence: A Clinician's Approach*, Philadelphia: 2003, Butterworth Heinemann.
2. Swoboda KJ, Saul JP, McKenna CE, Speller NB, et al: Aromatic L-amino acid decarboxylase deficiency: Overview of clinical features and outcomes, *Ann Neurol* 54(Suppl 6):S49-S55, 2003.
3. Korenke GC, Christen HJ, Hyland K, Hunneman DH, et al: Aromatic L-amino acid decarboxylase deficiency: An extrapyramidal movement disorder with oculogyric crises, *Eur J Paediatr Neurol* 1:67-71, 1997.
4. Swoboda KJ, Hyland K, Goldstein DS, Kuban KC, et al: Clinical and therapeutic observations in aromatic L-amino acid decarboxylase deficiency, *Neurology* 53:1205-1211, 1999.
5. Pons R, Ford B, Chiriboga CA, Clayton PT, et al: Aromatic L-amino acid decarboxylase deficiency: Clinical features, treatment, and prognosis, *Neurology* 62:1058-1065, 2004.
6. Abdenur JE, Abeling N, Specola N, Jorge L, et al: Aromatic L-amino acid decarboxylase deficiency: Unusual neonatal presentation and additional findings in organic acid analysis, *Mol Genet Metab* 87:48-53, 2006.
7. Letarte J, Garagorri JM: Congenital hypothyroidism: Laboratory and clinical investigation of early detected infants. In Collu R, Ducharme JR, Guyda HJ, editors: *Pediatric Endocrinology*, 2nd ed, New York: 1989, Raven Press.
8. Fisher DA: Screening for congenital hypothyroidism, *Trends Endocrinol Metab* 2:129-133, 1991.
9. Fisher DA, Dussault JH, Foley TP Jr, Klein AH, et al: Screening for congenital hypothyroidism: Results of screening one million North American infants, *J Pediatr* 94:700-705, 1979.
10. Klein RZ: New England congenital hypothyroidism collaborative, effects of neonatal screening for hypothyroidism: Prevention of mental retardation by treatment before clinical manifestations, *Lancet* 2:1095-1097, 1981.
11. Price DA, Ehrlich RM, Walfish PG: Congenital hypothyroidism: Clinical and laboratory characteristics in infants detected by neonatal screening, *Arch Dis Child* 56:845-851, 1981.
12. Alm J, Hagenfeldt L, Larsson A, Lundberg K: Incidence of congenital hypothyroidism: Retrospective study of neonatal laboratory screening versus clinical symptoms as indicators leading to diagnosis, *Br Med J (Clin Res Ed)* 289:1171-1175, 1984.
13. Holm VA, Cassidy SB, Butler MG, Hanchett JM, et al: Prader-Willi syndrome: Consensus diagnostic criteria, *Pediatrics* 91:398-402, 1993.
14. Aughton DJ, Cassidy SB: Physical features of Prader-Willi syndrome in neonates, *Am J Dis Child* 144:1251-1254, 1990.
15. Greenberg F, Elder FB, Ledbetter DH: Neonatal diagnosis of Prader-Willi syndrome and its implications, *Am J Med Genet* 28:845-856, 1987.
16. Wharton RH, Bresnan MJ: Neonatal respiratory depression and delay in diagnosis in Prader-Willi syndrome, *Dev Med Child Neurol* 31:231-236, 1989.
17. Cassidy SB: Prader-Willi syndrome, *Curr Probl Pediatr* 14:1-55, 1984.
18. Stephenson JBP: Neonatal presentation of Prader-Willi syndrome, *Am J Dis Child* 146:151-152, 1992.
19. Butler MG: Prader-Willi syndrome: Current understanding of cause and diagnosis, *Am J Med Genet* 35:319-332, 1990.
20. Hamabe J, Fukushima Y, Harada N, Abe K, et al: Molecular study of the Prader-Willi syndrome: Deletion, RFLP, and phenotype analyses of 50 patients, *Am J Med Genet* 41:54-63, 1991.
21. Chu CE, Cooke A, Stephenson J, Tolmie JL, et al: Diagnosis in Prader-Willi syndrome, *Arch Dis Child* 71:441-442, 1994.
22. Sone S: Muscle histochemistry in the Prader-Willi syndrome, *Brain Dev* 16:183-188, 1994.
23. Ehara H, Ohno K, Takeshita K: Frequency of the Prader-Willi syndrome in the San-in district, Japan, *Brain Dev* 17:324-326, 1995.
24. Dubowitz V: *Muscle Disorders in Childhood*, 2nd ed, Philadelphia: 1995, Saunders.
24a. Russman BS: Spinal muscular atrophy: clinical classification and disease heterogeneity, *J Child Neurol* 22:946-951, 2007.
25. Miller SP, Riley P, Shevell MI: The neonatal presentation of Prader-Willi syndrome revisited, *J Pediatr* 134:226-228, 1999.
26. L'Hermine AC, Aboura A, Brisset S, Cuisset L, et al: Fetal phenotype of Prader-Willi syndrome due to maternal disomy for chromosome 15, *Prenat Diagn* 23:938-943, 2003.
27. Stevenson DA, Anaya TM, Clayton-Smith J, Hall BD, et al: Unexpected death and critical illness in Prader-Willi syndrome: Report of ten individuals, *Am J Med Genet A* 124:158-164, 2004.
28. Dykens EM, Sutcliffe JS, Levitt P: Autism and 15q11-q13 disorders: Behavioral, genetic, and pathophysiological issues, *Ment Retard Dev Disabil Res Rev* 10:284-291, 2004.

29. Butler MG, Bittel DC, Kibiryeva N, Talebizadeh Z, et al: Behavioral differences among subjects with Prader-Willi syndrome and type I or type II deletion and maternal disomy, *Pediatrics* 113:565-573, 2004.

30. Thomson AK, Glasson EJ, Bittles AH: A long-term population-based clinical and morbidity review of Prader-Willi syndrome in Western Australia, *J Intellect Disabil Res* 50:69-78, 2006.

31. Yoshii A: Abnormal cortical development shown by 3D MRI in Prader-Willi syndrome, *Neurology* 59:644-645, 2002.

32. Lee S, Walker CL, Karten B, Kuny SL, et al: Essential role for the Prader-Willi syndrome protein necdin in axonal outgrowth, *Hum Mol Genet* 14:627-637, 2005.

33. Sarnat HB, Alcalá H: Human cerebellar hypoplasia: A syndrome of diverse causes, *Arch Neurol* 37:300-305, 1980.

34. Werdnig G: Zwei fruhinfantile hereditare falle von progressiver Muskelatrophie unter dem Bilde der Dystrophie, aber auch neurotischer Grundlage, *Arch Psychiatr Nervenkr* 22:437, 1891.

35. Werdnig G: Die fruhinfantile progressive spinale Amyotrophie, *Arch Psychiatr Nervenkr* 26:706, 1894.

36. Hoffmann J: Ueber chronische spinale Muskelatrophie im Kindesalter auf familiarer Basis, *Dtsch Z Nervenheilkd* 3:427, 1893.

37. Hoffmann J: Ueber die hereditare progressive spinale Muskelatrophie im Kindesalter, *München Med Wochenschr* 47:1649, 1900.

38. Dubowitz V: Very severe spinal muscular atrophy (SMA type 0): An expanding clinical phenotype, *Eur J Paediatr Neurol* 3:49-51, 1999.

39. Macleod MJ, Taylor JE, Lunt PW, Mathew CG, et al: Prenatal onset spinal muscular atrophy, *Eur J Paediatr Neurol* 3:65-72, 1999.

40. Garcia-Cabezas MA, Garcia-Alix A, Martin Y, Gutierrez M, et al: Neonatal spinal muscular atrophy with multiple contractures, bone fractures, respiratory insufficiency and 5q13 deletion, *Acta Neuropathol (Berl)* 107:475-478, 2004.

41. Brandt S: *Werdnig-Hoffman's Progressive Muscular Atrophy*, Copenhagen: 1950, Ejnar Munksgaard.

42. Hausmanowa-Petrusewicz I, Fidzianska-Dolot A: Clinical feature of infantile and juvenile spinal muscular atrophy. In Gamstorp I, Sarnat HB, editors: *Progressive Spinal Muscular Atrophies*, New York: 1984, Raven Press.

43. Crawford TO: Infantile botulism. In Jones HR Jr, DeVivo DC, Darras BT, editors: *Neuromuscular Disorders of Infancy, Childhood, and Adolescence: A Clinician's Approach*, Philadelphia: 2003, Butterworth Heinemann.

44. Swoboda KJ, Prior TW, Scott CB, McNaught TP, et al: Natural history of denervation in SMA: Relation to age, SMN2 copy number, and function, *Ann Neurol* 57:704-712, 2005.

45. Thomas NH, Dubowitz V: The natural history of type 1 (severe) spinal muscular atrophy, *Neuromuscul Disord* 4:497-502, 1994.

46. Hausmanowa-Petrusewicz I, Modrzycka BB, Ryniewicz B: On chaos in classification of childhood spinal muscular atrophy, *Neuromuscul Disord* 2:429-430, 1992.

47. Munsat TL: International SMA collaboration, *Neuromuscul Disord* 1:81-86, 1991.

48. Russman BS, Iannacone ST, Buncher CR, Samaha FJ, et al: Spinal muscular atrophy: New thoughts on the pathogenesis and classification schema, *J Child Neurol* 7:347-353, 1992.

49. Iannaccone ST, Browne RH, Samaha FJ, Buncher CR: Prospective study of spinal muscular atrophy before age 6 years, *Pediatr Neurol* 9:187-193, 1993.

50. Parano E, Fiumara A, Falsaperla R, Pavone L: A clinical study of childhood spinal muscular atrophy in Sicily: A review of 75 cases, *Brain Dev* 16:104-107, 1994.

51. Ignatius J: The natural history of severe spinal muscular atrophy: Further evidence for clinical subtypes, *Neuromuscular Disord* 4:527-528, 1994.

52. Zerres K, Wirth B, Rudnik-Schoneborn S: Spinal muscular atrophy: Clinical and genetic correlations, *Neuromuscul Disord* 7:202-207, 1997.

53. Soler-Botija C, Ferrer I, Gich I, Baiget M, et al: Neuronal death is enhanced and begins during foetal development in type I spinal muscular atrophy spinal cord, *Brain* 125:1624-1634, 2002.

54. Kyllerman M: Infantile spinal muscular dystrophy (morbus Werdnig-Hoffmann) causing neonatal asphyxia, *Neuropadiatrie* 8:53-56, 1977.

55. Dubowitz V: *Muscle Disorders in Childhood*, 2nd ed, Philadelphia: 1978, Saunders.

56. Byers RK, Banker BQ: Infantile muscular atrophy, *Arch Neurol* 5:140-164, 1961.

57. Gamstorp I: Historical review of the progressive spinal muscular atrophy (atrophies) with onset in infancy or early childhood, *Progressive Spinal Muscular Atrophies*, New York: 1984, Raven Press.

58. Bingham PM, Shen N, Rennert H, Rorke LB, et al: Arthrogryposis due to infantile neuronal degeneration associated with deletion of the SMN^T gene, *Neurology* 49:848-851, 1997.

59. Devriendt K, Lammens M, Schollen E, Van Hole C, et al: Clinical and molecular genetic features of congenital spinal muscular atrophy, *Ann Neurol* 40:731-738, 1996.

60. Gordon N: Arthrogryposis multiplex congenita, *Brain Dev* 20:507-511, 1998.

61. Novelli G, Capon F, Tamisari L, Grandi E, et al: Neonatal spinal muscular atrophy with diaphragmatic paralysis is unlinked to 5q11.2-q13, *J Med Genet* 32:216-219, 1995.

62. Rudnik-Schoneborn S, Forkert R, Hahnen E, Wirth B, et al: Clinical spectrum and diagnostic criteria of infantile spinal muscular atrophy: Further delineation on the basis of SMN gene deletion findings, *Neuropediatrics* 27:8-15, 1996.

63. Gorgen-Pauly U, Sperner J, Reiss I, Gehl H, et al: Familial pontocerebellar hypoplasia type 1 with anterior horn cell disease, *Eur J Paediatr Neurol* 3:33-38, 1999.

64. Mercuri E, Goodwin F, Sewry C, Dubowitz V, et al: Diaphragmatic spinal muscular atrophy with bulbar weakness, *Eur J Paediatr Neurol* 4:69-72, 2000.

65. Munsat TL, Skerry L, Korf B, Pobert B, et al: Phenotypic heterogeneity of spinal muscular atrophy mapping to chromosome 5q11.2-13.3 (SMA 5q), *Neurology* 40:1831-1836, 1990.

66. Zerres K, Rudnik-Schoneborn S: Natural history in proximal spinal muscular atrophy: Clinical analysis of 445 patients and suggestions for a modification of existing classifications, *Arch Neurol* 52:518-523, 1995.

66a. Oskoui M, Levy G, Garland CJ, Gray JM, et al: The changing nature history of spinal muscular atrophy type 1, *Neurology* 69:1931-1936, 2007.

67. Dubowitz V: Infantile muscular atrophy: A prospective study with particular reference to a slowly progressive variety, *Brain* 87:707-718, 1964.

68. Munsat TL, Woods R, Fowler W, Pearson CM: Neurogenic muscular atrophy of infancy with prolonged survival, *Brain* 92:9-24, 1969.

69. Pearn JH, Wilson J: Chronic generalized spinal muscular atrophy of infancy and childhood, *Arch Dis Child* 48:768-774, 1973.

70. Russell JW, Afifi AK, Ross MA: Predictive value of electromyography in diagnosis and prognosis of the hypotonic infant, *J Child Neurol* 7:387-391, 1992.

71. Jones HR, Bolton CF, Harper C Jr: *Pediatric Clinical Electromyography*, Philadelphia: 1996, Lippincott-Raven.

72. Moosa A, Dubowitz V: Motor nerve conduction velocity in spinal muscular atrophy of childhood, *Arch Dis Child* 51:974-977, 1976.

73. Hergerberg M, Glatzel M, Capone A, Achermann S, et al: Deletions in the spinal muscular atrophy gene region in a newborn with neuropathy and extreme generalized muscular weakness, *Eur J Pediatr Neurol* 4:35-38, 2000.

74. Rudnik-Schoneborn S, Goebel HH, Scholote W, Molaian S, et al: Classical infantile spinal muscular atrophy with SMN deficiency causes sensory neuronopathy, *Neurology* 60:983-987, 2003.

75. Anagnostou E, Miller SP, Guiot MC, Karpati G, et al: Type I spinal muscular atrophy can mimic sensory-motor axonal neuropathy, *J Child Neurol* 20:147-150, 2005.

76. Osborne JP, Murphy EG, Hill A: Thin ribs on chest X-ray: A useful sign in the differential diagnosis of the floppy newborn, *Dev Med Child Neurol* 25:343-345, 1983.

77. Rodriguez JI, Garcia-Alix A, Palacios J, Paniagua R: Changes in the long bones due to fetal immobility caused by neuromuscular disease: A radiographic and histological study, *J Bone Joint Surg Am* 70:1052-1060, 1988.

78. Rodriguez JI, Palacios J, Garcia-Alix A, Pastor I, et al: Effects of immobilization on fetal bone development: A morphometric study in newborns with congenital neuromuscular diseases with intrauterine onset, *Calcif Tissue Int* 43:335-339, 1988.

79. Heckmatt JZ, Dubowitz V: Diagnosis of spinal muscular atrophy with pulse echo ultrasound. In Gamstorp I, Sarnat HB, editors: *Progressive Spinal Muscular Atrophies*, New York: 1984, Raven Press.

80. Fidzianska-Dolot A, Hausmanowa-Petrusewicz I: Morphology of the lower motor neuron and muscle. In Gamstorp I, Sarnat HB, editors: *Progressive Spinal Muscular Atrophies*, New York: 1984, Raven Press.

81. Murayama S, Bouldin TW, Suzuki K: Immunocytochemical and ultrastructural studies of Werdnig-Hoffman disease, *Acta Neuropathol (Berl)* 81:408-417, 1991.

82. Yamanouchi Y, Yamanouchi H, Becker LE: Synaptic alterations of anterior horn cells in Werdnig-Hoffman disease, *Pediatr Neurol* 15:32-35, 1996.

83. Crawford TO, Pardo CA: The neurobiology of childhood spinal muscular atrophy, *Neurobiol Dis* 3:97-110, 1996.

84. Chou SM, Nonaka I: Werdnig-Hoffmann disease: Proposal of a pathogenetic mechanism, *Acta Neuropathol (Berl)* 41:45, 1978.

85. Ghatak NR: Spinal roots in Werdnig-Hoffmann disease, *Acta Neuropathol (Berl)* 41:1, 1978.

86. Omran H, Ketelsen UP, Heinen F, Sauer M, et al: Axonal neuropathy and predominance of type II myofibers in infantile spinal muscular atrophy, *J Child Neurol* 13:327-331, 1998.

87. Brzustowicz LM, Lehner T, Castilla LH: Genetic mapping of childhood-onset spinal muscular atrophy to chromosome 5q11.2-13.3, *Nature* 344:540-541, 1990.

88. Gilliam TC, Brzustowicz LM, Castilla LH: Genetic homogeneity between acute (SMA I) and chronic (SMA II & III) forms of spinal muscular atrophy, *Nature* 345:823-825, 1990.

89. Morrison KE: Advances in SMA research: Review of gene deletions, *Neuromuscul Disord* 6:397-408, 1996.

90. Crawford TO: From enigmatic to problematic: The new molecular genetics of childhood spinal muscular atrophy, *Neurology* 46:335-340, 1996.

91. Stewart H, Wallace A, McGaughran J, Mountford R, et al: Molecular diagnosis of spinal muscular atrophy, *Arch Dis Child* 78:531-535, 1998.

92. Talbot K: What's new in the molecular genetics of spinal muscular atrophy? *Eur J Paediatr Neurol* 5:149-155, 1998.

93. Somerville MJ, Hunter AG, Aubry HL, Korneluk RG, et al: Clinical application of the molecular diagnosis of spinal muscular atrophy: Deletions of neuronal apoptosis inhibitor protein and survival motor neuron genes, *Am J Med Genet* 69:159-165, 1997.
94. Wang CH, Carter TA, Das K, Xu J, et al: Extensive DNA deletion associated with severe disease alleles on spinal muscular atrophy homologues, *Ann Neurol* 42:41-49, 1997.
95. Matthijs G, Devriendt K, Fryns JP: The prenatal diagnosis of spinal muscular atrophy, *Prenat Diagn* 18:607-610, 1998.
96. Erdem H, Pehlivan S, Topaloglu H, Ozguc M: Deletion analysis in Turkish patients with spinal muscular atrophy, *Brain Dev* 21:86-89, 1999.
97. Biros I, Forrest S: Spinal muscular atrophy: Untangling the knot? *J Med Genet* 36:1-8, 1999.
98. Cusco I, Barcelo J, del Rio E, Baiget M, et al: Detection of novel mutations in the SMN Tudor domain in type I SMA patients, *Neurology* 63:146-149, 2004.
99. Monani UR: Spinal muscular atrophy: A deficiency in a ubiquitous protein, a motor neuron-specific disease, *Neuron* 48:885-896, 2005.
100. Cusco I, Barcelo MJ, Rojas-Garcia R, Illa I, et al: SMN2 copy number predicts acute or chronic spinal muscular atrophy but does not account for intrafamilial variability in siblings, *J Neurol* 253:21-25, 2006.
100a. Sumner CJ: Molecular mechanisms of spinal muscular atrophy, *J Child Neurol* 22:979-989, 2007.
100b. Prior TW: Spinal muscular atrophy diagnostic, *J Child Neurol* 22:952-956, 2007.
101. Kerr DA, Nery JP, Traystman RJ, Chau BN, et al: Survival motor neuron protein modulates neuron-specific apoptosis, *Proc Natl Acad Sci U S A* 97:13312-13317, 2000.
102. Feng W, Gubitz AK, Wan L, Battle DJ, et al: Gemins modulate the expression and activity of the SMN complex, *Hum Mol Genet* 14:1605-1611, 2005.
103. Rossoll W, Jablonka S, Andreassi C, Kroning AK, et al: SMN, the spinal muscular atrophy-determining gene product, modulates axon growth and localization of beta-actin mRNA in growth cones of motoneurons, *J Cell Biol* 163:801-812, 2003.
104. Wan L, Battle DJ, Yong J, Gubitz AK, et al: The survival of motor neurons protein determines the capacity for snRNP assembly: Biochemical deficiency in spinal muscular atrophy, *Mol Cell Biol* 25:5543-5551, 2005.
105. Eggert C, Chari A, Laggerbauer B, Fischer U: Spinal muscular atrophy: The RNP connection, *Trends Mol Med* 12:113-121, 2006.
105a. Kolb SJ, Battle DJ, Dreyfuss G: Molecular function of the SMN complex, *J Child Neurol* 22:990-994, 2007.
106. Gordon N: The spinal muscular atrophies, *Dev Med Child Neurol* 33:930-938, 1991.
107. Iannaccone ST, Guilfoile T: Long-term mechanical ventilation in infants with neuromuscular disease, *J Child Neurol* 3:30-32, 1988.
108. Gilgoff IS, Kahlstrom E, MacLaughlin E, Keens TG: Long-term ventilatory support in spinal muscular atrophy, *J Pediatr* 115:904-909, 1989.
109. Birnkrant DJ, Pope JF, Martin JE, Repucci AH, et al: Treatment of type I spinal muscular atrophy with noninvasive ventilation and gastrostomy feeding, *Pediatr Neurol* 18:407-410, 1998.
110. Gilgoff RL, Gilgoff IS: Long-term follow-up of home mechanical ventilation in young children with spinal cord injury and neuromuscular conditions, *J Pediatr* 142:476-480, 2003.
111. Sritippayawain S, Kun SS, Keens TG, Davidson Ward SL: Initiation of home mechanical ventilation in children with neuromuscular diseases, *J Pediatr* 142:481-485, 2003.
111a. Iannaccone ST: Modern management of spinal muscular atrophy, *J Child Neurol* 22:974-978, 2007.
111b. Wang CH, Finkel RS, Bertini ES, Schroth MK, et al: Consensus statement for standard of care in spinal muscular atrophy, *J Child Neurol* 22:1027-1049, 2007.
112. Mercuri E, Bertini E, Messina S, Pelliccioni M, et al: Pilot trial of phenylbutyrate in spinal muscular atrophy, *Neuromuscul Disord* 14:130-135, 2004.
113. Grzeschik SM, Ganta M, Prior TW, Heavlin WD, et al: Hydroxyurea enhances SMN2 gene expression in spinal muscular atrophy cells, *Ann Neurol* 58:194-202, 2005.
114. Brichta L, Holker I, Haug K, Klockgether T, et al: In vivo activation of SMN in spinal muscular atrophy carriers and patients treated with valproate, *Ann Neurol* 59:970-975, 2006.
115. Mercuri E, Bertini E, Messina S, Solari A, et al: Randomized, double-blind, placebo-controlled trial of phenylbutyrate in spinal muscular atrophy, *Neurology* 68:51-55, 2007.
116. Grohmann K, Varon R, Stolz P, Schuelke M, et al: Infantile spinal muscular atrophy with respiratory distress Type 1 (SMARD1), *Ann Neurol* 54:719-724, 2003.
117. Appleton RE, Hubner C, Grobmann K, Varon R: Congenital peripheral neuropathy presenting as apnoea and respiratory insufficiency: Spinal muscular atrophy with respiratory distress type 1 (SMARD1) [letter], *Dev Med Child Neurol* 46:576, 2004.
118. Sangiuolo F, Filareto A, Giardina E, Nardone AM, et al: Prenatal diagnosis of spinal muscular atrophy with respiratory distress (SMARM) in a twin pregnancy, *Prenat Diagn* 24:839-841, 2004.
119. Rudnik-Schoneborn S, Stolz P, Varon R, Grohmann K, et al: Long-term observations of patients with infantile spinal muscular atrophy with respiratory distress type 1 (SMARD1), *Neuropediatrics* 35:174-182, 2004.
120. Tachi N, Kikuchi S, Kozuka N, Nogami A: A new mutation of IGHMBP2 gene in spinal muscular atrophy with respiratory distress type 1, *Pediatr Neurol* 32:288-290, 2005.
121. Muntoni F, Goodwin F, Sewry C, Cox P, et al: Clinical spectrum and diagnostic difficulties of infantile ponto-cerebellar hypoplasia type 1, *Neuropediatrics* 30:243-248, 1999.
122. Ryan MM, Cooke-Yarborough CM, Orocopis PG, Ouvrier RA: Anterior horn cell disease and olivopontocerebellar hypoplasia, *Pediatr Neurol* 23:180-184, 2000.
123. Salman MS, Blaser S, Buncic JR, Westall CA, et al: Pontocerebellar hypoplasia type 1: New leads for an earlier diagnosis, *J Child Neurol* 18:220-225, 2003.
124. Rudnik-Schoneborn S, Sztriha L, Aithala GR, Houge G, et al: Extended phenotype of pontocerebellar hypoplasia with infantile spinal muscular atrophy, *Am J Med Genet A* 117:10-17, 2003.
125. Kizilates SU, Talim B, Sel K, Kose G, et al: Severe lethal spinal muscular atrophy variant with arthrogryposis, *Pediatr Neurol* 32:201-204, 2005.
126. Felderhoff-Mueser U, Harder A, Stadelmann C, Zerres K, et al: Severe spinal muscular atrophy variant associated with congenital bone fractures, *J Child Neurol* 17:718-721, 2002.
127. Van Toorn R, Dvies J, Wilmshurst JM: Spinal muscular atrophy with congenital fractures: Postmortem analysis, *J Child Neurol* 17:721-723, 2002.
128. Mercuri E, Messina S, Kinali M, Cini C, et al: Congenital form of spinal muscular atrophy predominantly affecting the lower limbs: A clinical and muscle MRI study, *Neuromuscul Disord* 14:125-129, 2004.
129. Darwish H, Sarnat H, Archer G, Brownell K, et al: Congenital cervical spinal atrophy, *Muscle Nerve* 4:106-110, 1981.
130. Hageman G, Ramaekers VT, Hilhorst BG, Rozeboom AR: Congenital cervical spinal muscular atrophy: A non-familial, non-progressive condition of the upper limbs, *J Neurol Neurosurg Psychiatry* 56:365-368, 1993.
131. Fleury P, Hageman G: A dominantly inherited lower motor neuron disorder presenting at birth with associated arthrogryposis, *J Neurol Neurosurg Psychiatry* 48:1037-1048, 1985.
132. Kaiboriboon K, Hayat GR: Congenital cervical spinal atrophy: An intrauterine hypoxic insult, *Neuropediatrics* 32:330-334, 2001.
133. Narbona J, Mestre M, Beguiristain JL, Martinez-Lage JM: Intramedullary telangiectasis causing congenital cervical spinal atrophy, *Muscle Nerve* 5:256, 1982.
134. Sarnat HB: Neuromuscular disorders in the neonatal period. In Korobkin R, Guilleminault C, editors: *Advances in Perinatal Neurology*, New York: 1979, Spectrum Publications.
135. Tsukamoto H, Inagaki M, Tomita Y, Ohno K: Congenital caudal spinal atrophy: A case report, *Neuropediatrics* 23:260-262, 1992.
136. Hogan GR, Gutmann L, Schmidt R, Gilbert E: Pompe's disease, *Neurology* 19:894-900, 1969.
137. DiMauro S, Eastwood AB: Disorders of glycogen and lipid metabolism. In Griggs RC, Moxley RT, editors: *Treatment of Neuromuscular Diseases*, New York: 1977, Raven Press.
138. Howell RR, Williams JC: The glycogen storage diseases. In Stanbury JB, Wyngaarden JB, Frederickson DS, editors: *The Metabolic Basis of Inherited Diseases*, New York: 1983, McGraw-Hill.
139. Hirschhorn R: Glycogen storage disease type II: Acid α-glucosidase (acid maltase) deficiency. In Scriver CR, Beaudet AL, Sly WS, et al, editors: *The Metabolic and Molecular Bases of Inherited Disease*, 7th ed, New York: 1995, McGraw-Hill.
140. van den Hout HMP, Hop WC, van Diggelen OP, Smeithink JAM, et al: The natural course of infantile Pompe's disease: 20 original cases compared with 133 cases from the literature, *Pediatrics* 112:332-340, 2003.
141. Kishnani PS, Hwu W-L, Mandel H, Nicouno M, et al: A retrospective, multinational, multicenter study on the natural history of infantile-onset Pompe disease, *J Pediatr* 148:671-676, 2006.
142. Chien YH, Lee NC, Peng SF, Hwu WL: Brain development in infantile-onset Pompe disease treated by enzyme replacement therapy, *Pediatr Res* 60:349-352, 2006.
143. Harriman DG: Diseases of muscle. In Blackwood W, Corsellis JAN, editors: *Greenfield's Neuropathology*, Chicago: 1977, Year Book.
144. Crome L, Stern J: Inborn lysosomal enzyme deficiencies. In Blackwood W, Corsellis JAN, editors: *Greenfield's Neuropathology*, Chicago: 1977, Year Book.
145. Hers HG: The concept of inborn lysosomal disease *Lysosomes and Storage Diseases*, New York: 1973, Academic Press.
146. Hirschhorn R, Reuser AJJ: Glycogen storage disease type II: Acid α-glucosidase (acid maltase) deficiency. In Schriver CR, Beaudet AT, Valle D, editors: *The Metabolic and Molecular Bases of Inherited Disease*, 8th ed, New York: 2001, McGraw-Hill.
147. Brown BI, Brown DH, Jeffrey PL: Simultaneous absence of alpha-1,4-glucosidase and alpha-1,6-glucosidase activities (pH 4) in tissues of children with type II glycogen storage diseases, *Biochemistry* 9:1423-1428, 1970.
148. Hug G, Schubert WK, Soukup S: Ultrastructure and enzyme deficiency of fibroblast cultures in type II glycogenesis, *Pediatr Res* 5:107, 1971.

149. Malatack JJ, Consolini DM, Bayever E: The status of hematopoietic stem cell transplantation in lysosomal storage disease, *Pediatr Res* 29:391-403, 2003.

150. Wilcox WR: Lysosomal storage disorders: The need for better pediatric recognition and comprehensive care, *J Pediatr* 144(Suppl):S3-S14, 2004.

151. Kishnani PS, Corzo D, Nicolino M, Byrne B, et al: Recombinant human acid α-glucosidase: Major clinical benefits in infantile-onset Pompe disease, *Neurology* 68:99-109, 2007.

152. Wagner KR: Enzyme replacement for infantile Pompe disease: The first step toward a cure, *Neurology* 68:88-89, 2007.

153. Bergeisen GH, Bauman RJ, Gilmore RL: Neonatal paralytic poliomyelitis: A case report, *Arch Neurol* 43:192-194, 1986.

154. Beausoleil J, Nordgren RE, Modlin JF: Vaccine-associated paralytic poliomyelitis, *J Child Neurol* 9:334-335, 1994.

155. Baskin J, Soule EH, Mills SD: Poliomyelitis of the newborn, *Am J Dis Child* 80:10-21, 1950.

156. Schaeffer M, Fox MJ, Pi CP: Intrauterine poliomyelitis infection: Report of a case, *JAMA* 155:248-250, 1954.

157. Bates T: Poliomyelitis in pregnancy, fetus, and newborn, *Am J Dis Child* 90:189-195, 1955.

158. Elliott GB, McAllister JE: Fetal poliomyelitis, *Am J Obstet Gynecol* 72:896-902, 1956.

159. Barsky P, Beale AJ: The transplacental transmission of poliomyelitis, *J Pediatr* 51:207-211, 1957.

160. Hagberg B, Lyon G: Pooled European series of hereditary peripheral neuropathies in infancy and childhood: A correspondence workshop report of the European Federation of Child Neurology Societies (EFCNS), *Neuropediatrics* 12:9-17, 1981.

161. Byers RK, Taft LT: Chronic multiple peripheral neuropathy in childhood, *Pediatrics* 20:517-537, 1957.

162. Chambers R, MacDermot V: Polyneuritis as a cause of amyotonia congenita, *Lancet* 1:397-401, 1957.

163. Dyck PJ, Lambert EH: Lower motor and primary sensory neuron disease with peroneal muscular atrophy. I. Neurologic, genetic, and electrophysiologic findings in hereditary polyneuropathies, *Arch Neurol* 18:603-618, 1968.

164. Lyon G: Ultrastructural study of a nerve biopsy from a case of early infantile chronic neuropathy, *Acta Neuropathol (Berl)* 13:131-142, 1969.

165. Gamstorp I: Characteristic clinical findings in some neurogenic myopathies and in some myogenic myopathies causing muscular weakness, hypotonia and atrophy in infancy and early childhood, *Birth Defects Orig Artic Ser* 7:72-81, 1971.

166. Anderson RM, Dennett X, Hopkins IJ, Shield LK: Hypertrophic interstitial polyneuropathy in infancy, *J Pediatr* 82:619-624, 1973.

167. Joosten E, Gabreels F, Gabreels-Festen A, Vrensen G, et al: Electron microscopic heterogeneity of onion-bulb neuropathies of the Dejerine-Sottas type: Two patients in one family with the variant described by Lyon (1969), *Acta Neuropathol (Berl)* 27:105-118, 1974.

168. Karch SB, Urich H: Infantile polyneuropathy with defective myelination: An autopsy study, *Dev Med Child Neurol* 17:504-511, 1975.

169. Kasman M, Bernstein L, Schulman S: Chronic polyradiculoneuropathy of infancy, *Neurology* 26:565-573, 1976.

170. Kennedy WR, Sung JH, Berry JF: A case of congenital hypomyelination neuropathy, *Arch Neurol* 34:337-345, 1977.

171. Moss RB, Sriram S, Kelts A, Forno LS, et al: Chronic neuropathy presenting as a floppy infant with respiratory distress, *Pediatrics* 64:459-464, 1979.

172. Zimmerman AW: Congenital demyelinative neuropathy. Paper presented at the Child Neurology Society Annual Meeting, Hanover, New Hampshire, 1979.

173. Towfighi J: Congenital hypomyelination neuropathy: Glial bundles in cranial and spinal nerve roots, *Ann Neurol* 10:570-573, 1981.

174. Ulrich J, Hirt HR, Kleihues P, Oberholzer M: Connatal polyneuropathy: A case with proliferated microfilaments in Schwann cells, *Acta Neuropathol (Berl)* 55:39-46, 1981.

175. Guzzetta F, Ferriere G, Lyon G: Congenital hypomyelination polyneuropathy: Pathological findings compared with polyneuropathies starting later in life, *Brain* 105:395-416, 1982.

176. Ono J, Senba E, Okada S: A case report of congenital hypomyelination, *Eur J Pediatr* 138:265-270, 1982.

177. Hakamada S, Kumagai T, Hara K: Congenital hypomyelination neuropathy in a newborn, *Neuropediatrics* 14:182-183, 1983.

178. Hagberg B, Westerberg B, Hagne I, Sellden U: Hereditary motor and sensory neuropathies in Swedish children. III. De- and remyelinating type in 10 sporadic cases, *Acta Paediatr Scand* 72:537-544, 1983.

179. Hagberg B, Westerberg B: Hereditary motor and sensory neuropathies in Swedish children. I. Prevalence and distribution by disability groups, *Acta Paediatr Scand* 72:379-383, 1983.

180. Hagberg B, Westerberg B: The nosology of genetic peripheral neuropathies in Swedish children, *Dev Med Child Neurol* 25:3-18, 1983.

181. Tachi N, Ishikawa Y, Minami R: Two cases of congenital hypomyelination neuropathy, *Brain Dev* 6:560-565, 1984.

182. Balestrini MR, Cavaletti G, D'Angelo A, Tredici G: Infantile hereditary neuropathy with hypomyelination: Report of two siblings with different expressivity, *Neuropediatrics* 27:65-70, 1991.

183. Harati Y, Butler I: Congenital hypomyelinating neuropathy, *J Neurol Neurosurg Psychiatry* 48:1269-1276, 1985.

184. Ouvrier RA, McLeod JG, Conchin TE: The hypertrophic forms of hereditary motor and sensory neuropathy: A study of hypertrophic Charcot-Marie-Tooth disease (HMSN type I) and Dejerine-Sottas disease (HMSN type III) in childhood, *Brain* 110:121-148, 1987.

185. Ouvrier R, McLeod JC, Pollard J: *Peripheral Neuropathy in Childhood*, New York: 1990, Raven Press.

186. Lutschg J, Vassella F, Boltshauser, E, et al: Heterogeneity of congenital motor and sensory neuropathies, *Neuropediatrics* 16:33-38, 1985.

187. Vital A, Vital C, Couquet M, Hernandorena X, et al: Congenital hypomyelination with axonopathy, *J Pediatr* 148:470-472, 1989.

188. Vital A, Vital C, Riviere JP, Brechenmacher C, et al: Variability of morphological features in early infantile polyneuropathy with defective myelination, *Acta Neuropathol (Berl)* 73:295-300, 1987.

189. Vallat JM, Gil R, Leboutet MJ, Hugon J, et al: Congenital hypo- and hypermyelination neuropathy, *Acta Neuropathol (Berl)* 74:197-201, 1987.

190. Boylan KB, Ferriero DM, Greco CM, Sheldon RA: Congenital hypomyelination neuropathy with arthrogryposis multiplex congenita, *Ann Neurol* 31:337-340, 1992.

191. Sghirlanzoni A, Pareyson D, Balestrini MR, Bellone E, et al: HMSN III phenotype due to homozygous expression of a dominant HMSN II gene, *Neurology* 42:2201-2204, 1992.

192. Hagberg B: Polyneuropathies in paediatrics, *Eur J Pediatr* 149:296-305, 1990.

193. Nara T, Akashi M, Nonaka I, Nakanishi Y, et al: Muscle and intramuscular nerve pathology in congenital hypomyelination neuropathy, *J Neurol Sci* 129:170-174, 1995.

194. Sawaishi Y, Hayasaka K, Goto A, Kawamura K, et al: Congenital hypomyelination neuropathy: Decreased expression of the P2 protein in peripheral nerve with normal DNA sequence of the coding region, *J Neurol Sci* 134:150-159, 1995.

195. Warner LE, Hilz MJ, Appel SH, Killian JM, et al: Clinical phenotypes of different MPZ (P0) mutations may include Charcot-Marie-Tooth type 1B, Dejerine-Sottas, and congenital hypomyelination, *Neuron* 17:451-460, 1996.

196. Ouvrier RA, Nicholson GA: Advances in the genetics of hereditary hypertrophic neuropathy in childhood, *Brain Dev* 17:31-38, 1995.

197. Ionasescu VV, Ionasescu R, Searby C, Neahring R: Dejerine-Sottas disease with de novo dominant point mutation of the PMP 22 gene, *Neurology* 45:1766-1767, 1995.

198. Ionasescu VV, Searby CC, Ionasescu R, Chatkupt S, et al: Dejerine-Sottas neuropathy in mother and son with same point mutation of PMP22 gene, *Muscle Nerve* 20:97-99, 1997.

199. Ghamdi M, Armstrong DL, Miller G: Congenital hypomyelinating neuropathy: A reversible case, *Pediatr Neurol* 16:71-73, 1997.

200. Levy BK, Fenton GA, Loaiza S, Hayat GR: Unexpected recovery in a newborn with severe hypomyelinating neuropathy, *Pediatr Neurol* 16:245-248, 1997.

201. Tyson J, Ellis D, Fairbrother U, King RH, et al: Hereditary demyelinating neuropathy of infancy: A genetically complex syndrome, *Brain* 120:47-63, 1997.

202. Marques W, Thomas PK, Sweeney MG, Carr L, et al: Dejerine-Sottas neuropathy and PMP22 point mutations: A new base pair substitution and a possible "hot spot" on Ser72, *Ann Neurol* 43:680-683, 1998.

203. Phillips JP, Warner LE, Lupski JR, Garg BP: Congenital hypomyelinating neuropathy: Two patients with long-term follow-up, *Pediatr Neurol* 20:226-232, 1999.

204. Mandich P, Mancardi GL, Varese A, Soriani S, et al: Congenital hypomyelination due to myelin protein zero Q215X mutation, *Ann Neurol* 45:676-678, 1999.

205. Parman Y, Plante-Bordeneuve V, Guiochon-Mantel A, Eraksoy M, et al: Recessive inheritance of a new point mutation of the PMP₂₂ gene in Dejerine-Sottas disease, *Ann Neurol* 45:518-522, 1999.

206. Lupski JR: Charcot-Marie-Tooth polyneuropathy: Duplication, gene dosage, and genetic heterogeneity, *Pediatr Res* 45:159-165, 1999.

207. Wilmshurst JM, Pollard JD, Nicholson G, Antony J, et al: Peripheral neuropathies of infancy, *Dev Med Child Neurol* 45:408-414, 2003.

208. Parman Y, Battaloglu E, Baris I, Bilir B, et al: Clinicopathological and genetic study of early-onset demyelinating neuropathy, *Brain* 127:2540-2550, 2004.

209. Szigeti K, Saifi GM, Armstrong DC, Belmont JW, et al: Disturbance of muscle fiber differentiation in congenital hypomyelinating neuropathy caused by a novel myelin protein zero mutation, *Ann Neurol* 54:398-402, 2003.

210. Kochanski A, Kabzinska D, Drac H, Ryniewicz B, et al: Early onset Charcot-Marie-Tooth type 1B disease caused by a novel Leu190fs mutation in the myelin protein zero gene, *Eur J Paediatr Neurol* 8:221-224, 2004.

211. Nelis E, Erdem S, Van den Bergh PY, Belpaire-Dethiou MC, et al: Mutations in GDAP1: Autosomal recessive CMT with demyelination and axonopathy, *Neurology* 59:1865-1872, 2002.

212. Gabreels-Festen A, Gabreels F: Congenital and early infantile neuropathies. In Jones HR Jr, DeVivo DC, Darras BT, editors: *Neuromuscular Disorders of Infancy, Childhood, and Adolescence: A Clinician's Approach*, Philadelphia: 2003, Butterworth Heinemann.

213. Kochanski A, Drac H, Kabzinska D, Ryniewicz B, et al: A novel MPZ gene mutation in congenital neuropathy with hypomyelination, *Neurology* 62:2122-2123, 2004.

214. Le N, Nagarajan R, Wang JY, Araki T, et al: Analysis of congenital hypomyelinating Egr2Lo/Lo nerves identifies Sox2 as an inhibitor of Schwann cell differentiation and myelination, *Proc Natl Acad Sci U S A* 102:2596-2601, 2005.

215. Inoue K, Shilo K, Boerkoel CF, Crowe C, et al: Congenital hypomyelinating neuropathy, central dysmyelination, and Waardenburg-Hirschsprung disease: Phenotypes linked by SOX10 mutation, *Ann Neurol* 52:836-842, 2002.

216. Jones HR: Pediatric electromyography. In Brown WF, Bolton CF, editors: *Clinical Electromyography*, 2nd ed, Boston: 1993, Butterworth Heinemann.

217. Birouk N, Azzedine H, Dubourg O, Muriel M-P, et al: Phenotypical features of a Moroccan family with autosomal recessive Charcot-Marie-Tooth disease associated with the S194X mutation in the GDAP1 gene, *Arch Neurol* 60:598-604, 2003.

218. Goikhman I, Meer J, Zelnik N: Hereditary neuropathy with liability to pressure palsies in infancy, *Pediatr Neurol* 28:307-309, 2003.

219. Gabreels-Festen AAW, Joosten EMG, Gabreels FJM, Stegeman DF, et al: Congenital demyelinating motor and sensory neuropathy with focally folded myelin sheaths, *Brain* 113:1629-1643, 1990.

220. Sladky JT, Brown MJ, Berman PH: Chronic inflammatory demyelinating polyneuropathy of infancy: A corticosteroid-responsive disorder, *Ann Neurol* 20:76-81, 1986.

221. Gabreels-Festen AA, Hageman AT, Gabreels FJ, Joosten EM, et al: Chronic inflammatory demyelinating polyneuropathy in two siblings, *J Neurol Neurosurg Psychiatry* 49:152-156, 1986.

222. Pasternak JF, Hageman J, Adams MA: Exchange transfusion in neonatal myasthenia, *J Pediatr* 99:644-646, 1981.

223. Majumdar A, Hartley L, Manzur AY, King RH, et al: A case of severe congenital chronic inflammatory demyelinating polyneuropathy with complete spontaneous remission, *Neuromuscul Disord* 14:818-821, 2004.

224. Pearce J, Pitt M, Martinez A: A neonatal diagnosis of congenital chronic inflammatory demyelinating polyneuropathy, *Dev Med Child Neurol* 47:489-492, 2005.

225. Yuill GM, Lynch PG: Congenital non-progressive peripheral neuropathy with arthrogryposis multiplex, *J Neurol Neurosurg Psychiatry* 37:316-323, 1974.

226. Westerberg B, Hagne I, Sellden U: Hereditary motor and sensory neuropathies in Swedish children. II. Neuronal-axonal types, *Acta Paediatr Scand* 72:685-693, 1983.

227. Breningstall GN, Smith SA, Kennedy WR: Congenital axonal neuropathy in the neonate. Paper presented at the Child Neurology Society Annual Meeting, Phoenix, Arizona, 1984.

228. Goebel HH, Zeman W, DeMyer W: Peripheral motor and sensory neuropathy of early childhood, simulating Werdnig-Hoffmann disease, *Neuropaediatrie* 7:182-195, 1976.

229. Guzzetta F, Ferriere G: Congenital neuropathy with prevailing axonal changes, *Acta Neuropathol (Berl)* 68:185-190, 1985.

230. Appleton R, Riordan A, Tedman B, MacKenzie J, et al: Congenital peripheral neuropathy presenting as apnoea and respiratory insufficiency, *Dev Med Child Neurol* 36:545-553, 1994.

231. Diers A, Kaczinski M, Grohmann K, Hubner C, et al: The ultrastructure of peripheral nerve, motor end-plate and skeletal muscle in patients suffering from spinal muscular atrophy with respiratory distress type 1 (SMARD1), *Acta Neuropathol (Berl)* 110:289-297, 2005.

232. Sarnat HB: Pathology of spinal muscular atrophy. In Gamstorp I, Sarnat HB, editors: *Progressive Spinal Muscular Atrophies*, New York: 1984, Raven Press.

233. Shishikura K, Hara M, Sasaki Y, Misugi K: A neuropathologic study of Werdnig-Hoffmann disease with special reference to the thalamus and posterior roots, *Acta Neuropathol (Berl)* 60:99-106, 1983.

234. Towfighi J, Young RS, Ward RM: Is Werdnig-Hoffmann disease a pure lower motor neuron disorder? *Acta Neuropathol (Berl)* 65:270-280, 1985.

235. Bargeton E, Nezelof C, Guran P, Job JC: Étude anatomique d'un cas d'arthrogrypose multiple congenitale et familiale, *Rev Neurol* 104:479-489, 1961.

236. Pena CE, Miller F, Budzilovich GN, Feigin I: Arthrogryposis multiplex congenita: Report of two cases of radicular type with familial incidence, *Neurology* 18:920-930, 1968.

237. Carpenter S, Karpati G, Rothman S: Pathological involvement of primary sensory neurons in Werdnig-Hoffmann disease, *Acta Neuropathol (Berl)* 42:91-97, 1978.

238. Probst A, Ulrich J, Bischoff A, Boltshauser E: Sensory ganglioneuropathy in infantile spinal muscular atrophy: Light and electron microscopic findings in two cases, *Neuropediatrics* 12:215-231, 1981.

239. Swift TR: Commentary: Electrophysiology of progressive spinal muscular atrophy. In Gamstorp I, Sarnat HB, editors: *Progressive Spinal Muscular Atrophies*, New York: 1984, Raven Press.

240. Imai T, Minami R, Nagaoka M, Ishikawa Y, et al: Proximal and distal motor nerve conduction velocities in Werdnig-Hoffman disease, *Pediatr Neurol* 6:82-86, 1990.

241. Chien YY, Nonaka I: Peripheral nerve involvement in Werdnig-Hoffman disease, *Brain Dev* 11:221-229, 1989.

242. Korinthenberg R, Sauer M, Ketelsen UP, Hanemann CO, et al: Congenital axonal neuropathy caused by deletions in the spinal muscular atrophy region, *Ann Neurol* 42:364-368, 1997.

243. Kimura S, Kobayashi T, Sasaki Y, Hara M, et al: Congenital polyneuropathy in Walker-Warburg syndrome, *Neuropediatrics* 23:14-17, 1992.

244. Lieberman JS, Oshtory M, Taylor RG, Dreyfus PM: Perinatal neuropathy as an early manifestation of Krabbe's disease, *Arch Neurol* 37:446-447, 1980.

245. Namiki H: Subacute necrotizing encephalomyelopathy: Case report with special emphasis on associated pathology of peripheral nervous system, *Arch Neurol* 12:98-107, 1965.

246. Robinson F, Solitaire GB, Lamarche JB, Levy LL: Necrotizing encephalomyelopathy of childhood, *Neurology* 17:472-484, 1967.

247. Dunn HG, Dolman CL: Necrotizing encephalomyelopathy: Report of a case with relapsing polyneuropathy and hyperalaninemia and with manifestations resembling Friedreich's ataxia, *Neurology* 19:536-550, 1969.

248. Moosa A: Peripheral neuropathy in Leigh's encephalomyelopathy, *Dev Med Child Neurol* 17:621-624, 1975.

249. Stickler DE, Valenstein E, Neiberger RE, Perkins LA, et al: Peripheral neuropathy in genetic mitochondrial diseases, *Pediatr Neurol* 34:127-131, 2006.

250. Carpenter S, Karpati G, Andermann F, Gold R: Giant axonal neuropathy: A clinically and morphologically distinct neurological disease, *Arch Neurol* 31:312-316, 1974.

251. Koch T, Schultz P, Williams R, Lampert P: Giant axonal neuropathy: A childhood disorder of microfilaments, *Ann Neurol* 1:438-451, 1977.

252. Larbrisseau A, Jasmin G, Hausser C: Generalized giant axonal neuropathy: A case with features of Fazio-Londe disease, *Neuropaediatrie* 10:76-86, 1979.

253. Mizuno Y, Otsuka S, Takano Y: Giant axonal neuropathy: Combined central and peripheral nervous system disease, *Arch Neurol* 36:107-108, 1979.

254. Ouvrier RA: Giant axonal neuropathy: A review, *Brain Dev* 11:207-214, 1989.

255. Kumar K, Barre P, Nigro M, Jones MZ: Giant axonal neuropathy: Clinical, electrophysiologic, and neuropathologic features in two siblings, *J Child Neurol* 5:229-234, 1990.

256. Stollhoff K, Albani M, Goebel HH: Giant axonal neuropathy and leukodystrophy, *Pediatr Neurol* 7:69-71, 1991.

257. Richen P, Tandan R: Giant axonal neuropathy: Progressive clinical and radiologic CNS involvement, *Neurology* 42:2220-2222, 1992.

258. Flanigan KM, Crawford TO, Griffin JW, Goebel HH, et al: Localization of the giant axonal neuropathy gene to chromosome 16q24, *Ann Neurol* 43:143-148, 1998.

259. Brunno C, Bertini E, Federico A, Tonoli E, et al: Clinical and molecular findings in patients with giant axonal neuropathy (GAN), *Neurology* 62:13-16, 2004.

260. Gordon N: Giant axonal neuropathy, *Dev Med Child Neurol* 46:717-719, 2004.

261. Kinney RB, Gottfried MR, Hodson AK, Autillo-Gambetti L, et al: Congenital giant axonal neuropathy, *Arch Pathol Lab Med* 109:639-641, 1985.

262. Maia M, Pires MM, Guimaraes A: Giant axonal disease: Report of three cases and review of the literature, *Neuropediatrics* 19:10-15, 1988.

263. Pena SD: Giant axonal neuropathy: Intermediate filament aggregates in cultured skin fibroblasts, *Neurology* 31:1470-1473, 1981.

264. Pena SD: Giant axonal neuropathy: An inborn error of organization of intermediate filaments, *Muscle Nerve* 5:166-172, 1982.

265. Dyck PJ, Ohta M: Neuronal atrophy and degeneration predominantly affecting peripheral sensory neurons. In Dyck PJ, editor: *Peripheral Neuropathy II*, Philadelphia: 1975, Saunders.

266. Dyck PJ, Mellinger JF, Reagan TJ: Not "indifference to pain" but varieties of hereditary sensory and autonomic neuropathy, *Brain* 106:373-390, 1983.

267. Ferriere G, Guzzetta F, Kulakowski S, Evrard P: Nonprogressive type II hereditary sensory autonomic neuropathy: A homogeneous clinicopathologic entity, *J Child Neurol* 7:364-370, 1992.

268. Murray TJ: Congenital sensory neuropathy, *Brain* 90:387-394, 1973.

269. Barry JE, Hopkins IJ, Neal BW: Congenital sensory neuropathy, *Arch Dis Child* 49:128-132, 1974.

270. Axelrod FB, Pearson J: Congenital sensory neuropathies, *Am J Dis Child* 138:947-954, 1984.

271. Suarez GA: Autonomic neuropathies. In Jones HR Jr, DeVivo DC, Darras BT, editors: *Neuromuscular Disorders of Infancy, Childhood, and Adolescence: A Clinician's Approach*, Philadelphia: 2003, Butterworth Heinemann.

272. Axelrod FB, Cash R, Pearson J: Congenital autonomic dysfunction with universal pain loss, *J Pediatr* 103:60-64, 1983.

273. Hansen A, Guerina N: Central apnea in a child with congenital autonomic dysfunction and universal pain loss, *J Child Neurol* 11:162-164, 1996.

274. Axelrod FB, Pearson J, Tepperberg J, Ackerman BD: Congenital sensory neuropathy with skeletal dysplasia, *J Pediatr* 102:727-730, 1983.

275. Swanson AG, Buchan GC, Alvord ED Jr: Absence of Lissauer's tract and small dorsal root axons in familial, congenital, universal insensitivity to pain, *Trans Am Neurol Assoc* 88:99-103, 1963.

276. Pinsky L, DiGeorge AM: Congenital familial sensory neuropathy with anhidrosis, *J Pediatr* 68:1-13, 1966.

277. Rafel E, Alberca R, Bautista J: Congenital insensitivity to pain with anhidrosis, *Muscle Nerve* 3:216-220, 1980.

278. Itoh Y, Yagishita S, Nakajima S, Nakano T: Congenital insensitivity to pain with anhidrosis: Morphological and morphometrical studies on the skin and peripheral nerves, *Neuropediatrics* 17:103-110, 1986.
279. Rosemberg S, Marie SK, Kliemann S: Congenital insensitivity to pain with anhidrosis (hereditary sensory and autonomic neuropathy type IV), *Pediatr Neurol* 11:50-56, 1994.
280. Tachi N, Ohya K, Nihira H, Minagawa K: Muscle involvement in congenital insensitivity to pain with anhidrosis, *Pediatr Neurol* 12:264-266, 1995.
281. Ismail EAR, Al-Shammart N, Anim JT, Moosa A: Congenital insensitivity to pain with anhidrosis: Lack of eccrine sweat gland innervation confirmed, *J Child Neurol* 13:243-246, 1998.
282. Berkovitch M, Copeliovitch L, Tauber T, Vaknin Z, et al: Hereditary insensitivity to pain with anhidrosis, *Pediatr Neurol* 19:227-229, 1998.
283. Toscano E, della Casa R, Mardy S, Gaetaniello L, et al: Multisystem involvement in congenital insensitivity to pain with anhidrosis (CIPA), a nerve growth factor receptor (Trk A)-related disorder, *Neuropediatrics* 31:39-41, 2000.
284. Ohto T, Iwasaki N, Fujiwara J, Ohkoshi N, et al: The evaluation of autonomic nervous function in a patient with hereditary sensory and autonomic neuropathy type IV with novel mutations of the TRKA gene, *Neuropediatrics* 35:274-278, 2004.
285. Barone R, Lempereur L, Anastasi M, Parano E, et al: Congenital insensitivity to pain with anhidrosis (NTRK1 mutation) and early onset renal disease: Clinical report on three sibs with a 25-year follow-up in one of them, *Neuropediatrics* 36:270-273, 2005.
286. Pavone L, Huttenlocher P, Siciliano L, Micali G, et al: Two brothers with a variant of hereditary sensory neuropathy, *Neuropediatrics* 23:92-95, 1992.
287. Axelrod FB, Chelimsky GG, Weese-Mayer DE: Pediatric autonomic disorders, *Pediatrics* 118:309-321, 2006.
288. Perlman M, Benady S, Saggi E: Neonatal diagnosis of familial dysautonomia, *Pediatrics* 63:238-241, 1979.
289. Pearson J: Familial dysautonomia: A brief review, *J Autonom Nerv Syst* 1:119-126, 1979.
290. Amir N, Chemke J, Shapira Y: Familial dysautonomia manifesting as neonatal nemaline myopathy, *Pediatr Neurol* 1:245-247, 1985.
291. Guzzetta F, Tortorella G, Cardia E, Ferriere G: Familial dysautonomia in a non-Jewish girl, with histological evidence of progression in the sural nerve, *Dev Med Child Neurol* 28:62-76, 1986.
292. Axelrod FB, Porges RF, Sein ME: Neonatal recognition of familial dysautonomia, *J Pediatr* 110:946-948, 1987.
293. Axelrod FB: Familial dysautonomia, *Muscle Nerve* 29:352-363, 2004.
294. Casella EB, Bousso A, Corvello CM, Fruchtengarten LV, et al: Episodic somnolence in an infant with Riley-Day syndrome, *Pediatr Neurol* 32:273-274, 2005.
295. Carroll JE, Jedziniak M, Guggenheim MA: Guillain-Barré syndrome: Another cause of the "floppy infant," *Am J Dis Child* 131:699-700, 1977.
296. Al-Qudah AA, Shahar E, Logan WJ, Murphy EG: Neonatal Guillain-Barré syndrome, *Pediatr Neurol* 4:255-256, 1988.
297. Gilmartin RC, Chien LT: Guillain-Barré syndrome with hydrocephalus in early infancy, *Arch Neurol* 34:567-569, 1977.
298. Luijckx GJ, Vies J, de Baets M, Buchwald B, et al: Guillain-Barré syndrome in mother and newborn child, *Lancet* 349:27, 1997.
299. Jackson AH, Baquis GD, Shah BL: Congenital Guillain-Barré syndrome, *J Child Neurol* 11:407-410, 1996.
300. Buchwald B, de Baets M, Luijckx G-J, Toyka KV: Neonatal Guillain-Barré syndrome: Blocking antibodies transmitted from mother to child, *Neurology* 53:1246-1253, 1999.
301. Attarian S, Azulay JP, Chabrol B, Escande-Beillard N, et al: Neonatal lower motor neuron syndrome associated with maternal neuropathy with anti-GM1 IgG, *Neurology* 63:379-381, 2004.
302. Bamford N, Trojaborg W, Sherbany AA, De Vivo DC: Congenital Guillain-Barré syndrome associated with maternal inflammatory bowel disease is responsive to intravenous immunoglobulin, *Eur J Paediatr Neurol* 6:115-119, 2002.
303. Millichap JG, Dodge PR: Diagnosis and treatment of myasthenia gravis in infancy, childhood, and adolescence, *Neurology* 10:1007, 1960.
304. Seybold ME, Lindstrom JM: Myasthenia gravis in infancy, *Neurology* 31:476-480, 1981.
305. Roach ES, Buono G, McLean WT: Early-onset myasthenia gravis, *J Pediatr* 108:193-197, 1986.
306. Evans OB, Vig V, Parker CC: Prematurity and early-onset juvenile myasthenia gravis, *Pediatr Neurol* 8:51-53, 1992.
307. Strickroot FL, Schaeffer RL, Bergo HL: Myasthenia gravis occurring in an infant born of a myasthenic mother, *JAMA* 120:1207, 1942.
308. Namba T, Brown SB, Grob D: Neonatal myasthenia gravis: Report of two cases and review of the literature, *Pediatrics* 45:488-504, 1970.
309. Papazian O: Transient neonatal myasthenia gravis, *J Child Neurol* 7:135-141, 1992.
310. Batocchi AP, Majolini L, Evoli A, Lino MM, et al: Course and treatment of myasthenia gravis during pregnancy, *Neurology* 52:447-452, 1999.
311. Tellez-Zenteno JF, Hernandez-Ronquillo L, Salinas V, Estanol B, et al: Myasthenia gravis and pregnancy: Clinical implications and neonatal outcome, *BMC Musculoskelet Disord* 5:42, 2004.
312. Podciechowski L, Brocka-Nitecka U, Dabrowska K, Bielak A, et al: Pregnancy complicated by myasthenia gravis: Twelve years experience, *Neuro Endocrinol Lett* 26:603-608, 2005.
313. Hoff JM, Daltveit AK, Gilhus NE: Myasthenia gravis: Consequences for pregnancy, delivery, and the newborn, *Neurology* 61:1362-1366, 2003.
314. Morel E, Eymard B, Vernet-der Garabedian B, Pannier C, et al: Neonatal myasthenia gravis: A new clinical and immunologic appraisal on 30 cases, *Neurology* 38:138-142, 1988.
315. Heckmatt JZ, Placzek M, Thompson AH, Dubowitz V, et al: An unusual case of neonatal myasthenia, *J Child Neurol* 2:63-66, 1987.
316. Vial C, Charles N, Chauplannaz G, Bady B: Myasthenia gravis in childhood and infancy: Usefulness of electrophysiologic studies, *Arch Neurol* 48:847-849, 1991.
317. Hays RM, Michaud LJ: Neonatal myasthenia gravis: Specific advantages of repetitive stimulation over edrophonium testing, *Pediatr Neurol* 4:245-247, 1988.
318. Gardnerova M, Eymard B, Morel E, Faltin M, et al: The fetal/adult acetylcholine receptor antibody ratio in mothers with myasthenia gravis as a marker for transfer of the disease to the newborn, *Neurology* 48:50-54, 1997.
319. Bassan H, Muhlbaur B, Tomer A, Spirer Z: High-dose intravenous immunoglobin in transient neonatal myasthenia gravis, *Pediatr Neurol* 18:181-183, 1998.
320. Andrews PI, Sanders DB: Juvenile myasthenia gravis. In Jones HR Jr, DeVivo DC, Darras BT, editors: *Neuromuscular Disorders of Infancy, Childhood, and Adolescence: A Clinician's Approach*, Philadelphia: 2003, Butterworth Heinemann.
321. Carr SR, Gilchrist JM, Abuelo DN, Clark D: Treatment of antenatal myasthenia gravis, *Obstet Gynecol* 78:485-489, 1991.
322. Moutard-Codou ML, Delleur MM, Doulac O, Morel E, et al: Myasthenie néo-natale sévère avec arthrogrypose, *Presse Med* 16:615-618, 1987.
323. Dulitzky F, Sirota L, Landman J, Homburg R: An infant with multiple deformations born to a myasthenic mother, *Helv Paediatr Acta* 42:173-176, 1987.
324. Shepard MK: Arthrogryposis multiplex congenita in sibs, *Birth Defects Orig Artic Ser* 7:127, 1971.
325. Holmes LB, Driscoll SG, Bradley WG: Contractures in a newborn infant of a mother with myasthenia gravis, *J Pediatr* 96:1067-1069, 1980.
326. Wise GA, McQuillen MP: Transient neonatal myasthenia, *Arch Neurol* 22:556-565, 1970.
327. Koenigsberger MR, Patten B, Lovelace RE: Studies of neuromuscular function in the newborn. I. A comparison of myoneural function in full term and premature infants, *Neuropaediatrie* 4:350-361, 1973.
328. Drachman DB: The biology of myasthenia gravis, *Annu Rev Neurosci* 4:195-225, 1981.
329. Almon RR, Andrew CG, Appel SH: Serum globulin in myasthenia gravis: Inhibition of alpha-bungarotoxin binding to acetylcholine receptors, *Science* 186:55-57, 1974.
330. Toyka KB, Drachman DB, Pestronk A: Myasthenia gravis: Passive transfer from man to mouse, *Science* 190:397, 1975.
331. Appel SH, Anwyl R, McAdams MW, Elias S: Accelerated degradation of acetylcholine receptor from cultured rat myotubes with myasthenia gravis sera and globulins, *Proc Natl Acad Sci U S A* 74:2130-2134, 1977.
332. Heinemann S, Merlie J, Lindstrom J: Modulation of acetylcholine receptors in rat diaphragm by anti-receptors sera, *Nature* 274:65-68, 1978.
333. Reiness CG, Weinberg CB, Hall ZW: Antibody to acetylcholine receptor increases degradation of junctional and extrajunctional receptors in adult muscle, *Nature* 274:68-70, 1978.
334. Lennon VA, Lambert EH: Myasthenia gravis induced by monoclonal antibodies to acetylcholine receptors, *Nature* 285:238-240, 1980.
335. Kao I, Drachman DB: Myasthenic immunoglobulin accelerates acetylcholine receptor degradation, *Science* 196:527-529, 1977.
336. Engel AG, Lambert EA, Howard FM: Immune complexes (IgG and C3) at the motor endplate in myasthenia gravis, *Mayo Clin Proc* 52:267-280, 1977.
337. Keesey J, Lindstrom J, Cokely H: Anti-acetylcholine receptor antibody in neonatal myasthenia gravis, *N Engl J Med* 296:55, 1977.
338. Nakao K, Nishitani H, Suzuki M, Ohta M, et al: Anti-acetylcholine receptor IgG in neonatal myasthenia gravis, *N Engl J Med* 297:169-170, 1977.
339. Donaldson JO, Penn AS, Lisak RP, Abramsky O, et al: Anti-acetylcholine receptor antibody in neonatal myasthenia gravis, *Am J Dis Child* 125:222-226, 1981.
340. Ohta M, Matsubara F, Hayashi K, Nakao K, et al: Acetylcholine receptor antibodies in infants of mothers with myasthenia gravis, *Neurology* 31:1019-1022, 1981.
341. Olanow CW, Lane RJ, Hull KL, Roses AD: Neonatal myasthenia gravis in the infant of an asymptomatic thymectomized mother, *Can J Neurol Sci* 9:85-87, 1982.
342. Lefvert AK, Osterman PO: Newborn infants to myasthenic mothers: A clinical study and an investigation of acetylcholine receptor antibodies in 17 children, *Neurology* 33:133-138, 1983.
343. Donat JF, Donat JR, Lennon VA: Exchange transfusion in neonatal myasthenia gravis, *Neurology* 31:911-912, 1981.
344. Rider LG, Sherry DD, Glass ST: Neonatal lupus erythematosus simulating transient myasthenia gravis at presentation, *J Pediatr* 118:417-419, 1991.

345. Lefvert AK, Bergstrom K, Matell G, Osterman PO, et al: Determination of acetylcholine receptor antibody in myasthenia gravis: Clinical usefulness and pathogenic implications, *J Neurol Neurosurg Psychiatry* 41:394-403, 1978.

346. Elias SB, Butler I, Appel SH: Neonatal myasthenia gravis in the infant of a myasthenic mother in remission, *Ann Neurol* 6:72-75, 1979.

347. Tagber RJ, Baumann R, Desai N: Failure of intravenously administered immunoglobulin in the treatment of neonatal myasthenia gravis, *J Pediatr* 134:233-235, 1999.

348. Engel AG, Ohno K, Milone M, Sine SM: Congenital myasthenic syndromes caused by mutations in acetylcholine receptor genes, *Neurology* 48:S28-S35, 1997.

349. Engel AG, Ohno K, Sine SM: Congenital myasthenic syndromes, *Arch Neurol* 56:163-167, 1999.

350. Ohno K, Engel AG: Congenital myasthenic syndromes, *Eur J Paediatr Neurol* 7:227-228, 2003.

351. Engel AG, Ohno K, Harper CM: Congenital myasthenic syndromes. In Jones HR Jr, DeVivo DC, Darras BT, editors: *Neuromuscular Disorders of Infancy, Childhood, and Adolescence: A Clinician's Approach*, Philadelphia: 2003, Butterworth Heinemann.

352. Engel AG, Ohno K, Sine SM: Congenital myasthenic syndromes: Progress over the past decade, *Muscle Nerve* 27:4-25, 2003.

353. Harper CM: Congenital myasthenic syndromes, *Semin Neurol* 24:111-123, 2004.

354. Cornblath DR: Disorders of neuromuscular transmission in infants and children, *Muscle Nerve* 9:606-611, 1986.

355. Engel AG: Congenital myasthenic syndromes, *J Child Neurol* 3:233-246, 1988.

356. Misulis KE, Fenichel GM: Genetic forms of myasthenia gravis, *Pediatr Neurol* 5:205-210, 1989.

357. Lecky BR, Morgan-Hughes JA, Murray NM, Landon DN, et al: Congenital myasthenia: Further evidence of disease heterogeneity, *Muscle Nerve* 9:233-242, 1986.

358. Vajsar J, Sloane A, MacGregor DL, Ronen GM, et al: Arthrogryposis multiplex congenita due to congenital myasthenic syndrome, *Pediatr Neurol* 12:237-241, 1995.

359. Anlar B, Ozdirim E, Renda Y, Yalaz K, et al: Myasthenia gravis in childhood, *Acta Paediatr* 85:838-842, 1996.

360. Zammarchi E, Donati MA, Masi S, Sarti A, et al: Familial infantile myasthenia: A neuromuscular cause of respiratory failure, *Child Nerv Syst* 10:347-349, 1994.

361. Ohno K, Hutchinson DO, Milone M, Brengman JM, et al: Congenital myasthenic syndrome caused by prolonged acetylcholine receptor channel openings due to a mutation in the M2 domain of the ε subunit, *Proc Natl Acad Sci U S A* 92:758-762, 1995.

362. Sieb JP, Dorfler P, Tzartos S, Wewer UM, et al: Congenital myasthenic syndromes in two kinships with end-plate acetylcholine receptor and u-trophin deficiency, *Neurology* 50:54-61, 1998.

363. Harper CM, Engel AG: Quinidine sulfate therapy for the slow-channel congenital myasthenic syndrome, *Ann Neurol* 43:480-484, 1998.

364. Ohno K, Anlar B, Ozdirim E, Brengman JM, et al: Myasthenic syndromes in Turkish kinships due to mutations in the acetylcholine receptor, *Ann Neurol* 44:234-241, 1998.

365. Shen XM, Ohno K, Fukudome T, Tsujino A, et al: Congenital myasthenic syndrome caused by low-expressor fast-channel AChR delta subunit mutation, *Neurology* 59:1881-1888, 2002.

366. Zafeiriou DI, Pitt M, de Sousa C: Clinical and neurophysiological characteristics of congenital myasthenic syndromes presenting in early infancy, *Brain Dev* 26:47-52, 2004.

367. Gurnett CA, Bodnar JA, Neil J, Connolly AM: Congenital myasthenic syndrome: Presentation, electrodiagnosis, and muscle biopsy, *J Child Neurol* 19:175-182, 2004.

368. Webster R, Brydson M, Croxen R, Newsom-Davis J, et al: Mutation in the AChR ion channel gate underlies a fast channel congenital myasthenic syndrome, *Neurology* 62:1090-1096, 2004.

369. Barisic N, Muller JS, Paucic-Kirincic E, Gazdik M, et al: Clinical variability of CMS-EA (congenital myasthenic syndrome with episodic apnea) due to identical CHAT mutations in two infants, *Eur J Paediatr Neurol* 9:7-12, 2005.

370. Burke G, Cossins J, Maxwell S, Robb S, et al: Distinct phenotypes of congenital acetylcholine receptor deficiency, *Neuromuscul Disord* 14:356-364, 2004.

371. Bowman JR: Myasthenia gravis in young children, *Pediatrics* 1:472, 1948.

372. Fenichel GM: Clinical syndromes of myasthenia in infancy and childhood, *Arch Neurol* 35:97-103, 1978.

373. Simpson JF, Westerberg MR, Magee KR: Myasthenia gravis: An analysis of 295 cases, *Acta Neurol Scand Suppl* 42:1-27, 1966.

374. Barisic N, Schmidt C, Sidorova OP, Herczegfalvi A, et al: Congenital myasthenic syndrome (CMS) in three European kinships due to a novel splice mutation (IVS7-2A/G) in the epsilon acetylcholine receptor (AChR) subunit gene, *Neuropediatrics* 33:249-254, 2002.

375. Sieb JP, Kraner MS, Schrank B, Reitter B, et al: Severe congenital myasthenic syndrome due to homozygosity of the 1293insG epsilon-acetylcholine receptor subunit mutation, *Ann Neurol* 48:379-383, 2000.

376. Burke G, Cossins J, Maxwell S, Owens G, et al: Rapsyn mutations in hereditary myasthenia: Distinct early- and late-onset phenotypes, *Neurology* 61:826-828, 2003.

377. Ioos C, Barois A, Richard P, Eymard B, et al: Congenital myasthenic syndrome due to rapsyn deficiency: Three cases with arthrogryposis and bulbar symptoms, *Neuropediatrics* 35:246-249, 2004.

378. Muller JS, Baumeister SK, Rasic VM, Krause S, et al: Impaired receptor clustering in congenital myasthenic syndrome with novel *RAPSN* mutations, *Neurology* 67:1159-1164, 2006.

379. Namba T, Brunner NG, Brown SB, Muguruma M, et al: Familial myasthenia gravis: Report of 27 patients in 12 families and review of 164 patients in 73 families, *Arch Neurol* 25:49-60, 1971.

380. Engel AG: Myasthenia gravis and myasthenic syndromes, *Ann Neurol* 16:519-534, 1984.

381. Vincent A, Cull-Candy SG, Newsom-Davis J, Trautmann A, et al: Congenital myasthenia: Endplate acetylcholine receptors and electrophysiology in five cases, *Muscle Nerve* 4:306-318, 1981.

382. Nichols P, Croxen R, Vincent A, Rutter R, et al: Mutation of the acetylcholine receptor ε-subunit promotor in congenital myasthenic syndrome, *Ann Neurol* 45:439-443, 1999.

383. Ohno K, Anlar B, Engel AG: Congenital myasthenic syndrome caused by a mutation in the Ets-binding site of the promoter region of the acetylcholine receptor epsilon subunit gene, *Neuromuscul Disord* 9:131-135, 1999.

384. Triggs WJ, Beric A, Butler IJ, Roongta SM: A congenital myasthenic syndrome refractory to acetylcholinesterase inhibitors, *Muscle Nerve* 15:267-272, 1992.

385. Palace J, Wiles CM, Newsom-Davis J: 3,4-Diaminopyridine in the treatment of congenital (hereditary) myasthenia, *J Neurol Neurosurg Psychiatry* 54:1069-1072, 1991.

386. Greer M, Schotland M: Myasthenia gravis in the newborn, *Pediatrics* 26:101-108, 1960.

387. Conomy JP, Levinsohn M, Fanaroff A: Familial infantile myasthenia gravis: A cause of sudden death in young children, *J Pediatr* 87:428-430, 1975.

388. Robertson WC, Chun RW, Kornguth SE: Familial infantile myasthenia, *Arch Neurol* 37:117-119, 1980.

389. Albers JW, Faulkner JA, Dorovini-Zis K, Barald KF, et al: Abnormal neuromuscular transmission in an infantile myasthenic syndrome, *Ann Neurol* 16:28-34, 1984.

390. Gieron MA, Korthals JK: Familial infantile myasthenia gravis: Report of three cases with follow-up until adult life, *Arch Neurol* 42:143-144, 1985.

391. Matthes JW, Kenna AP, Fawcett PRW: Familial infantile myasthenia: A diagnostic problem, *Dev Med Child Neurol* 33:912-929, 1991.

392. Mora M, Lambert E, Engel AG: Synaptic vesicle abnormality in familial infantile myasthenia, *Neurology* 37:206-214, 1987.

393. Lipsitz PJ: The clinical and biochemical effects of excess magnesium in the newborn, *Pediatrics* 47:501-509, 1971.

394. Lipsitz PJ, English IC: Hypermagnesemia in the newborn infant, *Pediatrics* 40:856-862, 1967.

395. Sokal MM, Koenigsberger MR, Rose JS, Berdon WE, et al: Neonatal hypermagnesemia and the meconium-plug syndrome, *N Engl J Med* 286:823-825, 1972.

396. Gutierrez AR, Bodensteiner J, Gutmann L: Electrodiagnosis of infantile botulism, *J Child Neurol* 9:362-366, 1994.

397. Brady JP, Williams HC: Magnesium intoxication in a premature infant, *Pediatrics* 40:100-103, 1967.

398. Percy AK, Saef EC: An unusual complication of retrograde pyelography: Neuromuscular blockade, *Pediatrics* 39:603-606, 1967.

399. McQuillen MP, Cantor HE, O'Rourke JF: Myasthenic syndrome associated with antibiotics, *Arch Neurol* 18:402-415, 1968.

400. Wright EA, McQuillen MP: Antibiotic-induced neuromuscular blockade, *Ann N Y Acad Sci* 183:358-368, 1971.

401. Jones WP: Calcium treatment for ineffective respiration resulting from administration of neomycin, *JAMA* 170:943-944, 1959.

402. Hokkanen E: The aggravating effect of some antibiotics on the neuromuscular blockade in myasthenia gravis, *Acta Neurol Scand* 40:346-352, 1964.

403. Pickett J, Berg B, Chaplin E, Brunstetter-Shafer M: Syndrome of botulism in infancy: Clinical and electrophysiologic study, *N Engl J Med* 295:770-772, 1976.

404. Grover WD, Peckman GJ, Berman PH: Recovery following cranial nerve dysfunction and muscle weakness in infancy, *Dev Med Child Neurol* 16:163-171, 1974.

405. Arnon SS: Infant botulism, *Annu Rev Med* 31:541-560, 1980.

406. Arnon SS, Damus K, Chin J: Infant botulism: Epidemiology and relation to sudden infant death syndrome, *Epidemiol Rev* 3:45-66, 1981.

407. Arnon SS, Chin J: Infant botulism. In Wehrle PF, Top F, editors: *Communicable and Infectious Diseases*, St. Louis, MO: 1981, Mosby.

408. Arnon SS: Infant botulism: A Pan-Pacific perspective, *Med J Aust* 8:404-405, 1983.

409. Long SS: Epidemiologic study of infant botulism in Pennsylvania: Report of the infant botulism study group, *Pediatrics* 75:928-934, 1985.

410. Long SS, Gajewski JL, Brown LW, Gilligan PH: Clinical, laboratory, and environmental features of infant botulism in southeastern Pennsylvania, *Pediatrics* 75:935-941, 1985.

411. Spika JS, Shaffer N, Hargrett-Bean N: Risk factors for infant botulism in the United States, *Am J Dis Child* 143:828-832, 1989.

412. Schreiner MS, Field E, Ruffy R: Infant botulism: A review of 12 years' experience at the Children's Hospital of Philadelphia: *Pediatrics* 87:159-165, 1991.

413. Graf WD, Hays RM, Astley SJ, Mendelman PM: Electrodiagnosis reliability in the diagnosis of infant botulism, *J Pediatr* 120:747-749, 1992.

414. Hurst DL, Marsh WW: Early severe infantile botulism, *J Pediatr* 122:909-911, 1993.

415. Thilo EH, Townsend SF: Infant botulism at 1 week of age: Report of two cases, *Pediatrics* 92:151-153, 1993.

416. Cochran DP, Appleton RE: Infant botulism: Is it that rare? *Dev Med Child Neurol* 37:274-278, 1995.

417. Sheth RD, Lotz BP, Hecox KE, Waclawik AJ: Infantile botulism: Pitfalls in electrodiagnosis, *J Child Neurol* 14:156-158, 1999.

418. Keet CA, Fox CK, Margeta M, Marco E, et al: Infant botulism, type F, presenting at 54 hours of life, *Pediatr Neurol* 32:193-196, 2005.

419. Fox CK, Keet CA, Strober JB: Recent advances in infant botulism, *Pediatr Neurol* 32:149-154, 2005.

420. Thompson JA, Filloux FM, Van Orman CB, Swoboda K, et al: Infant botulism in the age of botulism immune globulin, *Neurology* 64:2029-2032, 2005.

421. Clay SA, Ramseyer JC, Fishman LS, Sedgwick RP: Acute infantile motor unit disorder, *Arch Neurol* 34:236-243, 1977.

422. Arnon SS, Midura TF, Clay SA, Wood RM, et al: Infant botulism: Epidemiological, clinical and laboratory aspects, *JAMA* 237:1946-1951, 1977.

423. Arnon SS, Damus K, Midura TF, Wood RM, et al: Intestinal infection and toxin production by *Clostridium botulinum* as one cause of sudden infant death syndrome, *Lancet* 1:1273-1277, 1978.

424. Turner HD, Brett EM, Gilbert RJ, Ghosh AC, et al: Infant botulism in England, *Lancet* 1:1277-1278, 1978.

425. Arnon SS, Midura TJ, Damus K, Thompson B, et al: Honey and other environmental risk factors for infant botulism, *J Pediatr* 94:331-336, 1979.

426. Johnson RO, Clay SA, Arnon SS: Diagnosis and management of infant botulism, *Am J Dis Child* 133:586-593, 1979.

427. Cornblath DR, Sladky JT, Sumner AJ: Clinical electrophysiology of infantile botulism, *Muscle Nerve* 6:448, 1983.

428. Arnon SS, Schechter R, Maslanka SE, Jewell NP, et al: Human botulism immune globulin for the treatment of infant botulism, *N Engl J Med* 354:462-471, 2006.

428a. Arnon SS: Creation and development of the public service orphan drug human botulism immune globulin, *Pediatrics* 119:785-789, 2007.

429. Glauser TA, Maguire HC, Sladky JT: Relapse of infant botulism, *Ann Neurol* 28:187-189, 1990.

430. Ravid S, Maytal J, Eviatar L: Biphasic course of infant botulism, *Pediatr Neurol* 23:338-340, 2000.

431. Peterson DR, Eklund MW, Chinn NM: The sudden infant death syndrome and infant botulism, *Rev Infect Dis* 1:630-636, 1979.

432. Sonnabend O, Sonnabend W: Different types of *Clostridium botulinum* (A, D and G) found at autopsy in humans. II. Pathological and epidemiological findings in 12 sudden and unexpected deaths. In Lewis GE, editor: *Biomedical Aspects of Botulism: Proceedings of an International Conference*, New York: 1981, Academic Press.

433. Brown LW: Infant botulism, *Adv Pediatr* 28:141-157, 1981.

434. Gurwith MJ, Langston C, Citron DM: Toxin-producing bacteria in infants: Lack of association with sudden infant death syndrome, *Am J Dis Child* 135:1104-1106, 1981.

435. Engel WK: Brief, small, abundant motor unit action potentials: A further critique of electromyographic interpretation, *Neurology* 25:173-176, 1975.

436. Ambache N: The peripheral action of Clostridium botulinum toxin, *J Physiol* 108:127-141, 1949.

437. Brooks VB: The action of botulinum toxin on motor-nerve filaments, *J Physiol* 134:264-277, 1956.

438. Thesleff S: Neurophysiologic aspects of botulism poisoning. In Lewis GE, editor: *Biomedical Aspects of Botulism: Proceedings of an International Conference*, New York: 1981, Academic Press.

439. Montecucco C: How do tetanus and botulinum toxins bind to neuronal membranes? *Trends Biochem Sci* 11:314-317, 1986.

440. Dressler D, Saberi FA: Botulinum toxin: Mechanisms of action, *Eur Neurol* 53:3-9, 2005.

441. L'Hommedieu C, Stough R, Brown L, Kettrick R, et al: Potentiation of neuromuscular weakness in infant botulism by aminoglycosides, *J Pediatr* 95:1065-1070, 1979.

Chapter 19

Neuromuscular Disorders: Muscle Involvement and Restricted Disorders

Muscle, the final component of the motor system, is the site of abnormalities with those essential clinical manifestations of hypotonia and weakness that unify the other disorders of the motor system (see Chapter 18). In this chapter, I deal with important myopathic disorders in the neonatal patient. In addition, certain restricted disorders of the motor system are reviewed.

LEVEL OF THE MUSCLE

Disorders of muscle account for a substantial proportion of infants affected with hypotonia and weakness. Although a relatively large number of myopathic disorders may cause manifestations in the neonatal period, only a few disorders account for most of the cases observed. Myotonic dystrophy is the most frequent (see subsequent sections). However, more of the myopathic disorders can be detected in the neonatal period if the physician's index of suspicion is appropriately high. Detection is valuable for purposes of genetic counseling, determination of prognosis, and institution of therapy.

The major myopathic disorders of interest in newborns may be categorized into two broad groups: those in which the histology, although sometimes impressive, is not distinctive enough to be diagnostic, and those in which the histology is distinctive enough to be diagnostic (with some qualifications) (Table 19-1). In the following discussions, major emphasis is placed on the most common disorders.

Myopathic Disorders with Nondiagnostic Histology

Several disorders are characterized by neonatal hypotonia and weakness and by muscle histological findings that are sometimes impressive, although not distinctive enough to be diagnostic. This category includes the most frequently encountered examples of myopathic disease with clinical manifestations evident in the neonatal period. Myotonic dystrophy is the most common of all, although congenital muscular dystrophy (CMD) is not rare (see Table 19-1). Facioscapulohumeral dystrophy (FSHD) rarely manifests in the neonatal period but is important to recognize. Polymyositis is a rare but treatable muscle disorder in the newborn. Congenital myopathy with minimal or no change as determined by current laboratory investigation (i.e., minimal change myopathy) represents a shrinking group as diagnostic techniques improve.

Congenital Myotonic Dystrophy

Congenital myotonic dystrophy is an inherited disorder of muscle that exhibits numerous distinctive differences from myotonic dystrophy of adult patients. The disorder may be associated with muscle weakness so severe that death results in the newborn period. The hallmark of congenital myotonic dystrophy is hypotonia, rather than myotonia, as observed in adult patients. The congenital form of myotonic dystrophy was first described clearly by Vanier in 1960.[1]

Clinical Features. The disorder is usually apparent in the first hours and days of life. Certain characteristics of the pregnancy often precede the neonatal disorder (Table 19-2) and tend to be prominent in the most severely affected cases. Thus, spontaneous abortion or premature birth occurs in the most severely affected infants.[2-7] Polyhydramnios is a common characteristic of the pregnancy (see Table 19-2). Indeed, this sign is almost invariable in the most severely affected infants and is thought to be caused by the disturbance in swallowing.[3,8-12] Polyhydramnios in a mother with myotonic dystrophy is a fairly reliable indicator of serious involvement of the fetus. Abnormalities of labor, which may be either prolonged or abbreviated, have been attributed to maternal uterine muscle involvement.[2,9]

The *clinical features in the neonatal* period are usually marked and characteristic (see Table 19-2).[1,3-5,8,12-26] In the well-established case, the most striking clinical features are facial diplegia, respiratory and feeding difficulties, arthrogryposis (especially of the lower extremities), and hypotonia. The facial diplegia imparts the characteristic tent-shaped appearance to the upper lip (Fig. 19-1). The respiratory difficulties relate to weakness of respiratory muscles, impaired swallowing and handling of secretions, and occasionally diaphragmatic disturbance (Fig. 19-2). At least 80% of patients require mechanical ventilation. The respiratory impairment may be so severe that the newborn infant fails to establish adequate ventilation and suffers an asphyxial episode that so dominates the clinical syndrome that the myopathic origin of the respiratory failure is overlooked. The feeding difficulties involve both sucking and swallowing and are related particularly to weakness

TABLE 19-1	Hypotonia and Weakness: Level of the Muscle

Histology Not Diagnostic
Congenital myotonic dystrophy
Congenital muscular dystrophy
Facioscapulohumeral dystrophy
Polymyositis
Minimal change myopathy

Histology Diagnostic
Central core disease
Nemaline (rod body) myopathy
Myotubular (centronuclear) myopathy
Congenital fiber type disproportion
Multi-minicore disease
Mitochondrial myopathies
  Cytochrome c oxidase deficiency
  Mitochondrial DNA depletion
Metabolic myopathies
  Glycogen disorders
  Lipid disorders

TABLE 19-2	Clinical Features of Congenital Myotonic Dystrophy

Clinical Feature	Cases Exhibiting Feature*
Reduced fetal movements	68%
Polyhydramnios	80%
Premature birth (< 36 wk)	52%
Facial diplegia	100%
Feeding difficulties	92%
Hypotonia	100%
Atrophy	100%
Hyporeflexia or areflexia	87%
Respiratory distress	88%
Arthrogryposis	82%
Edema	54%
Elevated right hemidiaphragm	49%
Transmission by mother	100%[†]
Neonatal mortality	41%
Mental retardation in survivors	100%

*See text for references.
†Paternal transmission has been documented, albeit very rarely.

of the facial, masticatory, and pharyngeal musculature. (A role for myotonia of pharyngeal muscles is possible.[11]) A disturbance of gastric motility, a manifestation of the smooth muscle involvement in this disorder, may contribute in a major way to the feeding difficulties in some infants.[27] Arthrogryposis (Fig. 19-3) is almost invariable and usually involves at least the ankles. Indeed, in one large series of arthrogryposis multiplex congenita, 50% of the patients with cases related to muscle disease had congenital myotonic dystrophy.[28] Hypotonia also is essentially invariable, accompanied by weakness and, in approximately 90% of the cases, by areflexia or marked hyporeflexia. Atrophy is usually obvious, especially after the first days of life, when edema, which is often excessive in these infants, subsides.[3] Clinical myotonia, elicited by percussion of such muscles as the deltoid, has been detected as early as 3 hours of age,[14] but it usually is not readily elicited until much later in infancy.

Less severely affected infants may go undetected in the newborn period. Facial weakness and hypotonia are the two most common manifestations in such patients.

The *clinical course* relates clearly to the severity of the disease. Neonatal mortality is generally approximately 15% to 20%, but it is as high as approximately 40% in severely affected patients. Feeding difficulties, which initially may require institution of tube feedings, usually improve, at least in reported survivors.[4,5,8,11,12,25,26] However, approximately 20% of infants surviving to adolescence and young adulthood have major gastrointestinal symptoms (e.g., diarrhea and abdominal pain), presumably reflecting smooth muscle involvement.[2,17,29] Moreover, the persistence of some degree of pharyngeal and palatal weakness leads to recurrent otitis media in approximately 25%, occasionally with accompanying hearing loss.[17] Like the neonatal feeding difficulties, the respiratory difficulties subside over the ensuing weeks. However, approximately one third of

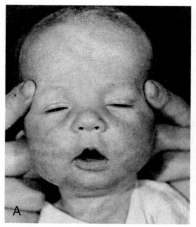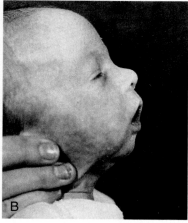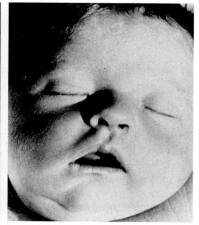

Figure 19-1   Congenital myotonic dystrophy: facial appearance in the neonatal period. A, Note the bilateral ptosis and facial diplegia with tent-shaped appearance of upper lip. **B,** Note retrognathia caused by muscle weakness but often mistakenly attributed to a structural anomaly. **C,** Another affected infant; note the facial diplegia, tented upper lip, and retrognathia. *(A and B, From Dodge PR, Gamstorp I, Byers RK, Russell P: Myotonic dystrophy in infancy and childhood,* Pediatrics *35:3–19, 1965; C, from Swift TR, Ignacio OJ, Dyken PR: Neonatal dystrophia myotonica,* Am J Dis Child *129:734-737, 1975.)*

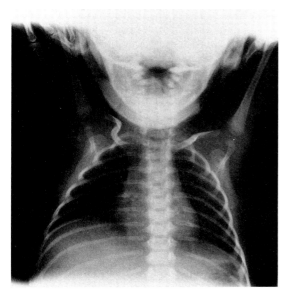

Figure 19-2 Congenital myotonic dystrophy: diaphragmatic involvement. This radiograph of the chest is from a newborn with congenital myotonic dystrophy. The right hemidiaphragm is elevated and paralyzed. Note also the thin ribs, characteristic of severe congenital neuromuscular disease. *(From Sarnat HB: Neuromuscular disorders in the neonatal period. In Korobkin R, Guilleminault C, editors: Advances in Perinatal Neurology, vol 1, New York: 1978, Spectrum Publications.)*

patients require mechanical ventilation for longer than 30 days.[26] Even after cessation of mechanical ventilation, ventilatory reserve may be compromised in severely affected infants, and death secondary to respiratory complications in association with anesthesia or aspiration may occur later in infancy.[5,17,26] Unlike the general improvement in neonatal feeding and in respiratory difficulties, facial diplegia usually becomes more obvious as "baby fat" disappears; ptosis often becomes apparent as well. Muscle weakness, which initially is generalized or more marked proximally, begins to assume the *distal* preponderance characteristic of the adult disease. Clinical myotonia becomes elicitable later in infancy (Fig. 19-4) and is present in the majority of patients after the age of 5 years.[15] Cardiac muscle involvement, manifested by electrocardiographic

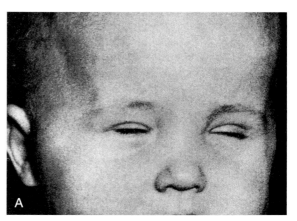
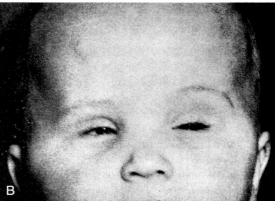

Figure 19-4 Clinical myotonia in an 11-month-old infant. A, Blinking was precipitated by a bright flash of light. **B,** This photograph was taken approximately 15 seconds later. Note the persisting partial closure of the eyelids caused by myotonia of the orbicularis oculi muscles and also the temporal hollowing, suggesting atrophy. *(From Dodge PR, Gamstorp I, Byers RK, Russell P: Myotonic dystrophy in infancy and childhood, Pediatrics 35:3-19, 1965.)*

abnormalities, also becomes more prominent later in infancy. However, in very severely affected newborns, cardiomyopathy may be apparent in the newborn period and may contribute to neonatal demise.[30,31] (Cataracts, baldness, gonadal atrophy, and marked facial atrophy develop later in adult life.)

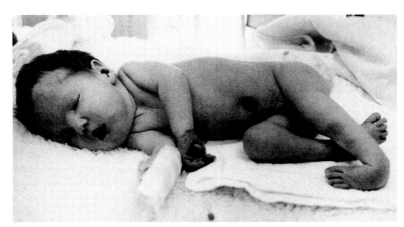

Figure 19-3 Congenital myotonic dystrophy: arthrogryposis. This affected newborn exhibits contractures at the hips, knees, and ankles. Note also the facial diplegia with a tented upper lip. *(From Sarnat HB, O'Connor T, Byrne PA: Clinical effects of myotonic dystrophy on pregnancy and the neonate, Arch Neurol 33:459-465, 1976.)*

Impairment of motor and intellectual development is apparent in the first weeks of life (see Table 19-2). Mental retardation is essentially invariable in infants with congenital myotonic dystrophy who survive the neonatal period.[4,5,12,32] Intelligence quotient (IQ) scores in the 50 to 65 range have been generally observed. The disturbance of intellectual development is nonprogressive. The only available data on relatively long-term follow-up (i.e., ≈10 to 30 years) indicated that only 2 of 42 patients managed "normal education," and only one was "gainfully employed."[17] Some improvement in motor function occurs in late infancy and childhood.[26]

Transmission of myotonic dystrophy in patients with the neonatal form of the disease is essentially *always through the mother* (see Table 19-2). Only approximately seven cases of congenital myotonic dystrophy transmitted through an affected father have been reported.[33-38] At any rate, it is critical for the physician to be cognizant of the disorder as it appears in adults. Indeed, it is common for the mother with an affected infant to be unaware that she has the disease.[3-5,25,39] Most helpful in recognition of the disease in the mother is the typical facies of myotonic dystrophy (Fig. 19-5), characterized by atrophy of the masseter and temporalis muscles, ptosis, and a straight, stiff smile. Myotonia is prominent and readily elicited. Thus, active myotonia is seen in the affected woman when she closes her eyes tightly and then is unable to open them fully for several seconds or more, or when she clenches her fist tightly and then cannot extend her fingers immediately on command. Passive myotonia is demonstrable by percussion of such muscles as the deltoid, thenar eminence, and tongue, and by observation of the prolonged dimpling caused by sustained muscle contraction. Other characteristics (e.g., cataracts, disturbance of intellect, and cardiac abnormality) may also be present. The essential point is that the physician should examine the mother when this diagnosis is considered in a newborn.

Laboratory Studies. Serum creatine kinase (CK) level, cerebrospinal fluid (CSF) protein concentration, and nerve conduction velocities are normal. Slender ribs are observed commonly on chest radiographs (see Fig. 19-2) and may suggest the diagnosis in an infant thought initially to have primary asphyxia.[40,41] This finding can be observed with other congenital myopathic disorders, as well as with Werdnig-Hoffmann disease.[41]

The diagnosis is supported particularly by demonstrating myotonic discharges on the electromyogram (EMG). These discharges are difficult to elicit in the neonatal period, although they have been observed as early as 5 days of age.[14,39] Electrical myotonia is elicited by movement of the recording needle or by direct percussion of the recorded muscle; this procedure results in repetitive electrical potentials of up to 100/second that wax and wane in frequency and amplitude (Fig. 19-6).[4,14,25] These potentials produce the characteristic "dive bomber" sound. Later in infancy, particularly after the age of 2 to 3 years, myotonia is elicited more easily, and small-amplitude, short-duration, and polyphasic potentials, typical of myopathic disease, also can be demonstrated.[16] Fibrillation potentials also may be observed.[25]

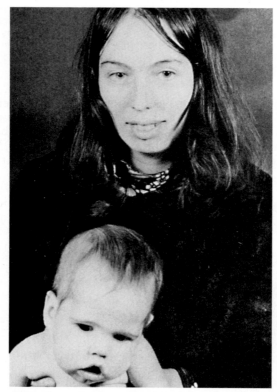

Figure 19-5 **Congenital myotonic dystrophy: infant and mother.** The mother exhibits the typical facial features of myotonic dystrophy, as described in the text. Note also in the affected infant the facial diparesis with a tent-shaped upper lip. *(From Dubowitz V: Muscle Disorders in Childhood, Philadelphia: 1978, Saunders.)*

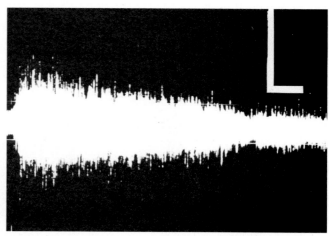

Figure 19-6 **Electromyogram from an infant with congenital myotonic dystrophy at 5 days of age.** The movement of the needle produces a burst of electrical discharges that then subside over several seconds. Calibration: 200 μV, 1 second. *(From Swift TR, Ignacio OJ, Dyken PR: Neonatal dystrophia myotonica, Am J Dis Child 129:734-737, 1975.)*

Ventricular dilation has been observed in approximately 80% of newborns studied by ultrasonography, computed tomography (CT), or magnetic resonance imaging (MRI).[4,5,42-44] In one study, macrocephaly was present in approximately 70% of the infants in the presence or absence of ventricular dilation.[43] However, head circumference within the upper one half of the normal range is more common than is overt macrocephaly.[5] The ventricular dilation is nonprogressive and is not accompanied by rapid head growth or signs of increased intracranial pressure. The occasional occurrence of periventricular echodensities on ultrasound scans or hyperintensity on subsequent T2-weighted MRI scans may reflect periventricular leukomalacia occurring in association with neonatal respiratory disturbance.[42-46] However, this white matter change also could reflect an abnormality of myelination. A small corpus callosum was documented in four of seven infants studied by MRI in another study.[44] The possibility of an abnormality in neuronal development was raised by the demonstration by MR spectroscopy of decreased levels of *N*-acetylaspartic acid, a neuronal marker (see Chapter 4), in five infants and children with congenital myotonic dystrophy.[47]

Pathology. *Muscle pathology* in congenital myotonic dystrophy is different from that observed in the adult with the disease and consists particularly of features of immaturity.[4,25,30,48,49] In a detailed postmortem analysis of three infants, Sarnat and Silbert and others[48,50-52] demonstrated particular involvement of limb muscles around arthrogrypotic joints, pharyngeal muscles, and the diaphragm. The features indicative of a disturbance of maturation included small round muscle fibers with large internal nuclei and sparse myofibrils, reminiscent of fetal myotubes (Fig. 19-7). Moreover, differentiation of fibers into distinct histochemical types was incomplete. Similarly, electron microscopy showed dilated transverse tubules that were aligned longitudinally, as in fetal myotubes, as well as poorly formed Z-bands, simple mitochondria, peripheral halo of absent mitochondria, and many satellite cells, which are also features of immature muscle. Investigators have suggested that these changes principally represent an arrest in fetal muscle maturation.[48,51] Others have viewed these changes as signs of abnormal development.[30] Pathological findings in pancreas (nesidioblastosis), kidney (persistent renal blastemia), and other organs (cryptorchidism and patent ductus arteriosus) support the concept of a disturbance of maturation.[53]

The *neuropathological substrate* for the intellectual failure is unclear. A study of three adult patients with subnormal IQ scores by Rosman and Rebeiz[54] revealed pachygyria in two and disordered cortical architectonics with neuronal heterotopias in all three. These findings were not observed in a later study of four infants from the same institution.[53] However, another report from a different institution also described cerebral cortical neuronal heterotopias in four infants and neuronal heterotopias in two studied post mortem.[43] Thus, the neuropathological basis for the consistent impairment of intellect currently is not established conclusively. It seems reasonable to postulate that an aberration of maturation, as in muscle and other organs, is present. A study of the organizational aspects of brain development (see Chapter 2) would be of interest.

Pathogenesis and Etiology. The disorder is inherited as an *autosomal dominant* trait, in virtually every case through *the mother*. Additionally, the risk of congenital myotonic dystrophy bears a distinct relationship with the disease in the mother.[55] The earlier the onset and the more severe the maternal disease, the greater is the risk for the severe congenital form of myotonic dystrophy in the child. This phenomenon is consistent with

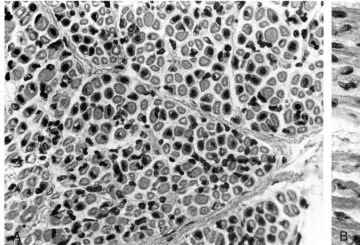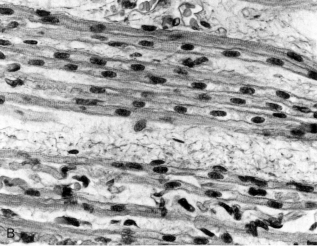

Figure 19-7 Congenital myotonic dystrophy: muscle pathology. These specimens were obtained at autopsy from an affected infant who never established spontaneous respiration and who died at 14 days of age. Many of the histological features are those of immature muscle. **A**, Cross section of rectus abdominis. The muscle fibers are small, round, and loosely arranged, and most contain a single, large internal nucleus or a central pale space (hematoxylin and eosin [H & E] stain, ×400). **B**, Longitudinal section of diaphragm. The large vesicular internal nuclei are aligned in rows within the muscle fibers, with clear vacuolated spaces between them. The sarcomeric striations are poorly distinguished (H & E stain, × 400). *(From Sarnat HB, Silbert SW: Maturational arrest of fetal muscle in neonatal myotonic dystrophy, Arch Neurol 33:466-474, 1976.)*

TABLE 19-3 Molecular Genetics of Congenital Myotonic Dystrophy*

The disease is associated with an abnormally high number of CTG trinucleotide reports in the 3'-untranslated region of the myotonic dystrophy protein kinase gene (MDPK) on chromosome 19q13.3.

The increased number of repeats correlates approximately with earlier onset and more severe disease.

The mutation is "dynamic" (i.e., does not remain of constant size within a pedigree or across generations).

Maternal transmission is associated with expansion (i.e., increased number) of the repeat region and with more severe disease in the infant (i.e., "anticipation").

The extent of repeat expansion varies among tissues (i.e., "somatic mosaicism"); thus, determination of the number of repeats in DNA in blood or chorionic villus cannot predict severity of disease in muscle or other tissues with absolute accuracy.

The function of MDPK is unknown, but the gene likely affects the function of ion channels; multiple biologic effects may relate to sequestration of multiple RNA and DNA binding proteins by the region of multiple repeats.

*See text for references.

anticipation (i.e., the occurrence of progressively earlier onset and more severe disease in successive generations).[55,56]

Molecular genetic studies have provided major insight into the reasons for anticipation and related aspects of congenital myotonic dystrophy (Table 19-3).[4,23-25,55-69] Thus, myotonic dystrophy has been shown to be associated with an increase in the number of specific (CTG) trinucleotide repeats in an unstable DNA region of the 3' untranslated region of the myotonic dystrophy gene, which is located at chromosome 19q13.3. Moreover, the number of repeats increases with maternal transmission of the gene and a correlation of the number of repeats (i.e., the extent of the so-called expansion of the triplet repeat region on chromosome 19) exists with severity and early onset of the disease in the infant. This molecular genetic phenomenon underlies anticipation. Current data suggest that *paternal* transmission of the unstable trinucleotide repeat is associated with reduced amplification or even contraction of the region of repeats, in contrast to the situation with maternal transmission.[36,70] This feature of paternal transmission may be related to negative selection of sperm with large repeat numbers and may explain the exclusively maternal transmission of congenital myotonic dystrophy. At any rate, determination of the number of repeats from a DNA sample of a woman can be used to estimate the likelihood of transmitting severe congenital myotonic dystrophy, and, in an affected infant, such a determination can be used to estimate the likely severity of the disorder. However, correlations are not perfect, in part because of somatic mosaicism (i.e., the extent of repeat expansion varies from tissue to tissue). Somatic mosaicism has been documented in congenital myotonic dystrophy,[30,71] although it is less pronounced than in the adult form of the disease.

The gene affected in myotonic dystrophy *(MDPK)* encodes a protein kinase that appears to result in altered function of sodium, chloride and potassium channels.[24,66,68] Sodium channel defects underlie such later-onset pediatric myotonic syndromes as paramyotonia congenita and hyperkalemic periodic paralysis with myotonia.[24,25] Recent data suggest that MDPK does not lead directly to disturbance of channel function. The features of congenital myotonic dystrophy appear to be related to a toxic RNA gain of function.[69] Thus, the trinucleotide repeats appear to bind and sequester multiple RNA and DNA-binding proteins and thereby to lead to multiple deleterious effects (see Table 19-3).

Management. Management of the affected infant is, in considerable part, an ethical decision. For optimal development, adequate nutrition and ventilation must be ensured, and respiratory support and tube feedings may be needed for days to weeks.[4,12,26] Survivors usually are able to suck and swallow adequately for oral nutrition by 8 to 12 weeks of age.[4,12] When ventilatory support is required for more than 3 to 4 weeks, the mortality rate exceeds 25%.[12,18,26,72] However, the use of nasal continuous positive airway pressure has facilitated weaning in affected infants after such prolonged mechanical ventilation.[73] In infants with particularly poor gastric motility, metoclopramide, which decreases the smooth muscle threshold for the action of acetylcholine, may be especially useful.[27]

Subsequent problems relate to both the muscle and central nervous system (CNS). Supportive measures for the myopathy are required. Most of the joint deformities often can be managed with a nonsurgical approach, although more aggressive management of the foot and ankle deformities may prevent gait disturbances.[17]

Congenital Muscular Dystrophy

The term *congenital muscular dystrophy* (CMD) refers to a group of disorders that share clinical and myopathological features. In older patients, the term *muscular dystrophy* has been used for a group of progressive, inherited disorders of muscle that share a striking myopathology. Although some of the reported cases of CMD do not exhibit definite progression, and a familial nature cannot always be established, the disorder indeed does conform generally to an inherited (autosomal recessive) involvement of muscle, progressing prenatally (and ultimately also postnatally) and sharing a myopathology similar to that of later onset dystrophies.

Classification of CMDs has become particularly difficult, because in the past few years, largely through molecular genetic studies, increasing numbers of clinical phenotypes and responsible genes have been recognized.[74,75] I have elected to use a fundamentally clinical categorization, and I focus on those disorders that may manifest in the neonatal period (Table 19-4). I find it most useful to distinguish those CMD disorders that involve primarily muscle (i.e., without overt CNS abnormalities, e.g., manifested by major neurological deficits) from those CMD disorders that are

TABLE 19-4	Congenital Muscular Dystrophy: Major Neonatal Types	
Disease	**Gene Symbol**	**Protein**
CMD *without* Overt CNS Abnormalities		
Merosin-deficient CMD		
Primary merosin-deficiency	*LAMA2*	Laminin alpha-2 chain
Secondary merosin deficiency	?	?
Merosin-positive CMD		
Classic (pure) CMD	?	?
Ullrich CMD	*COL6A*	Collagen VI
Rigid spine syndrome	*SEPN1*	Selenoprotein N, 1
CMD *with* Overt CNS Abnormalities		
Fukuyama CMD	*FCMD*	Fukutin (protein glycosylation)
Walker-Warburg syndrome	*POMT1*	Protein-*O*-mannosyl-transferase
Muscle-Eye-Brain disease	*POMGnT1*	Protein-*O*-mannosyl-*N*-acetylglucosaminyl-transferase
CMD with *FKRP* mutations	*FKRP*	Fukutin-related protein (protein-glycosylation)

CMD, congenital muscular dystrophy; CNS, central nervous system.

accompanied by overt CNS abnormalities (with such associated deficits as mental retardation; see Table 19-4). I focus on those disorders that are most likely to be associated with a clear neonatal presentation (i.e., primary, merosin-deficient CMD, classic merosin-positive CMD, and the four CMDs with overt CNS abnormalities; see Table 19-4). I describe only briefly those disorders that are particularly unusual or that do not generally result in marked neonatal features (i.e., Ullrich syndrome and rigid spine syndrome).

Congenital Muscular Dystrophy without Overt Central Nervous System Abnormalities. *CMD caused by a primary deficiency of merosin* (i.e., laminin

alpha-2 chain; see later), accounts for approximately 40% to 50% of cases of CMD (see Table 19-4). In 1979, an initial series of five infants with CMD was reported with no clinical sign of CNS disease (except for one with seizures) but with marked hypodensity of cerebral white matter on CT.[76] Over the next decade, subsequent reports of a similar relationship between CMD and abnormal cerebral white matter, primarily on CT scans, were published.[77-88] With the discovery that this disorder is associated with a deficiency of a critical basement membrane component (i.e., the laminin alpha-2 chain), recognition of the relative frequency of this disorder increased dramatically.[74,75,89-108] The disorder differs considerably from "classic" or "pure" merosin-positive CMD, as discussed later (Tables 19-5 and 19-6). The clinical presentation with weakness and hypotonia in merosin-deficient CMD is more severe than in classic or pure merosin–positive CMD. Indeed, motor function usually does not evolve past sitting or standing with orthotic support; ambulation is hardly ever achieved. Contractures are common, although severe neonatal arthrogryposis is rare. Nevertheless, in my experience, merosin-deficient CMD and congenital myotonic dystrophy are the two most common muscle disorders leading to multiple congenital contractures. Facial weakness is often prominent. Disturbance of chewing and swallowing, with a tendency for aspiration, is very

TABLE 19-5	Distinguishing Features: Merosin-Deficient and Merosin-Positive ("Classic") Congenital Muscular Dystrophy*	
Distinguishing Features	**Merosin-Deficient**	**Merosin-Positive**
Clinical severity	Marked	Moderate
Ambulation	Rare	Usual
Creatine kinase elevation	Marked	Mild or None
Myopathology	Severe	Moderate
Nerve conduction velocity	Slow	Normal
White matter abnormality	Marked	None
Cerebral visual evoked and somatosensory evoked responses	Abnormal	Normal
Epilepsy	≈20%	None
Chromosomal locus	6q2	Unknown (likely heterogenous)
Laminin alpha-2 (merosin)	Absent†	Present

*See text for references.
†Partial but not total deficiency of laminin alpha-2 chain is associated with less severe phenotype (see text).

TABLE 19-6	Clinical Features of Congenital Muscular Dystrophy (Merosin-Positive)
Common	
Facial weakness	
Hypotonia	
Axial weakness, neck and trunk	
Limb weakness, proximal > distal	
Contractures	
Nonprogressive or slowly progressive course	
Less Common	
Dysphagia	
Respiratory difficulty	

common. As many as 20% to 30% die of cardiopulmonary complications in the first year or so of life. A less severe phenotype, associated with *partial deficiency of merosin*, has been reported more recently.[96,99,100,107-113]

Despite the uniform occurrence of diffusely abnormal cerebral white matter by brain imaging in merosin-deficient CMD (see later discussion), clinical neurological abnormalities are unusual. Approximately 20% to 30% of patients develop seizure disorders, usually later in childhood, and approximately 5% to 10% of patients exhibit cognitive deficits.

CMD with secondary deficiency of merosin is rare in the neonatal period and likely represents a heterogenous disorder (see Table 19-4). Formerly, the best characterized of this group was CMD related to *FKRP* mutations (see later). However, the more recent recognition that this disorder is associated with overt CNS abnormalities makes it more appropriate to discuss later.

Merosin-positive CMD encompasses multiple clinical phenotypes, but the three most likely to be encountered in the neonatal period are classic (pure) CMD, Ullrich syndrome, and rigid spine syndrome (see Table 19-4). *Classic merosin-positive CMD* is a heterogenous disorder that is shrinking in number as molecular genetic studies characterize distinct disorders. In general, the illness is apparent at birth and usually manifests neonatally as a typical myopathic disorder (see Table 19-6).[4,76,87,91,94,96,97,114-136] The *most common* features are facial weakness, variable in severity, and diffuse hypotonia and weakness. The weakness particularly involves the neck, and defective head control, especially of flexion, is a very consistent feature. Limb weakness often exhibits the pattern typical of muscle disease (i.e., proximal more than distal affection). Contractures often are present at birth, and severe arthrogryposis multiplex congenita has been described, albeit uncommonly.[28,123,137] *Less common* features have included disturbances of swallowing and ventilatory function. Extraocular muscle function is spared.

The *clinical course* in classic CMD has ranged from slow improvement to inexorable progression to death.* However, it is likely that many earlier studies, before molecular testing, included merosin-deficient cases among those with classic CMD. Improvement of function during infancy and early childhood may be greater than would have been predicted from the neonatal clinical (or myopathological) findings (Fig. 19-8). However, in one large study (24 patients) with a long follow-up (most between 8 and 16 years), the disease was reported to be ultimately progressive in all.[122] Thus, of 15 infants who eventually walked independently (mean age, 2.6 years), only 6 remained ambulant.[122] Involvement of the diaphragm and intercostal muscles developed later in infancy and childhood, and approximately one third of these patients ultimately died of respiratory failure. In another large series, 10% of patients died of

respiratory failure between the ages of 3 months and 12 years, 32% developed spine deformities, and all patients older than 20 years exhibited clearly progressive muscle weakness.[128] CNS phenomena (e.g., seizures and impaired intellectual development) are generally absent. Such phenomena would suggest one of the syndromes of CMD with CNS involvement (see later). Indeed, in the series of McMenamin and co-workers[122] of cases of CMD without CNS involvement, intellectual development was normal in all patients. Classic merosin-positive CMD exhibits marked differences from merosin-deficient CMD (see Table 19-5).

Ullrich CMD is a type of merosin-positive CMD with a characteristic clinical phenotype (see Table 19-4).[74,75,140-147a] Neonatal presentation with hypotonia, weakness, proximal joint contractures, torticollis, hip dislocation, spine kyphosis, and marked distal hyperlaxity is characteristic. Subsequent motor development is severely delayed, and walking independently occurs in the minority. The defect involves the gene *(COL6A)* for collagen VI, an extracellular matrix protein. Most neonatal onset cases are autosomal recessive.

Rigid spine syndrome is a third merosin-positive CMD that usually presents clinically after the neonatal period with hypotonia and axial weakness.[74,75] Neonatal onset has been reported. Subsequently, the characteristic spinal extensor contractures become apparent, with resulting spinal rigidity, scoliosis, and restrictive respiratory disease. The defect involves the gene *(SEPN1)* for an endoplasmic reticulum protein, selenoprotein N, the function of which is unknown.

Congenital Muscular Dystrophy with Overt Central Nervous System Abnormalities. CMD may be accompanied by prominent involvement of the CNS, manifested by severe neurological deficits (e.g., mental retardation; see Table 19-4). Although primary merosin deficiency is associated with a morphological disturbance of cerebral white matter (see later), no clinical neurological abnormalities occur in most cases. The four entities in this category are associated with disorders of neuronal migration, cerebral white matter abnormalities, hindbrain anomalies, and marked clinical neurological abnormalities and are termed Fukuyama CMD, Walker-Warburg syndrome, muscle-eye-brain disease, and CMD with *FKRP* mutations (see Table 19-4). Because these disorders are related to abnormalities of glycosylation of alpha-dystroglycan, they are often grouped as *dystroglycanopathies*. (A fifth such CMD disorder, related to a deficit in the *LARGE* gene, another putative glycosyltransferase, was reported in a single case with presentation beyond the neonatal period and is not discussed here).[148]

Fukuyama CMD (see Table 19-4) has been described in several hundred Japanese children and in a much smaller number of children in North America, Europe, and Australia.[74,75,96,123,124,149-165] The disorder exhibits the same basic clinical features referable to muscle involvement as the CMDs without CNS involvement: (1) onset in the neonatal period, (2) marked diffuse weakness and hypotonia, (3) facial weakness, and (4)

---

*See references 4,76,87,94,96,97,116,117,120-124,128,130-134, 138,139.

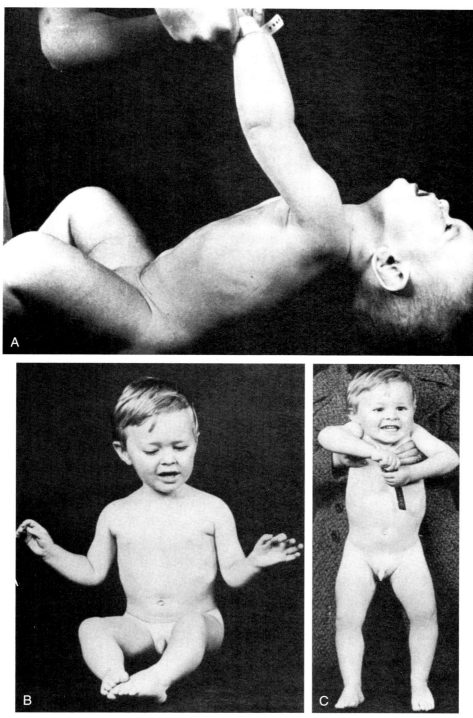

Figure 19-8 Clinical improvement in congenital muscular dystrophy. A, A 9-month-old boy with weakness and hypotonia from birth. Note the marked head lag with pull to sit. The infant cannot sit without support or support his body weight on his legs. **B** and **C,** The same child at 2 years of age. He can sit without support and can bear considerable weight when standing with support. *(From Dubowitz V: Muscle Disorders in Childhood, Philadelphia: 1978, Saunders.)*

joint contractures that develop particularly in infancy after the neonatal period. The *clinical course* of the motor function is characterized generally by slow acqui-sition of skills, usually the ability to crawl or to stand with support, until approximately the age of 8 years, when motor functions begin to deteriorate, ultimately to a lower level. The progression relates both to worsening of contractures and to apparent increasing weakness. Most patients become bedridden by the age of 10 years, and life expectancy is usually approximately 20 years.[96]

The hallmark of Fukuyama CMD is the evidence of major CNS disease. *Mental retardation* is essentially con-stant, and the usual IQ level is between 30 and

50.[74,75,123,149,161,162,165] Moreover, *febrile and afebrile seizures* occur in approximately 60% of the cases. CT and, especially, MRI scanning and neuropathological studies (see subsequent discussions of diagnosis and pathology) establish the causes of these neural phenomena, i.e., major neuronal migrational and other abnormalities.

Walker-Warburg syndrome is the more severe of the two CMDs with prominent ocular as well as CNS abnormalities (see Chapter 2).[74,75,166] Indeed, the life expectancy in this disorder is less than 3 years. In the newborn, the muscle disorder is often overshadowed by the severe CNS (cobblestone lissencephaly, pontocerebellar hypoplasia, severe white matter abnormality) and ocular (microphthalmia, hypoplastic optic nerves, colobomata, retinal detachment) abnormalities. Severe disturbances of feeding and tube or gastrostomy feeding are nearly invariable.

Muscle-eye-brain disease is a similar CMD, with ocular and CNS abnormalities, although it is milder than Walker-Warburg syndrome (see Table 19-4). Thus, an initial report from Finland described 18 affected patients with the clinical features referable to CMD, mental retardation of variable severity in 15 of the 18 reported patients, "occasional" seizures, and, distinctively, a wide variety of ocular abnormalities.[167] These ocular defects included high myopia, congenital or infantile glaucoma, hypoplasia of the retina and optic nerve, coloboma of the optic nerve, and cataracts.[167,168] Many subsequent reports further delineated this type of CMD.[74,75,96,123,166,169-190]

Although patients with muscle-eye-brain disease that is overt at birth may exhibit severe abnormalities, in general the features of this disorder are milder than those observed with Walker-Warburg syndrome, and both these cerebro-ocular types of CMD exhibit differences from Fukuyama CMD (Table 19-7).

The most recently described CMD with overt CNS abnormalities is related to defects in the FKRP gene, which encodes a fukutin-related protein (see Table 19-4). Although this disorder usually manifests beyond the neonatal period and is not considered in detail, neonatal onset is well documented.[74,75,108,191,192,192a] Weakness and hypotonia are apparent in the first weeks or months of life, although a phenotype as severe as primary deficiency of merosin has been observed. Subsequent motor development is markedly impaired, and respiratory muscle weakness leading to ventilatory failure occurs in the first or second decade of life. In neonatal-onset cases, severe cognitive deficits are common. Muscle biopsy shows a partial deficiency of laminin alpha-2 protein, and thus this disorder previously was classified as CMD with secondary deficiency of merosin. However, the principal defect involves fukutin-related protein, presumed to be a phosphosugar transferase, with alpha-dystroglycan the likely substrate. More recently, more than half of 25 reported cases with *FKRP* mutations have had prominent CNS abnormalities and thus should be included with the CMD group shown in Table 19-4 with overt CNS abnormalities.[193,194] The neurological abnormalities have included mental retardation, and the CNS structural deficits have included subependymal heterotopias, focal pachygyria, white matter abnormalities, cerebellar cysts, marked cerebellar dysplasia, and pontine hypoplasia. These CNS deficits are consistent, at least in part, with neuronal migrational disturbance and overlap with those observed in Fukuyama CMD, Walker-Warburg syndrome, and muscle-eye-brain disease. This similarity is noteworthy because, as discussed earlier, the latter three types of CMD with overt CNS abnormalities all also involve disturbances of glycosylation of alpha-dystroglycan. More data will be of great interest.

Laboratory Studies. When all types of CMD (see Table 19-4) are considered, the serum CK level is elevated in most cases, particularly early in the course of the disease. However, the presence and degree of elevation vary with the type of disorder. In the largest series of cases ($n = 50$) of *merosin-positive classic (pure) CMD*, 54% of infants had elevated CK level, and the

TABLE 19-7 Distinguishing Features among Major Syndromes of Congenital Muscular Dystrophy with Overt Central Nervous System Abnormalities

	TYPE OF CMD		
Clinical Feature	**Fukuyama**	**Walker-Warburg**	**Muscle-Eye-Brain**
Neurological deficits	+	+	+
Microcephaly	+	−	−
Macrocephaly	−	+	+
Hypotonia	+	+	+
Ocular abnormalities (severe)	−	+	+
White matter abnormality on neuroimaging (persistent or progressive)	+	+	−
Lissencephaly-pachygyria	+	+	+
Cortical mantle thin	±	+	−
Corpus callosum absent	±	+	−
Hydrocephalus	−	+	±
Encephalocele	−	+*	−
Cerebellar malformation	−	+	±

*Characteristic when present, but described in less than 50% of cases.
+, prominent feature; −, not a prominent feature; ±, variable feature; CMD, congenital muscular dystrophy.

average elevation was approximately three times the upper limit of normal.[128] In another series of 24 cases, CK elevation was 2.5-fold above the normal upper limit.[122] The important clinical point is that a normal CK level does not exclude the diagnosis. By contrast, in *merosin-negative CMD*, the CK levels are consistently and markedly elevated to approximately 10-fold to 20-fold higher than the upper limit of normal.[89-93,95,96,123,138] In Fukuyama CMD, CK levels generally range from 10-fold to 50-fold higher than the normal upper limit. Levels are similarly very high in muscle-eye-brain disease and in Walker-Warburg syndrome. In all cases, CK levels tend to decline with the patient's age. The EMG reveals the changes of myopathy (see Table 17-7), including small-amplitude, brief-duration, and polyphasic motor unit potentials.

CT and MRI scans of the head are useful in identification of the cerebral white matter abnormality characteristic of primary *merosin-deficient CMD* (Fig. 19-9). The appearance on CT is decreased attenuation of cerebral white matter and on MRI is increased signal on T2-weighted images. The cerebral white matter is affected diffusely, and the cerebellar white matter is unaffected. The cerebral white matter abnormality generally is not apparent in the first weeks of life and becomes apparent by approximately 6 months of life (see Fig. 19-9).[74,75,95,195] However, utilization of T2-weighted images with a fast spin-echo sequence has demonstrated the white matter abnormality at 5 days of age.[196] The abnormal white matter signal is most prominent in structures myelinated after birth (e.g., cerebral white matter), rather than in those structures myelinated before birth (e.g., brain stem and cerebellar white matter).[197] Thus, the abnormality may reflect a delay or arrest in myelination, and the finding in the affected white matter of abnormally increased apparent diffusion coefficients, characteristic of immature white matter, is perhaps consistent with this notion.[198] Although the cerebral white matter abnormality is the unifying feature of the primary merosin-negative cases, several reports documented the occurrence of cortical gyral dysplasia, especially in the occipital region, in isolated cases.[105,186,199-203] Hypoplasia of the cerebellum was observed by MRI to varying degrees in 6 of 14 well-studied cases[103] and associated cerebellar cysts have also been described.[204]

In *Fukuyama CMD*, the most striking abnormality is the gyral disturbance (Fig. 19-10). The two major findings detectable by MRI are as follows: (1) a thick cortex with shallow sulci in the frontal regions, consistent with polymicrogyria; and (2) a thick cortex with a smooth surface in the temporo-occipital regions, consistent with lissencephaly-pachygyria.[163] These findings correlate well with the neuropathology (see later discussion). Additional consistent features are white matter changes similar to those described earlier for merosin-deficient CMD. However, distinction of these two entities by MRI is straightforward because of the marked gyral abnormalities in Fukuyama CMD. Moreover, the white matter abnormality in the latter diminishes with age. The corpus

callosum is slightly hypoplastic in most of the Fukuyama cases.[162]

In *Walker-Warburg syndrome and muscle-eye-brain disease*, the dominant finding is the gyral abnormality. In its full form, as in Walker-Warburg syndrome, the appearance of type II lissencephaly ("cobblestone" lissencephaly) and pachygyria is striking and is associated with diffuse white matter abnormality of the type observed in merosin-deficient CMD. Again, the distinction by MRI from the latter disorder is straightforward because of the presence of the gyral disturbance, as well as marked dysgenesis of cerebellum and hypoplasia of the pons, especially in Walker-Warburg syndrome.

Additional laboratory studies of interest include measurements of cerebral visual and somatosensory evoked responses and of peripheral nerve conduction velocities in merosin-deficient CMD (see Table 19-5). Thus, for somatosensory evoked responses, latencies have been delayed in all patients studied, and for visual evoked responses, latencies have been delayed in approximately 90% of patients.[74,75,195,205,206] Nerve conduction velocity studies showed moderately slow values in more than 80% of merosin-deficient cases studied thus far.[195,207,208] One infant studied in the newborn period had normal values but exhibited slowed conduction when studied again at 6 months of age.[195] No abnormalities in cerebral evoked responses or motor nerve conduction velocities have been observed in merosin-positive CMD.

The demonstration of laminin alpha-2 deficiency in skin biopsy and in cultured fibroblasts in primary merosin-deficient cases indicates the potential value of this approach for the diagnosis of merosin-deficient CMD. Additionally, the prenatal demonstration of merosin deficiency in trophoblastic tissue obtained from chorionic villus samples indicates the value of this approach (with simultaneous linkage analysis) in prenatal diagnosis.[209-211]

Pathology. *Muscle biopsy* in all types of CMD shows striking changes, consistent with a dystrophic process.[4,16,123] Notable are marked variation in fiber size in a nongrouped distribution, internal nuclei, and marked replacement of muscle by fat and connective tissue (Fig. 19-11).[4,74,75,94,122-124,138,149,212,213] Necrosis of fibers and evidence of regeneration are common. Striking changes not apparent on initial biopsies may appear on subsequent biopsies. The fiber type pattern is retained (see Fig. 19-11); the muscle does not exhibit the prominent signs of maturational disturbance observed in myotonic dystrophy (see earlier discussion). Although comparisons are difficult, the myopathic changes reported in primary merosin-deficient CMD are more striking than those in merosin-positive CMD.[4,93,94,127,214] Several reports have emphasized the presence of inflammatory cellular infiltrates, especially early in the disease and perhaps related to necrosis[215-217]; this finding should not lead to the mistaken diagnosis of infantile polymyositis, a treatable and self-limited disorder (see later discussion). The diagnostic feature critical for merosin-deficient

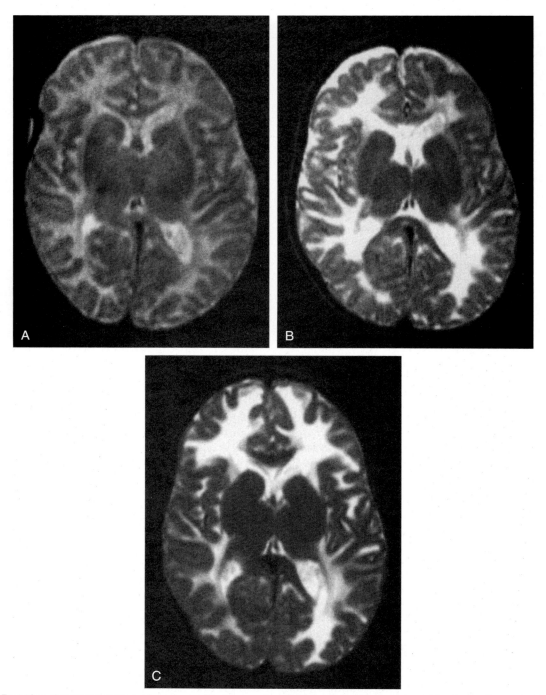

Figure 19-9   **Evolution of cerebral white matter abnormality in merosin-deficient congenital muscular dystrophy, as demonstrated by magnetic resonance imaging (T2-weighted images). A,** At 3 weeks of age, the appearance of cerebral white matter was within normal limits. **B,** At 6 months of age, abnormal signal intensity in cerebral white matter was clearly apparent. **C,** At 12 months of age, the white matter was extremely abnormal. *(From Mercuri E, Pennock J, Goodwin F, Sewry C, et al: Sequential study of central and peripheral nervous system involvement in an infant with merosin-deficient congenital muscular dystrophy,* Neuromuscul Disord *6:425-429, 1996.)*

CMD is the lack of staining for this molecule on immunocytochemical study (Fig. 19-12). Partial absence is observed in the infants with the less severe, partial type of merosin-deficient CMD or in secondary merosin deficiencies.[74,75,97,99,100,109-111]

The *neuropathology* in infants with the *merosin-deficient CMD with cerebral white matter abnormalities* is not clearly known. The little neuropathological information

available is inconclusive.[78,79] The findings that the white matter abnormality becomes most apparent later in infancy and is associated with disturbances of visual and somatosensory evoked potentials and the MRI findings suggesting a defect in postnatal myelin development (see earlier discussions) suggest that myelination is altered in some way. Laminin alpha-2 chain is expressed in the basement membrane of blood

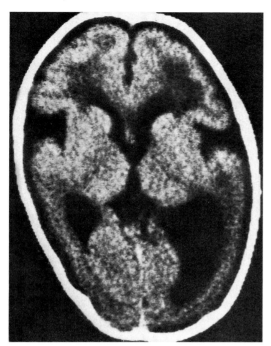

Figure 19-10 Computed tomography scan of a 3-year-old-child with Fukuyama congenital muscular dystrophy. Note the following: the paucity of the cortical gyri, most marked in the temporal, parietal, and occipital lobes; hypodensity of the cerebral white matter, especially in the frontal region; prominent sylvian fissures; and asymmetrical dilation of the occipital horns. *(From McMenamin JB, Becker LE, Murphy EG: Fukuyama-type congenital muscular dystrophy, J Pediatr 101:580-582, 1982.)*

vessels that form the blood-brain barrier and also along developing axonal tracts where interaction with oligodendrocytes may occur.[75] Disturbances at either or both loci could lead to disturbed myelin development and the abnormal signal with increased water diffusion on MRI or the "edema" by MR spectroscopy.[75a]

The *neuropathology* in infants with *Fukuyama CMD* is striking.[123,149,151-154,159,178-180,218-226] The dominant finding is cerebral gyral abnormality, most consistently polymicrogyria (Fig. 19-13A), pachygyria, or agyria (type II lissencephaly). The disorder indicates a disturbance of neuronal migration, as described in Chapter 2. Other neuropathological abnormalities include subpial neuronal-glial heterotopias, cerebellar polymicrogyria (Fig. 19-13B), aberrant myelinated fascicles over the surface of the cerebellum, hypoplasia and aberrant course of the pyramidal tracts, leptomeningeal thickening, and occasional hydrocephalus. No distinct changes have been described in cerebral white matter, except for a delay in myelination, and hence the basis for the white matter abnormality detected by CT or MRI is unclear (see earlier discussion).

The *neuropathology* in *the two CMDs with prominent ocular* and *brain abnormalities* has been described.[74,75,169,170,174,175,178-180,185] The findings bear similarities to those described in Fukuyama CMD, including the following: type II lissencephaly; polymicrogyria, pachygyria, and heterotopias in the basal meninges; hypoplasia of the pyramidal tracts; and aqueductal stenosis. Distinguishing features in the more severe form of cerebro-ocular CMD, Walker-Warburg syndrome, include more severe cortical migrational disturbances, hydrocephalus, cerebellar dysplasia-hypoplasia (including absence of vermis), and encephalocele (see Table 19-7). In general, the findings in muscle-eye-brain disease are milder than in Walker-Warburg syndrome.

Pathogenesis and Etiology. The pathogenesis and etiology of this group of disorders focus on the sarcolemma membrane and the related proteins that link the extracellular matrix to the actin filaments of the myocytic cytoskeleton.[74,75,96,97,227,228] The key

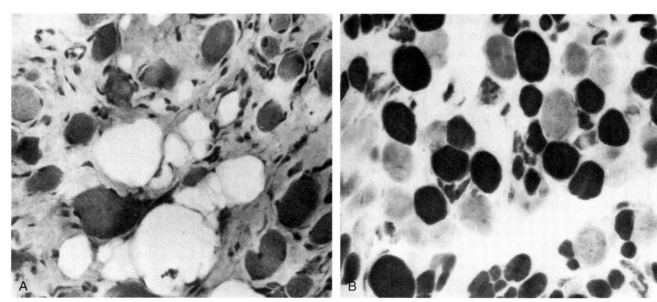

Figure 19-11 Congenital muscular dystrophy: muscle pathology. These biopsy specimens are from the child shown in Figure 19-8. **A,** Note nongrouped changes with marked variation in fiber size and extensive replacement of muscle by connective tissue *(gray areas)* and fat *(clear areas)* (Verhoeff–van Gieson stain, ×250). **B,** Histochemical preparation shows retention of fiber type pattern (adenosine triphopsphatase stain, pH 4.6, ×250). *(From Dubowitz V: Muscle Disorders in Childhood, Philadelphia: 1978, Saunders.)*

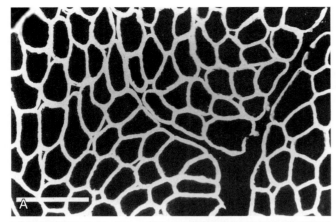

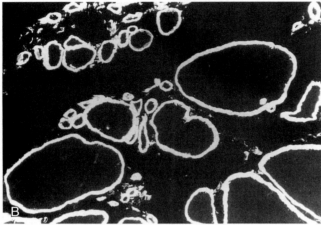

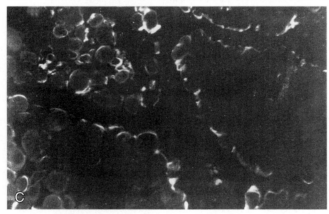

Figure 19-12 **Immunofluorescence analysis for merosin. A,** Normal muscle. **B** and **C,** Muscle from two infants with congenital muscular dystrophy. **A,** Normal muscle shows strong, continuous staining around the periphery of the myofibers. **B,** Similar staining is evident in one of the infants with congenital muscular dystrophy, despite the marked variation in fiber size and increased connective tissue. Thus, this infant has classic merosin-positive congenital muscular dystrophy. In **C,** however, minimal staining for merosin is apparent. This infant has merosin-deficient congenital muscular dystrophy. *(From North KN, Specht LA, Sethi RK, Shapiro F, et al: Congenital muscular dystrophy associated with merosin deficiency, J Child Neurol 11:291-295, 1996.)*

sarcolemma protein involved in linking to the extracellular matrix is alpha-dystroglycan; the latter interacts with the key extracellular matrix protein, laminin, which, in turn, interacts with collagen type VI. The intracellular connection is mediated by the interaction

of alpha-dystroglycan with the sarcolemma proteins, sarcoglycans, which are linked to dystrophin and thereby to the actin cytoskeleton. In the CMDs, the key proteins affected are *alpha-dystroglycan, laminin,* and *collagen type VI,* defects of which interrupt the vital relationship between the extracellular matrix and the muscle cytoskeleton and result in the muscle degeneration of CMD.

The molecular basis of primary *merosin-deficient CMD* is well established.[74,75,95-97,138,227-229] Laminin-2 or merosin is the critical alpha-dystroglycan-binding, basement membrane protein of the muscle extracellular matrix. The critical laminin alpha-2 chain of laminin 2 is encoded by the *LAMA2* gene on chromosome 6q2, and this is the gene defective in merosin-deficient CMD. Laminin alpha-2 chain is also present in basement membrane of Schwann cells, and thus its lack may underlie the defect of peripheral nerve described earlier. Moreover, as noted earlier, laminin alpha-2 is present in blood vessels and along developing axons in human brain (see earlier). How these observations relate to the cerebral white matter abnormality remains to be clearly elucidated. Demonstration of the deficient protein in muscle and skin facilitates diagnosis in the infant, and demonstration of the defect in chorionic villus samples facilitates prenatal diagnosis.

The molecular basis of *classic (pure) merosin-positive CMD* is unclear and is likely to be heterogeneous. As the spectrum of phenotypes associated with the known genetic types of CMD expands further, this group will be better clarified. Moreover, the not infrequent autosomal recessive inheritance supports this notion as well as the likelihood that continued molecular genetic studies will elucidate new disorders with this myopathic phenotype. Isolated cases of male infants with CMD with dystrophin deficiency, as in Duchenne-Becker muscular dystrophy, have been reported.[94,230-232]

The molecular basis of *Ullrich CMD* involves the gene *(COL6A)* for collagen VI (see earlier). This defect results in a prominent loss of the basal lamina of muscle fibers and interrupts the vital link between the extracellular space and the intracellular cytoskeleton, as described earlier.

The molecular basis of *rigid spine syndrome* involves a deficiency of the gene *(SEPN1)* selenoprotein N, an endoplasmic reticulum protein (see earlier). The function of this protein is unknown.

The molecular bases for the four CMDs with overt CNS abnormalities (i.e., *Fukuyama CMD, Walker-Warburg syndrome, muscle-eye-brain disease* and *CMD with* FKRP *mutations),* the dystroglycanopathies, all involve defects in genes involved in the O-linked glycosylation of alpha-dystroglycan (see Table 19-4).[74,75,138,189,224,225,233] In Walker-Warburg syndrome, the defective gene *(POMT1)* encodes the protein O-mannosyl transferase and in muscle-eye-brain disease, *POMGnT1* encodes the protein O-mannosyl-N-acetylglucosaminyl transferase. Multiple O-linked glycosylation sites are present in certain serine-threonine rich domains of alpha-dystroglycan. Fukuyama CMD is caused by a defect in a gene *(FCMD)* that

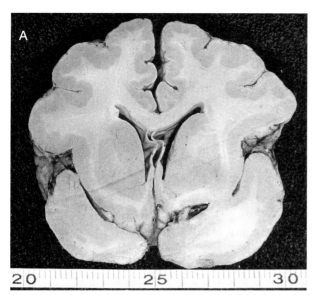
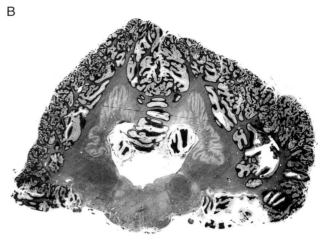

Figure 19-13   Fukuyama congenital muscular dystrophy, with associated encephalopathy (migrational disturbance). This cerebrum and cerebellum are from a child with severe hypotonia and weakness from birth and severe mental retardation. The child died at 6 years, 5 months of age; the muscle pathology was consistent with congenital muscular dystrophy. **A**, Coronal section of cerebrum. Note the polymicrogyric cortex involving the superomedial and lateral convexity, the pachygyric cortex involving the lateral convexity, and the agyric cortex involving the temporal lobes. **B**, Horizontal section of cerebellum and brain stem. Note the marked and diffuse polymicrogyria involving the cerebellar cortex. *(From Kamoshita S, Konishi Y, Segawa M, Fukuyama Y: Congenital muscular dystrophy as a disease of the central nervous system, Arch Neurol 33:513-516, 1976.)*

encodes fukutin, a putative glycosyltransferase, the exact function of which is yet unclear. Disturbances in glycosylation of alpha-dystroglycan impair its interaction with laminin and with sarcolemmal proteins, especially beta-dystroglycan. Muscle degeneration is the result. Because alpha-dystroglycan also is present in the basement membrane of the glia limitans in the developing cerebral cortex, defective glycosylation results in the disturbances in neuronal migration that underlie the occurrence of cobblestone lissencephaly (see Chapter 2). As noted earlier, more than one half of cases of CMD related to *FKRP* mutations and fukutin-related protein deficiency, which exhibit CNS abnormalities milder but mechanistically similar to those of the three disorders discussed here, are relevant in this context, because the fukutin-related protein also appears to be a glycosyltransferase for alpha-dystroglycan.[193]

Management. Because the course in most patients with any of the types of CMD is nonprogressive for many months to years, it is important to attempt to correct existing contractures by physical therapy (i.e., passive stretching or serial splints) and to prevent the development of contractures by active and passive exercises. The development of fixed deformities is often more deleterious to future motor abilities than is muscle weakness. Although no specific therapies are available, more details concerning supportive management are available in specialized sources.[138]

Facioscapulohumeral Dystrophy

FSHD is usually recognized as an autosomal dominantly inherited myopathy with prominent involvement of the face and upper extremities, onset in adolescence or early adulthood, and a slowly progressive or apparently static course.[4,234] A rare type of FSHD with onset in early infancy and a more severe course has been delineated.[234-246]

Clinical Features. The *clinical syndrome* is characterized by onset in early infancy of facial weakness.[234-246] The weakness is distinctive, in that most patients are unable to move the upper lip and later have a peculiar horizontal smile. Difficulty in closing the eyes is prominent, and the infant may sleep with the eyes open. The whole face tends to be smooth and expressionless. Difficulty in sucking is common. However, motor milestones usually are not significantly delayed, and 8 of 11 patients in the largest series walked alone by 15 months of age.[235] Later in infancy and early childhood, progressive weakness and wasting of axial and limb muscles supervene, particularly in the proximal upper extremities, but then also in the lower extremities. Of 5 patients who had reached 15 years of age or more, 4 were no longer walking, and the remaining patient was walking with difficulty. A similarly progressive disease course has been documented by other investigators.[237,239,242,243] In a report of 7 infantile-onset cases, the mean duration between onset of first symptoms and wheelchair dependency was 9.9 years.[246] The other clinical accompaniment, observed in the series of Carroll and Brooke,[235] was sensorineural hearing loss in 6 of 11 children; this loss was severe in 2 children. Approximately 50% of subsequently reported cases have exhibited sensorineural hearing loss.[234,239-244] Later in childhood, some patients have developed retinal telangiectasia, exudation, and detachment (in addition to sensorineural hearing loss).[238,239,241,243,247] Mental retardation was observed in 30% of cases in one series,[239] and it was also documented in other cases.[244]

Laboratory Studies. The serum CK level is moderately elevated in nearly all patients.[235-239,242,244] The EMG reveals low-amplitude and short-duration potentials, indicative of myopathy. Nerve conduction velocities are normal.

Pathology. Muscle pathology was striking in six of the nine patients studied in detail by Carroll and Brooke,[235] and it exhibited an *inflammatory* response suggestive of polymyositis (Fig. 19-14). Inflammatory changes in FSHD have been noted by others.[235,238,241,244,248,249] This finding may lead to treatment with steroids, which results in no objective benefit. Indeed, it is clear from the relative frequencies of infantile FSHD and of polymyositis (see later) that inflammatory changes in muscle in an infant should raise the question of FSHD rather than polymyositis, especially if the face is particularly involved.

Pathogenesis and Etiology. The genetic abnormality in this dominantly inherited disease is located at chromosome 4q35.[239,240,242,243,246] The frequency of new mutations is high. However, as many as one half of apparently sporadic cases were found to have an affected parent on careful examination. The defect is particularly interesting and involves a reduction in the number of repeats of a 3.3-kb repeat sequence at the 4q35 locus. Normal individuals carry 11 or more repeats; patients with FSHD have 10 copies or fewer.[234] The mechanism by which this genetic change causes FSHD and the genes involved is unclear. A deleterious gain of function of genes located close to the site of the reduced repeats is likely.[234,243] Molecular diagnosis is possible by examination of leukocyte DNA.

Management. Management is similar to that of progressive myopathy in late childhood and adolescence.[4] Of importance for the physician evaluating the newborn with facial weakness is the recognition that FSHD may be present; family members must be examined and perhaps have their leukocyte DNA evaluated. The parents should be counseled that, although the disorder in the affected parent is mild, a distinct possibility exists of a more severe form in their children (i.e., the phenomenon of anticipation).[234,235,238,240,243,245]

Polymyositis

Previously reported in infants no younger than 3 months of age, *polymyositis* was described in two newborns in 1982.[250] The newborns exhibited marked hypotonia and weakness, weak cry, and poor sucking and feeding ability. Neck flexors were affected markedly, as in older patients with polymyositis. Particularly striking were markedly elevated levels of creatine phosphokinase (CK; 2500 and 3600 mU/mL) and muscle biopsy findings that included lymphocytic infiltration as well as myopathic changes. Improvement in overall strength and decrease in CK levels followed treatment with steroids at 6 and 15 months of age. The observations

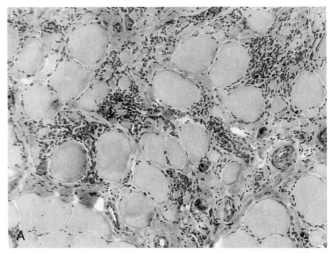
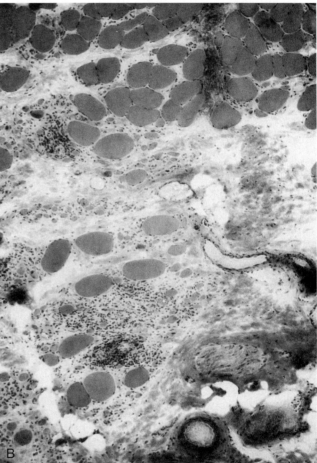

Figure 19-14 Infantile facioscapulohumeral dystrophy: muscle pathology. A and B, Striking inflammatory response in muscle from two affected children. In addition, random fiber loss and an increase in connective tissue are evident (**A**, hematoxylin and eosin stain, ×74; **B**, Gomori trichrome stain, × 74). *(Courtesy of Dr. James E. Carroll.)*

suggested that polymyositis may occur in the newborn, that the diagnosis should be suspected with the findings of markedly elevated CK levels and inflammatory cells in the muscle biopsy specimens, and that treatment with steroids may be beneficial.

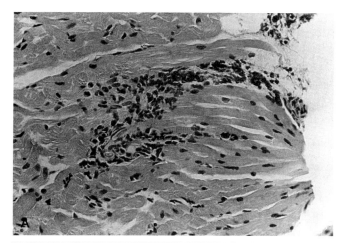

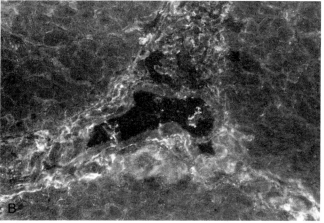

Figure 19-15 Congenital polymyositis: muscle pathology. A, Muscle biopsy shows focal inflammation. **B,** Immunofluorescence microscopy for immunoglobulin G documents immune complex deposition in a ringlike pattern around individual atrophic muscle fibers. *(From Roddy SM, Ashwal S, Peckham N: Infantile myositis: A case diagnosed in the neonatal period,* Pediatr Neurol *2:241-244, 1986.)*

Subsequent reports supported these general conclusions.[251-256] The myopathic changes are consistent with an inflammatory myopathy with an immunological basis (Fig. 19-15). The finding of perifascicular myopathy, generally considered a feature of such autoimmune myopathies as dermatomyositis, is particularly characteristic.[254-256] It is important to rule out other neonatal myopathic disorders with inflammatory changes (e.g., FSHD or merosin-deficient CMD), but other features of these latter disorders should make this distinction possible (see earlier discussions).

Minimal Change Myopathy

Minimal change myopathy, or *nonspecific congenital myopathy*, is the designation used for those infants with congenital hypotonia and weakness who exhibit minor (or even no) abnormalities of serum enzyme levels, EMG, or muscle biopsy.[4,257,258] Myopathic illness is inferred from the clinical features (e.g., proximal more than distal weakness, preserved tendon reflexes, normal sensation, and absence of fasciculations), as well as from the occasional myopathic changes observed on the EMG (e.g., small amplitude, brief duration, and

polyphasic potentials) and abnormal muscle biopsy (e.g., modest variation in fiber size). The clinical features are not as prominent as those observed in more common myopathies (e.g., congenital myotonic dystrophy) and in most cases of CMD. Many of these infants have good prognoses and improve over time. With continuing improvements in delineation of genetic myopathies, this category is becoming less common.

Myopathic Disorders with Diagnostic Histology

The *histology diagnostic* myopathic disorders are characterized by histological changes so striking and distinctive that a specific diagnosis usually can be made. An enormous literature has developed in this area since the 1970s, and several books and reviews deal with the details and complexities of the problem.[4,121,247,259-269] Because most of the designations for these disorders are derived from histological and not clinical criteria, the clinical syndromes associated with each histological change vary. Moreover, considerable overlap exists among the disorders on both clinical and histological grounds. Nevertheless, certain specific congenital myopathies are well defined clinically, morphologically, and genetically, and several conclusions relevant to the neonatal patient can be drawn.

In the following discussion, I emphasize the most common features of each disorder, particularly those disorders with prominent clinical manifestations in the neonatal period. Of the seven categories listed in Table 19-1, the first five refer to the disorders with morphologically distinctive changes by standard histological and histochemical techniques (i.e., *specific congenital myopathies*). Certain features are commonly observed among these disorders (Table 19-8). Central core disease, nemaline myopathy, myotubular myopathy, and congenital fiber type disproportion are emphasized because, albeit uncommon, they are the most common in this category (Table 19-9). Multi-minicore myopathy is rare in the newborn and is described only briefly. The *mitochondrial myopathies* may be suspected by standard histological techniques, but electron microscopic studies are needed to define the distinctive mitochondrial abnormalities. Biochemical studies may identify a specific abnormality of a mitochondrial enzyme. The *metabolic myopathies* may show no

TABLE 19-8	Specific Congenital Myopathies: Certain Common Features
Inheritance: autosomal dominant > recessive > X-linked recessive	
Onset in neonatal period	
Recognition often after the neonatal period	
Hypotonia	
Weakness: proximal > distal	
Tendon reflexes decreased in proportion to weakness	
Muscle enzymes: normal	
Electromyogram: myopathic	
Muscle biopsy: diagnostic	

TABLE 19-9 Specific Congenital Myopathies: Major Neonatal Types

Disease	Gene Symbols	Proteins
Central core disease*	RYR1	Ryanodine receptor
Nemaline myopathy*	NEM2	Nebulin
	ACTA1	alpha-Actin
	TPM3	alpha-Tropomyosin
	TPM2	beta-Tropomyosin
	TNNT1	Troponin T, slow
Myotubular myopathy*	MTM1	Myotubularin
Congenital fiber type disproportion†	ACTA1	alpha-Actin
Multi-minicore disease	SEPN1	Selenoprotein N
	RYR1	Ryanodine receptor

*Most common in the neonatal period.
†Genetically heterogeneous.

distinctive morphological change, and thus one could argue that these myopathies should be classified as *histology not diagnostic*. However, they are included here because the biopsy specimen indicates glycogen or lipid deposition in muscle, which is usually the critical initial finding in the definition of the specific biochemical lesion.

Central Core Disease

Central core disease, originally described in 1956,[270] was the first of the specific congenital myopathies to be defined. Subsequent reports further delineated a fairly discrete clinical syndrome.[4,121,259,262-269,271-278]

Clinical Features. The *clinical syndrome* consists of hypotonia and weakness, apparent usually in the neonatal period. However, many infants are not recognized as exhibiting muscle disease until months later. Muscle weakness is usually more prominent in the proximal extremities, and tendon reflexes are usually preserved, although diminished in proportion to the weakness.

Congenital hip dislocation is also common. Mild facial weakness is not unusual. Ptosis, extraocular muscle weakness, dysphagia, and respiratory difficulties have *not* been features.

The *course* of the disease is usually nonprogressive, and infants attain motor milestones, albeit at a slow rate. Slow progression of weakness may occur, but even without this progression, contractures and kyphoscoliosis may result. In a series of 11 patients followed to the age of 4 to 20 years, 2 were unable to walk alone, and 2 had difficulty climbing stairs.[265] An increased risk of malignant hyperthermia (e.g., during anesthesia) must be recognized to avoid unexpected death.

Laboratory Studies. Laboratory investigations, aside from muscle biopsy, are not particularly helpful. The serum CK level is usually normal, and the EMG shows myopathic changes, although frequently minor.

Pathology. Muscle pathology is distinctive and diagnostic in the presence of the clinical findings.[4,121,266] Many muscle fibers (20% to 100%) exhibit cores that are central or somewhat eccentric in location (Fig. 19-16). Single or multiple cores may be observed in a given fiber and are well demonstrated with the histochemical stains for oxidative enzymes (e.g., reduced nicotinamide adenine dinucleotide-tetrazolium reductase [NADH-TR]), which are absent in the core region. Indeed, electron microscopy shows an absence of mitochondria in the core region. The cores have a particular predilection for type I fibers and, in some cases, type I fibers predominate or are the only fiber type observable.

Pathogenesis and Etiology. The pathogenesis relates to a genetic defect that is usually inherited in an autosomal dominant manner, although rarely autosomal recessive inheritance has been documented.[266-269, 278-280] The gene involved is *RYR1*, which is located on chromosome 19q13.1 and encodes the skeletal muscle ryanodine receptor. The latter is a ligand-related release

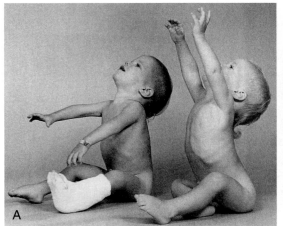
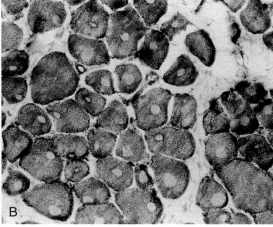

Figure 19-16 **Central core disease. A,** Photograph of twins, one of whom has the disease. Note the weakness of the proximal upper extremities. **B,** Muscle biopsy from the affected twin. Note the numerous central cores with decreased oxidative enzyme activity (reduced nicotinamide adenine dinucleotide-tetrazolium reductase [NADH-TR] stain, × 200). *(From Cohen ME, Duffner PK, Heffner R: Central core disease in one of identical twins, J Neurol Neurosurg Psychiatry 41:659-663, 1978.)*

channel for internally stored calcium and thereby plays a crucial role in excitation-contraction coupling.

Management. Management is the same as that of nonprogressive or slowly progressive myopathy. The prevention of contractures is important.

Nemaline Myopathy

Nemaline (rod body) myopathy, described initially by Shy and colleagues in 1963,[281] was the second of the specific congenital myopathies to be defined. The term *nemaline* is derived from the Greek word *nema*, meaning "thread." Numerous subsequent reports emphasized a considerable variation in clinical expression.[4,121,259,262-264,266,267,269,282-325a]

Clinical Features. The *clinical presentation* in infants with manifestations from the neonatal period can be divided into three syndromes. First, as in typical central core disease, hypotonia and weakness are relatively mild and are sometimes even overlooked in the newborn period. This variety is termed *typical congenital nemaline myopathy*. Second, marked neonatal hypotonia and weakness occur with no spontaneous movements or respiration at birth. Severe contractures and sometimes fractures complete this syndrome of *severe congenital nemaline myopathy*. Third, marked neonatal hypotonia and weakness occur, but with some movement and respiratory effort and no severe contractures. This serious disorder, although not so marked as the "severe" cases, is termed *intermediate congenital nemaline myopathy*. In one large series of nemaline myopathy ($n = 143$), approximately 50% of patients presented in the neonatal period, and of these, 35% had the severe congenital form, 45% had the intermediate congenital form, and 20% had the typical congenital form.[320] Accompanying the severe and intermediate forms were marked facial diplegia and feeding disturbances. The milder, typical form is associated with varying degrees of facial diparesis. Various skeletal anomalies, including high-arched palate, long dysmorphic face, prognathism malocclusion, pectus excavatum, and "pigeon chest," may be seen. In surviving infants, pes cavus, kyphoscoliosis, and lumbar lordosis evolve.

The *course* of the typical, milder nemaline myopathy is considered generally to be nonprogressive or slowly progressive.[266] However, in a study with a 5- to 25-year follow-up, 10 of 12 patients exhibited clinical deterioration, and only 8 of 12 were walking unsupported.[294] Ten of 12 patients had developed scoliosis. Similar findings with 3- to 24-year follow-up were reported in a later study.[265]

The *course* in those infants with the two more severe forms of the disease (i.e., the severe and intermediate forms) is generally unfavorable.[269,320-325] Thus, in one series, 74% of patients with severe congenital cases died, generally before 1 year of age, and 28% of patients with intermediate congenital cases died.[320] Among the infants with the severe form, a requirement for ventilation at birth or in the first month was followed by death in more than 90% of cases. Such infants fail to establish adequate ventilation after birth because of weakness of respiratory muscles. This weakness results in failure of full expansion of lungs and, secondary to difficulty with secretions, aspiration often is added. Infants usually die in the neonatal period or in the first months of life. However, longterm survival in these patients, who are usually bedridden and are receiving mechanical ventilation, has been observed.[290,293,299] Moreover, rare affected infants with the need for mechanical ventilation at birth, severe weakness, and markedly impaired feeding have improved over the ensuing 2 to 3 years to become independent of mechanical ventilation and to achieve the ability to stand or even walk.[297,309]

Laboratory Studies. Laboratory investigations have included either normal or slightly elevated values for the serum CK level. The EMG often exhibits shortduration and small-amplitude potentials of myopathy, but signs of denervation have also been observed, particularly late in the disease.[4,121,266,288,291,300,307,315] Nerve conduction velocities are normal.

Pathology. Muscle pathology is distinctive and diagnostic in the presence of the clinical features.[4,121,264,266,315] Although the rod bodies are readily overlooked on routine hematoxylin and eosin staining, Gomori trichrome, toluidine blue, and other selected stains demonstrate them well (Fig. 19-17). Predominance of type I fibers, which also are small, is consistent.[16,121,262,263,266,290,292,299,315]

The rod body is derived from lateral expansion of the Z-disk, the band found normally at either end of the sarcomere.[262,263,266,283,299,315,322,326-329] Thus, the rod bodies have been shown by electron microscopy to be in structural continuity with the Z-disk. The rod's major protein component is alpha-actin, the main protein of the Z-disk, and the bodies are penetrated by actin filaments, which normally penetrate the Z-disk. The rods are surrounded by desmin, the structural component of muscle-specific intermediate filaments.[315] Intranuclear rods have been detected in

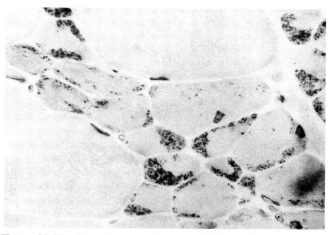

Figure 19-17 **Nemaline myopathy: muscle biopsy from an affected twin**. Note the rod bodies, principally subsarcolemmal in location and occurring in the smaller, atrophic fibers (Gomori trichrome stain, × 580). *(From Dubowitz V: Muscle Disorders in Childhood, Philadelphia: 1978, Saunders.)*

TABLE 19-10   Specific Congenital Myopathies: Distinguishing Clinical Features

	Neonatal Hypotonia and Weakness	Severe Form with Neonatal Death	Facial Weakness	Ptosis	Extraocular Muscular Weakness
Central core disease	+	0	±	0	0
Nemaline myopathy	+	+	+	0	0
Myotubular myopathy	+	+	+	+	+
Congenital fiber type disproportion	+	±	±	0	+

+, often a prominent feature; ±, variably a prominent feature; 0, not a prominent feature.

some severe fatal neonatal cases.[266,308,322,330,331] In general, the severity of the myopathological features correlate only imperfectly with the clinical course.[322]

Pathogenesis and Etiology. The pathogenesis of nemaline myopathy relates to defects in one of five genes encoding proteins of skeletal muscle thin filaments (see Table 19-9).[315,316,318,319,321-325] Approximately 60% to 75% of cases of severe congenital nemaline myopathy are related to defects of *ACTA1*, the gene for alpha-actin.[323,324,325a] Most of the remaining cases are related to nebulin defects and are principally autosomal recessive. Mutations in the genes for alpha-tropomyosin, beta-tropomyosin, and troponin are rare causes of severe disease.

Management. Management of the typical, nonprogressive, or slowly progressive form of nemaline myopathy depends principally on physical therapy and related techniques. However, respiratory failure may occur during infancy, rapidly and unexpectedly, with a fatal outcome, even in apparently stable or improving patients.[266,289,292,293,302,303,312] Thus, careful follow-up is necessary. Infants with the severe neonatal form require prompt recognition and vigorous ventilatory and nutritional support if they are to survive. However, on the basis of the data available, appreciable improvement, despite diligent supportive care, is unlikely.

Myotubular Myopathy

Myotubular myopathy, described initially in 1966 by Spiro and co-workers,[332] was the third specific congenital myopathy to be described. The name is derived from the morphological appearance of the affected muscle fibers, which resemble fetal myotubes. Subsequent reports described considerable variation in clinical expression.[4,121,259,263-267,269,316,333-363]

Clinical Features. The clinical features of myotubular myopathy can be divided roughly into two syndromes. Less commonly, hypotonia and weakness are relatively mild and are sometimes overlooked in the newborn period. These autosomal varieties generally do not manifest in the neonatal period. The more common disorder affects male infants and is characterized by marked hypotonia and weakness with respiratory failure. Many examples of this severe, malignant, X-linked neonatal form of myotubular myopathy have been described.[265-267,269,316,333,336,338-350,352,354-361,363]

Polyhydramnios and decreased fetal movement are noted in 50% to 60% during the pregnancy, failure to breathe effectively at birth often leads to asphyxia (and the mistaken diagnosis of hypoxic-ischemic encephalopathy for the subsequent motor deficits), and striking impairments of neonatal axial, appendicular, and facial movement, sucking, and breathing are apparent. Ptosis is common, and extraocular muscle weakness also is often present. Indeed, the constellation of marked facial weakness, ptosis, and ophthalmoplegia with generalized hypotonia and weakness is highly suggestive of myotubular myopathy, rather than other congenital myopathies (Table 19-10) of either the mild or severe varieties.

The *course* in the severely affected male infants with the X-linked syndrome has been considered to be nearly uniform evolution to a fatal outcome. However, a more recent series of 55 affected male infants showed that 64% survived beyond 1 year of age, although 60% of these long-term survivors were entirely ventilator dependent.[360] Only 13% of the long-term survivors did not require at least intermittent mechanical ventilation. Similar data have been reported in other series.[363] In the severely affected infant, because of the failure of lung expansion and the superimposed aspiration secondary to swallowing difficulties, atelectasis and pneumonia are the usual causes of death in the first days or weeks of life. Motor outcome in long-term survivors is very unfavorable in most, who often are bedridden or in wheelchairs. However, in a series of 36 patients, 3 were said to exhibit "no significant disability at 6 months, 5 years, and 7 years, respectively,"[356] and in another group of 55 cases, 7 had only slightly delayed motor milestones.[360]

Laboratory Studies. Laboratory investigations have included only an occasionally elevated serum CK level. The EMG is usually myopathic, although not impressively so; as with nemaline myopathy, fibrillation potentials are occasionally observed.[266,342,347] Chest radiographs often show very thin ribs.[41,348,349]

Pathology. The muscle pathology is distinctive and diagnostic in the presence of the clinical findings.* Muscle fibers contain one or more centrally placed nuclei, usually surrounded by an area devoid of myofibrils. With adenosine triphosphatase staining, the region around the nucleus appears as a clear zone or halo (Fig. 19-18). Ultrastructurally, the muscle fibers

---

*See references 4,52,121,266,346,348,351,356-359,363,364

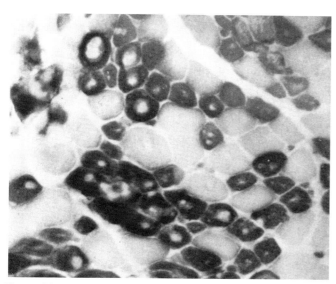

Figure 19-18 Myotubular myopathy. This muscle biopsy is from a child with deficits from birth. The central nuclei occur in both fiber types (difficult to see in the light, type I fibers) and leave a clear zone with adenosine triphosphatase (ATPase) reactions (ATPase stain, pH 9.4, × 250). *(From Dubowitz V: Muscle Disorders in Childhood, Philadelphia: 1978, Saunders.)*

bear some resemblance to fetal myotubes, with each fiber containing a longitudinal chain of central nuclei (Fig. 19-19). Consistent with these findings suggestive of a disturbance of maturation are other features characteristic of fetal but not mature muscle (i.e., abundant vimentin and desmin [filamentous proteins], neural cell adhesion molecules, and intracytoplasmic distribution of dystrophin).[357-359] Type I fibers tend to be small, and this type I fiber hypotrophy usually is a very prominent feature.[262,263,333,346,348,363,364]

Pathogenesis and Etiology. The pathogenesis of myotubular myopathy is not entirely understood; a maturational arrest has been suggested because of the

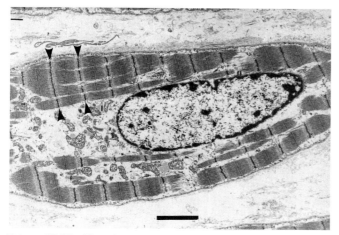

Figure 19-19 Myotubular myopathy. This electron micrograph is from a muscle biopsy of a term infant with myotubular myopathy. A central nucleus surrounded by mitochondria is shown. Z-bands are in register *(arrowheads)*, unlike fetal myotubes. *(From Sarnat HB: Myotubular myopathy: Arrest of morphogenesis of myofibres associated with persistence of fetal vimentin and desmin. Four cases compared with fetal and neonatal muscle, Can J Neurol Sci 17:109-123, 1990.)*

resemblance of the abnormal fibers to fetal myotubes and the persistence of other features of fetal myotubes, as noted in the previous section. Insight into the potential mechanism of this maturational defect has been gained by identification of the gene at Xq28 *(MTM1)*. *MTM1* encodes a protein, myotubularin, that is a phosphatidylinositol phosphatase.[363,365,366] Phosphoinositides, the products of the phosphatase, are involved in diverse cellular functions, including survival, differentiation, vesicle trafficking, and actin rearrangement. Which of these functions is altered and how the disturbance leads to the disease remain unclear.

Management. Management of the severe X-linked form of myotubular myopathy is as discussed for the severe congenital forms of nemaline myopathy (see previous section). The ethical issues concerning ventilatory support of the severely affected infants are obvious.

Congenital Fiber Type Disproportion

Congenital fiber type disproportion, initially described by Brooke in 1973,[367] was the fourth identified among the relatively common specific congenital myopathies. Subsequent reports confirmed and amplified the original observations of Brooke.[4,248,263-265,368-392] Indeed, variability of the clinical spectrum has been demonstrated conclusively.

Clinical Features. The *clinical syndrome* of the more than 70 reported cases has included particularly hypotonia and weakness of limbs, neck, and respiratory, trunk, facial, bulbar, and extraocular muscles. The last feature, ophthalmoparesis, is present in more than half of the patients who are overtly symptomatic in the neonatal period but in fewer than 10% of those who present later.[389] In most cases, the deficits in the early neonatal-onset cases are severe. Other musculoskeletal abnormalities are common, such as limb contractures, congenital hip dislocations, foot deformities, torticollis, and, later, scoliosis. These abnormalities represent primarily postural deformities, generated either prenatally or postnatally.

The *course* is variable, but in general, varies according to the time of onset. Thus, among the infants with overt neonatal-onset disease, fully 40% have died because of the combination of bulbar and respiratory muscle weakness. Most surviving infants have had a static course, with generally severe weakness. Infants with slightly later onset are more likely to have the static and then improving course, often considered characteristic of the disorder, or more precisely, group of disorders.

Laboratory Studies. The serum CK level is usually normal. The EMG usually exhibits myopathic changes, albeit often not severe.

Pathology. Muscle pathology establishes the diagnosis. The essential features are the predominance of type I fibers (i.e., type I fibers account for more than 55% of the total [normally, type I fibers account for 30% to

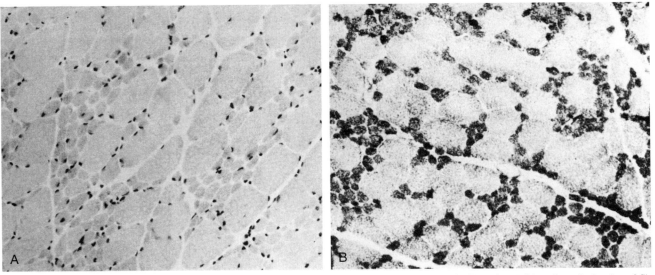

Figure 19-20 Congenital fiber type disproportion. This muscle biopsy is from an affected child. **A,** Note the striking disparity in size of fibers (hematoxylin and eosin stain, × 150). **B,** Histochemical preparation shows that the small fibers give a strong reaction for oxidative enzymes (i.e, type I fibers) (reduced nicotinamide adenine dinucleotide-tetrazolium reductase [NADH-TR] stain, × 150). *(From Dubowitz V: Muscle Disorders in Childhood, Philadelphia: 1978, Saunders.)*

55% of the total]) and the small size of type I fibers (i.e., a disparity of 12% or more in the mean diameters of type I and II fibers [normally, the diameters are approximately equal]; Fig. 19-20). Subsequently, hypertrophy of type II fibers appears to occur, and the discrepancy between the size of the fibers may become marked. (In several cases, type II fibers were hypotrophic.[379,380,383,384])

Fiber type disproportion of the variety observed with congenital fiber type disproportion may be observed with *other congenital myopathies,* particular nemaline myopathy, myotubular myopathy, and congenital myotonic dystrophy. However, in these disorders, additional changes in muscle coexist and serve to emphasize the nosological status of the disorders, as well as to lead to the correct diagnosis. Moreover, fiber type disproportion has been observed with *CNS disorders;* in one series, cerebellar hypoplasia was the most common CNS abnormality.[377]

Pathogenesis and Etiology. The pathogenesis of congenital fiber type disproportion is likely heterogeneous. A functional abnormality in maturation of the motor unit has been suggested for several reasons: (1) similar myopathology can be produced by denervation or cross innervation; (2) type IIc fibers, the fetal precursor of types IIa and IIb fibers, often are present in increased numbers; and (3) fiber type disproportions of various types may occur with developmental disturbances of brain.[375,377] The nature of the postulated disturbance in motor unit development is unclear. Numerous documentations of normal anterior horn cells and peripheral nerves in congenital fiber type disproportion are available.[372,377]

Approximately 45% of cases have a positive family history; approximately two thirds of these suggest autosomal dominant inheritance, and one third suggest autosomal recessive.[389,392] In a recent series of

neonatal-onset cases (*n* = 3), mutations in the *ACTA1* gene (different from those for nemaline myopathy) were detected (see Table 19-9).[390,390a] The clinical features were similar to the severely affected cases noted earlier, except for the absence of ophthalmoparesis. A report of eight cases with onset in the first year or later in infancy and childhood noted defects in the *SEPN1* gene (see the description of multi-minicore disease next).[393]

Management. The most essential aspect of management is recognition that this disorder may be associated with improvement. Thus, even severely affected infants should receive vigorous supportive care, and every effort should be expended to prevent contractures.

Multi-Minicore Disease

Multi-minicore disease should be discussed briefly in this context of specific congenital myopathies. Although other rare distinctive myopathies have been described (e.g., desmin-related [myofibrillar] myopathies, Bethlem myopathy), presentation in the neonatal period is not typical. However, the classic form of multi-minicore disease typically has its *clinical onset* in the neonatal period or early infancy.[266,267,269,394-396] Neonatal hypotonia and weakness, although generalized, tend to predominate in the axial muscles. Mild facial weakness is common. Respiratory difficulties generally appear later, as do spinal abnormalities, especially scoliosis. Motor development is prominently delayed. The clinical *course* is static in most patients, although approximately 20% of patients exhibit mild progression. The *pathology* is distinctive and consists of the occurrence of multifocal corelike areas, seen best as areas of reduced activity on oxidative enzyme stains.

Pathogenesis is likely heterogeneous with primarily sporadic and autosomal recessive cases reported. In separate cohorts, defects in the *SEPN1* gene, the gene mutated in rigid spine syndrome (see discussion of CMD earlier) and in some later-onset forms of congenital fiber type disproportion, and in the *RYR1* gene, the gene mutated in central core disease, have been identified (see Table 19-9). The clinical overlap with CMD with rigid spine syndrome and the histological overlap with central core disease are consistent with these initial genetic findings.

Mitochondrial Myopathies

Mitochondrial myopathy, in this context, refers to a disorder with prominent involvement of muscle and a *primary* (not secondary) abnormality of mitochondrial structure and function. Abnormalities of mitochondrial structure sometimes can be demonstrated initially on muscle biopsy by the modified Gomori trichrome stain, which reveals accumulations of red staining material within the fibers (i.e., "ragged red fibers").[4,397,398] Further definition of the structural disturbance in mitochondrial number, configuration, or both, is made by electron microscopy.[398-402] Of additional importance is documentation of the abnormalities in mitochondrial biochemical *function* that occur in mitochondrial myopathies.[398,402-407] Finally, as discussed later, study of the ratio of mitochondrial to nuclear DNA is important in identification of the mitochondrial DNA depletion syndrome.

Classification of mitochondrial myopathies according to biochemical defects is valuable, and clear definition of such defects has progressed rapidly. The major metabolic functions of mitochondria in muscle can be categorized relatively simply as follows: (1) substrate transport, (2) substrate utilization, (3) function of the Krebs cycle, and (4) function of the respiratory (electron transport) chain (Table 19-11).[398,400,402-410] Of these, only myopathic disease related to defects in the respiratory chain is clearly relevant to the newborn (see subsequent discussion).

Substrate Transport. Of particular importance is transport into mitochondria of the two major substrates for energy production through acetyl-coenzyme A (i.e., pyruvate from glucose metabolism and fatty acids). Disturbance of fatty acid transport occurs with carnitine deficiency but is discussed later with lipid myopathies because the lipid deposition dominates the myopathology.

Substrate Utilization. Pyruvate dehydrogenase deficiency usually results in a disorder with prominent CNS phenomena, rather than myopathic features (see Chapter 15). However, the enzymatic defect is demonstrable in muscle.[411] A major disorder of fatty acid utilization with occasional clinical presentation in the newborn period is medium-chain acyl-coenzyme A dehydrogenase. Because encephalopathic features also are usually present, in addition to hypotonia, this disorder is discussed in Chapter 15.

Krebs Cycle. No such disease primarily of muscle has yet been described in the newborn.

Respiratory Chain. Disturbances of the mitochondrial respiratory chain may lead to a striking neonatal myopathy syndrome with hypotonia and weakness. Defects primarily of complex IV (cytochrome oxidase), but also of complexes I, II, III, and V, sometimes in combination, and mitochondrial DNA depletion with impairment of multiple enzymes of the respiratory chain have been associated with this syndrome.[4,401,403,404-407,412-456] Disturbance of *cytochrome c oxidase* is the most common cause of this serious neonatal syndrome. The clinical features have been striking (Table 19-12): onset in the first days or weeks of life of severe hypotonia and weakness, with involvement of limbs, trunk, face, and sucking, but only rarely of eye movements. Tendon reflexes are usually absent. Hepatomegaly is common. Additional features have included de Toni-Fanconi-Debré renal syndrome in approximately two thirds and, occasionally, myocardiopathy.

TABLE 19-11   Mitochondrial Disorders Characterized by Presentation with Hypotonia or Weakness in the Neonatal Period

	CLINICAL FEATURES	
Biochemical Disorder	Primarily Myopathy	Primarily Encephalopathy
Substrate Transport		
Carnitine deficiency	+	−
Substrate Utilization		
Pyruvate carboxylase	−	+
Pyruvate dehydrogenase complex	−	+
Fatty acid oxidation	−	+
Krebs Cycle		
Fumarase deficiency	−	+
Respiratory Chain		
Complex I	+	+
Complex II	+	+
Complex III	+	+
Complex IV (cytochrome c oxidase)	+	+
Complex V (adenosine triphosphate synthase)	+	+
Multiple defects (mitochondrial DNA depletion)	+	+

TABLE 19-12   Major Features of Infantile Cytochrome c Oxidase Deficiency

Onset, first days or weeks
Hypotonia and weakness: axial, appendicular, and facial
Hyporeflexia, areflexia
Respiratory failure, death in early infancy
Hepatomegaly
de Toni-Fanconi-Debré syndrome
Lactic acidosis
"Ragged red" fibers, mitochondrial abnormalities, and absent staining for cytochrome c oxidase

Macroglossia has been noted occasionally. The *course* has been progressive, with death in the first year.

A remarkable *benign form* of cytochrome c oxidase deficiency has been delineated.[403-407,417,426-428,444,457] The newborns present clinically as in the fatal form of the disease but then, over the ensuing weeks and months, exhibit clinical, myopathological, and biochemical improvement. By 2 to 4 years of age, the infants are normal. Distinction of this benign form from the fatal form of cytochrome c oxidase deficiency in the *newborn period*, crucial for determining prognosis and formulating therapy, requires muscle immunohistochemistry (see discussion of muscle biopsy).

Laboratory studies have demonstrated lactic acidosis consistently (see Table 19-12). This finding is an important clue to the diagnosis. When evaluated, the serum pyruvate level also has been elevated. The serum CK level is only slightly elevated, and the EMG is usually normal. In those patients with the Fanconi renal abnormality, glycosuria, proteinuria, phosphaturia, and generalized aminoaciduria are present.

Muscle biopsy reveals abnormal accumulations of red staining material on modified Gomori trichrome stain and abnormalities of mitochondrial structure on electron microscopy. Accumulations of lipid and glycogen also are detected readily by appropriate stains (these *secondary* metabolic changes separate this disorder from the primary abnormalities of lipid and glycogen metabolism, described later). Histochemical staining for cytochrome c oxidase demonstrates the enzymatic deficiency (Figs. 19-21 and 19-22).

In infants with the benign form of cytochrome c oxidase deficiency, the deficiency of staining, instead of worsening, resolves (Fig. 19-23 to 19-25).

Immunohistochemistry with antibodies directed against individual subunits of cytochrome c oxidase differentiates the two disorders: the fatal infantile myopathy is characterized by absence of the nuclear DNA-encoded subunit VIIa,b of the enzyme, whereas in the benign myopathy, *both* the VIIa,b subunit *and* the mitochondrial DNA-encoded subunit II are absent (see Figs. 19-21 to 19-24).[407,428]

The *pathogenesis* of the myopathic disturbance relates to the impairment of energy production caused by the defect in cytochrome c oxidase. DiMauro and co-workers[423] used immunochemical techniques to demonstrate that the deficiency of enzymatic activity results from a decrease in the quantity of enzyme protein, rather than a disturbance in catalytic efficiency. The defect in the respiratory chain results in the lactic acidosis because of decreased utilization of pyruvate (which is converted to lactate by lactate dehydrogenase) and in the accumulation of lipid and glycogen because of decreased utilization of fatty acids and glycogen.

The enzymatic defect in the infantile form of cytochrome c oxidase deficiency appears to be inherited as an *autosomal recessive* disorder. Thus, children of both sexes have been affected, parents have been asymptomatic, and siblings with the disorder have been identified in several families.

Management requires intensive supportive therapy, particularly because of the possibility of the reversible form of cytochrome c oxidase deficiency. Infants afflicted with the latter disorder in early infancy are severely affected clinically, morphologically, and biochemically. Muscle immunohistochemistry is needed to distinguish the reversible and fatal forms *in the neonatal period.*

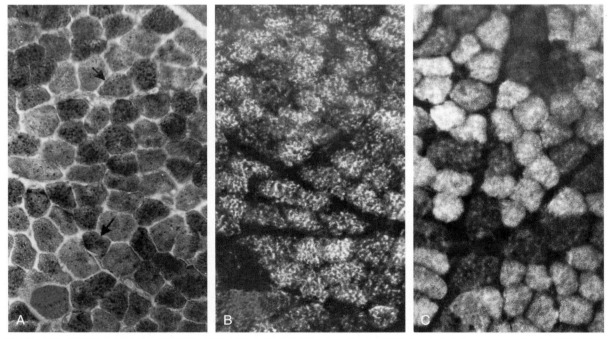

Figure 19-21 **Cytochrome c oxidase–deficient myopathies: cytochrome c oxidase (COX) in control human muscle. A**, COX histochemistry shows type I *(arrow)* and type II fibers. **B**, COX-II and, **C**, COX-VIIa,b immunostains show particulate immunoreaction of muscle mitochondria (× 350). *(From Tritschler HJ, Bonilla E, Lombes A, Andreetta F, et al: Differential diagnosis of fatal and benign cytochrome c oxidase–deficient myopathies of infancy, Neurology 41:300-305, 1991.)*

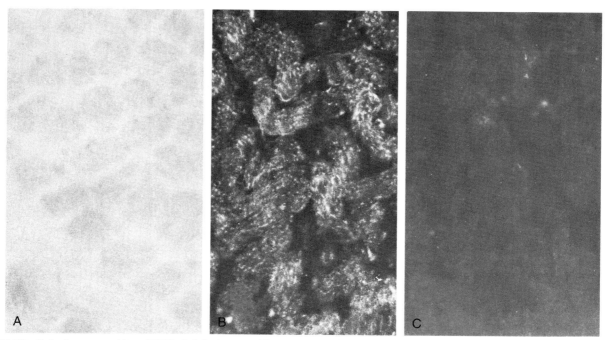

Figure 19-22   **Cytochrome c oxidase (COX)–deficient myopathies, severe form: muscle biopsies, fatal myopathy. A**, COX histochemistry shows lack of enzymatic activity in all fibers. **B**, COX-II shows particulate immunostain of mitochondria. **C**, COX-VIIa,b shows lack of immunostain in all fibers (× 350). *(From Tritschler HJ, Bonilla E, Lombes A, Andreetta F, et al: Differential diagnosis of fatal and benign cytochrome c oxidase–deficient myopathies of infancy,* Neurology *41:300-305, 1991.)*

Mitochondrial DNA depletion is a disorder with features similar to those just described for cytochrome c oxidase deficiency.[416,438,439,445,446,456,458-463] Thus, approximately 65% of infants with the reported cases have presented in the neonatal period with weakness (limbs and face), hypotonia, and hyporeflexia. Occasional features have been ophthalmoplegia, liver failure, Fanconi syndrome, and seizures. Lactic acidosis has been noted in approximately 50% of cases. Approximately 60% have had elevated values for CK, ranging from 2 to as high as 30 times the upper limit of normal. Of patients with neonatal onset, most have

died in the first year of life. Muscle biopsy shows ragged red fibers in the minority of cases, but consistent features are a decrease in the content of mitochondrial DNA and a deficiency of multiple mitochondrial enzymes, especially cytochrome c oxidase (complex IV) and combinations of complexes I, II, or III. In infantile-onset cases, the disorder appears to be autosomal recessive. The molecular genetic disturbances are likely multiple. At least one recognized gene is involved in DNA metabolism (i.e., thymidine kinase 2 *[TK2]*).[405,456] Other examples will likely be delineated. Recall that Alpers syndrome can be caused by

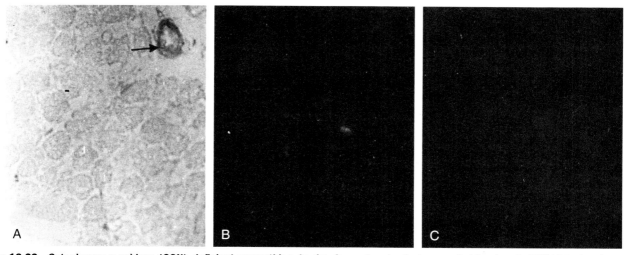

Figure 19-23   **Cytochrome c oxidase (COX)–deficient myopathies, benign form at early stage: muscle biopsies. A**, COX histochemistry shows lack of activity in all fibers. Enzymatic activity *(arrow)* is present in the arterial wall. **B**, COX-II and, **C**, COX VIIa,b show lack of immunostain in all fibers (× 350 before 14% reduction). *(From Tritschler HJ, Bonilla E, Lombes A, Andreetta F, et al: Differential diagnosis of fatal and benign cytochrome c oxidase–deficient myopathies of infancy,* Neurology *41:300-305, 1991.)*

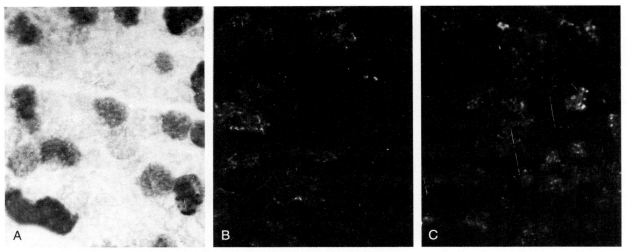

Figure 19-24 **Cytochrome c oxidase (COX)–deficient myopathies, benign form during recovery: muscle biopsies.** **A,** COX histochemistry shows activity in scattered fibers. **B,** COX-II and, **C,** COX-VIIa,b immunostains show particulate mitochondrial stain in scattered fibers (× 350 before 14% reduction). *(From Tritschler HJ, Bonilla E, Lombes A, Andreetta F, et al: Differential diagnosis of fatal and benign cytochrome c oxidase–deficient myopathies of infancy, Neurology 41:300-305, 1991.)*

mitochondrial DNA depletion resulting from a mitochondrial DNA-specific polymerase gamma gene *(POLG1;* see Chapter 16).

Metabolic Myopathies

Metabolic myopathy, in this context, refers to a disorder with prominent involvement of muscle and a *primary* abnormality of glycogen or lipid metabolism. Because glycogen and lipid metabolism also are affected *secondarily* by mitochondrial abnormalities (see previous section), a certain overlap of clinical and morphological features is to be expected. Glycogen (through glucose) and lipid (through fatty acids) are important for energy production and for structural maintenance and growth in muscle (see Chapter 17). Disorders of glycogen and lipid metabolism are classified here among myopathies that have diagnostic histology because appropriate fixation and staining (e.g., periodic

acid-Schiff [PAS] for glycogen and oil red O for lipid) usually demonstrate accumulation of the appropriate material and stimulate the search for the specific metabolic defect.

Disorders of Glycogen Metabolism. Disorders of glycogen metabolism are shown in Figure 18-7.[464-467] Disorders known to exhibit neuromuscular disease in early infancy are alpha-glucosidase (acid maltase) deficiency or Pompe disease (type II), debrancher deficiency (type III), brancher deficiency (type IV), muscle phosphorylase (type V) and phosphorylase kinase (type VIII) deficiencies, and phosphofructokinase deficiency (type VII; Table 19-13). Other glycogenoses may be associated with hypotonia secondary to hypoglycemia (e.g., glucose-6-phosphatase deficiency, Von Gierke disease type I, glycogen synthetase deficiency).

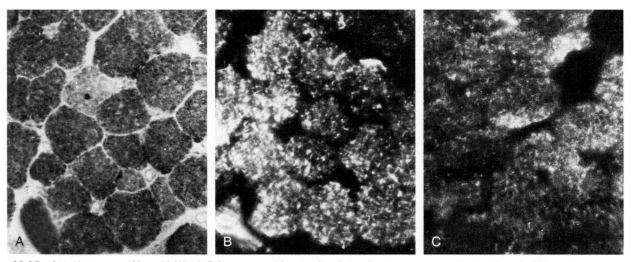

Figure 19-25 **Cytochrome c oxidase (COX)–deficient myopathies, benign form after recovery: muscle biopsies.** **A,** COX histochemistry shows activity in all fibers. **B,** COX-II and, **C,** COX-VIIa,b immunostains show particulate mitochondrial stain in all fibers (× 350 before 14% reduction). *(From Tritschler HJ, Bonilla E, Lombes A, Andreetta F, et al: Differential diagnosis of fatal and benign cytochrome c oxidase–deficient myopathies of infancy, Neurology 41:300-305, 1991.)*

TABLE 19-13	Neonatal Neuromuscular Disease and Disordered Glycogen Metabolism

Acid maltase deficiency (type II, Pompe disease)
Debrancher deficiency (type III)
Brancher deficiency (type IV)
Muscle phosphorylase deficiency (type V)
Muscle phosphorylase kinase deficiency (type VIII)
Phosphofructokinase deficiency (type VII)

Type II Glycogen Storage Disease (Pompe Disease). This disease is the prototype of the glycogenoses with onset in the first weeks of life and is discussed in detail in Chapter 18 regarding disorders at the level of the lower motor neuron. The disorder involves skeletal muscle, but involvement of anterior horn cells tends to dominate the clinical syndrome.

Type III Glycogen Storage Disease (Debrancher Deficiency). This disorder affects liver as well as muscle. Because debrancher enzyme is involved in the major metabolic pathway for the degradation of glycogen to glucose, hypoglycemia may occur and may be a prominent aspect of the clinical syndrome. Hepatomegaly is impressive, and, indeed, hepatic disease may be severe. Hypotonia and weakness from the neonatal period have been reported, albeit rarely.[4,468]

Type IV Glycogen Storage Disease (Brancher Deficiency). This disorder classically presents in infancy as progressive cirrhosis of the liver. However, several cases of glycogen storage disease type IV, brancher enzyme deficiency, have been associated with lethal myopathy, sometimes with cardiomyopathy and anterior horn cell glycogen accumulation.[469-471]

Type V Glycogen Storage Disease (Muscle Phosphorylase Deficiency). This disorder, better known as McArdle disease, usually manifests around the time of puberty with exercise intolerance, muscle cramps, fatigue, and myoglobinuria. However, three patients with a fatal infantile form were reported.[472-474] The infants exhibited severe, generalized weakness and hypotonia from the neonatal period. Two infants had evidence of prenatal onset because of congenital contractures at the elbows, hips, and knees.[473,474] In all three infants, the disorder progressed rapidly to death by respiratory failure at 16 days, 12 weeks, and 13 weeks.[472,473] The diagnosis of glycogen myopathy was suggested by the finding of subsarcolemmal vacuoles on muscle biopsy (Fig. 19-26), which were PAS positive. Electron microscopy demonstrated large subsarcolemmal deposits of glycogen that were not membrane bound (unlike the lysosomal-bound deposits of Pompe disease). No phosphorylase staining was apparent on histochemical reaction of muscle. In two cases studied biochemically, the glycogen content of muscle was found to be increased threefold.[472,474] Other enzymes of glycogen metabolism were normal, and immunochemical techniques demonstrated absence of phosphorylase protein. The occurrence of parental consanguinity in one of the two cases suggests that the disorder is autosomal recessive.[473]

Type VIII Glycogen Storage Disease (Muscle Phosphorylase Kinase Deficiency). A different defect at the phosphorylase step has been described in two infants. One had moderate hypotonia and weakness and delayed motor development from birth (sitting but not walking at 19 months of age).[475] Although total phosphorylase activity was normal in vitro in both cases, the proportion of the active ("a") form was markedly depressed, thus indicating that in vivo most of muscle phosphorylase was present as the inactive ("b") form. A defect in the phosphorylase kinase necessary for activation of phosphorylase caused the disorder. A second infant exhibited more severe weakness and hypotonia and died at 7 months of age.[476]

Type VII Glycogen Storage Disease (Phosphofructokinase Deficiency). This disorder, like McArdle disease, is associated characteristically with later onset of

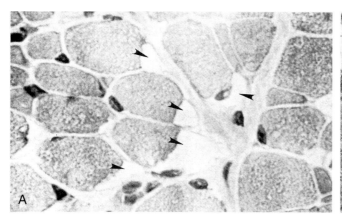
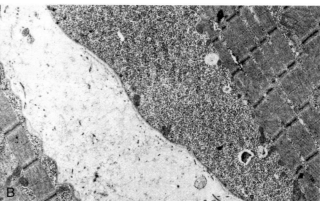

Figure 19-26 **Infantile muscle phosphorylase deficiency: muscle biopsy from an affected infant who died at 13 weeks of age. A,** Transverse section shows many fibers containing subsarcolemmal vacuoles *(arrowheads)* (modified Gomori trichrome stain, × 500). **B,** Electron micrograph of longitudinal section shows granular, subsarcolemmal glycogen deposit (× 7500). *(From DiMauro S, Hartlage PL: Fatal infantile form of muscle phosphorylase deficiency,* Neurology *28:1124-1129, 1978.)*

exercise intolerance, muscle cramps, fatigue, and myoglobinuria. However, several examples of a severe infantile form of phosphofructokinase deficiency were reported.[477-481] In the initial report, two siblings, born to related parents, were described with hypotonia and weakness, worse in the upper extremities, from the first days of life. Muscle contractures developed rapidly. One infant died at 6 months of age with respiratory complications, and the other, alive at 14 months at the time of report, could not sit without support. In subsequent reports, three infants were described with progressive weakness and hypotonia, with death at 7, 21, and 21 months, respectively.[479,480] One infant exhibited cortical blindness and seizures, and another had mental retardation.[478,479] The third infant was treated with a ketogenic diet from 4 months of age and was alive and improving at 2 years of age.[481] Muscle specimens showed subsarcolemmal vacuoles that were PAS positive. Glycogen accumulation was demonstrated by biochemical techniques, and muscle phosphofructokinase activity was severely depressed.

Disorders of Lipid Metabolism. Defects in the utilization of fatty acids, the steps for which are outlined in Table 19-14, result in several disorders with hypotonia and weakness in the neonatal period or early infancy.[4,398,466,482-494]

Most of the patients reported with all the defects listed in Table 19-14 exhibit clinical features long after the neonatal period. Even those with neonatal onset manifest, in addition to hypotonia, more prominent features such as stupor or coma, cardiac failure, or congenital malformations (see Chapter 15). Moreover, all but one of the disorders include features more characteristic of a metabolic disorder (hypoketotic hypoglycemia, hyperammonemia) and are discussed as such in Chapter 15. However, the defect of the carnitine transporter (i.e., primary carnitine deficiency) manifests clinically primarily as myopathy involving skeletal and cardiac muscle and thus is discussed here.

TABLE 19-14 Metabolic Defects in Fatty Acid Oxidation

Carnitine transporter*
Carnitine palmitoyltransferase I
Carnitine-acylcarnitine translocase
Carnitine palmitoyltransferase II
Very-long-chain acyl-CoA dehydrogenase*
Long-chain acyl-CoA dehydrogenase
Medium-chain acyl-CoA dehydrogenase*
Short-chain acyl-CoA dehydrogenase*
Multiple acyl-CoA dehydrogenase*
Long-chain 3-hydroxy acyl-CoA dehydrogenase
Short-chain 3-hydroxy acyl-CoA dehydrogenase
Acetoacetyl-CoA thiolase (beta-ketothiolase)*
3-Oxoacid: CoA transferase
Hydroxymethylglutaryl-CoA lyase*

See text for references.
*Prominent hypotonia and weakness may occur in the neonatal period.
CoA, coenzyme A.

Primary Carnitine Deficiency (Carnitine Transporter Deficiency). This disorder is usually characterized by the onset of cardiomyopathy in late infancy or early childhood, but onset in the first 2 months of life is well documented.[398,484,485,493,495,496] The major features of this disorder are weakness, hypotonia, and cardiomyopathy. Decreasing fasting ketosis or hypoketotic hypoglycemia may develop. Progression to death may occur if treatment with carnitine is not instituted. Muscle histology demonstrates subsarcolemmal and intermyofibrillar vacuoles that contain lipid (Fig. 19-27). Carnitine levels in muscle and serum are depressed.

The nature of the defect in primary carnitine deficiency involves impairment of transport of carnitine into muscle.[483] Studies of cultured fibroblasts showed a defect in the specific high-affinity, carrier-mediated carnitine uptake mechanism (i.e., the carnitine transporter).[398,484,486,493,496] *Management* of primary carnitine deficiency is based particularly on treatment with oral carnitine.[398,484,487] Prolonged duration of therapy is necessary.

RESTRICTED NEUROMUSCULAR DISORDERS

Several disorders of the neuromuscular apparatus are restricted to a small portion of the motor system. Some restricted disorders are clearly related to traumatic insults and are discussed in Chapter 22. *Restricted disorders that are not established as caused principally by trauma are considered next.*

Congenital Ptosis

Clinical Features. *Ptosis* is the most common of the congenital nonprogressive neuromuscular syndromes restricted to the ocular region that are likely to manifest in the newborn period (Table 19-15). The disorder is usually familial and is transmitted in an autosomal dominant or an X-linked dominant manner. In both cases, male and female infants are affected equally. Involvement is unilateral in approximately 75% of cases. Patterns of weakness are consistent within families; thus, in one pedigree, left unilateral predominance was striking.[497] In a large pedigree of 96 people, 49 had congenital ptosis, and 92% of those had bilateral involvement.[498] Superior rectus weakness also may be present; when this weakness accompanies the ptosis, it is on the same side as the levator palpebrae weakness.

Pathology. The anatomical locus of the defect generally is considered to be in the muscle of the levator palpebrae, rather than in the third nerve or nucleus thereof. In support of the myogenic theory are the histological abnormalities in the levator muscle and the lack of abnormalities in other structures (e.g., pupil[499]) innervated by the third nerve.[499,500] However, the possibility that the primary abnormality involves an impairment of the caudal central subnucleus of the third nerve with secondary changes in muscle has not been clarified.

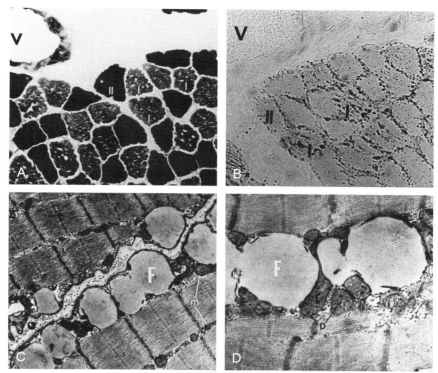

Figure 19–27 Muscle carnitine deficiency with lipid myopathy: muscle biopsy from an affected infant who died at 28 months of age. **A**, Histochemical preparation shows that vacuoles are predominantly in type I fibers (II, type II fibers; V, blood vessels) (adenosine triphosphatase stain, pH 9.3, × 200). **B**, Vacuoles stain positively for lipid (oil red O stain, × 200). **C**, Electron micrograph shows numerous fat vacuoles in the subsarcolemmal area (F, fat; m, mitochondria) (× 14,600). **D**, Electron micrograph shows rows of lipid vacuoles (F) in intermyofibrillar spaces. Multiple electron-dense granules (D) are visible in some of the mitochondria (× 45,000). *(From Hart ZH, Chang CH, DiMauro S, Farooki Q, et al: Muscle carnitine deficiency and fatal cardiomyopathy, Neurology 28:147-151, 1978.)*

Pathogenesis and Etiology. The pathogenesis of the disorder in the typical autosomal dominant case involves a gene on chromosome 1 *(PTOS1)*.[501,502] The X-linked locus is at chromosome Xq24-q27.1 *(PTOS2)*.[501,502]

Management. No specific therapy exists. In examples of severe congenital ptosis with the risk of secondary amblyopia, a surgical corrective procedure for the lid is carried out between 6 months and 5 years of age.[501]

Congenital Unilateral Third Nerve Palsy

Clinical Features. The designation *congenital unilateral third nerve palsy* refers to those cases of unilateral and isolated third nerve palsies apparent from birth. This lesion is not common, although it is frequently not recognized until after the neonatal period. In contrast to congenital ptosis, only uncommonly is congenital third nerve palsy familial (2 of 16 cases in one series).

TABLE 19-15	Congenital Nonprogressive Ocular Syndromes
Ptosis	
Unilateral third nerve palsy	
Congenital fibrosis of the extraocular muscles	
Duane retraction syndrome	
Other ocular disorders (see text)	

A very small proportion of cases can be related to orbital trauma (1 of 16 cases in one series).[503] The lateral deviation of the affected eye may be confused with comitant exotropia. The usual position of the eye, however, is downward as well as outward. The oculomotor deficits involve medial and upward gaze particularly, and, in addition, ptosis and pupillary dilation are present in the majority of cases. Later in infancy, signs of aberrant reinnervation of third nerve structures are apparent (e.g., constriction of pupil on attempted upward gaze or widening of the palpebral fissure on attempted medial gaze).

Pathology. The anatomical locus of the lesion in the common unilateral case often is considered to be outside the brain stem because of the general absence of other signs of brain stem involvement (e.g., contralateral hemiparesis) and the presence of aberrant regeneration.[503] However, a disturbance of development of the neurons of the nucleus, as in the congenital fibrosis syndromes (see later), is certainly possible. The usual involvement of the entire third nerve complex excludes a lesion after the bifurcation within the orbit, and the absence of concomitant involvement of the fourth and sixth nerves also suggests that the portion within the cavernous sinus is not the site. Thus, the lesion probably involves the third nerve nucleus or nerve between its exit from the brain stem and its entrance into the cavernous sinus. The pathological substrate is unclear.

Rarely, a prenatal mesencephalic infarct produces a congenital nuclear syndrome of the oculomotor nerve, with contralateral hemiparesis and aberrant regeneration.[504] In addition, a rare bilateral case of congenital partial third nerve palsy secondary to a mesencephalic malformation was reported.[505]

Pathogenesis and Etiology. The pathogenesis of the usual case is unknown, but the possibility has been raised that the nerve is injured by cranial deformations during labor and delivery, perhaps at the site of its course over the tentorial edge.[503] As just noted, a prenatal ischemic lesion of the brain stem or mesencephalic anomaly rarely is responsible.[504,505]

Management. Management may include surgical correction of the ptosis, which can be severe, and of the lateral eye deviation. It is critical in the neonatal period to be sure that an intracranial process, such as a supratentorial lesion (e.g., hematoma) leading to herniation of temporal lobe through the tentorial notch and compression of the third nerve, is not present.

Congenital Fibrosis of the Extraocular Muscles

Clinical Features. Congenital fibrosis of the extraocular muscles (CFEOM) syndromes are characterized by congenital, bilateral ptosis, and a *restrictive* external ophthalmoplegia, with eyes partially or completely fixed in a strabismic position.[501,502,506-508] Limitation of extraocular movement in both eyes is pronounced, and forced duction tests reveal marked restriction of globe movement in all directions. The limitations are nonprogressive. When affected infants develop consistent visual fixation and following, the head is held in an extended position to compensate for the marked ptosis. Two clinical phenotypes are most common, designated CFEOM1 and CFEOM2. CFEOM1 is characterized by congenital bilateral ptosis and external ophthalmoplegia, (with pupillary sparing, i.e., not internal ophthalmoplegia). The primary position of the eyes is downward, and patients have a restricted upward gaze and a variably restricted horizontal gaze. In CFEOM2, in addition to the bilateral ptosis, marked exotropia occurs, with severely limited horizontal and vertical eye movements. The only normally functioning extraocular muscle is the abducens-innervated lateral rectus that allows outward movement of each eye.

Pathology. Because of the marked fibrosis of the extraocular muscles, it was assumed until the past 10 years that these disorders were basically myopathic. In CFEOM1, careful neuropathological study showed an absence of the superior divisions of the third cranial nerves and corresponding alpha motor neurons in midbrain, with presumably secondary abnormalities of the superior rectus and levator palpebrae superioris muscles, normally innervated by this branch and responsible for elevation of the eye and eyelid.[506,508] In CFEOM2, it appears likely that abnormal development

of both the oculomotor and trochlear nuclei is responsible for all eye movements except abduction.[508]

Pathogenesis and Etiology. The pathological defects suggest that these disorders reflect *abnormality in the development of the extraocular muscle lower motor neuron system.*[506,508] CFEOM1, an autosomal dominant disorder, is related to heterozygous mutations in *K1F21A*, a developmental kinesin.[508] Kinesins are molecular motors that transport molecules along microtubules. The CFEOM1 defect appears to be in axonal targeting to the extraocular muscles. CFEOM2, an autosomal recessive disorder, is caused by mutations in *PHOX2A*, which encodes a homeodomain transcription factor necessary for development of the oculomotor and trochlear nerves.

Management. Management is difficult and primarily involves surgical attempts to improve the bilateral ptosis.

Duane Retraction Syndrome

Clinical Features. *Duane syndrome* is an uncommon congenital disorder of ocular motility with the following characteristics: (1) limitation of abduction of the eye and (2) retraction of the eye into the orbit and consequent narrowing of the palpebral fissure on adduction.[500,501,509] Thus, this disorder is another type of congenital *restrictive* ophthalmoparesis, akin to CFEOM. Additional oculomotor findings may include protrusion of the globe and widening of the palpebral fissure on attempted abduction and downward or upward deviation of the eyes with adduction. Approximately 80% of cases are unilateral. The left eye is involved approximately twice as commonly as the right.[500] Approximately 5% to 10% of cases are familial, and inheritance in such cases is autosomal dominant.[510,511]

At least one other congenital malformation accompanies approximately 33% of cases, and 8% of patients have three or more additional anomalies.[511] The anomalies are principally skeletal, auricular, or ocular.[511-513] Major skeletal anomalies include vertebral, palatal, and upper extremity defects (e.g., Klippel-Feil anomaly, cervical spina bifida, cleft palate, and anomalies of thumb, radius, and ulna). Auricular anomalies include malformed pinna, auricular appendages, and malformed inner ear with accompanying deafness. Ocular defects include microphthalmia, coloboma, heterochromia iridis, and congenital cataract. Several syndromes are recognized with varying combinations of these anomalies in association with Duane syndrome.[501,502,508,508a]

Pathology. Analogous to the abnormality in CFEOM (see earlier discussion), Duane syndrome is associated with an absence of the abducens nerve and its corresponding abducens nucleus in the pons, with presumably secondary abnormalities in the lateral rectus muscle, the abductor of the eye.[508,514,515] The fibrosis of the lateral rectus has been thought to cause the retraction of the globe on attempted adduction. The Chiari I malformation was reported in two episodic cases of Duane retraction syndrome, perhaps through involvement of the abducens nerve.[508,516,517]

Pathogenesis and Etiology. As in CFEOM, the pathological defect suggests that Duane retraction syndrome and its several variants are related to an abnormality in the development of the extraocular muscle lower motor neuron system. The occasional familial occurrence and the not infrequent association with anomalies of certain skeletal, auricular, and ocular structures also are consistent with a defect in embryogenesis. Cross and Pfaffenbach[512] emphasized that the sixth nerves and nuclei are developing between the fourth and eighth weeks of gestation, during a period when the eyes, auditory structures, palate, vertebrae, and distal upper extremities are also evolving. Identification of the genes responsible for several of the syndromic variants of Duane syndrome suggests that the disorders relate to disturbances of nuclear development and axonal targeting.[508,518]

Management. Management should include a careful evaluation of skeletal, auditory, and ocular structures to detect accompanying abnormalities.

Other Ocular Disorders

Other ocular disorders may be observed in the neonatal period but are generally rare. Congenital Horner syndrome, unassociated with brachial plexus palsy (see Chapter 22), may occur[519]; association with cervical neuroblastoma has been reported.[520,521] Congenital abducens (lateral rectus palsy) may be observed as an isolated finding, although association with Duane retraction syndrome or Möbius syndrome is common.[522] Congenital fourth nerve palsy usually escapes detection in the neonatal period (the eye is deviated vertically and medially); anomaly of the brain stem may be present.[523]

Möbius Syndrome

Clinical Features. *Möbius syndrome*, or *congenital facial diplegia syndrome*, described in 1888 by Möbius,[524] consists of facial diplegia and abducens palsies, which are usually bilateral (Table 19-16). Although the essential features of the syndrome are rather restricted, the disorder is accompanied by a variety of neuromuscular and other abnormalities. At first glance, confusion may exist with other disorders of the motor unit with prominent facial weakness (e.g., myasthenias, congenital myotonic dystrophy, CMD, FSHD, nemaline myopathy, myotubular myopathy, congenital fiber type disproportion, and cytochrome c oxidase deficiency [mitochondrial myopathy]). However, associated features usually allow clinical distinction in the newborn period.

The *clinical findings* are striking (see Table 19-16).[525-547] The *facial weakness* is essentially always bilateral and severe. In approximately one third of patients, the face

TABLE 19-16	Clinical Features of Möbius Syndrome*	
Clinical Feature		**Percentage of Total**
Congenital facial diplegia		100%
Upper = lower†		35%
Upper > lower		63%
Lower > upper		2%
Abducens palsy		100%
Total external ophthalmoplegia		10%
Oculomotor palsy		20%
Ptosis (bilateral)		10%
Tongue weakness		75%
Talipes equinovarus		30%
Hand or arm malformation		40%
Pectoralis hypoplasia		10%

*See text for references.
†Usually complete or near-complete facial paralysis.

is essentially immobile. In at least 60% of patients, the upper part of the face is affected more severely than the lower. The eyes cannot be closed, and the face is smooth and expressionless. The severe involvement of the face prevents formation of a proper seal around the nipple, and feeding difficulty in the newborn period is a major problem.

Abducens palsy, present essentially invariably, is almost always bilateral. In a smaller percentage of cases, total external ophthalmoplegia is present, and, in some patients, lateral gaze palsies (i.e., conjugate weakness) appear to be present. Oculomotor nerve involvement is apparent in 20% and bilateral ptosis in 10% of patients. Involvement of tongue is relatively common, associated with atrophy and bilateral in approximately half of patients.

Other neuromuscular abnormalities are frequent. Thus, talipes equinovarus occurs in approximately one third; in a few patients, more widespread arthrogryposis may be present. Hypoplasia of the pectoralis muscle, always unilateral, occurs in approximately 10% to 15% of patients, and when it is associated with syndactyly of the hand, it constitutes *Poland syndrome*. Hand and arm malformations (e.g., brachydactyly and syndactyly) are present in approximately 40% of patients. Rarer patients with Möbius syndrome have the marked micrognathia of the Robin sequence, congenital myopathy, developmental delay, and other features of Carey-Fineman-Ziter syndrome.[548-551] Central respiratory dysfunction requiring mechanical ventilation was observed in 13 patients with Möbius syndrome, 7 of whom died because of respiratory failure.[542] Mental retardation has been reported in 10% to 30% of infants. Autistic spectrum disorders have been observed in 25% to 40%.[546] This finding is of particular note because brain stem disturbance has been postulated as a pathogenic mechanism in autism.[546]

Pathology. The anatomical sites of the pathological features are diverse and may include cranial nerve nuclei, roots, nerves, or muscle. Involvements of cranial nerve nuclei have included apparent developmental hypoplasia or aplasia and

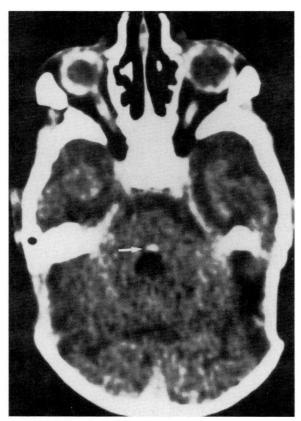

Figure 19-28 Möbius syndrome. This computed tomography scan shows symmetric dorsal pontine calcifications *(arrow)*. *(From D'Cruz OF, Swisher CN, Jaradeh S, Tang T, et al: Mobius syndrome: Evidence for a vascular etiology,* J Child Neurol *8:260-265, 1993.)*

destructive lesions.[526,527,529,532-534,538-540,543,545,547,552-562] By far the leading abnormalities have been aplasia or hypoplasia of cranial nerve nuclei, sometimes in combination with brain stem hypoplasia, or focal necroses, usually with calcification, involving cranial nerve nuclei. Primary involvement of peripheral nerve or muscle is very uncommon. Abnormalities of brain stem conduction times with testing of brain stem auditory evoked responses, and other electrophysiological measures, have provided in vivo functional correlates of the neuropathology.[526,540,563] CT may show calcification at the site of ischemic necrosis in brain stem, usually in the region of the dorsal pons (Fig. 19-28). MRI provides details of brain stem morphology, including hypoplasia or necroses. Involvement of cranial nerves has included apparent developmental hypoplasia or aplasia (with normal cranial nerve nuclei) and possible demyelinative neuropathy.[564,565] Involvement of muscle has included apparent primary hypoplasia or aplasia.[566]

Pathogenesis and Etiology. The pathogenesis of the syndrome is undoubtedly heterogenous, understandable in view of the multiple sites of pathology. Both developmental aberrations and destructive processes appear to be operative. The latter appear to be more common and include intrauterine ischemic brain stem injury, for which neuropathological and brain

imaging data are abundant (see earlier discussion). An ischemic event at approximately 5 to 6 weeks of gestation appears to be very important. Thus, one case occurred after a maternal overdose of ergotamine on day 39 of gestation. Exposure to a similar agent in the first 2 months of gestation was associated with Möbius syndrome or limb reduction deficits, or both, in seven other cases.[567] Also supportive of an insult during the fourth to eighth weeks, especially at 5 to 6 weeks of gestation, is the presence of muscle, limb defects, and heart anomalies. It is relevant in this context that the brain stem forms and differentiates rapidly during weeks 5 and 6 and that blood flow changes from the primitive trigeminal circulation to the vertebral arteries. Investigators have hypothesized that, during this period, the pontomesencephalic and pontomedullary tegmental areas, the sites of the affected cranial nerve nuclei, become watershed areas and are thereby vulnerable to ischemic insult.[540] It is quite possible that most cases are related to vascular disturbance, with hypoplasias and aplasias the response early in utero and necrosis and calcification later, when fetal inflammatory mechanisms develop.

A few cases have been familial, including autosomal dominant and, perhaps, autosomal recessive inheritance.[502,568,569] A pedigree described with seven affected members and a reciprocal translocation between chromosomes 1 and 13, demonstrable by banding techniques, suggested that cytogenetic investigation should be considered in the evaluation of affected patients.[570] Several other loci have been identified, but responsible genes have not been identified.[571] A disturbance of rhombencephalic development is suggested by some of the neuropathological features, and such lesions represent good candidates for defects in homeobox genes. This notion received support by the description of a rare, Möbius-like syndrome characterized by bilateral Duane syndrome, facial weakness, sensorineural hearing loss, hypoventilation, mental retardation, and autism spectrum disorder in association with aberrant hindbrain segmentation. The gene involved was *HOXA1*, which functions in hindbrain patterning.[508,508a,572] As postulated in Möbius syndrome, abnormalities of vascular development were demonstrated.[572]

Management. Management requires particular attention to feeding techniques. In addition, poor eye closure may result in conjunctival irritation, and thus appropriate eye drops are needed. Later, surgical correction for the severe facial paralysis may be beneficial.[501,573]

Congenital Hypoplasia of Depressor Anguli Oris Muscle

Clinical Features. *Congenital hypoplasia of the depressor anguli oris muscle* is characterized by an asymmetrical crying facies (Fig. 19-29). The defect is present in approximately 0.5% to 1.0% of newborn infants.[574-576a] The essential clinical finding is a failure of one corner of the mouth to move downward and outward,

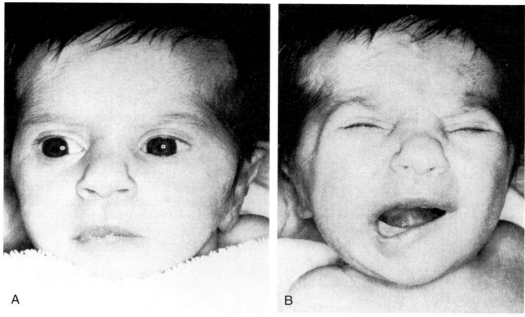

A   B

Figure 19-29 **Asymmetrical crying facies. A,** At rest, the infant's face is symmetrical. **B,** During crying, left corner of the mouth fails to move down and laterally. (From Pape KE, Pickering D: Asymmetric crying facies: An index of other congenital anomalies, J Pediatr 81:21-30, 1972.)

particularly during cry or grimace.[576-580] Other functions of the facial muscles, such as frowning, eye closure, and nasolabial fold depth, are normal. The left side of the face is affected in nearly 80% of cases.[580] The appearance of the face during cry or grimace may lead to the mistaken notion that the patient has facial palsy on the side *opposite* the defect, because the normally functioning muscles, in pulling the corner of the mouth downward and outward, may cause the appearance of lower facial drooping on that normal side. On follow-up, the defect may be less obvious as smiling and other aspects of facial expression become more prominent. A very broad smile or grimace is necessary to elicit the defect in the older child or adult.

The major clinical significance relates to an *association of the lesion with major congenital anomalies*, especially in the cardiovascular system.[566,574,576,576a,580-588] Although the reported incidence of the facial defect and the associated anomalies have varied according to the selection of patients, a prospective study of 6487 newborn infants resulted in 44 cases.[575] Of these, 3 (6.8%) had cardiac defects (versus 0.45% of controls). The total number with congenital anomalies was 9 (20%), compared with 2.7% of controls. In a hospital-based population, the incidence of anomalies was 70%, and the most common of these were generally minor anomalies of ear and face.[580] The proportion with cardiac anomalies in this more selected population was 44%. The cardiac anomalies have been diverse; approximately 50% have consisted of ventricular septal defect (15% to 25%), tetralogy of Fallot, patent ductus arteriosus, and coarctation of the aorta.[576a,580,583] Most of the remaining 50% have been atrial septal defects. Other reported anomalies

include genitourinary, musculoskeletal (especially vertebral), and, rarely, CNS defects. The latter include agenesis of the corpus callosum, mega cisterna magna, and cerebral and cerebellar atrophy.[576,576a,585,588]

The occurrence of the defect in 5% to 10% of infants with congenital heart disease led to the designation *cardiofacial syndrome*.[566] Cayler cardiofacial syndrome is one of a group of conditions linked to a microdeletion in the long arm of chromosome 22.[586,587] These syndromes are grouped by the term CATCH22 (Cardiac defects, Abnormal facies, Thymic hyperplasia, Cleft palate, and Hypocalcemia) and include DiGeorge velocardiofacial and Takas syndromes.[586]

Pathology. The anatomical locus of the defect is the depressor anguli oris muscle and probably represents hypoplasia, although no pathological documentation is available. The EMG reveals paucity of motor units but no fibrillations or other signs of disease of nerve or anterior horn cell. The likelihood of muscle hypoplasia or aplasia is supported further by the occurrence in one family of a mother with aplasia of the left tensor fasciae latae muscle, a child with right hemidiaphragmatic hypoplasia, and another child with aplasia of left depressor anguli oris muscle.[579]

Pathogenesis and Etiology. The pathogenesis is unclear. The possibility of an inherited defect was suggested by reports of familial occurrence with autosomal dominant characteristics.[575] This defect is readily overlooked unless family members are specifically examined for the lesion. Moreover, the occurrence in one family of a mother and two children with aplasia or hypoplasia of different muscles (including the depressor anguli oris; see previous section) further supports the possibility of autosomal dominant inheritance with variable expression. In Cayler syndrome, 94% of probands have a de novo deletion of 22q11.2, and 6% have inherited the deletion from a parent.[586] Thus, fluorescent in situ hybridization analysis should be carried out on patients with asymmetric crying facies and cardiac anomalies, and the parents' karyotypes should be evaluated if a deletion is found in the infant.

Management. Management essentially is based on ensuring that no other major congenital anomaly is present. An abdominal ultrasound scan to look for visceral anomaly or a neuroblastoma also may be appropriate.

Vocal Cord Paralysis

Vocal cord paralysis, or so-called *laryngeal paralysis*, is a relatively common neonatal disorder.[589-593] Most descriptions of clinical features, etiology, natural history, and therapy are contained in the otolaryngological literature, and surprisingly few descriptions are contained in the pediatric literature. Data for newborn patients, distinct from older patients, are difficult to obtain, but a reasonable synthesis of current information follows.

Clinical Features. The major presenting sign is stridor, which is inspiratory and crowing and is present in approximately 70% of cases. Severe airway obstruction with a need for immediate intubation occurs in approximately 45% of affected infants. Dysphonia, notable with crying, dysphagia, and aspiration are less common. Approximately 40% to 50% of cases are unilateral, and, when unilateral, the left side is affected in 80% to 90% of cases. The course of the disorder relates largely to cause (see "Pathogenesis and Etiology"). The diagnosis is established by laryngoscopy.

Pathology. The anatomical locus of the pathology is diverse, although few precise data are available. Consideration of probable causes (Table 19-17) suggests that disease at several levels of the neuraxis may be responsible, and levels vary from bilateral upper motor neuron, cranial nuclear (nucleus ambiguus), cranial nerve root (vagal nerve roots), and peripheral nerve (vagus nerve and laryngeal branches).

Pathogenesis and Etiology. The major causes of vocal cord paralysis in the newborn are shown in Table 19-17. Most commonly, no clear cause is apparent. Most such cases resolve spontaneously over a period of weeks or months.[589] Chiari type 2 malformation associated with myelomeningocele accounts for approximately 20% of cases. In these patients, the syndrome most often evolves several weeks after birth, after correction of the myelomeningocele, in association with the development of hydrocephalus with intracranial hypertension. Vocal cord paralysis often

TABLE 19-17	Etiology of Vocal Cord Paralysis in the Newborn*	
Cause		**Percentage of Total**
Unknown		35%
Chiari type 2 malformation with myelomeningocele		20%
Associated with miscellaneous neurological disorders		20%
Associated with laryngeal anomalies		10%
Birth trauma		10%
Other		5%

*Based on 208 cases.
Data from Holinger LD, Holinger PC, Holinger PH: Etiology of bilateral abductor vocal cord paralysis: A review of 389 cases, *Ann Otol Rhinol Laryngol* 85:428–436, 1976; and Cohen SR, Birns JW, Geller KA, Thompson JW: Laryngeal paralysis in children: A long-term retrospective study, *Ann Otol Rhinol Laryngol* 91:417-424, 1982.

improves after placement of ventriculoperitoneal shunt and is presumably related to the deformation of the lower brain stem (see Chapter 1). Approximately 20% of infants with vocal cord paralysis have miscellaneous neurological disorders (e.g., cerebral developmental anomalies and Möbius syndrome), which appear to account for the paralysis (see Table 19-17). The 10% of affected infants with associated laryngeal anomalies presumably have a developmental disturbance of the peripheral neuromuscular apparatus in the larynx. The infants with birth trauma usually exhibit signs earliest (i.e., in the first days of life).[590] The likelihood of recovery is good (see Chapter 22). Among other causes worthy of note are the association of unilateral vocal cord paralysis with congenital heart defects complicated by pulmonary hypertension and presumed compression of the recurrent laryngeal nerve by the enlarged, tense pulmonary artery *(cardiovocal syndrome)*.[594] Injury to the recurrent laryngeal nerve or vagus nerve, or both, in association with the neck dissection required for the institution of extracorporeal membrane oxygenation has been reported in approximately 3% of infants undergoing this procedure.[591] In this circumstance, the paralysis is on the right side (i.e., the side of the dissection), unlike the predominantly left-sided paralysis in most cases of unilateral vocal cord paralysis (see earlier discussion). Familial cases are rare, but autosomal dominant, X-linked recessive, and autosomal recessive examples have been observed.[593]

Management. Unilateral paralysis generally requires no treatment, and, even when recovery does not occur, compensation by the normal vocal cord allows adequate phonation. Bilateral paralysis requires very close surveillance. An artificial airway should be placed if ventilatory compromise appears imminent. Infants with bilateral vocal cord paralysis may die unexpectedly, particularly if the lesion is taken lightly. A need for long-term tracheostomy is not unusual.

Congenital Isolated Pharyngeal Dysfunction

Clinical Features. Severe impairment of swallowing in a newborn is a life-threatening event. Causes of such impairment include structural malformations of the nasal-oral cavity (e.g., choanal atresia, cleft palate), esophageal or tracheal-esophageal anomalies (e.g., tracheoesophageal fistula, esophageal stenosis, aberrant vessels related to the aortic arch), and a variety of neurological disorders (e.g., bilateral cerebral disorder, Chiari type II malformation, Möbius syndrome, myasthenia, merosin-deficient CMD, myotonic dystrophy, nemaline myopathy, myotubular myopathy). However, nearly all the neurological disorders are characterized by other, generally obvious neurological abnormalities. However, one striking defect (i.e., congenital isolated pharyngeal dysfunction) is confined to the pharyngeal musculature. Approximately 30 cases have been reported,[584,595-598] but the disorder may be overlooked frequently. Approximately half of all reported cases have been in premature infants. Because the disorder is transient, with spontaneous recovery reported in 2 to 40 months, it is crucial to recognize its presence and to institute measures to prevent aspiration and pneumonia, which have resulted in the death of several of the reported infants.

The usual presentation is the development of cyanosis and respiratory distress at the first attempts at feeding. The neurological examination is entirely unremarkable except for the total lack of spontaneous or elicited movements of the pharyngeal muscles and soft palate. Video fluoroscopy of swallowing demonstrates a normal oral propulsive phase but no pharyngeal movement and passive aspiration of contrast medium into the trachea. MRI has revealed no abnormality. The EMG of pharyngeal muscles has been normal.

Pathology. Careful study of the brain stem nuclei crucial for swallowing (e.g., nucleus ambiguus, dorsal nucleus of the vagus, nuclei of cranial nerves V, X, and XII, nucleus of the tractus solitarius, and adjacent ventromedian reticular formation in the medulla) has revealed no abnormality. Moreover, no abnormality of other central structures, cranial nerves, or muscles has been detected.

Pathogenesis and Etiology. The basic nature of congenital isolated pharyngeal dysfunction is unclear. An abnormality in the functioning of the nucleus ambiguus appears most likely. The abnormality may be at the receptor level, as shown by Kinney and co-workers in the arcuate nucleus of the ventral medulla in sudden infant death syndrome.[599]

Management. Cessation of attempts at oral feeding and institution of nasogastric tube feedings are crucial. I recommend a period of observation of at least 3 to 6 months with a nasogastric tube before placement of a gastrostomy or jejunostomy tube because more than one half of all affected infants, especially premature infants, recover within 6 months. Clinical improvement precedes radiological improvement,

and thus follow-up studies with barium swallow or video fluoroscopy may not provide an early indication of recovery.[598]

Congenital Torticollis

Clinical Features. *Congenital torticollis* is characterized by contracture of the sternocleidomastoid muscle, with resultant lateral flexion of the neck toward the lesion and slight rotation of the neck with the chin away from the side of the lesion.[4,600-607] The prominent feature of the syndrome is the head tilt. In association with the tilt of the head, asymmetries of the face and skull usually evolve and include flattening of the face and ear on the side of the lesion and flattening of the occiput on the opposite side (the side of contact of the skull with the bed; see Chapter 3). The rhomboidal skull (i.e., plagiocephaly) usually improves spontaneously with rapid brain and skull growth in the first 5 to 6 months of life if active motility and physical therapy supervene. Most infants can hold the head in the midline position after several weeks.[608] Only occasionally do patients have localized swelling of the sternocleidomastoid muscle in the neonatal period, but, when present, this fusiform mass may be quite prominent after 2 to 4 weeks. Although the mass is not usually apparent in the newborn, ultrasonography reveals findings consistent with fibrosis.[606] The mass usually disappears gradually by approximately 6 to 8 months of age. In the neonatal period, the muscle often appears shortened, may feel fibrous, and may resist stretch.

Pathology. The anatomical locus of the disease is usually confined to the sternocleidomastoid muscle, although occasionally the deep cervical muscles and trapezius appear to be involved (manifested by retraction of the head and elevation of the shoulder). The pathological features consist of fibrotic replacement of muscle tissue, but the remaining muscle appears normal.

Pathogenesis and Etiology. The pathogenesis of the disorder in previous years was considered most often to be hemorrhage within the muscle with subsequent fibrosis, but no histological proof of hemorrhage exists. The cause of such hemorrhage is not clear, although birth trauma is often cited. In a study of 311 infants, among those who presented within the first 6 weeks of life with a sternomastoid mass ($n = 195$), 52% had a history of breech presentation, forceps delivery, or vacuum extraction.[607] In another study of 510 infants, the infants with the most severe degree of torticollis had been born after breech presentation in 25% and after "vacuum extraction/forceps delivery" in 41%.[605] However, trauma is often difficult to document, and Eng[601] suggested that any difficulties observed with delivery relate to the already established intrauterine deformity secondarily disturbing engagement of the head during labor. This possibility could underlie the high frequency of breech presentations reported. In a careful study of 34 patients with congenital torticollis, good evidence indicated that the deformity resulted from *aberrant intrauterine positioning* in 29%, and evidence was suggestive in an additional 41%.[608] Further support for intrauterine constraint as the major cause of congenital torticollis is derived from a well-studied infant born to a mother with a large uterine leiomyoma.[609] Hemorrhage into the sternocleidomastoid from vascular anomaly may account for the 18% of infants with congenital torticollis with cavernous hemangioma of face and neck in one series.[608]

Management. Management consists of physical therapy, with emphasis on two basic exercises: (1) stretching of the clavicular portion of the sternocleidomastoid muscle by lateral flexion of the head to the opposite side and (2) stretching of the sternal portion of the muscle by rotation of the chin toward the affected side. Performance of the exercises in the prone position is easier than in the supine position and is preferable.[4] Active stretching exercises may be tolerated more readily than the passive stretching exercises just described; the former exercises involve encouraging the infant to rotate the neck to bottle or breast (when the infant's shoulders are stabilized) through visual cues of the nipple or bottle and rooting reflex.[608] Faithful physical therapy is successful in preventing facial and skull deformities and in relieving the contracture in most cases. In one large series ($n = 311$), 95% of infants experienced total resolution by 6.5 months.[607] Early onset of physical therapy is important. Rarely, botulinum toxin (Botox) injections may be considered. Neglected patients may require tenotomy and develop deformities. Plagiocephaly that persists after 5 to 6 months can be improved markedly by fitting the infant with an individualized plastic helmet to use the remaining brain growth to redirect head growth over approximately the next 6 months (see Chapter 3).[608]

Isolated Diaphragmatic Myopathy

Although most examples of isolated diaphragmatic paralysis in the newborn are related to trauma (see Chapter 22) or to aplasia, at least one case has been described in which a disorder of muscle appeared to be restricted to the diaphragm.[610] The infant exhibited respiratory distress with excessive movement of ribs but no movement of diaphragm. The EMG and the serum CK level were normal. Plication of the diaphragm was attempted at 2 months of age, but the infant died at 3 months. At postmortem examination, no abnormality of anterior horn cells, spinal nerve roots, or phrenic nerves could be found. Histological examination of a variety of peripheral muscles was normal. However, the diaphragm, which was very atrophic, exhibited marked random variation in fiber size and degenerating and necrotic muscle fibers. The findings were compatible with a myopathic process. Seven similar cases have been described recently.[610a] The possibility of myopathy restricted to the diaphragm should thus be considered in infants with respiratory distress secondary to diaphragmatic dysfunction.

Congenital Central Hypoventilation Syndrome

Congenital central hypoventilation syndrome (CCHS), or *Ondine's curse*, is a disorder of ventilation, particularly during sleep, and is categorized here because the syndrome is manifested as a restricted defect of a motor function. However, the essential defect involves a critical *afferent* component of the ventilatory system, rather than of the neuromuscular apparatus per se. Many cases have been recorded in the literature.[611-637]

Clinical Features. The essential *clinical features* are as follows: (1) decreased ventilatory drive during sleep, with impaired response to hypercarbia and hypoxemia, and (2) no recognizable disease of brain stem (e.g., myelomeningocele), spinal cord (e.g., traumatic transection), or cardiopulmonary system to account for the ventilatory defect. Most patients present in the first days of life with the respiratory disturbance (i.e., hypoventilation), apnea with cyanosis, or both, particularly during sleep. Blood gas studies confirm the presence of hypoxemia and hypercarbia. The respiratory disturbance is most apparent during quiet (non-rapid eye movement [REM]) sleep when the ventilatory drive is most dependent on the response of medullary chemoreceptors to carbon dioxide. This basic defect of unresponsiveness of medullary chemoreceptors to carbon dioxide, however, is also often apparent in these infants during REM sleep. Indeed, some patients also hypoventilate during wakefulness.

Associated abnormalities have included Hirschsprung disease in at least 20% of cases and ganglioneuroblastoma or neuroblastoma in approximately 5%. Indeed CCHS, Hirschsprung disease, and neural crest-derived tumors constitute the major neurocristopathies (see later). Associated disturbances of swallowing, sometimes preceded by polyhydramnios, sensorineural hearing loss, and various ocular abnormalities (e.g., ptosis, pupillary dilation) occur in a distinct minority of infants. Additionally, careful studies of heart rate variability delineated abnormalities in all 12 cases in a series.[631] These findings enhance the notion of a disturbance in derivatives of the neural crest (i.e., autonomic neurons, sensory neurons, adrenal medullary neurons).

Not only is the relationship of the ventilatory syndrome with Hirschsprung disease an excellent example of this common pathogenesis, but also the combination probably accounts for more cases than previously suspected.[633] Indeed, CCHS complicates 1.5% of all cases of Hirschsprung disease and fully 10% of *severe* cases with total colonic aganglionosis. Approximately 15% to 20% of patients with CCHS and Hirschsprung disease have an associated neuroblastoma or ganglioneuroblastoma.[633]

Diagnosis. The diagnosis is established by the characteristic clinical features and by documentation of the ventilatory abnormalities and resulting blood gas derangements. In contrast to the lack of responsiveness of medullary chemoreceptors to carbon dioxide, the ventilatory response to oxygen through peripheral chemoreceptors is normal. Detailed evaluation to rule out structural disease of brain stem, spinal cord, phrenic nerves, diaphragm, intercostal muscles, and cardiopulmonary system is important. A search for neuroblastoma or ganglioneuroblastoma also is appropriate. Any suggestion of gastrointestinal dysfunction should lead to rectal biopsy to evaluate the possibility of Hirschsprung disease. Functional MRI studies have shown deficits in pontomedullary regions.[638]

Etiology. *Pathological studies*, in general, have demonstrated no consistent abnormalities. In a few cases, an ill-defined decrease in the number of medullary neurons or medullary gliosis has been noted.

Molecular genetic studies have clarified the *etiology* of the disorder. Thus, the gene involved is *PHOX2B* (a homeobox gene), which is crucial in the development of all autonomic neural crest derivatives. Although most cases are related to sporadic de novo mutations, the heterozygous genetic defect behaves as an autosomal dominant. *PHOX2B* is involved in Hirschsprung disease and in neuroblastoma.

Management. Management must begin with prompt detection and careful surveillance. It is important to correct both the hypoxemia and the hypercarbia to prevent the development of pulmonary hypertension and cor pulmonale. Treatment commonly has consisted of *mechanical ventilation*, particularly during sleep. *Diaphragmatic pacing* by stimulation of phrenic nerves has improved treatment while allowing the patient normal mobility and the parents convenient management at home. The apparatus consists of an external radio frequency transmitter, a subcutaneously implanted receiver to convert the radio frequency signal to an electrical current, and a stimulatory electrode on the phrenic nerve.[621,628,639] The effectiveness of this approach has been improved by using bilateral rather than unilateral pacing, by minimizing electrical injury to the phrenic nerve, and by using pacing only when necessary (e.g., during sleep) rather than continuously.[614,616,619,621,623,628] In the largest experience with diaphragmatic pacing, emphasis was placed on the complementary roles of phrenic nerve pacing and intermittent positive pressure ventilation, and the latter was used in patients with superimposed respiratory illness or inadequate ventilation while awake as well as asleep.

DISTINGUISHING FEATURES OF DISORDERS OF THE MOTOR SYSTEM

Definition of the anatomical level of the abnormality and of the likely pathology in neonatal disorders of the motor system is possible when one keeps in mind the relatively few distinguishing features (Table 19-18). Thus, the levels to be defined include those above the lower motor neuron (i.e., central), the anterior horn cell, the peripheral nerve, the neuromuscular junction, and the muscle. Distinguishing clinical features include the pattern of weakness,

the activity of tendon reflexes, the presence of fasciculations or sensory loss, CSF findings, the level of muscle enzymes in serum, the pattern on the EMG, nerve conduction velocities, and the histological appearance of the muscle biopsy (or, less commonly, nerve biopsy).

Disorders related to *central* causes (e.g., hypoxic-ischemic encephalopathy) are characterized by weakness of limbs (degree of weakness usually less striking than degree of hypotonia), relatively preserved tendon reflexes (which become hyperactive after the first months of life), and absence of fasciculations or abnormalities on examination of CSF, serum enzymes, EMG, nerve conduction velocities, and muscle biopsy. Other indicators of central disease (e.g., seizures, hemiparesis, and developmental failure) are important to identify. Disease of the *anterior horn cell (especially spinal muscular atrophy type I or Werdnig-Hoffmann disease)* is characterized by generalized weakness, *absent* reflexes, and *fasciculations* (especially of tongue) but normal sensory function, CSF examination, and serum enzyme levels. The EMG shows fasciculations, fibrillations, and other signs of denervation, and muscle biopsy demonstrates marked panfascicular atrophy (only uncommonly type grouping or grouped atrophy). Disease of *peripheral nerve* is characterized by weakness that often has a distal preponderance, depressed reflexes, *abnormal sensory examination, elevated CSF protein concentration*, and *depressed nerve conduction velocities.* Muscle biopsy demonstrates signs of denervation, and *nerve biopsy* shows usually hypomyelinative changes, with or without onion bulb formation. Disease of *neuromuscular junction* (e.g., myasthenia gravis) is characterized by weakness that involves the *face* and, perhaps, *extraocular* muscles, but normal reflexes (usually), sensory function, CSF examination, and serum enzyme levels are present. The *EMG* reveals the characteristic decremental response to repetitive stimulation. In botulism, the absence of *pupillary* reactions and the presence of an incremental response, the brief-duration, small-amplitude, overly abundant motor unit potentials pattern, or both, on the *EMG* are characteristic. Disease of *muscle* is characterized by weakness that often is greater in *proximal* limbs. Involvement of the *face* is prominent in several such disorders (e.g., myotonic dystrophy, CMD, FSHD, central core disease, nemaline myopathy, myotubular myopathy, congenital fiber type disproportion, and cytochrome c oxidase deficiency [mitochondrial myopathy]). Tendon reflexes are depressed in proportion to the weakness; no fasciculations or sensory or CSF abnormalities are present. *Muscle enzyme* concentrations in serum may be elevated, although in the slowly progressive disorders, this often is not detectable. The *EMG* exhibits myopathic changes and, perhaps, more distinctive abnormalities (e.g., myotonia). *Muscle biopsy* demonstrates myopathic changes and, in certain disorders, abnormalities that are diagnostic (e.g., central cores, rod bodies, myotubular fibers, disproportionate distribution and size of muscle fiber types, multi-minicores, abnormal mitochondria, or accumulation of glycogen or lipid).

TABLE 19-18   Distinguishing Features of Disorders of the Motor System

Locus of Lesion	WEAKNESS				Deep Tendon Reflexes	EMG	Muscle Biopsy	Other
	Face	Arms	Legs	Proximal-Distal				
Central	0	+	+	> or =	Normal or increased	Normal	Normal	Seizures, hemiparesis, and delayed development
Anterior horn cell	Late	++++	++++	> or =	0	Fasciculations and fibrillations	Denervation pattern	Fasciculations (tongue)
Peripheral nerve	0	+++	+++	<	Decreased	Fibrillations	Denervation pattern	Sensory deficit, elevated cerebrospinal fluid protein, depressed nerve conduction velocity, abnormal nerve biopsy
Neuromuscular junction	+++	+++	+++	=	Normal	Decremental response (myasthenia); incremental response and BSAP (botulism)	Normal	Response to neostigmine or edrophonium (myasthenia); constipation and fixed pupils (botulism)
Muscle	Variable (+ to ++++)	++	+	>	Decreased	Short duration, small amplitude motor unit potentials and myopathic polyphasic potentials	Myopathic pattern*	Elevated muscle enzyme levels (variable)

+ to ++++, varying degrees of severity; EMG, electromyography.

*May also show unique features, such as in central core disease, nemaline myopathy, myotubular myopathy, congenital fiber type disproportion, and multi-minicore disease.

Thus, with the aforementioned distinguishing features in mind, the clinician should be able to define the level of the lesion in the neuromuscular apparatus that accounts for the hypotonia and weakness in the infant. This critical initial accomplishment usually leads rapidly to the correct pathological and etiological diagnosis. Appropriate therapeutic intervention, specific or nonspecific, then becomes a relatively straightforward next step.

REFERENCES

1. Vanier TM: Dystrophia myotonica in childhood, *Br Med J* 2:1284-1288, 1960.
2. Sarnat HB, O'Connor T, Byrne PA: Clinical effects of myotonic dystrophy on pregnancy and the neonate, *Arch Neurol* 33:459-465, 1976.
3. Pearse RG, Howeler CJ: Neonatal form of dystrophia myotonica, *Arch Dis Child* 54:331-338, 1979.
4. Dubowitz V: *Muscle Disorders in Childhood*, 2nd ed, Philadelphia: 1995, Saunders.
5. Roig M, Balliu PR, Navarro C, Brugera R, et al: Presentation, clinical course, and outcome of the congenital form of myotonic dystrophy, *Pediatr Neurol* 11:208-213, 1994.
6. Erikson A, Forsberg H, Drugge U, Holmgren G: Outcome of pregnancy in women with myotonic dystrophy and analysis of CTG gene expansion, *Acta Paediatr* 84:416-418, 1995.
7. Rudnik-Schoneborn S, Nicholson GA, Morgan G, Rohrig D, et al: Different patterns of obstetric complications in myotonic dystrophy in relation to the disease status of the fetus, *Am J Med Genet* 80:314-321, 1998.
8. Dodge PR, Gamstorp I, Byers RK, Russell P: Myotonic dystrophy in infancy and childhood, *Pediatrics* 35:3-19, 1965.
9. Shore RN, MacLachlan TB: Pregnancy with myotonic dystrophy, *Obstet Gynecol* 38:448-454, 1971.
10. Dunn LJ, Dierker LI: Recurrent hydramnios in association with myotonia dystrophica, *Obstet Gynecol* 42:104-106, 1973.
11. Moosa A: The feeding difficulty in infantile myotonic dystrophy, *Dev Med Child Neurol* 16:824-825, 1974.
12. Hageman A, Gabreels F, Liem KD, Renkawek K, et al: Congenital myotonic dystrophy: A report on 13 cases and a review of the literature, *J Neurol Sci* 115:95-101, 1993.
13. Watters GV, Williams TW: Early onset myotonic dystrophy, *Arch Neurol* 17:137-152, 1967.
14. Swift TR, Ignacio OJ, Dyken PR: Neonatal dystrophia myotonica, *Am J Dis Child* 129:734-737, 1975.
15. Harper PS: Congenital myotonic dystrophy in Britain. I. Clinical aspects, *Arch Dis Child* 50:505-513, 1975.
16. Dubowitz V: *Muscle Disorders in Childhood*, Philadelphia: 1978, Saunders.
17. O'Brien TA, Harper PS: Course, prognosis and complications of childhood-onset myotonic dystrophy, *Dev Med Child Neurol* 26:62-67, 1984.

18. Connolly MB, Roland EH, Hill A: Clinical features for prediction of survival in neonatal muscle disease, *Pediatr Neurol* 8:285-294, 1992.
19. Fujii T, Yorifuji T, Okuno T, Toyokuni S, et al: Congenital myotonic dystrophy with progressive edema and hypoproteinemia, *Brain Dev* 13:58-60, 1991.
20. Curry CJ, Chopra D, Finer NN: Hydrops and pleural effusions in congenital myotonic dystrophy, *J Pediatr* 113:555-557, 1988.
21. Nicholson A, Rivlin E, Sims DG, Chiswick ML, et al: Developmental delay in congenital myotonic dystrophy after neonatal intensive care, *Early Hum Dev* 22:99-103, 1990.
22. Wesstrom G, Bensch J, Schollin J: Congenital myotonic dystrophy, *Acta Paediatr Scand* 75:849-854, 1986.
23. Harper PS, Rudel R: Myotonic dystrophy. In Engel AG, Franzini-Armstrong C, editors: *Myology*, New York: 1994, McGraw-Hill.
24. Moxley RT: Myotonic disorders in childhood: Diagnosis and treatment, *J Child Neurol* 12:116-129, 1997.
25. Moxley RT: Channelopathies affecting skeletal muscle: Myotonic disorders including myotonic dystrophy and periodic paralysis. In Jones HR Jr, DeVivo DC, Darras BT, editors: *Neuromuscular Disorders of Infancy, Childhood, and Adolescence: A Clinician's Approach*, Philadelphia: 2003, Butterworth Heinemann.
26. Campbell C, Sherlock R, Jacob P, Blayney M: Congenital myotonic dystrophy: Assisted ventilation duration and outcome, *Pediatrics* 113:811-816, 2004.
27. Bodensteiner JB, Grunow JE: Gastroparesis in neonatal myotonic dystrophy, *Muscle Nerve* 7:486, 1984.
28. Darin N, Kimber E, Kroksmark A-K, Tulinius M: Multiple congenital contractures: Birth prevalence, etiology, and outcome, *J Pediatr* 140:61-67, 2002.
29. Lenard HG, Goebel HH, Weigel W: Smooth muscle involvement in congenital myotonic dystrophy, *Neuropaediatrie* 8:42-52, 1977.
30. Joseph JT, Richards CS, Anthony DC, Upton M, et al: Congenital myotonic dystrophy pathology and somatic mosaicism, *Neurology* 49:1457-1460, 1997.
31. Igarashi H, Momoi MY, Yamagata T, Shiraishi H, et al: Hypertrophic cardiomyopathy in congenital myotonic dystrophy, *Pediatr Neurol* 18:366-369, 1998.
32. Dyken PR, Harper PS: Congenital dystrophia myotonica, *Neurology* 23:465-473, 1973.
33. Nakagawa M, Yamada H, Higuchi I, Kaminishi Y, et al: A case of paternally inherited congenital myotonic dystrophy, *J Med Genet* 31:397-400, 1994.
34. Ohya K, Tachi N, Chiba S, Sato T, et al: Congenital myotonic dystrophy transmitted from an asymptomatic father with a DM-specific gene, *Neurology* 44:1958-1960, 1994.
35. Tachi N, Ohya K, Yamagata H, Miki T, et al: Haplotype analysis of congenital myotonic dystrophy patients from asymptomatic DM father, *Pediatr Neurol* 16:315-318, 1997.
36. de Die-Smulders CE, Smeets HJ, Loots W, Anten HB, et al: Paternal transmission of congenital myotonic dystrophy, *J Med Genet* 34:930-933, 1997.
37. Tanaka Y, Suzuki Y, Shimozawa N, Nanba E, et al: Congenital myotonic dystrophy: Report of paternal transmission, *Brain Dev* 22:132-134, 2000.
38. Zeesman S, Carson N, Whelan DT: Paternal transmission of the congenital form of myotonic dystrophy type 1: A new case and review of the literature, *Am J Med Genet* 107:222-226, 2002.
39. Kuntz NL: Clinical and electrophysiologic profile of congenital myotonic dystrophy, *Ann Neurol* 19:931-939, 1984.
40. Chassevent J, Sauvegrain J, Besson-Leaud M, Kalifa G: Myotonic dystrophy (Steinert's disease) in the neonate, *Pediatr Radiol* 127:747-749, 1978.
41. Osborne JP, Murphy EG, Hill A: Thin ribs on chest x-ray: A useful sign in the differential diagnosis of the floppy newborn, *Dev Med Child Neurol* 25:343-345, 1983.
42. Regev R, de Vries LS, Heckmatt JZ, Dubowitz V: Cerebral ventricular dilation in congenital myotonic dystrophy, *J Pediatr* 111:372-376, 1987.
43. Garcia-Alix A, Cabanas F, Morales C, Pellicer A, et al: Cerebral abnormalities in congenital myotonic dystrophy, *Pediatr Neurol* 7:28-32, 1991.
44. Hashimoto T, Tayama M, Miyazaki M, Murakawa K, et al: Neuroimaging study of myotonic dystropy. I. Magnetic resonance imaging of the brain, *Brain Dev* 17:24-27, 1995.
45. Tanabe Y, Iai M, Tamai K, Fujimoto N, et al: Neuroradiological findings in children with congenital myotonic dystrophy, *Acta Paediatr* 81:613-617, 1992.
46. Kuo HC, Hsiao KM, Chen CJ, Hsieh YC, et al: Brain magnetic resonance image changes in a family with congenital and classic myotonic dystrophy, *Brain Dev* 27:291-296, 2005.
47. Hashimoto T, Tayama M, Yoshimoto T, Miyazaki M, et al: Proton magnetic resonance spectroscopy of brain in congenital myotonic dystrophy, *Pediatr Neurol* 12:335-340, 1995.
48. Sarnat HB, Silbert SW: Maturational arrest of fetal muscle in neonatal myotonic dystrophy, *Arch Neurol* 33:466-474, 1976.
49. Tachi N, Kozuka N, Ohya K, Chiba S, et al: CTG repeat size and histologic findings of skeletal muscle from patients with congenital myotonic dystrophy, *J Child Neurol* 11:430-432, 1996.
50. Farkas E, Tome FM, Fardeau M, Arsenio-Nunes ML, et al: Histochemical and ultrastructural study of muscle biopsies in three cases of dystrophia myotonica in the newborn child, *J Neurol Sci* 21:273-288, 1974.
51. Farkas-Bargeton E, Barbet JP, Dancea S, Wehrle R, et al: Immaturity of muscle fibers in the congenital form of myotonic dystrophy: Its consequences and its origin, *J Neurol Sci* 83:145-159, 1988.
52. Sarnat HB: New insights into the pathogenesis of congenital myopathies, *J Child Neurol* 9:193-201, 1994.
53. Young RS, Gang DL, Zalneraitis EL, Krishnamoorthy KS: Dysmaturation in infants of mothers with myotonic dystrophy, *Arch Neurol* 38:716-719, 1981.
54. Rosman NP, Rebeiz JJ: The cerebral defect and myopathy in myotonic dystrophy, *Neurology* 17:1106-1112, 1976.
55. Koch MC, Grimm T, Harley HG, Harper PS: Genetic risks for children of women with myotonic dystrophy, *Am J Hum Genet* 48:1084-1091, 1991.
56. Harper PS, Harley HG, Reardon W, Shaw DJ: Anticipation in myotonic dystrophy: New light on an old problem, *Am J Hum Genet* 51:10-16, 1992.
57. Speer MC, Pericak-Vance MA, Yamaoka L, Hung WY, et al: Presymptomatic and prenatal diagnosis in myotonic dystrophy by genetic linkage studies, *Neurology* 40:671-676, 1990.
58. Hunter A, Jacob P, O'Hoy K, MacDonald I, et al: Decrease in the size of the myotonic dystrophy CTG repeat during transmission from parent to child: Implications for genetic counselling and genetic anticipation, *Am J Med Genet* 45:401-407, 1993.
59. Fu YH, Pizzuti A, Fenwick RG Jr, King J, et al: An unstable triplet repeat in a gene related to myotonic dystrophy, *Science* 255:1256-1258, 1992.
60. Andrews PI, Wilson J: Relative disease severity in siblings with myotonic dystrophy, *J Child Neurol* 7:161-167, 1992.
61. Ashizawa T, Dubel JR, Dunne PW, Dunne CJ, et al: Anticipation in myotonic dystrophy. II. Complex relationships between clinical findings and structure of the GCT repeat, *Neurology* 42:1877-1883, 1992.
62. Shelbourne P, Davies J, Buxton J, Anvret M, et al: Direct diagnosis of myotonic dystrophy with a disease-specific DNA marker, *N Engl J Med* 328:471-475, 1993.
63. Buxton J, Shelbourne P, Davies J, Jones C, et al: Detection of an unstable fragment of DNA specific to individuals with myotonic dystrophy, *Nature* 355:547-548, 1992.
64. Mahadevan M, Tsilfidis C, Sabourin L, Shutler G, et al: Myotonic dystrophy mutation: An unstable CTG repeat in the 3' untranslated region of the gene, *Science* 255:1253-1255, 1992.
65. Aslanidis C, Jansen G, Amemiya C, Shutler G, et al: Cloning of the essential myotonic dystrophy region and mapping of the putative defect, *Nature* 355:548-551, 1992.
66. Ptacek LJ, Johnson KJ, Griggs RC: Mechanisms of disease: Genetics and physiology of the myotonic muscle disorders, *N Engl J Med* 328:482-489, 1993.
67. Gennarelli M, Pavoni M, Amicucci P, Angelini C, et al: Reduction of the DM-associated homeo domain protein (DMAHP) mRNA in different brain areas of myotonic dystrophy patients, *Neuromuscul Disord* 9:215-219, 1999.
68. Bernareggi A, Furling D, Mouly V, Ruzzier F, et al: Myocytes from congenital myotonic dystrophy display abnormal Na⁺ channel activities, *Muscle Nerve* 31:506-509, 2005.
69. Mooers BHM, Logue JS, Berglund JA: The structural basis of myotonic dystrophy from the crystal structure of CUG repeats, *Proc Natl Acad Sci U S A* 102:16626-16631, 2005.
70. Mulley JC, Staples A, Donnelly A, Gedeon AK, et al: Explanation for exclusive maternal origin for congenital form of myotonic dystrophy, *Lancet* 341:236-237, 1993.
71. Tachi N, Ohya K, Chiba S, Sato T, et al: Minimal somatic instability of CTG repeat in congenital myotonic dystrophy, *Pediatr Neurol* 12:81-83, 1995.
72. Rutherford MA, Heckmatt JZ, Dubowitz V: Congenital myotonic dystrophy: Respiratory function at birth determines survival, *Arch Dis Child* 64:191-195, 1989.
73. Keller C, Reynolds A, Lee B, Garcia-Prats J: Congenital myotonic dystrophy requiring prolonged endotracheal and noninvasive assisted ventilation: Not a uniformly fatal condition, *Pediatrics* 101:704-706, 1998.
74. Kirschner J, Bonnemann CG: The congenital and limb-girdle muscular dystrophies: Sharpening the focus, blurring the boundaries, *Arch Neurol* 61:189-199, 2004.
75. Muntoni F, Voit T: The congenital muscular dystrophies in 2004: A century of exciting progress, *Neuromuscul Disord* 14:635-649, 2004.
75a. Brockmann K, Dechent P, Bonnemann C, Schreiber G, et al: Quantitative proton MRS of cerebral metabolites in laminin alpha2 chain deficiency, *Brain Dev* 29:357-364, 2007.
76. Bernier JP, Brooke MH, Naidich TP, Carroll JE: Myoencephalopathy: Cerebral hypomyelination revealed by CT scan of the head in a muscle disease, *Ann Neurol* 6:165-172, 1979.
77. Nogen AG: Congenital muscular disease and abnormal findings on computerized tomography, *Dev Med Child Neurol* 22:658-663, 1980.
78. Egger J, Kendall BE, Erdohazi M: Involvement of the central nervous system in congenital muscular dystrophies, *Dev Med Child Neurol* 25:32-42, 1983.
79. Echenne B, Pages M, Marty-Double C: Congenital muscular dystrophy with cerebral white matter spongiosis, *Brain Dev* 6:491-495, 1984.

80. Echenne B, Arthuis M, Billard C, Campos-Castello J, et al: Congenital muscular dystrophy and cerebral CT scan anomalies, *J Neurol Sci* 75:7-22, 1986.

81. Topaloglu H, Yalax K, Kale G, Ergin M: Congenital muscular dystrophy with cerebral involvement: Report of a case of "occidental type cerebromuscular dystrophy"?, *Neuropediatrics* 21:53-54, 1990.

82. Topaloglu H, Yalaz K, Renda Y, Gaglar M, et al: Occidental type cerebromuscular dystrophy: A report of eleven cases, *J Neurol Neurosurg Psychiatry* 54:226-229, 1991.

83. Tanaka J, Mimaki T, Okada S, Fujimura H: Changes in cerebral white matter in a case of congenital muscular dystrophy (non-Fukuyama type), *Neuropediatrics* 21:183-186, 1990.

84. Streib EW, Lucking CH: Congenital muscular dystrophy with leukoencephalopathy, *Eur Neurol* 29:211-215, 1989.

85. Yoshioka M, Kuroki S, Mizue H: Congenital muscular dystrophy and non-Fukuyama type with characteristic CT images, *Brain Dev* 9:316-318, 1987.

86. Kao KP, Lin KP: Congenital muscular dystrophy of a non-Fukuyama type with white matter hyperlucency on CT scan, *Brain Dev* 14:420-422, 1992.

87. Pihko H, Louhimo T, Valanne L, Donner M: CNS in congenital muscular dystrophy without mental retardation, *Neuropediatrics* 23:116-122, 1992.

88. Trevisan CP, Carollo C, Segalla P, Angelini C, et al: Congenital muscular dystrophy: Brain alterations in an unselected series of Western patients, *J Neurol Neurosurg Psychiatry* 54:330-334, 1991.

89. Leyten QH, Gabreëls FJ, Renier WO, van Engelen BG, et al: White matter abnormalities in congenital muscular dystrophy, *J Neurol Sci* 129:162-169, 1995.

90. Vainzof M, Marie SK, Reed UC, Schwartzman JS, et al: Deficiency of merosin (laminin M or α2) in congenital muscular dystrophy associated with cerebral white matter alterations, *Neuropediatrics* 26:293-297, 1995.

91. Philpot J, Sewry C, Pennock J, Dubowitz V: Clinical phenotype in congenital muscular dystrophy, correlation with expression of merosin in skeletal muscle, *Neuromuscul Disord* 5:301-305, 1995.

92. Fardeau M, Tome FM, Helbling-Leclerc A, Evangelista T, et al: Congenital muscular dystrophy with merosin deficiency: Clinical, histopathological, immunocytochemical and genetic study, *Rev Neurol (Paris)* 152:11-19, 1996.

93. Reed UC, Marie SK, Vainzof M, Salum PB, et al: Congenital muscular dystrophy with cerebral white matter hypodensity: Correlation of clinical features and merosin deficiency, *Brain Dev* 18:51-58, 1996.

94. Connolly AM, Pestronk A, Planer GJ, Yue J, et al: Congenital muscular dystrophy syndromes distinguished by alkaline and acid phosphatase, merosin, and dystrophin staining, *Neurology* 46:810-814, 1996.

95. Pegoraro E, Marks H, Garcia CA, Crawford T, et al: Laminin α2 muscular dystrophy: Genotype/phenotype studies of 22 patients, *Neurology* 51:101-110, 1998.

96. Voit T: Congenital muscular dystrophies: 1997 update, *Brain Dev* 20:65-74, 1998.

97. Tome FM: The saga of congenital muscular dystrophy, *Neuropediatrics* 30:55-65, 1999.

98. Farina L, Morandi L, Milanesi I, Ciceri E, et al: Congenital muscular dystrophy with merosin deficiency: MRI findings in five patients, *Neuroradiology* 40:807-811, 1998.

99. Cohn RD, Herrmann R, Sorokin L, Wewer UM, et al: Laminin α2 chain-deficient congenital muscular dystrophy: Variable epitope expression in severe and mild cases, *Neurology* 51:94-101, 1998.

100. Morandi L, DiBlasi C, Farina L, Sorokin L, et al: Clinical correlations in 16 patients with total or partial laminin α2 deficiency characterized using antibodies against 2 fragments of the protein, *Arch Neurol* 56:209-215, 1999.

101. Caro PA, Scavina M, Hoffman E, Pegoraro E, et al: MR imaging findings in children with merosin-deficient congenital muscular dystrophy, *AJNR Am J Neuroradiol* 20:324-326, 1999.

102. Cohn RD, Mayer U, Saher G, Herrmann R, et al: Secondary reduction of α7B integrin in laminin α2 deficient congenital muscular dystrophy supports an additional transmembrane link in skeletal muscle, *J Neurol Sci* 163:140-152, 1999.

103. Philpot J, Cowan F, Pennock J, Sewry C, et al: Merosin-deficient congenital muscular dystrophy: The spectrum of brain involvement on magnetic resonance imaging, *Neuromuscul Disord* 9:81-85, 1999.

104. Philpot J, Bagnall A, King C, Dubowitz V, et al: Feeding problems in merosin deficient congenital muscular dystrophy, *Arch Dis Child* 80:542-547, 1999.

105. Taratuto A, Lubieniecki F, Diaz D, Schultz M, et al: Merosin-deficient congenital muscular dystrophy associated with abnormal cerebral cortical gyration: An autopsy study, *Neuromuscul Disord* 9:86-94, 1999.

106. Pegoraro E, Fanin M, Trevisan CP, Angelini C, et al: A novel laminin α2 isoform in severe laminin α2 deficient congenital muscular dystrophy, *Neurology* 55:1128-1134, 2000.

107. Jones KJ, Morgan G, Johnston H, Tobias V, et al: The expanding phenotype of laminin α2 chain (merosin) abnormalities: Case series and review, *J Med Genet* 38:649-657, 2001.

108. Di Blasi C, Piga D, Brioschi P, Moroni I, et al: LAMA2 gene analysis in congenital muscular dystrophy: New mutations, prenatal diagnosis, and founder effect, *Arch Neurol* 62:1582-1586, 2005.

109. Herrmann R, Straub V, Meyer K, Kahn T, et al: Congenital muscular dystrophy with laminin alpha 2 chain deficiency: Identification of a new intermediate phenotype and correlation of clinical findings to muscle immunohistochemistry, *Eur J Pediatr* 155:968-976, 1996.

110. Tachi N, Kamimura S, Ohya K, Chiba S, et al: Congenital muscular dystrophy with partial deficiency of merosin, *J Neurol Sci* 151:25-27, 1997.

111. Naom IS, D'Alessandro M, Topaloglu H, Sewry C, et al: Refinement of the laminin alpha 2 chain locus to human chromosome 6q2 in severe and mild merosin deficient congenital muscular dystrophy, *J Med Genet* 34:99-104, 1997.

112. He Y, Jones KJ, Morgan G, Vignier N, et al: Congenital muscular dystrophy with primary partial laminin α2 chain deficiency: Molecular study, *Neurology* 57:1319-1322, 2001.

113. Prandini P, Berardinelli A, Fanin M, Morello F, et al: LAMA2 loss-of-function mutation in a girl with a mild congenital muscular dystrophy, *Neurology* 63:1118-1121, 2004.

114. Pearson CM, Fowler WG: Hereditary non-progressive muscular dystrophy inducing arthrogryposis syndrome, *Brain* 86:75-88, 1963.

115. Gubbay SS, Walton JN, Pearce GW: Clinical and pathological study of a case of congenital muscular dystrophy, *J Neurol Neurosurg Psychiatry* 29:500-509, 1966.

116. Zellweger H, Afifi A, McCormick WF, Mergner W: Benign congenital muscular dystrophy: A special form of congenital hypotonia, *Clin Pediatr* 6:655-663, 1967.

117. Zellweger H, McCormick WF, Mergner W: Severe congenital muscular dystrophy, *Am J Dis Child* 114:591, 1967.

118. Fowler MC, Manson JI: Congenital muscular dystrophy with malformation of the central nervous system. In Kakulas BA, editor: *Clinical Studies in Myology*, New York: 1973, Elsevier.

119. Donner M, Rapola J, Somer H: Congenital muscular dystrophy: A clinicopathological and followup study of 15 patients, *Neuropaediatrie* 6:239-258, 1975.

120. Kamoshita S, Konishi Y, Segawa M, Fukuyama Y: Congenital muscular dystrophy as a disease of the central nervous system, *Arch Neurol* 33:513-516, 1976.

121. Brooke MH, Carroll JE, Ringel SP: Congenital hypotonia revisited, *Muscle Nerve* 2:84-100, 1979.

122. McMenamin JB, Becker LE, Murphy EG: Congenital muscular dystrophy: A clinicopathologic report of 24 cases, *J Pediatr* 100:692-697, 1982.

123. Leyten QH, Gabreels FJ, Reiner WO, Ter Laak JH, et al: Congenital muscular dystrophy, *J Pediatr* 115:214-221, 1989.

124. Banker BQ: The congenital muscular dystrophies. In Engel AG, Franzini-Armstrong C, editors: *Myology*, New York: 1994, McGraw-Hill.

125. Parano E, Pavone L, Fiumara A, Falsaperia R, et al: Congenital muscular dystrophies: Clinical review and proposed classification, *Pediatr Neurol* 13:97-103, 1995.

126. Topaloglu H, Kale G, Yalnzoglu D, Tasdemir AH, et al: Analysis of "pure" congenital muscular dystrophies in thirty-eight cases: How different is the classical type 1 from the occidental type cerebromuscular dystrophy? *Neuropediatrics* 25:94-100, 1994.

127. North KN, Specht LA, Sethi RK, Shapiro F, et al: Congenital muscular dystrophy associated with merosin deficiency, *J Child Neurol* 11:291-295, 1996.

128. Kobayashi O, Hayashi Y, Arahata K, Ozawa E, et al: Congenital muscular dystrophy: Clinical and pathologic study of 50 patients with the classical (Occidental) merosin-positive form, *Neurology* 46:815-818, 1996.

129. Al-Qudah AA, Tarawneh M: Congenital muscular dystrophy in Jordanian children, *J Child Neurol* 13:383-386, 1998.

130. Voit T, Cohn RD, Sperner J, Leube B, et al: Merosin-positive congenital muscular dystrophy with transient brain dysmyelination, pontocerebellar hypoplasia and mental retardation, *Neuromuscul Disord* 9:95-101, 1999.

131. Reed UC, Tsanaclis AM, Vainzof M, Marie SK, et al: Merosin-positive congenital muscular dystrophy in two siblings with cataract and slight mental retardation, *Brain Dev* 21:274-278, 1999.

132. Salih MA, Al Rayess M, Cutshall S, Urtizberea JA, et al: A novel form of familial congenital muscular dystrophy in two adolescents, *Neuropediatrics* 29:289-293, 1998.

133. Mahjneh I, Bushby K, Anderson L, Muntoni F, et al: Merosin-positive congenital muscular dystrophy: A large inbred family, *Neuropediatrics* 30:22-28, 1999.

134. Philpot J, Pennock J, Cowan F, Sewry CA, et al: Brain magnetic resonance imaging abnormalities in merosin-positive congenital muscular dystrophy, *Eur J Paediatr Neurol* 4:109-114, 2000.

135. Flanigan KM, Kerr L, Bromberg MB, Leonard C, et al: Congenital muscular dystrophy with rigid spine syndrome: A clinical pathological, radiological, and genetic study, *Ann Neurol* 47:152-161, 2000.

136. Tetreault M, Duquette A, Thiffault I, Bherer C, et al: A new form of congenital muscular dystrophy with joint hyperlaxity maps to 3p23-21, *Brain* 129:2077-2084, 2006.

137. Banker BQ, Victor M, Adams RD: Arthrogryposis multiplex due to congenital muscular dystrophy, *Brain* 80:319-334, 1957.

138. Jones K, North K: Congenital muscular dystrophies. In Jones HR Jr, DeVivo DC, Darras BT, editors: *Neuromuscular Disorders of Infancy, Childhood, and Adolescence: A Clinician's Approach*, Philadelphia: 2003, Butterworth Heinemann.

139. Korematsu S, Imai K, Sato K, Maeda T, et al: Congenital neuromuscular disease with uniform type-1 fibers, presenting early stage dystrophic muscle pathology, *Brain Dev* 28:63-66, 2006.

140. Bertini E, Pepe G: Collagen type VI and related disorders: Bethlem myopathy and Ullrich scleroatonic muscular dystrophy, *Eur Paediatr Neurol* 6:193-198, 2002.

141. Higuchi I, Shiraishi T, Hashiguchi T, Suehara M, et al: Frameshift mutation in the collagen VI gene causes Ullrich's disease, *Ann Neurol* 50:261-265, 2001.

142. Ishikawa H, Sugie K, Murayama K, Awaya A, et al: Ullrich disease due to deficiency of collagen VI in the sarcolemma, *Neurology* 62:620-623, 2004.

143. Demir E, Ferreiro A, Sabatelli P, Allamand V, et al: Collagen VI status and clinical severity in Ullrich congenital muscular dystrophy: Phenotype analysis of 11 families linked to the COL6 loci, *Neuropediatrics* 35:103-112, 2004.

144. Baker NL, Morgelin M, Peat R, Goemans N, et al: Dominant collagen VI mutations are a common cause of Ullrich congenital muscular dystrophy, *Hum Mol Genet* 14:279-293, 2005.

145. Giusti B, Lucarini L, Pietroni V, Lucioli S, et al: Dominant and recessive COL6A1 mutations in Ullrich scleroatonic muscular dystrophy, *Ann Neurol* 58:400-410, 2005.

146. Kirschner J, Hausser I, Zou YQ, Schreiber G, et al: Ullrich congenital muscular dystrophy: Connective tissue abnormalities in the skin support overlap with Ehlers-Danlos syndromes, *Am J Med Genet A* 132:296-301, 2005.

147. Pepe G, Lucarini L, Zhang RZ, Pan TC, et al: COL6A1 genomic deletions in Bethlem myopathy and Ullrich muscular dystrophy, *Ann Neurol* 59:190-195, 2006.

147a. Okada M, Kawahara G, Noguchi S, Sugie K, et al: Primary collagen VI deficiency is the second most common congenital muscular dystropy in Japan, *Neurology* 69:1035-1042, 2007.

148. Longman C, Brockington M, Torelli S, Jimenez-Mallebrera C, et al: Mutations in the human LARGE gene cause MDC1D, a novel form of congenital muscular dystrophy with severe mental retardation and abnormal glycosylation of alpha-dystroglycan, *Hum Mol Genet* 12:2853-2861, 2003.

149. Fukuyama Y, Osawa M, Suzuki H: Congenital progressive muscular dystrophy of the Fukuyama type: Clinical, genetic and pathological considerations, *Brain Dev* 3:1-29, 1981.

150. Fukuyama Y, Osawa M: A genetic study of the Fukuyama type congenital muscular dystrophy, *Brain Dev* 6:373, 1984.

151. Krijgsman JB, Barth PG, Stam FC, Slooff JL, et al: Congenital muscular dystrophy and cerebral dysgenesis in a Dutch family, *Neuropaediatrie* 11:108-120, 1980.

152. McMenamin JB, Becker LE, Murphy EG: Fukuyama-type congenital muscular dystrophy, *J Pediatr* 101:580-582, 1982.

153. Goebel HH, Fidzianska A, Lenard HG, Osse G, et al: A morphological study of non-Japanese congenital muscular dystrophy associated with cerebral lesions, *Brain Dev* 5:292-301, 1983.

154. Peters AC, Bots CT, Roos RA, van Gelderen HH: Fukuyama type congenital muscular dystrophy: Two Dutch siblings, *Brain Dev* 6:406-416, 1984.

155. Ishikawa A: Fukuyama-type congenital muscular dystrophy, *Arch Neurol* 39:671, 1982.

156. Kumura S, Kobayashi T, Amemiya F, Sasaki Y, et al: Diaphragm muscle pathology in Fukuyama type congenital muscular dystrophy, *Brain Dev* 12:779-783, 1990.

157. Sugino S, Miyatake M, Ohtani Y, Yoshioka K, et al: Vascular alterations in Fukuyama type congenital muscular dystrophy, *Brain Dev* 13:77-81, 1991.

158. Takada K, Nakamura H, Takashima S: Cortical dysplasia in Fukuyama congenital muscular dystrophy (FCMD): A Golgi and angioarchitectonic analysis, *Acta Neuropathol (Berl)* 76:170-178, 1988.

159. Takada K: Fukuyama congenital muscular dystrophy as a unique disorder of neuronal migration: A neuropathological review and hypothesis, *Yonago Acta Med* 31:1-16, 1988.

160. Yoshioka M, Saiwai S: Congenital muscular dystrophy (Fukuyama type): Changes in the white matter low density on CT, *Brain Dev* 10:41-44, 1988.

161. Aihara M, Tanabe Y, Kato K: Serial MRI in Fukuyama type congenital muscular dystrophy, *Neuroradiology* 34:396-398, 1992.

162. Wang Z-P, Osawa M, Fukuyama Y: Morphometric study of the corpus callosum in Fukuyama type congenital muscular dystrophy by magnetic resonance imaging, *Brain Dev* 17:104-110, 1995.

163. Aida N, Tamagawa K, Takada K, Yagishita A, et al: Brain MR in Fukuyama congenital muscular dystrophy, *AJNR Am J Neuroradiol* 17:605-613, 1996.

164. Hino N, Kobayashi M, Shibata N, Yamamoto T, et al: Clinicopathological study on eyes from cases of Fukuyama type congenital muscular dystrophy, *Brain Dev* 23:97-107, 2001.

165. Matsumoto H, Hayashi YK, Kim DS, Ogawa M, et al: Congenital muscular dystrophy with glycosylation defects of alpha-dystroglycan in Japan, *Neuromuscul Disord* 15:342-348, 2005.

166. Cormand B, Pihko H, Mayes M, Valanne L, et al: Clinical and genetic distinction between Walker-Warburg syndrome and muscle-eye-brain disease, *Neurology* 56:1059-1069, 2001.

167. Raitta C, Lamminen M, Santavuori P, Leisti J: Ophthalmological findings in a new syndrome with muscle, eye and brain involvement, *Acta Ophthalmol* 56:465-472, 1978.

168. Santavuori P, Leisti J, Kruus S, Raitta C: Muscle, eye and brain disease: A new syndrome, *Doc Ophthalmol* 17:393, 1978.

169. Korinthenberg R, Palm D, Schlake W, Klein J: Congenital muscular dystrophy, brain malformation and ocular problems (muscle, eye and brain disease) in two German families, *Eur J Pediatr* 142:64-68, 1984.

170. Pavone L, Gullotta F, Grasso S, Vannucchi C: Hydrocephalus, lissencephaly, ocular abnormalities and congenital muscular dystrophy: A Warburg syndrome variant? *Neuropediatrics* 17:206-211, 1986.

171. Heyer R, Ehrich J, Goebel H-H, Christen H-J, et al: Congenital muscular dystrophy with cerebral and ocular malformations (cerebro-oculomuscular syndrome), *Brain Dev* 8:614-618, 1986.

172. Heggie P, Grossniklaus HE, Roessmann U, Chou SM, et al: Cerebro-ocular dysplasia: Muscular dystrophy syndrome, *Arch Ophthalmol* 105:520-524, 1987.

173. Tachi N, Tachi M, Sasaki K, Tanabe C, et al: Walker-Warburg syndrome in a Japanese patient, *Pediatr Neurol* 4:236-240, 1988.

174. Santavuori P, Somer H, Sainio K, Rapola J, et al: Muscle-eye-brain disease (MEB), *Brain Dev* 1989:147-153, 1989.

175. Federico A, Dotti MT, Malandrini A, Guazzi GC: Cerebro-ocular dysplasia and muscular dystrophy: Report of two cases, *Neuropediatrics* 19:109-112, 1988.

176. Leyten QH, Renkawek K, Reiner WO, Gabreëls FJM, et al: Neuropathological findings in muscle-eye-brain disease (MEB-D), *Acta Neuropathol (Berl)* 83:55-60, 1991.

177. Leyten QH, Gabreels FJM, Renier WO, Renkawek K, et al: Congenital muscular dystrophy with eye and brain malformations in six Dutch patients, *Neuropediatrics* 23:316-320, 1992.

178. Takada K: Fukuyama-type congenital muscular dystrophy and the Walker-Warburg syndrome: Commentary, *Brain Dev* 15:244-245, 1993.

179. Dobyns WB: Classification of the cerebro-oculo-muscular syndrome(s): Commentary, *Brain Dev* 15:242-244, 1993.

180. Kumura S, Sasaki Y, Kobayashi T, Ohtsuki N, et al: Fukuyama-type congenital muscular dystrophy and the Walker-Warburg syndrome, *Brain Dev* 15:182-191, 1993.

181. Wewer UM, Durkin ME, Zhang X, Laursen H, et al: Laminin β2 chain and adhalin deficiency in the skeletal muscle of Walker-Warburg syndrome (cerebro-ocular dysplasia-muscular dystrophy), *Neurology* 45:2099-2101, 1995.

182. Pihko H, Lappi M, Raitta C, Sainio K, et al: Ocular findings in muscle-eye-brain (MEB) disease: A follow-up study, *Brain Dev* 17:57-61, 1995.

183. Warburg M: Muscle-eye brain disease and Walker-Warburg syndrome: Phenotype-genotype speculations. Commentary to Pihko's paper (pp. 57-61), *Brain Dev* 17:62-63, 1995.

184. Topaloglu H, Cila A, Tasdemir AH, Saatci I: Congenital muscular dystrophy with eye and brain involvement: The Turkish experience in two cases, *Brain Dev* 17:271-275, 1995.

185. Haltia M, Leivo I, Somer H, Pihko H, et al: Muscle-eye-brain disease: A neuropathological study, *Ann Neurol* 41:173-180, 1997.

186. van der, Knaap MS, Smit LM, Barth PG, Catsman-Berrevoets CE, et al: Magnetic resonance imaging in classification of congenital muscular dystrophies with brain abnormalities, *Ann Neurol* 42:50-59, 1997.

187. Santavuori P, Valanne L, Autti T, Haltia M, et al: Muscle-eye-brain disease: Clinical features, visual evoked potentials and brain imaging in 20 patients, *Eur J Paediatr Neurol* 1:41-47, 1998.

188. Kanoff RJ, Curless RG, Petito C, Siatkowski RM, et al: Walker-Warburg syndrome: Neurologic features and muscle membrane structure, *Pediatr Neurol* 18:76-80, 1998.

189. Vervoort VS, Holden KR, Ukadike KC, Collins JS, et al: POMGnT1 gene alterations in a family with neurological abnormalities, *Ann Neurol* 56:143-148, 2004.

190. Longman C, Mercuri E, Cowan F, Allsop J, et al: Antenatal and postnatal brain magnetic resonance imaging in muscle-eye-brain disease, *Arch Neurol* 61:1301-1306, 2004.

191. Topaloglu H, Brockington M, Yuva Y, Talim B, et al: FKRP gene mutations cause congenital muscular dystrophy, mental retardation, and cerebellar cysts, *Neurology* 60:988-992, 2003.

192. Mercuri E, Brockington M, Straub V, Quijano-Roy S, et al: Phenotypic spectrum associated with mutations in the fukutin-related protein gene, *Ann Neurol* 53:537-542, 2003.

192a. MacLeod H, Pytel P, Wollmann R, Chelmicka-Schorr E, et al: A novel FKRP mutation in congenital muscular dystrophy disrupts the dystrophin glycoprotein complex, *Neuromuscul Disord* 17:285-289, 2007.

193. Mercuri E, Topaloglu H, Brockington M, Berardinelli A, et al: Spectrum of brain changes in patients with congenital muscular dystrophy and FKRP gene mutations, *Arch Neurol* 63:251-257, 2006.

194. Quijano-Roy S, Marti-Carrera I, Makri S, Mayer M, et al: Brain MRI abnormalities in muscular dystrophy due to FKRP mutations, *Brain Dev* 28:232-242, 2006.

195. Mercuri E, Pennock J, Goodwin F, Sewry C, et al: Sequential study of central and peripheral nervous system involvement in an infant with merosin-deficient congenital muscular dystrophy, *Neuromuscul Disord* 6:425-429, 1996.

196. Mercuri E, Rutherford M, DeVile C, Counsell S, et al: Early white matter changes on brain magnetic resonance imaging in a newborn affected by merosin-deficient congenital muscular dystrophy, *Neuromuscul Disord* 11:297-299, 2001.

197. Gilhuis HJ, ten Donkelaar HJ, Tanke RB, Vingerhoets DM, et al: Nonmuscular involvement in merosin-negative congenital muscular dystrophy, *Pediatr Neurol* 26:30-36, 2002.

198. Leite CC, Reed UC, Otaduy MC, Lacerda MT, et al: Congenital muscular dystrophy with merosin deficiency: H-1 MR spectroscopy and diffusion-weighted MR imaging, *Radiology* 235:190-196, 2005.

199. Sunada Y, Edgar TS, Lotz BP, Rust RS, et al: Merosin-negative congenital muscular dystrophy associated with extensive brain abnormalities, *Neurology* 45:2084-2089, 1995.

200. Pini A, Merlini L, Tome FM, Chevallay M, et al: Merosin-negative congenital muscular dystrophy, occipital epilepsy with periodic spasms and focal cortical dysplasia: Report of three Italian cases in two families, *Brain Dev* 18:316-322, 1996.

201. Mackay MT, Kornberg AJ, Shield L, Phelan E, et al: Congenital muscular dystrophy, white-matter abnormalities, and neuronal migration disorders: The expanding concept, *J Child Neurol* 13:481-487, 1998.

202. Tsao CY, Mendell JR, Rusin J, Luquette M: Congenital muscular dystrophy with complete laminin-α2-deficiency, cortical dysplasia, and cerebral white-matter changes in children, *J Child Neurol* 13:253-256, 1998.

203. Brett FM, Costigan D, Farrell MA, Heaphy P, et al: Merosin-deficient congenital muscular dystrophy and cortical dysplasia, *Eur J Paediatr Neurol* 2:77-82, 1998.

204. Triki C, Louhichi N, Meziou M, Choyakh F, et al: Merosin-deficient congenital muscular dystrophy with mental retardation and cerebellar cysts, unlinked to the LAMA2, FCMD, MEB and CMD1B loci, in three Tunisian patients, *Neuromuscul Disord* 13:4-12, 2003.

205. Mercuri E, Muntoni F, Berardinelli A, Pennock J, et al: Somatosensory and visual evoked potentials in congenital muscular dystrophy: Correlation with MRI changes and muscle merosin status, *Neuropediatrics* 26:3-7, 1995.

206. Mercuri E, Anker S, Philpot J, Sewry C, et al: Visual function in children with merosin-deficient and merosin-positive congenital muscular dystrophy, *Pediatr Neurol* 18:399-401, 1998.

207. Shorer Z, Philpot J, Muntoni F, Sewry C, et al: Demyelinating peripheral neuropathy in merosin-deficient congenital muscular dystrophy, *J Child Neurol* 10:472-475, 1995.

208. Matsumura K, Yamada H, Saito F, Sunada Y, et al: Peripheral nerve involvement in merosin-deficient congenital muscular dystrophy and dy mouse, *Neuromuscul Disord* 7:7-12, 1997.

209. Naom I, Sewry C, D'Allesandro M, Tapaloglu H, et al: Prenatal diagnosis in merosin-deficient congenital muscular dystrophy, *Neuromuscul Disord* 7:176-179, 1997.

210. Marbini A, Bellanova MF, Ferrari A, Lodesani M, et al: Immunohistochemical study of merosin-negative congenital muscular dystrophy: Laminin α2 deficiency in skin biopsy, *Acta Neuropathol (Berl)* 94:103-108, 1997.

211. Sewry CA, D'Allessandro M, Wilson LA, Sorokin LM, et al: Expression of laminin chains in skin in merosin-deficient congenital muscular dystrophy, *Neuropediatrics* 28:217-222, 1997.

212. Nonaka I, Sugita H, Takada K, Kumagai K: Muscle histochemistry in congenital muscular dystrophy with central nervous system involvement, *Muscle Nerve* 5:102-106, 1982.

213. Matsumura K, Nonaka I, Campbell KP: Abnormal expression of dystrophin-associated proteins in Fukuyama-type congenital muscular dystrophy, *Lancet* 341:521-522, 1993.

214. Osari S-I, Kobayashi O, Yamashita Y, Matsuishi T, et al: Basement membrane abnormality in merosin-negative congenital muscular dystrophy, *Acta Neuropathol (Berl)* 91:332-336, 1996.

215. Fadic R, Waclawik AJ, Lewandoski PJ, Lotz BP: Muscle pathology and clinical features of the sarcolemmopathies, *Pediatr Neurol* 16:79-82, 1997.

216. Pegararo E, Mancias P, Swerdlow SH, Raikow RB, et al: Congenital muscular dystrophy with primary laminin α2 (merosin) deficiency presenting as inflammatory myopathy, *Ann Neurol* 40:782-791, 1996.

217. Mrak RE: The pathologic spectrum of merosin deficiency, *J Child Neurol* 13:513-516, 1998.

218. Takada K, Nakamura H, Tanaka J: Cortical dysplasia in congenital muscular dystrophy with central nervous system involvement (Fukuyama type), *J Neuropathol Exp Neurol* 43:395-407, 1984.

219. Takada K, Nakamura H, Suzumori K, Ishikawa T, et al: Cortical dysplasia in a 23-week fetus with Fukuyama congenital muscular dystrophy (FCMD), *Acta Neuropathol (Berl)* 74:300-306, 1987.

220. Takashima S, Becker LE, Chan F, Takada K: A Golgi study of the cerebral cortex in Fukuyama-type congenital muscular dystrophy, Walker-type "lissencephaly," and classical lissencephaly, *Brain Dev* 9:621-626, 1987.

221. Itoh H, Houdou S, Kawahara H, Ohama E: Morphological study of the brainstem in Fukuyama type congenital muscular dystrophy, *Pediatr Neurol* 15:327-331, 1996.

222. Yamamoto T, Topyoda C, Kobayashi M, Kondo E, et al: Pial-glial barrier abnormalities in fetuses with Fukuyama congenital muscular dystrophy, *Brain Dev* 19:35-42, 1997.

223. Yamamoto T, Armstrong D, Shibata N, Kanazawa M, et al: Immature astrocytes in Fukuyama congenital muscular dystrophy: An immunohistochemical study, *Pediatr Neurol* 20:31-37, 1999.

224. Saito Y, Mizuguchi M, Oka A, Takashima S: Fukutin protein is expressed in neurons of the normal developing human brain but is reduced in Fukuyama-type congenital muscular dystrophy brain, *Ann Neurol* 47:756-764, 2000.

225. Yamamoto T, Kato V, Karita M, Kawaguchi M, et al: Expression of genes related to muscular dystrophy with lissencephaly, *Pediatr Neurol* 31:183-190, 2004.

226. Yamamoto T, Kato Y, Kawaguchi M, Shibata N, et al: Expression and localization of fukutin, POMGnT1, and POMT1 in the central nervous system: Consideration for functions of fukutin, *Med Electron Microsc* 37:200-207, 2004.

227. Campbell KP: Three muscular dystrophies: Loss of cytoskeleton extracellular matrix linkage, *Cell* 80:675-679, 1995.

228. Muntoni F, Sewry CA: Congenital muscular dystrophy, *Neurology* 51:14-16, 1998.

229. Tome FMS, Evangelista T, Lechere A: Congenital muscular dystrophy with merosin deficiency, *CR Acad Sci (Paris)* 317:351-357, 1994.

230. Prelle A, Medori R, Moggio M, Chan HW, et al: Dystrophin deficiency in a case of congenital myopathy, *J Neurol* 239:76-78, 1992.

231. Kyriakides T, Gabriel G, Drousiotou A, Meznanicpetrusa M, et al: Dystrophinopathy presenting as congenital muscular dystrophy, *Neuromuscul Disord* 4:387-392, 1994.

232. Cordone G, Bado M, Morreale G, Pedemonte M, et al: Severe dystrophinopathy in a patient with congenital hypotonia, *Childs Nerv Syst* 12:466-469, 1996.

233. Biancheri R, Bertini E, Falace A, Pedemonte M, et al: POMGnT1 mutations in congenital muscular dystrophy: Genotype-phenotype correlation and expanded clinical spectrum, *Arch Neurol* 63:1491-1495, 2006.

234. Orrell RW, Darras BT, Griggs RC: Facioscapulohumeral dystrophy, scapuloperoneal syndromes, and distal myopathies. In Jones HR Jr, DeVivo DC, Darras BT, editors: *Neuromuscular Disorders of Infancy, Childhood, and Adolescence: A Clinician's Approach*, Philadelphia: 2003, Butterworth Heinemann.

235. Carroll JE, Brooke MH: Infantile facioscapulohumeral dystrophy. In Serratrice G, Roux TH, editors: *Peroneal Atrophies and Related Disorders*, New York: 1979, Masson.

236. Hanson PA, Rowland LP: Mobius syndrome and facioscapulohumeral muscular dystrophy, *Arch Neurol* 24:31-39, 1971.

237. Korf BR, Bresnan MJ, Shapiro F, Sotrel A, et al: Facioscapulohumeral dystrophy presenting in infancy with facial diplegia and sensorineural deafness, *Ann Neurol* 17:513-516, 1985.

238. Yasukohchi S, Yagi Y, Akabane T, Terauchi A, et al: Facioscapulohumeral dystrophy associated with sensorineural hearing loss, tortuosity of retinal arterioles, and an early onset and rapid progression of respiratory failure, *Brain Dev* 10:319-324, 1988.

239. Brouwer OF, Padberg GW, Bakker E, Wijmenga C, et al: Early onset facioscapulohumeral muscular dystrophy, *Muscle Nerve* 2:S67-S72, 1995.

240. Tawil R, Forrester J, Griggs RC, Mendell J, et al: Evidence for anticipation and association of deletion size with severity in facioscapulohumeral muscular dystrophy, *Ann Neurol* 39:744-748, 1996.

241. Nakagawa M, Higuchi I, Yoshidome H, Isashiki Y, et al: Familial facioscapulohumeral muscular dystrophy: Phenotypic diversity and genetic abnormality, *Acta Neurol Scand* 93:189-192, 1996.

242. Okinaga A, Matsuoka T, Umeda J, Yanagihara I, et al: Early-onset facioscapulohumeral muscular dystrophy: Two case reports, *Brain Dev* 19:563-567, 1997.

243. Tawil R, Figlewicz DA, Griggs RC, Weiffenbach B, et al: Facioscapulohumeral dystrophy: A distinct regional myopathy with a novel molecular pathogenesis, *Ann Neurol* 43:279-282, 1998.

244. Miura K, Kumagai T, Matsumoto A, Irlyama E, et al: Two cases of chromosome 4q35-linked early onset facioscapulohumeral muscular dystrophy with mental retardation and epilepsy, *Neuropediatrics* 29:239-241, 1998.

245. Dorobek M, Kabzinska D: A severe case of facioscapulohumeral muscular dystrophy (FSHD) with some uncommon clinical features and a short 4q35 fragment, *Eur J Paediatr Neurol* 8:313-316, 2004.

246. Klinge L, Eagle M, Haggerty ID, Roberts CE, et al: Severe phenotype in infantile facioscapulohumeral muscular dystrophy, *Neuromuscul Disord* 16:553-558, 2006.

247. Dubowitz V: *The Floppy Infant*, Philadelphia: 1980, JB Lippincott.

248. Sarnat HB: Neuromuscular disorders in the neonatal period. In Korobkin R, Guilleminault C, editors: *Advances in Perinatal Neurology*, New York: 1979, Spectrum Publications.

249. Munsat TL, Piper D, Cancilla P: Inflammatory myopathy with facioscapulohumeral distribution, *Neurology* 22:335-347, 1972.

250. Thompson CF: Infantile myositis, *Dev Med Child Neurol* 24:307-311, 1982.

251. Shevell M, Rosenblatt B, Silver K, Carpenter S, et al: Congenital inflammatory myopathy, *Neurology* 40:1111-1114, 1990.

252. Roddy SM, Ashwal S, Peckham N: Infantile myositis: A case diagnosed in the neonatal period, *Pediatr Neurol* 2:241-244, 1986.

253. Nagai T, Hasegawa T, Saito M, Hayashi S, et al: Infantile polymyositis: A case report, *Brain Dev* 14:167-169, 1992.

254. Vajsar J, Jay V, Babyn P: Infantile myositis presenting in the neonatal period, *Brain Dev* 18:415-419, 1996.

255. Nevo Y, Pestronk A: Neonatal perifascicular myopathy, *Pediatr Neurol* 15:150-152, 1996.

256. McNeil SM, Woulfe J, Ross C, Tarnopolsky MA: Congenital inflammatory myopathy: A demonstrative case and proposed diagnostic classification, *Muscle Nerve* 25:259-264, 2002.

257. Nonaka I, Nakamura Y, Tojo M, Sugita H, et al: Congenital myopathy without specific features (minimal change myopathy), *Neuropediatrics* 14:237-241, 1983.

258. Jong YJ, Shishikura K, Aoyama M, Kitahara H, et al: Nonspecific congenital myopathy (minimal change myopathy): A case report, *Brain Dev* 9:61-64, 1987.

259. Gamstorp I: Non-dystrophic, myogenic myopathies with onset in infancy or childhood: A review of some characteristic syndromes, *Acta Paediatr Scand* 71:881-886, 1982.

260. Kinoshita M: Congenital and metabolic myopathies, *Brain Dev* 5:116, 1983.

261. Fardeau M: Relevance of morphological studies in the classification and pathophysiology of congenital myopathies. In Serratrice G, editor: *Neuromuscular Diseases*, New York: 1984, Raven Press.

262. Goebel HH: Neuropathological aspects of congenital myopathies. In Zimmerman M, editor: *Progress in Neuropathology*, New York: 1986, Raven Press.

263. Fardeau M: Congenital myopathies. In Mastaglia FL, Detchant LW, editors: *Skeletal Muscle Pathology*, 2nd ed, New York: 1992, Churchill Livingstone.

264. Fardeau M, Tome FM: Congenital myopathies. In Engel AG, Franzini-Armstrong C, editors: *Myology*, New York: 1994, McGraw-Hill.

265. Akiyama C, Nonaka I: A follow-up study of congenital non-progressive myopathies, *Brain Dev* 18:404-408, 1996.

266. North K, Goebel HH: Congenital myopathies. In Jones HR Jr, DeVivo DC, Darras BT, editors: *Neuromuscular Disorders of Infancy, Childhood, and Adolescence: A Clinician's Approach*, Philadelphia: 2003, Butterworth Heinemann.

267. Jungbluth H, Sewry CA, Muntoni F: What's new in neuromuscular disorders? The congenital myopathies, *Eur J Paediatr Neurol* 7:23-30, 2003.

268. Goebel HH: Congenital myopathies at their molecular dawning, *Muscle Nerve* 27:527-548, 2003.

269. Goebel HH: Congenital myopathies in the new millennium, *J Child Neurol* 20:94-101, 2005.

270. Shy GM, Magee KR: A new congenital nonprogressive myopathy, *Brain* 79:610-621, 1956.

271. Dubowitz V, Roy S: Central core disease of muscle: Clinical, histochemical, and electron microscopic studies of an affected mother and child, *Brain* 93:133-146, 1970.

272. Mrozek K, Strugalska M, Fidzianska A: A sporadic case of central core disease, *J Neurol Sci* 10:339-348, 1970.

273. Armstrong RM, Koenigsberger R, Mellinger J, Lovelace RE: Central core disease with congenital hip dislocation, *Neurology* 21:369-376, 1971.

274. Bethlem J, van Wijngaarden GK, Meijer AE, Fleury P: Observations on central core disease, *J Neurol Sci* 14:293-299, 1971.

275. Saper JR, Itabashi HH: Central core disease: A congenital myopathy, *Dis Nerv Syst* 37:649-653, 1976.

276. Cohen ME, Duffner PK, Heffner R: Central core disease in one of identical twins, *J Neurol Neurosurg Psychiatry* 41:659-663, 1978.

277. Tojo M, Ozawa M, Nonaka I: Central core disease and congenital neuromuscular disease with uniform type 1 fibers in one family, *Brain Dev* 22:262-264, 2000.

278. Wu S, Ibarra MC, Malicdan MC, Murayama K, et al: Central core disease is due to RYR1 mutations in more than 90% of patients, *Brain* 129:1470-1480, 2006.

279. Jungbluth H, Muller CR, Halliger-Keller B, Brockington M, et al: Autosomal recessive inheritance of RYR1 mutations in a congenital myopathy with cores, *Neurology* 59:284-287, 2002.

280. Ferreiro A, Monnier N, Romero NB, Leroy J-P, et al: A recessive form of central core disease, transiently presenting as multi-minicore disease, is associated with a homozygous mutation in the ryanodine receptor type 1 gene, *Ann Neurol* 51:750-759, 2002.

281. Shy GM, Engel WK, Somers JE, Wanko T: Nemaline myopathy: A new congenital myopathy, *Brain* 86:793-810, 1963.

282. Kolin IS: Nemaline myopathy: A fatal case, *Am J Dis Child* 114:95-100, 1967.

283. Shafiq SA, Dubowitz V, Peterson H de C, Milhorat AT: Nemaline myopathy: Report of a fatal case, with histochemical and electron microscopic studies, *Brain* 90:817-828, 1967.

284. Karpati G, Carpenter S, Andermann F: A new concept of childhood nemaline myopathy, *Arch Neurol* 24:291-304, 1971.

285. Kuitunen P, Rapola J, Noponen AL, Donner M: Nemaline myopathy: Report of four cases and review of the literature, *Acta Paediatr Scand* 61:353-361, 1972.

286. Neustein HB: Nemaline myopathy: A family study with three autopsied cases, *Arch Pathol* 96:192-195, 1973.

287. Gilles C, Raye J, Vasan R: Nemaline (rod) myopathy, *Arch Pathol Lab Med* 103:1-14, 1979.

288. McComb RD, Markesbery WR, O'Connor WN: Fatal neonatal nemaline myopathy with multiple congenital anomalies, *J Pediatr* 94:47-51, 1979.

289. Kondo K, Yuasa T: Genetics of congenital nemaline myopathy, *Muscle Nerve* 3:308-315, 1980.

290. Nonaka I, Tojo M, Sugita H: Fetal muscle characteristics in nemaline myopathy, *Neuropediatrics* 14:47-52, 1983.

291. Norton P, Ellison P, Sulaiman AR, Harb J: Nemaline myopathy in the neonate, *Neurology* 33:351-356, 1983.

292. McMenamin JB, Curry B, Taylor GP, Becker LE, et al: Fatal nemaline myopathy in infancy, *Can J Neurol Sci* 11:305-309, 1984.

293. Shahar E, Tervo R, Murphy EG: Heterogeneity of nemaline myopathy, *Pediatr Neurosci* 14:236-240, 1988.

294. Wallgren-Pettersson C: Congenital nemaline myopathy: A clinical follow-up study of twelve patients, *J Neurol Sci* 89:1-14, 1989.

295. Nonaka I, Ishiura S, Arahata K, Ishibashi-Ueda H, et al: Progression in nemaline myopathy, *Acta Neuropathol (Berl)* 78:484-491, 1989.

296. Schmalbruch H, Kamieniecka Z, Arroe M: Early fatal nemaline myopathy: Case report and review, *Dev Med Child Neurol* 29:784-804, 1987.

297. Roig M, Harnandez MA, Salcedo S: Survival from symptomatic nemaline myopathy in the newborn period, *Pediatr Neurosci* 13:95-97, 1987.

298. Wallgren-Pettersson C, Arjomaa P, Holmberg C: α-Actinin and myosin light chains in congenital nemaline myopathy, *Pediatr Neurol* 6:171-174, 1990.

299. Shimomura C, Nonaka I: Nemaline myopathy: Comparative muscle histochemistry in the severe neonatal, moderate congenital, and adult-onset forms, *Pediatr Neurol* 5:25-31, 1989.

300. Wallgren-Pettersson C, Sainio K, Salmi T: Electromyography in congenital nemaline myopathy, *Muscle Nerve* 12:587-593, 1989.

301. Fidzianska A, Goebel HH, Kleine M: Neonatal form of nemaline myopathy, muscle immaturity, and a microvascular injury, *J Child Neurol* 5:122-126, 1990.

302. Logghe K, Wit JM, Jennekens F, Pruijs JE: Respiratory deterioration during growth hormone therapy in a case of congenital nemaline myopathy, *Eur J Pediatr* 150:69-71, 1990.

303. Sasaki M, Yoneyama H, Nonaka I: Respiratory muscle involvement in nemaline myopathy, *Pediatr Neurol* 6:425-427, 1990.

304. Van Antwerpen CL, Gospe SM, Dentinger MP: Nemaline myopathy associated with hypertrophic cardiomyopathy, *Pediatr Neurol* 4:306-308, 1988.

305. Ishibashi-Ueda H, Imakita M, Yutani C, Takahashi S, et al: Congenital nemaline myopathy with dilated cardiomyopathy: An autopsy study, *Hum Pathol* 21:77-82, 1990.

306. Laing NG, Majda BT, Akkari PA, Layton MG, et al: Assignment of a gene (NEMI) for autosomal dominant nemaline myopathy to chromosome-I, *Am J Hum Genet* 50:576-583, 1992.

307. Colamaria V, Zanetti R, Simeone M, Tomelleri G, et al: Minipolymyoclonus in congenital nemaline myopathy: A nonspecific clinical marker of neurogenic dysfunction, *Brain Dev* 13:358-362, 1991.

308. Rifai Z, Kazee AM, Kamp C, Griggs RC: Intranuclear rods in severe congenital nemaline myopathy, *Neurology* 43:2372-2377, 1993.

309. Banwell BL, Singh NC, Ramsay DA: Prolonged survival in neonatal nemaline rod myopathy, *Pediatr Neurol* 10:335-337, 1994.

310. Vendittelli F, Manciet-Labarchede C, Gilbert-Dussardier B: Nemaline myopathy in the neonate: Two case reports, *Eur J Pediatr* 155:502-505, 1996.

311. Wada H, Nishio H, Kugo M, Waku S, et al: Severe neonatal nemaline myopathy with delayed maturation of muscle, *Brain Dev* 18:135-138, 1996.

312. Sasaki M, Takeda M, Kobayashi K, Nonaka I: Respiratory failure in nemaline myopathy, *Pediatr Neurol* 16:344-346, 1997.

313. Lammens M, Moerman P, Fryns JP, Lemmens F, et al: Fetal akinesia sequence caused by nemaline myopathy, *Neuropediatrics* 28:116-119, 1997.

314. Itakura Y, Ogawa Y, Murakami N, Nonada I: Severe infantile congenital myopathy with nemaline and cytoplasmic bodies: A case report, *Brain Dev* 20:112-115, 1998.

315. North KN, Laing NG, Wallgren-Pettersson C, Akkari A, et al: Nemaline myopathy: Current concepts, *J Med Genet* 34:705-713, 1997.

316. Wallgren-Pettersson C: Genetics of the nemaline myopathies and the myotubular myopathies, *Neuromuscul Disord* 8:401-404, 1998.

317. Skyllouriotis ML, Marx M, Ksyllouriotis P, Bittner R, et al: Nemaline myopathy and cardiomyopathy, *Pediatr Neurol* 20:319-321, 1999.

318. Pelin K, Hilpela P, Donner K, Sewry C, et al: Mutations in the nebulin gene associated with autosomal recessive nemaline myopathy, *Proc Natl Acad Sci U S A* 96:2305-2310, 1999.

319. Wallgren-Pettersson C, Pelin K, Hilpela P, Donner K, et al: Clinical and genetic heterogeneity in autosomal recessive nemaline myopathy, *Neuromuscul Disord* 9:564-572, 1999.

320. Ryan MM, Schnell C, Strickland CD, Shield LK, et al: Nemaline myopathy: A clinical study of 143 cases, *Ann Neurol* 50:312-320, 2001.

321. Wallgren-Pettersson C, Donner K, Sewry C, Bijlsma E, et al: Mutations in the nebulin gene can cause severe congenital nemaline myopathy, *Neuromuscul Disord* 12:674-679, 2002.

322. Ryan MM, Ilkovski B, Strickland CD, Schnell C, et al: Clinical course correlates poorly with muscle pathology in nemaline myopathy, *Neurology* 60:665-673, 2003.

323. Wallgren-Pettersson C, Pelin K, Nowak KJ, Muntoni F, et al: Genotype-phenotype correlations in nemaline myopathy caused by mutations in the genes for nebulin and skeletal muscle alpha-actin, *Neuromuscul Disord* 14:461-470, 2004.

324. Agrawal PB, Strickland CD, Midgett C, Morales A, et al: Heterogeneity of nemaline myopathy cases with skeletal muscle alpha-actin gene mutations, *Ann Neurol* 56:86-96, 2004.

325. Corbett MA, Akkari PA, Domazetovska A, Cooper ST, et al: An alpha-tropomyosin mutation alters dimer preference in nemaline myopathy, *Ann Neurol* 57:42-49, 2005.

325a. Nowak KJ, Sewry CA, Navarro C, Squier W, et al: Nemaline myopathy caused by absence of alpha-skeletal muscle actin, *Ann Neurol* 61:175-184, 2007.

326. Nienhuis AW, Coleman RF, Brown JW: Nemaline myopathy: A histopathologic and histochemical study, *Am J Clin Pathol* 48:1-13, 1967.

327. Yamaguchi M, Robson RM, Stromer MH, Dahl DS: Actin filaments form the backbone of nemaline myopathy rods, *Nature* 271:265-267, 1978.

328. Jennekens FG, Roord JJ, Veldman H: Congenital nemaline myopathy. I. Defective organization of alpha-actinin is restricted to muscle, *Muscle Nerve* 6:61-68, 1983.

329. Stuhlfauth I, Jennekens FG, Willemse J, Jockusch BM: Congenital nemaline myopathy. II. Quantitative changes in alpha-actinin and myosin in skeletal muscle, *Muscle Nerve* 6:69-74, 1983.

330. Barohn RJ, Jackson CE, Kaganhallet KS: Neonatal nemaline myopathy with abundant intranuclear rods, *Neuromuscular Disord* 4:513-520, 1994.

331. Goebel HH, Pursoo A, Warlo I, Schofer O, et al: Infantile intranuclear rod myopathy, *J Child Neurol* 12:22-30, 1997.

332. Spiro AJ, Shy GM, Gonatas NK: Myotubular myopathy, *Arch Neurol* 14:1-14, 1966.

333. Engel WK, Gold GN, Karpati G: Type I fiber hypotrophy with internal nuclei, *Arch Neurol* 18:435-444, 1968.

334. Badurska B, Fidzianska A, Kamieniecka Z, Prot J, et al: Myotubular myopathy, *J Neurol Sci* 8:563-571, 1969.

335. Bethlem J, van Wijngaarden GK, Meijer AE, Hulsmann WC: Neuromuscular disease with type I fiber atrophy, central nuclei and myotube-like structures, *Neurology* 19:705-710, 1969.

336. Campbell MJ, Rebeiz JJ, Walton JN: Myotubular centronuclear or pericentronuclear myopathy? *J Neurol Sci* 8:425-443, 1969.

337. Munsat TL, Thompson LR, Coleman RF: Centronuclear (myotubular) myopathy, *Arch Neurol* 20:120-131, 1969.

338. Van Wijngaarden GK, Fleury P, Bethlem J, Meijer AE: Familial myotubular myopathy, *Neurology* 19:901-908, 1969.

339. Torres CF, Griggs RC, Goetz JP: Severe neonatal centronuclear myopathy with autosomal dominant inheritance, *Arch Neurol* 42:1011-1014, 1985.

340. Barth PG, van Wijngaarden GK, Bethlem J: X-linked myotubular myopathy with fatal neonatal asphyxia, *Neurology* 25:531-536, 1975.

341. Coers C, Telerman-Toppet N, Gerard JM, Szliwowski H, et al: Changes in motor innervation and histochemical patterns of muscle fibers in some congenital myopathies, *Neurology* 26:1046-1053, 1976.

342. Raju TN, Vidyasagar D, Reyes M, Chokroverty S: Centronuclear myopathy in the newborn period causing severe respiratory distress, *Pediatrics* 59:29-34, 1977.

343. Reitter B, Mortier W, Wille L: Neonatal respiratory insufficiency due to centronuclear myopathy, *Acta Paediatr Scand* 68:773-778, 1979.

344. Askanas V, Engel WK, Reddy PG, Barth PG, et al: X-linked recessive congenital muscle fiber hypotrophy with central nuclei, *Arch Neurol* 36:604-609, 1979.

345. Torres CF, Merritt TA, Vandyke DH: Myotubular myopathy with type I fiber hypotrophy and neuropathy, *Neurology* 29:572-576, 1979.

346. Sarnat HB, Roth SI, Jimenez JF: Neonatal myotubular myopathy: Neuropathy and failure of postnatal maturation of fetal muscle, *Can J Neurol Sci* 8:313-320, 1981.

347. Elder GB, Dean D, McComas AJ, Paes B, et al: Infantile centronuclear myopathy: Evidence suggesting incomplete innervation, *J Neurol Sci* 60:79-88, 1983.

348. Ambler MW, Neave C, Tutschka BG, Pueschel SM, et al: X-linked recessive myotubular myopathy. I. Clinical and pathologic findings in a family, *Human Pathol* 15:566-574, 1984.

349. Bruyland M, Liebaers I, Sacre L, Vandeplas Y, et al: Neonatal myotubular myopathy with a probable X-linked inheritance: Observations on a new family with a review of the literature, *J Neurol* 231:220-222, 1984.

350. Starr J, Lamont M, Iselius L, Harvey J, et al: A linkage study of a large pedigree with X-linked centronuclear myopathy, *J Med Genet* 27:281-283, 1990.

351. Sawchak JA, Sher JH, Norman MG, Kula RW, et al: Centronuclear myopathy heterogeneity: Distinction of clinical types by myosin isoform patterns, *Neurology* 41:135-140, 1991.

352. De Angelis MS, Palmucci L, Leone M, Doriguzzi C: Centronuclear myopathy: Clinical morphological and genetic characters. A review of 288 cases, *J Neurol Sci* 103:2-9, 1991.

353. Sandler DL, Burchfield DJ, McCarthy JA, Rojiani AM, et al: Early-onset respiratory failure caused by severe congenital neuromuscular disease, *J Pediatr* 124:636-638, 1994.

354. Waclawik AJ, Edgar TS, Lotz BP, Lewandoski BS, et al: Congenital myopathy with ringlike distribution of myonuclei and mitochondria and accumulation of nemaline rods: A variant of centronuclear myopathy? *Pediatr Neurol* 12:370-373, 1995.

355. Joseph M, Pai GS, Holden KR, Herman G: X-linked myotubular myopathy: Clinical observations in ten additional cases, *Am J Med Genet* 59:168-173, 1995.

356. Wallgren-Pettersson C, Clarke A, Samson F, Fardeau M, et al: The myotubular myopathies: Differential diagnosis of the X linked recessive, autosomal dominant, and autosomal recessive forms and present state of DNA studies, *J Med Genet* 32:673-679, 1995.

357. Mora M, Morandi L, Merlini L, Vita G, et al: Fetus-like dystrophin expression and other cytoskeletal protein abnormalities in centronuclear myopathies, *Muscle Nerve* 17:1176-1184, 1994.

358. Fidzianska A, Warlo I, Goebel HH: Neonatal centronuclear myopathy with N-CAM decorated myotubes, *Neuropediatrics* 25:158-161, 1994.

359. Lerman-Sagie T, Berns L, Tomer A, Glick B, et al: Central nervous system involvement in X-linked myotubular myopathy, *J Child Neurol* 12:70-72, 1997.

360. Herman GE, Finegold M, Zhao W, de Gouyan B, et al: Medical complications in long-term survivors with X-linked myotubular myopathy, *J Pediatr* 134:206-214, 1999.

361. de Goede CG, Kelsey A, Kingston H, Tomlin PI, et al: Muscle biopsy without centrally located nuclei in a male child with mild X-linked myotubular myopathy, *Dev Med Child Neurol* 47:835-837, 2005.

362. Jeannet PY, Bassez G, Eymard B, Laforet P, et al: Clinical and histologic findings in autosomal centronuclear myopathy, *Neurology* 62:1484-1490, 2004.

363. Pierson CR, Tomczak K, Agrawal P, Moghadaszadeh B, et al: X-linked myotubular and centronuclear myopathies, *J Neuropathol Exp Neurol* 64:555-564, 2005.

364. Sarnat HB: Myotubular myopathy: Arrest of morphogenesis of myofibres associated with persistence of fetal vimentin and desmin. Four cases compared with fetal and neonatal muscle, *Can J Neurol Sci* 17:109-123, 1990.

365. Laporte J, Hu LJ, Kretz C, Mandel JL, et al: A gene mutated in X-linked myotubular myopathy defines a new putative tyrosine phosphatase family conserved in yeast, *Nat Genet* 13:175-182, 1996.

366. Noguchi S, Fujita M, Murayama K, Kurokawa R, et al: Gene expression analyses in X-linked myotubular myopathy, *Neurology* 65:732-737, 2005.

367. Brooke MH: A neuromuscular disease characterized by fiber type disproportion. In Kakulas BA, editor: *Clinical Studies in Myology*, New York: 1973, Elsevier.

368. Fardeau M, Harpey JP, Caille B: Disproportion congenitale des différentes types de fibre musculaire avec petitesse relative des fibres de type I, *Rev Neurol (Paris)* 131:745-766, 1975.

369. Kinoshita M, Satoyoshi E, Kumagai M: Familial type I fiber atrophy, *J Neurol Sci* 25:11-17, 1975.

370. Lenard HG, Goebel HH: Congenital fiber type disproportion, *Neuropaediatrie* 6:220-228, 1975.

371. Curless RG, Nelson MB: Congenital fiber type disproportion in identical twins, *Ann Neurol* 2:455-459, 1977.

372. Cavanagh NP, Lake BD, McMeniman P: Congenital fiber type disproportion myopathy, *Arch Dis Child* 54:735-743, 1980.

373. Clancy RR, Kelts KA, Oehlert JW: Clinical variability in congenital fiber type disproportion, *J Neurol Sci* 46:257-266, 1980.

374. Sandyk R: Congenital fibre type disproportion: A case report, *S Afr Med J* 60:833-834, 1981.

375. Argov Z, Gardner-Medwin D, Johnson MA, Mastaglia FL: Patterns of muscle fiber-type disproportion in hypotonic infants, *Arch Neurol* 41:53-57, 1984.

376. Glick B, Shapira Y, Stern A. Congenital muscle fiber type disproportion myopathy: A follow-up study of 20 cases. Paper presented at the Child Neurology Society Annual Meeting, Phoenix, Arizona, 1984.

377. Sarnat HB: Cerebral dysgeneses and their influence on fetal muscle development, *Brain Dev* 8:495-499, 1986.

378. Mizuno Y, Komiya K: A serial muscle biopsy study in a case of congenital fiber-type disproportion associated with progressive respiratory failure, *Brain Dev* 12:431-436, 1990.

379. Yoshioka M, Kuroki S, Ohkura K, Itagaki Y, et al: Congenital myopathy with type II muscle fiber hypoplasia, *Neurology* 37:860-863, 1987.

380. Gallanti A, Prelle A, Chianese L, Barbieri S, et al: Congenital myopathy with type-2A muscle fiber uniformity and smallness, *Neuropediatrics* 23:10-13, 1992.

381. Jong YJ, Huang SC, Liu GC, Chiang CH: Mental retardation in congenital nonprogressive myopathy with uniform type 1 fibers, *Brain Dev* 13:444-446, 1991.

382. Gerdes AM, Petersen MB, Schroder HD, Wulff K, et al: Congenital myopathy with fiber type disproportion: A family with a chromosomal translocation t(10;17) may indicate candidate gene regions, *Clin Genet* 45:11-16, 1994.

383. Jung EY, Hattori H, Higuchi Y, Mitsuyoshi I, et al: Brain atrophy in congenital neuromuscular disease with uniform type 1 fibers, *Pediatr Neurol* 16:56-58, 1998.

384. Muranaka H, Osari SI, Fujita H, Kimura Y, et al: Congenital familial myopathy with type 2 fiber hypoplasia and type 1 fiber predominance, *Brain Dev* 19:362-365, 1997.

385. Nakagawa E, Ozawa M, Yamanouchi H, Sugai K, et al: Severe central nervous system involvement in a patient with congenital fiber-type disproportion myopathy, *J Child Neurol* 11:71-73, 1996.

386. Banwell BL, Becker LE, Jay V, Taylor GP, et al: Cardiac manifestations of congenital fiber-type disproportion myopathy, *J Child Neurol* 14:83-87, 1999.

387. Tsuji M, Higuchi Y, Shiraishi K, Mitsuyoshi I, et al: Congenital fiber type disproportion: Severe form with marked improvement, *Pediatr Neurol* 21:658-660, 1999.

388. Imoto C, Nonaka I: The significance of type 1 fiber atrophy (hypotrophy) in childhood neuromuscular disorders, *Brain Dev* 23:298-302, 2001.

389. Clarke NF, North KN: Congenital fiber type disproportion: 30 years on, *J Neuropathol Exp Neurol* 62:977-989, 2003.

390. Laing NG, Clarke NF, Dye DE, Liyanage K, et al: Actin mutations are one cause of congenital fibre type disproportion, *Ann Neurol* 56:689-694, 2004.

390a. Clarke NF, Ilkovski B, Cooper S, Valova VA, et al: The pathogenesis of ACTA1-related congenital fiber, *Ann Neurol* 61:552-561, 2007.

391. Clarke NF, Smith RL, Bahlo M, North KN: A novel X-linked form of congenital fiber-type disproportion, *Ann Neurol* 58:767-772, 2005.

392. Sobrido MJ, Fernandez JM, Fontoira E, Perez-Sousa C, et al: Autosomal dominant congenital fibre type disproportion: A clinicopathological and imaging study of a large family, *Brain* 128:1716-1727, 2005.

393. Clarke NF, Kidson W, Quijano-Roy S, Estournet B, et al: SEPN1: Associated with congenital fiber-type disproportion and insulin resistance, *Ann Neurol* 59:546-552, 2006.

394. Ferreiro A, Estourner B, Chateau D, Romero NB, et al: Mult-minicore disease—searching for boundaries: Phenotype analysis of 38 cases, *Ann Neurol* 48:745-757, 2000.

395. Jungbluth H, Sewry C, Brown SC, Manzur AY, et al: Minicore myopathy in children: A clinical and histopathological study of 19 cases, *Neuromuscul Disord* 10:264-273, 2000.

396. Jungbluth H, Zhou H, Hartley L, Halliger-Keller B, et al: Minicore myopathy with ophthalmoplegia caused by mutations in the ryanodine receptor type 1 gene, *Neurology* 65:1930-1935, 2005.

397. Black JT, Judge D, Demers L, Gordon S: Ragged-red fibers: A biochemical and morphological study, *J Neurol Sci* 26:479, 1975.

398. DeVivo DC: The expanding clinical spectrum of mitochondrial diseases, *Brain Dev* 15:1-22, 1993.

399. Shy GM, Gonatas NK, Perez M: Two childhood myopathies with abnormal mitochondria. I. Megaconial myopathy. II. Peoconial myopathy, *Brain* 89:133-158, 1966.

400. Sengers RC, Stadhouders AM, Trijbels JM: Mitochondrial myopathies: Clinical, morphological and biochemical aspects, *Eur J Pediatr* 141:192-207, 1984.

401. DiMauro S, Bonilla E, Zeviani M: Mitochondrial myopathies, *Ann Neurol* 17:521-538, 1985.

402. Morgan-Hughes JA: Mitochondrial diseases. In Engel AG, Franzini-Armstrong C, editors: *Myology*, New York: 1994, McGraw-Hill.

403. Robinson BH: Human cytochrome oxidase deficiency, *Pediatr Res* 48:581-585, 2000.

404. DiMauro S, Schon EA: Mechanisms of disease: Mitochondrial respiratory-chain diseases, *N Engl J Med* 348:2657-2668, 2003.

405. Zeviani M, Di Donato S: Mitochondrial disorders, *Brain* 127:2153-2172, 2004.

406. DiMauro S, Hirano M: Mitochondrial encephalomyopathies: An update, *Neuromuscul Disord* 15:276-286, 2005.

407. DeVivo DC, Bonilla E, DiMauro S: Mitochondrial diseases. In Jones HR Jr, DeVivo DC, Darras BT, editors: *Neuromuscular Disorders of Infancy, Childhood, and Adolescence: A Clinician's Approach*, Philadelphia: 2003, Butterworth Heinemann.

408. Aprille JR: Mitochondrial cytopathies and mitochondrial DNA mutations, *Curr Opin Pediatr* 3:1045-1054, 1991.

409. DiMauro S, Moraes CT, Schon EA: Mitochondrial encephalomyopathies: Problems of classification. In Sato T, DiMauro S, editors: *Progress in Neuropathology*, New York: 1991, Raven Press, Ltd.

410. Moraes CT, Schon EA, DiMauro S: Mitochondrial diseases: Toward a rational classification. In Appel SH, editor: *Current Neurology*, St. Louis, MO: 1991, Mosby.

411. Toshima K, Kuroda Y, Miyao M, Suehiro T, et al: Histological changes of muscle in a patient with pyruvate dehydrogenase deficiency, *Brain Dev* 5:571-576, 1983.

412. Van Biervliet JP, Bruinvis L, Ketting D, De Bree PK, et al: Hereditary mitochondrial myopathy with lactic acidemia, a de Toni-Fanconi-Debre syndrome, and a defective respiratory chain in voluntary striated muscles, *Pediatr Res* 11:1088-1093, 1977.

413. DiMauro S, Mendell JR, Sahenk Z, Bachman D, et al: Fatal infantile mitochondrial myopathy and renal dysfunction due to cytochrome-c-oxidase deficiency, *Neurology* 30:795-804, 1980.

414. Heiman-Patterson TD, Bonilla E, DiMauro S, Foreman J, et al: Cytochrome-c-oxidase deficiency in a floppy infant, *Neurology* 32:898-901, 1982.

415. Rimoldi M, Bottacchi E, Rossi L, Cornelio F, et al: Cytochrome-c-oxidase deficiency in muscles of a floppy infant without mitochondrial myopathy, *J Neurol* 227:201-207, 1982.

416. Boustany RN, Aprille JR, Halperin J: Mitochondrial cytochrome deficiency presenting as a myopathy with hypotonia, external ophthalmoplegia, and lactic acidosis in an infant and a fatal hepatopathy in a second cousin, *Ann Neurol* 14:462-470, 1983.

417. DiMauro S, Nicholson JF, Hays AP, Eastwood AB, et al: Benign infantile mitochondrial myopathy due to reversible cytochrome c oxidase deficiency, *Ann Neurol* 14:226-234, 1983.

418. Muller-Hocker J, Pongratz D, Deufel T, Trijbels JM, et al: Fatal lipid storage myopathy with deficiency of cytochrome c oxidase and carnitine: A contribution to the combined cytochemical-fine-structural identification of cytochrome-c-oxidase in long-term frozen muscle, *Virchows Arch A Pathol Anat Histopathol* 399:11-23, 1983.

419. Minchom PE, Dormer RL, Hughes IA, Stansbie D, et al: Fatal infantile mitochondrial myopathy due to cytochrome c oxidase deficiency, *J Neurol Sci* 60:453-463, 1983.

420. Trijbels JM, Sengers R, Monnens L: A patient with lactic acidemia and cytochrome oxidase deficiency, *J Inherit Metab Dis* 6:127, 1983.

421. Behbehani AW, Goebel H, Osse G, Gabriel M, et al: Mitochondrial myopathy with lactic acidosis and deficient activity of muscle succinate cytochrome-c-oxidoreductase, *Eur J Pediatr* 143:67-71, 1984.

422. Sengers RC, Trijbels JM, Bakkeren JA, Ruitenbeek W, et al: Deficiency of cytochromes b and aa3 in muscle from a floppy infant with cytochrome oxidase deficiency, *Eur J Pediatr* 141:178-180, 1984.

423. Bresolin N, Zeviani M, Bonilla E, Miller RH, et al: Fatal infantile cytochrome c oxidase deficiency: Decrease of immunologically detectable enzyme in muscle, *Neurology* 35:802-812, 1985.

424. Zeviani M, Nonaka I, Bonilla E, Okino E, et al: Fatal infantile mitochondrial myopathy and renal dysfunction due to cytochrome c oxidase deficiency: Immunological studies in a new patient, *Ann Neurol* 17:414-417, 1985.

425. Roodhooft AM, Van Acker KJ, Martin JJ, Ceuterick C, et al: Benign mitochondrial myopathy with deficiency of NADH-CoQ reductase and cytochrome c oxidase, *Neuropediatrics* 17:221-226, 1986.

426. Salo MK, Rapola J, Somer H, Pihko H, et al: Reversible mitochondrial myopathy with cytochrome c oxidase deficiency, *Arch Dis Child* 67:1033-1035, 1992.

427. Zeviani M, Peterson P, Servidei S, Bonilla E, et al: Benign reversible muscle cytochrome c oxidase deficiency: A second case, *Neurology* 37:64-67, 1987.

428. Tritschler HJ, Bonilla E, Lombes A, Andreetta F, et al: Differential diagnosis of fatal and benign cytochrome c oxidase–deficient myopathies of infancy, *Neurology* 41:300-305, 1991.

429. Griebel V, Krageloh-Mann I, Ruitenbeek W, Trijbels JM, et al: A mitochondrial myopathy in an infant with lactic acidosis, *Dev Med Child Neurol* 32:528-548, 1990.

430. Muller-Hocker J, Droste M, Kadenbach B, Pongratz D, et al: Fatal mitochondrial myopathy with cytochrome-c-oxidase deficiency and subunit-restricted reduction of enzyme protein in two siblings: An autopsy-immunocytochemical study, *Hum Pathol* 20:666-672, 1989.

431. Zheng X, Shoffner JM, Lott MT, Voljavec AS, et al: Evidence in a lethal infantile mitochondrial disease for a nuclear mutation affecting respiratory complex I and IV, *Neurology* 39:1203-1209, 1989.

432. Tulinius MH, Eriksson BO, Hjalmarson O, Holme E, et al: Mitochondrial myopathy and cardiomyopathy in siblings, *Pediatr Neurol* 5:182-188, 1989.

433. Takayanagi T, Inoue M, Tomimasu K, Shimomura C, et al: Infantile cytochrome c oxidase deficiency with neonatal death, *Pediatr Neurol* 5:179-181, 1989.

434. Oldfors A, Sommerland H, Holme E, Tulinius M, et al: Cytochrome c oxidase deficiency in infancy, *Acta Neuropathol (Berl)* 77:267-275, 1989.

435. Nonaka I, Koga Y, Okino E, Kikuchi A, et al: Defects in muscle fiber growth in fatal infantile cytochrome c oxidase deficiency, *Brain Dev* 10:223-230, 1988.

436. Zeviani M, Van Dyke D, Servidei S, Bauserman SC, et al: Myopathy and fatal cardiopathy due to cytochrome c oxidase deficiency, *Arch Neurol* 43:1198-1202, 1986.

437. Nagai T, Tuchiya Y, Taguchi Y, Sakuta R, et al: Fatal infantile mitochondrial encephalomyopathy with Complex I and IV deficiencies, *Pediatr Neurol* 9:151-154, 1993.

438. Macmillan CJ, Shoubridge EA: Mitochondrial DNA depletion: Prevalence in a pediatric population referred for neurologic evaluation, *Pediatr Neurol* 14:203-210, 1996.

439. Vu TH, Sciacco M, Tanji K, Nichter C, et al: Clinical manifestations of mitochondrial DNA depletion, *Neurology* 50:1783-1790, 1998.

440. Rubio-Gozalbo ME, Smeitink JA, Ruitenbeek W, Ter Laak H, et al: Spinal muscular atrophy-like picture, cardiomyopathy, and cytochrome c oxidase deficiency, *Neurology* 52:383-386, 1999.

441. Darras BT, Friedman NR: Metabolic myopathies: A clinical approach. I, *Pediatr Neurol* 22:87-97, 2000.

442. Sue CM, Karadimas C, Checcarelli N, Tanji K, et al: Differential features of patients with mutations in two COX assembly genes, SURF-1 and SCO2, *Ann Neurol* 47:589-595, 2000.

443. Absolon MJ, Harding CO, Fain DR, Mack KJ: Leigh syndrome in an infant resulting from mitochondrial DNA depletion, *Pediatr Neurol* 24:60-63, 2001.

444. Darin N, Oldfors A, Moslemi AR, Holme E, et al: The incidence of mitochondrial encephalomyopathies in childhood: Clinical features and morphological, biochemical, and DNA abnormalities, *Ann Neurol* 49:377-383, 2001.

445. Filiano J, Goldenthal M, Mamourian A, Hall C, et al: Mitochondrial DNA depletion in Leigh syndrome, *Pediatr Neurol* 26:239-242, 2002.

446. Mancuso M, Salviati L, Sacconi S, Otaegui D, et al: Mitochondrial DNA depletion: Mutations in thymidine kinase gene with myopathy and SMA, *Neurology* 59:1197-1202, 2002.

447. Darin N, Moslemi AR, Lebon S, Rustin P, et al: Genotypes and clinical phenotypes in children with cytochrome-c oxidase deficiency, *Neuropediatrics* 34:311-317, 2003.

448. Sacconi S, Salviati L, Sue CM, Shanske S, et al: Mutation screening in patients with isolated cytochrome c oxidase deficiency, *Pediatr Res* 53:224-230, 2003.

449. Von Kleist-Retzow JC, Cormeir-Dare V, Viot G, Goldenberg A, et al: Antenatal manifestations of mitochondrial respiratory chain deficiency, *J Pediatr* 143:208-212, 2003.

450. Meulemans A, Lissens W, Coster RV, Meirleir LD, et al: Analysis of the mitochondrial encoded subunits of complex I in 20 patients with a complex I deficiency, *Eur J Paediatr Neurol* 8:299-306, 2004.

451. Coenen MJ, van den Heuvel LP, Ugalde C, Ten Brinke M, et al: Cytochrome c oxidase biogenesis in a patient with a mutation in COX10 gene, *Ann Neurol* 56:560-564, 2004.

452. McFarland R, Kirby DM, Fowler KJ, Ohtake A, et al: De Novo mutations in the mitochondrial ND3 gene as a cause of infantile mitochondrial encephalopathy and complex I deficiency, *Ann Neurol* 55:58-64, 2004.

453. Bohm M, Pronicka E, Karczmarewicz E, Pronicki M, et al: Retrospective, multicentric study of 180 children with cytochrome C oxidase deficiency, *Pediatr Res* 59:21-26, 2006.

454. Dinopoulos A, Cecil KM, Schapiro MB, Papadimitriou A, et al: Brain MRI and proton MRS findings in infants and children with respiratory chain defects, *Neuropediatrics* 36:290-301, 2005.

455. Esteitie N, Hinttala R, Wibom R, Nilsson H, et al: Secondary metabolic effects in complex I deficiency, *Ann Neurol* 58:544-552, 2005.

456. Galbiati S, Bordoni A, Papadimitriou D, Toscano A, et al: New mutations in TK2 gene associated with mitochondrial DNA depletion, *Pediatr Neurol* 34:177-185, 2006.

457. Wada H, Woo M, Nishio H, Nagaki S, et al: Vascular involvement in benign infantile mitochondrial myopathy caused by reversible cytochrome c oxidase deficiency, *Brain Dev* 18:263-268, 1996.

458. Bodnar AG, Cooper JM, Holt IJ, Leonard JV, et al: Nuclear complementation restores mtDNA levels in cultured cells from a patient with mtDNA depletion, *Am J Hum Genet* 53:663-669, 1993.

459. Moraes CT, Shanske S, Tritschler HJ: mDNA depletion with variable tissue expression: A novel genetic abnormality in mitochondrial disease, *Am J Hum Genet* 48:492-501, 1991.

460. Telerman-Toppet N, Biarent D, Boulton JM: Fatal cytochrome c oxidase-deficient myopathy of infancy associated with mDNA depletion. Differential involvement of skeletal muscle and cultured fibroblasts, *J Inherit Metab Dis* 15:323-326, 1992.

461. Tritschler H-J, Andreetta F, Moraes CT: Mitochondrial myopathy of childhood associated with depletion of mitochondrial DNA, *Neurology* 42:209-217, 1992.

462. Mazziotta M, Ricci E, Bertini E: Fatal infantile liver failure associated with mitochondrial DNA depletion, *J Pediatr* 121:896-901, 1992.

463. Marin-Garcia J, Goldenthal MJ: Mitochondrial biogenesis defects and neuromuscular disorders, *Pediatr Neurol* 22:122-129, 2000.

464. Engel AG, Hirschhorn R: Acid maltase deficiency. In Engel AG, Franzini-Armstrong C, editors: *Myology*, New York: 1994, McGraw-Hill.

465. DiMauro S, Tsujino S: Nonlysosomal glycogenoses. In Engel AG, Franzini-Armstrong C, editors: *Myology*, New York: 1994, McGraw-Hill.

466. Darras BT, Friedman NR: Metabolic myopathies: A clinical approach. II, *Pediatr Neurol* 22:171-181, 2000.

467. Bruno C, Hays AP, DiMauro S: Glycogen storage diseases of muscle. In Jones HR Jr, DeVivo DC, Darras BT, editors: *Neuromuscular Disorders of Infancy, Childhood, and Adolescence: A Clinician's Approach*, Philadelphia: 2003, Butterworth Heinemann.

468. Tsao CY, Boesel CP, Wright FS: A hypotonic infant with complete deficiencies of acid maltase and Debrancher enzyme, *J Child Neurol* 9:90-91, 1994.

469. Tang TT, Segura AD, Chen YT, Ricci LM, et al: Neonatal hypotonia and cardiomyopathy secondary to type IV glycogenosis, *Acta Neuropathol (Berl)* 87:531-536, 1994.

470. Nambu M, Kawabe K, Fukuda T, Okuno TB, et al: A neonatal form of glycogen storage disease type IV, *Neurology* 61:392-394, 2003.

471. Tay SK, Akman HO, Chung WK, Pike MG, et al: Fatal infantile neuromuscular presentation of glycogen storage disease type IV, *Neuromuscul Disord* 14:253-260, 2004.

472. DiMauro S, Hartlage PL: Fatal infantile form of muscle phosphorylase deficiency, *Neurology* 28:1124-1129, 1978.

473. Milstein JM, Herron TM, Haas JE: Fatal infantile muscle phosphorylase deficiency, *J Child Neurol* 4:186-188, 1989.

474. Buhrer C, van Landeghem F, Bruck W, Feiderhoff-Muser U, et al: Fetal-onset severe skeletal muscle glycogenosis associated with phosphorylase-b kinase deficiency, *Neuropediatrics* 31:104-106, 2000.

475. Ohtani Y, Matsuda I, Iwamasa T, Tamari H, et al: Infantile glycogen storage myopathy in a girl with phosphorylase kinase deficiency, *Neurology* 32:833-838, 1982.

476. Sahin G, Gungor T, Rettwitz-Volk W, Schlote W, et al: Infantile muscle phosphorylase-b-kinase deficiency: A case report, *Neuropediatrics* 29:48-50, 1998.

477. Guibaud P, Carrier H, Mathieu M, Dorche C, et al: Observation familiale de dystrophie musculaire congenitale par deficit en phosphofructokinase, *Arch Fr Pediatr* 35:1105-1115, 1978.

478. Danon MJ, Carpenter S, Manaligod JR, Schliselfeld LH: Fatal infantile glycogen storage disease: Deficiency of phosphofructokinase and phosphorylase beta-kinase, *Neurology* 31:1303-1307, 1981.

479. Servidei S, Bonilla E, Diedrich RG, Kornfeld M, et al: Fatal infantile form of muscle phosphofructokinase deficiency, *Neurology* 36:1465-1470, 1986.

480. Amit R, Bashan N, Abarbanel JM, Shapira Y, et al: Fatal familial infantile glycogen storage disease: Multisystem phosphofructokinase deficiency, *Muscle Nerve* 15:455-458, 1992.

481. Swoboda KJ, Specht L, Jones HR, Shapiro F, et al: Infantile phosphofructokinase deficiency with arthrogryposis: Clinical benefit of a ketogenic diet, *J Pediatr* 131:932-934, 1997.

482. Di Mauro S, Trevisan C, Hays A: Disorders of lipid metabolism in muscle, *Muscle Nerve* 3:369-388, 1980.

483. Rebouche CJ, Engel AG: Carnitine metabolism and deficiency syndromes, *Mayo Clin Proc* 58:533-540, 1983.

484. Tein I, DeVivo DC, Bierman F, Pulver P, et al: Impaired skin fibroblast carnitine uptake in primary systemic carnitine deficiency manifested by childhood carnitine-responsive cardiomyopathy, *Pediatr Res* 28:247-255, 1990.

485. DeVivo DC, Tein I: Primary and secondary disorders of carnitine metabolism, *Int Pediatr* 5:134-141, 1990.

486. Hale DE, Bennett MJ: Fatty acid oxidation disorders: A new class of metabolic diseases, *J Pediatr* 121:1-11, 1992.

487. Shapira Y, Glick B, Harel S, Vattin JJ, et al: Infantile idiopathic myopathic carnitine deficiency: Treatment with L-carnitine, *Pediatr Neurol* 9:35-38, 1993.

488. Wilcken B, Carpenter KH, Hammond J: Neonatal symptoms in medium chain acyl coenzyme-A dehydrogenase deficiency, *Arch Dis Child* 69:292-294, 1993.

489. Rinaldo P, Stanley CA, Hsu BY, Sanchez LA, et al: Sudden neonatal death in carnitine transporter deficiency, *J Pediatr* 131:304-305, 1997.

490. Stanley CA: Dissecting the spectrum of fatty acid oxidation disorders, *J Pediatr* 132:384-386, 1998.

491. Tein I, Haslam RHA, Rhead WJ, Bennett MJ, et al: Short-chain acyl-CoA dehydrogenase deficiency: A cause of ophthalmoplegia and multicore myopathy, *Neurology* 52:366-372, 1999.

492. Pons R, Cavadini P, Baratta S, Invernizzi F, et al: Clinical and molecular heterogeneity in very-long-chain acyl-coenzyme A dehydrogenase deficiency, *Pediatr Neurol* 22:98-105, 2000.

493. Tein I: Lipid storage muscular disorders. In Jones HR Jr, DeVivo DC, Darras BT, editors: *Neuromuscular Disorders of Infancy, Childhood, and Adolescence: A Clinician's Approach*, Philadelphia: 2003, Butterworth Heinemann.

494. Longo N, Amat di San Filippo C, Pasquali M: Disorders of carnitine transport and the carnitine cycle, *Am J Med Genet C Semin Med Genet* 142:77-85, 2006.

495. Hart ZH, Chang CH, DiMauro S, Farooki Q, et al: Muscle carnitine deficiency and fatal cardiomyopathy, *Neurology* 28:147-151, 1978.

496. Roe CR, Coates PM: Mitrochondrial fatty acid oxidation disorders. In Scriver CR, Beaudet AL, Sly WS, et al, editors: *The Metabolic and Molecular Bases of Inherited Disease*, New York: 1995, McGraw-Hill.

497. Pavone P, Barbagallo M, Parano E, Pavone L, et al: Clinical heterogeneity in familial congenital ptosis: Analysis of fourteen cases in one family over five generations, *Pediatr Neurol* 33:251-254, 2005.

498. Cohen HB: Congenital ptosis: A new pedigree and classification, *Arch Ophthalmol* 87:161-163, 1972.

499. Berke RN, Wadsworth JA: Histology of levator muscle in congenital and acquired ptosis, *Arch Ophthalmol* 53:413-428, 1955.

500. In Nelson LB, Calhoun JH, Harley RD, editors: *Pediatric Ophthalmology*, 3rd ed, Philadelphia: 1991, Saunders.

501. Ryan MM, Stasheff SF, Engle EC: Disorders of the ocular motor cranial nerves and extraocular muscles. In Jones HR Jr, DeVivo DC, Darras BT, editors: *Neuromuscular Disorders of Infancy, Childhood, and Adolescence: A Clinician's Approach*, Philadelphia: 2003, Butterworth Heinemann.

502. Gutowski NJ, Bosley TM, Engle EC: 110th ENMC International Workshop: The congenital cranial dysinnervation disorders (CCDDs), Naarden, the Netherlands, 25-27 October, 2002, *Neuromuscul Disord* 13:573-578, 2003.

503. Victor DI: The diagnosis of congenital unilateral third-nerve palsy, *Brain* 99:711-718, 1976.

504. Prats JM, Monzon MJ, Zuazo E, Garaizar C: Congenital nuclear syndrome of oculomotor nerve, *Pediatr Neurol* 9:476-478, 1993.

505. Parmeggiani A, Posar A, Leonardi M, Rossi PG: Neurological impairment in congenital bilateral ptosis with ophthalmoplegia, *Brain Dev* 14:107-109, 1992.

506. Engle EC, Goumnerov BC, McKeown CA, Schatz M, et al: Oculomotor nerve and muscle abnormalities in congenital fibrosis of the extraocular muscles, *Ann Neurol* 41:314-325, 1997.

507. Wang SM, Zwaan J, Mullaney PB, Jabak MH, et al: Congenital fibrosis of the extraocular muscles type 2, an inherited exotropic strabismus fixus, maps to distal 11q13, *Am J Hum Genet* 63:517-525, 1998.

508. Engle EC: The genetic basis of complex strabismus, *Pediatr Res* 59:343-348, 2006.

508a. Bosley TM, Salih MA, Alorainy IA, Oystreck DT, et al: Clinical characterization of the HOXA1 syndrome BSAS variant, *Neurology* 69:1245-1253, 2007.

509. Duane A: Congenital deficiency of abduction, association with impairment of adduction, retraction movements, contraction of the palpebral fissure and oblique movements of the eye, *Arch Ophthalmol* 34:133, 1905.

510. Duke-Elder S: *System of Ophthalmology*, London: 1964, Henry Kimptom.

511. Pfaffenbach DD, Cross HE, Kearns TP: Congenital anomalies in Duane's retraction syndrome, *Arch Ophthalmol* 88:635-639, 1972.

512. Cross HE, Pfaffenbach DD: Duane's retraction syndrome and associated congenital malformations, *Am J Ophthalmol* 73:442-450, 1972.

513. Okihiro MM, Tasaki T, Nakano KK, Bennett BK: Duane syndrome and congenital upper-limb anomalies, *Arch Neurol* 34:174-179, 1977.

514. Hotchkiss MG, Miller NR, Clark AW, Green WG: Bilateral Duane's retraction syndrome: A clinical-pathological case report, *Arch Ophthalmol* 98:870-874, 1980.

515. Miller NR, Kiel SM, Green WR, Clark AW: Unilateral Duane's retraction syndrome (type 1), *Arch Ophthalmol* 100:1468-1472, 1982.

516. Yamanouchi H, Iwasaki Y, Mukuno K: Duane retraction syndrome associated with Chiari I malformation, *Pediatr Neurol* 9:327-329, 1993.

517. Prats JM, Garaizar C: Duane retraction syndrome associated with Chiari I malformation, *Pediatr Neurol* 10:340, 1994.

518. Bosley TM, Salih MAM, Jen JC, Lin DDM, et al: Neurologic features of horizontal gaze palsy and progressive scoliosis with mutations in ROBO3, *Neurology* 64:1196-1203, 2005.

519. Morrison DA, Bibby K, Woodruff G: The "harlequin" sign and congenital Horner's syndrome, *J Neurol Neurosurg Psychiatry* 62:626-628, 1997.

520. Gibbs J, Appleton RE, Martin J, Findlay G: Congenital Horner syndrome associated with non-cervical neuroblastoma, *Dev Med Child Neurol* 34:642-644, 1992.

521. Zafeiriou DI, Economou M, Koliouskas D, Triantafyllou P, et al: Congenital Horner's syndrome associated with cervical neuroblastoma, *Eur J Paediatr Neurol* 10:90-92, 2006.

522. Afifi AK, Bell WE, Menezes AH: Etiology of lateral rectus palsy in infancy and childhood, *J Child Neurol* 7:295-299, 1992.

523. Bale JF, Scott WE, Yuh W, Sato Y, et al: Congenital fourth nerve palsy and occult cranium bifidum, *Pediatr Neurol* 4:320-321, 1988.

524. Möbius PJ: Ueber angeborene doppelseitigne Abducens-Facialis-Laehmung, *Munch Med Wochenschr* 35:91, 1888.

525. Henderson JL: The congenital facial diplegia syndrome: Clinical features, pathology and etiology, *Brain* 62:381, 1939.

526. Sudarshan A, Goldie WD: The spectrum of congenital facial diplegia (Moebius syndrome), *Pediatr Neurol* 1:180-184, 1985.

527. Govaert P, Vanhaesebrouck P, De Praeter C, Frankel U, et al: Moebius sequence and prenatal brainstem ischemia, *Pediatrics* 84:570-573, 1989.

528. Raroque HG, Hershewe GL, Snyder RD: Mobius syndrome and transposition of the great vessels, *Neurology* 38:1894-1895, 1988.

529. Erro MIG, Correale J, Arberas C, Muchnik S, et al: Familial congenital facial diplegia: Electrophysiologic and genetic studies, *Pediatr Neurol* 5:262-264, 1989.

530. Kawai M, Momoi T, Fujii T, Nakano S, et al: The syndrome of Mobius sequence, peripheral neuropathy and hypogonadotropic hypogonadism, *Am J Med Genet* 37:578-583, 1990.

531. Gilmore RL, Falace P, Kanga J, Baumann R: Sleep-disordered breathing in Mobius syndrome, *J Child Neurol* 6:73-77, 1991.

532. Fujita I, Koyanagi T, Kukita J, Yamashita H, et al: Moebius syndrome with central hypoventilation and brainstem calcification: A case report, *Eur J Pediatr* 150:582-583, 1991.

533. Hatanaka T, Yoshijima S, Hayashi N, Owa K, et al: Electrophysiologic studies in an infant with Möbius syndrome, *J Child Neurol* 8:182-185, 1993.

534. Byerly KA, Pauli RM: Cranial nerve abnormalities in CHARGE association, *Am J Med Genet* 45:751-757, 1993.

535. Kankirawatana P, Tennison MB, D'Cruz O, Greenwood RS: Mobius syndrome in infant exposed to cocaine in utero, *Pediatr Neurol* 9:71-72, 1993.

536. Schimke RN, Collins DL, Hiebert JM: Congenital nonprogressive myopathy with Mobius and Robin sequence—the Carey-Fineman-Ziter syndrome: A confirmatory report, *Am J Med Genet* 46:721-723, 1993.

537. Singh B, Shahwan SA, Singh P, Al-Deeb SM, et al: Mobius syndrome with basal ganglia calcification, *Acta Neurol Scand* 85:436-438, 1992.

538. St. Charles S, Dimario FJ, Grunnet ML: Mobius sequence: Further in vivo support for the subclavian artery supply disruption sequence, *Am J Med Genet* 47:289-293, 1993.

539. D'Cruz OF, Swisher CN, Jaradeh S, Tang T, et al: Mobius syndrome: Evidence for a vascular etiology, *J Child Neurol* 8:260-265, 1993.

540. Jaradeh S, D'Cruz O, Howard JF, Haberkamp TJ, et al: Mobius syndrome: Electrophysiologic studies in seven cases, *Muscle Nerve* 19:1148-1153, 1996.

541. Graf WD, Shepard TH: Uterine contraction in the development of Mobius syndrome, *J Child Neurol* 12:225-227, 1997.

542. Igarashi M, Rose DF, Storgion SA: Moebius syndrome and central respiratory dysfunction, *Pediatr Neurol* 16:237-240, 1997.

543. Lammens M, Moerman P, Fryns JP, Schroder JM, et al: Neuropathological findings in Moebius syndrome, *Clin Genet* 54:136-141, 1998.

544. Stromland K, Sjogreen L, Miller M, Gillberg C, et al: Mobius sequence: A Swedish multidicipline study, *Eur J Paediatr Neurol* 6:35-45, 2002.

545. Verzijl HT, van der Zwaag B, Cruysberg JR, Padberg GW: Mobius syndrome redefined: A syndrome of rhombencephalic maldevelopment, *Neurology* 61:327-333, 2003.

546. Johansson M, Wentz E, Fernell E, Stromland K, et al: Autistic spectrum disorders in Mobius sequence: A comprehensive study of 25 individuals, *Dev Med Child Neurol* 43:338-345, 2001.

547. Verzijl HT, Valk J, de Vries R, Padberg GW: Radiologic evidence for absence of the facial nerve in Mobius syndrome, *Neurology* 64:849-855, 2005.

548. Maheshwari A, Calhoun DA, Lacson A, Pereda L, et al: Pontine hypoplasia in Carey-Fineman-Ziter (CFZ) syndrome, *Am J Med Genet Part A* 127A:288-290, 2004.

549. Carey JC: The Carey-Fineman-Ziter syndrome: Follow-up of the original siblings and comments on pathogenesis, *Am J Med Part A* 127A:294-297, 2004.

550. Dufke A, Riethmuller J, Enders H: Severe congenital myopathy with Mobius, Robin, and Poland sequences: New aspects of the Carey-Fineman-Ziter syndrome, *Am J Med Genet Part A* 127A:291-293, 2004.

551. Verloes A, Bitoun P, Heuskin A, Amrom D, et al: Mobius sequence, Robin complex, and hypotonia: Severe expression of brainstem disruption spectrum versus Carey-Fineman-Ziter syndrome, *Am J Med Genet A* 127:277-287, 2004.

552. Richter RB: Congenital hypoplasia of the facial nucleus, *J Neuropathol Exp Neurol* 17:520, 1958.

553. Thakkar N, O'Neil W, Duvally J, Liu C, et al: Mobius syndrome due to brain stem tegmental necrosis, *Arch Neurol* 34:124-126, 1977.

554. Towfighi J, Marks K, Palmer E, Vannucci R: Mobius syndrome: Neuropathologic observations, *Acta Neuropathol (Berl)* 48:11-17, 1979.

555. Wilson ER, Mirra SS, Schwartz JF: Congenital diencephalic and brain stem damage: Neuropathologic study of three cases, *Acta Neuropathol (Berl)* 57:70-74, 1982.

556. Pedraza S, Gamez J, Rovira A, Zamora A, et al: MRI findings in Mobius syndrome: Correlation with clinical features, *Neurology* 55:1058-1060, 2000.

557. Peleg D, Nelson GM, Williamson RA, Widness JA: Expanded Mobius syndrome, *Pediatr Neurol* 24:306-309, 2001.

558. Verzijl HT, van der Zwaag B, Lammens M, ten Donkelaar HJ, et al: The neuropathology of hereditary congenital facial palsy vs Mobius syndrome, *Neurology* 64:649-653, 2005.

559. Ouanounou S, Saigal G, Birchansky S: Mobius syndrome, *AJNR Am J Neuroradiol* 26:430-432, 2005.

560. Rerecich A, Alfonso I: Brain calcification in Mobius syndrome, *Pediatr Neurol* 31:236-237, 2004.

561. Dooley JM, Stewart WA, Hayden JD, Therrien A: Brainstem calcification in Mobius syndrome, *Pediatr Neurol* 30:39-41, 2004.

562. Sarnat HB: Watershed infarcts in the fetal and neonatal brainstem: An aetiology of central hypoventilation, dysphagia, Mobius syndrome and micrognathia, *Eur J Pediatr Neurol* 8:71-87, 2004.

563. Verzijl HT, Padberg GW, Zwarts MJ: The spectrum of Mobius syndrome: An electrophysiological study, *Brain* 128:1728-1736, 2005.

564. Hanissian AS, Fuste F, Hayes WT, Duncan JM: Mobius syndrome in twins, *Am J Dis Child* 120:472-475, 1970.

565. Rubinstein AE, Lovelace RE, Behrens MM, Weisberg LA: Moebius syndrome in Kallmann syndrome, *Arch Neurol* 32:480-482, 1975.

566. Cayler GG, Blumenfeld CM, Anderson RL: Further studies of patients with cardiofacial syndrome, *Chest* 60:161-165, 1971.

567. Gonzalez CH, Vargas FR, Perez AB: Limb deficiency with or without Mobius sequence in seven Brazilian children associated with misoprostol use in the first trimester of pregnancy, *Am J Med Genet* 47:59-64, 1993.

568. McKusick VA: *Mendelian Inheritance in Man*, Baltimore: 1975, Johns Hopkins University Press.

569. Becker-Christensen F, Lund HT: A family with Mobius syndrome, *J Pediatr* 84:115-117, 1974.

570. Ziter FA, Wiser WC, Robinson A: Three-generation pedigree of a Mobius syndrome variant with chromosome translocation, *Arch Neurol* 34:437-442, 1977.

571. Van der Zwaag B, Verzijl HT, Wichers KH, Beltran-Valero de Bernabe D, et al: Sequence analysis of the PLEXIN-D1 gene in Mobius syndrome patients, *Pediatr Neurol* 31:114-118, 2004.

572. Tischfield MA, Bosley TM, Salih MA, Alorainy IA, et al: Homozygous HOXA1 mutations disrupt human brainstem, inner ear, cardiovascular and cognitive development, *Nat Genet* 37:1035-1037, 2005.

573. Puckett CL, Beg SA: Facial reanimation in Mobius syndrome, *South Med J* 71:1498-1501, 1978.

574. Alexiou D, Manolidis C, Papaevangellou G, Nicopoulos D, et al: Frequency of other malformations in congenital hypoplasia of depressor anguli oris muscle syndrome, *Arch Dis Child* 51:891-893, 1976.

575. Papadatos C, Alexiou D, Nicolopoulos D, Mikropoulos H, et al: Congenital hypoplasia of depressor anguli oris muscle: A genetically determined condition? *Arch Dis Child* 49:927-931, 1974.

576. Sapin SO, Miller AA, Bass HN: Neonatal asymmetric crying facies: A new look at an old problem, *Clin Pediatr (Phila)* 44:109-119, 2005.

576a. Dubnov-Raz G, Merlob P, Geva-Dayan K, Blumenthal D, et al: Increased rate of major birth malformations in infants with neonatal "asymmetric crying face": A hospital-based cohort study, *Am J Med Genet A* 143A:305-310, 2007.

577. Nelson KB, Eng G: Congenital hypoplasia of the depressor anguli oris muscle: Differentiation from congenital facial palsy, *J Pediatr* 81:16-20, 1972.

578. Lenarsky C, Shewmon DA, Shaw A, Feig SA: Occurrence of neuroblastoma and asymmetric crying facies: Case report and review of the literature, *J Pediatr* 107:268-270, 1985.

579. Meberg A, Skogen P: Three different manifestations of congenital muscular aplasia in a family, *Acta Paediatr Scand* 76:375-377, 1987.

580. Lin DS, Huang FY, Lin SP, Chen MR, et al: Frequency of associated anomalies in congenital hypoplasia of depressor anguli oris muscle: A study of 50 patients, *Am J Med Genet* 71:215-218, 1997.

581. Cayler GG: Cardiofacial syndrome: Congenital heart disease and facial weakness, a hitherto unrecognized association, *Arch Dis Child* 44:69-75, 1969.

582. Pape KE, Pickering D: Asymmetric crying facies: An index of other congenital anomalies, *J Pediatr* 81:21-30, 1972.

583. Levin SE, Silverman NH, Milner S: Hypoplasia or absence of the depressor anguli oris muscle and congenital abnormalities, with special reference to the cardiofacial syndrome, *S Afr Med J* 61:227-231, 1982.

584. Renault F, Quijano-Roy S: Congenital and acquired facial palsies. In Jones HR Jr, DeVivo DC, Darras BT, editors: *Neuromuscular Disorders of Infancy, Childhood, and Adolescence: A Clinician's Approach*, Philadelphia: 2003, Butterworth Heinemann.

585. Voudris KA, Skardoutsou A, Vagiakou EA: Congenital asymmetric crying facies and agenesis of corpus callosum, *Brain Dev* 25:133-136, 2003.

586. Rioja-Mazza D, Lieber E, Kamath V, Kalpatthi R: Asymmetric crying facies: A possible marker for congenital malformations, *J Matern Fetal Neonatal Med* 18:275-277, 2005.

587. Akcakus M, Ozkul Y, Gunes T, Kurtoglu S, et al: Associated anomalies in asymmetric crying facies and 22q11 deletion, *Genet Couns* 14:325-330, 2003.

588. Caksen H, Odabas D, Tuncer O, Kirimi E, et al: A review of 35 cases of asymmetric crying facies, *Genet Couns* 15:159-165, 2004.

589. Holinger LD, Holinger PC, Holinger PH: Etiology of bilateral abductor vocal cord paralysis: A review of 389 cases, *Ann Otol Rhinol Laryngol* 85:428-436, 1976.

590. Cohen SR, Birns JW, Geller KA, Thompson JW: Laryngeal paralysis in children: A long-term retrospective study, *Ann Otol Rhinol Laryngol* 91:417-424, 1982.

591. Schumacher RE, Weinfeld IJ, Bartlett RH: Neonatal vocal cord paralysis following extracorporeal membrane oxygenation, *Pediatrics* 84:793-796, 1989.

592. Chaten FC, Lucking SE, Young ES, Mickell JJ: Stridor: Intracranial pathology causing postextubation vocal cord paralysis, *Pediatrics* 87:39-43, 1991.

593. Koppel R, Friedman S, Fallet S: Congenital vocal cord paralysis with possible autosomal recessive inheritance: Case report and review of the literature, *Am J Med Genet* 64:485-487, 1996.

594. Condon LM, Katkov H, Singh A, Helseth HK: Cardiovocal syndrome in infancy, *Pediatrics* 76:22-25, 1985.

595. Ardran GM, Benson PF, Butler NR, Ellis HL, et al: Congenital dysphagia resulting from dysfunction of the pharyngeal musculature, *Dev Med Child Neurol* 7:157-166, 1965.

596. Bellmaine SP, McCredie J, Storey B: Pharyngeal incoordination from birth to three years, with recurrent bronchopneumonia and ultimate recovery, *Aust Paediatr J* 8:137-139, 1972.

597. Mbonda E, Claus D, Bonnier C, Evrard P, et al: Prolonged dysphagia caused by congenital pharyngeal dysfunction, *J Pediatr* 126:923-927, 1995.

598. Inder TE, Volpe JJ: Recovery of congenital isolated pharyngeal dysfunction: Implications for early management, *Pediatr Neurol* 19:222-224, 1998.

599. Kinney HC, Filiano JJ, Sleeper LA, Mandell F, et al: Decreased muscarinic receptor binding in the arcuate nucleus in sudden infant death syndrome, *Science* 269:1446-1450, 1995.

600. Ford FR: *Diseases of the Nervous System in Infancy, Childhood, and Adolescence*, Springfield, IL: 1960, Charles C Thomas.

601. Eng GD: Neuromuscular diseases. In Avery GB, editor: *Neonatology, Pathophysiology and Management of the Newborn*, Philadelphia: 1994, JB Lippincott.

602. Davids JR, Wenger DR, Mubarak SJ: Congenital muscular torticollis: Sequela of intrauterine or perinatal compartment syndrome, *J Pediatr Orthop* 13:141-147, 1993.

603. Cheng JC, Au AW: Infantile torticollis: A review of 624 cases, *J Pediatr Orthop* 14:802-808, 1994.

604. Entel RJ, Carolan FJ: Congenital muscular torticollis: Magnetic resonance imaging and ultrasound diagnosis, *J Neuroimaging* 17:128-130, 1997.

605. Cheng JC, Tang SP, Chen TM: Sternocleidomastoid pseudotumor and congenital muscular torticollis in infants: A prospective study of 510 cases, *J Pediatr* 134:712-716, 1999.

606. Chen MM, Chang HC, Hsieh CF, Yen MF, et al: Predictive model for congenital muscular torticollis: Analysis of 1201 infants with sonography, *Arch Phys Med Rehabil* 86:2199-2203, 2005.

607. Tatli B, Aydinli N, Caliskan M, Ozmen M, et al: Congenital muscular torticollis: Evaluation and classification, *Pediatr Neurol* 34:41-44, 2006.

608. Clarren SK: Plagiocephaly and torticollis: Etiology, natural history, and helmet treatment, *J Pediatr* 98:92-95, 1981.

609. Romero R, Chervenak FA, DeVore G: Fetal head deformations and congenital torticollis associated with a uterine tumor, *Am J Obstet Gynecol* 141:839-840, 1981.

610. Bergen BJ, Sangalang VE, Aterman K: Isolated myopathic involvement of the diaphragmatic musculature in a neonate, *Ann Neurol* 1:403-407, 1977.

610a. Hartley L, Kinali M, Knight R, Mercuri E, et al: A congenital myopathy with diaphragmatic weakness not linked to the SMARD1 locus, *Neuromuscul Disord* 17:174-179, 2007.

611. Mellins RB, Balfour HH, Turino GM, Winters RW: Failure of automatic control of ventilation (Ondine's curse): Report of an infant born with this syndrome and review of the literature, *Medicine (Baltimore)* 49:487-504, 1970.

612. Deonna T, Arczynska W, Torrado A: Congenital failure of autonomic ventilation (Ondine's curse): A case report, *J Pediatr* 84:710-714, 1974.

613. Shannon DC, Marsland DW, Gould JB, Callahan B, et al: Central hypoventilation during quiet sleep in two infants, *Pediatrics* 57:342-346, 1976.

614. Hunt CE, Matalon SV, Thompson TR, Demuth S, et al: Central hypoventilation syndrome: Experience with bilateral phrenic nerve pacing in three neonates, *Am Rev Respir Dis* 118:23-28, 1978.

615. Phillipson EA: Control of breathing during sleep, *Am Rev Respir Dis* 118:909-939, 1978.

616. Coleman M, Boros SJ, Huseby TL, Brennom WS: Congenital central hypoventilation syndrome: A report of successful experience with bilateral diaphragmatic pacing, *Am J Dis Child* 55:901-903, 1980.

617. Fleming PJ, Cade D, Bryan MH, Bryan AC: Congenital central hypoventilation and sleep states, *Pediatrics* 66:425-428, 1980.

618. Wells HH, Kattwinkel J, Morrow JD: Control of ventilation in Ondine's curse, *J Pediatr* 96:865-867, 1980.

619. Ilbawi MN, Hunt CE, DeLeon SY, Idriss FS: Diaphragm pacing in infants and children: Report of a simplified technique and review of experience, *Ann Thorac Surg* 31:61-65, 1981.

620. Guilleminault C, McQuitty J, Ariagno RL, Challamel MJ, et al: Congenital central alveolar hypoventilation syndrome in six infants, *Pediatrics* 70:684-694, 1982.

621. Brouillette RT, Ilbawi MN, Hunt CE: Phrenic nerve pacing in infants and children: A review of experience and report on the usefulness of phrenic nerve stimulation studies, *J Pediatr* 102:32-39, 1983.

622. Guilleminault C, Challamel MJ: Congenital central hypoventilation syndrome (CCHS): Independent syndrome or generalized impairment of the autonomic nervous system? In Korobkin R, Guilleminault C, editors: *Progress in Perinatal Neurology*, Baltimore: 1981, Williams & Wilkins.

623. Ruth V, Pesonen E, Raivio KO: Congenital central hypoventilation syndrome treated with diaphragm pacing, *Acta Paediatr Scand* 72:295-297, 1983.

624. Poceta JS, Strandjord T, Badura R, Milstein JM: Ondine curse and neurocristopathy, *Pediatr Neurol* 3:370-372, 1987.

625. Khalifa MM, Flavin MA, Wherrett BA: Congenital central hypoventilation syndrome in monozygotic twins, *J Pediatr* 113:853-855, 1988.

626. Alvord EC, Shaw CM: Congenital difficulties with swallowing and breathing associated with maternal polyhydramnios: Neurocristopathy or medullary infarction? *J Child Neurol* 4:299-306, 1989.

627. Marcus CL, Jansen MT, Poulsen MK, Keens SE, et al: Medical and psychosocial outcome of children with congenital central hypoventilation syndrome, *J Pediatr* 119:888-895, 1991.

628. Weese-Mayer DE, Hunt CE, Brouillette RT, Silvestri JM: Diaphragm pacing in infants and children, *J Pediatr* 120:1-8, 1992.

629. Weese-Mayer DE, Silvestri JM, Menzies LJ, Morrowkenny AS, et al: Congenital central hypoventilation syndrome: Diagnosis, management, and long-term outcome in 32 children, *J Pediatr* 120:381-387, 1992.

630. Silvestri JM, Weesemayer DE, Nelson MN: Neuropsychologic abnormalities in children with congenital central hypoventilation syndrome, *J Pediatr* 120:388-393, 1992.

631. Woo MS, Woo MA, Gozal D, Jansen MT, et al: Heart rate variability in congenital central hypoventilation syndrome, *Pediatr Res* 31:291-296, 1992.

632. Weese-Mayer DE, Silvestri JM, Marazita ML, Hoo JJ: Congenital central hypoventilation syndrome: Inheritance and relation to sudden infant death syndrome, *Am J Med Genet* 47:360-367, 1993.

633. Croaker GD, Shi E, Simpson E, Cartmill T, et al: Congenital central hypoventilation syndrome and Hirschsprung's disease, *Arch Dis Child* 78:316-322, 1998.

634. Todd ES, Weinberg SM, Berry-Kravis EM, Silvestri JM, et al: Facial phenotype in children and young adults with PHOX2B-determined congenital central hypoventilation syndrome: Quantitative pattern of dysmorphology, *Pediatr Res* 59:39-45, 2006.

635. Gaultier C, Trang H, Dauger S, Gallego J: Pediatric disorders with autonomic dysfunction: What role for PHOX2B? *Pediatr Res* 58:1-6, 2005.

636. Gaultier C: Functional brain deficits in congenital central hypoventilation syndrome, *Pediatr Res* 57:471-472, 2005.

637. Chiaretti A, Zorzi G, Di Rocco C, Genovese O, et al: Neurotrophic factor expression in three infants with Ondine's curse, *Pediatr Neurol* 33:331-336, 2005.

638. Woo MA, Macey PM, Macey KE, Keen TG, et al: FMRI responses to hyperoxia in congenital central hypoventilation syndrome, *Pediatr Res* 57:510-518, 2005.

639. Chen ML, Tablizo MA, Kun S, Keens TG: Diaphragm pacers as a treatment for congenital central hypoventilation syndrome, *Expert Rev Med Devices* 2:577-585, 2005.

INTRACRANIAL INFECTIONS

Chapter 20

Viral, Protozoan, and Related Intracranial Infections

The central nervous system (CNS) and its covering membranes may become involved in a variety of infectious processes, with devastating effects on structure and function. Infections may occur during intrauterine development, in association with the birth process, or in the first postnatal days or weeks. Microbial organisms implicated include several viruses, a protozoan *(Toxoplasma gondii)*, a spirochete *(Treponema pallidum)*, and numerous bacteria and fungi. In this and the following chapter, I review the major features of infections caused by these agents. Because some excellent sources review the microbiological aspects of these infections,[1,2] the emphasis of the following discussion is principally on the neurological and neuropathological features.

In this chapter, infections of the CNS by viruses, *Toxoplasma*, and *Treponema* are reviewed. The major infections in this group are frequently designated by the term *TORCH syndrome*, in which *T* stands for toxoplasmosis, *O is* for others (i.e., syphilis and human immunodeficiency virus [HIV] infection), *R* is for rubella, *C* is for cytomegalovirus (CMV) infection, and *H* represents herpes simplex. I prefer the term *SCRATCHES*, in which *S* stands for syphilis, *C* is for CMV infection, *R* is for rubella, *A* is for acquired immunodeficiency syndrome (AIDS) or HIV infection, *T* is for toxoplasmosis, *C* is for chickenpox or varicella, *H* stands for herpes simplex, and *ES* is for enterovirus infections. Some of the essential features of this group are described in Table 20-1. Most are examples of infection by transplacental passage of the microorganism, usually consequent to infection within the maternal bloodstream. Serious illness resulting from herpes simplex virus (HSV) infection is an exception to this rule because most such cases are contracted around the time of birth, either as an ascending infection just before birth or during passage through an infected birth canal. HIV is transmitted to the fetus by both mechanisms; the relative importance is not entirely clear. With most infections within each group, patients are asymptomatic in the neonatal period, although the neonatal neurological syndromes that do occur are quite dramatic. An exception to this rule, again, is HSV infection, which is rarely accompanied by an asymptomatic neonatal period.

In addition to the TORCH group of microbes, enterovirus infections, varicella, and lymphocytic choriomeningitis may cause fetal or neonatal illness, with significant neurological consequences. The neonatal disorders caused by these organisms are reviewed after the discussion of the TORCH syndromes.

DESTRUCTIVE VERSUS TERATOGENIC EFFECTS

Although the mechanisms involved in the production of the neuropathological processes associated with these nonbacterial disorders are discussed in more detail in relation to specific infections, two different types of lesions can be distinguished. The first relates to *inflammatory, destructive effects* and the second relates to *developmental derangements* (i.e., *teratogenic effects*). It may be difficult to separate these two types of effects, because destructive processes affecting the developing brain often cause *coincident* tissue loss *and* subsequent anomalous development. The distinction is made still more difficult by the relatively limited capacity of early fetal brain to respond to injury; thus, the neuropathologist, evaluating the brain later, finds it difficult to identify signs of parenchymal inflammation and destruction.

In contrast, conventional means of identifying intrauterine viral infection (e.g., neonatal virus isolation or antibody response) may not be adequate to detect an infection during early brain development that is completed before the fetus is capable of mounting a humoral antibody response ($\approx$20 weeks of gestation) or is subjected to viral isolation procedures.[3] Such early viral infection has been shown to cause serious brain anomalies in animals. That a similar phenomenon may occur in human infants is suggested by studies in which investigators used a sensitive immunological indicator of early fetal virus exposure (i.e., detection of increased *cell-mediated* immune response [lymphocyte blastogenesis]).[3] Employing this approach, Thompson and Glasgow[3] demonstrated early intrauterine exposure to virus in 8 of 23 human infants with several congenital anomalies of the CNS. No elevation of humoral antibody to the viruses involved (mumps and HSV) could be demonstrated. Mumps accounted for seven of the eight cases. These observations require confirmation and elaboration but suggest the possibility that early fetal viral infection may be a more important cause of developmental aberration of the human nervous system than is currently recognized.

Although destructive and teratogenic effects overlap, and the precise quantitative contributions of each effect

TABLE 20-1   Central Nervous System Involvement by the TORCH Group

Organism or Disease	Major Route of Infection	Usual Time of Infection*	NEONATAL NEUROLOGICAL ILLNESS	
			Symptomatic	Asymptomatic
Cytomegalovirus	Transplacental	T1, T2	+	++++
Herpes simplex	Ascending and/or parturitional	Birth	++++	+
Rubella	Transplacental	T1	++	+++
Toxoplasmosis	Transplacental	T1, T2	+	++++
Syphilis	Transplacental	T2, T3	+	++++
Human immunodeficiency virus	Transplacental/parturitional	T2, T3, Birth	+	++++

*For occurrence of neonatal neurological disease; T1, T2, and T3 refer to the first, second, and third trimesters of gestation, respectively.
+, 0% to 25%; ++, 26% to 50%; +++, 51% to 75%; ++++, 76% to 100%; TORCH: T, toxoplasmosis; O, others (i.e., syphilis and human immunodeficiency virus); R, rubella; C, cytomegalovirus; H, herpes simplex.

are not always clear, I attempt to retain a separation of these two basic concepts. The recurring theme regarding destructive effects is varying degrees of inflammation, often with tissue injury (i.e., meningoencephalitis). Regarding teratogenic effects, the theme is more varied, although aberrations of neuronal proliferation and migration have been recognized. Defects in organizational events may be significant but require further study for documentation.

TORCH INFECTIONS

Cytomegalovirus Infection

CMV infection of the infant occurs in utero by transplacental mechanisms (congenital infection). CMV infection is the most common and serious congenital infection. In the United States, approximately 35,000 to 45,000 infants with CMV infection are born yearly.[4-7] This number could increase in societies similar to the United States, where mothers with young children work and have their children in day care. Approximately 25% to 75% of such children acquire CMV infection, and 50% of all family members then acquire the infection from them.[4,5,7,8] A minority of infants infected in utero exhibit overt neurological or systemic signs in the neonatal period. A majority of infants with congenital infection are asymptomatic, but many of these infants exhibit important sequelae. Still larger numbers of infants acquire CMV infection at the time of birth, during passage through an infected birth canal, or in the first weeks of life, through breast milk or, less commonly, through blood transfusion or other sources.[2,5,7,9-16] These infants appear to escape without serious neurological injury.

Pathogenesis

Fetal Infection. Clinically significant infection with CMV occurs during intrauterine life by transplacental passage of the virus.[2,7,9,14,17,18] The organism is transmitted to the fetus usually during a primary maternal infection (less commonly during recurrent infection) with viremia and subsequent placentitis.[7,19] The maternal infection is usually asymptomatic but may be manifested by a mononucleosis-like illness (≈10%) or a more serious systemic illness.[7,9] Maternal infection is

very common; cytomegaloviruria occurs in 3% to 6% of unselected pregnant women.[7,9,20] Cervical CMV infection is several times more common than cytomegaloviruria but tends to occur late in pregnancy and is probably less likely to result in significant fetal infection. Clinically significant fetal CMV infection probably occurs principally in the first or second trimesters, particularly if CNS disease is the outcome measure.[7,14,17,21] The possibility of CNS involvement after CMV infection in the third trimester was suggested by a study of seven children, but the exact timing of the fetal infection was established in only one case (at 27 weeks of gestation).[22] Moreover, the nature of the neuropathological features in some infected infants is also consistent with CNS involvement secondary to infection relatively late in pregnancy (see later discussion).[23,24]

Approximately 30% to 40% of infants whose mothers experience primary infection during pregnancy develop congenital infection.[2,7,18,20,25-27] Cytomegaloviruria has been observed in approximately 0.5% to 2% of infants in the neonatal period.[3,6,7,10,28-31] Because a period of approximately 4 to 8 weeks is required between the time of infection and the viruria,[32] these neonatal examples reflect intrauterine infection and not perinatal acquisition from parturitional or postnatal exposure. In these cases of congenital CMV infection, involvement of the CNS may be overt in the neonatal period or may not become apparent for months or years thereafter (see later discussion). In a prospective series of more than 12,000 pregnant women, primary CMV infection was complicated by congenital infection in 41% of infants, and only 12% of the affected infants were overtly symptomatic at birth.[20] Severe, clinically apparent congenital infection rarely occurs following recurrent (nonprimary) infection (i.e., infection in women with preexisting seroimmunity).[2,5,7,21,33-35] However, this generally very low risk is increased if the recurrent maternal infection involves a strain of CMV different from that resulting in the preexisting seroimmunity.[36]

Parturitional and Postnatal Infections. Parturitional and postnatal exposures cause an additional 10% to 15% of infants to acquire CMV infection in the first 4 to 8 weeks of life.[7,10-13,17] Breast milk is probably the

TABLE 20-2	Neuropathology of Congenital Cytomegalovirus Infection Symptomatic in the Neonatal Period

Meningoencephalitis
Germinal matrix necrosis/cysts
Periventricular cerebral calcification
Cerebral white matter cysts/calcification with atrophy and
   ventriculomegaly
Cerebral cortical atrophy
Microcephaly
Migrational disturbances: polymicrogyria, lissencephaly/
   pachygyria, schizencephaly
Cerebellar hypoplasia

single most important source of CMV exposure in premature infants.[7,37-41] Blood transfusion has been a particularly important source in low-birth-weight infants.[15] Although the results of one study raised the possibility of an increased risk of neurological sequelae in premature infants who acquire CMV infection during the first 8 weeks of life,[13] most data have indicated that CNS involvement does not occur with parturitional or early postnatal infection.[2,7,10-13,16,17,41] The reasons for the difference in propensity to affect the CNS between early prenatal versus natal or postnatal acquisitions of CMV remain to be determined.

Neuropathology

Congenital CMV infection may be associated with asymptomatic or symptomatic neurological presentations in the neonatal period (see subsequent discussion). The symptomatic presentation is uncommon but serves as the prototype for the neuropathology produced by primary infection of the developing CNS by this virus. Evidence both for inflammation and destruction and for teratogenicity can be observed

TABLE 20-3	Neuropathological Features of Congenital Cytomegalovirus Infection in 15 Preterm Infants*	
Neuropathological Feature		**Percentage of Infants Affected**
Microcephaly		87%
Meningoencephalitis		75%
Calcifications		80%
Periventricular		73%
Cortical		40%
Both		40%
Polymicrogyria		33%
Lissencephaly		7%
Ventriculomegaly		27%
Cerebellar hypoplasia		33%
Periventricular leukomalacia or porencephaly		20%

*Nine infants (mean birth weight, 2350 g; mean gestational age, 33 weeks) died in the neonatal period; 6 infants (mean birth weight, 1145 g; mean gestational age, 33 wks) were stillborn.
Data from Perlman JM, Argyle C: Lethal cytomegalovirus infection in preterm infants: Clinical, radiological, and neuropathological findings, *Ann Neurol* 31:64-68, 1992.

(Table 20-2). The spectrum of the neuropathology was well illustrated by a large neuropathological study of 15 premature infants who died with congenital CMV infection (Table 20-3).

Meningoencephalitis. *Meningoencephalitis* is characterized by the following features: (1) inflammatory cells in the meninges; (2) perivascular infiltrates with inflammatory cells; (3) necrosis of brain parenchyma, with all cellular elements affected, especially in the periventricular region, and often associated with calcification; (4) reactive microglial and astroglial proliferation; and (5) occurrence of enlarged cells (neuronal and glial elements) with intranuclear inclusions (Fig. 20-1).[25,32,42-45] Electron microscopic studies have revealed virions in brain tissue, a finding attesting to the primary infection of the CNS by the organism.[46] Recovery of virus from brain confirmed this conclusion.[9] A role for the inflammatory response itself in causing tissue destruction is suggested by the disparity between the detection of cytomegaloviral DNA by in situ hybridization and the extent of the tissue necrosis.[47]

The *cellular and regional targets of the meningoencephalitis* include especially the *germinal matrix, cerebral white matter*, and *cerebral cortex*.[24,25,32,42-45,48-54] Germinal matrix necrosis and cysts are prominent. Subsequent matrix calcification is important in determining the *periventricular* distribution of *calcifications*. Periventricular cerebral white matter also is a site of injury, sometimes with cyst formation and subsequent calcification. A predilection for the *parietal white matter* may mimic periventricular leukomalacia. In addition, a predilection for *anterior temporal white matter* is particularly suggestive of CMV infection. Cerebral cortical atrophy is a later feature.

Microcephaly. *Microcephaly* is a common feature in the neonatal period and is still more prominent later in infancy. The small size of the brain appears to relate to the encephaloclastic effects of the virus and probably also to a disturbance of cell proliferation in the developing brain. The latter disturbance relates to the propensity of the virus to affect the subependymal germinal matrix (see earlier). A predilection for involvement of proliferative cells is also suggested by the frequency of intrauterine growth retardation in congenital CMV infection and by the observation in a variety of tissues of a decrease in absolute number of cells.[55-58]

Disturbances of Neuronal Migration. Disturbances of neuronal migration have been described repeatedly in congenital CMV infection.[23,24,42-45,48,50-52,54,59-72] Indeed, polymicrogyria has been documented in approximately 65% of well-studied cases. The polymicrogyria may involve cerebellar (Fig. 20-2) as well as cerebral cortex. Although polymicrogyria has been observed most commonly, lissencephaly, pachygyria, schizencephaly, and neuronal heterotopias have also been reported.[23,24,45,64,65,69-72] These observations demonstrate the teratogenic potential of CMV and suggest the occurrence of infection in the latter part of the first trimester and in the second trimester, when

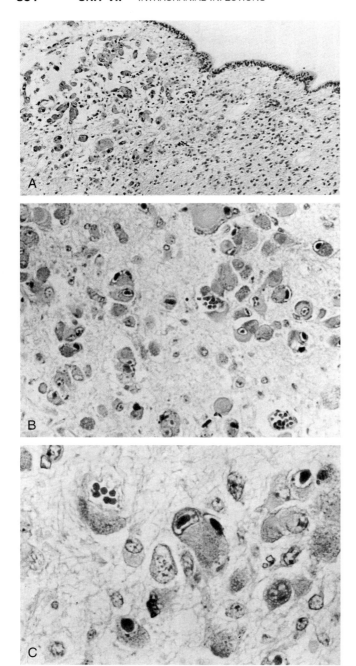

Figure 20-1 Congenital cytomegalovirus infection: encephalitis, from an infant who died at 10 weeks of age. A, Region of necrosis in the subependymal germinal matrix (ependyma is at the *upper right*). Note enlargement of cells, many with intranuclear inclusions. **B**, Higher-power view of the same region showing the enlarged cells with prominent intranuclear inclusions. **C**, A closer view of the inclusions; note the clear halo around the inclusions and the nuclear chromatin displaced to the periphery (Cowdry type A inclusions). *(From Bell WE, McCormick WF: Neurologic Infections in Children, Philadelphia: 1975, Saunders.)*

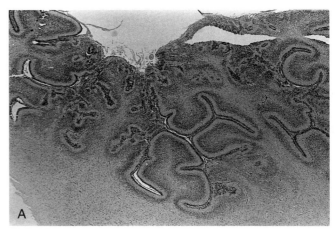

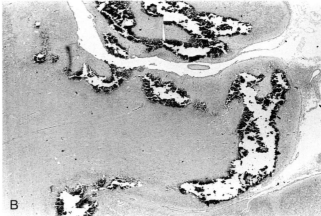

Figure 20-2 Congenital cytomegalovirus infection: neuronal migrational disturbance. A, Microgyric cerebellar cortex from a preterm infant with congenital cytomegalovirus infection. **B**, Section of the same microgyric cerebellar cortex shown in **A**, illustrating the distribution of calcification within the malformed cerebellar cortex and suggesting the coexistence of destructive and teratogenic effects. *(From Perlman JM, Argyle C: Lethal cytomegalovirus infection in preterm infants: Clinical, radiological, and neuropathological findings, Ann Neurol 31:64-68, 1992.)*

neuronal migration begins and then becomes active (see Chapter 2). The usual coexistence of inflammatory, destructive lesions indicates persistent infection by the organism. These cases also may be relevant to the notion that cerebral cortical neuronal injury late in the second trimester may underlie other examples of polymicrogyria (see Chapter 2). One careful study of four affected brains from infants with congenital CMV infection provided evidence of neuronal destruction in the lower cortical layers within areas of polymicrogyria and suggested that the cortical neuronal injury led ultimately to the gyral abnormality.[44] At any rate, CMV infection is the only one of the congenital infections that is associated with overt disturbances of gyral development, and the pathogenesis thereof may include a combination of teratogenic and encephaloclastic mechanisms.

Cerebellar Hypoplasia. Cerebellar hypoplasia, best detected by magnetic resonance imaging (MRI), is a feature in at least 50% of symptomatic cases. This finding likely is primarily a proliferative disturbance, although, as noted earlier, migrational disturbances may also be seen in the cerebellum. The finding of cerebellar hypoplasia in the clinical setting of an intrauterine infection is highly suggestive of congenital CMV.

Other Findings. Porencephaly, hydranencephaly, hydrocephalus, focal subcortical cysts, impaired myelination, and more diffuse cerebral calcifications also have been described to variable extents in congenital CMV infection.

Clinical Aspects

Incidence of Clinically Apparent Infection. Although congenital CMV infection occurs frequently, clinical manifestations thereof do not. Indeed, available data indicate that approximately 90% of affected infants are asymptomatic in the newborn period.[2,7,20,28,31,56,57,73-78]

Clinical Features. The most frequent clinical features of symptomatic congenital CMV infection are shown in Table 20-4.[2,7,9,14,17-19,56,57,79-84] The most common findings relate to disturbance of the reticuloendothelial system. Hepatosplenomegaly and a petechial rash, usually related to thrombocytopenia, are encountered very frequently. Infants are often small for gestational age; moreover, approximately one third of affected infants have a gestational age of 37 weeks or less. Inguinal hernia is a helpful clinical sign when present (≈25% of cases).

The *neurological syndrome* is variable in presentation. Seizures may be prominent, although only approximately 10% of symptomatic patients exhibit overt neonatal seizures. Microcephaly is a most consistent manifestation in patients with severe disease and appears in approximately 50% of all symptomatic patients. Cerebral calcification, usually periventricular in location, occurs in 50% to 60% of cases. Cerebrospinal fluid (CSF) findings of encephalitis (e.g., pleocytosis, elevated protein content) are found in the majority of patients, but precise data are not available.

The *clinical course* is most commonly that of a static process. However, evidence of progressive encephaloclastic disease, documented by computed tomography (CT) scan, was provided by a report of two such cases.[85] Similarly, postnatal evolution of cerebral calcification and of subependymal necrosis has been documented.[45,86] Moreover, progression of hearing loss during infancy and early childhood has been described clearly (see later).[7,18,20,78,83,84,87-90] The observation that virus is still recoverable in urine in 50% of cases at 5 years of age[91] demonstrates persistence of infection and further raises the possibility of progressive disease.

Clinical Diagnosis. The diagnosis of congenital CMV infection may be suspected with a high degree of accuracy on the basis of certain clinical features. These features include the periventricular locus of the cerebral calcification, microcephaly, CSF pleocytosis, and intrauterine growth retardation. Cerebellar hypoplasia and neuronal migrational abnormality are also distinctive features. The absence of the "salt-and-pepper" chorioretinitis of congenital rubella and the relative infrequency of the grossly scarring chorioretinitis of congenital toxoplasmosis are also helpful.

Laboratory Evaluation

Virus Isolation. Identification of the microbial agent is based principally on viral cultures and detection of viral genetic material.[2,7,9,14,17,18,92] The organism is cultured most readily from the urine but also can be grown from the throat and occasionally from the CSF. The detection of virus in urine remains a highly specific and sensitive test for the diagnosis of congenital CMV infection. Infectivity of urine is retained after storage at 4°C (not at room temperature and not frozen) for as long as 7 days.[93] A period of 2 to 4 weeks is required to detect the characteristic cytopathic effects in tissue culture. The detection of DNA of CMV in urine by the *polymerase chain reaction* (PCR) allows for diagnosis of infection in 1 day.[7,94] The increase in sensitivity of this test to virtually 100% by the removal of inhibitory materials in urine by glass filter paper absorption helped make this technique the ideal test for detection of infection.[92] PCR has also been shown to detect the virus in CSF, serum, and specimens of umbilical cord, although the sensitivity and specificity in these sites remain to be established.[95-98] Immunofluorescent procedures that permit *demonstration of specific CMV antigens* in the nuclei of tissue culture cells inoculated with infected urine are positive in 90% to 100% of cases.[93,99,100] This approach provides diagnostic information in 1 to 3 days.

Serological Studies. Many serological tests have been used, but the complement fixation test, enzyme-linked immunosorbent assay (ELISA), and fluorescent antibody test are used most commonly.[7,9,56,57] The commonly used complement fixation test depends on immunoglobulin G (IgG), and because this fraction is primarily derived by passive transfer from the infected mother, titers are high in the neonatal period. *Persistence* of an

TABLE 20-4	Clinical Features of Symptomatic Congenital Cytomegalovirus Infection*	
Clinical Feature		**Approximate Frequency**
Pregnancy		
Intrauterine growth retardation		21%–50%
Premature birth		21%–50%
Central Nervous System		
Meningoencephalitis		51%–75%
Microcephaly		21%–50%
Cerebral calcification		51%–75%
Eye		
Chorioretinitis		0%–20%
Reticuloendothelial System		
Hepatosplenomegaly		51%–75%
Hyperbilirubinemia		51%–75%
Hemolytic and other anemias		21%–50%
Thrombocytopenia		51%–75%
Petechiae or ecchymoses		51%–75%
Other		
Inguinal hernias		21%–50%
Pneumonitis		0%–20%

*See text for references.

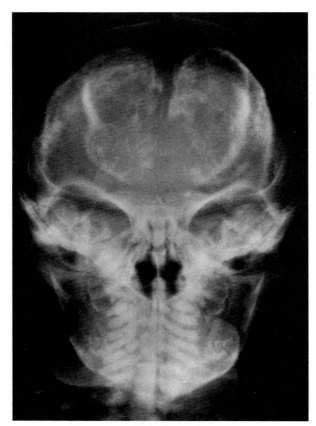

Figure 20-3 **Congenital cytomegalovirus infection: periventricular calcification.** This skull radiograph is from an affected 5-day-old infant with microcephaly. *(From Bell WE, McCormick WF: Neurologic Infections in Children, 2nd ed, Philadelphia: 1981, Saunders.)*

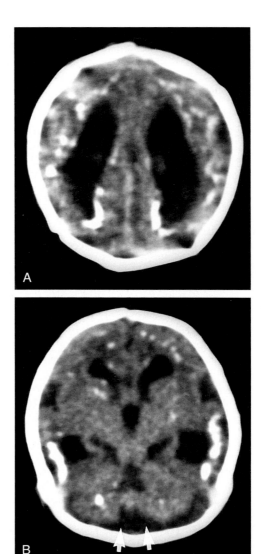

Figure 20-4 **Congenital cytomegalovirus infection: computed tomography scans.** These scans are from a 5-day-old infant with congenital cytomegalovirus infection. **A,** Periventricular and diffuse cerebral calcifications and ventriculomegaly are apparent. **B,** In addition to calcifications and ventriculomegaly, note the cerebellar hypoplasia and large cisterna magna *(arrows).*

elevated titer in the neonate suggests infection of the infant, because passively transferred maternal antibody is degraded with an approximate half-life of 23 days.[9]

A faster and more useful test depends on the detection of CMV-specific immunoglobulin M (IgM), which is primarily derived from the infected fetus and infant.[7] This specific IgM fraction is detected best by ELISA or a solid-phase radioimmunoassay that has improved the sensitivity and specificity of detection of CMV-specific IgM.[7,17]

Diagnostic Studies. *CSF* characteristically exhibits the findings of meningoencephalitis. In a study of 18 infants with neurological manifestations, the mean white blood cell count was 42, including predominantly lymphocytes, and the mean protein content was 192 mg/dL.[101] In a later series of nine newborns with neurological involvement, all had elevated cell counts and protein levels.[102] In a later study of 56 infants (which included 30% with no CT abnormalities), CSF protein exceeded 120 mg/dL in 50%.[82]

Skull radiographs formerly were used to demonstrate the periventricular calcifications (Fig. 20-3). However, *CT scanning* is more sensitive than skull radiography for detection of calcifications (Fig. 20-4), and CT also provides information on the extent and severity of the cerebral injury.[69-71,82,101,103,104] In a series of 41 infants

with symptomatic congenital CMV infection, a CT-detected abnormality was present in 78%. Of those with abnormalities, periventricular calcifications occurred in 75%, varying degrees of cortical and white matter abnormalities were seen in 30%, and ventriculomegaly was reported in 40%.[104] In a smaller series (*n* = 15), similar findings were reported.[101] Occasionally, lissencephaly-pachygyria or diffuse polymicrogyria may be apparent by CT scan (Fig. 20-5).

Cranial ultrasound scans frequently demonstrate abnormalities.[45,48,101,103,105-115] These findings consist of periventricular cysts, especially in the region of the subependymal germinal matrix (see Fig. 20-5), ventriculomegaly, periventricular (and more diffuse) calcifications, and periventricular echolucencies (consistent with cerebral white matter cysts) (Figs. 20-6 and 20-7). The correlations with neuropathological

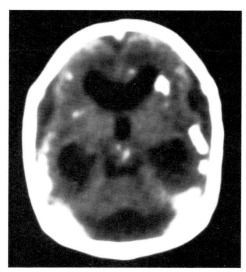

Figure 20-5 Congenital cytomegalovirus infection: computed tomography scan. This scan was performed on the first postnatal day shows smooth cerebral cortex, characteristic of lissencephaly, in addition to periventricular and more diffuse calcifications, ventriculomegaly, and cerebellar hypoplasia.

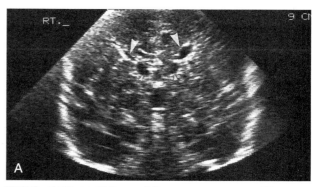

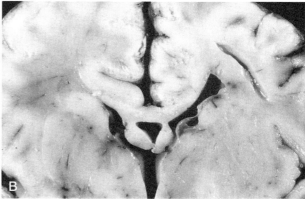

Figure 20-6 Congenital cytomegalovirus infection: periventricular cyst in subependymal germinal matrix demonstrated by cranial ultrasound scan. A, This scan performed at 1 day of age demonstrates the bilateral cysts *(small arrowheads)*. The ventricles are indicated by the *large arrowheads*. **B,** Coronal section of brain shows both cysts in the subependymal regions. *(Courtesy of Dr. Gary Shackelford.)*

findings (see previous discussion) are obvious. An additional ultrasonographic finding, overt in approximately one third of cases, is the presence of *branched echodensities in basal ganglia and thalamus* (Fig. 20-8).[103,110-114] That the echodensities represent arteries has been shown by Doppler ultrasound examination.[111,112,114] In two series, 15% to 40% of infants with such echodensities had CMV infection. (Other diagnoses included congenital rubella, congenital syphilis, trisomy 13, trisomy 21, fetal alcohol syndrome, and "neonatal asphyxia.") One pathological study defined hypercellular vessel walls and a mineralizing vasculopathy, probably secondary to perivascular inflammation (Fig. 20-9).[110]

MRI is of particular value for detection of the disorders of neuronal migration, cerebral parenchymal destruction, delays in myelination, and cerebellar

hypoplasia observed with congenital CMV (Figs. 20-10 to 20-12).[23,24,48,52-54,69-72] In a carefully studied series of 11 infants with congenital CMV infection, polymicrogyria was present in 5 and lissencephaly in 4.[23] In a series of MRI-documented lissencephaly-pachygyria, CMV infection was present in 6 of 23 cases.[69] In a related study of 10 infants with MRI-identified migrational disorders, especially polymicrogyria, 4 were found to have

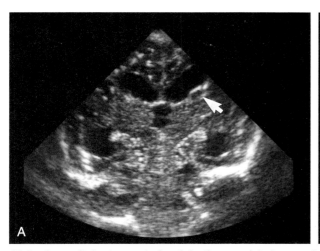

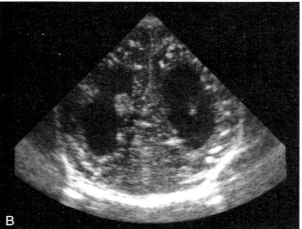

Figure 20-7 Congenital cytomegalovirus infection: cranial ultrasound scan. A and **B,** Coronal scans in a 1-day-old infant show periventricular echodensities with associated echolucencies, consistent with calcification and white matter injury, dilation of lateral and third ventricles, and a subependymal cyst *(arrow in **A**)*.

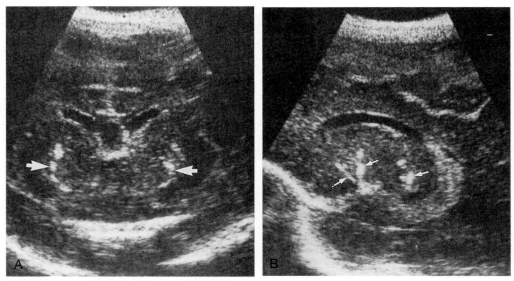

Figure 20-8   Congenital cytomegalovirus infection: cranial ultrasound scan. A, Coronal and, **B,** sagittal scans of newborn known to have cytomegalovirus infection demonstrate bright vessels *(arrows)* in the region of the basal ganglia and thalami. *(From Teele RL, Hernanz-Schulman M, Sotrel A: Echogenic vasculature in the basal ganglia of neonates: A sonographic sign of vasculopathy,* Radiology *169:423-427, 1988.)*

CMV.[52] Delays in myelination and increased signal on T2-weighted images (see Figs. 20-11 and 20-12) have been observed in approximately one half of infants with CMV studied by MRI.[23,24,48,53,54,69-71] Indeed, the predilection of abnormal cerebral white matter signal, including cystic change, for posterior parietal regions may mimic periventricular leukomalacia. Thus, in an MRI series of 152 infants (mean age, 22 months) with "static leukoencephalopathy of unknown etiology," 10% were found to have congenital CMV, based on retrospective PCR testing of neonatal blood spots.[53] Cerebellar hypoplasia, a finding in 40% to 70% of infants, is detected best by MRI scanning. Notably, MRI is *less* sensitive than CT for detection of cerebral calcifications.

Testing of *brain stem auditory evoked responses in the neonatal period and subsequently* demonstrates the high likelihood of sensorineural hearing loss, including the delayed onset and the postnatal progression of this loss. In 4 series of 281 infants with symptomatic congenital CMV infections, 50% to 75% exhibited hearing loss on

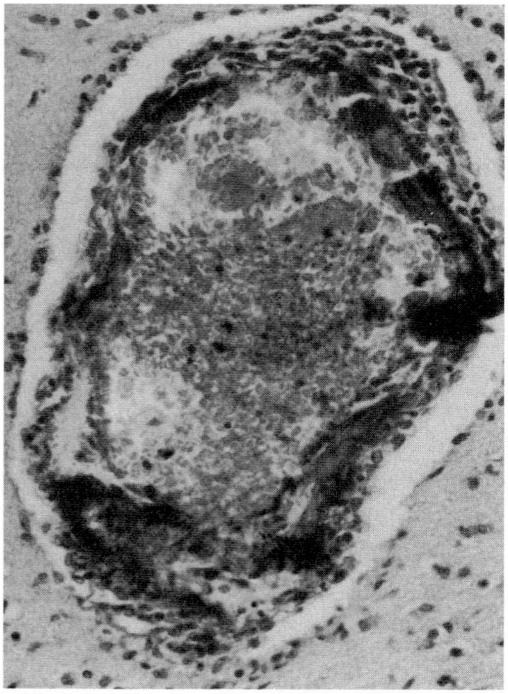

Figure 20-9   Congenital cytomegalovirus infection: photomicrograph of small vessel. Note the thickened wall, focal globular subendothelial deposits of mineralized material, mononuclear infiltrates in adventitia, and perivascular reactive astrocytosis (hematoxylin and eosin, Luxol fast blue, × 250). *(From Teele RL, Hernanz-Schulman M, Sotrel A: Echogenic vasculature in the basal ganglia of neonates: A sonographic sign of vasculopathy,* Radiology *169:423-427, 1988.)*

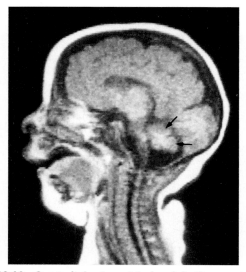

Figure 20-10   Congenital cytomegalovirus infection: magnetic resonance imaging scan. Note the striking cerebellar hypoplasia on this sagittal view *(arrows)*. *(Courtesy of Dr. Klaus Sartor.)*

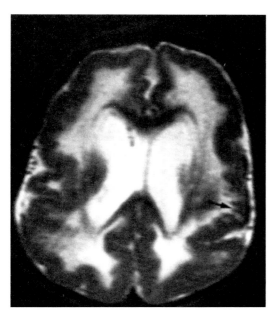

Figure 20-11 Congenital cytomegalovirus infection: magnetic resonance imaging scan. This axial T2-weighted image shows markedly high signal intensity in cerebral white matter and diffusely thickened cerebral cortex with undulating appearance of the cortical–white matter junction, *(arrow)*; the latter finding is characteristic of polymicrogyria. *(From Titelbaum DS, Hayward JC, Zimmerman RA: Pachygyriclike changes: Topographic appearance at MR imaging and CT and correlation with neurologic status, Radiology 173:663-667, 1989.)*

follow-up.[84,89,104,116] Although approximately 60% of those with hearing loss had hearing loss at birth or in the neonatal period, fully 40% had *delayed-onset* loss (i.e., not apparent until months after the neonatal period). Additionally, *progressive* hearing loss was noted in approximately 60% of the infants with hearing loss.[89] Progression of hearing loss has also been observed in infants with *asymptomatic* CMV infection. Thus, in one series, 3% of such patients had hearing loss detected in the neonatal period, but by the age of 6 years, 11% of the previously asymptomatic patients had hearing loss.[83] *The value and importance of serial studies throughout infancy are obvious.*

Prognosis

Relation to Neonatal Clinical Syndrome. The outcome relates to the severity of the neuropathological findings, and these findings correlate with the neonatal clinical syndrome (Table 20-5).* Although the data depicted in Table 20-5 are based on a sample that was selected to a certain degree, the observations are useful regarding the relationship between the neonatal clinical signs and the neurological outcome in congenital CMV infection. Thus, of those infants with the overt neurological syndrome (i.e., microcephaly, intracranial calcifications, or chorioretinitis), approximately 95% had major neurological sequelae (e.g., mental retardation, seizures, deafness, and motor deficits) or died. Infants with less obvious

("other") neurological phenomena had slightly better prognoses. Approximately 70% of these infants with neonatal neurological signs also experienced systemic phenomena. In the large series ($n = 80$) of MacDonald and Tobin,[27] of the group of infants with systemic signs but no neonatal neurological deficits, approximately 50% were normal, and only 16% exhibited major neurological sequelae or died (see Table 20-5). Data from a later series (34 infants) are approximately similar, except the lack of neurological abnormalities in the newborn period was not clearly associated with more favorable outcomes.[117] The major neurological deficits include pronounced cognitive deficits, most commonly with intelligence quotient (IQ) scores lower than 70, spastic motor deficits, seizure disorders, and bilateral hearing loss.[17,27,78,81,82,87,89,104,117-119] In 2 series of 97 infants with symptomatic congenital CMV infection, mental retardation (IQ < 70) developed in 45% (IQ < 50 in 36%), cerebral palsy in 45%, seizures in 11%, and sensorineural hearing loss in 60%.[82,104]

Outcome with Asymptomatic Congenital Infection. The asymptomatic group has been the particular focus of several investigators.[7,35,78,83,84,90,120-127] In these studies, the most consistent sequela was sensorineural hearing loss (Table 20-6). Approximately 11% of the infants developed bilateral hearing loss, with moderate to profound loss in 6%. Often, hearing deficits were not detected until serious impairment of language development occurred. Indeed, as noted with symptomatic disease, with more frequent serial measurements, it became clear that hearing impairment often did not become clearly apparent until, and progressed during, infancy and early childhood (see earlier discussion). In a large longitudinal study of 307 infants, 7.2% exhibited sensorineural hearing loss, and among these infants, 50% exhibited progression (median age at onset of progression, 18 months), and 18% exhibited delayed onset (median age of detection, 27 months).[127] In a later study of 388 infants, as noted earlier, 3% of asymptomatic infants had sensorineural hearing loss in the first month, and 11% had hearing loss by 6 years of age.[83] In a more recent series of 300 affected infants born after nonprimary ($n = 124$) or primary ($n = 176$) infection, although bilateral hearing loss occurred equally in both groups (10% to 11%), infants born after primary maternal infection were more likely to have severe or profound hearing loss (63% versus 15%).[90] The diagnosis of hearing loss was made earlier in the infants born after primary maternal infection (mean age, 13 months versus 39 months). Histopathological and immunofluorescent studies of the inner ear in two affected infants revealed destruction of cells of the organ of Corti and the neurons of the eighth nerve, as well as the presence of viral antigen.[122] Thus, involvement of cochlear structures with congenital CMV infection and the consequent disturbance of hearing may be an enormous public health problem, in view of the prevalence of the infection.

The possibility of subtle disturbances of intellectual function was initially suggested by studies conducted by Hanshaw and co-workers,[121] who demonstrated a

---

*See references 7,14,17,18,27,78,81,82,87,89,104,117-120.

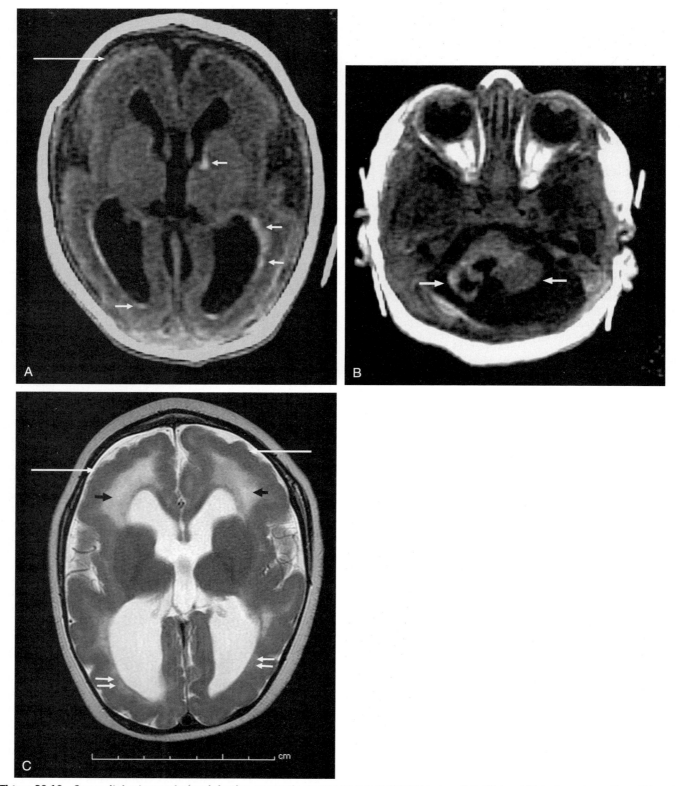

Figure 20-12   Congenital cytomegalovirus infection, magnetic resonance imaging (MRI) scans. This 16-day-old infant was born after a 31-week gestation with congenital cytomegalovirus infection identified in utero. The axial T1-weighted MRI scan shows in **A**, increased signal in the periventricular regions *(short arrows)*, consistent with calcification, and diffuse polymicrogyria *(long arrow)*; in **B**, note the striking cerebellar hypoplasia *(arrows)*. At 6 months of age, the axial T2-weighted MRI scan **(C)** shows diffuse frontal polymicrogyria *(long arrows)*, abnormal high signal intensity in cerebral white matter *(short black arrows)*, and marked paucity of parieto-occipital cerebral white matter *(double white arrows)*. *(Courtesy of Dr. Omar Khwaja.)*

TABLE 20-5   Relationship between Neonatal Clinical Signs and Neurological Outcome in Congenital Cytomegalovirus Infection*

| Neonatal Signs | NEUROLOGICAL SEQUELAE[†] | | | |
	Normal	Major	Minor	Death
Neurological				
Microcephaly, intracranial calcifications, or chorioretinitis	7%	79%	0%	14%
Other	40%	50%	0%	10%
Systemic				
Jaundice, hepato-splenomegaly, or purpura, but no neurological signs	48%	12%	36%	4%
No Neurological or Systemic Signs	81%	3%	16%	0%

*Based on 80 infants.
[†]Expressed as percentage of those with designated neonatal clinical signs.
Data from MacDonald H, Tobin HO: Congenital cytomegalovirus infection: A collaborative study on epidemiological, clinical and laboratory findings, *Dev Med Child Neurol* 20:471-478, 1978.

statistically significant lower mean IQ score in asymptomatic patients versus matched controls (102 versus 112). Subsequent large-scale studies did not document definite impairment of intellectual function in asymptomatic infants,[123,124,128] particularly when hearing-impaired children were excluded.[120,125] Intellectual outcome in hearing impaired children has not yet been studied in detail; outcome in this setting is important to define separately because the virus clearly has entered the CNS in this subgroup of infected infants. Nevertheless, several reports suggest that an asymptomatic neonatal period may be followed by varying combinations of developmental delay, microcephaly, ataxia, sensorineural hearing loss, and seizures, usually recognized in the first year of life.[22,23,52-54] CT or MRI may show cerebral calcification, abnormal cerebral white matter signal, delayed myelination, polymicrogyria, focal subcortical areas of abnormality, or cerebellar

TABLE 20-6   Subsequent Hearing Loss in Infants with Asymptomatic Congenital Cytomegalovirus Infection

| Type | HEARING LOSS | |
	Severity*	Affected
Bilateral		11%
	Mild	5%
	Moderate to profound	6%
Unilateral		8%
	Mild	4%
	Moderate to profound	4%

*Mild hearing loss, 22 to 55 dB; moderate to profound, ≥ 55 dB.
Data from references 121 to 124.

hypoplasia. The possibility of late intrauterine acquisition of infection has been suggested in some of these infants. *The important clinical point is that CMV infection should be considered later in infancy in the presence of such neurological or neuroradiological features, or both, even if the neonatal period was unremarkable.* More data are needed on these issues.

Management

Prevention. Congenital CMV infection is related to primary infection of the pregnant woman, presumably early in pregnancy. Two preventive approaches may be used: one to prevent or treat the primary infection and the other to terminate the pregnancy. Prevention of the primary maternal infection by vaccination has received initial investigation, with variable results.[5,7,129,130] However, more information is needed about the effectiveness, hazards, and feasibility of this approach.[5,7,9,131-133a] Treatment of the primary maternal infection with hyperimmune gamma globulin is a possibility, but the difficulty in detecting most maternal infections has been a major problem with this approach. Termination of a pregnancy complicated by a primary maternal infection has been difficult for a similar reason and also because the exact risks of fetal infection are not entirely known. Detection of the infected fetus by amniocentesis and identification of the virus or DNA by culture or PCR, respectively, comprise the principal approach.[7,49,130,134-138] The sensitivity for detection of fetal infection increases markedly after 21 weeks of gestation. The fetal condition then can be assessed further by ultrasonography, which may show intracranial calcification or other evidence of parenchymal disease, and, if desired, by cordocentesis, with evaluation of fetal blood for abnormal liver function tests, CMV-specific IgM, anemia, or thrombocytopenia. In one series, the risk of identification of *neonatal* neurological abnormality by neurological examination, cranial ultrasonography, or hearing assessment was only 19% when no *prenatal* ultrasonographic abnormalities were present.[49] Ultrasonographic abnormalities were detected prenatally in 21%, and nearly all these pregnancies were terminated.

Supportive Therapy. From the neonatal neurological standpoint, supportive therapy consists principally of control of seizures.

Antimicrobial Therapy. Several antiviral agents, including adenine arabinoside (Ara-A), 5-iodo-2′-deoxyuridine (IDU), cytosine arabinoside (Ara-C), and acyclovir, have been studied because of their effectiveness in vitro.[9,132,133] Ara-A and acyclovir are the least toxic of these agents, but early trials did not provide reason for optimism. Ganciclovir, an acyclovir derivative, has been shown to be effective in prophylaxis and treatment of CMV infections in immunocompromised adults and children.[7,139-142] Initial data with infants are promising.[143] An earlier study of 12 infants with congenital CMV infection suggested distinct clinical benefit (e.g., loss of hepatosplenomegaly, improvement in

TABLE 20-7	**Effect of Ganciclovir Therapy on Hearing in Symptomatic Cytomegalovirus Disease***	
Hearing from Neonatal Period to ≥ 1 Year	**Ganciclovir**	**No Treatment**
No deficit: both periods	23%	22%
Deficit: improved	25%	0%
Deficit: unchanged	31%	17%
Deficit: worsened	21%	61%

*Total number of infants, 43; 24 received ganciclovir and 19 had no treatment. Values are percentages of all ears tested in each group.
Data from Kimberlin DW, Lin CY, Sanchez PJ, Demmler GJ, et al: Effect of ganciclovir therapy on hearing in symptomatic congenital cytomegalovirus disease involving the central nervous system: A randomized, controlled trial, *J Pediatr* 143:16-25, 2003.

tone) with a 3-month course of therapy.[102] The most impressive data with ganciclovir involved a randomized controlled trial of the effect of the agent on hearing in symptomatic congenital CMV disease involving the CNS (Table 20-7).[116] The treated infants received ganciclovir, 6 mg/kg per dose administered intravenously every 12 hours for 6 weeks. Hearing deficits either improved or remained static in 56% of the ears of treated infants versus only 17% of those of the control infants (see Table 20-7). Progression of deficits occurred in only 21% in the ganciclovir group versus 61% in the control group. The beneficial effect of ganciclovir was accompanied by significant neutropenia in approximately 65% of treated infants. The need for an agent that has less toxicity and can be administered orally is apparent. Valganciclovir, shown to be effective in adults with CMV retinitis, may prove to be such an agent. A recent case report described an effective systemic response in symptomatic neonatal CMV infection to a 6-week course of this drug.[144] Ultimately, treatment of asymptomatic infants would be ideal, if the risk-to-benefit ratio of the agent could be favorable.

It is perhaps unlikely, although not proven, that postnatal therapy would benefit the CNS, because the injury appears to occur principally in utero. However, more data are needed on this issue.

Toxoplasmosis

Intrauterine infection with *T. gondii*, a protozoan parasite, causes congenital toxoplasmosis. This congenital infection is second only to congenital CMV infection in terms of frequency and clinical importance. As with infection with CMV, congenital toxoplasmosis is acquired in utero by transplacental mechanisms, and most affected newborn infants are asymptomatic. However, with careful clinical evaluation and a high index of suspicion, this infection is more readily identified in the infected newborn than is CMV infection.

Pathogenesis

Fetal Infection. Clinically significant infection with toxoplasmosis occurs during intrauterine life by transplacental passage of the parasite.[2,145-147] The sequence of events is (1) primary infection of the mother, (2)

parasitemia, (3) placentitis, and (4) hematogenous spread to the fetus.[145,148] The organism can be cultured consistently from the placenta when the fetus is infected.[149] As with CMV, the mother infected with toxoplasmosis is usually asymptomatic.[150-152] The most common clinical presentation of the mother is localized or generalized lymphadenopathy, sometimes with fever and other features suggestive of infectious mononucleosis.[150]

The incidence of primary maternal infection during pregnancy varies around the world. In Paris, when consumption of undercooked meat was relatively common, the value was as high as 5 per 100 pregnancies.[148-150] At a comparable time, the rate in the United States was approximately 1.1 per 1000 pregnancies.[151] More recent incidences are 0.5 to 2.0 per 1000 pregnancies in Western Australia, Europe, and the United States.[145,146,153-155] These rates should be contrasted with the approximately tenfold-higher rates for CMV infection during pregnancy (see earlier discussion). A study of congenital infection, based on a serological study of filter paper blood specimens for neonatal metabolic screening in Massachusetts, yielded an incidence of only approximately 1 per 10,000.[156-158]

The unusual susceptibility of the human fetus and newborn to severe infection with *T. gondii* appears to relate, in large part, to inadequate cellular defenses.[145,159] Mononuclear phagocytes are the principal defense against such infection, and a decreased generation of macrophage-activating material by fetal lymphocytes has been demonstrated. Moreover, the response to this activating material by macrophages in the neonate is also deficient. Unchecked replication of the organism is the expected result.

Importance of Time of Maternal Infection. The likelihood and severity of congenital toxoplasmosis bear a distinct relation to the time of maternal infection (Table 20-8). Only approximately 20% to 25% of infants will be infected if the maternal infection occurs in the first or second trimester, especially the

TABLE 20-8	**Relationship between the Incidence and Severity of Congenital Toxoplasmosis and the Time of Maternal Infection***		
		CONGENITAL TOXOPLASMOSIS†	
Maternal Infection: Trimester of Pregnancy	**Infants Infected**	**Severe**	**Asymptomatic or Mild**
First	17%	60%	40%
Second	25%	30%	70%
Third	65%	0%	100%

*Based on 145 pregnancies.
†Percentage of infected infants with severe disease (central nervous system and ocular involvement) or those with asymptomatic disease or isolated ocular involvement (mild).
Data from Desmonts G, Couvreur J: Toxoplasmosis in pregnancy and its transmission to the fetus, *Bull N Y Acad Med* 50:146-159, 1974.

second to sixth months of gestation, versus approximately 65% if maternal infection occurs in the third trimester.[145,150,160] In a large series of 603 women with confirmed maternal toxoplasmosis, the maternal-fetal transmission rate was only 6% with infection at 13 weeks but increased to 72% with infection at 36 weeks.[160] However, although fetal infection is less likely earlier in pregnancy, the *severity* of the disease is greater. Indeed, most infants infected in the first trimester exhibit severe disease, manifested by CNS and ocular involvement (see Table 20-8). As a result of these counterbalancing effects, in one large series the highest risk of bearing an infected infant with early clinical manifestations (10%) occurred in women who seroconverted at 24 to 30 weeks of gestation.[160] A CT study of 31 infants further documented the severity of the CNS lesions as a function of the time of intrauterine infection.[161] Therefore, it appears that although a fetal-maternal barrier to infection may be operative early in pregnancy, once fetal infection is established at that time, it is a potentially devastating disease. Treatment of the infected mother alters both the likelihood of fetal transmission and the severity of the disease (see later discussion).

Neuropathology

As with CMV infection, congenital toxoplasmosis may be associated with asymptomatic or symptomatic neurological presentations in the newborn period (see later discussion). Although the symptomatic neurological presentation is relatively uncommon, I describe it here because it serves as the prototype for the neuropathology produced by infection with this organism. Toxoplasmosis does not appear to possess the teratogenic potential of CMV infection, and essentially all the neuropathological features are related to tissue inflammation and destruction (Table 20-9).[42,43,145,162-164]

Meningoencephalitis. The meningoencephalitis of toxoplasmosis has a striking multifocal, necrotizing, granulomatous quality and is characterized by the following: (1) inflammatory cells in the meninges, especially over focal lesions; (2) perivascular infiltrates with inflammatory cells, the latter often including eosinophils; (3) multifocal and diffuse necroses of brain parenchyma, with all cellular elements affected, involving cerebrum, brain stem and spinal cord, and often associated with calcification; (4) reactive microglial and

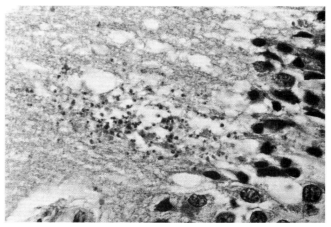

Figure 20-13   Congenital toxoplasmosis: encephalitis. Photomicrograph of a region of necrosis containing many free *Toxoplasma* organisms (note small, darkly stained nuclei to the left of larger, preserved neurons). Although this lesion was from an older child with *Toxoplasma* encephalitis who was receiving immunosuppressive therapy, the organisms are identical in appearance to those of the congenital form. *(From Bell WE, McCormick WF: Neurologic Infections in Children, Philadelphia: 1975, Saunders.)*

astroglial proliferation; and (5) miliary granulomas, containing large epithelioid cells and free, intracellular, or encysted organisms (Fig. 20-13).

Porencephaly and Hydranencephaly. With particularly severe, diffuse, cerebral destructive disease, porencephalic cysts or hydranencephaly may develop.[67,165] Of the 33 fetuses with congenital toxoplasmosis studied by Hohlfeld and co-workers,[163] all exhibited areas of brain necrosis, the initial lesions that evolve to porencephaly and hydranencephaly. The development of these large areas of tissue dissolution is particularly likely if aqueductal block and increased intraventricular pressure are associated.

Hydrocephalus. Two processes appear to be operative in the periventricular region with toxoplasmosis and may underlie the propensity for aqueductal block and consequent hydrocephalus in this disorder. First, the inflammation with toxoplasmosis has a predilection for the periventricular region, as with CMV infection (although in toxoplasmosis more severe diffuse disease is present elsewhere, and calcified areas of necrosis are present throughout the cerebrum). Second, it is believed that *Toxoplasma* organisms enter the ventricular system from the parenchymal lesions and disseminate there. This highly antigenic ventricular fluid then seeps through the damaged ependyma to periventricular blood vessels, where an antigen-antibody reaction may occur at the vessel wall, thereby causing thrombosis and periventricular infarction.[162] This additional necrosis apparently causes the serious aqueductal block that results in the common complication, hydrocephalus. Among 33 infected fetuses identified in utero by Hohlfeld and co-workers,[163] 19 (58%) had ventricular dilation at autopsy after elective termination of pregnancy.

TABLE 20-9	**Neuropathology of Congenital Toxoplasmosis Overtly Symptomatic in the Neonatal Period**

Meningoencephalitis, granulomatous
Diffuse cerebral necrosis, sometimes with porencephaly and hydranencephaly
Diffuse cerebral calcifications
Periventricular inflammation and necrosis, especially periaqueductal
Hydrocephalus

Microcephaly. Although hydrocephalus is a more common result of congenital infection with *T. gondii* and is more frequent in this variety of congenital infection than in any other, microcephaly does occur in a significant percentage of patients, approximately 15% (see subsequent discussion). The microcephaly relates to the multifocal necrotizing encephalitis, particularly of the cerebral hemispheres. Indeed, even in those patients with hydrocephalus, it is clear that a serious loss of brain substance, in addition to the effects of the hydrocephalus, invariably has occurred.

Clinical Aspects

Incidence of Clinically Apparent Infection. As with
CMV, clinically asymptomatic cases of congenital toxoplasmosis outnumber symptomatic cases. However, a larger proportion of infants with congenital toxoplasmosis than with congenital CMV infection can be detected clinically in the newborn period. Of 156 children with congenital toxoplasmosis who were monitored prospectively from the time of maternal infection, approximately 18% had CNS and ocular involvement, 2% had CNS involvement without ocular involvement, 12% had ocular involvement only, and 68% were asymptomatic.[145] Thus, 20% of infants with congenital toxoplasmosis had observable CNS involvement in the newborn period in this study. The incidence of subclinical infection is higher in infants of women treated during pregnancy than in infants of women not treated (see later discussion).

Clinical Features. Symptomatic patients (not treated in utero) often can be divided into those with predominantly neurological syndromes and those with predominantly systemic syndromes (Table 20-10 shows combined data for both syndromes).[2,145,146,164,166,167] The *neurological syndrome* accounts for approximately two thirds of the cases and consists principally of abnormal CSF and other signs of meningoencephalitis, seizures, diffuse intracranial calcification, hydrocephalus, or, less commonly, microcephaly (see Table 20-10). At least 90% of these patients exhibit chorioretinitis. In congenital toxoplasmosis, chorioretinitis is typically bilateral and prominent in the macular regions (Fig. 20-14) and is of major diagnostic importance.[145] Initially, the lesion appears in the fundus as yellowish white, cotton-like patches with indistinct margins. These patches evolve over the ensuing months into sharply demarcated, "punched-out," pigmented lesions, often accompanied by optic atrophy. Although the chorioretinopathy is most commonly apparent in the newborn period, particularly by indirect ophthalmoscopy, it may not develop for months.[145,146,163,168]

The *systemic syndrome* of congenital toxoplasmosis is dominated by signs referable to the reticuloendothelial system, especially hepatosplenomegaly, hyperbilirubinemia, and anemia (see Table 20-10). A petechial rash may occur but is less common than with CMV infection. Overt clinical evidence of neurological involvement is often lacking in these patients, but CSF abnormalities, frequently with a disproportionately elevated protein

TABLE 20-10	Clinical Features of Symptomatic Congenital Toxoplasmosis	
Clinical Feature		**Approximate Frequency**
Pregnancy		
Prematurity, intrauterine growth retardation, or both		0%–20%
Central Nervous System		
Seizures		21%–50%
Meningoencephalitis		51%–75%
Intracranial calcification		51%–75%
Hydrocephalus		21%–50%
Microcephaly		0%–20%
Eye		
Chorioretinitis		76%–100%
Reticuloendothelial System		
Hepatosplenomegaly		21%–50%
Hyperbilirubinemia		21%–50%
Anemia		51%–75%
Petechiae		0%–20%
Other		
Pneumonitis		0%–20%

Data from Remington JS, McLeod R, Thulliez P, Desmonts G: Toxoplasmosis. In Remington JS, Klein JO, Wilson CB, et al, editors: *Infectious Diseases of the Fetus and Newborn Infant*, 6th ed, Philadelphia: 2006, Elsevier Saunders; and Eichenwald H: A study of congenital toxoplasmosis. In Siim JC, editor: *Human Toxoplasmosis*, Copenhagen, 1970, Munksgaard.

content for the degree of pleocytosis, occur in approximately 85% and reflect concomitant meningoencephalitis.[56,57] Chorioretinitis is observed in at least two thirds of patients with systemic cases, and this finding underscores the importance of careful evaluation of the fundus, especially by indirect ophthalmoscopy, when congenital toxoplasmosis is possible.

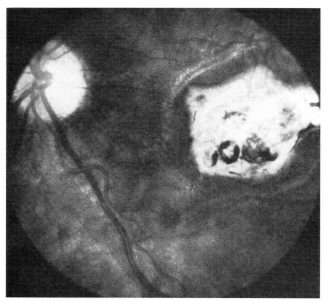

Figure 20-14 Congenital toxoplasmosis: chorioretinitis. Note the striking lesion at the macula *(right)*, as well as optic atrophy *(left)*. *(From Bell WE, McCormick WF: Neurologic Infections in Children, Philadelphia: 1975, Saunders.)*

An unknown but probably very considerable number of infants with no neurological or systemic signs of congenital toxoplasmosis (i.e., *asymptomatic disease*) will exhibit chorioretinitis, detectable in the newborn period by indirect ophthalmoscopy. Although most of the retinal lesions observed later probably develop in the weeks and months after delivery (see subsequent discussion), further data are needed regarding the proportion detectable in the newborn period. In a series of 48 asymptomatic infants in whom infection was detected by newborn blood screening, 2 had active chorioretinitis, and 7 others had retinal scars; thus, 19% had retinal disease.[158] Moreover, approximately 20% had cerebral calcifications detectable by CT, and 25% had CSF findings consistent with encephalitis. The later development of neurological deficits and visual loss is appreciable and is discussed in the "Prognosis" section.

The *clinical course* of the disease is not readily predicted, and indeed, evidence of progression of retinal and cerebral disease has been presented.[146,163,168-171] Because many patients with symptomatic congenital toxoplasmosis exhibit very severe neurological deficits from the neonatal period, the frequency of progression is difficult to quantitate.

Clinical Diagnosis. Certain clinical features are helpful in suggesting the diagnosis of congenital toxoplasmosis. A particularly noteworthy constellation of features includes evidence of meningoencephalitis, focal and multifocal cerebral necroses, diffuse cerebral calcification, hydrocephalus, and scarring chorioretinopathy in the macular regions. Intrauterine growth retardation or prematurity is generally not a prominent feature, as in infants with congenital CMV or rubella infections, and microcephaly is less common than in congenital CMV infection. The systemic syndrome may cause confusion when differentiating toxoplasmosis from other congenital infections, but a petechial rash is relatively less common in congenital toxoplasmosis.

Laboratory Evaluation

Toxoplasma Isolation. Determination of *T. gondii* as the responsible microbe in the newborn with congenital toxoplasmosis depends principally on serological tests, rather than isolation of the organism per se. Nevertheless, the organism or associated DNA can be isolated from placental tissue, ventricular or lumbar CSF, and blood.[145] The tissue extracts or fluids can be injected into either mice or tissue culture preparations.[145,172,173] Parasitemia is more readily demonstrated in the first week after birth (71%) than in the second to fourth weeks (33%), and it is detected most easily in generalized rather than in neurological disease.[145] The isolation procedures for toxoplasmosis require specialized techniques and an experienced, skilled laboratory staff. Detection of *T. gondii* in amniotic fluid by PCR with a sensitivity of 80% has suggested that this rapid test (result available in ≤6 hours) could become very important in the diagnosis when the technique is applied to biological fluids of the newborn infant.[145,174] However, available data suggest

that the sensitivity of PCR on placental tissue is only approximately 60%.[175]

Serological Studies. The identification of most cases of congenital toxoplasmosis is established by serological techniques. The two most commonly used tests are the Sabin-Feldman dye test and the IgM-fluorescent antibody test. The *Sabin-Feldman dye test*, perhaps the single most reliable test, is performed by mixing live organisms with the test serum (and a human serum component, the accessory factor) and then exposing the mixture to methylene blue. Parasites exposed to the antibody-containing serum are modified and stained. The antibodies for the dye test are passively transferred, and the maternal component does not decrease significantly for several months after birth. Persistence of high titers is necessary for diagnosis and obviously is time consuming. Moreover, the dye test requires hazardous live organisms, and the accessory factor is sometimes difficult to obtain. The *Toxoplasma-specific IgM-fluorescent antibody technique* is faster and more specific.[2,56,57,145,146,176] This test measures fetally produced IgM antibody to the organism. Killed organisms are used to bind specific IgM, which is then detected by exposure to fluorescein-antiserum to human IgM. The reliability of this test is hindered by certain factors that impair both sensitivity and specificity.[153,157] The more recently developed *IgM-capture ELISA*, which isolates and concentrates the infant's IgM, increases the sensitivity markedly (90% of infected infants are detected), and false-positive reactions are unusual.[157] This test has been adapted to filter paper blood specimens.[157] More recent data suggest value for analysis of IgA or IgE in neonatal blood.[145,175] However, sensitivities for all the latter tests are very low for infants infected in the first 20 weeks of gestation, when severe disease is the most likely result.

Neurodiagnostic Studies. Neurodiagnostic studies that particularly suggest congenital toxoplasmosis are evaluations of CSF and brain imaging. Pleocytosis and elevated protein content of CSF indicate meningoencephalitis and may be observed in asymptomatic as well as symptomatic patients. Particularly characteristic of congenital toxoplasmosis is the finding of a very high protein content in the ventricular fluid, usually reflecting the aqueductal obstruction and stagnation of infection within the lateral ventricles. Although skull radiographs are effective in demonstrating the diffuse and periventricular cerebral calcification (Fig. 20-15), *CT scan* is more effective and, in addition, provides information on the extent and severity of cerebral injury (Fig. 20-16).[161] CT data indicate that calcifications of the basal ganglia are more common than previously suspected.[161] The calcifications associated with congenital toxoplasmosis, especially of the periventricular type or of the basal ganglia, also can be detected by *cranial ultrasound scan* (Fig. 20-17).[105,108] Moreover, I have observed in congenital toxoplasmosis the echogenic thalamic vasculature described earlier (see "Cytomegalovirus Infection") (Fig. 20-18). *MRI scan* provides the most detailed assessment of parenchymal necroses.

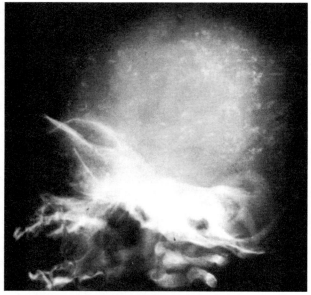

Figure 20-15 Congenital toxoplasmosis: diffuse calcification shown on skull radiograph. This is a lateral skull film of an infant with hydrocephalus, chorioretinitis, and multiple, punctate calcifications scattered diffusely in brain. *(From Bell WE, McCormick WF: Neurologic Infections in Children, Philadelphia: 1975, Saunders.)*

Prognosis

Relation to Neonatal Clinical Syndrome. As with CMV, the outcome of untreated congenital toxoplasmosis relates to the severity of the neuropathology, which correlates to a modest extent with the neonatal clinical syndrome (Table 20-11). Infants with congenital toxoplasmosis with prominent neonatal *neurological*

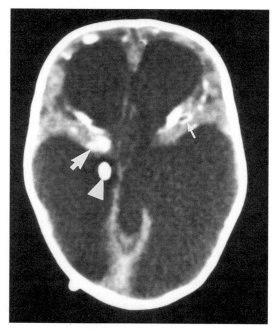

Figure 20-16 Congenital toxoplasmosis: computed tomography scan. This scan performed at 3 months of age shows cerebral calcifications, both periventricular and diffuse, including involvement of thalamus *(large arrow)* and basal ganglia *(small arrow)*. A shunt catheter *(arrowhead)* is in the lateral ventricle.

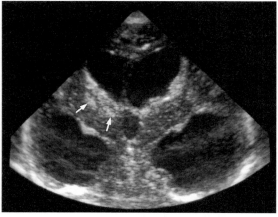

Figure 20-17 Congenital toxoplasmosis: cranial ultrasound scan. This coronal scan performed at 3 days of age shows marked hydrocephalus and evidence of calcification in basal ganglia *(arrows)* and subependymal regions.

features do poorly; only 9% are normal on follow-up. Most of the remaining infants exhibit serious disturbances of cerebral function (i.e., mental retardation, seizures, and spastic motor deficits). Essentially all such patients have chorioretinitis and may also have optic atrophy; as a consequence, approximately 70% have severe visual impairment.

Somewhat unlike congenital CMV infection, congenital toxoplasmosis with a neonatal syndrome characterized by prominent *systemic* signs, if untreated, also results in a poor neurological outcome. Approximately 50% of such patients with CMV are normal on follow-up, whereas only approximately 16% of patients with congenital toxoplasmosis are normal (see Table 20-11). Although the nature of the study populations differs, it seems reasonable to conclude that CNS involvement in congenital toxoplasmosis is more prominent than in congenital CMV infection when non-neurological features dominate the neonatal syndrome. Again, chorioretinitis

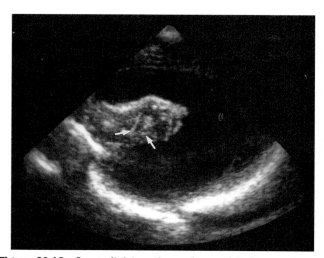

Figure 20-18 Congenital toxoplasmosis: cranial ultrasound scan. This parasagittal scan obtained at 3 days of age shows marked hydrocephalus and echogenic vessels *(arrows)* in thalamus. The latter are consistent with the lenticulostriate vasculopathy seen in congenital cytomegalovirus infection (compare Fig. 20-8).

TABLE 20-11   Relationship between Neonatal Clinical Signs and Neurological Outcome in Symptomatic Congenital Toxoplasmosis

Neurological Outcome	NEONATAL SIGNS*	
	Neurological	Systemic
Mental retardation	89%	81%
Seizures	83%	77%
Spastic motor deficits	76%	58%
Severe visual impairment	69%	42%
Deafness	17%	10%
Normal	9%	16%

*Values for each neurological outcome are expressed as percentage of infants who exhibited the designated neonatal signs (i.e., neurological [n = 108] or systemic [n = 44]).

Data from Remington JS, McLeod R, Thulliez P, Desmonts G: Toxoplasmosis. In Remington JS, Klein JO, Wilson CB, et al, editors: *Infectious Diseases of the Fetus and Newborn Infant*, 6th ed, Philadelphia: 2006, Elsevier Saunders; and Eichenwald H: A study of congenital toxoplasmosis. In Siim JC, editor: *Human Toxoplasmosis*, Copenhagen, 1970, Munksgaard.

is found in the majority of such patients with toxoplasmosis, and severe visual impairment occurs in approximately 40%. Antiparasitic treatment, begun in the first 2½ months of life, has a beneficial effect on outcome in symptomatic congenital toxoplasmosis (see later discussion).

Outcome with Asymptomatic Congenital Infection.

Infants with subclinical infection (i.e., the majority of cases of congenital toxoplasmosis) comprise an important group. For example, in the United States, approximately 3000 such infants are affected yearly.[171] Previous studies emphasized that such infants had a relatively high frequency of chorioretinitis and a modest impairment of intellect.[122,145,157,177,178] A prospective study of 13 asymptomatic infants identified by serological screening in the newborn period and evaluated by particularly detailed serial, ocular, neurological, and audiological follow-up studies indicated that few such asymptomatic children escape without deficits

TABLE 20-12   Subsequent Deficits with Asymptomatic Congenital Toxoplasmosis

Subsequent Deficit	Number Affected* (Total n = 13)
None	2
Chorioretinitis	11
Bilateral	8
Unilateral	3
Neurological sequelae	5
Major	1
Minor	4
Mean intelligence quotient	89 ± 23
Sensorineural hearing loss	3

*Based on 13 infants identified by serological screening in the newborn period and studied prospectively.

Data from Wilson CB, Remington JS, Stagno S, Reynolds DW: Development of adverse sequelae in children born with subclinical congenital toxoplasma infection, *Pediatrics* 66:767-774, 1980.

(Table 20-12).[65] Thus, 11 infants in this study developed chorioretinitis (3 with unilateral blindness), and 5 had neurological sequelae (1 with severe mental retardation and microcephaly). The neurological sequelae were always associated with chorioretinitis. The mean IQ score for the group was only 89. Sensorineural hearing loss occurred in 3 of 10 infants so tested, although in none was moderate or severe bilateral loss observed. However, diagnosis by neonatal screening and prompt institution of therapy result in a markedly better outcome (see later discussion).

Management

Prevention. Three major approaches to prevention include (1) avoidance of primary maternal infection, (2) treatment of maternal infection, and (3) abortion in the presence of maternal infection. The first of these approaches is the most important. Pregnant women who have seronegative test results *must avoid primary acquisition of Toxoplasma* infection; the two measures necessary are avoiding ingestion of infective cysts (e.g., in raw meat) and contact with sporulating oocysts (e.g., in animal intestine and feces).[145,146,157,171,179] Ingestion of infective cysts occurs when infected meat is undercooked. It is recommended that consumption of raw or undercooked meat be completely avoided and that handling of raw meat be done with gloves on or followed by careful hand washing. Contact with sporulating oocysts is principally through household cats that carry oocysts in their intestines. It is recommended that pregnant women avoid contact with cat feces and that contact with soil or other materials potentially contaminated with cat feces be avoided or performed while wearing gloves. Cost-to-benefit analyses (relative to other approaches to prevention) demonstrate the particular desirability of a health education campaign to encourage these practices.[180]

Primary maternal infection has been treated with the antibiotic spiramycin.[2,145,146,148,163,171,171a] In one large series, a significant reduction in cases of congenital infection was observed in treated (24%) versus untreated (45%) mothers.[148] The approximately 50% decrease in incidence of congenital toxoplasmosis was confirmed by subsequent data.[163,171,171a] Moreover, a more recent multicenter study showed a marked decrease in the incidence of neonatal chorioretinitis and intracranial lesions when prenatal treatment (spiramycin) was instituted *within but not after* 4 weeks of diagnosis of maternal infection.[181]

Abortion has been performed in women who have exhibited serological evidence for primary infection during early pregnancy. This approach is less desirable for several reasons, one of which is the finding that only 17% to 25% of women infected in the first and second trimesters transmit the infection to the fetus (see Table 20-8). However, initial work by Desmonts and co-workers,[149] and subsequently by others,[145,163,182-189] demonstrated the feasibility of prenatal diagnosis of congenital toxoplasmosis. Thus, the evaluation of pregnant women for possible fetal infection with toxoplasmosis is based principally on sampling amniotic fluid by amniocentesis and detection

TABLE 20-13   Neonatal Outcome of Liveborn Infants with Congenital *Toxoplasma* infection in the Periods before (1972 to 1981) and after (1982 to 1988) Fetal Treatment*

| | TIME OF MATERNAL INFECTION (TRIMESTER) | | | | | |
| | FIRST | | SECOND | | THIRD | |
Neonatal Outcome[†]	1972–1981	1982–1988	1972–1981	1982–1988	1972–1981	1982–1988
Subclinical	10%	67%	37%	77%	68%	100%
Benign	50%	22%	45%	23%	29%	0%
Severe	40%	11%	18%	0%	3%	0%

*See text for details of prenatal and postnatal treatment. Groups are not entirely comparable, and study was not controlled; data, however, provide an approximation of the effect in the second epoch of prenatal and postnatal treatment with spiramycin (100%) plus pyrimethamine and sulfonamide (85%).

[†]Subclinical, no symptoms. Benign form, infants with chorioretinitis but no visual impairment or with intracerebral calcifications but no neurological impairment. Severe form, infants with hydrocephalus, microcephaly, bilateral chorioretinitis with visual impairment, and abnormal neurological status.

Data from Hohlfeld P, Daffos F, Thulliez P, Aufrant C, et al: Fetal toxoplasmosis: Outcome of pregnancy and infant follow-up after in utero treatment, *J Pediatr* 115:765-769, 1989.

of the organism's DNA by PCR. Sampling of fetal blood by cordocentesis under ultrasound guidance for serological indicators of infection is less useful. Ultrasonography of the fetal cranium at approximately 19 to 20 weeks of gestation provides information concerning cerebral abnormality. Fetal cranial ultrasonography may show ventriculomegaly, evidence of tissue necrosis, and cerebral calcifications. The diagnosis of fetal infection has also been made by isolation of the organism from fetal blood or from amniotic fluid and by identification in fetal blood of hematological abnormalities (e.g., eosinophilia, thrombocytopenia), elevated gamma-glutamyltransferase activity, and *Toxoplasma*-specific IgM.

The positive identification of fetal infection provides the possibility of *treatment of the fetus*.[2,145,163,171a] In the classic study of Hohlfeld and co-workers,[163] fetal treatment consisted of administration to the mother of alternating 3-week courses of spiramycin and of pyrimethamine, sulfadiazine, and folinic acid (see later discussion). (The latter three agents are not used before the 18th week of gestation because of the teratogenic potential of pyrimethamine.) The beneficial effect on the *severity* of fetal infection was dramatic (Table 20-13). Although, as in pretreatment years, the incidence

TABLE 20-14   Postnatal Evolution of Chorioretinitis in 327 Children with Congenital Toxoplasmosis Treated from Birth*

Time of Assessment	Diagnosis of First Lesion
1st mo	3%
2nd–12th mo	9%
2nd yr	2%
3rd–6th yr	5%
7th–9th yr	4%
9th–13th yr	1%
Total	24%

*Infants were treated for approximately the first postnatal year, as described in the text. Eighty-four percent of the mothers had also received therapy in utero.

Data from Wallon M, Kodjikian L, Binquet C, Garweg J, et al: Long-term ocular prognosis in 327 children with congenital toxoplasmosis, *Pediatrics* 113:1567-1572, 2004.

of severe fetal infection increased the earlier in pregnancy the infection was acquired, only 11% of first trimester infections treated in utero resulted in severe manifestations in the neonatal period. Moreover, of the third trimester fetal infections treated in utero, all resulted in *asymptomatic* newborns. Continuation of antimicrobial therapy postnatally in 53 infants was accompanied after relatively short-term follow-up by normal neurological development and examination in 52 (98%) and by the development of peripheral chorioretinitis, with no visual impairment, in 5 (9%). These favorable outcomes represent a dramatic improvement when compared with outcomes in the pretreatment era (see Table 20-11). A longer-term study confirmed the favorable effects of combined fetal and postnatal therapy, although delayed onset of chorioretinitis was shown (Table 20-14).[168] Thus, by the age of 13 years, 24% of children had developed chorioretinitis, with one half of the lesions appearing after the first year of life and some as late as 13 years. Severe bilateral visual impairment, however, did not occur. Nevertheless, careful long-term follow-up is imperative.

Supportive Therapy. Such therapy is carried out as described for congenital CMV infection.

Antimicrobial Therapy. Although significant injury has already occurred in many cases of congenital toxoplasmosis by the time of birth, good evidence indicates that some of this injury is reversible and continuing postnatal injury is preventable by therapy directed against the organism.* The drugs of choice are pyrimethamine and sulfadiazine, with the addition of folinic acid to counteract the folic acid antagonistic effect of pyrimethamine on the bone marrow. Pyrimethamine is highly effective in experimental infection with *Toxoplasma* and, because of its high lipid solubility, appears to be concentrated in brain.[145] Sulfadiazine acts synergistically with

---

*See references 2,145,146,157,158,163,164,166,168,177,184,190-192.

TABLE 20-15	Effect of Postnatal Treatment on Clinically Symptomatic and Asymptomatic Congenital Toxoplasmosis
Clinically Symptomatic*	
Motor deficits	20%–25%
Intelligence quotient < 70	25%
Retinopathy	90% (81% present in neonatal period)
Asymptomatic†	
Motor deficits	2%
Severe cognitive deficits	2%
Retinopathy	29% (19% present in neonatal period)

*Data from Roizen N, Swisher CN, Stein MA, Hopkins J, et al: Neurologic and developmental outcome in treated congenital toxoplasmosis, *Pediatrics* 95:11-20, 1995 (*n* = 34); and McLeod R, Boyer K, Karrison T, Kasza K, et al: Outcome of treatment for congenital toxoplasmosis, 1981-2004: The National Collaborative Chicago-Based, Congenital Toxoplasmosis Study, *Clin Infect Dis* 42:1383-1394, 2006 (*n* = 120).

†Data from Guerina NG, Hsu HW, Meissner HC, Maguire JH, et al: Neonatal serologic screening and early treatment for congenital *Toxoplasma gondii* infection, *N Engl J Med* 330:1858-1863, 1994 (*n* = 50).

pyrimethamine, such that their combined activity is eight times that expected if additive effects were operative.[193,194] Caution must be exercised with sulfadiazine, particularly in infants with hyperbilirubinemia. The combination of pyrimethamine and sulfadoxine (Fansidar) is more convenient because it can be administered every 2 weeks rather than daily. Thrombocytopenia is a particularly early manifestation of pyrimethamine toxicity, and folinic acid is particularly effective in correcting this phenomenon. These antimicrobials kill actively multiplying parasites but not resistant cyst stages. Therefore, treatment must begin promptly and must continue until the infant's immune system has matured sufficiently to control the infection. The total recommended duration of therapy in both symptomatic and asymptomatic disease is 1 year.[145,163] In infants with evidence of severe inflammation, manifested by markedly elevated CSF protein ($\geq$1 g/dL) or by severe chorioretinitis, corticosteroids have been recommended. Doses and modes of administration of these various agents are discussed elsewhere.[145] The beneficial effects of postnatal onset of therapy in congenital toxoplasmosis, either clinically symptomatic or detected by newborn blood screening ("asymptomatic"), are illustrated by the data in Table 20-15.

Rubella

Congenital infection of the infant with rubella occurs in utero by transplacental mechanisms. Before the institution of rubella vaccination, congenital rubella, especially in epidemic years, was a common and devastating disease of the newborn. With the widespread use of rubella vaccination, the frequency of the disorder has diminished markedly. For example, the incidence in the United States is less than 1 per 1 million live births.[2,195] There were 47 cases reported in the United States in

1991, and 22 of these occurred in a cluster in southern California.[196] Nevertheless, rubella remains a common illness in many parts of the world, and as a consequence congenital rubella syndrome is not rare (e.g., in Morocco annual rates of congenital rubella syndrome are approximately 1 per 10,000 live births).[197] The relationship between intrauterine infection with rubella and congenital defects was first clearly recognized in 1941 by Gregg.[198]

Pathogenesis

Fetal Infection. Clinically significant infection with rubella virus occurs during intrauterine life by transplacental passage of the virus.[2,9,195] As with CMV infection and toxoplasmosis, the sequence of events is primary maternal infection, viremia, placental infection, and, finally, fetal infection. Cases of asymptomatic maternal infection are common, outnumbering those of symptomatic infection by nearly 2 to 1.[56,57,195] Viremia occurs during the week before the onset of clinical manifestations, which include fever, cervical adenopathy, and a maculopapular rash lasting 3 days.

Importance of Time of Maternal Infection. The likelihood and the severity of fetal infection are functions of the time of maternal infection.[2,195,199-201] The risk to the fetus begins when the rash in the mother appears at least 12 days after the last menstrual period (i.e., the likely time of conception); in a series of 38 carefully studied pregnancies in the periconceptional period, no cases of fetal infection occurred when the rash appeared at 11 days or less after the last menstrual period.[202] In general, *both* the frequency of occurrence of infection *and* the severity of clinical disease are greater the earlier in pregnancy the maternal infection occurs (Table 20-16). Thus, it is different from the situation with toxoplasmosis, in which the likelihood of infection is less but the severity of disease greater when acquired early in pregnancy. With congenital rubella, *ocular* and *cardiac* defects are particularly common when infection occurs in the first and second months, but they become essentially nonexistent when infection occurs after the first trimester. However, *hearing loss*, although most common with early infection, is still found in approximately half of infants infected in the fourth month; later maternal infection appears not to be dangerous in this regard. *Neurological deficits*, especially intellectual retardation and motor deficits, are most common with infection in the first 2 months and are not observed with infection past the fourth month.

The *most critical gestational periods* concerning the major defects have been defined particularly closely.[200] In a series of 55 children from carefully dated, affected pregnancies, cataracts were observed with maternal infection between 26 and 57 days of gestational age; heart disease occurred in maternal infection between 25 and 93 days of gestational age; deafness occurred in maternal infection between 16 and 131 days of gestational age; and severe mental retardation occurred in maternal infection between 26 and 45 days of gestational age. The placenta may play the greatest role in

TABLE 20-16   **Relationship between the Clinical Manifestations of Congenital Rubella and the Time of Maternal Infection**

	MATERNAL INFECTION: MONTH OF PREGNANCY*				
Clinical Manifestation	**First**	**Second**	**Third**	**Fourth**	**> Fourth**
Ocular defect	50%	29%	7%	0%	0%
Cardiac defect	57%	58%	21%	5%	6%
Deafness	83%	72%	67%	49%	0%
Neurological deficit	57%	59%	24%	26%	0%

*Values for each clinical manifestation are expressed as the percentage of infants affected after maternal infection during the designated month. Data from Cooper LZ, Ziring PR, Ockerse AB, Fedun BA, et al: Rubella, *Am J Dis Child* 118:18-29, 1969.

determining the decreasing incidence of fetal infection with progression of gestation. Maturational factors of host tissue may be most important in determining the concomitant changes in organ susceptibility.

Neuropathology

As with congenital CMV infection and toxoplasmosis, the neuropathology of congenital rubella is characterized by considerable inflammation and tissue necrosis (Table 20-17).[2,42,195,203-205] In addition, rubella also appears to interfere with cellular proliferation in the developing brain and, as a consequence, causes microcephaly and, perhaps, impaired myelination.

Meningoencephalitis. The meningoencephalitis of rubella infection is similar in certain respects to the other neonatal encephalitides and is characterized by the following: (1) inflammatory cells in the meninges; (2) perivascular infiltrates with inflammatory cells; (3) necrosis of brain parenchyma, with all cellular elements affected; and (4) reactive microglial and astroglial proliferation.

Vasculopathy. An additional, prominent, and distinctive feature of rubella infection is vasculopathy. Involvement of blood vessels is observed in many organs and prominently in the brain.[203] In the well-studied series of Rorke and Spiro,[203] involvement of large leptomeningeal vessels and, particularly, smaller intraparenchymal vessels and capillaries was defined. Destruction of one or more layers of the vessel wall occurs, with replacement by deposits of amorphous granular material (Fig. 20-19). Associated with these vascular lesions are focal areas of ischemic necrosis, especially in the cerebral white matter (centrum semi-ovale, periventricular regions, and corpus callosum) and in the basal ganglia. The vascular abnormalities may account for the echogenic vessels observable on cranial ultrasonography of the affected newborn (see later discussion).

TABLE 20-17   **Neuropathology of Congenital Rubella Symptomatic in the Neonatal Period**

Meningoencephalitis
Vasculopathy with focal ischemic necrosis
Microcephaly
Delayed myelination

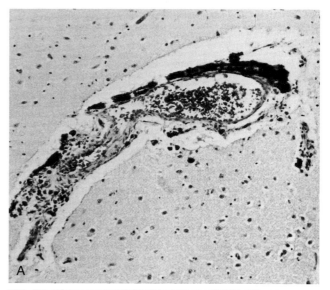

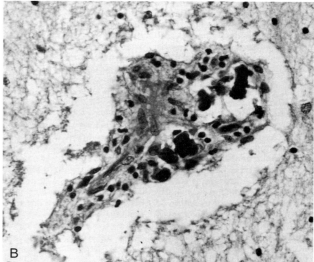

Figure 20-19   **Congenital rubella infection: vasculopathy. A** and **B,** Cerebral vessels from a 10-week-old infant with a birth weight of 2250 g and involvement of multiple organs. Note the destruction of vessel walls with replacement by deposits of amorphous granular material, which is evident especially in **A.** Surrounding ischemic changes are also present, especially in **B.** *(From Bell WE, McCormick WF: Neurologic Infections in Children, Philadelphia: 1975, Saunders.)*

Microcephaly and Impaired Myelination. Two additional features of congenital rubella (i.e., microcephaly and impaired myelination) may relate to the effect of the virus on cellular replication. Microcephaly does not appear to be accounted for readily by destructive disease and, indeed, is often not prominent until months after birth. The possibility that the decreased brain mass is related to a decrease in the number of neurons and glia is supported by the observations that rubella disturbs mitotic activity of human fetal cells in culture and also causes a reduced number of cells in a variety of organs in affected infants.[2,206,207] In addition to the microcephaly, a cellular deficit may account for the moderately impaired myelination observed by Rorke and Spiro[203] and by Kemper and co-workers.[208] Indeed, although quantitative data are lacking, an apparent decrease in oligodendrocytes has been observed in association with the retardation of myelination.[203]

Clinical Aspects

Incidence of Clinically Apparent Infection. The devastating rubella pandemic of the mid-1960s afforded the opportunity to define the enormous clinical spectrum of congenital rubella.[2,9,32,43,56,57,195,209-221] Because the largest portion of available data was derived from studies of infants identified at birth, the spectrum of manifestations as a function of *maternal infection* has been more difficult to define than for congenital CMV infection or toxoplasmosis. Nevertheless, it does appear that the likelihood of asymptomatic congenital rubella infection is more nearly comparable to that of congenital toxoplasmosis than to that of congenital CMV infection. Thus, approximately two thirds of patients are asymptomatic in the neonatal period.[218] However, most of these infants do develop evidence of disease in the first several years of life, a finding imparting clinical significance to observations that prolonged viral replication is an important feature of this disease.[2,210,217]

Clinical Features. The clinical features in symptomatic patients are shown in Table 20-18.[9,56,57,195,214] Intrauterine growth retardation (followed by postnatal growth failure) is a particularly common feature. Disturbances of the reticuloendothelial system are also prominent and are characterized particularly by hepatosplenomegaly and thrombocytopenia with or without purpura.[9] The purpura should be distinguished from the peculiar dermal erythropoiesis that results in the small purple lesions of the "blueberry muffin" syndrome. Cardiovascular defects are characteristic and consist principally of peripheral pulmonic stenoses and patent ductus arteriosus.[209,215] Myocardial injury can be demonstrated in a few patients by abnormal electrocardiographic findings, as well as pathologically,[211] and it may contribute to the occurrence of congestive heart failure. Other lesions, apparent in 20% to 50% of patients, are linear areas of radiolucency of the metaphyses of long bones (i.e., "celery stalk lesions"), prominent especially around the knee, and interstitial pneumonitis.[212] The latter abnormalities usually subside in the first few months of life.

TABLE 20-18   **Clinical Features of Symptomatic Congenital Rubella**

Clinical Feature	Approximate Frequency
Pregnancy	
Intrauterine growth retardation	51%–75%
Central Nervous System	
Meningoencephalitis	51%–75%
Full anterior fontanelle	21%–50%
Lethargy	21%–50%
Irritability	21%–50%
Hypotonia	21%–50%
Opisthotonos-retrocollis	0%–20%
Seizures	0%–20%
Eye	
Cataracts	21%–50%
Chorioretinitis	21%–50%
Microphthalmia	0%–20%
Hearing	
Suspected or definite hearing loss	21%–50%
Cardiovascular System	
Peripheral pulmonic stenoses	51%–75%
Patent ductus arteriosus	21%–50%
Myocardial necrosis	0%–20%
Reticuloendothelial System	
Hepatosplenomegaly	51%–75%
Hyperbilirubinemia	0%–20%
Thrombocytopenia ± purpura	21%–50%
Anemia	0%–20%
Dermal erythropoiesis ("blueberry muffin")	0%–20%
Other	
Bony radiolucencies	21%–50%
Pneumonitis	21%–50%

Data from Alford CA Jr: Chronic congenital and perinatal infections. In Avery GB, editor: *Neonatology: Pathophysiology and Management of the Newborn*, 3rd ed, Philadelphia: 1987, JB Lippincott; and Desmond MM, Wilson GS, Melnick JL, Singer DB, et al: Congenital rubella encephalitides, *J Pediatr* 71:311-331, 1967.

Neurological phenomena in the newborn period are prominent in approximately 50% to 75% of the cases (see Table 20-18).[32,43,56,57,77,214,222] The most common manifestations relate to meningoencephalitis, seen most clearly in most patients by elevated levels of CSF protein and mononuclear cells.[214] The anterior fontanelle is full in 25% to 50% of patients. The most common initial neurological features are "lethargy" and hypotonia, accompanied and followed shortly by prominent irritability. The irritability may relate to meningeal irritation, which probably also accounts for the occurrence of retrocollis and opisthotonos. These signs of meningeal irritation may worsen in the first weeks or months of life. Seizures appear in approximately 10% to 15% of infants.[214] Definite microcephaly is unusual at birth. Most of the acute clinical features subside over the first several months and evolve to the sequelae outlined subsequently.

The *ocular lesions* consist principally of cataracts, usually white or pearly, especially centrally, and chorioretinitis.[2,9,223] Chorioretinitis may be more common than was previously appreciated. Indirect ophthalmoscopy is especially helpful to demonstrate the characteristic spotty pigmentation (i.e., "salt-and-pepper") appearance, which may be particularly prominent peripherally.[213] Microphthalmia is sometimes difficult to appreciate when it is bilateral and is associated particularly with cataract.

The *auditory lesion* may be difficult to demonstrate in the newborn, although the application of brain stem evoked response audiometry has improved detection. In one series, approximately 20% of infants had suspected or definite hearing loss by behavioral testing in the neonatal period.[220] The basis for the hearing loss in congenital rubella is a cochlear inflammatory and destructive lesion.[219] A significant minority of infants subsequently will exhibit disturbances in response to sound that appear to be on a "central" basis,[216] although the locus of this central pathology is unclear. In a detailed study of hearing loss in children with congenital rubella, the hearing deficit was usually uniform over all frequencies, symmetrical, and severe (mean threshold, 93 dB).[224] As many as 60% to 80% of infants with congenital rubella are found later to have hearing loss as children.[2,195,214,224] This increase in incidence from early infancy to childhood relates to a combination of inadequate testing in infancy with delayed diagnosis and progression of disease in the auditory apparatus; the relative importance of each of these factors remains unclear.

Clinical Diagnosis. Clinical features that favor the diagnosis of congenital rubella are intrauterine growth retardation, CSF pleocytosis, salt-and-pepper chorioretinopathy, cataracts, cardiovascular defects, and skeletal lesions. The absences of prominent cerebral calcification, hydrocephalus, overt microcephaly, and vesicular rash are the clinical features that best differentiate congenital rubella from congenital toxoplasmosis, CMV infection, and HSV infection.

Laboratory Evaluation

Virus Isolation. Determination of rubella virus as the responsible microbe depends particularly on isolation of the virus and serological tests.[2,9,195,205] The virus can be isolated best from the nasopharynx and urine, but it can also be isolated from stool and CSF (and various tissues, including lens and brain). Approximately 55% to 85% of patients exhibit positive cultures.[2,214] Performance of multiple cultures increases the yield appreciably. The virus has been isolated from approximately 30% to 45% of CSF samples examined.[211,214] This relatively high frequency of isolation of virus from CSF is unlike other congenital viral encephalitides. The chronicity of rubella infection is emphasized by the finding of positive CSF cultures in infants as old as 18 months.[214] A similar conclusion can be derived from isolation of virus from the cataractous lens of a child aged 2 years, 11 months.[221] Moreover, as many as one third of infants with congenital rubella are still excreting virus at 8 months of age.[9]

Serological Studies. Serological diagnosis may be based on the persistence of hemagglutination inhibition or neutralization antibody titers after 4 to 6 months of age, when passively transferred antibody is usually undetectable. However, the fastest and most useful test is determination of IgM-specific antibody; this is the most definitive serological diagnostic test in the first few weeks of life.

Neurodiagnostic Studies. No specific neurodiagnostic tests are available, although a high rate of viral isolation from the CSF and the frequency of *CSF signs of inflammation* are very helpful in diagnosis. *CT scan* is useful in the detection of the focal areas of ischemic necrosis secondary to the vasculopathy and the less common calcification in basal ganglia.[71,109] CT scans performed between 1 and 3 years of age have demonstrated cerebral white matter hypodensity and multiple calcified nodules in the centrum semiovale,[225] presumably reflecting the impaired myelination and focal ischemic lesions described earlier in the section on neuropathology. *MRI scan* is most useful for detection of the presumed ischemic lesions in cerebral white matter and impairment of myelination.[109] *Cranial ultrasound scan* may show focal areas of calcification,[108] subependymal cysts,[106,109,226] and echogenic vessels in the basal ganglia and thalamus.[106,109,110,227] In a series of 12 infants with echogenic vessels in basal ganglia, 2 patients had congenital rubella.[110]

Prognosis

Relation to Neonatal Clinical Syndrome. Although the outcome is related to the neonatal clinical features, the relationships are not so obvious as with congenital CMV infection and toxoplasmosis. This fact may relate to the particular chronicity of congenital rubella, as well as to the relative infrequency of completely asymptomatic neonatal disease. In a population of 100 infants carefully studied, 90% of whom were overtly symptomatic in the neonatal period and very early infancy, only 9% appeared to be free of deficits at 18 months (Table 20-19).[214] Neuromotor deficits (i.e., spastic motor deficits and delayed neurological development) were severe in approximately 50% of the patients. Fully 81% of these infants had microcephaly, and 72% had definite hearing loss or other apparent disturbances related to auditory perception. In a subsequent report of the same population, of patients followed to 16 to 18 years of age, 28% exhibited mental retardation, and an additional 25% exhibited low-average intelligence.[228] Of 14 children with "suspect" hearing loss at 18 months, 13 were definitely hearing impaired. In another prospective series of infants with congenital rubella, approximately similar outcomes were observed; approximately 45% of such infants exhibited "psychomotor retardation," and 50% of these infants were moderately or severely affected.[199]

Long-Term Hearing Deficits and Other Sequelae. Even those infants who appear to be less severely affected often show evolution of disabling auditory, motor, behavioral, and learning deficits as they grow

TABLE 20-19	Outcome at Age 18 Months of Survivors of Congenital Rubella Syndrome	
Outcome		**Percentage Affected**
Neuromotor Deficits		
None		31%
Mild		22%
Severe		47%
Microcephaly		81%
Hearing Loss		
None		28%
Definite		45%
Poor speech, inconsistent response to sound		27%
Ocular Manifestations		
Cataract		47%
Chorioretinitis		31%
No Hearing, Speech, or Visual Problem		9%

Data from Desmond MM, Wilson GS, Melnick JL, Singer DB, et al: Congenital rubella encephalitides, *J Pediatr* 71:311-331, 1967.

older (Table 20-20).[2,195,220] A multidisciplinary, longitudinal study of 29 "nonretarded" infants with congenital rubella demonstrated definite hearing loss in 1 infant in the first 2 months, in 12 infants by 12 months, in 22 infants by 24 months, in 25 infants by 48 months, and in an additional 2 infants by 11 years, for a total of 27, or 93% of the children. This accretion of patients with definite hearing loss may reflect continuing cochlear injury. The analogy with the delayed onset of hearing loss in congenital CMV infection and of chorioretinopathy in congenital toxoplasmosis is apparent.

In the longitudinal study just mentioned, early disturbances of motor development and of tone were followed by impairments of motor coordination and muscle weakness in approximately 50% of the children.[220] Behavioral disturbances, which in the early years included impaired attention span and hyperkinesis, evolved to emotional irritability and persisting distractibility in approximately 50%. A propensity for congenital rubella infection to lead to impairment of

TABLE 20-20	Identification of Hearing Loss in 29 Nonretarded, Longitudinally Studied Children with Congenital Rubella Syndrome	
	HEARING LOSS	
Age	**Suspected**	**Diagnosed**
Birth–2 mo	5	1
3–12 mo	10	11
13–24 mo	2	10
25–48 mo	2	3
4–11 yr	—	2
		27 (93%)

Data from Desmond MM, Fisher ES, Vorderman AL, Schaffer HG, et al: The longitudinal course of congenital rubella encephalitis in nonretarded children, *J Pediatr* 93:584-591, 1978.

behavioral and emotional development is also apparent in other studies by a 6% incidence of subsequent autism.[195] Moreover, although IQ scores remained within the normal range in the study of Desmond and co-workers,[220] learning deficits and visual-perceptual-motor deficits were prominent in approximately 50%. These abnormalities had major impacts on the adaptation of the children to educational and home environments and underscore the necessity for careful follow-up and appropriate interventions in infants with congenital rubella.

An interesting relationship between the rate of linear growth and cognitive outcome was apparent in a 20-year follow-up of 105 cases of congenital rubella syndrome.[229] Children with normal growth had normal cognitive development, and those whose linear growth was at less than the fifth percentile exhibited moderate to severe mental retardation.

Late Progressive Panencephalitis. A rare complication of congenital rubella, the precise frequency and importance of which are not clear, is the occurrence of progressive panencephalitis with onset, usually in the second decade, of intellectual and motor deterioration, elevated CSF protein levels, and elevated antibody titers to rubella virus in serum and CSF.[195,230] The virus has been isolated from the brain.[231] Whether this disorder represents reactivated infection or bears a relation to the role of measles virus in subacute sclerosing panencephalitis, or both, remains to be determined.

Management

Prevention. Preventive measures present the realistic hope of eradication of congenital rubella. Of the three major approaches to prevention (avoidance of maternal infection, treatment of maternal infection, and abortion in the presence of maternal infection), the first has been accomplished in large part through vaccination.

Active immunization with a live attenuated rubella vaccine has been accomplished by two major approaches.[2,9,195,232] In the United States, mass vaccination of all children aged 1 year to puberty has been used to limit the spread of infection to the pregnant woman by curtailing circulation of virus in the community. In the United Kingdom and in many other European countries, selected immunization, especially of girls from ages 11 to 14 years, was used initially to provide protection for the childbearing years.[233,234] Mass vaccination of all children in the second year of life was instituted in the United Kingdom in 1988. The policy in the United States has been effective; the incidence of congenital rubella declined by approximately fivefold in the decade following the initiation of this vaccination regimen.[9,232] Indeed, as noted earlier, the current incidence of congenital rubella in the United States is less than 1 per 1 million live births.[223] However, some questions still remain concerning how long vaccine-induced protection will last or whether inapparent reinfection of the mother with transmission to the fetus may occur.

Passive immunization with immune globulin may be useful in the special case of a susceptible pregnant woman exposed to rubella. The effectiveness of this approach is controversial, but it is necessary to recognize that passive immunization is useful to prevent viremia and fetal infection and therefore must be given promptly.

Abortion in the woman infected with rubella requires understanding of the risks of fetal infection as they relate to the timing of the infection in pregnancy. The demonstration of prenatal diagnosis by fetal blood sampling in the 20th week of gestation may help to prevent abortion of the unaffected fetus.[235]

Supportive Therapy. Supportive therapy is carried out principally as described for congenital CMV infection. In addition, recognition and prompt control of cardiac failure are critical, particularly in view of cerebral vasculopathy and therefore already compromised cerebral perfusion. Careful auditory assessment, with brain stem evoked response audiometry as well as with behavioral studies, is critical to detect hearing loss and to provide appropriate intervention as early as possible. Similarly, detection of cataract is important because delay of surgery into the second and third years of life prevents useful vision. However, opinions differ about the optimal time of therapy. Nevertheless, the infant with auditory and visual deficits is at great risk for subsequent disturbances of language and other aspects of neurological development, and the earliest interventions regarding vision and audition are critical.

Antimicrobial Therapy. No known effective chemotherapeutic agents of value exist in the treatment of congenital (or postnatal) rubella infection.

Herpes Simplex

Neonatal HSV infection, in most cases, is acquired during passage through an infected birth canal. Less commonly, ascending infection near the time of birth is the means of acquisition of the virus. Still less commonly, transplacental passage of virus causes intrauterine infection, or postnatal acquisition of virus from infected adults or infants causes severe postnatal illness. Neonatal HSV infection is very much less common than the other major neonatal infection caused by a herpes virus, CMV infection. However, unlike CMV infection, essentially all examples of neonatal HSV infection are symptomatic, often with serious neurological concomitants apparent in the newborn period. The premature infant is apparently more susceptible than the full-term infant and accounts for as many as 25% to 35% of cases.[2,236-242]

The incidence of neonatal HSV infection increased pari passu with the increase in incidence of genital HSV infection in adults in the United States over the several decades before the decline of the past few years.[2,239,241,243] In detailed studies from King County, Washington, the incidence of neonatal HSV infection increased progressively from a rate of 2.6 per 100,000 live births during the years 1966 through 1969

to 28.2 per 100,000 live births in 1982.[244] A twofold increase over the last 4 years of the study suggested that the incidence was continuing to rise rapidly. Later data indicated that the prevalence of HSV type 2 (HSV-2) in the United States was approximately 20% to 30% in adults, with the highest values (40% to 60%) in black women of childbearing age.[245,246] However, more recent data suggest that the trajectory of increasing seroprevalence of HSV, especially HSV-2, in the United States has ceased.[243] Thus, in a study of more than 11,000 adults, the seroprevalences in 1999 to 2004 versus those in 1988 to 1994 were, for HSV-2, 17.0% versus 21.0%, and for HSV-1, they were 57.7% versus 62.0%.[243]

Pathogenesis

Parturitional and Ascending Infection. Most infants with neonatal HSV infection acquire the infection during passage through an infected birth canal near or at the time of birth. The markedly higher rate of neonatal HSV infection in infants born to mothers shedding virus at delivery when delivery is by the vaginal route than by cesarean section is consistent with this notion (Table 20-21).[241] In the classic case, the virus is acquired by direct contact of the infant's skin, eye, or oral cavity with the virus in the mother's birth canal. (Overt maternal herpetic lesions are uncommonly present.) Because of the importance of direct contact, it is understandable that the vesicular lesions that result in the infant are usually over the scalp and face in cephalic presentations and over the buttocks in breech presentations.[2,237,239,241] Vivid demonstrations of the relation of contact to the site of herpetic lesions are provided by the several reports of vesicular lesions (and serious neonatal disease) at the sites of placement of fetal scalp electrodes for intrapartum

TABLE 20-21	**Risk Factors for Development of Neonatal Herpes Simplex Virus Infection***	
Risk Factor	**No. of Infants with Neonatal Herpes Simplex Virus Infection/No. of Deliveries**	***P* Value**
Type of Delivery		
Cesarean	1/85 (1.2%)	0.47
Vaginal	9/117 (7.7%)	
Invasive Monitors		
Yes	8/79 (10.1%)	.02
No	2/123 (1.6%)	
Type Isolated		
HSV-1	5/16 (31.3%)	<.001
HSV-2	5/186 (2.7%)	
First Episode		
Yes	8/26 (30.8%)	<.001
No	2/151 (1.3%)	

*Based on study of 40,023 deliveries with cultures. Data shown concern the 202 deliveries complicated by neonatal herpes simplex virus infection.

Data from Brown ZA, Wald A, Morrow RA, Selke S, et al: Effect of serologic status and cesarean delivery on transmission rates of herpes simplex virus from mother to infant, *JAMA* 289:203-209, 2003.

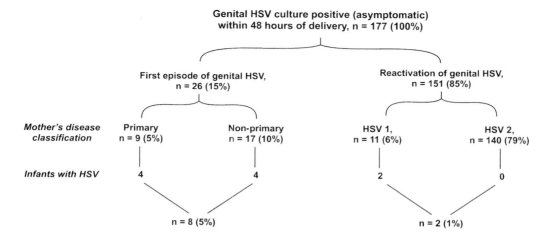

Figure 20-20   **Neonatal herpes simplex virus (HSV) infection in relation to asymptomatic maternal infection at the time of labor.** Infection was determined by viral culture at the time of delivery. Classification of maternal disease was made by type-specific serological testing. Primary genital infection was diagnosed in culture-positive women without antibodies to HSV-1 or HSV-2 in the initial serum sample, obtained at the time of delivery, who then became seropositive for one of the virus types in the subsequent sample obtained 6 to 8 weeks later. Nonprimary genital infection was diagnosed in culture-positive women with antibodies to HSV-1 (or HSV-2) in the initial sample from whom HSV-2 (or HSV-1) then was isolated in early labor and who were seropositive on the subsequent sample. *(Adapted from Brown ZA, Wald A, Morrow RA, Selke S, et al: Effect of serologic status and cesarean delivery on transmission rates of herpes simplex virus from mother to infant, JAMA 289:203-209, 2003.)*

monitoring.[242,247-254] In a large study of women with asymptomatic infection with HSV at delivery, fetal scalp electrodes were used in 25 infants, of whom 5 developed neonatal herpes, versus 0 cases of neonatal herpes in the 25 deliveries in which fetal scalp electrodes were not used.[253] A larger study later confirmed the importance of invasive monitoring (see Table 20-21).[241] In general, approximately 50% to 75% of neonatal infections are caused by HSV-2, which usually infects the maternal genital tract, and the remainder are caused by HSV-1, which usually infects nongenital sites. A recent report from Canada ($n = 58$) showed that HSV-1 now accounts for the majority of the cases (62%) in that country.[242] The risk of transmission to the newborn is more than 10-fold greater when the mother is shedding HSV-1 than HSV-2 at delivery (see Table 20-21).[241]

Large-scale studies of neonatal HSV infection in relation to the type of maternal infection have been of great interest.[2,239,241,242,253,255-257] It is clear that in most cases, neonatal infection occurs in children of *asymptomatic* rather than symptomatic mothers. Moreover, the serological status of the mother is a critical determinant of the risk of neonatal infection (Fig. 20-20).[241,253] Of 177 women with positive HSV cultures within 48 hours of delivery, 26 (15%) had evidence of a recently acquired first episode of infection. *Nearly one third of these pregnancies resulted in neonatal HSV infection, and fully 80% of neonatal HSV infection in the entire cohort occurred in this subset of infected women.* No difference in risk of transmission was noted in the first episode group whether the infection was primary (mother had no antibodies to HSV) or nonprimary (mother had antibodies to HSV-1 with HSV-2 infection or to HSV-2 with HSV-1 infection). In the large group of women ($n = 151$) with reactivated infection, 85% of the total group, the risk of transmission of neonatal HSV infection was very low (i.e., only ≈1%). Although most of the reactivated maternal infections

involved HSV-2, the risk of transmission of virus to the infant was confined to the small group with reactivated HSV-1 (see Table 20-21). Indeed, none of 140 reactivated maternal HSV-2 infections resulted in neonatal HSV, whereas 2 of 11 reactivated maternal HSV-1 infections were transmitted.

Symptomatic primary infection is characterized by fever, pain, and vesiculoulcerative lesions of the vagina and cervix. The risk of infection for a newborn delivered vaginally in the presence of clinically visible maternal genital infection in an antibody-negative woman may approach 50% (a much higher risk than in the much more common circumstance of an antibody-positive woman).[237,258]

Ascending infection of the fetus can occur after rupture of the membranes. Indeed, available data suggest that the risk of fetal infection in the presence of *clinically visible* maternal genital infection is greater by the ascending route than by parturitional contact (Table 20-22). This finding may relate to a larger inoculum of virus and exposure at multiple sites with ascending versus parturitional infection.[56,57] The current rarity of this clinical situation is illustrated by a recent study of 58 cases of neonatal HSV infection; only 1 mother had intrapartum genital lesions.[242]

Fetal (Transplacental) Infection. Prenatal acquisition of HSV through transplacental mechanisms is a rare cause of fetal infection. Isolated examples have been reported in single case reports.[2,239,256,259-265] However, in a study of 155 cases of neonatal HSV infection, 8 (5%) had evidence of acquisition of infection during early gestation.[266] Of these 8 infants, all were premature. Clinical manifestations have included skin lesions at birth, chorioretinitis, microphthalmia, microcephaly, hydranencephaly, multicystic encephalomalacia, cerebral calcifications, and other CNS abnormalities on CT scan. The clinical features of intrauterine HSV

TABLE 20-22   Risk of Herpes Simplex Virus Infection of the Infant as a Function of the Type of Delivery from a Mother with Clinically Apparent Genital Infection*

Type of Delivery	No. of Infants Infected/Total No. of Deliveries
Vaginal	10/20
Cesarean section	
After membrane rupture (>6 hr)	6/7
Before or within 4 hr of membrane rupture	1/16

*The antibody status of these women was not known, and the risk of neonatal infection depends markedly on this status (see text for details).

Data from Whitley RJ, Nahmias AJ, Visintine AM, Fleming CL, et al: The natural history of herpes simplex virus infection of mother and newborn, *Pediatrics* 66:489-494, 1980.

infection as a function of estimated time of acquisition of the virus are summarized in Table 20-23.

Postnatal Infection. Postnatal acquisition of HSV by the newborn is an uncommon but documented occurrence.[2,239,267] Of 24 infants described in a review as having acquired infection shortly after birth, 13 acquired the infection from mothers with oral herpetic lesions, 9 from other adults (including hospital personnel), and 2 from other infected infants.[267] As in other examples of HSV infection of the newborn, the infection was serious, and 67% of the children died. These data have important implications for prevention of exposure of the newborn to sources of HSV.

Role of Host Factors. Host factors must play some role in explaining the malignancy of HSV infection in

TABLE 20-23   Clinical Features of Intrauterine Herpes Simplex Virus Infection

	PRESUMED TIMING OF INFECTION	
	First or Second Trimester	Late Second to Third Trimester
Number of Infants	6	14
Premature Delivery	60%	75%
Organ Involvement at Birth		
Skin	84%	100%
Brain	84%*	29%*
Eye	84%	29%
Microcephaly	100%	—
Outcome		
Neonatal death	20%	46%
Developmental delay	80%	16%
Normal	—	38%

*Includes hydranencephaly, porencephalies, multicystic leukomalacia, and cerebral calcification.

Data from Christie JD, Rakusan TA, Martinez MA, Lucia HL, et al: Hydranencephaly caused by congenital infection with herpes simplex virus. *Pediatr Infect Dis* 5:473-478, 1986.

the perinatal period. Indeed, in older patients who are immunologically competent, severe disseminated disease is rare. The likelihood of neonatal disturbances in the response to HSV infection has been delineated.[239,268-274] Defects in the infant's response to simplex infection can be divided into those response mechanisms involved in the initial "containment" phase, during which the virus is localized to a limited anatomical area, and those mechanisms active in the later specific "curative" phase, during which localized infection is eliminated.[272,273] Defects in the initial containment phase involve operation of the alveolar-macrophage barrier, expression of natural killer cytotoxicity, and production of interferon-alpha and tumor necrosis factor. Defects in the later elimination phase involve antibody production, both of the neutralizing type and that responsible for antibody-dependent cellular (leukocyte) cytotoxicity, T-cell proliferation, and interferon-gamma production.

Neuropathology

Neonatal HSV infections may result in a wide range of involvement of the CNS, from no abnormality to devastating brain destruction. Significant involvement is most common and consists of inflammation and destruction (Table 20-24). Whether the few infants with intrauterine infection by transplacental acquisition have, in addition, aberrations of developmental events remains to be established. In this regard, microcephaly is a consistent feature of early intrauterine infection (see Table 20-23).

Meningoencephalitis. The meningoencephalitis is characterized by (1) inflammatory cells in the meninges, (2) perivascular infiltrates with inflammatory cells, (3) severe multifocal necrosis of all cellular elements of brain parenchyma (only very uncommonly is the involvement greatest in the temporal and inferior frontal regions as in older patients with HSV encephalitis), (4) reactive microglial and astroglial proliferation, and (5) occurrence of Cowdry type A intranuclear inclusions in neuronal and glial, especially oligodendroglial, cells. The nucleus containing the inclusions is characteristically distorted with clumping of nuclear chromatin and undulation of the nuclear membrane.[42] These pathological findings are often accompanied by a considerable degree of brain swelling, and hemorrhage in the areas of necrosis may occur, in part because of associated endothelial involvement.[42]

Neuropathological Sequelae. The result of HSV infection of the perinatal brain most commonly is a devastating effect on neural structure and function. Subsequent failure of brain growth and microcephaly

TABLE 20-24   Neuropathology of Neonatal Herpes Simplex Virus Infection

Meningoencephalitis
Multifocal parenchymal necrosis, occasionally hemorrhagic
Brain swelling
Multicystic encephalomalacia

(after the neonatal period) are the rule. Multicystic encephalomalacia has been documented repeatedly (Fig. 20-21).[268-271,275-283] Indeed, the destruction may be so complete that hydranencephaly is the result. These lesions can be demonstrated readily by CT and MRI scans (see later).

Clinical Aspects

Incidence of Clinically Apparent Infection. Neonatal HSV infection is distinctive among the organisms of the TORCH complex in the essentially uniform occurrence of *symptomatic* disease. The clinical spectrum varies from infection localized to a few vesicles on the skin to dissemination to every major organ (Table 20-25).[2,9,237-240,242,254,257,283-289] A major distinction is made between disseminated and localized HSV disease. Disseminated disease is associated with evidence for involvement of multiple systems, particularly the reticuloendothelial system. Hepatoadrenal necrosis is the hallmark of the disorder.[9,237,239] Localized disease

TABLE 20-25   Clinical Spectrum and Outcome of *Untreated* Neonatal Herpes Simplex Virus Infection*

| | | OUTCOME | | |
Clinical Type	No. of Patients	Died	Neurological Sequelae	No Apparent Sequelae
Disseminated	116	77%	11%	12%
Localized				
Central nervous system	61	37%	51%	12%
Ocular	13	0%	31%	69%
Skin	39	10%	26%	64%
Oral	4	0%	0%	100%
Asymptomatic	2	0%	0%	100%

*Excludes infants who received antiviral therapy.
Data from Nahmias AJ, Keyserling HL, Kerrick GM: Herpes simplex. In Remington JS, Klein JO, editors: *Infectious Diseases of the Fetus and Newborn Infant*, 2nd ed, Philadelphia: 1983, Saunders.

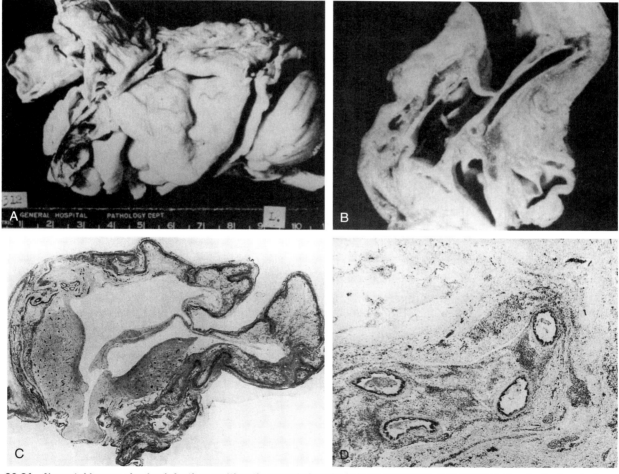

Figure 20-21   **Neonatal herpes simplex infection: multicystic encephalomalacia in an infant who died at 24 weeks of age.** Onset of recognized disease at approximately 21 days of age with seizures was followed by rapid progression to electrocerebral silence at 34 days of age and subsequent vegetative state. **A,** Left lateral view of brain showing thickened covering membranes and severe destruction of cerebral hemispheres. **B,** Coronal section of cerebral hemispheres showing parenchymal destruction with cavitation. **C,** Photomicrograph of coronal section of cerebral hemispheres stained with hematoxylin and eosin. Note destruction of cerebral cortex and subcortical white matter and replacement by astrocytic glial stroma and dramatic masses of foamy macrophages. The macrophages are particularly striking in the superior aspects of the cerebral convexity. **D,** Higher-power view showing the cavitation, necrotic debris, and masses of macrophages, especially around blood vessels. *(From Young GF, Knox DL, Dodge PR: Necrotizing encephalitis and chorioretinitis in a young infant: Report of a case with rising herpes simplex antibody titers, Arch Neurol 13:15-24, 1965.)*

TABLE 20-26 **Clinical Features of Disseminated Neonatal Herpes Simplex Virus Infection***

Clinical Feature	Approximate Frequency
Central Nervous System	
Meningoencephalitis	51%–75%
Seizures	21%–50%
Coma	21%–50%
Tense anterior fontanelle	0%–50%
Skin and Oral Cavity	
Vesicular exanthem	51%–75%
Vesicular enanthem	0%–20%
Eye	
Conjunctivitis	0%–20%
Keratitis	0%–20%
Chorioretinitis	0%–20%
Reticuloendothelial System	
Hepatomegaly	21%–50%
Hyperbilirubinemia	21%–50%
Bleeding	21%–50%
Hemolytic and other anemias	0%–20%
Other	
Fever	21%–50%
Pneumonitis	0%–20%
Rapidly fatal course (untreated)	76%–100%

*See text for references.

is associated with involvement confined to a single site; if multiple sites are involved, the term *localized* is still used if the reticuloendothelial system and other visceral organs are not included. A distinction is made between disease localized to the CNS (a serious form) and that localized to skin, eye, or mouth (a less serious form). Ten or more years ago, disseminated disease accounted for approximately 40% to 70% of all cases. More recently, the approximate distribution of clinical types has been as follows: disseminated disease, 30% to 40%; localized CNS disease, 30% to 40%; and localized skin-eye-mouth disease, 20% to 40%.[2,239,240,254,257,286,287] Overlap of the latter two localized forms is not uncommon. The relative decrease in disseminated disease and the increase in skin-eye-mouth disease appear to relate to earlier diagnosis and the use of antiviral therapy.

Clinical Features of Disseminated Disease. The early signs of disseminated HSV infection occur in most cases by the end of the first week of life.* In a series of 186 infected infants, approximately 10% of patients were reported to exhibit signs of illness on the first postnatal day. The usual mode of onset includes lethargy and cessation of feeding. This is followed promptly in approximately half of the cases by a neurological syndrome characterized by stupor, irritability, and seizures (often focal), with progression to coma and opisthotonos (Table 20-26).[56,57,240]

---

*See references 2,9,43,56,57,237-240,253,254,285-287,289-291.

CSF pleocytosis (sometimes with red blood cells) and elevated protein content are present. In approximately one third of patients with disseminated cases, overt CNS signs are not present. However, CSF pleocytosis and elevated protein content may be observed in such cases, and the occurrence of neurological residua in survivors indicates that CNS involvement is frequently present in these infants, even though overt neonatal neurological signs are not apparent.

In disseminated disease, hepatomegaly, hyperbilirubinemia, and bleeding are common (see Table 20-26). The bleeding relates to a combination of hepatic disease and, often, disseminated intravascular coagulation, and it may be very severe. Skin vesicles are present in approximately 50% to 60% of patients with disseminated disease. The vesicles often appear *after* the clinical onset of the disease and evolve from macules to papules before formation of the vesicles, which often resemble pustules. Disseminated HSV infection is a devastating disorder (see Table 20-25); before the era of therapy, approximately 80% of children died, frequently in a matter of a few days, and approximately 50% of the survivors exhibited serious neurological sequelae, predictable on the basis of the neuropathology (see the previous section).

Clinical Features of Localized Disease. Localized HSV infection is characterized by the absence of clinical or laboratory evidence of visceral involvement.[2,237,239,240,252,283,288] The sites most commonly affected are the CNS, skin, eye, and oral cavity (see Table 20-25).[2,237-239,242,254,287,290] The age of onset of localized involvement of the *CNS* is *later* than for disseminated disease (i.e., usually the second or third week of life). In one carefully studied series, the mean age of onset was 16 days.[291] Indeed, because relatively more term infants exhibit localized CNS disease than disseminated disease,[280] the infant with this variety of neonatal HSV infection usually already has been discharged from the hospital before the illness begins. The usual signs are stupor and irritability, which evolve to seizures (often focal) and, perhaps, coma (Table 20-27). In the past several years, I have seen infants who presented clinically with focal seizures and a normal level of consciousness. As with disseminated disease, many infants ($\approx$35%) do not exhibit mucocutaneous lesions.[240,283,287,290,291] CSF pleocytosis and elevated protein are characteristic, and depressed CSF glucose is also common.[283] The outcome is unfavorable but better than with disseminated disease. Before antiviral therapy, approximately 60% of these infants survived,

TABLE 20-27 **Major Clinical Features of Localized Neonatal Herpes Simplex Virus Infection of the Central Nervous System**

Stupor and irritability
Seizures (often focal)
Vesicular exanthem
Cerebrospinal fluid pleocytosis, elevated protein

although approximately 80% of *survivors* exhibited serious neurological sequelae (see Table 20-25).

HSV infection clinically localized to the skin, eye, or mouth presents in the latter part of the first week or second week of life.[254,287,291] The progression from macules to vesicles occurs over 24 to 48 hours, often at sites of trauma (e.g., site of scalp electrodes or presenting body part). The vesicles may be obscured by overlying hair. The presence of a vesicle in a newborn should be considered an HSV infection until ruled out by appropriate diagnostic studies as soon as possible (see later). Progression to CNS or disseminated disease occurs in 75% of untreated cases. Indeed, clinical localization of lesions to skin, eye, or mouth does not imply that the CNS is not also affected (see Table 20-25). Before therapy, approximately 30% of such patients exhibited neurological sequelae on follow-up.[237]

Clinical Diagnosis. Of the congenital infections, neonatal HSV infection may be the most distinctive. The presence of a vesicular rash, keratoconjunctivitis, seizures, tense anterior fontanelle, and CSF evidence of meningoencephalitis is characteristic. However, the skin and ocular manifestations are present at the *onset* of the illness in only the *minority* of cases. Additional information of value is epidemiological, regarding HSV infection in the mother or her sexual contact. Important negative differential diagnostic information includes the rarity *in the neonatal period* of microcephaly, hydrocephalus, intracranial calcification, and cardiovascular defects.

Laboratory Evaluation

Cytological Techniques. Identification of HSV infection is based principally on cytological techniques, isolation of the virus, or detection of viral DNA.[9,32,56,57,237,239,291-295] A high index of suspicion of the disease is crucial. Certainly, any infant with a vesicular lesion should be considered to have an HSV infection and should be evaluated appropriately. However, nonspecific signs (e.g., lethargy, cessation of feeding, or other features suggestive of bacterial sepsis) should raise the possibility of neonatal HSV infection. Cytological techniques are readily available and are a rapid means of establishing a presumptive diagnosis of neonatal HSV infection. Scrapings can be obtained from the base of vesicular lesions of the skin or oral cavity or from conjunctival lesions. Smears are fixed in alcohol and stained immediately, according to the Papanicolaou method. The typical morphological changes are multinucleated giant cells and intranuclear inclusions. Viral particles may also be observed by electron microscopic examination of material from lesions and from urine and CSF.[296] HSV antigens have also been detected in CSF leukocytes by using immunofluorescence techniques.[297]

Virus Isolation and Detection of Viral DNA. Isolation of the virus is a definitive means for establishing the diagnosis and is best accomplished from observable lesions, but isolation is also possible from throat, stool, urine, and CSF. In one series, pharyngeal swab was the source with the highest detection rate (79%).[285] In appropriate media, samples can be transported at room temperature.[298,299] Cytopathic changes in inoculated tissue cultures are usually detectable within 1 to 3 days.[237] The virus not uncommonly is difficult to isolate from CSF very early in localized CNS disease.

A major advance in diagnosis of neonatal HSV infection is application of PCR to amplify the very small quantities of viral DNA, which then can be detected by conventional methods (e.g., DNA hybridization).[239,292-295,300,301] PCR assay has been shown in the newborn to be clearly superior to culture and is highly sensitive and specific for CNS involvement when CSF is studied. However, HSV DNA in CSF may be undetectable in 30% of cases early in the disease, and serial sampling is required to reach nearly 100% sensitivity in HSV encephalitis.

Importance of Maternal Evaluation. Isolation of the virus from mothers (or their sexual contacts) with genital infection is a valuable adjunct to diagnosis of the neonatal disorder. Because most cases of genital herpes in pregnant women are subclinical, cultures or PCR assays, or both, are usually necessary to establish the diagnosis.[239,295,302] Viral cultures of genital secretions and serological studies of maternal serum by Western blot are the most convenient and effective approaches.[2,253,257,302,303] Detection of viral DNA in genital specimens by PCR is a highly sensitive approach, but its value for routine use in obstetrics is not yet established.

Serological Studies. Serological studies for diagnosis of neonatal infection with HSV are less useful than for other congenital infections. This finding relates to the masking of the infant's own IgG response by passively transferred maternal antibody and the 1- to 2-week delay in the rise in specific IgM antibody generated by the infant. Specific HSV IgM antibody can be detected rapidly by an immunofluorescence test.[252,304] Because the antibody persists for 6 to 12 months, this test is useful in survivors of the neonatal infection.

Neurodiagnostic Studies. Neurodiagnostic studies of value include, particularly, examination of the CSF, electroencephalogram (EEG), and brain imaging findings. Brain biopsy no longer is a frequent diagnostic consideration.

The *CSF* exhibits the findings of meningoencephalitis (i.e., pleocytosis and elevated protein content). Polymorphonuclear cells occasionally are predominant, and in severely affected cases, the pleocytosis includes many red blood cells. The CSF glucose level may be depressed.[252,278,279,281-284,305] In one series, mean CSF glucose in the first week of the disease was 39 mg/dL; in the second week, it was 32 mg/dL; and in the third to fifth weeks, it was 28 mg/dL. Protein level is elevated consistently and often exceeds 100 to 150 mg/dL as the disease progresses. Any infant with a CSF formula suggestive of encephalitis (i.e., pleocytosis and elevated protein) should be considered to have

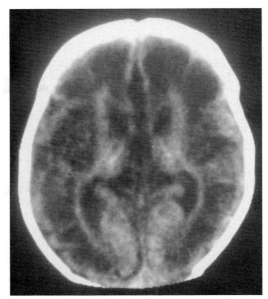

Figure 20-22 Neonatal herpes simplex infection: multicystic encephalomalacia. This computed tomography scan is from an affected 6-week-old infant who had onset of neurological signs at 7 days of age. Note the large lucent areas, representing regions of cystic necrosis, scattered throughout the cerebral hemispheres. *(Courtesy of Dr. Charles Abramson.)*

HSV encephalitis until proven otherwise. The virus can be isolated from the CSF, but as noted in the previous section, the cultures often are negative early in the disease. *PCR assay* clearly is the optimal method to identify the virus in CSF rapidly. As noted earlier, the sensitivity early in the disease is approximately 50% to 75% and increases to nearly 100% with later CSF samples.[283,294,295]

CT scan is of value to demonstrate the extent and severity of the brain injury (Fig. 20-22). Progression of abnormalities to multicystic encephalomalacia is documented readily by serial studies. *Cranial ultrasound scan* also is useful in the detection of parenchymal changes.[306] Multicystic encephalomalacia is detected readily by cranial ultrasonography. *MRI scan* is the most useful approach for identification of the parenchymal lesions. Diffusion-weighted MRI is the most sensitive imaging modality for the early detection of CNS disease[306a] (Fig. 20-23). The rapid evolution to multicystic encephalomalacia is clearly delineated by MRI (Fig. 20-24).

The *EEG* usually shows striking and characteristic changes (Fig. 20-25).[283-286,307] These changes are principally focal or multifocal paroxysmal, periodic, or quasiperiodic discharges, consisting of repetitive sharp-slow wave complexes.[284] The occurrence of prolonged periods (1 to 2 minutes) of such discharges was associated with death or major neurological sequelae in 9 of 10 affected infants in a reported series.[307] A normal EEG was associated with normal outcome in all five infants in another series.[286] The EEG is one of the most sensitive noninvasive laboratory studies in the diagnosis of herpes infection (Table 20-28). In the study of Mikati and co-workers,[284] EEG was abnormal when CT and ultrasonographic studies were normal in

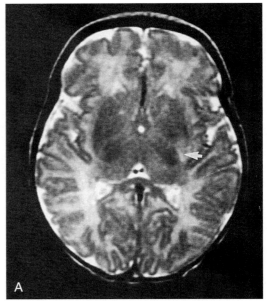

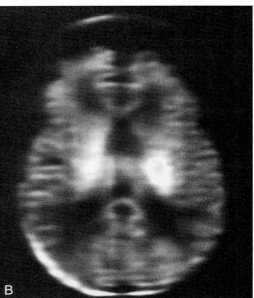

Figure 20-23 Neonatal herpes simplex encephalitis: magnetic resonance imaging (MRI) scans. **A,** T2-weighted and, **B,** diffusion-weighted MRI scans in neonatal herpes simplex encephalitis. This infant had onset of right focal seizures at 5 days of age. Note on the T2-weighted scan (**A**) a subtle lesion in the left putamen and deep cerebral white matter *(arrow)*. By contrast, the diffusion-weighted scan (**B**) shows a substantial lesion as well as an abnormality on the right.

the first 4 days of the illness in seven infants who had both EEG and an imaging study.

Prognosis

Relation to the Neonatal Clinical Syndrome. The outcome in affected infants is related clearly to the nature of the neonatal clinical syndrome (as discussed earlier) and is depicted in Table 20-25 for infants not treated with antiviral therapy. The mortality rate is highest with disseminated disease (≈80%) and lowest with localized skin involvement (no deaths). Survivors exhibit neurological sequelae predictable from the

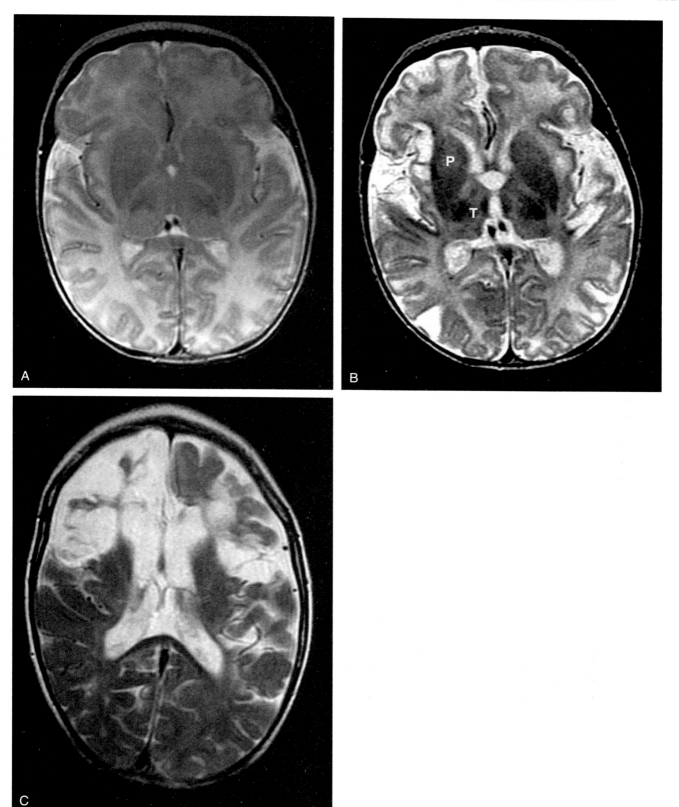

Figure 20-24 **Neonatal herpes simplex infection: magnetic resonance imaging (MRI) scans.** An axial T2-weighted MRI scan on the second postnatal day **(A)** showed no definite abnormality (although the diffusion-weighted scan exhibited abnormal signal in basal ganglia). By 1 month of age **(B)**, the axial T2-weighted scan showed evidence of diffuse cerebral cortical and white matter injury with early cystic changes, as well as lesions in putamen (P) and thalamus (T). At 6 months of age, an axial T2-weighted MRI scan **(C)** showed multicystic encephalomalacia, most prominent in the right frontal region. *(Courtesy of Dr. Omar Khwaja.)*

22 d♀; 3rd Day of illness

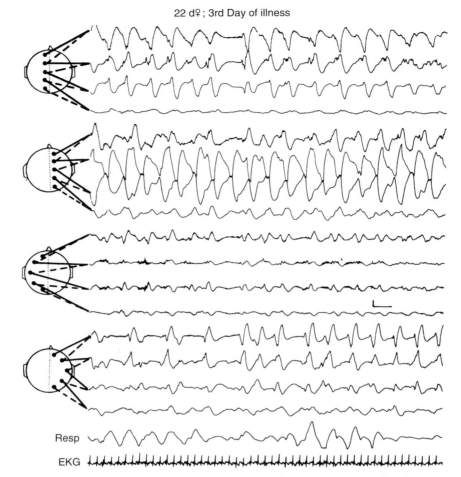

Figure 20-25   **Electroencephalographic tracings from an infant with neonatal herpes simplex infection.** The tracings were obtained with two different electrode arrays. The upper two tracings were obtained from one array, and the lower two tracings were from a second array. Foci of periodic lateralized epileptiform activity are apparent in both hemispheres. *(From Mizrahi EM, Tharp BR: A characteristic EEG pattern in neonatal herpes simplex encephalitis,* Neurology *32:1215-1220, 1982.)*

neuropathology (i.e., intellectual retardation, seizures, multifocal spastic motor deficits, and microcephaly). These sequelae are not uncommon in infections clinically localized to sites outside the CNS (e.g., ocular and skin) and indicate subclinical involvement of the CNS. The relatively high rate of neurological sequelae (31%) in patients with localized ocular disease may relate, in

part, to direct transmission of virus into the CNS from the eye, demonstrated experimentally.[308] Moreover, the observation that the incidence of chorioretinal scars on follow-up of infants infected with HSV as newborns increased from 4% in the neonatal period to 28% suggests that the virus may continue to cause injury in this region postnatally.[286]

Later data indicate a decrease in the proportion of disseminated HSV infection and an increase in the proportion of disease localized to skin, eye, and mouth (see earlier discussion). This change in clinical spectrum relates to both earlier diagnosis and onset of antiviral therapy.[2,239,257] Currently, the most favorable outcome is with skin-eye-mouth disease (no mortality, 95% to 100% normal), intermediate with localized CNS disease (15% mortality, 30% of survivors normal), and worst with disseminated disease (30% to 60% mortality, although 80% of survivors were normal; see later).[2,239,240,252,285-287,309]

Management

Prevention. Most cases of neonatal HSV infection are acquired close to the time of delivery, and, thus, the

TABLE 20-28	Electroencephalographic Findings in Neonatal Herpes Simplex Encephalitis		
		FINDINGS	
Days of Illness	**No.**	**Abnormal Background***	**Paroxysmal***
1–4	8	7	7
5–11	13	13	11
≥12	10	9	2

*Background abnormalities consisted primarily of low-voltage activity; paroxysmal activity consisted primarily of focal or multifocal periodic abnormalities.
Data from Mikati MA, Feraru E, Krishnamoorthy K, Lombroso CT: Neonatal herpes simplex meningoencephalitis: EEG investigations and clinical correlates, *Neurology* 40:1433-1437, 1990.

major issues are prevention of maternal infection and, if infection is present, detection thereof and management of delivery.[2,77,237,239,252,257,258,287,310] *Prevention of maternal infection* currently depends principally on advice to pregnant women to avoid sexual contact, especially in the later part of the pregnancy, with men who have genital herpes. Indeed, current data indicate that prevention of transmission of HSV infection from the male partner to the susceptible pregnant woman can reduce the incidence of neonatal HSV by 60% to 80%.[302]

Because the acquisition of most neonatal HSV infections is around the time of delivery, determination of the infected pregnant woman and, in particular, the woman with a *first episode of genital infection* is crucial (see Fig. 20-20).[2,239,241,253,258,287,311] Routine screening of pregnant women with viral cultures in the third trimester has failed to identify the women infected at the time of delivery.[287] The optimal approach for screening pregnant women is identification of the mother with primary infection at the time of labor. Serological testing is of importance in this context. Detection of genital shedding of virus can be made by viral cultures or PCR. The latter approach is the most sensitive and rapid.[239,241,312,313] The risk of HSV in the woman with a first episode of genital infection is 31% versus 1% in the woman with reactivated infection.[241] Indeed, among women with reactivated infection, those whose infection is with HSV-2 (i.e., mother has antibodies to HSV-2), although common, *rarely* transmit HSV-2 to their infants. However, reactivated infection with HSV-1 (i.e., mother has antibodies to HSV-1) is followed by transmission to the infant in approximately 20% of cases. These points concerning the risks of first episode of genital infection and of HSV-1 versus HSV-2 reactivated infection will help to determine whether antiviral suppressive therapy of the mother should be considered.

The *management of delivery* in the women with genital infection is based, in considerable part, on the markedly lower risk of transmission to the infant with cesarean section versus vaginal delivery (see earlier; see Table 20-22). Moreover, the risk of ascending infection after membranes have ruptured is significant and time related (see Table 20-22). Although the risk of neonatal infection increases with duration of ruptured membranes, cesarean section is recommended regardless of duration of amniorrhexis,[314] because it cannot be assumed that every infant has already acquired the virus through ascending infection (note the small number for cesarean section more than 6 hours after amniorrhexis in Table 20-22). In general, membrane rupture for up to 24 hours has been considered a duration still appropriate for cesarean section.[315] All these comments must be interpreted with the awareness that the serological status of the woman is most crucial in determining the potential value of cesarean section (see Fig. 20-20).

Supportive Therapy. Supportive therapy emphasizes the management of seizures. Although brain swelling is significant with severe involvement of the CNS, no evidence indicates that steroids or hyperosmolar solutions are generally useful. Avoidance of fluid overload, however, is important. Management of disseminated intravascular coagulation, bleeding, ventilation, circulation, and the like is reviewed in standard writings of neonatology.

Antimicrobial Therapy. Specific antiviral therapy is available for neonatal HSV infection. Although the outlook for treated patients remains serious (see subsequent discussion), the value of therapy is established. The decision of *whom to treat* is sometimes difficult. Optimal benefit requires prompt institution of therapy.[2,237-240,289,291,309] Indeed, in one study, involvement of additional organ systems by HSV was noted in 57% of infants between the time of presentation to medical personnel and diagnosis.[244] In another report, the mean time of onset of therapy was 5 to 6 days after onset of symptoms.[240] The difficulties in establishing the diagnosis rapidly in some infants are described earlier in "Laboratory Evaluation." I believe that antiviral therapy for suspected HSV infection of the newborn should be instituted in the same fashion as antibiotic therapy for suspected bacterial meningitis. Thus, I favor treatment after the culture or PCR specimens (including CSF) have been obtained for infants with the suspicious clinical features described previously (e.g., CSF findings suggestive of encephalitis) or vesicles in a clinically sick infant. With proven infection, it is universally recognized that infants with disseminated disease and localized CNS involvement should be treated immediately in view of the poor outcome. It is sometimes not so well recognized that even infants with localized skin-eye-mouth disease also require prompt therapy. Thus, infants with localized mucocutaneous or ocular disease on *initial* presentation progress to disseminated disease, overt CNS involvement, or both, in more than 50% of cases without therapy (Table 20-29).[236-239] Therefore, prompt antiviral therapy is indicated even when herpetic disease is apparently localized to mucocutaneous or ocular structures. In addition, because serial assessments of survivors of herpetic disease have demonstrated recurrence of disease in 10% to 30% of cases, including development of chorioretinitis and perhaps of neurological deficits during later infancy, the possibility of *progressive* disease (as with the other infections of the TORCH group) suggests an indication for intermittent later therapy or prolonged initial therapy.[2,239,286,295,316,317]

Four *antiviral drugs* (IDU, Ara-C, Ara-A or vidarabine, and acyclovir) have been shown to inhibit HSV in vitro by inhibiting DNA synthesis and have been used clinically since the 1980s.[237,239,291,309,318-321] IDU and Ara-C proved to be too toxic because of effects on such rapidly dividing cells as the gastrointestinal tract and hemopoietic systems. Moreover, Ara-C has a potent antimitotic effect on dividing brain cells, at least in the rat. A considerable degree of DNA synthesis, especially by glial cells, occurs in human brain in the perinatal period and potentially could be seriously deranged by this drug.

TABLE 20-29 Outcome of *Untreated* Neonatal Herpes Simplex Virus Infection Manifested Initially by Skin Vesicles Only*

| | | OUTCOME | | |
Neonatal Clinical Course	No. of Patients	Died	Neurological Sequelae	No Apparent Sequelae
Vesicles progressed to				
Disseminated disease	21	57%	24%	19%
Local central nervous system disease	10	30%	60%	10%
Local ocular disease	2	0%	50%	50%
Vesicles remained localized to skin	28	0%	29%	71%
Total	**61**	**24%**	**33%**	**43%**

*Infants were managed prior to availability of antiviral therapy.
Data from Nahmias AJ, Keyserling HL, Kerrick GM: Herpes simplex. In Remington JS, Klein JO, editors: *Infectious Diseases of the Fetus and Newborn Infant,* 2nd ed, Philadelphia: 1983, Saunders.

Vidarabine, a purine nucleotide, proved to be beneficial in reducing mortality and morbidity of neonatal HSV infections in controlled studies.[291,315,318,322,323] The drug crosses the blood-brain barrier efficiently and exerts its antiviral activity with less systemic toxicity than Ara-C. Even with severe disease (i.e., disseminated or localized CNS involvement), a sharp decrease in both mortality and morbidity (an approximately three-fold increase in normal survivors) was observed. Major disadvantages of vidarabine are the relatively low solubility of the drug and the need for administration of relatively large volumes of fluid with each dose.

Acyclovir represented an advance in therapy because of limited toxicity, high specificity, and greater activity against the virus than vidarabine.[239,291,307] The drug is a deoxyguanosine analogue that is activated by a herpes-specific thymidine kinase and inhibits viral DNA polymerase and thereby viral replication.[291,321] Controlled studies of HSV encephalitis in adults indicated greater benefit in relation to both mortality and morbidity for acyclovir than for vidarabine.[320,324] A controlled multi-institutional study of acyclovir versus vidarabine in the treatment of neonatal HSV infection demonstrated no appreciable difference in efficacy between the two.[291,315] However, acyclovir is preferred because of its higher solubility and relatively low toxicity.

One study compared outcome in infants with neonatal HSV disease treated with either acyclovir in standard dose (30 mg/kg/day) or high dose (60 mg/kg/day), administered intravenously for 21 days.[309] Concerning mortality, a markedly beneficial effect of high dose versus low dose was seen in children with disseminated HSV disease; the mortality rate was 60% to 70% for the standard dose (historical controls) versus 31% for high dose. For CNS disease, a beneficial effect on mortality rate was suggested but did not reach statistical significance; for standard-dose therapy, the mortality rate was approximately 20% versus 6% for high-dose treatment. Concerning morbidity, both treated groups showed striking beneficial effects compared with untreated historical controls (Fig. 20-26; compare Table 20-25). Compared with standard-dose therapy, high-dose therapy was associated with a better outcome in disseminated disease; 83% of infants treated with high-dose therapy were normal versus 60% of infants treated with standard-dose therapy. For localized skin-eye-mouth disease, no mortality occurred, and the outcome was essentially uniformly favorable with both therapy groups (see Fig. 20-26). Intravenous high-dose acyclovir is given daily in three divided doses of 20 mg/kg for 21 days; the dose is lowered in the presence of renal or hepatic dysfunction.

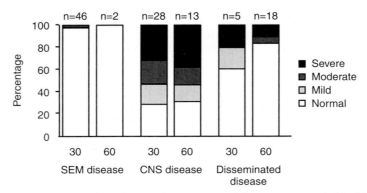

Figure 20-26 **Neonatal herpes simplex infection: effect of acyclovir on outcome.** Infants were treated with either 30 mg/kg/day (low-dose) or 60 mg/kg/day (high-dose) acyclovir. See text for details. SEM, skin-eye-mouth. *(From Kimberlin DW, Lin CY, Jacobs RF, Powel DA, et al: Safety and efficacy of high-dose intravenous acyclovir in the management of neonatal herpes simplex virus infections,* Pediatrics *108:230-238, 2001.)*

TABLE 20-30 Outcome of Pregnancy as a Function of Stage of Untreated Maternal Syphilis*

Maternal Status	OUTCOME OF PREGNANCY			
	Congenital Syphilis	Perinatal Death	Premature Infant	Normal Infant
Untreated syphilis				
Primary or secondary	50%	— — — — 50% — — — —		0%
Early latency	40%	20%	20%	20%
Late	10%	11%	9%	70%
No syphilis	0%	1%	8%	91%

*Adapted from Ingall D, Norins L: Syphilis. In Remington JS, Klein JO, editors: *Infectious Diseases of the Fetus and Newborn Infant*, 2nd ed, Philadelphia: 1983, Saunders.

Congenital Syphilis

Congenital infection with *T. pallidum* occurs by transplacental mechanisms, principally in the second and third trimesters of gestation. In the preantibiotic era, this disorder occurred with exceeding frequency; with the advent of penicillin treatment and improved public health measures, the disease became a rarity. However, in the mid-1980s, associated with some relaxation of surveillance techniques and a variety of social changes, syphilitic infection of women of childbearing age increased in frequency; with this, so did congenital syphilis.[325-328] In the later 1980s and early 1990s, these increases became dramatic and paralleled the increases in use of illegal drugs, especially cocaine, and in HIV infection.[77,325,328-334] Although congenital syphilis rarely is associated with *overt* neurological phenomena in the newborn period, involvement of the CNS appears to be relatively common and, in large part, curable. Thus, it is imperative for the perinatal physician to be aware of the features of the disorder.

Pathogenesis

Fetal Infection. Congenital syphilis results from intrauterine infection of the fetus with *T. pallidum* by transplacental mechanisms.[325,328,329,335] The fetus is infected during maternal spirochetemia, with resulting placentitis and, then, hematogenous spread of the organisms to multiple fetal organs. Maternal spirochetemia occurs during primary, secondary, and early latency stages of the maternal infection.[56,57,325,328,329,336] The primary infection is represented by a painless chancre at the portal of entry and is followed by the secondary stage of the disease approximately 6 weeks later, when mucocutaneous lesions and generalized lymphadenopathy often occur. This stage is followed by a variable period of 2 to 4 years during which spirochetemia, often asymptomatic, may recur.[328,337] Most infants acquire the infection in utero from an asymptomatic mother in the early latency stage, when diagnosis by serological testing is a reliable means of detecting the maternal infection.[328,338] Fetal syphilis can be suspected by the finding in approximately 65% of cases of hepatomegaly on intrauterine ultrasound examination; the diagnosis can be established by detection of *T. pallidum* DNA by PCR in amniotic fluid or of fetal antitreponemal IgM and abnormal hepatic transaminases in fetal blood.[336]

Importance of Stage and Timing of Maternal Infection. Two factors are of particular importance in determining fetal outcome: the stage of maternal infection and the time of fetal exposure to this infection. The risk to the fetus, according to the *stage of untreated maternal infection*, is depicted in Table 20-30. The later the stage of the maternal syphilitic process, the better the fetal outcome will be. This finding may relate to a protective effect of maternal immunity acquired with increasing duration of infection.[325,328] The *time of fetal exposure* to maternal infection is also important; fetal infection rarely occurs before approximately 16 to 20 weeks of gestation. This characteristic has been attributed historically to a protective effect of the Langhans cell layer of the early placenta, and infection is most likely after approximately 24 weeks, when complete atrophy of this layer is said to occur.[338-340] More recent electron microscopic studies showed persistence of the Langhans cell layer throughout pregnancy. A role for other factors (e.g., immunological) is likely.

Neuropathology

Congenital syphilis affects the CNS in most cases, although the involvement is confined to the meninges in most patients. Congenital syphilis is divided, somewhat arbitrarily, into early and late stages: those manifestations apparent in the first 2 years of life are designated early, and those apparent after 2 years are termed late. The neuropathological aspects of each stage are shown in Table 20-31.

Acute and Subacute Meningitis. The most common lesion, syphilitic meningitis, which occurs in acute or

TABLE 20-31 Neuropathology of Congenital Neurosyphilis

Early
Acute and subacute meningitis
Chronic meningovascular syphilis
    Cranial neuropathies
    Hydrocephalus
    Cerebrovascular lesions, primarily infarction

Late
Optic atrophy and auditory nerve injury
Juvenile general paresis
Juvenile tabes dorsalis

subacute form, has its onset as early as the newborn period but more often at 4 to 5 months of age.[42,341-343] It is characterized by inflammatory infiltration of the leptomeninges with mononuclear cells. These cells principally include lymphocytes, plasma cells, and macrophages. The infiltrates are often greatest in the basilar meninges, involving the sheaths of cranial nerves, and around blood vessels. Indeed, the perivascular cellular infiltrates may extend through the Virchow-Robin space into the brain parenchyma. Distinct parenchymal lesions are uncommon, although superficial layers of the cerebral cortex may be involved by the inflammatory infiltrates.

Chronic Meningovascular Syphilis. Presumably, an extension of acute-subacute meningitis, chronic meningovascular syphilis, may develop (see Table 20-31). In this disorder, the involvement of basilar meninges becomes marked and may result in two major consequences. The first includes cranial nerve abnormalities (i.e., optic atrophy and involvement of facial, oculomotor, and, probably, auditory nerves). The second consequence of the chronic arachnoiditis is hydrocephalus, usually apparent between approximately the fourth and the ninth months of life.[42,341] The vasculitis may become so severe that obliteration of vessels occurs with resulting cerebral infarction, usually between 1 and 2 years of life. Rarely, involvement of blood vessels results in aneurysm formation and cerebral hemorrhage.

Juvenile General Paresis and Tabes Dorsalis. The late CNS consequences of congenital syphilis, in addition to persistent optic atrophy and auditory nerve injury, are juvenile general paresis and tabes dorsalis. These latter two, relatively rare parenchymal lesions appear usually at approximately 10 to 15 years of age and are discussed in standard writings on pediatric neurology.[341]

Clinical Aspects

Incidence of Clinically Apparent Infection. Congenital syphilis is particularly likely to be asymptomatic, at least regarding *neurological* illness, *in the neonatal period*.[56,57,325,327,328,333,334,344,345] Depending on the mode of ascertainment, between approximately 65% to 90% of cases are totally asymptomatic in the neonatal period.[329,346,347] Premature infants are more likely to exhibit clinical phenomena (usually hepatosplenomegaly) during their stay in the nursery, because of either more severe disease or a longer period in the neonatal unit.[56,57]

Clinical Features: Early Congenital Syphilis. The clinical features of congenital syphilis, symptomatic in the first 2 years of life (i.e., early), are shown in Table 20-32.[56,57,325,326,331,345-350] The major portions of the clinical syndrome are apparent in the first months of life but usually *not until* after the first 2 weeks.[328,351,352] The most prominent features relate to the skin and the reticuloendothelial and skeletal systems. Characteristic rashes include vesiculobullous or papulosquamous

TABLE 20-32	Clinical Features of Symptomatic Early Congenital Syphilis*	
Clinical Feature	**Approximate Frequency**
Pregnancy	
Prematurity	21%–50%
Central Nervous System	
Meningitis	51%–75%
Seizures	0%–20%
Cranial nerve palsies	0%–20%
Hydrocephalus	0%–20%
Cerebrovascular accident	0%–20%
Reticuloendothelial System	
Hepatosplenomegaly	51%–75%
Hyperbilirubinemia	21%–50%
Lymphadenopathy	51%–75%
Hemolytic and other anemias	51%–75%
Skin	
Pleomorphic rashes	51%–75%
Mucocutaneous lesions	21%–50%
Bone	
Osteochondritis	76%–100%
Periostitis	51%–75%
Other	
Pneumonitis	0%–20%

*See text for references.

lesions, with a predilection for the face and the oral and anogenital regions (Fig. 20-27).[43,56,57,325,328,353] A prominent mucocutaneous lesion is associated with a mucopurulent discharge, referred to as *snuffles*. Involvement of the reticuloendothelial system is characterized particularly by hepatosplenomegaly, lymphadenopathy, and anemia. Hyperbilirubinemia and other signs of hepatic disease are common. Involvement of bone is extremely common and is characterized by diagnostic changes of the distal metaphyses (osteochondritis) with associated periosteal elevations (periostitis).[354-357] In cases with particularly early onset of clinical disease, bony changes are more common in affected premature infants than in term newborns.[356] Bone changes also have been observed in approximately 20% of clinically asymptomatic newborns.[355]

Involvement of the *CNS* is characterized by CSF pleocytosis and elevated protein content in most symptomatic cases. In the series of Platou and co-workers,[358] CSF was abnormal in 76% of 58 infants younger than 3 months of age. Among clinically asymptomatic newborns, however, the incidence of abnormal CSF findings depends on the definitions of normal values. Thus, nearly all infants identified in large series had CSF leukocyte values of 5/mm³ or higher and protein levels of 40 mg/dL or greater (the Centers for Disease Control and Prevention thresholds).[359,360] However, in a study of 67 infants born to untreated or inadequately treated seropositive women, and thereby designated as presumptive congenital syphilis by Centers for Disease Control and Prevention criteria, mean CSF values of leukocytes (7.7/mm³) and protein content (98 mg/dL) did not

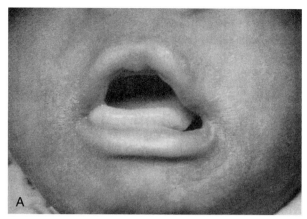

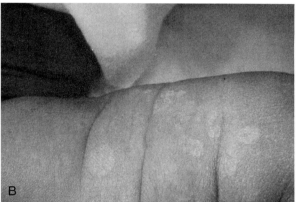

Figure 20-27   **A 6-week-old infant with congenital syphilis. A,** Note the papular scaling perioral lesions. Later radial scars, termed *rhagades*, develop at this site. **B,** Note the ovoid, annular scaly lesions. *(From Tunnessen WW: Congenital syphilis,* Am J Dis Child *146:115-116, 1992.)*

differ from values in control infants.[359] Neurological signs are *very* unusual in the first weeks of life, and, indeed, such signs are uncommon among all patients with early congenital syphilis. This is true even in the presence of abnormal CSF; in a series of 106 infants with abnormal CSF, only 6 had neurological signs.[358] However, the following are occasionally observed: seizures; cranial nerve palsies, especially of cranial nerve VII but also of nerves III, IV, and VI; hydrocephalus; signs of increased intracranial pressure (e.g., bulging anterior fontanelle); and focal neurological deficits (see Table 20-32). These phenomena are seen in association with acute and subacute syphilitic meningitis and chronic meningovascular syphilis, as described in the "Neuropathology" section.

Clinical Features: Late Congenital Syphilis. Later clinical manifestations of congenital syphilis include the following: abnormalities of the teeth, especially the upper central incisors (Hutchinson teeth) and the first lower molars (mulberry molars); interstitial keratitis; optic atrophy and visual loss; sensorineural deafness; and signs of cerebral disease (general paresis) or spinal cord disease (tabes dorsalis).[325,328,329] For the most part, these features are unusual and are discussed in standard writings of pediatric neurology.[341]

Clinical Diagnosis. The diagnosis of congenital syphilis in the neonatal period is difficult to establish on clinical grounds because of the paucity of clinical phenomena. Particularly helpful when present are vesiculobullous and papulosquamous eruptions, mucocutaneous lesions, hepatosplenomegaly, lymphadenopathy, and osteochondritis. CSF signs of inflammation further support the diagnosis.

Laboratory Evaluation

***Treponema* Identification.** Determination of *T. pallidum* as the responsible microbe in congenital syphilis depends particularly on serological techniques, although in the evaluation of any infant suspected of having the disease because of clinical phenomena or a history of a mother with a positive serological test for syphilis, search for the organisms, spirochetal antigen, or DNA should be carried out as well. Dark-field microscopic examination of specimens obtained from skin or mucocutaneous lesions, nasal discharge, placenta, umbilical cord, or amniotic fluid is an effective means for identification of the organism.[325,328,361] The most highly sensitive technique for detection of the organism is by inoculation of clinical specimens into rabbits (rabbit infectivity test), but this test is not routinely available.[328,361] The application of PCR to CSF to amplify the DNA of the organism has shown a sensitivity of 65% and a specificity of 97% in detection of CSF infection.[343] PCR testing in serum or blood was more sensitive (94%) but not as specific, with a positive predictive value of 73%. Combinations of tests are needed.

Serological Studies. Serological techniques are critical in diagnosis. Two basic types are used: nontreponemal and treponemal techniques.[325,328,329,345,362-365] In the former type, *nonspecific or reagin antigens* are used; the most widely used assay for antibody against these antigens is the Venereal Disease Research Laboratory (VDRL) test. A major disadvantage of assay of these antibodies is, as one would expect, the relative frequency of false-positive reactions.[56,57,325,328] *Specific treponemal antibody assays* largely circumvent the problem of false-positive reactions; of the tests available, the fluorescence treponemal antibody-absorbed (FTA-ABS) assay is highly specific and sensitive.[56,57,325,328] In the FTA-ABS assay, serum antibody is complexed to specific treponemal antigen and is then detected by fluorescein-labeled antihuman gamma globulin. (The term *absorbed* refers to the initial step of removing antibodies directed against treponemes other than *T. pallidum* from the serum.) This test is especially useful to identify the infected mother at delivery and thereby the infant at risk for congenital syphilis.[364] Because VDRL and FTA-ABS reactivity can be found in the IgG as well as in the IgM classes of antibody, confirmation of fetal infection necessitates the demonstration of persistence of reactivity beyond the time that passively transferred antibody would be expected.[345,366,367] However, *specific IgM treponemal antibody* is synthesized by the infected fetus and is not passively transferred. A fluorescein-labeled antihuman IgM (FTA-ABS-IgM) has been used in a procedure for detecting *specific IgM antibody against T. pallidum.*[368] This test was shown to be sensitive as an indicator of neonatal syphilitic infection.[328,329,362,363,369-371] More recent improvements in this technique have increased the sensitivity to 75% and specificity to 100%. Currently, the Centers for Disease Control and Prevention defines a *presumptive case* of congenital syphilis as either an infant whose mother had untreated or inadequately treated syphilis at delivery (regardless of findings in the infant) or an infant who has a reactive treponemal test for syphilis and any of the following: (1) evidence for congenital syphilis on physical examination or on long bone radiographs, (2) reactive CSF VDRL, (3) elevated CSF cell count or protein, (4) nontreponemal serological titers in the infant that are fourfold higher than in the mother, or (5) a reactive test for fluorescent treponemal antibody absorption-19S IgM antibody.[328,361,365]

Neurodiagnostic Studies. The most important neurodiagnostic study is examination of the CSF. The high frequency of CSF pleocytosis and elevated protein content in symptomatic disease has already been mentioned. However, these abnormal CSF findings may not be striking, and interpretation in the newborn may be difficult. Another important test is CSF VDRL reactivity; a positive test result is considered diagnostic of CNS involvement, whether or not the patient is symptomatic. However, the test is relatively insensitive (22% to 69%). More than one abnormal CSF result (pleocytosis, protein content, VDRL) has an 82% sensitivity.[343] Indeed, because of the poor sensitivity of the available diagnostic tests for neurosyphilis, the Centers for Disease Control and Prevention has recommended that all infants with systemic evidence of congenital syphilis be treated for a minimum of 10 days with crystalline penicillin G or procaine penicillin G to ensure adequate therapy to sterilize the CSF.[77,328,329]

Prognosis

The outlook in congenital syphilis depends principally on the severity of the injury that has been incurred before the onset of therapy. Unfortunately, however, the precise relationships between the *timing* and *adequacy of treatment* of early congenital syphilis and the long-term outcome are not well documented.[325,365] Nevertheless, certain conclusions are justified. Untreated infection in utero may result in abortion or stillbirth in a substantial minority of patients (see "Pathogenesis"). Infection that is symptomatic in the early neonatal period is more likely to result in sequelae than is infection that is not symptomatic until after the first months of life.[325,328] The earlier therapy is initiated, the more likely a satisfactory response will be.[345,372] Neurological sequelae are relatively uncommon but can be severe; more important, such sequelae are preventable by early therapy. Indeed, the essential issues regarding outcome in congenital syphilis are early detection and prompt therapy, and these aspects are reviewed next.

Management

Prevention. Preventive measures center on three major approaches: avoidance of maternal infection, treatment of maternal infection, and treatment of fetal infection. The first approach is an important public health issue that is not appropriate to discuss in detail here. Particular attention must be paid to young, unmarried women of minority groups, who, with no prenatal care, constitute more than 50% of mothers of infants with congenital syphilis in the United States.[328,343,365] Prompt detection is begun by assay of maternal serum for reagin antibody (e.g., VDRL) at the first prenatal visit.[2,56,57,325,328,362,364] However, such serological tests are poor tools early in the co-urse of maternal disease. More specific antibody studies also miss detection of a significant minority of infected women. Careful examination of women in labor for evidence of primary syphilis is very important. The syphilitic woman should be treated with 2.4 million units of benzathine penicillin; if this therapy is accomplished in the first 16 weeks of pregnancy, fetal infection will be avoided. Of course, this statement is made on the assumption that reinfection does not occur. After the 16th week, eradication of fetal infection is achieved in most cases with the same regimen.[373] Because of an approximately 14% failure rate in this group of pregnant women, some authorities recommend a second dose of benzathine penicillin or a 10 to 14-day course of procaine penicillin G, 600,000 units/day.[328]

Supportive Therapy. From the neurological standpoint, the neonatal syndrome rarely presents therapeutic problems. Supportive measures directed toward involvement of extraneural systems are important.

Antimicrobial Therapy. Penicillin is the drug of choice in the treatment of congenital syphilis. The major questions faced in the neonatal period are *whom to treat and how to treat.* Detection of the infant with congenital syphilis requires a high index of suspicion and a careful evaluation. Particularly important are historical data related to the mother, maternal serology at delivery, and careful clinical radiographic, metabolic, and serological studies of the infant. Because maternal antibody response may occur so late in pregnancy that the infant's VDRL test is negative, positive maternal serology should provoke careful evaluation of the infant and consideration for treatment as outlined in Table 20-33. The mode of penicillin therapy depends largely on the adequacy of treatment of the mother during pregnancy (see Table 20-33). When the mother has had no or inadequate treatment during pregnancy, the infant is treated with a full 10 to 14-day course of either crystalline or procaine penicillin G in the doses shown in Table 20-33, whether the infant is asymptomatic or symptomatic and whether infection of the infant is confirmed or not. The dose schedule described in Table 20-33 results in adequate spirocheticidal levels in CSF,[374,375] although some data indicate that crystalline penicillin G is superior to

TABLE 20-33 Treatment of Infants Born to Mothers with Syphilis

Maternal Treatment	Neonatal Clinical Findings	Penicillin G	Dose and Duration
None or inadequate	Present or absent	Crystalline	100,000–150,000 units/kg/day IV every 8–12 hr for 10–14 days (50,000 units every 12 hr for 7 days; every 8 hr after 7 days)
		Procaine	50,000 units/kg/day IM once daily for 10–14 days
Adequate	Absent	Benzathine (only if follow-up cannot be ensured and cerebrospinal fluid is normal)	500,000 units/kg IM, one dose

IM, intramuscularly; IV, intravenously.
Data from Ingall D, Norins L: Syphilis. In Remington JS, Klein JO, editors: *Infectious Diseases of the Fetus and Newborn Infant*, 2nd ed, Philadelphia: 1983, Saunders; and Ikeda MK, Jenson HB: Evaluation and treatment of congenital syphilis, *J Pediatr* 117:843-852, 1990.

procaine penicillin.[376] The importance of treating all confirmed or presumptive cases of congenital syphilis with the higher doses relates to the finding that the CNS may be infected without demonstrable abnormalities of CSF and may serve as an incubating reservoir of infection that culminates in relapse and neurosyphilis.[329]

For infants who are asymptomatic, who have normal physical examinations and laboratory evaluations, and whose mothers have been adequately treated, the risk of congenital syphilis is very low.[328,329] Treatment is not compulsory if close follow-up can be ensured.[329] However, if follow-up cannot be ensured, administration of a single dose of benzathine penicillin G is recommended (see Table 20-33). Whether follow-up can be ensured or not, the CSF should be examined, and if there is any suspicion of CNS involvement, a 10 to 14-day course of crystalline or procaine penicillin G should be administered.

OTHER VIRUSES

Human Immunodeficiency Virus

HIV infection of the fetus and newborn is a problem of enormous public health importance. Pediatric HIV infection is prevalent around the world. Regions affected most include sub-Saharan Africa, many Asian countries, India, and parts of Latin America.[2,377] The median HIV prevalence in antenatal clinics in southern African countries is 24%. In South Africa alone, of a total population of 44 million, 5.3 million have HIV infection. In 2003, 700,000 children were newly infected with HIV in developing countries.[378] In the United States, approximately 1000 new cases of pediatric AIDS, most acquired perinatally, were recorded in 2002. With the advent of measures to prevent mother-to-child transmission and the development of effective antiretroviral therapeutic programs, the yearly number of children diagnosed with AIDS in the United States has declined to approximately 100. Nevertheless, in the United States, currently approximately 950,000 people have HIV infection, and of individuals over 13 years of age with HIV-1, 29% are female. Thus, perinatal HIV infection remains an important issue in the United States and other developed countries, but the disorder is of truly extraordinary importance in developing countries.

Transmission of HIV to the fetus accounts for more than 90% of all cases of HIV infection in children in the United States, and mother-to-infant transmission is the principal means of acquisition of pediatric disease worldwide. However, neurological manifestations of HIV infection *in the newborn period* are rare. Indeed, the incidence of symptomatic neurological disease in the HIV-infected newborn is the lowest of all the major infectious disorders described in this chapter. Nevertheless, the importance of the infection for *subsequent* neurological disability and mortality requires its consideration in this chapter.

Pathogenesis

Transmission of HIV from the infected pregnant woman to her fetus is very common. Before major programs to prevent transmission, published rates varied from 10% to 40%.[248,379-410] In general, rates were lower in European and North American populations (generally 15% to 20%) than in African, Indian, or Thai populations (generally 25% to 40%). As discussed later, marked decreases in transmission rates have occurred in the last few years, especially in developed countries, with the advent of preventive measures (see later).[2,377]

Fetal and Parturitional Infection. The relative importance of transplacental and parturitional mechanisms of infection in transmission of HIV from mother to infant is not yet established conclusively, but it has been clarified considerably in recent years. Both mechanisms appear to be operative.* Concerning *transplacental infection*, although demonstration of virus by PCR is unusual in first trimester specimens, a growing body of data supports the occurrence of infection in the second and third trimester. The risk of such intrauterine transmission appears greatest with high plasma titers of HIV, and thus pregnant women with recently acquired primary HIV infection or those with advanced disease are most at risk for transmission to the fetus. Placental inflammation and disruption of the trophoblastic barrier (e.g., by infections such as

---

*See references 2,77,379,381,387-390,392,393,398-400,402,404, 405,407,411-419.

syphilis) may be additionally important. Overall, approximately 20% of vertically transmitted HIV is thought to occur before 36 weeks of gestation.

Concerning *parturitional infection*, the balance of current data suggests that this mode is the most important mechanism of vertical transmission of this virus and accounts for approximately 80% of cases. For the sake of this discussion, I include the last several weeks of pregnancy in this time period. Not uncommonly, infants born to seropositive mothers and subsequently shown to exhibit the clinical and immunological features of HIV infection are negative by PCR in the neonatal period and do not become positive until weeks later. Rather than a reflection of methodological deficiency of the PCR assay, these data suggest infection of infants very late in gestation or in the intrapartum period. The period from 36 weeks of gestation to the onset of labor is now considered particularly important, perhaps because the placenta begins to separate from the uterine wall.[419] As much as 50% of vertically transmitted HIV may occur during this period. The intrapartum period has long been considered important in transmission. The observations that first-born twins exhibit a more than twofold greater likelihood of perinatal transmission than second-born twins and that vaginally delivered first-born twins exhibit higher rates of transmission than do first-born (or second-born) twins delivered by cesarean section support the notion that acquisition of HIV during passage through the infected birth canal is important. Also consistent with parturitional acquisition is the increase in rate of vertical transmission with prolonged rupture of membranes (approximately twofold higher transmission rate in infants with membranes ruptured more than 4 hours versus infants with membranes ruptured less than 4 hours, and a rate of nearly 50% with membranes ruptured more than 24 hours). Potential mechanisms of parturitional acquisition are ingestion of maternal blood, maternal-fetal placental transfusion, or direct exposure of the fetus to infected cervical and vaginal secretions. Currently, at least 30% of vertically transmitted HIV occurs during this brief period.[419] Others consider the intrapartum period to account for more than 50% of all vertically transmitted disease.[377]

Postnatal Infection. Transmission of HIV from mother to infant by breast-feeding is an established means of infection.[2,377,381,394,406,407,418,420-430] The additional risk of infection through breast-feeding is between 10% and 25% and in general doubles the overall vertical transmission rate. HIV has been isolated from colostrum and breast milk and has been particularly associated with the macrophages contained in these secretions.[431,432] Because colostrum and early milk are particularly rich in such cells, the danger of transmission to the infant may be greatest in the early phases of breast-feeding. However, infection may also occur months later in the infant breast-fed by a mother who acquires primary infection in the postpartum period or who has established infection and transmits the infection only after many months of breast-feeding.

The data clearly have important public health implications.

Neuropathology

The neuropathology of HIV infection differs from that for the TORCH group in that the brain injury primarily occurs without conventional signs of inflammation and appears to relate in considerable part to the immune response of the host to the virus. Moreover, with few exceptions (see later discussion), the brain abnormalities are not apparent for several months or years after the neonatal period. That HIV does infect the brain is apparent from several related findings: recovery of HIV from CSF and brain,[433-435] increased levels of HIV-specific antibody in CSF (indicative of synthesis within the blood-brain barrier),[436] demonstration of HIV nucleotide sequences in brain by in situ hybridization,[434,437] localization of HIV in brain monocytes-macrophages particularly (and to a lesser extent, astrocytes by immunocytochemistry [absence of HIV in neurons, oligodendrocytes, and endothelial cells]),[438-446] identification of viral particles within multinucleated giant cells and macrophages by electronmicroscopy,[440,447,448] and demonstration of HIV-DNA by Southern blot analysis[437,440,449] or PCR.[449] The major neuropathological features of HIV infection in the infant are shown in Table 20-34.

Meningoencephalitis. The pathological manifestations of meningoencephalitis are less prominent in HIV encephalopathy than in infections of brain caused by the TORCH organisms. Thus, although (1) inflammatory cells within the meninges, (2) perivascular infiltration with inflammatory cells, and (3) areas of brain necrosis may be observed, these findings are usually not prominent. Indeed, the dominant cellular manifestations of HIV infection are abundant multinucleated giant cells (Fig. 20-28), often in syncytial formations, and macrophages.[433,438,439,441,448,450-458] The multinucleated cells appear to be derived from brain macrophages and have been shown to contain the virus. Indeed, macrophages and microglia are the predominant cell types infected by HIV.[434,444] The relative lack of the typical inflammatory characteristics of meningoencephalitis is consistent with the finding of CSF pleocytosis in living infants in only the minority of cases (see later discussion).

Cerebral Atrophy. Cerebral atrophy, secondary to loss of both neurons and myelin, is a prominent feature of

TABLE 20-34	Neuropathology in Infants with Human Immunodeficiency Virus Infection

Meningoencephalitis
Cerebral atrophy: neuronal and myelin loss, dendritic abnormalities
Cerebral calcification: basal ganglia and white matter
Calcific vasculopathy
Spinal cord myelin loss
Rare: central nervous system lymphoma, opportunistic infection, stroke

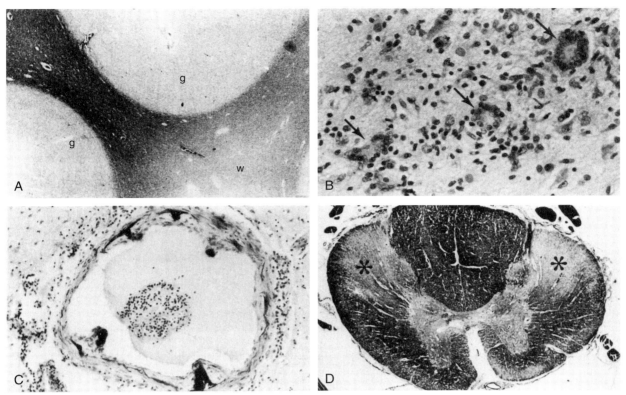

Figure 20-28   Congenital human immunodeficiency virus infection: neuropathology. A, Section of deep cerebral white matter (w) shows pallor on myelin stain; g indicates gray matter (Luxol fast blue, original magnification × 20). **B,** Section of basal ganglia shows three multinucleated giant cells *(arrows)* (hematoxylin and eosin [H & E], original magnification × 320). **C,** Large artery in basal ganglia shows multifocal intimal proliferation with dystrophic calcification (H & E, original magnification × 200). **D,** Spinal cord cross section with myelin stain shows pallor in both lateral *(asterisks)* and anterior funiculi (Luxol fast blue, original magnification × 8). *(From Belman AL, Diamond G, Dickson D, Horoupian D, et al: Pediatric acquired immunodeficiency syndrome,* Am J Dis Child *142:29-35, 1988.)*

the disease (Fig. 20-29). The result is micrencephaly, secondary to loss of both gray and white matter.[459,460] Neuronal loss particularly affects basal ganglia and cerebral cortex. The mechanism of the neuronal death is unclear. Experimental studies suggest that products of the immune system (i.e., cytokines) and of the virus may lead to cell death.[440,458,461-472] Thus, the coat protein of HIV, gp120, has been shown to be toxic to cultured neurons and to lead to cell death by causing an increase in cytosolic calcium. Moreover, the coat protein appears to sensitize neurons to glutamate-induced cell death mediated at the N-methyl-D-aspartate (NMDA) receptor. An additional HIV protein, designated Tat, also produces this effect.[472] The potentiating effect of specific HIV peptides on NMDA-mediated neuronal death has also been shown in vivo in the perinatal rat.[471-473] The crucial role of the gp120 coat protein in the genesis of the brain injury in HIV infection is supported particularly by the demonstration, in transgenic mice generated to produce gp120 in brain, of neuronal and glial changes similar to those observed in the disease.[474]

"Neurotoxins" (e.g., arachidonic acid metabolites, reactive oxygen species, glutamate, cytokines) released from infected macrophages and astrocytes also have been shown to lead to activation of the NMDA receptor.[440,458,467-470] Protection of neurons from cell death caused by the HIV coat protein or by the "toxins"

released from infected macrophages by NMDA antagonists and by a calcium channel antagonist is consistent with these observations concerning important roles for glutamate and calcium and raises interesting possibilities regarding therapy.[464,467,472,475-477]

The demonstration that inhibitors of nitric oxide synthase prevent the neurotoxicity of gp120 suggests that calcium activation of nitric oxide synthase and synthesis of nitric oxide may be the final common path to neuronal death, as described in Chapter 6 for excitotoxic cell death.[470,478,479] Thus, the sequence in HIV infection would be infection of brain macrophages (and perhaps astrocytes) by HIV, induction by gp120 of release of arachidonic metabolites, reactive oxygen species, and cytokines that act synergistically with endogenous glutamate to activate glutamate receptors, entry of calcium, nitric oxide synthesis, and cell death by free radical generation from nitric oxide.[478,479]

The cerebral cortical atrophy in HIV infection may relate also to dendritic abnormalities as well as neuronal death.[441,480,481] Such abnormalities have been delineated in adult patients and could be particularly important (and overlooked by conventional neuropathology) in infants, in view of the active dendritic development that occurs normally (see Chapter 2).

White matter loss in HIV encephalopathy can be marked (see Fig. 20-28). The myelin involvement may be diffuse or multifocal.[433,440,448,456,457,459] The

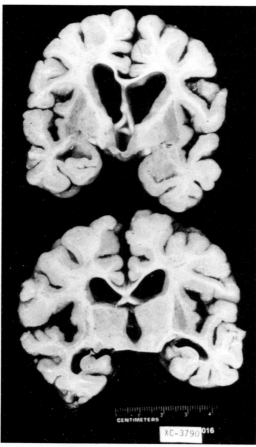

Figure 20-29 **Congenital human immunodeficiency virus infection: neuropathology.** Coronal sections of cerebrum show atrophy of both cerebral cortex and white matter. Note the marked sulcal widening and dilated ventricles. *(From Belman AL, Diamond G, Dickson D, Horoupian D, et al: Pediatric acquired immunodeficiency syndrome, Am J Dis Child 142:29-35, 1988.)*

mechanism of the myelin loss is unclear, although the finding of marked reactive astrocytosis within the areas of myelin loss suggests that the process is destructive rather than a disturbance of myelin formation. The frequent occurrence of calcification in white matter also supports a destructive rather than a developmental abnormality. The demonstration that the HIV coat protein gp120 injures developing oligodendrocytes in culture supports this formulation and links the deleterious role of the coat protein to *both* neuronal *and* oligodendroglial injury. The particular vulnerability of developing oligodendrocytes to reactive oxygen species, as delineated in Chapter 6, further links the final common pathway to cell death in both neurons and oligodendroglia in HIV infection of the brain.

Calcific Vasculopathy. A striking feature of HIV encephalopathy is calcific degeneration of blood vessels (see Fig. 20-28).[433,440,448,451,456,457] This finding is most striking in basal ganglia but is also often prominent in cerebral white matter. Involvement of blood vessels is manifested clinically later in the disease by the occurrence of hemorrhagic or ischemic stroke (see later discussion).

Spinal Cord Myelin Loss. Although relatively uncommonly examined, the spinal cord frequently exhibits myelin loss, particularly of the lateral cortical-spinal tracts.[433,438,439,451,452,456,482] Indeed, spastic motor deficits are an important component of neurological deficits observed later in some children with HIV infection (see later).[460] Approximately half of patients appear to exhibit only myelin loss, whereas the other half exhibit both myelin and axonal loss. The findings are unlike the vacuolar myelopathy of adults with HIV infection both in microscopic appearance and in topographic distribution (i.e., lateral cortical-spinal tracts rather than posterior columns as in vacuolar myelopathy).

Central Nervous System Lymphoma, Opportunistic Infections, Stroke. Only approximately 10% to 15% of cases of HIV infection of infants examined at autopsy exhibit neoplastic or infectious complications of HIV.[433,436,452,456,457,459] Nevertheless, CNS lymphoma or toxoplasmosis, CMV infection, or fungal (especially *Candida*) infection has been described. Evidence of cerebrovascular disease has been reported in up to 25% of autopsy cases[456,457,459,483,484]; lesions have included ischemic and hemorrhagic infarcts associated with arteriopathy and aneurysmal dilation of vessels.

Clinical Aspects

Incidence of Clinically Apparent Infection. The incidence of clinically recognizable neurological features in the neonatal period in HIV-infected infants is extremely small. Before the modern era of antiretroviral therapy during pregnancy and infancy, *onset of neurological disease was generally between approximately 2 months and 5 years.*[433,438,439,448,450-452,485-500] Approximately 20% of infected infants developed prominent encephalopathy by the age of 5 years, and approximately half of these occured by the age of 12 months (Fig. 20-30).[497,499] However, single case reports of infants with neonatal meningoencephalitis[501] and neonatal seizures with brain "atrophy" by cranial ultrasonography[454] have been recorded. Three of 41 infected infants in a reported series had microcephaly at birth,[502] and in large series, mean head circumference is approximately 1 cm lower in HIV-infected newborns than in appropriate control infants.[503] An HIV-infected newborn with cytomegaloviruria in the neonatal period died of fulminating cytomegalovirus encephalitis at 6 months of age.[504] A 2-month-old infant with HIV exhibited focal seizures and a hemorrhagic infarct in the distribution of the middle cerebral artery.[505]

Clinical Features. Before the era of antiretroviral therapy during pregnancy and infancy, the major *neurological syndromes* in infants with HIV disease were readily categorized as progressive encephalopathy and static encephalopathy.* The progressive encephalopathy is

---

*See references 433,438,439,448,450-452,460,488-494,496-500,502,506-519.

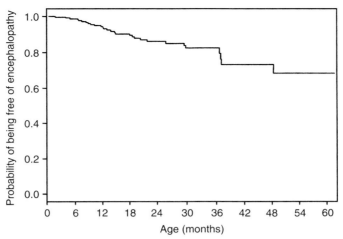

Figure 20-30 **Kaplan-Meier plot of development of encephalopathy among human immunodeficiency virus–infected infants (*n* = 128).** This study was conducted in the era before antiretroviral therapy. *(From Cooper ER, Hanson C, Diaz C, Mendez H, et al: Encephalopathy and progression of human immunodeficiency virus disease in a cohort of children with perinatally acquired human immunodeficiency virus infection, J Pediatr 132:808-812, 1998.)*

the less common but more serious of the two syndromes.

Progressive encephalopathy formerly was reported in approximately 20% of cases and developed in a rapid or subacute fashion in an infant who generally had exhibited a slowing or plateau of the rate of neurological development. In approximately 50% of affected infants, the onset was in the first year of life (see Fig. 20-30). The syndrome included a dementing process, decreasing rate of head growth, and, ultimately, microcephaly, spastic motor deficits, and, less commonly, extrapyramidal and cerebellar deficits. Seizures were uncommon and often reflected complicating illness, such as opportunistic infection or stroke. Occasionally, CNS lymphoma led to a progressive neurological syndrome.[520] Nearly all infants with the progressive encephalopathy exhibited prominent systemic features of HIV, usually apparent at the onset of the encephalopathy. The syndrome, not unexpectedly, was associated with particularly high levels of virus.[460,497,521] Median age of survival after diagnosis was 14 months, and in most infants the neurological syndrome progressed in parallel with the systemic disorder.

With the advent of the use of antiretroviral therapy during pregnancy and postnatally (see later), the progressive disorder now is rare. The incidence in most centers with such intervention has declined to less than 2%.[460,516,518,522] Moreover, in the rare instances of occurrence, the disorder presents later, is less severe, and does not progress to severe disability and death.

Before antiretroviral therapy during pregnancy and infancy, *static encephalopathy* became apparent in approximately an additional 20% to 25% of infants with HIV infection. The principal clinical characteristic is primarily cognitive impairment and motor dysfunction, usually not severe. The contribution of HIV-related factors (e.g., intrauterine drug exposure, other congenital infection, poor nutrition, systemic illness, poor environment) in the pathogenesis of the static encephalopathy is still unknown. This disorder is less

pronounced and has become less common in recent years.[460,500,522,523,523a] However, currently this syndrome is the principal neurological feature of perinatally acquired HIV infection.

Laboratory Evaluation

Virus Isolation. Identification of virus by culture or by detection of viral DNA provides definitive diagnosis of HIV infection.[2,377,379,400,407,414,524-540] Viral culture is performed on the infant's peripheral blood mononuclear cells, which are co-cultivated with peripheral blood mononuclear cells from an uninfected individual.

The PCR technique, which can be carried out on dried blood spots, detects HIV proviral DNA and is preferable to viral culture because the result is available in 1 day, as opposed to 1 to 4 weeks for viral culture.* PCR is slightly more sensitive than culture, but detection at birth is possible in only approximately 25% to 35% of infants later proved to be infected. The detection rate by PCR increases to 80% to 90% at 2 weeks, and to 90% to 95% at 3 weeks, and nearly all cases are detected by 1 month. This delay in the time of first positive result relates less to the difficulties with the PCR technique and more to the finding that approximately 75% of infections are acquired late in pregnancy and in the intrapartum period (see earlier discussion). As a consequence, the early tests are carried out at a previremic phase of the disease or when viral levels are very low.

Serological Studies. The serological diagnosis of HIV infection in the newborn is complicated by the passage of maternal IgG across the placenta and by the persistence of this IgG for as long as 15 months.[400,526,541] Determination of HIV-specific IgM in the newborn has not provided consistent diagnostic information.[377,407,538-541] After 18 months of life, detection of

---

*See references 2,377,379,400,407,414,525,526,532,536-540.

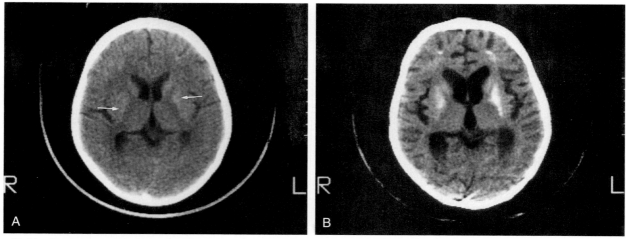

Figure 20-31 **Congenital human immunodeficiency virus infection: computed tomography (CT) scans**. **A,** CT scan shows mild cerebral atrophy and questionable bilateral calcification in basal ganglia *(arrows)* and frontal white matter (at the cortical-white matter junction). **B,** Eight months later, CT scan shows progressive cerebral cortical and white matter atrophy and pronounced basal ganglia calcification. Frontal white matter calcification is now obvious. *(From Belman AL, Diamond G, Dickson D, Horoupian D, et al: Pediatric acquired immunodeficiency syndrome, Am J Dis Child 142:29-35, 1988.)*

antibodies directed at envelope or core proteins is useful diagnostically.

Neurodiagnostic Studies. Detection of involvement of brain in the neonatal period is very difficult. CSF is usually normal.[438,439] Neuroradiological abnormalities primarily develop after the neonatal period, as may be predicted by the evolution of clinical phenomena (see earlier discussion). CT is most useful for detection of the basal ganglia and cerebral calcifications (Fig. 20-31), but MRI is superior for detection of the cerebral atrophy and white matter abnormalities.

Prognosis

The neurological syndromes just described should be viewed in the context of the overall prognosis of HIV infection of the newborn. Indeed, the overall prognosis now is recognized to be considerably more favorable than that based on earlier studies of selected populations.* *In centers where antiretroviral therapy during pregnancy and infancy is implemented, approximately 90% of infants with perinatally acquired HIV infection are alive at 6 years. From the neurological perspective, the incidence of the severe progressive encephalopathy has declined to 1% to 2%. Fewer than 25% of infants exhibit overt neurodevelopmental disturbances.* The best outlook is for infants treated with highly active antiretroviral therapy (HAART), which consists of a combination of at least a protease inhibitor, a nucleoside reverse transcriptase inhibitor, and a non-nucleoside reverse transcriptase inhibitor.[460]

Management

Prevention. Prevention of transmission of HIV infection from the pregnant woman to her fetus involves prevention of the maternal infection and management

of the infected woman. *Prevention of HIV infection* in the woman of childbearing age and detection of that infection are topics beyond the scope of this book.[2,377,544,545]

Management of the infected woman to prevent mother-to-infant transmission focuses most importantly on the use of antiretroviral therapy targeted to cover the major time periods of transmission (i.e., antenatal, intrapartum, and postnatal).[378,407,417,546-562] The initial dramatic breakthrough in this area came with the findings of a controlled study of *administration of zidovudine* initiated at 14 to 34 weeks of gestation and continued throughout pregnancy, intravenous zidovudine during labor, and oral zidovudine postpartum for 6 weeks. The result was a reduction from 26% to 8% in vertical transmission.[563] This beneficial effect was confirmed by several later reports.[407,546-548,564-569] Some reports indicated that benefit from the use of zidovudine is apparent with abbreviated perinatal regimens (Table 20-35).[409,410,567,570] Moreover, a study in

TABLE 20-35	Prevention of Mother-to-Infant Transmission of Human Immunodeficiency Virus by Zidovudine Prophylaxis*	
Time of Initiation of Zidovudine		**Rate of HIV Infection**
Prenatal		6.1%[†]
Intrapartum		10.0%[†]
≤48 hr of birth		9.3%[†]
≥3 days of age		18.4%
No zidovudine		28.6%

*n = 939.
[†]P <.05 in comparison with no zidovudine.
HIV, human immunodeficiency virus.
Data from Wade NA, Birkhead GS, Warren BL, Charbonneau TT, et al: Abbreviated regimens of zidovudine prophylaxis and perinatal transmission of the human immunodeficiency virus, *N Engl J Med* 339:1409-1414, 1998.

*See references 2,377,460,488,490,492-498,503,514,516,518,519,523a, 542,543.

TABLE 20-36	Prevention of Mother-to-Infant Transmission of Human Immunodeficiency Virus during the Era of Highly Active Antiretroviral Therapy

HAART therapy involves combinations of agents that interrupt both early and late steps in HIV replication.

Usual HAART therapy involves at least a nucleoside analogue (e.g., zidovudine, a reverse transcriptase inhibitor), a non-nucleoside analogue (e.g., nevirapine, a reverse transcriptase inhibitor), and a protease inhibitor (e.g., indinavir).

HAART therapy during pregnancy causes marked reduction in viral load at delivery.

The rate of mother-to-infant transmission is reduced to 1% to 2%.

The addition of elective cesarean section reduces transmission further to 0.5% to 1.0%.

HAART, highly active antiretroviral therapy; HIV, human immunodeficiency virus.

Data primarily from European Collaborative Study: Mother-to-child transmission of HIV infection in the era of highly active antiretroviral therapy, *Clin Infect Dis* 40:458-465, 2005.

Uganda showed that intrapartum and neonatal single-dose, oral administration of the antiretroviral agent nevirapine was nearly 50% more effective than zidovudine in prophylaxis.[570] These exciting data indicated major value for antiretroviral prophylaxis, even when begun in the intrapartum period or the first 2 days of life. Subsequent studies confirmed the benefits of shorter periods of therapy.[556,557] No adverse effects of the administration of zidovudine have been detected with follow-up as long as 5 to 6 years later.[571] The most impressive results have been observed with HAART (Table 20-36). This approach is designed to use a combination of drugs chosen to affect both early stages of HIV replication (reverse transcriptase inhibitors) and later stages (protease inhibitors). A large collaborative study in Europe indicated that this approach, which causes a remarkable reduction in maternal viral load, leads to a reduction in maternal to infant transmission to 1% to 2% (see Table 20-36).

A second approach for prevention of mother-to-infant HIV transmission is the use of *cesarean section*, before the onset of labor, to avoid many of the critical parturitional factors in viral transmission (see earlier discussion). Several studies showed a beneficial effect, with a reduction in HIV transmission of at least 50%.[378,407,417,548,562,572-575] The beneficial effect of cesarean section generally is not observed in infants who received *emergency* cesarean sections *after complicated labor*.[562,576] In one meta-analysis of 15 prospective studies, among mother-child pairs receiving full antiretroviral prophylaxis, the rates of vertical transmission were only 2.0% among mothers who underwent elective cesarean section versus 7.3% among those with other modes of delivery.[574] With the HAART approach (see Table 20-36) elective cesarean section led to reductions of transmission to 1% or less.

Because postnatal acquisition of HIV by breast-feeding is important in transmission to the infant (see earlier discussion), the U.S. Committee on Pediatric AIDS

recommended that "women who are known to be HIV infected must be counseled not to breast-feed or provide their milk for the nutrition of their own or other infants."[377,424] In many developing countries, no alternatives to breast-feeding exist. Under such circumstances, cessation of breast-feeding by approximately 6 months of age minimizes the *late* postnatal transmission that occurs with prolonged breast-feeding.[425,549] However, the complicated issue of breast-feeding in relation to HIV infection involves many competing considerations discussed in more specialized sources.[2,429]

Supportive Therapy. Because neurological phenomena are vanishingly rare in the neonatal period, supportive therapy is confined to non-neural phenomena and is discussed elsewhere.[2,377,544,577]

Antimicrobial Therapy. The possibility of specific antimicrobial therapy of the infected newborn (i.e., the infant in whom perinatal transmission was not prevented) was raised initially by the promising findings in studies of treatment of older infants and children with zidovudine.[546,578-586] Improvement of cognition, decrease of CT evidence of brain atrophy, decrease of CSF protein, improvement of auditory brain stem responses, and immunological improvement were documented. One infected infant treated from as early as 6 months of age exhibited over 6 months marked improvement in neurological examination, decrease in brain stem latencies on testing of auditory brain responses, and lessening of brain atrophy by CT.[582] Still more favorable responses have been observed with the combination therapy of the HAART approach (see earlier discussion). A striking reduction of at least 96% in plasma levels of HIV-1 RNA in infected infants 2 to 16 months of age treated with zidovudine, didanosine, and nevirapine was documented.[587] These data are important from the neurological perspective because zidovudine and nevirapine penetrate the CNS well. This property may explain the marked reduction in HIV encephalopathy in infants treated with HAART (see earlier).

Enteroviruses

Infection of the infant with one of the enteroviruses (e.g., poliovirus, coxsackieviruses A and B, and echovirus) may occur prenatally by transplacental mechanisms, during parturition from an infected mother, and postnatally by human contacts. Although poliovirus now is a rare cause of perinatal infection, nonpolio enteroviruses are relatively common causes of such infection.[588-592] Based on a 4-year study by the Centers for Disease Control and Prevention, a prevalence of 12 symptomatic cases per 100,000 infants less than 2 months of age was derived.[588] In view of the high (but not precisely quantifiable) ratio of asymptomatic to symptomatic cases of enteroviral disease, this prevalence represents a large underestimate of the actual prevalence of enteroviral infection in young infants. Infection tends to be seasonal (i.e., highest rates in late summer and early fall) and may occur in epidemic form, especially in nursery populations. The following discussion is concerned with coxsackievirus and echovirus infections; poliovirus infection is reviewed in Chapter 18.

Pathogenesis

Fetal Infection. Clinically significant infection with enterovirus may occur by transplacental, parturitional, or postnatal mechanisms. Transplacental acquisition of virus is associated with maternal viremia near the time of delivery and may cause symptoms of infection in the infant at birth.[591,593,594] No conclusive evidence exists for intrauterine infection with coxsackievirus or echovirus during the first or second trimesters of pregnancy. The recent demonstration that coxsackievirus B targets proliferating neuronal stem cells in immature mice may be relevant in this context.[595] Moreover, in a study of 28 newborns with congenital hydrocephalus or hydranencephaly, the ventricular fluid of four contained antibody to a coxsackievirus B serotype.[596] The finding is of interest because hydranencephaly and porencephaly have been identified in neonatal mice after intracranial injection of a coxsackievirus B. More data are needed.

Parturitional Infection. Although unequivocal evidence is lacking, it is probable that enteroviral infection may be acquired during parturition.[591,597] Approximately 4% of mothers excrete enterovirus in feces sampled near the time of delivery.[598] The demonstration that 63% of 61 infants with perinatal echovirus infection had onset of symptoms between the third and fifth days of life suggests that exposure to such maternal sources of virus as cervical and vaginal secretions and perineum at delivery is an important mechanism for fetal infection. (Recall that the incubation period for enteroviral infection in older children and adults is usually 5 to 8 days, with a range of 2 to 12 days.)

Postnatal Infection. Acquisition of enterovirus during the neonatal period is probably common, yet clinical illness is quite uncommon.[591,599] The main factor in postnatal spread of virus in infants, as in older patients, is human-to-human contact. Several epidemics of coxsackievirus B infection in neonatal nursery populations have been reported.[591,592,597-605] The most frequent mode of onset of such nursery infection is transmission from a mother to her infant. This contact then is followed by infant-to-infant transmission, through nursery personnel. Although most serious enteroviral nursery epidemics have involved coxsackievirus B, epidemics associated with neonatal disease have also been described for echovirus infection.[604-609]

Role of Host Factors. Although symptomatic enteroviral infections of the fetus and the newborn are less common than asymptomatic infections, it is apparent that, once established, infections are more severe in young patients than in older patients.[591,592] The precise reasons for this finding are unknown. An important role for deficient levels of antiviral antibody in vertically transmitted disease is apparent, because illness is more common in the newborn whose mother developed the illness within a week or less of delivery, before transplacental passage of sufficient antibody was possible.[604] Moreover, studies in animals suggest that a critical factor is the inability of cells of the immature animal to elaborate interferon.[610] Other possibilities suggested from experimental work include a relation to transplacentally acquired, increased concentrations of adrenocortical hormones or to a progressive, age-related loss of cells with receptors capable of allowing binding and infection by enterovirus.[611-613]

Neuropathology

Overview of Effects of Virus on the Central Nervous System. Understanding the neuropathology of enteroviral infection of the fetus and the newborn requires an awareness of the several possible effects of virus on the CNS in general. Numerous terms, particularly *meningoencephalitis*, are used in reports of perinatal enteroviral infection with little apparent regard for the precise neuropathology. In general, a virus may affect the CNS by leading to (1) acute toxic encephalopathy (e.g., Reye's syndrome), (2) meningitis, (3) primary viral encephalitis, (4) postinfectious encephalitis, or (5) acute necrotizing hemorrhagic leukoencephalitis. *Acute toxic encephalopathy* is not caused by direct infection of the CNS by virus but results from unknown metabolic mechanisms. This syndrome is characterized neuropathologically by cerebral edema and may complicate enteroviral infection later in infancy and childhood. *Meningitis* almost certainly is caused by primary viral infection of the meninges and is characterized by inflammatory infiltration of the pia-arachnoid, predominantly by mononuclear cells. This is the *most common neurological presentation for enteroviral infection in the neonatal period* as well as at later ages. *Primary viral encephalitis* is caused by primary viral infection of brain parenchyma and is characterized particularly by foci of parenchymal necrosis with glial proliferation (as with congenital or neonatal infection with CMV, rubella, HSV). This characteristic has been documented most clearly among nonpolio enteroviruses only for perinatal coxsackievirus B infection.[614-619] *Postinfectious encephalitis* is not caused by direct infection of the CNS by virus but results from immunological phenomena; it is characterized particularly by foci of perivenular demyelination. Postinfectious encephalitis has not been documented in *perinatal* enteroviral infection. *Acute necrotizing hemorrhagic leukoencephalitis* is not caused by direct infection of the CNS by virus; it can be considered analogous to severe postinfectious encephalitis with the addition of necrotizing vasculitis and is characterized particularly by demyelination, hemorrhage, edema, and necrosis. This disorder has not been reported in the perinatal period.

Perinatal Enteroviral Intracranial Infection. Of the five aforementioned disorders, viral ("aseptic") meningitis is the most common manifestation of enteroviral infection of the CNS in the perinatal period (Table 20-37).

TABLE 20-37	Neuropathology of Enteroviral Infections

Meningitis (coxsackievirus A and B, echovirus)
Meningoencephalitis (coxsackievirus B, echovirus, enterovirus)

In the large epidemiological survey of enteroviral infections in infants younger than 2 months of age reported by Morens,[588] approximately 47% of 338 cases had "aseptic meningitis" by CSF criteria. In a large series of documented neonatal coxsackievirus B infections, 48 of 77 infants had the CSF findings of meningitis.[619] Much less common is *primary viral encephalitis*, and, indeed, the best documented examples involve coxsackievirus B infections (see following section). Clinical and brain imaging data raise the possibility of a primary viral encephalitis with other enteroviruses (see later discussion).[609,620] In the series of Morens,[588] only 3% of infants with enteroviral infections were said to exhibit "encephalitis," and the criteria for this diagnosis were apparently clinical and were therefore not entirely reliable. Whether perinatal enteroviral infection may result also in acute toxic encephalopathy, postinfectious encephalitis, or acute necrotizing hemorrhagic leukoencephalopathy remains to be established. The dependence of the last two conditions on brisk immunological responses makes it unlikely that they would occur in the perinatal period.

Coxsackievirus B Meningoencephalitis. Primary viral encephalitis is an important feature of some infants with infections caused by coxsackievirus B.[591,592,614-619,621-624] The encephalitis has the three major features of a primary viral infection of brain: (1) infiltration of the meninges with inflammatory cells, predominantly mononuclear; (2) perivascular cuffing with inflammatory cells; and (3) multifocal lesions, characterized by parenchymal and primarily *neuronal* necrosis, with collections of microglia, macrophages, and, later, astrocytes. These essential features, coupled with the isolation of virus from CNS parenchyma[614,616,617,621] (and not the latter feature alone), indicate that the neuropathology is related to primary viral infection of brain.

The topography of coxsackievirus B encephalitis is moderately distinctive,[591,614-617,619,621,623] and it may explain the relative absence of cerebral signs (e.g., seizures) in affected patients (see following discussion). The brain regions most frequently and severely affected have been spinal cord (anterior horn cells), medulla (especially inferior olivary nuclei), pons, and cerebellum. The cerebrum is less regularly affected. The most consistently involved structure has been the inferior olivary nucleus. This is a helpful feature in distinguishing coxsackievirus B encephalitis from poliovirus infection, which also causes predominant involvement of spinal cord and parts of the brain stem.

Clinical Aspects

Although clinical distinctions on the basis of virological type are very difficult to make, for the sake of discussion the major nonpolio enteroviral groups are considered separately. The most prominent neurological features are observed with coxsackievirus B infections.

Coxsackievirus A. Coxsackievirus A infections appear to be the least common of the enteroviral infections of early infancy. Indeed, in the series of infants of younger than 2 months of age reported by Morens,[588] only 4% of the infections were related to coxsackievirus A. Several infants with sudden infant death syndrome were shown to harbor coxsackievirus A; Gold and coworkers[625] recovered coxsackievirus A4 from the brains of six infants with this syndrome. However, no pathological abnormalities were observed in the brain or spinal cord, even with reevaluation of the tissue sections after the results of the viral isolations were known. Thus, at present, coxsackievirus A does not appear to be associated with neurological disease in the newborn period. A 3-month-old infant with acute onset of seizures and hemiparesis and coxsackievirus A9 cultured from CSF developed a focal necrotic cerebral lesion with subsequent porencephaly.[626] Whether this occurrence represented a primary infection of brain is unclear.

Coxsackievirus B. Infection with coxsackievirus B in utero at or near the time of delivery or in the neonatal period can be associated with serious neurological disease. The most prominent clinical manifestations are myocarditis and meningitis, with or without encephalitis. Myocarditis is more common than encephalitis. Among coxsackievirus B subtypes, coxsackievirus B5 infections are particularly likely to be complicated by meningitis or encephalitis.[591]

Those infants with prominent myocarditis exhibit the clinical features depicted in Table 20-38.[591,599,600,619] Common initial features are feeding difficulties and fever. Cardiac signs (e.g., tachycardia and electrocardiographic changes of myocarditis) are common. Respiratory distress and cyanosis may be on a similar basis. CNS signs occur in only approximately one fourth of patients and are often not well defined. The course is biphasic in approximately one third of patients.

TABLE 20-38	Clinical Features of Neonatal Coxsackievirus B Myocarditis
Clinical Features	**Frequency**
Feeding difficulty	84%
Cardiac signs	81%
Respiratory distress	75%
Cyanosis	72%
Fever	70%
Pharyngitis	64%
Hepatosplenomegaly	53%
Central nervous system signs	27%
Jaundice	13%
Diarrhea	8%

Data from Cherry JD: Enterovirus and parechovirus infections. In Remington JS, Klein JO, Wilson CB, et al, editors: *Infectious Diseases of the Fetus and Newborn Infant*, 6th ed, Philadelphia: 2006, Elsevier Saunders.

TABLE 20-39	Neurological Features of Neonatal Coxsackievirus B Encephalitis
Neurological Feature	**Approximate Frequency**
Depressed level of consciousness	Common
Hypotonia	Common
Seizures	Uncommon
Focal motor deficits	Rare

The outlook for preservation of cardiac function is good, and the mortality rate is on the order of only 10%.[599,600]

Infants with prominent encephalitis are of interest for two reasons. First, at least in the isolated fatal cases reported, a predominance of infection in the mothers occurs either just before or at the time of labor.[614-616,618,619,623] This finding suggests the possibility that infection acquired in utero during maternal viremia results in particularly severe disease, perhaps the result of diffuse dissemination of a large inoculum of virus. Second, a paucity of neurological phenomena is referable to the cerebrum (Table 20-39). In the 12 infants studied in a nursery epidemic by Eilard and co-workers,[603] seizures were noted in a single patient with heart failure (a finding suggesting a possible relation of seizures to cerebral ischemia), and the remaining infants exhibited principally a depressed level of consciousness or hypotonia, or both. Similar phenomena have been observed in fatal cases.[614-618,623] Whether the depressed level of consciousness relates to involvement of brain stem reticular formation and whether the hypotonia relates to anterior horn cell involvement are intriguing possibilities (see "Neuropathology"), but they remain to be established. The relative paucity of cerebral phenomena (e.g., seizures and focal motor deficits) presumably is associated with the scarcity of cerebral neuropathological changes.

Echovirus. Infection with the many types of echovirus is relatively common in the neonatal period. In the study of Morens,[588] 51% of infants less than 2 months of age infected with enterovirus exhibited echovirus infection. The clinical syndromes are legion and include asymptomatic infection, febrile illness without specific symptoms, gastroenteritis, pneumonia, hepatic disease, and meningitis.[591] In a review of 61 cases of neonatal echovirus infection, hepatitis was the dominant clinical feature in 67%.[604] In the same series, 26% exhibited clinical evidence of "meningitis or meningoencephalitis."[604] One half of these "neurological" cases had infection with echovirus 11.

Several reports have led to the suggestion that primary viral encephalitis may occur with perinatal echovirus or other noncoxsackievirus enteroviral infection.[604,609,620,627-635] The best-documented cases are noteworthy because cerebral white matter necrosis was the prominent feature. Thus, one full-term infant in whom echovirus (not typed) was cultured from CSF exhibited evidence by MRI of focal cerebral white necrosis (Fig. 20-32).[620] No CSF pleocytosis was observed. However, the asymmetry of the necrosis, the gestational age of the infant, and the lack of overt ischemic insult suggested that the lesion did not represent periventricular leukomalacia and could be secondary to primary infection of brain by echovirus. A recent report described five infants with prominent neurological features, including seizures, onset a few days to weeks after birth, a family history of recent enteroviral type infection, occurrence during the summer, presence of a rash in four infants, positive enteroviral cultures from CSF in four infants, CSF pleocytosis in three infants, and abnormal signal in cerebral white matter in all five infants, with cysts in three (Fig. 20-33).[609] Although no pathological material was available, the findings suggest a true encephalitis with a predilection for white matter. Two of the five infants had spastic motor deficits on follow-up. Further data will be of considerable interest.

Clinical Diagnosis. The clinical features of enteroviral infection are so diverse that it is difficult to define distinctive features. Indeed, this finding should raise the possibility of such infection in *any patient* with a CSF pleocytosis and elevated protein content indicative of

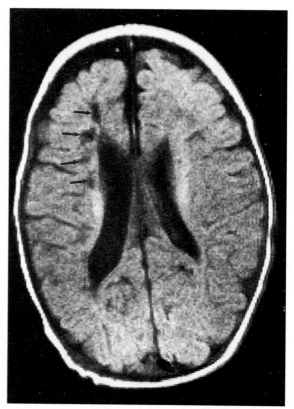

Figure 20-32 **Possible neonatal echovirus encephalitis: magnetic resonance imaging scan.** This scan was performed at 1 month of age in a previously healthy term infant who had onset of a febrile illness at 5 days of age, subsequent focal seizures, and two cerebrospinal fluid cultures positive for echovirus (not typed). The child recovered by 25 days of age. Note the focal areas of white matter necrosis *(arrows)*. *(From Haddad J, Messer J, Gut JP, Chaigne D, et al: Neonatal echovirus encephalitis with white matter necrosis, Neuropediatrics 21:215-217, 1990.)*

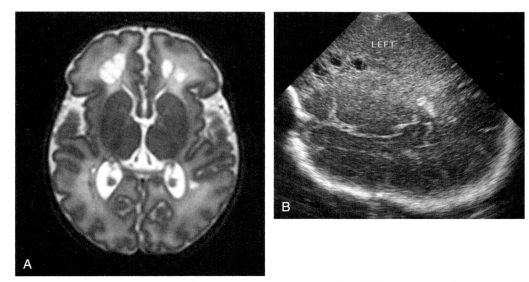

Figure 20-33 Neonatal enteroviral meningoencephalitis: magnetic resonance imaging (MRI) scan. Axial T2-weighted MRI scan (**A**) 3 weeks after the onset of enteroviral infection shows large cystic lesions in the frontal white matter (detectable by ultrasound scan [**B**]) and smaller lesions in the parieto-occipital periventricular region. *(From Verboon-Maciolek MA, Groenendaal F, Cowan F, Govaert P, et al: White matter damage in neonatal enterovirus meningoencephalitis, Neurology 66:1267-1269, 2006.)*

aseptic meningitis. The most prominent systemic signs in one series of newborns with enteroviral infection were fever (93%) and diarrhea (81%).[636] Certainly, the presence of signs of myocarditis and encephalitis in a newborn should suggest coxsackievirus B infection. Time of year is helpful because enteroviral infections are particularly prevalent in summer and fall in temperate climates. In the series of Morens[588] of infants younger than 2 months of age, a striking peak of prevalence was observed in August, with most infections occurring between June and October. Knowledge of exposures and incubation periods is particularly helpful, and careful history of maternal illness, however slight, or illness in nursery personnel is critical to elicit and to document. In a large review of reported cases of fatal neonatal coxsackievirus B infection, 60% of mothers had signs of a viral-like infection between 10 antepartum and 5 postpartum days.[619]

Laboratory Evaluation

Virus Isolation. The most critical laboratory aid in diagnosis is isolation of the virus or detection of enteroviral RNA by PCR. Because disease in newborns tends to be generalized, collection of material from multiple sites is indicated, particularly from the throat, stool, blood, urine, and CSF.[591] Tissue culture evidence of enteroviral infection is documented readily by most clinical laboratories and is apparent usually within a few days, in most cases, in less than a week.[591,637] The detection of enteroviral RNA by PCR in CSF from patients with enteroviral meningitis is an important diagnostic approach.[591,592,638] It has been recommended that "the general workup for febrile neonates hospitalized for possible sepsis should include PCR for enterovirus in blood and CSF."[591] I would add a similar recommendation for the general workup of neonatal seizures of unknown cause.

Serological Studies. Serological techniques are usually not of major value in the primary diagnosis of neonatal enteroviral disease. The disorder is acquired near or shortly after the time of birth, and a rise in antibody titer over 2 to 4 weeks is needed to demonstrate infection.

Neurodiagnostic Studies. Neurodiagnostic studies should center on the analysis of the CSF. Identification of the CSF formula for meningitis with or without encephalitis and attempts to isolate the virus or genetic material from CSF are important. EEG may be useful in suggesting cerebral involvement.[639] CT or MRI is effective for evaluation of parenchymal disease.

Prognosis

In general, the prognosis with neonatal coxsackievirus and echovirus infections is relatively good. Exceptions are the severe cases of coxsackievirus B myocarditis and encephalitis, which constitute a very small proportion of the total group of affected cases. The possibility of neurological or cognitive deficits after enteroviral infection in early infancy has been raised in several relatively *small* studies.[591,599] One report, often cited as evidence for an unfavorable outcome, does not clearly relate to neonatal infection.[640] Thus, a group of 13 infants with onset of enteroviral disease at ages "less than 1 year" and "evidence of CNS involvement" were shown at follow-up to have a lower mean IQ score than a control group (97 versus 115); only 58% were said to be free of detectable neurological abnormality. However, in this series, the youngest affected infant was 1 month of age, and no data are presented to determine whether the infants experienced neurological sequelae as a consequence of complicating disturbances (e.g., ventilation and perfusion) or to determine what constituted the likely neuropathological diagnosis. These data do not appear to be applicable to the newborn with enteroviral infection. A later study of 45 children in whom enteroviral "meningitis" developed between the ages of 4 days and 12 months found no evidence of impairments of neurological or cognitive function on follow-up.[641] In a group of 15 children who had neonatal meningoencephalitis secondary to coxsackievirus B infection, only 2 had neurological deficits (spasticity, cognitive deficits) at follow-up at the age of 6 years.[642] In the recent series of 5 infants described earlier with apparent neonatal enteroviral white matter necrosis and encephalitis, 2 exhibited "cerebral palsy" subsequently.[609]

Management

Prevention. Two major approaches to prevention can be recommended. First, maternal infection should be sought with a high index of suspicion, and if infection is present, delivery should not be encouraged. Cesarean section may increase the risk of severe disease by decreasing the time for maternal synthesis and transplacental transfer of protective IgG antibody.[604] Second, nursery procedures should be strict regarding enteroviral infection. For example, infants with suspected disease should be isolated. Nursery personnel who may be infected should be detected and should not be allowed contact with patients. If illness is demonstrated, the nursery is probably best closed to new admissions.[600]

Supportive Care. The considerations outlined for other congenital infections are appropriate regarding seizures, but seizures are uncommon, even in overt coxsackievirus B encephalitis.

Antimicrobial Therapy. No antiviral therapy is known at the present time for perinatal enteroviral infections.

Varicella

Varicella infection of the infant occurs in utero by transplacental mechanisms. Postnatal acquisition of the virus may occur in the newborn period, but this is rare and is not of neurological importance. Two syndromes related to intrauterine acquisition of varicella should be distinguished: *congenital varicella syndrome*, caused by maternal-fetal infection primarily in the first 20 weeks of pregnancy; and *perinatal varicella*, caused by maternal-fetal infection within approximately 21 days of delivery (the upper range of the duration of the incubation period for varicella). Both disorders are rare but are important to recognize, in part because appropriate intervention may attenuate or prevent serious disease in the infant (see later discussion).

Perinatal Varicella

Perinatal varicella in this context refers to infection of the fetus acquired near the time of delivery and clinically apparent within the first 10 postnatal days. This disorder is rare, principally because varicella infection is rare during pregnancy (most women have natural immunity

because of childhood infection). The incidence of varicella during pregnancy is 0.7 per 1000 pregnancies.[9,77,643,644] In the United States, this incidence should decline as women who received the vaccine as infants begin to reach childbearing age. Approximately 25% of infants born to mothers with varicella during the last 21 days of pregnancy develop the disease.[77,278,645-652]

Pathogenesis. The virus is acquired in utero by *transplacental passage* as a consequence of maternal viremia.[278,652] The incubation period, defined as the interval between the onset of the rash in the mother and onset in the newborn (or fetus), is usually 9 to 15 days.[653] The reason for this slightly shorter than usual incubation period is not clearly understood.

Maternal antibody transferred to the fetus has the capacity to modify the disease.[278,652] As discussed subsequently, those infants with early onset of disease (during the first 4 days of life) have milder disease than those with later onset (from 5 to 10 days of life). In later-onset cases, antibody titers at birth are considerable in the mother and are either absent or much lower in the infant, whereas in early-onset cases, antibody titers in maternal and cord blood are similar.[654] These data suggest that several days are needed before maternal IgG antibodies against varicella virus cross the placenta and equilibrate with the fetal circulation. This evidence of a protective effect of maternal antibody has implications for the management of the pregnant woman with varicella near the time of delivery (see later discussion).

Neuropathology. The pathological changes in the most severe (i.e., fatal) cases of perinatal varicella include inflammation and necrosis in the lungs, liver, adrenal glands, gastrointestinal tract, kidney, and spleen.[2,278,592,652] The predilection for liver and adrenals is reminiscent of neonatal infection with another virus of the herpes group, HSV. Of five brains examined, only one was said to show areas of necrosis; the necrotic areas were associated with dissolution of all tissue elements and with calcification.[655] The lesions were said to be similar to those of toxoplasmosis, but no *Toxoplasma* organisms were seen. No serological studies were available, and the possibility of a dual infection was not excluded. Thus, it remains unclear whether a primary viral encephalitis occurs with perinatal varicella; even if so, such an occurrence is exceedingly rare.

Clinical Aspects. Perinatal varicella is characterized by a vesicular rash that may be hemorrhagic in severe cases. The spectrum of severity varies from a few vesicles to a nearly confluent eruption. The severity of disease relates particularly to the time of onset of the maternal illness in relation to delivery (Table 20-40).[2,9,645-648,651,652,656,657] Early-onset neonatal disease is benign, whereas later-onset disease is associated with a significant mortality (i.e., ≈30%). The latter statistic relates to the severe systemic manifestations.

TABLE 20-40	Perinatal Varicella: Relation to Maternal Infection and Outcome*			
Onset of Maternal Rash	Onset of Neonatal Disease	No. of Neonatal Cases	Mortality	
≥5 days before delivery	0–4 days	27	0%	
≤4 days before delivery	5–10 days	23	30%	

*See text for references.

The *diagnosis* is usually readily apparent in the presence of a vesicular rash and the maternal history. If the latter is unavailable, confusion with HSV is possible, and the distinction is important. In HSV infection, vesicles tend to occur in clusters, rather than in the more even distribution of varicella infection.

Laboratory Evaluation. The laboratory procedures of most value initially are *culture of the virus from the lesion, detection of viral antigen by immunofluorescence, or viral DNA by PCR.* Serological studies also provide diagnostic information; varicella-specific IgM antibodies usually are detectable early in the disease but disappear shortly after birth.

Prognosis. The difference in prognosis as a function of the time of maternal illness has been outlined (see Table 20-40).

Management. Modification of the neonatal disease can be accomplished by *passive immunization* with varicella-zoster immune globulin (Table 20-41).[2,9,278,592,651,652,656,658-660] Passive immunization, however, does not decrease the clinical attack rate.[77,278,279,651,660] When the onset of maternal varicella is less than 5 days before delivery, a considerable risk exists that (1) varicella was acquired by the fetus too near the time of delivery for significant passive transfer of maternal antibody, and (2) serious neonatal disease, with a 30% fatality rate, will result. Thus, for the infant delivered less than 5 days after onset of maternal varicella (some investigators suggest <7 days),[660] varicella-zoster immune globulin (1.25 mL) should be administered intramuscularly

TABLE 20-41	Management of the Newborn Exposed to Varicella In Utero*
Time of Maternal Infection	Newborn Management
6–20 days before delivery	Isolation from mother until no longer clinically infectious
<5 days before delivery	Varicella-zoster immune globulin and isolation from mother†
<2 days after delivery	Varicella-zoster immune globulin and isolation from mother†

*See text for references.
†Acyclovir should be considered if varicella develops in the infant (see text).

(see Table 20-41). Similarly, if the mother contracts varicella within the first few days (2 days is the period recommended by the Centers for Disease Control and Prevention) after delivery, the infant is at risk for having acquired varicella transplacentally in utero before significant passive transfer of maternal antibody. Such an infant should receive varicella-zoster immune globulin and should be isolated from the mother. Finally, if the infant acquires the disease and the manifestations appear to be becoming severe, a course of intravenous acyclovir should be instituted.[592,652]

Congenital Varicella Syndrome

Congenital varicella syndrome is a rare constellation of stigmata caused by intrauterine infection with varicella virus acquired during the first, second, or, perhaps, early third trimesters. Individual case reports have established that a distinctive clinical constellation is associated, albeit rarely, with varicella infection, usually in the first 20 weeks.[9,77,278,650-652,656,661-675] The risk of congenital varicella in most studies is approximately 2% (range, 1% to 2%).[2,651,652,656,676-679] In a prospective study of 1373 women, the risk of congenital varicella was 0.4% with maternal disease from 0 to 12 weeks of pregnancy and 2% with maternal disease from 13 to 20 weeks.[677] The risk is minimal with maternal infection after 20 weeks.

Pathogenesis. The pathogenesis of the congenital varicella syndrome is presumed to be fetal infection acquired by transplacental passage of virus in association with maternal viremia. Detection of the virus in amniotic fluid and in fetal blood has been accomplished by PCR.[678,679] The similarity of some of the neuropathology to later infection by herpes zoster (see later discussion) and the occurrence of disseminated disease with zoster in immunocompromised individuals are of interest, because before 18 to 20 weeks of pregnancy, the fetus exhibits many features of a deficient immune response. Unlike infection with CMV, the fetal infection is not chronic, and, indeed, isolation of the virus after birth has not been accomplished. The nature of the lesions indicates that inflammation and destruction of tissue underlie most of the major defects observed.

Neuropathology. The neuropathology was well described in an infant who died at 6½ months of age.[666] The major features included meningoencephalitis, myelitis, dorsal root ganglionitis, and denervation (and hypoplasia) of muscle in a *segmental* distribution (Table 20-42). *Primary viral encephalitis* was suggested by a necrotizing parenchymal process with inflammatory

TABLE 20-42	Neuropathology of Congenital Varicella Syndrome

Meningoencephalitis
Myelitis, especially affecting anterior horn cells
Dorsal root ganglionitis
Denervation atrophy (and hypoplasia) of muscle in segmental distribution

cells in the meninges and throughout the brain. Indeed, the cerebral hemispheres were said to be "replaced by an extensive fluid-filled cyst enclosed by a semilucent yellowish membrane of varying thickness."[666] Evidence of a focal destructive ependymitis in the floor of the fourth ventricle was particularly obvious. Less severe degrees of parenchymal necrosis with perivascular cuffing with inflammatory cells have been described.[672,674] *Dorsal root ganglia* in the lumbar region, as well as lumbar *spinal cord* and, particularly, the anterior horn cells, exhibited inflammatory and necrotic changes. In association with the predominant involvement of anterior horn cells of the left lumbar segments was *marked deficiency of muscle* in the atrophic left lower extremity, the muscular lesion corresponding to the segmental regions particularly affected in the spinal cord. The neuropathological data indicated a severe, inflammatory, destructive process affecting all levels of the CNS, including anterior horn cells and their associated sites of innervation, as well as the dorsal root ganglia of the peripheral nervous system. The involvement of dorsal root ganglia is particularly interesting in view of the tendency for varicella-zoster virus to remain latent at that site and to become reactivated as herpes zoster infection in adult life. Indeed, herpes zoster cutaneous lesions have been observed postnatally at 2 weeks,[680] 3 months,[673] and at 17 months[681] of age after intrauterine exposure to varicella.

Although neuropathological information is not available for other cases of congenital varicella, ultrasound or CT scans in several other infants have revealed such findings as microcephaly, dilated lateral ventricles, and cerebral calcifications, indicative of a destructive process.[661-663,670,672,674,676,682,683] Active inflammation at the time of birth is not common, as evidenced by several patients with normal CSF analysis.[665,666,668] These data further support the notion that

TABLE 20-43	Clinical Features of Congenital Varicella Syndrome*	
Clinical Feature	**Approximate Frequency**
Maternal infection	
8–12 wk	51%–75%
13–20 wk	26%–50%
>20 wk	0%–25%
Small for dates or prematurity or both	51%–75%
Cutaneous scars (dermatome distribution)	76%–100%
Ocular abnormality	76%–100%
Limb abnormality	51%–75%
Hypoplastic muscle	51%–75%
Deformity	51%–75%
Bulbar signs	26%–50%
Muscle weakness	26%–50%
Microcephaly	26%–50%
Seizures (survivors)	26%–50%
Retarded neurological development (survivors)	51%–75%
Death in infancy	26%–50%

*See text for references.

congenital varicella syndrome is related to a discrete, acute attack by varicella in utero and is not associated with the type of chronic infection observed with such congenital infections as rubella, CMV, and syphilis.

Clinical Aspects. The clinical presentation is dramatic and distinctive (Table 20-43). In the majority of cases, the mothers of the affected infants had varicella between 8 and 20 weeks of gestation. In a few cases, first or second trimester zoster infection was responsible.[2,9] The mother of the least severely affected infant had varicella in the 28th week of pregnancy.[667] Cutaneous scars, characteristically depressed, are nearly invariable (Fig. 20-34). The lesions occur in a *segmental* distribution and often exhibit the zigzag

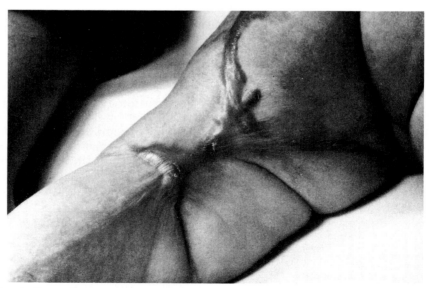

Figure 20-34 Congenital varicella syndrome: cutaneous scar in an infant whose mother had varicella-zoster infection in the 12th week of pregnancy. Note the severe scar over the posterior aspect of the lower extremity in the distribution of the first sacral segment. The limb was also hypoplastic. *(From Hanshaw JB, Dudgeon JA: Viral Disease of the Fetus and Newborn, Philadelphia: 1973, Saunders.)*

appearance observed in herpes zoster infections in adults. The limb abnormalities consist of atrophy or hypoplasia of muscle, associated usually with a limb deformity (e.g., talipes equinovarus, hypoplastic limb). Rarely, patients exhibit hypoplastic of the face, neck, or abdomen, and not the limbs.

Neurological features have been prominent in nearly every case. Bulbar signs, especially serious difficulty in swallowing, have occurred in many patients, thus bringing to mind the neuropathological observation of particular destruction in the floor of the fourth ventricle (see previous discussion). Muscle weakness is associated with the segmental hypoplasia or atrophy of muscle and presumably is related to anterior horn cell involvement. Sensation was diminished to pinprick in the one case in which this aspect of the neurological examination is mentioned specifically; in view of the involvement of dorsal root ganglia, it is reasonable to suspect that this was present but not elicited in other cases. Cerebral involvement is reflected by the frequent occurrence of microcephaly, seizures, and retarded neurological development (see Table 20-43).

Ocular abnormalities have been present in nearly every case and consist most commonly of chorioretinitis, but also microphthalmia, cataracts, optic atrophy, anisocoria, or Horner syndrome.[2,9,278,279,652,665,679,683] The presence of Horner syndrome suggests involvement of cervical sympathetic ganglion or cells of the intermediate column of the spinal cord.

The clinical constellation is distinctive enough to suggest the *diagnosis*. The maternal history of varicella confirms the impression.

Laboratory Evaluation. No consistent means of establishing the virological diagnosis in the newborn has been identified. In rare cases, viral particles and multinucleated giant cells obtained from vesicular fluid were compatible with varicella[664,679]; however, the virus was not isolated. Other attempts to isolate virus from CSF, eye, and other tissues have not been successful.[9,278,644,650,662,664,666] However, detection of viral DNA in CSF by PCR has been reported in the newborn.[652,674] As noted earlier, viral DNA has been detected in amniotic fluid and fetal blood by PCR.[678,679] Detection of varicella-specific IgM in cord blood obtained in utero by cordocentesis also has been reported.[672]

Serological studies, albeit usually not extensive, have been compatible with fetal infection in approximately 75% of cases.[9,278,644,650] In most instances, this conclusion is based on the persistence of varicella-zoster antibody, measured by complement fixation, beyond the age at which maternal antibody should be expected to have disappeared. A cell-mediated immune response to varicella-zoster virus was detected in two infants.[9] Varicella-specific IgM also has been identified in approximately one half of infants studied.[652]

Prognosis. The unfavorable outlook regarding mortality, retardation of neurological development, occurrence of seizures, and other neurological signs is reviewed in Table 20-43. Nevertheless, approximately 20% of reported patients develop normally in the first year

of life.[650,668] A 27-year-old woman with congenital varicella was normal except for a motor deficit related to limb hypoplasia.[671]

Management. *Prevention* of this disorder is difficult. However, the low risk of transmission of infection to the fetus must be considered when counseling the parents. Thus, the risk for symptomatic intrauterine varicella-zoster infection after maternal varicella in the first 20 weeks of gestation is only approximately 2% (see earlier discussion). Intrauterine diagnosis appears to be possible early in pregnancy. Varicella-zoster–specific IgM has been detected in fetal blood, and virus has been identified by PCR in amniotic fluid, chorionic villus samples, and fetal blood.[2,652,672,678,679] Varicella-zoster immune globulin administered to the susceptible mother after exposure to varicella prevents or modifies her disease, but it is not definitely known whether this therapy decreases the risk of transmission to the fetus.[2,652,679] A similar conclusion applies to treatment of the maternal disease with acyclovir.

Supportive management for the affected infant should include control of seizures. A particular problem is maintenance of adequate nutrition in those infants who have difficulty swallowing. Tube feedings have been required in early infancy. Appropriate training for infants with serious visual impairment secondary to ocular abnormality has been accompanied by normal development.[668]

Lymphocytic Choriomeningitis

Lymphocytic choriomeningitis virus has been associated in approximately 50 cases with intrauterine infection and the development of chorioretinitis, hydrocephalus, and cerebral calcifications.[2,684-690b] Infection in the mother generally has occurred in the first and second trimesters of pregnancy. Acquisition of virus by the mother has been shown or assumed to be related to exposure to domestic or other rodents, which commonly harbor the virus.[239,690a] The clinical features in most of the neonatal cases have included microcephaly (70%) and chorioretinitis (100%).[690a] Gyral abnormalities occur in 45% and periventricular calcifications in 80%. Subsequently, visual impairment, motor deficits, seizures, and mental retardation occur in most infants.[690a] The disorder likely is much more common than previously expected. Thus, in a review of 14 infants identified with chorioretinitis over a 3-year period at a major children's hospital, 3 infants had elevated antibody titers to lymphocytic choriomeningitis but not to CMV, *Toxoplasma*, rubella, or HSV.[689] Moreover, 2 of 4 children with chorioretinitis or chorioretinal scars at a home for the severely mentally retarded had similar findings. The diagnosis has been made serologically by determination of lymphocytic choriomeningitis virus antibody levels by immunofluorescent or ELISA determinations. PCR techniques may be useful in the future. Management consists of attempts at prevention by counseling pregnant women to avoid contact with pets, laboratory and household mice, and hamsters, as well as avoidance of aerosolized excreta.

Adenovirus

The possibility that adenovirus should be added to the short list of viruses that can infect the neonatal brain was raised by the report of a fatal neonatal case of encephalitis from which adenovirus type 11 was cultured from brain tissue.[691] The neuropathological examination showed frequent perivascular cuffing with inflammatory cells; brain edema and reactive astrocytosis also were noted.[691] Among at least 14 previous cases of fatal adenoviral illness characterized primarily by pneumonia, depressed level of consciousness has been common, and seizures were noted in 3 of these patients. However, no previous examples of neuropathology consistent with encephalitis (see earlier discussion) or isolation of virus or viral antigen from brain had been reported. More data will be of interest.

West Nile Virus

West Nile virus, first isolated from a febrile woman in the West Nile province of Uganda in 1937, was recognized in a cluster of cases of encephalitis in New York in 1999. It is now apparent that this virus can be transmitted from mother to fetus and can cause fetal disease. The virus has spread throughout North America.[692] Five cases of maternal-fetal transmission have been documented with maternal infections from 16 to 28 weeks of gestation. One infant exhibited chorioretinitis and cerebral parenchymal destruction.[692] Diagnosis in the mother can be made by PCR or serology. The affected infant exhibited West Nile virus–specific IgM and viral nucleic acid by PCR in placenta and umbilical cord tissue. With the dramatic increase in numbers of cases of West Nile viral disease (4000 cases reported to the Centers for Disease Control in the United States in 2002), this disorder could evolve as an important cause of fetal infection. The demonstration that the virus also can be transmitted by breast-feeding further supports an enhanced suspicion of West Nile infection in early infancy.[692]

REFERENCES

1. Remington JS, Klein JO, Wilson CB, Baker CJ: *Infectious Diseases of the Fetus and Newborn Infant*, 6th ed, Philadelphia: 2006, Elsevier Saunders.
2. Freij BJ, Sever JL: Viral and protozoal infections. In MacDonald MG, Mullett MD, Seshia MM, editors: *Avery's Neonatology, Pathophysiology, and Management of the Newborn*, 6th ed, Philadelphia: 2005, Lippincott Williams & Wilkins.
3. Thompson JA, Glasgow LA: Intrauterine viral infection and the cell-mediated immune response, *Neurology* 30:212-215 1980.
4. Yow MD: Congenital cytomegalovirus disease: A NOW problem, *J Infect Dis* 159:163-167 1989.
5. Yow MD, Demmler GJ: Congenital cytomegalovirus disease: 20 years is long enough [editorial], *N Engl J Med* 326:702-703 1992.
6. Murph JR, Souza IE, Dawson JD, Benson P, et al: Epidemiology of congenital cytomegalovirus infection: Maternal risk factors and molecular analysis of cytomegalovirus strains, *Am J Epidemiol* 147:940-947, 1998.
7. Stagno S, Britt WJ: Cytomegalovirus infections. In Remington JS, Klein JO, Wilson CB, et al, editors: *Infectious Diseases of the Fetus and Newborn Infant*, 6th ed, Philadelphia: 2006, Elsevier Saunders.
8. Tookey PA, Ades AE, Peckham CS: Cytomegalovirus prevalence in pregnant women: The influence of parity, *Arch Dis Child* 67:779-783, 1992.
9. Hanshaw JB, Dudgeon JA, Marshall WC: *Viral Diseases of the Fetus and Newborn*, Philadelphia: 1985, Saunders.
10. Ahlfors K, Ivarsson SA, Johnsson T, Svensson I: Congenital and acquired cytomegalovirus infections, *Acta Paediatr Scand* 67:321-328, 1978.
11. Ballard RA, Drew WL, Hufnagle KG, Riedel PA: Acquired cytomegalovirus infection in preterm infants, *Am J Dis Child* 133:482-485, 1979.
12. Spector SA, Schmidt K, Ticknor W, Grossman M: Cytomegaloviruria in older infants in intensive care nurseries, *J Pediatr* 95:444-446, 1979.
13. Paryani SG, Yeager AS, Hosford-Dunn H, Johnson SJ, et al: Sequelae of acquired cytomegalovirus infection in premature and sick term infants, *J Pediatr* 107:451-456, 1985.
14. Zaia JA, Lang DJ: Cytomegalovirus infection of the fetus and neonate, *Neurol Clin* 2:387-410, 1984.
15. Griffin MP, O'Shea M, Brazy JE, Koepke J, et al: Cytomegalovirus infection in a neonatal intensive care unit, *Am J Dis Child* 142:1188-1193, 1988.
16. Gentile MA, Boll TJ, Stagno S, Pass RF: Intellectual ability of children after perinatal cytomegalovirus infection, *Dev Med Child Neurol* 31:782-786, 1989.
17. Stagno S, Pass RF, Dworsky ME, Alford CA: Congenital and perinatal cytomegalovirus infections, *Semin Perinatol* 7:31-42, 1983.
18. Bale JF: Human cytomegalovirus infection and disorders of the nervous system, *Arch Neurol* 41:310-320, 1984.
19. Boppana SB, Fowler KB, Britt WJ, Stagno S, et al: Symptomatic congenital cytomegalovirus infection in infants born to mothers with preexisting immunity to cytomegalovirus, *Pediatrics* 104:55-60, 1999.
20. Stagno S, Pass RF, Britt WJ, Alford CA: Consequences of primary maternal CMV infection (P-CMV), *Pediatr Res* 19:305A, 1985.
21. Britt WJ, Vugler LG: Antiviral antibody responses in mothers and their newborn infants with clinical and subclinical congenital cytomegalovirus infections, *J Infect Dis* 161:214-219, 1990.
22. Steinlin MI, Nadal D, Eich GF, Martin E, et al: Late intrauterine cytomegalovirus infection: Clinical and neuroimaging findings, *Pediatr Neurol* 15:249-253, 1996.
23. Barkovich AJ, Lindan CE: Congenital cytomegalovirus infection of the brain: Imaging analysis and embryologic considerations, *AJNR Am J Neuroradiol* 15:703-715, 1994.
24. Barkovich AJ: *Pediatric Neuroimaging*, 4th ed, Philadelphia: 2005, Lippincott Williams & Wilkins.
25. Haymaker W, Girdany BR, Stephens J, Lillie RD, et al: Cerebral involvement with advanced periventricular calcification in generalized cytomegalic inclusion disease in the newborn, *J Neuropathol Exp Neurol* 13:562-586, 1954.
26. Monif GR, Egan EA 2nd, Held B, Eitzman DV: The correlation of maternal cytomegalovirus infection during varying stages in gestation with neonatal involvement, *J Pediatr* 80:17-20, 1972.
27. MacDonald H, Tobin HO: Congenital cytomegalovirus infection: A collaborative study on epidemiological, clinical and laboratory findings, *Dev Med Child Neurol* 20:471-480, 1978.
28. Starr JG, Bart RD, Gold E: Inapparent congenital cytomegalovirus infection: Clinical and epidemiologic characteristics in early infancy, *N Engl J Med* 282:1075-1078, 1970.
29. Hanshaw JB: Congenital cytomegalovirus infection: A fifteen year perspective, *J Infect Dis* 123:555-561, 1971.
30. Hanshaw JB: Congenital cytomegalovirus infection, *N Engl J Med* 288:1406-1407, 1973.
31. Murph JR, Bale JF: Congenital cytomegalovirus infection in the Midwest, *Pediatr Res* 33:171A, 1992.
32. Griffith JF: Nonbacterial infections of the fetus and newborn, *Clin Perinatol* 4:117-130, 1977.
33. Gaytant MA, Rours CI, Steegers EAP, Galama JM, et al: Congenital cytomegalovirus infection after recurrent infection: Case reports and review of the literature, *Eur J Pediatr* 162:248-253, 2003.
34. Lazzarotto T, Varani S, Guerra B, Nicolosi A, et al: Prenatal indicators of congenital cytomegalovirus infection, *J Pediatr* 137:90-95, 2000.
35. Prober CG, Enright AM: Congenital cytomegalovirus (CMV) infections: Hats off to Alabama, *J Pediatr* 143:4-6, 2003.
36. Boppana SB, Rivera LB, Fowler KB, Mach M, et al: Intrauterine transmission of cytomegalovirus to infants of women with preconceptional immunity, *N Engl J Med* 344:1366-1371, 2001.
37. Yasuda A, Kimura H, Hayakawa M, Ohshiro M, et al: Evaluation of cytomegalovirus infections transmitted via breast milk in preterm infants with a real-time polymerase chain reaction assay, *Pediatrics* 111:1333-1336, 2003.
38. Mussi-Pinhata MM, Yamamoto AY, Do Carmo Rego MA, Pinto PC, et al: Perinatal or early-postnatal cytomegalovirus infection in preterm infants under 34 weeks gestation born to CMV-seropositive mothers within a high-seroprevalence population, *J Pediatr* 145:685-688, 2004.
39. Bryant P, Morley C, Garland S, Curtis N: Cytomegalovirus transmission from breast milk in premature babies: Does it matter? *Arch Dis Child Fetal Neonatal Ed* 87:F75-F77 2002.
40. Doctor S, Friedman S, Dunn MS, Asztalos EV, et al: Cytomegalovirus transmission to extremely low-birthweight infants through breast milk, *Acta Paediatr* 94:53-58, 2005.
41. Neuberger P, Hamprecht K, Vochem M, Maschmann J, et al: Case-control study of symptoms and neonatal outcome of human milk–transmitted cytomegalovirus infection in premature infants, *J Pediatr* 148:326-331, 2006.
42. Friede RL: *Developmental Neuropathology*, 2nd ed, New York: 1989, Springer-Verlag.
43. Bell WE, McCormick WF: *Neurologic Infections in Children*, 2nd ed, Philadelphia: 1981, Saunders.
44. Dias MJ, Harmant-van Rijckevorsel G, Landrieu P, Lyon G: Prenatal cytomegalovirus disease and cerebral microgyria: Evidence for perfusion

failure, not disturbance of histogenesis, as the major cause of fetal cytomegalovirus encephalopathy, *Neuropediatrics* 15:18-24, 1984.

45. Perlman JM, Argyle C: Lethal cytomegalovirus infection in preterm infants: Clinical, radiological, and neuropathological findings, *Ann Neurol* 31:64-68, 1992.
46. Anzil AP, Blinzinger K, Dozic S: Cerebral form of generalized cytomegaly of early infancy: Light and electron microscopic findings, *Virchows Arch A Pathol Pathol Anat* 351:233-247, 1970.
47. Bale JF, O'Neil ME, Hart MN, Harris JD, et al: Human cytomegalovirus nucleic acids in tissues from congenitally infected infants, *Pediatr Neurol* 5:216-220, 1989.
48. De Vries LS, Gunardi H, Barth PG, Bok LA, et al: The spectrum of cranial ultrasound and magnetic resonance imaging abnormalities in congenital cytomegalovirus infection, *Neuropediatrics* 35:113-119, 2004.
49. Lipitz S, Achiron R, Zalel Y, Mendelson E, et al: Outcome of pregnancies with vertical transmission of primary cytomegalovirus infection, *Obstet Gynecol* 100:428-433, 2002.
50. Malinger G, Lev D, Zahalka N, Ben-Aroia Z, et al: Fetal cytomegalovirus infection of the brain: The spectrum of sonographic findings, *AJNR Am J Neuroradiol* 24:28-32, 2003.
51. Guibaud L, Attia-Sobol J, Buenerd A, Foray P, et al: Focal sonographic periventricular pattern associated with mild ventriculomegaly in foetal cytomegalic infection revealing cytomegalic encephalitis in the third trimester of pregnancy, *Prenat Diagn* 24:727-732, 2004.
52. Zucca C, Binda S, Borgatti R, Triulzi F, et al: Retrospective diagnosis of congenital cytomegalovirus infection and cortical maldevelopment, *Neurology* 61:710-712, 2003.
53. van der Knaap MS, Vermeulen G, Barkhof F, Hart AA, et al: Pattern of white matter abnormalities at MR imaging: Use of polymerase chain reaction testing of Guthrie cards to link pattern with congenital cytomegalovirus infection, *Radiology* 230:529-536, 2004.
54. Tatli B, Ozmen M, Aydinli N, Caliskan M: Not a new leukodystrophy but congenital cytomegalovirus infection, *J Child Neurol* 20:525-527, 2005.
55. Naeye RL: Cytomegalic inclusion disease: The fetal disorder, *Am J Clin Pathol* 47:738-744, 1967.
56. Reynolds DW, Stagno S, Alford CA: Chronic congenital and perinatal infections. In Avery GB, editor: *Neonatology: Pathophysiology and Management of the Newborn*, 2nd ed, Philadelphia: 1981, JB Lippincott.
57. Alford CA Jr: Chronic congenital and perinatal infections. In Avery GB, editor: *Neonatology: Pathophysiology and Management of the Newborn*, 3rd ed, Philadelphia: 1987, JB Lippincott.
58. Shinmura Y, Kosugi I, Aiba-Masago S, Baba S, et al: Disordered migration and loss of virus-infected neuronal cells in developing mouse brains infected with murine cytomegalovirus, *Acta Neuropathol (Berl)* 93:551-557, 1997.
59. Diezel PB: Mikrogyrie infolge cerebraler Speicheldrusenvirusinfektion im Rahmen einer generalisierten Cytomegalie bei einem Saugling, *Virchows Arch* 325:109-130, 1954.
60. Crome L, France NE: Microgyria and cytomegalic inclusion disease in infancy, *J Clin Pathol* 12:427-434, 1959.
61. Wolf A, Cowen D: Perinatal infections of the central nervous system, *J Neuropathol Exp Neurol* 18:191-243, 1959.
62. Bignami A, Appicciutoli L: Micropolygyria and cerebral calcification in cytomegalic inclusion disease, *Acta Neuropathol (Berl)* 4:127-133, 1964.
63. Navin JJ, Angevine JM: Congenital cytomegalic inclusion disease with porencephaly, *Neurology* 18:470, 1968.
64. Becroft DM: Prenatal cytomegalovirus infection and muscular deficiency (eventration) of the diaphragm, *J Pediatr* 94:74-79, 1969.
65. Wayne ER, Burrington JD, Myers DN, Cotton E, et al: Bilateral eventration of the diaphragm in a neonate with congenital cytomegalic inclusion disease, *J Pediatr* 83:164-165, 1973.
66. Ceballos R, Ch'ien LT, Whitley RJ, Brans YW: Cerebellar hypoplasia in an infant with congenital CMV infection, *Pediatrics* 57:155-157, 1976.
67. Friede RL, Mikolasek J: Postencephalitic porencephaly, hydranencephaly or polymicrogyria. A review, *Acta Neuropathol (Berl)* 43:161-168, 1978.
68. Bale JF, Reiley TT, Bray PF, Kelsey DK: CMV and dual infection in infants, *Arch Neurol* 37:236-238, 1980.
69. Titelbaum DS, Hayward JC, Zimmerman RA: Pachygyriclike changes: Topographic appearance at MR imaging and CT and correlation with neurologic status, *Radiology* 173:663-667, 1989.
70. Sugita K, Ando M, Makino M, Takanashi J, et al: Magnetic resonance imaging of the brain in congenital rubella virus and cytomegalovirus infections, *Neuroradiology* 33:239-242, 1991.
71. Shaw D, Cohen WA: Viral infections of the CNS in children: Imaging features, *AJR Am J Roentgenol* 160:125-133, 1993.
72. Iannetti P, Nigro G, Spalice A, Faiella A, et al: Cytomegalovirus infection and schizencephaly: Case reports, *Ann Neurol* 43:123-127, 1998.
73. Melish ME, Hanshaw JB: Congenital cytomegalovirus infection: Developmental progress of infants detected by routine screening, *Am J Dis Child* 126:190, 1973.
74. Stern H, Tucker SM: Prospective study of cytomegalovirus infection in pregnancy, *Br Med J* 2:268-270, 1973.
75. Reynolds DW, Stagno S, Stubbs KG: Inapparent congenital cytomegalovirus infection with elevated cord IgM levels: Causal relation with auditory and mental deficiency, *N Engl J Med* 290:291-296, 1974.

76. Nankervis GA, Kumar ML, Cox FE, Gold E: A prospective study of maternal cytomegalovirus infection and its effect on the fetus, *Am J Obstet Gynecol* 149:435-440, 1984.
77. Freij BJ, Sever JL: Chronic infections. In Avery GB, Fletcher MA, MacDonald MG, editors: *Neonatology: Pathophysiology and Management of the Newborn*, 5th ed, Philadelphia: 1999, Lippincott Williams & Wilkins.
78. Williamson WD, Demmler GJ, Percy AK, Catlin FI: Progressive hearing loss in infants with asymptomatic congenital cytomegalovirus infection, *Pediatrics* 90:862-866, 1992.
79. Stagno S: Cytomegalovirus. In Remington JS, Klein JD, editors: *Infectious Diseases of the Fetus and Newborn Infant*, 3rd ed, Philadelphia: 1990, Saunders.
80. Mena W, Royal S, Pass RF, Whitley RJ, et al: Diabetes insipidus associated with symptomatic congenital cytomegalovirus infection, *J Pediatr* 122:911-913, 1993.
81. Boppana SB, Fowler KB, Pass RF, Britt WJ: Newborn findings and outcome in children with symptomatic congenital CMV infection (SX-CMV), *Pediatr Res* 29:158A, 1992.
82. Boppana SB, Fowler KB, Vaid Y, Hedlund G, et al: Neuroradiographic findings in the newborn period and long-term outcome in children with symptomatic congenital cytomegalovirus infection, *Pediatrics* 99:409-414, 1997.
83. Fowler KB, Dable AJ, Boppana SB, Pass RF: Newborn hearing screening: Will children with hearing loss caused by congenital cytomegalovirus infection be missed? *J Pediatr* 135:60-64, 1999.
84. Boppana SB, Fowler KB, Pass RF, Rivera LB, et al: Congenital cytomegalovirus infection: Association between virus burden in infancy and hearing loss, *J Pediatr* 146:817-823, 2005.
85. Bray PF, Bale JF, Anderson RE, Kern ER: Progressive neurological disease associated with chronic cytomegalovirus infection, *Ann Neurol* 9:499-502, 1981.
86. Bale JF, Sato Y, Eisert D: Progressive postnatal subependymal necrosis in infant with congenital cytomegalovirus infection, *Pediatr Neurol* 2:367-370, 1986.
87. Williamson WD, Desmond MM, LaFevers N, Taber LH, et al: Symptomatic congenital cytomegalovirus: Disorders of language, learning and hearing, *Am J Dis Child* 136:902-905, 1982.
88. Remington JS, Klein JO: *Infectious Diseases of the Fetus and Newborn Infant*, 4th ed, Philadelphia: 1995, Saunders.
89. Rivera LB, Boppana SB, Fowler KB, Britt WJ, et al: Predictors of hearing loss in children with symptomatic congenital cytomegalovirus infection, *Pediatrics* 110:762-767, 2002.
90. Ross SA, Fowler KB, Ashrith G, Stagno S, et al: Hearing loss in children with congenital cytomegalovirus infection born to mothers with preexisting immunity, *J Pediatr* 148:332-336, 2006.
91. Pass RF, Stagno S, Britt WJ, Alford CA: Specific cell-mediated immunity and the natural history of congenital infection with cytomegalovirus, *J Infect Dis* 148:953-961, 1983.
92. Sokol DM, Demmler GJ, Troendle JF, Buffone GJ: Glass filter paper (GFP), polymerase chain reaction (PCR) to screen newborns for congenital cytomegalovirus (CMV) infection, *Pediatr Res* 29:282A, 1992.
93. Stagno S, Pass RF, Reynolds DW, Moore MA, et al: Comparative study of diagnostic procedures for congenital cytomegalovirus infection, *Pediatrics* 65:251-257, 1980.
94. Demmler GJ, Buffone GJ, Schimbor CM, May RA: Detection of cytomegalovirus in urine from newborns by using polymerase chain reaction DNA amplification, *J Infect Dis* 158:1177-1184, 1988.
95. Atkins JT, Demmler GJ, Williamson WD, McDonald JM, et al: Polymerase chain reaction to detect cytomegalovirus DNA in the cerebrospinal fluid of neonates with congenital infection, *J Infect Dis* 169:1334-1337, 1994.
96. Darin N, Bergstrom T, Fast A, Kyllerman M: Clinical, serological and PCR evidence of cytomegalovirus infection in the central nervous system in infancy and childhood, *Neuropediatrics* 25:316-322, 1995.
97. Numazaki K, Asanuma H, Ikehata M, Chiba S: Detection of cytokines and cytomegalovirus DNA in serum as test for congenital infection, *Early Hum Dev* 52:43-48, 1998.
98. Ikeda S, Tsuru A, Moriuchi M, Moriuchi H: Retrospective diagnosis of congenital cytomegalovirus infection using umbilical cord, *Pediatr Neurol* 34:415-416, 2006.
99. Alpert G, Plotkin SA: Rapid detection of human cytomegalovirus, *Pediatr Res* 19:286, 1985.
100. Weber B, Hamann A, Ritt B, Rabenau H, et al: Comparison of shell viral culture and serology for the diagnosis of human cytomegalovirus infection in neonates and immunocompromised subjects, *Clin Invest* 70:503-507, 1992.
101. Bale JF, Bray PF, Bell WE: Neuroradiographic abnormalities in congenital cytomegalovirus infection, *Pediatr Neurol* 1:42-47, 1985.
102. Nigro G, Scholz H, Bartmann U: Ganciclovir therapy for symptomatic congenital cytomegalovirus infection in infants: A two-regimen experience, *J Pediatr* 124:318-322, 1994.
103. Grant EG, Williams AL, Schellinger D, Slovis TL: Intracranial calcification in the infant and neonate: Evaluation by sonography and CT, *Radiology* 157:63-68, 1985.

104. Noyola DE, Demmler GJ, Nelson CT, Griesser C, et al: Early predictors of neurodevelopmental outcome in symptomatic congenital cytomegalovirus infection, *J Pediatr* 138:525-531, 2001.

105. Dykes FD, Ahmann PA, Lazzara A: Cranial ultrasound in the detection of intracranial calcifications, *J Pediatr* 100:406-408, 1982.

106. Shackelford GD, Fulling KH, Glasier CM: Cysts of the subependymal germinal matrix: Sonographic demonstration with pathologic correlation, *Radiology* 149:117-121, 1983.

107. Butt W, Mackay RJ, de Crespigny LC: Intracranial lesions of congenital cytomegalovirus infection detected by ultrasound scanning, *Pediatrics* 73:611-614, 1984.

108. Levene MI, Williams JL, Fawer CL: *Ultrasound of the Infant Brain*, London: 1985, Blackwell Scientific.

109. Yamashita Y, Matsuishi T, Murakami Y, Shoji H, et al: Neuroimaging findings (ultrasonography, CT, MRI) in 3 infants with congenital rubella syndrome, *Pediatr Radiol* 21:547-549, 1991.

110. Teele RL, Hernanz-Schulman M, Sotrel A: Echogenic vasculature in the basal ganglia of neonates: A sonographic sign of vasculopathy, *Radiology* 169:423-427, 1988.

111. Ries M, Deeg KH, Heininger U, Stehr K: Brain abscesses in neonates: Report of 3 cases, *Eur J Pediatr* 152:745-746, 1993.

112. Toma P, Magnano GM, Mezzano P, Lazzini F, et al: Cerebral ultrasound images in prenatal cytomegalovirus infection, *Neuroradiology* 31:278-279, 1989.

113. Hughes P, Weinberger E, Shaw DW: Linear areas of echogenicity in the thalami and basal ganglia of neonates: An expanded association, *Radiology* 179:103-105, 1991.

114. Cabanas F, Pellicer A, Morales C, Garcia-Alix A, et al: New pattern of hyperechogenicity in thalamus and basal ganglia studied by color Doppler flow imaging, *Pediatr Neurol* 10:109-116, 1994.

115. Ancora G, Lanari M, Lazzarotto T, Venturi V, et al: Cranial ultrasound scanning and prediction of outcome in newborns with congenital cytomegalovirus infection, *J Pediatr* 150:157-161, 2007.

116. Kimberlin DW, Lin CY, Sanchez PJ, Demmler GJ, et al: Effect of ganciclovir therapy on hearing in symptomatic congenital cytomegalovirus disease involving the central nervous system: A randomized, controlled trial, *J Pediatr* 143:16-25, 2003.

117. Pass RF, Stagno S, Myers GJ, Alford CA: Outcome of symptomatic congenital cytomegalovirus infection: Results of long-term longitudinal follow-up, *Pediatrics* 66:758-762, 1980.

118. Ramsay ME, Miller E, Peckham CS: Outcome of confirmed symptomatic congenital cytomegalovirus infection, *Arch Dis Child* 66:1068-1069, 1991.

119. Bale JF, Blackman JA, Sato Y: Outcome in children with symptomatic congenital cytomegalovirus infection, *J Child Neurol* 5:131-136, 1989.

120. Ivarsson SA, Lernmark B, Svanberg L: Ten-year clinical, developmental, and intellectual follow-up of children with congenital cytomegalovirus infection without neurologic symptoms at one year of age, *Pediatrics* 99:800-803, 1997.

121. Hanshaw JB, Scheiner AP, Moxley AW: School failure and deafness after "silent" congenital cytomegalovirus infection, *N Engl J Med* 295:468-470, 1976.

122. Stagno S, Reynolds DW, Amos CS, Dahle AJ, et al: Auditory and visual defects resulting from symptomatic and subclinical congenital cytomegaloviral and toxoplasma infections, *Pediatrics* 59:669-678, 1977.

123. Saigal S, Lunyk O, Larke RP, Chernesky MA: The outcome in children with congenital cytomegalovirus infection: A longitudinal follow-up study, *Am J Dis Child* 136:896-901, 1982.

124. Kumar ML, Nankervis GA, Jacobs IB, Ernhart CB, et al: Congenital and postnatally acquired cytomegalovirus infections: Long-term follow-up, *J Pediatr* 104:674-679, 1984.

125. Conboy TJ, Pass RF, Stagno S, Britt WJ, et al: Intellectual development in school-aged children with asymptomatic congenital cytomegalovirus infection, *Pediatrics* 77:801-806, 1986.

126. Hicks T, Fowler K, Richardson M, Dahle A, et al: Congenital cytomegalovirus infection and neonatal auditory screening, *J Pediatr* 123:779-782, 1993.

127. Fowler KB, McCollister FP, Dahle AJ, Boppana S, et al: Progressive and fluctuating sensorineural hearing loss in children with asymptomatic congenital cytomegalovirus infection, *J Pediatr* 130:624-630, 1997.

128. Conboy TJ, Pass RF, Stagno S: Congenital cytomegalovirus (CMV) infection and intellectual development, *Pediatr Res* 19:116, 1985.

129. Fowler KB, Stagno S, Pass RF, Britt WJ, et al: The outcome of congenital cytomegalovirus infection in relation to maternal antibody status, *N Engl J Med* 326:663-667, 1992.

130. Bodeus M, Hubinont C, Bernard P, Bouckaert A, et al: Prenatal diagnosis of human cytomegalovirus by culture and polymerase chain reaction: 98 pregnancies leading to congenital infection, *Prenat Diagn* 19:314-317, 1999.

131. Elek SD, Stern H: Vaccination against cytomegalovirus [letter], *Lancet* 1:171, 1974.

132. Plotkin S: Prevention of cytomegalovirus disease, *Pediatr Infect Dis* 3:1-4, 1984.

133. Plotkin S, Michelson S, Alford C, Starr SE, et al: The pathogenesis and prevention of human cytomegalovirus infection, *Pediatr Infect Dis* 3:67-74, 1984.

133a. Schleiss MR: Prospects for development and potential impact of a vaccine against congenital cytomegalovirus (CMV) infection, *J Pediatr* 151:564-570, 2007.

134. Lamy ME, Mulongo KN, Gadisseux JF, Lyon G, et al: Prenatal diagnosis of fetal cytomegalovirus infection, *Am J Obstet Gynecol* 166:91-94, 1992.

135. Grose C, Weiner CP: Prenatal diagnosis of congenital cytomegalovirus infection: Two decades later, *Am J Obstet Gynecol* 163:447-450, 1990.

136. Hohlfeld P, Vial Y, Maillard-Brignon C, Vaudaux B, et al: Cytomegalovirus fetal infection: Prenatal diagnosis, *Obstet Gynecol* 78:615-618, 1991.

137. Lynch L, Daffos F, Emanuel D, Giovangrandi Y, et al: Prenatal diagnosis of fetal cytomegalovirus infection, *Am J Obstet Gynecol* 165:714-718, 1991.

138. Hogge WA, Buffone GJ, Hogge JS: Prenatal diagnosis of cytomegalovirus (CMV) infection: A preliminary report, *Prenat Diagn* 13:131-136, 1993.

139. Gudnason T, Belani KK, Balfour HH: Ganciclovir treatment of cytomegalovirus disease in immunocompromised children, *Pediatr Infect Dis J* 8:436-440, 1989.

140. Schmidt GM, Horak DA, Niland JC, Duncan SR, et al: A randomized, controlled trial of prophylactic ganciclovir for cytomegalovirus pulmonary infection in recipients of allogeneic bone marrow transplants, *N Engl J Med* 324:1005-1011, 1991.

141. Goodrich JM, Mori M, Gleaves CG, Du Mond C, et al: Early treatment with ganciclovir to prevent cytomegalovirus disease after allogeneic bone marrow transplantation, *N Engl J Med* 325:1601-1607, 1991.

142. Studies of Ocular Complications of AIDS Research Group: Mortality in patients with the acquired immunodeficiency syndrome treated with either foscarnet or ganciclovir for cytomegalovirus retinitis, *N Engl J Med* 326:213-220, 1992.

143. Smets K, De Coen K, Dhooge I, Standaert L, et al: Selecting neonates with congenital cytomegalovirus infection for ganciclovir therapy, *Eur J Pediatr* 165:885-890, 2006.

144. Schulzke S, Buhrer C: Valganciclovir for treatment of congenital cytomegalovirus infection, *Eur J Pediatr* 165:575-576, 2006.

145. Remington JS, McLeod R, Thulliez P, Desmonts G: Toxoplasmosis. In Remington JS, Klein JO, Wilson CB, et al, editors: *Infectious Diseases of the Fetus and Newborn Infant*, 6th ed, Philadelphia: 2006, Elsevier Saunders.

146. Gordon N: Toxoplasmosis: A preventable cause of brain damage, *Dev Med Child Neurol* 35:567-573, 1993.

147. Lynfield R, Eaton RB: Congenital toxoplasmosis, *Teratology* 52:176-180, 1995.

148. Desmonts G, Couvreur J: Congenital toxoplasmosis: A prospective study of 378 pregnancies, *N Engl J Med* 290:1110-1116, 1974.

149. Desmonts G, Daffos F, Forestier F, Capella-Pavlovsky M, et al: Prenatal diagnosis of congenital toxoplasmosis, *Lancet* 1:500-504, 1985.

150. Desmonts G, Couvreur J: Toxoplasmosis in pregnancy and its transmission to the fetus, *Bull N Y Acad Med* 50:146-159, 1974.

151. Sever JL, Ellenberg JH, Ley AC, Madden DL, et al: Toxoplasmosis: Maternal and pediatric findings in 23,000 pregnancies, *Pediatrics* 82:181-192, 1988.

152. Remington JS, McLeod R, Desmonts G: Toxoplasmosis. In Remington JS, Klein JO, editors: *Infectious Diseases of the Fetus and Newborn Infant*, 4th ed, Philadelphia: 1995, Saunders.

153. Stagno S: Congenital toxoplasmosis, *Am J Dis Child* 134:635-637, 1980.

154. Walpole IR, Hodgen N, Bower C: Congenital toxoplasmosis: A large survey in Western Australia, *Med J Aust* 154:720-724, 1991.

155. Lebech M, Andersen O, Christensen NC, Hertel J, et al: Feasibility of neonatal screening for toxoplasma infection in the absence of prenatal treatment, *Lancet* 353:1834-1837, 1999.

156. Hsu HW, Grady GF, Maguire JH, Weiblen BJ, et al: Newborn screening for congenital toxoplasma infection: Five years experience in Massachusetts, USA, *Scand J Infect Dis* 84:59-64, 1992.

157. Hoff R, Weiblen J, Reardon LA, Maguire JH: Screening for congenital toxoplasma infection, *Trans Dis Perinat Detect Treat Manage* 14: 169–182, 1990.

158. Guerina NG, Hsu HW, Meissner HC, Maguire JH, et al: Neonatal serologic screening and early treatment for congenital *Toxoplasma gondii* infection, *N Engl J Med* 330:1858-1863, 1994.

159. Wilson CB, Haas JE: Cellular defenses against *Toxoplasma gondii* in newborns, *J Clin Invest* 73:1606-1616, 1984.

160. Dunn D, Wallon M, Peyton F, Petersen E, et al: Mother-to-child transmission of toxoplasmosis: Risk estimates for clinical counselling, *Lancet* 353:1829-1833, 1999.

161. Diebler C, Dusser A, Dulac O: Congenital toxoplasmosis: Clinical and neuroradiological evaluation of the cerebral lesions, *Neuroradiology* 27:125-130, 1985.

162. Frenkel JK: Pathology and pathogenesis of congenital toxoplasmosis, *Bull N Y Acad Med* 50:182-191, 1974.

163. Hohlfeld P, Daffos F, Thulliez P, Aufrant C, et al: Fetal toxoplasmosis: Outcome of pregnancy and infant follow-up after in utero treatment, *J Pediatr* 115:765-769, 1989.

164. Roizen N, Swisher CN, Stein MA, Hopkins J, et al: Neurologic and developmental outcome in treated congenital toxoplasmosis, *Pediatrics* 95:11-20, 1995.

165. Altshuler G: Toxoplasmosis as a cause of hydranencephaly, *Am J Dis Child* 125:251, 1973.

166. Eichenwald H: A study of congenital toxoplasmosis. In Siim JC, editor: *Human Toxoplasmosis*, Copenhagen: 1970, Munksgaard.

167. Freeman K, Oakley L, Pollak A, Buffolano W, et al: Association between congenital toxoplasmosis and preterm birth, low birthweight and small for gestational age birth, *Br J Obstet Gynaecol* 112:31-37, 2005.

168. Wallon M, Kodjikian L, Binquet C, Garweg J, et al: Long-term ocular prognosis in 327 children with congenital toxoplasmosis, *Pediatrics* 113:1567-1572, 2004.

169. Robinson RO, Baumann RJ: Late cerebral relapse of congenital toxoplasmosis, *Arch Dis Child* 55:231-232, 1980.

170. Wilson CB, Remington JS, Stagno S, Reynolds DW: Development of adverse sequelae in children born with subclinical congenital toxoplasma infection, *Pediatrics* 66:767-774, 1980.

171. Wilson CB, Remington JS: What can be done to prevent congenital toxoplasmosis? *Am J Obstet Gynecol* 138:357-363, 1980.

171a. The SYROCOT (Systematic Review on Congenital Toxoplasmosis) Study Group: Effectiveness of prenatal treatment for congenital toxoplasmosis: A meta-analysis of individual patients' data, *Lancet* 369:115-122, 2007.

172. Verlinde JD, Makstenieks O: Repeated isolation of Toxoplasma from the cerebrospinal fluid and from the blood, and the antibody response in four cases of congenital toxoplasmosis, *Antonie van Leeuwenhoek* 16:366-372, 1950.

173. Chang CH, Stulberg C, Bollinger RO: Isolation of Toxoplasma gondii in tissue culture, *J Pediatr* 81:790-791, 1972.

174. Cazenave J, Forestier F, Bessieres MH, Broussin B, et al: Contribution of a new PCR assay to the prenatal diagnosis of congenital toxoplasmosis, *Prenat Diagn* 12:119-127, 1992.

175. Naessens A, Jenum PA, Pollak A, Decosler A, et al: Diagnosis of congenital toxoplasmosis in the neonatal period: A multicenter evaluation, *J Pediatr* 135:714-719, 1999.

176. Remington JS, Desmonts G: Congenital toxoplasmosis: Variability in the IgM-fluorescent antibody response and some pitfalls in diagnosis, *J Pediatr* 83:27-30, 1973.

177. Saxon SA, Knight W, Reynolds DW, Satgno S, et al: Intellectual deficits in children born with subclinical congenital toxoplasmosis: A preliminary report, *J Pediatr* 82:792-797, 1973.

178. Koppe JG, Kloosterman GJ, de Roever-Bonnet H: Toxoplasmosis and pregnancy with a long-term follow-up of the children, *Eur J Obstet Gynecol Reprod Biol* 4:101-109, 1974.

179. Frenkel JK: Congenital toxoplasmosis: Prevention or palliation? *Am J Obstet Gynecol* 141:359-361, 1981.

180. Henderson JB, Beattie CP, Hale EG, Wright T: The evaluation of new services: Possibilities for preventing congenital toxoplasmosis, *Int J Epidemiol* 13:65-72, 1984.

181. Gras L, Wallon M, Pollak A, Cortina-Borja M, et al: Association between prenatal treatment and clinical manifestations of congenital toxoplasmosis in infancy: A cohort study in 13 European centres, *Acta Paediatr* 94:1721-1731, 2005.

182. Foulon W, Naessens A, Mahler T, DeWaele M, et al: Prenatal diagnosis of congenital toxoplasmosis, *Obstet Gynecol* 76:769-772, 1990.

183. Foulon W, Naessens A, de Catte L, Amy JJ: Detection of congenital toxoplasmosis by chorionic villus sampling and early amniocentesis, *Am J Obstet Gynecol* 63:1511-1513, 1990.

184. Daffos F, Forestier F, Capella-Pavovsky M, Thulliez P, et al: Prenatal management of 746 pregnancies at risk for congenital toxoplasmosis, *N Engl J Med* 318:271-275, 1988.

185. Foulon W: Congenital toxoplasmosis: Is screening desirable, *Scand J Infect Dis* 84:11-17, 1992.

186. Thulliez P, Daffos F, Forestier F: Diagnosis of toxoplasma infection in the pregnant woman and the unborn child: Current problems, *Scand J Infect Dis* 84:18-22, 1992.

187. Berrebi A, Kobuch WE, Bessieres MH, Bloom MC, et al: Termination of pregnancy for maternal toxoplasmosis, *Lancet* 344:36-39, 1994.

188. Foulon W, Pinon JM, Stray-Pedersen B, Pollak A, et al: Prenatal diagnosis of congenital toxoplasmosis: A multicenter evaluation of different diagnostic parameters, *Am J Obstet Gynecol* 181:843-847, 1999.

189. Hezard N, Marx-Chemla C, Foudrinier F, Villena I, et al: Prenatal diagnosis of congenital toxoplasmosis in 261 pregnancies, *Prenat Diagn* 17:1047-1054, 1997.

190. Roizen N, Swisher C, Boyer K, Patel D, et al: Developmental and neurologic function in treated congenital toxoplasmosis, *Pediatr Res* 29:353A, 1992.

191. Friedman S, Ford-Jones LE, Toi A, Ryan G, et al: Congenital toxoplasmosis: Prenatal diagnosis, treatment and postnatal outcome, *Prenat Diagn* 19:330-333, 1999.

192. McLeod R, Boyer K, Karrison T, Kasza K, et al: Outcome of treatment for congenital toxoplasmosis, 1981–2004: The National Collaborative Chicago-Based, Congenital Toxoplasmosis Study, *Clin Infect Dis* 42:1383-1394, 2006.

193. Eyles DE, Coleman M: Synergistic effect of sulfadiazine and Daraprim against experimental toxoplasmosis in the mouse, *Antibiotics Chemother* 3:483, 1953.

194. Sheffield HG, Melton ML: Effect of pyrimethamine and sulfadiazine on the fine structure and multiplication of Toxoplasma gondii in cell cultures, *J Parasitol* 61:704-712, 1975.

195. Cooper LZ, Alford CAJ: Rubella. In Remington JS, Klein JO, Wilson CB, et al, editors: *Infectious Diseases of the Fetus and Newborn Infant*, 6th ed, Philadelphia: 2006, Elsevier Saunders.

196. Lee SH, Ewert DP, Frederick PD, Mascola L: Resurgence of congenital rubella syndrome in the 1990s: Report on missed opportunities and failed prevention policies among women of childbearing age, *JAMA* 267:2616-2620, 1992.

197. Bloom S, Rguig A, Berraho A, Zniber L, et al: Congenital rubella syndrome burden in Morocco: A rapid retrospective assessment, *Lancet* 365:135-141, 2005.

198. Gregg NM: Congenital cataract following German measles in the mother, *Trans Ophthalmol Soc Aust* 3:34, 1941.

199. Cooper LZ, Ziring PR, Ockerse AB, Fedun BA, et al: Rubella, *Am J Dis Child* 118:18-29, 1969.

200. Ueda K, Nishida Y, Oshima K, Shepard TH: Congenital rubella syndrome: Correlation of gestational age at time of maternal rubella with type of defect, *J Pediatr* 94:763-765, 1979.

201. Miller E, Cradock-Watson JE, Pollock TM: Consequences of confirmed maternal rubella at successive stages of pregnancy, *Lancet* 2:781-784, 1982.

202. Enders G, Miller E, Nickeri-Pacher U, Crodock-Watson JE: Outcome of confirmed periconceptional maternal rubella, *Lancet*:1445–1448, 1988.

203. Rorke LB, Spiro AJ: Cerebral lesions in congenital rubella syndrome, *J Pediatr* 70:243-245, 1967.

204. Singer DB, Rudolph AJ, Rosenberg HS, Rawls WE, et al: Pathology of the congenital rubella syndrome, *J Pediatr* 71:665-675, 1967.

205. Waxham MN, Wolinsky JS: Rubella virus and its effects on the central nervous system, *Neurol Clin* 2:367-385, 1984.

206. Plotkin SA, Boue A, Boue JG: The in vitro growth of rubella virus in human embryo cells, *Am J Epidemiol* 81:71-85, 1965.

207. Naeye RL, Blanc W: Pathogenesis of congenital rubella, *JAMA* 194:1277-1283, 1965.

208. Kemper TL, Lecours AR, Gates MJ, Yakovlev PI: Retardation of the myelo- and cytoarchitectonic maturation of the brain in the congenital rubella syndrome, *Res Publ Assoc Res Nerv Ment Dis* 51:23-62, 1973.

209. Campbell M: Place of maternal rubella in the aetiology of congenital heart disease, *Br Med J* 1:691-696, 1961.

210. Sheridan MD: Final report of a prospective study of children whose mothers had rubella in early pregnancy, *Br Med J* 2:536-539, 1964.

211. Korones SB, Ainger LE, Monif GR: Congenital rubella syndrome: New clinical aspects with recovery of virus from affected infants, *J Pediatr* 67:166-177, 1965.

212. Rudolph AJ, Singleton EB, Rosenberg HS, Singer DB, et al: Osseous manifestations of the congenital rubella syndrome, *Am J Dis Child* 110:428-433, 1965.

213. Roy FH, Hiatt RL, Korones SB, Roane J: Ocular manifestations of congenital rubella syndrome, *Arch Ophthalmol* 75:601-607, 1966.

214. Desmond MM, Wilson GS, Melnick JL, Singer DB, et al: Congenital rubella encephalitides, *J Pediatr* 71:311-331, 1967.

215. Hastreiter AR, Joorabchi B, Pujatti G, van der Horst RL, et al: Cardiovascular lesions associated with congenital rubella, *J Pediatr* 71:59-65, 1967.

216. Ames MD, Plotkin SA, Winchester RA, Atkins TE: Central auditory imperception: A significant factor in congenital rubella deafness, *JAMA* 213:419-421, 1970.

217. Forrest JM, Menser MA: Congenital rubella in school children and adolescents, *Arch Dis Child* 45:63-69, 1970.

218. Schiff GM, Sutherland J, Light I: Congenital rubella. In Thalhammer O, editor: *Prenatal Infections*, Stuttgart: 1971, Springer-Verlag.

219. Friedmann I: Cochlear pathology in viral disease, *Adv Otorhinolaryngol* 20:155-177, 1973.

220. Desmond MM, Fisher ES, Vorderman AL, Schaffer HG, et al: The longitudinal course of congenital rubella encephalitis in nonretarded children, *J Pediatr* 93:584-591, 1978.

221. Menser MA, Harley JD, Hertzberg R, Dorman DC, et al: Persistence of virus in lens for three years after prenatal rubella, *Lancet* 2:387-388, 1967.

222. Cooper LZ, Preblud SR, Alford CA: Rubella. In Remington JS, Klein JO, editors: *Infectious Diseases of the Fetus and Newborn Infant*, 4th ed, Philadelphia: 1995, Saunders.

223. Preblud SR, Alford CA Jr: Rubella. In Remington JS, Klein JO, editors: *Infectious Diseases of the Fetus and Newborn Infant*, 3rd ed, Philadelphia: 1990, Saunders.

224. Wild NJ, Sheppard S, Smithells RW, Holzel H, et al: Onset and severity of hearing loss due to congenital rubella infection, *Arch Dis Child* 64:1280-1283, 1989.

225. Ishikawa A, Murayama T, Sakuma N: Computed cranial tomography in congenital rubella syndrome, *Arch Neurol* 39:420-421, 1982.

226. Beltinger C, Saule H: Sonography of subependymal cysts in congenital rubella syndrome, *Eur J Pediatr* 148:206-207, 1988.

227. Ben-Ami T, Yousefzadeh D, Backus M, Reichman B, et al: Lenticulostriate vasculopathy in infants with infections of the central

nervous system sonographic and Doppler findings, *Pediatr Radiol* 20:575-579, 1990.

228. Desmond MM, Wilson GW, Murphy MA: Congenital rubella children at adolescence: Developmental status, *Pediatr Res* 19:117-129, 1985.

229. Chirboga-Klein S, Oberfield SE, Casullo AM, Halahan N, et al: Growth in congenital rubella syndrome and correlation with clinical manifestations, *J Pediatr* 115:251-255, 1989.

230. Townsend JJ, Wolinsky JS, Baringer JR: The neuropathology of progressive rubella panencephalitis of late onset, *Brain* 99:81-90, 1976.

231. Weil ML, Itabashi H, Cremer NE, Oshiro L: Chronic progressive panencephalitis due to rubella virus simulating subacute sclerosing panencephalitis, *N Engl J Med* 292:994-998, 1975.

232. Bart K, Orenstein W, Preblud S, Hinman AR, et al: Elimination of rubella and congenital rubella from the United States, *Pediatr Infect Dis* 4:14-21, 1985.

233. Banatvala JE: Rubella: Continuing problems, *Br J Obstet Gynaecol* 92:193-196, 1985.

234. Gudmundsdottir S, Antonsdottir A, Gudnadottir S, Elefsen S, et al: Prevention of congenital rubella in Iceland by antibody screening and immunization of seronegative females, *Bull WHO* 63:83-92, 1985.

235. Daffos F, Forestier F, Grangeot-Keros L, Capella Pavlovsky M, et al: Prenatal diagnosis of congenital rubella, *Lancet* 2:1-3, 1984.

236. Nahmias AJ, Visintine AM: Herpes simplex. In Remington JS, Klein JD, editors: *Infectious Diseases of the Fetus and Newborn Infant*, Philadelphia: 1976, Saunders.

237. Nahmias AJ, Keyserling HL, Kerrick GM: Herpes simplex. In Remington JS, Klein JO, editors: *Infectious Diseases of the Fetus and Newborn Infant*, 2nd ed, Philadelphia: 1983, Saunders.

238. Whitley RJ, Nahmias AJ, Visintine AM, Fleming CL, et al: The natural history of herpes simplex virus infection of mother and newborn, *Pediatrics* 66:489-494, 1980.

239. Arvin AM, Whitley RJ, Gutierrez KM: Herpes simplex virus infections. In Remington JS, Klein JO, Wilson CB, et al, editors: *Infectious Diseases of the Fetus and Newborn Infant*, 6th ed, Philadelphia: 2006, Elsevier Saunders.

240. Kimberlin DW, Lin CY, Jacobs J, Powell DA, et al: Natural history of neonatal herpes simplex virus infections in the acyclovir era, *Pediatrics* 108:223-229, 2001.

241. Brown ZA, Wald A, Morrow RA, Selke S, et al: Effect of serologic status and cesarean delivery on transmission rates of herpes simplex virus from mother to infant, *JAMA* 289:203-209, 2003.

242. Kropp RY, Wong T, Cormier L, Ringrose A, et al: Neonatal herpes simplex virus infections in Canada: Results of a 3-year national prospective study, *Pediatrics* 117:1955-1962, 2006.

243. Xu F, Sternberg MR, Kottiri BJ, McQuillan GM, et al: Trends in herpes simplex virus type 1 and type 2 seroprevalence in the United States, *JAMA* 296:964-973, 2006.

244. Sullivan-Bolyai J, Hull HF, Wilson C, Corey L: Neonatal herpes simplex virus infection in King County, Washington: Increasing incidence and epidemiologic correlates, *JAMA* 250:3059, 1983.

245. Johnson RE, Nahmias AJ, Magder LS, Lee FK, et al: A seroepidemiologic survey of the prevalence of herpes simplex virus type 2 infection in the United States, *N Engl J Med* 321:7-12, 1989.

246. Fleming DT, McQuillan GM, Johnson RE, Nahmias AJ, et al: Herpes simplex virus type 2 in the United States, 1976 to 1994, *N Engl, J, Med* 337:1105-1111, 1997.

247. Adams G, Purohit DM, Bada HS, Andrews BF: Neonatal infection by Herpesvirus hominis type 2, a complication of intrapartum fetal monitoring, *Pediatr Res* 9:337, 1975.

248. Golden SM, Merenstein GB, Todd WA, Hill JM: Disseminated herpes simplex neonatorum: A complication of fetal monitoring, *Am J Obstet Gynecol* 129:917-918, 1977.

249. Parvey LS, Ch'ien LT: Neonatal herpes simplex virus infection introduced by fetal-monitor scalp electrode, *Pediatrics* 65:1150-1153, 1980.

250. Kaye EM, Dooling EC: Neonatal herpes simplex meningoencephalitis associated with fetal monitor scalp electrodes, *Neurology* 31:1045-1047, 1981.

251. Goldkrand JW: Intrapartum inoculation of herpes simplex virus by fetal scalp electrode, *Obstet Gynecol* 59:263-265, 1982.

252. Whitley RJ, Arvin AM: Herpes simplex virus infections. In Remington JS, Klein JO, editors: *Infectious Diseases of the Fetus and Newborn Infant*, 4th ed, Philadelphia: 1995, Saunders.

253. Brown ZA, Benedetti J, Ashley R, Burchett S, et al: Neonatal herpes simplex virus infection in relation to asymptomatic maternal infection at the time of labor, *N Engl J Med* 324:1247-1252, 1991.

254. Malm G, Berg U, Forsgren M: Neonatal herpes simplex: Clinical findings and outcome in relation to type of maternal infection, *Acta Paediatr* 84:256-260, 1995.

255. Prober CG, Sullender WM, Yasukawa LL, Au DS, et al: Low risk of herpes simplex virus infections in neonates exposed to the virus at the time of vaginal delivery to mothers with recurrent genital herpes simplex virus infections, *N Engl J Med* 316:240-244, 1987.

256. Brown ZA, Vontver LA, Benediti J, Critchlow CW, et al: Effects on infants of a first episode of genital herpes during pregnancy, *N Engl J Med* 317:1246-1251, 1987.

257. Carmack MA, Prober CG: Neonatal herpes: Vexing dilemmas and reasons for hope, *Pediatrics* 5:21-28, 1993.

258. Randolph AG, Washington AE, Prober CG: Cesarean delivery for women presenting with genital herpes lesions: Efficacy, risks, and costs, *JAMA* 270:77-82, 1993.

259. South MA, Tompkins WA, Morris CR, Rawls WE: Congenital malformation of the central nervous system associated with genital type (type 2) herpesvirus, *J Pediatr* 75:13-18, 1969.

260. Schaffer AJ, Avery ME: *Diseases of the Newborn*, Philadelphia: 1971, Saunders.

261. Florman AL, Gershon AA, Blackett PR, Nahmias AJ: Intrauterine infection with herpes simplex virus, *JAMA* 225:129-132, 1973.

262. Montgomery JR, Flanders RW, Yow MD: Congenital anomalies and herpesvirus infection, *Am J Dis Child* 126:364-366, 1973.

263. Dublin AB, Merten DF: Computed tomography in the evaluation of herpes simplex encephalitis, *Radiology* 125:133-134, 1977.

264. Reynolds JD, Griebel M, Mallory S, Steele R: Congenital herpes simplex retinitis, *Am J Ophthalmol* 102:33-36, 1986.

265. Duin LK, Willekes C, Baldewijns MM, Robben SG, et al: Major brain lesions by intrauterine herpes simplex virus infection: MRI contribution, *Prenat Diagn* 27:81-84, 2007.

266. Hutto C, Willett L, Yeager A, Whitley R: Congenital herpes simplex virus (HSV) infection: Early versus late gestational acquisition, *Pediatr Res* 19:296-299, 1985.

267. Light IJ: Postnatal acquisition of herpes simplex virus by the newborn infant: A review of the literature, *Pediatrics* 63:480-482, 1979.

268. Hirsch MS, Zisman B, Allison AC: Macrophages and age-dependent resistance to herpes simplex virus in mice, *J Immunol* 104:1160-1165, 1970.

269. Zisman B, Hirsch MS, Allison AC: Selective effects of antimacrophages. I. An analysis of the cell-virus interaction, *J Exp Med* 133:19, 1971.

270. Kohl S, Loo LS: Defective production of anti-herpes simplex virus (HSV) antibody in neonatal mice, *Pediatr Res* 19:277, 1985.

271. Kohl S, James AR: Herpes simplex virus encephalitis during childhood: Importance of brain biopsy diagnosis, *J Pediatr* 107:212-215, 1985.

272. Kohl S: The neonatal human's immune response to herpes simplex virus infection: A critical review, *Pediatr Infect Dis J* 8:67-74, 1989.

273. Kohl S, West S, Prober CG, Sullender WM, et al: Neonatal antibody-dependent cellular cytotoxic antibody levels are associated with the clinical presentation of neonatal herpes simplex virus infection, *J Infect Dis* 160:770-776, 1989.

274. Burchett SK, Corey L, Mohan KM, Westall J, et al: Diminished interferon-gamma and lymphocyte proliferation in neonatal and postpartum primary herpes simplex virus infection, *J Infect Dis* 165:813-818, 1992.

275. Haynes RE, Azimi PH, Cramblett HG: Fatal herpes virus hominis (herpes simplex virus) infections in children, *JAMA* 206:312-319, 1968.

276. Charnock EL, Cramblett HG: 5-Diodo-2-deoxyiuridine in neonatal herpes virus hominis encephalitis, *J Pediatr* 76:459-463, 1970.

277. Mirra JM: Aortitis and malacoplakia-like lesions of the brain in association with neonatal herpes simplex, *Am J Clin Pathol* 56:104-111, 1971.

278. Young NA, Gershon AA: Chickenpox, measles and mumps. In Remington JS, Klein JO, editors: *Infectious Diseases of the Fetus and Newborn Infant*, 2nd ed, Philadelphia: 1983, Saunders.

279. Gershon AA: Chickenpox, measles and mumps. In Remington JS, Klein JO, editors: *Infectious Diseases of the Fetus and Newborn Infant*, 3rd ed, Philadelphia: 1990, Saunders.

280. Smith JB, Groover RV, Klass DW, Houser OW: Multicystic cerebral degeneration in neonatal herpes simplex virus encephalitis, *Am J Dis Child* 131:568-572, 1977.

281. Chutorian AM, Michener RC, Defendini R, Hilal SK, et al: Neonatal polycystic encephalomalacia: Four new cases and review of the literature, *J Neurol Neurosurg Psychiatry* 42:154-160, 1979.

282. Dubois PJ, Heinz ER, Wessel HB, Zaias BW: Multiple cystic encephalomalacia of infancy: Computed tomographic findings in two cases with associated intracerebral calcification, *J Comput Assist Tomogr* 3:97-102, 1979.

283. Toth C, Harder S, Yager J: Neonatal herpes encephalitis: A case series and review of clinical presentation, *Can J Neurol Sci* 30:36-40, 2003.

284. Mikati MA, Feraru E, Krishnamoorthy K, Lombroso CT: Neonatal herpes simplex meningoencephalitis: EEG investigations and clinical correlates, *Neurology* 40:1433-1437, 1990.

285. Koskiniemi M, Happonen JM, Jarvenpaa AL, Pettay O, et al: Neonatal herpes simplex virus infection: A report of 43 patients, *Pediatr Infect Dis J* 8:30-35, 1989.

286. Malm G, Forsgren M, el Azaz M, Persson A: A follow-up study of children with neonatal herpes simplex virus infections with particular regard to late nervous disturbances, *Acta Paediatr Scand* 80:226-234, 1991.

287. Arvin AM, Prober CG: Herpes simplex virus infections: The genital tract and the newborn, *Pediatr Rev* 13:11-15, 1992.

288. Kimura H, Futamura M, Ito Y, Ando Y, et al: Relapse of neonatal herpes simplex virus infection, *Arch Dis Child Fetal Neonatal Ed* 88:F483-F486, 2003.

289. Fidler KJ, Pierce CM, Cubitt WD, Novelli V, et al: Could neonatal disseminated herpes simplex virus infections be treated earlier? *J Infect* 49:141-146, 2004.

290. Arvin AM, Yeager AS, Bruhn FW, Grossman M: Neonatal herpes simplex infection in the absence of mucocutaneous lesions, *J Pediatr* 100:715-721, 1982.

291. Whitley RJ, Gnann JW: Acyclovir: A decade later, *N Engl J Med* 327:782-789, 1992.

292. Kimura H, Futamura M, Kito H, Ando T, et al: Detection of viral DNA in neonatal herpes simplex virus infections: Frequent and prolonged presence in serum and cerebrospinal fluid, *J Infect Dis* 164:289-293, 1991.

293. Troendle-Atkins J, Demmier G, Buffone GJ: Rapid diagnosis of herpes simplex virus encephalitis by using the polymerase chain reaction, *J Pediatr* 123:376-380, 1993.

294. Malm G, Forsgren M: Neonatal herpes simplex virus infections: HSV DNA in cerebrospinal fluid and serum, *Arch Dis Child Fetal Neonatal Ed* 81:F24-F29, 1999.

295. Frenkel L, Maldonado H, Delorenzi A: Retrieval improvement is induced by water shortage through angiotensin II, *Neurobiol Learn Mem* 83:173-177, 2005.

296. Lee FK, Nahmias AJ, Stagno S: Rapid diagnosis of cytomegalovirus infection in infants by electron microscopy, *N Engl J Med* 299:1266-1270, 1978.

297. Dayan AD, Stokes MI: Rapid diagnosis of encephalitis by immunofluorescent examination of cerebrospinal fluid cells, *Lancet* 1:177-179, 1973.

298. Nahmias A, Wickliffe C, Pipkin J: Transport media for herpes simplex virus types 1 and 2, *Appl Environ Microbiol* 122:451-454, 1971.

299. Rodin P, Hare MJ, Barwell CF, Withers MJ: Transport of herpes simplex virus in Stuart's medium, *Br J Vener Dis* 47:198-199, 1971.

300. Rowley AH, Whitley RJ, Lakeman FD, Wolinsky S: Rapid detection of herpes-simplex-virus DNA in cerebrospinal fluid of patients with herpes simplex encephalitis, *Lancet* 335:440-441, 1990.

301. Gressens P, Langston C, Mitchell WJ, Martin JR: Detection of viral DNA in neonatal herpes encephalitis autopsy tissues by solution-phase PCR: Comparison with pathology and immunohistochemistry, *Brain Pathol* 3:237-250, 1993.

302. Baker DA: Risk factors for herpes simplex virus transmission to pregnant women: A couples study, *Am J Obstet Gynecol* 193:1887-1888, 2005.

303. Koutsky LA, Stevens CE, Holmes KK, Ashley RL, et al: Underdiagnosis of genital herpes by current clinical and viral-isolation procedures, *N Engl J Med* 326:1533-1539, 1992.

304. Nahmias AJ, Dowdle WR, Josey WE, Naib ZM, et al: Newborn infection with herpesvirus hominis types 1 and 2, *J Pediatr* 75:1194-1203, 1969.

305. Mikati MA, Krishnamoorthy KS: Hypoglycorrhachia in neonatal herpes simplex virus meningoencephalitis, *J Pediatr* 107:746-748, 1985.

306. Matsumoto N, Yano S, Miyao M: Two-dimensional ultrasonography of the brain: Its diagnostic usefulness in herpes simplex encephalitis and cytomegalic inclusion disease, *Brain Dev* 5:327-333, 1983.

306a. Kubota T, Ito M, Maruyama K, Kato Y, et al: Serial diffusion-weighted imaging of neonatal herpes encephalitis: A case report, *Brain Dev* 29:171-173, 2007.

307. Sainio K, Granstrom ML, Pettay O, Donner M: EEG in neonatal herpes simplex encephalitis, *Electroencephalogr Clin Neurophysiol* 56:556-561, 1983.

308. Baringer JR, Griffith JF: Experimental herpes simplex encephalitis: Early neuropathological changes, *J Neuropathol Exp Neurol* 29:89-104, 1970.

309. Kimberlin DW, Lin CY, Jacobs RF, Powel DA, et al: Safety and efficacy of high-dose intravenous acyclovir in the management of neonatal herpes simplex virus infections, *Pediatrics* 108:230-238, 2001.

310. Roberts SW, Cox SM, Dax J, Wendel GD, et al: Genital herpes during pregnancy: No lesions, no cesarean, *Obstet Gynecol* 85:261-264, 1995.

311. Gardella C, Brown Z, Wald A, Selke S, et al: Risk factors for herpes simplex virus transmission to pregnant women: A couples study, *Am J Obstet Gynecol* 193:1891-1899, 2005.

312. Rogers BB, Josephson SL, Sweeney PJ: Polymerase chain reaction amplification of herpes simplex virus DNA from clinical samples, *Obstet Gynecol* 79:464-469, 1992.

313. Cone RW, Hobson AC, Brown Z, Ashley R, et al: Frequent detection of genital herpes simplex virus DNA by polymerase chain reaction among pregnant women, *JAMA* 272:792-796, 1994.

314. Robichaux AG, Grossman JH: Obstetric management of herpes simplex infections. In Nelson NM, editor: *Current Therapy in Neonatal-Perinatal Medicine*, St. Louis, MO: 1985, Mosby.

315. Whitley RJ: Herpes simplex. In Remington JS, Klein JO, editors: *Infectious Diseases of the Fetus and Newborn Infant*, 3rd ed, Philadelphia: 1990, Saunders.

316. Bergstrom T, Trollfors B: Recurrent herpes simplex virus type 2 encephalitis in a preterm neonate, *Acta Paediatr Scand* 80:878-881, 1991.

317. Rudd C, Rivadeneira ED, Gutman LT: Dosing considerations for oral acyclovir following neonatal herpes disease, *Acta Paediatr* 83:1237-1243, 1994.

318. Whitley RJ, Yeager A, Kartus P: Neonatal herpes simplex virus infection: Follow-up evaluation of vidarabine therapy, *Pediatrics* 72:778-785, 1983.

319. Hirsch MS, Schooley RT: Treatment of herpes virus infections. I, *N Engl J Med* 309:1034-1039, 1983.

320. Skoldenberg B, Forsgren M, Alestig K, Bergstrom T, et al: Acyclovir versus vidarabine in herpes simplex encephalitis: Randomised multicentre study in consecutive Swedish patients, *Lancet* 2:707-711, 1984.

321. Englund JA, Fletcher CV, Balfour HH: Acyclovir therapy in neonates, *J Pediatr* 119:129-135, 1991.

322. Ch'ien LT, Whitley RJ, Nahmias AJ, Lewin EB, et al: Antiviral chemotherapy and neonatal herpes simplex virus infections: A pilot study experience with adenine arabinoside, *Pediatrics* 55:678-685, 1975.

323. Whitley RJ, Nahmias AJ, Soong SJ: Adenine arabinoside therapy of neonatal herpes viral simplex viral infection, *Pediatr Res* 14:566-575, 1980.

324. Whitley RJ, Alford CA, Hirsch MS, Schooley RT, et al: Vidarabine versus acyclovir therapy in herpes simplex encephalitis, *N Engl J Med* 314:144-149, 1986.

325. Ingall D, Norins L: Syphilis. In Remington JS, Klein JO, editors: *Infectious Diseases of the Fetus and Newborn Infant*, 2nd ed, Philadelphia: 1983, Saunders.

326. Mascola L, Pelosi R, Blount JH: Congenital syphilis: Why is it still occurring? *JAMA* 252:1719-1722, 1984.

327. Mascola L, Pelosi R, Blount J: Congenital syphilis revisited, *Am J Dis Child* 139:575-580, 1985.

328. Ingall D, Sanchez PJ, Baker CJ: Syphilis. In Remington JS, Klein JO, Wilson CB, et al, editors: *Infectious Diseases of the Fetus and Newborn Infant*, 6th ed, Philadelphia: 2006, Elsevier Saunders.

329. Ikeda MK, Jenson HB: Evaluation and treatment of congenital syphilis, *J Pediatr* 117:843-852, 1990.

330. Sison C, Ostrea EM, Reyes MP, Salari V: The resurgence of congenital syphilis is a drug related problem, *Neonat Epidemiol* 31:261A, 1992.

331. Ricci JM, Fojaco RM, O'Sullivan MJ: Congenital syphilis: The University of Miami/Jackson Memorial Medical Center experience, 1986–1988, *Obstet Gynecol* 74:687-693, 1989.

332. Klass PE, Brown ER, Pelton SI: Incidence of prenatal syphilis at the Boston City Hospital: A comparison across four decades, *Pediatrics* 94:24-28, 1994.

333. Sison CG, Ostrea EM, Reyes MP, Salari V: The resurgence of congenital syphilis: A cocaine-related problem, *J Pediatr* 130:289-290, 1997.

334. Mobley JA, McKeown RE, Jackson KL, Sy F, et al: Risk factors for congenital syphilis in infants of women with syphilis in South Carolina, *Am J Public Health* 88:597-602, 1998.

335. Wendel GD: Identification of *Treponema pallidum* in amniotic fluid and fetal blood from pregnancies complicated by congenital syphilis, *Obstet Gynecol* 78:890-895, 1991.

336. Hollier IM, Harstad TW, Sanchez PJ, Twickler DM, et al: Fetal syphilis: Clinical and laboratory characteristics, *Obstet Gynecol* 97:947-953, 2001.

337. Whipple DV, Dunham EC: Congenital syphilis. I. Incidence, transmission and diagnosis, *J Pediatr* 12:386, 1938.

338. Holder WR, Knox JM: Syphilis in pregnancy, *Med Clin North Am* 56:1151-1160, 1972.

339. Dippel AL: The relationship of congenital syphilis to abortion and miscarriage and the mechanism of intrauterine protection, *Am J Obstet Gynecol* 47:369, 1944.

340. Fiumara NJ: Venereal disease. In Charles D, Finland M, editors: *Obstetric and Perinatal Infections*, Philadelphia: 1973, Lea & Febiger.

341. Ford FR: *Diseases of the Nervous System in Infancy, Childhood, and Adolescence*, Springfield, IL: 1960, Charles C Thomas.

342. Wolf B, Kalangu K: Congenital neurosyphilis revisited, *Eur J Pediatr* 152:493-495, 1993.

343. Michelow IC, Wendel GD, Norgard MV, Zeray F, et al: Central nervous system infection in congenital syphilis, *N Engl J Med* 346:1792-1798, 2002.

344. Srinivasan G, Ramamurthy R, Bharathi A: Congenital syphilis: A diagnostic and therapeutic dilemma, *Pediatr Infect Dis* 2:436-441, 1983.

345. Schelonka RL, Freij BJ, McCracken GH Jr: Bacterial and fungal infections. In MacDonald MG, Mullett MD, Seshia MM, editors: *Avery's Neonatology, Pathophysiology, and Management of the Newborn*, 6th ed, Philadelphia: 2005, Lippincott Williams & Wilkins.

346. Rawstron SA, Jenkins S, Blanchard S, Li PW, et al: Maternal and congenital syphilis in Brooklyn, NY: Epidemiology, transmission, and diagnosis, *Am J Dis Child* 147:727-731, 1993.

347. Ingall D, Sanchez P, Musher DM: Syphilis. In Remington JS, Klein JO, editors: *Infectious Diseases of the Fetus and Newborn Infant*, 4th ed, Philadelphia: 1995, Saunders.

348. Platou RV: Treatment of congenital syphilis with penicillin, *Adv Pediatr* 4:39-53, 1949.

349. Chawla V, Pandit PB, Nkrumah FK: Congenital syphilis in the newborn, *Arch Dis Child* 63:1393-1394, 1988.

350. Daaboul JJ, Kartchner W, Jones KL: Neonatal hypoglycemia caused by hypopituitarism in infants with congenital syphilis, *J Pediatr* 123:983-985, 1993.

351. Woody NC, Sistrunk WF, Platou RV: Congenital syphilis: A laid ghost walks, *J Pediatr* 64:63-67, 1964.

352. Wilkinson RH, Heller RM: Congenital syphilis: Resurgence of an old problem, *Pediatrics* 47:27-30, 1971.

353. Tunnessen WW: Congenital syphilis, *Am J Dis Child* 146:115-116, 1992.

354. Dunn RA, Zenker PN: Why radiographs are useful in evaluation of neonates suspected of having congenital syphilis, *Radiology* 182:639-640, 1992.

355. Brion LP, Manuli M, Rai B, Kresch MJ, et al: Long-bone radiographic abnormalities as a sign of active congenital syphilis in asymptomatic newborns, *Pediatrics* 88:1037-1040, 1991.

356. Greenberg SB, Bernal DV: Are long bone radiographs necessary in neonates suspected of having congenital syphilis? *Radiology* 182:637-639, 1992.

357. Moyer VA, Schneider V, Yetman R, Garcia-Prats J, et al: Contribution of long-bone radiographs to the management of congenital syphilis in the newborn infant, *Arch Pediatr Adolesc Med* 152:353-357, 1998.

358. Platou RV, Hill AJ Jr, Ingraham NR Jr: Early congenital syphilis: Treatment of 252 patients with penicillin, *JAMA* 133:10-19, 1947.

359. Beeram MR, Chopde N, Dawood Y, Siriboe S, et al: Lumbar puncture in the evaluation of possible asymptomatic congenital syphilis in neonates, *J Pediatr* 128:125-129, 1996.

360. Risser WL, Hwang LY: Problems in the current case definitions of congenital syphilis, *J Pediatr* 129:499-505, 1996.

361. Souza IE, Bale JF: The diagnosis of congenital infections: Contemporary strategies, *J Child Neurol* 10:271-282, 1995.

362. Dorfman DH, Glaser JH: Congenital syphilis presenting in infants after the newborn period, *N Engl J Med* 323:1299-1302, 1990.

363. Bromberg K, Rawstron S, Tannis G: Diagnosis of congenital syphilis by combining *Treponema pallidum*–specific IgM detection with immunofluorescent antigen detection for *T. pallidum*, *J Infect Dis* 168:238-242, 1993.

364. Chhabra RS, Brion LP, Castro M, Freundlich L, et al: Comparison of maternal sera, cord blood, and neonatal sera for detecting presumptive congenital syphilis: Relationship with maternal treatment, *Pediatrics* 91:88-91, 1993.

365. Gutman LT: Syphilis. In Feigin RD, Cherry JD, editors: *Textbook of Pediatric Infectious Diseases*, 4th ed, Philadelphia: 1998, Saunders.

366. Julian AJ, Logan LC, Norins LC: Early syphilis: Immunoglobulins reactive in immunofluorescence and other serologic tests, *J Immunol* 102:1250-1259, 1969.

367. Julian AJ, Logan LC, Norins LC, Scotti A: Latent syphilis: Immunoglobulins reactive in immunofluorescence and other serologic tests, *J Immunol* 3:559-561, 1971.

368. Scotti AT, Logan L: A specific IgM antibody test in neonatal congenital syphilis, *J Pediatr* 73:242-243, 1968.

369. Alford CA Jr, Polt SS, Cassady GE, Straumfjord JV, et al: IgM-fluorescent treponemal antibody in the diagnosis of congenital syphilis, *N Engl J Med* 280:1086-1091, 1969.

370. Scotti A, Logan L, Caldwell JG: Fluorescent antibody test for neonatal congenital syphilis: A progress report, *J Pediatr* 75:1129-1134, 1969.

371. Mamunes P, Cave VG, Budell JW, Andersen JA, et al: Early diagnosis of neonatal syphilis: Evaluation of a gamma M-fluorescent treponema antibody test, *Am J Dis Child* 120:17-21, 1970.

372. Tan KL: The re-emergence of early congenital syphilis, *Acta Pediatr Scand* 62:601-607, 1973.

373. Idsoe O, Guthe T, Willcox RR: Penicillin in treatment of syphilis: The experience of three decades, *Bull WHO* 47:1-68, 1972.

374. McCracken GH Jr, Kaplan JM: Penicillin treatment for congenital syphilis: A critical reappraisal, *JAMA* 228:855-858, 1974.

375. Speer M, Mason E, Scharnberg J: Cerebrospinal fluid concentrations of aqueous procaine penicillin G in the neonate, *Pediatrics* 67:387-388, 1981.

376. Azimi PH, Janner D, Berne P, Fulroth R, et al: Concentrations of procaine and aqueous penicillin in the cerebrospinal fluid of infants treated for congenital syphilis, *J Pediatr* 124:649-653, 1994.

377. Maldonado YA: Acquired immunodeficiency syndrome in the infant. In Remington JS, Klein JO, Wilson CB, et al, editors: *Infectious Diseases of the Fetus and Newborn Infant*, 6th ed, Philadelphia: 2006, Elsevier Saunders.

378. Luzuriaga K, Sullivan JL: Prevention of mother-to-child transmission of HIV infection, *Clin Infect Dis* 40:466-467, 2005.

379. Rogers MF, Ou CY, Rayfield M, Thomas PA, et al: Use of the polymerase chain reaction for early detection of the proviral sequences of human immunodeficiency virus in infants born to seropositive mothers, *N Engl J Med* 320:1649-1654, 1989.

380. Pizzo PA, Butler K, Balis F, Brouwers E, et al: Dideoxycytidine alone and in an alternating schedule with zidovudine in children with symptomatic human immunodeficiency virus infection, *J Pediatr* 117:799-808, 1990.

381. Pizzo PA, Butler KM: In the vertical transmission of HIV, timing may be everything, *N Engl J Med* 325:652-654, 1991.

382. Ryder RW, Nsa W, Hassig SE: Use of the polymerase chain reaction for early detection of the proviral sequences of human immunodeficiency virus in infants born to seropositive mothers, *N Engl J Med* 320:1649-1654, 1989.

383. Blanche S, Calvez T, Rouzioux C, Ortigao MB, et al: Randomized study of two doses of didanosine in children infected with human immunodeficiency virus, *J Pediatr* 122:966-973, 1993.

384. Mayers MM, Davenny K, Schoenbaum EE, Feingold AR, et al: A prospective study of infants of human immunodeficiency virus seropositive and seronegative women with a history of intravenous drug use or of intravenous drug-using sex partners, in the Bronx, New York City, *Pediatrics* 88:1248-1256, 1991.

385. European Collaborative Study: Children born to women with HIV-1 infection: Natural history and risk of transmission, *Lancet* 337:253-260, 1991.

386. Italian Multicentre Study: Epidemiology, clinical features and prognostic factors of paediatric HIV infection, *Lancet* 2:1043-1045, 1988.

387. Katz SL, Wilfert CM: Human immunodeficiency virus infection of newborns, *N Engl J Med* 320:1687-1689, 1989.

388. Hutto C, Parks WP, Lai S, Mastrucci MT, et al: A hospital-based prospective study of perinatal infection with human immunodeficiency virus type 1, *J Pediatr* 118:347-353, 1991.

389. Ehrnst A, Lindgren S, Dictor M, Johansson B, et al: HIV in pregnant women and their offspring: Evidence for late transmission, *Lancet* 338:203-207, 1991.

390. Ehrnst A, Lindgren S, Belfrage E, Sonnerborg A, et al: Intrauterine and intrapartum transmission of HIV, *Lancet* 339:245-246, 1992.

391. Gabiano C, Tovo PA, de Martino M, Galli L, et al: Mother-to-child transmission of human immunodeficiency virus type-1: Risk of infection and correlates of transmission, *Pediatrics* 90:369-374, 1992.

392. Lepage P, Vandeperre P, Msellati P, Hitimana DG, et al: Mother-to-child transmission of human immunodeficiency virus type-1 (HIV-1) and its determinants: A cohort study in Kigali, Rwanda, *Am J Epidemiol* 137:589-599, 1993.

393. St Louis ME, Kamenga M, Brown C, Nelson AM, et al: Risk for perinatal HIV-1 transmission according to maternal immunologic, virologic, and placental factors, *JAMA* 269:2853-2859, 1993.

394. Ades AE, Davison CF, Holland FJ, Gibb DM, et al: Vertically transmitted HIV infection in the British Isles, *Br Med J* 306:1296-1299, 1993.

395. Johnson JP, Vink PE, Hines SE, Robinson B, et al: Vertical transmission of human immunodeficiency virus from seronegative or indeterminate mothers, *Am J Dis Child* 145:1239-1241, 1991.

396. Terragna A, Ferrazin A, Gotta C, Cirillo C, et al: Epidemiology of neonatal HIV-1 infection in Italy. In Melica F, editor: *AIDS and Human Reproduction*, Basel: 1992, Karger.

397. Kind C, Brändle B, Wyler CA, Calame A, et al: Epidemiology of vertically transmitted HIV-1 infection in Switzerland: Results of a nationwide prospective study, *Eur J Pediatr* 151:442-448, 1992.

398. Borkowsky W, Krasinski K: Perinatal human immunodeficiency virus infection: Ruminations on mechanisms of transmission and methods of intervention, *Pediatrics* 90:133-136, 1992.

399. Ukwu HN, Graham BS, Lambert JS, Wright PF: Perinatal transmission of human immunodeficiency virus-1 infection and maternal immunization strategies for prevention, *Obstet Gynecol* 80:458-468, 1992.

400. Newell ML, Peckham C: Risk factors for vertical transmission of HIV-1 and early markers of HIV-1 infection in children, *AIDS* 7:91-97, 1993.

401. The European Collaborative Study: Risk factors for mother-to-child transmission of HIV-1, *Lancet* 339:1007-1012, 1992.

402. Minkoff H, Burns DN, Landesman S, Youchah J, et al: The relationship of the duration of ruptured membranes to vertical transmission of human immunodeficiency virus, *Am J Obstet Gynecol* 173:585-589, 1995.

403. Working Group on Mother-to-Child Transmission of HIV: Rates of mother-to-child transmission of HIV-1 in Africa, America, and Europe: Results from 13 perinatal studies, *J Acquir Immune Defic Syndr Hum Retrovirol* 8:506-510, 1995.

404. Landesman SH, Kalish LA, Burns DN, Minkoff H, et al: Obstetrical factors and the transmission of human immunodeficiency virus type I from mother to child, *N Engl J Med* 334:1617-1623, 1996.

405. Mandelbrot L, Mayaux MJ, Bongain A, Berrebi A, et al: Obstetric factors and mother-to-child transmission of human immunodeficiency virus type 1: The French perinatal cohorts, *Am J Obstet Gynecol* 175:661-667, 1996.

406. Bulterys M, Lepage P: Mother-to-child transmission of HIV, *Curr Opin Pediatr* 10:143-150, 1998.

407. Newell ML: Mechanisms and timing of mother-to-child transmission of HIV-1, *AIDS* 12:831-837, 1998.

408. Stratton P, Tuomala RE, Abboud R, Rodriguez E, et al: Obstetric and newborn outcomes in a cohort of HIV-infected pregnant women: A report of the women and infants transmission study, *J Acquir Immune Defic Syndr Hum Retrovirol* 20:179-186, 1999.

409. Dabis F, Msellati P, Meda N, Welffens-Ekra C, et al: 6-month efficacy, tolerance, and acceptability of a short regimen of oral zidovudine to reduce vertical transmission of HIV in breastfed children in Cote d'Ivoire and Burkina Faso: A double-blind placebo-controlled multicentre trial, *Lancet* 353:786-792, 1999.

410. Wiktor SZ, Ekpini E, Karon JM, Nkengasong J, et al: Short-course oral zidovudine for prevention of mother-to-child transmission of HIV-1 in Abidjan, Cote d'Ivoire: A randomised trial, *Lancet* 353:781-785, 1999.

411. Mattern CFT, Murray K, Jensen A, Farzadegan H, et al: Localization of human immunodeficiency virus core antigen in term human placentas, *Pediatrics* 89:207-209, 1992.

412. Goedert JJ, Duliege A-M, Amos CI, Felton S, et al: High risk of HIV-1 for first-born twins, *Lancet* 338:1471-1475, 1991.

413. Mano H, Chermann J-C: Fetal human immunodeficiency virus type 1 infection of different organs in the second trimester, *AIDS Res Hum Retroviruses* 7:83-88, 1991.

414. Rogers MD, Ou CY, Kilbourne B, Schochetman G: Advances and problems in the diagnosis of human immunodeficiency virus infection in infants, *Pediatr Infect Dis J* 10:523-531, 1991.

415. Luzuriaga K, McQuilkin P, Alimenti A, Sullivan JL: Vertical HIV-1 infection: Intrauterine vs. intrapartum transmission, *Infect Dis* 34:169A, 1992.
416. Tovo PA: Caesarean section and perinatal HIV transmission: What next?, *Lancet* 342:630, 1993.
417. Newell ML, Gray G, Bryson YJ: Prevention of mother-to-child transmission of HIV-1 infection, *AIDS* 11:S165-S172, 1997.
418. Fowler MG, Simonds RJ, Roongpisuthipong A: Update on perinatal HIV transmission, *Pediatr Clin North Am* 47:21-38, 2000.
419. Kourtis AP, Bulterys M, Nesheim SR, Lee FK: Understanding the timing of HIV transmission from mother to infant, *JAMA* 285:709-712, 2001.
420. Van de Perre P, Simonon A, Msellati P, Hitimana DG, et al: Postnatal transmission of human immunodeficiency virus type 1 from mother to infant, *N Engl J Med* 325:593-598, 1991.
421. Stiehm ER, Vink P: Transmission of human immunodeficiency virus infection by breast-feeding, *J Pediatr* 118:410-412, 1991.
422. Dunn DT, Newell ML, Ades AE, Peckham CS: Risk of human immunodeficiency virus type-1 transmission through breastfeeding, *Lancet* 340:585-588, 1992.
423. Ruff AJ, Halsey NA, Coberly J, Boulos R: Breast-feeding and maternal-infant transmission of human immunodeficiency virus type 1, *J Pediatr* 121:325-329, 1992.
424. Committee on Pediatric AIDS: Human milk, breastfeeding, and transmission of human immunodeficiency virus in the United States, *Pediatrics* 96:977-979, 1995.
425. Ekpini ER, Wiktor SZ, Satten GA, Adjorlolo-Johnson GT, et al: Late postnatal mother-to-child transmission of HIV-1 in Abidjan, Cote d'Ivoire, *Lancet* 349:1054-1059, 1997.
426. Newell ML: Infant feeding and HIV-1 transmission, *Lancet* 354:442-443, 1999.
427. Nduati R, John G, Mbori-Ngacha D, Richardson B, et al: Effect of breast-feeding and formula feeding on transmission of HIV-1: A randomized clinical trial, *JAMA* 283:1167-1174, 2000.
428. Guay LA, Ruff AJ: HIV and infant feeding: An ongoing challenge, *JAMA* 286:2462-2464, 2001.
429. Breastfeeding and HIV International Transmission Study Group, Coutsoudis A, Dabis F, Fawzi W, et al: Late postnatal transmission of HIV-1 in breast-fed children: An individual patient data meta-analysis, *J Infect Dis* 189:2154-2166, 2004.
430. Bulterys M, Fowler MG, VanRompay KK, Kourtis AP: Prevention of mother-to-child transmission of HIV-1 through breast-feeding: Past, present, and future, *J Infect Dis* 189:2149-2153, 2004.
431. Thiry L, Sprecher-Goldberger S, Jonckheer T: Isolation of AIDS virus from cell-free breast milk of three healthy virus carriers, *Lancet* 2:891-892, 1985.
432. Vogt MW, Witt DJ, Craven DE: Isolation of HTLV-III/LAV from cervical secretions of women at risk for AIDS, *Lancet* 1:525-527, 1986.
433. Belman AL, Diamond G, Dickson D, Horoupian D, et al: Pediatric acquired immunodeficiency syndrome, *Am J Dis Child* 142:29-35, 1988.
434. Brinkmann R, Schwinn A, Narayan O, Zink C, et al: Human immunodeficiency virus infection in microglia: Correlation between cells infected in the brain and cells cultured from infectious brain tissue, *Ann Neurol* 31:361-365, 1992.
435. Jovaisas E, Koch MA, Schafer A: LAV/HTLV-III in 20 week fetus, *Lancet* 2:1129, 1985.
436. Epstein LG, Sharer LR, Oleske JM, et al: Neurologic manifestations of human immunodeficiency virus infection in children, *Pediatrics* 78:678-687, 1986.
437. Shaw GM, Harper ME, Hahn BH, et al: HTLV-III infection in brains of children and adults with AIDS encephalopathy, *Science* 227:177-181, 1985.
438. Belman AL: Central nervous system involvement in infants and children with symptomatic human immunodeficiency virus infection. *Transplacental Disorders: Perinatal Detection, Treatment and Management (Including Pediatric AIDS)*, New York: 1990, Liss.
439. Belman AL: Neurologic syndromes associated with symptomatic human immunodeficiency virus infection in infants and children. In Kozlowski PB, Snider DA, Vietze PM, et al, editors: *Brain in Pediatric AIDS*, Basel: 1990, Karger.
440. Epstein LG, Gendelman HE: Human immunodeficiency virus type I infection of the nervous system: Pathogenetic mechanisms, *Ann Neurol* 33:429-436, 1993.
441. Masliah E, Achim CL, Ge N, DeTeresa R, et al: Spectrum of human immunodeficiency virus–associated neocortical damage, *Ann Neurol* 32:321-329, 1992.
442. Tornatore C, Chandra R, Berger JR, Major EO: HIV-1 infection of subcortical astrocytes in the pediatric central nervous system, *Neurology* 44:481-487, 1994.
443. Saito Y, Sharer LR, Epstein LG, Michaels J, et al: Overexpression of *nef* as a marker for restricted HIV-1 infection of astrocytes in postmortem pediatric central nervous tissues, *Neurology* 44:474-481, 1994.
444. Takahashi K, Wesselingh SL, Griffin DE, McCarthur JC, et al: Localization of HIV-1 in human brain using polymerase chain reaction/in situ hybridization and immunocytochemistry, *Ann Neurol* 39:705-711, 1996.
445. Brack-Werner R: Astrocytes: HIV cellular reservoirs and important participants in neuropathogenesis, *AIDS* 13:1-22, 1999.

446. Hao HN, Lyman WD: HIV infection of fetal human astrocytes: The potential role of a receptor-mediated endocytic pathway, *Brain Res* 823:24-32, 1999.
447. Epstein LG, Sharer LR, Cho SE: HTLV-III/LAV-like retrovirus particles in the brains of patients with AIDS encephalopathy, *AIDS Res Hum Retroviruses* 1:447-454, 1985.
448. Epstein LG, Sharer LR, Goudsmit J: Neurological and neuropathological features of human immunodeficiency virus infection in children, *Ann Neurol* 23(Suppl):19-23, 1988.
449. Vazeux R, Lacroix CC, Blanche S, Cumont MC, et al: Low levels of human immunodeficiency virus replication in the brain tissue of children with severe acquired immunodeficiency syndrome encephalopathy, *Am J Pathol* 140:137-144, 1992.
450. Belman AL, Ultmann MH, Horoupian D, Novick B, et al: Neurological complications in infants and children with acquired immune deficiency syndrome, *Ann Neurol* 18:560-566, 1985.
451. Belman AL, Lantos G, Horoupian D, Novick BE, et al: AIDS: Calcification of the basal ganglia in infants and children, *Neurology* 36:1192-1199, 1986.
452. Belman AL: Acquired immunodeficiency syndrome and the child's central nervous system, *Pediatr Neurol* 39:691-714, 1992.
453. Davis SL, Halsted CC, Levy N, Ellis W: Acquired immune deficiency syndrome presenting as progressive infantile encephalopathy, *J Pediatr* 110:884-888, 1987.
454. Tovo PA, Gabiano C, Favro-Paris S, Palomba E, et al: Brain atrophy with intracranial calcification following congenital HIV infection, *Acta Paediatr Scand* 77:776-779, 1988.
455. Sharer LR: Central nervous system pathology in children with HIV-1 infection. In Fejerman N, Chamoles NA, editors: *New Trends in Pediatric Neurology*, Amsterdam: 1993, Elsevier Science.
456. Burns DK: The neuropathology of pediatric acquired immunodeficiency syndrome, *J Child Neurol* 7:332-346, 1992.
457. Bell JE, Lowrie S, Koffi K, Honde M, et al: The neuropathology of HIV-infected African children in Abidjan, Cote d'Ivoire, *J Neuropathol Exp Neurol* 56:686-692, 1997.
458. Speth C, Dierich MR, Sopper S: HIV-infection of the central nervous system: The tightrope walk of innate immunity, *Mol Immunol* 42:213-228, 2005.
459. Kozlowski PB, Brudkowska J, Kraszpulski M, Sersen EA, et al: Microencephaly in children congenitally infected with human immunodeficiency virus: A gross-anatomical morphometric study, *Acta Neuropathol (Berl)* 93:136-145, 1997.
460. Chiriboga CA, Fleishman S, Champion S, Gaye-Robinson L, et al: Incidence and prevalence of HIV encephalopathy in children with HIV infection receiving highly active anti-retroviral therapy (HAART), *J Pediatr* 146:402-407, 2005.
461. Pulliam L, Herndier BG, Tang N, McGrath MS: Human immunodeficiency virus–infected macrophages produce soluble factors that cause histological and neurochemical alterations in cultured human brains, *J Clin Invest* 87:503-512, 1991.
462. Lipton SA, Sucher NJ, Kaiser PK, Dreyer EB: Synergistic effects of HIV coat protein and NMDA receptor-mediated neurotoxicity, *Neuron* 7:111-118, 1991.
463. Brenneman DE, Westbrook GL, Fitzgerald SP, Ennist DL, et al: Neuronal cell killing by the envelope protein of HIV and its prevention by vasoactive intestinal peptide, *Nature* 335:639-642, 1988.
464. Dreyer EB, Kaiser PK, Offermann JT, Lipton SA: HIV-1 coat protein neurotoxicity prevented by calcium channel antagonists, *Science* 248:364-367, 1990.
465. Tyor WR, Glass JD, Griffin JW, Becker PS, et al: Cytokine expression in the brain during the acquired immunodeficiency syndrome, *Ann Neurol* 31:349-360, 1992.
466. Merrill JE, Chen ISY: HIV-1, macrophages, glial cells, and cytokines in AIDS nervous system disease, *FASEB J* 5:2391-2397, 1991.
467. Giulian D, Vaca K, Noonan CA: Secretion of neurotoxins by mononuclear phagocytes infected with HIV-1, *Science* 250:1593-1596, 1990.
468. Benos DJ, Hahn BH, Bubien JK, Ghosh SK, et al: Envelope glycoprotein gp120 of human immunodeficiency virus type 1 alters ion transport in astrocytes: Implications for AIDS dementia complex, *Proc Natl Acad Sci U S A* 91:494-498, 1994.
469. Lipton SA: HIV displays its coat of arms, *Nature* 367:113-114, 1994.
470. Gendelman HE, Lipton SA, Tardieu M, Bukrinsky MI, et al: The neuropathogenesis of HIV-1 infection, *J Leukocyte Biol* 56:389-398, 1994.
471. Barks JD, Sun R, Malinak C, Silverstein FS: Gp120, an HIV-1 protein, increases susceptibility to hypoglycemic and ischemic brain injury in perinatal rats, *Exp Neurobiol* 132:123-133, 1995.
472. Wang P, Barks JDE, Silverstein FS: Tat, a human immunodeficiency virus-1–derived protein, augments excitotoxic hippocampal injury in neonatal rats, *Neuroscience* 88:585-597, 1999.
473. Barks JD, Nair MP, Schwartz SA, Silverstein FS: Potentiation of N-methyl-D-aspartate-mediated brain injury by a human immunodeficiency virus-1–derived peptide in perinatal rodents, *Pediatr Res* 34:192-198, 1993.

474. Toggas SM, Masliah E, Rockenstein EM, Rall GF, et al: Central nervous system damage produced by expression of the HIV-1 coat protein gp120 in transgenic mice, *Nature* 367:188-193, 1994.

475. Lipton SA: Models of neuronal injury in AIDS: Another role for the NMDA receptor? *Trends Neurosci* 15:75-79, 1992.

476. Lipton SA: Memantine prevents HIV coat protein-induced neuronal injury in vitro, *Neurology* 42:1403-1405, 1992.

477. Lipton SA: Requirement for macrophages in neuronal injury induced by HIV envelope protein gp120, *Neuroreport* 3:913-915, 1992.

478. Dawson VL, Dawson TM, Uhl GR, Snyder SH: Human immunodeficiency virus type 1 coat protein neurotoxicity mediated by nitric oxide in primary cortical cultures, *Neurobiology* 90:3256-3259, 1993.

479. Dawson VL, Dawson TM, Bartley DA, Uhl GR, et al: Mechanisms of nitric oxide–mediated neurotoxicity in primary brain cultures, *J Neurosci* 13:2651-2661, 1993.

480. Masliah E, Ge N, Morey M, Deteresa R, et al: Cortical dendritic pathology in human immunodeficiency virus encephalitis, *Lab Invest* 66:285-291, 1992.

481. Kaufmann WE: Cerebrocortical changes in AIDS, *Lab Invest* 66:261-264, 1992.

482. Dickson DW, Belman AL, Kim TS, Horoupian DS, et al: Spinal cord pathology in pediatric acquired immunodeficiency syndrome, *Neurology* 39:227-235, 1989.

483. Park YD, Belman AL, Kim T-S, Kure K, et al: Stroke in pediatric acquired immunodeficiency syndrome, *Ann Neurol* 28:303-311, 1990.

484. Husson RN, Saini R, Lewis LL, Butler KM, et al: Cerebral artery aneurysms in children infected with human immunodeficiency virus, *J Pediatr* 121:927-930, 1992.

485. Tovo PA, Demartino M, Gabiano C, Cappello N, et al: Prognostic factors and survival in children with perinatal HIV-1 infection, *Lancet* 339:1249-1253, 1992.

486. Mintz M: Neurological manifestations and the results of treatment of pediatric HIV infection. In Fejerman N, Chamoles NA, editors: *New Trends in Pediatric Neurology*, Amsterdam: 1993, Elsevier Science.

487. Newell ML, Dunn D, Ciaquinto C, Truscia D, et al: Perinatal findings in children born to HIV-infected mothers, *Br J Obstet Gynecol* 101:136-141, 1994.

488. Belman AL, Muenz LR, Marcus JC, Goedert JJ, et al: Neurologic status of human immunodeficiency virus 1–infected infants and their controls: A prospective study from birth to 2 years, *Pediatrics* 98:1109-1118, 1996.

489. Gay CL, Armstrong FD, Cohen D, Lai S, et al: The effects of HIV on cognitive and motor development in children born to HIV-seropositive women with no reported drug use: Birth to 24 months, *Pediatrics* 96:1078-1082, 1995.

490. Nozyce M, Hittelman J, Muenz L, Durako SJ, et al: Effect of perinatally acquired human immunodeficiency virus infection on neurodevelopment in children during the first two years of life, *Pediatrics* 94:883-891, 1994.

491. Msellati P, Lepage P, Hitimana DG, Van Goethem C, et al: Neurodevelopmental testing of children born to human immunodeficiency virus type 1 seropositive and seronegative mothers: A prospective cohort study in Kigali, Rwanda, *Pediatrics* 92:843-848, 1993.

492. Tardieu M, Mayaux MJ, Seibel N, Funckbrentano I, et al: Cognitive assessment of school-age children infected with maternally transmitted human immunodeficiency virus type 1, *J Pediatr* 126:375-379, 1995.

493. Wolters PL, Brouwers P, Moss HA, Pizzo PA: Differential receptive and expressive language functioning of children with symptomatic HIV disease and relation to CT scan brain abnormalities, *Pediatrics* 95:112-119, 1995.

494. Barnhart HX, Caldwell B, Thomas P, Mascola L, et al: Natural history of human immunodeficiency virus disease in perinatally infected children: An analysis from the pediatric spectrum of disease project, *Pediatrics* 97:710-716, 1996.

495. Mayaux MJ, Burgard M, Teglas JP, Cottalorda J, et al: Neonatal characteristics in rapidly progressive perinatally acquired HIV-1 disease, *JAMA* 275:606-610, 1996.

496. Blanche S, Newell ML, Mayaux MJ, Dunn DT, et al: Morbidity and mortality in European children vertically infected by HIV-1: The French pediatric HIV infection study group and European collaborative study, *J Acquir Immune Defic Syndr Hum Retrovirol* 14:442-450, 1997.

497. Cooper ER, Hanson C, Diaz C, Mendez H, et al: Encephalopathy and progression of human immunodeficiency virus disease in a cohort of children with perinatally acquired human immunodeficiency virus infection, *J Pediatr* 132:808-812, 1998.

498. Tardieu M: HIV-1 and the developing central nervous system, *Dev Med Child Neurol* 40:843-846, 1998.

499. Tardieu M, Le Chenadec J, Persoz A, Meyer L, et al: HIV-1 related encephalopathy in infants compared with children and adults, *Neurology* 54:1089-1095, 2000.

500. Van Rie A, Harrington PR, Dow A, Robertson K: Neurologic and neurodevelopmental manifestations of pediatric HIV/AIDS: A global perspective, *Eur J Paediatr Neurol* 11:1-9, 2007.

501. Srugo I, Wittek AE, Israele V, Bruneill PA: Meningoencephalitis in a neonate congenitally infected with human immunodeficiency virus type 1, *J Pediatr* 120:93-95, 1992.

502. Schmitt B, Seeger J, Kreuz W, Enenkel S, et al: Central nervous system involvement of children with HIV infection, *Dev Med Child Neurol* 33:535-540, 1991.

503. Abrams EJ, Matheson PB, Thomas PA, Thea DM, et al: Neonatal predictors of infection status and early death among 332 infants at risk of HIV-1 infection monitored prospectively from birth, *Pediatrics* 96:451-458, 1995.

504. Belec L, Tayot J, Tron P, Mikol J, et al: Cytomegalovirus encephalopathy in an infant with congenital acquired immuno-deficiency syndrome, *Neuropediatrics* 21:124-129, 1990.

505. Visudtibhan A, Visudhiphan P, Chiemchanya S: Stroke and seizures as the presenting signs of pediatric HIV infection, *Pediatr Neurol* 20:53-56, 1999.

506. Diamond GW, Gurdin P, Wiznia AA, Belman AL, et al: Effects of congenital HIV infection on neurodevelopmental status of babies in foster care, *Dev Med Child Neurol* 32:999-1005, 1990.

507. Butler C, Hittelman J, Hauger SB: Approach to neurodevelopmental and neurologic complications in pediatric HIV infection, *J Pediatr* 119(Suppl):41-46, 1991.

508. Aylward EH, Butz AM, Hutton N, Joyner ML, et al: Cognitive and motor development in infants at risk for human immunodeficiency virus, *Am J Dis Child* 146:218-222, 1992.

509. Chamberlain MC, Nichols SL, Chase CH: Pediatric AIDS: Comparative cranial MRI and CT scans, *Pediatr Neurol* 7:357-362, 1991.

510. Levenson RL, Mellins CA, Zawadzki R, Kairam R, et al: Cognitive assessment of human immunodeficiency virus exposed children, *Am J Dis Child* 146:1479-1483, 1992.

511. Chamberlain MC: Pediatric AIDS: A longitudinal comparative MRI and CT brain imaging study, *J Child Neurol* 8:175-181, 1993.

512. DeCarli C, Civitello LA, Brouwers P, Pizzo PA: The prevalence of computed tomographic abnormalities of the cerebrum in 100 consecutive children symptomatic with the human immune deficiency virus, *Ann Neurol* 34:198-205, 1993.

513. Blanche S, Mayaux MJ, Rouzioux C, Teglas JP, et al: Relation of the course of HIV infection in children to the severity of the disease in their mothers at delivery, *N Engl J Med* 330:308-312, 1994.

514. Grubman S, Gross E, Lerner-Weiss N, Hernandez M, et al: Older children and adolescents living with perinatally acquired human immunodeficiency virus infection, *Pediatrics* 95:657-663, 1995.

515. Macmillan C, Magder LS, Brouwers P, Chase C, et al: Head growth and neurodevelopment of infants born to HIV-1–infected drug-using women, *Neurology* 57:1402-1411, 2001.

516. Sanchez-Ramon S, Resino S, Cano JM, Ramos JT, et al: Neuroprotective effects of early antiretrovirals in vertical HIV infection, *Pediatr Neurol* 29:218-221, 2003.

517. Llorente A, Brouwers P, Charurat M, Magder LS, et al: Early neurodevelopmental markers predictive of mortality in infants infected with HIV-1, *Dev Med Child Neurol* 45:76-84, 2003.

518. Berk DR, Falkovitz-Halpern MS, Hill DW, Albin C, et al: Temporal trends in early clinical manifestations of perinatal HIV infection in a population-based cohort, *JAMA* 293:2221-2231, 2005.

519. Foster C, Biggs R, Melvin D, Walters M, et al: Neurodevelopmental outcomes in children with HIV infection under 3 years of age, *Dev Med Child Neurol* 48:677-682, 2006.

520. Douek P, Bertrand Y, Tran-Minh VA, Patet JD, et al: Primary lymphoma of the CNS in an infant with AIDS: Imaging findings, *AJR Am J Roentgenol* 156:1037-1038, 1991.

521. Shearer WT, Quinn TC, LaRussa P, Lew JF, et al: Viral load and disease progression in infants infected with human immunodeficiency virus type 1, *N Engl J Med* 336:1337-1342, 1997.

522. Mitchell CD: HIV-1 encephalopathy among perinatally infected children: Neuropathogenesis and response to highly active antiretroviral therapy, *Ment Retard Dev Disabil Res Rev* 12:216-222, 2006.

523. Willen EJ: Neurocognitive outcomes in pediatric HIV, *Ment Retard Dev Disabil Res Rev* 12:223-228, 2006.

523a. Lindsey JC, Malee KM, Brouwers P, Hughes MD: Neurodevelopmental functioning in HIV-infected infants and young children before and after the introduction of protease inhibitor-based highly active antiretroviral therapy, *Pediatrics* 119:e681-693, 2007.

524. Husson RN, Comeau AM, Hoff R: Diagnosis of human immunodeficiency virus infection in infants and children, *Pediatrics* 86:1-10, 1990.

525. Krivine A, Yakudima A, Le May M, Pena-Cruz V, et al: A comparative study of virus isolation, polymerase chain reaction, and antigen detection in children of mothers infected with human immunodeficiency virus, *J Pediatr* 116:372-376, 1990.

526. Frenkel LD, Gaur S: Pediatric human immunodeficiency virus infection and disease, *Curr Opin Pediatr* 3:867-873, 1991.

527. Martin NL, Levy JA, Legg H, Weintrub PS, et al: Detection of infection with human immunodeficiency virus (HIV) type 1 in infants by an anti-HIV immunoglobulin A assay using recombinant proteins, *J Pediatr* 118:354-358, 1991.

528. Hutto C, Owens C, Dumond D, Saenz M, et al: Early detection of perinatal HIV-1 infection with polymerase chain reaction (PCR), virus culture and p24 antigen88, *Infect Dis* 34:164A, 1992.

529. Burgard M, Mayaux MJ, Blanche S, Ferroni A, et al: The use of viral culture and p24-antigen testing to diagnose human immunodeficiency virus infection in neonates, *N Engl J Med* 327:1192-1197, 1992.

530. Gwinn M, Redus MA, Granade TC, Hannon WH, et al: HIV-1 serologic test results for one million newborn dried-blood specimens: Assay performance and implications for screening, *J Acquir Immune Defic Syndr Hum Retrovirol* 5:505-512, 1992.

531. Fauvel M, Henrard D, Delage G, Lapointe N: Early detection of HIV in neonates, *N Engl J Med* 329:60-61, 1993.

532. Comeau AM, Hsu HW, Schwerzler M, Mushinsky G, et al: Identifying human immunodeficiency virus infection at birth: Application of polymerase chain reaction to Guthrie cards, *J Pediatr* 123:252-258, 1993.

533. Suarez MA, Bianco B, Brion LP, Schulman M, et al: A rapid test for the detection of human immunodeficiency virus antibodies in cord blood, *J Pediatr* 123:259-261, 1993.

534. Getchell JP, Hausler WJ, Ramirez MT, Susanin JM: HIV screening of newborns, *Biochem Med Metab Biol* 49:143-148, 1993.

535. Miles SA, Balden E, Magpantay L, Wei L, et al: Rapid serologic testing with immune-complex dissociated HIV p24 antigen for early detection of HIV infection in neonates, *N Engl J Med* 328:297-302, 1993.

536. Brandt CD, Rakusan TA, Sison AV, Saxena ES, et al: Human immunodeficiency virus infection in infants during the first 2 months of life, *Arch Pediatr Adolesc Med* 148:250-254, 1994.

537. Nelson RP, Price LJ, Halsey AB, Graven SN, et al: Diagnosis of pediatric human immunodeficiency virus infection by means of a commercially available polymerase chain reaction gene amplification, *Arch Pediatr Adolesc Med* 150:40-45, 1995.

538. Owens DK, Holodniy M, McDonald TW, Scott J, et al: A meta-analytic evaluation of the polymerase chain reaction for the diagnosis of HIV infection in infants, *JAMA* 275:1342-1348, 1996.

539. Bremer JW, Lew JF, Cooper E, Hillyer GV, et al: Diagnosis of infection with human immunodeficiency virus type 1 by a DNA polymerase chain reaction assay among infants enrolled in the Women and Infants' Transmission Study, *J Pediatr* 129:198-207, 1996.

540. Comeau AM, Pitt J, Hillyer GV, Landesman S, et al: Early detection of human immunodeficiency virus on dried blood spot specimens: Sensitivity across serial specimens, *J Pediatr* 129:111-118, 1996.

541. Nicholas SW, Sondheimer DL, Willoughby AD, Yaffe SJ, et al: Human immunodeficiency virus infection in childhood, adolescence, and pregnancy: A status report and national research agenda, *Pediatrics* 83:293-308, 1989.

542. Pliner V, Weedon J, Thomas PA, Steketee RW: Incubation period of HIV-1 in perinatally infected children, *AIDS* 12:759-766, 1998.

543. Liu KL, Peters V, Weedon J, Thomas P, et al: Sex differences in morbidity and mortality among children with perinatally acquired human immunodeficiency virus infection in New York city, *Arch Pediatr Adolesc Med* 158:1187-1188, 2004.

544. Falloon J, Pizzo PA: Acquired immunodeficiency syndrome in the infant. In Remington JS, Klein JD, editors: *Infectious Diseases in the Fetus and Newborn Infant*, Philadelphia: 1990, Saunders.

545. Task Force on Pediatric AIDS: Perinatal human immunodeficiency virus (HIV) testing, *Pediatrics* 89:791-794, 1992.

546. Mofenson L: Antiretroviral therapy and interruption of HIV perinatal transmission, *Immunol Allergy Clin North Am* 18:441-463, 1998.

547. Mofenson LM: Can perinatal HIV infection be eliminated in the United States? *JAMA* 282:577-579, 1999.

548. Gibb DM, Tess BH: Interventions to reduce mother-to-child transmission of HIV infection: New developments and current controversies, *AIDS* 13:S93-S102, 1999.

549. DeCock KM, Flowler MG, Mercier E, de VincenziI, et al: Prevention of mother-to-child HIV transmission in resource-poor countries: Translating research into policy and practice, *JAMA* 283:1175-1182, 2000.

550. Mandelbrot L, Landreau-Mascaro A, Rekacewicz C, Berrebi A, et al: Lamivudine-zidovudine combination for prevention of maternal-infant transmission of HIV-1, *JAMA* 285:2083-2093, 2001.

551. Lallemant M, Jourdain G, Le Coeur S, Kim S, et al: A trial of shortened zidovudine regimens to prevent mother-to-child transmission of human immunodeficiency virus type 1, *N Engl J Med* 343:982-990, 2000.

552. Dorenbaum A, Cunningham CK, Gelber RD, Culnane M, et al: Two-dose intrapartum/newborn nevirapine and standard antiretroviral therapy to reduce perinatal HIV transmission, *JAMA* 288:189-198, 2002.

553. Tuomala RE, Shapiro DE, Mofenson LM, Bryson Y, et al: Antiretroviral therapy during pregnancy and the risk of an adverse outcome, *N Engl J Med* 346:1863-1870, 2002.

554. Italian Register for Human Immunodeficiency Virus Infection in Children: Determinants of mother-to-infant human immunodeficiency virus 1 transmission before and after the introduction of zidovudine prophylaxis, *Arch Pediatr Adolesc Med* 156:915-921, 2002.

555. Moodley D, Moodley J, Coovadia H, Gray G, et al: A multicenter randomized controlled trial of nevirapine versus a combination of zidovudine and lamivudine to reduce intrapartum and early postpartum mother-to-child transmission of human immunodeficiency virus type 1, *J Infect Dis* 187:725-735, 2003.

556. Mofenson LM: Tale of two epidemics: The continuing challenge of preventing mother-to-child transmission of human immunodeficiency virus, *J Infect Dis* 187:721-724, 2003.

557. Taha TE, Kumwenda NI, Gibbons A, Broadhead RL, et al: Short post-exposure prophylaxis in newborn babies to reduce mother-to-child transmission of HIV-1: NVAZ randomised clinical trial, *Lancet* 362:1171-1177, 2003.

558. Cunningham CK, Balasubramanian R, Delke I, Maupin R, et al: The impact of race/ethnicity on mother-to-child HIV transmission in the United States in Pediatric AIDS Clinical Trials Group Protocol 316, *J Acquir Immune Defic Syndr Hum Retrovirol* 36:800-807, 2004.

559. Jourdain G, Ngo-Giang-Huong N, LeCoeur S, Bowonwatanuwong C, et al: Intrapartum exposure to Nevirapine and subsequent maternal responses to Nevirapine-based antiretroviral therapy, *N Engl J Med* 351:229-240, 2004.

560. Lallemant M, Jourdain G, LeCoeur S, Mary JY, et al: Single-dose perinatal nevirapine plus standard zidovudine to prevent mother-to-child transmission of HIV-1 in Thailand, *N Engl J Med* 351:217-228, 2004.

561. Coovadia H: Antiretroviral agents: How best to protect infants from HIV and save their mothers from AIDS, *N Engl J Med* 351:289-292, 2004.

562. European Collaborative Study: Mother-to-child transmission of HIV infection in the era of highly active antiretroviral therapy, *Clin Infect Dis* 40:458-465, 2005.

563. Connor EM, Sperling RS, Gelber R: Reduction of maternal-infant transmission of human immunodeficiency virus type 1 with zidovudine treatment, *N Engl J Med* 331:1773-1780, 1994.

564. Sperling RS, Shapiro DE, Coombs RW, Todd JA, et al: Maternal viral load, zidovudine treatment, and the risk of transmission of human immunodeficiency virus type 1 from mother to infant, *N Engl J Med* 335:1621-1629, 1996.

565. Mayaux M-J, Teglas J-P, Mandelbrot L, Berrebi A, et al: Acceptability and impact of zidovudine for prevention of mother-to-child human immunodeficiency virus-1 transmission in France, *J Pediatr* 131:857-862, 1997.

566. Fiscus SA, Adimora AA, Schoenbach VJ, Lim W, et al: Perinatal HIV infection and the effect of zidovudine therapy on transmission in rural and urban counties, *JAMA* 275:1483-1488, 1996.

567. Wade NA, Birkhead GS, Warren BL, Charbonneau TT, et al: Abbreviated regimens of zidovudine prophylaxis and perinatal transmission of the human immunodeficiency virus, *N Engl J Med* 339:1409-1414, 1998.

568. Lindergren ML, Byers RH, Thomas P, Davis SF, et al: Trends in perinatal transmission of HIV/AIDS in the United States, *JAMA* 282:531-538, 1999.

569. Mofenson LM, Lambert JS, Stiehm ER, Bethel J, et al: Risk factors for perinatal transmission of human immunodeficiency virus type 1 in women treated with zidovudine, *N Engl J Med* 341:385-393, 1999.

570. Guay LA, Musoke P, Fleming T, Bagenda D, et al: Intrapartum and neonatal single-dose nevirapine compared with zidovudine for prevention of mother-to-child transmission of HIV-1 in Kampala, Uganda: HIVMET 012 randomised trial, *Lancet* 354:795-802, 1999.

571. Culnane M, Fowler MG, Lee SS, McSherry G, et al: Lack of long-term effects of in utero exposure to zidovudine among uninfected children born to HIV-infected women, *JAMA* 281:151-157, 1999.

572. Maguire A, Sanchez E, Fortuny C, Casabona J, et al: Potential risk factors for vertical HIV-1 transmission in Catalonia, Spain: The protective role of Cesarean section, *AIDS* 11:1851-1857, 1997.

573. European Collaborative Study: Caesarean section and risk of vertical transmission of HIV-1 infection, *Lancet* 343:1464-1467, 1994.

574. International Perinatal HIV Group: The mode of delivery and the risk of vertical transmission of human immunodeficiency virus type 1: A meta-analysis of 15 prospective cohort studies, *N Engl J Med* 340:977-987, 1999.

575. Riley LE, Greene MF: Elective cesarean delivery to reduce the transmission of HIV, *N Engl J Med* 340:1032-1033, 1999.

576. Manderbrot L, Le Chenadec J, Berrebi A, Bongain A, et al: Perinatal HIV-1 transmission: Interaction between zidovudine prophylaxis and mode of delivery in the French Perinatal Cohort, *JAMA* 280:55-60, 1998.

577. Mueller BU, Pizzo PA: Acquired immunodeficiency syndrome in the infant. In Reminston JS, Klein JO, editors: *Infectious Diseases of the Fetus and Newborn Infant*, 4th ed, Philadelphia: 1995, Saunders.

578. Pizzo PA, Eddy J, Falloon J: Effect of continuous intravenous infusion of zidovudine (AZT) in children with symptomatic HIV infection, *N Engl J Med* 319:889-896, 1988.

579. McKinney RE, Maha MA, Connor EM, Feinberg J, et al: A multicenter trial of oral zidovudine in children with advanced human immunodeficiency virus disease, *N Engl J Med* 324:1018-1025, 1991.

580. Brouwers P, Moss H, Wolters P, Eddy J, et al: Effect of continuous-infusion zidovudine therapy on neuropsychologic functioning in children with symptomatic human immunodeficiency virus infection, *J Pediatr* 117:980-985, 1990.

581. DeCarli C, Fugate L, Falloon J, Eddy J, et al: Brain growth and cognitive improvement in children with human immunodeficiency virus–induced encephalopathy after 6 months of continuous infusion zidovudine therapy, *J Acquir Immune Defic Syndr Hum Retrovirol* 4:585-592, 1991.

582. Brivio L, Tornaghi R, Musetti L, Marchisio P, et al: Improvement of auditory brainstem responses after treatment with zidovudine in a child with AIDS, *Pediatr Neurol* 7:53-55, 1991.

583. Tudor-Williams G, St. Clair M, McKinney RE, Maha M, et al: HIV-1 sensitivity to zidovudine and clinical outcome in children, *Lancet* 339:15-19, 1992.

584. Working Group on Antiretroviral Therapy, Connor EM, Pizzo PA, Balis F, et al: Antiretroviral therapy and medical management of the human immunodeficiency virus–infected child, *Pediatr Infect Dis J* 12:513-522, 1993.

585. Hirsch MS, Daquila RT: Therapy for human immunodeficiency virus infection, *N Engl J Med* 328:1686-1695, 1993.

586. Husson RN, Mueller BU, Farley M, Woods L, et al: Zidovudine and didanosine combination therapy in children with human immunodeficiency virus infection, *Pediatrics* 93:316-322, 1994.

587. Luzuriaga K, Bryson Y, Krogstad P, Robinson J, et al: Combination treatment with zidovudine, didanosine, and nevirapine in infants with human immunodeficiency virus type 1 infection, *N Engl J Med* 336:1343-2349, 1997.

588. Morens DM: Enteroviral disease in early infancy, *J Pediatr* 92:374-377, 1978.

589. Berlin LE, Rorabaugh ML, Heldrich F, Roberts K, et al: Aseptic meningitis in infants <2 years of age: Diagnosis and etiology, *J Infect Dis* 168:888-892, 1993.

590. Rorabaugh ML, Berlin LE, Heldrich F, Roberts K, et al: Aseptic meningitis in infants younger than 2 years of age: Acute illness and neurologic complications, *Pediatrics* 92:206-211, 1993.

591. Cherry JD: Enterovirus and parechovirus infections. In Remington JS, Klein JO, Wilson CB, et al, editors: *Infectious Diseases of the Fetus and Newborn Infant*, 6th ed, Philadelphia: 2006, Elsevier Saunders.

592. Overall JC Jr: Viral infections of the fetus and neonate. In Feigin RD, Cherry JD, editors: *Textbook of Pediatric Infectious Diseases*, 4th ed, Philadelphia: 1998, Saunders.

593. Euscher E, Davis J, Holzman I, Nuovo GJ: Coxsackie virus infection of the placenta associated with neurodevelopmental delays in the newborn, *Obstet Gynecol* 98:1019-1026, 2001.

594. Sauerbrei A, Gluck B, Jung K, Bittrich H, et al: Congenital skin lesions caused by intrauterine infection with coxsackievirus B3, *Infection* 28:326-328, 2000.

595. Feuer R, Pagarigan RR, Harkins S, Liu F, et al: Coxsackievirus targets proliferating neuronal progenitor cells in the neonatal CNS, *J Neurosci* 25:2434-2444, 2005.

596. Gauntt CJ, Gudvangen RJ, Brans YW, Marlin AE: Coxsackievirus group B antibodies in the ventricular fluid of infants with severe anatomic defects in the central nervous system, *Pediatrics* 76:64-68, 1985.

597. Katz SL: Case records of the Massachusetts General Hospital, *N Engl J Med* 272:907, 1965.

598. Cherry JD, Soriano F, Johns CL: Search for perinatal viral infection: A prospective, clinical, virologic, and serologic study, *Am J Dis Child* 116:245, 1968.

599. Cherry JD: Enteroviruses. In Remington JS, Klein JO, editors: *Infectious Diseases of the Fetus and Newborn Infant*, 2nd ed, Philadelphia: 1983, Saunders.

600. Cherry JD: Enteroviruses. In Remington JS, Klein JO, editors: *Infectious Diseases of the Fetus and Newborn Infant*, 4th ed, Philadelphia: 1995, Saunders.

601. Javett SN, Heymann S, Mundel B: Myocarditis in the newborn infant: A study of an outbreak associated with Coxsackie group B virus infection in a maternity home in Johannesburg, *J Pediatr* 48:1-22, 1956.

602. Brightman VJ, Scott TF, Westphal M, Boggs TR: An outbreak of coxsackie B-5 virus infection in a newborn nursery, *J Pediatr* 69:179-192, 1966.

603. Eilard T, Kyllerman M, Wennerblom I, Eeg-Olofsson O, et al: An outbreak of Coxsackie virus type B2 among neonates in an obstetrical ward, *Acta Paediatr Scand* 63:103-107, 1974.

604. Modlin JF: Perinatal echovirus infection: Insights from a literature review of 61 cases of serious infection and 16 outbreaks in nurseries, *Infect Dis* 8:918-926, 1986.

605. Rabkin CS, Telzak EE, Ho M-S, Goldstein J, et al: Outbreak of echovirus 11 infection in hospitalized neonates, *Pediatr Infect Dis J* 7:186-190, 1988.

606. Eichenwald HF, Ababio A, Arky AM, Hartman AP: Epidemic diarrhea in premature and older infants caused by ECHO virus type 18, *JAMA* 166:1563-1566, 1958.

607. Miller DG, Gabrielson MO, Bart KJ: An epidemic of aseptic meningitis, primarily among infants, caused by echovirus 11, *Pediatrics* 41:77-90, 1968.

608. Cramblett HG, Haynes RE, Azimi PH, Hilty MD, et al: Nosocomial infection with echovirus type 11 in handicapped and premature infants, *Pediatrics* 51:603-607, 1973.

609. Verboon-Maciolek MA, Groenendaal F, Cowan F, Govaert P, et al: White matter damage in neonatal enterovirus meningoencephalitis, *Neurology* 66:1267-1269, 2006.

610. Heineberg H, Gold E, Robbins FC: Differences in interferon content in tissues of mice of various ages infected with Coxsackie B1 virus, *Proc Soc Exp Biol Med* 115:947-953, 1964.

611. Boring WD, Angevine DM, Walker DL: Factors influencing host-virus interactions. I. A comparison of viral multiplication and histopathology in infant, adult, and cortisone-treated adult mice infected with the Conn-5 strain, *J Exp Med* 102:753-766, 1955.

612. Kunin CM: Virus-tissue union and pathogenesis of enterovirus infections, *J Immunol* 88:556-569, 1962.

613. Kunin CM: Cellular susceptibility to enteroviruses, *Bacteriol Rev* 28:382-390, 1964.

614. Kibrick S, Benirschke K: Acute aseptic myocarditis and meningoencephalitis in the newborn child infected with coxsackie virus group B, type 3, *N Engl J Med* 255:883-889, 1956.

615. Moossy J, Geer JC: Encephalomyelitis, myocarditis and adrenal cortical necrosis in Coxsackie B virus infection, *Arch Pathol* 70:614-622, 1960.

616. McLean DM, Donohue WL, Snelling CE, Wyllie JC: Coxsackie B5 virus as a cause of neonatal encephalitis and myocarditis, *Can Med Assoc J* 85:1046-1051, 1961.

617. Fechner RE, Smith MG, Middelkamp JN: Coxsackie B virus infection of the newborn, *Am J Pathol* 42:493-505, 1963.

618. Richardson EP: Case records of the Massachusetts General Hospital, *N Engl J Med* 272:907-911, 1965.

619. Kaplan MH, Klein SW, McPhee J, Harper RG: Group B coxsackievirus infections in infants younger than three months of age: A serious childhood illness, *Rev Infect Dis* 5:1019-1032, 1983.

620. Haddad J, Messer J, Gut JP, Chaigne D, et al: Neonatal echovirus encephalitis with white matter necrosis, *Neuropediatrics* 21:215-217, 1990.

621. Delaney TB, Fukunaga FH: Myocarditis in a newborn infant with encephalomeningitis due to Coxsackie virus group B, type 5, *N Engl J Med* 259:234-236, 1958.

622. Schurmann W, Statz A, Mertens T, Gladtke E, et al: Two cases of coxsackie B2 infection in neonates: Clinical, virological, and epidemiological aspects, *Eur J Pediatr* 140:59-63, 1983.

623. Wong SN, Tam AY, Ng TK, Tong CY, et al: Fatal coxsackie B1 virus infection in neonates, *Pediatr Infect Dis J* 8:638-641, 1989.

624. Estes ML, Rorke LB: Liquefactive necrosis in Coxsackie B encephalitis, *Arch Pathol Lab Med* 110:1090-1092, 1986.

625. Gold E, Carver DH, Heineberg H: Viral infection: A possible cause of sudden unexpected death in infants, *N Engl J Med* 264:53-60, 1961.

626. Chalhub EG, DeVivo DC, Siegel BA, Gado MH, et al: Coxsackie A9 focal encephalitis associated with acute infantile hemiplegia and porencephaly, *Neurology* 27:574-579, 1977.

627. Eichenwald HF, Kostevalov I: Immunologic responses of premature and full-term infants to infection with certain viruses, *Pediatrics* 25:829-839, 1960.

628. Butterfield J, Moscovici C, Berry C, Kempe CH: Cystic emphysema in premature infants: A case report of an outbreak with isolation of type 19 ECHO virus in one case, *N Engl J Med* 268:18-21, 1963.

629. Rawls WE, Shorter RG, Herrmann EC: Fatal neonatal illness associated with ECHO 9 (Coxsackie A-23) virus, *Pediatrics* 33:278-280, 1964.

630. Haynes RE, Cramblett HG, Hilty MD, Azimi PH, et al: ECHO virus type 3 infections in children: Clinical and laboratory studies, *J Pediatr* 80:589-595, 1972.

631. Philip AG, Larson EJ: Overwhelming neonatal infection with ECHO 19 virus, *J Pediatr* 82:391-397, 1973.

632. Cho CT, Janelle JG, Behbehani A: Severe neonatal illness associated with ECHO 9 virus infection, *Clin Pediatr* 12:304-305, 1973.

633. Bose CL, Gooch WM 3rd, Sanders GO, Bucciarelli RL: Dissimilar manifestations of intrauterine infection with echovirus 11 in premature twins, *Arch Pathol Lab Med* 107:361-363, 1983.

634. Wreghitt TG, Gandy GM, King A, Sutehall G: Fatal neonatal echo 7 virus infection, *Lancet* 2:465, 1984.

635. Chow KC, Lee CC, Lin YY, Shen WC, et al: Congenital enterovirus 71 infection: A case study with virology and immunohistochemistry, *Clin Infect Dis* 31:509-512, 2000.

636. Lake AM, Lauer BA, Clark JC, Wesenberg RL, et al: Enterovirus infections in neonates, *J Pediatr* 89:787-791, 1976.

637. Herrmann EC Jr: Experience in providing a viral diagnostic laboratory compatible with medical practice. *Mayo Clin Proc* 42:112-123, 1967.

638. Glimaker M, Johansson B, Olcen P, Ehrnst A, et al: Detection of enteroviral RNA by polymerase chain reaction in cerebrospinal fluid from patients with aseptic meningitis. *Scand J Infect Dis* 25:547-557, 1993.

639. Kitamoto I, Nakayama M, Miyazaki C, Minami T, et al: Evoked potentials in neonates and infants with aseptic meningitis, *Pediatr Neurol* 5:342-346, 1989.

640. Sells CJ, Carpenter RL, Ray CG: Sequelae of central nervous system enterovirus infections, *N Engl J Med* 293:1-4, 1975.

641. Bergman I, Painter MJ, Wald ER, Chiponis D, et al: Outcome in children with enteroviral meningitis during the first year of life, *J Pediatr* 110:705-709, 1987.

642. Farmer K, MacArthur BA, Clay MM: A follow-up study of 15 cases of neonatal meningoencephalitis due to coxsackie virus B5, *J Pediatr* 87:568-571, 1975.

643. Sever J, White LR: Intrauterine viral infections, *Annu Rev Med* 19:471-486, 1968.

644. Gershon AA: Chickenpox, measles and mumps. In Remington JS, Klein JO, editors: *Infectious Diseases of the Fetus and Newborn Infant*, 4th ed, Philadelphia: 1995, Saunders.

645. Abler C: Neonatal varicella, *Am J Dis Child* 107:492, 1964.

646. Pearson HE: Parturition varicella-zoster, *Obstet Gynecol* 23:21-27, 1964.
647. Newman CG: Perinatal varicella, *Lancet* 2:1159-1161, 1965.
648. Brunell PA: Varicella-zoster infections in pregnancy, *JAMA* 199:315-317, 1967.
649. Meyers JD: Congenital varicella in term infants: Risk reconsidered, *J Infect Dis* 129:215-217, 1974.
650. Brunell PA: Fetal and neonatal varicella-zoster infections, *Semin Perinatol* 7:47-56, 1983.
651. Brunell PA: Varicella in pregnancy, the fetus, and the newborn: Problems in management, *J Infect Dis* 166(Suppl):S42-S47, 1992.
652. Gershon AA: Chickenpox, measles, and mumps. In Remington JS, Klein JO, Wilson CB, et al, editors: *Infectious Diseases of the Fetus and Newborn Infant*, 6th ed, Philadelphia: 2006, Elsevier Saunders.
653. Nankervis GA, Gold E: Varicella-zoster viruses. In Kaplan AS, editor: *The Herpesviruses*, New York: 1973, Academic Press.
654. Brunell PA: Placental transfer of varicella-zoster antibody, *Pediatrics* 38:1034-1038, 1966.
655. Garcia AG: Fetal infection in chickenpox and alastrim, with histopathologic study of the placenta, *Pediatrics* 32:895-901, 1963.
656. McIntosh D, Isaacs D: Varicella zoster virus infection in pregnancy, *Arch Dis Child* 68:1-2, 1993.
657. Pignotti MS, Indolfi G, Messineo A, Donzelli G: Aseptic meningitis in neonatal varicella complicated by *Escherichia coli* sepsis, *Eur J Pediatr* 163:343-344, 2004.
658. DeNicola LK, Hanshaw JB: Congenital and neonatal varicella, *J Pediatr* 94:175-176, 1979.
659. Preblud SR, Zaia JA, Nieberg PI: Management of pregnant patient exposed to varicella, *J Pediatr* 95:334-339, 1979.
660. Miller E, Cradock-Watson JE, Ridehalgh MK: Outcome in newborn babies given anti–varicella-zoster immunoglobulin after perinatal maternal infection with varicella-zoster virus, *Lancet* 2:371-373, 1989.
661. Laforet EG, Lynch CL Jr: Multiple congenital defects following maternal varicella, *N Engl J Med* 236:534-539, 1947.
662. Rinvik R: Congenital varicella encephalomyelitis in surviving newborn, *Am J Dis Child* 117:231-235, 1969.
663. McKendry JB, Bailey JD: Congenital varicella associated with multiple defects, *Can Med Assoc J* 108:66-68, 1973.
664. Dodion-Fransen J, Dekegel D, Thiry L: Congenital varicella-zoster infection related to maternal disease in early pregnancy, *Scand J Infect Dis* 5:149-153, 1973.
665. Savage MO, Moosa A, Gordon RR: Maternal varicella infection as a cause of fetal malformations, *Lancet* 1:352-354, 1973.
666. Srabstein JC, Morris N, Larke RP, DeSa DJ, et al: Is there a congenital varicella syndrome? *J Pediatr* 84:239-243, 1974.
667. Asha Bai PV, John TJ: Congenital skin ulcers following varicella in late pregnancy, *J Pediatr* 94:65-72, 1979.
668. Kotchmar GS Jr, Grose C, Brunell PA: Complete spectrum of the varicella congenital defects syndrome in 5-year-old child, *Pediatr Infect Dis* 3:142-145, 1984.
669. Randel RC, Kearns DB, Nespeca MP, Scher CA, et al: Vocal cord paralysis as a presentation of intrauterine infection with varicella-zoster virus, *Pediatrics* 97:127-128, 1996.
670. Wheatley R, Morton RE, Nicholson J: Chickenpox in mid-trimester pregnancy: Always innocent? *Dev Med Child Neurol* 38:455-466, 1996.
671. Schulze A, Dietzsch HJ: The natural history of varicella embryopathy: A 25-year follow-up, *J Pediatr* 137:871-874, 2000.
672. Petignat P, Vial Y, Laurini R, Hohlfeld P: Fetal varicella-herpes zoster syndrome in early pregnancy: Ultrasonographic and morphological correlation, *Prenat Diagn* 21:121-124, 2001.

673. Sauerbrei A, Pawlak J, Wutzler P: Intracerebral varicella-zoster virus reactivation in congenital varicella syndrome, *Dev Med Child Neurol* 45:837-840, 2003.
674. Mazzella M, Arioni C, Bellini C, Allegri AEM, et al: Severe hydrocephalus associated with congenital varicella syndrome, *CMAJ* 168:561-563, 2003.
675. Corbeel L: Congenital varicella syndrome, *Eur J Pediatr* 163:345-346, 2004.
676. Pastuszak AL, Levy M, Schick B, Zuber C, et al: Outcome after maternal varicella infection in the first 20 weeks of pregnancy, *N Engl J Med* 330:901-905, 1994.
677. Enders G, Miller E, Cradock-Watson J, Bolley L, et al: Consequences of varicella and herpes zoster in pregnancy: Prospective study of 1739 cases, *Lancet* 1:1548-1551, 1994.
678. Mouly F, Mirlesse V, Meritet JF, Rozenberg F, et al: Prenatal diagnosis of fetal varicella-zoster virus infection with polymerase chain reaction of amniotic fluid in 107 cases, *Am J Obstet Gynecol* 177:894-898, 1997.
679. Birthistle K, Carrington D: Fetal varicella syndrome: A reappraisal of the literature. A review prepared for the UK Advisory Group on Chickenpox on behalf of the British Society for the Study of Infection, *J Infect* 36(Suppl 1):25-29, 1998.
680. Bennet R, Forsgren M, Herin P: Herpes zoster in a 2-week-old premature infant with possible congenital varicella encephalitis, *Acta Paediatr Scand* 74:979-981, 1985.
681. Leis AA, Butler IJ: Infantile herpes zoster ophthalmicus and acute hemiparesis following intrauterine chickenpox, *Neurology* 37:1537-1538, 1987.
682. Scheffer IE, Baraitser M, Brett EM: Severe microcephaly associated with congenital varicella infection, *Dev Med Child Neurol* 33:912-929, 1991.
683. Alkalay AL, Pomerance JJ, Rimoin DL: Fetal varicella syndrome, *J Pediatr* 111:320-323, 1987.
684. Komrower GM, Williams BI, Stones PB: Lymphocytic choriomeningitis in the newborn: Probable transplacental infection, *Lancet* 1:697-698, 1955.
685. Ackermann R, Korver G, Turss R, Wonne R, et al: Prenatal infection with the lymphocytic choriomeningitis virus, *Dtsch Med Wochenschr* 13:629-632, 1974.
686. Sheinbergas MM: Hydrocephalus due to prenatal infection with the lymphocytic choriomeningitis virus, *Infection* 4:185-191, 1976.
687. Barton LL, Budd SC, Morfitt WS: Congenital lymphocytic choriomeningitis virus infection in twins, *Pediatr Infect Dis J* 12:942-946, 1993.
688. Larsen PD, Chartrand SA, Tomashek KM, Hauser LG, et al: Hydrocephalus complicating lymphocytic choriomeningitis virus infection, *Pediatr Infect Dis J* 12:528-531, 1993.
689. Mets MB, Barton LL, Khan AS, Ksiazek TG: Lymphocytic choriomeningitis virus: An underdiagnosed cause of congenital chorioretinitis, *Am J Ophthalmol* 130:209-215, 2000.
690. Barton LL, Mets MB, Beauchamp CL: Lymphocytic choriomeningitis virus: Emerging fetal teratogen, *Am J Obstet Gynecol* 187:1715-1716, 2002.
690a. Bonthius DJ, Wright R, Tseng B, Barton L, et al: Congenital lymphocytic choriomeningitis virus infection: spectrum of disease, *Ann Neurol* 62:347-355, 2007.
690b. Bonthius DJ, Nichols B, Harb H, Mahoney J, et al: Lymphocytic choriomeningitis virus infection of the developing brain: Critical role of host age, *Ann Neurol* 62:356-374, 2007.
691. Osamura T, Mizuta R, Yoshioka H, Fushiki S: Isolation of adenovirus type-11 from the brain of a neonate with pneumonia and encephalitis, *Eur J Pediatr* 152:496-499, 1993.
692. Hayes EB, O'Leary DR: West Nile virus infection: A pediatric perspective, *Pediatrics* 113:1375-1381, 2004.

Chapter 21

Bacterial and Fungal Intracranial Infections

Bacterial infections of the central nervous system (CNS) in the newborn are common and are of major clinical importance. By far the most frequent of these infections is neonatal bacterial meningitis, and this chapter deals with this disorder in detail. Other bacterial processes include primary intracranial infections (e.g., epidural and subdural empyema and brain abscess) and disorders in which involvement of the CNS is secondary to extraneural infection (e.g., subacute bacterial endocarditis with focal embolic encephalitis, neonatal botulism, and neonatal tetanus). Because most of these bacterial diseases are exceedingly rare, and one (botulism) is discussed in Chapter 18, I review briefly in this chapter only brain abscess and neonatal tetanus. Systemic candidiasis, a disseminated fungal infection, also is discussed briefly (rather than in Chapter 20) because the manifestations thereof, which include meningitis and brain abscess, are related more closely to the subject matter of this chapter.

BACTERIAL MENINGITIS

Bacterial meningitis is the most common and serious variety of neonatal intracranial bacterial infection. In most cases, bacterial meningitis is associated with recognizable bacteremia (i.e., sepsis). The disorder is usually fulminating in evolution but is amenable to therapeutic intervention. Indeed, prompt recognition and appropriate therapy of bacterial meningitis are major challenges in the care of the neonatal patient.

Early-Onset and Late-Onset Bacterial Sepsis and Meningitis

Certain basic and common themes recur in any discussion of neonatal bacterial sepsis and meningitis. Perhaps most prominent of these themes is the dual pattern of illness observed with the major etiological agents for neonatal bacterial meningitis (see following discussion). Thus, early-onset and late-onset disease often can be readily distinguished (Table 21-1).[1-19] In *early-onset disease* (i.e., onset usually in the first days of life), infection appears to be derived near the time of delivery from an infected birth canal. Understandably, obstetrical complications are common, and infants are often of low birth weight. Multisystemic manifestations are prominent. In *late-onset disease* (i.e., onset usually after the first few days of life), infection may still have been acquired from the mother but frequently is

acquired from contacts with infected medical personnel, other infants, contaminated equipment, and vascular access devices or other materials. Meningitis is often the dominant manifestation of late-onset disease.

The major bacterial causes of early- versus late-onset sepsis are shown in Table 21-2. Group B *Streptococcus* is the most prominent early-onset pathogen, whereas coagulase-negative *Staphylococcus* (CONS) (e.g., *Staphylococcus epidermidis*), becomes very prominent in late-onset sepsis, especially sepsis after very long hospital stays (> 30 days). These organisms are part of the normal skin and mucosal flora and induce infection in the presence of prolonged indwelling vascular catheters and related features of neonatal intensive care, especially of very premature infants. *Pseudomonas* and related gram-negative organisms that contaminate moist ventilatory equipment also become prominent in late-onset sepsis. *Escherichia coli* and *Klebsiella* species account for 20% to 25% of both early-onset and late-onset cases. Although the causes of neonatal meningitis reflect the causes of neonatal sepsis, the relative proportions for each organism differ somewhat because of the varying propensity to invade the CNS (see later).

In the ensuing discussion, I review the etiology, pathogenesis, neuropathology, clinical features, diagnostic aspects, prognosis, and management of neonatal bacterial *meningitis*. Particular emphasis is placed on aspects most relevant to neonatal neurology. Where relevant, the discussion centers on specific aspects related to a particular organism, but, in general, the features of neonatal bacterial meningitis caused by most organisms exhibit more similarities than differences.

Etiology

The major organisms associated with neonatal meningitis and their relative frequency as current etiological agents are shown in Table 21-3.[5,10,12,16,20-29] Although relative frequencies vary somewhat from one medical center to another and over time, the data are at least representative of cases largely in medical centers in North America. Group B *Streptococcus* is the single most commonly encountered organism, with *E. coli* second. *Listeria monocytogenes* is the third most common organism and accounts for approximately 5% of cases in most series in North America. The remaining cases are accounted for principally by other streptococcal and staphylococcal species, by other

TABLE 21-1   Major Features of Early-Onset and Late-Onset Bacterial Sepsis-Meningitis*

Major Feature	Early-Onset Disease	Late-Onset Disease
Usual age of onset	First 72 hours	> 7 days
Obstetrical complications	Common	Uncommon
Dominant clinical signs referable to sepsis and respiratory disease	Common	Uncommon
Dominant clinical signs referable to meningitis	Uncommon	Common
Mode of transmission	Mother to infant	Mother to infant
		Human contacts, equipment, vascular access devices, and so forth
Specific serotype	Uncommon	Common

*See text for references.

TABLE 21-2   Bacterial Etiology of Early-Onset and Late-Onset Neonatal Sepsis*

	PERCENTAGE OF TOTAL	
Organism	Early-Onset Sepsis	Late-Onset Sepsis
Group B beta-hemolytic streptococci	50%	5%
Group D streptococci	5%	10%
Coagulase-negative staphylococci	5%	40%[†]
Staphylococcus aureus	5%	10%
Escherichia coli, Klebsiella species	25%	20%
Pseudomonas, Serratia	0%	10%
Miscellaneous	10%	5%

*See text for references.
[†]More common in cases with onset after 30 days, especially in low-birth-weight infants.
Most data from references 14, 17, and 18.

TABLE 21-3   Bacterial Etiology of Neonatal Meningitis*

Bacterial Etiology	Percentage of Total
Group B *Streptococcus*	50%
Other streptococci and staphylococci (including especially group D streptococci, *Streptococcus pneumoniae, Staphylococcus epidermidis,*[†] and *Staphylococcus aureus*)	5%
Escherichia coli	25%
Other gram-negative enteric bacteria (including *Pseudomonas aeruginosa, Klebsiella* and *Enterobacter* species, *Proteus* species, *Citrobacter* species, and *Serratia marcescens*)	10%
Listeria monocytogenes	5%
Other (including *Haemophilus influenzae, Salmonella* species, and *Flavobacterium meningosepticum*)	5%

*See text for references.
[†]Coagulase-negative staphylococci are particularly common etiologies in very-low-birth-weight infants with late-onset meningitis.

gram-negative enteric bacilli, and by a variety of unusual organisms. Particular note should be made of the role of *Staphylococcus aureus* and *S. epidermidis* (CONS*)* in the presence of indwelling catheters, particularly in association with neurosurgical procedures, and the role of *Proteus* species, *Pseudomonas aeruginosa, Serratia marcescens,* and *Flavobacterium meningosepticum* in the presence of respiratory devices using moist inhalation. An occasional newborn infant develops meningitis secondary to *Haemophilus influenzae, Salmonella, Pasteurella multocida, Vibrio cholerae, Mycoplasma hominis,* or several other less commonly known organisms.[5,20-27,30-58]

Pathogenesis

Meningitis is more common in premature infants than in full-term infants and in the first months of life than in succeeding months.[16,32,51,53] Because the final common pathway in the pathogenetic sequence is almost always bacteremia leading to meningitis, a close association exists between the causes and rates of neonatal sepsis and neonatal meningitis. The association is not perfect, however, because certain organisms are particularly efficient at invading the CNS (see later). Sepsis occurs at a rate of approximately 1.5 per 1000 live births, and meningitis occurs at a rate of approximately 0.3 per 1000 live births.[51,53-55] Thus, neonatal meningitis is an enormously important problem, and understanding its pathogenesis will be critical for attempts to reduce the enormity of the problem in the future.

Factors Related to Pregnancy and Delivery

Most cases of neonatal sepsis and meningitis, especially those of early onset, are related to acquisition of bacteria during labor or delivery, after rupture of membranes. Acquisition is principally by parturitional exposure or, less commonly, ascending infection (e.g., after prolonged rupture of membranes). Thus, it is not surprising that important factors predisposing to sepsis and meningitis include a variety of complications of labor and delivery (especially fetal distress, obstetrical trauma, and placental abnormalities), maternal peripartum infection (especially of the genital or urinary tracts), prolonged rupture of membranes (> 24 hours), and chorioamnionitis (Table 21-4).[11,14,21,22,26,28,51,59-67a]

Maternal urinary tract infection associated with neonatal sepsis and meningitis is usually gram negative, and maternal genital infection associated with these neonatal disorders is usually with group B *Streptococcus*. Indeed, genital infection secondary to group B *Streptococcus* (usually asymptomatic) is identifiable at delivery in approximately 15% to 35% of women.[59,61,65,68-77] Approximately 40% to 70% of infants delivered to such women become colonized at one or more mucocutaneous sites (e.g., ear, throat, rectum, and umbilicus). Approximately 2% to 4% of such colonized infants exhibit invasive, early-onset group B streptococcal disease. The incidence is particularly high (8%) in those infants heavily colonized (i.e., found to have three to four positive mucocutaneous sites).

Factors related to pregnancy and delivery are also particularly important in the pathogenesis of early-onset neonatal listeriosis.[59,78-87] Thus, various obstetrical complications are present in the history of approximately half of such patients, and in most cases maternal isolates of serotypes identical to those infecting the infants have been found. In the majority of cases of early-onset neonatal listeriosis, a maternal history of flulike syndrome, unexplained fever, or urinary tract symptoms in the several days to weeks before delivery can be elicited. In keeping with probable fecal-oral transmission of this organism, epidemics of maternal infection during pregnancy and subsequent neonatal listeriosis have been associated with consumption of contaminated foods.[78,84,87] Indeed, unlike the other varieties of neonatal meningitis, listeriosis probably occurs commonly by transplacental passage, as evidenced by the finding of well-developed placentitis with recognizable organisms in carefully studied cases.[80,81,87]

Factors Related to the Infant

Significant host factors operative in the newborn period relate particularly to defense mechanisms versus bacterial infection. Relative defects in so-called *nonspecific* and *specific immunity* have been described in detail.

TABLE 21-4	Neonatal Sepsis-Meningitis: Predisposing Factors Related to Pregnancy and Delivery
Complications of labor and delivery	
Maternal peripartum infection, especially of the genital or urinary tract	
Prolonged rupture of membranes	
Chorioamnionitis	

Nonspecific immunity refers particularly to functions of granulocytic leukocytes and opsonins. *Specific immunity* refers particularly to the T-lymphocyte system and the B-lymphocyte–antibody system. Mononuclear phagocytes and natural killer cells bridge nonspecific and specific immunity. The innate immune system is mediated by the monocyte-macrophage series and is discussed later with regard to specific immunity.

Nonspecific Immunity. Deficiencies of nonspecific immunity include the following: impaired leukocyte chemotaxis, phagocytosis, and bactericidal activity; defective neutrophilic metabolic responses after phagocytosis (e.g., activation of hexose monophosphate shunt and, especially, oxidative metabolism, with diminished generation of the critical bactericidal hydroxyl radical); impaired chemotaxis of the mononuclear phagocyte system, secondary to a functional deficiency of the critical M_3 subset of mononuclear cells; and diminished concentrations of several complement components.[16,60,66,69,70,77,87-92] Moreover, lower fibronectin concentrations in the newborn appear to contribute to diminished opsonization and phagocytosis. These defects are accentuated and especially severe in premature infants and in infants subjected to illnesses of diverse types.

Specific Immunity. Deficiencies of specific humoral immunity have involved the immunoglobulin M (IgM) and immunoglobulin G (IgG) classes of antibodies.[66,92-97] The latter are transferred passively across the placenta, particularly in the third trimester.[95] Thus, some premature infants may have decreased levels of IgG antibodies.[94] IgM and immunoglobulin A (IgA) are not transferred passively across the placenta and are in very low concentrations in the normal newborn. IgM antibodies include several antibody types important in the defense against gram-negative bacteria, and deficiency of these antibodies in the newborn infant may play a role in the susceptibility to gram-negative bacteria.[93] IgA antibodies are abundant at later ages at mucosal surfaces (e.g., the respiratory and gastrointestinal tracts), and their deficiency in the newborn may explain in part the relative ease with which mucosal barriers are colonized and penetrated.[96] Newborn infants have diminished production of these antibodies because of both immaturity of the antibody-producing B cells and plasma cells and diminished T-cell help for antibody production. The deficiency in immune globulins led to clinical trials of the use of intravenous immune globulin in prophylaxis and treatment of bacterial infection in newborns, especially premature newborns.[92,98,99] This approach has not proven useful for general practice.

Of major importance is the function of the *innate immune system* and thereby the monocyte-macrophage defense mechanism. The brain microglial cell, which is derived from monocytes (see Chapter 6), is an important part of this defense. Activation of innate immune cells occurs by way of specific cell surface receptors (i.e., Toll-like receptors [TLRs]), which respond to specific molecular motifs shared by the products of large classes of microorganisms.[100–103] For example, TLR4 is the receptor that recognizes gram-negative bacterial lipopolysaccharide, and TLR2 is the receptor for gram-positive peptidoglycan and lipopeptides. Activation of these receptors triggers an inflammatory response by a mechanism that operates through nuclear factor (NF) kappaB and mitogen-activated protein kinase. A recent study of newborns showed that the basal expression of TLR2 (but not TLR4) is slightly lower in neonatal than in adult phagocytes.[103] In infants with sepsis, TLR2 is sharply up-regulated, unlike TLR4. A similar disturbance of TLR4 responsiveness was shown in neonatal monocytes as a function of gestational age.[104] Thus, the deficits in TLR2 and TLR4 may be relevant to the importance of such gram-positive organisms as group B *Streptococcus* and CONS and of such gram-negative organisms as *E. coli* in neonatal sepsis and meningitis.

Immunological Aspects of Group B Streptococcal Infection. Immunological studies of perinatal group B streptococcal infection illustrated the potential roles of both maternal and host defense factors in pathogenesis.[59,66,77] Thus, using a sensitive, radioactive antigen-binding assay, Baker and Kasper[105,106] showed that the prevalence of antibody to group B *Streptococcus* (capsular polysaccharide of the type III strain) in *mothers* with vaginal colonization was 76% for those whose infants did not develop group B streptococcal disease and only 5% for those whose infants did develop group B streptococcal sepsis or meningitis. These data suggest that this IgG antibody is important in protection of the infant and that passive transfer across the placenta did not occur because of maternal failure to synthesize the antibody. In addition, the infants with sepsis or meningitis had low levels of antibody *after* recovery, a finding suggesting that, in addition, these infants also failed to synthesize this IgG component. Similarly, infants who develop group B streptococcal sepsis have been shown to exhibit defective humoral (opsonic activity) and neutrophilic responses to their infecting strain.[107]

Factors Related to the Neonatal Environment

Certain factors related to the neonatal environment increase the risk of sepsis and meningitis, including the following: use of inhalation therapy equipment; use of aerosols; use of vascular, umbilical, and intraventricular indwelling catheters; and exposure to nursery personnel, parents, or other infants harboring pathogenic organisms.[3,14,16,22,51,66,108–110] Operation of some of these factors may be suggested by the organism causing the sepsis or meningitis, as discussed earlier. Horizontal (or nosocomial) transmission of an organism from human contacts has been studied, particularly for group B *Streptococcus*. Thus, nosocomial infection rates of up to 40% have been reported, particularly in medical centers in which high rates of newborns are already colonized at birth (by vertical transmission from mother) and in which high daily census rates are reported, thereby favoring cross-contamination of infants by nursery personnel.[59,111,112] The particular importance of factors related to neonatal intensive care is illustrated by the marked increase in CONS infections with increasing time in neonatal intensive care (see Table 21-2). This issue is particularly important in very premature infants, in whom later-onset sepsis is related primarily to CONS and of whom nearly 80% have a central vascular catheter in place at the time of infection.[14] In the subset of very-low-birth-weight infants, CONS are important etiological agents. Indeed, in a series of 134 very-low-birth-weight (< 1500 g) infants with meningitis, 76% of whom weighed less than 1000 g at birth, 29% had positive cerebrospinal fluid (CSF) and blood cultures for CONS.[113]

Factors Related to the Microorganism

Specific Serotypes Related to Meningitis. The propensity for specific strains of group B *Streptococcus*, *E. coli*, and *L. monocytogenes* to be most commonly responsible for neonatal meningitis suggests important pathogenetic roles for the microorganism itself. (Recall the earlier discussion concerning innate immunity and the risk of infection by gram-negative and gram-positive organisms.) Thus, serotype III of group B *Streptococcus*, K1 strains of *E. coli*, and serotype IVb of *L. monocytogenes* are the predominant specific types of these three bacteria that cause neonatal meningitis (Table 21-5).[1,51,59,66,67,82,85,114] Approximately 70% to 80% of all cases of neonatal meningitis are caused by these three bacterial types.

Importance of Capsular Polysaccharides. The likelihood that capsular polysaccharides reflect, to a considerable degree, an intrinsic virulence of these organisms is suggested by in vivo and in vitro observations.[51,59,66,77,87,114–117] Studies with immature rats demonstrated, for K1 strains of *E. coli* relative to other *E. coli* strains, a high virulence, particularly regarding

TABLE 21-5 Relationship between Severity of Neonatal Infection and Specific Strain of Group B *Streptococcus*, *Escherichia coli*, and *Listeria monocytogenes*

Organism	CLINICAL DISEASE*		
	Asymptomatic	Sepsis	Meningitis
Group B *Streptococcus* serotype III	36%	32%	85%
Escherichia coli K1 strain	12%	39%	84%
Listeria monocytogenes serotype IVb	?	42% (early-onset disease)	78% (late-onset disease)

*Data for each clinical disorder expressed as a percentage of total cases (caused by the indicated bacterium) resulting from the specific serotype. Data from references 1, 114, and 274.

TABLE 21-6 Outcome of Neonatal Meningitis Caused by K1 and Non-K1 Strains of *Escherichia coli*

Type of *Escherichia coli*	OUTCOME		
	Normal	Neurological Sequelae	Dead
Non-K1 strains	8 (89%)	1 (11%)	0
K1 strains	19 (40%)	14 (29%)	15 (31%)

n = 57.
Data from McCracken GH Jr, Sarff LD, Glode MP, Mize SG, et al: Relation between *Escherichia coli* K1 capsular polysaccharide antigen and clinical outcome in neonatal meningitis, *Lancet* 2:246–250, 1974.

bacteremia and meningitis, that was age related.[116] The younger the animal, the greater was the likelihood of serious disease. Moreover, investigators showed that group B *Streptococcus* type III and K1 strains of *E. coli* have distinctive capsules, which contain polysaccharide with sialic acid in high concentration (≥25% of total carbohydrate).[106,114,115,117] (This distinctive polysaccharide for *E. coli* is termed *K1*, hence the name *K1 strain*.) A relation of the capsular polysaccharide antigen to virulence is suggested by the different outcomes of *E. coli* meningitis secondary to K1 and non-K1 strains (Table 21-6).[118] In addition to a marked preponderance of cases secondary to K1 strains, whereas 60% of reported infants with meningitis secondary to K1 strains died or exhibited neurological sequelae, only 11% of infants with meningitis secondary to non-K1 strains exhibited the poor outcome (see Table 21-6). A protein component of the outer membrane of the K1 strain of *E. coli*, OmpA, was also shown to be critical for the capacity of this strain to penetrate brain endothelial cells and thus to cause intracranial infection.[119] The relation of the capsular polysaccharide antigen to virulence is supported further by the studies reviewed previously, relating the occurrence of group B streptococcal type III neonatal disease to the deficiency in the mother and in the newborn of antibody against the specific capsular polysaccharide of that organism.

Neuropathology

Major Features

The neuropathology of bacterial meningitis may be considered in terms of acute and chronic changes (Table 21-7). Moreover, certain additional histological features are particularly characteristic of infection with specific organisms, and these features are discussed separately.

Acute Changes

The acute changes of bacterial meningitis are dramatic and include arachnoiditis, ventriculitis, vasculitis, cerebral edema, infarction, and associated encephalopathy (see Table 21-7).[88,120-124] Because the hallmark of the disease is arachnoiditis, this aspect is discussed first; however, the neuropathological progression of neonatal bacterial meningitis probably begins with choroid plexitis and ventriculitis (Fig. 21-1). I discuss the arachnoiditis first, because it is the dominant feature of bacterial meningitis.

Arachnoiditis. The hallmark of bacterial meningitis is infiltration of the arachnoid with inflammatory cells.

TABLE 21-7 Major Neuropathological Features of Neonatal Bacterial Meningitis

Acute
Arachnoiditis
Ventriculitis: choroid plexitis
Vasculitis
Cerebral edema
Infarction
Associated encephalopathy (cortical neuronal necrosis, periventricular leukomalacia)

Chronic
Hydrocephalus
Multicystic encephalomalacia: porencephaly
Cerebral cortical and white matter atrophy
Cerebral cortical developmental (organizational) defects (?)

The exudate is predominant over the base of the brain in approximately one half of the cases and is distributed more evenly in most of the remainder (Fig. 21-2). The evolution of this inflammatory response was well described by Berman and Banker.[88]

In the acute state (i.e., *approximately the first week*), the predominant cells in the arachnoidal (and ventricular) exudate are polymorphonuclear leukocytes. Bacteria are visible, free, and within polymorphonuclear leukocytes and macrophages. The inflammatory exudate is particularly prominent around blood vessels and

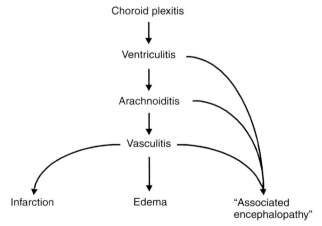

Figure 21-1 **Neuropathological progression of neonatal bacterial meningitis.** The process probably begins with choroid plexitis and ventriculitis. The pathogenesis of associated encephalopathy, especially cerebral cortical neuronal injury and periventricular leukomalacia, is detailed in Figure 21-9.

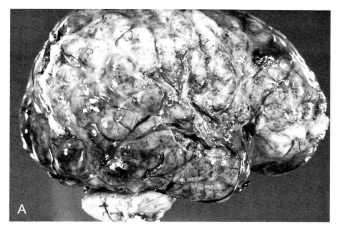

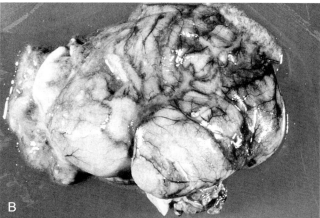

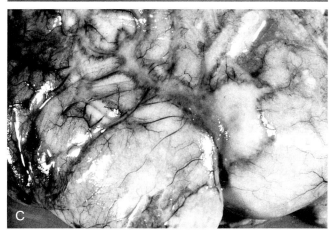

Figure 21-2 Neonatal bacterial meningitis: arachnoidal exudate.
A, From an infant with group B streptococcal meningitis who died at 12 days of age. This right lateral view of the cerebrum shows thick arachnoidal exudate. **B,** From an infant who died at 13 days of age with *Escherichia coli* meningitis. This left lateral view of the cerebrum shows thick arachnoidal exudate, especially prominent in the region of the sylvian fissure. **C,** Closer view of the exudate in the region of the sylvian fissure. *(A, From Bell WE, McCormick WF: Neurologic Infections in Children, Philadelphia: 1975, Saunders.)*

macrophages. Lymphocytes and plasma cells are present in relatively small numbers, and this paucity is a characteristic feature of neonatal meningitis. Whether this apparent deficiency of cells involved in the immunological response plays a role in the relative tenacity of neonatal bacterial meningitis remains to be determined but seems plausible. A prominent feature of this stage of the disease is infiltration of cranial nerve roots by the exudate; particular involvement occurs in the subarachnoid space of the posterior fossa and especially affects cranial nerves III through VIII. This involvement is clinically relevant (see subsequent discussion). *After approximately 3 weeks,* the exudate decreases in amount and consists of mononuclear cells. Thick strands of collagen become apparent as arachnoidal fibrosis begins to develop. This process is probably important in the genesis of the obstructions to CSF flow that result in hydrocephalus.

The characteristics of the arachnoiditis caused by different bacteria vary little. However, *early-onset group B streptococcal* meningitis is accompanied by *much less arachnoidal inflammation* than is late-onset meningitis.[59] Indeed, approximately 75% of cases of early-onset meningitis (i.e., positive culture results) are said to exhibit little or no evidence of "leptomeningeal inflammation" at autopsy.[59] It is not clear whether the relative lack of arachnoidal inflammatory response relates to rapidity of death after onset of symptoms or to immaturity of host responses to infection within the CNS of premature infants (who represent the largest proportion of fatal cases of early-onset group B streptococcal meningitis).

Ventriculitis. *Ventriculitis* (i.e., inflammatory exudate and bacteria in the ventricular fluid and lining) is a particularly common feature of neonatal meningitis. In the 50 brains studied by Berman and Banker[88] and by Gilles and co-workers,[122] overt ventriculitis was present in 44 (88%). In a collaborative study of 70 infants with meningitis caused by gram-negative bacteria in whom ventricular tap was performed at the time of diagnosis, 51 (73%) had ventriculitis, as manifested by positive cultures with pleocytosis in the ventricular fluid (comparable data are not available for group B streptococcal meningitis). Although precise, controlled data are not available, ventriculitis appears to be more common in neonatal meningitis than in meningitis at later ages.[125]

The ventriculitis is initially characterized by exudate most prominent in the *choroid plexus stroma and just external to the plexus* (Fig. 21-3).[69,88,122] Exudative excrescences from the ventricular surface can be visualized in vivo by cranial ultrasonography (see later discussion). In the second and third weeks of the disease course, the ventricular exudate is associated with active ependymitis, characterized by disruption of the ependymal lining and projections of glial tufts into the ventricular lumen. Later, glial bridges may develop and cause obstruction, particularly at the aqueduct of Sylvius (Fig. 21-4). Less commonly, septations in the lateral ventricle may produce a multiloculated state that is similar to abscess formation. The multiple ventricular

extends into the brain parenchyma along the Virchow-Robin space. In *the second and third weeks* of the disease, the proportion of polymorphonuclear leukocytes decreases gradually and constitutes approximately 25% of the cell population. The predominant cells are now mononuclear, mainly histiocytes and

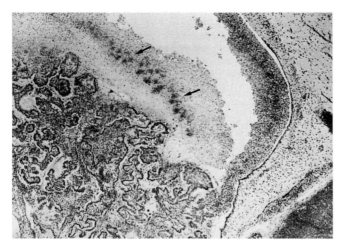

Figure 21-3 **Ventriculitis and choroid plexitis from an infant who died of bacterial meningitis in the first month of life.** Choroid plexus is in the left lower corner. Plexus stroma is filled with cellular exudate. The lateral ventricle contains mass of protein-rich cellular exudate and necrotic debris organized into layers. The middle layer *(arrows)* is composed of colonies of bacteria (hematoxylin and eosin, × 60). *(From Gilles FH, Jammes JL, Berenberg W: Neonatal meningitis: The ventricle as a bacterial reservoir,* Arch Neurol *34:560-562, 1977.)*

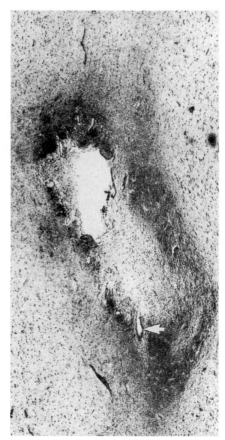

Figure 21-4 **Aqueductal obstruction subsequent to ventriculitis from an infant who died of neonatal bacterial meningitis.** Stain for glial fibers shows formation of glial bridges that have narrowed and partially occluded the aqueduct. The lower portion of the aqueduct is reduced to a small slit *(arrow)* (phosphotungstic acid hematoxylin × 100). *(From Berman PH, Banker BQ: Neonatal meningitis: A clinical and pathological study of 29 cases,* Pediatrics *38:6-24, 1966.)*

obstructions, in fact, may "isolate" portions of the lateral ventricles or the fourth ventricle, cause disproportionate and severe dilation of the affected ventricle, and present a difficult therapeutic problem.[126,127] Ventriculitis with obstructive hydrocephalus may manifest subacutely in newborns (with no history of acute meningitis) after several weeks, especially ventriculitis caused by group B streptococcal meningitis.[128]

The nearly uniform occurrence of ventriculitis in acute bacterial meningitis in the newborn has *pathogenetic and therapeutic implications.* Regarding *pathogenesis,* it appears reasonable to suggest that the initial sequence of events in bacterial invasion of the CNS is for hematogenously borne bacteria to localize first in the choroid plexus and to cause choroid plexitis, with subsequent entrance of bacteria into the ventricular system and later movement to the arachnoid through normal CSF flow (see Fig. 21-1). Gilles and co-workers[122] presented considerable data to support this view, including the high glycogen content of the neonatal choroid plexus, which provides an excellent medium for bacteria. Moreover, an age-related effect is suggested by the postnatal decrease in glycogen content of plexus epithelial cells.[129]

Experimental studies of bacterial meningitis produced in infant rhesus monkeys indicated that infection of the lateral ventricle is a *uniform* feature.[130] Moreover, when discordance between the amount of bacteria in ventricular and subarachnoid CSF samples was observed in these studies of rhesus monkeys, ventricular bacterial densities were greater. These observations further support the notion that the initial events in the genesis of bacterial meningitis are bacteremia and infection of the choroid plexus and lateral ventricles.

The *therapeutic implications* of these data concerning ventriculitis are important and are discussed later in "Management." Suffice it to say here that the ventricle may be a major reservoir of bacterial infection, inaccessible either to systemic antibiotics, which are unable to penetrate the purulent covering over the ventricular lining, or to intraventricular antibiotics, which are unable to reach the choroid plexus epithelium (and particularly inaccessible to intrathecal antibiotics, which are unable to reach the ventricles because of normal CSF flow). Moreover, if obstruction of the ventricular system is added (e.g., at the aqueduct), a closed infection, approximating an extraparenchymal abscess, will result.

Vasculitis. Vasculitis is an almost invariable feature of neonatal bacterial meningitis.[88] The involvement of both arteries and veins can be considered an extension of the inflammatory reaction in the arachnoid and within the ventricles. The arteritis is manifested particularly by inflammatory cells in the adventitia, although involvement of the intima is not uncommon.[20,131] Although the arterial lumen may be narrowed, only rarely is complete occlusion observed. Involvement of veins is severe and includes arachnoidal, cortical, and subependymal veins.[120] In contrast to arterial involvement, phlebitis is frequently complicated by thrombosis and complete occlusion. Multiple fibrin thrombi of adjacent veins are often observed in association with areas of hemorrhagic infarction (see "Infarction," later). The vasculitic changes are apparent in the *first days* of meningitis and become particularly prominent by the second and third weeks.

More similarities than differences exist among various bacteria with regard to the nature and severity of the vascular changes with meningitis. However, vasculitis with thrombosis or even hemorrhage is relatively frequent in early-onset group B streptococcal disease, despite the relatively modest arachnoidal inflammation.[59]

Cerebral Edema. Cerebral edema is a characteristic of the acute stage of neonatal bacterial meningitis (Fig. 21-5). Indeed, the swelling of brain parenchyma is often so severe that the ventricles are reduced to small slits. The difficulty and hazard of performing ventricular puncture in the acute stage are significant because of this phenomenon. The cause of the edema is related primarily to the vasculitis and increased permeability of blood vessels (i.e., vasogenic edema; see Fig. 21-1). This vasogenic component may be complicated by a cytotoxic component, when parenchymal injury occurs (e.g., through infarction), or when impairment of CSF flow results in development of interstitial edema (see later discussion).

Despite the edema, another feature of neonatal bacterial meningitis that is distinctive relative to disease at later ages is the rarity of evidence, clinical or pathological, for herniation of supratentorial structures through the tentorial notch or of cerebellar tonsils into the foramen magnum. This feature may relate to the distensibility of the neonatal cranium, especially because of the separable sutures. This factor also may prevent marked increases in intracranial pressure and therefore impaired cerebral perfusion; studies of intracranial pressure and cerebral blood flow velocity in neonatal bacterial meningitis supported this suggestion (see later discussion).[132] Nevertheless, lethal uncal and cerebellar tonsillar herniation has been documented in neonatal bacterial meningitis.[133] Moreover, the rare phenomenon of anterior fontanelle herniation has been reported to complicate neonatal meningitis.[134]

Infarction. Infarction may be a prominent and serious feature of neonatal bacterial meningitis (see Fig. 21-1). Studies of autopsy cases indicate an incidence of 30% to 50% (see Table 21-7).[88,120,124] More than one half of the cases in Friede's[120] neuropathological series sustained their lesions in the *first week* after the diagnosis of meningitis. Thus, although the vascular lesions become particularly prominent in the second and third weeks, infarction often may be an early event. The lesions most frequently are related to *venous* occlusions and are often hemorrhagic (characteristic of venous infarcts). Occlusion of *multiple adjacent* veins appears to be necessary to result in infarction, as evidenced by the usual demonstration of several thrombosed vessels contiguous to the infarct. The loci of the infarcts, most often, are cerebral cortex and underlying white matter (Fig. 21-6), although subependymal and deep white matter lesions are not uncommon. Involvement of major cerebral arteries may be more common than previously expected because brain imaging in living infants not uncommonly demonstrates lesions in an arterial distribution (see later discussion; Table 21-8).[135] The origin of the infarction is related particularly to the vasculitis, in combination with concomitant thrombotic effects of arachidonic acid metabolites (e.g., thromboxanes, platelet-activating factor), impaired cerebrovascular autoregulation, and decreased cerebral perfusion pressure (caused by systemic hypotension or increased intracranial pressure, or both; see later "Mechanisms of Brain Injury" section). Such a

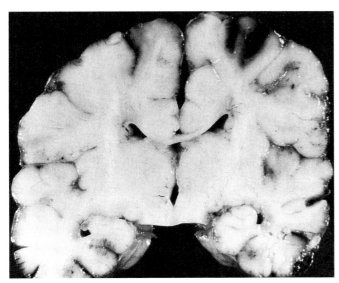

Figure 21-5 Cerebral edema with neonatal bacterial meningitis. Coronal section of the brain from the same infant shown in Figure 21-2A. Note the diffusely swollen appearance of the cerebral parenchyma, resulting in flattened gyri and small, slitlike ventricles. Purulent material is evident in the ventricles (medial aspect), and a hemorrhagic infarct is apparent in the parasagittal region. *(From Bell WE, McCormick WF: Neurologic Infections in Children, Philadelphia: 1975, Saunders.)*

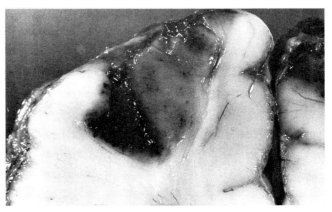

Figure 21-6 Infarction with neonatal bacterial meningitis. Same specimen as shown in Figure 21-5 but a higher-power view of the hemorrhagic infarct in the parasagittal region. The lesion was secondary to cortical vein thrombosis. *(From Bell WE, McCormick WF: Neurologic Infections in Children, Philadelphia: 1975, Saunders.)*

TABLE 21-8   Cerebral Infarction in Neonatal Bacterial Meningitis

≈30% to 50% of autopsy cases
Associated with thrombi in inflamed meningeal, cortical, and/or subependymal veins; venous sinuses; arteries ("arterial distribution" often suggested by brain imaging findings)
Related to a combination of vasculitis, endothelial injury, thrombotic effects of arachidonic acid metabolites, impaired autoregulation, decreased cerebral perfusion pressure

TABLE 21-9   Impaired Cerebral Blood Flow in Bacterial Meningitis

Vascular Narrowing or Obstruction
Vasculitis
Vasospasm
Thrombosis
Increased Intracranial Pressure
Vasogenic > cytotoxic > interstitial edema
Hydrocephalus
Systemic Hypotension
Septic shock
Impaired Cerebrovascular Autoregulation

combination of factors presumably could lead to infarction in the presence of vascular narrowing and not necessarily complete thrombotic occlusion.

Although venous or arterial infarction of cerebral structures predominates, involvement of spinal cord may occur. Indeed, spinal cord necrosis and the clinical picture of a segmental myelopathy may rarely develop.[136]

Associated Encephalopathy. Associated with neonatal bacterial meningitis are parenchymal changes (i.e., "associated encephalopathy") the causes of which have been elucidated increasingly in recent years (see later discussion in "Mechanisms of Brain Injury"). The major changes are (1) diffuse gliosis of regions subjacent to inflammatory exudate, (2) neuronal loss in cerebral cortex and several other brain regions, and (3) periventricular leukomalacia. The first change, parenchymal gliosis, is observed in cerebral cortex (molecular layer and superficial cortical layers), cerebellar cortex (molecular layer), brain stem and spinal cord (marginal white matter), and subependymal regions. These various regions are immediately subjacent to the inflammatory exudate and presumably are injured by the toxic and metabolic factors associated with the bacterial process (see later discussion). The clinical significance of the gliosis is not entirely clear. The second and third changes, involving cortical neurons and periventricular white matter, are similar in topography, in many ways, to hypoxic-ischemic encephalopathy. The cause of these neuronal and white matter lesions probably relates at least in part to *ischemia* (see later discussion; Table 21-9). Moreover, it is likely that concentrations of endotoxin and related cytokines in brain and ventricular fluid are high in gram-negative bacterial meningitis and that the endotoxin could injure cerebral white matter through *activation of innate immunity* in brain (see later and Chapter 6). A similar conclusion applies to the capsular polysaccharides and proteins of group B *Streptococcus*, which also have been shown to be neurotoxic (see Chapter 6). Further data are needed on these issues, because the clinical significance of the neuronal loss and of the white matter injury is almost certainly considerable.

Subdural Effusion and Empyema. One neuropathological feature of neonatal bacterial meningitis,

conspicuous by its relative lack of prominence, is subdural effusion.[88,121] The reason for the notable difference in incidence of significant subdural effusion between meningitis in the newborn and in the infant of 2 to 3 months of age and older is not clear.

Subdural empyema is a very rare acute feature of bacterial meningitis. I have seen three cases since the early 1970s.

Long-Term Changes

The major neuropathological sequelae of neonatal bacterial meningitis are hydrocephalus, multicystic encephalomalacia, and cerebral cortical and white matter atrophy (see Table 21-7).[88,121,123] Experimental observations suggest the possibility of a subsequent impairment in brain development, involving organizational events (see later discussion).

Hydrocephalus. In studies of postmortem material, hydrocephalus is apparent in approximately 50% of cases.[88] Of the 14 autopsy cases of hydrocephalus studied carefully by Berman and Banker,[88] the major obstruction to CSF flow appeared to be at the level of the aqueduct in 4, at the outflow of the fourth ventricle in 2, and in the subarachnoid space (i.e., communicating) in 8. Multiple sites of impairment in CSF flow are probable. Ventricular dilation secondary to obstruction to CSF flow should be distinguished from that secondary to loss of cerebral substance. Because both hydrocephalus and cerebral atrophy are usually present concurrently, this distinction may be difficult.

Multicystic Encephalomalacia and Porencephaly. Multicystic encephalomalacia and porencephaly are the end of the continuum of multifocal parenchymal injury secondary to neonatal bacterial meningitis. The single or multiple cystic areas of destruction in the cerebral hemispheres appear to reflect primarily residua of infarction (Fig. 21-7). In postmortem material, some of the cavities rarely appear to represent abscesses.[120] The implications of multicystic encephalomalacia for neurological outcome are obviously grave.

Cerebral Cortical and White Matter Atrophy. Most commonly, the major neuropathological sequela of neonatal bacterial meningitis is cerebral atrophy, manifested particularly by loss of cerebral cortical neurons

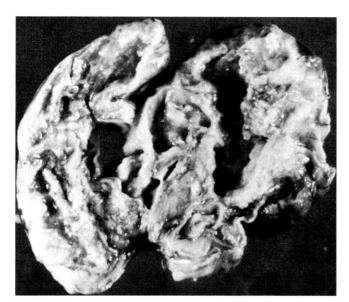

Figure 21-7 Multicystic encephalomalacia following neonatal bacterial meningitis: neuropathology. From an infant with neonatal gram-negative bacterial meningitis who died at 5 weeks of age. This coronal section of the cerebrum shows that the cerebral hemispheres have been converted into a necrotic mass with many cystic cavities of various sizes. The corpus callosum is necrotic, and the ventricles cannot be delineated from cystic spaces in the brain. *(From Bell WE, McCormick WF: Neurologic Infections in Children, Philadelphia: 1975, Saunders.)*

TABLE 21-10	Additional Neuropathological Changes Caused by Specific Microorganisms

***Citrobacter, Serratia marcescens, Proteus, Pseudomonas, Enterobacter* species**
Tissue necrosis, often hemorrhagic, and/or brain abscess
***Listeria monocytogenes* (Transplacental)**
Multifocal granulomata with or without microabscesses

and periventricular white matter. This state appears to be a sequela principally of the associated encephalopathy described previously. Neuronal loss in deep cortical layers and myelin loss in the periventricular region, both areas also infiltrated with glial fibers, are the major histological findings.

Possible Cerebral Cortical Developmental (Organizational) Defects. Experimental data suggest that more refined techniques may reveal subsequent aberrations of brain *development* following neonatal bacterial meningitis. In an infant rat model of bacterial meningitis, disturbances of subsequent dendritic arborization and synaptogenesis were observed.[137] Because of the timing of neonatal bacterial meningitis with regard to brain developmental events (see Chapter 2), it is reasonable to postulate that application of Golgi, immunocytochemical, and electron microscopic techniques to the study of cerebral cortex and myelin of infants who survive the acute state of neonatal meningitis would reveal impairment of cerebral organizational events and, perhaps, myelination. Further data in this regard would be of particular importance concerning the effects of neonatal bacterial meningitis on subsequent neurological outcome.

Neuropathological Changes Characteristic of Specific Microorganisms

Certain neuropathological changes are particularly characteristic of specific microorganisms (Table 21-10).

***Citrobacter* species, *Serratia marcescens, Proteus, Pseudomonas, Enterobacter* species.** These bacteria have a particular propensity to cause severe cerebral necrosis, usually hemorrhagic (see Table 21-10).[41,123,138-146] One consequence of this tissue necrosis, in the presence of bacteremia, is the occurrence of brain abscess. Indeed, the brain abscess may dominate the clinical syndrome, which occasionally may evolve in a less acute fashion than uncomplicated meningitis.[144] (The most common organism leading to meningitis complicated by brain abscess is *Citrobacter*, which is discussed later in the section "Brain Abscess.")

An even more dramatic and malignant form of neonatal bacterial meningitis is caused by *S. marcescens*.[123,147] Widespread hemorrhagic necrosis of cerebral cortex and white matter occurs (Fig. 21-8). Striking invasion of brain parenchyma by bacteria, which can be seen streaming from blood vessels (see Fig. 21-8), is a prominent feature.

Listeria monocytogenes. Although *L. monocytogenes* may cause typical bacterial meningitis in the newborn, especially in infants with late-onset disease, transplacental infection of the fetus may occur and may produce a particularly fulminating infection.[1,78-82,84-87,121,123,148,149] The latter may be manifest in utero and may result in fetal death or in an early-onset, septicemic type of syndrome. The pathological features of this multifocal variety of listeriosis are miliary granulomatous lesions in many organs, including the CNS (see Table 21-10).[121,123] The characteristic lesion is a necrotizing granuloma, which occurs particularly in the meninges, ventricular walls, and choroid plexus. Granulomata may form microabscesses, and organisms can be demonstrated in the necrotic portions of the lesions. As may be expected, this variety of infection is not readily accessible to antibiotics, and death occurs in 25% to 50% of cases, often in utero. Notably, however, treatment of the *mother* early in her infection can prevent infection and sequelae in the fetus and newborn.[87]

Mechanisms of Brain Injury

The neuropathological features of neonatal bacterial meningitis are caused by the action of a complex series of mechanisms summarized very broadly in Figure 21-1 and in detail in Figures 21-9 and 21-10. The mechanisms shown in Figures 21-9 and 21-10 represent a summary of more detailed physiological and biochemical processes, described briefly next and based on a variety of studies, primarily in animal models and cellular systems but also in human infants.[150-182a] Thus, the process begins with sepsis, followed by invasion of the CNS; the role of specific

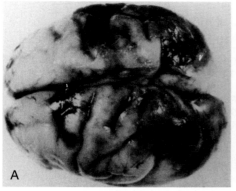
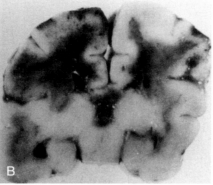
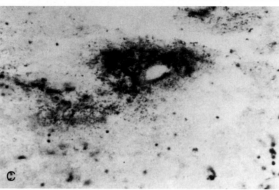

Figure 21-8 **Neonatal bacterial meningitis secondary to *Serratia marcescens*. A** and **B**, Note the regions of hemorrhagic necrosis involving both hemispheres. **C**, Gram-negative bacteria can be seen around a small vein and invading the surrounding parenchyma (cresyl violet). *(From Larroche JC:* Developmental Pathology of the Neonate, *New York: 1977, Excerpta Medica.)*

capsular polysaccharides in this invasion is crucial, as discussed earlier. The meningitic process begins with the action of specific bacterial components, especially in gram-positive bacteria, the peptidoglycan layers and the teichoic acid of the cell wall, and in gram-negative bacteria, the lipopolysaccharide molecules of the outer cell membrane. Among the early events induced by these products, of particular importance is activation

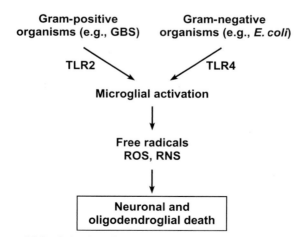

Figure 21-9 **Role of the innate immune response in the pathogenesis of neuronal and oligodendroglial death in bacterial meningitis.** Microglia contain the two Toll-like receptors that are activated by specific molecular components of gram-positive (TLR2) and gram-negative organisms (TLR4) (see text and Chapter 6). Microglial activation and release of toxic reactive oxygen species (ROS) and reactive nitrogen species (RNS) lead to cell death in both gray (neuronal) and white (oligodendroglial) matter. GBS, group B streptococci.

of the immediate immune response (i.e., the *innate immune response;* see Fig. 21-9). As noted earlier, these molecular products of gram-positive organisms (e.g., group B *Streptococcus*) and gram-negative organisms (e.g., *E. coli*) activate specific receptors on brain microglia (the immune cell of the CNS). For gram-positive organisms, the receptor is TLR2, and for gram-negative organisms, it is TLR4. The resulting microglial activation results in several effects, the most important of which is generation of free radicals, both reactive oxygen and nitrogen species. These reactive compounds ultimately lead to neuronal and oligodendroglial death (see also Chapter 6), the key feature of the associated encephalopathy of neonatal bacterial meningitis. Evidence of neonatal bacterial meningitis leading to generation of free radicals and periventricular leukomalacia has been obtained by direct serial measurements of markers of free radical attack in CSF and correlation of elevations of these markers with the occurrence of magnetic resonance imaging (MRI)–documented cerebral white matter lesions.[176]

The myriad deleterious biochemical and physiological events initiated by the bacterial products discussed earlier are shown in Figure 21-10. Thus, these components induce an increase in blood-brain barrier permeability and the early phases of the inflammatory response (i.e., the synthesis and secretion of cytokines, especially tumor necrosis factor from CNS macrophages [microglia] and astrocytes and interleukin-1beta from astrocytes and endothelial cells). The cytokines lead to the adhesion and interaction of leukocytes with endothelial cells by induction of specific cell surface molecules on both leukocytes and

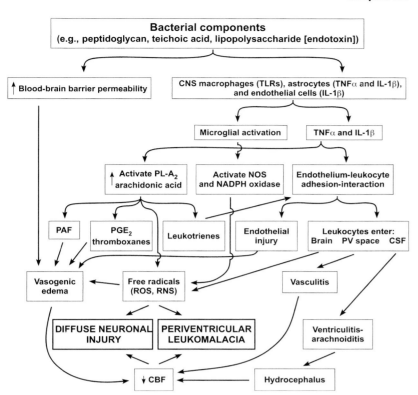

Figure 21-10 Major mechanisms leading to brain injury, especially diffuse cerebral cortical neuronal injury and periventricular white matter injury, in neonatal bacterial meningitis. See text for details. CBF, cerebral blood flow; CSF, cerebrospinal fluid; IL-1beta, interleukin-1beta; NADPH, reduced nicotinamide adenine dinucleotide phosphate; NOS, nitric oxide synthase; PL-A$_2$, phospholipase A$_2$; PAF, platelet-activating factor; PGE$_2$, prostaglandin E$_2$; PV space, perivascular space (Virchow-Robin space); ROS/RNS, reactive oxygen species/reactive nitrogen species; TLR, Toll-like receptor; TNF, tumor necrosis factor.

endothelial cells. The result is the ventriculitis, arachnoiditis, and vasculitis described earlier, the generation of free radicals by leukocytes, and the activated microglia just discussed (see Fig. 21-10). A second crucial effect of the cytokines is the activation of phospholipase A$_2$ and thereby arachidonic acid release and subsequent metabolism, the products of which include free radicals, platelet-activating factor, prostaglandins, thromboxanes, and leukotrienes. The interaction of these effects leading to diffuse neuronal injury, periventricular leukomalacia, and thrombotic cerebral infarction is shown in Figure 21-10. The importance of impaired cerebral blood flow is substantial, as discussed earlier. Impairment of cerebrovascular autoregulation is suggested by experimental data (Fig. 21-11), and the importance of systemic hypotension is implied by clinical observations. Ischemia as an important final common denominator is suggested further by the demonstrations of elevations of extracellular glutamate and reactive oxygen and nitrogen species in experimental models of bacterial meningitis.

Finally, activation of innate immunity and of many of the mechanisms shown in Figures 21-9 and 21-10 may occur *without* bacterial invasion of the CNS, as discussed in Chapters 6 and 8 concerning the roles of systemic infection in white matter and neuronal injury, especially in the premature infant. *Indeed, in a large study of more than 6000 premature infants (401 to 1000 g at birth), infants with sepsis alone (without meningitis) had 50% to 100% higher rates of cognitive deficits, cerebral palsy, visual impairment, hearing impairment, and neurodevelopmental disability when compared with rates of these outcomes in uninfected infants.*[183]

Clinical Features

Two Basic Syndromes

The clinical features of neonatal bacterial meningitis occur in the setting of two basic clinical syndromes, separable principally by age of onset: early-onset disease and late-onset disease (see Table 21-1). Both syndromes have been described with the three major

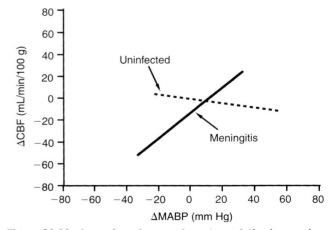

Figure 21-11 Loss of cerebrovascular autoregulation in experimental bacterial meningitis in rabbits. Change in cerebral blood flow (ΔCBF) as a function of change in mean arterial blood pressure (ΔMABP) in control and meningitic rabbits. Changes in MABP result in corresponding changes in CBF in infected rabbits (indicative of impaired autoregulation) but do not cause similar alterations in control (indicative of intact autoregulation). *(From Tureen JH, Dworkin RJ, Kennedy SL, et al: Loss of cerebrovascular autoregulation in experimental meningitis in rabbits, J Clin Invest 85:577-581, 1990.)*

organisms associated with neonatal bacterial meningitis: group B *Streptococcus, E. coli,* and *L. monocytogenes.**

Early-Onset Disease

Early-onset disease is associated with clinical phenomena usually in the first 72 hours of life. As noted earlier, a history of obstetrical complications and premature birth is common, and, understandably, the mode of transmission is primarily from mother to infant near the time of delivery. Specific serotypes are less likely to be involved, and the course may be fulminating. However, mortality rates in recent years are much lower than previously (see "Prognosis," later).

Dominance of Non-neurological Signs. The clinical presentation is dominated by *non-neurological signs* (i.e., signs related to sepsis and respiratory disease). The most common signs are hyperthermia, apnea, hypotension, disturbances of feeding, jaundice, hepatomegaly, and respiratory distress; less common signs are hypothermia, skin lesions (e.g., petechiae and sclerema), and overt focal infection (e.g., otitis media, omphalitis, arthritis, and osteomyelitis). Neurological signs are usually limited to stupor (usually termed *lethargy*) and irritability. Signs suggestive of meningitis (see later discussion) are unusual, in part because overt meningitis occurs in only approximately 30% of the patients with early-onset disease. Indeed, even those infants with culture-proven meningitis often do not exhibit striking CSF pleocytosis.

The respiratory manifestations of early-onset sepsis-meningitis may be particularly prominent with group B streptococcal infection and, indeed, may simultaneously present serious diagnostic problems and important diagnostic clues. Approximately 40% to 60% of infants with early-onset group B streptococcal disease have manifestations of prominent respiratory disease in the first 6 hours of life.[28,59,74,77,186] Only approximately 35% of these infants exhibit radiographic infiltrates suggestive of congenital pneumonia, whereas approximately 50% exhibit radiographic features of respiratory distress syndrome.[59] Distinction from nonbacterial respiratory disease is suggested by the history of premature rupture of membranes, low Apgar scores (< 4 at 1 minute in 85%), rapid progression of pulmonary disease, and low or declining absolute neutrophil counts in the first 24 hours of life.[59,187]

Late-Onset Disease

Late-onset bacterial sepsis-meningitis is much more likely to manifest as a neurological syndrome with overt signs of meningitis. Indeed, approximately 80% to 90% of affected infants have CSF findings clearly indicative of meningitis.[1,2,51,53,59] As noted earlier, unlike in early-onset disease, obstetrical complications and prematurity are uncommon, and onset is usually after the first week of life. The mode of transmission may be from mother to infant, but often horizontal transmission from human contacts,

indwelling catheters, or contaminated equipment can be documented. Specific serotypes are usually involved (serotype III for group B *Streptococcus,* IVb for *L. monocytogenes,* and K1 strains for *E. coli*); the course is not so fulminating as in early-onset disease, and the mortality rate is slightly lower.

Dominance of Neurological Signs. Although *neurological signs* associated with meningitis are *prominent in late-onset disease,* some of the signs prominent in early-onset disease are also common, especially fever and feeding disturbances. Most impressive, however, are the neurological signs (Table 21-11).[16,29,51,60,88,185] In my experience, most patients exhibit *impairment of consciousness,* manifested usually as varying degrees of stupor, with or without irritability. The disturbances of level of consciousness presumably relate to the cerebral edema and, perhaps, the associated encephalopathy (see "Neuropathology"). *Seizures* develop at some time in the illness in nearly 50% of cases, although these seizures may be predominantly subtle. The convulsive phenomena presumably relate to the cortical effects of the arachnoidal inflammatory infiltration. *Focal seizures* occur in approximately 50% of infants with seizures and may be prominent. These focal episodes may be related to ischemic vascular lesions. Similar bases are probable for the *focal cerebral signs* (e.g., hemiparesis and horizontal deviation of eyes), which are movable with the doll's eyes maneuver. These signs are reported only uncommonly in the literature, but, in my experience, they can be elicited with careful examination in nearly one half of cases. *Extensor rigidity* occurs in approximately one third of cases and may be so severe that opisthotonos occurs. These phenomena probably relate to the arachnoidal inflammation, especially in the posterior fossa. A similar basis is likely for the nuchal rigidity, which occurs in fewer than 25% of cases. Apparent in most patients, however, is a distinct increase in irritability, elicitable by flexion of the neck and, presumably, the neonatal counterpart of more overt nuchal rigidity. *Cranial nerve signs* involve usually the seventh, third, and sixth nerves, in that order of frequency, and are more common than often suggested in the literature. These signs relate to involvement of cranial nerve roots by the arachnoidal inflammation (see "Neuropathology"). A *bulging or full anterior fontanelle* is present, often later in the course of the disease, in approximately 35% to 50% of patients. This feature relates to an increase in

TABLE 21-11 Neurological Signs of Neonatal Bacterial Meningitis

Neurological Sign	Approximate Frequency
Stupor with or without irritability	76%–100%
Seizures	26%–50%
Bulging or full anterior fontanelle	26%–50%
Extensor rigidity, opisthotonos	26%–50%
Focal cerebral signs	26%–50%
Cranial nerve signs	26%–50%
Nuchal rigidity	0%–25%

*See references 2–4,10,16,21,23,26,28,29,59,74,77,82,87,184,185.

intracranial pressure (see following section). Rarely, anterior fontanelle herniation of cerebral tissue occurs and imparts a "doughy" consistency to the bulging fontanelle.[134] Moreover, very uncommonly, signs of segmental cord involvement (sensory level, flaccidity below the level of the lesion), secondary to myelopathy, may be present.[136]

Major Neurological Complications

The clinical course of neonatal bacterial meningitis may be *complicated* by the following four major and often interrelated events: (1) severe increase in intracranial pressure, (2) ventriculitis with localization of infection, (3) acute hydrocephalus, and (4) an intracerebral mass or extraparenchymal collection (e.g., abscess, hemorrhagic infarct, and subdural effusion) (Table 21-12).

Increased Intracranial Pressure. Intracranial pressure, although only uncommonly monitored, may be markedly increased in neonatal bacterial meningitis. Major causes include cerebral edema, hydrocephalus, and, uncommonly, formation of an intracranial mass or extracerebral collection (Table 21-13). Cerebral edema (vasogenic and cytotoxic) is a frequent feature in the first several days of the disease and may be aggravated by water retention secondary to inappropriate antidiuretic hormone secretion.[188-190] Increased intracranial pressure may persist or worsen in the ensuing days, with the development of acute hydrocephalus or an intracranial space-occupying lesion (see subsequent discussion).

The increased intracranial pressure rarely causes signs of transtentorial (e.g., unilateral dilated pupil) or cerebellar (e.g., apnea and bradycardia) herniation, but both these forms of herniation have been reported.[133] Although uncommon, the increased intracranial pressure may interfere with cerebral perfusion and may contribute to the associated encephalopathy described in the "Neuropathology" section. Clinical signs suggestive of increased intracranial pressure include a full or bulging anterior fontanelle, separated cranial sutures, and deterioration of the level of consciousness.

Ventriculitis with Localization of Infection. Ventriculitis complicated by localization of infection is caused by particularly exuberant inflammation of the ependymal lining, usually in association with obstruction to CSF flow, especially at the aqueduct. Occasionally, formation of glial septa may localize intraventricular infection in a particularly severe manner. No reliable clinical signs exist for these events, and the diagnosis must be suspected on the basis of the failure of clinical and bacterial responses to therapy (see "Management"). Ultrasound scanning may show signs suggestive of ventriculitis (see "Diagnosis") and may at least indicate the potential for sequestered infection.

Acute Hydrocephalus. Hydrocephalus occurs in an appreciable proportion of infants with neonatal bacterial meningitis who survive into the second and third weeks of life. The causes of hydrocephalus include obstruction to CSF flow, either inside the ventricular system, secondary to ventriculitis, or outside the

TABLE 21-12	Neurological Complications of Neonatal Bacterial Meningitis
Increased intracranial pressure	
Ventriculitis with localized, inaccessible infection	
Acute hydrocephalus	
Intracerebral mass or extracerebral collection	

ventricular system, secondary to arachnoiditis. The suggestive clinical signs are those of increased intracranial pressure, as just discussed, and acceleration of head growth. Diagnosis is made best with ultrasound or other brain modality (see "Diagnosis"), particularly because ventricular dilation develops *before* overt clinical signs.

Intracerebral Mass or Extracerebral Collection. Formation of an intracerebral mass or extracerebral collection of clinical significance is very uncommon in neonatal bacterial meningitis. *Brain abscess* can occur, particularly in necrotic brain tissue (e.g., infarction), and it should be suspected if existing clinical signs worsen, despite apparently adequate therapy, and if signs of increased intracranial pressure or focal cerebral disturbance develop (see later section on "Brain Abscess"). Sudden onset of a focal deficit with evidence for unilateral mass also may occur with a large *hemorrhagic infarct.* Abscess and massive infarction, although clinically very important, are very unusual in neonatal bacterial meningitis. *Subdural effusion* should be suspected in the presence of accelerated head growth and signs of increased intracranial pressure. Increased cranial transillumination can be helpful at the bedside. However, clinically significant subdural effusion is very uncommon in neonatal bacterial meningitis. Similarly, *subdural empyema* is a rare extracerebral collection that may cause signs of increased intracranial pressure in addition to fever and leukocytosis.

TABLE 21-13	Causes of Increased Intracranial Pressure in Neonatal Bacterial Meningitis
Cerebral Edema	
Vasogenic: endothelial effects of bacterial components, cytokines, arachidonate metabolites, free radicals, vasculitis	
Cytotoxic: cellular injury	
Water intoxication: inappropriate antidiuretic hormone secretion	
Hydrocephalus, Secondary to Obstruction of Cerebrospinal Fluid Flow	
Arachnoiditis and extraventricular block	
Ventriculitis and intraventricular block	
Intracerebral Mass or Extracerebral Collection	
Abscess	
Subdural effusion or empyema	
Other	

Diagnosis

Clinical Evaluation

The clinical suspicion of *sepsis* is based on a wide variety of *very common*, previously discussed, clinical signs. It is necessary to consider and distinguish not only virtually all nonbacterial infections (see Chapter 20), but also disorders of other organ systems as common as respiratory distress syndrome. Obstetrical and epidemiological factors are very important to evaluate. Indeed, the most significant point is that *a high index of clinical suspicion is critical* and should provoke the initiation of laboratory studies (reviewed in the next section).

Clinical suspicion of *meningitis*, of course, must always be raised when sepsis is suspected. In addition, certain neurological signs should suggest meningitis (see previous discussion). Unfortunately, too often these signs appear *after* significant disease is well established. Disturbances of the *level of consciousness* are the most nearly constant *initial* neurological signs; indeed, perhaps the most useful early clinical constellation that should lead to the suspicion of neonatal bacterial meningitis is the combination of stupor, even if slight, and irritability.

Laboratory Evaluation

The essential questions to be answered through laboratory studies in the evaluation of the infant suspected of having bacterial meningitis are principally the following:

1. Is meningitis present?
2. What is the cause?
3. What is the status of the CNS?

The answer to the first question is based principally on evaluation of the CSF, the answer to the second is based on the identification of the microorganism, and the answer to the third is based on several important neurodiagnostic studies.

Cerebrospinal Fluid Findings. I believe that examination of the CSF is indicated in any infant with suspected sepsis, even in the absence of overt neurological signs. Indeed, in one series, 37% of cases of primarily early-onset neonatal meningitis would have been missed or the diagnosis delayed if the decision to perform a lumbar puncture had been reserved for infants with "neurological signs" or proven bacteremia.[191] Similarly, in a series of 9461 very-low-birth-weight infants, *one third of those with meningitis had meningitis in the absence of sepsis.*[113] Because CSF cultures were performed only half as often as blood cultures, the discordance in blood and CSF culture results suggested that "meningitis may be underdiagnosed among very-low-birth-weight infants."[113]

Interpretation of the CSF findings in the newborn is difficult, especially when that interpretation is critical in making a diagnosis (i.e., bacterial meningitis) that requires urgent intervention. Among the many reasons for the difficulties in interpretation of the CSF findings, the most important relates to the uncertainty of normal values in the *specific population of infants at risk* for bacterial meningitis (see Chapter 4). Previously published studies dealt with normal or poorly defined populations.

Sarff and co-workers[192] described the *CSF findings in 117 high-risk infants* (87 term and 30 preterm, with 95% examined in the first week of life) without meningitis or other clinical evidence of viral or bacterial disease (Table 21-14). Mean values for term and preterm infants, respectively, were as follows: white blood cell (WBC) count, 8 and 9 cells/mm³ (60% polymorphonuclear leukocytes); protein concentration, 90 and 115 mg/dL; glucose concentration, 52 and 50 mg/dL; and ratio of CSF to blood glucose concentration, 81% and 74%. Although the ranges are wide, the values provided a useful framework. A later study by Rodriguez and co-workers[193] amplified these findings by focusing on very-low-birth-weight infants, 80% of whom were examined *after* the first week of life. CSF findings as a function of postconceptional age were defined (Table 21-15). CSF values for protein and glucose contents are highest in the most immature infants and may reflect an increased permeability of the blood-brain barrier in

TABLE 21-14 **Cerebrospinal Fluid Findings in High-Risk Newborns without Bacterial Meningitis***

CSF Findings	Term	Preterm
White Blood Cell Count (cells/mm³)		
Mean	8	9
Range	0–3	0–29
Protein Concentration (mg/dL)		
Mean	90	115
Range	20–170	65–150
Glucose Concentration (mg/dL)		
Mean	52	50
Range	34–119	24–63
CSF/Blood Glucose (%)		
Mean	81	74
Range	44–248	55–105

*95% of infants were examined *in the first week of life.*
CSF, cerebrospinal fluid.
Data from Sarff LD, Platt LH, McCracken GH Jr: Cerebrospinal fluid evaluation in neonates: Comparison of high-risk infants with and without meningitis, *J Pediatr* 88:473-477, 1976.

TABLE 21-15 **Cerebrospinal Fluid Findings in Infants Weighing Less than 1500 g as a Function of Postconceptional Age**[*]

| Postconceptional Age (wk) | CSF FINDINGS | | |
	WBCs/mm^3 (Mean ± SD)	Glucose (mg/dL) (Mean ± SD)	Protein (mg/dL) (Mean ± SD)
26–28 (n=17)	6 ± 10	85 ± 39	177 ± 60
29–31 (n=23)	5 ± 4	54 ± 18	144 ± 40
32–34 (n=18)	4 ± 3	55 ± 21	142 ± 49
35–37 (n=8)	6 ± 7	56 ± 21	109 ± 53
38–40 (n=5)	9 ± 9	44 ± 10	117 ± 33

[*]80% of infants were examined *after the first week of life.*
CSF, cerebrospinal fluid; WBCs, white blood cells.
Data from Rodriguez AF, Kaplan SL, Mason EO Jr: Cerebrospinal fluid values in the very-low-birth-weight infant, *J Pediatr* 116:971-974, 1990.

these infants (see Table 21-15 and Chapter 4). These additional features are important in assessing the CSF in the large numbers of very premature infants evaluated in modern neonatal intensive care units.

The CSF formula for neonatal bacterial meningitis is an elevated WBC count predominantly consisting of polymorphonuclear leukocytes, an elevated protein concentration, and a depressed glucose concentration, particularly in relationship to blood glucose concentration. The abnormalities tend to be more severe for late-onset than early-onset disease and for gram-negative enteric than group B streptococcal meningitis. Of 119 newborn infants with proven bacterial meningitis, more than 1000 WBCs/mm^3 were observed in the initial sample of CSF in approximately 75% of patients with gram-negative infection but in only approximately 30% with group B streptococcal infection.[192] Values in excess of 10,000 WBCs/mm^3 were observed in approximately 20% of gram-negative infections but were rare in group B streptococcal infections. Evaluation of the other end of the continuum is still more informative (Table 21-16). Thus, using the *ranges* determined in their high-risk newborns (see Table 21-14), Sarff and co-workers[192] showed that CSF values for WBC count were within the "normal" range for approximately 30% of infants with culture-proven group B streptococcal meningitis versus only 4% of infants with gram-negative meningitis. Values for CSF protein concentration and CSF to blood glucose ratio were within the "normal" range in nearly 50% of the infants with group B streptococcal meningitis versus

only 15% to 25% of the infants with gram-negative bacterial meningitis (see Table 21-16). The importance of evaluating *all* the CSF findings, and not just one isolated value, is emphasized by the finding that *only 1 of 119 infants had normal values for all three parameters in the initial lumbar puncture sample.*[192] Thus, the CSF findings should be evaluated in toto and in the context of other clinical, epidemiological, and laboratory data when assessing the possibility of meningitis. In the rare patient with a totally normal CSF examination but a continuing suspicion of meningitis, a second lumbar puncture is indicated.

Identification of the Microorganism in Cerebrospinal Fluid. Determination of the bacterial cause of meningitis obviously is made most readily and decisively by *culture of the CSF.* The yield in the previously untreated patient whose CSF is cultured promptly on the various media necessary to isolate the different microorganisms responsible for neonatal bacterial meningitis (including *Listeria*) approaches 100%. The result is usually available within 48 hours.

Faster techniques available for identifying microorganisms include Gram-stained smears, countercurrent immunoelectrophoresis, limulus lysate assay, and latex particle agglutination. *Stained smears* demonstrated bacteria on the initial CSF evaluation of 119 newborn infants with meningitis in 83% of patients with group B streptococcal meningitis and in 78% of those with gram-negative bacterial meningitis.[192] This universally available, simple procedure should be performed on every CSF sample. *Countercurrent immunoelectrophoresis*

TABLE 21-16 **Cerebrospinal Fluid Findings in Neonatal Bacterial Meningitis**

| CSF Finding | BACTERIAL ETIOLOGY OF MENINGITIS[*] | |
	Group B Streptococcus	Gram-Negative Organism
WBC count <32/mm^3	29%	4%
Protein concentration <170 mg/dL	47%	23%
CSF/blood glucose >44%	45%	15%

[*]Data expressed as *percentage* of total patients with indicated type of meningitis.
CSF, cerebrospinal fluid.
From Sarff LD, Platt LH, McCracken GH Jr: Cerebrospinal fluid evaluation in neonates: Comparison of high-risk infants with and without meningitis, *J Pediatr* 88:473-477, 1976.

is a sensitive and rapid technique that demonstrates the presence of bacterial antigen within approximately 2 hours. The test formerly was widely used particularly in the previously treated patient with possible nonviable bacteria in the CSF. Countercurrent immunoelectrophoresis requires specific antiserum, which is available for type III group B *Streptococcus* and K1 *E. coli* (among the common pathogens for neonatal meningitis).[51,53,194-198] Rapid detection of meningitis caused by gram-negative enteric organisms formerly was based particularly on the *limulus lysate assay*.[51,199] The latter two tests have been largely replaced by *latex particle agglutination tests*.[200] This approach is based on the agglutination of specific antibody-coated latex particles by bacterial antigen. The test is particularly useful for group B *Streptococcus* and *E. coli* K1. The assay can provide a result in minutes.

Identification of the Microorganism from Other Sites. Valuable supporting data and occasionally the only information concerning the precise bacterial cause of meningitis are derived from isolation of the organism or its antigens in body fluids other than CSF. *Blood cultures* are positive in approximately 50% to 80% of cases of neonatal bacterial meningitis.[28,32,60,113,201,202] Detection of bacterial antigen by *latex particle agglutination tests* can be made with serum or urine as well as with CSF. *Concentrated urine* specimens are the most productive for detection of group B streptococcal antigen.[59,203] In a cumulative series, 88% of concentrated urine specimens were antigen positive by countercurrent immunoelectrophoresis, and 96% were antigen positive by latex particle agglutination. Moreover, when urine, CSF, and serum are all studied, the likelihood of missing the infection is minimal. In the unusual case in which a suppurative focus (e.g., otitis media, arthritis, or skin abscess) is the source of the meningitic infection, *cultures and stains of aspirated material* are of obvious value. Isolation of an organism from surface cultures (e.g., skin, nose, throat, rectum, and umbilicus) indicates *colonization* but does not establish active systemic infection. Recent data suggest that rapid fluorescent real-time polymerase chain reaction testing for group B streptococcal DNA is highly sensitive for rapid detection of colonization by this organism.[204]

Adjunct Tests. Adjunct tests that support the diagnosis of bacterial infection include an increase in the absolute neutrophilic band count, and, particularly, the ratio of immature to total neutrophils.[66,198,205-207] Neutrophilic leukocytosis or leukopenia is demonstrable in 50% to 75% of cases. Other tests (e.g., determination of C-reactive protein, erythrocyte sedimentation rate, and IgM level) are somewhat less sensitive.[208,209] Several studies raise the possibility that detection of certain proinflammatory cytokines, chemokines, adhesion molecules, and cell surface markers may have value in early identification of neonatal bacterial sepsis (determinations in serum) or meningitis (determinations in CSF), even before the onset of clinical disease.[173,180,209-213] More data will be important.

Neurodiagnostic Studies

The status of the CNS in neonatal bacterial meningitis is evaluated best by careful clinical examination and by selected neurodiagnostic studies. Choice of studies depends particularly on the stage of the disease and, as a corollary, the neuropathological features to be assessed. The three neurodiagnostic tests, in addition to examination of CSF, that I consider most valuable are (1) measurement of CSF pressure, (2) ventricular puncture (in highly selected cases), and (3) brain imaging studies (ultrasound, computed tomography [CT], and MRI scans). The electroencephalogram is of definite adjunct value (see "Prognosis," later).

Cerebrospinal Fluid Pressure. CSF pressure may be a critical factor in determining outcome, and measurements of pressure, especially in the acute stage, are valuable. The initial lumbar puncture should include CSF pressure measurement, and CSF pressure in excess of normal (i.e., $\approx$50 mm H_2O) should be cause for concern. Continual or frequent intermittent monitoring of CSF pressure with an anterior fontanelle sensor, when available (see Chapter 4), can be useful in the evaluation of the degree of cerebral edema, the development of obstructive hydrocephalus, and the occurrence of a major intracerebral mass or extracerebral collection. Clear elevations of intracranial pressure should provoke further, more definitive diagnostic studies and appropriate intervention (see "Management"). Our initial studies of this issue demonstrated that intracranial hypertension with impaired cerebral blood flow velocity, measured at the anterior fontanelle by the Doppler technique (see Chapter 4), was more commonly a complication of bacterial meningitis *of older infants than of newborns*.[132] This observation concerning intracranial hypertension was confirmed in a later study.[214]

Ventricular Puncture. Ventricular puncture provides valuable information concerning intraventricular pressure and the presence of ventriculitis, particularly when associated with serious localized infection (Table 21-17). *Although only uncommonly necessary*, ventricular puncture should be performed in any newborn with bacterial meningitis who is not responding favorably to apparently appropriate antibiotic therapy, in terms *either* of clinical signs *or* of sterilization of lumbar CSF (see "Management"). Severe ventriculitis may be present in an infant with improved or even normal *lumbar* CSF WBC count.[215] Indeed, the constellation of a deteriorating clinical state (e.g., apnea or bradycardia, or both, and

TABLE 21-17	Ventriculitis

Definition: Ventricular inflammation with infection (often apparently inaccessible to systemically administered antibiotics)
Suspect if (1) persistence of infection in lumbar CSF at 4 days or (2) clinical deterioration or failure of clinical improvement, even with improvement of CSF pleocytosis and CSF sterilization

CSF, cerebrospinal fluid.

persistent fever) in the presence of decreasing CSF pleo-cytosis or even CSF sterilization should raise the suspicion of clinically important ventriculitis. Moreover, ventriculitis may evolve in a subacute fashion, with signs of increased intracranial pressure, either de novo or after apparent recovery from bacterial meningitis.[215,216] The presence in ventricular fluid of bacteria (Gram stain or culture) or bacterial antigen (latex particle agglutination) and a WBC count in excess of approximately 100 WBCs/mm³ indicates ventriculitis. Cranial ultrasonography often shows excrescences associated with the ependymal surface. Whether ventricular infection is localized and inaccessible to antibiotics depends on evaluation of a variety of factors. Favoring such a possibility is the presence of marked pleocytosis in ventricular CSF or evidence of intraventricular block of CSF flow (e.g., elevated intraventricular pressure and dilated ventricles) or both pleocytosis and CSF block. Management of such a situation is reviewed in subsequent discussions.

Ventricular puncture should be performed by a physician with expertise in the procedure and awareness of its hazards. In acute bacterial meningitis, the lateral ventricles are often small and may be tapped only with considerable difficulty. A CT scan or ultrasound scan before the procedure is important. Indeed, ventricular puncture with ultrasound guidance is recommended if the ventricles are small. Ventricular puncture may be followed by the development of a cystic cavity.[125,217,218] This development is particularly likely to occur if

obstruction to CSF flow and increased intraventricular pressure, common complications of bacterial ventriculitis, are present. The subsequent cavitation along the needle track relates most probably to the combination of disruption of edematous, poorly myelinated, readily separable brain parenchyma and transmission of elevated intraventricular pressure. In the large, older series studied by Lorber and Emery,[217] the approximately 50% of infants subjected to *multiple* ventricular punctures for the treatment of bacterial ventriculitis subsequently developed cystic cavities, demonstrable by ventriculography, at the sites of the taps. The incidence of significant cavity formation in infants with ventriculitis after a *single tap* is unknown but probably is relatively low. In my experience, although small diverticula from the lateral ventricles into the needle track are common after single taps, major cavity formation is very unusual.

Ultrasound Scan. Cranial ultrasound scan has proved very useful in the evaluation of infants with bacterial meningitis.[219-226] The spectrum of abnormalities has included both acute changes (e.g., evidence of ventriculitis [intraventricular strands attached to the ventricular surface and echogenic ependyma] [Fig. 21-12], echogenic sulci, abnormal parenchymal echogenicities [periventricular or focal cerebral] [Figs. 21-13 and 21-14], and extracellular fluid collection) and chronic changes (e.g., ventricular dilation [see Fig. 21-12] and multicystic parenchymal change). The neuropathological correlates of the

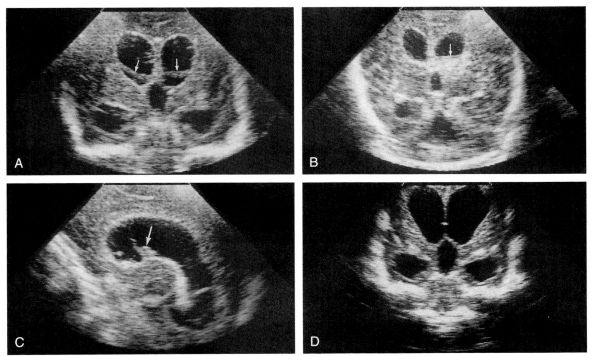

Figure 21-12 Cranial ultrasound scans in neonatal bacterial meningitis. A, Coronal scan obtained from a 27-day-old infant with group B streptococcal meningitis on the third hospital day. Note dense linear strands of echogenic material in the lateral ventricles *(arrows)*, apparently attached to the ependymal surface, and diffuse low-level echoes in both lateral ventricles. **B,** Coronal scan on the fourth hospital day. Note the collection of intraventricular material apparently attached to the ventricular wall *(arrow)*. **C,** Parasagittal view of the same scan as shown in **B.** Note abnormal intraventricular echoes *(arrow)* apparently contiguous with ventricular surface and choroid plexus. **D,** Note later development of hydrocephalus and disappearance of abnormal echoes.

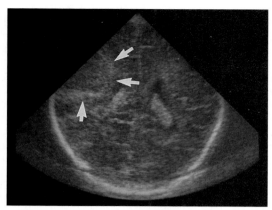

Figure 21-13   Neonatal bacterial meningitis: ultrasound scan. This coronal scan obtained from an infant with *Escherichia coli* meningitis shows an area of increased echogenicity *(arrows)* in the distribution of the middle cerebral artery, consistent with an infarction.

sonographic changes include essentially the entire spectrum of the neuropathology (see previous discussion). The particular value of cranial ultrasonography is the capacity to perform serial studies safely and at the patient's bedside and thus to define progression of complications. Such definition is of major benefit in formulating rational management.

Computed Tomography Scan. The CT scan is valuable at all stages of neonatal bacterial meningitis (Figs. 21-15 to 21-19). In the acute stage, CT scan may provide information regarding the degree of cerebral edema (small size of ventricles), the occurrence and site of block to CSF flow (dilated ventricles, according to the locus of the block), the occurrence of major infarction (cerebral areas of increased or decreased attenuation, depending on the hemorrhagic component to the infarction), the type of associated encephalopathy (e.g., periventricular hypoattenuation secondary to periventricular leukomalacia), and the unusual occurrence of abscess or subdural collection. Subsequently, in the course of bacterial meningitis, CT scan is used particularly for the detection of (1) ventricular dilation before

rapid head growth, (2) multicystic encephalomalacia, and (3) degree of cerebral cortical and white matter atrophy (through the size of the ventricles and the extracerebral subarachnoid space). In a careful study of 45 infants with neonatal gram-negative bacterial meningitis, CT findings were normal in only 30% and demonstrated hydrocephalus in 44%, changes consistent with ischemic lesions in 29%, abscess in 18%, and subdural effusion in 7%.[227]

Magnetic Resonance Imaging Scan. As for nearly all other forms of neonatal neuropathology, MRI scan provides important structural information. All the acute and chronic lesions of neonatal bacterial meningitis observable by CT scan (see earlier) are delineated very well by MRI scan (Fig. 21-20). In addition, diffusion-weighted MRI shows ischemic lesions and brain edema more effectively and earlier than does CT scan. A striking demonstration of increased diffusion consistent with vasogenic edema, a characteristic feature of bacterial meningitis, is shown in Figure 21-21.

Prognosis

Reservations Concerning Available Data

The prognosis for neonatal bacterial meningitis depends on the rapidity of diagnosis and the institution of appropriate therapy. Therapy is not perfect, and, indeed, in certain types of meningitis, it is often inadequate. In any assessment of outcome, it is necessary to recognize the inherent difficulty in extrapolating to a given infant with meningitis data that are generalized from large-scale studies, which are often based on populations with a broad spectrum of bacterial causes and followed for relatively brief durations.

Duration of follow-up is particularly important for two reasons. The first is obvious: disturbances of higher cortical function may not become apparent until the child is of school age. Similarly, deficits in certain sensory discriminations, particularly hearing, may be difficult to detect in infancy. The second reason for the importance of duration of follow-up relates to the not

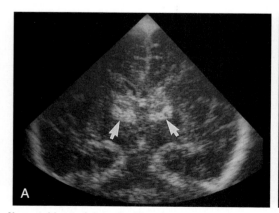
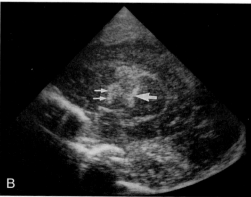

Figure 21-14   Neonatal bacterial meningitis: ultrasound scans. A, Coronal and, **B,** parasagittal ultrasound scans from a 2-week-old infant with bacterial meningitis show discrete areas of echogenicity, most consistent with deep venous infarction. Note on the coronal scan **(A)** bilateral symmetrical areas of involvement in the region of the basal ganglia (putamen and globus pallidus) *(arrows)*. On the parasagittal scan **(B)**, the involvement is seen not only in basal ganglia *(small arrows)* but also in thalamus (large arrow).

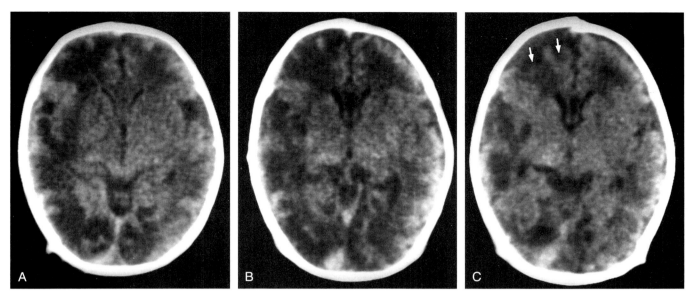

Figure 21-15 **Neonatal bacterial meningitis: computed tomography scans.** Scans were obtained from an infant with *Escherichia coli* meningitis on postnatal days, **A**, 9, **B**, 16, and, **C**, 26. Note the multiple areas of decreased attenuation involving both cerebral cortex and periventricular white matter, greater on the right than the left. By 26 days **(C)**, atrophic changes began to appear, especially in the right frontal region (*arrows* indicate the shrunken cerebral cortical surface).

infrequent, *transient* nature of neurological deficits after neonatal meningitis. Infants may improve for many months, and deficits that were striking shortly after the neonatal period may decrease markedly in severity or may disappear totally. The relation of these observations to the plasticity of developing brain is an interesting topic for future research. Nevertheless, with these reservations, useful estimates of prognosis can be derived from available data (see next sections).

Group B Streptococcal Infection

By far the most common gram-positive organism causing meningitis is group B *Streptococcus*, the outcome for which is shown in Table 21-18.[10,12,29,77,113,185,228] These data, derived from several large populations,

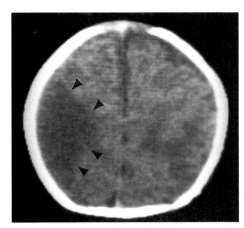

Figure 21-16 **Neonatal bacterial meningitis: computed tomography scan.** This scan from an infant with group B streptococcal meningitis shows triangular area of decreased attenuation (*arrowheads*) in the distribution of the middle cerebral artery, consistent with ischemic infarction.

included more later-onset cases and term infants than early-onset cases and premature infants. The overall fatality rate has declined in recent years to approximately 10% to 15%, with slightly higher rates for early-onset disease or premature infants and slightly lower rates for later-onset cases or term infants. Fifty percent of survivors are normal; approximately 40% have mild or moderate sequelae, and only approximately 10% exhibit severe deficits. These outcomes represent a decline in mortality rates and in morbidity among survivors, when compared with results of earlier reports.[24-26,59,74,229-235]

Gram-Negative Enteric Infections

Neonatal meningitis secondary to gram-negative enteric organisms has been considered more ominous than neonatal meningitis secondary to gram-positive organisms, particularly group B *Streptococcus*. More recent data suggested that this distinction may no longer be obvious (Table 21-19).[10,12,16,29,113,185] Thus, findings suggest that the outcome is nearly similar to that for group B streptococcal meningitis, especially among later-onset cases. Mortality rates and incidence of sequelae in survivors are slightly higher in early-onset cases or premature infants, or both. The most striking change in neonatal outcome with gram-negative bacterial meningitis in recent years has been continuation of a sharp decrease in mortality rate.*

Selected Prognostic Factors

Certain factors, readily identified in the newborn period, may have prognostic importance, at least regarding the likelihood of a fatal outcome or survival

---

*See references 10,12,16,21,24-26,29,51,113,185,227,236.

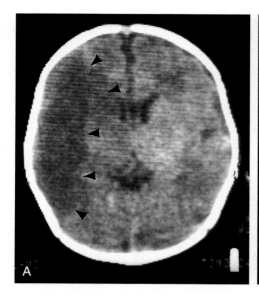

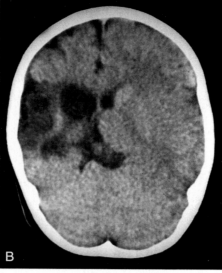

Figure 21-17 Neonatal bacterial meningitis: computed tomography scans. Scans were obtained from an infant with *Escherichia coli* meningitis at, **A**, 10 postnatal days and, **B**, 6 postnatal months. In the acute period (**A**), the area of decreased attenuation *(arrowheads)* is consistent with an infarction in the distribution of the middle cerebral artery. The follow-up scan (**B**) shows a much smaller area of atrophy *(with dilated frontal horn)*, indicating that a major portion of the acute lesion represented edema and other reversible changes.

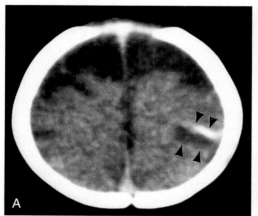

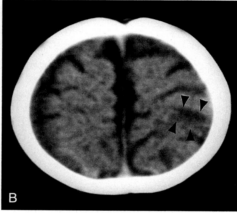

Figure 21-18 Neonatal bacterial meningitis: computed tomography scans. Scans obtained, **A**, after 5 days of meningitis and, **B**, 2 weeks later. **A**, Note the area of both decreased and increased attenuation *(arrowheads)*, consistent with hemorrhagic infarction, probably secondary to cortical vein thrombosis. **B**, A small area of cortical atrophy *(arrowheads)* is apparent on follow-up.

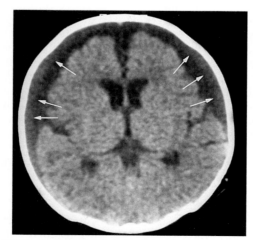

Figure 21-19 Neonatal bacterial meningitis: computed tomography scan. This scan was obtained 2 weeks after diagnosis and appropriate antibiotic treatment of *Escherichia coli* meningitis. Note the increased extracerebral fluid, the outer portion of which is of greater attenuation *(arrows)* than the inner portion. The appearance is consistent with a subdural effusion.

with severe neurological sequelae.* Thus, decreased survival rates and higher incidences of severe sequelae are associated with low birth weight, marked leukopenia or neutropenia, or both, coma or opisthotonos, persistent seizures (> 12 hours), and markedly elevated CSF protein content. Also of value with specific infections are the quantitative levels in CSF of the type III group B streptococcal or the K1 *E. coli* antigenic markers; these levels correlate directly with prognosis.[53] A careful study of the electroencephalogram during bacterial meningitis in 29 infants indicated value for the degree of background abnormality in prediction of outcome (Table 21-20).[238] A more recent study confirmed these initial findings.[228] Although not systematically analyzed, I find that the degree of injury on MRI scan performed late in the infant's course is useful prognostically. However, although these various associations are valuable, outcome in neonatal bacterial meningitis depends on the interplay of so many factors that

*See references 10,12,16,29,51,53,60,77,113,185,202,228,232,236, 237.

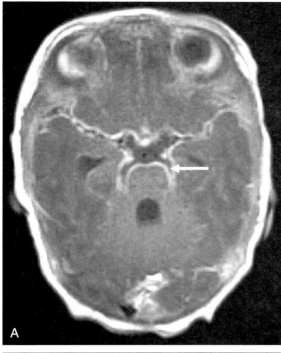

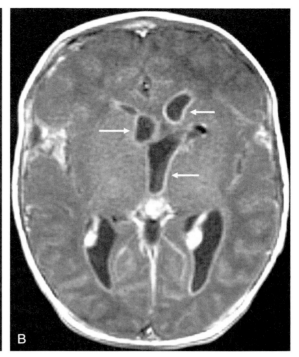

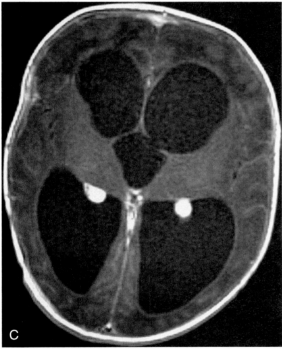

Figure 21-20 Neonatal bacterial meningitis: magnetic resonance imaging (MRI) scans. The initial MRI scan (**A** and **B**), obtained during the acute period, shows, after administration of gadolinium, leptomeningeal enhancement (*arrow* in **A**), consistent with leptomeningitis, ependymal enhancement (*arrows* in **B**), consistent with ventriculitis (with loculation), and evidence of diffuse cerebral white matter injury and more focal bifrontal lesions, possibly infarcts. Three weeks later (**C**), note marked dilation of the lateral and third ventricles, indicative of hydrocephalus (with a likely block at the aqueduct) and diffuse cerebral cortical and white matter injury, especially bifrontally. *(Courtesy of Dr. Omar Khwaja.)*

prognostic judgments in every case must be carefully individualized. Indeed, in my experience, in perhaps no other variety of neonatal neurological disease is dramatic recovery from a devastated clinical state more likely to be observed than in an infant with neonatal bacterial meningitis.

Management

The major issues in the management of neonatal bacterial meningitis relate to prevention, supportive care, neurological complications, antibiotics, and ventriculitis. Although many aspects of management are surrounded by unresolved problems, the basic fact remains that neonatal bacterial meningitis is a treatable disease.

Prevention (Group B Streptococcal Infection)

The most critical and challenging problem in the prevention of neonatal bacterial meningitis relates to group B streptococcal disease. Group B *Streptococcus* is the single most common organism implicated in

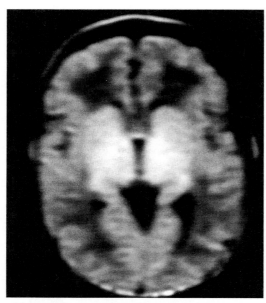

Figure 21-21 Diffusion-weighted magnetic resonance imaging **(DWI) scan in *Listeria* meningitis.** Computed tomography and conventional magnetic resonance imaging scans were not definitely abnormal (not shown). By contrast, the DWI scan shows a striking and diffuse *decrease* in signal intensity in cerebral white matter, indicative of *increased* diffusion, consistent with vasogenic edema.

intravenous ampicillin or penicillin during labor leads to a marked reduction in colonization of infants born to infected mothers and to a virtual elimination of early-onset group B streptococcal sepsis-meningitis. The most difficult issue has been whom to treat. The data depicted in Table 21-21 emanated from a classic study and showed the value of intrapartum chemoprophylaxis, especially in certain high-risk groups.[247] Indeed, in the years since the advent of widespread intrapartum chemoprophylaxis, the incidence of group B streptococcal disease has declined markedly: for early-onset sepsis-meningitis, it has declined from 1.7 in 1000 births to approximately 0.3 in 1000; and for late-onset disease, it has declined from 0.5/1000 births to 0.3 in 1000 births.[77] These and similar observations have led to the current recommendations of the Centers for Disease Control and Prevention: (1) a screening strategy with culture of pregnant women for group B *Streptococcus* at 35 to 37 weeks of gestation and administration of intrapartum penicillin G (or ampicillin) to all culture-positive women, whether or not they have a risk factor (see next); or (2) a non-screening approach with administration of intrapartum penicillin G (or ampicillin) to all women with a risk factor (previous delivery of an infant with group B streptococcal disease, history of group B streptococcal bacteremia during pregnancy, preterm labor < 37 weeks of gestation, rupture of membranes ≥ 18 hours before delivery, or intrapartum fever).

many medical centers (see earlier). The enormity of the public health problem associated with neonatal sepsis and meningitis caused by group B *Streptococcus* has been alluded to earlier (see "Pathogenesis"). Two basic approaches to prevention of neonatal disease have been proposed: chemoprophylaxis and immunoprophylaxis.

Chemoprophylaxis. Historically, chemoprophylaxis has been an attractive approach because of the susceptibility of group B *Streptococcus* to penicillin in vitro and the relative ease of administering such a relatively safe and well-known antibiotic. The three major chemoprophylactic approaches used since the late 1980s have included treatment of a colonized woman in the third trimester, or at delivery, and treatment of the newborn at birth.[59,72,75,77,239-252]

Among these approaches, *treatment of the colonized woman at delivery* has become the approach of choice.[72,75,77,200,239-242,245,247-251,253-255] The findings in several controlled studies showed conclusively that

Immunoprophylaxis. Immunoprophylaxis is potentially of greater value than chemoprophylaxis because the approach would be less complex and would be most likely to prevent late-onset as well as early-onset disease.[59,77,242,256,257] Because of the protective value of antibody directed against the capsular polysaccharide of group B *Streptococcus, passive immunization* of antibody-deficient women or newborns with intravenous gamma globulin is a reasonable consideration.[59] Given that transplacental transfer of antibody does not occur until after the 34th week of gestation, this approach requires timing late in pregnancy. The value of intravenous human globulin administration was demonstrated in a newborn animal model of group B streptococcal sepsis.[258] Of greatest promise is *active immunization* with purified group B streptococcal polysaccharide. The type III polysaccharide was shown to be immunogenic in adult volunteers,

TABLE 21-18 Outcome of Meningitis Caused by Group B Streptococcal Infection*

Status	Percentage of Survivors	Percentage of Total
Dead		10%–15%
Normal	50%	
Mild or moderate sequelae (borderline or mild mental retardation, unilateral sensorineural hearing loss, arrested hydrocephalus, and spastic monoparesis)	40%	
Severe sequelae (uncontrolled seizures, cortical blindness, spastic quadriparesis, mental retardation [excluding mild cases], severe microcephaly, and hydrocephalus)	10%	

*See text for references.

TABLE 21-19	Outcome of Meningitis Caused by Gram-Negative Enteric Organisms*		
Status		**Percentage of Survivors**	**Percentage of Total**
Dead			15%
Normal		50%	
Mild or moderate sequelae (see Table 21-18)		40%	
Severe sequelae (see Table 21-18)		10%	

*See text for references.

TABLE 21-20	Relationship between Electroencephalographic Background Activity and Outcome*		
	OUTCOME		
Most Abnormal Background	**Normal or Mildly Abnormal**	**Severely Abnormal**	**Death**
Normal or mildly abnormal	9	0	0
Moderately abnormal	5	3	1
Markedly abnormal[†]	0	5	6

Data from Chequer RS, Tharp BR, Dreimane D, Hahn JS, et al: Prognostic value of EEG in neonatal meningitis: Retrospective study of 29 infants, *Pediatr Neurol* 8:417-422, 1992.
*From a study of 29 infants, 15 of whom were less than 38 weeks of gestational age.
[†]Markedly abnormal: markedly excessive discontinuity for postconceptional age, burst suppression, markedly excessive interhemispheric asynchrony or asymmetry, diffusely slow background, extremely low voltage (<5 μV for all states), or isoelectric.

TABLE 21-21	Effect of Intrapartum Chemoprophylaxis on Early-Onset Neonatal Group B Streptococcal Disease		
	NEONATAL EARLY-ONSET DISEASE		
Perinatal Risk Factor	**Ampicillin**	**Control**	
None	0/85 (0%)	5/1170 (0.4%)	
Gestation <37 wk or membrane rupture >12 hr	0/167 (0%)	12/305 (4.0%)	
Intrapartum fever	0/80 (0%)	3/23 (13.0%)	
Total	0/320 (0%)	20/1493 (1.3%)	

Data from Boyer KM, Gotoff SP: Prevention of early-onset neonatal group B streptococcal disease with selective intrapartum chemoprophylaxis, *N Engl J Med* 314:1665-1669, 1986.

including pregnant women, and to be protective of neonatal infection in a mouse model of maternal immunization.[59,77,250,256,257,259-261] More refined vaccines are under development.[77] More data are needed about the optimal vaccine preparation, the degree of immunogenicity, and the prophylactic benefit of available vaccine preparations before widespread use can be recommended, but the approach appears to be very promising.

Supportive Care

Because most infants with neonatal bacterial meningitis exhibit bacteremia and, to varying degrees, multisystem disease, vigorous supportive care is often a major factor in determining outcome. Diligent attention must be paid to ventilation, perfusion, temperature, metabolic state, and complications such as disseminated intravascular coagulation and the development of focal areas of suppurative infection.

Particular importance for vigorous treatment of systemic hypotension relates to the danger of decreases in cerebral blood flow and the consequent occurrence of ischemic neuronal and white matter injury. Thus, the combination of increased intracranial pressure (see Table 21-13) and impaired cerebrovascular autoregulation (see Fig. 21-11) may lead to impaired cerebral blood flow particularly easily with systemic hypotension. A careful clinical study of the occurrence of periventricular leukomalacia in infants with group B streptococcal infection supported this conclusion.[234]

Neurological Disturbances

The major neurological disturbances that must be dealt with in these infants are seizures, inappropriate antidiuretic hormone secretion, cerebral edema, acute hydrocephalus, subdural effusion, and brain abscess.

Seizures. Seizures associated with neonatal bacterial meningitis are notoriously difficult to manage, particularly in the early phases of the disease. Seizures that occur later in the disease, often related to vasculitis and ischemic events, are controlled more readily. In the newborn, phenobarbital is the drug of choice, and the dosage regimen, mode of administration, and other aspects of anticonvulsant management are described in Chapter 5.

Inappropriate Antidiuretic Hormone Secretion. Inappropriate secretion of antidiuretic hormone should be suspected in the infant who exhibits hyponatremia and hypo-osmolality with inappropriately concentrated urine. The diagnosis can be suggested by measurements of serum and urine osmolality, urine volume, fluid intake, and body weight. A radioimmunoassay for antidiuretic hormone can corroborate the diagnosis.[189,190]

The syndrome may lead to a degree of hyponatremia and hypo-osmolality that results in deterioration of the level of consciousness and seizures, as well as aggravation of increased intracranial pressure. Therapy consists principally of fluid restriction.

Cerebral Edema. Cerebral edema is common early in the disease but rarely is severe enough to cause life-threatening herniation of temporal lobe through the tentorial notch or cerebellar tonsils through the foramen magnum. However, this occurrence has been documented in the newborn.[133] Elevation of intracranial pressure is a common accompaniment, but when arterial blood pressure is maintained, the degree of intracranial hypertension alone is not usually severe enough to raise the likelihood of impaired cerebral perfusion. Measurements of cerebral blood flow velocity in patients with neonatal bacterial meningitis support this conclusion.[132] Nevertheless, intracranial pressure should be determined, and, as noted earlier, control of arterial blood pressure is crucial.

Specific treatment of suspected cerebral edema must not be instituted without good reason. Indeed, considerable concern exists that use of hyperosmolar solutions (e.g., mannitol) could cause more difficulties than benefits because of increased movement of the material across the inflamed and permeable blood-brain barrier. Nevertheless, study of a rabbit model of bacterial meningitis showed, after bolus infusion of mannitol, not only a decline in elevated intracranial pressure, but also a decrease in elevated CSF lactate and hypoxanthine concentrations, consistent with an improvement in cerebral perfusion.[262] More data are needed on this issue.

Corticosteroids (dexamethasone) are worthy of consideration because of their value in management of some forms of vasogenic edema (e.g., in association with brain tumors) and bacterial meningitis in older infants and children (particularly that caused by *H. influenzae*).[263–268] In the latter situation, corticosteroids (dexamethasone) administered *at the onset* of antibiotic therapy have been associated with a decreased incidence of neurological or audiological sequelae, perhaps through inhibition of cytokine production and action. However, a randomized clinical trial of 54 infants with neonatal meningitis showed *no apparent benefit of dexamethasone* (0.15 mg/kg/day for 4 days from onset of antibiotic treatment).[269] Administration of fluids at minimal maintenance levels is usually adequate in the management of cerebral edema with neonatal bacterial meningitis.

Acute Hydrocephalus. *Acute* hydrocephalus is a serious, although uncommon, complication. This complication should be suspected when signs of increased intracranial pressure appear in the latter part of the first week and in the second and third weeks of the disease (see also "Clinical Signs" and "Diagnosis"). When prompt decompression is needed, ventriculostomy is the most effective and the safest treatment. Because acute hydrocephalus is often related to marked ventriculitis with localized infection that may be inaccessible to systemic antibiotics, ventriculostomy may also be used for instillation of antibiotic (see "Ventriculostomy"). Occasionally, intraventricular infection and inflammation subside, and the hydrocephalus does not progress after removal of the ventriculostomy. More commonly, a ventriculoperitoneal shunt is subsequently required for long-term treatment of the hydrocephalic state.

Subdural Effusion. Subdural effusion is rarely of clinical significance in neonatal meningitis (i.e., it is not associated with increased intracranial pressure, localized infection, or development of craniocerebral disproportion).[53,270] This complication can be detected from the clinical evaluation, coupled with transillumination, or, in the more suggestive case, by CT or MRI scan. In the absence of signs of increased intracranial pressure, localized infection, or imminent development of craniocerebral disproportion, a patient with subdural effusion detected by imaging should not be subjected to repeated taps, because the natural history of the lesion is to resolve spontaneously.[270,271]

Brain Abscess. Brain abscess may occur with neonatal bacterial meningitis (see earlier discussion), and management thereof is discussed in a separate section later. The diagnosis is best made by CT or MRI scan.

Antibiotics

The central goal in the treatment of neonatal bacterial meningitis is eradication of microorganisms from the CSF. To accomplish this goal, the appropriate antibiotic must be chosen and administered in adequate doses and by an effective route. In general, the CSF in meningitis secondary to gram-positive organisms (e.g., group B *Streptococcus* and *L. monocytogenes*) is more readily sterilized than in meningitis secondary to gram-negative organisms. Thus, with group B *Streptococcus* or *L. monocytogenes*, negative cultures are usually attained after 24 to 48 hours of treatment, whereas with coliform bacilli, negative cultures generally are not obtained until after 2 to 5 days of treatment.[198,227,236,272,273] To a considerable degree, this time difference relates to the relative ease of attaining adequate CSF concentrations of ampicillin versus an aminoglycoside.

Initial Treatment. The optimal initial treatment in a newborn with bacterial meningitis of unknown cause is a combination of ampicillin and an aminoglycoside.[16,22,51,53,66,198,200,273–277] The choice of aminoglycoside among gentamicin, kanamycin, amikacin, and tobramycin depends particularly on the susceptibility of gram-negative bacteria likely to be found in a given nursery population, but gentamicin is used most

TABLE 21-22 **Antibiotics Preferred in Neonatal Meningitis According to Organism**

Organism	Antibiotics
Group B *Streptococcus*	Ampicillin (or penicillin G) and aminoglycoside (gentamicin)
Escherichia coli and other coliforms	Aminoglycoside and ampicillin or third-generation cephalosporin (cefotaxime) with or without aminoglycoside
Aminoglycoside-resistant coliforms	Third-generation cephalosporin (cefotaxime)
Listeria monocytogenes	Ampicillin with or without aminoglycoside
Group D *Streptococcus* (nonenterococcal)	Ampicillin
Group D *Streptococcus* (enterococcal)	Ampicillin and aminoglycoside
Staphylococcus epidermidis	Vancomycin
Staphylococcus aureus	Methicillin or vancomycin
Pseudomonas aeruginosa	Ceftazidime and aminoglycoside
Citrobacter diversus	Third-generation cephalosporin (cefotaxime), gentamicin, trimethoprim-sulfamethoxazole (or meropenem or imipenem-cilastatin)

commonly. Although more readily demonstrated in vitro than in vivo, the combination of ampicillin and an aminoglycoside has been shown to be synergistic versus several common gram-negative and gram-positive organisms.[32,278-280] The *usual doses, before results of cultures*, are, for ampicillin, 150 mg/kg/day in the first week of life and 200 mg/kg/day after the first week, and, for gentamicin, 5 mg/kg/day in the first week and 7.5 mg/kg/day after the first week.[281] The drugs can be administered intramuscularly, but intravenous administration is preferred. Standard sources should be consulted for recent changes in preferred antibiotics and dosing.[281]

Specific Treatment. When a definitive bacteriological diagnosis is established and appropriate susceptibilities are determined, more specific antibiotic treatment can be instituted. The usual organisms and the respective, preferred antibiotics are shown in Table 21-22.* Thus, a penicillin (ampicillin or penicillin G) and an aminoglycoside (see later section) are preferred for group B *Streptococcus*, ampicillin and an aminoglycoside or cefotaxime with or without an aminoglycoside are preferred for *E. coli* and most other coliforms, a third-generation cephalosporin (e.g., cefotaxime) is preferred for aminoglycoside-resistant coliform bacteria, ampicillin alone or with an aminoglycoside is preferred for *L. monocytogenes* and nonenterococcal group D *Streptococcus* (ampicillin and an aminoglycoside are used for enterococcal group D *Streptococcus*), vancomycin is used for *S. epidermidis* (a common organism in infants with indwelling vascular catheters) infections, methicillin or vancomycin is given for *S. aureus* (almost always beta-lactamase positive) infections, and a third-generation cephalosporin (ceftazidime) and an aminoglycoside are preferred for *P. aeruginosa*. (Meningitis caused by *Pseudomonas* should be treated with intraventricular instillation of gentamicin in addition to the parenteral route, in view of the gravity of this infection.) Treatment of *Citrobacter diversus* is very difficult and consists of a third-generation cephalosporin (cefotaxime),

gentamicin, and trimethoprim-sulfamethoxazole; imipenem-cilastatin may be a useful alternative to the last of these agents. Standard sources should be consulted for recent changes in preferred antibiotics and dosing.[281]

Duration of Treatment. The duration of treatment in neonatal bacterial meningitis is based on the clinical condition of the patient, as well as on the bacteriological response to therapy. Bacteriological response to therapy is monitored by sampling of CSF approximately every 2 to 3 days in the first week after initiation of therapy or until the CSF is sterile. In general, meningitis caused by gram-negative organisms is treated for at least 2 weeks after sterilization of the CSF or for a total of 3 weeks, whichever is greater. Meningitis resulting from gram-positive organisms most prudently is treated also for 3 weeks, although the infant with a rapid bacteriological response and good clinical status could be treated for 2 weeks after bacteria can no longer be cultured from the CSF. A repeat examination of the CSF is indicated 48 hours after discontinuation of antibiotic therapy.

Treatment Failure. Treatment failure, for the purposes of this discussion, refers to abnormal persistence of a positive CSF culture or clinical deterioration, or both. Failure to sterilize the CSF in meningitis is much more common with gram-negative than with gram-positive organisms and is related principally to (1) inadequate delivery of antibiotic to the site of the infection within the subarachnoid and ventricular spaces, (2) the presence of an organism that is not sensitive to the usually attainable concentration of antibiotic in the CSF, (3) the presence of a site of infection that is inaccessible to antibiotic, and (4) host factors. Evaluation of these factors requires assessment of antibiotic levels in at least lumbar (and, perhaps, ventricular) CSF, of inhibitory and bactericidal susceptibilities of the organism to the antibiotics used, and of a possible site of sequestered infection (e.g., ventriculitis; see the next section).

Ventriculitis

Ventriculitis is considered an important cause of the difficulty in sterilizing the CSF, and as a corollary, of

---

*See references 16,22,51,53,59,66,77,198,273,275,281-286.

the relatively poor prognosis in neonatal bacterial meningitis, particularly that resulting from infection with gram-negative organisms, for two major reasons. First, as I described earlier, involvement of the ventricular lining is a nearly uniform occurrence.[88,122,272] Second, as noted by experienced clinicians and as reported in earlier uncontrolled series of infants with ventriculitis and persistence of infection in the CSF after treatment with systemic antibiotics, intraventricular instillation of antibiotics appears to be beneficial in *selected* cases.[125,198,287-289]

Inadequacy of Intrathecal Therapy. Intrathecal antibiotic therapy is not an adequate means of sterilizing ventricular CSF or improving outcome in gram-negative neonatal bacterial meningitis. In a controlled study of 117 infants with meningitis caused by gram-negative organisms, the effect of the addition of intrathecal gentamicin to a regimen of systemic ampicillin and gentamicin was evaluated.[236] No benefit of intrathecal antibiotic was observed. The failure to demonstrate any benefit from the intrathecal therapy was considered to suggest that adequate concentrations of antibiotic were not delivered throughout the CNS and, particularly, the ventricular system. Failure of intrathecal administration of antibiotic to enter and sterilize the ventricular CSF has been demonstrated in older patients.[290,291] These latter observations are entirely compatible with the unidirectional flow of CSF out of the ventricular system.

Inadequacy of Routine Intraventricular Therapy. A cooperative study of 70 infants with meningitis caused by gram-negative organisms was carried out to evaluate the role of *intraventricular* instillation of gentamicin (in addition to systemic ampicillin and gentamicin).[272] Fifty-one infants had evidence of ventriculitis (i.e., ventricular CSF containing > 200 WBCs/mm³ or organisms on stained smear or culture); the results of treatment of that group are displayed in Table 21-23. No difference between the two groups in the time required to sterilize the CSF was observed. Still more impressive, the mortality rate in the infants treated with parenteral therapy alone was lower than in those treated with parenteral therapy and intraventricular therapy. Thus, *routine* intraventricular therapy of meningitis produced by gram-negative organisms had no beneficial effect and may have had a deleterious effect. (If the latter is true, the cause of such a deleterious effect is unclear,

although injury to myelin and axons in brain stem of an adult human patient and in brain stem and spinal cord of rabbits administered gentamicin by the intrathecal route has been described.[292] Deleterious neurological and neuropathological effects of gentamicin also have been demonstrated in rabbits administered gentamicin intraventricularly.[293]) However, in view of the generally favorable outcome in the control group, it is apparent that ventriculitis only very uncommonly results in a site of infection inaccessible to systemic antibiotics. To determine conclusively whether intraventricular antibiotics are useful in the small subset of patients with such inaccessible intraventricular infection, a much larger study would be required (this requirement may not be possible to fulfill, because the study of McCracken and co-workers[272] included 10 institutions). Our approach to this subset of patients is described later in "Ventriculostomy."

Indications for Diagnostic Ventricular Puncture. The failure to improve the prognosis of meningitis caused by gram-negative bacteria with routine intraventricular therapy raises two important questions in the management of neonatal bacterial meningitis:

1. When should the lateral ventricle be tapped?
2. How should the information obtained be used?

As discussed earlier in "Diagnosis," I believe that the indications for evaluating the lateral ventricles in the infant are as follows: (1) bacteriological (i.e., persistence of infection in the lumbar CSF at 4 days) or (2) clinical (i.e., failure of clinical improvement or, still more importantly, the appearance of clinical deterioration, even if lumbar CSF cell count is improving and CSF sterilization occurs). If these indications are present and *antibiotic therapy has been appropriate in terms of susceptibilities of the organism, doses of the drugs, and, if available, concentrations of the critical drugs in the CSF*, an ultrasound scan or CT or MRI scan should be obtained. If the ventricles are not too small, a ventricular tap should be performed. If the ventricular fluid exhibits marked pleocytosis and organisms demonstrable on smear or culture, it is likely that the systemically administered antibiotics, usually aminoglycosides in meningitis caused by gram-negative bacteria, are not eradicating a reservoir of infection within the ventricular system.

Ventriculostomy. Ventriculostomy (with intermittent intraventricular instillation of an antibiotic, usually through a reservoir) is indicated when the ventricular

TABLE 21-23 **Effect of Intraventricular Therapy on Neonatal Meningitis and Ventriculitis Caused by Gram-Negative Enteric Organisms***

Mode of Therapy	Days CSF Culture Positive	Mortality Rate	Normal (Percentage of Survivors)
Parenteral†	3.6	13%	54%
Parenteral† and intraventricular‡	3.4	44%	60%

CSF, cerebrospinal fluid.
Data from McCracken GH Jr, Mize SG, Neonatal Cooperative Study Group: Intraventricular therapy of neonatal meningitis caused by gram-negative enteric bacilli, *Pediatr Res* 13:464, 1979.
*Based on 51 cases.
†Ampicillin and gentamicin.
‡Gentamicin.

TABLE 21-24 Intraventricular Antibiotics for Ventriculitis		
Antibiotic	**Dose (mg)**	**Desired Peak Cerebrospinal Fluid Concentration (μg/mL)**
Gentamicin	1–5	80–120*
Vancomycin	4–5	80–100
Polymyxin	1–2	Unknown

*Histological change in white matter observed with concentrations >150 μg/mL.
Data from Smith AL, Haas J: Neonatal bacterial meningitis. In Scheld WM, Whitley RJ, Durack DT, editors: *Infections of the Central Nervous System*, New York: 1991, Raven Press.

tap demonstrates *purulent fluid with persistent infection*.[198] Antibiotics should be instilled in concentrations that generally exceed those usually sought in serum. Table 21-24 shows the commonly used intraventricular antibiotics and the concentrations sought.[198] Serial measurements of the CSF concentrations of the antibiotics are important. The best approach is to administer the agent at a dose calculated to produce a concentration approximately 20-fold greater than the measured minimal bactericidal concentration.[198]

Ventriculostomy, with external drainage, may be required in neonatal bacterial meningitis when ventriculitis has caused obstruction to CSF flow and acute hydrocephalus, manifested by increased intracranial pressure and dilated lateral ventricles. This condition may develop despite eradication of the ventricular infection by the systemic antibiotics and therefore with a sterile ventricular CSF. In such a circumstance, intraventricular instillation of antibiotic is not needed, and the task is management of the intracranial hypertension by CSF drainage, as described in Chapter 11 in relation to rapidly progressive posthemorrhagic hydrocephalus.

BRAIN ABSCESS

Brain abscess is an uncommon and devastating, although potentially treatable, disorder in the neonatal period (Table 21-25). Most examples of neonatal brain abscess occur as a complication of bacterial meningitis, especially that resulting from particularly virulent gram-negative organisms.[41,146,294-310] However, approximately 25 cases of neonatal brain abscesses have been reported that were apparently not the consequence of meningitis.[144,303,311-318]

Etiology

The most commonly reported organisms associated with brain abscess have been those with the particular capacity to invade nervous tissue and cause necrosis. Gram-negative organisms have been implicated most often, especially *Citrobacter*, but also *Proteus, Pseudomonas, Serratia*, and other coliform bacilli (see previous discussion of bacterial meningitis).[41,145,146,295-298,301-306,308-310,319] *Citrobacter* and, to a lesser extent, *Proteus* and *Serratia* are the most commonly identified pathogens. Gram-positive organisms are involved much less often, although group B *Streptococcus* and *S. aureus* have been identified in isolated cases.[109,316,320-322] Spinal epidural abscess secondary to *S. aureus* also has been reported.[323] Still rarer, three cases of neonatal brain abscess secondary

to *M. hominis* have been recorded.[314,318,320] Finally, as noted in the following section, certain fungi, especially *Candida*, may cause brain abscess, usually multiple and small, especially in very-low-birth-weight infants.

Pathogenesis

The common conditions for the development of brain abscess are *cerebral necrosis and bacteremia*. In bacterial meningitis, the parenchymal necrosis that may become infected to form an abscess is usually caused initially by vasculitis with infarction. It is not surprising, then, that the organisms associated with brain abscess are those that produce severe vasculopathy with the meningitis. This point was demonstrated vividly by the study of Foreman and co-workers.[324] Severe vasculitis with infarction and with numerous organisms present around inflamed blood vessels and in cerebral parenchyma was shown in two infants who died within 2 days of clinical onset of meningitis caused

TABLE 21-25 Brain Abscess in the Newborn*
Occurrence without Bacterial Meningitis
≈33% of cases of neonatal brain abscess *not* accompanied by bacterial meningitis
Relation to Bacterial Meningitis
≈15% of *gram-negative* bacterial meningitis complicated by abscess
Most Common Organisms
Citrobacter diversus, Proteus species, *Serratia* species
Neuropathology
Abscesses usually large, multiple (≈60%), frontal (≈70%), and not well encapsulated
Onset of Clinical Features
Average age, 9 days
Clinical Presentation
Seizures > nonspecific signs of sepsis > increasing head circumference
Complications
Hydrocephalus requiring shunt placement (35%): only in patients with meningitis
Treatment
Aspiration (ultrasound-guided) and antibiotics generally effective; antibiotics alone may lead to cure
Prognosis
Mortality rate, ≈15%; cognitive deficits, ≈75%; epilepsy, ≈60%

*See text for references.

by *Citrobacter*.[324] Presumably, the next phase of the illness would have been infection of necrotic tissue and abscess formation, a feature of approximately 50% to 80% of reported cases of *Citrobacter* meningitis.[16,295,296,301-303,308,310] In the rarer cases of brain abscess not associated with primary meningitis, the initial injury to brain is not always clear but often has appeared to be hypoxic-ischemic cerebral injury, periventricular hemorrhagic infarction, or septic embolus.

Neuropathology

The distinguishing features of brain abscess in the newborn have been threefold: (1) relatively large size of lesions, (2) relatively poor capsule formation, and (3) multiple number. The lesions have been located almost uniformly in the cerebral hemispheres, most often the frontal lobes, and often have encompassed several lobes. Occasionally, the abscess has been tapped inadvertently at the time of ventricular or subdural puncture. Detailed microscopic data are not available, but hemorrhage and necrosis usually have been noted with the purulence.

Clinical Features

Two major clinical syndromes have been described with neonatal brain abscess: (1) an acute to subacute evolution of signs of cerebral parenchymal involvement, especially seizures (less commonly, hemiparesis), often accompanied by signs of increased intracranial pressure (vomiting, bulging anterior fontanelle, separated sutures, and enlarging head); and (2) an acute onset of fulminating bacterial meningitis. The *first syndrome* is more common, has its onset from the first few days to weeks of life, and often occurs in association with acute or ongoing bacterial meningitis. The initial diagnosis occasionally has been congenital hydrocephalus. The *second syndrome* differs little from later-onset neonatal bacterial meningitis (see previous section).

Diagnosis

Clinical Evaluation

The diagnosis of brain abscess should be considered in any infant with the acute or subacute evolution of signs of increased intracranial pressure or possible hydrocephalus. In the absence of meningitis, fever is not a feature; in the six well-studied cases of Hoffman and co-workers,[312] four infants were afebrile. In an infant with bacterial meningitis, brain abscess should be suspected when seizures or prominent focal cerebral signs develop, a poor clinical response to antibiotic therapy occurs, or the CSF formula does not appear to be compatible with the clinical syndrome (e.g., several hundred WBCs in the CSF of a gravely ill infant, or, in a child with "meningitis" and a few hundred WBCs in the initial CSF, the sudden appearance of several thousand polymorphonuclear WBCs in a subsequent CSF examination and marked clinical deterioration). (The latter

occurrence develops with rupture of the brain abscess into the lateral ventricle or subarachnoid space.)

Laboratory Evaluation

Peripheral White Blood Cell Count. The combination of clinical features just described, without fever but with a high peripheral WBC count, is common in brain abscess without meningitis. In the series of Hoffman and co-workers,[312] the peripheral WBC count ranged from 18,000 to 34,000.

Cerebrospinal Fluid. In the infant without bacterial meningitis, the CSF usually contains pleocytosis consisting predominantly of mononuclear cells and usually numbering less than a few hundred. CSF protein content is elevated, usually to approximately 75 to 150 mg/100 mL. Unless bacterial meningitis is also present, the organism will not be apparent on Gram stain or culture. The sudden appearance of clinical deterioration and thousands of polymorphonuclear leukocytes in the CSF is characteristic of rupture of the abscess into the ventricular system.

Brain Imaging. The diagnosis of brain abscess is raised most conclusively by CT or, especially, MRI scan and, occasionally, by ultrasound scan. On CT scan, a variably circumscribed region of decreased attenuation is apparent, often much greater in extent than the abscess itself, because of the presence of cerebritis with surrounding edema. The rim of the abscess usually enhances after the injection of contrast material (Fig. 21-22). MRI scanning provides better resolution than does CT scanning (Figs. 21-23 and 21-24).

Cranial ultrasound scan has proved somewhat useful in diagnosis of cerebral abscess in the newborn. Thus, in experimental brain abscess, ultrasound scanning was as effective as CT in identification of the early stages. An echogenic rim with a hypoechogenic center was characteristic.[325] Such an appearance has been observed in neonatal brain abscess.[300,304,322,326,327]

Identification of the Organism. The organism occasionally can be isolated from blood, but aspiration of the abscess cavity is usually necessary to obtain a definite bacteriological diagnosis. (In the presence of meningitis, the organism can be isolated from CSF.) Aspiration can be carried out with ultrasonographic guidance (see "Management"). Because some of the responsible organisms require special techniques for isolation and identification, the material should be handled in an especially careful manner.

Prognosis

The prognosis has been poor for those infants in whom correct diagnosis and appropriate treatment were delayed. Overall, approximately 15% of newborns with brain abscess have died of the acute illness, and of the survivors, 75% have experienced mental deficiency (intelligence quotient or development quotient <80), and 60% have developed epilepsy.[16,145,295,296,300-306,308,310,312,316] Perhaps the most

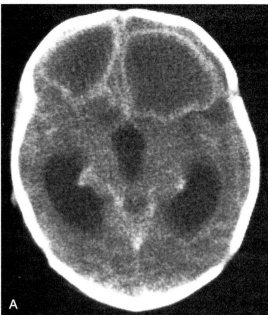

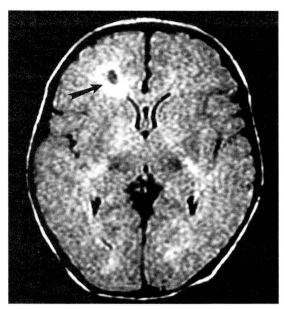

Figure 21-23 Brain abscess: magnetic resonance imaging (MRI) scan. This 2-week-old infant had *Citrobacter* meningitis. This fluid-attenuated inversion-recovery MRI scan shows a circumscribed lesion in the right frontal white matter *(arrow)*, with surrounding edema, consistent with an abscess. The lesion enhanced after injection of gadolinium (not shown). Resolution of the presumed abscess occurred after antibiotic therapy only.

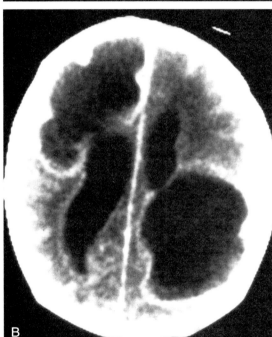

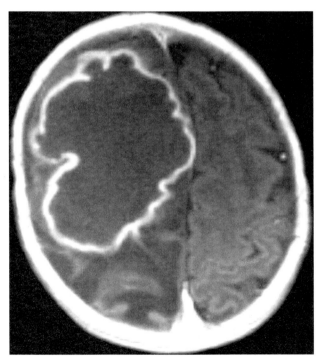

Figure 21-22 Brain abscess: computed tomography scans. Scans were obtained from infants with *Citrobacter diversus* meningitis, after injection of contrast material. Note the areas of decreased attenuation surrounded by a rim of increased attenuation in, **A**, bilateral frontal areas and, **B**, right frontal and left parietal areas. *(Courtesy of Dr. Mark W. Kline.)*

unfavorable outcome has been in infants with abscess and *C. diversus* meningitis; the mortality rate has been 30%, and only 20% of survivors have been normal on follow-up.

Management

The most essential issue concerning management is prompt diagnosis. In the infant with meningitis,

Figure 21-24 Brain abscess: magnetic resonance imaging (MRI) scan, after gadolinium contrast. This 5-week-old infant had focal seizures, *Proteus* sepsis, and a complicated congenital cardiac lesion, including an atrioventricular canal defect. This axial MRI scan shows a striking ring-enhancing cerebral lesion, consistent with brain abscess. Craniotomy with drainage of the abscess was performed. *(Courtesy of Dr. Omar Khwaja.)*

particularly that caused by *Citrobacter, Proteus*, or *Serratia*, serial brain imaging is indicated to detect abscess as early as possible. In the infant without meningitis, a high index of clinical suspicion is critical, and appropriate imaging procedures are essential.

No consensus exists for therapy for brain abscess in the neonatal period. The three principal approaches are (1) medical therapy alone, (2) aspirations through a burr hole or through the percutaneous route, and (3) open surgical drainage and extirpation. The demonstration of cure early in the disease with systemic antibiotics has been observed in newborns as in older children.[146,305,306,308,317,318,322,328-332] Whether antibiotics with potent bactericidal activity, broad antibacterial spectrum, and good penetration into the CNS (e.g., third-generation cephalosporins) will prove most useful in this regard remains to be determined. In the case of *C. diversus*, the addition to the antibiotic regimen of a drug that is concentrated in phagocytes (i.e., trimethoprim-sulfamethoxazole) or to which the organism is especially sensitive (i.e., meropenem or imipenem) may be particularly important.[281,301,302,310]

Despite the multiple reports of "medical cure" of brain abscess, drainage is necessary in selected cases. Of the two approaches to drainage (i.e., serial aspirations and open surgical drainage), the advent of ultrasound-guided aspirations suggests that this method is of particular value, even for multiple lesions.[326,327] CT-guided aspiration also can be used, but this approach is less convenient. Needle aspiration is useful not only for initial diagnosis and drainage, but also for determination of antibiotic levels in the abscess cavity.

Open surgical drainage is the most definitive therapeutic approach for brain abscess. However, if the infant's condition is not deteriorating and the responsible organism has been identified, a trial of intensive antibiotic therapy, followed, if necessary, by serial ultrasound-guided needle aspirations, is reasonable. Careful serial brain imaging should be performed to ensure that the lesion (or lesions) is (are) not worsening. In such a circumstance, prompt open surgical drainage is necessary.

DISSEMINATED FUNGAL INFECTION

Disseminated fungal infection in the newborn may cause meningitis, often with microabscesses. I discuss this category of nonbacterial disease in this chapter rather than in Chapter 20 because the clinical features often mimic those of bacterial sepsis and the neuropathological features are similar to those of bacterial meningitis and brain abscess. Although several fungi (e.g., *Cryptococcus, Coccidioides*, and *Aspergillus*) have been reported to cause meningitis or abscess, or both, in the newborn, systemic infection by *Candida*, especially *Candida albicans* and, more recently, *Candida parapsilosis*, particularly in the very-low-birth-weight newborn, is by far the most common neonatal disseminated fungal infection.[333-358] Earlier studies of somewhat selected cases indicated that at least one third of cases of systemic candidiasis in premature infants exhibited involvement of the CNS.[336,340,344] More recent data show that approximately 10% to 25% of cases exhibit CNS involvement.[349,352-355] However, the magnitude of the problem is substantial because approximately 10% to 20% of all infants weighing less than 1000 g at birth develop candidiasis, as do approximately 25% of infants of 23 to 24 weeks of gestational age.[351,355,357,359] The major features of systemic candidiasis in the newborn are summarized in Table 21-26.

Pathogenesis

The reasons that the newborn, particularly the premature newborn, is vulnerable to disseminated fungal infection are not entirely known but involve a combination of multiple immune deficiencies and insufficient anatomical barriers to infection, in a setting of intensive medical interventions for systemic illness.[333,340,356,357,360] The common historical findings of prolonged use of indwelling vascular catheters, endotracheal intubation, necrotizing enterocolitis, and surgery indicate possible portals of entry for the organism.[333,335,337,338,340,350,356,357,360] The retrograde medication syringes of total parenteral nutrition systems were important sites for infection in one large study.[347] The prior use of multiple courses of broad-spectrum antibiotics in most patients is a likely cause of disrupted microbial flora and enhances the potential for fungal infection.[340,357,360,361]

Neuropathology

Neuropathological studies of neonatal systemic candidiasis are not abundant.[349,357] However, the principal

---

TABLE 21-26   Major Features of Systemic Candidiasis

Very-low-birth-weight infant (<1500 g), especially extremely-low-birth-weight infant (<1000 g)
History of *broad-spectrum antibiotic therapy* and *indwelling vascular catheters*; also, total parenteral nutrition, steroid therapy, necrotizing enterocolitis, and abdominal or cardiac surgery
Acute or subacute evolution of respiratory deterioration, temperature instability, apnea and bradycardia, abdominal distention, guaiac-positive stools, and hyperglycemia
Diagnosis by identification of organism (usually *Candida albicans*) by Gram stain and culture
Neuropathology of meningitis and brain abscesses
Treatment by combination of amphotericin B and flucytosine
Outcome in promptly identified and treated patients improving: 70%–85% survive but ≈50% of survivors have neurodevelopmental impairments

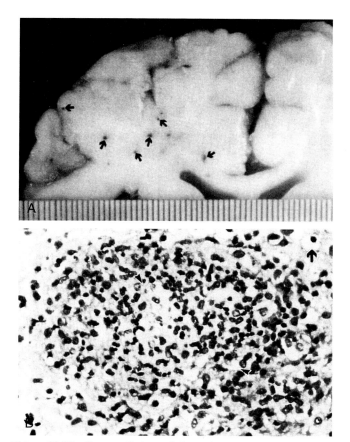

features have included meningitis, ventriculitis, and cerebral or cerebellar microabscesses. The abscesses are characterized by a necrotic center with a rim of inflammatory cells and edema (Fig. 21-25). Fungal filaments are common in the lesion. With subacute lesions, a more granulomatous appearance develops, and endothelial proliferation is often prominent. The microabscesses may become confluent and may create prominent mass lesions.

Clinical Features

Like bacterial sepsis, systemic candidiasis does not produce a distinct clinical syndrome. However, certain features are common (see Table 21-26), such as insidious more often than abrupt onset, mean age of approximately 2 to 4 weeks (albeit with an overall wider range), respiratory deterioration (often requiring reinstitution of ventilatory therapy), apnea and bradycardia, abdominal signs suggestive of necrotizing enterocolitis (e.g., abdominal distention and guaiac-positive stools), and carbohydrate intolerance with hyperglycemia and

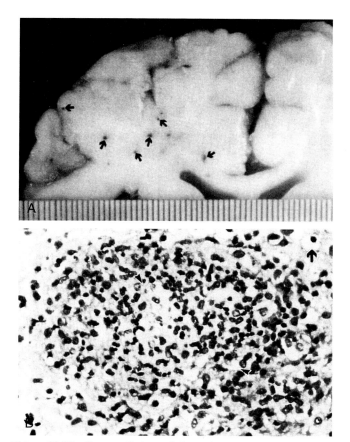

Figure 21-25 Neuropathology of disseminated candidiasis in a premature infant (29 weeks of gestation) who died at 3 months of age. Note the microabscesses *(arrows)* in **A**, a coronal section of cerebrum. **B**, Photomicrograph of a microabscess shows a slightly necrotic center with infiltrating leukocytes *(arrowheads)* and surrounding swollen astrocytes *(arrows)*. *(From Huang CC, Chen CY, Yang HB, Wang SM, et al: Central nervous system candidiasis in very low-birth-weight premature neonates and infants: US characteristics and histopathologic and MR imaging correlates in five patients, Radiology 209:49-56, 1998.)*

glycosuria.[335-338,340,348,349,353-355,357,360] Many infants exhibit a generalized macular erythematous rash shortly after onset of the systemic illness; skin abscesses are apparent somewhat less commonly.[335,340,360]

Diagnosis

A high index of suspicion and a persistent approach to diagnosis are critical. *Identification of the organism in blood, CSF, or urine* is the most common means of establishing the diagnosis.[333,335,337,338,340,348,357,360] Gram stain of urine or CSF, especially urine, is a particularly useful means of diagnosis. The presence of gram-positive, small, oval, budding yeast cells, and sometimes hyphae with budding yeast cells attached along their length, is typical.[333,338] Culture then results in growth of the organism in 2 to 3 days; however, cultures may be positive only intermittently, and frequent cultures are necessary.

Careful *study of the CSF* shows abnormalities, albeit often not marked, in most patients with CNS involvement. In a study of 13 patients, the WBC count was greater than $10/mm^3$ in 10 patients (range, 2 to $260/mm^3$), the protein concentration was greater than 100 mg/dL in 11 (range, 84 to 825 mg/dL), and the CSF-to-serum glucose ratio was less than 0.60 in 4 patients (range, 0.35 to 0.70).[336] At least one of these abnormalities was present in all 13 patients. In a later study of 5 infants, the CSF WBC count ranged from 31 to $399/mm^3$, the protein concentration ranged from 127 to 259 mg/dL, and the glucose concentration ranged from 10 to 58 mg/dL.[349] In a more recent study, of 16 infants, the median WBC count was $52/mm^3$, and the protein level 226 mg/dL.[354] However, it is not unusual to observe overt *Candida* meningitis by cranial imaging with unremarkable CSF findings. Moreover, cerebral abscesses have been reported in multiple infants with negative CSF cultures or CSF examinations, and often both.[334,335,353]

The structural pathology is shown particularly well by ultrasound, CT, and MRI scanning.[349] Ultrasound scan is especially effective in demonstrating the intraventricular septa and periventricular echogenicity of the ventriculitis (Fig. 21-26). Moreover, the multiple echogenic foci of microabscesses may be seen in cerebral parenchyma, basal ganglia, and cerebellum. MRI is particularly sensitive for the demonstration of the microabscesses and the meningitis, especially in the posterior fossa (Fig. 21-27).

Prognosis

The outcome is not entirely clear because of the relatively recent advent of prompt diagnosis and therapy. In previous years, most affected infants with CNS involvement either were first detected at postmortem examination or died before therapy could be instituted. However, with prompt diagnosis and therapy (see following section), approximately 70% to 85% of premature infants have survived, although approximately 50% of survivors exhibit cognitive or motor deficits, or both.[335-338,340,349,358,360,362] The outcome is distinctly better in term than in premature infants.[352-355,357,360] Substantial numbers of deaths in the premature infants have been related to complicating illnesses (e.g., chronic pulmonary disease).

Management

Prevention is a major goal, and, surely, injudicious use of indwelling vascular catheters and broad-spectrum antibiotics should be avoided. In recent years, promising data have been presented concerning the use of fluconazole prophylaxis in premature infants in neonatal intensive care facilities.[359,362-364a] A reduction in colonization and systemic *Candida* infection and decreased rates of progression from initial colonization to systemic disease have been shown. In one study, prophylactic fluconazole was targeted to infants administered broad-spectrum antibiotics for more than 3 days; the incidences of invasive fungal infection were 6.3% in the control group versus 1.1% in the treated group.[362]

Treatment of documented infection should be prompt. It is critical to remove central catheters promptly.[355] Amphotericin B remains the drug of choice for systemic candidiasis.[348,357] The initial dose is 0.5 mg/kg and is increased promptly to 1 mg/kg/day if no toxicity is observed. For CNS disease, a cumulative dose of 25 to 30 mg/kg is usually necessary. The major adverse effect in newborns is renal toxicity; hepatic toxicity is much less common in infants than in older patients. Careful monitoring of blood levels and reduction in dosage at the first signs of toxicity are important and effective.[337,338] The addition of 5-fluorocytosine (flucytosine, 50 to 100 mg/kg/day) has been advocated for patients with CNS disease.[337,338,344,346,348,357] This agent exhibits hepatotoxicity but acts synergistically with amphotericin B in treatment of the disease. Moreover, the excellent penetration into the CSF of flucytosine, as opposed to amphotericin B, suggests that this is the particularly critical drug for intracranial

disease. In apparently resistant infection, caspofungin, a newer antifungal agent, has been effective.[365]

TETANUS NEONATORUM

Neonatal tetanus is a rare disorder in the United States, primarily because of widespread immunization programs and effective obstetrical care. Three cases have been reported in the United States in the past 25 years.[366] However, in many developing countries, the disease is very common and is a major cause of neonatal death. In a careful study conducted in a town in Sudan, 1 in every 110 infants died of neonatal tetanus.[367] In Bangladesh, Pakistan, and India, the rate of deaths caused by neonatal tetanus has been reported to be more than 20 per 1000 live births.[368] Such worldwide mortality rates from neonatal tetanus suggest that at least 260,000 lives are lost each year from neonatal tetanus in developing countries.[368-373]

Pathogenesis

Neonatal tetanus is caused by the exotoxin of the anaerobe *Clostridium tetani*, which usually gains entry through the umbilical stump. The umbilical cord usually has been cut at the time of birth with an unsterile instrument and occasionally has even been smeared with a variety of unsterile foreign materials. Any degree of passive transfer of immunity to the infant during gestation is rare. In an older series of 54 affected

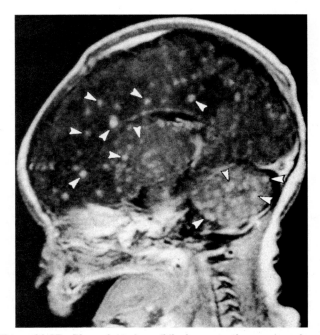

Figure 21-27 **Disseminated candidiasis: magnetic resonance imaging (MRI) scan.** This parasagittal T1-weighted MRI scan after gadolinium injection shows disseminated enhancing nodules *(arrowheads)*, consistent with microabscesses. *(From Huang CC, Chen CY, Yang HB, Wang SM, et al: Central nervous system candidiasis in very low-birth-weight premature neonates and infants: US characteristics and histopathologic and MR imaging correlates in five patients, Radiology 209:49-56, 1998.)*

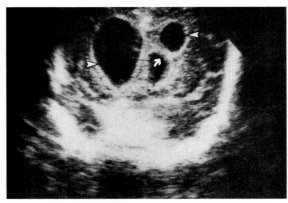

Figure 21-26 **Disseminated candidiasis: coronal ultrasound scan in a premature infant.** Note the echogenic ependyma *(arrowheads)* and the intraventricular septa *(arrow)*, both consistent with ventriculitis. *(From Huang CC, Chen CY, Yang HB, Wang SM, et al: Central nervous system candidiasis in very low-birth-weight premature neonates and infants: US characteristics and histopathologic and MR imaging correlates in five patients, Radiology 209:49-56, 1998.)*

infants reported from the United States, only 3 of the mothers had any form of tetanus toxoid immunization.[374] A similar experience, albeit with much greater magnitude, has been reported from developing countries.[369-373,375-378] In one large study in Bangladesh, the apparent risk of neonatal tetanus initially appeared to be no less in infants of mothers who had received tetanus toxoid previously; subsequent to the survey, it was discovered by a reference laboratory that the tetanus vaccine had "no potency."[370]

Tetanus toxin, a protein of 150,000 molecular weight, selectively inhibits *inhibitory* synaptic activity within the CNS.[379-382] The tetanus neurotoxin has been shown to be a zinc-dependent protease, the substrate for which is a membrane protein localized to the presynaptic nerve ending.[382] The latter protein serves as a docking site of synaptic vesicles before vesicular release. The proteolytic action of the tetanus neurotoxin on this vesicle-associated membrane protein releases the latter into the cytosol and prevents docking and thereby release of the neurotransmitter-containing vesicles. The *synaptic release* of inhibitory transmitters, particularly glycine and gamma-aminobutyric acid, is affected. The synapses are those of interneurons of polysynaptic pathways, especially in spinal cord and brain stem. Once fixed at the presynaptic membrane site, the toxin cannot be neutralized by antitoxin, and clinical recovery depends on the slow process of membrane turnover and synthesis of vesicle-associated membrane protein. The enhanced excitatory activity that characterizes the neurological features of neonatal tetanus presumably relates to an impairment of the normal balance between inhibitory and excitatory influences on the lower motor neurons in the brain stem and spinal cord.

Clinical Features

The major clinical features, depicted in Table 21-27, have been derived from the study of hundreds of affected infants reported from developing countries.[371,372,377,383-394] The usual incubation period is 5 to 10 days, and thus it is not surprising that most cases of neonatal tetanus begin in the latter part of the first week or early in the second week of life. The earlier the onset, the more severe are the clinical features and the greater is the risk of death. In the moderate to severe case, the course is characteristic. Diminished sucking or refusal to suck, impaired feeding, excessive crying, irritability, and rigid abdomen are the initial features. Fever is common and is a risk factor for a poor outcome. These signs are followed within 24 to 48 hours by the hallmarks of the disease, which are related to enhanced muscular activity (i.e., trismus, facial rigidity [risus sardonicus], generalized rigidity [retrocollis and opisthotonos in severe cases], and spasms). The trismus impairs feeding, and the infant exhibits certain features particularly characteristic of neonatal tetanus (i.e., the jaw often is held open, only to close tightly when stimulated by attempts to feed the infant orally). The generalized rigidity is usually accompanied by a characteristic, persistent flexion of the toes. The spasms are exacerbated by stimulation, may occur many times an hour, and may be

TABLE 21-27	Major Clinical Features of Neonatal Tetanus
Home delivery of infant	
Deficient or absent maternal immunization	
Fever	
Diminished suck or refusal to suck	
Impaired feeding	
Abnormal crying	
Rigid abdomen	
Trismus	
Cyanosis	
Facial rigidity (risus sardonicus)	
Opisthotonos	
Generalized rigidity	
Flexed toes; muscular spasms	

mistaken for seizures. Commonly, the spasms are accompanied by apnea and cyanosis. Indeed, respiratory failure resulting from repeated spasms is the most common cause of mortality and morbidity in this disease. The usual duration of disease in the patient with a moderate to severe case and who is effectively supported therapeutically is 3 to 5 weeks.

Diagnosis

Clinical Evaluation

The diagnosis of neonatal tetanus is based primarily on clinical findings. The setting of birth at home, inadequate management of the umbilical stump, nonimmunized mother, and characteristic neurological features should raise the suspicion of the diagnosis of tetanus. Initially, nuchal rigidity may suggest meningeal irritation and hence meningitis or intracranial hemorrhage. Moreover, the spasms are readily mistaken for convulsions and therefore a variety of cerebral conditions. These disorders should be ruled out, because more specific therapy may be needed urgently (e.g., therapy for bacterial meningitis).

Laboratory Evaluation

No convenient laboratory test identifies neonatal tetanus. Cultures of the umbilical stump, even when handled carefully for anaerobic organisms, are usually negative. Electromyographic findings of increased insertional activity in the form of trains of motor unit discharges can be helpful in diagnosis of the difficult case.[391]

Prognosis

Until recently, the mortality of neonatal tetanus in large series varied from 60% to 85%.[374,383-385,387] In an earlier study of 196 cases in India in the 1950s, the mortality rate was approximately 85%.[383] More recent studies suggest that, with improved management, mortality can be decreased to approximately 10%.[389,393,395,396] However, in many underdeveloped areas, the mortality rate remains high (i.e., 30% to 80%).[367,371,377,390,392,394] Approximately 10% to 30% of survivors exhibit neurological sequelae (e.g., mental retardation and spastic motor deficits), which are apparently secondary to hypoxic-ischemic injury sustained in association with severe muscular spasms. In a cumulative series of 138 infants, 19 (14%) exhibited mental retardation or an intelligence quotient lower than 80 on long-term follow-up.[388,390,396,397] However, in addition to this cerebral involvement, the demonstration of flaccid quadriparesis and a muscle biopsy indicative of denervation in one child raised the possibility of anterior horn cell injury by the toxin, at least in isolated cases.[398]

Management

Prevention

The most essential feature of management of tetanus neonatorum is prevention. This goal has been accomplished to a major degree in many countries by the widespread active immunization of the population, such that transplacental transfer of antitoxin is adequate. Immunization of women during pregnancy has proved highly effective in preventing the occurrence of disease in the infant.[372,375,376] Also of particular importance are delivery of infants and management of the newborn and the umbilical cord under aseptic conditions.

Treatment

The improved outcome for the newborn with tetanus in recent years appears to be related primarily to improved supportive care.[389,390,393-395] The major aspects of management are depicted in Table 21-28.

Supportive Care. Supportive care is paramount in the management of neonatal tetanus, and maintenance of adequate ventilation is most important of all. Nasotracheal intubation (rather than tracheostomy), mechanical ventilation, and a degree of muscular paralysis (with pancuronium bromide) sufficient to allow smooth ventilatory control have been shown to be highly effective.[395] Important therapeutic adjuncts include administration of intravenous fluids, enteric feeding by indwelling nasogastric tube, and control of temperature. These various measures are designed to prevent the respiratory failure, pulmonary disease, hyperpyrexia, pneumonia, and dehydration that may result in death.

The *sedative* drugs chosen to alleviate the muscular spasms most commonly have included primarily phenobarbital, chlorpromazine, and diazepam.[399] The use of doses of diazepam as high as 20 to 40 mg/kg/day (in association with intragastric phenobarbital) has been associated with a 90% survival.[389,396] The need for such doses was shown in pharmacokinetic and clinical studies.[390,400] Although management of infants not requiring mechanical ventilation should include reduction of environmental stimulation and some form of sedation, it appears that the most effective approach is to use mechanical ventilation early in the course of the disease and in association with the administration of a paralytic agent. This approach requires a skilled neonatal intensive care team, and, indeed, when rapid transfer of such infants to an appropriate facility can be accomplished, the use of dangerously high levels of sedative drugs can be avoided. Nevertheless, a skilled neonatal intensive care team with sophisticated equipment is usually unavailable in developing countries, where high-dose diazepam without routine use of mechanical ventilation is the mainstay of therapy.[389,390]

Antitoxin and Antimicrobial Therapy. The umbilical infection does not usually require local surgical therapy, but penicillin G is administered intravenously in a dose of 10,000 units/kg/day for 10 days.[395] Tetanus immune globulin, 500 units, is administered intramuscularly in divided doses to neutralize any unbound toxin. A controlled study demonstrated equivalent benefit for human tetanus immune globulin, 500 units, and equine tetanus antitoxin, 10,000 units.[401] Because tetanus immune globulin has a more sustained effect (i.e., half-life of ≈4 to 5 weeks versus 1 to 2 weeks for equine tetanus antitoxin) and is less frequently associated with adverse side effects, this preparation is preferred, when available.

TABLE 21-28	Management of Neonatal Tetanus

Intravenous fluids
Enteric feeding
Temperature control
Respiratory support, including mechanical ventilation and neuromuscular blockade
Sedation and muscle relaxation, especially with high-dose diazepam
Tetanus immune globulin
Penicillin G

REFERENCES

1. Albritton WL, Wiggins GL, Feeley JC: Neonatal listeriosis: Distribution of serotypes in relation to age at onset of disease, *J Pediatr* 88:481-483, 1976.
2. Perlman JM, Rollins N, Sanchez PJ: Late-onset meningitis in sick, very-low-birth-weight infants: Clinical and sonographic observations, *Am J Dis Child* 146:1297-1301, 1992.
3. Dobson SRM, Baker CJ: Enterococcal sepsis in neonates: Features by age at onset and occurrence of focal infection, *Pediatrics* 85:165-171, 1990.
4. Grauel EL, Halle E, Bollmann R, Buchholz P, et al: Neonatal septicaemia: Incidence, etiology and outcome. A 6-year analysis, *Acta Paediatr Scand Suppl* 360:113-119, 1989.
5. Synnott MB, Morse DL, Hall SM: Neonatal meningitis in England and Wales: A review of routine national data, *Arch Dis Child Fetal Neonatal Ed* 71:F75-F80, 1994.
6. Stoll BJ, Gordon T, Korones SB, Shankaran S, et al: Early-onset sepsis in very low birth weight neonates: A report from the National Institute of Child Health and Human Development Neonatal Research Network, *J Pediatr* 129:72-80, 1996.
7. Stoll BJ, Gordon T, Korones SB, Shankaran S, et al: Late-onset sepsis in very low birth weight neonates: A report from the National Institute of Child Health and Human Development Neonatal Research Network, *J Pediatr* 129:63-70, 1996.
8. Moses LM, Heath PT, Wilkinson AR, Jeffery HE, et al: Early onset group B streptococcal neonatal infection in Oxford 1985-96, *Arch Dis Child Fetal Neonatal Ed* 79:F148-F149, 1998.
9. Berger A, Salzer HR, Weninger M, Sageder B, et al: Septicaemia in an Austrian neonatal intensive care unit: A 7-year analysis, *Acta Paediatr* 87:1066-1069, 1998.
10. Holt DE, Halket S, de Louvois J, Harvey D: Neonatal meningitis in England and Wales: 10 years on, *Arch Dis Child Fetal Neonatal Ed* 84:F85-F89, 2001.

11. Mifsud AJ, Efstratiou A, Charlett A, McCartney AC: Early-onset neonatal group B streptococcal infection in London: 1990–1999, *Br J Obstet Gynaecol* 111:1006-1011, 2004.
12. Stevens JP, Eames M, Kent A, Halket S, et al: Long term outcome of neonatal meningitis, *Arch Dis Child* 88:179-184, 2003.
13. Makhoul I, Sujov P, Smolkin T, Lusky A, et al: Epidemiological, clinical, and microbiological characteristics of late-onset sepsis among very low birth weight infants in Israel: A national survey, *Pediatrics* 109:34-39, 2002.
14. Bizzarro MJ, Raskind C, Baltimore RS, Gallagher PG: Seventy-five years of neonatal sepsis at Yale: 1928–2003, *Pediatrics* 116:595-602, 2005.
15. Makhoul IR, Sujov P, Smolkin T, Lusky A, et al: Pathogen-specific early mortality in very low birth weight infants with late-onset sepsis: A national survey, *Clin Infect Dis* 40:218-224, 2005.
16. Palazzi DL, Klein JO, Baker CJ: Bacterial sepsis and meningitis. In Remington JS, Klein JO, Wilson CB, et al, editors: *Infectious Diseases of the Fetus and Newborn Infant*, 6th ed, Philadelphia: 2006, Elsevier Saunders.
17. Stoll BJ, Hansen N, Fanaroff AA, Wright LL, et al: Late-onset sepsis in very low birth weight neonates: The experience of the NICHD neonatal research network, *Pediatrics* 110:285-291, 2002.
18. Stoll BJ, Hansen N, Fanaroff AA, Wright LL, et al: Changes in pathogens causing early onset sepsis in very low birth weight infants, *N Engl J Med* 347:240-247, 2002.
19. Vergnano S, Sharland M, Kazembe P, Mwansambo C, et al: Neonatal sepsis: An international perspective, *Arch Dis Child Fetal Neonatal Ed* 90:F220-F224, 2005.
20. Thompson CM, Pappu L, Levkoff AH, Herbert KH: Neonatal septicemia and meningitis due to *Pasteurella multocida*, *Pediatr Infect Dis* 3:559-561, 1984.
21. Unhanand M, Mustafa MM, Mccracken GH, Nelson JD: Gram-negative enteric bacillary meningitis: A 21-year experience, *J Pediatr* 122:15-21, 1993.
22. Schaad UB: Etiology and management of neonatal bacterial meningitis. In Schonfeld H, Helwig H, editors: *Bacterial Meningitis*, Basel: 1992, Karger.
23. Tessin I, Trollfors B, Thiringer K: Incidence and etiology of neonatal septicaemia and meningitis in Western Sweden 1975–1986, *Acta Paediatr Scand* 79:1023-1030, 1990.
24. de Louvois J, Blackbourn J, Hurley R, Harvey D: Infantile meningitis in England and Wales: A two year study, *Arch Dis Child* 66:603-607, 1991.
25. Franco SM, Cornelius VE, Andrews BF: Long-term outcome of neonatal meningitis, *Am J Dis Child* 146:567-571, 1992.
26. Hristeva L, Booy R, Bowler I, Wilkinson AR: Prospective surveillance of neonatal meningitis, *Arch Dis Child* 69:14-18, 1993.
27. Hansen LN, Eschen C, Bruun B: Neonatal salmonella meningitis: Two case reports, *Acta Paediatr* 85:629-631, 1996.
28. Andersen J, Christensen R, Hertel J: Clinical features and epidemiology of septicaemia and meningitis in neonates due to *Streptococcus agalactiae* in Copenhagen county, Denmark: A 10 year survey from 1992 to 2001, *Acta Paediatr* 93:1334-1339, 2004.
29. Klinger G, Chin CN, Beyenne J, Perlman M: Predicting the outcome of neonatal bacterial meningitis, *Pediatrics* 106:477-482, 2000.
30. Mulcare RJ, Harter DH: Changing patterns of staphylococcal meningitis, *Arch Neurol* 7:114-120, 1962.
31. Wellman WE, Senft RA: Bacterial meningitis. III. Infections caused by *Staphylococcus aureus*, *Mayo Clin Proc* 39:263-269, 1964.
32. Feigin RD: Bacterial meningitis in the newborn infant, *Clin Perinatol* 4:103-116, 1977.
33. Pickering LK, Simon FA: *Haemophilus influenzae* infections of the newborn, *Perinatal Care* 2:20, 1978.
34. Baumgartner ET, Augustine RA, Steele RW: Bacterial meningitis in older neonates, *Am J Dis Child* 137:1052-1054, 1983.
35. Rabinowitz SG, MacLeod NR: Salmonella meningitis, *Am J Dis Child* 123:259-262, 1972.
36. Rubin LG, Altman J, Epple LK, Yolken RH: *Vibrio cholerae* meningitis in a neonate, *J Pediatr* 98:940-942, 1981.
37. McNaughton RD, Robertson JA, Ratzlaff VJ, Molberg CR: *Mycoplasma hominis* infection of the central nervous system in a neonate, *Can Med Assoc J* 129:353-354, 1983.
38. Waecker NJ, Davis CE, Bernstein G, Spector SA: *Plesiomonas shigelloides* septicemia and meningitis in a newborn, *Pediatr Infect Dis J* 7:877-879, 1988.
39. Vohra K, Torrijos E, Jhaveri R, Gordon H: Neonatal sepsis and meningitis caused by *Edwardsiella tarda*, *Pediatr Infect Dis J* 7:814-815, 1988.
40. Long JG, Preblud SR, Keyserling HL: *Clostridium perfringens* meningitis in an infant: Case report and literature review, *Pediatr Infect Dis J* 6:752-754, 1987.
41. Willis J, Robinson JE: *Enterobacter sakazakii* meningitis in neonates, *Pediatr Infect Dis J* 7:196-199, 1988.
42. Garland SM, Murton LJ: Neonatal meningitis caused by *Ureaplasma urealyticum*, *Pediatr Infect Dis J* 6:868-869, 1987.
43. McDonald JC, Moore DL: *Mycoplasma hominis* meningitis in a premature infant, *Pediatr Infect Dis J* 7:795-798, 1988.
44. Valencia GB, Banzon F, Cummings M, McCormack WM, et al: *Mycoplasma hominis* and *Ureaplasma urealyticum* in neonates with suspected infection, *Pediatr Infect Dis J* 12:571-573, 1993.
45. Dinsmoor MJ, Ramamurthy RS, Gibbs RS: Transmission of genital mycoplasmas from mother to neonate in women with prolonged membrane rupture, *Pediatr Infect Dis J* 8:483-487, 1989.
46. Dinsmoor MJ, Ramamurthy RS, Cassell GH, Gibbs RS: Neonatal serologic response at term to the genital mycoplasmas, *Pediatr Infect Dis J* 8:487-491, 1989.
47. Waites KB, Crouse DT, Nelson KG, Rudd PT, et al: Chronic *Ureaplasma urealyticum* and *Mycoplasma hominis* infections of central nervous system in preterm infants, *Lancet* 9:17-21, 1988.
48. Waites KB, Duffy LB, Crouse DT, Dworsky ME, et al: Mycoplasmal infections of cerebrospinal fluid in newborn infants from a community hospital population, *Pediatr Infect Dis J* 9:241-245, 1990.
49. Waites KB, Crouse DT, Cassell GH: *Ureaplasma* and *Mycoplasma* CNS infections in newborn babies, *Lancet* 335:658-659, 1990.
50. Shaw NJ, Pratt BC, Weindling AM: Ureaplasma and Mycoplasma infections of the central nervous system in preterm infants, *Lancet* 30:1530-1531, 1989.
51. Klein JO, Marcy SM: Bacterial sepsis and meningitis. In Remington JS, Klein JO, editors: *Infectious Diseases of the Fetus and Newborn Infant*, 4th ed, Philadelphia: 1995, Saunders.
52. Shinefield HR: Staphylococcal infections. In Remington JS, Klein JO, editors: *Infectious Diseases of the Fetus and Newborn Infant*, 4th ed, Philadelphia: 1995, Saunders.
53. Saez-Llorens X, McCracken GHJ: Perinatal bacterial diseases. In Feigin RD, Cherry JD, editors: *Textbook of Pediatric Infectious Diseases*, 4th ed, Philadelphia: 1998, Saunders.
54. Beardsall K, Thompson MH, Mulla RJ: Neonatal group B streptococcal infection in South Bedfordshire, 1993–1998, *Arch Dis Child Fetal Neonatal Ed* 82:F205-F207, 2000.
55. Schrag SJ, Zywicki S, Farley MM, Reingold AL, et al: Group B streptococcal disease in the era of intrapartum antibiotic prophylaxis, *N Engl J Med* 342:15-20, 2000.
56. Wolthers KC, Kornelisse RF, Platenkamp GJ, Schuurmanvander-Lem MI, et al: A case of *Mycoplasma hominis* meningo-encephalitis in a full-term infant: Rapid recovery after start of treatment with ciprofloxacin, *Eur J Pediatr* 162:514-516, 2003.
57. Hoffman JA, Mason EO, Schultze GE, Tan TQ, et al: *Streptococcus pneumoniae* infections in the neonate, *Pediatrics* 112:1095-1102, 2003.
58. Stoll BJ, Hansen N, Fanaroff AA, Lemons JA: *Enterobacter sakazakii* is a rare cause of neonatal septicemia or meningitis in VLBW infants, *J Pediatr* 144:821-823, 2004.
59. Baker CJ, Edwards MS: Group B streptococcal infections. In Remington JS, Klein JO, editors: *Infectious Diseases of the Fetus and Newborn Infant*, 4th ed, Philadelphia: 1995, Saunders.
60. Overall JC Jr: Neonatal bacterial meningitis: Analysis of predisposing factors and outcome compared with matched control subjects, *J Pediatr* 76:499-511, 1970.
61. Anthony BF: Carriage of group B streptococci during pregnancy: A puzzler, *J Infect Dis* 145:789-793, 1982.
62. Bell WE, McGuinness GA: Suppurative central nervous system infections in the neonate, *Semin Perinatol* 6:1-24, 1982.
63. Ancona RJ, Ferrieri P, Williams PP: Maternal factors that enhance the acquisition of group-B streptococci by newborn infants, *J Med Microbiol* 13:272-280, 1980.
64. Boyer KM, Gadzala CA, Burd LI, Fisher DE, et al: Selective intrapartum chemoprophylaxis of neonatal group B streptococcal early-onset disease. I. Epidemiologic rationale, *J Infect Dis* 148:795-801, 1983.
65. Boyer KM, Gadzala CA, Kelly PD, Burd LI, et al: Selective intrapartum chemoprophylaxis of neonatal group B streptococcal early-onset disease. II. Predictive value of prenatal cultures, *J Infect Dis* 148:802-809, 1983.
66. Davies PA, Gothefors LA: *Bacterial Infections in the Fetus and Newborn Infant*. Philadelphia: 1984, Saunders.
67. Mulder CJ, Zanen HC: Neonatal group B streptococcal meningitis, *Arch Dis Child* 59:439-443, 1984.
67a. Buhimschi CS, Buhimschi IA, Abdel-Razeq S, Rosenberg VA, et al: Proteomic biomarkers of intra-amniotic inflammation: Relationship with funisitis and early-onset sepsis in the premature neonate, *Pediatr Res* 61:318-324, 2007.
68. Baker CJ, Barrett FF: Transmission of group B streptococci among parturient women and their neonates, *J Pediatr* 83:919-925, 1973.
69. Anthony BF, Okada DM: The emergence of group B streptococci in infections of the newborn infant, *Annu Rev Med* 28:355-369, 1977.
70. Pass MA, Gray BM, Khare S, Dillon HC Jr: Prospective studies of group B streptococcal infections in infants, *J Pediatr* 95:437-443, 1979.
71. Yow MD, Leeds LJ, Thompson PK, Mason EO Jr, et al: The natural history of group B streptococcal colonization in the pregnant woman and her offspring. I. Colonization studies, *Am J Obstet Gynecol* 137:34-38, 1980.
72. Allardice JG, Baskett TF, Seshia MM, Bowman N, et al: Perinatal group B streptococcal colonization and infection, *Am J Obstet Gynecol* 142:617-620, 1982.
73. Hoogkamp-Korstanje JA, Gerards LJ, Cats BP: Maternal carriage and neonatal acquisition of group B streptococci, *J Infect Dis* 145:800-803, 1982.
74. Weisman LE, Stoll BJ, Cruess DF, Hall RT, et al: Early-onset group B streptococcal sepsis: A current assessment, *J Pediatr* 121:428-433, 1992.

75. American Academy of Pediatrics Committee on Infectious Diseases and Committee on Fetus and Newborn: Revised guidelines for prevention of early-onset group B streptococcal (GBS) infection, *Pediatrics* 99:489-496, 1997.

76. Locksmith GJ, Clark P, Duff P: Maternal and neonatal infection rates with three different protocols for prevention of group B streptococcal disease, *Am J Obstet Gynecol* 180:416-422, 1999.

77. Edwards MS, Nizet V, Baker CJ: Group B streptococcal infections. In Remington JS, Klein JO, Wilson CB, et al, editors: *Infectious Diseases of the Fetus and Newborn Infant*, 6th ed, Philadelphia: 2006, Elsevier Saunders.

78. Lennon D, Lewis B, Mantell C, Becroft D, et al: Epidemic perinatal listeriosis, *Pediatr Infect Dis* 3:30-34, 1984.

79. Bortolussi R: Neonatal listeriosis: Where do we go from here? *Pediatr Infect Dis* 4:228-229, 1985.

80. Evans JR, Allen AC, Stinson DA, Bortolussi R, et al: Perinatal listeriosis: Report of an outbreak, *Pediatr Infect Dis* 4:237-241, 1985.

81. Krause VW, Embree JE, MacDonald SW, Acker WC, et al: Congenital listeriosis causing early neonatal death, *Can Med Assoc J* 127:36-38, 1982.

82. Gellin BG, Broome CV, Bibb WF, Weaver RE, et al: The epidemiology of listeriosis in the United States: 1986, *Am J Epidemiol* 133:392-401, 1991.

83. Kessler SL, Dajani AS: Listeria meningitis in infants and children, *Pediatr Infect Dis J* 9:61-63, 1990.

84. Teberg AJ, Yonekura ML, Salminen C, Pavlova E: Clinical manifestations of epidemic neonatal listeriosis, *Pediatr Infect Dis J* 6:817-820, 1987.

85. Mulder CJJ, Zanen HC: *Listeria monocytogenes* neonatal meningitis in the Netherlands, *Eur J Pediatr* 145:60-62, 1986.

86. Boucher M, Yonekura ML: Perinatal listeriosis (early-onset): Correlation of antenatal manifestations and neonatal outcome, *Obstet Gynecol* 68:593-597, 1986.

87. Bortolussi R, Mailman TL: Listeriosis. In Remington JS, Klein JO, Wilson CB, et al, editors: *Infectious Diseases of the Fetus and Newborn Infant*, 6th ed, Philadelphia: 2006, Elsevier Saunders.

88. Berman PH, Banker BQ: Neonatal meningitis: A clinical and pathological study of 29 cases, *Pediatrics* 38:6-24, 1966.

89. Adinolfi M, Gardner B: Synthesis of beta-1E and beta-1C components of complement in human foetuses, *Acta Paediatr Scand* 56:450-454, 1967.

90. Coen R, Grush O, Kauder E: Studies of bactericidal activity and metabolism of the leukocyte in full term neonates, *J Pediatr* 75:400-406, 1969.

91. McCracken GH Jr, Eichenwald HF: Leukocyte function and the development of opsonic and complement activity in the neonate, *Am J Dis Child* 121:120-126, 1971.

92. Lewis DB, Wilson CB: Developmental immunology and role of host defenses in neonatal susceptibility to infection. In Remington JS, Klein JO, editors: *Infectious Diseases of the Fetus and Newborn Infant*, 4th ed, Philadelphia: 1995, Saunders.

93. Gitlin D, Rosen FS, Michael JG: Transient 19S gamma deficiency in the newborn infant and its significance, *Pediatrics* 31:197-208, 1963.

94. Yeung CY, Hobbs JR: Serum gamma-G-globulin levels in normal, premature, post-mature, and "small-for-dates" newborn babies, *Lancet* 1:1167-1170, 1968.

95. Alford CA: Immunoglobulin determinants in the diagnosis of fetal infections, *Pediatr Clin North Am* 18:102-112, 1971.

96. Ogra PL: Ontogeny of the local immune system, *Pediatrics* 64:765-774, 1979.

97. Schibler KR, Liechty KW, White WL, Rothstein G, et al: Defective production of interleukin-6 by monocytes: A possible mechanism underlying several host defense deficiencies of neonates, *Pediatr Res* 31:18-21, 1992.

98. Baker CJ, Melish ME, Hall RT, Casto DT, et al: Intravenous immune globulin for the prevention of nosocomial infection in low-birth-weight neonates, *N Engl J Med* 327:213-219, 1992.

99. Hill HR: Intravenous immunoglobulin use in the neonate: Role in prophylaxis and therapy of infection, *Pediatr Infect Dis J* 12:549-559, 1993.

100. Zhang GL, Ghosh S: Toll-like receptor-mediated NF-kappa B activation: A phylogenetically conserved paradigm in innate immunity, *J Clin Invest* 107:13-19, 2001.

101. Hallman M, Ramet M, Ezekowitz RA: Toll-like receptors as sensors of pathogens, *Pediatr Res* 50:315-321, 2001.

102. Ahrens P, Kattner E, Kohler B, Hartel C, et al: Mutations of genes involved in the innate immune system as predictors of sepsis in very low birth weight infants, *Pediatr Res* 55:652-656, 2004.

103. Viemann D, Dubbel G, Schleifenbaum S, Harms E, et al: Expression of Toll-like receptors in neonatal sepsis, *Pediatr Res* 58:654-659, 2005.

104. Forster-Waldl E, Sadeghi K, Tamandl D, Gerhold B, et al: Monocyte Toll-like receptor 4 expression and LPS-induced cytokine production increase during gestational aging, *Pediatr Res* 58:121-124, 2005.

105. Baker CJ, Kasper DL: Correlation of maternal antibody deficiency with susceptibility to neonatal group B streptococcal infection, *N Engl J Med* 294:753-756, 1976.

106. Baker CJ, Kasper DL: Immunological investigations of infants with septicemia or meningitis due to group B streptococcus, *J Infect Dis* 136(Suppl):S98-S104, 1977.

107. Hill HR, Shigeoka AO, Hall RT, Hemming VG: Neonatal cellular and humoral immunity to group B streptococci, *Pediatrics* 64:787-794, 1979.

108. Feigin RD, Shearer WT: Opportunistic infection. III. In the normal host, *J Pediatr* 87:852-866, 1975.

109. Orschein RC, Shinefield HR, St. Germe JW: Staphylococcal infections. In Remington JS, Klein JO, Wilson CB, et al, editors: *Infectious Diseases of the Fetus and Newborn Infant*, 6th ed, Philadelphia: 2006, Elsevier Saunders.

110. Fortunov RM, Hulten KG, Hammerman WA, Mason EO Jr, et al: Community-acquired *Staphylococcus aureus* infections in term and near-term previously healthy neonates, *Pediatrics* 118:874-881, 2006.

111. Aber RC, Allen N, Howell JT, Wilkensen HW: Nosocomial transmission of group B streptococci, *Pediatrics* 58:346-353, 1976.

112. Paredes A, Wong P, Mason EO, Taber LH, et al: Nosocomial transmission of group B streptococci in a newborn nursery, *Pediatrics* 59:679-682, 1977.

113. Stoll BJ, Hansen N, Fanaroff AA, Wright LL, et al: To tap or not to tap: High likelihood of meningitis without sepsis among very low birth weight infants, *Pediatrics* 113:1181-1186, 2004.

114. Robbins JB, McCracken GH Jr, Gotschlich EC, Orskov I, et al: *Escherichia coli* K1 capsular polysaccharide associated with neonatal meningitis, *N Engl J Med* 290:1216-1220, 1974.

115. Sarff LD, McCracken GH Jr, Schiffer MS: Epidemiology of *Escherichia coli* K1 in healthy and diseased newborns, *Lancet* 1:1099-1103, 1975.

116. Glode MP, Sutton A, Moxon ER, Robbins JB: Pathogenesis of neonatal *Escherichia coli* meningitis: Induction of bacteremia and meningitis in infant rats fed E coli K1, *Infect Immun* 16:75-78, 1977.

117. Siitonen A, Phlic A, Takala A, Ratiner YA, et al: Invasive *Escherichia coli* infections in children: Bacterial characteristics in different age groups and clinical entities, *Pediatr Infect Dis J* 12:606-612, 1993.

118. McCracken GH Jr, Sarff LD, Glode MP, Mize SG, et al: Relation between *Escherichia coli* K1 capsular polysaccharide antigen and clinical outcome in neonatal meningitis, *Lancet* 2:246-250, 1974.

119. Wang YH, Kim KS: Role of OmpA and IbeB in *Escherichia coli* K1 invasion of brain microvascular endothelial cells in vitro and in vivo, *Pediatr Res* 51:559-563, 2002.

120. Friede RL: Cerebral infarcts complicating neonatal leptomeningitis, *Acta Neuropathol (Berl)* 23:245-253, 1973.

121. Friede RL: *Developmental Neuropathology*, 2nd ed, New York: 1989, Springer-Verlag.

122. Gilles FH, Jammes JL, Berenberg W: Neonatal meningitis: The ventricle as a bacterial reservoir, *Arch Neurol* 34:560-562, 1977.

123. Larroche JC: *Developmental Neuropathology*, New York: 1975, Springer-Verlag.

124. Bortolussi R, Krishnan C, Armstrong D, Tovichayathamrong P: Prognosis for survival in neonatal meningitis: Clinical and pathologic review of 52 cases, *Can Med Assoc J* 118:165-168, 1978.

125. Salmon JH: Ventriculitis complicating meningitis, *Am J Dis Child* 124:35-40, 1972.

126. Schultz P, Leeds NE: Intraventricular septations complicating neonatal meningitis, *J Neurosurg* 38:620-626, 1973.

127. Kalsbeck JE, DeSousa AL, Kleiman MB, Goodman JM, et al: Compartmentalization of the cerebral ventricles as a sequela of neonatal meningitis, *J Neurosurg* 52:547-552, 1980.

128. Miyairi I, Causey KT, Devincenzo JP, Buckingham SC: Group B streptococcal ventriculitis: A report of three cases and literature review, *Pediatr Neurol* 34:395-399, 2006.

129. Kappers JA: Structural and functional changes in the telencephalic choroid plexus during human ontogenesis. In Wolstenholm GEW, O'Connor CM, editors: *The Cerebrospinal Fluid*, Boston: 1958, Little Brown.

130. Daum RS, Scheifele DW, Syriopoulou VP: Ventricular involvement in experimental *Haemophilus influenzae* meningitis, *J Pediatr* 93:927-930, 1978.

131. Gluck L, Wood HF, Fousek MD: Septicemia of the newborn, *Pediatr Clin North Am* 13:1131-1148, 1966.

132. McMenamin JB, Volpe JJ: Bacterial meningitis in infancy: Effects on intracranial pressure and cerebral blood flow velocity, *Neurology* 34:500-504, 1984.

133. Feske SK, Carrazana EJ, Kupsky WJ, Volpe JJ: Uncal herniation secondary to bacterial meningitis in a newborn, *Pediatr Neurol* 8:142-144, 1992.

134. Cueva JP, Egel RT: Anterior fontanel herniation in group B streptococcus meningitis in newborns, *Pediatr Neurol* 10:332-334, 1994.

135. Ment LR, Ehrenkranz RA, Duncan CC: Bacterial meningitis as an etiology of perinatal cerebral infarction, *Pediatr Neurol* 2:276-279, 1986.

136. Coker SB, Muraskas JK, Thomas C: Myelopathy secondary to neonatal bacterial meningitis, *Pediatr Neurol* 10:259-261, 1994.

137. Averill DR Jr, Moxon ER, Smith AL: Effects of *Haemophilus influenzae* meningitis in infant rats on neuronal growth and synaptogenesis, *Exp Neurol* 50:337-345, 1976.

138. Rance CP, Roy TE, Donohue WL, Sepp A, et al: An epidemic of septicemia with meningitis and hemorrhagic encephalitis in premature infants, *J Pediatr* 61:24-32, 1962.

139. Shortland-Webb WR: Proteus and coliform meningoencephalitis in neonates, *J Clin Pathol* 21:422-431, 1968.

140. Cussen LJ, Ryan GB: Hemorrhagic cerebral necrosis in neonatal infants with enterobacterial meningitis, *J Pediatr* 71:771-776, 1967.

141. Gross RJ, Rowe B, Easton JA: Neonatal meningitis caused by *Citrobacter koseri*, *J Clin Pathol* 26:138-139, 1973.

142. Gwynn CM, George RH: Neonatal Citrobacter meningitis, *Arch Dis Child* 48:455-458, 1973.
143. Tamborlane WV, Soto EV: *Citrobacter diversus* meningitis: A case report, *Pediatrics* 55:739-741, 1975.
144. Vogel LC, Ferguson L, Gotoff SP: *Citrobacter* infections of the central nervous system in early infancy, *J Pediatr* 93:86-88, 1978.
145. Lin PY, Devoe WF, Morrison C, Libonati J, et al: Outbreak of neonatal *Citrobacter diversus* meningitis in a suburban hospital, *Pediatr Infect Dis J* 6:50-56, 1987.
146. Kimpen JL, Brus F, Arends JP, de Vries-Hospers HG: Successful medical treatment of multiple *Serratia marcescens* brain abscesses in a neonate, *Eur J Pediatr* 155:916, 1996.
147. Ragazzini F, La Cauza C, Ferrucci I: Infection by *Serratia marcescens* in premature children, *Ann Pediatr* 205:289-300, 1965.
148. Bortolussi R, Schlech WF: Listeriosis. In Remington JS, Klein JO, editors: *Infectious Diseases of the Fetus and Newborn Infant*, 4th ed, Philadelphia: 1995, Saunders.
149. Robertson MH, Mussalli NG, Aizad T, Okaro JM, et al: Two cases of perinatal listeriosis, *Arch Dis Child* 54:549-551, 1979.
150. Fishman RA: Biochemical mechanisms underlying the encephalopathy of purulent meningitis, *Pediatr Infect Dis J* 6:1150-1151, 1987.
151. Smith AL: Neurologic sequelae of meningitis, *N Engl J Med* 319:1012-1013, 1988.
152. Scheld WM: Morphofunctional alterations of the blood-brain barrier during experimental meningitis, *Pediatr Infect Dis J* 6:1145-1146, 1987.
153. Tauber MG: Brain edema and intracranial pressure in experimental meningitis, *Pediatr Infect Dis J* 6:1147-1150, 1987.
154. Tureen JH, Stella FB, Clyman RI, Mauray F, et al: Effect of indomethacin on brain water content, cerebrospinal fluid white blood cell response and prostaglandin E2 levels in cerebrospinal fluid in experimental pneumococcal meningitis in rabbits, *Pediatr Infect Dis J* 6:1151-1153, 1987.
155. Kadurugamuwa JL, Hengstler B, Zak O: Effects of antiinflammatory drugs on arachidonic acid metabolites and cerebrospinal fluid proteins during infectious pneumococcal meningitis in rabbits, *Pediatr Infect Dis J* 6:1153-1154, 1987.
156. Sande MA, Scheld M, McCracken GH: Summary of a workshop: Pathophysiology of bacterial meningitis—implications for new management strategies, *Pediatr Infect Dis J* 6:1167-1171, 1987.
157. Williams PA, Bohnsack JF, Augustine NH, Drummond WK, et al: Production of tumor necrosis factor by human cells in vitro and in vivo, induced by group B streptococci, *J Pediatr* 123:292-300, 1993.
158. Shiga Y, Onodera H, Kogure K, Yamasaki Y, et al: Neutrophil as a mediator of ischemic edema formation in the brain, *Neurosci Lett* 125:110-112, 1991.
159. Ashwal S, Stringer W, Tomasi L, Schneider S, et al: Cerebral blood flow and carbon dioxide reactivity in children with bacterial meningitis, *J Pediatr* 117:523-530, 1990.
160. Guerra-Romero L, Tureen JH, Tauber MG: Pathogenesis of central nervous system injury in bacterial meningitis. In Schonfeld H, Helwig H, editors: *Bacterial Meningitis*, Basel: 1992, Karger.
161. De Bont ES, Martens A, Van Raan J, Samson G, et al: Tumor necrosis factor-α, interleukin-1β, and interleukin-6 plasma levels in neonatal sepsis, *Pediatr Res* 33:380-383, 1993.
162. Megyeri P, Abraham CS, Temesvari P, Kovacs J, et al: Recombinant human tumor necrosis factor-alpha constricts pial arterioles and increases blood brain barrier permeability in newborn piglets, *Neurosci Lett* 148:137-140, 1992.
163. Temesvari P, Abraham CS, Speer CP, Kovacs J, et al: *Escherichia coli* 0111 B4 lipopolysaccharide given intracisternally induces blood-brain barrier opening during experimental neonatal meningitis in piglets, *Pediatr Res* 34:182-186, 1993.
164. Berkowitz ID, Hayden WR, Traystman RJ, Jones MD: *Haemophilus influenzae* type B impairment of pial vessel autoregulation in rats, *Pediatr Res* 33:48-51, 1993.
165. McKnight AA, Keyes WG, Hudak ML, Jones MD: Oxygen free radicals and the cerebral arteriolar response to group B streptococci, *Pediatr Res* 31:640-644, 1992.
166. Quagliarello V, Scheld WM: Bacterial meningitis: Pathogenesis, pathophysiology, and progress, *N Engl J Med* 327:864-872, 1992.
167. Guerra-Romero L, Tureen H, Fournier MA, Makrides V, et al: Amino acids in cerebrospinal and brain interstitial fluid in experimental pneumococcal meningitis, *Pediatr Res* 33:510-513, 1993.
168. Perry VI, Young RSK, Aquila WJ, During MJ: Effect of experimental *Escherichia coli* meningitis on concentrations of excitatory and inhibitory amino acids in the rabbit brain: In vivo microdialysis study, *Pediatr Res* 34:187-191, 1993.
169. Ohga S, Aoki T, Okada K, Akeda H, et al: Cerebrospinal fluid concentrations of interleukin-1β, tumour necrosis factor-α, and interferon gamma in bacterial meningitis, *Arch Dis Child* 70:123-125, 1994.
170. Tureen J, Liu Q, Chow L: Near-infrared spectroscopy in experimental pneumococcal meningitis in the rabbit: Cerebral hemodynamics and metabolism, *Pediatr Res* 40:759-763, 1996.
171. Rudinsky BF, Lozon M, Bell A, Hipps R, et al: Group B streptococcal sepsis impairs cerebral vascular reactivity to acute hypercarbia in piglets, *Pediatr Res* 39:55-63, 1995.
172. Ling EW, De Noya FJ, Richard G, Beharry K, et al: Biochemical mediators of meningeal inflammatory response to group B streptococcus in the newborn piglet model, *Pediatr Res* 38:981-987, 1995.

173. Doellner H, Arntzen KJ, Haereid PE, Aag S, et al: Interleukin-6 concentrations in neonates evaluated for sepsis, *J Pediatr* 132:295-299, 1998.
174. Koedel U, Pfister HW: Oxidative stress in bacterial meningitis, *Brain Pathol* 9:57-67, 1999.
175. Pfister LA, Tureen JH, Shaw S, Christen S, et al: Endothelin inhibition improves cerebral blood flow and is neuroprotective in pneumococcal meningitis, *Ann Neurol* 47:329-335, 2000.
176. Inder TE, Mocatta T, Darlow B, Spencer C, et al: Markers of oxidative injury in the cerebrospinal fluid of a premature infant with meningitis and periventricular leukomalacia, *J Pediatr* 140:617-621, 2002.
177. Kastenbauer S, Koedel U, Becker BF, Pfister HW: Oxidative stress in bacterial meningitis in humans, *Neurology* 58:186-191, 2002.
178. Simon RP, Beckman JS: Why pus is bad for the brain, *Neurology* 58:167-168, 2002.
179. Schaper M, Gergely S, Lykkesfeldt J, Zbaren J, et al: Cerebral vasculature is the major target of oxidative protein alterations in bacterial meningitis, *J Neuropathol Exp Neurol* 61:605-613, 2002.
180. Verboon-Maciolek MA, Thijsen SF, Hemels MA, Menses M, et al: Inflammatory mediators for the diagnosis and treatment of sepsis in early infancy, *Pediatr Res* 59:457-461, 2006.
181. Lehnardt S, Lachance C, Patrizi S, Lefebvre S, et al: The Toll-like receptor TLR4 is necessary for lipopolysaccharide-induced oligodendrocyte injury in the CNS, *J Neurosci* 22:2478-2486, 2002.
182. Lehnardt S, Henneke P, Lien E, Kasper DL, et al: A mechanism for neurodegeneration induced by group B streptococci through activation of the TLR2/MyD88 pathway in microglia, *J Immunol* 177:583-592, 2006.
182a. Hoffmann O, Braun JS, Becker D, Halle A, et al: TLR2 mediates neuroinflammation and neuronal damage, *J Immunol* 178:6476-6481, 2007.
183. Stoll BJ, Hansen NI, Adams-Chapman I, Fanaroff AA, et al: Neurodevelopmental and growth impairment among extremely low-birth-weight infants with neonatal infection, *JAMA* 292:2357-2365, 2004.
184. Payne NR, Burke BA, Day DL, Christenson PD, et al: Correlation of clinical and pathologic findings in early onset neonatal group B streptococcal infection with disease severity and prediction of outcome, *Pediatr Infect Dis J* 7:836-847, 1988.
185. de Louvois J, Halket S, Harvey D: Neonatal meningitis in England and Wales: Sequelae at 5 years of age, *Eur J Pediatr* 164:730-734, 2005.
186. Baker CJ: Early onset group B streptococcal disease, *J Pediatr* 93:124-125, 1978.
187. Menke JA, Giacoia GP, Jockin H: Group B beta-hemolytic streptococcal sepsis and the idiopathic respiratory distress syndrome: A comparison, *J Pediatr* 94:467-471, 1979.
188. Reynolds DW, Dweck HS, Cassady G: Inappropriate antidiuretic hormone secretion in a neonate with meningitis, *Am J Dis Child* 123:251-253, 1972.
189. Kaplan SL, Feigin RD: The syndrome of inappropriate secretion of antidiuretic hormone in children with bacterial meningitis, *J Pediatr* 92:758-761, 1978.
190. Padilla G, Ervin G, Roos MG, Leake RD: Vasopressin levels in infants during the course of aseptic and bacterial meningitis, *Am J Dis Child* 145:991-993, 1991.
191. Wiswell TE, Baumgart S, Gannon CM, Spitzer AR: No lumbar puncture in the evaluation for early neonatal sepsis: Will meningitis be missed?, *Pediatrics* 95:803-806, 1995.
192. Sarff LD, Platt LH, McCracken GH Jr: Cerebrospinal fluid evaluation in neonates: Comparison of high-risk infants with and without meningitis, *J Pediatr* 88:473-477, 1976.
193. Rodriguez AF, Kaplan SL, Mason EO Jr: Cerebrospinal fluid values in the very low birth weight infant, *J Pediatr* 116:971-974, 1990.
194. Dajani AS: Rapid identification of beta hemolytic streptococci by counterimmunoelectrophoresis, *J Immunol* 110:1702-1705, 1973.
195. Hill HR, Riter ME, Menge SK, Johnson DR, et al: Rapid identification of group B streptococci by counterimmunoelectrophoresis, *J Clin Microbiol* 1:188-191, 1975.
196. Siegel JD, McCracken GH Jr: Detection of group B streptococcal antigens in body fluids of neonates, *J Pediatr* 93:491-492, 1978.
197. Edwards MS, Baker CJ: Prospective diagnosis of early onset group B streptococcal infection by countercurrent immunoelectrophoresis, *J Pediatr* 94:286-288, 1979.
198. Smith AL, Haas J: Neonatal bacterial meningitis. In Scheld WM, Whitley RJ, Durack DT, editors: *Infections of the Central Nervous System*, New York: 1991, Raven Press.
199. Levin J, Poore TE, Zauber NP, Oser RS: Detection of endotoxin in the blood of patients with sepsis due to gram-negative bacteria, *N Engl J Med* 283:1313-1316, 1970.
200. Schelonka RL, Freij BJ, McCracken GH Jr: Bacterial and fungal infections. In MacDonald MG, Mullett MD, Seshia MM, editors: *Avery's Neonatology: Pathophysiology and Management of the Newborn*, 6th ed, Philadelphia: 2005, Lippincott Williams & Wilkins.
201. Fosson AR, Fine RN: Neonatal meningitis, *Clin Pediatr* 7:404-410, 1968.
202. Fitzhardinge PM, Kazemi M, Ramsay M, Stern L: Long-term sequelae of neonatal meningitis, *Dev Med Child Neurol* 16:3-8, 1974.
203. Stechenberg BW, Schreiner RL, Grass SM, Shackelford PG: Countercurrent immunoelectrophoresis in group B streptococcal disease, *Pediatrics* 64:632-634, 1970.

204. Natarajan G, Johnson YR, Zhang F, Chen KM, et al: Real-time polymerase chain reaction for the rapid detection of group B streptococcal colonization in neonates, *Pediatrics* 118:14-22, 2006.
205. Klein JO, Marcy SM: Bacterial sepsis and meningitis. In Remington JS, Klein JO, editors: *Infectious Diseases of the Fetus and Newborn Infant*, 3rd ed, Philadelphia: 1990, Saunders.
206. Manroe BL, Rosenfeld CR, Weinberg AG, Browne R: The differential leukocyte count in the assessment and outcome of early-onset neonatal group B streptococcal disease, *J Pediatr* 91:632-637, 1977.
207. Speer CP, Hauptmann D, Stubbe P, Gahr M: Neonatal septicemia and meningitis in Gottingen, West Germany, *Pediatr Infect Dis* 4:36-41, 1985.
208. Doellner H, Arntzen KJ, Haereid PE, Aag S, et al: Increased serum concentrations of soluble tumor necrosis factor receptors p55 and p75 in early onset neonatal sepsis, *Early Hum Dev* 52:251-261, 1998.
209. Messer J, Eyer D, Donato L, Gallati H, et al: Evaluation of interleukin-6 and soluble receptors of tumor necrosis factor for early diagnosis of neonatal infection, *J Pediatr* 129:574-580, 1996.
210. Dulkerian SJ, Kilpatrick L, Costarino AT, McCawley L, et al: Cytokine elevations in infants with bacterial and aseptic meningitis, *J Pediatr* 126:872-876, 1995.
211. Kuster H, Weiss M, Willeitner AE, Detlefsen S, et al: Interleukin-1 receptor antagonist and interleukin-6 for early diagnosis of neonatal sepsis 2 days before clinical manifestation, *Lancet* 352:1271-1277, 1998.
212. Ng PC: Diagnostic markers of infection in neonates, *Arch Dis Child Fetal Neonatal Ed* 89:F229-F235, 2004.
213. Harris MC, D'Angio CT, Gallagher PR, Kaufman D, et al: Cytokine elaboration in critically ill infants with bacterial sepsis, necrotizing enterocolitis, or sepsis syndrome: Correlation with clinical parameters of inflammation and mortality, *J Pediatr* 147:462-468, 2005.
214. Minns RA, Engleman HM, Stirling H: Cerebrospinal fluid pressure in pyogenic meningitis, *Arch Dis Child* 64:814-820, 1989.
215. Baker JP, Chalhub EG, Shackelford PG: Ventriculitis in group B streptococcal (GBS) meningitis, *Pediatr Res* 12:549-550, 1978.
216. McCrory JH, Au-Yeung YB, Sugg VM, Chiu TT, et al: Recurrent group B streptococcal infection in an infant: Ventriculitis complicating type 1b meningitis, *J Pediatr* 92:231-233, 1978.
217. Lorber J, Emery JL: Intracerebral cysts complicating ventricular needling in hydrocephalic infants: A clinico-pathological study, *Dev Med Child Neurol* 6:125-139, 1964.
218. Bell WE, McCormick WF: *Neurologic Infections in Children*, 2nd ed, Philadelphia: 1981, Saunders.
219. Horbar JD, Philip AG, Lucey JF: Ultrasound scan in neonatal ventriculitis, *Lancet* 1:976, 1980.
220. Hill A, Shackelford GD, Volpe JJ: Ventriculitis with neonatal bacterial meningitis: Identification by real-time ultrasound, *J Pediatr* 99:133-136, 1981.
221. Edwards MK, Brown DL, Chua GT: Complicated infantile meningitis: Evaluation by real-time sonography, *AJNR Am J Neuroradiol* 3:431-434, 1982.
222. Reeder JD, Sanders RC: Ventriculitis in the neonate: Recognition by sonography, *AJNR Am J Neuroradiol* 4:37-41, 1983.
223. Stannard MW, Jimenez JF: Sonographic recognition of multiple cystic encephalomalacia, *AJNR Am J Neuroradiol* 4:1111-1115, 1983.
224. Han BK, Babcock DS, McAdams L: Bacterial meningitis in infants: Sonographic findings, *Radiology* 154:645-650, 1985.
225. Rosenberg HK, Levine RS, Stoltz K, Smith DR: Bacterial meningitis in infants: Sonographic features, *AJNR Am J Neuroradiol* 4:822-825, 1983.
226. Raghav B, Goulatia RK, Gupta AK, Misra NK, et al: Giant subdural empyema in an infant, *Neuroradiology* 32:154-155, 1990.
227. McCracken GH, Threlkeld N, Mize S: Moxalactam therapy for neonatal meningitis due to gram-negative enteric bacilli, *JAMA* 252:1427-1432, 1984.
228. Klinger G, Chin C-N, Otsubo H, Beyene J, et al: Prognostic value of EEG in neonatal bacterial meningitis, *Pediatr Neurol* 24:28-31, 2001.
229. Baker CJ, Barrett FF, Gordon RC, Yow MD: Suppurative meningitis due to streptococci of Lancefield group B: A study of 33 infants, *J Pediatr* 82:724-729, 1973.
230. Barton LL, Feigin RD, Lins R: Group B beta hemolytic streptococcal meningitis in infants, *J Pediatr* 82:719-723, 1973.
231. Horn KA, Zimmerman RA, Knostman JD, Meyer WT: Neurological sequelae of group B streptococcal neonatal infection, *Pediatrics* 53:501-504, 1974.
232. Haslam RH, Allen JR, Dorsen MM, Kanofsky DL, et al: The sequelae of group B beta-hemolytic streptococcal meningitis in early infancy, *Am J Dis Child* 131:845-849, 1977.
233. Chin KC, Fitzhardinge PM: Sequelae of early-onset group B hemolytic streptococcal neonatal meningitis, *J Pediatr* 106:819-822, 1985.
234. Faix RG, Donn SM: Association of septic shock caused by early-onset group B streptococcal sepsis and periventricular leukomalacia in the preterm infant, *Pediatrics* 76:415-419, 1985.
235. Wald ER, Bergman I, Taylor G, Chiponis D, et al: Long-term outcome of group B streptococcal meningitis, *Pediatrics* 77:217-221, 1986.
236. McCracken GH, Mize SG: A controlled study of intrathecal antibiotic therapy in gram-negative enteric meningitis in infancy, *J Pediatr* 89:66, 1976.
237. De Praeter C, Vanhaesebrouck P, Govaert P, Delanghe J, et al: Creatine kinase isoenzyme BB concentrations in the cerebrospinal fluid of newborns: Relationship to short-term outcome, *Pediatrics* 88:1204-1210, 1991.
238. Chequer RS, Tharp BR, Dreimane D, Hahn JS, et al: Prognostic value of EEG in neonatal meningitis: Retrospective study of 29 infants, *Pediatr Neurol* 8:417-422, 1992.
239. Boyer KM, Gadzala CA, Kelly PD, Gotoff SP: Selective intrapartum chemoprophylaxis of neonatal group B streptococcal early-onset disease. III. Interruption of mother-to-infant transmission, *J Infect Dis* 148:810-816, 1983.
240. Gotoff SP: Chemoprophylaxis of early onset of group B streptococcal disease, *Pediatr Infect Dis* 3:401-403, 1984.
241. Boyer KM, Gotoff SP, Gadzala CA: Selective intrapartum chemoprophylaxis of early-onset group B streptococcal disease, *Pediatr Res* 19:288A, 1985.
242. Siegel J: Prevention and treatment of group B streptococcal infections, *Pediatr Infect Dis* 4(Suppl):S33-S36, 1985.
243. Morales WJ, Lim DV, Walsh AF: Prevention of neonatal group B streptococcal sepsis by the use of a rapid screening test and selective intrapartum chemoprophylaxis, *Am J Obstet Gynecol* 155:979-983, 1986.
244. Minkoff H, Mead P: An obstetric approach to the prevention of early-onset streptococcal sepsis, *Am J Obstet Gynecol* 154:973-977, 1986.
245. Gotoff SP, Boyer KM: Prevention of group B streptococcal early onset sepsis: 1989, *Pediatr Infect Dis J* 8:268-270, 1989.
246. Tuppurainen N, Hallman M: Prevention of neonatal group B streptococcal disease: Intrapartum detection and chemoprophylaxis of heavily colonized parturients, *Obstet Gynecol* 73:583-587, 1989.
247. Boyer KM, Gotoff SP: Prevention of early-onset neonatal group B streptococcal disease with selective intrapartum chemoprophylaxis, *N Engl J Med* 314:1665-1669, 1986.
248. Boyer KM: Perinatal group B streptococcal infection: Clinical significance and preventive strategies. In *Transplacental Disorders: Perinatal Detection, Treatment and Management*, New York: 1990, Liss.
249. Mohle-Boetani JC, Schuchat A, Plikaytis BD, Smith JD, et al: Comparison of prevention strategies for neonatal group-B streptococcal infection: A population-based economic analysis, *JAMA* 270:1442-1448, 1993.
250. Boyer KM: Neonatal group B streptococcal infections, *Curr Opin Pediatr* 7:13-18, 1995.
251. Halsey N, Schuchat A, Oh W, Baker CJ: The 1997 AAP guidelines for prevention of early-onset group B streptococcal disease, *Pediatrics* 100:383-384, 1997.
252. Freij BJ, McCracken GH: Acute infections. In Avery GB, Fletcher MA, MacDonald MG, editors: *Neonatology: Pathophysiology and Management of the Newborn*, Philadelphia: 1999, Lippincott Williams & Wilkins.
253. Yow MD, Mason EO, Leeds LJ: Ampicillin prevents intrapartum transmission of group B streptococcus, *JAMA* 241:1245-1247, 1979.
254. Pylipow M, Gaddis M, Kinney JS: Selective intrapartum prophylaxis for group B streptococcus colonization: Management and outcome of newborns, *Pediatrics* 93:631-635, 1994.
255. Hickman ME, Rench MA, Ferrieri P, Baker CJ: Changing epidemiology of group B streptococcal colonization, *Pediatrics* 104:203-209, 1999.
256. Baker CJ, Rench MA, Kasper DL: Response to type II polysaccharide in women whose infants have had invasive group B streptococcal infection, *N Engl J Med* 322:1857-1860, 1990.
257. Coleman RT, Sherer DM, Maniscalco WM: Prevention of neonatal group-B streptococcal infections: Advances in maternal vaccine development, *Obstet Gynecol* 80:301-309, 1992.
258. Christensen RD, Hill HR, Rothstein G, Harper TE: Intravenous human immunoglobulin prevents neutropenia, neutrophil supply exhaustion and death in experimental group B streptococcal sepsis, *Pediatr Res* 19:289A, 1985.
259. Baker CJ, Kasper DL: Group B streptococcal vaccines, *Rev Infect Dis* 7:458-467, 1985.
260. Eisenstein TK, De Cueninck BJ, Resavy D, Shickman GD, et al: Quantitative determination in human sera of vaccine-induced antibody to type-specific polysaccharides of group B streptococci using an enzyme-linked immunosorbent assay, *J Infect Dis* 147:847-856, 1983.
261. Baker CJ, Edwards MS, Rench MA, Kasper DL: Neonatal immunity to type III group B streptococcal (III-GBS) polysaccharide from maternal third trimester vaccination, *Pediatr Res* 19:287A, 1985.
262. Syrogiannopoulos GA, Olsen KD, McCracken GH: Mannitol treatment in experimental *Haemophilus influenzae* type B meningitis, *Pediatr Res* 22:118-122, 1987.
263. Lebel MH, Freij BJ, Syrogiannopoulos GA: Dexamethasone therapy for bacterial meningitis: Results of two double-blind, placebo-controlled trials, *N Engl J Med* 319:964-971, 1988.
264. McCracken GH, Lebel MH: Dexamethasone therapy for bacterial meningitis in infants and children, *Am J Dis Child* 143:287-289, 1989.
265. Plotkin SA, Halsey NA, Lepow ML, Marcuse EK, et al: Dexamethasone therapy for bacterial meningitis in infants and children, *Pediatrics* 86:130-133, 1990.
266. Schaad UB, Lips U, Gnehm HE, Blumberg A, et al: Dexamethasone therapy for bacterial meningitis in children, *Lancet* 342:457-461, 1993.
267. Syrogiannopoulos GA, Lourida AN, Theodoridou MC, Pappas IG, et al: Dexamethasone therapy for bacterial meningitis in children: 2- versus 4-day regimen, *J Infect Dis* 169:853-858, 1994.
268. McIntyre PB, Berkey CS, King SM, Schaad UB, et al: Dexamethasone as adjunctive therapy in bacterial meningitis, *JAMA* 278:925-931, 1997.
269. Daoud AS, Batieha A, Al-Sheyyab M, Abuekteish F, et al: Lack of effectiveness of dexamethasone in neonatal bacterial meningitis, *Eur J Pediatr* 158:230-233, 1999.

270. Syrogiannopoulos GA, Nelson JD, McCracken GH: Subdural collections of fluid in acute bacterial meningitis: A review of 136 cases, *Pediatr Infect Dis* 5:343-352, 1986.
271. Rabe EF, Flynn RE, Dodge PR: Subdural collections of fluid in infants and children: A study of 62 patients with special reference to factors influencing prognosis and the efficacy of various forms of therapy, *Neurology* 18:559-570, 1968.
272. McCracken GH Jr, Mize SG, Neonatal Cooperative Study Group: Intraventricular therapy of neonatal meningitis caused by gram-negative enteric bacilli, *Pediatr Res* 13:464, 1979.
273. McCracken GH: New developments in the management of children with bacterial meningitis, *Pediatr Infect Dis* 3(Suppl):S32-S34, 1984.
274. Baker CJ, Edwards MS: Group B streptococcal infections. In Remington JS, Klein JO, editors: *Infectious Diseases of the Fetus and Newborn Infant*, 3rd ed, Philadelphia: 1990, Saunders.
275. Starr SE: Antimicrobial therapy of bacterial sepsis in the newborn infant, *J Pediatr* 106:1043-1048, 1985.
276. McCracken GH, Nelson JD, Kaplan SL, Overturf GD, et al: Consensus report: Antimicrobial therapy for bacterial meningitis in infants and children, *Pediatr Infect Dis J* 6:501-505, 1987.
277. Word BM, Klein JO: Current therapy of bacterial sepsis and meningitis in infants and children: A poll of directors of programs in pediatric infectious diseases, *Pediatr Infect Dis J* 7:267-270, 1988.
278. Weinstein AJ, Moellering RC Jr: Penicillin and gentamicin therapy for enterococcal infections, *JAMA* 223:1030-1032, 1973.
279. Broughton DD, Mitchell WG, Grossman M, Hadley WK, et al: Recurrence of group B streptococcal infection, *J Pediatr* 89:182-185, 1976.
280. Schauf V, Deveikis A, Riff L, Serota A: Antibiotic-killing kinetics of group B streptococci, *J Pediatr* 89:194-198, 1976.
281. Saez-Llorens X, McCracken GH Jr: Clinical pharmacology of antibacterial agents. In Remington JS, Klein JO, Wilson CB, et al, editors: *Infectious Diseases of the Fetus and Newborn Infant*, 6th ed, Philadelphia: 2006, Elsevier Saunders.
282. McCracken GH Jr, Freij BJ: Clinical pharmacology of antimicrobial agents. In Remington JS, Klein JO, editors: *Infectious Diseases of the Fetus and Newborn Infant*, 3rd ed, Philadelphia: 1990, Saunders.
283. Eichenwald HF: Antimicrobial therapy in infants and children: Update 1976–1985, *J Pediatr* 107:161-168, 1985.
284. McCracken GH: New antimicrobial agents for pediatricians, *Pediatr Infect Dis* 4(Suppl):S10-S12, 1985.
285. Powell KR, Pincus PH: Five years of experience with the exclusive use of amikacin in a neonatal intensive care unit, *Pediatr Infect Dis J* 6:461-466, 1987.
286. Haimi-Cohen Y, Amir J, Weinstock A, Varsano I: The use of imipenem-cilastatin in neonatal meningitis caused by *Citrobacter diversus*, *Acta Paediatr* 82:530-532, 1993.
287. Lee EL, Robinson MJ, Thong ML: Intraventricular chemotherapy in neonatal meningitis, *J Pediatr* 91:991-995, 1977.
288. Corbeel L, de Boeck K, Logghe N, Eggermont E, et al: Treatment of purulent meningitis in infants, *Lancet* 1:622, 1979.
289. Wright PF, Kaiser AB, Bowman CM, McKee KT Jr: The pharmacokinetics and efficacy of an aminoglycoside administered into the cerebral ventricles in neonates: Implications for further evaluation of this route of therapy in meningitis, *J Infect Dis* 143:141-147, 1981.
290. Moellering RC, Fischer EG: Relationship of intraventricular gentamicin levels to cure of meningitis, *J Pediatr* 81:534-537, 1972.
291. Kaiser AB, McGee ZA: Aminoglycoside therapy of gram-negative bacillary meningitis, *N Engl J Med* 293:1215-1220, 1975.
292. Watanabe I, Hodges GR, Dworzack DL: Neurotoxicity of intrathecal gentamicin: A case report and experimental study, *Ann Neurol* 4:564-572, 1978.
293. Hodges GR, Watanabe I, Singer P, Rengachary S, et al: Central nervous system toxicity of intraventricularly administered gentamicin in adult rabbits, *J Infect Dis* 143:148-155, 1981.
294. Smith ML, Mellor D: *Proteus mirabilis* meningitis and cerebral abscess in the newborn period, *Arch Dis Child* 55:308-310, 1980.
295. Curless RG: Neonatal intracranial abscess: Two cases caused by Citrobacter and a literature review, *Ann Neurol* 8:269-272, 1980.
296. Graham DR, Band JD: *Citrobacter diversus* brain abscess and meningitis in neonates, *JAMA* 245:1923-1925, 1981.
297. Graham DR, Anderson RL, Ariel FE, Ehrenkranz NJ, et al: Epidemic nosocomial meningitis due to *Citrobacter diversus* in neonates, *J Infect Dis* 144:203-209, 1981.
298. Shahar E, Brand N, Barzilay Z: Fatal neonatal central nervous system infection caused by *Citrobacter diversus*, *Isr J Med Sci* 17:370-371, 1981.
299. Butler NR, Barrie H, Paine KW: Cerebral abscess as a complication of neonatal sepsis, *Arch Dis Child* 32:461-465, 1975.
300. Sutton DL, Ouvrier RA: Cerebral abscess in the under 6 month age group, *Arch Dis Child* 58:901-905, 1983.
301. Kline MW, Kaplan SL: *Citrobacter diversus* and neonatal brain abscess, *Pediatr Neurol* 3:178-180, 1987.
302. Kline MW: Citrobacter meningitis and brain abscess in infancy: Epidemiology, pathogenesis, and treatment, *J Pediatr* 113:430-434, 1988.
303. Renier D, Flandin C, Hirsch E, Hirsch J-F: Brain abscesses in neonates: A study of 30 cases, *J Neurosurg* 69:877-882, 1988.
304. Ries M, Deeg KH, Heininger U, Stehr K: Brain abscesses in neonates: Report of 3 cases, *Eur J Pediatr* 152:745-746, 1993.
305. Berger A, Rohrmeister K, Haiden N, Assadian O, et al: *Serratia marcescens* in the neonatal intensive care unit: Re-emphasis of the potentially devastating sequelae, *Wien Klin Wochenschr* 114:1017-1022, 2002.
306. Messerschmidt A, Prayer D, Olischar M, Pollak A, et al: Brain abscesses after *Serratia marcescens* infection on a neonatal intensive care unit: Differences on serial imaging, *Neuroradiology* 46:148-152, 2004.
307. Makhoul IR, Epelman M, Kassis I, Daitzchman M, et al: *Escherichia coli* brain abscess in a very low birthweight premature infant, *Isr Med Assoc J* 4:727-728, 2002.
308. Goodkin K, Harper MB, Pomeroy SL: Intracerebral abscess in children: Historical trends at Children's Hospital Boston, *Pediatrics* 113:1765-1770, 2004.
309. Heep A, Schaller C, Rittmann N, Himbert U, et al: Multiple brain abscesses in an extremely preterm infant: Treatment surveillance with interleukin-6 in the CSF, *Eur J Pediatr* 163:44-45, 2004.
310. Agrawal D, Mahapatra AK: Vertically acquired neonatal *Citrobacter* brain abscess: Case report and review of the literature, *J Clin Neurosci* 12:188-190, 2005.
311. Eberhard SJ: Diagnosis of brain abscesses in infants and children: A retrospective study of twenty-six cases, *N C Med J* 30:301-313, 1969.
312. Hoffman HJ, Hendrick EB, Hiscox JL: Cerebral abscesses in early infancy, *J Neurosurg* 33:172-177, 1970.
313. Samson DS, Clark K: A current review of brain abscess, *Am J Med* 54:201-210, 1973.
314. Siber GR, Alpert S, Smith AL, Lin JS, et al: Neonatal central nervous system infection due to *Mycoplasma hominis*, *J Pediatr* 90:625-627, 1977.
315. Darby CP, Conner E, Kyong CU: *Proteus mirabilis* brain abscess in a neonate, *Dev Med Child Neurol* 20:366-368, 1978.
316. Koot RW, Reedijk B, Tan WF, De Sonnaville-De Roy Van Zuide ML: Neonatal brain abscess: Complication of fetal monitoring, *Obstet Gynecol* 93:857, 1999.
317. Tsutsumi S, Arai H, Hishii M, Suzuki K, et al: A case of neonatal cerebellar abscess, *Childs Nerv Syst* 19:683-685, 2003.
318. Rao RP, Ghanayem NS, Kaufman BA, Kehl KS, et al: *Mycoplasma hominis* and *Ureaplasma* species brain abscess in a neonate, *Pediatr Infect Dis J* 21:1083-1085, 2002.
319. Joaquin A, Khan S, Russel N, al Fayez N: Neonatal meningitis and bilateral cerebellar abscesses due to *Citrobacter freundii*, *Pediatr Neurosurg* 17:23-24, 1991.
320. Fischer EG, McLennan JE, Suzuki Y: Cerebral abscess in children, *Am J Dis Child* 135:746-749, 1981.
321. Garijo JA, Gomila DT, Mengual MV: Cerebellar abscess in early infancy, *Child's Brain* 5:540-542, 1979.
322. Daniels SR, Price JK, Towbin RB, McLaurin R: Nonsurgical cure of brain abscess in a neonate, *Childs Nerv Syst* 1:346-348, 1985.
323. Palmer JJ, Kelly WA: Epidural abscess in a 3-week-old infant: Case report, *Pediatrics* 50:817-820, 1972.
324. Foreman SD, Smith EE, Ryan NJ, Hogan GR: Neonatal *Citrobacter* meningitis: Pathogenesis of cerebral abscess formation, *Ann Neurol* 16:655-659, 1984.
325. Enzmann DR, Britt RH, Lyons B, Carroll B, et al: High-resolution ultrasound evaluation of experimental brain abscess evolution: Comparison with computed tomography and neuropathology, *Radiology* 142:95-102, 1982.
326. Theophilo F, Burnett A, Filho GJ, Adler A, et al: Ultrasound-guided brain abscess aspiration in neonates, *Childs Nerv Syst* 3:371-374, 1987.
327. Obana WG, Cogen PH, Callen PW, Edwards MS: Ultrasound-guided aspiration of a neonatal brain abscess, *Childs Nerv Syst* 7:272-274, 1991.
328. Levy RL, Saunders RL: *Citrobacter* meningitis and cerebral abscess in early infancy: Cure by moxalactam, *Neurology* 31:1575-1577, 1981.
329. Rennels MB, Woodward CL, Robinson WL, Gumbinas MT, et al: Medical cure of apparent brain abscesses, *Pediatrics* 72:220-224, 1983.
330. Ferriero DM, Derechin M, Edwards MS, Berg BO: Outcome of brain abscess treatment in children: Reduced morbidity with neuroimaging, *Pediatr Neurol* 3:148-152, 1987.
331. Marcus MG, Atluru VL, Epstein NE: Conservative management of *Citrobacter diversus* meningitis with brain abscess, *N Y State J Med* 84:252-254, 1984.
332. Sener RN: Diffusion MRI findings in neonatal brain abscess, *J Neuroradiol* 31:69-71, 2004.
333. Miller MJ: Fungal infections. In Remington JS, Klein JO, editors: *Infectious Diseases of the Fetus and Newborn Infant*, 4th ed, Philadelphia: 1995, Saunders.
334. Haruda F, Bergman MA, Headings D: Unrecognized *Candida* brain abscess in infancy: Two cases and a review of the literature, *Johns Hopkins Med J* 147:182-185, 1980.
335. Baley JE, Kliegman RM, Fanaroff AA: Disseminated fungal infections in very low-birth-weight infants: Clinical manifestations and epidemiology, *Pediatrics* 73:144-152, 1984.
336. Faix RG: Systemic *Candida* infections in infants in intensive care nurseries: High incidence of central nervous system involvement, *J Pediatr* 105:616-622, 1984.
337. Johnson DE, Thompson TR, Green TP, Ferrieri P: Systemic candidiasis in very low-birth-weight infants (< 1,500 grams), *Pediatrics* 73:138-143, 1984.

338. Smith H, Congdon P: Neonatal systemic candidiasis, *Arch Dis Child* 60:365-369, 1985.

339. Golden SE, Morgan CM, Bartley DL, Campo RV: Disseminated coccidioidomycosis with chorioretinitis in early infancy, *Pediatr Infect Dis* 5:272-274, 1986.

340. Faix RG, Kovarik SM, Shaw TR, Johnson RV: Mucocutaneous and invasive candidiasis among very low birth weight (< 1,500 grams) infants in intensive care nurseries: A prospective study, *Pediatrics* 83:101-107, 1989.

341. Lenoir P, DeMeirleir L, Bougatef A, Marchand J, et al: Unexpected diagnosis of *candida albicans* meningitis in a premature neonate, *Pediatr Neurol* 5:370-372, 1989.

342. Eppes SC, Troutman JL, Gutman LT: Outcome of treatment of candidemia in children whose central catheters were removed or retained, *Pediatr Infect Dis J* 8:99-104, 1989.

343. Bhandari V, Narang A: Oral itraconazole therapy for disseminated candidiasis in low birth weight infants, *J Pediatr* 120:330, 1992.

344. Baley JE, Meyers C, Kliegman RM, Jacobs MR, et al: Pharmacokinetics, outcome of treatment, and toxic effects of amphotericin B and 5-fluorocytosine in neonates, *J Pediatr* 116:791-797, 1990.

345. Lackner H, Schwinger W, Urban C, Muller W, et al: Liposomal amphotericin-B (AmBisome) for treatment of disseminated fungal infections in two infants of very low birth weight, *Pediatrics* 89:1259-1262, 1992.

346. Butler KM, Rench M, Baker CJ: Amphotericin B as a single agent in the treatment of systemic candidiasis in neonates, *Pediatr Infect Dis J* 9:51-56, 1990.

347. Sherertz RJ, Gledhill KS, Hampton KD, Pfaller MA, et al: Outbreak of *Candida* bloodstream infections associated with retrograde medication administration in a neonatal intensive care unit, *J Pediatr* 120:455-461, 1992.

348. Sanchez PJ: Miscellaneous infections of the newborn. In Feigin RD, Cherry JD, editors: *Textbook of Pediatric Infectious Diseases*, 4th ed, Philadelphia: 1998, Saunders.

349. Huang CC, Chen CY, Yang HB, Wang SM, et al: Central nervous system candidiasis in very-low-birth-weight premature neonates and infants: US characteristics and histopathologic and MR imaging correlates in five patients, *Radiology* 209:49-56, 1998.

350. Campbell JR, Zaccaria E, Baker CJ: Systemic candidiasis in extremely low birth weight infants receiving topical petrolatum ointment for skin care: A case-control study, *Pediatrics* 105:1041-1045, 2000.

351. Johnsson H, Ewald U: The rate of candidaemia in preterm infants born at a gestational age of 23–28 weeks is inversely correlated to gestational age, *Acta Paediatr* 93:954-958, 2004.

352. Benjamin KDJ, Poole C, Steinbach WJ, Rowen JL, et al: Neonatal candidemia and end-organ damage: A critical appraisal of the literature using meta-analytic techniques, *Pediatrics* 112:634-640, 2003.

353. Friedman S, Richardson SE, Jacobs SE, O'Brien K: Systemic *Candida* infection in extremely low birth weight infants: Short term morbidity and long term neurodevelopmental outcome, *Pediatr Infect Dis J* 19:499-504, 2000.

354. Fernandez M, Moylett EH, Noyola DE, Baker CJ: Candidal meningitis in neonates: A 10-year review, *Clin Infect Dis* 31:458-463, 2000.

355. Benjamin DK Jr, Stoll BJ, Fanaroff AA, McDonald SA, et al: Neonatal candidiasis among extremely low birth weight infants: Risk factors, mortality rates, and neurodevelopmental outcomes at 18 to 22 months, *Pediatrics* 117:84-92, 2006.

356. Bendel CM: Nosocomial neonatal candidiasis, *Pediatr Infect Dis J* 24:831-832, 2005.

357. Bendel CM: Candidiasis. In Remington JS, Klein JO, Wilson CB, et al, editors: *Infectious Diseases of the Fetus and Newborn Infant*, 6th ed, Philadelphia: 2006, Elsevier Saunders.

358. Fridkin SK, Kaufman D, Edwards JR, Shetty S, et al: Changing incidence of *Candida* bloodstream infections among NICU patients in the United States: 1995–2004, *Pediatrics* 117:1680-1687, 2006.

359. Manzoni P, Arisio R, Mostert M, Leonessa M, et al: Prophylactic fluconazole is effective in preventing fungal colonization and fungal systemic infections in preterm neonates: A single-center, 6-year, retrospective cohort study, *Pediatrics* 117:e22-e32, 2006.

360. Weese-Mayer DE, Fondriest DW, Brouillette RT: Risk factors associated with candidemia in the neonatal intensive care unit: A case-control study, *Pediatr Infect Dis J* 6:190-196, 1987.

361. Cotten CM, McDonald S, Stoll B, Goldberg RN, et al: The association of third-generation cephalosporin use and invasive candidiasis in extremely low birth-weight infants, *Pediatrics* 118:717-722, 2006.

362. Uko S, Soghier LM, Vega M, Marsh J, et al: Targeted short-term fluconazole prophylaxis among very low birth weight and extremely low birth weight infants, *Pediatrics* 117:1243-1252, 2006.

363. Fanaroff AA: Fluconazole for the prevention of fungal infections: Get ready, get set, caution, *Pediatrics* 117:214-215, 2006.

364. Long SS, Stevenson DK: Reducing *Candida* infections during neonatal intensive care: Management choices, infection control, and fluconazole prophylaxis, *J Pediatr* 147:135-141, 2005.

364a. Manzoni P, Stolfi I, Pugni L, Decembrino L, et al: A multicenter, randomized trial of prophylactic fluconazole in preterm neonates, *N Engl J Med* 356:2483-2495, 2007.

365. Natarajan G, Lulic-Botica M, Rongkavilit C, Pappas A, et al: Experience with caspofungin in the treatment of persistent fungemia in neonates, *J Perinatol* 25:770-777, 2005.

366. Pascual FB, McGinley EL, Zanardi LR, Cortese MM, et al: Tetanus surveillance: United States, 1998–2000, *MMWR Surveill Summ* 52:1-8, 2003.

367. Woodruff AW, Grant J, El Bashir EA, Yugusuk AZ, et al: Neonatal tetanus: Mode of infection, prevalence, and prevention in southern Sudan, *Lancet* 1:378-379, 1984.

368. Galazka A, Cook R: Preventing neonatal tetanus: Failure of the possible, *Lancet* 1:789-790, 1984.

369. Hinman AR, Foster SO, Wassilak SG: Neonatal tetanus: Potential for elimination in the world, *Pediatr Infect Dis J* 6:813-816, 1987.

370. Hlady WG, Bennett JV, Samadi AR, Begum J, et al: Neonatal tetanus in rural Bangladesh: Risk factors and toxoid efficacy, *Am J Public Health* 82:1365-1369, 1992.

371. Gurses N, Aydin M: Factors affecting prognosis of neonatal tetanus, *Scand J Infect Dis* 25:353-355, 1993.

372. Weinstein LL, Harrison RE, Cherry JD: Tetanus. In Feigin RD, Cherry JD, editors: *Textbook of Pediatric Infectious Diseases*, 4th ed, Philadelphia: 1998, Saunders.

373. Lawn JE, Wilczynska-Ketende K, Cousens SN: Estimating the causes of 4 million neonatal deaths in the year 2000, *Int J Epidemiol* 35:1–13, 2006.

374. LaForce FM, Young LS, Bennett JV: Tetanus in the United States (1965–1966): epidemiologic and clinical features, *N Engl J Med* 280:569-574, 1969.

375. Glezen WP: Prevention of neonatal tetanus, *Am J Public Health* 88:871-872, 1998.

376. Demicheli V, Barale A, Rivetti A: Vaccines for women to prevent neonatal tetanus, *Cochrane Database Syst Rev* 4:CD002959, 2005.

377. Amsalu S, Lulseged S: Tetanus in a children's hospital in Addis Ababa: Review of 113 cases, *Ethiop Med J* 43:233-240, 2005.

378. Asekun-Olarinmoye EO, Lawoyin TO, Onadeko MO: Risk factors for neonatal tetanus in Ibadan, Nigeria, *Eur J Pediatr* 162:526-527, 2003.

379. Brooks VB, Curtis DR, Eccles JC: The action of tetanus toxin on the inhibition of motor neurones, *J Physiol* 135:655-672, 1957.

380. Mellanby J, Green J: How does tetanus toxin act? *Neuroscience* 6:281-300, 1981.

381. Montecucco C: How do tetanus and botulinum toxins bind to neuronal membranes?, *Trends Biochem Sci* 11:314-317, 1986.

382. Montecucco C, Schiavo G: Tetanus and botulism neurotoxins: A new group of zinc proteases, *Trends Biochem Sci* 18:324-327, 1993.

383. Patel JC, Joag GG: Grading of tetanus to evaluate prognosis, *Indian J Med Sci* 13:834-840, 1959.

384. Pinheiro D: Tetanus of the newborn infant: A review of 238 cases treated in the Hospital das Clinica, São Paulo, Brazil, *Pediatrics* 84:32-37, 1964.

385. Athavale VB, Pai PN: Tetanus neonatorum: Clinical manifestations, *J Pediatr* 67:649-656, 1965.

386. Marshall FN: Tetanus in the newborn: With special reference to experiences in Haiti, W.I., *Adv Pediatr* 15:65-110, 1968.

387. Nourmand A, Ghavami A, Ziai M, Tahernia AC: Tetanus neonatorum in Iran, *Clin Pediatr* 9:609-610, 1970.

388. Teknetzi P, Manios S, Katsouyanopoulos V: Neonatal tetanus: Long-term residual handicaps, *Arch Dis Child* 58:68-69, 1983.

389. Okuonghae HO, Airede AI: Neonatal tetanus: Incidence and improved outcome with Diazepam, *Dev Med Child Neurol* 34:448-453, 1992.

390. Okan M, Hacimustafaoglu M, Ildirim I, Donmez O, et al: Long-term neurologic and psychomotor sequelae after neonatal tetanus, *J Child Neurol* 12:270-272, 1997.

391. Khuraibet AJ, Neubauer D, Noor KZ, Haleem MA, et al: A case of neonatal tetanus with characteristic neurophysiological findings, *Muscle Nerve* 21:971-972, 1998.

392. Nida H: Neonatal tetanus in Awassa: Retrospective analysis of patients admitted over 5 years, *Ethiop Med J* 39:241-246, 2001.

393. Okoromah CN, Lesi FE, Egri-Okwaji MT, Iroha E: Clinical and management factors related to outcome in neonatal tetanus, *Niger Postgrad Med J* 10:92-95, 2003.

394. Ertem M, Cakmak A, Saka G, Ceylan A: Neonatal tetanus in the South-Eastern region of Turkey: Changes in prognostic aspects by better health care, *J Trop Pediatr* 50:297-300, 2004.

395. Adams JM, Kenny JD, Rudolph AJ: Modern management of tetanus neonatorum, *Pediatrics* 64:472, 1979.

396. Khoo H, Lee EL, Lam KL: Neonatal tetanus treated with high dosage diazepam, *Arch Dis Child* 53:737-738, 1978.

397. Anlar B, Yalaz K, Dizmen R: Long-term prognosis after neonatal tetanus, *Dev Med Child Neurol* 31:76-80, 1989.

398. Gadoth N, Dagan R, Sandbank U, Levy D, et al: Permanent tetraplegia as a consequence of tetanus neonatorum, *J Neurol Sci* 51:273-278, 1981.

399. Okoromah CN, Lesi FE: Diazepam for treating tetanus, *Cochrane Database of Systematic Reviews* 1:1–17, 2006.

400. Tekur U, Gupta A, Tayal G, Agrawal KK: Blood concentrations of diazepam and its metabolites in children and neonates with tetanus, *J Pediatr* 102:145-147, 1983.

401. McCracken GH Jr, Dowell DL, Marshall FN: Double blind trial of equine antitoxin and human immune globulin in tetanus neonatorum, *Lancet* 1:1146-1149, 1971.

PERINATAL TRAUMA

Injuries of Extracranial, Cranial, Intracranial, Spinal Cord, and Peripheral Nervous System Structures

The terms *perinatal trauma* and *birth injury* have been given definitions so broad as to be confusing and nearly meaningless. Indeed, one commonly used definition of birth injury is any condition that affects the fetus adversely during labor or delivery. In this discussion, however, *perinatal trauma* refers to those adverse effects on the fetus during labor or delivery and in the neonatal period that are caused *primarily* by *mechanical* factors. Thus, specifically excluded are the disturbances of labor and delivery that lead principally to *hypoxic-ischemic* brain injury (see Chapters 6 to 9). (Nevertheless, overlap between mechanical trauma and the occurrence of hypoxic-ischemic cerebral injury is important to recognize because perinatal mechanical insults may result in primarily hypoxic-ischemic cerebral injury, probably secondary to disturbances of placental or cerebral blood flow.[1,2])

The incidence of traumatic brain injury, as defined for this chapter, is difficult to establish. This difficulty is related, in large part, to the frequent concurrence of hypoxic-ischemic injury as a sequela to perinatal trauma. Nevertheless, the incidence of traumatic injuries to central and peripheral nervous structures has been drastically reduced, primarily because of improved obstetrical management. Specific examples are apparent in the subsequent discussions, but recurring themes are the rational use of cesarean section and improved techniques of manual and instrumental vaginal deliveries.

MAJOR VARIETIES OF PERINATAL TRAUMA

The major varieties of perinatal trauma are outlined in Table 22-1. These include extracranial hemorrhage, skull fracture, intracranial hemorrhage, cerebral contusion, cerebellar contusion, spinal cord injury, and several types of injury to the peripheral nervous system (e.g., nerve roots and cranial or peripheral nerves). The injuries to extracranial, cranial, and central nervous system structures are discussed first.

INJURY TO EXTRACRANIAL, CRANIAL, AND CENTRAL NERVOUS SYSTEM STRUCTURES

Extracranial Hemorrhage

The three major varieties of extracranial hemorrhage are caput succedaneum, subgaleal hemorrhage, and cephalhematoma. These lesions occur in different tissue planes between the skin and the cranial bone (Fig. 22-1 and Table 22-2).

Caput Succedaneum

This term *caput succedaneum* refers to the hemorrhagic edema that is observed very commonly after vaginal delivery. Compression on the presenting part, exerted by the uterus or cervix, is the most common pathogenesis. Caput succedaneum and related scalp injuries occur in 20% to 40% of deliveries by vacuum extraction.[3] The usual site of caput formation is the vertex, and marked molding of the head is a common accompaniment. The edema is soft, superficial, and pitting, and it crosses sites of suture lines (see Table 22-2). The lesion steadily resolves over the first days of life, and no intervention is necessary.

Subgaleal Hemorrhage

Subgaleal hemorrhage refers to hemorrhage beneath the aponeurosis covering the scalp and connecting the frontal and occipital components of the occipitofrontalis muscle (see Fig. 22-1).[4] (Understandably, this lesion also is termed *subaponeurotic hemorrhage*.) Blood may spread beneath the entire scalp and may even dissect into the subcutaneous tissue of the neck. The pathogenesis of subgaleal hematoma is related to a combination of external compressive and dragging forces, occasionally aided by a coagulation disturbance (e.g., vitamin K deficiency).[5-7] A strong association with delivery by vacuum extraction is suggested by available data.[6-8] In one series, approximately 90% of the lesions were associated with vacuum extraction.[9] In a prospective series of 71 infants with subgaleal hemorrhage and delivery by vacuum extraction, a strong relationship

TABLE 22-1 Perinatal Traumatic Lesions	
Extracranial Hemorrhage	**Cerebral Contusion**
Caput succedaneum	**Cerebellar Contusion**
Subgaleal hemorrhage	**Spinal Cord Injury**
Cephalhematoma	**Peripheral Nervous System Injury**
Skull Fracture	Brachial plexus
Linear	Phrenic nerve (diaphragmatic
Depressed	paralysis)
Occipital osteodiastasis	Facial nerve
	Laryngeal nerve
Intracranial Hemorrhage	Median nerve
Epidural	Radial nerve
Subdural	Lumbosacral plexus
Primary subarachnoid	Sciatic nerve
Intraventricular	Peroneal nerve
Intracerebral	
Intracerebellar	

TABLE 22-2 Major Varieties of Traumatic Extracranial Hemorrhage

Lesion	Features of External Swelling	Increases After Birth	Crosses Suture Lines	Marked Acute Blood Loss
Caput succedaneum	Soft, pitting	No	Yes	No
Subgaleal hematoma	Firm, fluctuant	Yes	Yes	Yes
Cephalhematoma	Firm, tense	Yes	No	No

was observed with maternal multiparity, placement of the vacuum cup over the sagittal suture, or cup placement less than 3 cm from the anterior fontanelle.[7] The latter two factors would cause the vacuum extractor to exert traction forces with slanting or shearing effects on the scalp, considered to be central to the rupture of the emissary veins in the subgaleal space. The infants presented at 1 hour of age and had a relatively high incidence of hypovolemic shock (10%), requirement for volume expansion or inotropic support (35%), need for transfusion for anemia (35%), secondary coagulopathy (50%), and hyperbilirubinemia (35%). In a unique study of 27 infants evaluated by computed tomography (CT) scan, 14 infants demonstrated various angulation abnormalities of the parietal bones; such abnormalities suggest that the lesion can result from bleeding caused by one or more of three mechanisms (linear skull fracture, suture diastasis, fragmentation of the superior margin of the parietal bone), as illustrated in Figure 22-2.[8] This lesion is much less common than caput succedaneum, although the precise incidence is

unknown. In contrast to uncomplicated caput, subgaleal hematoma manifests as a firm, fluctuant mass, increases in size after birth, and it may be present in the subcutaneous tissue of the posterior side of the neck (see Table 22-2). Because of the findings noted earlier, infants must be watched carefully for signs of blood loss, coagulopathy, and the development of hyperbilirubinemia. Urgent blood transfusion may be necessary. After the acute phase, the lesion resolves over 2 to 3 weeks.

Cephalhematoma

Cephalhematoma refers to a circumscribed region of hemorrhage overlying the skull and confined by cranial sutures.

Incidence. Cephalhematoma occurs in approximately 1% to 2% of live births.[8] The lesion is more frequent in children of primiparous than multiparous mothers. The use of forceps or vacuum assist in delivery sharply increases the incidence.[10-12] In two large series, the incidence of cephalhematoma after the use of outlet forceps was 4.3%; after low forceps, it was 7.4%; after midforceps delivery, it was 9.5%[11]; and after the use of vacuum assist, it was 10.8%.[12a]

Pathology. The hemorrhage is subperiosteal in cephalhematoma, as opposed to the edema and blood in

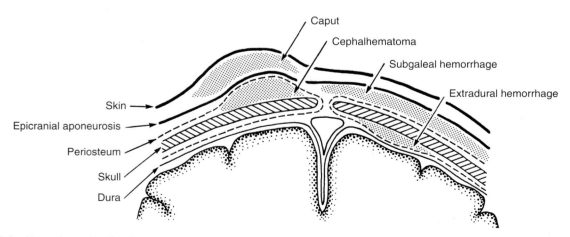

Figure 22-1 **Sites of extracranial (and extradural) hemorrhages in the newborn.** Schematic diagram of important tissue planes from skin to dura. *(Adapted from Pape KE, Wigglesworth JS:* Haemorrhage, Ischaemia and the Perinatal Brain, *Philadelphia: 1979, JB Lippincott.)*

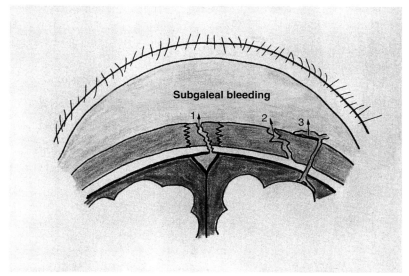

Figure 22-2 **Schematic drawing of the potential events that lead to subgaleal hemorrhage.** *1,* Suture diastasis, *2,* skull fracture, and, *3,* fragmentation of the superior margin of the parietal bone with ruptured emissary vein. *(From Govaert P, Vanhaesebrouck P, Depraeter C, Moens K, et al: Vacuum extraction, bone injury and neonatal subgaleal bleeding,* Eur J Pediatr *151:532-535, 1992.)*

caput succedaneum and subgaleal hemorrhage, which are located over the periosteum in either the subcutaneous or subaponeurotic spaces (see Fig. 22-1). The subperiosteal locus explains the confinement of the hematoma by cranial sutures (see Table 22-2). By far the most common locus of cephalhematoma is over the parietal bone and unilateral. The rare occipital cephalhematoma, midline in location because of confinement by the lambdoid sutures, may mimic occipital encephalocele. (Cranial ultrasound scan is a convenient means to make this distinction.[13]) An underlying linear skull fracture is detected in 10% to 25% of patients with cephalhematoma.[14,15]

Pathogenesis. Cephalhematoma is caused by mechanical forces (i.e., it is clearly a traumatic lesion in nearly all cases). The most reasonable formulation for pathogenesis implicates generally unavoidable obstetrical factors, relating to the size of skull and birth canal and to the use of forceps, thus causing tight apposition of subcutaneous structures to the periosteum but separation of periosteum from bone by external dragging forces.[16]

Clinical Features. The lesion usually increases in size after birth and manifests as a firm, tense mass that does not transilluminate (see Table 22-2; Fig. 22-3). The elevated periosteum palpable at the margin of the hematoma causes the palpating finger to appreciate a ridge at the margin of the lesion and a recessed center. This finding is readily mistaken for a depressed skull fracture. Cephalhematoma is rarely of clinical significance from the neurological standpoint unless a complicating intracranial lesion is present. I have seen one infant with an infected cephalhematoma and meningitis. Rare additional complications are hyperbilirubinemia, late onset anemia, and osteomyelitis.[17-20]

Essentially, all these lesions resolve in a few weeks to months. The few lesions that calcify and result initially in hard skull protuberances gradually disappear over many months of skull growth and remodeling.

Management. No specific therapy is indicated. The degree of acute blood loss rarely requires urgent intervention. Evacuation of the lesion is contraindicated. Treatment of the rare complications noted previously is necessary.

Skull Fracture

Three principal bony lesions of the newborn are categorized appropriately under the designation *skull fracture.* These lesions are linear and depressed skull fractures and occipital osteodiastasis (see Table 22-1). In fact, only with linear skull fracture does loss of bony continuity and therefore true fracture exist.

Linear Fracture

Linear skull fracture refers to a nondepressed fracture and is most commonly parietal in location (Fig. 22-4).

Incidence. Linear skull fractures are relatively common in newborns; however, the incidence is difficult to determine precisely because identification of the lesion depends particularly on the frequency of radiographic studies and the diligence of examination. In one series reported in 1975, the incidence was 10%.[15]

Pathology. Linear skull fracture may be associated with extracranial (e.g., cephalhematoma) and intracranial (e.g., epidural and subdural hemorrhage and cerebral contusion) complications. However, the more serious, intracranial complications are *rare* concomitants of linear skull fracture in the newborn. Also rarely, the fracture is associated with a tear of the

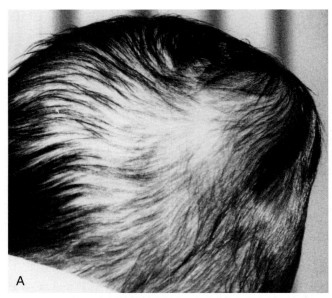

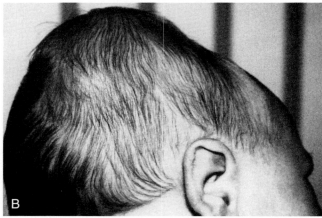

Figure 22-3 Parietal cephalhematoma: clinical appearance from a 10-day-old infant delivered with the aid of midforceps. A, Posterior view. **B,** Right lateral view. Note prominent swelling that extends medially to the sagittal suture, posteriorly to the lambdoid suture, and laterally to the squamosal suture.

dura and subsequent development of a leptomeningeal cyst. Leptomeningeal cyst also may occur after an unusual type of linear fracture (i.e., coronal suture diastasis), particularly secondary to vacuum extraction.[21]

Pathogenesis. Linear skull fracture is a traumatic lesion. Direct compressive effects are probably most important in genesis of the fracture.

Clinical Features. No clinical feature is associated with the fracture per se. The important clinical point is that the fracture should alert the physician to the possibility, however remote, of a more serious intracranial traumatic lesion. The development of a leptomeningeal cyst over the weeks or months subsequent to fracture can be easily detected at the bedside by the finding of increased transillumination of the affected region or, in more detail, by CT or magnetic resonance imaging (MRI) scan.

Management. No therapy is indicated. Follow-up skull radiographs at several months of age are useful to document that healing has occurred and that a widened defect indicative of an enlarging leptomeningeal cyst has not developed.

Depressed Fracture

Depressed skull fracture in the newborn usually refers to the "ping-pong" lesion associated with inward buckling of the unusually resilient neonatal bone, generally without loss of bony continuity (Fig. 22-5).

Incidence. In a large series of 270 infants "injured at birth," 32 exhibited depressed skull fracture.[22] The use of forceps is almost invariable; thus, in 28 of these 32 patients, forceps were known to have been used. In a more recent series, 50 of 68 cases of depressed skull fracture occurred after instrument-related delivery.[23]

Pathology. The most common site of depressed fracture is the parietal bone. Although in most cases no fracture is visible, occasionally bone fragments may be seen. Rarely, epidural or subdural hemorrhage or cerebral contusion is associated with this fracture type.

Pathogenesis. Depressed fracture is almost certainly a result of localized compression of skull. The compressing force is generated by either forceps or pressure against maternal pelvic structures during labor. A prolonged second stage of labor followed by forceps delivery was the most common sequence in one large series.[23] Rarely, depressed skull fracture may occur in utero.[24]

Clinical Features. The obvious and palpable bony defect calls immediate attention to the lesion (Fig. 22-6). Neurological accompaniments are unusual and relate to associated intracranial traumatic complications. Neurological complications are rare in spontaneous depressed skull fracture but are common in depressed skull fractures related to forceps deliveries. Indeed, in the latter group, epidural or subdural hemorrhage complicates 30% of cases, and subsequent neurological sequelae occur in 4%.[23]

Management. Traditionally, depressed fractures were considered an indication for neurosurgical elevation.[25] This view was challenged by the observation in several cases of spontaneous elevation of the deformity.[26-28] Indeed, the natural history of neonatal depressed skull fracture is unclear, and the incidence of spontaneous elevation is unknown. This fact and the reports of elevation by digital pressure,[29] use of breast pump,[30] and obstetrical vacuum extractor[31,32] suggest that neurosurgical intervention may be indicated less commonly than is currently assumed. The combination of a transparent breast pump shield attached to a vacuum extractor appears to be particularly useful (Fig. 22-7). Nevertheless, 85% of 68 patients in one series were said to "require neurosurgery."[23]

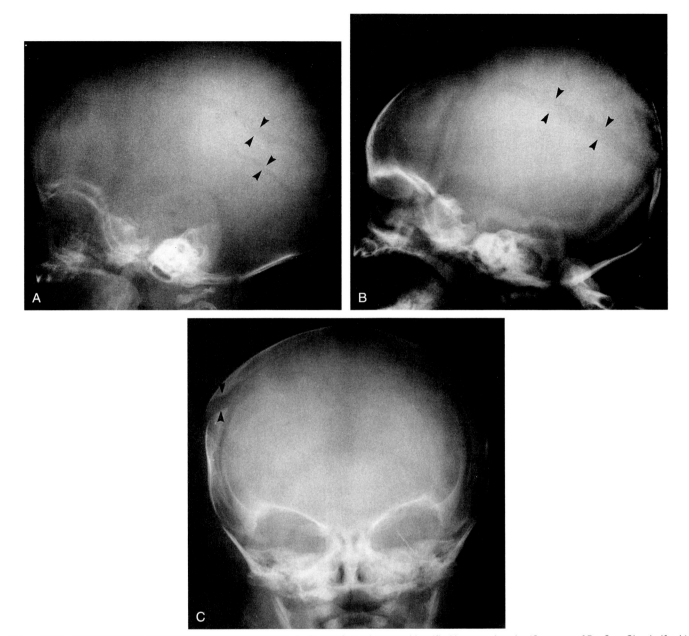

Figure 22-4   **Linear skull fractures in neonatal radiographs. A, B**, and **C**, Lesions are identified by *arrowheads*. *(Courtesy of Dr. Gary Shackelford.)*

The most reasonable approach to depressed fracture is careful radiological assessment of the lesion, including CT scan, to rule out the presence of extradural or subdural clot or bone fragments, and careful neurological surveillance to ensure that acute complications do not develop. This approach can then be followed by a trial of the nonsurgical modalities noted previously. If the nonsurgical trial is unsuccessful, consideration of neurosurgical intervention is then appropriate. However, small, uncomplicated "ping-pong" fractures, on the basis of current information, do not seem to warrant prompt neurosurgical intervention.

Occipital Osteodiastasis

Occipital osteodiastasis, defined as separation of the squamous and lateral parts of the occipital bone, may result in posterior fossa subdural hemorrhage, cerebellar contusion, and cerebellar-medullary compression without hemorrhage or gross contusion.[4] The evolution of the lesion by skull radiography is shown in Figure 22-8.[33] Its consequences are discussed primarily in Chapter 10.

Intracranial Hemorrhage

Major Varieties

The major varieties of intracranial hemorrhage associated with cranial trauma in the perinatal period include epidural hemorrhage, subdural hemorrhage (acute, subacute, and chronic), primary subarachnoid hemorrhage, intraventricular hemorrhage, intracerebral hemorrhage, and intracerebellar hemorrhage (see Table 22-1). Pathogeneses other than trauma play

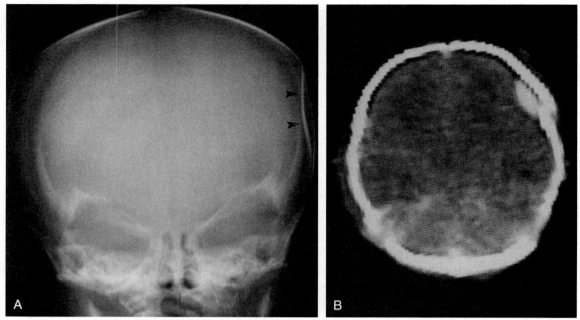

Figure 22-5 **Depressed skull fracture: radiograph and computed tomography (CT) scan. A,** Conventional skull radiograph showing the typical depressed, "ping-pong" fracture of the newborn *(arrowheads).* **B,** CT scan from another infant showing a less common depressed "fracture" in which the right coronal suture has been disrupted, thereby causing the parietal bone to be sharply depressed. An underlying small epidural hematoma exhibits the characteristic convex configuration.(**A,** Courtesy of Dr. Gary Shackelford.)

more important roles in several of these varieties of intracranial hemorrhage. Trauma plays the dominant pathogenetic role in epidural and subdural hemorrhage and may contribute to pathogenesis of the other varieties of intracranial hemorrhage. Except for epidural hemorrhage, the neuropathology, clinical features, management, and other features of neonatal intracranial hemorrhage are discussed in detail in Chapters 10 and 11.

Epidural Hemorrhage

Epidural hemorrhage refers to hemorrhage in the plane between the bone and the periosteum on the inner

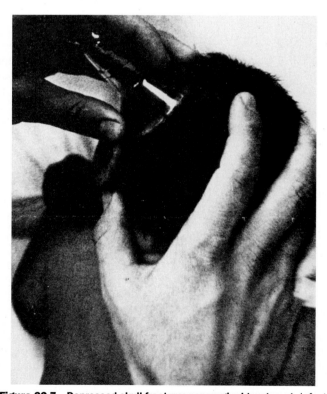

Figure 22-7 **Depressed skull fracture: nonsurgical treatment.** Infant with a "ping-pong" fracture is shown with a transparent plastic breast pump shield applied over the left frontal lesion. The transparent shield, which allows visualization of the elevation of the depression, is attached to an obstetrical vacuum extractor. *(From Saunders BS, Lazoritz S, McArtor RD, Marshall P: Depressed skull fracture in the neonate: Report of three cases,* J Neurosurg *50:512-514, 1979.)*

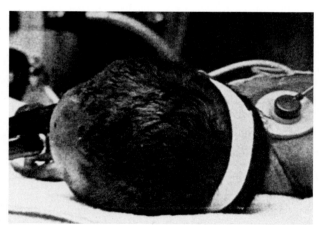

Figure 22-6 **Depressed skull fracture: clinical appearance.** From an infant with the typical "ping-pong" fracture shown in Figure 22-5A. Note the depression in the right parietal region. *(From Saunders BS, Lazoritz S, McArtor RD, Marshall P: Depressed skull fracture in the neonate: Report of three cases,* J Neurosurg *50:512-514, 1979.)*

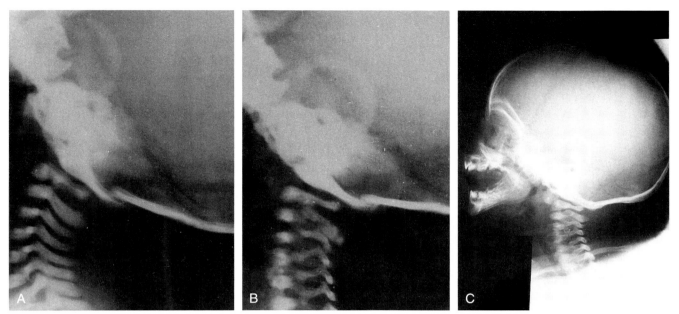

Figure 22-8 Lateral skull radiographs showing occipital osteodiastasis. A, In the seventh day of life, **B**, at 2½ months, and, **C**, at 1 year. Note the gradual improvement in the neonatal period and the normal appearance at 1 year. *(From Roche MC, Velez A, Garcia Sanchez P: Occipital osteodiastasis: A rare complication in cephalic delivery,* Acta Paediatr Scand *79:380-382, 1990.)*

surface of the skull (see Fig. 22-1).[4] It represents the intracranial analogue of a cephalhematoma (which is often associated).

Incidence. Epidural hemorrhage is a rare lesion in the newborn and constitutes only approximately 2% of all cases of neonatal intracranial hemorrhage observed at autopsy.[34] This relative rarity may relate to the finding that the dura in the newborn is unusually thick and is largely contiguous with the inner periosteum.[34]

Pathology. Bleeding into the epidural space is derived either from branches of the middle meningeal artery or from major veins or venous sinuses. Fractures across suture lines are likely to be associated with the venous sinuses. Linear skull fracture is present in the majority of cases, but not all.[34] Cephalhematoma is also a frequent accompaniment.[35,36]

Pathogenesis. When epidural hemorrhage is accompanied by linear skull fracture, overriding of fracture segments and tearing of branches of the middle meningeal artery or a large venous sinus are the probable reasons for the hemorrhage. In the infant without fracture, the reason for the hemorrhage is unclear. The dura can be separated from the bone when "the skull is bent inward or outward" at autopsy, and it is possible that this separation in vivo could cause tears of arteries running in the richly vascularized dural-periosteal layer of the neonatal cranium.[34]

Clinical Features. Most affected infants have experienced a traumatic labor or delivery and exhibit signs of increased intracranial pressure (bulging anterior fontanelle) from the first hours of life. A delay in onset of

signs also may occur,[36] perhaps when a venous origin is present. In two of the five cases reported by Takagi and co-workers, seizures were also present.[34] Signs of uncal herniation (e.g., fixed, dilated ipsilateral pupil) may occur. Suspicion of the lesion is an indication for emergency CT scan, which should demonstrate the hemorrhage effectively. The convex, lentiform appearance of the lesion is characteristic (see Fig. 22-5B; Fig. 22-9A). Untreated infants often die within 24 to 48 hours, although surgical evacuation and survival have been reported.[34,35] Moreover, survival after nonsurgical therapy also has been documented (see Fig. 22-9).[36]

Management. Although epidural hemorrhage is a rare lesion, it should be considered in any infant who has experienced a traumatic labor or delivery or who exhibits signs of increased intracranial pressure in the first day of life. Rapid diagnosis by CT scan and prompt intervention should improve the outcome. Although surgical evacuation has been the most common therapy, in one series, three infants treated by aspiration of an accompanying cephalhematoma recovered without sequelae.[36] In each case, the epidural hematoma disappeared after the aspiration of the cephalhematoma, apparently because of communication of the two lesions through a fracture site (see Fig. 22-9). In a fourth patient without cephalhematoma, the hematoma resolved with no direct therapy.[36]

Cerebral Contusion

Cerebral contusion refers to a focal region of necrosis and hemorrhage, usually involving the cerebral cortex and subcortical white matter.[4]

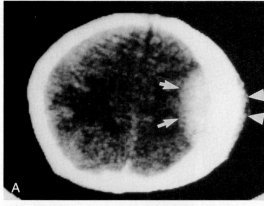

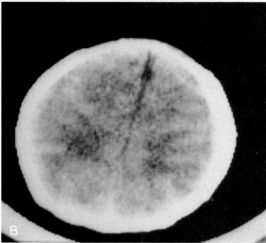

Figure 22-9   Computed tomography (CT) scans of a newborn with epidural hematoma. **A**, Before and, **B**, after aspiration of an overlying cephalhematoma. The epidural hematoma, apparent as a lentiform high-density area *(arrows)*, disappeared after aspiration of the cephal-hematoma *(arrowheads)*. A similar resolution occurred without aspiration in another infant with no cephalhematoma. *(From Negishi H, Lee Y, Itoh K, Suzuki J, et al: Nonsurgical management of epidural hematoma in neonates, Pediatr Neurol 5:253-256, 1989.)*

Incidence

Cerebral contusion is an apparently uncommon lesion in the newborn, although the precise incidence is unknown because of past difficulty in establishing the diagnosis in vivo. The reason for the relatively low incidence relates to the uncommon occurrence in the perinatal period of focal blunt trauma and to the relative resiliency of the neonatal cranium and cerebral mantle. These properties render less likely acceleration-deceleration movements of brain, which result in cerebral contusion at later ages.

Pathology

The term *cerebral contusion* describes the pathology typically observed in older children of focal necrosis and hemorrhage, involving particularly cerebral cortex and subcortical white matter. Such lesions are usually found in coup and contrecoup, as well as inferior orbital, frontal, and temporal locations. This characteristic topography is observed only rarely in the newborn.

Another variety of cerebral contusion described in newborns and young infants consists of slitlike tears in hemispheric white matter that may extend into the cerebral cortex or even the walls of the lateral ventricle.[37]

Pathogenesis

Focal areas of cortical necrosis and hemorrhage result from direct compressive effects in the newborn. Studies in neonatal rat pups implicated excitotoxic effects, mediated at the N-methyl-D-aspartate receptor, in the final pathway to tissue injury and showed protective effects of N-methyl-D-aspartate antagonists administered 30 minutes or 1 hour after the insult.[38] The tears of white matter are attributed to shearing forces within subcortical cerebral parenchyma produced by rapid and extreme deformation of brain.[37] The latter is made possible by the pliability of the newborn skull. An additional predisposing factor may relate to the relative lack of myelin in the developing cerebral white matter.

Clinical Features

Cerebral contusion probably constitutes the substrate for many of the cerebral signs associated with serious perinatal traumatic injury. Thus, seizures, often focal, motor deficits, especially hemiparesis or monoparesis, and deviation of eyes to the side of the lesion (but movable with the doll's eyes maneuver) represent particularly characteristic cerebral signs. Diagnosis is possible by CT or MRI.

Management

No specific therapy is indicated.

Cerebellar Contusion

Cerebellar contusion may occur with occipital osteodiastasis. More often, the contusion that results is associated with infratentorial subdural hematoma or intracerebellar hemorrhage. These lesions are discussed in Chapter 10.

Spinal Cord Injury

Spinal cord injury incurred during delivery results from excessive traction or rotation and is unlike the compression injury that is characteristic of most spinal cord injuries encountered in older patients. Spinal cord injury secondary to obstetrical disturbance, a moderately common lesion, is distinguished readily from the rare spinal cord injuries encountered in the neonatal period in association with vascular occlusion, observed with umbilical artery catheterization or accidental injection of air into a peripheral vein.[39-42]

Incidence

The true incidence of spinal cord injury is difficult to determine because the spinal cord is examined at autopsy only uncommonly. It is likely that significant injury to the spinal cord is more common than expected. Indeed, in one early series reported in 1923,

TABLE 22-3	**Pathology of Neonatal Spinal Cord Injury**
Major Sites of Injury	
Lower cervical and upper thoracic regions (especially breech delivery)	
Upper and midcervical regions (especially cephalic delivery)	
Major Neuropathological Changes	
Acute: hemorrhage (epidural and intraspinal), edema, laceration, disruption, and/or transection of cord	
Chronic: fibrosis of dura, arachnoid, and cord; focal areas of necrosis, often cystic; syringomyelia; disrupted architecture; and vascular occlusions with infarction	

Pierson[43] identified intraspinal hemorrhages in 46% of infants of breech deliveries examined at autopsy. The clinical significance of such lesions is not clear. The most widely cited observations are those of Towbin,[44,45] who concluded in the 1960s that spinal cord injury was a causal factor in approximately 10% of neonatal deaths. Friede[46] cautioned against overinterpretation of these data and suggested a distinction of clearly clinically significant lesions from "the often observed minor perivascular petechiae in the cord and from the extreme congestion or hemorrhagic imbibition of the epidural adipose tissue of newborns," presumably of little clinical importance.

Pathology

Two major sites of injury can be identified (Table 22-3). One site occurs principally with breech delivery and involves the lower cervical and upper thoracic regions[46-50a]; the other site occurs principally with cephalic delivery and involves the upper to midcervical regions.[46,48,49,50a,51-56] In one large series, the latter site was involved more than twice as often as the former.[49]

The dominant *acute lesions* are hemorrhages, especially epidural and intraspinal, and edema. The intraspinal hemorrhages particularly involve dorsal and central gray matter. These hemorrhagic lesions are usually associated with varying degrees of stretching, laceration, and disruption, or total transection. The dura not infrequently is torn, but complete spinal cord transection may occur with an intact dura.[47] Only uncommonly do lesions of the vertebral column appear.[46,50] These lesions consist of vertebral fractures or dislocations and separation of the vertebral epiphysis.[50,50a,57]

The acute lesions of spinal cord are followed by striking subacute and *chronic changes* (e.g., formation of fibrotic adhesions between dura, leptomeninges, and spinal cord; focal areas of necrosis with cystic cavities within the cord; syringomyelia; drastically disrupted architecture of the cord; and, often, total separation of transected cord segments). Vascular occlusions, perhaps developing as a post-traumatic event, may cause ischemic infarction of spinal cord segments caudal to the level of the primary lesion (Fig. 22-10).[58,59] This "post-traumatic vasopathy" may be related causally to the persistence of the clinical state of "spinal shock" in certain patients (see subsequent section).

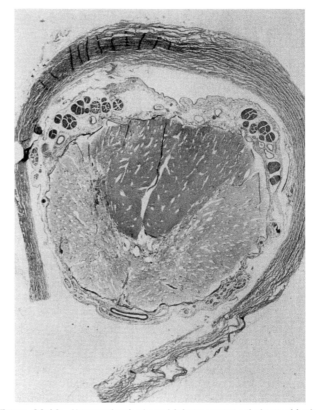

Figure 22-10   Neonatal spinal cord injury: neuropathology of ischemic infarction below the level of the traumatic lesion. Horizontal section of spinal cord at the upper thoracic level from an infant who died at 6 months of age after a neonatal cervical cord transection at the level of C2. Note the striking pallor, consistent with infarction, in the distribution of the anterior spinal artery.

Pathogenesis

Central to the pathogenesis of neonatal spinal cord injury is the finding that most cases are associated with *excessive longitudinal or lateral traction of the spine or excessive torsion.* Traction is more important in breech deliveries, which now account for the minority of cases, and torsion is more important in cephalic deliveries, which now account for the majority of cases.

The critical factors in pathogenesis relate to the *relative elasticities* of the vertebral column with its associated ligamentous and muscular structures, the dura, and the spinal cord. In the newborn, the bony vertebral column is nearly entirely cartilaginous and is very elastic, as are the associated ligaments.[60-62] Similarly, the muscles are relatively hypotonic, and the tone may be depressed further by maternal drugs or anesthesia. The dura is somewhat less elastic. However, least elastic is the neonatal spinal cord, which is anchored above by the medulla and the roots of the brachial plexus and below by the cauda equina. Thus, it is easy to understand why excessive longitudinal traction results in marked stretching of the vertebral column and rupture of the dura (the "snap" often heard at delivery of the aftercoming head in such cases) and the spinal cord. The cord ruptures at the sites of particular mobility and anchoring (i.e., in the lower cervical to upper thoracic region). With extreme rotational maneuvers, as with forceps rotation in difficult cephalic deliveries, the site of particular spinal cord mobility and most frequent rupture is in the upper to midcervical region. In a series of 15 cases of high cervical cord injury, the nearly invariable feature was forceps rotation of 90 degrees or more from the occipitoposterior to occipitotransverse position.[55] The infant's spine is particularly susceptible to rotational forces because the bony processes ("uncinate processes") of one vertebral body that articulate with corresponding processes of the adjacent vertebral body and thereby limit rotation are not well developed in the newborn.[48]

Insight into pathogenesis at the vascular, cellular, and molecular levels has been gained from studies of adult animals and humans.[63-72] Thus, early post-traumatic disturbance in spinal cord perfusion may result from local disturbances in spinal cord microcirculation and from systemic hypotension. Release of excitatory amino acids from injured neurons may lead to local excitotoxic mechanisms of cell death, as described in Chapter 6. The final common pathway of ischemic and neurotransmitter injury includes increases in cytosolic calcium, release of arachidonic acid, production of vasoactive prostanoids and free radicals, lipid peroxidation, membrane injury, and cell death. Potential interventions (e.g., glutamate blockers, corticosteroids, lipid peroxidation inhibitors) are suggested from these findings, and one such intervention, early steroid therapy, has been shown to be of some benefit in human adults (see "Management").

Clinical Features

Clinical Settings. Of paramount importance in the clinical setting are obstetrical factors, particularly breech or midforceps deliveries, which are present in the majority of recognized neonatal spine injuries.[48-50,50a,56,73-77] In addition, a frequent contributing feature is fetal depression, secondary to maternal drugs or anesthesia or to intrauterine asphyxia.[56,78]

Basic Clinical Syndromes. The clinical syndromes of spinal cord injury in the newborn are principally three-fold (Table 22-4).[50,56,79] First, stillbirth or rapid neonatal death with failure to establish adequate respiratory function occurs, particularly in cases with lesions involving the upper cervical cord or lower brain stem,

or both. Second, severe respiratory failure may develop in the first days of life and may lead to death. (This development may be delayed by mechanical ventilation, which presents major ethical difficulties in the ensuing weeks.) Third, the infant may exhibit neurological phenomena in the neonatal period but may survive, with weakness and hypotonia of limbs as the prominent features. The nature of the *neonatal* neurological syndrome may not be recognized, and the possibility of a neuromuscular disorder or transient hypoxic-ischemic encephalopathy is often considered. Most of these infants later develop spasticity and may be mistakenly considered to have cerebral lesions ("cerebral palsy").

Neurological Features. The typical infant is born after a difficult delivery. In lower cervical-upper thoracic injury, the following neurological features are apparent to varying degrees in the first hours or days of life: flaccid weakness with areflexia of lower extremities and variable involvement of upper extremities (see subsequent discussion); sensory level in the region of the lower neck or upper trunk; respiratory disturbance with diaphragmatic breathing and "paradoxical" respiratory movements or even diaphragmatic paralysis; paralyzed abdominal muscles with a soft, sometimes bulging abdomen; atonic anal sphincter; and distended bladder that empties usually with gentle suprapubic pressure (see Table 22-4).[48,49,51,56,62,80] Involvement of the upper extremities may reflect concomitant brachial plexus injuries or, if only distal portions of the upper extremities are affected, injury to anterior horn cells at the segmental levels of the spinal cord injury. Horner syndrome is occasionally present and relates to either involvement of cord neurons in the intermediate column of gray matter or exiting roots (especially T1) destined for the sympathetic ganglia. The major additional neurological feature with middle or upper cervical injury is respiratory failure with the need for mechanical ventilation because innervation of the diaphragm emanates from cervical segments 3, 4, and 5, especially 4.

Detection of a sensory level is critical and is accomplished readily if the examiner observes both the quantity and quality of movement and the presence of grimace or affective facial response elicited by pinprick. Stimulation should be performed slowly, and low-level reflex movements without facial response, probably mediated at a spinal level, should be recognized.

Coexistence of the clinical features of hypoxic-ischemic encephalopathy (see Chapter 9) in the acute neonatal period is not unusual in those infants with upper cervical lesions and a need for mechanical ventilation. In the largest series of such cases reported to date (*n* = 14), nine infants exhibited such signs.[49] Similarly, cognitive deficits were observed later in approximately 40% of infants with upper cervical spinal injury who survived more than 3 months.[49]

Subsequent Course. The neonatal neurological syndrome is followed primarily by one of two courses. First, and less commonly, the state just described, sometimes characterized as spinal shock, persists.

TABLE 22-4	Neonatal Clinical Features of Spinal Cord Injury
Three Basic Clinical Syndromes	
Stillbirth or rapid neonatal death	
Neonatal respiratory failure	
Neonatal weakness and hypotonia → spasticity ("cerebral palsy")	
Neurological Features	
Motor: weakness, hypotonia, areflexia of lower extremities (perhaps also upper extremities), and diaphragmatic breathing (or paralysis)	
Sensory: sensory level	
Sphincters: distended bladder and patulous anus	
Other: Horner syndrome	

This state may relate to secondary ischemia (post-traumatic vasopathy, described earlier) or to degenerative changes in the caudal segment of cord. Second, and more commonly, as edema and hemorrhage subside over the ensuing several weeks to months, the state of spinal shock subsides and evolves to a state of enhanced reflex activity. Hypotonia gives way to spasticity, and lower limbs are maintained in a position of "triple flexion" (i.e., flexion of hips, knees, and ankles). Tendon reflexes become hyperactive, and Babinski signs appear. Changes in upper extremities depend on the level of the lesion. When anterior horn cells or brachial plexus are involved, these limbs remain flaccid and areflexic. When the lesion is midcervical or higher, spasticity and hyperreflexia supervene in upper extremities as in lower extremities. Persistent respiratory failure and need for mechanical ventilation also are present in such middle or upper cervical cases. Reflex emptying of bladder occurs, often as part of mass reflex activity elicited by cutaneous or other stimulation. Higher-level motor or affective responses to sensory stimulation below the level of the lesion, however, do not develop. Disturbances of autonomic function (e.g., sweating and vasomotor phenomena) may lead to wide fluctuations in body temperature, especially in young infants. Trophic disturbances of muscle and bone may become prominent. The orthopedic and urinary tract complications that dominate the clinical course of these patients in the years after infancy are appropriately discussed in other texts.

Diagnosis

The diagnosis is often not difficult in the typical case. In less severely affected newborns, differentiation is necessary from an occult dysraphic state (see Chapter 1), an intravertebral, extramedullary mass (e.g., abscess, neuroblastoma, or hemorrhage),[81] an intramedullary lesion (e.g., syringomyelia, hemangioblastoma,[82] apparent intrauterine traumatic lesions,[83,84] or infarction occurring prenatally or caused by a vascular catastrophe associated with an indwelling catheter),[39-42,85] and a neuromuscular disorder (see Chapters 18 and 19).[49,62,77,86] Radiographs of the spine and a search for cutaneous dimples, sinus tracts, hemangioma, and abnormal hair should aid in the differential diagnosis of occult dysraphic state. Demonstration of the sensory level rules out a neuromuscular disorder (e.g., Werdnig-Hoffmann disease). Somatosensory evoked potentials are useful in documenting a sensory level in infants with equivocal results on clinical examination. Differentiation from an extramedullary or intramedullary lesion requires an imaging study.

The principal choices for imaging the spinal cord are ultrasonography, CT, and MRI. Ultrasonography is useful because the infant need not be moved, and the modality demonstrates spinal cord size and configuration and echogenic blood or edema within the spinal cord or blood in the extramedullary space.[49,75,77,87] Although blood is more echogenic than is edema, this critical distinction can be difficult with ultrasonography. Serial studies are carried out readily. I consider ultrasonography the *initial* imaging modality of choice

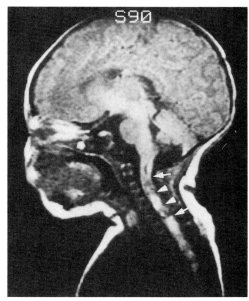

Figure 22-11 **Neonatal spinal cord injury: magnetic resonance imaging scan obtained at 5 days of age**. Sagittal plane of cervical cord on T1-weighted scan. Oval, high-intensity areas and surrounding low-intensity areas are observed in the lower cervical cord. *(From Minami T, Keiko I, Kukita J, Koyanagi T, et al: A case of neonatal spinal cord injury: Magnetic resonance imaging and somatosensory evoked potentials, Brain Dev 16:57-60, 1994.)*

in the acute situation. However, MRI provides superior resolution and should be used subsequently.[49,56,76,88-90] In the acute period, hemorrhage and edema can be distinguished by utilization of gradient-echo-acquisition sequences.[56] In the subacute and chronic periods, MRI provides superb resolution of parenchymal changes (Figs 22-11 and 22-12*A*). CT is useful when bony detail is required. CT or air myelography is generally no longer used because of the superiority of MRI. Newer diffusion tensor MRI techniques show promise for delineation of fiber tracts in the neonatal spinal cord.[91] Current MRI data indicate that the worst *prognosis* for subsequent cord function is associated with the finding of intramedullary hemorrhage.[88] The prognosis is better with edema over several segments and best with edema involving one segment or less.[56,88]

Management

Prevention. The most important element of management is prevention (Table 22-5). Of paramount importance is *appropriate management of breech presentations* and any other obstetrical situation that could lead to *dysfunctional labor*. Particularly, pharmacological augmentation of dysfunctional labor, ill-advised use of instrumentation, and the production of *fetal depression* by inappropriate use of maternal drugs or anesthesia should be avoided. Because many neonatal spinal cord injuries are associated with breech delivery, careful radiographic assessment of fetal position and size and of maternal pelvis is necessary.

Hyperextension of the fetal head represents a fetal position that carries a very high risk for the development of spinal cord injury, if the infant is delivered by the vaginal route.[92-97] It is critical to recognize that

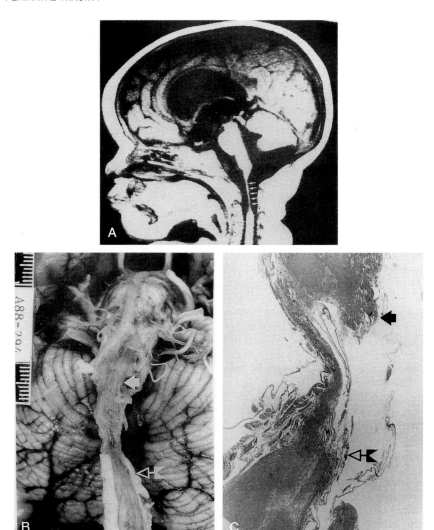

Figure 22-12   Neonatal spinal cord injury. A, Neonatal spinal cord injury: magnetic resonance imaging (MRI) scan at 4 months of age. Midline sagittal T1-weighted (TR, 500 milliseconds; TE, 15 milliseconds) MRI showing marked attenuation of cord caliber from the level of the caudal medulla to the level of C3 to C4 *(arrows)*. **B** and **C**, Pathological specimen of the infant whose MRI is shown in **A**. The infant died at 15 months of age. In **B**, note the gross specimen demonstrating complete disruption between the lower medulla *(arrow)* and the upper cervical cord *(open arrow)*. In **C**, note the microscopic section of upper cervical cord showing discontinuity between the lower medulla *(arrow)* and the upper cervical cord *(open arrow)*. The segment *between the two arrows* contains no neural elements, only leptomeninges and minimal scar tissue (hematoxylin and eosin, original magnification ×1.5). *(From Lanska MJ, Roessman U, Wiznitzer M: Magnetic resonance imaging in cervical cord birth injury, Pediatrics 85:760-764, 1990.)*

approximately 5% of all breech presentations are associated with hyperextended fetal head.[97-99] (This dangerous fetal position may also be present with a transverse lie.) Vaginal delivery of a fetus with hyperextended head and breech presentation is associated with death or survival with severe spinal cord injury in approximately 20% to 25% of cases. Thus, in a composite series of 73 such infants delivered vaginally, 15 experienced significant spinal cord injury, whereas none of 35 infants delivered by cesarean section experienced such injury.[97] Thus, the beneficial role of cesarean section in prevention of spinal cord injury is exemplified exceptionally well in this clinical setting. Nevertheless, a few infants with hyperextended fetal head in utero may sustain serious spinal cord injury *before* delivery and may exhibit quadriplegia and

respiratory failure despite cesarean section.[48,100-104] A decrease in fetal movement in the last weeks of gestation may herald the occurrence of spinal cord injury in the fetus with a hyperextended fetal head.[48] The spinal cord lesions have been upper cervical in location, and one careful neuropathological study suggested intrauterine vascular injury.[103] The likely intrauterine mechanisms (see "Pathogenesis") are subluxation and dislocation of upper cervical vertebrae, shown at autopsy to occur with hyperextension of the head, with compromise of the vertebral arteries, the vascular supply for upper cervical cord through the anterior spinal artery.[105] Thus, although cesarean section for the fetus in breech position with hyperextended head is critically important, spinal cord injury rarely may already have occurred. Indeed, other examples of

TABLE 22-5	Management of Spinal Cord Injury in the Neonatal Period
Prevention	
Appropriate management of breech presentations and dysfunctional labor	
Avoidance of fetal depression	
Cesarean section for hyperextension of fetal head	
Therapy	
Rule out surgically correctable lesion	
Supportive care	

spinal cord injury occurring in utero and observed after cesarean section have been recorded.[83,84,104]

Therapy. When a newborn infant has already sustained a serious spinal cord injury, no specific therapy can be offered (see Table 22-5). It is critical to rule out a surgically approachable lesion (e.g., an occult dysraphic state, vertebral fracture or dislocation, or other extramedullary lesion), as previously indicated. Careful history, physical examination, radiography of the spine, and ultrasonography may be sufficient to rule out such lesions. However, when any doubt exists about the nature of the lesion or the possible presence of an extramedullary block, MRI should be performed. Intramedullary block, usually secondary to marked spinal cord edema, is demonstrable in a few cases, but surgical intervention is generally not indicated. In the rare case of extramedullary block, exploration may be reasonable to rule out a surgically remediable lesion or a major epidural hemorrhage that could be contributing seriously to a traumatic lesion of the spinal cord. Nevertheless, little evidence indicates that laminectomy and decompression have anything to offer these unfortunate infants, in view of the basic nature of the spinal cord lesion. Further data, however, are needed on this issue.

A potential role for methylprednisolone in the acute management of spinal cord injury is suggested by the results of randomized, controlled trials in adult patients.[66,67,72] Individuals who received methylprednisolone as a bolus dose of 3 mg/kg within 8 hours of injury, and as a maintenance infusion of 5.4 kg/hour for 23 hours, had increased survival rates and better neurological recovery than placebo-injected or naloxone-treated controls. Because the glucocorticoid has been shown to prevent the early decline in spinal cord blood flow and the deleterious metabolic events, including lipid peroxidation, described earlier in experimental models, a clear rationale for benefit is apparent. In a subsequent study, the beneficial effect of methylprednisolone was confirmed, and additionally it was shown that patients treated between 3 and 8 hours after injury had as favorable a response to therapy as those treated within 3 hours of injury if the former patients were treated for 48 hours instead of only 24 hours.[72] Proof of benefit (without major risk) is difficult to obtain in infants because of the relatively small number of cases available for study. Moreover, the

correct diagnosis is usually delayed for many hours or days in infants (see earlier discussion).

Supportive therapy is important and is directed at ventilation, maintenance of body temperature, and prevention of urinary tract infection and contractures. At least initially, the bladder can be emptied by gentle use of the Credé maneuver, with the hope of subsequent development of automatic bladder function.[51] The possibility that prolonged treatment with monosialotetrahexosylganglioside (GM-1 ganglioside) can lead to improved recovery was suggested by a study of adults with spinal cord injury treated and followed for 1 year (first dose administered in the first 72 hours of injury).[65] In experimental models, GM-1 ganglioside led to increased neuronal survival and function of myelinated tracts. Study of this agent in models of spinal cord injury of immature animals would be of considerable interest. Moreover, current experimental studies concerning the use of stem cells, trophic factors, and related molecules in models of spinal cord regeneration may ultimately prove relevant in this context.

Major ethical issues are raised when infants are unable to sustain adequate ventilation without mechanical support. *Prediction of outcome in the neonatal period* is very difficult and is clearly essential for decisions to withdraw life support. Certain tentative conclusions can be made at 24 hours of age and at 30 days of age. Thus, in one series of nine infants with spinal cord injury above the level of C4 who required mechanical ventilation *and who survived at least 3 months*, the only two patients who survived with a favorable outcome (independent daytime breathing, good motor function) had *breathing movements on day 1*.[49] Of the seven survivors who took their first breath after the first day of life, all still required mechanical ventilation (except one infant who required only nocturnal mechanical ventilation) 8 months to 9 years later.[49] All four survivors who were *totally apneic beyond 30 days of age* required long-term mechanical ventilation and had severe motor disability.[49] (In this study, five additional patients with upper cervical spinal lesions had no respiratory movements in the first days of life and had life support withdrawn at 4 to 10 days of age.) Nevertheless, although these data are useful in predicting outcome, the numbers of infants studied are relatively small, and conclusions remain tentative. Moreover, some rehabilitative centers report that improvements in home mechanical ventilatory systems have been associated long term with relatively low mortality rates and intercurrent morbidities and with successful reintegration into schools and the community.[106]

INJURY TO PERIPHERAL NERVOUS SYSTEM STRUCTURES

Traumatic injury to peripheral structures (e.g., nerve roots, plexuses, and peripheral and cranial nerves) may result in serious and sometimes fatal disorders. In this section, I first review the four most common or serious of these injuries (i.e., brachial plexus palsies, diaphragmatic paralysis, facial paralysis, and median nerve injury). Next, I review a variety of less common peripheral traumatic injuries of nerve roots, plexuses, and trunks.

Brachial Plexus Injury

Brachial plexus injury refers to weakness or total paralysis of muscles innervated by the nerve roots that supply the brachial plexus (i.e., cervical roots 5 to 8 [C5 to C8] and thoracic root 1 [T1]).

Incidence

Brachial plexus injury is distinctly more common than spinal cord injury. In the largest reported series of traumatic birth injuries, brachial plexus injuries occurred 10 to 20 times more commonly than did spinal cord injuries.[107,108] The incidence generally varies between 0.5 and 2 per 1000 live births.[109-124] Because the lesion is virtually confined to the full-term newborn, the incidence in such infants is somewhat higher; in a representative report, brachial plexus injury was observed in 2.6 per 1000 live full-term infants in a major teaching hospital.[125] Attesting further to the relatively common occurrence, albeit not necessarily severe, of brachial plexus injury, I have been impressed with the relative frequency with which subtle but definite evidence for plexus injury can be ascertained by meticulous examination of infants at risk for such traumatic injury (see "Pathogenesis"). This observation has not been made in a systematic or quantitative fashion, and, indeed, the clinical significance is probably minimal, because the subtle deficits invariably resolve in a matter of days.

Pathology

Although the term *brachial plexus injury* is consistently used, the major disorder often involves the nerve *roots* that supply the plexus, particularly at the site where the roots form the trunks of the plexus (a similar site is observed in "stretch" injuries to brachial "plexus" in adults).[126] In the most severe neonatal lesions, actual avulsion of the root from the spinal cord and, often, associated spinal cord injury are present. In the much more common, less severe lesions, hemorrhage and edema consequent to injury to the nerve sheath or axon are prominent.[62,116,127,128] In the most common form of brachial plexus palsy, involvement of the proximal upper extremity (i.e., Erb palsy) is caused particularly by a lesion at the point (the Erb point) where the fifth and sixth cervical nerve roots unite to form the upper trunk of the brachial plexus. Involvement of the distal upper extremity (i.e., Klumpke palsy) is caused particularly by a lesion at the point where the eighth cervical and first thoracic nerve roots unite to form the lower trunk of the plexus.

The general relationships between the nature of the gross pathology and outcome are summarized in Table 22-6. Injury to the nerve sheath with associated hemorrhage and edema but with intact axons *(neurapraxia)* secondarily impairs axonal function, primarily by compression, but recovery is complete. *Severance of axons or roots is more serious.* Rupture of roots is associated with essentially no chance of spontaneous recovery.

TABLE 22-6   Relation of Pathology to Likelihood of Spontaneous Recovery in Brachial Plexus Injury

Severity of Lesion	Nerve Sheath	Axons	Roots	Likelihood of Spontaneous Recovery
Mild	Intact*	Intact	Intact	Good
Moderate	Intact	Severed	Intact	Fair
Severe	Severed	Severed	Intact	Poor
Severe	Intact	Intact	Severed	Poor

*Nerve sheath intact but injured; injury usually consists of edema and hemorrhage with secondary impairment of axonal function.

Similarly, axonal rupture when associated with severance of the nerve sheath and thus loss of a "guide" for regenerating axons *(neurotmesis)* is associated with a poor spontaneous outcome. However, axonal rupture with an intact nerve sheath is intermediate in severity; axonal regeneration occurs at a rate of approximately 1.8 mm/day,[129] somewhat faster than the rate of approximately 1 mm/day in older individuals.

Pathogenesis

Brachial plexus injury is thought to result from stretching of the brachial plexus, with its roots anchored to the cervical cord, by extreme lateral traction. The traction is exerted by the shoulder, in the process of delivering the head with breech deliveries, and by the head, in the process of delivering the shoulder in cephalic deliveries. The upper roots of the plexus are most vulnerable, but with marked traction, all roots are affected and total paralysis results. The relatively rare occurrence of intrauterine injury to the brachial plexus has been secondary to abnormalities of fetal position or of uterine structure.[118,130-132]

The pathogenetic events just mentioned occur secondary to, especially, *obstetrical factors* and *large fetal size.*[12,110,112-115,117-125,127,133-135a] Thus, in a large, essentially unselected series reported by Gordon and colleagues,[110] abnormal presentations occurred in 56% of cases; this group consisted of 14% breech and 42% abnormal vertex presentations (occiput posterior and occiput transverse). Shoulder dystocia was present in 51% of all vertex deliveries and in 30% of all breech deliveries. Labor was augmented in 50% of these cases. In the large series (*n* = 276) studied in the United Kingdom and Ireland, 65% had shoulder dystocia.[120] In several series of shoulder dystocia, approximately 20% of infants sustained some degree of brachial plexus injury.[115,124,135] Birth weight of affected infants exceeds 3500 g in 50% to 85% of cases.[110,114,115,120,122-124,133,135-137] In a large Swedish series, the incidence of brachial plexus palsy was 45-fold greater at a birth weight of more than 4500 g than at a birth weight of less than 3500 g.[117] In an older study, intrauterine asphyxia with fetal depression was suggested by the signs of fetal distress in 44% and Apgar score at 1 minute of less than 4 in 39%.[110] Thus, a large, depressed infant after abnormal labor and delivery appears to be at added risk.

Clinical Features

Clinical Setting. The typical clinical setting comprises obstetrical and fetal factors that predispose the infant to traumatic injury, particularly by excessive traction. Thus, as noted previously, abnormal presentations, dysfunctional labor, augmented labor, large fetal size, and perhaps fetal depression occur to varying degrees in most cases of brachial plexus injury.

Neonatal Varieties. In standard writings on brachial plexus injury, two basic types are recognized: the upper type, or Erb palsy, and the lower type, or Klumpke palsy. In neonatal patients, approximately 90% of cases of brachial plexus injury involve the proximal upper limb and correspond to Erb palsy.[110,112,120,133,138-140] True Klumpke palsy (i.e., weakness of distal upper extremity *only*), in my experience, does not occur in the newborn period; infants with distal involvement *also* exhibit proximal involvement. Essentially *total* brachial plexus palsy in neonates is often classified, appropriately or not, as *Klumpke palsy*.

The nerve roots involved in the common, upper, Erb palsy emanate from cervical segments 5 and 6 in at least 50% of such cases, with the addition of cervical segment 7 in the other 50%.[133] The additional roots involved in the patients with total brachial plexus injury emanate from cervical segment 8 and thoracic segment 1. In Erb palsy, involvement of the diaphragm may be associated if involvement extends to cervical roots 4 and, perhaps, 3. (The innervation to the diaphragm, as noted previously, is from cervical segments 3, 4, and 5, with most input from C4.) Involvement of ipsilateral diaphragm is present in approximately 5% of cases of Erb palsy. In total plexus injury, involvement of sympathetic outflow from thoracic root 1 may result in Horner syndrome, manifested in the newborn by ptosis and miosis. An additional complication of this deficit of sympathetic innervation of the iris is a disturbance in pigment formation. Thus, the affected eye remains unpigmented (i.e., blue) for many months or years.[62]

Major Neurological Features. The major neurological features of Erb palsy and total plexus palsy are best considered in terms of effects on muscle function, tendon reflexes (especially the biceps), Moro and grasp reflexes, and sensory function (Tables 22-7 to 22-9). In general, the motor deficits are much more

striking than the sensory deficits because of the overlapping innervation of sensory dermatomes, the greater involvement of anterior than posterior roots, and the difficulty of precise assessment of sensation in the newborn. Based on clinical features, the lesion is bilateral in approximately 5% of cases.[96,120,133,134,138] One careful electrophysiological study of 18 cases showed *neurophysiological* abnormalities in the clinically unaffected arm in 5 cases.[141]

Erb Palsy. In Erb (upper) palsy, patients have weakness at the shoulder of abduction (deltoid, C5) and external rotation (spinatus, C5), at the elbow of flexion (biceps, brachioradialis, C5, C6) and supination (biceps, supinator, C5, C6), and to a variable extent at the wrist and fingers of extension (extensors of the wrist and long extensors of the fingers, C6, C7) (see Table 22-7). Thus, the limb assumes the characteristic "waiter's tip" posture because of preservation of shoulder abduction and internal rotation, elbow extension and pronation, and wrist and finger flexion (Fig. 22-13). The biceps (C5, C6) reflex is absent (see Table 22-9). (The brachioradialis and triceps reflexes [C6, C7, C8], which are sometimes difficult to elicit in the newborn, may be expected to be inconsistently disturbed.) The Moro reflex is disturbed because of the deficit in shoulder abduction (although hand movement is present). The grasp reflex is present because of the preserved finger flexion. I have found *sensory deficits* to pinprick (assessed primarily by observation of facial response) to be relatively common, contrary to the experience

TABLE 22-8 Major Additional Pattern of Weakness with Total Brachial Plexus Palsy

Weak Movement	Spinal Cord Segment	Resulting Position
Wrist flexion	C7, C8; T1	Extended
Finger flexion	C7, C8; T1	Extended
Finger abduction	C8, T1	Neutral position
Finger adduction	C8, T1	Neutral position
Dilator of iris	T1	Miosis
Full lid elevation	T1	Ptosis

TABLE 22-9 Reflex Abnormalities in Erb (Upper) and Total Brachial Plexus Palsies

Reflex	Spinal Cord Segment	Upper Palsy	Total Palsy
Biceps	C5, C6	Absent	Absent
Moro			
Shoulder abduction	C5	Absent	Absent
Hand movement	C8, T1	Present	Absent
Palmar grasp	C8, T1	Present	Absent

TABLE 22-7 Major Pattern of Weakness with Erb (Upper) Brachial Plexus Palsy

Weak Movement	Spinal Cord Segment	Resulting Position
Shoulder abduction	C5	Adducted
Shoulder external rotation	C5	Internally rotated
Elbow flexion	C5, C6	Extended
Supination	C5, C6	Pronated
Wrist extension	C6, C7	Flexed
Finger extension	C6, C7	Flexed
Diaphragmatic descent	C4, C5	Elevated

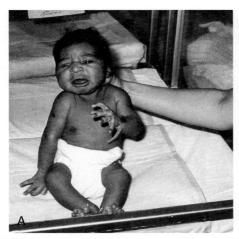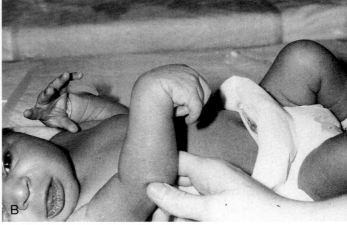

Figure 22-13   **Brachial plexus injury, upper or Erb type: clinical appearance. A,** Infant holds the upper extremity adducted, internally rotated, and pronated. **B,** "Waiter's tip" position of affected wrist and fingers. *(From Painter MJ, Bergman I: Obstetrical trauma to the neonatal central and peripheral nervous system,* Semin Perinatol *6:89-104, 1982.)*

recorded by many other investigators. The most consistent hypesthesia is over the lateral aspect of the proximal upper extremity (C5). *Diaphragmatic paralysis,* which should be looked for specifically, was associated with Erb palsy in 3 of the 55 cases studied by Gordon and co-workers.[110]

Total Plexus Palsy. In total plexus palsy, with involvement of lower as well as upper roots, the paralysis extends to the intrinsic muscles of the hand (C8, T1; see Table 22-8). (I have never seen a case of involvement of hand *alone,* although a report recorded 1 case among 57 cases of neonatal brachial plexus palsy.[113]) The grasp reflex is *absent* (see Table 22-8). The sensory loss is more extensive in these patients with total plexus involvement because of the loss of the overlapping sensory innervation. *Horner syndrome* has been reported in approximately 30% of these severely affected infants.[110,112,120,133,138]

Other Traumatic Lesions. Other traumatic lesions may be associated with brachial plexus injury. Thus, the approximate proportions of associated lesions are as follows: fractured clavicle (10%), fractured humerus (10%), subluxation of the shoulder (5% to 10%), subluxation of cervical spine (5%), cervical spinal cord injury (5% to 10%), and facial palsy (10%).[113,120,124,133]

Diagnosis

Delineation of the *clinical features* can be accomplished effectively by meticulous neurological examination. *Electromyographic (EMG) studies* have been recommended as adjuncts to the evaluation at approximately 1 and 3 months of age.[112,133,138-140,142] Signs of denervation (i.e., fibrillations) appear approximately 2 to 3 weeks after the injury. If fibrillations are absent, the likely lesion is neurapraxia, and the outlook is favorable. Nerve root avulsion and a poor outcome are indicated on the first study by diffuse fibrillations, unrecordable or scanty motor unit potentials, no muscle response with stimulation of motor nerves, and no improvement on the second EMG examination.

Definition of diaphragmatic paralysis can be made conclusively by *real-time ultrasound scan,* which demonstrates high placement of the diaphragm on the affected side and "seesaw" movements of the whole diaphragm with respiration. The latter results because on inspiration the paralyzed side ascends while the intact side descends; the opposite occurs with expiration. *MRI* may demonstrate pseudomeningoceles and other findings suggesting partial or complete avulsion of roots and hence a poor prognosis for spontaneous recovery (Fig. 22-14).[143,144] However, pseudomeningoceles may be absent in infants who ultimately have a poor outcome, and the presence of these lesions is not invariably followed by a poor outcome.[139] Occasionally, differentiation of brachial plexus injury from "pseudoparalysis" secondary to bony lesions presents a diagnostic problem. *Radiographs of cervical spine, clavicles, and humerus* are of value in this regard.

Prognosis

Prognosis relates to the severity and extent of the lesion. Reported rates of full recovery generally range from 65% to 90%.[110,115,117,120,121,124,133,145-151b] The variation in rates depends particularly on whether the population has been followed from the neonatal period and on whether full recovery is based on careful clinical examination and excludes good functional recovery, albeit with residual weakness. In populations followed from the neonatal period, recovery rates are generally higher than in populations later referred to a tertiary center. For example, in two series followed from the neonatal period, approximately 90% of patients were said to be "normal" at 6 months of age.[110,115] In a carefully studied population followed at a children's hospital (*n* = 116), only 33% were normal at 6 months of age, 45% were normal at 9 months, and 66% were normal at 15 months.[147] Early onset of recovery (i.e., within 2 to 4 weeks) is an excellent prognostic sign; in one series, all patients who recovered fully showed some improvement in arm function by 2 weeks.[152] The importance of serial assessments and, in particular, of the findings at 6 months in prediction of outcome is illustrated by

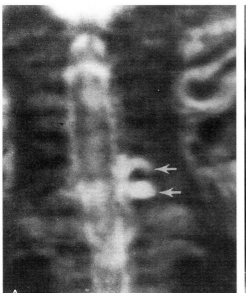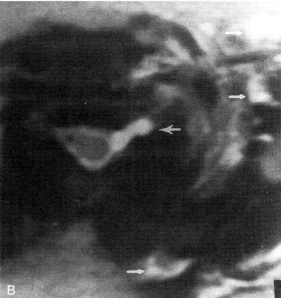

Figure 22-14   **Magnetic resonance imaging in a 6-day-old infant with left brachial plexus injury. A,** Reconstructed coronal T2-weighted image shows pseudomeningoceles of the left C7 and C8 roots *(arrows).* **B,** Axial T2-weighted image shows pseudomeningoceles of the left C8 root *(large arrow).* Note also soft tissue swelling and fluid in fascial planes of the left lower neck and shoulder *(small arrows). (From Francel PC, Koby M, Park TS, Lee B, et al: Fast spin-echo magnetic resonance imaging for radiological assessment of neonatal brachial plexus injury,* J Neurosurg *83:461-466, 1995.)*

the data in Table 22-10. Thus, infants with complete recovery recovered antigravity movement of biceps, triceps, and deltoid by 4.5 months (80% by 3 months); those patients with mild residual weakness recovered antigravity movement by 6 months; those with moderate residual weakness had failure of antigravity recovery at least in the deltoid by 6 months; and those with severe residua had no or trace recovery of wrist extensors by 6 months. Clearly, the last group had extensive plexus lesions. In an obstetrical series of 19 infants with C5 to T1 lesions, none made a full recovery, 68% had a partial recovery, and fully 32% made no recovery.[120]

TABLE 22-10   Outcome of Neonatal Brachial Plexus Palsy Relative to Examination at 6 Months

Muscle Strength at 6 Mo*	Patients	Final Outcome
≥3/5 in BTD *(also at 4.5 mo)*	53 (66%)	Complete recovery
≥3/5 in BTD	9 (11%)	Mild weakness
3/5 in B, T, or both, ***but not D***	7 (9%)	Moderate weakness
0–1/5 WE and/or ≤2/5 in BTD	11 (14%)	Severe weakness

*Muscle strength scale: 0, no contraction; 1, trace contraction; 2, active movement with gravity eliminated; 3, active movement against gravity; 4, active movement against gravity and resistance; 5, normal.
B, biceps; T, triceps; D, deltoid; WE, wrist extensors.
Data from Noetzel MJ, Park TS, Robinson S, Kaufman B: Prospective study of recovery following neonatal brachial plexus injury, *J Child Neurol* 16:488-492, 2001.

Management

The management of brachial plexus injury in the neonatal period has two major aspects. The first is prevention, and the second is care of the affected infant.

Prevention. Prevention of brachial plexus injury must be based on eliminating the opportunity for traction injury (see "Pathogenesis"). Reasoned obstetrical management of abnormal presentations and deliveries and the judicious use of maternal drugs and anesthesia to avoid fetal depression, especially in the presence of a large fetus, are critical.

Therapy. Management of the infant, once affected, is directed particularly toward prevention of the development of contractures, which worsen the degree of functional disability. After the diagnosis is made, the limb should be immobilized gently across the upper abdomen. Therapy should begin in the latter part of the first week with gentle, passive, range-of-motion exercises at shoulder, elbow, wrists, and small joints of the hands.[112,133,138] Supportive wrist splints to prevent flexion contractures and to stabilize the fingers are important. Not recommended is the former "Statue of Liberty" splint that placed the limb in a position at shoulder, elbow, and wrist that was opposite from that assumed by the unsupported limb. This type of splint carries considerable risk of causing contractures in the new position. Trophic disturbances of skin, muscle, and bone are particularly likely to develop in infants with *total* plexus involvement (which usually includes marked sensory involvement), and these disturbances are difficult to treat effectively. In addition, a few infants, even some with good sensorimotor recovery, "ignore and refuse to use" the affected limb.[133] This state has been attributed to a failure of development of appropriate cerebral motor patterns and organization of body image, secondary to the transient interruption of peripheral pathways, which is a conclusion with some experimental support.[153] Eng's considerable clinical experience led to the following conclusion: "Attempts at sensory stimulation, massage, calling the infant's attention to the arm have been questionably successful in minimizing this problem."[133] Orthopedic problems at the shoulder and elbow may require surgical intervention, as discussed elsewhere.[154]

The possibility of *surgical treatment* should be considered in selected patients after careful serial assessments over the first 6 months. The advent of the operating microscope and more recent success in microsurgical repair of brachial plexus lesions in adults led to surgical management of severely affected infants.[116,123,127,140,146,151,154-157] Surgical options depend on the specific findings but include removal of disruptive fibrous tissue at the site of the lesion, excision of neuroma, sural nerve graft at the site of axonal rupture, and local root grafts from intact roots at the site of root avulsions.[116,123,127,154] Improvement in function has been reported in the majority of operated infants.[116,123,127,140] The critical issue concerning *timing of the decision* to proceed to surgery is unresolved.[151,156,157] I consider particularly rational the approach based in considerable part on the data shown in Table 22-10.[147] Thus, infants with upper plexus palsies who attain antigravity movements of biceps, triceps, and deltoid by 6 months of age have a very high likelihood of excellent spontaneous recovery. However, the families of those infants destined for a poor outcome (see "severe weakness" in Table 22-10), including more severe upper plexus palsies and total plexus palsies, should be apprised of neurosurgical interventions at 4 to 6 months of age. EMG and MRI can provide additional useful information (see earlier). Neurosurgical intervention is probably best considered for infants aged 6 to 9 months.[147] For the small group of infants with total plexus palsies, some clinicians advocate neurosurgical intervention before this period.[151]

Diaphragmatic Paralysis

Diaphragmatic paralysis secondary to traumatic injury to cervical nerve roots supplying the phrenic nerve may occur as an isolated finding or in association with brachial plexus injury (Table 22-11).

Incidence

The incidence of neonatal diaphragmatic paralysis is related to the incidence of brachial plexus injury, because approximately 80% to 90% of cases are associated with such plexus injury, and approximately 5% of cases of brachial plexus injury are associated with diaphragmatic paralysis.[86,120,134,138,158-171] In medical centers that perform substantial numbers of major cardiac surgical procedures in newborns, diaphragmatic

TABLE 22-11	Diaphragmatic Paralysis in the Newborn: Clinical and Related Features
Relation to Brachial Plexus Injury ≈80% to 90% of cases with associated plexus injury; ≈5% of plexus injuries with diaphragmatic paralysis	
Cervical Roots Involved C3–C5, especially C4	
Onset First hours after birth	
Diagnosis Ultrasonography, chest fluoroscopy	
Prognosis Mortality in composite series ≈10%–15%	

paralysis secondary to phrenic nerve injury may be encountered in the absence of brachial plexus injury.[172] Finally, rarely chest drains abutting the mediastinum may lead to phrenic nerve injury in the newborn.[173]

Pathology

The pathogenesis of diaphragmatic paralysis appears to be similar in most cases to that described for brachial plexus injury. This conclusion is supported by the high frequency of similar obstetrical and fetal factors and of extreme lateral traction in the delivery of affected infants. Phrenic nerve injury is more common after breech than cephalic deliveries. The major sites of injury defined in anatomical studies are shown in Figure 22-15.[174]

Clinical Features

Clinical Syndrome. Although the clinical syndrome is somewhat variable, the most typical features can be summarized as follows.[86,158-169,171,174-176] The birth

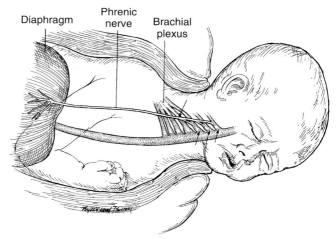

Figure 22-15 Schematic appearance of infant during vaginal delivery before lateral traction of the head and neck to deliver the right shoulder (*uppermost in the figure*). Sites where the phrenic nerve can be stretched and injured are indicated by the *four arrows.* (*From Alvord EC, Austin EJ, Larson CP: Neuropathologic observations in congenital phrenic nerve palsy, J Child Neurol 5:205-209, 1990.*)

occurs in a clinical setting that includes the obstetrical and fetal factors conducive to traumatic injury, in particular difficult breech delivery, as described previously for brachial plexus injury. Often, diaphragmatic paralysis appears to have a biphasic course. *In the first hours after birth*, the infant experiences respiratory difficulty, frequently with tachypnea, but with blood gas values suggestive of hypoventilation (e.g., hypoxemia, hypercapnia, and acidosis). In some cases, signs of gross ventilation-perfusion unevenness are suggested by hypoxemia without significant hypercapnia.[163] The occurrence of cyanosis with the respiratory difficulty often raises the possibility of congenital heart disease or primary pulmonary disease. *Over the next several days*, the infant may improve, or at least stabilize, with oxygen therapy and varying degrees of ventilatory support. The diagnosis of diaphragmatic paralysis may be missed during this period, despite radiographs of the chest, because the elevated hemidiaphragm commonly is not present or prominent early in the course, especially with positive pressure ventilation. In more severely affected infants, deterioration, sometimes insidious, of respiratory status occurs over the next days to weeks, often provoked by atelectasis or pulmonary infection. Indeed, in the four infants studied by Schifrin,[177] the diagnosis was not made before the sixth week. Of course, in the most severely affected infants, with bilateral involvement, respiratory failure is obvious from birth.

Diagnosis

The diagnosis is established by ultrasonographic or fluoroscopic examination of the chest, which reveals the elevated hemidiaphragm and the paradoxical movement of the affected side with breathing (see the previous "Brachial Plexus Injury" section). These radiographic abnormalities will not be present if the infant is receiving positive-pressure ventilation. Real-time ultrasonography is particularly useful in the detailed assessment of diaphragmatic function because of the lack of radiation and the capacity for serial study.[172,178] Approximately 80% of the lesions involve the right side, and fewer than 10% of lesions are bilateral.

Prognosis

The subsequent course of the infant's condition depends, in part, on the severity of the injury, but particularly on the quality of supportive care. The mortality rate for infants with the common unilateral lesions in composite series has been approximately 10% to 15%. However, most infants recover, usually in the first 6 to 12 months of life.[162,168,171,177] Clinical recovery may occur despite persistence of considerable weakness demonstrable by radiography.[177] The outcome is predictably poorer for the small number of infants with bilateral diaphragmatic paralysis.[168-171,175,176,179] In these infants, mortality has approached 50% with the prolonged ventilatory support required. However, advances in management are improving outcome (see the next section).

Management

Prevention. The comments on prevention of brachial plexus injury are appropriate here, because the mechanism of production of the root lesions is similar.

Therapy. Once diaphragmatic paralysis is documented in the newborn infant, careful surveillance of respiratory status and intervention, when appropriate, are critical. Clinical experience suggests that the newborn infant tolerates diaphragmatic paralysis less well than does the older child or adult. Reasons suggested for this difference in vulnerability in the newborn include the following: the usual recumbent posture, which leads to a greater reduction in vital capacity than does the upright posture; the relatively weaker intercostal muscles; the relatively greater risk of airway obstruction, secondary to proportionately smaller airways; and the relatively longer time spent in rapid eye movement sleep, when tone in such postural muscles as the intercostals is inhibited.[172,175,180] Management of the newborn with diaphragmatic paralysis may be divided into *nonsurgical, so-called expectant modalities* and *surgical plication of the diaphragm*.

The *nonsurgical modalities* have been characterized as "expectant" because their major purpose is to stabilize the infant and to provide adequate ventilation temporarily, until natural improvement of the neural injury occurs. These modalities have included the rocker bed, continuous positive airway pressure, intermittent negative pressure ventilation, and intermittent positive pressure ventilation (Table 22-12). Substantial benefit has been achieved with the use of a *rocker bed* in affected newborns, and this modality still may be useful for selected infants.[168] *Continuous positive airway pressure* through a nasal cannula (with the infant in a semiupright position) has been associated with some benefit and merits a trial, because it obviates the need for endotracheal intubation.[179] *Intermittent negative pressure ventilation* has also been useful[175]; this approach has the advantages of avoiding intubation and preventing trauma to airways. In recalcitrant cases, *intubation and intermittent positive pressure breathing* have been advocated.[168] In general, investigators have suggested that the trial of positive pressure ventilation be continued for at least 2 months until it is clear that no recovery is occurring.[175] If the latter is the case, then *plication of the affected diaphragm* is appropriate. In patients with bilateral lesions, it is recommended that, if possible, only the more severely involved hemidiaphragm be plicated.[175]

TABLE 22-12	**Management of Diaphragmatic Paralysis in the Newborn**
Nonsurgical Modalities	
Rocker bed (?)	
Continuous positive airway pressure	
Intermittent negative pressure ventilation	
Intermittent positive pressure ventilation	
Surgical Plication	

Autologous nerve transplantation was associated with improved diaphragmatic function in one reported bilateral case.[171]

Phrenic nerve stimulation (percutaneous) with surface recordings of diaphragmatic action potentials may provide important information for appropriate management.[86,171,181,182] Thus, extremely prolonged conduction latencies or marked reductions in amplitude or absent diaphragmatic action potentials suggest that spontaneous recovery will not occur and that surgical plication is necessary.

Facial Paralysis

Facial paralysis refers to weakness of facial muscles. In this context of perinatal trauma, the term indicates facial nerve injury and therefore involvement of the muscles of the upper as well as lower parts of the face.

Incidence

Facial weakness secondary to injury to facial nerve is the most common neurological manifestation of perinatal trauma. In 875 term infants examined for facial paresis on the second day of life in a series reported in 1951, the incidence was 6.4% (Table 22-13).[183] In a more recent series, the incidence was 0.75% of term infants.[125]

Pathology

The pathological basis for the typical traumatic injury to facial nerve is unknown. It is likely that the pathological features in most infants consist of hemorrhage or edema into the nerve sheath, rather than disruption of nerve fibers, in view of the nearly uniformly favorable prognosis (see "Prognosis"). The site of the lesion is almost certainly at or near the exit of the nerve from the stylomastoid foramen. The nerve divides into its two major branches: the temporofacial, to the zygomatic region, eye, and upper face; and the cervicofacial, to the mandibular region and platysma, shortly after exit from the foramen. Involvement of the nerve at more proximal sites (e.g., in the facial canal or posterior fossa) is rare in the newborn infant. However, compression against a fracture of the petrous temporal bone, identified at surgery, was reported in two infants.[184,185]

Pathogenesis

Hepner's[183] interesting 1951 study of 875 term infants examined on the second postnatal day presented strong evidence of the pathogenetic importance of intrauterine

TABLE 22-13	Incidence of Facial Paresis as a Function of Type of Delivery		
Type of Delivery	Deliveries (n)	Paresis (n)	Facial Incidence
Natural	159	10	6.3%
Forceps*	716	46	6.4%

*Not further characterized regarding low, middle, high, and so forth.
Data from Hepner WR Jr: Some observations on facial paresis in the newborn infant: Etiology and incidence, *Pediatrics* 8:494-497, 1951.

TABLE 22-14	Relation of Side of Facial Paresis to Intrauterine Position		
Infants (n)	Type of Delivery	Side of Facial Paresis	Intrauterine Position
6	Natural	Left	Occiput left transverse
4	Natural	Right	Occiput right transverse
34	Forceps	Left	Occiput left transverse or anterior
12	Forceps	Right	Occiput right anterior, transverse, or posterior

Data from Hepner WR Jr: Some observations on facial paresis in the newborn infant: Etiology and incidence, *Pediatrics* 8:494-497, 1951.

pressure on the facial nerve by the sacral promontory (see Table 22-13; Table 22-14).[183] No difference in incidence of facial palsy was noted, whether forceps were used in the delivery or not, and more important, in each of the 56 cases of facial paralysis, a direct correlation existed between the side of face affected and the position of the head in utero. Thus, the 40 infants with left facial paresis were born from the occiput left transverse or left anterior obstetrical positions, and the 16 infants with right facial paresis were born from similar obstetrical positions on the right. The common denominator was the position of the face on the sacral promontory. Thus, compression of the nerve as the face is pressed against this bony protuberance appeared to cause the injury.

The pathogenetic formulation just described is not to deny cases in which compression by intrauterine position of head and neck (e.g., angle of jaw against the shoulder) or by forceps blade is the source of the pressure. Indeed, in a study of nearly 14,000 singleton live term infants at a major teaching hospital, those with facial nerve injury were delivered with forceps in 72% of cases (midforceps in 28%) versus 33% (midforceps in 4%) in the control group.[125] One study of 357 vertex deliveries by forceps extraction clearly showed a relationship of the incidence of facial palsy with the level of forceps delivery (Table 22-15).[11] Moreover, although more data are needed, I have the impression that the incidence of *marked* facial weakness is greater in difficult midforceps extractions than in low-forceps or outlet-forceps extractions or natural deliveries. Consistent with these findings, a more recent study of more than 4000 infants delivered by forceps or vacuum extraction showed a fourfold higher risk of facial nerve palsy in the forceps-delivered infants.[186] However, in a large retrospective series of children (*n* = 61) with *permanent* congenital facial nerve palsy who were evaluated by a plastic surgery service, the incidence of forceps-assisted delivery in the affected children was no different from controls.[187] Thus, it appears that *permanent* congenital facial nerve palsy, which is much rarer than the typical neonatal facial palsy emphasized in this section, is not

TABLE 22-15	Incidence of Facial Paresis as a Function of Level of Forceps Delivery

	LEVEL OF FORCEPS DELIVERY*		
	Outlet	Low	Middle
Number of infants	116	178	63
Percentage with facial palsy	0.8%	1.7%	9.5%

*The level of forceps delivery is based on the revised definition of level in which midforceps is the highest level (i.e., the term "high forceps" is not used).
Data from Hagadorn-Freathy AS, Yeomans ER, Hankins GD: Validation of the 1988 ACOG forceps classification system, *Obstet Gynecol* 77:356-360, 1991.

predominantly related to forceps-assisted delivery but rather primarily to intrauterine factors, including genetic factors.[188-190]

Clinical Features

Clinical Setting. The clinical setting often is not that of an overtly traumatic birth, although forceps deliveries are overrepresented (see "Pathogenesis"). The traumatic nature of the lesion is emphasized by the almost invariable relationship between the side of the facial weakness and the side of the face that was apposed in utero to the sacral promontory or encountered by a forceps blade. The forceps blade may leave a distinct mark on the face near the underlying stylomastoid foramen. Less commonly, the infant appears to exhibit evidence of an abnormal fetal posture (i.e., firm apposition of the angle of the jaw to the shoulder).

Clinical Syndrome. By far the most common syndrome of neonatal facial nerve palsy is related to involvement of the nerve after it exits the stylomastoid foramen; therefore, the typical features include weakness of both upper and lower facial muscles (Fig. 22-16). At rest, the palpebral fissure is wider on the affected side, the nasolabial fold is flattened, and the subtle nuances of facial expression are absent. With elicited movement, it is apparent that the infant is unable to wrinkle the brow, close the eye firmly, or move the corner of the mouth or lower face into an effective grimace. Moreover, liquid often dribbles from the corner of the mouth during feeding. Approximately 75% of cases involve the left side of the face, a finding perhaps reflecting the relative frequencies of intrauterine positions (see previous discussion).

Diagnosis

The differential diagnosis in the newborn with facial palsy is discussed in Chapter 3. Most infants with overt paralysis of *upper and lower* face (i.e., a "peripheral" lesion) have sustained the apparently traumatic injury discussed in this section. Peripheral facial nerve lesions at other sites (e.g., posterior fossa subdural or intracerebellar hemorrhage, lesions within the brain stem [e.g., hemorrhage, ischemia]), and central lesions (e.g., hypoxic-ischemic injury and cerebral contusions) are distinctly uncommon or have other

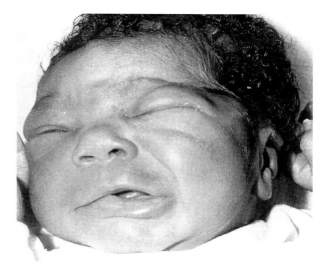

Figure 22-16 Right facial paralysis: clinical appearance. Note that lack of movement on the right leads to the appearance of the face being "pulled" to the left with cry. The right nasolabial fold is flattened. *(From Painter MJ, Bergman I: Obstetrical trauma to the neonatal central and peripheral nervous system, Semin Perinatol 6:89-104, 1982.)*

identifying neurological features. Disorders of muscle (myotonic dystrophy), myoneural junction (myasthenia gravis), and nucleus of facial nerve (Möbius syndrome), although potentially involving both upper and lower face, are usually bilateral and exhibit the ancillary features described in Chapters 18 and 19. The unilateral weakness of the depressor of the corner of the mouth (see Chapter 19) is a more restricted deficit and is readily distinguished from typical peripheral facial paralysis.

I generally do not use electrodiagnostic tests to evaluate these infants. However, in infants with marked involvement, such testing may be useful.[184,185,188] Thus, in typical traumatic facial nerve paresis, transdermal stimulation of the facial nerve at the stylomastoid foramen usually reveals normal facial nerve function in the first 48 hours of life, because the distal nerve is still capable of conduction. The percentage of decrease of this facial nerve function over time provides useful prognostic information.[188] The presence of fibrillations after 2 to 3 weeks indicates denervation of muscle fibers. However, these abnormalities do not necessarily preclude excellent functional recovery, and, thus, electrodiagnostic abnormalities must be interpreted with caution and in the context of personal experience.

Prognosis

The prognosis of affected infants is very good. Most infants recover completely within 1 to 3 weeks, and only rarely do infants have any detectable deficit after several months.[11,86,187,191] Regeneration of the nerve in the unusual case with severe degeneration takes place at the rate of "approximately 1 inch a month."[191] Unusual sequelae of facial paralysis include contracture and synkinesis (mass facial motion).[192]

Management

Therapy generally is restricted to the use of artificial tears and, if necessary, taping of the involved eye to prevent corneal injury. No controlled data indicate a value for massage, electrical stimulation, or early surgical intervention. Some investigators have advocated surgical exploration in patients with severe persistent findings of denervation; rarely, a petrous temporal fracture may compress the nerve.[184] I have not encountered this situation. Indeed, the lesion usually resolves before any therapy can be attempted.

Laryngeal Nerve Palsy

Disturbance of branches of the laryngeal nerve may affect swallowing and breathing, and this occurrence has led to the descriptive term *duosyndrome of the laryngeal nerve*.[193] The disorder appears to result in many cases from an intrauterine posture in which the head is rotated slightly and is flexed laterally. It also is likely that similar head and neck movements during delivery, when marked, may injure the laryngeal nerve and may account for the approximately 10% of examples of vocal cord paralysis attributed to "birth trauma" (see Chapter 19).[194,195] Similarly, such head and neck movements may occur during deliveries that result in brachial plexus injuries, because approximately 2% of the latter are accompanied by evidence of laryngeal nerve involvement (e.g., stridor).[138] The lateral neck flexion causes the rigid thyroid cartilage of the larynx to compress the superior branch of the laryngeal nerve against the hyoid bone above or the recurrent branch against the cricoid cartilage below. The result is disturbance of swallowing (because of involvement of the superior branch) or of vocal cord closure with resulting dyspnea (because of involvement of the recurrent branch). A similar syndrome may be observed as a result of either direct trauma during cannulation of neck vessels for extracorporeal membrane oxygenation or injury with intubation. The vocal cord paralysis is the dominant and most dangerous feature of the syndrome. Because the rotation of head causes the face to be compressed against the pelvic wall, contralateral facial paresis may be associated. Moreover, if the lateral flexion of neck is severe, the phrenic nerve may be affected, and diaphragmatic paresis may occur.[177,193] Similarly, the nearby hypoglossal nerve may be injured and may result in paralysis of tongue.[196,197] The diagnosis of the laryngeal involvement is best made by direct laryngoscopic examination.

Treatment is symptomatic. In patients with severe lesions, gavage feeding or tracheotomy may be required. Noisy breathing and the threat of aspiration may last a year or longer, although affected patients usually recover by 6 to 12 months of life.[193]

Median Nerve Injury

Injury to the median nerve has been described at two sites (i.e., the antecubital fossa and the wrist), both related to percutaneous arterial punctures, of the brachial artery and the radial artery, respectively (Table 22-16). The median nerve is derived from the brachial plexus, courses through the antecubital fossa into the forearm, where it supplies muscles that principally pronate the

TABLE 22-16	Arterial Puncture and Median Nerve Injury in the Neonatal Period
Site of Injury	**Artery Punctured**
Antecubital fossa	Brachial (usually right)
Wrist	Radial

forearm and flex the wrist and fingers, and then proceeds over the radial aspect of the wrist and through the carpal tunnel to the hand, where it supplies muscles that oppose, flex, and adduct the thumb.

Antecubital Fossa and Brachial Artery

Injury to the median nerve in the antecubital fossa was described in one study in 13% of low-birth-weight infants (≤1500 g) examined at 18 months after term.[198] Median nerve dysfunction was identified clinically on the basis of impaired pincer grasp, which depends on flexion of the index finger and adduction, opposition, and flexion of the thumb. A characteristic posture of the hand was observed in affected patients (Fig. 22-17). Evidence of injury was most frequent in the smallest infants; 30% of infants weighing less than 1000 g were affected versus 8% of infants weighing 1000 to 1500 g.

Two observations suggested that injury to the median nerve in the antecubital fossa was responsible for the clinical deficits. First, all affected infants had obviously visible scarring in the antecubital fossa related to frequent percutaneous brachial artery punctures. Because the right brachial artery is preferred for arterial puncture (to avoid contamination from ductal

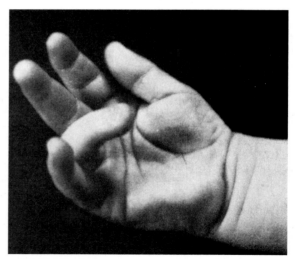

Figure 22-17 Median nerve injury: clinical appearance. The right hand of an infant, approximately 24 months of age, who weighed less than 1500 g at birth and who sustained median nerve injury secondary to brachial artery puncture in the neonatal period. Note the position of the hand, assumed because of weakness of flexion of the proximal phalanx of the first three fingers and the distal phalanx of the thumb and weakness of adduction and opposition of the thumb; all these functions are mediated by the median nerve. Note also the slight atrophy of the thenar eminence. *(From Pape KE, Armstrong DL, Fitzhardinge PM: Peripheral median nerve damage secondary to brachial arterial blood gas sampling,* J Pediatr 93:852-856, 1978.)

shunting), the right hand and antecubital fossa were affected in all 18 infants. In 5 of these infants, bilateral deficits were present, as were bilateral scarring and histories of left as well as right punctures. The second observation was derived from block sections of the cubital fossa at autopsy on 12 randomly selected low-birth-weight infants who had one or more percutaneous brachial artery punctures during life; perineural hemorrhage and axonal injury with wallerian degeneration were observed in 8 infants.

Further data are needed to define the frequency of the aforementioned deficits of the *dominant* hand in the low-birth-weight infant and, more importantly, the long-term functional consequences. The data suggest that percutaneous brachial artery puncture should be avoided, if possible, in the very small infant.

Wrist and Radial Artery

Radial artery puncture has been shown to cause injury to the median nerve in the newborn infant. Two infants exhibited prolonged median nerve conduction velocity and distal motor latency after radial artery punctures for determination of arterial blood gas values.[199] Postmortem examination in one infant demonstrated compression of the median nerve by hematoma. The other infant had a diminished grasp on the affected side, but electrical and clinical functions became normal after 4 weeks. This compressive neuropathy could go undetected in the neonatal period without careful clinical and electrical testing. These data again raise the question whether long-term effects on hand function occur in graduates of neonatal intensive care facilities as a result of median nerve injury.

Radial Nerve Injury

Injury to the radial nerve has been associated most often with apparent compression of the nerve, the latter caused in utero by restricted fetal position (e.g., secondary to passively acquired sedative drugs or constricting uterine bands), during difficult labor or delivery by forceps, or both, and postnatally by such factors as blood pressure cuffs.[62,86,200-208] An indurated area with underlying fat necrosis, usually over the distal course of the nerve around the humerus above the radial epicondyle, often marks the site of compression. Less common etiological factors are humeral fracture or subcutaneous abscess. The clinical features are distinctive and consist of weakness of the extensors of wrist, fingers, and thumb, the normal distal innervations of the radial nerve (Fig. 22-18). Thus, wrist drop calls attention to the injury. On cursory examination, the patient's deficits could be mistaken for a lower brachial plexus lesion, but the preservation of grasp and function of other intrinsic muscles of the hand rules out this diagnosis. EMG examination indicates fibrillations in the affected muscles after a still to be defined interval, although probably at least 1 week.[204] Of the approximately 21 reported patients with adequate follow-up data, all except 1 recovered in the first weeks or months of life. The sole exception had apparently long-standing intrauterine compression.

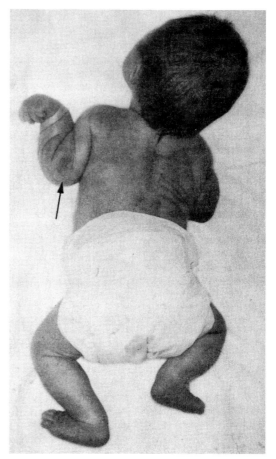

Figure 22-18 Radial nerve injury in a newborn: clinical features. Note the evidence of weakness of extensors of wrist and fingers, with the appearance of wrist drop. Because the lesion in this case was proximal to the triceps branch of the nerve, the limb is also held in flexion at the elbow. The *arrow* points to an area of subcutaneous fat necrosis overlying the radial nerve, an appearance consistent with local intrauterine pressure, perhaps secondary to the umbilical cord. *(From Ross D, Jones HR, Fisher J, Konkol RJ: Isolated radial nerve lesion in the newborn, Neurology 33:1354-1356, 1983.)*

Lumbosacral Plexus Injury

Injury to lumbosacral roots is exceedingly uncommon. In Eng's[191] series of "128 neonatal peripheral palsies," only 3 such cases were observed. The injury involves roots of both the lumbar plexus (L2 to L4) and the sacral plexus (L4 to S3) and is related to traction, primarily with frank breech deliveries. The clinical features essentially include total paralysis of the involved lower extremity. One infant with involvement principally of the lumbar component exhibited particular weakness of knee extension (quadriceps function) and an absent knee jerk.[209] Differentiation of lumbosacral plexus injury from sciatic nerve injury and occult dysraphic state with asymmetry is necessary (see "Sciatic Nerve Injury"). Sciatic nerve injury spares motor functions of the femoral and obturator nerves (L2 to L4), and, thus, hip flexion, adduction, and external rotation are present. Occult dysraphic states in most cases are associated with cutaneous, subcutaneous, and skeletal stigmata and are rarely, if ever, entirely confined to one limb. The outcome in an infant with lumbosacral plexus injury is difficult to generalize from the small numbers reported, but in Eng's[191] series, "none of the recoveries … was complete." In the single patient whom I have studied, although only minimal function was present at 2 months of age, rapid recovery commenced thereafter, and at 3 years of age, only minor disability remained.

Sciatic Nerve Injury

Sciatic nerve injury in the newborn has been observed principally after misplaced injection of drugs into the buttocks, but also after prolonged paralysis (induced by pancuronium) with pressure necrosis of the skin overlying the buttock,[205,206] as well as after injection of hypertonic glucose or certain other agents into the umbilical artery.[86,210-213] The mechanism of the effect in the latter instance is presumed to be spasm or thrombosis in the inferior gluteal artery that supplies the sciatic nerve. Traction injury with difficult breech deliveries may also lead to sciatic nerve injury.[214] The clinical features include deficits of abduction at the hip and of all movements at more distal joints. (Necrosis of buttock tissue may be an obvious accompaniment.) Distinction from lumbosacral plexus injury is based primarily on the sparing of hip flexion, adduction, and external rotation in sciatic nerve injury. Distinction from peroneal nerve injury (see next section) may be difficult because preferential involvement of the superficially and laterally placed fibers destined for the peroneal nerve often occurs, and foot drop may be the prominent neurological abnormality.

Prognosis is variable. Many infants have failed to recover after misplaced intramuscular injections, whereas the prognosis appears to be better from the small number of cases reported secondary to umbilical artery injections.

Peroneal Nerve Injury

Several reports of *injury to the peroneal nerve* of the newborn have been recorded.[214-220] The common pathogenetic factor has been compression, whether in utero by uterine bands or postnatally by footboard or infiltrated intravenous solution. The site of injury is the superficial course of the nerve around the fibular head. The clinical feature that calls attention to the lesion is *foot drop*, which is caused by weakness of ankle dorsiflexion and eversion, functions of the peroneal nerve. Determinations of nerve conduction velocities can establish the site of the injury.[216,218] The demonstration of fibrillations on the first day of life established the intrauterine timing of the injury in two cases.[219,220] The reported patients have recovered within 3 to 6 months.

REFERENCES

1. Baethmann M, Kahn T, Lenard HG, Voit T: Fetal CNS damage after exposure to maternal trauma during pregnancy, *Acta Paediatr* 85:1331-1338, 1996.
2. Hope P, Breslin S, Lamont L, Lucas A, et al: Fatal shoulder dystocia: A review of 56 cases reported to the Confidential Enquiry into Stillbirths and Deaths in Infancy, *Br J Obstet Gynaecol* 105:1256-1261, 1998.
3. Chenoy R, Johanson R: A randomized prospective study comparing delivery with metal and silicone rubber vacuum extractor cups, *Br J Obstet Gynaecol* 99:360-363, 1992.
4. Pape KE, Wigglesworth JS: *Haemorrhage, Ischaemia and the Perinatal Brain*, Philadelphia. JB: 1979, Lippincott.
5. Robinson RJ, Rossiter MA: Massive subaponeurotic hemorrhage in babies of African origin, *Arch Dis Child* 43:684-687, 1968.
6. Fortune PM, Thomas RM: Sub-aponeurotic haemorrhage: A rare but life-threatening neonatal complication associated with ventouse delivery, *Br J Obstet Gynaecol* 106:868-870, 1999.
7. Boo NY, Foong KW, Mahdy ZA, Yong SC, et al: Risk factors associated with subaponeurotic haemorrhage in full-term infants exposed to vacuum extraction, *Br J Obstet Gynaecol* 112:1516-1521, 2005.
8. Govaert P, Vanhaesebrouck P, Depraeter C, Moens K, et al: Vacuum extraction, bone injury and neonatal subgaleal bleeding, *Eur J Pediatr* 151:532-535, 1992.
9. Ng PC, Siu YK, Lewindon PJ: Subaponeurotic haemorrhage in the 1990s: A 3-year surveillance, *Acta Paediatr* 84:1065-1069, 1995.
10. Churchill JA, Stevenson L, Habhab G: Cephalhematoma and natal brain injury, *Obstet Gynecol* 27:580-584, 1966.
11. Hagadorn-Freathy AS, Yeomans ER, Hankins GD: Validation of the 1988 ACOG forceps classification system, *Obstet Gynecol* 77:356-360, 1991.
12. Hankins GD, Leicht T, Van Hook J, Uckan EM: The role of forceps rotation in maternal and neonatal injury, *Am J Obstet Gynecol* 180:231-234, 1999.
12a. Simonson C, Barlow P, Dehennin N, Sphel M, et al: Neonatal complications of vacuum-assisted delivery, *Obstet Gynecol* 109:626-633, 2007.
13. Levene MI, Williams JL, Fawer CL: *Ultrasound of the Infant Brain*, London: 1985, Blackwell Scientific.
14. Kendall N, Woloshin H: Cephalhematoma associated with fracture of the skull, *J Pediatr* 41:125-132, 1952.
15. Gresham EL: Birth trauma, *Pediatr Clin North Am* 22:317-328, 1975.
16. Hartley JB, Burnett CW: An inquiry into the causation and characteristics of cephalohematoma, *Br J Radiol* 17:33, 1944.
17. Leonard S, Anthony B: Giant cephalhematoma of newborn, *Am J Dis Child* 101:170-173, 1961.
18. Rausen AR, Diamond LK: Enclosed hemorrhage and neonatal jaundice, *Am J Dis Child* 101:164-169, 1961.
19. Ellis SS, Montgomery JR, Wagner M, Hill RM: Osteomyelitis complicating neonatal cephalhematoma, *Am J Dis Child* 127:100-102, 1974.
20. Mohon RT, Mehalic TF, Grimes CK, Philip AG: Infected cephalhematoma and neonatal osteomyelitis of the skull, *Pediatr Infect Dis* 5:253-256, 1986.
21. Djientcheu VD, Rilliet B, Delavelle J, Argyropoulo M, et al: Leptomeningeal cyst in newborns due to vacuum extraction: Report of two cases, *Childs Nerv Sys* 12:399-403, 1996.
22. Harwood-Nash DC, Hendrick EB, Hudson AR: The significance of skull fracture in children: A study of 1,187 patients, *Radiology* 101:151-156, 1971.
23. Dupuis O, Silveira R, Dupont C, Mottolese C, et al: Comparison of "instrument-associated" and "spontaneous" obstetric depressed skull fractures in a cohort of 68 neonates, *Am J Obstet Gynecol* 192:165-170, 2005.
24. Nakahara T, Sakoda K, Uozumi T, Takeda T, et al: Intrauterine depressed skull fracture, *Pediatr Neurosci* 15:121-124, 1989.
25. Matson D: *Neurosurgery of Infancy and Childhood*, Springfield, IL: 1969, Charles C. Thomas.
26. Natelson SE, Sayers MP: The fate of children sustaining severe head trauma during birth, *Pediatrics* 51:169-174, 1973.
27. Loeser JD, Kilburn HL, Jolley T: Management of depressed skull fracture in the newborn, *J Neurosurg* 44:62-64, 1976.
28. Steinbok P: Intrauterine depressed skull fracture, *Pediatr Neurosci* 15:317, 1989.
29. Raynor R, Parsa M: Nonsurgical elevation of depressed skull fracture in an infant, *J Pediatr* 72:262-264, 1968.
30. Schrager GO: Elevation of depressed skull fracture with a breast pump, *J Pediatr* 77:300-301, 1970.
31. Tan KL: Elevation of congenital depressed fractures of the skull by the vacuum extractor, *Acta Paediatr Scand* 63:562-564, 1974.
32. Saunders BS, Lazoritz S, McArtor RD, Marshall P: Depressed skull fracture in the neonate: Report of three cases, *J Neurosurg* 50:512-514, 1979.
33. Roche MC, Velez A, Garcia Sanchez P: Occipital osteodiastasis: A rare complication in cephalic delivery, *Acta Paediatr Scand* 79:380-382, 1990.
34. Takagi T, Nagai R, Wakabayashi S, Mizawa I, et al: Extradural hemorrhage in the newborn as a result of birth trauma, *Childs Brain* 4:306-318, 1978.
35. Gama CH, Fenichel GM: Epidural hematoma of the newborn due to birth trauma, *Pediatr Neurol* 1:52-53, 1985.
36. Negishi H, Lee Y, Itoh K, Suzuki J, et al: Nonsurgical management of epidural hematoma in neonates, *Pediatr Neurol* 5:253-256, 1989.
37. Lindenberg R, Freytag E: Morphology of brain lesions from blunt trauma in early infancy, *Arch Pathol* 87:298-305, 1969.

38. Ikonomidou C, Qin Q, Labruyere J, Kirby C, et al: Prevention of trauma-induced neurodegeneration in infant rat brain, *Pediatr Res* 39:1020-1027, 1996.
39. Aziz EM, Robertson AF: Paraplegia: A complication of umbilical artery catheterization, *J Pediatr* 82:1051-1052, 1973.
40. Krishnamoorthy KS, Fernandex RJ, Todres ID, DeLong GR: Paraplegia associated with umbilical artery catheterization in the newborn, *Pediatrics* 58:443-445, 1976.
41. Willis J, Duncan C, Gottschalk S: Paraplegia due to peripheral venous air embolus in a neonate: A case report, *Pediatrics* 67:472-473, 1981.
42. Munoz ME, Roche C, Escriba R, Martinez-Bermejo A, et al: Flaccid paraplegia as complication of umbilical artery catheterization, *Pediatr Neurol* 9:401-403, 1993.
43. Pierson RN: Spinal and cranial injuries of the baby in breech deliveries: A clinical and pathological study of thirty-eight cases, *Surg Gynecol Obstet* 37:802, 1923.
44. Towbin A: Spinal cord and brain stem injury at birth, *Arch Pathol* 77:620-632, 1964.
45. Towbin A: Latent spinal cord and brain stem injury in newborn infants, *Dev Med Child Neurol* 11:54-68, 1969.
46. Friede RL: *Developmental Neuropathology*, 2nd ed, New York: 1989, Springer-Verlag.
47. Byers RK: Transection of the spinal cord in the newborn: Case with autopsy and comparison with normal cord at the same age, *Arch Neurol Psychiatry* 27:585-594, 1932.
48. Rossitch E, Oakes WJ: Perinatal spinal cord injury: Clinical, radiographic and pathologic features, *Pediatr Neurosurg* 18:149-152, 1992.
49. MacKinnon JA, Perlman M, Kirpalani H, Rehan V, et al: Spinal cord injury at birth: Diagnostic and prognostic data in twenty-two patients, *J Pediatr* 122:431-437, 1993.
50. Caird MS, Reddy S, Ganley TJ, Drummond DS: Cervical spine fracture-dislocation birth injury: Prevention, recognition, and implications for the orthopaedic surgeon, *J Pediatr Orthop* 25:484-486, 2005.
50a. Vialle R, Pietin-Vialle C, Ilharreborde B, Dauger S, et al: Spinal cord injuries at birth: A multicenter review of nine cases, *J Matern Fetal Neonatal Med* 20:435-440, 2007.
51. Byers RK: Spinal-cord injuries during birth, *Dev Med Child Neurol* 17:103-110, 1975.
52. Shulman ST, Madden JD, Esterly JR, Shanklin DR: Transection of spinal cord: A rare obstetrical complication of cephalic delivery, *Arch Dis Child* 46:291-294, 1971.
53. Norman MC, Wedderburn LC: Fetal spinal cord injury with cephalic delivery, *Obstet Gynecol* 42:355-358, 1973.
54. Gould SJ, Smith JF: Spinal cord transection, cerebral ischaemic and brain stem injury in a brain following a Kjelland's forceps rotation, *Neuropathol Appl Neurobiol* 10:151-158, 1984.
55. Menticoglou SM, Perlman M, Manning FA: High cervical spinal cord injury in neonates delivered with forceps: Report of 15 cases, *Obstet Gynecol* 86:589-594, 1995.
56. Mills JF, Dargaville PA, Coleman LT, Rosenfeld JV, et al: Upper cervical spinal cord injury in neonates: The use of magnetic resonance imaging, *J Pediatr* 138:105-108, 2001.
57. Couvelaire A: Hemorrhagies du système nerveux central des nouveau-nés, *Ann Gynecol Obstet* 59:253, 1903.
58. Jellinger K, Schwingshackl A: Birth injury of the spinal cord: Report of two necropsy cases with several weeks survival, *Neuropaediatrie* 4:111-123, 1973.
59. Yamano T, Fujiwara S, Matsukawa S, Aotani H, et al: Cervical cord birth injury and subsequent development of syringomyelia: A case report, *Neuropediatrics* 23:327-328, 1992.
60. Crothers B: The effect of breech extraction on the central nervous system of the fetus, *Med Clin North Am* 5:1287, 1922.
61. Crothers B: Injury of the spinal cord in breech extraction as an important cause of fetal death and paraplegia in childhood, *Am J Med Sci* 165:94, 1923.
62. Ford FR: *Diseases of the Nervous System in Infancy, Childhood, and Adolescence*, Springfield, IL: 1960, Charles C Thomas.
63. Tator CH, Fehlings MG: Review of the secondary injury theory of acute spinal cord trauma with emphasis on vascular mechanisms, *J Neurosurg* 75:15-26, 1991.
64. Walker MD: Acute spinal-cord injury, *N Engl J Med* 324:1885-1887, 1991.
65. Geisler FH, Dorsey FC, Coleman WP: Recovery of motor function after spinal-cord injury: A randomized, placebo-controlled trial with GM-1 ganglioside, *N Engl J Med* 324:1829-1838, 1991.
66. Bracken MD, Shepard MJ, Collins WF, Holford TR, et al: A randomized, controlled trial of methylprednisolone or naloxone in the treatment of acute spinal-cord injury, *N Engl J Med* 322:1405-1411, 1990.
67. Bracken MD, Shepard MJ, Collins WF, Holford TR, et al: Methylprednisolone or naloxone treatment after acute spinal cord injury: 1-year follow-up data, *J Neurosurg* 76:23-31, 1992.
68. Holtz A, Gerdin B: MK 801, an N-methyl-D-aspartate channel blocker, does not improve the functional recovery nor spinal cord blood flow after spinal cord compression in rats, *Acta Neurol Scand* 84:334-338, 1991.
69. Demediuk P, Daly MP, Faden AI: Effect of impact trauma on neurotransmitter and nonneurotransmitter amino acids in rat spinal cord, *J Neurochem* 52:1529-1536, 1989.
70. Faden AI, Simon RP: A potential role for excitotoxins in the pathophysiology of spinal cord injury, *Ann Neurol* 23:623-626, 1988.
71. Faden AI, Lemke M, Simon RP, Noble LJ: N-Methyl-D-aspartate antagonist MK801 improves outcome following traumatic spinal cord injury in rats: Behavioral, anatomic, and neurochemical studies, *J Neurotrauma* 5:33-45, 1988.
72. Bracken MB, Shepard MJ, Holford TR, Leo-Summers L, et al: Administration of methylprednisolone for 24 or 48 hours or tirilazad mesylate for 48 hours in the treatment of acute spinal cord injury, *JAMA* 277:1597-1604, 1997.
73. Stern WE, Rand RW: Birth injuries to the spinal cord: A report of 2 cases and review of the literature, *Am J Obstet Gynecol* 78:498-512, 1959.
74. Adams C, Babyn PS, Login WJ: Spinal cord birth injury: Value of computed tomographic myelography, *Pediatr Neurol* 4:105-109, 1988.
75. Babyn PS, Chuang SH, Daneman A, Davidson GS: Sonographic evaluation of spinal cord birth trauma with pathologic correlation, *AJR Am J Roentgenol* 9:765-768, 1988.
76. Lanska MJ, Roessman U, Wiznitzer M: Magnetic resonance imaging in cervical cord birth injury, *Pediatrics* 85:760-764, 1990.
77. Rehan VK, Seshia MM: Spinal cord birth injury: Diagnostic difficulties, *Arch Dis Child* 69:92-94, 1993.
78. De Souza SW, Davis JA: Spinal cord damage in the newborn infant, *Arch Dis Child* 49:70-71, 1974.
79. Allen JP, Meyers GG, Condon VR: Laceration of the spinal cord related to breech delivery, *JAMA* 208:1019-1022, 1969.
80. Leventhal HR: Birth injuries of the spinal cord, *J Pediatr* 56:447-453, 1960.
81. Blount J, Doughty K, Tubbs RS, Wellons JC, et al: In utero spontaneous cervical thoracic epidural hematoma imitating spinal cord birth injury, *Pediatr Neurosurg* 40:23-27, 2004.
82. Roig M, Ballesca M, Navarro C, Ortega A, et al: Congenital spinal cord haemangioblastoma: Another cause of spinal cord section syndrome in the newborn, *J Neurol Neurosurg Psychiatry* 51:1091-1093, 1988.
83. Morgan C, Newell SJ: Cervical spinal cord injury following cephalic presentation and delivery by caesarean section, *Dev Med Child Neurol* 43:274-276, 2001.
84. Hedderly T, Chalmers S, Fox G, Hughes E: Extensive cervical spinal cord lesion with late foetal presentation, *Acta Paediatr* 94:245-247, 2005.
85. Ebinger F, Boor R, Bruhl K, Reitter B: Cervical spinal cord atrophy in the atraumatically born neonate: One form of prenatal or perinatal ischaemic insult?, *Neuropediatrics* 34:45-51, 2003.
86. Schaffer AJ, Avery ME: *Diseases of the Newborn*, Philadelphia: 1971, Saunders.
87. Simanovsky N, Stepensky P, Hiller N: The use of ultrasound for the diagnosis of spinal hemorrhage in a newborn, *Pediatr Neurol* 31:295-297, 2004.
88. Barkovich AJ: *Pediatric Neuroimaging*, 4th ed, Philadelphia: 2005, Lippincott Williams & Wilkins.
89. Dimario FJ, Wood BP: Radiological case of the month: Transsection of the spinal cord associated with breech delivery, *Am J Dis Child* 146:351-352, 1992.
90. Minami T, Keiko I, Kukita J, Koyanagi T, et al: A case of neonatal spinal cord injury: Magnetic resonance imaging and somatosensory evoked potentials, *Brain Dev* 16:57-60, 1994.
91. Murphy BP, Zientara GP, Huppi PS, Maier SE, et al: Line scan diffusion tensor MRI of the cervical spinal cord in preterm infants, *J Magn Reson Imaging* 13:949-953, 2001.
92. Lazar MR, Salvaggio AT: Hyperextension of the fetal head in breech presentation, *Obstet Gynecol* 14:198-199, 1959.
93. Hellstrom B, Sallmander U: Prevention of spinal cord injury in hyperextension of the fetal head, *JAMA* 204:1041-1044, 1968.
94. Bhagwanani SG, Price HV, Laurence KM, Ginz B: Risks and prevention of cervical cord injury in the management of breech presentation with hyperextension of the fetal head, *Am J Obstet Gynecol* 115:1159-1161, 1973.
95. Bresnan MJ, Abroms IF: Neonatal spinal cord transection secondary to intrauterine hyperextension of the neck in breech presentation, *J Pediatr* 84:734-737, 1974.
96. Daw E: Hyperextension of the head in breech presentation, *Am J Obstet Gynecol* 119:564-565, 1974.
97. Caterini H, Langer A, Sama JC, Devanesan M, et al: Fetal risk in hyperextension of the fetal head in breech presentation, *Am J Obstet Gynecol* 123:632-636, 1975.
98. Wilcox HL: The attitude of the fetus in breech presentation, *Am J Obstet Gynecol* 58:478, 1949.
99. Westgren M, Grundsell H, Ingemarsson I, Muhlow A, et al: Hyperextension of the fetal head in breech presentation: A study with long-term follow-up, *Br J Obstet Gynecol* 88:101-104, 1981.
100. Maekawa K, Masaki T, Kokubun Y: Fetal spinal-cord injury secondary to hyperextension of the neck: No effect of cesarean section, *Dev Med Child Neurol* 18:229-232, 1976.
101. Cattamanchi GR, Tamaskar V, Egel RT, Singh RS, et al: Intrauterine quadriplegia associated with breech presentation and hyperextension of fetal head: A case report, *Am J Obstet Gynecol* 140:831-833, 1981.

102. Weinstein D, Margalioth EJ, Navot D, Mor-Yosef S, et al: Neonatal fetal death following cesarean section secondary to hyperextended head in breech presentation, *Acta Obstet Gynecol Scand* 62:629-631, 1983.

103. Young RS, Towfighi J, Marks KH: Focal necrosis of the spinal cord in utero, *Arch Neurol* 40:654-655, 1983.

104. Kobayashi S, Kanda K, Yokochi K, Ohki S: A case of spinal cord injury that occurred in utero, *Pediatr Neurol* 35:367-369, 2006.

105. Gilles FH, Bina M, Sotrel A: Infantile atlanto-occipital instability: The potential danger of extreme extension, *Am J Dis Child* 133:30-37, 1979.

106. Gilgoff RL, Gilgoff IS: Long-term follow-up of home mechanical ventilation in young children with spinal cord injury and neuromuscular conditions, *J Pediatr* 142:476-480, 2003.

107. Crothers B, Putnam MC: Obstetrical injuries of the spinal cord, *Medicine (Baltimore)* 6:41, 1927.

108. Rubin A: Birth injuries: Incidence, mechanisms and end results, *Obstet Gynecol* 23:218-221, 1964.

109. Adler JB, Patterson RL: Erb's palsy: Long-term results of treatment in eighty-eight cases, *J Bone Joint Surg Am* 49:1052-1064, 1967.

110. Gordon M, Rich H, Deutschberger J, Green M: The immediate and long-term outcome of obstetric birth trauma. I. Brachial plexus paralysis, *Am J Obstet Gynecol* 117:51-56, 1973.

111. Specht EE: Brachial plexus palsy in the newborn: Incidence and prognosis, *Clin Orthop Relat Res* 110:32-34, 1975.

112. Molnar GE: Brachial plexus injury in the newborn infant, *Pediatr Rev* 6:110-115, 1984.

113. Al-Rajeh S, Corea JR, Al-Sibai MH, Al-Umran K, et al: Congenital brachial palsy in the eastern province of Saudi Arabia, *J Child Neurol* 5:35-38, 1990.

114. McFarland LV, Raskin M, Daling JR, Benedetti TJ: Erb/Duchenne's palsy: A consequence of fetal macrosomia and method of delivery, *Obstet Gynecol* 68:784-788, 1986.

115. Nocon JJ, McKenzie DK, Thomas LJ, Hansell RS: Shoulder dystocia: An analysis of risks and obstetric maneuvers, *Am J Obstet Gynecol* 168:1732-1739, 1993.

116. Laurent JP, Lee RT: Birth-related upper brachial plexus injuries in infants: Operative and nonoperative approaches, *J Child Neurol* 9:111-117, 1994.

117. Bager B: Perinatally acquired brachial plexus palsy: A persisting challenge, *Acta Paediatr* 86:1214-1219, 1997.

118. Gherman RB, Ouzounian JG, Goodwin TM: Brachial plexus palsy: An in utero injury?, *Am J Obstet Gynecol* 180:1303-1307, 1999.

119. Donnelly V, Foran A, Murphy J, McParland P, et al: Neonatal brachial plexus palsy: An unpredictable injury, *Am J Obstet Gynecol* 187:1209-1212, 2002.

120. Evans-Jones G, Kay SP, Weindling AM, Cranny G, et al: Congenital brachial palsy: Incidence, causes, and outcome in the United Kingdom and Republic of Ireland, *Arch Dis Child* 88:185-189, 2003.

121. Pondaag W, Malessy MJ, van Dijk JG, Thomeer RT: Natural history of obstetric brachial plexus palsy: A systematic review, *Dev Med Child Neurol* 46:138-144, 2004.

122. Mollberg M, Hagberg H, Bager B, Lilja H, et al: Risk factors for obstetric brachial plexus palsy among neonates delivered by vacuum extraction, *Obstet Gynecol* 106:913-918, 2005.

123. Piatt JH: Birth injuries of the brachial plexus, *Pediatr Clin North Am* 51:421-440, 2004.

124. Chauhan SP, Rose CH, Gherman RB, Magann EF, et al: Brachial plexus injury: A 23-year experience from a tertiary center, *Am J Obstet Gynecol* 192:1795-1802, 2005.

125. Levine MG, Holroyde J, Woods JR, Siddiqi TA, et al: Birth trauma: Incidence and predisposing factors, *Obstet Gynecol* 63:792-795, 1984.

126. Kline DG, Judice DJ: Operative management of selected brachial plexus lesions, *J Neurosurg* 58:631-649, 1983.

127. Laurent JP, Shenaq S, Lee R, Parke J, et al: Upper brachial plexus birth injuries: A neurosurgical approach, *Concepts Pediatr Neurosurg* 10:156-178, 1990.

128. Vredeveld JW, Blaauw G, Slooff BA, Richards R, et al: The findings in paediatric obstetric brachial palsy differ from those in older patients: A suggested explanation, *Dev Med Child Neurol* 42:158-161, 2000.

129. Kwast O: Electrophysiological assessment of maturation of regenerating motor nerve fibres in infants with brachial plexus palsy, *Dev Med Child Neurol* 31:56-65, 1989.

130. Gherman RB, Goodwin TM, Ouzounian JG, Miller DA, et al: Brachial plexus palsy associated with cesarean section: An in utero injury?, *Am J Obstet Gynecol* 177:1162-1164, 1997.

131. Alfonso I, Papazian O, Shuhaiber H, Yaylali I, et al: Intrauterine shoulder weakness and obstetric brachial plexus palsy, *Pediatr Neurol* 31:225-227, 2004.

132. Alfonso I, Diaz-Arca G, Alfonso DT, Shuhaiber HH, et al: Fetal deformations: A risk factor for obstetrical brachial plexus palsy?, *Pediatr Neurol* 35:246-249, 2006.

133. Eng GD: Brachial plexus palsy in newborn infants, *Pediatrics* 48:18-28, 1971.

134. Ubachs JMH, Slooff ACJ, Peters LLH: Obstetric antecedents of surgically treated obstetric brachial plexus injuries, *Br J Obstet Gynaecol* 102:813-817, 1995.

135. Gherman RB, Ouzounian JG, Satin AJ, Goodwin TM, et al: A comparison of shoulder dystocia-associated transient and permanent brachial plexus palsies, *Obstet Gynecol* 102:544-548, 2003.

135a. Weizsaecker K, Deaver JE, Cohen WR: Labour characteristics and neonatal Erb's palsy, *BJOG* 114:1003-1009, 2007.

136. Jennett RJ, Tarby TJ, Kreinick CJ: Brachial plexus palsy: An old problem revisited, *Am J Obstet Gynecol* 166:1673-1677, 1992.

137. Poggi SH, Stallings SP, Ghidini A, Spong CY, et al: Intrapartum risk factors for permanent brachial plexus injury, *Am J Obstet Gynecol* 189:725-729, 2003.

138. Eng GD, Binder H, Getson P, O'Donnell R: Obstetrical brachial plexus palsy (OBPP) outcome with conservative management, *Muscle Nerve* 19:884-891, 1996.

139. Yilmaz K, Caliskan M, Oge E, Aydmli N, et al: Clinical assessment, MRI, and EMG in congenital brachial plexus palsy, *Pediatr Neurol* 21:705-710, 1999.

140. Jones K, North K: Congenital muscular dystrophies. In Jones HR Jr, DeVivo DC, Darras BT, editors: *Neuromuscular Disorders of Infancy, Childhood, and Adolescence: A Clinician's Approach*, Philadelphia: 2003, Butterworth Heinemann.

141. Scarfone H, McComas AJ, Pape K, Newberry R: Denervation and reinnervation in congenital brachial palsy, *Muscle Nerve* 22:600-607, 1999.

142. Paradiso G, Granana N, Maza E: Prenatal brachial plexus paralysis, *Neurology* 49:261-262, 1997.

143. Francel PC, Koby M, Park TS, Lee B, et al: Fast spin-echo magnetic resonance imaging for radiological assessment of neonatal brachial plexus injury, *J Neurosurg* 83:461-466, 1995.

144. Miller SF, Glasier CM, Griebel ML, Boop FA: Brachial plexopathy in infants after traumatic delivery: Evaluation with MR imaging, *Radiology* 189:481-484, 1993.

145. Sundholm LK, Eliasson AC, Forssberg H: Obstetric brachial plexus injuries: Assessment protocol and functional outcome at age 5 years, *Dev Med Child Neurol* 40:4-11, 1998.

146. Strombeck C, Krumlinde-Sundholm L, Forssberg H: Functional outcome at 5 years in children with obstetrical brachial plexus palsy with and without microsurgical reconstruction, *Dev Med Child Neurol* 42:148-157, 2000.

147. Noetzel MJ, Park TS, Robinson S, Kaufman B: Prospective study of recovery following neonatal brachial plexus injury, *J Child Neurol* 16:488-492, 2001.

148. DiTaranto P, Campagna L, Price AE, Grossman JAI: Outcome following nonoperative treatment of brachial plexus birth injuries, *J Child Neurol* 19:87-90, 2004.

149. Hoeksma AF, ter Steeg AM, Nelissen RG, van Ouwerkerk WJ, et al: Neurological recovery in obstetric brachial plexus injuries: An historical cohort study, *Dev Med Child Neurol* 46:76-83, 2004.

150. Smith NC, Rowan P, Benson LJ, Ezaki M, et al: Neonatal brachial plexus palsy: Outcome of absent biceps function at three months of age, *J Bone Joint Surg Am* 86:2163-2170, 2004.

151. Grossman JA: Early operative intervention for selected cases of brachial plexus birth injury, *Arch Neurol* 63:1031-1032, 2006.

151a. Strombeck C, Krumlinde-Sundholm L, Remahl S, Sejersen T: Long-term follow-up of children with obstetric brachial plexus palsy. I: Functional aspects, *Dev Med Child Neurol* 49:198-203, 2007.

151b. Strombeck C, Remahl S, Krumlinde-Sundholm L, Sejersen T: Long-term follow-up of children with obstetric brachial plexus palsy. II: Neurophysiological aspects, *Dev Med Child Neurol* 49:204-209, 2007.

152. Bennett GC, Harrold AJ: Prognosis and early management of birth injuries to the brachial plexus, *Br Med J* 1:1520-1527, 1970.

153. Zalis OS, Zalis AW, Barron KD, Oester YT: Motor patterning following transitory sensory and motor deprivation, *Arch Neurol* 13:487-494, 1965.

154. Hunt D: Surgical management of brachial plexus birth injuries, *Dev Med Child Neurol* 30:821-828, 1988.

155. Gilbert A, Tassin JL: Surgical repair of the brachial plexus in obstetric paralysis, *Chirurgie* 110:70-75, 1984.

156. Roach ES: Surgery for brachial plexus palsy: Does timing matter?, *Arch Neurol* 63:1034-1035, 2006.

157. Sparagana SP, Ezaki M: Microneurosurgery for neonatal brachial plexus palsy: The need for more information, *Arch Neurol* 63:1033-1034, 2006.

158. Dyson JE: Paralysis of right diaphragm in newborn due to phrenic nerve injury, *JAMA* 88:94-97, 1927.

159. Tyson R, Bowman J: Paralysis of the diaphragm in the newborn, *Am J Dis Child* 46:30, 1933.

160. Blattner R: Unilateral paralysis of the diaphragm without involvement of the brachial plexus, *J Pediatr* 20:223, 1942.

161. Bingham JA: Two cases of unilateral paralysis of the diaphragm in the newborn treated surgically, *Thorax* 9:248-252, 1954.

162. France NE: Unilateral diaphragmatic paralysis and Erb's palsy in the newborn, *Arch Dis Child* 29:357-359, 1954.

163. Adams FH, Gyepes MT: Diaphragmatic paralysis in the newborn infant simulating cyanotic heart disease, *J Pediatr* 78:119-121, 1971.

164. Harris GB: Unilateral paralysis of the diaphragm in the newborn, *Postgrad Med* 50:51-54, 1971.

165. Sethi G, Reed WA: Diaphragmatic malfunction in neonates and infants: Diagnosis and treatment, *J Thorac Cardiovasc Surg* 62:138-143, 1971.

166. Smith BT: Isolated phrenic nerve palsy in the newborn, *Pediatrics* 49:449-451, 1972.
167. Anagnostakis D, Economou-Mavrou E, Moschos A, Vlachos P, et al: Diaphragmatic paralysis in the newborn, *Arch Dis Child* 48:977-979, 1973.
168. Greene W, L'Heureux P, Hunt CE: Paralysis of the diaphragm, *Am J Dis Child* 129:1402-1405, 1975.
169. Yasuda R, Nishioka T, Fukumasu H, Yokota Y: Bilateral phrenic nerve palsy in the newborn infant, *J Pediatr* 89:986-987, 1976.
170. Painter MJ, Bergman I: Obstetrical trauma to the neonatal central and peripheral nervous system, *Semin Perinatol* 6:89-104, 1982.
171. Zifko U, Hartmann M, Girsch W, Zoder G, et al: Diaphragmatic paresis in newborns due to phrenic nerve injury, *Neuropediatrics* 26:281-284, 1995.
172. Epelman M, Navarro OM, Daneman A, Miller SF: M-mode sonography of diaphragmatic motion: Description of technique and experience in 278 pediatric patients, *Pediatr Radiol* 35:661-667, 2005.
173. Williams O, Greenough A, Mustfa N, Haugen S, et al: Extubation failure due to phrenic nerve injury, *Arch Dis Child Fetal Neonatal Ed* 88:F72-F73, 2003.
174. Alvord EC, Austin EJ, Larson CP: Neuropathologic observations in congenital phrenic nerve palsy, *J Child Neurol* 5:205-209, 1990.
175. Aldrich TK, Herman JH, Rochester DF: Bilateral diaphragmatic paralysis in the newborn infant, *J Pediatr* 97:988-991, 1980.
176. Rubaltelli FF, Orzali A, Audino G, Laverda AM: Bilateral diaphragmatic paralysis, *J Pediatr* 99:667-668, 1981.
177. Schifrin N: Unilateral paralysis of the diaphragm in the newborn infant due to phrenic nerve injury, with and without associated brachial palsy, *Pediatrics* 9:69-76, 1952.
178. Ambler R, Gruenewald S, John E: Ultrasound monitoring of diaphragm activity in bilateral diaphragmatic paralysis, *Arch Dis Child* 60:170-172, 1985.
179. Bucci G, Marzetti G, Picece-Bucci S, Nodari S, et al: Phrenic nerve palsy treated by continuous positive pressure breathing by nasal canula, *Arch Dis Child* 49:230-232, 1974.
180. Muller NL, Bryan AC: Chest wall mechanics and respiratory muscles in infants, *Pediatr Clin North Am* 26:503-516, 1979.
181. Brouillette RT, Ilbawi MN, Hunt CE: Phrenic nerve pacing in infants and children: A review of experience and report on the usefulness of phrenic nerve stimulation studies, *J Pediatr* 102:32-39, 1983.
182. Wright FS, Ashwal S: *Phrenic Nerve Studies in Diaphragmatic Paralysis*, Charlottesville, VA: 1977, Child Neurology Society.
183. Hepner WR Jr: Some observations on facial paresis in the newborn infant: Etiology and incidence, *Pediatrics* 8:494-497, 1951.
184. Renault F, Quijano-Roy S: Congenital and acquired facial palsies. In Jones HR Jr, DeVivo DC, Darras BT, editors: *Neuromuscular Disorders of Infancy, Childhood, and Adolescence: A Clinician's Approach*, Philadelphia: 2003, Butterworth Heinemann.
185. Renault F: Facial electromyography in newborn and young infants with congenital facial weakness, *Dev Med Child Neurol* 43:421-427, 2001.
186. Caughey AB, Sandberg PL, Zlatnik MG, Thiet MP, et al: Forceps compared with vacuum: Rates of neonatal and maternal morbidity, *Obstet Gynecol* 106:908-912, 2005.
187. Hamish M, Laing E, Harrison DH, Jones BM, et al: Is permanent congenital facial palsy caused by birth trauma?, *Arch Dis Child* 74:56-58, 1996.
188. Shapiro NL, Cunningham MJ, Parikh SR, Eavey RD, et al: Congenital unilateral facial paralysis, *Pediatrics* 97:261-264, 1996.
189. Kondev L, Bhadelia RA, Douglass LM: Familial congenital facial palsy, *Pediatr Neurol* 30:367-370, 2004.
190. Toelle SP, Boltshauser E: Long-term outcome in children with congenital unilateral facial nerve palsy, *Neuropediatrics* 32:130-135, 2001.
191. Eng GD: *Neonatology*, Philadelphia: 1981, JB Lippincott.
192. Manning J, Adour K: Facial paralysis in children, *Pediatrics* 1:102-109, 1972.
193. Chapple CC: A duosyndrome of the laryngeal nerve, *Am J Dis Child* 91:14-18, 1956.
194. Holinger LD, Holinger PC, Holinger PH: Etiology of bilateral abductor vocal cord paralysis: A review of 389 cases, *Ann Otol* 85:428-436, 1976.
195. Cohen SR, Birns JW, Geller KA, Thompson JW: Laryngeal paralysis in children: A long-term retrospective study, *Ann Otol Rhinol Laryngol* 91:417-424, 1982.
196. Haenggeli CA, Lacourt G: Brachial plexus injury and hypoglossal paralysis, *Pediatr Neurol* 5:197-198, 1989.
197. Greenberg SJ, Kandt RS, D'Souza BJ: Birth injury-induced glossolaryngeal paresis, *Neurology* 37:533-535, 1987.
198. Pape KE, Armstrong DL, Fitzhardinge PM: Peripheral median nerve damage secondary to brachial arterial blood gas sampling, *J Pediatr* 93:852-856, 1978.
199. Koenigsberger MR, Moessinger AC: Iatrogenic carpal tunnel syndrome in the newborn infant, *J Pediatr* 91:443-445, 1977.
200. Lightwood R: Radial nerve palsy associated with localized subcutaneous fat necrosis in the newborn, *Arch Dis Child* 26:436-437, 1951.
201. Feldman GV: Radial nerve palsies in the newborn, *Arch Dis Child* 32:469-471, 1957.
202. Tollner U, Bechinger D, Pohlandt F: Radial nerve palsy in a premature infant following long-term measurement of blood pressure, *J Pediatr* 96:921-922, 1980.
203. Weeks PM: Radial, median, and ulnar nerve dysfunction associated with a congenital constricting band of the arm, *Plast Reconstr Surg* 69:333-336, 1982.
204. Ross D, Jones HR, Fisher J, Konkol RJ: Isolated radial nerve lesion in the newborn, *Neurology* 33:1354-1356, 1983.
205. Jones HR: Compressive neuropathy in childhood: A report of 14 cases, *Muscle Nerve* 9:720-723, 1986.
206. Jones HR, Bolton CF, Harper C Jr: *Pediatric Clinical Electromyography*, Philadelphia: 1996, Lippincott-Raven.
207. Hayman M, Roland EH, Hill A: Newborn radial nerve palsy: Report of four cases and review of published reports, *Pediatr Neurol* 21:648-651, 1999.
208. Felice KJ, Jones HR Jr: Upper extremity mononeuropathies. In Jones HR Jr, DeVivo DC, Darras BT, editors: *Neuromuscular Disorders of Infancy, Childhood and Adolescence: A Clinician's Approach*, Philadelphia: 2003, Butterworth Heinemann.
209. Hope EE, Bodensteiner JB, Thong N: Neonatal lumbar plexus injury, *Arch Neurol* 42:94-95, 1985.
210. Curtiss PH, Tucker HJ: Sciatic palsy in premature infants, *JAMA* 174:1586-1588, 1960.
211. Gilles FH, Matson DD: Sciatic nerve injury following misplaced gluteal injection, *J Pediatr* 76:247-254, 1970.
212. San Augustin M, Nitowsky HM, Borden JN: Neonatal sciatic palsy after umbilical vessel injection, *J Pediatr* 60:408-413, 1962.
213. Purohit DM, Levkoff AH, DeVito PC: Gluteal necrosis with foot drop: Complications associated with umbilical artery catheterization, *Am J Dis Child* 132:897-899, 1978.
214. Escolar DM, Ryan MM, Jones HR Jr: Lower extremity mononeuropathies. In Jones HR Jr, DeVivo DC, Darras BT, editors: *Neuromuscular Disorders of Infancy, Childhood, and Adolescence: A Clinician's Approach*, Philadelphia: 2003, Butterworth Heinemann.
215. Craig WS, Clark JM: Of peripheral nerve palsies in newly born, *J Obstet Gynecol Br Emp* 65:229-237, 1958.
216. Crumrine P, Koenigsberger MR, Chutorian AM: Foot drop in the neonate with neurologic and electrophysiologic data, *Pediatrics* 86:779-780, 1975.
217. Fischer AQ, Straburger MD: Footdrop in the neonate secondary to the use of footboards, *J Pediatr* 101:1003-1004, 1982.
218. Kreusser KL, Volpe JJ: Peroneal palsy produced by intravenous fluid infiltration in a newborn, *Dev Med Child Neurol* 26:522-524, 1984.
219. Jones HR, Herbison GJ, Jacobs SR, Kollros PR, et al: Intrauterine onset of a mononeuropathy: Peroneal neuropathy in a newborn with electromyographic findings at age one day compatible with prenatal onset, *Muscle Nerv* 19:88-91, 1996.
220. Yilmaz Y, Oge AE, Yilmaz-Degpirmenci S, Say A: Peroneal nerve palsy: The role of early electromyography, *Eur J Paediatr Neurol* 4:239-242, 2000.

INTRACRANIAL
MASS LESIONS

Chapter 23

Brain Tumors and Vein of Galen Malformations

In this chapter, I discuss brain tumors and vein of Galen malformations. These disorders are considered in the same chapter because they represent important intracranial mass lesions and share certain clinical features. I do not review in detail management, which is considered in depth in standard neurosurgical writings. However, for both lesions, as noted later, improvements in management in recent years have made the prognosis of these serious disorders considerably more favorable than in the past. Because arachnoid cysts are intracranial mass lesions increasingly identified antenatally, a brief discussion of them concludes the chapter.

BRAIN TUMORS

Brain tumors manifesting either at birth (or in utero) or within the first 2 months of life account for approximately 1% to 2% of all brain tumors encountered in the pediatric age group.[1-9] Although in most major reviews neonatal brain tumors are grouped with tumors manifesting in the first 1 to 2 years of life, brain tumors appearing at birth (or in utero) or in the first 2 postnatal months are sufficiently distinctive in histological and clinical characteristics to be considered separately. In this chapter, I discuss only tumors manifesting at birth (or in utero) and in the first 2 postnatal months.

I do not discuss etiological considerations, because very little is currently known about the origin of either neonatal or later-appearing pediatric brain tumors. Derangements in the control of cell proliferation and differentiation are central to etiology, and abnormalities of genes encoding proteins that function as growth factors (e.g., platelet-derived growth factor), as stimulators of cell proliferation (e.g., oncogenes), or as suppressors of cell proliferation (e.g., tumor suppressor genes) have been identified in various tumors.[7] Additionally, abnormal genetic material inserted into the human genome by certain viruses may induce tumor formation; polymerase chain reaction technology has been used to show the presence of DNA sequences of simian virus 40, one member of a family of viruses (polyomaviruses) that induces tumors in laboratory animals.[10] These sequences were observed in 10 of 20 choroid plexus tumors and in 10 of 11 ependymomas in children; both these tumors are relatively common in the neonatal period (see later discussion). More data on these issues will be of major importance.

Neuropathology

Histological Types

The histological types of neonatal brain tumors differ considerably according to the time of clinical presentation (Table 23-1).[1,3-9,11-28] Thus, teratomas are the predominant tumors in infants who present clinically in fetal life or at birth, whereas tumors of neuroepithelial origin predominate in the first 2 postnatal months. The high proportion of teratomas shown in Table 23-1 is based on two large series (cumulative total, 425).[1,7] These lesions are usually very large (Fig. 23-1). Indeed, approximately 35% to 60% are so large that the site of origin in the supratentorial compartment cannot be determined.[1,7,9] Nearly 20% of neonatal teratomas originate from the region of the lateral ventricle, and another approximately 10% to 20% originate from the region of the third ventricle. Only uncommonly do neonatal teratomas originate from the pineal region, the site of most intracranial teratomas that manifest clinically after the neonatal period.

The major types of *nonteratomatous tumors* (i.e., neuroepithelial and mesenchymal tumors) are shown in Table 23-2.[1,7] Astrocytoma is the most common single category. Medulloblastoma, choroid plexus papilloma (and carcinoma), and ependymoma (and ependymoblastoma) are also relatively common. The remaining tumors encountered include primitive neuroectodermal tumors (not medulloblastoma), ganglioglioma, oligodendroglioma, mixed gliomas, and pineoblastoma. Of the neuroepithelial tumors, choroid plexus papilloma has the most consistent site of origin (i.e., the lateral ventricle in most cases). Among other tumors, craniopharyngioma is the most common single type, although sarcoma, fibroma, hemangioblastoma, hemangioma, and meningioma have been documented.[1,6,7,29-34]

Particularly unusual, additional examples of neonatal brain tumors include intracranial chordoma, derived from midline remnants of notochord, gliomatosis cerebri, mixed neural tissue masses extending into the oropharynx, hypothalamic hamartoma, lipoma of corpus callosum, multiple lipomata, and subependymal giant cell astrocytoma associated with tuberous sclerosis.[1,6,7,35-44a] The astrocytomas associated with tuberous sclerosis are usually accompanied in the newborn by cardiac rhabdomyoma, and, indeed, the latter may be the principal clue to the diagnosis of tuberous sclerosis in the neonatal period in such patients (see Chapter 2). The cardiac tumor may lead

TABLE 23-1 Neonatal Brain Tumors: Histological Types*

	Percentage of Tumors with Presentation at Birth or in Utero	Percentage of Tumors with Presentation in First 2 Mo
Teratoma	47%	26%
Neuroepithelial	40%	65%
Other	13%	9%

*n = 200 in study of Wakai and colleagues.
Data from Wakai S, Arai T, Nagai M: Congenital brain tumors, *Surg Neurol* 21:597–609, 1984; and Isaacs H: I. Perinatal brain tumors: A review of 250 cases, *Pediatr Neurol* 27:249–261, 2002.

TABLE 23-2 Types of Nonteratomatous Neonatal Brain Tumors*

	Percentage of Total Nonteratomatous Tumors
Neuroepithelial	
Astrocytoma	29%
Medulloblastoma	14%
Choroid plexus papilloma (and carcinoma)	14%
Ependymoma, ependymoblastoma	13%
Miscellaneous neuroepithelial (e.g., primitive neuroectodermal tumor, ganglioglioma, oligodendroglioma, pineoblastoma, mixed gliomas)	7%
Other	
Craniopharyngioma	12%
Mesenchymal (meningioma, sarcoma)	10%
Miscellaneous (hemangioblastoma)	1%

*n = 225.
Data from Isaacs H: I. Perinatal brain tumors: A review of 250 cases, *Pediatr Neurol* 27:249–261, 2002.

to cardiac complications (e.g., arrhythmia) that can be life-threatening at the time of surgery for the subependymal astrocytoma.

Location

The *location of neonatal brain tumors* is distinctly different from that observed in pediatric patients in late infancy and childhood (Table 23-3).[1,4-9,15,16] Thus, *supratentorial* predominance is apparent. This predominance is marked for teratomas, which are nearly always supratentorial in location. In contrast, medulloblastoma is the one type of neonatal brain tumor with consistent predominance in the infratentorial compartment. If only neuroepithelial tumors are considered, the ratio of supratentorial to infratentorial lesions is 1.7:1 for tumors manifesting at birth and 2.4:1 for those appearing in the first 2 postnatal months. If all neonatal brain tumors are considered (i.e., teratomas and mesenchymal tumors, as well as neuroepithelial tumors), the supratentorial predominance is even more marked (see Table 23-3).

Clinical Features

The clinical features of neonatal brain tumors can be divided essentially into four major syndromes (Table 23-4).[1-3,5-9,14,16,17,21,27,36,45-55] The *first syndrome* is characterized by a mass lesion that is so large in fetal life that severe macrocrania results in cranial-pelvic disproportion, dystocia, stillbirth, or premature labor. This "obstetrical" syndrome is characteristic of teratomas (Fig. 23-2), but it may also be observed with large neuroepithelial tumors (see Table 23-4). Commonly, other features related to displacement of intracranial

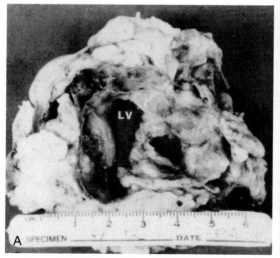
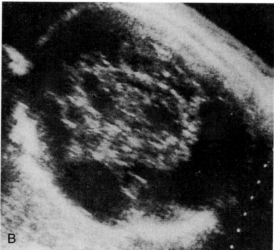

Figure 23-1 Intracranial teratoma: gross neuropathology. A, Multicystic mass replaces most of normal brain; the dilated lateral ventricle (LV) is visible. **B,** Intrauterine ultrasound scan shows a multicystic mass replacing normal brain; no normal intracranial structures could be identified. *(From Lipman SP, Pretorius DH, Rumack CM, Manco-Johnson ML: Fetal intracranial teratoma: US diagnosis of three cases and a review of the literature,* Radiology *157:491–494, 1985.)*

TABLE 23-3 **Supratentorial and Infratentorial Locations of Neonatal Brain Tumors**

	PRESENTATION AT BIRTH		PRESENTATION IN FIRST 2 MO	
	Supratentorial	Infratentorial	Supratentorial	Infratentorial
Teratoma	44	0	18	1
Neuroepithelial				
Medulloblastoma	2	7	1	8
Astrocytoma	5	3	9	2
Choroid plexus papilloma	6	0	9	0
Ependymoma, ependymoblastoma	4	0	7	2
Other neuroepithelial	10	6	8	2
Total of all neuroepithelial tumors	27	16	34	14
Supratentorial-to-infratentorial ratio for neuroepithelial tumors	1.7:1		2.4:1	
Supratentorial-to-infratentorial ratio for all tumors (teratoma, neuroepithelial, mesenchymal)	5.2:1		3.4:1	

Data from Wakai S, Arai T, Nagai M: Congenital brain tumors, *Surg Neurol* 21:597–609, 1984.

tissue by tumor (e.g., local skull swelling, proptosis, or epignathus) may be present in this syndrome. The *second syndrome* is characterized predominately by macrocrania and bulging fontanelle, often secondary to hydrocephalus. This syndrome may accompany the features just described for teratomas and may occur for tumors that manifest at birth or in the first 2 postnatal months (see Table 23-4). The *third syndrome* consists of specific neurological features related to the particular type and location of the tumor and is particularly characteristic of tumors manifesting after birth, in the first 2 postnatal months. These neurological features include seizures, present in 15% to 25% of patients with neonatal brain tumors, hemiparesis or quadriparesis, cranial nerve abnormalities, and signs of increased intracranial pressure, often secondary to hydrocephalus. The last of these characteristics is a consistent feature of choroid plexus papilloma. Specific neurological features of spinal cord tumors include torticollis with high

cervical spinal cord lesions, usually astrocytoma, and weakness of lower extremities with disturbance of sphincter function in lumbosacral-coccygeal lesions, usually teratoma.[9,54-56] The spinal cord lesions are particularly important to identify promptly, because abrupt neurological deterioration may occur spontaneously or after mild trauma (e.g., neck manipulation). The *fourth clinical syndrome* associated with neonatal brain tumors is abrupt onset of intracranial hemorrhage (Figs. 23-3 and 23-4).[1,6-9,18,22,45,47,53,57] Hemorrhage with brain tumor is more common in neonatal lesions than in tumors at later ages and develops in approximately 8% to 18% of cases, more commonly in patients with neuroepithelial lesions or vascular tumors (e.g., cavernous hemangioma) than in patients with teratomas (Table 23-5). More often, the hemorrhage is an incidental finding at the time of diagnostic brain imaging, surgery, or autopsy, but occasionally it is large enough to be the presenting clinical feature. Indeed, any infant with an intraparenchymal hemorrhage with no readily identifiable cause (see Chapter 10) should be evaluated for the presence of brain tumor.

TABLE 23-4 **Neonatal Brain Tumors: Initial Signs and Symptoms***

Signs and Symptoms	PRESENTATION AT BIRTH		Presentation in First 2 Months
	Teratoma	Others	
Dystocia	45%	20%	—
Stillborn	40%	15%	—
Prematurity	30%	20%	—
Large head and/ or bulging fontanelle	70%	55%	70%
Epignathus	10%	—	—
Local skull swelling	10%	5%	2%
Proptosis	8%	1%	—
Seizure	—	2%	15%
Vomiting	—	1%	30%

*n = 200 in reference 1, n = 250 in reference 7, and n = 534 in reference 9. Numbers are rounded off.
Data from references 1, 7, and 9.

Diagnosis

The diagnosis is based on a high index of clinical suspicion. The need for evaluation for brain tumor is straightforward in the infant with macrocrania, bulging anterior fontanelle, hydrocephalus of unknown cause, or focal neurological deficit. Sometimes overlooked is the need to consider tumor in the infant with unexplained intracranial hemorrhage (see earlier discussion), seizures, irritability, or persistent vomiting. The diagnostic approach should begin with a brain imaging procedure, and cranial ultrasonography is the best initial choice. This noninvasive modality demonstrates tumors in and near the lateral and third ventricles especially well (Figs. 23-5 and 23-6).[6,7,30,39] The addition of Doppler evaluation of blood flow within the tumor is useful in the identification of choroid plexus papilloma, a strikingly hypervascular tumor (Fig. 23-7).[58]

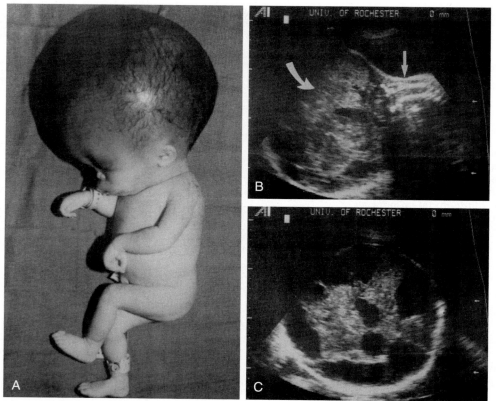

Figure 23-2 **Teratoma with intrauterine presentation. A,** Newborn exhibits massive craniomegaly secondary to intracranial teratoma. The infant died at 90 minutes of age. **B** and **C,** Intrauterine ultrasonography of the same infant. Note in **B,** a midsagittal view of the fetus, the solid echogenic mass *(curved arrow)* in the cranium above the level of the cervical spine *(straight arrow).* In **C,** a transverse view of fetal vertex shows the absence of normal symmetrical intracranial anatomy and the presence of a solid echogenic core surrounded by cystic structures. *(From Sherer DM, Abramowicz JS, Eggers PC, Metlay LA, et al: Prenatal ultrasonographic diagnosis of intracranial teratoma and massive craniomegaly with associated high-output cardiac failure,* Am J Obstet Gynecol *168:97–99, 1993.)*

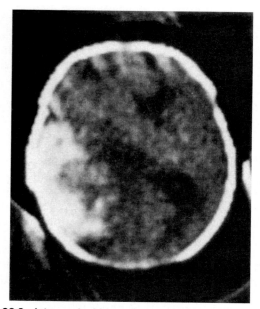

Figure 23-3 **Intracerebral hemorrhage associated with an astrocytoma: computed tomography scan from a 2-week-old infant with a 9-day history of vomiting, left focal seizures, and left hemiparesis.** Note the large hemorrhagic mass in the right cerebral hemisphere with surrounding edema and shift of ventricles to the left. A fibrillary astrocytoma was identified at surgery. *(From Rothman SM, Nelson JS, DeVivo DC, Coxe WS: Congenital astrocytoma presenting with intracerebral hematoma,* J Neurosurg *51:237–239, 1979.)*

In general, however, computed tomography (CT) and magnetic resonance imaging (MRI) are the mainstays of the diagnostic evaluation (see Fig. 23-4; Figs. 23-8 to 23-12).[2,22,59] MRI is preferred for all lesions, especially for those in the posterior fossa and spinal cord (see Fig. 23-12).

Prognosis

The outcome of patients with neonatal brain tumors depends on the size and location of the lesion, the time of diagnosis, and particularly on the histological type of the tumor. General conclusions concerning prognosis of the most common neonatal brain tumors are summarized in Table 23-6.*

Teratomas are associated with a poor outcome. Mortality rates in these patients generally exceed 90%, principally because the lesions are usually very extensive at the time of identification. In the largest experience (*n* = 73), the 1-year survival rate for patients with teratomas was 7.2%.[1]

Medulloblastoma manifesting at birth or in the first 2 postnatal months is also associated with a poor

_____

*See references 1,5-9,14,16,17,21-23,26,27,45,46,50,52,53,56,60-62.

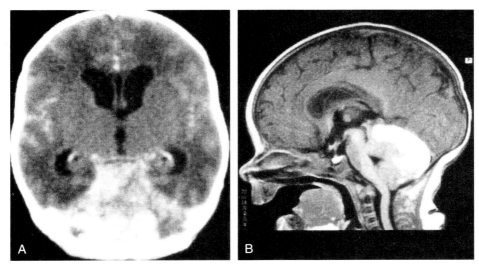

Figure 23-4   Posterior fossa hemorrhage in a newborn with a medulloblastoma. A, Axial computed tomography scan shows an apparent posterior fossa hemorrhage in a term infant who presented at 6 hours of age with signs of brain stem compression. **B,** Sagittal magnetic resonance imaging scan shows posterior fossa subdural hemorrhage, apparently originating in the cerebellar vermis. Six months later, a large midline medulloblastoma was detected. *(From Perrin RG, Rutka JT, Drake JM, Meltzer H, et al: Management and outcomes of posterior fossa subdural hematomas in neonates,* Neurosurgery *40:1190–1200, 1997.)*

outcome, with mortality rates exceeding 80%. In a series of 19 cases of perinatal medulloblastoma, only 1 survivor was reported.[7]

Choroid plexus papilloma has the most favorable outcome. With rare exceptions, all infants are cured and have a normal outcome. Choroid plexus carcinoma, which accounts for approximately 5% to 10% of neonatal choroid plexus tumors, had been associated with a poor chance for survival until recently, when improvements in chemotherapy appreciably increased the chance of prolonged survival.

Astrocytomas and ependymomas are associated with variable outcomes, depending primarily on the degree of differentiation of the tumor and its location. Markedly anaplastic lesions and deep diencephalic and brain stem locations are rarely curable.

Management

Major Modalities of Treatment

Major modalities of treatment of brain tumors in children are surgery, chemotherapy, and radiation therapy. *Surgery* is by far the most important of these modalities in the management of neonatal brain tumors. Indeed, improvements in localization of lesions by modern brain imaging, the advances in pediatric neuroanesthesia and intensive care, and the advent of

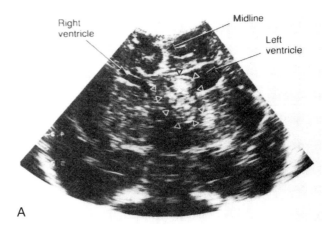

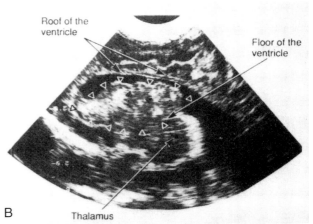

Figure 23-5   Cranial ultrasonography: neonatal subependymal astrocytoma. A, Coronal and, **B,** sagittal ultrasound scans obtained from the anterior fontanelle show a large intraventricular mass in the left lateral ventricle *(outlined with open arrowheads)* with midline shift and dilation of the left lateral ventricle. *Closed arrowheads* indicate some areas of calcification. This infant had tuberous sclerosis. *(From Hahn JS, Bejar R, Gladson CL: Neonatal subependymal giant cell astrocytoma associated with tuberous sclerosis: MRI, CT, and ultrasound correlation,* Neurology *41:124–128, 1991.)*

TABLE 23-5	Association of Hemorrhage with Neonatal Brain Tumors*	
Histological Type	**Incidence of Hemorrhage**
Teratoma	8%
Neuroepithelial and other	18%
All tumors	14%

*See text for references.

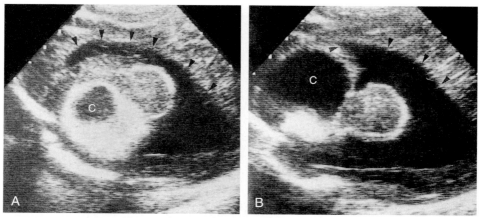

Figure 23-6 **Cranial ultrasonography: neonatal craniopharyngioma. A** and **B**, Sagittal ultrasound scans show cystlike regions of tumor (C) with internal echoes. Adjacent to the cystlike regions are focal echogenic areas with shadowing, consistent with calcification. The lateral ventricle *(arrowheads)* is dilated. *(From Hurst RW, McIlhenny J, Park TS, Thomas WO: Neonatal craniopharyngioma: CT and ultrasonographic features,* J Comput Assist Tomogr *12:858–861, 1988.)*

microneurosurgical techniques have markedly reduced the operative mortality of patients with even large tumors. Indeed, aggressive resection, including subtotal hemispherectomy, has been advocated for large tumors.[6,7,14,53,63]

Chemotherapy in the neonatal period is hindered by the immaturity of the infant's hepatic and renal mechanisms for metabolism and excretion of these agents.[60] However, in recent years, improved *multiagent chemotherapy after surgery* has been advocated to delay or obviate the need for radiation therapy, a modality of high risk in the young infant.[64,65]

Radiation therapy is the most problematic and controversial approach in the treatment of neonatal brain tumors.[14,53,64-67] Indeed, few data are available for newborns and very young infants, but in a series of 13 infants treated for brain tumors at less than 2 years of age, 10 later had below-normal intelligence

quotient and impaired growth.[67] Such adverse neurological and endocrinological effects have been replicated in infants and young children treated with craniospinal irradiation for prophylaxis for acute lymphoblastic leukemia.[68-70] Indeed, many clinicians consider radiation to be "absolutely contraindicated in the neonate"[53] and to be used only for recurrent disease after aggressive surgery and, when indicated, chemotherapy.[14] The advent of stereotactically applied, highly focused radiation (radiation surgery), which provides radiation to the tumor with a minimum of involvement of normal brain in the management of pediatric brain tumors, raises the possibility of ultimate application of this technique to young infants.[71,72] Unfortunately, the frequent presence of infiltrating tumor borders in neonatal brain tumors may limit the applicability of even this promising approach.

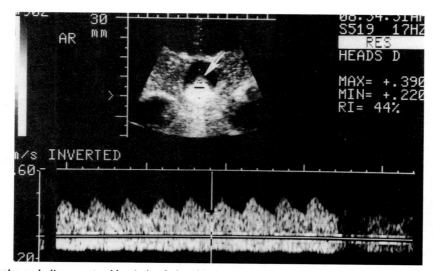

Figure 23-7 **Cranial Doppler and ultrasonographic study of choroid plexus papilloma.** This coronal study shows a dilated third ventricle within which is an echogenic mass *(arrow)*. Dilated lateral ventricles and temporal horns also are visible. The Doppler tracing *(lower portion of figure)* from the mass indicates hypervascularity with high blood flow. *(From Harmon BH, Yap MA: One-month-old infant with increasing head size,* Invest Radiol *25:862–864, 1990.)*

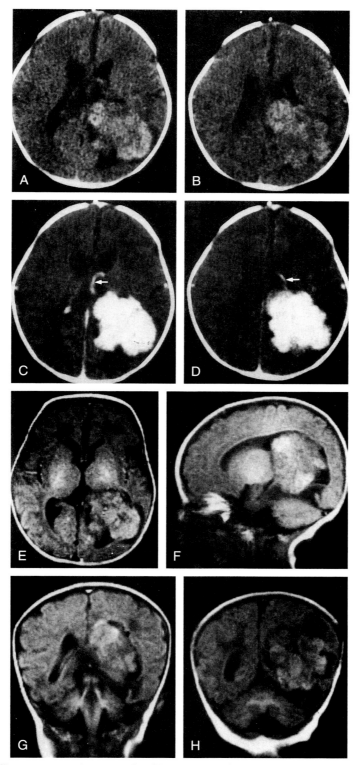

Figure 23-8 **Choroid plexus papilloma: computed tomography (CT) and magnetic resonance imaging (MRI) scans from an 11-day-old infant with macrocrania.** **A** to **D**, Axial CT sections before (**A** and **B**) and following (**C** and **D**) contrast enhancement reveal a large, lobulated, partially calcified, hyperdense mass that is near a dilated choroidal vessel (*arrows* in **C** and **D**). The mass expands the ventricle and extends into the surrounding parenchyma. **E** to **H**, Spin-echo T1-weighted MRI scans in axial (**E**), sagittal (**F**), and coronal (**G** and **H**) planes demonstrate mixed high and low signal intensity of the mass within the ventricle and periventricular tissue. *(From Radkowski MA, Naidich TP, Tomita T, Byrd SE, et al: Neonatal brain tumors: CT and MR findings,* J Comput Assist Tomogr *12:10–20, 1988.)*

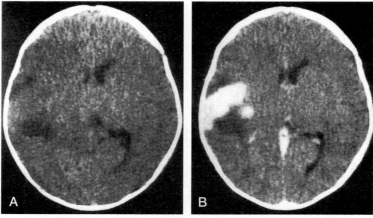

Figure 23-9 **Gliosarcoma in a 26-day-old infant: computed tomography (CT) scan.** Axial CT sections, **A**, before and, **B**, following contrast enhancement reveal an isodense, densely enhancing temporoparietal mass, associated edema, and compression of the right lateral ventricle. The tumor itself reaches the pial surface of the brain (confirmed by surgery). *(From Radkowski MA, Naidich TP, Tomita T, Byrd SE, et al: Neonatal brain tumors: CT and MR findings,* J Comput Assist Tomogr *12:10–20, 1988.)*

Treatment of Specific Tumors

Concerning *treatment of specific tumors*, teratomas are managed essentially entirely by surgery. Unfortunately, usually only partial resections are possible because of the very large size of these lesions. Medulloblastoma is treated with partial or total resection and, in recent years, by chemotherapy. Radiation therapy, if used at all, is instituted most often later in infancy for recurrent disease. Choroid plexus papilloma is treated with total surgical resection, and choroid plexus carcinoma is treated with surgery and chemotherapy. Astrocytoma and ependymoma are treated with aggressive surgery, the former with more success than the latter, particularly because of more favorable locations with astrocytoma. Multiagent chemotherapy has had some postoperative benefit for anaplastic astrocytomas but not particularly for ependymomas.[64,65]

Limited-volume radiation therapy is under investigation for these lesions.[64,65]

VEIN OF GALEN MALFORMATION

Vein of Galen malformation is discussed best in this context because, like brain tumor, the disorder constitutes an intracranial mass lesion and manifests in the newborn in approximately 60% of all pediatric examples of this malformation (Table 23-7).[73-77] Moreover, certain features of the clinical presentation (e.g., macrocephaly and hydrocephalus) can be similar to the clinical presentation of brain tumors. Notably, however, the clinical presentation more commonly does not mimic brain tumor and is quite distinctive (see later discussion). Vein of Galen malformation continues to be a great therapeutic challenge. Despite advances in radiological diagnosis, neonatal intensive care, and

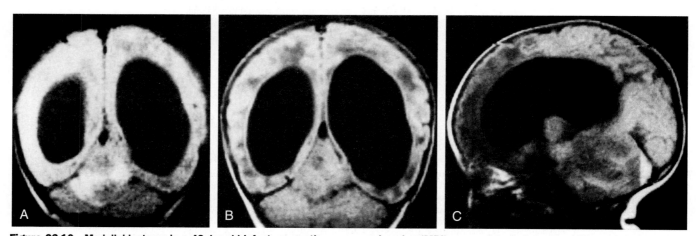

Figure 23-10 **Medulloblastoma in a 49-day-old infant: magnetic resonance imaging (MRI) scans.** A to **C**, Spin-echo MRI scans in the coronal plane at TR 1000, TE 30 milliseconds (**A** and **B**) and in the sagittal plane at TR 550, TE 30 milliseconds (**C**) reveal a large superior vermian mass that compresses the fourth ventricle and brain stem, invades the tectum to obliterate the aqueduct (causing hydrocephalus), and grows exophytically to overlie the cerebellar hemispheres. *(From Radkowski MA, Naidich TP, Tomita T, Byrd SE, et al: Neonatal brain tumors: CT and MR findings,* J Comput Assist Tomogr *12:10–20, 1988.)*

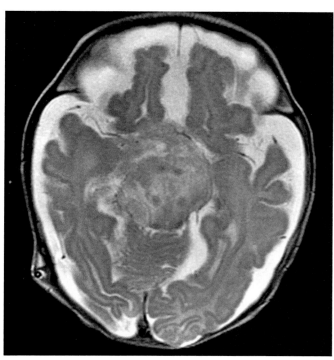

Figure 23-11 Glioma: magnetic resonance imaging scan. This 2-month-old infant had a large, heterogenous mass (undifferentiated glioma) in the diencephalic–upper midbrain region. Disseminated tumor was present in extracerebral spaces, which are markedly widened. *(Courtesy of Dr. Omar Khwaja.)*

TABLE 23-6	General Conclusions Concerning Prognosis of Most Common Neonatal Brain Tumors
Teratomas	>90% mortality rate
Astrocytoma	65% mortality rate (however, prognosis can vary from uniformly poor for poorly differentiated supratentorial tumor to potentially curable for cystic cerebellar astrocytoma)
Medulloblastoma	>90% mortality rate
Choroid Plexus Papilloma	Minimal mortality rate and high likelihood of normal outcome
Ependymoma	Variable prognosis, as stated for astrocytoma, but less commonly curable

microneurosurgical and endovascular techniques, this disorder, when it is severe enough to appear in the newborn, remains a major therapeutic problem.

Neuropathology

The essential feature of the vein of Galen malformation is aneurysmal dilation of the venous structure generally characterized as the vein of Galen. The most common feeding arterial vessels into this dilated venous structure are, in order of frequency, the posterior choroidal artery, the anterior cerebral (pericallosal) artery, the

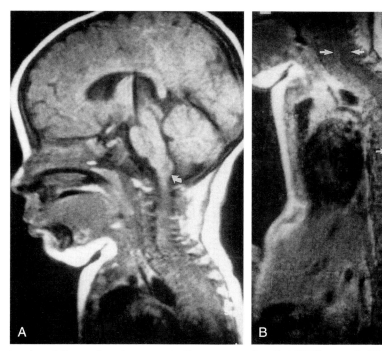

Figure 23-12 Spinal cord and medullary astrocytoma: magnetic resonance imaging (MRI) scan. A, Midsagittal MRI, T1-weighted (TR 600/TE 15), unenhanced. The tumor can be appreciated in the medulla *(curved arrow).* Additional signal sequences (not shown) had no indication of a fluid cavity or enhancement. **B,** Midsagittal MRI, T1-weighted (TR 770, TE 15), gadolinium enhanced. The entire spinal cord is diffusely expanded by a nonenhancing, noncystic mass *(arrows).* (From Kaufman BA, Park TS: Congenital spinal cord astrocytomas, Childs Nerv Syst *8:389–393, 1992.)*

TABLE 23-7   Vein of Galen Malformation with Presentation in the Neonatal Period

Neonatal Presentation
≈60% of all pediatric cases of vein of Galen malformation

Most Common Arterial Feeding Vessels
Choroidal arteries (posterior and anterior), anterior and middle cerebral arteries, and proximal posterior cerebral arteries

Clinical Presentation
High-output congestive heart failure in virtually all neonatal cases; hydrocephalus present in ≈15%

Diagnosis
Made most readily by ultrasonography, Doppler studies of cerebral vessels and peripheral arteries, computed tomographic angiography, and magnetic resonance imaging

Outcome
In previous years, nearly 100% mortality; more recently, ≈40% to 65% have favorable outcome

Therapy
Most commonly embolization, either by selective arterial infusion with liquid adhesive agents or microcoils or by transvenous-transtorcular embolization with metallic coils

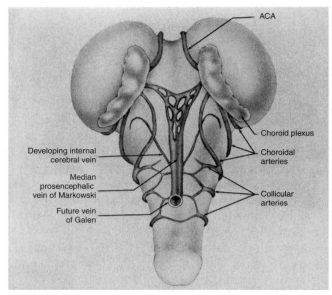

Figure 23-13   Artist's rendering of the early vascularization of the choroid plexuses. Just before the growth of the neural tube induces the development of the intrinsic vascularization, the meninx primitiva invaginates into the ventricular lumen to produce the choroid plexuses. The arterial afferents are the choroidal arteries, including the terminal branch of the anterior cerebral artery (ACA). The venous blood drains through the median prosencephalic vein of Markowski. This single midline vein forms by collecting blood from the plexuses at the level of the paraphysis and courses backward toward the dorsal (interhemispheric) dural plexus. Simultaneously, the development of the collicular plate is accompanied by development of quadrigeminal (collicular) arteries. Later, when the intrinsic vascularization develops in the basal ganglia and thalamus, the internal cerebral veins develop to drain them. These join with the posterior end of the median prosencephalic vein to form what will become the vein of Galen. Progressively, the internal cerebral veins replace the median prosencephalic vein for choroidal venous drainage; the median prosencephalic vein attenuates and disappears, and the vein of Galen develops. *(From Raybaud CA, Strother CM, Hald JK: Aneurysms of the vein of Galen: Embryonic considerations and anatomical features relating to the pathogenesis of the malformation,* Neuroradiology *31:109–128, 1989.)*

middle cerebral artery (especially thalamoperforating branches), the anterior choroidal artery, and the posterior cerebral artery (see Table 23-7).[74,76,78,79] Although the vein of Galen is considered in most writings to be the vein that is dilated, careful anatomical study suggests that the so-called *median prosencephalic vein of Markowski*, a transitory venous structure that normally disappears by the 11th week of gestation, is the vein involved (Figs. 23-13 and 23-14).[78] During early development, this vein drains directly into the vein of Galen, and after 11 weeks, it is replaced by the internal cerebral veins. The median prosencephalic vein is involved particularly in venous drainage from the choroid plexus.[78,80] The frequent position of the aneurysmally dilated vein anterior to the position of the vein of Galen further supports the notion that the involved vein is the primitive median prosencephalic vein. The frequent association of abnormal venous channels, including the so-called *falcine sinus*, a normally transient fetal vessel, is additionally consistent with this hypothesis.[78] Nevertheless, the term *vein of Galen malformation* is entrenched in the medical literature, and I continue to use it to characterize this entity.

The *associated neuropathological findings* observed with vein of Galen malformation consist of a variety of ischemic, hemorrhagic, and mass effects of the malformation.[74-76,78-92] Thus, in a carefully analyzed series of 13 infants who died in the first 6 weeks of life, *ischemic lesions* included cerebral infarction (focal vascular and border zone lesions) in 4 infants, basal ganglia or other infarction in 3, periventricular leukomalacia in 7, pontosubicular necrosis in 3, and selective neuronal necrosis of cerebral cortex or brain stem, or both, in 4 infants. *Hemorrhagic lesions* included

subarachnoid hemorrhage in 3 infants, germinal matrix–intraventricular hemorrhage in 2, and intracerebral hemorrhage in 2. Venous thrombosis was present in 3 infants. *Mass effects* included hydrocephalus secondary to obstruction, usually at the level of quadrigeminal plate and the aqueduct, in 2 infants, and compression of other structures (e.g., cerebral peduncles) in 1 infant. The mechanisms of these lesions are multifactorial and are summarized in Table 23-8.

The ischemic phenomena are related primarily to a combination of intracranial "steal" phenomena, caused by the absence or even the reverse of diastolic cerebral blood flow, and congestive heart failure. The heart failure is caused principally by the remarkably high cardiac output, secondary to both the marked decrease in cerebrovascular resistance and the increased venous return to the heart, and by marked cardiac ischemia. The latter results from decreased coronary blood flow, which normally occurs predominately during diastole, because of the low diastolic pressure associated with the vein of Galen malformation.

TABLE 23-8 Major Mechanisms of Brain Injury with the Vein of Galen

Intracranial "steal" phenomena because of diastolic "run-off," resulting in cerebral ischemia

Congestive heart failure (secondary to high cardiac output and myocardial ischemia, because of low diastolic pressure and, as a consequence, impaired coronary flow), resulting in cerebral ischemia

Thrombosis of the dilated vein of Galen with hemorrhagic infarction or intraventricular hemorrhage, or both

Vascular rupture with massive hemorrhage

Atrophy secondary to compression of adjacent structures by the dilated vein of Galen

Hydrocephalus secondary to aqueductal obstruction (by compression)

Clinical Features

The clinical manifestations of the vein of Galen malformation in the neonatal period reflect the large size of the lesions and consist predominately of congestive heart failure (see Table 23-7).[73-77,79,87,89-102] Thus, of the approximately 130 cases with adequate clinical data, 80% to 95% of infants presented with congestive heart failure. The remaining infants presented with hydrocephalus, subarachnoid hemorrhage, or intraventricular hemorrhage. The features accompanying the congestive failure aid in diagnosis and include a cranial bruit and bounding carotid pulses. The cranial bruit differs from the benign systolic bruit of infancy and early childhood by its continuous nature and by the frequent localization over the posterior cranium rather than the anterior cranium. The marked carotid pulses may be accompanied by prominent peripheral pulses, but in the presence of overt congestive heart failure, the peripheral pulses may be depressed, whereas the carotid pulses remain prominent. A consequence of congestive heart failure, prerenal azotemia, was observed in 11 of 15 infants in a reported series.[73] Seizures and other neurological signs are very unusual.

The clinical presentation of neonatal cases differs from that in older infants and children with vein of Galen malformation. Thus, older infants present most commonly with hydrocephalus, and children present most commonly with neurological signs (perhaps secondary to intracranial "steal" phenomena), headache, and, occasionally, subarachnoid hemorrhage.

The subsequent course in newborns with an untreated vein of Galen malformation who survive the

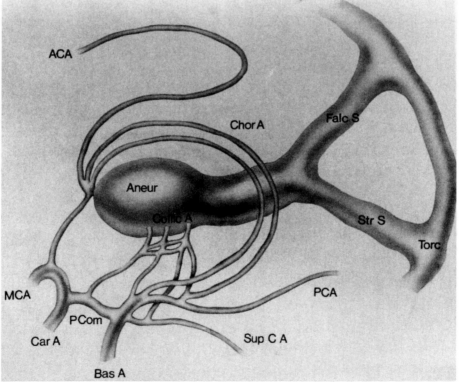

Figure 23-14 Artist's rendering of a vein of Galen malformation. This drawing is based on two anatomical dissections. Two fistula sites are present in the aneurysmal sac (Aneur). The anterior fistula receives blood from the choroidal vessels (anterior cerebral artery [ACA], choroidal branches (Chor A) of the posterior cerebral artery [PCA]) and from posterior perforators of the middle cerebral artery (MCA). The inferior fistula receives blood from an arterioarterial subarachnoid maze formed by anastomoses between the collicular arteries (branches of the superior cerebellar arteries [Sup C A], the PCA, and the posteromedial choroidal arteries). Posterior thalamoperforating arteries also may be involved. The aneurysmal sac is usually drained by dural sinuses, either the normal straight sinus (Str S) or a persistent fetal falcine sinus (Falc S), or both, as shown here. Bas A, basilar artery; Car A, carotid artery; PCom, posterior communicating artery; Torc, torcular. *(From Raybaud CA, Strother CM, Hald JK: Aneurysms of the vein of Galen: Embryonic considerations and anatomical features relating to the pathogenesis of the malformation,* Neuroradiology *31:109–128, 1989.)*

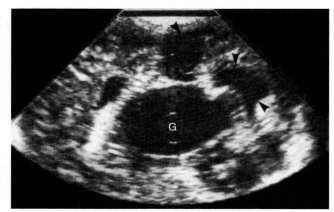

Figure 23-15   Ultrasound scan of an arteriovenous malformation in an infant with cardiac failure. This coronal ultrasound scan shows large, circular, midline, aneurysmal vein of Galen (G); the areas of echolucency in the left hemisphere represent regions of necrosis (arrowheads). *(Courtesy of Dr. Gary D. Shackelford.)*

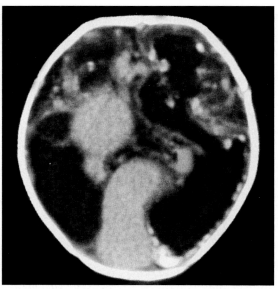

Figure 23-16   Computed tomography scan of an arteriovenous malformation from an infant with cardiac failure. The scan shows the midline aneurysmal vein of Galen and large areas of necrosis and calcification in both hemispheres, probably secondary to a "steal" phenomenon.

neonatal period and whose congestive heart failure is stabilized medically is dominated by the development of neurological disturbances and progressive hydrocephalus. The neurological disturbances include delayed development and development of major neurological deficits, presumably secondary to the intracranial ischemic and hemorrhagic phenomena (see later discussion).

Diagnosis

The diagnosis of the vein of Galen malformation should be suspected in any newborn with unexplained congestive heart failure, especially high-output heart failure, or with unexplained intracranial hemorrhage or hydrocephalus. The initial diagnostic

evaluation should be performed using cranial ultrasonography.[76,79,85-87,98,103-110] The aneurysmally dilated vein appears as a large, echolucent region in the region of the vein of Galen (Fig. 23-15). The addition of Doppler study of flow velocity in the arterial feeders and in the vein further defines the hemodynamics and the anatomy of the lesion.[108,110]

CT is useful for assessment of parenchymal ischemic injury or intracranial hemorrhage (Figs. 23-16 and 23-17). In infants with intraventricular hemorrhage, a clue that a vein of Galen malformation is the source of

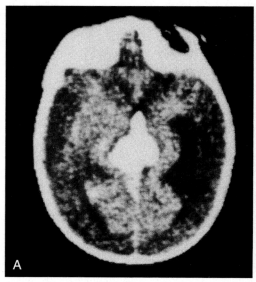
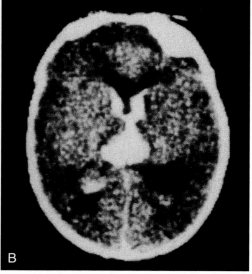

Figure 23-17   Computed tomography scans of intracranial hemorrhage secondary to an arteriovenous malformation, involving the vein of Galen. These scans are from a full-term infant with abrupt onset of seizures and opisthotonic posturing on the fourth day of life. **A**, Note the large amount of blood distending the posterior third ventricle. **B**, A relatively small amount of blood has extended into the lateral ventricles and is visible over the head of the caudate nuclei and in the occipital horns. *(From Schum TR, Meyer GA, Grausz JP, Glaspey JC: Neonatal intracranial ventricular hemorrhage due to an intracranial arteriovenous malformation: A case report, Pediatrics 64:242–244, 1979.)*

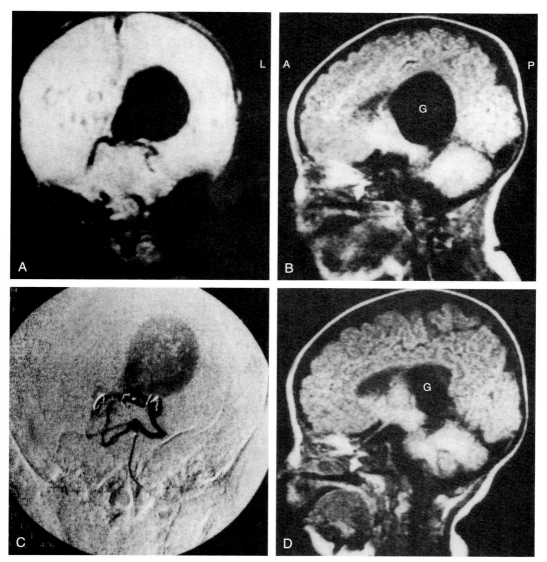

Figure 23-18   Vein of Galen malformation: magnetic resonance imaging (MRI) scan. A, Coronal and, **B,** sagittal MRI scans of a newborn before, and, **D,** sagittal image 2 months after, embolization show a marked decrease in the size of the aneurysmal dilation (G). In **A,** feeding arteries are demonstrated in the coronal plane. **C,** Anteroposterior view of a left vertebral angiogram showing microcoils within feeding arteries from the posterior cerebral arteries (8 days of age). *(From Yamashita Y, Abe T, Ohara N, Maruoka T, et al: Successful treatment of neonatal aneurysmal dilation of the vein of Galen: The role of prenatal diagnosis and trans-arterial embolization,* Neuroradiology *34:457–459, 1992.)*

the hemorrhage is a dilated third ventricle filled with blood in the absence of a large amount of blood in the lateral ventricles.[97] The major current value of CT is to identify the vascular details with spiral CT angiography.[79]

MRI is especially effective not only in the evaluation of the brain parenchyma and the aneurysmally dilated vein but also in the demonstration of major arterial feeding vessels (Fig. 23-18). MR angiography is also an effective noninvasive means of delineating the vascular supply and drainage of the malformation.

Angiography is used to define the anatomical details of the vein of Galen malformation. Delineation of the crucial arterial feeders and of the size and location of the aneurysmally dilated vein is crucial for determination of intervention (see later discussion).

Prognosis

The natural history of the vein of Galen malformation with clinical presentation in the newborn period is apparent from the review of Hoffman and co-workers[74] in 1982 of 16 personal cases and 45 reported by others. Thus, no difference in outcome between those treated and not treated was reported. Overall, of the 61 cases, 51 (84%) died, usually in early infancy, 8 (13%) survived with neurological impairment, and only 2 (3%) were normal on follow-up. Survival with neurological impairment principally reflected the ischemic and hemorrhagic phenomena that complicate the lesion, and some of these pathological features were shown to occur in utero.

The development and application of endovascular therapies for this lesion in the late 1980s and 1990s

TABLE 23-9   Outcome of Neonatal Vein of Galen Malformation after Endovascular Treatment*

Outcome	Percentage of Total
Death	19%
Developmental evaluation	
No permanent disability	43%[†]
Permanent disability	57%
Neurological examination	
No/mild abnormality	43%
Severe abnormality	57%
Epilepsy	33%

*n = 21. The median length of follow-up was 4.5 years.
[†]Value was 38% for the 16 infants who had congestive heart failure and 60% for the 5 infants without congestive heart failure.
Data from Fullerton HJ, Aminoff AR, Ferrierio DM, Gupta N, et al: Neurodevelopmental outcome after endovascular treatment of vein of Galen malformations, *Neurology* 61:1386–1390, 2003.

brought an increasing improvement in outcome.[75,76,99,101] The outcome in the largest neonatal series (n = 21) with the longest duration of follow-up (4.5 years) after neonatal endovascular therapy is shown in Table 23-9. Thus, 80% of the infants survived, and nearly one half had a normal or nearly normal outcome.[91] Similarly promising results have been reported by other investigators.[79,90,92]

Management

Management of a vein of Galen malformation large enough to manifest clinically in the neonatal period is a major therapeutic challenge. Medical management requires vigorous therapy of cardiac failure. Aggressive use of beta-adrenergic agents (dobutamine, dopamine) may worsen cardiac output. Best results appear to occur with use of low-dose dopamine in combination with a systemic vasodilator (e.g., a phosphodiesterase inhibitor).[92]

Concerning the approach to the vein of Galen malformation, in many centers no intervention is chosen if the infant already exhibits evidence of severe cerebral injury.[76] Direct neurosurgical attack is made extraordinarily difficult by the large size and complicated nature of the lesions and by the vulnerability of the infant in congestive heart failure and with a compromised myocardium (see earlier discussion). Indeed, the possibility of hypotension in association with surgery greatly increases the risk of fatal myocardial ischemia because of the already low diastolic flow and thereby impaired coronary circulation resulting from the malformation. Currently, the treatment of choice is an endovascular approach (see next).

The *principal approaches to treatment* in the newborn involve attempts to eliminate the high flow through the vascular lesion, either by arterial embolization, usually with a liquid adhesive (glue-forming) agent (e.g., bucrylate or related polymerizing compound) or microcoils, or by venous embolization, usually by retrograde catheterization through femoral or jugular access or by a transtorcular approach with placement of microcoils.* Technological advances may further improve treatment and outcome. Currently, the most common initial therapeutic intervention is the transarterial femoral approach with delivery of a liquid adhesive agent.[79] Multiple procedures are usually necessary. In the large series shown in Table 23-9, three procedures per patient, on average, were required.[91]

ARACHNOID CYSTS

Arachnoid cysts, although fundamentally developmental anomalies, are best discussed briefly in this context because their clinical presentation in the newborn most closely mimics a space-occupying lesion. These *congenital* or *primary* arachnoid cysts should be distinguished from arachnoidal cystic collections secondary to hemorrhage or infection. The clinical distinction is usually straightforward. Recognition of arachnoid cysts in the neonatal period has increased markedly in recent years because of the widespread use of fetal cranial ultrasonography and neonatal imaging, especially MRI.

Pathology

Arachnoid cysts are derived from the developing arachnoid and appear to arise by splitting or duplication of the arachnoid.[115] The fine structure of the lining is similar to that of normal arachnoidal cells, which secrete cerebrospinal fluid and cause the expansion often observed in vivo. In some cases, a one-way ball-valve mechanism between the cyst and the subarachnoid space may contribute to the expansion.[116]

The *principal loci* of arachnoid cysts include regions particularly rich in arachnoid, often cisterns. The reported distribution of loci differs according to the age of the infant or child, the means of identification, and the clinical features, if any. Approximately 50% of these cysts are located in the *region of the sylvian fissure* and are often associated with underdevelopment of the anterior superior surface of the temporal lobe.[59,115-118] Whether the temporal abnormality is an associated developmental anomaly or occurs secondary to compression is unknown. Other common sites include the following: the *suprasellar region*, often associated with displacement of the pituitary stalk, hypothalamus, and optic chiasm; the *interhemispheric fissure*, often with agenesis of the corpus callosum; the *supracollicular area*, with tectal compression; the *cerebellopontine angle*, with congenital peripheral nerve paralysis and other signs; and *supracerebellar and infracerebellar areas*, sometimes confused with Dandy-Walker complex (see Chapter 1).[59,115-117,119,120]

Clinical Features

Arachnoid cysts identified in the fetal and neonatal period most often cause no clinical abnormalities. Clinical features, when present, usually consist of

---

*See references 73,75-77,79,83,84,87,89-92,99,101,111-114.

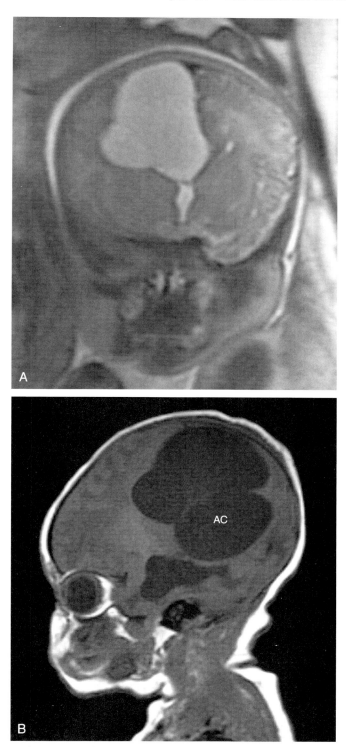

Figure 23-19   Arachnoidal cyst, magnetic resonance imaging (MRI) scans. A, Coronal scan performed in utero at 33 weeks of gestation shows a large arachnoidal cyst in the interhemispheric fissure. **B,** On this postnatal sagittal MRI, the lesion was shown to be continuous with a multilobulated cyst (AC) in the suprasellar region.

various combinations of macrocrania, hydrocephalus, signs of increased intracranial pressure, or, least commonly, neurological abnormalities related to the locus of the cyst (see earlier). Slight to moderate hemiparesis related to the presence of a cyst in the region of the sylvian fissure or elsewhere in the middle cranial fossa is the most common of these abnormalities.[116,117]

The *diagnosis* is often suspected by screening intrauterine or neonatal ultrasonography. The finding of a large, fluid-filled space may mimic an epidermoid lesion or a cystic tumor (e.g., cystic astrocytoma) (Fig. 23-19).

The *prognosis* of arachnoid cysts is largely unknown, because the natural history is obscure. Lesions may regress antenatally.[116] Many other cysts remain stationary and do not cause neurological symptoms. Nevertheless, some arachnoid cysts clearly increase in size and lead to macrocephaly or hydrocephalus, or both, or to parenchymal signs, progressive hemiparesis, intractable epilepsy, hypothalamic syndromes, or posterior fossa disorders, according to the site of the lesion.

Management

Management of arachnoid cysts is controversial because of uncertainties about natural history. However, in the neonatal period, the clearest indications for intervention are signs of increased intracranial pressure (vomiting, bulging fontanelle, rapid head growth) and prominent or progressive parenchymal signs. Currently, the two leading neurosurgical interventions are craniotomy, usually with fenestration of the cyst to produce communication with the subarachnoid space, and cyst-peritoneal shunt, especially with a programmable valve.[116,117] These approaches have eliminated signs of increased intracranial pressure, have restored normal head growth, and have often reversed or at least halted the progression of parenchymal signs.

REFERENCES

1. Wakai S, Arai T, Nagai M: Congenital brain tumors, *Surg Neurol* 21:597-609, 1984.
2. Radkowski MA, Naidich TP, Tomita T, Byrd SE, et al: Neonatal brain tumors: CT and MR findings, *J Comput Assist Tomogr* 12:10-20, 1988.
3. Fort DW, Rushing EJ: Congenital central nervous system tumors, *J Child Neurol* 12:157-164, 1997.
4. Rickert CH, Probst-Cousin S, Gullotta F: Primary intracranial neoplasms of infancy and early childhood, *Childs Nerv Syst* 13:507-513, 1997.
5. Rickert CH: Neuropathology and prognosis of foetal brain tumours, *Acta Neuropathol* 98:567-576, 1999.
6. Isaacs H: II. Perinatal brain tumors: A review of 250 cases, *Pediatr Neurol* 27:333-342, 2002.
7. Isaacs H: I. Perinatal brain tumors: A review of 250 cases, *Pediatr Neurol* 27:249-261, 2002.
8. Erman T, Gocer IA, Erdogan S, Gunes Y, et al: Congenital intracranial immature teratoma of the lateral ventricle: A case report and review of the literature, *Neurol Res* 27:53-56, 2005.
9. Isaacs H Jr: Perinatal (fetal and neonatal) germ cell tumors, *J Pediatr Surg* 39:1003-1013, 2004.
10. Bergsagel DJ, Finegold MJ, Butel JS, Kupsky WJ, et al: DNA sequences similar to those of simian virus 40 in ependymomas and choroid plexus tumors of childhood, *N Engl J Med* 326:988-993, 1992.
11. Janisch W, Haas JF, Schreiber D, Gerlach H: Primary central nervous system tumors in stillborns and infants, *J Neurooncol* 2:113-116, 1984.
12. Jellinger K, Sunder-Plassman M: Connatal intracranial tumors, *Neuropadiatrie* 4:46-63, 1973.
13. Lipman SP, Pretorius DH, Rumack CM, Manco-Johnson ML: Fetal intracranial teratoma: US diagnosis of three cases and a review of the literature, *Radiology* 157:491-494, 1985.
14. Haddad SF, Menezes AH, Bell WE, Godersky JC, et al: Brain tumors occurring before 1 year of age: A retrospective review of 22 cases in an 11-year period (1977-1987), *Neurosurgery* 29:8-13, 1991.
15. Kumar R, Tekkok IH, Jones RA: Intracranial tumours in the first 18 months of life, *Childs Nerv Syst* 6:371-374, 1990.
16. DiRocco C, Iannelli A, Ceddia A: Intracranial tumors of the first year of life, *Childs Nerv Syst* 7:150-153, 1991.
17. Galassi E, Godano U, Cavallo M, Donati R, et al: Intracranial tumors during the 1st year of life, *Childs Nerv Syst* 5:288-298, 1989.
18. Arnstein LH, Boldrey E, Naffziger HC: A case report and survey of brain tumors during the neonatal period, *J Neurosurg* 8:315-319, 1951.
19. Takaku A, Kodama N, Ohara H, Hori S: Brain tumor in newborn babies, *Childs Brain* 4:365-375, 1978.
20. Raskind R, Beigel F: Brain tumors in early infancy: Probably congenital in origin, *J Pediatr* 65:727-732, 1964.
21. Sherer DM, Abramowicz JS, Eggers PC, Metlay LA, et al: Prenatal ultrasonographic diagnosis of intracranial teratoma and massive craniomegaly with associated high-output cardiac failure, *Am J Obstet Gynecol* 168:97-99, 1993.
22. Anderson DR, Falcone S, Bruce JH, Mejidas AA, et al: Radiologic-pathologic correlation. Congenital choroid plexus papillomas, *AJNR Am J Neuroradiol* 16:2072-2076, 1995.
23. DiRocco C, Iannelli A: Poor outcome of bilateral congenital choroid plexus papillomas with extreme hydrocephalus, *Eur Neurol* 37:33-37, 1997.
24. Costa JM, Ley L, Claramunt E, Lafuente J: Choroid plexus papillomas of the III ventricle in infants: Report of three cases, *Childs Nerv Syst* 13:244-249, 1997.
25. Narita T, Kurotaki H, Hashimoto T, Ogawa Y: Congenital oligodendroglioma: A case report of a 34th-gestational week fetus with immunohistochemical study and review of the literature, *Hum Pathol* 28:1213-1217, 1997.
26. Rickert CH, Probst-Cousin S, Louwen F, Feldt B, et al: Congenital immature teratoma of the fetal brain, *Childs Nerv Syst* 13:556-559, 1997.
27. Chien YH, Tsao PN, Lee WT, Peng SF, et al: Congenital intracranial teratoma, *Pediatr Neurol* 22:72-74, 2000.
28. Mazouni C, Porcu-Buisson G, Girard N, Sakr R, et al: Intrauterine brain teratoma: A case report of imaging (US, MRI) with neuropathologic correlations, *Prenat Diagn* 23:104-107, 2003.
29. Chadduck WM, Boop FA, Blankenship JB, Husain M: Meningioma and sagittal craniosynostosis in an infant: Case report, *Neurosurgery* 30:441-442, 1992.
30. Hurst RW, McIlhenny J, Park TS, Thomas WO: Neonatal craniopharyngioma: CT and ultrasonographic features, *J Comput Assist Tomogr* 12:858-861, 1988.
31. Richmond BK, Schmidt JH: Congenital cystic supratentorial hemangioblastoma: Case report, *J Neurosurg* 82:113-115, 1995.
32. Hundt C, Auberger K, Munch G, Willemsen UF, et al: Brain hemangiomas of infancy, *J Neuroimaging* 7:81-85, 1997.
33. Winters JL, Wilson D, Davis DG: Congenital glioblastoma multiforme: A report of three cases and a review of the literature, *J Neurol Sci* 188:13-19, 2001.
34. Trehan G, Bruge H, Vinchon M, Khalil C, et al: MR imaging in the diagnosis of desmoplastic infantile tumor: Retrospective study of six cases, *AJNR Am J Neuroradiol* 25:1028-1033, 2004.
35. Oexle K, Dammann O, Bechmann B, Vortmeyer AO, et al: Intracranial chordoma in a neonate, *Eur J Pediatr* 151:336-338, 1992.
36. Alfonso I, Lopez PF, Cullen RF, Martin-Jimenez R, et al: Spinal cord involvement in encephalocranio-cutaneous lipomatosis, *Pediatr Neurol* 2:380-384, 1986.
37. Barth PG, Stam FC, Hack W, Delemarre-van de Waal HA: Gliomatosis cerebri in a newborn, *Neuropediatrics* 19:197-200, 1988.
38. Painter MJ, Pang D, Ahdab-Barmada M, Bergman I: Connatal brain tumors in patients with tuberous sclerosis, *Neurosurgery* 14:570-573, 1984.
39. Hahn JS, Bejar R, Gladson CL: Neonatal subependymal giant cell astrocytoma associated with tuberous sclerosis: MRI, CT, and ultrasound correlation, *Neurology* 41:124-128, 1991.
40. Boechat MI, Kangarloo H, Diament MJ, Krauthamer R: Lipoma of the corpus callosum: Sonographic appearance, *J Clin Ultrasound* 11:447-448, 1983.
41. Wakai S, Nakamura K, Arai T, Nagai M: Extracerebral neural tissue mass in the middle cranial fossa extending into the oropharynx in a neonate, *J Neurosurg* 59:692-696, 1983.
42. Oikawa S, Sakamoto K, Kobayashi N: A neonatal huge subependymal giant cell astrocytoma: Case report, *Neurosurgery* 35:748-750, 1994.
43. Saxonhouse MA, Yachnis AT, Burchfield DJ, Quisling R, et al: Neonatal hypothalamic hamartoma: A differentiating nonlethal hamartoblastoma, *J Neurosurg* 103:277-281, 2005.
44. Thompson WD Jr, Kosnik EJ: Spontaneous regression of a diffuse brainstem lesion in the neonate: Report of two cases and review of the literature, *J Neurosurg* 102:65-71, 2005.
44a. Brat DJ, Shehata BM, Castellano-Sanchez AA, Hawkins C, et al: Congenital glioblastoma: a clinicopathologic and genetic analysis, *Brain Pathol* 17:276-281, 2007.
45. Jooma R, Kendall BE, Hayward RD: Intracranial tumors in neonates: A report of seventeen cases, *Surg Neurol* 21:165-170, 1984.
46. Roosen N, Deckert M, Nicola N, Wechsler W, et al: Congenital anaplastic astrocytoma with favorable prognosis, *J Neurosurg* 69:604-609, 1988.
47. Rothman SM, Nelson JS, DeVivo DC, Coxe WS: Congenital astrocytoma presenting with intracerebral hematoma, *J Neurosurg* 51:237-239, 1979.
48. Rutledge SL, Snead OC, Morawetz R, Chandra-Sekar B: Brain tumors presenting as a seizure disorder in infants, *J Child Neurol* 2:214-219, 1987.
49. Ellams ID, Neuhauser G, Agnoli AL: Congenital intracranial neoplasms, *Childs Nerv Syst* 2:165-168, 1986.
50. Tomita T, McLone DG, Flannery AM: Choroid plexus papillomas of neonates, infants and children, *Pediatr Neurosci* 14:23-30, 1988.
51. Lippa C, Abroms JF, Davidson R, DeGiorlami U: Congenital choroid plexus papilloma of the fourth ventricle, *J Child Neurol* 4:127-130, 1989.
52. Asai A, Hoffman HJ, Hendrick EB, Humphreys RP, et al: Primary intracranial neoplasms in the first year of life, *Childs Nerv Syst* 5:230-233, 1989.
53. Venes JL: A proposal for management of congenital brain tumors. In Marlin AE, editor: *Concepts in Pediatric Neurosurgery*, Basel: 1985, Karger.
54. Shafrir Y, Kaufman BA: Quadriplegia after chiropractic manipulation in an infant with congenital torticollis caused by a spinal cord astrocytoma, *J Pediatr* 120:266-269, 1992.
55. Pascual-Castroviejo I: Congenital tumors or malformations. In Pascual-Castroviejo I, editor: *Spinal Tumors in Children and Adolescents*, New York: 1990, Raven Press.

56. Kaufman BA, Park TS: Congenital spinal cord astrocytomas, *Childs Nerv Syst* 8:389-393, 1992.

57. Sandbank U: Congenital astrocytoma, *J Pathol Bacteriol* 84:226-228, 1962.

58. Harmon BH, Yap Ma: One-month-old infant with increasing head size. In Brogdon BG, editor: *Cases from the Wards*. Philadelphia: 1990, JB Lippincott.

59. Barkovich AJ: *Pediatric Neuroimaging*, 4th ed. Philadelphia: 2005, Lippincott Williams & Wilkins.

60. Cohen ME, Duffner PK: Brain tumors in children less than 2 years of age. In Familusi J, Fukuyama Y, editors: *Brain Tumors in Children*, New York: 1984, Raven Press.

61. Johnson DL: Management of choroid plexus tumors in children, *Pediatr Neurosci* 15:195-206, 1989.

62. Ventureyra EC, Herder S: Neonatal intracranial teratoma, *J Neurosurg* 59:879-883, 1983.

63. Rivera-Luna R, Medina-Sanson A, Leal-Leal C, Pantoja-Guillen F, et al: Brain tumors in children under 1 year of age: Emphasis on the relationship of prognostic factors, *Childs Nerv Syst* 19:311-314, 2003.

64. Geyer JR, Sposto R, Jennings M, Boyett JM, et al: Multiagent chemotherapy and deferred radiotherapy in infants with malignant brain tumors: A report from the Children's Cancer Group, *J Clin Oncol* 23:7621-7631, 2005.

65. Kalifa C, Grill J: The therapy of infantile malignant brain tumors: Current status, *J Neurooncol* 75:279-285, 2005.

66. Ellenberg L, McComb JG, Siegel SE, Stowe S: Factors affecting intellectual outcome in pediatric brain tumor patients, *Neurosurgery* 21:638-644, 1987.

67. Spunberg JJ, Chang CH, Goldman M, Auricchio E, et al: Quality of long-term survival following irradiation for intracranial tumors in children under the age of two, *Int J Radiat Oncol Biol Phys* 7:727-736, 1981.

68. Meadows AT, Massari DJ, Fergusson J, Gordon J, et al: Declines in I.Q. scores and cognitive dysfunctions in children with acute lymphocytic leukaemia treated with cranial irradiation, *Lancet* 2:1015-1018, 1981.

69. Waber DP, Urion DK, Tarbell NJ, Niemeyer C, et al: Late effects of central nervous system treatment of childhood acute lymphoblastic leukemia are sex-dependent, *Dev Med Child Neurol* 32:238-248, 1990.

70. Waber DP, Gioia G, Paccia J, Sherman B, et al: Sex differences in cognitive processing in children treated with CNS prophylaxis for acute lymphoblastic leukemia (ALL), *J Pediatr Psychol* 15:105-122, 1990.

71. Loeffler JS, Rossitch E, Siddon R, Moore MR, et al: Role of stereotactic radiosurgery with a linear accelerator in treatment of intracranial arteriovenous malformations and tumors in children, *Pediatrics* 85:774-782, 1990.

72. Pollack IF: Brain tumors in children, *N Engl J Med* 331:1500-1507, 1994.

73. Wisoff JH, Berenstein A, Choi IS, Friedman D, et al: Management of vein of Galen malformations. In Marlin AE, editor: *Concepts in Pediatric Neurosurgery*, Basel: 1990, Karger.

74. Hoffman HJ, Chuang S, Hendrick B, Humphreys RP: Aneurysms of the vein of Galen: Experience at the Hospital for Sick Children, *J Neurosurg* 57:316-322, 1982.

75. Lylyk P, Vinuela F, Dion JE, Duckwiler G, et al: Therapeutic alternatives for vein of Galen vascular malformations, *J Neurosurg* 78:438-445, 1993.

76. Lasjaunias P: *Vascular Diseases in Neonates, Infants, and Children*, Berlin: 1997, Springer-Verlag.

77. Johnston IH, Whittle IR, Besser M, Morgan MK: Vein of Galen malformation: Diagnosis and management, *Neurosurgery* 20:747-758, 1987.

78. Raybaud CA, Strother CM, Hald JK: Aneurysms of the vein of Galen: Embryonic considerations and anatomical features relating to the pathogenesis of the malformation, *Neuroradiology* 31:109-128, 1989.

79. Gailloud P, O'Riordan DP, Burger I, Levrier O, et al: Diagnosis and management of vein of Galen aneurysmal malformations, *J Perinatol* 25:542-551, 2005.

80. Lasjaunias P, Garcia-Monaco R, Rodesch G, Terbrugge K: Deep venous drainage in great cerebral vein (vein of Galen) absence and malformations, *Neuroradiology* 33:234-238, 1991.

81. Takashima S, Becker LE: Neuropathology of cerebral arteriovenous malformations in children, *J Neurol Neurosurg Psychiatry* 43:380-385, 1980.

82. Norman MG, Becker LE: Cerebral damage in neonates resulting from arteriovenous malformations in the vein of Galen, *J Neurol Neurosurg Psychiatry* 37:252-258, 1974.

83. Yamashita Y, Abe T, Ohara N, Maruoka T, et al: Successful treatment of neonatal aneurysmal dilation of the vein of Galen: The role of prenatal diagnosis and trans-arterial embolization, *Neuroradiology* 34:457-459, 1992.

84. Lasjaunias P, Garcia-Monaco R, Rodesch G, Ter Brugge K, et al: Vein of Galen malformation: Endovascular management of 43 cases, *Childs Nerv Syst* 7:360-367, 1991.

85. Yamashita Y, Nakamura Y, Okudera T, Nishiyori A, et al: Neuroradiological and pathological studies on neonatal aneurysmal dilation of the vein of Galen, *J Child Neurol* 5:45-48, 1990.

86. Baenziger O, Martin E, Willi U, Fanconi S, et al: Prenatal brain atrophy due to a giant vein of Galen malformation, *Neuroradiology* 35:105-106, 1993.

87. Horowitz BM, Jungreis CA, Quisling RG, Pollack I: Vein of Galen aneurysms: A review and current perspective, *AJNR Am J Neuroradiol* 15:1486-1496, 1994.

88. de Koning TJ, Meijboom EJ, de Vries LS, Gooskens R, et al: Arteriovenous malformation of the vein of Galen in three neonates: Emphasis on associated early ischaemic brain damage, *Eur J Pediatr* 156:228-229, 1997.

89. Nakano S, Agid R, Klurfan P, dos Santos Souza MP, et al: Limitations and technical considerations of endovascular treatment in neonates with high-flow arteriovenous shunts presenting with congestive heart failure: Report of two cases, *Childs Nerv Syst* 22:13-17, 2006.

90. Wong FY, Mitchell PJ, Tress BM, Dargaville PA, etal: Hemodynamic disturbances associated with endovascular embolization in newborn infants with vein of Galen malformation, *J Perinatol* 26:13-17, 2006.

91. Fullerton HJ, Aminoff AR, Ferriero DM, Gupta N, et al: Neurodevelopmental outcome after endovascular treatment of vein of Galen malformations, *Neurology* 61:1386-1390, 2003.

92. Frawley GP, Dargaville PA, Mitchell PJ, Tress BM, et al: Clinical course and medical management of neonates with severe cardiac failure related to vein of Galen malformation, *Arch Dis Child Fetal Neonatal Ed* 87:F144-F149, 2002.

93. Hirano A, Solomon S: Arteriovenous aneurysm of the vein of Galen, *Arch Neurol* 3:589-593, 1960.

94. Gomez MR, Shitten CF, Nolke A: Aneurysmal malformation of the great vein of Galen causing heart failure in early infancy: Report of five cases, *Pediatrics* 31:400-411, 1963.

95. Watson DG, Smith RR, Brann AW: Arteriovenous malformation of the vein of Galen, *Am J Dis Child* 130:520-525, 1976.

96. Iannucci AM, Buonanno F, Rizzuto N: Arteriovenous aneurysm of the vein of Galen, *J Neurol Sci* 40:29-37, 1979.

97. Schum TR, Meyer GA, Grausz JP, Glaspey JC: Neonatal intracranial ventricular hemorrhage due to an intracranial arteriovenous malformation: A case report, *Pediatrics* 64:242-244, 1979.

98. O'Donnabhain D, Duff DF: Aneurysms of the vein of Galen, *Arch Dis Child* 64:1612-1617, 1989.

99. Rodesch G, Hui F, Alvarez H, Tanaka A, et al: Prognosis of antenatally diagnosed vein of Galen aneurysmal malformations, *Childs Nerv Syst* 10:79-83, 1994.

100. Lasjaunias PL, Alvarez H, Rodesch G, Garcia-Monaco R, et al: Aneurysmal malformations of the vein of Galen, *Interv Neuroradiol* 2:15-26, 1996.

101. Friedman DM, Verma R, Madrid M, Wisoff JH, et al: Recent improvement in outcome using transcatheter embolization techniques for neonatal aneurysmal malformations of the vein of Galen, *Pediatrics* 91:583-586, 1993.

102. Meyers PM, Halbach VV, Phatouros CP, Dowd CF, et al: Hemorrhagic complications in vein of Galen malformations, *Ann Neurol* 47:748-755, 2000.

103. Mullaart RA, Daniels O, Hopman JC: Ultrasound detection of congenital arteriovenous aneurysm of the great cerebral vein of Galen, *Eur J Pediatr* 139:195, 1982.

104. Schwechheimer K, Kuhl G: Arteriovenous angioma of the vein of Galen causing cardiac failure in the neonate, *Neuropediatrics* 14:184, 1983.

105. Cubberley DA, Jaffe RB, Nixon GW: Sonographic demonstration of galenic arteriovenous malformations in the neonate, *AJNR Am J Neuroradiol* 3:435-439, 1982.

106. Langer R, Kaufmann HJ: Arteriovenous malformation of the great cerebral vein of Galen in a newborn, *Eur J Pediatr* 146:87-89, 1987.

107. Abbitt PL, Hurst RW, Ferguson RDG, McIlhenny J, et al: The role of ultrasound in the management of vein of Galen aneurysms in infancy, *Neuroradiology* 32:86-89, 1990.

108. Deeg KH, Scharf J: Colour Doppler imaging of arteriovenous malformation of the vein of Galen in a newborn, *Neuroradiology* 32:60-63, 1990.

109. Vaksmann G, Decoulx E, Mauran P, Jardin A, et al: Evaluation of vein of Galen arteriovenous malformations in newborns by two-dimensional ultrasound, pulsed and colour Doppler method, *Eur J Pediatr* 148:510-512, 1989.

110. Tessler FN, Dion J, Vinuela F, Perrella RR, et al: Cranial arteriovenous malformations in neonates: Color Doppler imaging with angiographic correlation, *AJR Am J Roentgenol* 153:1027-1030, 1989.

111. McCord FB, Shields MD, McNeil A, Halliday HL, et al: Cerebral arteriovenous malformation in a neonate: Treatment by embolisation, *Arch Dis Child* 62:1273-1275, 1987.

112. King WA, Wackym PA, Vinuela F, Peacock W: Management of vein of Galen aneurysms: Combined surgical and endovascular approach, *Childs Nerv Syst* 5:208-211, 1989.

113. Miller VS, Roach ES: Embolization and radiosurgical treatment of cerebral arteriovenous malformations, *Int Pediatr* 7:173-180, 1992.

114. Swanstrom S, Flodmark O, Lasjaunias P: Conditions for treatment of cerebral arteriovenous malformation associated with ectasia of the vein of Galen in the newborn, *Acta Paediatr* 83:255-257, 1994.

115. Harding BN, Surtees R: Metabolic and neurodegenerative diseases of childhood. In Graham DI, Lantos PL, editors: *Greenfield's Neuropathology*, 7, London: 2002, Arnold Publishers.

116. Gosalakkal JA: Intracranial arachnoid cysts in children: A review of pathogenesis, clinical features, and management, *Pediatr Neurol* 26:93-98, 2002.

117. Germano A, Caruso G, Caffo M, Baldari S, et al: The treatment of large supratentorial arachnoid cysts in infants with cyst-peritoneal shunting and Hakim programmable valve, *Childs Nerv Syst* 19:166-173, 2003.

118. Arriola G, Castro P, Verdu A: Familial arachnoid cysts, *Pediatr Neurol* 33:146-148, 2005.

119. Balsubramaniam C, Laurent J, Rouah E, Armstrong D, et al: Congenital arachnoid cysts in children, *Pediatr Neurosci* 15:223-228, 1989.

120. Erman T, Demirhindi H, Gocer AI, Akgul E, et al: Congenital peripheral facial palsy associated with cerebellopontine angle arachnoid cyst, *Pediatr Neurosurg* 40:297-300, 2004.

DRUGS AND THE DEVELOPING NERVOUS SYSTEM

Chapter 24

Teratogenic Effects of Drugs and Passive Addiction

Drugs may exert a major impact on the developing central nervous system (CNS) in a variety of direct and indirect ways. The two most important mechanisms are *teratogenic effects* and the development of *passive addiction*. In this chapter, I consider, under the term *teratogenic effect*, any disturbance of CNS development. In many instances, the precise nature of the disturbance remains to be defined. *Passive addiction* refers to the state of physical dependence that develops in the fetus exposed to a maternal source of drug. The hallmark of this dependence is the occurrence of a withdrawal syndrome after birth and the consequent cessation of the maternal supply of the drug.

MAJOR DRUGS IMPLICATED IN TERATOGENIC EFFECTS ON THE CENTRAL NERVOUS SYSTEM AND DEVELOPMENT OF PASSIVE ADDICTION

Numerous neuroactive drugs can be implicated in the genesis of neural teratogenic effects, in the development of passive addiction, or in both processes (Table 24-1). Teratogenic effects are observed most clearly after maternal ingestion of several anticonvulsants, alcohol, the vitamin A analogue, isotretinoin, and cocaine. (Although disturbances of brain development or later cognitive function, or both, have been suggested to follow maternal exposure to tobacco, tobacco smoke, and polychlorinated biphenyls, more data are needed to establish the direct neurological teratogenicity of these agents.[1-4])

Passive addiction is observed particularly prominently as a result of maternal ingestion of certain narcotic-analgesics, especially heroin and methadone, but also of selective serotonin reuptake inhibitors (SSRIs) and certain sedative-hypnotics, especially barbiturates (see Table 24-1). Less commonly recognized causes of passive addiction are other sedative antianxiety agents (e.g., diazepam [Valium], chlordiazepoxide [Librium], hydroxyzine [Atarax], and ethchlorvynol [Placidyl]), tricyclic antidepressants, analgesics (e.g., propoxyphene [Darvon], pentazocine [Talwin], and codeine), and combinations of drugs (e.g., "T's and blues," which are pentazocine [T for Talwin] and tripelennamine). The most commonly used drug of all, alcohol, also can result in passive addiction.

DRUGS WITH TERATOGENIC EFFECTS

Anticonvulsant Drugs

Anticonvulsant drugs administered to the mother may exert three major adverse effects on the fetal and neonatal CNS (Table 24-2): (1) a teratogenic effect, manifested by a constellation of specific defects (dependent, in part, on the specific class of anticonvulsant drug); (2) a coagulation disturbance, manifested by neonatal hemorrhage, including intracranial hemorrhage; and (3) passive addiction, manifested by a neonatal withdrawal syndrome when the supply of drug (i.e., barbiturate) is eliminated by the process of birth. The first of these effects is the subject of this section, and the last is the subject of a later section. However, before reviewing the teratogenic syndromes associated with certain anticonvulsant drugs, I briefly review the second of these three adverse effects (i.e., the coagulation disturbance and its role in the genesis of neonatal hemorrhage).

Neonatal Hemorrhage

Neonatal hemorrhage is a recognized complication of the maternal administration of anticonvulsant drugs.[5-25] The drugs incriminated are hepatic enzyme inducers and have included *hydantoins, barbiturates, primidone* (which is metabolized to phenobarbital in vivo) and *carbamazepine*. In a series of 111 infants born to epileptic women who were treated with phenytoin or phenobarbital, 8 infants exhibited "severe" bleeding.[19] In this syndrome, the infant develops hemorrhage shortly after birth. This *early onset* is unlike hemorrhagic disease of the newborn secondary to vitamin K deficiency. Sites of hemorrhage are, in order of decreasing frequency, skin, liver, gastrointestinal tract, intracranial sites, and thorax. *Intracranial hemorrhage* has been reported in 20% to 25% of patients with hemorrhage. The course may be fulminating, and approximately 40% of reported infants have died. Clotting studies demonstrate diminution of the vitamin K–dependent clotting factors (factors II, VII, IX, and X), with prolongation of either the prothrombin time or partial thromboplastin time, or both. Vitamin K levels in cord blood are depressed, as evidenced by the presence of PIVKA-II (a protein, induced by vitamin K absence), an incompletely carboxylated, functionally defective form of factor II (prothrombin).[26,27] Indeed, in a

TABLE 24-1	Major Drugs Implicated in Teratogenic Effects on the Central Nervous System and Passive Addiction

Teratogenic Effects
Anticonvulsant drugs
    Hydantoins, barbiturates, primidone, carbamazepine, trimethadione, paramethadione
    Valproate
Alcohol
Isotretinoin
Cocaine

Passive Addiction
Heroin-methadone
Selective serotonin reuptake inhibitors
Barbiturates
Alcohol
Diazepam
Chlordiazepoxide
Tricyclic antidepressants
Ethchlorvynol
Propoxyphene
Pentazocine
"T's and blues"
Codeine

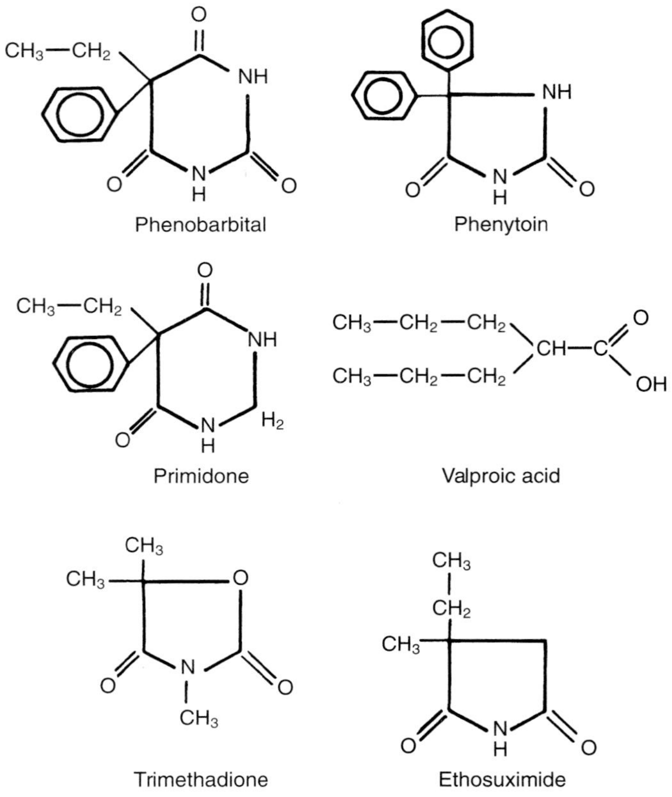

Figure 24-1 Chemical structures of important anticonvulsant drugs. Note the structural similarity of phenobarbital, phenytoin, and primidone; each is composed of a basic five- or six-membered ring and a side chain substitution containing phenol groups. Carbamazepine, not shown in the figure, shares structural similarities. Trimethadione and ethosuximide differ from these drugs by virtue of the aliphatic side chain substitutions. Valproic acid differs markedly from the other anticonvulsant drugs and is essentially a short-chain fatty acid.

study of 24 infants born to mothers who were receiving anticonvulsant therapy during pregnancy, 13 infants (54%) had detectable levels of PIVKA-II, and when the 4 infants exposed to valproate (none of whom had detectable levels of PIVKA-II) were excluded, the incidence was 65%. Moreover, vitamin K levels also were depressed in these infants.[26,27] The findings suggested increased degradation of vitamin K with impaired action of vitamin K on hepatic production of pro-thrombin. The latter results because of insufficient carboxylation of the glutamic acid residues of pro-thrombin, a post-translational event that requires vitamin K. The pathogenetic mechanism by which the anticonvulsants lead to vitamin K deficiency may relate primarily to increased degradation of vitamin K by fetal hepatic microsomal mixed-function oxidase enzymes, known to be inducible by phenytoin, pheno-barbital, primidone, and carbamazepine.[26,27] The similarity in structure of these so-called enzyme-inducible anticonvulsant agents is shown in Figure 24-1.

Nevertheless, *this disorder appears to have become rare*.[28-30] Three reports (total numbers of patients, 105, 204, and 662) showed no increased incidence of

TABLE 24-2	Major Adverse Effects of Anticonvulsant Drugs, Administered during Pregnancy, on the Fetal and Neonatal Central Nervous System

Teratogenic effect, with constellation of specific defects
Coagulation disturbance, with neonatal (intracranial) hemorrhage
Passive addiction, with neonatal withdrawal syndrome (barbiturates)

hemorrhagic complications among women treated with various combinations of phenobarbital, phenytoin, primidone, and carbamazepine during pregnancy. The women were not treated with vitamin K during pregnancy (although the infants received vitamin K at birth). Whether the decline in incidence in this disorder relates to the diminishing use of polytherapy or the increasing use of alternative drugs or related factors is unclear.

Previous *management* of newborn infants whose mothers had been taking anticonvulsant drugs during pregnancy was recommended as follows: (1) consideration of delivery by cesarean section *if* a difficult or traumatic delivery was anticipated, (2) administration of oral vitamin K (10 mg/day) to the mother before delivery during the last month of pregnancy (with parenteral vitamin K administered as soon as possible after the onset of labor if oral vitamin K was not given), (3) administration of vitamin K to the infant intravenously immediately after birth, (4) administration of fresh frozen plasma to the infant if clotting studies were distinctly abnormal, and (5) consideration of exchange transfusion if hemorrhage ensued.[17,19,20,22,23]

Oral supplementation of vitamin K_1 to the mother for 2 to 4 weeks before delivery prevented neonatal coagulation defects in one study,[19] and it prevented the occurrence of detectable levels of PIVKA-II and depressed vitamin K levels in another.[27] However, in view of the more recent studies that indicated no clearly enhanced risk of hemorrhage in infants whose mothers did not receive vitamin K during pregnancy, the need for prenatal vitamin K has been questioned.[29,30] A more selective approach may be preferable (i.e., in pregnancies with a high likelihood of trauma or prematurity or a related risk factor for hemorrhage, prenatal vitamin K could be used).

Teratogenic Potential of Anticonvulsant Drugs

Current information indicates a teratogenic effect of anticonvulsant drugs on the developing fetus. However, establishing this fact, determining the quantitative aspects thereof, and defining the mechanisms involved have been exceptionally difficult for several reasons. First, the prevalence of epilepsy among pregnant women is relatively low. In a series from the Mayo Clinic of Rochester, Minnesota, that spanned 35 years, only approximately 4 of 1000 live births were to women with active epilepsy.[31] Second, the incidence of congenital malformations is relatively low, and the reported incidence for a given malformation varies, depending on the length of the follow-up period and the vigor with which the malformation is sought. Third, the dose of the drug and the timing of its administration during pregnancy are probably critical and are not always known. Fourth, multiple anticonvulsant drugs (i.e., polytherapy) commonly are used in the treatment of the epileptic patient. Delineation of the teratogenic potential of each drug or combinations of drugs can be very difficult. Fifth, maternal seizures and their attendant metabolic consequences may play an alternative or additive deleterious role. Sixth, genetic factors relating to the cerebral disorder underlying the epilepsy may be considerable. Seventh, genetic factors in maternal or fetal disposition of anticonvulsant drugs or in important metabolic effects of the drugs may also be considerable. Other factors could be cited, although the aforementioned are probably the most important. Despite these problems, certain conclusions seem justified.

A relationship between the maternal ingestion of anticonvulsant drugs and the occurrence of major congenital malformations was suggested initially by results of careful epidemiological studies in the 1970s and 1980s.[16,22-24,32-53] Early work, based largely on retrospective methods but with patient numbers measured in the thousands, suggested a slightly greater than twofold higher incidence of major malformations in the children of epileptic women who were taking anticonvulsant drugs versus those not taking medication or in nonepileptic women. Subsequent studies in the 1990s supported the initial work.[22,24,32,47-51] The earlier work also showed no increase in major malformations in the children of epileptic women who were not taking antiepileptic therapy or who were treated later than the first trimester.

TABLE 24-3   **Major Congenital Malformations as a Function of Maternal Ingestion of Anticonvulsant Drugs***

Drug Exposure	MCM Rate	Adjusted Odds Ratio (95% CI)	P Value
None	3.5%	1.0	—
Monotherapy	3.7%	1.03 (0.49–2.17)	.94
Carbamazepine	2.2%	1.0	—
Valproate	6.2%	2.97 (1.65–5.35)	.001
Lamotrigine	3.2%	1.71 (0.88–3.32)	.114
Phenytoin	3.7%	1.60 (0.43–5.95)	.484
Polytherapy	6.0%	1.76 (0.80–3.86)	.16
Valproate/ carbamazepine	8.8%	N/A	N/A
Valproate/ lamotrigine	9.6%	N/A	N/A
Carbamazepine/ lamotrigine	0.0%	N/A	N/A

*Total population was 3607.
CI, confidence interval; MCM, major congenital malformation; N/A, not available.
Data from Morrow J, Russell A, Guthrie E, Parsons L, et al: Malformation risks of antiepileptic drugs in pregnancy: A prospective study from the UK Epilepsy and Pregnancy Register, *J Neurol Neurosurg Psychiatry* 77:193–198, 2006.

The advent in recent years of large registries of pregnant epileptic women in North America, Europe, the United Kingdom, and elsewhere has begun to clarify the risk of major malformations in the children of epileptic women treated with anticonvulsant drugs.[54-64a] Although the data are not perfectly consistent, several conclusions appear justified (Table 24-3). Thus, the risk of monotherapy in the genesis of major malformations ("involving an abnormality of essential embryonic structure requiring significant treatment and present at birth or discovered during the first 6 weeks of life") is nil or relatively minor, except for *valproate* (see later). Moreover, *polytherapy* accentuates the risk of major malformations, but this accentuation has been noted only with regimens that included valproate (see Table 24-3).[63,64a]

The most common *major malformations* reported in recent large series are neural tube defects, cardiac anomalies, facial clefts, hypospadias and other genitourinary anomalies, gastrointestinal anomalies, and skeletal deficits (Table 24-4).[54,63,64,64a] This distribution of malformations confirms earlier reports based on generally smaller populations studied.[22-24,32,46,50]

These epidemiological studies have been of major importance in defining *individual* major malformations associated with the use of anticonvulsant drugs. However, the nature of such large surveys, which usually and necessarily involve many observers and the determination of abnormal findings by various methodologies, makes difficult the detection of a *constellation or cluster of abnormalities*, such as the so-called *fetal hydantoin syndrome*. This syndrome is a sequela to the use of major anticonvulsant drugs during pregnancy and provides insight into the teratogenic mechanisms of these agents.

TABLE 24-4   **Types of Major Congenital Malformation by Antiepileptic Drugs**

Drug	Cases (*N*)	PERCENTAGE WITH MALFORMATION			
		NTD	Cardiac	Facial Cleft	Hypospadias/Gut
Carbamazepine	900	0.2%	0.7%	0.4%	0.2%
Valproate	715	1.0%	0.7%	1.5%	1.3%
Lamotrigine	647	0.2%	0.6%	0.2%	0.9%
Phenytoin	82	0.0%	1.2%	1.2%	0.0%

NTD, neural tube defect.
Data from Morrow J, Russell A, Guthrie E, Parsons L, et al: Malformation risks of antiepileptic drugs in pregnancy: A prospective study from the UK Epilepsy and Pregnancy Register, *J Neurol Neurosurg Psychiatry* 77:193–198, 2006.

Fetal Hydantoin Syndrome

Although the results of the epidemiological studies just reviewed emphasized the occurrence of specific major malformations (e.g., congenital heart disease and cleft lip or palate), careful observation of individual cases led to the early recognition of a constellation of anomalies that appeared to be characteristic of intrauterine exposure to certain major anticonvulsant drugs.[16,65] In subsequent studies, the syndrome was defined in more detail, with emphasis on the occurrence of mild to moderate growth disturbance, delayed neurological development, a characteristic craniofacial appearance, and hypoplastic distal phalanges and nails.[22,24,54,66-75] Although most of the patients in the cases initially reported were exposed to phenytoin in combination with barbiturates or, less commonly, primidone, the syndrome (or at least many of the features thereof) has been observed with exposure to phenytoin alone, and hence the term *fetal hydantoin syndrome* has been used commonly. However, the observation of a similar clinical syndrome in 22 infants exposed to barbiturates but not to phenytoin,[76,77] in several infants exposed to primidone alone,[78-80] and in infants exposed to carbamazepine[81-83] suggests that the so-called fetal hydantoin syndrome can be caused by at least these additional anticonvulsants. Valproic acid, which can interfere with the metabolism of these drugs (see later discussion), may potentiate their teratogenic potential, although more data are needed on this issue. The structural similarities of phenytoin, phenobarbital, primidone, and carbamazepine are noteworthy (see Fig. 24-1), and primidone is metabolized, in part, to phenobarbital in vivo. *For the sake of simplicity, I use the term fetal hydantoin syndrome rather than the more inclusive term fetal hydantoin-barbiturate-primidone-carbamazepine syndrome or the less precise terms fetal antiepileptic drug syndrome, fetal anticonvulsant drug syndrome, and anticonvulsant embryopathy.*

Incidence. The incidence of the fetal hydantoin syndrome is not entirely known, but it is likely to be less than that recorded in earlier reports. In a prospective study of 35 children born to 23 women who were treated with hydantoin anticonvulsant drugs with or without barbiturates, 11% of the children had sufficient features to be classified as having fetal hydantoin syndrome.[68] An *additional* 31% exhibited some features compatible with the prenatal effect of hydantoin.

A matched control evaluation of 104 children, whose mothers had epilepsy and were treated with hydantoins with or without barbiturates, and who were part of the Collaborative Perinatal Project of the National Institute of Neurological and Communicative Disorders and Stroke, resulted in detection of 11 children with the fetal hydantoin syndrome (i.e., a similar percentage to that observed with the smaller prospective study).[68] In another series, 7% of children exposed to phenytoin were affected.[84] Subsequent work has shown that the incidence of the full-blown syndrome is approximately 5% to 10%, although this value remains controversial.[22-24,48,54,75,85-93]

Clinical Features. The clinical features of the fetal hydantoin syndrome include abnormalities of prenatal and postnatal growth, CNS function, craniofacial appearance, and distal limbs (Table 24-5 and Fig. 24-2).[22,39-46,54,65-68,71,73-76,79,85,93-96] Perhaps the most characteristic combination is a relatively small head, ocular hypotelorism, epicanthal folds, midface hypoplasia with broad or depressed nasal bridge, short nose, long upper lip, and flattened maxilla. Ocular hypotelorism and the hypoplastic nails were considered particularly characteristic of phenytoin exposure in prospective studies.[93] The magnitude of the cognitive deficits remains to be determined decisively in large populations, but data suggest that a significant disturbance of intellectual function is not rare. In a recent study of 80 infants exposed in utero to anticonvulsant drugs, the strongest correlation of intelligence with the physical features of the exposed children was the presence of microcephaly, which was associated with a deficit of 23.7 points in full-scale intelligence quotient (IQ).[75] Marginally significant defects in IQ accompanied midface hypoplasia and digital hypoplasia.[75]

Neuropathology. The neuropathological findings of the fetal hydantoin syndrome have not been defined. In the one case with detailed neuropathological study, "generalized gliosis" in the cerebrum may have related to the severe congestive heart failure caused by cardiac anomalies; however, migrational disturbances in the cerebellum were also observed and are of interest in view of the tendency for phenytoin to cause cerebellar injury at more advanced ages.[70] Microcephaly has been reported in 5% to 30% of affected patients, but the cause of the small brain is unknown.

TABLE 24-5 **Clinical Features of 63 Cases of the Fetal Hydantoin Syndrome**

Clinical Features	Percentage Affected*
Growth	
Prenatal growth deficiency	19%
Postnatal growth deficiency	26%
Central Nervous System	
Microcephaly	29%
Developmental delay or mental deficiency	38%[†]
Craniofacial	
Large anterior and posterior fontanel	42%
Metopic ridging	27%
Medial epicanthal folds	46%
Ocular hypertelorism	23%
Broad and/or depressed nasal bridge	54%
Cleft lip and/or palate	5%
Limb	
Nail and/or distal phalangeal hypoplasia	32%
Fingerlike thumb	14%
Other	
Short neck with or without low hairline	18%
Inguinal hernia	14%
Bifid or shawl scrotum	33%
Cardiac defect	8%

*Data are expressed as percentage of those patients for whom information is available.
[†]Includes only those patients 4 years of age or older.
Data from Hill RM, Verniaud WM, Horning MG, McCulley LB, et al: Infants exposed in utero to antiepileptic drugs, *Am J Dis Child* 127:645–653, 1974; and Hanson JW, Smith DW: The fetal hydantoin syndrome, *J Pediatr* 87:285–290, 1975

Pathogenesis. The occurrence of developmental anomalies after intrauterine exposure to major anticonvulsant drugs could relate to maternal seizures, a genetic factor related to epilepsy, or a teratogenic effect related to the action of the anticonvulsant drugs. As indicated previously, the epidemiological data support the notion of a teratogenic effect of anticonvulsant drugs. Hydantoins may be more teratogenic than other agents, but this point is not firmly established. The teratogenic capacity of at least phenytoin and barbiturates is supported by the demonstration that these agents can lead to abnormalities in the rodent that are similar to abnormalities in the human.[22,97-105] Dose-dependent effects can be demonstrated. The possibility that a genetic predisposition contributes to the development of the syndrome is suggested by animal studies,[98,106-109] and it is suggested in the human by the observation of quite variable degrees of the fetal hydantoin syndrome occurring in trizygotic triplets and in heteropaternal dizygotic twins.[72,110] In a careful study of 62 families with fetal hydantoin exposure during two or more pregnancies, in 15 of the families (25%), 1 or more infants were affected, and in the remaining 47 families, none of the infants

was affected.[89] More important, mothers who had a single affected child appeared to be at a much higher risk for having subsequently affected children (9 of 10) than were mothers whose first-born child was unaffected by the hydantoin exposure (1 of 48).

The *mechanism of the teratogenic effect* of phenytoin, phenobarbital, primidone, and carbamazepine may relate to a metabolite of these drugs. Thus, these agents are metabolized to an epoxide by a microsomal monooxygenase that can be induced by the drugs themselves (i.e., autoinduction) (Fig. 24-3).[88,106,107] Epoxides are highly reactive oxidative metabolites that can bind to nucleic acids and can impair developmental processes. These highly reactive compounds are detoxified by epoxide hydrolase, the product of which is the harmless dihydrodiol metabolite. The possibility that low fetal levels of epoxide hydrolase could lead to enhanced levels of the dangerous epoxide and teratogenicity was suggested by the work of Buehler and co-workers.[88,107,111] In a prospective study of 19 pregnancies in women treated with phenytoin monotherapy and monitored by amniocentesis, the occurrence of the fetal hydantoin syndrome was documented in 4 cases with hydrolase activities less than 30% of the standard value, whereas the 15 fetuses with activities more than 30% of the standard value were unaffected (Fig. 24-4). In a later study, the threshold level of activity was suggested to be 35%.[111] The data suggested that infants with lower levels of epoxide hydrolase, perhaps genetically determined, are at markedly increased risk of development of teratogenic levels of the dangerous epoxide derivative. This possibility, as well as the teratogenic potential of the epoxide metabolites, was supported by studies in animals.[107,109] The possible potentiating effect of valproate in the teratogenicity of phenytoin, phenobarbital, primidone, and carbamazepine, suggested by clinical data (see earlier discussion), could relate to the demonstration that valproate can lead to inhibition of the epoxide hydrolase. The data raise the possibility that the fetus especially susceptible to the teratogenic effects of the hydantoin group of drugs could be identified in utero by examination of cultured amniocytes.

Other potential mechanisms of teratogenesis from phenytoin and related anticonvulsant drugs have included disturbances of folate metabolism.[22,24,112] Such a mechanism could underlie the approximately 1% risk of neural tube defects in infants treated with carbamazepine. Folate metabolism may be particularly important in the teratogenic effect of valproate on neural tube formation (see later discussion). Other investigators have suggested a disturbance in certain homeodomain transcription factors.[75]

Management. The major issue in management of fetal hydantoin syndrome is *prevention* and, specifically, counseling of young epileptic women about hydantoin, carbamazepine, and barbiturate use during pregnancy. The importance of preventing seizures during pregnancy is recognized, as is continuation of anticonvulsant medication when the risk of recurrent seizures is considerable (see the later discussion "Guidelines

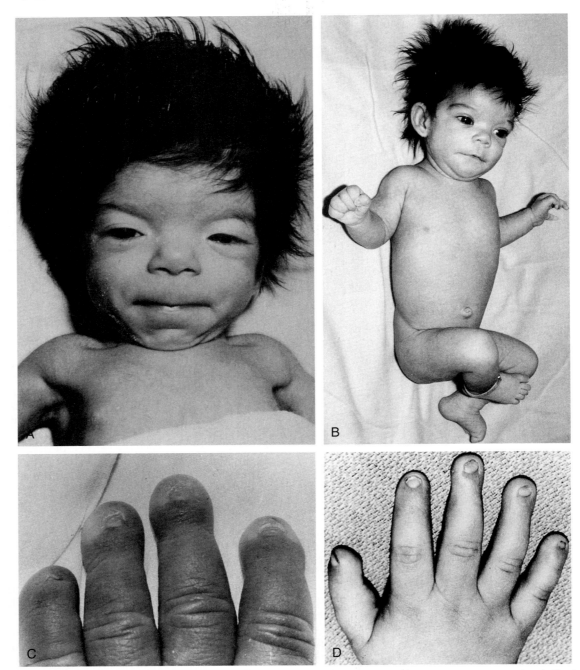

Figure 24-2   **Fetal hydantoin syndrome: clinical appearance**. **A** and **B**, Two different infants with the syndrome; note the similar facial appearance, especially the broad, depressed nasal bridge, the widely spaced eyes, the epicanthal folds, the low hairline at the forehead, and the short neck. **C**, Hand of an affected newborn. Note hypoplasia of nails and distal phalanges. **D**, Hand of an affected child at 1 year of age; some nail growth is evident. *(From Hill RM, Verniaud WM, Horning MG, McCulley LB, et al: Infants exposed in utero to antiepileptic drugs, Am J Dis Child 127:645-653, 1974.)*

Concerning Use of Antiepileptic Drugs during Pregnancy'').

Fetal Trimethadione Syndrome

Fetal trimethadione syndrome refers to the constellation of developmental defects associated with intrauterine exposure to oxazolidine derivatives, usually trimethadione, but also paramethadione; it consists of intrauterine growth retardation, disturbed CNS development, a characteristic craniofacial appearance, and

cardiac, genitourinary, and, to a lesser extent, other anomalies.[16,46,69,113-123] *This syndrome now is rare* because trimethadione and paramethadione have been supplanted by other anticonvulsant drugs. The teratogenic capacity of oxazolidines, particularly trimethadione, is very pronounced, and it is curious that this capacity was not recognized until approximately 1970.[113] This delay may have related to two major factors. First, petit mal seizures are infrequent in adult patients, and thus, in contrast to phenytoin

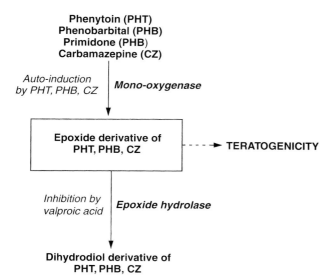

Phenytoin (PHT)
Phenobarbital (PHB)
Primidone (PHB)
Carbamazepine (CZ)

*Auto-induction
by PHT, PHB, CZ* | **Mono-oxygenase**

Epoxide derivative of
PHT, PHB, CZ ----→ TERATOGENICITY

*Inhibition by
valproic acid* | ***Epoxide hydrolase***

Dihydrodiol derivative of
PHT, PHB, CZ

Figure 24-3 Potential mechanism of teratogenic effect of major anticonvulsant drugs. Generation of epoxide derivative is catalyzed by a mono-oxygenase that is induced by the drugs themselves (i.e., autoinduction). The potentially teratogenic epoxide derivative must be degraded by a hydrolase to the apparently harmless dihydrodiol derivative. Impaired activity of the hydrolase, because of either genetic variability or exogenous factors (e.g., valproic acid), could cause the epoxide derivative to accumulate and exert teratogenic effects.

and phenobarbital, trimethadione is a medication not commonly used by women of childbearing age. Second, other drugs have supplanted oxazolidines in the treatment of petit mal seizures.

Incidence. The incidence of the syndrome after intrauterine exposure to oxazolidines is very high. Indeed, of the 53 reported pregnancies in which such a drug was used, 13 (24%) resulted in spontaneous abortions; of

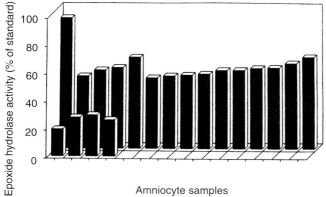

Figure 24-4 Epoxide hydrolase activity in amniocyte samples from 19 prospectively monitored fetuses whose mothers were administered phenytoin during the pregnancy. The samples from the 4 fetuses subsequently noted postnatally to exhibit the clinical features of fetal hydantoin syndrome are shown in the *front row of bars*, and the 15 samples from fetuses subsequently confirmed not to have the characteristic features of the syndrome are shown in the *rear row of bars*. Note the markedly lower epoxide hydrolase activities in the fetal samples from infants who exhibited the clinical features of fetal hydantoin syndrome. *(From Buehler BA, Delimont D, Van Waes M, Finnell RH: Prenatal prediction of risk of the fetal hydantoin syndrome,* N Engl J Med *322:1567–1572, 1990.)*

TABLE 24-6	**Clinical Features of 40 Children Exposed to Trimethadione or Paramethadione in Utero**
Clinical Features	**Percentage Affected***
Growth	
Prenatal growth deficiency	50%
Postnatal growth deficiency	53%
Central Nervous System	
Microcephaly	50%
Mental retardation	29%
Developmental delay	53%
Speech disturbance	47%
Facial	
V-shaped eyebrows	44%
Epicanthal folds	35%
Broad nasal bridge	43%
Malformed ears	70%
Palatal anomaly	57%
Cleft lip and/or palate	28%
Limbs	
Single transverse palmar crease	30%
Clinodactyly	17%
Cardiac	
Major anomaly	50%
Genitourinary	
Major anomaly	30%
Renal anomaly	13%
Hypospadias	21%
Other	
Tracheoesophageal defects	13%
Inguinal hernia	22%

*See text for references. Includes those cases for which data are available.

the 40 survivors, 33 (83%) had at least one major congenital anomaly characteristic of the fetal trimethadione syndrome.[120] Thus, only 17% of the children reported with exposure to trimethadione or paramethadione in utero were born without a major defect. Of the 8 children exposed only to trimethadione, 7 had the features of the syndrome.

Clinical Features. The clinical features of the fetal trimethadione syndrome include aberrations of prenatal and postnatal growth, CNS function, craniofacial appearance, and cardiovascular, genitourinary, and other structures (Table 24-6).[16,113-123] The syndrome was clearly described initially by Zackai and co-workers.[119] The two most helpful diagnostic features are the V-shaped eyebrows and the malformed ears, which are characterized by low placement, posterior rotation, and anteriorly folded helices (Fig. 24-5).

The disturbances of the CNS have not been defined in detail. Nevertheless, approximately 50% of the infants exhibit microcephaly and a definite delay of neurological development, and 29% of the older patients have had overt mental retardation, almost invariably mild. Disturbances of speech, usually not well described, are present in approximately one half of the patients.

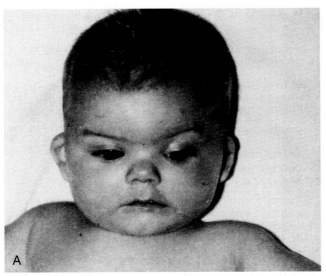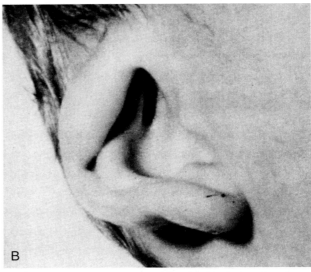

Figure 24-5   **Fetal trimethadione syndrome: clinical appearance**. An affected infant at 5 months of age. **A**, Note the V-shaped eyebrow and broad nasal bridge. **B**, Note the malformed right ear with small superior aspect of helix and cupped, overlapping helical fold. *(From Zackai EH, Mellman WJ, Neiderer B, Hanson JW: The fetal trimethadione syndrome, J Pediatr 87:280–284, 1975.)*

The anomalies of the *cardiovascular system, genitourinary tract*, and *tracheoesophageal structures* are frequent and very serious. The rate of occurrence of both the cardiac and genitourinary anomalies is approximately 50%, and that of the tracheoesophageal structures is approximately 15%. The anomalies together account for the relatively high neonatal mortality rate (nearly 40% of affected infants) and consist of such disorders as hypoplastic left heart, tetralogy of Fallot, transposition of the great vessels, absent or anomalous kidneys, common laryngotracheoesophagus, and large tracheoesophageal fistulas.[121]

Neuropathology. The neuropathological findings of the fetal trimethadione syndrome have not been defined. The occurrence of microcephaly in 50% of infants indicates a significant impairment of brain growth.

Pathogenesis. The mechanism of the teratogenic effect of oxazolidines is unknown. The drugs do cross the placenta and also were shown to be teratogenic when they were injected directly into the chick embryo.[124] Oxazolidines exhibit structural similarities to the major anticonvulsant drugs (e.g., phenytoin and phenobarbital), which also have teratogenic effects, as described earlier (see Fig. 24-1).

Management. *Prevention* is the critical aspect of management. Smith[69] recommended that women of childbearing age who are taking trimethadione or paramethadione "should be informed of their high teratogenicity, should ideally be taking birth control measures as long as they receive these drugs, and should have the option of terminating any pregnancy that occurs while receiving these agents." If the absence seizure disorder requires continuation of therapy, then use of a drug without the basic structure shown in Figure 24-1 could be a rational alternative.

However, valproic acid, a structurally different drug (see Fig. 24-1) with efficacy against absence seizures, also exhibits teratogenic capacity (see the next section). Ethosuximide (Zarontin), currently the most popular drug of first choice for petit mal seizures, is structurally very similar to trimethadione and paramethadione (see Fig. 24-1). This close structural similarity raises the possibility that ethosuximide may have the same teratogenic potential as trimethadione or paramethadione; however, initial epidemiological data do not suggest major teratogenic potential.[32]

Valproate

Valproic acid (see Fig. 24-1) is a widely used anticonvulsant drug. Valproate has teratogenic capability in the human and, concerning the nervous system, has been associated with an increased risk for neural tube defects. The drug also has been associated with the occurrence of systemic major and minor malformations, and the term *fetal valproate syndrome* has been used.

Neural Tube Defects. A relationship between the ingestion of valproate in the first weeks of gestation and the subsequent occurrence of *neural tube defects* was demonstrated both by a series of individual case reports and by large-scale epidemiological studies.[22,24,48,58,60,61,125-139] In a large prospective series of 96 women with epilepsy who were treated with valproate during pregnancy, 6 infants (including a set of monozygotic twins) developed open spina bifida, for an incidence of 6.3% (5.4% when the twins were counted as a single infant).[137] Other reports, most retrospective, suggested that the overall risk of neural tube defects after valproate exposure is 1% to 3%.[22-24,58,60,61,138-140] A role for genetic factors is suggested by the demonstration that the risk for neural tube defect after intrauterine exposure to valproate is considerably greater if a maternal or paternal family history

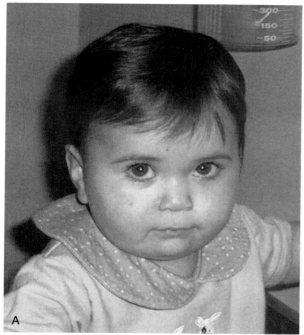
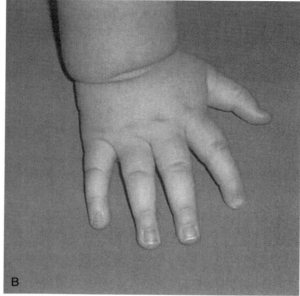

Figure 24-6 **Fetal valproate syndrome, clinical appearance.** Infant (10 months old) whose gestation was complicated by administration of 2000 mg of valproate daily to the mother: note the microbrachycephaly, apparent hypertelorism, broad flat nasal bridge, small mouth with thin lips **(A)**, and thin, tapering fingers **(B)**. *(From Schorry EK, Oppenheimer SG, Saal HM: Valproate embryopathy: Clinical and cognitive profile in 5 siblings, Am J Med Genet A 133:202–206, 2005.)*

of such a defect is present.[136] Moreover, a direct relationship between risk of neural tube defect and maternal dose of valproate is clear.[137] Thus, with daily doses of valproate of less than 1000 mg/day, the risk for neural tube defect was 0/54, with doses of 1000 to 1500 mg/day, it was 2/30, and with doses of more than 1500 mg/day, it was 3/8. In a later, larger study (*n* = 110), the risk increased sharply, with doses exceeding 1400 mg/day.[138] A dose-response effect has also been observed for major systemic congenital malformation.[64]

The *pathogenesis* of the occurrence of neural tube defects after valproate exposure may relate to an abnormality of folate metabolism.[141-144] Thus, the lesion can be produced in a rodent model by exposure to valproate during the time of primary neurulation, a process established to be vulnerable to folate deficiency (see Chapter 1). Moreover, valproate has been shown to mediate inhibition of glutamate formyltransferase, the enzyme responsible for generation of folate metabolites important in the actions of folate.[144] Administration of the product of the inhibited enzyme prevents the teratogenic effect of valproate.

Other Malformations: Fetal Valproate Syndrome.
The possibility of a constellation of major and minor anomalies caused by fetal exposure to valproate (i.e., *a fetal valproate syndrome* reminiscent of the syndrome described earlier in relation to exposure to phenytoin-phenobarbital-primidone or to trimethadione) now seems established. More than 100 cases have been reported.[24,59,134,135,140,145-157]

The *clinical features* include craniofacial abnormalities (i.e., a broad nasal bridge, apparent hypertelorism, epicanthal folds, long, flat philtrum, and thin upper lip) (Fig. 24-6).[157] Long, thin tapering fingers, and hypoplastic fifth toenails are also common. Cardiac, genital, and musculoskeletal defects occur in approximately 20% of patients. Neurological disturbances are common.[59,140,156,158-160] Depressed verbal IQ and autistic disorders occur in a substantial minority of valproate-exposed infants. Overt mental retardation is present in approximately 10%.

Guidelines Concerning Use of Antiepileptic Drugs during Pregnancy

The multiple issues involved in decisions about how to manage anticonvulsant therapy during the pregnancy of the woman with epilepsy are not all resolved, and thus definition of guidelines for management is very difficult. A revised practice parameter is in preparation by the American Academy of Neurology. Reasonable guidelines should include optimization of antiepileptic therapy before conception, avoidance of valproate if possible, use of monotherapy, monitoring of drug levels, administration of the lowest effective dose, and use of folic acid supplementation.

Alcohol

Fetal Alcohol Syndrome

The term *fetal alcohol syndrome* refers to a constellation of neural and extraneural anomalies and of impaired prenatal or postnatal brain and body growth that occurs in infants born to women with chronic alcoholism. The disorder was described in France in 1968 by Lemoine and co-workers,[161] and then it was reported in particular detail in 1973 by Jones and co-workers.[162,163] Subsequent work showed that maternal exposure to ethanol may not lead to the full expression of the fetal alcohol syndrome, but rather may result in a variety of less pronounced dysmorphic, cognitive, and behavioral effects, often termed *fetal alcohol effects* (see later discussion).[164] *Fetal alcohol spectrum disorders* is now used as an umbrella term to include the continuum of alcohol-related disorders, with the fetal alcohol syndrome as the most severe.[165-167] At the other end of the continuum, the neurological and behavioral features of fetal alcohol spectrum disorders may occur without apparent dysmorphic disturbance (see later).

Incidence. The incidence and prevalence of the fetal alcohol syndrome and the less pronounced fetal alcohol effects are not entirely known but are likely to be high. The overt fetal alcohol syndrome, clearly a more readily defined endpoint than so-called fetal alcohol effects, is one of the most common causes of mental retardation in the world. Prevalence rates in the United States are 0.5 to 2.0 per 1000 live births.[166,167] However, rates are as high as 9 per 1000 in certain Native American populations in the United States, and rates of 40 to 50 per 1000 live births have been reported in South Africa. The incidence of the entire group of fetal alcohol spectrum disorders is unknown but has been estimated to be as high as 1% of all live births in the United States.[167]

The amount, pattern, and timing of alcohol exposure are crucial in determining the likelihood and the severity of alcohol teratogenicity. For example, the incidence varies as a function of the incidence of chronic alcoholism. The rate of occurrence of the fetal alcohol syndrome in women with chronic alcoholism is probably 20% to 40%.[162,164,166-169] Moderate drinkers have a lower incidence of newborns with clinical features of fetal alcohol syndrome (i.e., ≈10%).[168] The level of alcohol that is harmless during pregnancy is unknown, and the possibility of a continuum of severity of clinical features is high.[166,167,170] The balance of data[166,167,169,171] supports the earlier conclusion of Smith[69] in 1979 that "ethanol is the most common chemical teratogen presently causing problems of malformation and mental deficiency in the human."

Quantitative relationships between the amount, pattern, and timing of maternal alcohol consumption and adverse fetal outcome have been difficult to delineate precisely. However, available data, although not always entirely congruent, support the following conclusions.[164,166-200] First, a distinct relationship exists between the amount of alcohol consumed by the mother, particularly around the time of conception and early in pregnancy, and the subsequent occurrence of full-blown fetal alcohol syndrome. For example, in one series of mothers who consumed 2 or more ounces of absolute alcohol per day before recognition of pregnancy, 19% delivered children with features consistent with the fetal alcohol syndrome. Of those who consumed between 1 to 2 ounces per day, 11% delivered abnormal children with such features.[168] Of those who consumed less than 1 ounce per day, only 2% had infants with features of the fetal alcohol syndrome.[168] Second, alcohol consumption in the second and third trimesters of pregnancy is *not* harmless and is associated with definite cognitive and behavioral deficits. Third, binge drinking, especially around the time of conception, is particularly dangerous, perhaps because of the high concentrations of blood alcohol achieved.

Genetic differences in fetal susceptibility to alcohol may be important, as they are in the effects of certain other teratogens (see earlier discussion of anticonvulsant drugs). Thus, the rate of concordance for occurrence of the dysmorphic effects of alcohol exposure and for impairment of intelligence is much greater for monozygotic than dizygotic twins.[201] However, even with dizygotic twins, a difference in phenotypic outcome can be pronounced, presumably because of genetic differences in susceptibility.[202] A dramatic recent finding delineated an important determinant of genetic susceptibility (i.e., the maternal *ADH1B*3* allele at the ADH1B locus, the locus of alcohol dehydrogenase).[200,203] The latter enzyme, the first step in alcohol degradation, catalyzes the oxidation of alcohol to acetaldehyde. The *ADH1B*3* allele encodes an isoenzyme that rapidly oxidizes alcohol to acetaldehyde and thereby maintains a relatively low blood alcohol concentration. This allele is unique to African Americans, occurs with a population frequency of 22%, and is associated with a reduced susceptibility to fetal alcohol effects.[203] The data emphasize that genetic factors may play a key role in determining the risk to the fetus at a given level of alcohol consumption during pregnancy.

Clinical Features. The clinical features of the fetal alcohol syndrome are distinctive (Table 24-7).[161-163,165,167-170,182,186,192,197,204-240a] The particularly defining features are *growth disturbance, characteristic facial anomalies,* and *neurological abnormalities*. A prominent disturbance of *growth* is the hallmark of the disorder. At birth, these infants have a distinctive pattern of growth retardation, with length often affected more than weight (the opposite pattern from that expected with intrauterine undernutrition). The growth deficiency persists postnatally, but weight gain becomes more disturbed than linear growth. The abnormalities of growth are not altered appreciably by attempts to change environmental variables, such as nutritional factors and the home setting.

The disturbance of the *CNS* is the most serious feature of the syndrome. Microcephaly is present in nearly all cases, and this reflection of disturbed brain growth is accompanied by delayed neurological development in approximately 90% of patients. The severity of the mental deficiency correlates most closely with the severity of the dysmorphic features. In one series, infants with the most severe dysmorphic manifestations of fetal alcohol syndrome had a mean IQ of 55, those with moderate manifestations had a mean IQ of 68, and those with mild manifestations had a mean IQ of 82. Mean IQ in reported series generally has varied

TABLE 24-7	Clinical Features of the Fetal Alcohol Syndrome*	
Clinical Features		**Approximate Frequency**
Growth		
Prenatal growth deficiency		95%
Postnatal deficiency		95%
Central Nervous System		
Microcephaly		95%
Developmental delay		90%
Facial		
Short palpebral fissures		90%
Epicanthal folds		50%
Midfacial hypoplasia		65%
Short, upturned nose		75%
Hypoplastic long or smooth philtrum		90%
Thin vermilion of upper lip		90%
Limb		
Abnormal palmar creases		55%
Joint abnormalities		50%
Cardiac		
Cardiac defects		50%
Other		
Ear anomalies		25%
Conductive hearing loss		75%
Sensorineural hearing loss		10%
Optic nerve hypoplasia		75%
External genital anomalies		30%
Cutaneous hemangioma		25%

*See text for references. Numbers are rounded off to nearest 5%.

between 65 and 85. The relationship between the severity of dysmorphogenesis and intellectual defect is not invariable; indeed, in some well-documented infants of mothers with chronic alcoholism, neurological disturbance appeared to be the only apparent abnormality, both clinically and neuropathologically.[241,242] Moreover, a distinctive abnormality of the electroencephalogram (EEG), termed *excessive hypersynchrony*, identified by spectral analysis of power on the EEG, was observed in infants in whom dysmorphic features were minor or apparently absent.[218,243-245] Similarly, diffusion tensor magnetic resonance imaging (MRI) detected microstructural alterations, especially in corpus callosum, in infants clinically less obviously affected.[246]

Subsequent school performance in these children is disturbed not only by the defective intellectual function but also by the very frequent accompaniments of hyperactivity, distractibility, and restricted attention span. Particular involvement of speech and language development, verbal more than nonverbal learning and memory, visuospatial abilities, and executive functioning have been emphasized. Subsequent performance on intelligence tests or in school does not change appreciably as a function of the child's environment. In addition to the serious cognitive deficits, the behavioral disturbances and the impaired communication skills, later maladaptive social function, manifested by lack of reciprocal friendships, impulsive behavior,

anxiety, and dysphoria, leads to a far-reaching, pervasive state of disability.

The *facial* abnormalities are characteristic (Fig. 24-7). The typical facies includes short palpebral fissures, epicanthal folds, a low nasal bridge with a short or upturned nose, midface hypoplasia, a smooth philtrum, and a long upper lip with a narrow vermilion border. The constellation of short palpebral fissures, smooth philtrum, and thin vermilion border of the upper lip is particularly characteristic. Minor ear anomalies are present in approximately one fourth of these children. Less common anomalies are strabismus, ptosis, micrognathia, and cleft palate.

Various *limb* anomalies occur. Approximately one half of the infants exhibit abnormal palmar creases and minor joint abnormalities. The latter include an inability to extend the elbows completely, camptodactyly, and clinodactyly.

Cardiac lesions occur in approximately one half of the infants, but these lesions are usually not severe. Most consist of septal defects (atrial more often than ventricular defects).

Numerous *additional features* occur in a minority of patients, including ear anomalies, ocular anomalies, cutaneous hemangioma, and minor abnormalities of the external genitalia. Although hearing loss, primarily conductive, occurs in 75% of infants, the severity is relatively mild. Optic nerve hypoplasia also occurs in 75% of infants, but disturbances of visual acuity are not marked.

Neuropathology. The essential nature of the neural disturbance in the fetal alcohol syndrome is *impairment of brain development* (Table 24-8). Several aspects of the developmental program appear to be involved, based on neuropathological analysis of approximately 20 affected infants.[190,242,247-252] In keeping with the microcephaly, micrencephaly is common. The most striking additional abnormalities reported appear to involve neuronal and glial migration. Thus, in the series of Clarren and co-workers,[242] the most frequent abnormality was leptomeningeal neuroglial heterotopia that took the form of a sheet of aberrant neuronal and glial cells covering portions of the cerebral, cerebellar, and brain stem surfaces (Fig. 24-8). Aberrations of brain stem and cerebellar development, in large part related to faulty migration, also have been particularly frequent.[242,247] Schizencephaly and polymicrogyria are other migrational disturbances observed.[247] In addition, disordered midline prosencephalic formation (e.g., agenesis of the corpus callosum, septo-optic dysplasia, and incomplete holoprosencephaly) has been documented.[249,251,252] Other developmental defects have included anencephaly, lumbar meningomyelocele, lumbosacral and sacral meningomyelocele, absent olfactory bulbs or "arrhinencephaly," and disturbances of dendritic development.[247,250,253,254]

Thus, it appears that multiple aspects of CNS development can be affected, including (in chronological order) neurulation, canalization and retrogressive differentiation, prosencephalic development, neuronal proliferation, neuronal migration, and organizational

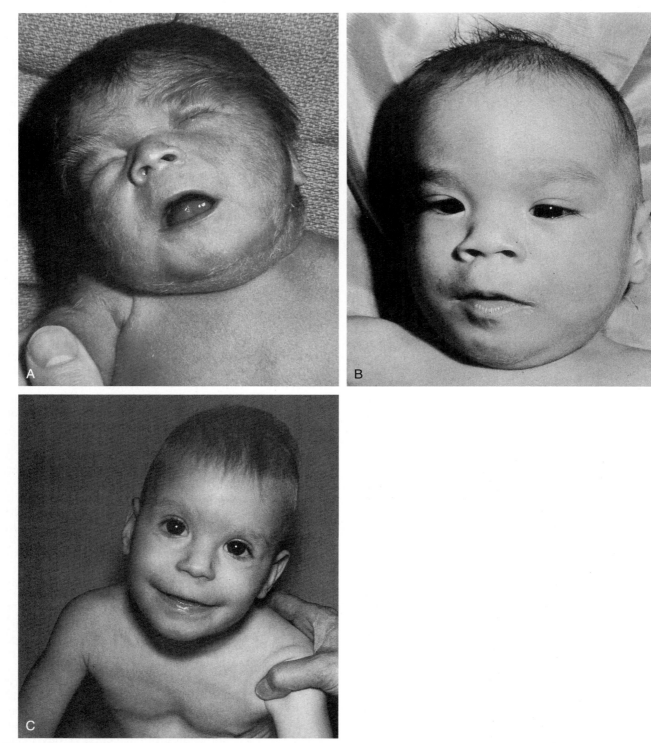

Figure 24-7   Fetal alcohol syndrome: clinical appearance. Two children: one, **A**, in the newborn period and, **B**, at the age of 6 months and, **C**, the other at the age of 16 months. Note the short palpebral fissures, especially prominent in the newborn **(A)**, and the low nasal bridge with short, upturned nose, epicanthal folds, long, hypoplastic philtrum, and convex upper lip with narrow vermilion border. *(A and B, From Jones KL, Smith DW: Recognition of the fetal alcohol syndrome in early infancy, Lancet 2:999–1001, 1973; C, from Hanson JW, Jones KL, Smith DW: Fetal alcohol syndrome: Experience with 41 patients, JAMA 235:1458–1460, 1976.)*

events (see Chapter 2). The time periods of the most frequently reported occurrences (i.e., disorders of neuronal proliferation and migration and of midline prosencephalic development) range from the second to the fifth month of gestation, and hence the teratogens could be acting either *during these time periods or, of course, earlier.* These data are entirely compatible with those from studies relating time of maternal alcohol intake during pregnancy to subsequent fetal outcome (see subsequent discussion). However, few data are

TABLE 24-8 Major Neuropathological Features of Fetal Alcohol Syndrome*

In Order of Decreasing Frequency:
Micrencephaly
Migrational abnormalities: neuronal > glial
Midline prosencephalic abnormalities: agenesis of the corpus callosum, septo-optic dysplasia, incomplete holoprosencephaly
Dendritic abnormalities
Disorders of neural tube formation

*See text for references.

TABLE 24-9 Major Central Nervous System Alterations Defined by Magnetic Resonance Imaging in Fetal Alcohol Spectrum Disorders*

Decreased brain size
Disproportionately reduced volume of parietal, temporal (perisylvian) and inferior frontal lobes
Disproportionate reduction of white matter in areas of reduced volume
Decreased volume of basal ganglia
Decreased volume of cerebellum
Abnormal corpus callosum: agenesis or hypoplasia, especially most anterior and posterior regions

*See text for references.

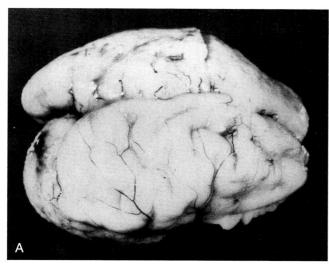

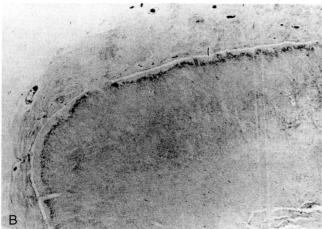

Figure 24-8 Fetal alcohol syndrome: neuropathology. Brain from a 6-week-old infant who was born after a 32-week gestation. **A**, Right superolateral view of the cerebrum. Note that nearly all of the left hemisphere is covered by a massive sheet of tissue that crosses the midline and extends onto the superior and medial aspect of the right frontal lobe. **B**, Section through the cerebral cortex covered by the aberrant tissue. Extending through a break in the pial surface (upper left of cortex) is the heterotopic sheet of tissue composed of neuronal, glial, and pial elements that have covered the true cortex. (A much smaller break in the pial surface is evident in the *lower left* of the figure.) *(From Jones KL, Smith DW: The fetal alcohol syndrome, Teratology 12:1–10, 1975.)*

available concerning the status of neuronal differentiation and other aspects of organizational events in infants of mothers with alcoholism. Disturbance of dendritic development has been documented,[250] and epidemiological data indicate impaired cognition in infants exposed to alcohol late in pregnancy (see later discussion) when organizational events are active. Moreover, experimental studies have demonstrated distinct disturbances of neuronal development (see "Pathogenesis").

Advanced MRI techniques (e.g., volumetric MRI) have been used to define further the neuropathology of fetal alcohol spectrum disorders (Table 24-9).[167,227,246,255-257] Some of the findings confirm those defined post mortem (see earlier), but *regional* disturbances of *cerebral* underdevelopment, disproportionate involvement of *white matter*, particular involvement of *basal ganglia* and *cerebellum*, and *regional* details of the *corpus callosal* abnormalities have been identified. These findings have correlates in the neurocognitive deficits described earlier. Thus, the verbal memory defect may relate to the temporal disturbances, the impulsiveness and defective inhibition may relate to frontal involvement, the visuospatial deficits may relate to parietal abnormality, the intermodal learning deficits may relate to callosal abnormality, and the motor and perhaps some of the learning deficits may relate to cerebellar abnormality.

Pathogenesis. The pathogenesis of the disturbances of CNS development has been studied in a variety of experimental models. The basis for the deleterious effect of ethanol on neuronal cell number may relate to a disturbance both of *neuronal proliferation*, particularly in the ventricular zone, and of programmed cell death (i.e., *apoptosis*).[190,196,258-266] The impairment of *neuronal migration* may be associated with both impairment of cell-cell adhesion and a loss of radial glial guides, the apparent result of either the premature differentiation of radial glial cells to astrocytes or a direct deleterious effect on astrocytic function.[196,262,267-269] Disturbances of *organizational events* in experimental models have included impaired synaptogenesis and development of neurotransmitter systems, including receptors, uptake mechanisms, synthetic and catabolic enzymes, and transduction mechanisms.[270-273]

The affected neurotransmitters have included gluta-mate, serotonin, dopamine, norepinephrine, acetylcho-line, and histamine. Additionally, disturbances of both astrocytic and oligodendroglial development have been defined in cell culture models.[274,275] A particular vul-nerability of cerebral white matter was shown in a fetal sheep model.[276] The disturbances of organizational events, particularly neuronal development, may be cru-cial, and search for potential human correlates of these disturbances is a fertile area for future research.

The fundamental mechanisms whereby ethanol administration leads to the disturbances of CNS development have not been delineated definitively. Current evidence favors the concept that ethanol or a metabolic product thereof is responsible for the tera-togenic effects expressed in the fetal alcohol syn-drome.[190,196,258,262-264,267,268,277-298] Alcohol rapidly crosses the placenta and the blood-brain barrier of the fetus. Indeed, a dose-dependent relationship between maternal alcohol intake in the first weeks of human pregnancy and the appearance of certain fea-tures of the fetal alcohol syndrome has been demon-strated (see earlier discussion).

Whether ethanol acts directly on target organs or indirectly is unknown. Suggested pathogenetic mech-anisms have included direct molecular effects of alcohol or its metabolites (e.g., acetaldehyde), maternal under-nutrition or malnutrition (e.g., vitamin or trace metal deficiencies), fetal hypoglycemia, and fetal hypoxia-is-chemia.[196,264,265,268,273,288,294,295,297-304] The last of these mechanisms is based on the demonstrations that (1) maternal ethanol exposure caused a striking impairment of uterine blood flow with resulting fetal hypoxia and acidosis in the third trimester fetal monkey, (2) ethanol induced vasoconstriction of uter-ine vessels in vitro, and (3) maternal ethanol exposure near term in sheep caused fetal hypoglycemia, a decrease in fetal cerebral metabolic rates for oxygen and glucose, and suppressed fetal breathing move-ments and electrocorticographic activity.[302,305-307] However, the deleterious effects of maternal ethanol exposure on fetal cerebral blood flow and metabolism did *not* occur in immature sheep,[308] a stage of develop-ment when the teratogenic effects of alcohol presum-ably are operative.

Several direct molecular effects of alcohol may be involved in the deleterious effects on the developing nervous system. The first of these may involve *fetal zinc* deficiency caused by decreased maternal supply, in turn related to the induction by alcohol of the zinc binding protein metallothionein in maternal liver, with subsequent sequestration of zinc by metallothionein and redistribution in the liver.[304] Zinc is necessary for many CNS developmental events including neurogen-esis, neuronal migration, and synaptogenesis. Notably, in a mouse model of fetal alcohol effects, prenatal zinc treatment limited the functional neural deficits pro-duced by maternal ethanol exposure.[304] A second molecular mechanism may involve the *generation of free radicals* with subsequent disturbances of neural development.[303,309-311] Prevention of these effects by antioxidant interventions is under investigation.

A third mechanism could involve *disturbance of glutamate receptor* function. For example, blockade of the *N*-methyl-D-aspartate (NMDA) type of glutamate receptor during a period in the rat corresponding to the third trimester of human gestation resulted in widespread apoptotic neurodegeneration.[264] Ethanol is a potent NMDA antagonist, and thus exposure to ethanol may lead to diminished cell number by deprivation of glu-tamate activation, crucial for neuronal survival.[264] Other deleterious effects of ethanol involve alteration of NMDA receptor subunit expression and potential enhancement of excitotoxicity.[312,313] A fourth mecha-nism involves inhibition by ethanol of the synthesis of retinoic acid.[297,298] Retinoic acid, a vitamin A metabo-lite, plays an essential role in many aspects of develop-ment through an effect on transcription of multiple genes.[314,315] Ethanol is a competitive inhibitor of the alcohol dehydrogenase that catalyzes the conversion of retinol (vitamin A) to retinal, which, in turn, is con-verted to retinoic acid by an aldehyde dehydrogenase. The *alcohol* dehydrogenase is the rate-limiting step in the synthesis of retinoic acid. The developmental role of retinoic acid is focused particularly on epithelial cell–derived tissues, and thus CNS, limbs, and face (sites characteristically affected in fetal alcohol syndrome) are especially involved. Because of the far-reaching effects of retinoic acid in development, the defect in retinoic acid synthesis could be a final common path-way for many of the teratogenic effects of alcohol on both neural and extraneural systems. A fifth mecha-nism may be particularly important in the impairment of neuronal migration, a central feature of the fetal alcohol syndrome (see "Neuropathology" earlier). Thus, ethanol has been shown to inhibit neural cell-cell adhesion at levels readily attained by "social drinking."[268] Such a disturbance could be crucial by disrupting the critical cell-cell interactions that are obligatory for neuronal and glial migration. A sixth mechanism could involve an effect on apoptosis. Ethanol in immature mice triggered activation of caspase-3 and widespread apoptotic neuronal death in forebrain.[265] This effect could be relevant to the occur-rence of micrencephaly. Notably, nicotinamide, which inhibits caspase-3, protects against this ethanol-induced apoptotic neurodegeneration. Similarly, ery-thropoietin, which has antiapoptotic properties, was neuroprotective in another model of ethanol-induced apoptosis in immature brain.[311]

Management. Management clearly consists primarily of *prevention*. It is critical that women be advised con-cerning the risks to the fetus as early in pregnancy as possible because the risk of malformations is greatest when the fetus is exposed during the first weeks and months of gestation. Indeed, advice ideally should be rendered *before pregnancy*, because most women do not begin prenatal care until after the important first weeks of pregnancy have passed. In a recent report from the Centers for Disease Control, more than half of the women of childbearing age in the United States consumed alcohol in the month before the survey, 15% of these were moderate or heavy drinkers, and approximately 15% continued to use alcohol during their pregnancy.[166,167] Reduction or cessation of alcohol consumption during pregnancy has been shown to have major beneficial preventive effects.* When this restriction is initiated very early in pregnancy, growth retardation and malformations are prevented. When it is carried out in midpregnancy, although, as would be expected, malformations are not prevented, growth retardation is clearly diminished. Thus, benefit is gained, even if cessation of drinking is delayed.

The degree of reduction in alcohol consumption necessary to prevent adverse effects is unknown. Moreover, because clinical and experimental data suggest a dose-dependent relationship (see earlier discussion), total abstinence continues to be recommended in the United States and in at least seven other countries.[164,166,321-323]

Future interventions may follow from the experimental studies described earlier (see "Pathogenesis"). Thus, such compounds as antioxidants, zinc, nicotinamide, and erythropoietin could ultimately play a role. The potential role of genotyping for alleles involved in determining susceptibility (e.g., *ADH1*3* allele, discussed earlier) remains to be clarified.

Isotretinoin

The vitamin A analogue isotretinoin (Accutane) was identified as the teratogenic agent in reports of more than 100 infants exposed in the first weeks of pregnancy.[324-334] The magnitude of the problem is potentially great because isotretinoin is used widely for treatment of severe acne, and more than one third of all isotretinoin prescribed is consumed by female patients 13 to 19 years old.[329]

The *clinical features* are characterized by a distinctive craniofacial appearance, cleft palate, CNS defects, and congenital heart lesions. The most distinctive and frequent craniofacial feature is anomalous ear development, consisting usually of small, malformed, or absent ears and atretic ear canals (Fig. 24-9). The congenital heart lesions have included, particularly, anomalies of the great vessels (conotruncal and aortic arch abnormalities) and septal defects. The CNS abnormalities have included, most notably, hydrocephalus (with aqueductal stenosis or obstruction of the outflow of the fourth ventricle), focal cerebral cortical migrational defects (pachygyria, agyria, and neuronal and glial heterotopias), micrencephaly, absent cerebellar vermis, and migrational abnormalities in cerebellum and brain stem. The CNS malformations are the most consistent of the anomalies reported and occur in at least 85% of affected infants.

Pathogenesis involves the teratogenic effect of isotretinoin, a vitamin A analogue (13-*cis*-retinoic acid). The syndrome has been identified after exposure to similar retinoid analogues of vitamin A (e.g., acitretin).[335] Anomalies similar to the human syndrome were

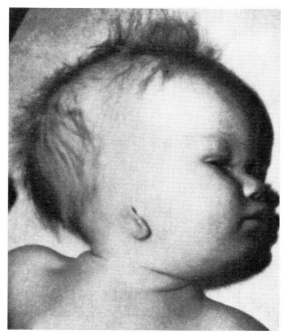

Figure 24-9 Fetal isotretinoin syndrome: clinical appearance. This patient at 8 months had a high forehead, hypoplastic nasal bridge, and, particularly, abnormal ears, including microtia. *(From Lott IT, Bocian M, Pribram HW, Leitner M: Fetal hydrocephalus and ear anomalies associated with maternal use of isotretinoin, J Pediatr 105:597–600, 1984.)*

produced in various experimental animals, including subhuman primates, exposed to excessive retinoic acid or vitamin A itself during early development.[336-338] Indeed, the pattern of defects observed in infants born to women who had consumed high levels of vitamin A (>10,000 units daily) before the seventh week of gestation bears important similarities to the pattern of defects observed in the isotretinoin-exposed infant.[339,340] The molecular mechanism appears to relate to an impairment of the normal role of retinoic acid in development of epithelial cells, including particularly the cephalic neural crest cells. The latter are of particular importance in promotion of differentiation of craniofacial structures. The site of the molecular disturbance bears close similarities to that proposed for alcohol (see previous section), except in the case of isotretinoin exposure, excessive levels of retinoic acid may be present, as opposed to the postulated depressed levels in alcohol exposure. The teratogenicity of retinoic acids may relate in particular to an effect on the expression of the homeobox gene *Hoxb-1* that regulates axial patterning in the embryo.[341,342]

Management consists primarily of prevention. The gravity of exposure to isotretinoin during pregnancy is emphasized by the high incidence of either spontaneous abortion or malformed infants in women who have taken the drug. Indeed, in a prospective series of 36 isotretinoin-exposed pregnancies (first trimester), only 64% of infants were born without major malformations.[326] The remaining 36% of pregnancies resulted in spontaneous abortion (22%), stillbirth of a malformed infant (3%), or birth of an infant with major malformations (11%), as described earlier. In a *retrospective* series of pregnancies exposed to isotretinoin in the first trimester, 80% to 90% ended in spontaneous abortion, stillbirth, or live birth with malformations. Because the first trimester, and probably early in this trimester, is the vulnerable period, it is important that women of childbearing age take measures to avoid becoming pregnant while taking the drug. Moreover, with inadvertent exposure to the agent while pregnant, the desirability of continuing the pregnancy should be addressed. *Topical* retinoic acid (tretinoin, also used in the treatment of acne) administered in the first trimester of pregnancy has been associated with the occurrence of ear and cerebral anomalies,[343] although the frequency of this relationship is unknown.[344] A more recent review of 106 pregnant women with first trimester exposure to topical tretinoin identified no examples of ear or cerebral anomalies.[345] Thus, the risk of using topical tretinoin is unclear. The possibility should be considered that some women and fetuses are genetically susceptible or uniquely capable of absorbing relatively high doses of tretinoin after topical application.[345] Finally, because of the similarity in phenotypic expression of the teratogenicity of high maternal vitamin A intake, it is recommended that women who are or who may become pregnant not consume daily supplements of more than 8000 IU of vitamin A.[340]

Cocaine

The effect on the fetus, and thereby the newborn, of cocaine use by the pregnant woman is a topic of major public health importance, in considerable part because of the relatively high incidence of cocaine abuse worldwide (see later discussion). Cocaine has profound effects on the central and peripheral neural systems of the adult and may have the potential to cause, directly and indirectly, adverse alterations in neurological, cognitive, and behavioral functions and brain structure in the fetus.

Delineation of the effects of intrauterine exposure to cocaine on the fetus and the newborn is difficult for several reasons, and these *methodological difficulties* must be considered in any analysis of the available information on this topic. First, accurate determination of which infants have been exposed to cocaine in utero awaits development of a simple, sensitive, and specific test. Currently, infant exposure to cocaine in utero often is ascertained initially by maternal urine analysis for cocaine and its metabolites, by maternal interview, or both. The importance of *both* these approaches is well illustrated by the data of Zuckerman and co-workers (Table 24-10).[346-348] In a prospective study of 1226 mothers, cocaine use was determined by maternal interview and urine analysis. Based on a maternal interview alone, 24% of exposed infants would have been missed; urine analysis alone would have missed 47% of exposed infants. Moreover, because neonatal urine analysis provides evidence only of recent cocaine exposure (within $\approx$1 week), the *duration* of intrauterine exposure cannot be determined. The importance of this issue was emphasized by the observation that

TABLE 24-10	Estimation of Frequency of Cocaine Use during Pregnancy, According to Method of Ascertainment	
	MATERNAL INTERVIEW	
Neonatal Urine Assay	**Positive**	**Negative**
Positive	20%	24%
Negative	47%	—

Data from Zuckerman B, Frank DA, Hingson R, Amaro H, et al: Effects of maternal marijuana and cocaine use on fetal growth, *N Engl J Med* 320:762–768, 1989.

deleterious effects on the fetus could not be documented in women who used light or moderate amounts of cocaine and who decreased drug use during their pregnancies.[349] Indeed, a dose-dependent effect of cocaine on the fetus was quantitated in a careful study.[350] The determination of cocaine metabolites in *meconium*[351,352] is an excellent addition or alternative to urine analysis.[352-358] Analyses of meconium provide information on the degree of cocaine exposure over many weeks during pregnancy following onset of meconium production (i.e., 14 to 16 weeks). Investigators have suggested that serial analyses of meconium may provide information about timing, with the initial sample of meconium relevant to early pregnancy and later samples relevant to later in pregnancy. The demonstration of a cocaine metabolite in hair from adult cocaine users, the correlation of hair levels with reported quantity of cocaine used, and the ability to detect changes in content along the hair shaft as a function of the time of cocaine use suggested that analysis of hair may be particularly valuable.[359] Cocaine metabolite has been detected in *hair of newborn infants* of women who used cocaine during pregnancy,[359,360] and available data suggest that detection of fetal exposure during the last trimester of pregnancy is possible.[354] Relevant neonatal hair samples may be obtained for approximately 3 postnatal months.[360] A more readily applied approach in the newborn period may be analysis of *maternal hair* samples shortly after delivery.[350]

The second difficulty in determining the effects of intrauterine exposure to cocaine is the frequent presence of many potentially deleterious, confounding variables in the prenatal and postnatal periods of the infants.[348,358,361-364] Thus, pregnant women who abuse cocaine commonly also abuse other illicit drugs, smoke cigarettes or marijuana, or both, drink alcohol, have poor nutrition, fail to seek prenatal care, transmit to the fetus such infections as syphilis or human immunodeficiency virus, and provide the newborn with a poor postnatal nutritional and social environment.[169,358,361-363,365-379] Indeed, in a study of 619 mothers who reported abusing cocaine, only 2% reported no use of other drugs, and 77% used cocaine and at least two other drugs.[358]

A third difficulty relates to the choice of outcome measures for infants exposed to cocaine in utero. *The neural systems most likely to be affected by cocaine are involved in neurological and behavioral functions that are not readily quantitated, particularly by standard measures of infant*

TABLE 24-11   Incidence of Cocaine Use in a Suburban U.S. Hospital

	Private (*n* = 366)	Clinic (*n* = 134)
Cocaine use (meconium)	6.3%	26.9%
Cocaine use (maternal report)	0%	4.0%

Data from Schutzman DL, Frankenfield CM, Clatterbaugh HE, Singer J: Incidence of intrauterine cocaine exposure in a suburban setting, *Pediatrics* 88:825–827, 1991.

development and cognition. Such functions relate to attention, arousal, motivation, and social interaction, among others (see later discussions).

A fourth difficulty relates to selection bias for the reporting of positive rather than negative results in studies of the effects of intrauterine exposure to cocaine.[380] Among abstracts submitted to the Society for Pediatric Research from 1980 to 1989, only 11% of those describing no effect of cocaine were accepted for presentation versus 57% of those describing a positive effect. Indeed, I suspect that I have been guilty of this bias in attempting to prepare a succinct section in this book, although I have tried to minimize this bias.

Incidence

Of women cared for at urban teaching hospitals, 5% to 45% use cocaine during their pregnancies.[346, 350-352,356,358,365,379,381-390] The problem of fetal cocaine exposure is not confined to urban hospital populations; in one study, 6% of infants born to women at a private suburban hospital had a cocaine metabolite in meconium (Table 24-11).[391] In a study of more than 29,000 women delivering in California, the percentage of positive urine assays for cocaine and its metabolites, and therefore an indication of exposure only in approximately the last week of pregnancy, was 1.1%.[169]

Pharmacology

Cocaine Preparations and Metabolism. Cocaine is benzoylmethylecgonine, an alkaloid derived from the leaves of the *Erythroxylon* plant species.[392,393] It is available in two forms: cocaine hydrochloride and highly purified cocaine alkaloid (free base).[392-401] The latter is derived from the former principally by alkali extraction. Cocaine hydrochloride is heat labile but water soluble and therefore is generally administered by nasal insufflation, orally, or intravenously. Cocaine alkaloid is heat stable but highly water insoluble and therefore is generally administered by inhalation (smoking). The cocaine alkaloid preparation is also called "crack" because of the popping sound made by the heated crystals. The activities of the cocaine-metabolizing cholinesterases and therefore elimination of cocaine are relatively low in the pregnant female, fetus, and newborn rodent.[400] However, systematic data in humans are lacking. Infants born to mothers who used cocaine 1 or 2 days before delivery excrete cocaine for 12 to 24 hours after delivery and benzoylecgonine for as long as 5 to 7 days.[397,402] Another metabolite,

hydroxybenzoylecgonine, when detected in meconium, is a highly sensitive indicator of fetal exposure.[358]

Mechanisms of Action. Cocaine has pronounced effects on both the peripheral and central neural systems. First, it impairs the reuptake of norepinephrine and epinephrine by presynaptic nerve endings, and consequently, these neurotransmitters accumulate at synapses.[169,392-394,403-406] The result is a striking activation of adrenergic systems, and it is indeed the pronounced stimulation of the sympathetic nervous system that causes the most dramatic acute effects of the drug in the adult (e.g., hypertension, tachycardia, vasoconstriction). Second, cocaine impairs the reuptake of dopamine by binding to the dopamine transporter, the reuptake carrier.[407] Dopamine therefore accumulates in synaptic clefts and activates dopaminergic systems. This activation is crucial for the sense of euphoria that follows acute cocaine ingestion and involves mesolimbic or mesocortical pathways, or both.[403] Activation of mesolimbocortical dopaminergic pathways also accounts for the strong reinforcing qualities of the drug.[407,408] However, with longer-term use, dopamine becomes progressively depleted from nerve endings, and this depletion may lead to the dysphoria so prominent during withdrawal and to the subsequent craving for the drug. Third, cocaine impairs the homeostasis of serotonin by blocking the uptake of both tryptophan, its precursor, and serotonin itself.[392,409-411] The result may account for the striking acute alteration in sleep-wake cycling (i.e., the decreased need for sleep) and may enhance the central excitatory effects of dopamine. Fourth, cocaine acts on peripheral nerves to prevent the increase in permeability of sodium ions required for initiation and propagation of nerve impulses.[394] This effect underlies the local anesthetic action of cocaine.

Clinical Features

Maternal-Fetal Effects. Cocaine use during pregnancy may have deleterious effects on both the mother and the fetus.[169,350,379,412-420] The specific features and the magnitude of these effects are relatively consistent among reported studies. For example, in one large, multisite, prospective randomized study, compared with nonexposed infants, cocaine-exposed infants had lower birth weights, lower gestational age, higher rate of prematurity, shorter length, smaller head circumference, and increased likelihood to be small for gestational age (Table 24-12).[379]

The *mechanisms* of the adverse effects just mentioned are undoubtedly multiple and interrelated (Fig. 24-10). However, the occurrence of premature labor and delivery relates, at least in part, to the increased uterine contractility associated with the increase in catecholamines stimulated by cocaine.[421-423] A direct effect of cocaine on human myometrial contractile activity also is likely.[424] The increased uterine contractility also may underlie the higher risk of abruptio placentae reported in some studies.[412] An important factor in the pathogenesis of the impairment of fetal growth is a disturbance in nutrient transfer to the fetus, probably

TABLE 24-12	Selected Perinatal Outcomes for Cocaine Exposed versus Nonexposed during Pregnancy		
	Cocaine Exposed (*n* = 717)	Nonexposed (*n* = 7442)	*P* Value
Birth weight (mean ± SD, g)	2,531±695	3,067±776	<.001
Gestational age (mean ± SD, cm)	37.1±3.4	38.3±3.0	<.001
Small for gestational age (%)*	29.4%	13.5%	<.001
Length at birth (mean ± SD, cm)	46.3±4.4	48.9±4.5	<.001
Head circumference at birth (mean ± SD, cm)	31.9±2.8	33.4±2.7	<.001

*Defined as less than 10th percentile.
Data from Bauer CR, Langer JC, Shankaran S, Bada HS, et al: Acute neonatal effects of cocaine exposure during pregnancy, Arch Pediatr Adolesc Med 159:824–834, 2005.

secondary, in part, to impaired placental blood flow.[421,425-427] Additionally, the increase in catecholamines may raise metabolism and may thereby deplete nutrient stores in the fetus.[425,428] The crucial disturbance of brain growth, manifested by decreased head circumference (see Table 24-12), is discussed in more detail in the next section.

Teratogenic Effects on the Central Nervous System. This section concerns the effects of cocaine on the *development* of the brain or regions thereof (i.e., teratogenic effects). Those effects that are primarily destructive (i.e., associated with the histopathological hallmarks of a destructive process such as dissolution of tissue with a reactive cellular response) are considered later. It may be difficult to distinguish developmental from destructive effects in the fetus because a destructive process that occurs in rapidly developing tissue may cause both derangement of subsequent development and injury to an already developed structure. Additionally, the reactive cellular response to tissue destruction may be less vigorous during early development, and hence evidence of a primarily destructive event may be absent or barely detectable morphologically. The major abnormalities of CNS development reported after intrauterine cocaine exposure and the developmental event apparently affected (see Chapters 1 and 2) are summarized in Table 24-13.[365,412,425,429-444]

Microcephaly. An impairment of intrauterine brain growth, manifested as diminished head circumference at birth is the most common brain abnormality in infants of cocaine-abusing mothers.* Indeed, in one large study, 16% of newborns exposed to cocaine in

utero (compared with 6% of control newborns) had microcephaly.[412] The conclusion that the impaired brain growth reflects primarily an intrauterine effect of cocaine, rather than associated factors (e.g., maternal undernutrition, intrauterine infection, use of other illicit drugs during pregnancy, and smoking during pregnancy), is supported by persistence of the decreased head circumference in analyses in which the confounding variables were controlled. Moreover, in one study based on analysis of maternal hair, a clear dose-dependent relationship was shown between risk for head size less than the 10th percentile and level of cocaine exposure.[350]

Disturbances of Midline Prosencephalic Development and Neuronal Migration. An earlier study of a selected group of seven infants with abnormal neurological or ocular findings suggested that disorders of midline prosencephalic development or neuronal migration may be associated with intrauterine cocaine exposure.[437] Three of the seven infants had varying combinations of agenesis of the corpus callosum, absence of septum pellucidum, septo-optic dysplasia, schizencephaly, and neuronal heterotopias, and two of the three also had optic nerve hypoplasia and blindness.[437] The remaining four infants had evidence of destructive cerebral lesions. Subsequent reports confirmed these findings and documented the occurrence of schizencephaly, lissencephaly, pachygyria, and neuronal heterotopias as manifestations of disorders of neuronal migration.[436,442-444] Funduscopic examination of cocaine-exposed infants revealed optic nerve dysgenesis, coloboma, hypoplasia, and atrophy.[441,444,451] The possibility that both the disorders of midline prosencephalic development and neuronal migration and of optic nerve development are more common than is currently known is real because cranial ultrasonography and computed tomography may not detect some of these abnormalities, and careful funduscopic examinations are not often done in newborn infants. Nevertheless, in a recent and careful study of 717 cocaine-exposed infants, cranial ultrasonography failed to detect *any abnormalities* of prosencephalic development or overt migrational disturbance.[379]

Neuronal Differentiation. The possibility that cocaine exposure disturbs neuronal differentiation in cerebral, diencephalic, and brain stem structures was suggested by a series of neuroanatomical, neurobehavioral, neuropharmacological, neurochemical, and physiological studies, primarily in rats but also in subhuman primates and, more recently, in human infants.[434,452-478] Thus, prenatal cocaine exposure in rats and monkeys resulted in persistent defects in learning and memory. Moreover, Dow-Edwards and co-workers,[452,453] using radioactive 2-deoxyglucose autoradiography, found that *adult* rats exposed to cocaine *prenatally* had impaired glucose metabolism in the following: the hippocampus, a structure crucial for memory and learning; the nigrostriatal pathway, important in regulation of movement; the mesolimbic dopaminergic system, important for the reinforcing effects of drugs such as cocaine; and the hypothalamus, important for reproductive function, growth

---

*See references 346,350,379,412,416,419,420,425,430-433,437-440,444-450.

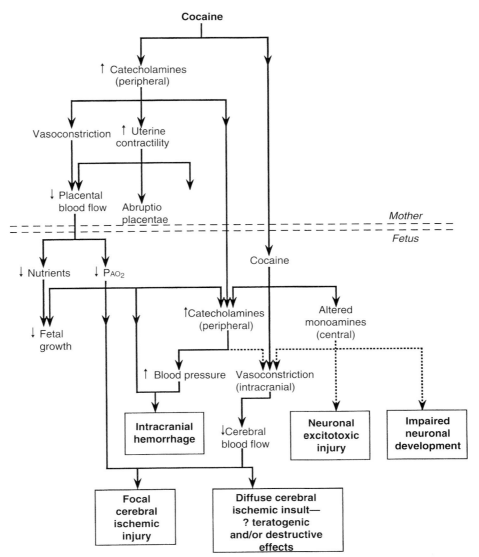

Figure 24-10   **Scheme for the potentially deleterious effects of cocaine taken by pregnant women on their fetuses**. Effects on the maternal side of the placenta are shown in the *upper portion* of the figure and on the fetus in the *lower portion*. Effects that appear plausible on the basis of current information but that require more supporting information are indicated by *interrupted lines*.

regulation, and osmotic balance. Thus, exposure to cocaine during the earliest phases of neuronal differentiation in the experimental animal led to profound and permanent effects on the function of many crucial neuronal systems. These effects should be considered teratogenic because it appears that permanent derangement of neuronal development resulted. The correlate, if any, in humans remains to be defined, but one report noted disturbances of neuronal differentiation demonstrated by immunocytochemical and histological techniques in cerebral cortex of three infants exposed to cocaine in utero.[436] Very similar findings were observed in the cerebral cortex of newborn rats exposed to cocaine in utero.[465,466,473] Recent studies using advanced MRI showed a relationship between prenatal cocaine exposure and impaired development of both frontal white matter pathways[479] and caudate volume.[479a]

Destructive Effects on the Central Nervous System.
Cocaine is distinctive among the drugs (see Table 24-1) that produce teratogenic effects on the CNS in its additional capacity to lead to *destructive* neural effects. Indeed, distinction of the destructive effects from the teratogenic is difficult, in part because these effects may coexist in the same infant.

Cerebral Infarction and Intracranial Hemorrhage.
Exposure of the fetus to cocaine may lead to serious destructive lesions in the brain. The first clearly documented example was the demonstration of infarction in the distribution of the middle cerebral artery in a newborn infant whose mother used cocaine by nasal insufflation in large doses during the 3 days before delivery.[480] The presence of hemiparesis *at birth* and the appearance of the lesion on computed tomography indicated that the infarct occurred shortly before birth, presumably during the period of

TABLE 24-13	Major Developmental Disturbances Reported after Intrauterine Cocaine Exposure and Developmental Event Presumably Affected*
Abnormality Reported after Cocaine Exposure[†]	**Developmental Event Presumably Affected**
Micrencephaly	Neuronal proliferation
Agenesis of corpus callosum; agenesis of septum pellucidum; septo-optic dysplasia	Prosencephalic development
Schizencephaly, lissencephaly, pachygyria, neuronal heterotopias	Neuronal migration
Abnormal cortical neuronal differentiation (preliminary data)	Neuronal differentiation
Myelomeningocele, encephalocele	Neural tube formation

*See text for references.
[†]Abnormalities are listed in order of decreasing frequency.

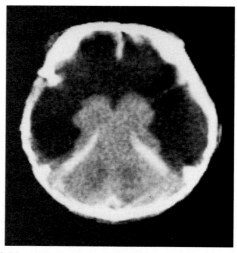

Figure 24-11   Hydranencephaly in an infant exposed to cocaine in utero. This computed tomography scan shows evidence of severe destruction of cerebral hemispheres in the distribution of the middle and anterior cerebral arteries. The appearance is consistent with severe ischemic insult in utero. *(Courtesy of Dr. Elke Roland.)*

cocaine exposure. Subsequently, numerous infants exposed to cocaine in utero, with cerebral infarction in the distribution of major cerebral vessels, usually the middle cerebral artery, were identified.[402,429,437,440,481-485] In one series, 6% of cocaine-exposed infants exhibited cerebral infarction. Although all such lesions appear to have been prenatal in origin, the timing of the infarctions based on radiographic and clinical criteria varied from hours to months before delivery. Thus, in the four affected newborns in the series of Dominguez and co-workers,[437] three had well-established porencephaly, compatible with an event occurring weeks or months previously, and one had findings (edema) compatible with an acute event. A similar prenatal origin was apparent in an infant with hydranencephaly, related to destruction of the cerebral hemispheres in the distribution of the middle and anterior cerebral arteries, noted at birth after a pregnancy marked by cocaine exposure (Fig. 24-11). However, the reported cases were selected and were not identified in a prospective manner. In a prospective study of 717 cocaine-exposed infants, cranial ultrasonography, although not the optimal imaging modality, did not identify cerebral infarction.[379]

Smaller areas of apparent infarction were described in basal ganglia, periventricular white matter and brain stem by some investigators.[440,444,486,487] However, it is unclear that such lesions are more common in cocaine-exposed infants than in appropriately chosen control infants.[379,449,488,489]

Intracranial *hemorrhage* was described in approximately 10% of primarily full-term cocaine-exposed infants in one series,[440] as well as in approximately 30% to 70% of very low-birth-weight, cocaine-exposed infants in three other series.[379,450,489,490] The lesions in the more mature infants were not of major clinical importance, and the incidence of the larger, clinically significant intraventricular hemorrhages in the very low-birth-weight infants did not appear to be accentuated by the cocaine exposure.[379,449,490]

In summary, the available data derived from studies of cocaine-exposed newborns by brain imaging lead to the tentative conclusion that both ischemic and hemorrhagic lesions may occur. However, available data indicate that the infarctions directly attributable to cocaine are likely rare, and the hemorrhagic lesions probably relate largely to the degree of prematurity.

Neonatal Neurological and Neurophysiological Features. The *neonatal features* of infants exposed to cocaine in utero are not characterized by a distinctive constellation of craniofacial or other anomalies, but neurological features are not uncommon.* The most consistent findings have been neurobehavioral and motor. The neurobehavioral features consist principally of altered sleep-wake states, impaired visual and auditory attentiveness, and increased periods of agitated behavior. The motor features consist of extensor hypertonicity, hyperreflexia, coarse tremor, and increased motor activity. Neither syndrome generally requires therapy, and the features subside usually over weeks to months. The likelihood that at least the motor syndrome is related to a direct effect of cocaine is supported by the demonstration of a dose-dependent relationship between the severity of these features and the results of maternal hair cocaine toxicology.[350] Newborns exposed in utero to cocaine also have abnormalities of the EEG and brain stem auditory evoked responses, which generally disappear after 1 to 6 months.[497,502,514-518] Audiological follow-up, however, is indicated. More sophisticated studies of EEGs, based on quantified EEGs, have shown persistence of abnormalities after 12 months.[519]

---

*See references 187,350,363,379,385,386,402,416,429,430,432,435, 437-440,445,449,450,481,491-514a.

Prognosis

In the first weeks and months of life, cocaine-exposed infants are at increased risk for the occurrence of *sudden infant death syndrome (SIDS)*. In an early study of 66 infants exposed to cocaine in utero, 10 died of SIDS, an incidence of 15%.[495] In several subsequent studies, the incidences, although lower, were relatively high (i.e., 0.5%,[520] 0.8%,[521] 0.9%,[522] 0.4%,[523] and 1.4%[413]). In general, the risk of SIDS in cocaine-exposed infants has been significantly greater statistically than the risk in control infants, with a range of increased risk from approximately threefold to seven-fold. Both clinical and laboratory data suggest that regulation of respiration and arousal is impaired in cocaine-exposed infants, and such impairment could presage the occurrence of SIDS.[521,524-527]

Neurological and cognitive outcomes of infants exposed to cocaine in utero have been addressed in many reports.[363,444,448,490,528-559] Nearly all reports that evaluated the study infants by the Bayley Scales of Infant Development or other conventional measures, except perhaps for measures of language development, detected no significant differences between cocaine-exposed and appropriately selected control infants. *However, it is important to ask whether conventional tests of neurological and cognitive development are suitable to detect the potential abnormalities in cocaine-exposed infants.* Thus, consideration of the experimental data concerning the monoaminergic systems most likely to be affected by prenatal cocaine exposure leads to the suggestion that the function of the limbic, hypothalamic, and extrapyramidal systems should be examined especially closely. However, most of the tests used in conventional follow-up studies do not quantify effectively arousal, attention, emotional control, and higher-level motor functions.[560] Such functions are crucial for effective adaptation to social and educational environments, and abnormalities therein could be disabling. Indeed, reports that addressed such neurobehavioral and motor capacities on follow-up generally delineated distinct deficits in older infants and young children exposed to cocaine in utero (Table 24-14).[444,448,490,511,543-548,552,557,558]

Pathogenesis

Cocaine exerts its effects on the developing nervous system through teratogenic effects and destructive effects. Although these two types of effects may exist in the same infant, they are discussed separately next.

TABLE 24-14	**Neurological Outcome in Cocaine-Exposed Newborns***
No consistent deficits in cognitive abilities measured by conventional measures (e.g., Bayley Scales) when confounders (e.g., other drugs, alcohol, intrauterine infection) are considered	
Deficits in neurobehavioral features (e.g., attention, emotional control, aggressiveness, emotional expressivity) and in higher motor functions	
Deficits ameliorated by enriched postnatal environment	

*See text for references.

Mechanisms of Teratogenic Effects. The balance of available data suggests that the teratogenic effects of cocaine relate to direct effects of the drug and are not secondary to destructive effects. The most common teratogenic manifestation of cocaine exposure (i.e., micrencephaly, as discussed earlier) may involve neuronal proliferation and differentiation. Cocaine administration to neonatal rats resulted in inhibition of DNA synthesis and alterations of membrane lipids in all brain regions,[561,562] consistent with the direct effects shown in nonneural tissues.[563,564] Deleterious effects on neuronal differentiation in rodent models were also observed.[474,477,478] Moreover, the disturbances in neuronal number and differentiation were observed in primate models.[474-476] Whether the effects on neuronal proliferation and differentiation relate to perturbation of the action of critical genes, including immediate early genes, is an intriguing possibility that requires further study.[467,468]

The mechanism of the effects of cocaine on neuronal differentiation and on development of crucial neuronal pathways in the cerebrum, diencephalon, and brain stem (subsequent to neuronal proliferation) could relate to the fundamental mechanisms of action of cocaine on neurotransmitters. The neuronal pathways involved either use several monoamines (e.g., norepinephrine, dopamine, serotonin) as neurotransmitters or are the targets of neurons that use monoamines as neurotransmitters. The derangements of homeostasis of these neurotransmitters by cocaine are, of course, the principal mechanisms of action of the drug in the adult brain. The specific nature of the derangements in the fetus requires further definition but appears similar. Although increased levels of these neurotransmitters may be expected, at least initially, long-term exposure to cocaine could lead to their depletion, as shown in experimental models and in adult humans.[392,565-569] The findings of reduction in striatal dopamine in neonatal rabbits exposed to cocaine in utero and diminished cerebrospinal fluid levels of homovanillic acid, the principal metabolite of dopamine, in cocaine-exposed newborns supports this possibility.[569,570] These neurotransmitters appear very early in brain development and *play important regulatory roles in development of neuronal circuitry*.[469,474,571-581] Indeed, because these monoaminergic systems, which originate especially in the brain stem, have widely distributed contacts in the basal ganglia, cerebral cortex, hypothalamus, and elsewhere, disturbances in their function during development could have very far-reaching effects. For example, neurons containing norepinephrine in the locus ceruleus (a pigmented nucleus in the pons) give rise to ascending monosynaptic pathways that are distributed widely in the cerebral cortex and diencephalon. These pathways are considered to have primarily activating influences. A prominent dopaminergic system originates in the substantia nigra of the midbrain and terminates in the striatum. These connections are important in regulation of movement and tone. Other dopaminergic systems terminate in limbic and cortical structures and are crucial not only for the reinforcing actions of drugs such as cocaine but

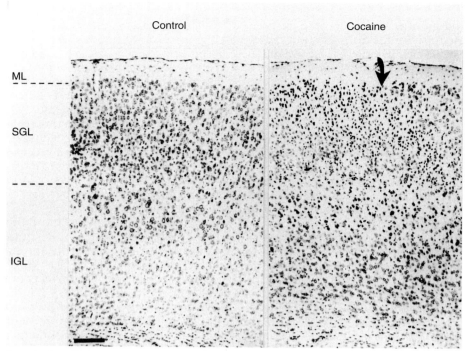

Figure 24-12 **Impaired cerebral cortical neuronal organization (in the adult rat) after intrauterine cocaine exposure.** Animals were exposed to saline (control) or cocaine from intrauterine day E8 through E18 and sacrificed at 40 days after birth. Cresyl violet staining of the molecular layer (ML), supragranular layers (SGL), and infragranular layers (IGL) of cerebral cortex is shown. The severe disorganization of the cortical layering in the cocaine-exposed animals contrasts with the regular lamination in the control animals. In particular, note the inversion of nuclear staining intensity between the SGL and IGL and the focal heterogeneity of nuclear size within the SGL *(arrow). (From Nassogne MC, Gressens P, Evrard P, Courtoy PJ: In contrast to cocaine, prenatal exposure to methadone does not produce detectable alterations in the developing mouse brain,* Dev Brain Res *110:61–67, 1998.)*

also for motivational-attentional functions. Prominent serotoninergic systems originate in the raphe nuclei of the brain stem, project widely, and are essential for regulation of sleep and level of alertness. However, because disturbances of the development of neuronal circuitry do not leave a readily identifiable, morphological stamp and require highly sensitive immunochemical and neuropharmacological techniques for detection, identification of such neural abnormalities in humans is very difficult. However, impairment of subsequent cerebral cortical development by prenatal cocaine exposure during the period in which monoamines influence neural development was shown in primate as well as rodent cerebral cortex.[465,469,473,475,476] Careful study of cerebral cortical development in the rat showed, in the *adult* cortex, abnormalities of neuronal lamination and dendritic morphology after *prenatal* exposure to cocaine (Fig. 24-12).[473,477]

Mechanisms of Destructive Effects. The mechanism of the ischemic and hemorrhagic CNS lesions associated with intrauterine cocaine exposure, albeit unusual, is probably multifactorial (see Fig. 24-9). Regarding the genesis of any *hemorrhagic lesions,* it is likely that fetal hypoxemia produced by restricted placental blood flow impairs fetal cerebrovascular autoregulation, as has been demonstrated in animal models[582,583] and thereby renders the fetus exquisitely vulnerable to changes in arterial blood pressure. The abrupt increases in blood pressure caused by both placentally transferred

catecholamines and elevated fetal catecholamine secretion because of the action of placentally transferred cocaine and fetal hypoxemia may encourage hemorrhages. Such hemorrhages could also occur in the immediate neonatal period, because elevations of blood pressure[584,585] and of cerebral blood flow velocity[449,586] have been documented on the first and second postnatal days in infants exposed to cocaine in utero.

Regarding the genesis of the *ischemic lesions,* vasospasm may be crucial, as it is in the genesis of ischemic cerebral vascular phenomena in adults (see Fig. 24-10). Several studies showed that application of cocaine directly to pial arteries of the neonatal piglet and the fetal and neonatal lamb caused a decrease in vessel diameter.[587-590] Studies of cerebrovascular resistance in fetal sheep documented an increase in cerebrovascular resistance in the minutes following cocaine administration.[591] The molecular mechanism of the vasoconstrictive effect of cocaine remains to be established, although cocaine-induced vasospasm leading to ischemic stroke in adult patients is well known.[592] Moreover, infants exposed to cocaine in utero have shown evidence of ischemic injury to heart, skeletal structures, and intestine.[593-595] The possibility that ischemic effects secondary to vasoconstriction may occur in a focal manner requires consideration in view of the demonstration in fetal and newborn sheep that cocaine did not decrease global cerebral blood flow.[591,596,597]

The *state of development of cerebral vessels in the human fetus* may explain the *distribution* of the ischemic lesions. The extraparenchymal, leptomeningeal arteries begin to develop a distinct muscularis in the second trimester and have a well-developed muscularis in the third trimester of gestation,[598] the time of occurrence of the cerebral infarcts reported in cocaine-exposed infants. Thus, the middle cerebral artery, the vessel affected in most cocaine-induced strokes, presumably does not develop the capacity to undergo spasm until the third trimester.

Neuronal excitotoxicity is a possible additional mechanism of neuronal injury in the cocaine-exposed fetus (see Fig. 24-10). Thus, in neuronal cell cultures, catecholamines can lead to neuronal death, principally by acting as glutamate agonists, especially in dopaminergic neurons and their projection targets.[599-602] Moreover, glutamate receptor antagonists markedly reduced the occurrence of cocaine-induced seizures, other neurological phenomena, and death in mice.[603,604]

Management

Prevention of cocaine exposure in utero is the cornerstone of management. In many respects, this aspect of management relates most closely to socioeconomics and education, topics discussed more appropriately elsewhere. The beneficial value of prenatal care has been documented.[169,605] In the neonatal period, no specific pharmacological intervention is warranted. An enriched *postnatal environment* over the first several years appears crucial in modulating any effects of cocaine on the infant's cognitive and behavioral development.[551-554,556,559]

DRUGS CAUSING PASSIVE ADDICTION

Passive addiction of the newborn refers to addiction acquired through a mother who, during pregnancy, used neuroactive drugs (e.g., narcotic analgesics such as heroin and methadone, SSRIs, sedative-hypnotics such as barbiturates, alcohol, and a variety of other medications). When the infant is deprived of this supply of drug by the process of birth, a withdrawal syndrome develops that shares many of the features seen in withdrawal in older patients. However, the *hallmark* of *neonatal withdrawal* is a striking disorder of movement, most aptly termed "jitteriness." The following sections include a discussion of neonatal drug withdrawal, with particular attention given to narcotic analgesics, which have been the best-studied causes of passive addiction. For several drugs, the possibility of a concomitant teratogenic effect has been raised (see later discussions), but the postnatal withdrawal syndrome *dominates* the clinical syndromes associated with maternal abuse of these agents.

Heroin

Passive addiction to heroin serves as the prototype for passive addiction to narcotic analgesics. Indeed, the principles of passive addiction to heroin apply in many respects to passive addiction to all neuroactive drugs. Thus, passive addiction of the newborn to this still commonly abused drug is appropriately discussed first and in greatest detail.

Incidence

The incidence of newborns passively addicted to narcotic analgesics among the total newborn population varies greatly from one medical center to another. In some large urban hospitals, where addicts (particularly heroin addicts) are found in great numbers, the incidence has been as high as 2% to 3% of all births.[606] In a study of 29,494 women delivering infants in California in the early 1990s, 1.5% of the women had a positive urine test for opiates.[169] Approximately 6000 to 10,000 newborns are born yearly to opiate-addicted women.[389]

Clinical Features

Infants who are born to heroin-addicted mothers most consistently have two major features. They are often *infants of low birth weight*, and they usually have a characteristic *withdrawal syndrome*.[169,171,389,606-621]

Low Birth Weight. The incidence of low birth weight (i.e., <2500 g) among newborns of heroin-addicted women, reported in earlier studies, was approximately 50%. In a composite series of reported cases gathered from those years, 260 of 521 infants born to heroin addicts weighed less than 2500 g (i.e., an ≈50% incidence).[608-611] In a more recent study, the mean values for opiate-exposed infants were 2651g birth weight and 37.3 weeks for gestational age.[555] Fully 42% of infants had a birth weight of less than 2500 g, and 31% were small for gestational age, thus indicating a role for *intrauterine growth retardation*. In one extensive study, the mean gestational age for heroin-addicted infants was 38 weeks; the mean birth weight was 2490 g (Table 24-15).[612] Infants born to mothers with a documented history of heroin abuse but who were drug free during the index pregnancy (i.e., ex-addicts) had a mean birth weight of only 2615 g, with a mean gestational age of 38.6 weeks (see Table 24-15). This occurrence of intrauterine growth retardation in infants of ex-addicts is reminiscent of experimental studies that demonstrated growth retardation in progeny of female rats given

TABLE 24-15   Mean Birth Weight and Gestational Age of Infants with Different Drug Exposure during Gestation

Maternal Drug Use	No. of Infants	Birth Weight: Mean (g)	Gestational Age: Mean (wk)
Heroin	61	2,490	38.0
Ex-addict	33	2,616	38.6
Heroin and methadone	59	2,535	38.3
Methadone	106	2,961	39.4
Control	66	3,176	40.0

Adapted from Kandall SR, Albin S, Lowinson J, Berle B, et al: Differential effects of maternal heroin and methadone use on birth weight, *Pediatrics* 58:681–685, 1976.

morphine *before* but not after conception.[622] However, it is also possible that other factors (e.g., related to nutrition or infection) were present in the mothers before and after addiction.

An additional and disturbing feature of the intrauterine growth retardation in infants passively addicted to heroin is a potential disturbance of brain growth, manifested by *small head size*. Thus, in a series of 40 infants, 40% of the babies exhibited a head circumference less than the 10th percentile for gestational age.[609] However, because of the methodological difficulties associated with studies of infants born to substance-abusing mothers (see earlier discussion of methodological difficulties in section on cocaine), definitive conclusion of impaired brain growth caused by heroin per se is difficult. The cause of the disturbances in intrauterine growth is not entirely clear, and the relative roles of intrauterine undernutrition, infection, and toxic effects of other drugs and exogenous materials remain to be elucidated. Although a direct effect of narcotic analgesics on cell number was suggested by experimental studies (see later), analysis of human infants is more supportive of an indirect effect related to impaired maternal nutrition or other factors related to maternal addiction.[378] Supportive of this notion is a recent study of 1227 infants whose head circumference was similar in opiate-exposed and non–opiate-exposed infants; many of the latter were exposed to other drugs, alcohol, and other variables.[555]

Withdrawal Syndrome. The incidence of the second major feature observed among newborns of heroin-addicted mothers, the characteristic withdrawal syndrome, varies with certain factors discussed subsequently. However, the overall incidence is approximately 70%, ranging from approximately 60% to 90%.[169,171,389,607-617,619,620,623-625]

The *likelihood of withdrawal symptoms* in an infant born to a heroin-addicted mother seems to relate primarily to four factors, namely, the amount of the maternal dose, the length of time from the last dose to birth, the duration of maternal addiction to the drug, and the gestational age of the infant.[169,171,607,611,613,614,617] Withdrawal symptoms in the passively addicted newborn are more likely if the maternal dose was high, if the last dose was within 24 hours of the time of birth, if the mother was a long-term addict, and if the infant was born at term.

The *time of onset* of the withdrawal syndrome in the newborn delivered to a heroin-addicted woman is usually quite early (Table 24-16). Approximately 65% of infants present within the first 24 hours of life; an additional approximately 20% present on the second day of life; and the remainder, or approximately 15%, present on the third and fourth days.[611] This temporal pattern of onset is a very helpful clinical point in differentiating the jitteriness of drug withdrawal from that resulting from other important causes (see Chapter 5). For example, hypocalcemia associated with jitteriness is usually manifested later (i.e., in the latter part of the first week or in the second week of life).

The *initial and dominant symptoms and signs* of the withdrawal syndrome relate primarily to disturbance of the *CNS* (Table 24-17). A virtually invariable feature is jitteriness. As discussed in Chapter 5, the movements of jitteriness are characterized primarily by tremulousness. They are exquisitely stimulus sensitive, are rhythmic, and usually are of equal rate and amplitude, and they can be induced to cease by gentle passive flexion of the limb. Unlike seizure, jitteriness is accompanied neither by abnormalities of gaze or extraocular movement nor by clonic jerking of limbs. The tremulous movements in infants passively addicted to heroin are usually quite dramatic and have a coarse, flapping quality. The babies are very irritable and frequently are extremely active and hypertonic. Sleep periods are markedly diminished, and the cry is often high pitched and shrill. Sucking is excessive, and often "frantic sucking" of the fists or fingers is noted. These frequent clinical features (75% to 100% of symptomatic cases) are very helpful in making the clinical distinction of the jitteriness of drug withdrawal from that resulting from other important causes (e.g., hypoglycemia and hypoxia). Hypoglycemia can cause jitteriness in the first 24 to 48 hours of life, but in hypoglycemia, the infant is almost always stuporous as well, quite unlike the hyperalert, hyperactive infant with withdrawal symptoms. Similarly, hypoxic-ischemic encephalopathy characteristically causes jitteriness in the first 24 to 48 hours of life, but such infants almost always have the characteristic history of a perinatal hypoxic-ischemic insult, are significantly stuporous, and very frequently exhibit seizures. The clinical picture may be complicated by concomitant passive addiction and hypoxic encephalopathy; in several series, fully 20% to 40% of addicted infants exhibited signs of fetal distress, Apgar scores of 6 or less at 1 or 5 minutes, or both.[389,626,627]

TABLE 24-16 **Time of Onset of Withdrawal Syndrome in Infants Passively Addicted to Heroin**

Time after Birth (hr)	No. of Infants	Percentage of Total*
0–12	76	29%
12–24	88	34%
24–48	56	21%
48–96	39	15%

*Total is all infants with withdrawal syndrome (i.e., 259 of 384, or 67.4% of complete series of infants born to heroin addicts).
Adapted from Zelson C, Rubio E, Wasserman E: Neonatal narcotic addiction: 10-year observation, *Pediatrics* 48:178–189, 1971.

TABLE 24-17 **Signs of Withdrawal from Heroin**

RELATIVE FREQUENCY (PERCENTAGE OF TOTAL)			
75%–100%	**25%–75%**	**<25%**	**Rare**
Jitteriness	Poor feeding	Fever	Seizures
Irritability	Vomiting		
Hyperactivity-hypertonicity	Diarrhea		
Decreased sleeping	Sneezing		
Shrill cry	Tachypnea		
Excessive sucking	Sweating		

Next in frequency of occurrence is a series of symptoms relating especially to *gastrointestinal* disturbance (see Table 24-17). Poor feeding is the most prominent of these features (one that, in fact, may reflect more of a neurological than a gastrointestinal disturbance). Despite the initially excessive sucking described previously, the infant decreases sucking rapidly with feeding. Dyscoordination of sucking, swallowing, and respiration is very common.[621] Regurgitation of feedings is also a relatively common feature. Diarrhea occurs in as many as 30% to 50% of these infants and can contribute to dehydration and electrolyte disturbances. These latter gastrointestinal phenomena tend to appear later (i.e., days 4 to 6) than those related to the CNS.[389,607,610,613]

Sneezing and tachypnea are less common disturbances (see Table 24-17). Still less common, but disturbing when they do occur, are *fever* and *sweating*. Fever must always raise the possibility of infection, and the diagnosis should be ruled out by appropriate studies. Although sweating is uncommon, it can be a helpful diagnostic sign, because it is very unusual to see sweating in newborns, especially small newborns.

Seizures are a distinctly uncommon manifestation of neonatal withdrawal to heroin (see Table 24-17). The reported incidence is approximately 1% to 2% of cases.[606,611] It is, in fact, difficult to be convinced from published data that any of the examples of seizure associated with withdrawal to heroin were not related to complicating factors (e.g., hypoxia-ischemia or metabolic disease) or were not examples of particularly marked jitteriness. This conclusion is compatible with the finding that seizures are not a feature of withdrawal to heroin in adult patients. (Seizures may be more common in the newborn in methadone withdrawal; see "Methadone.") Thus, passive addiction to heroin should be low on the list of considerations when one is faced with a newborn with seizures, and even in the infant who is definitely passively addicted to heroin, seizure phenomena should raise the possibility of a serious complicating illness and should provoke appropriate diagnostic studies.

Pathogenesis

Basic Theories. The pathogenesis of dependence to narcotic analgesics, and particularly the clinical syndrome that results on withdrawal of these drugs, is complex and probably involves the endogenous opiate receptors, cyclic guanosine monophosphate and cyclic adenosine monophosphate metabolism, intracellular signal transduction mechanisms, and, ultimately, effects on ion channels and several major neurotransmitter systems.[169,404,618,628-641] In their simplest form, two basic theories of withdrawal can be described: *disuse hypersensitivity* and *development of alternate pathways*.

The theory of *disuse hypersensitivity* notes that a drug may depress certain neural systems and may render their targets hypersensitive to their usual stimuli. When the depressing drug is removed, rebound hypersensitivity of the affected targets is apparent, and the withdrawal syndrome results. The hypersensitivity phenomenon may be caused, at least in certain circumstances, by an increase in synthesis of receptors. However, more complex intracellular effects also likely occur.

The theory of *alternate pathways* notes that a drug may depress a primary neural pathway, and as a result, alternate pathways, normally of minor activity, become prominent in an attempt to compensate. When the drug is removed, both the primary and alternate pathways are operative in an additive fashion and cause the withdrawal syndrome.

Probably both the pathways just mentioned are operative in passive addiction of the fetus and neonatal narcotic withdrawal syndrome. Endogenous opiates and opiate receptors of several types are important in the developing central and autonomic nervous systems.[618] However, the cellular and molecular mechanisms provoked by these receptors and operative in the addicted newborn remain largely unknown. As noted earlier, studies in mature neural models suggest that the most critical final step involves *neuronal norepinephrine release* in the locus ceruleus in brain stem.[641-643] Thus, opiates activate opiate receptors in the locus ceruleus, thereby causing, sequentially, a decrease in cyclic adenosine monophosphate production, an increase in potassium efflux, a decrease in calcium influx and, as a consequence, a reduction in norepinephrine release. With long-term opiate use, this effect is diminished as tolerance develops, and on opiate withdrawal, this inhibiting effect is lost, and a supranormal increase in norepinephrine levels occurs.[643]

Management

The three major facets to the management of the infant passively addicted to heroin are recognition, supportive therapy, and drug therapy (Table 24-18).

Recognition. First, the diagnosis must be considered. Perhaps it is trite to include this discussion, but so often the diagnosis is overlooked for a day or more because the obstetrician's account of the maternal history or the history from the pediatrician, often obtained only from the infant's father, did not suggest that the mother may have taken narcotics during pregnancy. The newborn's physician must ask specific questions about drug use, preferably directly to the mother, and,

TABLE 24-18	Management of Withdrawal Syndrome in Infants Passively Addicted to Heroin
Recognition	
Supportive therapy	
Drug therapy	
Narcotic agent*: tincture of opium, methadone, morphine	
Phenobarbital†	
Chlorpromazine	
Diazepam	

*Treatment of first choice.
†Combination of opiate and phenobarbital may be superior to opiate alone (see text).

when possible, should personally examine the mother for needle marks or other signs of drug use. A maternal history of hepatitis, thrombophlebitis, or other complications of illicit drug usage should also be sought. Suitable screening of urine and especially meconium, as described earlier for cocaine, is useful.[171,352,353,357,358,360,389]

Supportive Therapy. *Supportive therapy* is clearly the most critical aspect of the management of these infants. Pulmonary complications (aspiration pneumonia, including meconium aspiration, and hyaline membrane disease), infection, dehydration, and various metabolic derangements often complicate the clinical course. In a large series of 830 infants passively addicted to heroin (with or without methadone), 22 died; of these infants, 64% died of either severe hyaline membrane disease (41%) or meconium aspiration (23%), and "no death occurred secondary to narcotic withdrawal."[627] These complications must be watched for diligently and treated vigorously when they occur.

Drug Therapy. The third major aspect of the therapeutic program is the choice of the drug to be used for treatment, primarily, of the CNS and gastrointestinal disturbances. Of particular concern are marked jitteriness and hyperactivity, minimal sleeping, impaired feeding, and persistent vomiting and diarrhea. Most addicted newborns require such therapy. The four major drugs administered in the past and currently used in various medical centers are narcotic agents, phenobarbital, chlorpromazine, and diazepam.[169,171,389,609-613,624,625,643-648]

Narcotic agents used for this purpose have included paregoric, tincture of opium (or laudanum USP), and methadone. *Paregoric* has been a commonly used drug in this context. It is highly effective in treating both the CNS and gastrointestinal disturbances. However, this agent is no longer recommended because of potentially toxic additives (camphor, benzoic acid, anise oil).[643] Diluted tincture of opium (DTO) is preferred over paregoric. DTO (0.4 mg/mL of morphine equivalent) is administered in a dose of 0.05 to 0.1 mL/kg given orally.[169,625] The dose can be increased by 0.05- to 0.10-mL increments every 3 to 4 hours until the symptoms are controlled. The usual dose for infants ranges from 0.2 to 0.5 mL every 3 to 4 hours. Tincture of opium, unlike paregoric, does not contain camphor, a CNS stimulant. The symptoms usually disappear after days, but therapy is relatively long (i.e., many weeks on the average) because the dose must be diminished gradually to avoid recurrence of withdrawal symptoms.[389,645] In one controlled study, the duration of DTO use was 76±22 days.[625] When this drug was combined with phenobarbital, the duration of treatment with DTO was reduced to 35±21 days, and the duration of hospitalization diminished from 79 days to 38 days.[624,625] Methadone has been used in treatment of addicted infants; the initial dose is 0.05 to 0.10 mg/kg given every 6 to 12 hours, with increases of 0.05 mg/kg until symptoms are controlled. Methadone can be administered every 12 to 24 hours because of its relatively long half-life.[169] Morphine also has been effective,[648] but methadone may be preferable because of better oral bioavailability.[643] Of these agents, I have had most experience with tincture of opium.

Phenobarbital is effective in treating the CNS phenomena. A loading dose of 20 to 30 mg/kg is administered and followed by a dose of approximately 5 mg/kg/day, although the clinical response should determine the maintenance dose. Most patients exhibit marked improvement within 24 hours, and when phenobarbital is used with DTO, the durations of therapy and of hospitalization are less than for DTO alone.[624,625] However, vomiting and diarrhea are *not* benefited by phenobarbital, and poor sucking and feeding may, in fact, be made worse.[649] Thus, phenobarbital is not an ideal single agent.

Chlorpromazine therapy was satisfactory in several series. It was used exclusively in the largest single series reported, involving 178 treated infants.[611] The drug is effective in treating both the CNS and gastrointestinal phenomena. The recommended dose is 2 to 3 mg/kg/day, administered in divided doses every 6 hours.[389,609,611] The drug may be given orally. Marked improvement usually occurs within 24 hours, and the duration of therapy is 2 to 3 weeks. This drug carries the uncommon risks of causing extrapyramidal phenomena and hematological abnormalities in the newborn and of lowering the seizure threshold.

Diazepam (Valium) has been used in the treatment of narcotic withdrawal and is apparently effective in the control of some of the CNS phenomena. Its advantage, if any, has been claimed to be a decrease in the time needed for treatment to approximately 1 week.[650] However, this conclusion is based on a single small series. Although no controlled data exist from comparisons between diazepam and opiates, phenobarbital, or chlorpromazine, available information suggests that diazepam is not as effective as opiates.[606,643,645]

At the present time, I recommend *DTO as the drug of first choice* in therapy. *Phenobarbital* should be added if CNS phenomena are marked, and the balance of current data suggests that the combination of DTO and phenobarbital is the preferred treatment for neonatal narcotic withdrawal.

Prognosis

The prognosis of passive addiction to heroin may be considered in terms of the acute neonatal withdrawal syndrome, the development of the so-called *subacute withdrawal syndrome*, the occurrence of SIDS, and the long-term outlook.

Acute Withdrawal Syndrome. The acute prognosis relates primarily to the care of the newborn with the withdrawal syndrome. Morbidity and mortality are related principally to the aforementioned complications. By the 1990s, the mortality rate had been reduced to less than 5%.[169,171,389,609-611,627] Currently, with modern neonatal intensive care, it is reasonable to expect that no infant should die of narcotic withdrawal per se.

Subacute Withdrawal Syndrome. An interesting syndrome of subacute withdrawal was defined.[607,608,615,616] In one series, this phenomenon occurred in approximately 80% of babies who had withdrawal symptoms in the neonatal period.[608] The usual course was for the child to be discharged from the nursery after at least considerable improvement or even apparent recovery from neonatal drug withdrawal. Shortly after discharge, symptoms exacerbated or recurred. Patients exhibited restlessness, agitation, and tremors; the tremors were extremely sensitive to external stimuli, especially sound. In addition, these infants greatly stressed the tolerance of their mothers because of very brief sleep periods, excessive milk intake, colic, and vomiting. Not infrequently, the addicted mother who took her child home was unable to cope with such an infant and transferred the infant to foster care.[389,607,608] The syndrome persisted for 3 to 6 months and tended to disappear gradually without therapy.

Sudden Infant Death Syndrome. Prenatal exposure to opiates is associated with a sharply increased risk for SIDS.[169,171,389,522,651-654] In a large study of 1760 cases of SIDS in New York City, the rate of the syndrome in the no-drug group was 1.39 per 1000; in contrast, in the heroin-exposed infants, it was 5.83 per 1000.[654] The cause of this severalfold increased risk is unknown, but the risk has been highest in those infants who exhibited moderate to severe withdrawal syndromes as newborns.

Long-Term Intellectual Development. The long-term outcome of infants passively addicted to heroin has been variable but, in general, not consistently or clearly abnormal.[378,389,555,607,608,619,623,655-658] On balance, the data indicate that during the first 2 years of life and at the time of school age, neurological development and cognitive function are within the normal range, although sometimes slightly lower in narcotic-exposed infants than in control infants. However, as discussed for cocaine (see earlier section), it is not conclusively established that the conventional outcome measures evaluate those behavioral and cognitive phenomena most likely to be affected by prenatal exposure to narcotics. Indeed, abnormalities of behavior, state control, visual and auditory orientation, and consolability were observed on limited follow-up of narcotic-exposed infants.[169] Many studies in developing animals of opiate exposure suggest deleterious effects on neuronal and glial proliferation and differentiation.[607,618,659-672] However, a careful study of cortical development in the mouse showed no detectable alteration in animals treated prenatally with narcotic-analgesic.[473]

Currently, the most appropriate formulation appears to be that CNS abnormalities noted on follow-up evaluations are related not to the heroin exposure but to associated factors, such as poor prenatal care, maternal undernutrition, intrauterine infection (e.g., 27% of infants in one series of pregnant heroin addicts had syphilis),[555,658,673] toxic materials in street drug preparations, postnatal undernutrition, and otherwise defective home environment. Indeed, regression analysis of data derived from one carefully studied group led to the conclusions that the amount of prenatal care and prenatal disturbances (e.g., poor nutrition), as well as the home environment, were "most predictive of intellectual performance," and that "the degree of maternal narcotic use was not a significant factor."[378]

Methadone

Incidence

The other narcotic analgesic primarily associated with passive addiction of the newborn is methadone. Indeed, the most popular and effective mode of therapy currently available for addiction to heroin in the pregnant woman is maintenance with oral methadone. In fact, at present, methadone is probably the major drug of importance in passive addiction of the newborn. In the late 1970s, numerous programs in large urban medical centers were instituted in which pregnant heroin addicts were placed on methadone maintenance and were provided intensive medical and psychosocial support. These programs are the source of the most valuable information regarding the effects of methadone on the fetus and newborn.[169,378,389,612-614,617,646,673-693]

Clinical Features

Although methadone maintenance programs have had a beneficial effect on *mothers*, major prenatal difficulties remain.[169,378,389,626,673,680,686,689] Thus, medical diseases (e.g., syphilis) are detected and treated frequently. Good nutritional status is encouraged and is sometimes improved. Obstetrical complications (e.g., toxemia) are often controlled. Post partum, most mothers usually remain in the program, and most women keep their infants.[673] Nevertheless, important prenatal problems have persisted. In one careful study, methadone-treated women resembled untreated heroin addicts more than a control group in terms of nutritional status, weight gain, and amount of smoking.[378] Moreover, *total* narcotic usage (methadone and heroin) reported by methadone-treated mothers was *greater* than that of untreated heroin users.[378]

The *newborns* of methadone-treated mothers exhibit distinct effects of the passive addiction. (Nevertheless, the methadone programs were instituted primarily to decrease the *maternal* and *fetal* complications associated with illicit heroin use.) The two characteristic features of passive addiction of the newborn to narcotic analgesics, low birth weight and the withdrawal syndrome, are still very much apparent in methadone-addicted infants.

Low Birth Weight. The incidence of low birth weight (i.e., <2500 g) varies between 10% and 35%. Between 10% and 40% of these low-birth-weight infants are small for gestational age. However, in a large series of 106 such infants, mean birth weight was

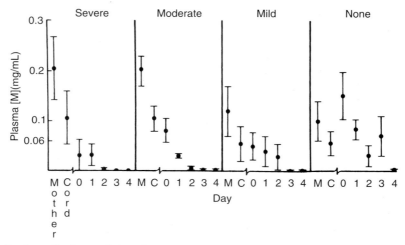

Figure 24-13　**Passive addiction to methadone: relation of occurrence and severity of signs of withdrawal to rate of elimination of methadone.** Data derived from study of 31 infants born to mothers receiving methadone during pregnancy. The fastest declines in plasma methadone (M) concentrations correlated with occurrence of the most severe signs. *(From Rosen TS, Pippenger CE: Pharmacologic observations on the neonatal withdrawal syndrome, J Pediatr 88:1044–1048, 1976.)*

significantly higher in methadone-addicted infants than in heroin-addicted infants (see Table 24-15).[612] The value of 2961 g was significantly lower than that in the control group (i.e., 3176 g).

Withdrawal Syndrome. The *incidence* of the withdrawal syndrome in infants born to mothers receiving methadone maintenance therapy is similar to the incidence recorded for infants of heroin-addicted mothers and varies from 50% to 95%.* The *likelihood of occurrence* of the syndrome relates particularly to the concentration of methadone in cord blood and to the rate of elimination of methadone in the infants.[684,686,694] Maternal dose during pregnancy does *not* appear to be a critical determinant,[691-693] although cord blood levels are inversely related to the occurrence of a neonatal withdrawal syndrome requiring therapy.[692] This relationship is likely related to the second factor (i.e., the postnatal rate of elimination of methadone). Thus, the likelihood of neonatal withdrawal features directly correlates with faster rates of decline of neonatal methadone levels.[688] Moreover, the *severity* of symptoms also relates particularly to the rate of elimination (Fig. 24-13). This finding is entirely consistent with an observation in adult patients (i.e., a rapid decrease in the drug level in blood causes more frequent and more severe symptoms).

The *onset* of the withdrawal symptoms with methadone is generally slightly later than with heroin. Thus, most infants have the onset of overt symptoms on the second day of life (Table 24-19), not on the first day as with heroin. The median onset of therapy in one study was 35 hours.[692] Ten to 15% of infants born to methadone-treated mothers have the onset of their

neurological syndrome *after* day 3.[626,673,695] This late onset is rare in infants who are passively addicted to heroin. The delay in onset correlates with the administration of the last dose of methadone before the time of delivery (Fig. 24-14). Indeed, withdrawal symptoms in infants passively addicted to methadone may occur initially or may recur as late as 2 to 4 weeks or more after birth.[389,695] In fact, an occasional infant has died before the nature of this later syndrome was recognized.

The reasons for the delayed onset and prolonged duration may relate to the pharmacokinetics of methadone elimination in the newborn.[688,694] It is well known in adults that the withdrawal syndrome in methadone addiction develops more slowly (peak 6 days) and lasts longer than with heroin.[638] Good evidence is available for avid tissue binding of methadone with gradual and slow release on withdrawal.[696] The critical point is that the clinician must be alert to this possibility of delayed onset in the infant of age 1 week or more who develops jitteriness, diarrhea, and other signs of withdrawal.

TABLE 24-19	Time of Onset of Withdrawal Syndrome in Infants Passively Addicted to Methadone	
Time after Birth (hr)	**No. of Infants**	**Percentage of Total***
0–12	0	—
12–24	8	27%
24–48	16	53%
48–72	3	10%
>72	3	10%

*Total is all infants with withdrawal syndrome.
Adapted from Stimmel B, Adamsons K: Narcotic dependency in pregnancy, *JAMA* 235:1121–1124, 1976.

---

*See references 169,171,612-614,617,626,673,676,677,680-686,689, 691-693.

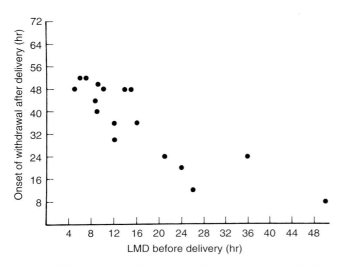

Figure 24-14   **Passive addiction to methadone: relation of the time of the last maternal methadone dose (LMD) to the time of onset of neonatal withdrawal.** The interval between onset of withdrawal and time of last maternal dose did not vary markedly and approximated 48 hours. *(From Rosen TS, Pippenger CE: Pharmacologic observations on the neonatal withdrawal syndrome,* J Pediatr *88:1044–1048, 1976.)*

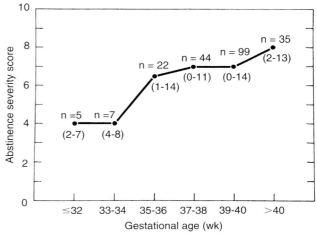

Figure 24-15   **Relationship between the severity of the neonatal withdrawal syndrome after passive addiction to methadone and the gestational age of the infant.** Scores are expressed as median values, with ranges in parentheses. Note the increase in severity with advancing gestational age. *(From Doberczak TM, Kandall SR, Wilets I: Neonatal opiate abstinence syndrome in term and preterm infants,* J Pediatr *118:933–937, 1991.)*

The *basic features of methadone-related withdrawal syndrome* are similar to those in heroin-addicted infants.* The likelihood and severity of the syndrome differ as a function of gestational age.[617] Thus, in a series of 178 term and 34 preterm infants, 50% and 16% of the term infants exhibited moderate and severe symptoms, respectively, whereas 21% and none of the premature infants exhibited moderate and severe symptoms, respectively.[617] The severity of the withdrawal syndrome as a function of gestational age is shown in Figure 24-15. The less severe manifestations in the preterm infant may relate to a lower total methadone exposure or to diminished neural capacity for clinical expression, or both factors. The *incidence of seizures* with passive addiction to methadone is *greater* than with heroin.[606,617,673,694] In the careful study of Herzlinger and co-workers,[606] 10 of 127 (8%) of infants passively addicted to methadone exhibited seizures. Seizures were a late manifestation of withdrawal, with a mean age of onset of 10 days. Paroxysmal phenomena were observed on the EEG preceding the onset of, as well as during, clinical seizures.[606] A direct relation of the seizures to the passive addiction to methadone, rather than to a complicating factor, was supported not only by the clinical data but also by the better response of the seizures to paregoric than to the anticonvulsant drug diazepam. A relation of the occurrence of seizures in methadone-exposed infants to gestational age is indicated by the occurrence of seizures in 7.3% of the term infants but in only 2.9% of the premature infants in the series of Doberczak and co-workers.[617] A second interesting difference between infants passively addicted to methadone and those addicted to heroin, reported in earlier studies, was a *more severe disturbance of the rate and effectiveness of nutritive sucking* in the methadone patients.[649] This disturbance, in part, may have been the cause of the particularly severe weight loss that can occur in these infants.[683] More recently, with prompt recognition and treatment of the withdrawal syndrome, the excessive sucking has become effective and hyperphagia is common, especially by the second postnatal week.[690]

Pathogenesis

The pathogenesis of passive addiction and the withdrawal syndrome with methadone is similar in basic principles to that described for heroin. The reason for the apparently increased incidence of seizures in methadone-addicted, as opposed to heroin-addicted, infants is unknown.

Management

Management of methadone-addicted infants is not different from that discussed earlier for heroin-addicted infants. A particularly important additional feature with the methadone-addicted babies is the need to be alert for delayed onset of the withdrawal syndrome, which may have very deleterious consequences. If treatment of the withdrawal syndrome is necessary, I consider DTO to be the drug of choice, with supplementation with phenobarbital if needed, as described for heroin. Indeed, the reports that showed the superiority of DTO and phenobarbital over DTO alone included cohorts that included more methadone-exposed than heroin-exposed infants.[624,625] In one comparative study of paregoric, phenobarbital, and diazepam as single therapeutic agents, paregoric was effective as a single agent in 91% of infants, phenobarbital in 47%, and diazepam in none.[646] A careful study of nutritive sucking in methadone-addicted infants

---

*See references 169,389,612-614,617,626,673,676,677,686,689,690, 697.

demonstrated a beneficial effect of paregoric and a very marked deleterious effect of diazepam.[649] Phenobarbital had an intermediate effect. As noted earlier, paregoric has been replaced by DTO.

Prognosis

Withdrawal Syndrome. The prognosis for methadone-dependent infants in the *newborn period* is similar in many ways to that described for heroin-dependent infants. The importance of management of complicating factors, as well as the withdrawal syndrome per se, cannot be overemphasized. Subacute evolution of abnormal behavioral features can be observed, as with heroin-addicted infants (see previous discussion).[389,607,614]

Sudden Infant Death Syndrome. As observed with prenatal heroin exposure, infants exposed to methadone in utero are at increased risk for SIDS in the first weeks and months of life.[627,654] In the study of 1760 cases of SIDS referred to earlier, the rate of deaths resulting from SIDS after prenatal methadone exposure was 9.66 per 1000 versus 1.39 per 1000 in the no-drug group and 5.83 per 1000 in the heroin-exposed group.[654]

Long-Term Intellectual Development. Intense interest in the long-term outcome of infants exposed to methadone in utero is understandable in view of the large numbers of these children. Some studies showed lower than normal head circumference in the neonatal period and low average mean scores in such developmental measures as the Bayley Scales of Infant Development and the McCarthy Cognitive Scales.* However, when comparison groups consisted of children of women with similarly poor prenatal status and postnatal home environment, the children generally scored as low as the children who were methadone-addicted infants. Indeed, as described earlier for heroin-addicted infants, methadone-maintained women often showed no advantage in terms of nutritional status, nicotine use, and other adverse factors during pregnancy.[378] Thus, it seems likely that the impairment in intellectual outcome in the methadone-dependent infants relates principally to other deleterious prenatal and postnatal factors and not directly to the effects of the narcotic analgesic on brain development.

Selective Serotonin Reuptake Inhibitors

Fetal exposure to SSRIs administered to pregnant women has been associated with a neonatal neurobehavioral syndrome. SSRIs are currently the drugs of choice for treatment of depression and anxiety disorders. Their mode of action is inhibition of serotonin uptake at the presynaptic nerve ending, resulting in increased serotonin concentrations in the synaptic cleft and thereby potentiated serotonergic neurotransmission. In general, no consistent evidence indicates an increased occurrence of major congenital anomalies

after intrauterine exposure to SSRIs, except perhaps for *slightly* increased risks for individual SSRIs.[698,698a,698b] By contrast, multiple reports since the mid-1990s clearly document a neonatal neurobehavioral syndrome.[699-714] The potential magnitude of this issue relates to the findings that the disorder requires neonatal intensive care in approximately 15% to 20% of cases, generally prolongs hospitalization, and is likely to be quite prevalent. Approximately 10% to 20% of pregnant women exhibit signs of depression, and as many as 35% receive pharmacological intervention. Thus, the number of women potentially involved is measured in the tens of thousands. As noted earlier, SSRIs currently are the drugs of choice for depression and anxiety.

Incidence

The incidence of a neonatal neurobehavioral syndrome after intrauterine exposure to SSRIs is not entirely known, but it is likely to be as high as 30% to 60%.[709,711,714] Thus, in view of the relatively high frequency of SSRI therapy of pregnant women with depression (see earlier), the prevalence of the neonatal syndrome is likely to be high. Because of the nature of the syndrome (see later) and its generally self-limited course, it is likely that the disorder has been overlooked or misdiagnosed, or both.

Clinical Features

Although fetal exposure to SSRIs is associated with neonatal clinical phenomena (see later), these drugs have no consistent effect on fetal development. Moreover, an effect on fetal growth, if present, is mild. Several reports recorded a slight decrease ($\approx$1 week) in gestational age and birth weight ($\approx$150 g).[699,706-708,713] This effect does not seem related to the neonatal syndrome.

A *neonatal neurobehavioral syndrome*, usually characterized as a withdrawal syndrome, is relatively consistent.[699-711,713,714] The history most commonly includes exposure to an SSRI, most commonly paroxetine (Paxil) or fluoxetine (Prozac), at least for the third trimester of pregnancy. Onset of the syndrome is in the first 2 days of life and consists principally of the features shown in Table 24-20. Approximately 30% of infants have a constellation that is prominent enough to be characterized as a moderate or severe *neonatal abstinence syndrome*. The principal clinical features are neurobehavioral, respiratory, and gastrointestinal. The neurobehavioral findings include irritability, agitation, high-pitched cry, sleep disturbances, tremor/jitteriness, shivering, hypertonicity, and, rarely, seizures. Seizures, generally, have been reported in fewer than 5% of infants, most often in approximately 1%.[708,711,713] The respiratory features include, most notably, tachypnea and respiratory distress. The gastrointestinal disturbances include exaggerated sucking, poor feeding, vomiting, and diarrhea. Hypoglycemia (blood glucose <40 mg/dL) has been observed in approximately 5% of cases and may relate to hyperinsulinism (SSRIs can cause maternal hyperglycemia, which could lead to fetal hyperinsulinism). Most infants recover over

*See references 169,378,389,555,607,613,614,623,674-679,687.

TABLE 24-20 Clinical Phenomena in Newborns Exposed to SSRIs In Utero*

Clinical Feature	SSRI-Exposed Infants (n = 60)	Control Infants (n = 60)
Neonatal abstinence syndrome*	18	0
High-pitched cry	18	0
Sleep disturbance	21	2
Tremor	37	11
Hypertonicity or myoclonus	14	1
Convulsions	2	0
Tachypnea	12	0
Gastrointestinal disturbance	34	2
Hypoglycemia	3	0

*Finnegan score of 4 or higher.
SSRIs, selective serotonin reuptake inhibitors.
Data from Levinson-Castiel R, Merlob P, Linder N, Sirota L, et al: Neonatal abstinence syndrome after in utero exposure to selective serotonin reuptake inhibitors in term infants, *Arch Pediatr Adolesc Med* 160:173–176, 2006.

several days to weeks. However, these infants not infrequently require neonatal intensive care and prolonged hospitalization, relative to normal term infants. Specific therapy generally is not required, although chlorpromazine has been used effectively in several cases.[704]

Prognosis

The *short-term outcome* is generally favorable. However, some of the neurobehavioral features may persist. I have recently seen six infants exposed in utero to SSRIs and referred for evaluation of "benign neonatal sleep myoclonus." Although the infants had very prominent neonatal sleep myoclonus, myoclonic jerks and tremors also were present during drowsiness as well. Resolution of these phenomena by 3 months of age has been the rule.

The *long-term outcome* is also generally favorable. Thus, when compared with nonexposed infants, SSRI-exposed infants have had no significant differences in Bayley Mental Developmental Index scores, temperament, mood, arousability, activity levels, distractibility, or behavior problems after 1 to 7 years.[709,715,716] In one report, a lower Bayley Psychomotor Development Index score (but not Mental Development Index score) was observed at 6 to 40 months.[716]

The nature of the neonatal disorder (i.e., *whether withdrawal or toxicity*) is unclear. The neonatal syndrome has features of *both* the withdrawal and "serotonin-toxic" syndromes observed in adults. In the absence of serial measurements of SSRIs in neonatal blood, it is difficult to resolve this issue. In one recent population-based series, in general "peak symptoms did not occur on the first day,"[711] and hence serotonin toxicity seems less likely. Further data are needed.

Barbiturates

Passive addiction of the newborn to barbiturates has been documented for shorter-acting derivatives (e.g., secobarbital, amylbarbital, and butabarbital) and for longer-active derivatives (e.g., phenobarbital). The clinical syndromes differ for these two types of barbiturates and are described separately.

Shorter-Acting Barbiturates

Incidence. The incidence of passive addiction of the newborn to shorter-acting barbiturates is unknown. Although described in only a few cases, the frequent use of such agents in the adult population raises the question of whether many cases are undetected.

Clinical Features. The *withdrawal syndrome* in a well-studied infant who was passively addicted to secobarbital was characterized principally by CNS signs in the first hours of life.[717] These signs consisted of jitteriness, hyperactivity, and hyperreflexia. Poor sucking and vomiting also were present. On the second postnatal day, generalized clonic *seizures* appeared. This evolution of jitteriness to seizures in 24 to 48 hours is similar to that observed in adults addicted to shorter-acting barbiturates. (Indeed, in the case reported, the mother, who was addicted to secobarbital, exhibited withdrawal symptoms with seizures in the postpartum period.) In another infant who was passively addicted to a shorter-acting barbiturate, butabarbital, a similar neonatal syndrome was described.[718] In view of the widespread use of analgesic preparations for "tension headache" that contain butabarbital, this observation is of particular interest. In the case reported, the mother took one tablet of such a preparation three times daily for the last 2 months of pregnancy.[718] In both cases, the seizures responded to the administration of phenobarbital.

Although passive addiction of the newborn is more frequent with narcotic analgesics than with shorter-acting barbiturates, *seizure* in a newborn who is passively addicted to a drug should raise more strongly the possibility of addiction to a shorter-acting barbiturate. The relatively brief list of other drugs associated with neonatal seizures as part of passive addiction and withdrawal is shown in Table 24-21.

Longer-Acting Barbiturates

Incidence. The incidence of passive addiction of the newborn to longer-acting barbiturates, particularly phenobarbital, is unknown. Although only 11 such cases have been clearly described, the relatively late onset of the syndrome may allow many other cases to escape detection.[389,719]

TABLE 24-21 Major Drugs Associated with Neonatal Seizures after Passive Addiction

Narcotic analgesic: methadone
Selective serotonin reuptake inhibitors
Barbiturates: shorter acting
Alcohol
Tricyclic antidepressants
Propoxyphene
"T's and blues" (pentazocine [Talwin] and tripelennamine [Pyribenzamine])

The magnitude of this problem could be considerable, given the relatively large numbers of pregnant women who receive phenobarbital, particularly for sedation. The lack of description of such a syndrome in relatively large series of infants whose mothers were treated with phenobarbital to control neonatal hyperbilirubinemia[720-722] may be considered an important point in favor of the supposition that phenobarbital withdrawal is rare. Two major factors rule against such a firm conclusion. First, in the latter studies, maternal treatment was generally less prolonged than in the mothers of infants described with the withdrawal syndrome. Second, most infants with phenobarbital withdrawal syndrome exhibited the onset of symptoms at approximately 7 days of life (i.e., frequently after discharge from the hospital). Thus, passive addiction to the commonly used longer-acting barbiturate phenobarbital may be more frequent than is currently recognized.

Clinical Features. Unlike the situation with narcotic analgesics, infants passively addicted to longer-acting barbiturates are *not* undergrown. Moreover, as previously noted, the *withdrawal syndrome* characteristically has its onset later in the neonatal period, approximately 7 days of age on the average.[389,719] This delay in onset is understandable in view of the slow elimination of phenobarbital in the immediate neonatal period (half-life of several days). The major features consist primarily of CNS phenomena (i.e., jitteriness, overactivity, disturbed sleeping, excessive crying, hyperreflexia, and disturbed sucking). Overt gastrointestinal phenomena (e.g., diarrhea) may occur but usually are not prominent. The symptoms may appear after the infant is discharged from the hospital, and the infant's irritability may be mistaken for colic or some other extraneural cause. Symptoms often worsen over several weeks and may persist for several *months*.[719] Therapy should consist of minimizing sensory overstimulation, and, if necessary, phenobarbital should be administered in a dose of 3 to 4 mg/kg/day and then tapered very slowly, over months, when symptoms are controlled.

Alcohol

Alcohol withdrawal is a well-known phenomenon in adults.[723] Alcohol withdrawal in a newborn infant born to a woman with chronic alcoholism was described first by Schaeffer[724] in 1962. Subsequently, many cases have been described.[171,209,210,725-729] Approximately 50% of the reported infants have also exhibited the fetal alcohol syndrome (see "Fetal Alcohol Syndrome"). The possibility has been raised that the tremulousness and irritability noted in many infants with the fetal alcohol syndrome reflect, in fact, alcohol withdrawal. The precise magnitude of the problem of neonatal alcohol withdrawal remains to be determined. The critical determinants for the occurrence of the syndrome appear to relate to the chronicity of maternal alcoholism and the proximity of alcohol ingestion to the time of delivery. In a study of more than 29,000 women delivering infants in California,

fully 6.7% had positive urine assays for alcohol at delivery.[169]

The infants described in the reports just mentioned exhibited *intrauterine growth retardation* (often not marked) in addition to the *withdrawal syndrome*.[171,209,210,724-729] The onset of the withdrawal syndrome usually was in the first 24 hours, often within 6 to 12 hours after delivery. In many cases, the mothers either were overtly intoxicated or had alcohol "on their breath" at the time of delivery, findings indicating that alcohol ingestion continued until near the time of birth. The newborn's initial symptoms were jitteriness, irritability, hyperreflexia, hypertonia, and hypersensitivity to sensory stimulation, especially sound. A marked disturbance of sleep states was apparent. Notably in this regard, studies of near-term pregnant women documented disorganized fetal behavioral state organization and decreased fetal breathing activity in the 2 hours after maternal consumption of two glasses of wine.[730] Generalized *seizures* are relatively common in the most overtly symptomatic patients and occur shortly after the onset of the tremulous movements; this evolution of tremor to seizures is characteristic of adult patients experiencing alcohol withdrawal.[723] I have seen one infant with seizures secondary to withdrawal after prenatal exposure to alcohol. Thus, among syndromes of passive addiction of the newborn, alcohol withdrawal is another in which seizures may occur (see Table 24-21). The clinical syndrome dissipates in a week or less. Therapy consists of the avoidance of sensory overstimulation and the administration of phenobarbital for generalized seizures.

Diazepam

Incidence

Diazepam (Valium) is one of the most commonly prescribed drugs in the world. Indeed, the extensive use of this drug in pregnancy and in labor has been accompanied by the occurrence in newborn infants of hypothermia, hyperbilirubinemia, and CNS depression.[731-736] However, only a few reports of a withdrawal syndrome secondary to passive addiction of the newborn to diazepam have been published.[389,735-738] The incidence of the syndrome may be very considerable, but, for the moment, it remains unknown. Mothers of the passively addicted infants reported were receiving standard doses of the drug for at least the last 3 months of pregnancy.

Clinical Features

The infants described with passive addiction to diazepam exhibited a *withdrawal syndrome* that mimics features of withdrawal to narcotic analgesics, and indeed the latter type of withdrawal was the major initial diagnostic consideration in several reported cases. Onset of the withdrawal syndrome to diazepam was in the first hours of life, usually 2 to 6 hours of age. Features consisted of jitteriness, irritability, hyperactivity, and hypertonicity. Diarrhea and vomiting were unusual features. In the best-described cases, symptoms responded to phenobarbital, and phenobarbital therapy was continued for approximately 2 to 4 weeks. However, some degree of jitteriness persisted, usually for 2 to 6 weeks.[738] One infant died of SIDS after discharge from the hospital, an occurrence reminiscent of infants addicted to narcotic analgesics (see earlier discussion). The observations emphasize the importance of careful observation of infants of any woman who has ingested diazepam during at least the latter part of pregnancy.

The occurrence of neonatal withdrawal to diazepam is understandable given that the drug is a small, highly lipid-soluble molecule that readily crosses the placenta and accumulates in fetal tissues, especially adipose tissue.[389,739] The drug, with a half-life of 54 hours, is eliminated slowly by the newborn.[740] The reason for the early onset of symptoms, despite the relatively long half-life, probably relates to the interval from the last maternal dose of the drug to the time of birth, which has varied from 2 to 14 days.[738] The limited ability of the newborn to mobilize, metabolize, and excrete diazepam results in the appearance of drug metabolites in the urine for many weeks[740] and probably accounts for the prolonged duration of symptoms.

The possibility of a teratogenic syndrome related to diazepam and other benzodiazepines is raised by studies from a single group of investigators.[735,736,741,742] Thus, dysmorphic characteristics resembling those of the fetal alcohol syndrome, with hypotonia, episodes of opisthotonos, and abnormal patterns on the EEG (not further characterized), were described in approximately 20 infants. A transient withdrawal syndrome was a common accompaniment. Slight delay in neurological development persisted at 18 months of age. The brain of the one infant studied at autopsy showed neuronal migrational defects. Data obtained from a separate group of investigators suggested that only approximately 9% of infants exposed to benzodiazepines in utero exhibited the dysmorphic characteristics just described, and in these cases, the confounding role of maternal alcohol ingestion could not be eliminated.[743] Further research will be of interest.

Chlordiazepoxide

Chlordiazepoxide (Librium), like diazepam, is a benzodiazepine that is in wide use. Twin infants born to a mother who was taking a therapeutic dose of chlordiazepoxide before and during her entire pregnancy exhibited a withdrawal syndrome that was probably secondary to passive addiction to the drug.[744] Jitteriness and irritability were first noted in both twins at 21 days of age and persisted for 5 days, despite therapy with phenobarbital. Institution of diazepam caused marked improvement, and after 9 days the drug was discontinued. The reason for the delayed onset of symptoms in the affected infants may relate in some way to the twin pregnancy or particularly to delayed mobilization, metabolism, and excretion of the drug.

Tricyclic Antidepressants

Tricyclic antidepressants are used widely for management of depressive illness. As noted earlier, SSRIs are now used more commonly. Passive addiction and neonatal withdrawal symptoms were described initially in three infants whose mothers were treated with the tricyclic antidepressant clomipramine during pregnancy.[745,746] Two of the infants developed *seizures* (onset at 7 and 8 hours of age), as well as jitteriness, irritability, and hypertonicity. Phenobarbital (dose not reported) did not control the seizures effectively; intravenous clomipramine administration was effective in the one patient so treated.[746] The two infants with seizures had initial levels of clomipramine that were 5-fold to 10-fold higher than the one infant who exhibited jitteriness without seizures.[745,746] Seizures in the first 12 hours of life may prove to be a distinctive finding of neonatal withdrawal from tricyclic antidepressants, among other syndromes of passive addiction with seizures (see Table 24-21). In a later population-based study, approximately 1% of 400 infants exposed in utero to tricyclic antidepressants exhibited seizures.[708] Additionally, 6% exhibited neonatal hypoglycemia, perhaps related to hyperinsulinism (like SSRIs, tricyclic antidepressants have a diabetogenic effect in the pregnant woman, perhaps leading to fetal hyperinsulinism).

Ethchlorvynol

Ethchlorvynol (Placidyl) is a sedative-hypnotic drug that was implicated in passive addiction of a newborn born to a woman who had taken the recommended dose of the medication at bedtime for the last 3 months of pregnancy.[747] The withdrawal syndrome that resulted had its onset in the first 24 hours and consisted particularly of jitteriness and irritability. Worsening of the symptoms led to the institution of phenobarbital therapy, which was effective in controlling the signs. Jitteriness dissipated after the fourth day of life, when urinary samples no longer contained the ethchlorvynol.

Propoxyphene

Propoxyphene (Darvon) is one of the most commonly prescribed analgesic drugs in the world. Drug dependency and a withdrawal syndrome have been described in adults addicted to this medication.[748-750] This dependency and its related withdrawal syndrome are not surprising because the structure of propoxyphene is nearly identical to that of methadone.

Two reports described a withdrawal syndrome in infants passively addicted to propoxyphene.[751,752] One mother took the drug for just 6 weeks before delivery. The onset of symptoms in the infant occurred in the first hours of life, and the syndrome was characterized by jitteriness, hypertonicity, hyperactivity, shrill cry, and diarrhea. One infant also experienced generalized tonic-clonic *seizures* (see Table 24-21), which responded to phenobarbital and phenytoin. Recovery was complete by 3 days of age in one infant and by 10 days in the other.[751,752] The striking withdrawal syndrome and the marked similarity in structure of propoxyphene and methadone indicate that this drug may have considerable potential for producing passive addiction in the newborn.

Pentazocine

Pentazocine (Talwin) was introduced originally as a potent but nonaddicting analgesic. Not long after its appearance, however, drug dependence and a withdrawal syndrome were described in adults.[753] Passive addiction of the newborn has also been described.[754,755]

A typical and well-described case report concerned an infant, small for gestational age, born to a mother who had taken oral pentazocine for low back pain throughout her pregnancy.[662] In addition to intrauterine growth retardation, the syndrome of passive addiction to pentazocine is similar to that observed with narcotic analgesics (e.g., heroin) in other respects as well. Thus, the onset of symptoms is in the first day of life, and symptoms consist of jitteriness, irritability, hyperactivity, hypertonicity, hyperreflexia, shrill cry, and vomiting.[754-758] Symptoms respond to tincture of opium and usually dissipate within 2 weeks. SIDS (reminiscent of that recorded with passive addiction to narcotic analgesics) has been observed after discharge from the hospital.[754]

"T's and Blues"

The combination of pentazocine (Talwin), the narcotic-analgesic just discussed, and tripelennamine (Pyribenzamine), an antihistamine, has been a popular form of drug abuse in the United States and produces a striking syndrome of passive addiction in the newborn.[759,760] The term "T's and blues" is derived from the brand name of pentazocine and the color of the tripelennamine tablets, which can be purchased over the counter. Intravenous injection of a solution of the crushed tablets is said to provide a "rush" similar to that of intravenous heroin and to potentiate and prolong the euphoria attributed to pentazocine.

Among infants of women who abuse "T's and blues" throughout their pregnancy, a *withdrawal syndrome* is almost invariable.[759,760] The time of onset and the basic qualities of this syndrome are similar to those of methadone withdrawal. In published reports, approximately one third of infants had onset of the syndrome on the first day of life, one third had onset on the second day, and one third manifested the syndrome between 3 and 7 days of age. Jitteriness, irritability, and hyperactivity were consistent findings, and approximately one half had poorly sustained suck, poor feeding, and vomiting.[759,760] Although not recorded in the two previously reported series (total of 28 infants with withdrawal), I have seen two infants who were passively addicted to "T's and blues" and who had *seizures* at approximately 24 hours of age, near the onset of their withdrawal syndrome. The seizures may represent a toxic (rather than withdrawal) effect of the tripelennamine, an antihistamine with epileptogenic properties. Indeed, the occurrence of

seizures promptly after injection of "T's and blues" is the most common CNS complication of abuse of this drug combination in adults.[761] At any rate, "T's and blues" should be added to the short list of drugs that may cause seizures in the passively addicted newborn (see Table 24-21). Most infants with passive addiction to "T's and blues" are asymptomatic within 10 days. Treatment with paregoric has been used for the minority of infants whose jitteriness and other signs require intervention. However, as discussed earlier, paregoric may have adverse effects in the newborn. DTO would be preferable. Phenobarbital is necessary for the infants who also exhibit seizures.

Codeine

Codeine, a commonly used analgesic, has been associated with passive addiction and a withdrawal syndrome in three infants.[762,763] The potent addictive potential of this drug is emphasized by the occurrence of addiction in infants after maternal use for *as few as 10 days before delivery.* The neonatal withdrawal syndrome began in the first 24 hours of life and was characterized by jitteriness, irritability, poor feeding, vomiting, and diarrhea. The affected infants responded promptly to paregoric, codeine, or phenobarbital. Because codeine is a frequent component of mixed preparations used for treatment of cough or pain, the physician should inquire about *any* medication taken at home before delivery and should determine whether codeine is contained therein.

REFERENCES

1. Drews CD, Murphy CC, Yeargin-Allsopp M, Decoufle P: The relationship between idiopathic mental retardation and maternal smoking during pregnancy, *Pediatrics* 97:547-553, 1996.
2. Gospe SM, Zhous SS, Pinkerton KE: Effects of environmental tobacco smoke exposure in utero and/or postnatally on brain development, *Pediatr Res* 39:494-498, 1996.
3. Huisman M, Koopman-Esseboom C, Fidler V, Hadders-Algra M, et al: Perinatal exposure to polychlorinated biphenyls and dioxins and its effect on neonatal neurological development, *Early Hum Dev* 41:111-127, 1995.
4. Jacobson JL, Jacobson SW: Intellectual impairment in children exposed to polychlorinated biphenyls in utero, *N Engl J Med* 335:783-789, 1996.
5. Van Creveld S: Nouveaux aspects de la maladie hemorragique du nouveau-né, *Arch Fr Pediatr* 15:721-735, 1958.
6. Lawrence A: Antiepileptic drugs and the foetus, *Br Med J* 2:1267, 1963.
7. Douglas H: Haemorrhage in the newborn, *Lancet* 1:816-818, 1966.
8. Kohler HG: Haemorrhage in the newborn of epileptic mothers, *Lancet* 1:267, 1966.
9. Alagille D, Odievre M, Houllemare L, Viterbo G, et al: Avitaminose K néonatalle sévère chez 2 enfants nés de mère traitée par des anticomitaux, *Arch Fr Pediatr* 25:31-41, 1968.
10. Monnet P, Rosenberg D, Bouvier-Lapierre M: Therapeutique anticomitale administrée pedant la grossesse et maladie hemorragique du nouveau-né, *Rev Fr Gynecol Obstet* 63:695-702, 1968.
11. Davis PP: Coagulation defect due to anticonvulsant drug treatment in pregnancy, *Lancet* 1:413-415, 1970.
12. Evans AR, Forrester RM, Discombe C: Neonatal hemorrhage following maternal anticonvulsant therapy, *Lancet* 1:517-518, 1970.
13. Mountain KR, Hirsh J, Gallus AS: Neonatal coagulation defect due to anticonvulsant drug treatment in pregnancy, *Lancet* 1:265-268, 1970.
14. Stevenson MM, Gilbert EF: Anticonvulsants and hemorrhagic diseases of the newborn infant, *J Pediatr* 77:516, 1970.
15. Margolis DG, Kantor NM: Hemorrhagic disease of the newborn: An unusual case related to maternal ingestion of antiepileptic drug, *Clin Pediatr* 11:59-66, 1972.
16. Speidel BD, Meadow SR: Maternal epilepsy and abnormalities of the fetus and newborn, *Lancet* 2:839-843, 1972.

17. Bleyer WA, Skinner AL: Fetal neonatal hemorrhage after maternal anticonvulsant therapy, *JAMA* 235:626, 1976.
18. Allen RW Jr, Ogden B, Bentley FL, Jung AL: Fetal hydantoin syndrome, neuroblastoma, and hemorrhagic disease in a neonate, *JAMA* 244:1464-1465, 1980.
19. Deblay MF, Vert P, Andre M, Marchal F: Transplacental vitamin K prevents haemorrhagic disease of infant of epileptic mother, *Lancet* 1:1247, 1982.
20. Srinivasan G, Seeler RA, Tiruvury A, Pildes RS: Maternal anticonvulsant therapy and hemorrhagic disease of the newborn, *Obstet Gynecol* 59:250-252, 1982.
21. Laosombat V: Hemorrhage disease of the newborn after maternal anticonvulsant therapy: A case report and literature review, *J Med Assoc Thai* 71:643-648, 1988.
22. Morrell MJ: Guidelines for the care of women with epilepsy, *Neurology* 51:S21-S27, 1998.
23. Report of the Quality Standards Subcommittee of the American Academy of Neurology: Practice parameter: Management issues for women with epilepsy (summary statement), *Neurology* 51:944-948, 1998.
24. Zahn CA, Morrell MJ, Collins SD, Labiner DM, et al: Management issues for women with epilepsy: A review of the literature, *Neurology* 51:949-956, 1998.
25. Renzulli P, Tuchschmid P, Eich G, Fanconi S, et al: Early vitamin K deficiency bleeding after maternal phenobarbital intake: Management of massive intracranial haemorrhage by minimal surgical intervention, *Eur J Pediatr* 157:663-665, 1998.
26. Cornelissen M, Steegerstheunissen R, Kollee L, Eskes T, et al: Increased incidence of neonatal vitamin-K deficiency resulting from maternal anticonvulsant therapy, *Am J Obstet Gynecol* 168:923-928, 1993.
27. Cornelissen M, Steegerstheunissen R, Kollee L, Eskes T, et al: Supplementation of vitamin-K in pregnant women receiving anticonvulsant therapy prevents neonatal vitamin-K deficiency, *Am J Obstet Gynecol* 168:884-888, 1993.
28. Hey E: Effect of maternal anticonvulsant treatment on neonatal blood coagulation, *Arch Dis Child Fetal Neonatal Ed* 81:F208-F210, 1999.
29. Kaaja E, Kaaja R, Matila R, Hiilesmaa V: Enzyme-inducing antiepileptic drugs in pregnancy and the risk of bleeding in the neonate, *Neurology* 58:549-553, 2002.
30. Choulika S, Grabowski E, Holmes LB: Is antenatal vitamin K prophylaxis needed for pregnant women taking anticonvulsants? *Am J Obstet Gynecol* 190:882-883, 2004.
31. Annegers JF, Elveback LR, Hauser WA, Kurland LT: Do anticonvulsants have a teratogenic effect? *Arch Neurol* 31:364-373, 1974.
32. Nakane Y, Okuma T, Takahashi R, Sato Y, et al: Multi-institutional study on the teratogenicity and fetal toxicity of antiepileptic drugs: A report of a collaborative study group in Japan, *Epilepsia* 21:663-680, 1980.
33. Elshove J, van Eck JH: Aangeboren misvormingen, met name gespleten lip met of zondergespleten verhemelte, bij kinderen van moeders met epilepsie, *Ned Tijdschr Geneeskd* 115:1371-1375, 1971.
34. South J: Teratogenic effects of anticonvulsants, *Lancet* 2:1154, 1972.
35. Fedrick J: Epilepsy and pregnancy: A report from the Oxford record linkage study, *Br Med J* 2:442-448, 1973.
36. Loughnan PM, Gold H, Vance JC: Phenytoin teratogenicity in man, *Lancet* 1:70-72, 1973.
37. Lowe CR: Congenital malformations among infants born to epileptic women, *Lancet* 1:9-10, 1973.
38. Meyer JG: The teratological effects of anticonvulsants and the effects on pregnancy and birth, *Eur Neurol* 10:179-190, 1973.
39. Monson RR, Rosenberg L, Hartz SC, Shapiro S, et al: Diphenylhydantoin and selected congenital malformations, *N Engl J Med* 289:1049-1052, 1973.
40. Barry JE, Danks DM: Anticonvulsants and congenital abnormalities [letter], *Lancet* 2:48-49, 1974.
41. Janz D: The teratogenic risk of antiepileptic drugs, *Epilepsia* 16:159-169, 1975.
42. Hill RM: Fetal malformations and antiepileptic drugs, *Am J Dis Child* 130:923-925, 1976.
43. Shapiro S, Hartz SC, Siskind V, Mitchell AA, et al: Anticonvulsants and parental epilepsy in the development of birth defects, *Lancet* 1:272-275, 1976.
44. Smithells RW: Environmental teratogens of man, *Br Med Bull* 32:27-33, 1976.
45. Prensky AL, Dodson WE: Prenatal factors affecting future development. In Thompson RA, Green JR, editors: *Pediatric Neurology and Neurosurgery*, New York: 1978, Spectrum.
46. Paulson GW, Paulson RB: Teratogenic effects of anticonvulsants, *Arch Neurol* 38:140-143, 1981.
47. Kaneko S, Otani K, Kondo T, Fukushima Y, et al: Malformation in infants of mothers with epilepsy receiving antiepileptic drugs, *Neurology* 42:68-74, 1992.
48. Dravet C, Julian C, Legras C, Magaudda A, et al: Epilepsy, antiepileptic drugs, and malformations in children of women with epilepsy: A French prospective cohort study, *Neurology* 42:75-82, 1992.
49. Lindhout D, Meinardi H, Meijer JW, Nau H: Antiepileptic drugs and teratogenesis in two consecutive cohorts: Changes in prescription policy paralleled by changes in pattern of malformations, *Neurology* 42:94-110, 1992.
50. Oguni M, Dansky L, Andermann E, Sherwin A, et al: Improved pregnancy outcome in epileptic women in the last decade: Relationship to maternal anticonvulsant therapy, *Brain Dev* 14:371-380, 1992.
51. Kaneko S, Battino D, Andermann E, Wada K, et al: Congenital malformations due to antiepileptic drugs, *Epilepsy Res* 33:145-158, 1999.
52. Wide K, Winbladh B, Tomson T, Sars-Zimmer K, et al: Psychomotor development and minor anomalies in children exposed to antiepileptic drugs in utero: A prospective population-based study, *Dev Med Child Neurol* 42:87-92, 2000.
53. Fonager K, Larsen H, Pedersen L, Sorensen HT: Birth outcomes in women exposed to anticonvulsant drugs, *Acta Neurol Scand* 101:289-294, 2000.
54. Holmes LB, Harvey EA, Coull BA, Huntington KB, et al: The teratogenicity of anticonvulsant drugs, *N Engl J Med* 344:1132-1138, 2001.
55. Fonager K, Larsen H, Pedersen L, Sorensen HT: Birth outcomes in women exposed to anticonvulsant drugs, *Acta Neurol Scand* 101:289-294, 2000.
56. Diav-Citrin O, Schechtman S, Arnon J, Ornoy A: Is carbamazepine teratogenic? A prospective controlled study of 210 pregnancies, *Neurology* 57:321-324, 2001.
57. Tomson T, Perucca T, Battino T: Navigating toward fetal and maternal health: The challenge of treating epilepsy in pregnancy, *Epilepsia* 45:1171-1175, 2004.
58. Artama M, Auvinen A, Raudaskoski T, Isojarvi I, et al: Antiepileptic drug use of women with epilepsy and congenital malformations in offspring, *Neurology* 64:1874-1878, 2005.
59. Moore SJ, Turnpenny P, Quinn A, Glover S, et al: A clinical study of 57 children with fetal anticonvulsant syndromes, *J Med Genet* 37:489-497, 2000.
60. Kaaja E, Kaaja R, Hiilesmaa V: Major malformations in offspring of women with epilepsy, *Neurology* 60:575-579, 2003.
61. Wide K, Winbladh B, Kallen B: Major malformations in infants exposed to antiepileptic drugs in utero, with emphasis on carbamazepine and valproic acid: A nation-wide, population-based register study, *Acta Paediatr* 93:174-176, 2004.
62. Cunnington M, Tennis P: Lamotrigine and the risk of malformations in pregnancy, *Neurology* 64:955-960, 2005.
63. Morrow J, Russell A, Guthrie E, Parsons L, et al: Malformation risks of antiepileptic drugs in pregnancy: A prospective study from the UK Epilepsy and Pregnancy Register, *J Neurol Neurosurg Psychiatry* 77:193-198, 2006.
64. Meador KJ, Baker GA, Finnell RH, Kalayjian LA, et al: In utero antiepileptic drug exposure: Fetal death and malformations, *Neurology* 67:407-412, 2006.
64a. Atkinson DE, Brice-Bennett S, D'Souza SW: Antiepileptic medication during pregnancy: Does fetal genotype affect outcome? *Pediatr Res* 62:120-127, 2007.
65. Meadow SR: Anticonvulsant drugs and congenital abnormalities, *Lancet* 2:1296, 1968.
66. Hill RM, Verniaud WM, Horning MG, McCulley LB, et al: Infants exposed in utero to antiepileptic drugs, *Am J Dis Child* 127:645-653, 1974.
67. Hanson JW, Smith DW: The fetal hydantoin syndrome, *J Pediatr* 87:285-290, 1975.
68. Hanson JW, Myrianthopoulos NC, Harvey MA, Smith DW: Risks to the offspring of women treated with hydantoin anticonvulsants, with emphasis on the fetal hydantoin syndrome, *J Pediatr* 89:662-668, 1976.
69. Smith DW: Fetal drug syndromes: Effects of ethanol and hydantoins, *Pediatr Rev* 1:165-178, 1979.
70. Mallow DW, Herrick MK, Gathman G: Fetal exposure to anticonvulsant drugs, *Arch Pathol Lab Med* 104:215-218, 1980.
71. Hanson JW, Buehler BA: Fetal hydantoin syndrome: Current status, *J Pediatr* 101:816-818, 1982.
72. Phelan MC, Pellock JM, Nance WE: Discordant expression of fetal hydantoin syndrome in heteropaternal dizygotic twins, *N Engl J Med* 307:99-101, 1982.
73. Albengres E, Tillement JP: Phenytoin in pregnancy: A review of the reported risks, *Biol Res Pregnancy Perinatol* 4:71-74, 1983.
74. Dessens AB, Cohen-Kettenis PT, Mellenbergh GJ, Koppe JG, et al: Association of prenatal phenobarbital and phenytoin exposure with small head size at birth and with learning problems, *Acta Paediatr* 89:533-541, 2000.
75. Holmes LB, Coull BA, Dorfman J, Rosenberger PB: The correlation of deficits in IQ with midface and digit hypoplasia in children exposed in utero to anticonvulsant drugs, *J Pediatr* 146:118-122, 2005.
76. Bethenod M, Frederich A: Les enfants des antiépileptiques, *Pediatrie* 30:227-248, 1975.
77. Seip M: Growth retardation, dysmorphic facies and minor malformations following massive exposure to phenobarbitone in utero, *Acta Paediatr Scand* 65:617-621, 1976.
78. Myhre SA, Williams R: Teratogenic effects associated with maternal primidone therapy, *J Pediatr* 99:160-162, 1981.
79. Krauss CM, Holmes LB, VanLang Q, Keith DA: Four siblings with similar malformations after exposure to phenytoin and primidone, *J Pediatr* 105:750-755, 1984.
80. Hoyme HE, Clericuzio CL: Fetal primidone effects, *Pediatr Res* 19:326A, 1985.
81. Jones KL, Lacro RV, Johnson KA, Adams J: Pattern of malformations in the children of women treated with carbamazepine during pregnancy, *N Engl J Med* 320:1661-1666, 1989.
82. Niesen M, Froscher W: Finger- and toenail hypoplasia after carbamazepine monotherapy in late pregnancy, *Neuropediatrics* 16:167-168, 1985.
83. Vestermark V, Vestermark S: Teratogenic effect of carbamazepine, *Arch Dis Child* 66:641-642, 1991.
84. Majewski F, Steger M, Richter B, Gill J, et al: The teratogenicity of hydantoins and barbiturates in humans, with considerations on the etiology of

malformations and cerebral disturbances in children of epileptic parents, *Int J Biol Res Pregnancy* 2:37-45, 1981.

85. Hanson JW: Teratogen update: Fetal hydantoin effects, *Teratology* 33:349-353, 1986.

86. Adams J, Vorhees CV, Middaugh LD: Developmental neurotoxicity of anticonvulsants: Human and animal evidence on phenytoin, *Neurotoxicol Teratol* 12:203-214, 1990.

87. Gaily E, Kantola-Sorsa E, Granstrom ML: Intelligence of children of epileptic mothers, *J Pediatr* 113:677-684, 1988.

88. Buehler BA, Delimont D, Van Waes M, Finnell RH: Prenatal prediction of risk of the fetal hydantoin syndrome, *N Engl J Med* 322:1567-1572, 1990.

89. Van Dyke DC, Hodge SE, Heide F, Hill LR: Family studies in fetal phenytoin exposure, *J Pediatr* 113:301-306, 1988.

90. Tanganelli P, Regesta G: Epilepsy, pregnancy, and major birth anomalies: An Italian prospective, controlled study, *Neurology* 42:89-93, 1992.

91. Granstrom ML, Gaily E: Psychomotor development in children of mothers with epilepsy, *Neurology* 42:144-148, 1992.

92. Delgado-Escueta AV, Janz D: Consensus guidelines: Preconception counseling management, and care of the pregnant woman with epilepsy, *Neurology* 42:149-160, 1992.

93. Yerby MS, Leavitt A, Erickson DM, McCormick KB, et al: Antiepileptics and the development of congenital anomalies, *Neurology* 42:132-140, 1992.

94. Anderson RC: Cardiac defects in children of mothers receiving anticonvulsant therapy during pregnancy, *J Pediatr* 89:318-319, 1976.

95. Scolnik D, Nulman I, Rovert J, Gladstone D, et al: Neurodevelopment of children exposed in utero to phenytoin and carbamazepine monotherapy, *JAMA* 271:767-770, 1994.

96. Reinisch JM, Sanders SA, Mortensen EL, Rubin DB: In utero exposure to phenobarbital and intelligence deficits in adult men, *JAMA* 274:1518-1525, 1995.

97. Massey KM: Teratogenic effects of diphenylhydantoin sodium, *J Oral Ther* 2:380-385, 1966.

98. Gibson JE, Becker BA: Teratogenic effects of diphenylhydantoin in Swiss-Webster and A/J mice, *Proc Soc Exp Biol Med* 128:905-909, 1968.

99. Harbison RD, Becker BA: Relation of dosage and time of administration of diphenylhydantoin to its teratogenic effect in mice, *Teratology* 2:305-311, 1969.

100. Harbison RD, Becker BA: Effect of phenobarbital and SKF 525A pretreatment on diphenylhydantoin teratogenicity in mice, *J Pharmacol Exp Ther* 175:283-288, 1970.

101. Mackler B: Studies of the development of congenital anomalies in rats. III. Effects of inhibition of mitochondrial energy systems on embryonic development, *Teratology* 12:291-296, 1975.

102. Paulson RB, Paulson GW, Jreissaty S: Phenytoin and carbamazepine in production of cleft palates in mice, *Arch Neurol* 36:832-836, 1979.

103. Finnell RH: Phenytoin-induced teratogenesis: A mouse model, *Science* 211:483-484, 1981.

104. Lorente CA, Tassinari MS, Keith DA: The effects of phenytoin on rat development: An animal model system for fetal hydantoin syndrome, *Teratology* 24:169-180, 1981.

105. Bruckner A, Lee YJ, O'Shea KS, Henneberry RC: Teratogenic effects of valproic acid and diphenylhydantoin on mouse embryos in culture, *Teratology* 27:29-42, 1983.

106. Lindhout D: Pharmacogenetics and drug interactions: Role in antiepileptic-drug-induced teratogenesis, *Neurology* 42:43-47, 1992.

107. Finnell RH, Buehler BA, Kerr BM, Ager PL, et al: Clinical and experimental studies linking oxidative metabolism to phenytoin-induced teratogenesis, *Neurology* 42:25-31, 1992.

108. Hartsfield JK, Holmes LB, Morel JG: Phenytoin embryopathy: Effect of epoxide hydrolase inhibitor on phenytoin exposure in utero in C57BL/6J mice, *Biochem Mol Med* 56:131-143, 1995.

109. Hartsfield JK, Benford SA, Hilbelink DR: Induction of microsomal epoxide hydrolase activity in inbred mice by chronic phenytoin exposure, *Biochem Mol Med* 56:144-151, 1995.

110. Bustamante SA, Stumpff LC: Fetal hydantoin syndrome in triplets: A unique experiment of nature, *Am J Dis Child* 132:978-979, 1978.

111. Raymond GV, Buehler BA, Finnell RH, Holmes LB: Anticonvulsant teratogenesis. III. Possible metabolic basis, *Teratology* 51:55-56, 1995.

112. Dansky LV, Rosenblatt DS, Andermann E: Mechanisms of teratogenesis: Folic acid and antiepileptic therapy, *Neurology* 42:32-42, 1992.

113. German J, Kowal A, Ehlers KH: Trimethadione and human teratogenesis, *Teratology* 3:349-362, 1970.

114. Pashayan H, Pruzansky D, Pruzansky S: Are anticonvulsants teratogenic? *Lancet* 2:702-703, 1971.

115. Rutman JY: Anticonvulsants and fetal damage, *N Engl J Med* 289:696-697, 1973.

116. Nichols MM: Fetal anomalies following maternal trimethadione ingestion, *J Pediatr* 82:885-886, 1973.

117. Biale Y, Lewenthal H, Aderet NB: Congenital malformations due to anticonvulsive drugs, *Obstet Gynecol* 45:439-442, 1975.

118. Lawrence TY, Stiles QR: Persistent fifth aortic arch in man, *Am J Dis Child* 129:1229-1231, 1975.

119. Zackai EH, Mellman WJ, Neiderer B, Hanson JW: The fetal trimethadione syndrome, *J Pediatr* 87:280-284, 1975.

120. Feldman GL: The fetal trimethadione syndrome, *Am J Dis Child* 131:1389-1392, 1977.

121. Rosen RC, Lightner ES: Phenotypic malformations in association with maternal trimethadione therapy, *J Pediatr* 92:240-244, 1978.

122. Clifford DB: Seizures and pregnancy, *Am Fam Physician* 29:271-275, 1984.

123. Farrar HC, Blumer JL: Fetal effects of maternal drug exposure, *Annu Rev Pharmacol Toxicol* 31:525-547, 1991.

124. Rifkind AB: Teratogenic effects of trimethadione and dimethadione in the chick embryo, *Toxicol Appl Pharmacol* 30:452-457, 1974.

125. Gomez MR: Possible teratogenicity of valproic acid, *J Pediatr* 98:508-509, 1981.

126. Stanley OH, Chambers TL: Sodium valproate and neural tube defects, *Lancet* 2:1282-1283, 1982.

127. Blaw ME, Woody RC: Valproic acid embryopathy? *Neurology* 33:255, 1983.

128. Bjerkedal T, Czeizel A, Goujard J, Kallen B, et al: Valproic acid and spina bifida, *Lancet* 2:1096, 1982.

129. Jeavons PM: Summary of 39 pregnancies with abnormal outcome where the mother had taken sodium valproate, *Lancet* 2:1283-1284, 1982.

130. Mastroiacovo P, Bertollini R, Morandini S, Segni G: Maternal epilepsy, valproate exposure, and birth defects, *Lancet* 2:1499, 1983.

131. Lindhout D, Meinardi H: Spina bifida and in utero exposure to valproate, *Lancet* 2:396, 1984.

132. Weinbaum PJ, Cassidy SB, Vintzileos AM, Campbell WA, et al: Prenatal detection of a neural tube defect after fetal exposure to valproic acid, *Obstet Gynecol* 67:31S-33S, 1986.

133. Lindhout D, Schmidt D: In utero exposure to valproate and neural tube defects, *Lancet* 1:1392-1393, 1986.

134. Lammer EJ, Sever LE, Oakley GP: Teratogen update: Valproic acid, *Teratology* 35:465-473, 1987.

135. Laegreid L, Kyllerman M, Hedner T, Hagberg B, et al: Benzodiazepine amplification of valproate teratogenic effects in children of mothers with absence epilepsy, *Neuropediatrics* 24:88-92, 1993.

136. Lindhout D, Omtzigt JG, Cornel MC: Spectrum of neural-tube defects in 34 infants prenatally exposed to antiepileptic drugs, *Neurology* 42:111-118, 1992.

137. Omtzigt JG, Los FJ, Grobbee DE, Pijpers L, et al: The risk of spina bifida aperta after first-trimester exposure to valproate in a prenatal cohort, *Neurology* 42:119-125, 1992.

138. Vajda FJ, Eadie MJ: Maternal valproate dosage and foetal malformations, *Acta Neurol Scand* 112:137-143, 2005.

139. Wyszynski DF, Nambisan M, Surve T, Alsdorf RM, et al: Increased rate of major malformations in offspring exposed to valproate during pregnancy, *Neurology* 64:961-965, 2005.

140. Kozma C: Valproic acid embryopathy: Report of two siblings with further expansion of the phenotypic abnormalities and a review of the literature, *Am J Med Genet* 98:168-175, 2001.

141. Ehlers K, Sturje H, Merker HJ, Nau H: Valproic acid-induced spina bifida: A mouse model, *Teratology* 45:145-154, 1992.

142. Vorhees CV, Acuff-Smith KD, Weisenburger WP, Minck DR, et al: Lack of teratogenicity of trans-2-ene-valproic acid compared to valproic acid in rats, *Teratology* 43:583-590, 1991.

143. Hansen DK, Grafton TF: Lack of attenuation of valproic acid-induced effects by folinic acid in rat embryos in vitro, *Teratology* 43:575-582, 1991.

144. Wegner C, Nau H: Alteration of embryonic folate metabolism by valproic acid during organogenesis: Implications for mechanism of teratogenesis, *Neurology* 42:17-24, 1992.

145. DiLiberti JH, Farndon PA, Dennis NR, Curry CJR: The fetal valproate syndrome, *Am J Med Genet* 19:473-481, 1984.

146. Dalens B, Raynaud EJ, Gaulme J: Teratogenicity of valproic acid, *J Pediatr* 97:332, 1980.

147. Clay SA, McVie R, Chen H: Possible teratogenic effect of valproic acid, *J Pediatr* 99:828, 1981.

148. Hanson JW, Ardinger HH, DiLiberti JH: Effects of valproic acid on the fetus, *Pediatr Res* 18:306-307, 1984.

149. Jager-Roman E, Deichl A, Jakob S, Hartman AM, et al: Fetal growth, major malformations, and minor anomalies in infants born to women receiving valproic acid, *J Pediatr* 108:997-1004, 1986.

150. Chitayat D, Farrell K, Anderson L, Gall JG: Congenital abnormalities in two sibs exposed to valproic acid in utero, *Am J Med Genet* 31:369-373, 1988.

151. Verloes A, Frikiche A, Gremillet C, Paquay T, et al: Proximal phocomelia and radial ray aplasia in fetal valproic syndrome, *Eur J Pediatr* 149:266-267, 1990.

152. Thisted E, Ebbesen F: Malformations, withdrawal manifestations, and hypoglycemia after exposure to valproate in utero, *Arch Dis Child* 69:288-291, 1993.

153. Christianson AL, Chesler N, Kromberg JG: Fetal valproate syndrome: Clinical and neurodevelopmental features in two sibling pairs, *Dev Med Child Neurol* 36:357-369, 1994.

154. Barrera MN, Campos MR, Ribed MLS: Partial hydranencephaly in a child coincident with intrauterine exposure to sodium valproate, *Neuropediatrics* 25:334-335, 1995.

155. Malm H, Kajantie E, Kivirikko S, Kaariainen H, et al: Valproate embryopathy in three sets of siblings: Further proof of hereditary susceptibility, *Neurology* 59:630-633, 2002.

156. Adab N, Kini U, Vinten J, Ayres J, et al: The longer term outcome of children born to mothers with epilepsy, *J Neurol Neurosurg Psychiatry* 75:1575-1583, 2004.

157. Schorry EK, Oppenheimer SG, Saal HM: Valproate embryopathy: Clinical and cognitive profile in 5 siblings, *Am J Med Genet A* 133:202-206, 2005.

158. Rasalam AD, Hailey H, Williams JHG, Moore SJ, et al: Characteristics of fetal anticonvulsant syndrome associated autistic disorder, *Dev Med Child Neurol* 47:551-555, 2005.

159. Williams G, King J, Cunningham M, Stephan M, et al: Fetal valproate syndrome and autism: Additional evidence of an association, *Dev Med Child Neurol* 43:202-206, 2001.

160. Vinten J, Adab N, Kini U, Gorry J, et al: Neuropsychological effects of exposure to anticonvulsant medication in utero, *Neurology* 64:949-954, 2005.

161. Lemoine P, Harrousseau H, Borteyru JP: Les enfants de parents alcooliques: Anomalies observées. À propos de 127 cas, *Ouest Med* 25:477, 1968.

162. Jones KL, Smith DW, Ulleland CN, Streissguth AP: Pattern of malformation in offspring of chronic alcoholic mothers, *Lancet* 1:1267-1271, 1973.

163. Jones KL, Smith DW: Recognition of the fetal alcohol syndrome in early infancy, *Lancet* 2:999-1001, 1973.

164. Committee on Substance Abuse: Fetal alcohol syndrome and fetal alcohol effects, *Pediatrics* 91:1004-1006, 1993.

165. Hoyme HE, May PA, Kalberg WO, Kodituwakku P, et al: A practical clinical approach to diagnosis of fetal alcohol spectrum disorders: Clarification of the 1996 institute of medicine criteria, *Pediatrics* 115:39-47, 2005.

166. Floyd RL, O'Connor MJ, Sokol RJ, Bertrand J, et al: Recognition and prevention of fetal alcohol syndrome, *Obstet Gynecol* 106:1059-1064, 2005.

167. Riley EP, McGee CL: Fetal alcohol spectrum disorders: An overview with emphasis on changes in brain and behavior, *Exp Biol Med* 230:357-365, 2005.

168. Hanson JW, Streissguth AP, Smith DW: The effects of moderate alcohol consumption during pregnancy on fetal growth and morphogenesis, *J Pediatr* 92:457-460, 1978.

169. Martinez A, Partridge JC, Bean X, Taeusch HW: Perinatal substance abuse. In Taeusch HW, Ballard RA, editors: *Avery's Diseases of the Newborn*, 7th ed, Philadelphia: 1998, Saunders.

170. Testa M, Quigley BM, Das Eiden R: The effects of prenatal alcohol exposure on infant mental development: A meta-analytical review, *Alcohol Alcohol* 38:295-304, 2003.

171. Ostrea EM, Lucena JL, Silvestre MA: The infant of the drug-dependent mother. In Avery GB, Fletcher MA, MacDonald MG, editors: *Neonatology: Pathophysiology and Management of the Newborn*, 4th ed, Philadelphia: 1994, JB Lippincott.

172. Zuckerman BS, Hingson R: Alcohol consumption during pregnancy: A critical review, *Dev Med Child Neurol* 28:649-661, 1986.

173. Ernhart CB, Sokol RJ, Martier S, Moron P, et al: Alcohol teratogenicity in the human: A detailed assessment of specificity, critical period, and threshold, *Am J Obstet Gynecol* 157:33-39, 1987.

174. Mills JL, Graubard BI: Is moderate drinking during pregnancy associated with an increased risk for malformations? *Pediatrics* 80:309-314, 1987.

175. Streissguth AP: Prenatal alcohol-induced brain damage and long-term postnatal consequences: Introduction to the symposium, *Alcohol Clin Exp Res* 14:648-649, 1990.

176. Driscoll CD, Streissguth AP, Riley EP: Prenatal alcohol exposure: Comparability of effects in humans and animal models, *Neurotoxicol Teratol* 12:231-237, 1990.

177. Werler MM, Lammer EJ, Rosenberg L, Mitchell AA: Maternal alcohol use in relation to selected birth defects, *Am J Epidemiol* 134:691-698, 1991.

178. Russell M, Czarnecki DM, Cowan R, McPherson E, et al: Measures of maternal alcohol use as predictors of development in early childhood, *Alcohol Clin Exp Res* 15:991-1000, 1991.

179. Day NL, Goldschmidt L, Robles N, Richardson G, et al: Prenatal alcohol exposure and offspring growth at 18 months of age: The predictive validity of two measures of drinking, *Alcohol Clin Exp Res* 15:914-918, 1991.

180. Hill RM, Hegemier S, Tennyson LM: The fetal alcohol syndrome: A multihandicapped child, *Neurotoxicology* 10:585-596, 1989.

181. Streissguth AP, Barr HM, Sampson PD: Moderate prenatal alcohol exposure: Effects on child IQ and learning problems at age 7 1/2 years, *Alcohol Clin Exp Res* 14:662-669, 1990.

182. Nanson JL, Hiscock M: Attention deficits in children exposed to alcohol prenatally, *Alcohol Clin Exp Res* 14:656-661, 1990.

183. Day NL, Richardson G, Robles N, Sambamoorthi U, et al: Effect of prenatal alcohol exposure on growth and morphology of offspring at 8 months of age, *Pediatrics* 85:748-752, 1990.

184. Autti-Rämö I, Granström ML: The effect of intrauterine alcohol exposition in various durations on early cognitive development, *Neuropediatrics* 22:203-210, 1991.

185. Forrest F, Florey CV, Taylor D, McPherson F, et al: Reported social alcohol consumption during pregnancy and infants' development at 18 months, *BMJ* 303:22-26, 1991.

186. Coles CD, Brown RT, Smith IE, Platzman KA, et al: Effects of prenatal alcohol exposure at school age. I. Physical and cognitive development, *Neurotoxicol Teratol* 13:357-367, 1991.

187. Coles CD, Platzman KA, Smith I, James ME, et al: Effects of cocaine and alcohol use in pregnancy on neonatal growth and neurobehavioral status, *Neurotoxicol Teratol* 14:23-33, 1992.

188. Coles CD: Prenatal alcohol exposure and human development. In Miller MW, editor: *Development of the Central Nervous System: Effects of Alcohol and Opiates*, New York: 1992, Wiley-Liss.

189. Walpole I, Zubrick S, Pontre J, Lawrence C: Low to moderate maternal alcohol use before and during pregnancy, and neurobehavioural outcome in the newborn infant, *Dev Med Child Neurol* 33:875-883, 1991.

190. West JR, Ward GR: Effects of alcohol on the developing brain. In Miller G, Ram JC, editors: *Static Encephalopathies of Infancy and Childhood*, New York: 1992, Raven Press.

191. Jacobson JL, Jacobson SW, Sokol RJ, Martier SS, et al: Teratogenic effects of alcohol on infant development, *Alcohol Clin Exp Res* 17:174-183, 1993.

192. Autti-Rämö I, Gaily E, Granstrom ML: Dysmorphic features in offspring of alcoholic mothers, *Arch Dis Child* 67:712-716, 1992.

193. Clarren SK, Astley SJ, Gunderson VM, Spellman D: Cognitive and behavioral deficits in nonhuman primates associated with very early embryonic binge exposures to ethanol, *J Pediatr* 121:789-796, 1992.

194. Autti-Rämö I, Granstrom ML: The psychomotor development during the first year of life of infants exposed to intrauterine alcohol of various duration: Fetal alcohol exposure and development, *Neuropediatrics* 22:59-64, 1991.

195. Autti-Rämö I, Korkman M, Hilakivi-Clarke L, Lehtonen M, et al: Mental development of 2-year-old children exposed to alcohol in utero, *J Pediatr* 120:740-746, 1992.

196. West JR, Chen W, Pantazis NJ: Fetal alcohol syndrome: The vulnerability of the developing brain and possible mechanisms of damage, *Metab Brain Dis* 9:291-322, 1994.

197. Streissguth AP, Barr HM, Sampson PD, Bookstein FL: Prenatal alcohol and offspring development: The first fourteen years, *Drug Alcohol Depend* 36:89-99, 1994.

198. Jacobson SW, Chiodo LM, Sokol RJ, Jacobson JL: Validity of maternal report of prenatal alcohol, cocaine, and smoking in relation to neurobehavioral outcome, *Pediatrics* 109:815-825, 2002.

199. May PA, Gossage JP, White-Country M, Goodhart K, et al: Alcohol consumption and other maternal risk factors for fetal alcohol syndrome among three distinct samples of women before, during, and after pregnancy: The risk is relative, *Am J Med Genet C Semin Med Genet* 127:10-20, 2004.

200. Jones KL: The role of genetic susceptibility for maternal alcohol metabolism in determining pregnancy outcome, *J Pediatr* 148:5-6, 2006.

201. Streissguth AP, Dehaene P: Fetal alcohol syndrome in twins of alcoholic mothers: Concordance of diagnosis and IQ, *Am J Med Genet* 47:857-861, 1993.

202. Riikonen RS: Difference in susceptibility to teratogenic effects of alcohol in discordant twins exposed to alcohol during the second half of gestation, *Pediatr Neurol* 11:332-336, 1994.

203. Jacobson SW, Carr LG, Croxford J, Sokol RJ, et al: Protective effects of the alcohol dehydrogenase-ADH1B allele in children exposed to alcohol during pregnancy, *J Pediatr* 148:30-37, 2006.

204. Hall BD, Orenstein WA: Noonan's phenotype in an offspring of an alcoholic mother, *Lancet* 1:680-681, 1974.

205. Palmer RH, Oullette EM, Warner L, Leichtman SR: Congenital malformations in offspring of a chronic alcoholic mother, *Pediatrics* 53:490-494, 1974.

206. Jones KL, Smith DW: The fetal alcohol syndrome, *Teratology* 12:1-10, 1975.

207. Root AW, Reiter EO, Andriola M, Duckett G: Hypothalamic-pituitary function in the fetal alcohol syndrome, *J Pediatr* 87:585-588, 1975.

208. Hanson JW, Jones KL, Smith DW: Fetal alcohol syndrome: Experience with 41 patients, *JAMA* 235:1458-1460, 1976.

209. Mulvihill JJ, Klimas JT, Stokes DC, Risemberg HM: Fetal alcohol syndrome: Seven new cases, *Am J Obstet Gynecol* 125:937-941, 1976.

210. Beyers N, Moosa A: The fetal alcohol syndrome, *Afr Med J* 54:575-578, 1978.

211. Nitowsky HM: Teratogenic effects of ethanol in human beings, *Neurobehav Toxicol Teratol* 2:151-162, 1980.

212. Streissguth AP, Clarren SK, Jones KL: Natural history of the fetal alcohol syndrome: A 10-year follow-up of eleven patients, *Lancet* 2:85-91, 1985.

213. Tanaka H, Arima M, Suzuki N: The fetal alcohol syndrome in Japan, *Brain Dev* 3:305-311, 1981.

214. Beattie JO, Day R, Cockburn F, Garg RA: Alcohol and the fetus in the west of Scotland, *Br Med J (Clin Res Ed)* 287:17-20, 1983.

215. Aronson M, Kyllerman M, Sabel KG, Sandin B, et al: Children of alcoholic mothers: Developmental, perceptual and behavioral characteristics as compared to matched controls, *Acta Paediatr Scand* 74:27-35, 1985.

216. Kyllerman M, Aronson M, Sabel KG, Karlberg E, et al: Children of alcoholic mothers: Growth and motor performance compared to matched controls, *Acta Paediatr Scand* 74:20-26, 1985.

217. Church MW: Chronic in utero alcohol exposure affects auditory function in rats and in humans, *Alcohol* 4:231-239, 1987.

218. Ioffe S, Chernick V: Prediction of subsequent motor and mental retardation in newborn infants exposed to alcohol in utero by computerized EEG analysis, *Neuropediatrics* 21:11-17, 1990.

219. Little BB, Snell LM, Ropsenfeld CR, Gilstrap LC, et al: Failure to recognize fetal alcohol syndrome in newborn infants, *Am J Dis Child* 144:1142-1146, 1990.

220. Jackson IT, Hussain K: Craniofacial and oral manifestations of fetal alcohol syndrome, *Plast Reconstr Surg* 85:505-512, 1990.

221. Conry J: Neuropsychological deficits in fetal alcohol syndrome and fetal alcohol effects, *Alcohol Clin Exp Res* 14:650-655, 1990.

222. Brown RT, Coles CD, Smith IE, Platzman KA, et al: Effects of prenatal alcohol exposure at school age. II. Attention and behavior, *Neurotoxicol Teratol* 13:369-376, 1991.

223. Astley SJ, Clarren SK, Little RE, Sampson PD, et al: Analysis of facial shape in children gestationally exposed to marijuana, alcohol, and/or cocaine, *Pediatrics* 89:67-77, 1992.

224. Stromland K, Hellstrom A: Fetal alcohol syndrome: An ophthalmological and socioeducational prospective study, *Pediatrics* 97:845-850, 1996.

225. Holzman C, Paneth N, Little R, Pinto-Martin J, et al: Perinatal brain injury in premature infants born to mothers using alcohol in pregnancy, *Pediatrics* 95:66-73, 1995.

226. Astley SJ, Clarren SK: A case definition and photographic screening tool for the facial phenotype of fetal alcohol syndrome, *J Pediatr* 129:33-41, 1996.

227. Johnson VP, Swayze VW, Sato Y, Andreasen NC: Fetal alcohol syndrome: Craniofacial and central nervous system manifestations, *Am J Med Genet* 61:329-339, 1996.

228. Rossig C, Wasser S, Oppermann P: Audiologic manifestations in fetal alcohol syndrome assessed by brainstem auditory-evoked potentials, *Neuropediatrics* 25:245-249, 1994.

229. Autti-Ramo I: Twelve-year follow-up of children exposed to alcohol in utero, *Dev Med Child Neurol* 42:406-411, 2000.

230. Clark CM, Li D, Conry J, Conry R, et al: Structural and functional brain integrity of fetal alcohol syndrome in nonretarded cases, *Pediatrics* 105:1096-1099, 2000.

231. Moore ES, Ward RE, Jamison PL, Morris CA, et al: The subtle facial signs of prenatal exposure to alcohol: An anthropometric approach, *J Pediatr* 139:215-219, 2001.

232. Stoler JM, Holmes LB: Recognition of facial features of fetal alcohol syndrome in the newborn, *Am J Med Genet C Semin Med Genet* 127:21-27, 2004.

233. Kvigne VL, Leonardson GR, Neff-Smith M, Brock E, et al: Characteristics of children who have full or incomplete fetal alcohol syndrome, *J Pediatr* 145:635-640, 2004.

234. Larroque B, Kaminski M, Dehaene P, Subtil D, et al: Prenatal alcohol exposure and signs of minor neurological dysfunction at preschool age, *Dev Med Child Neurol* 42:508-514, 2000.

235. Steinhausen HC, Willms J, Metzke CW, Spohr HL: Behavioural phenotype in foetal alcohol syndrome and foetal alcohol effects, *Dev Med Child Neurol* 45:179-182, 2003.

236. Narberhaus A, Segarra D, Gimenez M, Caldu X, et al: Differential cerebral and neuropsychological consequences in dizygotic twins with prenatal alcohol exposure, *Alcohol Alcohol* 39:321-324, 2004.

237. Malisza KL, Allman AA, Shiloff D, Jakobson L, et al: Evaluation of spatial working memory function in children and adults with fetal alcohol spectrum disorders: A functional magnetic resonance imaging study, *Pediatr Res* 58:1150-1157, 2005.

238. Carter RC, Jacobson SW, Molteno CD, Chiodo LM, et al: Effects of prenatal alcohol exposure on infant visual acuity, *J Pediatr* 147:473-479, 2005.

239. Astley SJ: Comparison of the 4-digit diagnostic code and the Hoyme diagnostic guidelines for fetal alcohol spectrum disorders, *Pediatrics* 118:1532-1545, 2006.

240. Spohr HL, Willms J, Steinhausen HC: Fetal alcohol spectrum disorders in young adulthood, *J Pediatr* 150:175-179, 2007.

240a. Bookstein FL, Connor PD, Huggins JE, Barr HM, et al: Many infants prenatally exposed to high levels of alcohol show one particular anomaly of the corpus callosum, *Alcohol Clin Exp Res* 31:868-879, 2007.

241. Jones KL, Smith DW, Streissguth AP, Myrianthopoulos NC: Outcome in offspring of chronic alcoholic women, *Lancet* 1:1076-1078, 1974.

242. Clarren SK, Alvord EC Jr, Sumi SM, Streissguth AP, et al: Brain malformations related to prenatal exposure to ethanol, *J Pediatr* 92:64-67, 1978.

243. Chernick V, Childiaeva R, Ioffe S: Effects of maternal alcohol intake and smoking on neonatal electroencephalogram and anthropometric measurements, *Am J Obstet Gynecol* 146:41-47, 1983.

244. Ioffe S, Childiaeva R, Chernick V: Prolonged effects of maternal alcohol ingestion on the neonatal electroencephalogram, *Pediatrics* 74:330-337, 1984.

245. Ioffe S, Chernick V: Development of the EEG between 30 and 40 weeks gestation in normal and alcohol-exposed infants, *Dev Med Child Neurol* 30:797-807, 1988.

246. Wozniak JR, Mueller BA, Chang PN, Muetzel RL, et al: Diffusion tensor imaging in children with fetal alcohol spectrum disorders, *Alcohol Clin Exp Res* 30:1799-1806, 2006.

247. Peiffer J, Majewski F, Fischbach H: Alcohol embryo and fetopathy: Neuropathology of 3 children and 3 fetuses, *J Neurol Sci* 41:125-137, 1979.

248. Wisniewski K, Dambska M, Sher JH, Qazi Q: A clinical neuropathological study of the fetal alcohol syndrome, *Neuropediatrics* 14:197-201, 1983.

249. Jones KL: Aberrant neuronal migration in the fetal alcohol syndrome, *Birth Def Orig Artic Ser* 7:131-132, 1975.

250. Ferrer I, Galofre E: Dendritic spine anomalies in fetal alcohol syndrome, *Neuropediatrics* 18:161-163, 1987.

251. Clarren SK: Central nervous system malformations in two offspring of alcoholic women, *Birth Def Orig Artic Ser* 13:151-153, 1977.

252. Coulter CL, Leech RW, Schaefer GB, Scheithauer BW, et al: Midline cerebral dysgenesis, dysfunction of the hypothalamic-pituitary axis, and fetal alcohol effects, *Arch Neurol* 50:771-775, 1993.

253. Clarren SK: Neural tube defects and fetal alcohol syndrome, *J Pediatr* 95:328, 1979.

254. Goldstein G, Arulanantham K: Neural tube defect and renal anomalies in a child with fetal alcohol syndrome, *J Pediatr* 93:636-637, 1978.

255. Archibald SL, Fennema-Notestine C, Gamst A, Riley EP, et al: Brain dysmorphology in individuals with severe prenatal alcohol exposure, *Dev Med Child Neurol* 43:148-154, 2001.

256. Riley EP, McGee CL, Sowell ER: Teratogenic effects of alcohol: A decade of brain imaging, *Am J Med Genet C Semin Med Genet* 127:35-41, 2004.

257. Bookheimer SY, Sowell ER: Brain imaging in FAS: Commentary on the article by Malisza et al, *Pediatr Res* 58:1148-1149, 2005.

258. West JR, Goodlett CR, Bonthius DJ, Hamre KM, et al: Cell population depletion associated with fetal alcohol brain damage: Mechanisms of BAC-dependent cell loss, *Alcohol Clin Exp Res* 14:813-818, 1990.

259. Miller MW: Effects of prenatal exposure to ethanol on neocortical development. II. Cell proliferation in the ventricular and subventricular zones of the rat, *J Comp Neurol* 287:326-338, 1989.

260. Kotch LE, Sulik KK: Experimental fetal alcohol syndrome: Proposed pathogenic basis for a variety of associated facial and brain anomalies, *Am J Med Genet* 44:168-176, 1992.

261. Bonthius DJ, West JR: Permanent neuronal deficits in rats exposed to alcohol during the brain growth spurt, *Teratology* 44:147-163, 1991.

262. Gressens P, Lammens M, Picard JJ, Evrard P: Ethanol-induced disturbances of gliogenesis and neuronogenesis in the developing murine brain: An in vitro and in vivo immunohistochemical and ultrastructural study, *Alcohol Alcohol* 27:219-226, 1992.

263. Miller MW: Effects of prenatal exposure to ethanol on cell proliferation and neuronal migration. In Miller MW, editor: *Development of the Central Nervous System: Effects of Alcohol and Opiates*, New York: 1992, Wiley-Liss.

264. Ikonomidou C, Bosch F, Miksa M, Bittigau P, et al: Blockade of NMDA receptors and apoptotic neurodegeneration in the developing brain, *Science* 283:70-74, 1999.

265. Ieraci A, Herrera DG: Nicotinamide protects against ethanol-induced apoptotic neurodegeneration in the developing mouse brain, *PLoS Med* 3:e101, 2006.

266. Rubert G, Minana R, Pascual M, Guerri C: Ethanol exposure during embryogenesis decreases the radial glial progenitor pool and affects the generation of neurons and astrocytes, *J Neurosci Res* 84:483-496, 2006.

267. Miller MW: Migration of cortical neurons is altered by gestational exposure to ethanol, *Alcohol Clin Exp Res* 17:304-314, 1993.

268. Charness ME, Safran RM, Perides G: Ethanol inhibits neural cell-cell adhesion, *J Biol Chem* 269:9304-9309, 1994.

269. Valles S, Sancho-Tello M, Minana R, Climent E, et al: Glial fibrillary acidic protein expression in rat brain and in radial glia culture is delayed by prenatal ethanol exposure, *J Neurochem* 67:2425-2433, 1996.

270. Tanaka H, Nasu F, Inomata K: Fetal alcohol effects: Decreased synaptic formations in the field CA3 of fetal hippocampus, *Int J Dev Neurosci* 9:509-517, 1991.

271. Savage DD, Queen SA, Sanchez CF, Paxton LL, et al: Prenatal ethanol exposure during the last third of gestation in rat reduces hippocampal NMDA agonist binding site density in 45-day-old offspring, *Alcohol* 9:37-41, 1992.

272. Druse MJ: Effects of in utero ethanol exposure on the development of neurotransmitter systems. In Miller MW, editor: *Development of the Central Nervous System: Effects of Alcohol and Opiates*, New York: 1992, Wiley-Liss.

273. Zhou FC, Sari Y, Powrozek TA: Fetal alcohol exposure reduces serotonin innervation and compromises development of the forebrain along the serotonergic pathway, *Alcohol Clin Exp Res* 29:141-149, 2005.

274. Lokhorst DK, Druse MJ: Effects of ethanol on cultured fetal astroglia, *Alcohol Clin Exp Res* 17:810-815, 1993.

275. Bass T, Volpe JJ: Ethanol in clinically relevant concentrations enhances expression of oligodendroglial differentiation but has no effect on astrocytic differentiation or DNA synthesis in primary cultures, *Dev Neurosci* 11:52-64, 1989.

276. Watari H, Born DE, Gleason CA: Effects of first trimester binge alcohol exposure on developing white matter in fetal sheep, *Pediatr Res* 59:560-564, 2006.

277. West JR, Hodges CA, Black AC: Prenatal exposure to ethanol alters the organization of hippocampal mossy fibers in rats, *Science* 211:957-959, 1981.

278. Corrigan GE: The fetal alcohol syndrome, *Tex Med* 72:72-74, 1976.

279. Papara-Nicholson D, Telford IR: Effects of alcohol on reproduction and fetal development in the guinea pig, *Anat Rec* 127:438, 1957.

280. Sandor S, Elias S: The influence of aethyl-alcohol on the development of the chick embryo, *Rev Roum Embryol Cytol Ser Embryol* 5:51, 1968.

281. Sandor S: The influence of aethyl-alcohol on the developing chick embryo. II, *Rev Roum Embryol Cytol Ser Embryol* 5:167, 1968.

282. Sandor S, Amels D: The action of ethanol on the prenatal development of albino rats: An attempt of multiphase screening, *Rev Roum Embryol Cytol Ser Embryol* 8:105, 1971.

283. Mann LI, Bhakthavathsalan A, Liv M, Makowski P: Placental transport of alcohol and the effect on maternal and fetal acid-base balance, *Am J Obstet Gynecol* 122:837-844, 1975.

284. Mann LI, Bhakthavathsalan A, Liv M, Makowski P: Effect of alcohol on fetal cerebral function and metabolism, *Am J Obstet Gynecol* 122:845-851, 1975.

285. Kronick JB: Teratogenic effects of ethyl alcohol administered to pregnant mice, *Am J Obstet Gynecol* 124:676-680, 1976.

286. Chernoff GF: The fetal alcohol syndrome in mice: An animal model, *Teratology* 15:223-229, 1977.

287. Abel EL, Dintcheff BA: Effects of prenatal alcohol exposure to growth and development in rats, *J Pharmacol Exp Ther* 207:916-921, 1978.

288. Randall CL, Taylor WJ: Prenatal ethanol exposure in mice: Teratogenic effects, *Teratology* 19:305-311, 1979.

289. Abel EL: Fetal alcohol syndrome: Behavioral teratology, *Psychol Bull* 87:29-50, 1980.

290. Abel EL, Dintcheff BA, Bush R: Effects of beer, wine, whiskey, and ethanol on pregnant rats and their offspring, *Teratology* 23:217-222, 1981.

291. Hammer RP, Scheibel AB: Morphologic evidence for a delay of neuronal maturation in fetal alcohol exposure, *Exp Neurol* 74:587-596, 1981.

292. Kennedy LA: The pathogenesis of brain abnormalities in the fetal alcohol syndrome: An integrating hypothesis, *Teratology* 29:363-368, 1984.

293. Abel EL: Prenatal effects of alcohol on growth: A brief overview, *Fed Proc* 44:2318-2322, 1985.

294. Randall CL, Ekblad U, Anton RF: Perspectives on the pathophysiology of fetal alcohol syndrome, *Alcohol Clin Exp Res* 14:807-812, 1990.

295. Schenker S, Becker HC, Randall CL, Phillips DK, et al: Fetal alcohol syndrome: Current status of pathogenesis, *Alcohol Clin Exp Res* 14:635-645, 1990.

296. Clarren SK, Astley SJ, Bowden DM, Lai H, et al: Neuroanatomic and neurochemical abnormalities in non-human primate infants exposed to weekly doses of ethanol during gestation, *Alcohol Clin Exp Res* 14:674-683, 1990.

297. DeJonge MH, Zachman RD: The effect of maternal ethanol ingestion on fetal rat heart vitamin A: A model for fetal alcohol syndrome, *Pediatr Res* 37:418-423, 1995.

298. Deltour L, Ang HL, Duester G: Ethanol inhibition of retinoic acid synthesis as a potential mechanism for fetal alcohol syndrome, *FASEB J* 10:1050-1057, 1996.

299. Erb L, Andresen BD: The fetal alcohol syndrome (FAS): A review of the impact of chronic maternal alcoholism on the developing fetus, *Clin Pediatr* 17:644-649, 1978.

300. Tanaka H, Nakazawa K, Suzuki N, Arima M: Prevention possibility for brain dysfunction in rat with the fetal alcohol syndrome: Low-zinc status and hypoglycemia, *Brain Dev* 4:429-438, 1982.

301. Keppen L, Pysher T, Rennert OM: Zinc deficiency potentiates ethanol embryopathy, *Pediatr Res* 19:327A, 1984.

302. Brien JF, Smith GN: Effects of alcohol (ethanol) on the fetus, *J Dev Physiol* 15:21-32, 1991.

303. Peng Y, Yang PH, Ng SS, Wong OG, et al: A critical role of Pax6 in alcohol-induced fetal microcephaly, *Neurobiol Dis* 16:370-376, 2004.

304. Summers BL, Rofe AM, Coyle P: Prenatal zinc treatment at the time of acute ethanol exposure limits spatial memory impairments in mouse offspring, *Pediatr Res* 59:66-71, 2006.

305. Mukherjee AB, Hodgen GD: Maternal ethanol exposure induces transient impairment of umbilical circulation and fetal hypoxia in monkeys, *Science* 218:700-702, 1982.

306. Altura BM, Altura BT, Carella A: Alcohol produces spasms of human umbilical blood vessels: Relationship of fetal alcohol syndrome (FAS), *Eur J Pharmacol* 86:311-312, 1982.

307. Richardson BS, Bousquet JE, Homan J, Brien JF: Cerebral metabolism in fetal lamb after maternal infusion of ethanol, *Am J Physiol* 249:R505-R509, 1985.

308. Gleason CA, Hotchkiss KJ: Cerebral responses to acute maternal alcohol intoxication in immature fetal sheep, *Pediatr Res* 31:645-648, 1992.

309. Smith AM, Zeve DR, Grisel JJ, Chen WJ: Neonatal alcohol exposure increases malondialdehyde (MDA) and glutathione (GSH) levels in the developing cerebellum, *Dev Brain Res* 160:231-238, 2005.

310. Cohen-Kerem R, Koren G: Antioxidants and fetal protection against ethanol teratogenicity. I. Review of the experimental data and implications to humans, *Neurotoxicol Teratol* 25:1-9, 2003.

311. Kumral A, Tugyan K, Gonenc S, Genc K, et al: Protective effects of erythropoietin against ethanol-induced apoptotic neurodegeneration and oxidative stress in the developing C57BL/6 mouse brain, *Dev Brain Res* 160:146-156, 2005.

312. Adde-Michel C, Hennebert O, Laudenbach V, Marret S, et al: Effect of perinatal alcohol exposure on ibotenic acid–induced excitotoxic cortical lesions in newborn hamsters, *Pediatr Res* 57:287-293, 2005.

313. Toso L, Poggi SH, Abebe D, Roberson R, et al: N-Methyl-D-aspartate subunit expression during mouse development altered by in utero alcohol exposure front matter, *Am J Obstet Gynecol* 193:1534-1539, 2005.

314. Keir WJ: Inhibition of retinoic acid synthesis and its implications in fetal alcohol syndrome, *Alcohol Clin Exp Res* 15:560-564, 1991.

315. Duester G: A hypothetical mechanism for fetal alcohol syndrome involving ethanol inhibition of retinoic acid synthesis at the alcohol dehydrogenase step, *Alcohol Clin Exp Res* 15:568-572, 1991.

316. Rosett HL, Weiner L, Edelin KC: Strategies for prevention of fetal alcohol effects, *Obstet Gynecol* 57:1-7, 1981.

317. Rosett HL, Weiner L: Prevention of fetal alcohol effects, *Pediatrics* 69:813-816, 1982.

318. Rosett HL, Weiner L, Lee A: Patterns of alcohol consumption and fetal development, *Obstet Gynecol* 61:539-546, 1983.

319. Larsson G, Bohlin AB, Tunell R: Prospective study of children exposed to variable amounts of alcohol in utero, *Arch Dis Child* 60:316-321, 1985.

320. Ingle D, Owen P, Jones L, Perry S, et al: Alcohol consumption and fetal alcohol syndrome awareness, *JAMA* 271:422-423, 1994.

321. Jones KL, Chambers CD, Hill LL, Hull AD, et al: Alcohol use in pregnancy: Inadequate recommendations for an increasing problem, *Br J Obstet Gynaecol* 113:967-968, 2006.

322. Surgeon General's advisory on alcohol and pregnancy. *FDA Drug Bull* 11:9-10, 1981.

323. Council on Scientific Affairs: Fetal effects of maternal alcohol use, *JAMA* 249:2517-2522, 1983.

324. Rosa FW: Teratogenicity of isotretinoin, *Lancet* 2:513, 1983.

325. Benke PJ: The isotretinoin teratogen syndrome, *JAMA* 251:3267-3269, 1984.

326. Lammer EJ, Chen DT, Hoar RM, Agnish ND, et al: Retinoic acid embryopathy, *N Engl J Med* 313:837-841, 1985.

327. De La Cruz E, Sun S, Vangvanichyakorn K, Desposito F: Multiple congenital malformations associated with maternal isotretinoin therapy, *Pediatrics* 74:428-430, 1984.

328. Fernhoff PM, Lammer EJ: Craniofacial features of isotretinoin embryopathy, *J Pediatr* 105:595-597, 1984.

329. Hall JG: Vitamin A: A newly recognized human teratogen. Harbinger of things to come?, *J Pediatr* 105:583-584, 1984.

330. Lott IT, Bocian M, Pribram HW, Leitner M: Fetal hydrocephalus and ear anomalies associated with maternal use of isotretinoin, *J Pediatr* 105:597-600, 1984.

331. Hansen LA, Pearl GS: Isotretinoin teratogenicity: Case report with neuropathologic findings, *Acta Neuropathol* 65:335-337, 1985.

332. Rosa F: Isotretinoin dose and teratogenicity, Lancet:1154, 1987.

333. Rizzo R, Lammer EJ, Parano E, Pavone L, et al: Limb reduction defects in humans associated with prenatal isotretinoin exposure, *Teratology* 44:599-604, 1991.

334. Morrison DG, Elsas FJ, Descartes M: Congenital oculomotor nerve synkinesis associated with fetal retinoid syndrome, *J AAPOS* 9:166-168, 2005.

335. Barbero P, Lotersztein V, Bronberg R, Perez M, et al: Acitretin embryopathy: A case report, *Birth Defects Res A Clin Mol Teratol* 70:831-833, 2004.

336. Geelen SA: Hypervitaminosis A induced teratogenesis, *CRC Crit Rev Toxicol* 6:351-359, 1979.

337. Newell-Morris L, Sirianni JE, Shepard TH, Fantel AG, et al: Teratogenic effects of retinoic acid in pigtail monkeys (*Macaca nemestrina*). II. Craniofacial features, *Teratology* 21:87-101, 1980.

338. Yip JE, Kokich VG, Shepard TH: The effect of high doses of retinoic acid on prenatal craniofacial development in *Macaca nemestrina*, *Teratology* 21:29-38, 1980.

339. Rothman KJ, Moore LI, Singer MR, Nguyen US, et al: Teratogenicity of high vitamin A intake, *N Engl J Med* 333:1369-1373, 1995.

340. Oakley GP, Erickson JD: Vitamin A and birth defects, *N Engl J Med* 333:1414-1415, 1995.

341. Marshall H, Studer M, Popperl H: A conserved retinoic acid response element required for early expression of the homeobox gene Hoxb-1, *Nature* 370:567-571, 1994.

342. Studer M, Popperl H, Marshall H, Kuriowa A, et al: Role of a conserved retinoic acid response element in rhombomere restriction of Hoxb-1, *Science* 265:1728-1732, 1994.

343. Selcen D, Seidman S, Nigro MA: Otocerebral anomalies associated with topical tretinoin use, *Brain Dev* 22:218-220, 2000.

344. Jick SS, Terris BZ, Jick H: First trimester topical tretinoin and congenital disorders, *Lancet* 341:1181-1182, 1993.

345. Loureiro KD, Kao KK, Jones KL, Alvarado S, et al: Minor malformations characteristic of the retinoic acid embryopathy and other birth outcomes in children of women exposed to topical tretinoin during early pregnancy, *Am J Med Genet A* 136:117-121, 2005.

346. Zuckerman B, Frank DA, Hingson R, Amaro H, et al: Effects of maternal marijuana and cocaine use on fetal growth, *N Engl J Med* 320:762-768, 1989.

347. Zuckerman B, Bresnahan K: Developmental and behavioral consequences of prenatal drug and alcohol exposure, *Pediatr Clin North Am* 38:1387-1406, 1991.

348. Frank DA, Zuckerman BS: Children exposed to cocaine prenatally: Pieces of the puzzle, *Neurotoxicol Teratol* 15:298-300, 1993.

349. Richardson GA, Day NL: Maternal and neonatal effects of moderate cocaine use during pregnancy, *Neurotoxicol Teratol* 13:455-460, 1991.

350. Chiriboga CA, Brust JCM, Bateman D, Hauser WA: Dose-response effect of fetal cocaine exposure on newborn neurologic function, *Pediatrics* 103:79-85, 1999.

351. Ostrea EM Jr, Brady MJ, Parks PM, Asensio DC, et al: Drug screening of meconium in infants of drug-dependent mothers: An alternative to urine testing, *J Pediatr* 115:474-477, 1989.

352. Ostrea EM Jr, Brady M, Gause S, Raymundo AL, et al: Drug screening of newborns by meconium analysis: A large-scale, prospective, epidemiologic study, *Pediatrics* 89:107-113, 1992.

353. Ostrea EM, Romero A, Yee H: Adaptation of the meconium drug test for mass screening, *J Pediatr* 124:152-154, 1993.

354. Callahan CM, Grant TM, Phipps P, Clark G, et al: Measurement of gestational cocaine exposure: Sensitivity of infants hair, meconium, and urine, *J Pediatr* 120:763-768, 1992.

355. Ostrea EM, Romero A, Knapp DK, Ostrea AR, et al: Postmortem analysis of meconium in early-gestation human fetuses exposed to cocaine: Clinical implications, *J Pediatr* 124:449-477, 1994.

356. Ostrea EM, Matias O, Keane C, Mac E, et al: Spectrum of gestational exposure to illicit drugs and other xenobiotic agents in newborn infants by meconium analysis, *J Pediatr* 133:513-515, 1998.

357. Ostrea EM, Knapp DK, Tannenbaum L, Ostrea AR, et al: Estimates of illicit drug use during pregnancy by maternal interview, hair analysis, and meconium analysis, *J Pediatr* 138:344-348, 2001.

358. Lester BM, El Sohly M, Wright LL, Smeriglio VL, et al: The maternal lifestyle study: Drug use by meconium toxicology and maternal self-report, *Pediatrics* 107:309-317, 2001.

359. Graham K, Koren G, Klein J, Schneiderman J, et al: Determination of gestational cocaine exposure by hair analysis, *JAMA* 262:3328-3330, 1989.

360. Bar-Oz B, Klein J, Karaskov T, Koren G: Comparison of meconium and neonatal hair analysis for detection of gestational exposure to drugs of abuse, *Arch Dis Child Fetal Neonatal Ed* 88:F98-F100, 2003.

361. Mayes LC, Granger RH, Bornstein MH, Zuckerman B: The problem of prenatal cocaine exposure. A rush to judgment, *JAMA* 267:406-408, 1992.

362. Lutiger B, Graham K, Einarson TR, Koren G: Relationship between gestational cocaine use and pregnancy outcome: A meta-analysis, *Teratology* 44:405-414, 1991.

363. Neuspiel DR, Hamel SC: Cocaine and infant behavior, *J Dev Behav Pediatr* 12:55-64, 1991.

364. Neuspiel DR: Cocaine and the fetus: Mythology of severe risk, *Neurotoxicol Teratol* 15:305-306, 1993.

365. Streissguth AP, Grant TM, Barr HM, Brown ZA, et al: Cocaine and the use of alcohol and other drugs during pregnancy, *Am J Obstet Gynecol* 164:1239-1243, 1991.

366. Fried PA: Cigarettes and marijuana: Are there measurable long-term neurobehavioral teratogenic effects? *Neurotoxicology* 10:577-583, 1989.

367. Rush D, Callahan KR: Exposure to passive cigarette smoking and child development: A critical review, *Ann N Y Acad Sci* 562:74-100, 1989.

368. Wilson GS: Clinical studies of infants and children exposed prenatally to heroin, *Ann N Y Acad Sci* 562:183-194, 1989.

369. Hans SL: Developmental consequences of prenatal exposure to methadone, *Ann N Y Acad Sci* 562:195-207, 1989.

370. Hutchings DE, Fifer WP: Neurobehavioral effects in human and animal offspring following prenatal exposure to methadone. In Riley EP, Vorhees CV, editors: *Handbook of Behavioral Teratology*, New York: 1986, Plenum Press.

371. Schultz S, Zweig M, Singh T: Congenital syphilis: New York City, 1986–1988, *MMRW Morb Mortal Wkly Rep* 38:825-829, 1989.

372. Shannon M, Lacouture PG, Roa J, Woolf A: Cocaine exposure among children seen at a pediatric hospital, *Pediatrics* 83:337-342, 1989.

373. Chaisson RE, Bacchetti P, Osmond D, Brodie B, et al: Cocaine use and HIV infection in intravenous drug users in San Francisco, *JAMA* 261:561-565, 1989.

374. Sterk C: Cocaine and HIV seropositivity [letter], *Lancet* 1:1052-1053, 1988.

375. Ultmann MH, Diamond GW, Ruff HA, Belman AL, et al: Developmental abnormalities in children with acquired immunodeficiency syndrome (AIDS): A follow-up study, *Int J Neurosci* 32:661-667, 1987.

376. Griffin ML, Weiss RD, Mirin SM, Lange U: A comparison of male and female cocaine abusers, *Arch Gen Psychiatry* 46:122-126, 1989.

377. Zuckerman B, Amaro H, Bauchner H, Cabral H: Depressive symptoms during pregnancy: Relationship to poor health behaviors, *Am J Obstet Gynecol*:1107-1111, 1989.

378. Lifschitz MH, Wilson GS, Smith EO, Desmond MM: Factors affecting head growth and intellectual function in children of drug addicts, *Pediatrics* 75:269-274, 1985.

379. Bauer CR, Langer JC, Shankaran S, Bada HS, et al: Acute neonatal effects of cocaine exposure during pregnancy, *Arch Pediatr Adolesc Med* 159:824-834, 2005.

380. Koren G, Graham K, Shear H, Einarson T: Bias against the null hypothesis: The reproductive hazards of cocaine, *Lancet* 2:1440-1442, 1989.

381. Amaro H, Zuckerman B, Cabral H: Drug use among adolescent mothers: Profile of risk, *Pediatrics* 84:144-151, 1989.

382. Chouteau M, Namerow PB, Leppert P: The effect of cocaine abuse on birth weight and gestational age, *Obstet Gynecol* 72:351-354, 1988.

383. Zuckerman BS, Amaro H, Aboagye K, Bauchner H, et al: Cocaine use during pregnancy: Prevalence and correlates, *Pediatrics* 82:888-895, 1988.

384. Little BB, Snell LM, Klein VR, Gilstrap Ld: Cocaine abuse during pregnancy: Maternal and fetal implications, *Obstet Gynecol* 73:157-160, 1989.

385. Neerhof MG, MacGregor SN, Retzky SS, Sullivan TP: Cocaine abuse during pregnancy: Peripartum prevalence and perinatal outcome, *Am J Obstet Gynecol* 161:633-638, 1989.

386. Osterloh JD, Lee BL: Urine drug screening in mothers and newborns, *Am J Dis Child* 143:791-793, 1989.

387. Gingras JL, Weesemayer DE, Hume RF, Odonnell KJ: Cocaine and development: Mechanisms of fetal toxicity and neonatal consequences of prenatal cocaine exposure, *Early Hum Dev* 31:1-24, 1992.

388. Kain ZN, Kain TS, Scarpelli EM: Cocaine exposure in utero: Perinatal development and neonatal manifestations—review, *J Toxicol Clin Toxicol* 30:607-636, 1992.

389. Ostrea EM, Lucena JL, Silvestre MA: The infant of the drug-dependent mother. In Avery GB, Fletcher MA, MacDonald MG, editors: *Neonatology: Pathophysiology and Management of the Newborn*, 4th ed, Philadelphia: 1994, JP Lippincott.

390. Vega WA, Kolody B, Hwang J, Noble A: Prevalence and magnitude of perinatal substance exposures in California, *N Engl J Med* 329:850-854, 1993.

391. Schutzman DL, Frankenfield CM, Clatterbaugh HE, Singer J: Incidence of intrauterine cocaine exposure in a suburban setting, *Pediatrics* 88:825-827, 1991.

392. Farrar HC, Kearns GL: Cocaine: Clinical pharmacology and toxicology, *J Pediatr* 115:665-675, 1989.

393. Woolverton WL, Johnson KM: Neurobiology of cocaine abuse, *Trends Pharmacol Sci* 13:193-200, 1992.

394. Van Dyke C, Byck R: Cocaine, *Sci Am* 246:128-141, 1982.

395. Ellenhorn M, Barceloux D: *Medical Toxicology: Diagnosis and Treatment of Human Poisoning*, New York: 1988, Elsevier Science.

396. Chow MJ, Ambre JJ, Ruo TI, Atkinson AJ Jr, et al: Kinetics of cocaine distribution, elimination, and chronotropic effects, *Clin Pharmacol Ther* 38:318-324, 1985.

397. Chasnoff IJ: Placental transfer of cocaine: Follow-up and outcome. In *Transplacental Disorders: Perinatal Detection, Treatment and Management (Including Pediatric AIDS)*, New York: 1990, Liss.

398. Mittleman RE, Cofino JC, Hearn WL: Tissue distribution of cocaine in a pregnant woman, *J Forensic Sci* 34:481-486, 1989.

399. Ambre JJ, Ruo TI, Smith GL, Backes D, et al: Ecgonine methyl ester, a major metabolite of cocaine, *J Anal Toxicol* 6:26-29, 1982.

400. Steward DJ, Inaba T, Lucassen M, Kalow W: Cocaine metabolism: Cocaine and norcocaine hydrolysis by liver and serum esterases, *Clin Pharmacol Ther* 25:464-468, 1979.

401. Inaba T, Stewart DJ, Kalow W: Metabolism of cocaine in man, *Clin Pharmacol Ther* 23:547-552, 1978.

402. Oro AS, Dixon SD: Perinatal cocaine and methamphetamine exposure: Maternal and neonatal correlates, *J Pediatr* 111:571-578, 1987.

403. Gawin FH, Ellinwood EH Jr: Cocaine and other stimulants: Actions, abuse, and treatment, *N Engl J Med* 318:1173-1182, 1988.

404. Nestler EJ: Molecular mechanisms of drug addiction, *J Neurosci* 12:2439-2450, 1992.

405. Giros B, El Mestikawy S, Bertrand L, Caron MG: Cloning and functional characterization of a cocaine-sensitive dopamine transporter, *FEBS Lett* 295:149-154, 1991.

406. Weaver DR, Rivkees SA, Reppert SM: Cocaine activates a dopamine system in the fetal biological clock, *Proc Natl Acad Sci U S A* 89:9201-9204, 1992.

407. Kuhar MJ, Ritz MC, Boja JW: The dopamine hypothesis of the reinforcing properties of cocaine, *Trends Neurosci* 14:299-302, 1991.

408. Goeders NE, Smith JE: Cortical dopaminergic involvement in cocaine reinforcement, *Science* 221:773-775, 1983.

409. Knapp S, Mandell AJ: Narcotic drugs: Effects on the serotonin biosynthetic systems of the brain, *Science* 177:1209-1211, 1972.

410. Lakoski JM, Cunningham KA: The interaction of cocaine with central serotonergic neuronal systems: Cellular electrophysiologic approaches. In *Mechanisms of Cocaine Abuse and Toxicity*, research monograph, Bethesda, MD: 1988, National Institute on Drug Abuse.

411. Ross SB, Renyi AL: Inhibition of the uptake of tritiated 5-hydroxytryptamine in brain tissue, *Eur J Pharmacol* 7:270-277, 1969.

412. Handler A, Kistin N, Davis F, Ferre C: Cocaine use during pregnancy: Perinatal outcomes, *Am J Epidemiol* 133:818-825, 1991.

413. Weathers WT, Crane MM, Sauvain KJ, Blackhurst DW: Cocaine use in women from a defined population: Prevalence at delivery and effects on growth in infants, *Pediatrics* 91:350-354, 1993.

414. Church MW, Kaufmann RA, Keenan JA, Martler SS, et al: Effects of prenatal cocaine exposure. In Watson RR, editor: *Biochemistry and Physiology of Substance Abuse*, Boca Raton, FL: 1991, CRC Press.

415. Slutsker L: Risks associated with cocaine use during pregnancy, *Obstet Gynecol* 79:778-789, 1992.

416. Fries MH, Kuller JA, Norton ME, Yankowitz J, et al: Facial features of infants exposed prenatally to cocaine, *Teratology* 48:413-420, 1993.

417. Kliegman RM, Madura D, Kiwi R, Eisenberg I, et al: Relation of maternal cocaine use to the risks of prematurity and low birth weight, *J Pediatr* 124:751-756, 1994.

418. Singer L, Arendt R, Song LY, Warshawsky E, et al: Direct and indirect interactions of cocaine with childbirth outcomes, *Arch Pediatr Adolesc Med* 148:959-964, 1994.

419. Bandstra ES, Morrow CE, Anthony JC, Churchill SS, et al: Intrauterine growth of full-term infants: Impact of prenatal cocaine exposure, *Pediatrics* 108:1309-1319, 2001.

420. Bada HS, Das A, Bauer CR, Shankaran S, et al: Gestational cocaine exposure and intrauterine growth: Maternal lifestyle study, *Obstet Gynecol* 100:916-924, 2002.

421. Moore TR, Sorg J, Miller L, Key TC, et al: Hemodynamic effects of intravenous cocaine on the pregnant ewe and fetus, *Am J Obstet Gynecol* 155:883-888, 1986.

422. Lederman RP, Lederman E, Work BA Jr, McCann DS: The relationship of maternal anxiety, plasma catecholamines, and plasma cortisol to progress in labor, *Am J Obstet Gynecol* 132:495-500, 1978.

423. Hurd WW, Smith AJ, Gauvin JM, Hayashi RH: Cocaine blocks extra-neuronal uptake of norepinephrine by the pregnant human uterus, *Obstet Gynecol* 78:249-253, 1991.

424. Monga M, Weisbrodt NW, Andres RL, Sanborn BM: The acute effect of cocaine exposure on pregnant human myometrial contractile activity, *Am J Obstet Gynecol* 169:782-785, 1993.

425. Frank DA, Bauchner H, Parker S, Huber AM, et al: Neonatal body proportionality and body composition after in utero exposure to cocaine and marijuana, *J Pediatr* 117:622-626, 1990.

426. Woods JR Jr, Plessinger MA, Clark KE: Effect of cocaine on uterine blood flow and fetal oxygenation, *JAMA* 257:957-961, 1987.

427. Dicke JM, Verges DK, Polakoski KL: Cocaine inhibits alanine uptake by human placental microvillous membrane vesicles, *Am J Obstet Gynecol* 169:515-521, 1993.

428. Chan K, Dodd PA, Day L, Kullama L, et al: Fetal catecholamine, cardiovascular, and neurobehavioral responses to cocaine, *Am J Obstet Gynecol* 167:1616-1623, 1992.

429. Chasnoff IJ, Griffith DR, MacGregor S, Dirkes K, et al: Temporal patterns of cocaine use in pregnancy: Perinatal outcome, *JAMA* 261:1741-1744, 1989.

430. Bingol N, Fuchs M, Diaz V, Stone RK, et al: Teratogenicity of cocaine in humans [published erratum appears in J Pediatr 110:350, 1987], *J Pediatr* 110:93-96, 1987.

431. Little BB, Snell LM: Brain growth among fetuses exposed to cocaine in utero: Asymmetrical growth retardation, *Obstet Gynecol* 77:361-364, 1991.

432. Fulroth R, Phillips B, Durand DJ: Perinatal outcome of infants exposed to cocaine and/or heroin in utero, *Am J Dis Child* 143:905-910, 1989.

433. Gillogley KM, Evans AT, Hansen RL, Samuels SJ, et al: The perinatal impact of cocaine, amphetamine, and opiate use detected by universal intrapartum screening, *Am J Obstet Gynecol* 163:1535-1542, 1990.

434. Dow-Edwards DL: Cocaine effects on fetal development: A comparison of clinical and animal research findings, *Neurotoxicol Teratol* 13:347-352, 1991.

435. Chasnoff IJ, Burns WJ, Schnoll SH, Burns KA: Cocaine use in pregnancy, *N Engl J Med* 313:666-669, 1985.

436. Kaufmann WE: Developmental cortical anomalies after prenatal exposure to cocaine, *Soc Neurosci Abstr* 16:305, 1990.

437. Dominguez R, Aguirre V, Coro A, Slopis JM, et al: Brain and ocular abnormalities in infants with in utero exposure to cocaine and other street drugs, *Am J Dis Child* 145:688-695, 1991.

438. Ryan L, Ehrlich S, Finnegan L: Cocaine abuse in pregnancy: Effects on the fetus and newborn, *Neurotoxicol Teratol* 9:295-299, 1987.

439. Hadeed AJ, Siegel SR: Maternal cocaine use during pregnancy: Effect on the newborn infant, *Pediatrics* 84:205-210, 1989.

440. Dixon SD, Bejar R: Echoencephalographic findings in neonates associated with maternal cocaine and methamphetamine use: Incidence and clinical correlates, *J Pediatr* 115:770-778, 1989.

441. Good WV, Ferriero DM, Golabi M, Kobori JA: Abnormalities of the visual system in infants exposed to cocaine, *Ophthalmology* 99:341-346, 1992.

442. Gomez-Anson B, Ramsey RG: Pachygyria in a neonate with prenatal cocaine exposure: MR features, *J Comput Assist Tomogr* 18:637-639, 1994.

443. Gieron-Korthals MA, Helal A, Martinez CR: Expanding spectrum of cocaine induced central nervous system malformations, *Brain Dev* 16:253-256, 1994.

444. Tsay CH, Partridge JC, Villarreal SF, Good WV, et al: Neurologic and ophthalmologic findings in children exposed to cocaine in utero, *J Child Neurol* 11:25-30, 1996.

445. Chiriboga CA, Bateman DA, Brust JCM, Hauser WA: Neurologic findings in neonates with intrauterine cocaine exposure, *Pediatr Neurol* 9:115-119, 1993.

446. Konkol RJ, Tikofsky RS, Wells R, Hellman RS, et al: Normal high-resolution cerebral ^{99m}Tc-HMPAO SPECT scans in symptomatic neonates exposed to cocaine, *J Child Neurol* 9:280-297, 1994.

447. Mirochnick M, Frank DA, Cabral H, Turner A, et al: Relation between meconium concentration of the cocaine metabolite benzoylecgonine and fetal growth, *J Pediatr* 126:636-638, 1995.

448. Nulman I, Rovet J, Altmann D, Bradley C, et al: Neurodevelopment of adopted children exposed in utero to cocaine, *Can Med Assoc J* 151:1591-1597, 1994.

449. King TA, Perlman JM, Laptook AR, Rollins N, et al: Neurologic manifestations of in utero cocaine exposure in near-term and term infants, *Pediatrics* 96:259-264, 1995.

450. Scafidi FA, Field TM, Wheeden A, Schanberg S, et al: Cocaine-exposed preterm neonates show behavioral and hormonal differences, *Pediatrics* 97:851-855, 1996.

451. Ferriero DM, Kobori JA, Good WV, Golabi M: Retinal defects in cocaine-exposed infants, *Ann Neurol* 26:458, 1989.

452. Dow-Edwards DL: Long-term neurochemical and neurobehavioral consequences of cocaine use during pregnancy, *Ann N Y Acad Sci* 562:280-289, 1989.

453. Dow-Edwards DL, Freed LA, Fico TA: Structural and functional effects of prenatal cocaine exposure in adult rat brain, *Brain Res Dev Brain Res* 57:263-268, 1990.

454. Raum WJ, McGivern RF, Peterson MA, Shryne JH, et al: Prenatal inhibition of hypothalamic sex steroid uptake by cocaine: Effects on neurobehavioral sexual differentiation in male rats, *Brain Res Dev Brain Res* 53:230-236, 1990.

455. Segal DS, Freed LA, Hughes HE, Milorat TH, et al: Alterations in 3H-SCH23390 binding in rat brain following perinatal exposure to cocaine [abstract], *Soc Neurosci Abstr* 519:19, 1989.

456. Spear LP, Kirstein CL, Frambes NA: Cocaine effects on the developing central nervous system: Behavioral, psychopharmacological, and neurochemical studies, *Ann N Y Acad Sci* 562:290-307, 1989.

457. Sobrian SK, Burton LE, Robinson NL, Ashe WK, et al: Neurobehavioral and immunological effects of prenatal cocaine exposure in rat, *Pharmacol Biochem Behav* 35:617-629, 1990.

458. Johns JM, Means MJ, Anderson DR, Means LW, et al: Prenatal exposure to cocaine. II. Effects on open-field activity and cognitive behavior in Sprague-Dawley rats, *Neurotoxicol Teratol* 14:343-349, 1992.

459. Heyser CJ, Spear NE, Spear LP: Effects of prenatal exposure to cocaine on conditional discrimination learning in adult rats, *Behav Neurosci* 106:837-845, 1992.

460. Akbari HM, Kramer HK, Whitaker-Azmitia PM, Separ LP, et al: Prenatal cocaine exposure disrupts the development of the serotonergic system, *Brain Res* 572:57-63, 1992.

461. Minabe Y, Ashby CR Jr, Heyser C, Spear LP, et al: The effects of prenatal cocaine exposure on spontaneously active midbrain dopamine neurons in adult male offspring: An electrophysiological study, *Brain Res* 586:152-156, 1992.

462. Seidler FJ, Slotkin TA: Fetal cocaine exposure causes persistent noradrenergic hyperactivity in rat brain regions: Effects on neurotransmitter turnover and receptors, *J Pharmacol Exp Ther* 263:413-421, 1992.

463. Dow-Edwards DL, Freed-Malen LA, Hughes HE: Long-term alterations in brain function following cocaine administration during the preweanling period, *Dev Brain Res* 72:309-313, 1993.

464. Cabrera TM, Yracheta JM, Li Q, Levy AD, et al: Prenatal cocaine produces deficits in serotonin mediated neuroendocrine responses in adult rat progeny: Evidence for long-term functional alterations in brain serotonin pathways, *Synapse* 15:158-168, 1993.

465. Gressens P, Kosofsky BE, Evrard P: Cocaine-induced disturbances of corticogenesis in the developing murine brain, *Neurosci Lett* 140:113-116, 1992.

466. Kosofsky BE, Wilkins AS, Gressens P, Evrard P: Transplacental cocaine exposure: A mouse model demonstrating neuroanatomic and behavioral abnormalities, *J Child Neurol* 9:234-241, 1994.

467. Kosofsky BE, Genova LM, Hyman SE: Postnatal age defines specificity of immediate early gene induction by cocaine in developing rat brain, *J Comp Neurol* 351:27-40, 1995.

468. Kosofsky BE, Genova LM, Hyman S: Substance P phenotype defines specificity of c-fos induction by cocaine in developing rat striatum, *J Com Neurol* 35:141-150, 1995.

469. Seidler FJ, Temple SW, McCook EC, Slotkin TA: Cocaine inhibits central noradrenergic and dopaminergic activity during the critical developmental period in which catecholamines influence cell development, *Brain Res Dev* 85:48-53, 1995.

470. Nassogne MC, Evrard P, Courtoy PJ: Selective neuronal toxicity of cocaine in embryonic mouse brain cocultures, *Proc Natl Acad Sci U S A* 92:11029-11033, 1995.

471. Lidow MS: Prenatal cocaine exposure adversely affects development of the primate cerebral cortex, *Synapse* 21:332-341, 1995.

472. Chai L, Choi WS, Ronnekleiv OK: Maternal cocaine treatment alters dynorphin and enkephalin mRNA expression in brains of fetal rhesus macaques, *J Neurosci* 17:1112-1121, 1997.

473. Nassogne MC, Gressens P, Evrard P, Courtoy PJ: In contrast to cocaine, prenatal exposure to methadone does not produce detectable alterations in the developing mouse brain, *Dev Brain Res* 110:61-67, 1998.

474. Dow-Edwards D, Mayes L, Spear L, Hurd Y: Cocaine and development: Clinical, behavioral, and neurobiological perspectives—a symposium report, *Neurotoxicol Teratol* 21:481-490, 1999.

475. Lidow MS, Song ZM: Primates exposed to cocaine in utero display reduced density and number of cerebral cortical neurons, *J Comp Neurol* 435:263-275, 2001.

476. Lidow MS: Consequences of prenatal cocaine exposure in nonhuman primates, *Brain Res Dev Brain Res* 147:23-36, 2003.

477. Lloyd SA, Wensley B, Faherty CJ, Smeyne RJ: Regional differences in cortical dendrite morphology following in utero exposure to cocaine, *Dev Brain Res* 147:59-66, 2003.

478. Yan QS, Zheng SZ, Yan SE: Prenatal cocaine exposure decreases brain-derived neurotrophic factor proteins in the rat brain, *Brain Res* 1009:228-233, 2004.

479. Warner TD, Behnke M, Eyler FD, Padgett K, et al: Diffusion tensor imaging of frontal white matter and executive functioning in cocaine-exposed children, *Pediatrics* 118:2014-2024, 2006.

479a. Avants BB, Hurt H, Giannetta JM, Epstein CL, et al: Effects of heavy in utero cocaine exposure on adolescent caudate morphology, *Pediatr Neurol* 37:275-279, 2007.

480. Chasnoff IJ, Bussey ME, Savich R, Stack CM: Perinatal cerebral infarction and maternal cocaine use, *J Pediatr* 108:456-459, 1986.

481. Kramer LD, Locke GE, Ogunyemi A, Nelson L: Neonatal cocaine-related seizures, *J Child Neurol* 5:60-64, 1990.

482. Hoyme HE, Jones KL, Dixon SD, Jewett T, et al: Prenatal cocaine exposure and fetal vascular disruption, *Pediatrics* 85:743-747, 1990.

483. Heier LA, Carpanzano CR, Mast J, Brill PW, et al: Maternal cocaine abuse: The spectrum of radiologic abnormalities in the neonatal CNS, *AJNR Am J Neuroradiol* 12:951-956, 1991.

484. Lavi E, Montone KT, Rorke LB, Kliman HJ: Fetal akinesia deformation sequence (Pena-Shokeir phenotype) associated with acquired intrauterine brain damage, *Neurology* 41:1467-1468, 1991.

485. Kankirawatana P, Tennison MB, D'Cruz O, Greenwood RS: Mobius syndrome in infant exposed to cocaine in utero, *Pediatr Neurol* 9:71-72, 1993.

486. Spires MC, Gordon EF, Choudhuri M, Maldonado E, et al: Intracranial hemorrhage in a neonate following prenatal cocaine exposure, *Pediatr Neurol* 5:324-326, 1989.

487. Puvabanditsin S, Garrow E, Augustin G, Titapiwatanakul R, et al: Poland-Mobius syndrome and cocaine abuse: A relook at vascular etiology, *Pediatr Neurol* 32:285-287, 2005.

488. Frank Da, McCarten K, Cabral H, Levenson SM, et al: Cranial ultrasounds in term newborns: Failure to replicate excess abnormalities in cocaine exposed, *Pediatr Res* 31:247A, 1992.

489. Dusick AM, Covert RF, Schreiber MD, Yee GT, et al: Risk of intracranial hemorrhage and other adverse outcomes after cocaine exposure in a cohort of 323 very low birth weight infants, *J Pediatr* 122:438-445, 1993.

490. Singer LT, Yamashita TS, Hawkins S, Cairns D, et al: Increased incidence of intraventricular hemorrhage and developmental delay in cocaine-exposed, very low birth weight infants, *J Pediatr* 124:765-771, 1994.

491. Madden JD, Payne TF, Miller S: Maternal cocaine abuse and effect on the newborn, *Pediatrics* 77:209-211, 1986.

492. Neuspiel DR, Hamel SC, Hochberg E, Greene J, et al: Maternal cocaine use and infant behavior, *Neurotoxicol Teratol* 13:229-233, 1991.

493. Anday EK, Cohen ME, Kelley NE, Leitner DS: Effect of in utero cocaine exposure on startle and its modification, *Dev Pharmacol Ther* 12:137-145, 1989.

494. Chaney NE, Franke J, Wadlington WB: Cocaine convulsions in a breast-feeding baby, *J Pediatr* 112:134-135, 1988.

495. Chasnoff IJ, Burns KA, Burns WJ: Cocaine use in pregnancy: Perinatal morbidity and mortality, *Neurotoxicol Teratol* 9:291-293, 1987.

496. Rivkin M, Gilmore HE: Generalized seizures in an infant due to environmentally acquired cocaine, *Pediatrics* 84:1100-1102, 1989.

497. Doberczak TM, Shanzer S, Senie RT, Kandall SR: Neonatal neurologic and electroencephalographic effects of intrauterine cocaine exposure, *J Pediatr* 113:354-358, 1988.

498. Hume RF Jr, O'Donnell KJ, Stanger CL, Killam AP, et al: In utero cocaine exposure: Observations of fetal behavioral state may predict neonatal outcome, *Am J Obstet Gynecol* 161:685-690, 1989.

499. Singer LT, Garber R, Kliegman R: Neurobehavioral sequelae of fetal cocaine exposure, *J Pediatr* 119:667-672, 1991.

500. Lester BM, Corwin MJ, Sepkoski C, Seifer R, et al: Neurobehavioral syndromes in cocaine-exposed newborn infants, *Child Dev* 62:694-705, 1991.

501. Eisen LN, Field TM, Bandstra ES, Roberts JP, et al: Perinatal cocaine effects on neonatal stress behavior and performance on the Brazelton scale, *Pediatrics* 88:477-480, 1991.

502. Legido A, Clancy RR, Spitzer AR, Finnegan LP: Electroencephalographic and behavioral-state studies in infants of cocaine-addicted mothers, *Am J Dis Child* 146:748-752, 1992.

503. Corwin MJ, Lester BM, Sepkoski C, McLaughlin S, et al: Effects of in utero cocaine exposure on newborn acoustical cry characteristics, *Pediatrics* 89:1199-1203, 1992.

504. Mayes LC, Granger RH, Frank MA, Schottenfeld R, et al: Neurobehavioral profiles of neonates exposed to cocaine prenatally, *Pediatrics* 91:778-783, 1993.

505. Hansen RL, Struthers JM, Gospe SM: Visual evoked potentials and visual processing in stimulant drug-exposed infants, *Dev Med Child Neurol* 35:798-805, 1993.

506. Gingras JL, Beibel JB, Dalley LB, Muelenaer A, et al: Maternal polydrug use including cocaine and postnatal sleep architecture: Preliminary observations and implications for respiratory control and behavior, *Early Hum Dev* 43:197-204, 1995.

507. Chiriboga CA, Vibbert M, Malouf R, Suarez MS, et al: Neurological correlates of fetal cocaine exposure: Transient hypertonia of infancy and early childhood, *Pediatrics* 96:1070-1077, 1995.

508. Napiorkowski B, Lester BM, Freier MC, Brunner S, et al: Effects of in utero substance exposure on infant neurobehavior, *Pediatrics* 98:71-75, 1996.

509. Delaney-Black V, Covington C, Ostrea E, Romero A, et al: Prenatal cocaine and neonatal outcome: Evaluation of dose-response relationship, *Pediatrics* 98:735-740, 1996.

510. Beltran RS, Coker SB: Transient dystonia of infancy, a result of intrauterine cocaine exposure? *Pediatr Neurol* 12:354-356, 1995.

511. Belcher HM, Shapiro BK, Leppert M, Butz AM, et al: Sequential neuromotor examination in children with intrauterine cocaine/polydrug exposure, *Dev Med Child Neurol* 41:240-246, 1999.

512. Lester BM, Tronick EZ, LaGasse L, Seifer R, et al: The maternal lifestyle study: Effects of substance exposure during pregnancy on neurodevelopmental outcome in 1-month-old infants, *Pediatrics* 110:1182-1192, 2002.

513. Singer LT, Arendt R, Minnes S, Farkas K, et al: Neurobehavioral outcomes of cocaine-exposed infants, *Neurotoxicol Teratol* 22:653-666, 2000.

514. Lester BM, LaGasse L, Seifer R, Tronick EZ, et al: The maternal lifestyle study (MLS): Effects of prenatal cocaine and/or opiate exposure on auditory brain response at one month, *J Pediatr* 142:279-285, 2003.

514a. John V, Dai H, Talati A, Charnigo RJ, et al: Autonomic alterations in cocaine-exposed neonates following orthostatic stress, *Pediatr Res* 61:251-256, 2007.

515. Shih L, Cone WB, Reddix B: Effects of maternal cocaine abuse on the neonatal auditory system, *Int J Pediatr Otorhinolaryngol* 15:245-251, 1988.

516. Salamy A, Eldredge L, Anderson J, Bull D: Brain-stem transmission time in infants exposed to cocaine in utero, *J Pediatr* 117:627-629, 1990.

517. Church MW, Overbeck GW: Sensorineural hearing loss as evidenced by the auditory brainstem response following prenatal cocaine exposure in the Long-Evans rat, *Teratology* 43:561-570, 1991.

518. Tan-Laxa MA, Sison-Switala C, Rintelman W, Ostrea EM: Abnormal auditory brainstem response among infants with prenatal cocaine exposure, *Pediatrics* 113:357-360, 2004.

519. Scher MS, Richardson GA, Day NL: Effects of prenatal cocaine/crack and other drug exposure on electroencephalographic sleep studies at birth and one year, *Pediatrics* 105:39-48, 2000.

520. Bauchner H, Zuckerman B, McClain M, Frank D, et al: Risk of sudden infant death syndrome among infants with in utero exposure to cocaine, *J Pediatr* 113:831-834, 1988.

521. Ward SL, Bautista D, Chan L, Derry M, et al: Sudden infant death syndrome in infants of substance-abusing mothers, *J Pediatr* 117:876-881, 1990.

522. Durand DJ, Espinoza AM, Nickerson BG: Association between prenatal cocaine exposure and sudden infant death syndrome, *J Pediatr* 117:909-911, 1990.

523. Kandall SR, Damus K, Gaines JJ, Habel L: Maternal substance use and sudden infant death syndrome (SIDS) in offspring, *Pediatr Res* 29:92A, 1991.

524. Chasnoff IJ, Hunt CE, Kletter R, Kaplan D: Prenatal cocaine exposure is associated with respiratory pattern abnormalities, *Am J Dis Child* 143:583-587, 1989.

525. Muelenaer A, Gingras J, McAdams L, O'Donnell K, et al: In utero cocaine exposure alters postnatal hypoxic arousal and ventilatory response to carbon dioxide, but not pneumograms, *Pediatr Res* 29:326A, 1991.

526. Ward SL, Bautista DB, Woo MS, Chang M, et al: Responses to hypoxia and hypercapnia in infants of substance-abusing mothers, *J Pediatr* 121:704-709, 1992.

527. Regalado MG, Schechtman VL, Del Angel AP, Bean XD: Cardiac and respiratory patterns during sleep in cocaine-exposed neonates, *Early Hum Dev* 44:187-200, 1996.

528. Belcher HM, Wallace PM: Neurodevelopmental evaluation of children with intrauterine cocaine exposure, *Pediatr Res* 29:7A, 1991.

529. Black VD, Roumell N: The effect of intrauterine cocaine exposure on neurologic status and Fagan Infantest at six months, *Pediatr Res* 29:253A, 1991.

530. Hurt H, Malmud E, Brodsky NG: Maternal cocaine use: Effect on infant developmental (DEV) outcome, *Pediatr Res* 29:257A, 1991.

531. Billman D, Nemeth P, Heimler R: Prenatal cocaine exposure (PCE): Advanced Bayley psychomotor scores, *Pediatr Res* 29:251A, 1991.

532. Chasnoff I, Griffith D, Azuma S: Intrauterine cocaine/polydrug exposure: Three year outcome, *Pediatr Res* 31:9A, 1992.

533. Chasnoff IJ, Griffith DR, Freier C, Murray J: Cocaine/polydrug use in pregnancy: Two-year followup, *Pediatrics* 89:284-289, 1992.

534. Hofkosh D, Hinderliter SA, Leviton LC, Schuh RG, et al: Impact of prenatal drug use on maternal and infant behavior, *Pediatr Res* 31:11A, 1992.

535. Hurt H, Brodsky N, Giannetta J, Belsky J: Comparison of play behaviors in cocaine (COC) exposed and control (CON) toddlers: A prospective study, *Pediatr Res* 31:11A, 1992.

536. Hurt H, Malmud E, Giannetta J: Prenatal exposure to cocaine (COC) has no effect on infant performance on Bayley Scales of Infant Development (BSID), *Pediatr Res* 31:251A, 1992.

537. Kaiser KM, Mooney KM, Anday EK: Effects of in utero cocaine exposure on early infant development, *Pediatr Res* 31:251A, 1992.

538. Katikaneni LD, Sallee FR, Ibrahim HM: Benzoylecogonine hair levels at birth in neonates following in utero cocaine exposure, *Pediatr Res* 31:251A, 1992.

539. Singer L, Arendt R, Yamashita T, Minnes S, et al: Development of infants exposed in utero to cocaine, *Pediatr Res* 31:260A, 1992.

540. Schneider JW, Chasnoff IJ: Motor assessment of cocaine/polydrug exposed infants at age 4 months, *Neurotoxicol Teratol* 14:97-101, 1992.

541. Hutchings DE: The puzzle of cocaine's effects following maternal use during pregnancy: Are there reconcilable differences? *Neurotoxicol Teratol* 15:281-286, 1993.

542. Azuma SD, Chasnoff IJ: Outcome of children prenatally exposed to cocaine and other drugs: A path analysis of three-year data, *Pediatrics* 92:396-402, 1993.

543. Mayes LC, Bornstein MH, Chawarska K, Granger RH: Information processing and developmental assessments in 3-month-old infants exposed prenatally to cocaine, *Pediatrics* 95:539-545, 1995.

544. Richardson GA, Conroy ML, Day NL: Prenatal cocaine exposure: Effects on the development of school-age children, *Neurotoxicol Teratol* 18:627-634, 1996.

545. Tronick EZ, Frank DA, Cabral H, Mirochnick M, et al: Late dose-response effects of prenatal cocaine exposure on newborn neurobehavioral performance, *Pediatrics* 98:76-83, 1996.

546. Jacobson SW, Jacobson JL, Sokol RJ, Martier SS, et al: New evidence for neurobehavioral effects of in utero cocaine exposure, *J Pediatr* 129:581-590, 1996.

547. Delaney-Black V, Covington C, Templin T, Martier S, et al: Prenatal cocaine exposure and child behavior, *Pediatrics* 102:945-950, 1998.

548. Arendt R, Angelopoulos J, Salvator A, Singer L: Motor development of cocaine-exposed children at age two years, *Pediatrics* 103:86-92, 1999.

549. Dempsey DA, Hajnal BL, Partridge C, Jacobson SN, et al: Tone abnormalities are associated with maternal cigarette smoking during pregnancy in in utero cocaine-exposed infants, *Pediatrics* 106:79-85, 2000.

550. Delaney-Black V, Covington C, Templin T, Ager J, et al: Teacher-assessed behavior of children prenatally exposed to cocaine, *Pediatrics* 106:782-791, 2000.

551. Singer LT, Arendt R, Minnes S, Salvator A, et al: Developing language skills of cocaine-exposed infants, *Pediatrics* 107:1057-1064, 2001.

552. Frank DA, Augustyn M, Knight WG, Pell T, et al: Growth, development, and behavior in early childhood following prenatal cocaine exposure, *JAMA* 285:1613-1625, 2001.

553. Frank DA, Jacobs RR, Beeghly M, Augustyn M, et al: Level of prenatal cocaine exposure and scores on the Bayley Scales of Infant Development: Modifying effects of caregiver, early intervention, and birth weight, *Pediatrics* 110:1143-1152, 2002.

554. Lewis BA, Singer LT, Short EJ, Minnes S, et al: Four-year language outcomes of children exposed to cocaine in utero, *Neurotoxicol Teratol* 26:617-627, 2004.

555. Messinger DS, Bauer CR, Das A, Seifer R, et al: The maternal lifestyle study: Cognitive, motor, and behavioral outcomes of cocaine-exposed and opiate-exposed infants through three years of age, *Pediatrics* 113:1677-1685, 2004.

556. Frank DA, Rose-Jacobs R, Beeghly M, Wilbur M, et al: Level of prenatal cocaine exposure and 48-month IQ: Importance of preschool enrichment, *Neurotoxicol Teratol* 27:15-28, 2005.

557. Bailey BN, Sood BG, Sokol RJ, Ager J, et al: Gender and alcohol moderate prenatal cocaine effects on teacher-report of child behavior, *Neurotoxicol Teratol* 27:181-189, 2005.

558. Sood BG, Bailey BN, Covington C, Sokol RJ, et al: Gender and alcohol moderate caregiver reported child behavior after prenatal cocaine, *Neurotoxicol Teratol* 27:191-201, 2005.

559. Hurt H, Brodsky NL, Roth H, Malmud E, et al: School performance of children with gestational cocaine exposure, *Neurotoxicol Teratol* 27:203-211, 2005.

560. Spear LP: Missing pieces of the puzzle complicate conclusions about cocaine's neurobehavioral toxicity in clinical populations: Importance of animal models, *Neurotoxicol Teratol* 15:307-309, 1993.

561. Anderson-Brown T, Slotkin TA, Seidler FJ: Cocaine acutely inhibits DNA synthesis in developing rat brain regions: Evidence for direct actions, *Brain Res* 537:197-202, 1990.

562. Leskawa KC, Jackson GH, Moody CA, Spear LP: Cocaine exposure during pregnancy affects rat neonate and maternal brain glycosphingolipids, *Brain Res Bull* 33:195-198, 1994.

563. Fantel AG, Person RE, Burroughs GC, Mackler B: Direct embryotoxicity of cocaine in rats: Effects on mitochondrial activity, cardiac function, and growth and development in vitro, *Teratology* 42:35-43, 1990.

564. el-Bizri H, Guest I, Varma DR: Effects of cocaine on rat embryo development in vivo and in cultures, *Pediatr Res* 29:187-190, 1991.

565. Wyatt RJ, Karoum F, Suddath R, Fawcett R: Persistently decreased brain dopamine levels and cocaine [letter], *JAMA* 259:2996, 1988.

566. Wilson RJ, Deck J, Shannak K: Markedly reduced striatal dopamine levels in brain of a chronic cocaine abuser [abstract], *Soc Neurosci Abstr* 16:252, 1990.

567. Dackis CA, Gold MS: New concepts in cocaine addiction: The dopamine depletion hypothesis, *Neurosci Biobehav Rev* 9:469-477, 1985.

568. Chen XL, Gupta M: Neuroanatomical studies of cocaine treatment on dopaminergic neurons: TH and GFAP immunocytochemical studies [abstract], *Soc Neurosci Abstr* 16:580, 1990.

569. Weese-Mayer DE, Silvestri JM, Lin D, Buhrfiend CM, et al: Effect of cocaine in early gestation on striatal dopamine and neurotrophic activity, *Pediatr Res* 34:389-392, 1993.

570. Needlman R, Zuckerman B, Anderson GM, Mirochnick M, et al: Cerebrospinal fluid monoamine precursors and metabolites in human neonates following in utero cocaine exposure: A preliminary study, *Pediatrics* 92:55-60, 1993.

571. Lauder JM, Krebs H: Effects of p-chlorophenylalanine on time of neuronal origin during embryogenesis in the rat, *Brain Res* 107:638-644, 1976.

572. Lauder JM, Towle AC, Patrick K, Henderson P, et al: Decreased serotonin content of embryonic raphe neurons following maternal administration of p-chlorophenylalanine: A quantitative immunocytochemical study, *Brain Res* 352:107-114, 1985.

573. Whitaker-Azmitia PM, Lauder JM, Shemmer A, Azmitia EC: Postnatal changes in serotonin receptors following prenatal alterations in serotonin levels: Further evidence for functional fetal serotonin receptors, *Brain Res* 430:285-289, 1987.

574. Shemer AV, Azmitia EC, Whitaker AP: Dose-related effects of prenatal 5-methoxytryptamine (5-MT) on development of serotonin terminal density and behavior, *Brain Res Dev Brain Res* 59:59-63, 1991.

575. Whitaker-Azmitia PM, Azmitia EC: Autoregulation of fetal serotonergic neuronal development: Role of high affinity serotonin receptors, *Neurosci Lett* 67:307-312, 1986.

576. Azmitia EC, Whitaker AP: Target cell stimulation of dissociated serotonergic neurons in culture, *Neuroscience* 20:47-63, 1987.

577. Whitaker-Azmitia PM, Quartermain D, Shemer AV: Prenatal treatment with a selective D1 receptor agonist (SKF 38393) alters adult [3H]paroxetine binding and dopamine and serotonin behavioral sensitivity, *Brain Res Dev Brain Res* 57:181-185, 1990.

578. Whitaker-Azmitia PM, Azmitia EC: Stimulation of astroglial serotonin receptors produces culture media which regulates growth of serotonergic neurons, *Brain Res* 497:80-85, 1989.

579. Gelbard HA, Teicher MH, Baldessarini RJ, Gallitano A, et al: Dopamine D1 receptor development depends on endogenous dopamine, *Brain Res Dev Brain Res* 56:137-140, 1990.

580. Liu JP, Lauder JM: Serotonin and nialamide differentially regulate survival and growth of cultured serotonin and catecholamine neurons, *Brain Res Dev Brain Res* 60:59-67, 1991.

581. Bar-Peled O, Gross IR, Ben HH, Hoskins I, et al: Fetal human brain exhibits a prenatal peak in the density of serotonin 5-HT$_{1A}$ receptors, *Neurosci Lett* 127:173-176, 1991.

582. Tweed A, Cote J, Lou H, Gregory G, et al: Impairment of cerebral blood flow autoregulation in the newborn lamb by hypoxia, *Pediatr Res* 20:516-519, 1986.

583. Tweed WA, Cote J, Pash M, Lou H: Arterial oxygenation determines autoregulation of cerebral blood flow in the fetal lamb, *Pediatr Res* 17:246-249, 1983.

584. Bada HS, Perry EH, Korones SB, Pourcyrous M, et al: Mean arterial blood pressure (MAP) in premature infants of cocaine abusing mothers, *Pediatr Res* 29:202A, 1991.

585. Horn PT: Persistent hypertension after prenatal cocaine exposure, *J Pediatr* 121:288-291, 1992.

586. van de Bor M, Walther FJ, Sims ME: Increased cerebral blood flow velocity in infants of mothers who abuse cocaine, *Pediatrics* 85:733-736, 1990.

587. Albuquerque ML, Kurth CD, Kim SJ, Wagerle LC: Cocaine-mediated cerebral vasoconstriction in newborn piglets, *Pediatr Res* 29:56A, 1991.

588. Lien R, Goplerud JM, Kurth CD, Wagerle LC, et al: Interaction of cocaine with sympathetic modulation of regional cerebral blood flow (RCBF) in newborn piglets, *Pediatr Res* 29:222A, 1991.

589. Albuquerque MLC, Kurth CD, Monitto CL, Shaw L, et al: Cocaine metabolites affect cerebrovascular tone in newborn piglets, *Pediatr Res* 31:57A, 1992.

590. Schreiber MD, Torgerson LJ, Covert RF, Madden JA: Cocaine and metabolite-induced vasoconstriction of isolated pressurized cerebral arteries from perinatal lambs, *Pediatr Res* 31:221A, 1992.

591. Gleason CA, Traystman RJ: Cerebral responses to maternal cocaine injection in immature fetal sheep, *Pediatr Res* 38:943-948, 1995.

592. Brown E, Prager J, Lee HY, Ramsey RG: CNS complications of cocaine abuse: Prevalence, pathophysiology, and neuroradiology, *AJR Am J Roentgenol* 159:137-147, 1992.

593. Hall TR, Zaninovic A, Lewin D, Barrett C, et al: Neonatal intestinal ischemia with bowel perforation: An in utero complication of maternal cocaine abuse—case report, *AJR Am J Roentgenol* 158:1303-1304, 1992.

594. Viscarello RR, Ferguson DD, Nores J, Hobbins JC: Limb-body wall complex associated with cocaine abuse: Further evidence of cocaine's teratogenicity, *Obstet Gynecol* 80:523-526, 1992.

595. Mehta S, Finkelhor RS, Anderson RL, Harcar-Sevcik RA, et al: Transient myocardial ischemia in infants prenatally exposed to cocaine, *J Pediatr* 122:945-949, 1993.

596. O'Brien T, Gleason CA, Jones MD, Cone EJ, et al: Cerebral responses to single and multiple cocaine injections in newborn sheep, *Pediatr Res* 35:339-343, 1994.

597. Pena AE, Burchfield DJ, Abrams RM: Myocardial and cerebral oxygen delivery are not adversely affected by cocaine administration to early-gestation fetal sheep, *Am J Obstet Gynecol* 174:1028-1032, 1996.

598. Kuban KC, Gilles FH: Human telencephalic angiogenesis, *Ann Neurol* 17:539-548, 1985.

599. Rosenberg PA: Catecholamine toxicity in cerebral cortex in dissociated cell culture, *J Neurosci* 8:2887-2894, 1988.

600. Rosenberg PA, Loring R, Xie Y, Zaleskas V, et al: 2,4,5-Trihydroxyphenylalanine in solution forms a non–N-methyl-D-aspartate glutamatergic agonist and neurotoxin, *Proc Natl Acad Sci U S A* 88:4865-4869, 1991.

601. Aizenman E, White WF, Loring RH, Rosenberg PA: A 3,4-dihydroxyphenylalanine oxidation product is a non–N-methyl-D-aspartate glutamatergic agonist in rat cortical neurons, *Neurosci Lett* 116:168-171, 1990.

602. Lipton SA, Kater SB: Neurotransmitter regulation of neuronal outgrowth, plasticity and survival, *Trends Neurosci* 12:265-270, 1989.

603. Rockhold RW, Oden G, Ho IK, Andrew M, et al: Glutamate receptor antagonists block cocaine-induced convulsions and death, *Brain Res Bull* 27:721-723, 1991.

604. Karler R, Calder LD: Excitatory amino acids and the actions of cocaine, *Brain Res* 582:143-146, 1992.

605. Racine A, Joyce T, Anderson R: The association between prenatal care and birth weight among women exposed to cocaine in New York City, *JAMA* 270:1581-1586, 1993.

606. Herzlinger RA, Kandall SR, Vaughan HG Jr: Neonatal seizures associated with narcotic withdrawal, *J Pediatr* 91:638-641, 1977.
607. Zagon IS, McLaughlin PJ: An overview of the neurobehavioral sequelae of perinatal opioid exposure. In Yanai J, editor: *Neurobehavioral Teratology*, New York: 1984, Elsevier Science.
608. Wilson GS, Desmond MM, Verniaud WM: Early development of infants of heroin-addicted mothers, *Am J Dis Child* 126:457-462, 1973.
609. Vargas GC, Pildes RS, Vidyasagar D, Keith LG: Effect of maternal heroin addiction on 67 liveborn neonates, *Clin Pediatr (Phila)* 14:751-753, 1975.
610. Reddy AM, Harper RG, Stern G: Observations on heroin and methadone withdrawal in the newborn, *Pediatrics* 48:353-358, 1971.
611. Zelson C, Rubio E, Wasserman E: Neonatal narcotic addiction: 10 year observation, *Pediatrics* 48:178-189, 1971.
612. Kandall SR, Albin S, Lowinson J, Berle B, et al: Differential effects of maternal heroin and methadone use on birthweight, *Pediatrics* 58:681-685, 1976.
613. Sweet AY: Narcotic withdrawal syndrome in the newborn, *Pediatr Rev* 3:285-295, 1982.
614. Finnegan LP: Effects of maternal opiate abuse on the newborn, *Fed Proc* 44:2314-2317, 1985.
615. Van Baar AL, Fleury P, Soepatmi S, Ultee CA, et al: Neonatal behaviour after drug dependent pregnancy, *Arch Dis Child* 64:235-240, 1989.
616. Van Baar AL, Fleury P, Ultee CA: Behaviour in first year after drug dependent pregnancy, *Arch Dis Child* 64:241-245, 1989.
617. Doberczak TM, Kandall SR, Wilets I: Neonatal opiate abstinence syndrome in term and preterm infants, *J Pediatr* 118:933-937, 1991.
618. DeCristofaro JD, LaGamma EF: Prenatal exposure to opiates, *Ment Retard Dev Disabil Res Rev* 1:177-182, 1995.
619. Bunikowski R, Grimmer I, Heiser A, Metze B, et al: Neurodevelopmental outcome after prenatal exposure to opiates, *Eur J Pediatr* 157:724-730, 1998.
620. O'Brien C, Hunt R, Jeffery HE: Measurement of movement is an objective method to assist in assessment of opiate withdrawal in newborns, *Arch Dis Child Fetal Neonatal Ed* 89:F305-F309, 2004.
621. Gewolb IH, Fishman D, Qureshi MA, Vice FL: Coordination of suck-swallow-respiration in infants born to mothers with drug-abuse problems, *Dev Med Child Neurol* 46:700-705, 2004.
622. Friedler G, Cochin J: Growth retardation in offspring of female rats treated with morphine prior to conception, *Science* 175:654-656, 1972.
623. Kaltenbach KA, Finnegan L: Prenatal opiate exposure: Physical, neurobehavioral, and developmental effects. In Miller MW, editor: *Development of the Central Nervous System: Effects of Alcohol and Opiates*, New York: 1992, Wiley-Liss.
624. Coyle MG, Ferguson A, LaGasse L, Liu J, et al: Neurobehavioral effects of treatment for opiate withdrawal, *Arch Dis Child Fetal Neonatal Ed* 90:F73-F74, 2005.
625. Coyle MG, Ferguson A, Lagasse L, Oh W, et al: Diluted tincture of opium (DTO) and phenobarbital versus DTO alone for neonatal opiate withdrawal in term infants, *J Pediatr* 140:561-564, 2002.
626. Stimmel B, Adamsons K: Narcotic dependency in pregnancy, *JAMA* 235:1121-1124, 1976.
627. Ostrea EM, Chavez CJ: Perinatal problems (excluding neonatal withdrawal) in maternal drug addiction: A study of 830 cases, *J Pediatr* 94:292-295, 1979.
628. Rosenman SJ, Smith CB: Catecholamine synthesis in mouse brain during morphine withdrawal, *Nature* 240:153-155, 1972.
629. Frederickson RC: Morphine withdrawal response and central cholinergic activity, *Nature* 257:131-132, 1975.
630. Huang YH, Redmond DE Jr, Snyder DR, Maas JW: In vivo location and destruction of the locus ceruleus in the stumptail macaque (*Macaca arctoides*), *Brain Res* 100:157-162, 1975.
631. Lal H: Narcotic dependence, narcotic action and dopamine receptors, *Life Sci* 17:483-495, 1975.
632. Merali Z, Singhal RL, Hrdina PD, Ling GM: Changes in brain cyclic AMP metabolism and acetylcholine and dopamine during narcotic dependence and withdrawal, *Life Sci* 16:1889-1894, 1975.
633. Takemori AE: Neurochemical bases for narcotic tolerance and dependence, *Biochem Pharmacol* 24:2121-2126, 1975.
634. Redmond DE Jr, Huang YH, Snyder DR, Maas JW: Behavioral effects of stimulation on the nucleus locus coeruleus in the stump-tailed monkey *Macaca arctoides*, *Brain Res* 116:502-510, 1976.
635. Gold MS, Redmond DE Jr, Kleber HD: Clonidine in opiate withdrawal, *Lancet* 1:929-930, 1978.
636. Gold MS, Redmond DE, Kleber HD: Clonidine blocks acute opiate-withdrawal symptoms, *Lancet* 2:599-602, 1978.
637. Snyder SH: Receptors, neurotransmitters and drug responses, *N Engl J Med* 300:465-472, 1979.
638. Jaffe JH: Drug addiction and drug abuse. In Goodman LA, Gilman A, editors: *The Pharmacological Basis of Therapeutics*, New York: 1980, MacMillan.
639. Di Chiara G, North RA: Neurobiology of opiate abuse, *Trends Pharmacol Sci* 13:185-193, 1992.
640. Koob GF: Neural substrates of opiate withdrawal, *Trends Neurosci* 15:186-190, 1992.
641. Wolf ME: Addiction. In Siegel GJ, Albers RW, Brady ST, et al, editors: *Basic Neurochemistry: Molecular, Cellular and Medical Aspects*, 7th ed, New York: 2006, Elsevier.

642. Koob GF, Sanna PP, Bloom FE: Neuroscience of addiction, *Neuron* 21:467-476, 1998.
643. Johnson K, Gerada C, Greenough A: Treatment of neonatal abstinence syndrome, *Arch Dis Child* 88:2-5, 2003.
644. Hill RM, Desmond MM: Management of the narcotic withdrawal syndrome in the neonate, *Pediatr Clin North Am* 10:67-86, 1963.
645. Finnegan LP: Neonatal abstinence. In Nelson NM, editor: *Current Therapy in Neonatal-Perinatal Medicine*, St. Louis, MO: 1985, Mosby.
646. Kaltenbach K, Finnegan L: Neonatal abstinence syndrome, pharmacotherapy and developmental outcome, *Neurobehav Toxicol Teratol* 8:353-355, 1986.
647. Wijburg FA, de Kleine MJ, Fleury P, Soepatmi S: Morphine as an antiepileptic drug in neonatal abstinence syndrome, *Acta Paediatr Scand* 80:875-877, 1991.
648. Jackson L, Ting A, McKay S, Galea P, et al: A randomised controlled trial of morphine versus phenobarbitone for neonatal abstinence syndrome, *Arch Dis Child Fetal Neonatal Ed* 89:F300-304, 2004.
649. Kron RE, Litt M, Phoenix MD, Finnegan LP: Neonatal narcotic abstinence: Effect of pharmacotherapeutic agents and maternal drug usage on nutritive sucking behavior, *J Pediatr* 88:637-641, 1976.
650. Nathenson G, Golden GS, Litt IF: Diazepam in the management of the neonatal narcotic withdrawal syndrome, *Pediatrics* 48:523-527, 1971.
651. Rajegowda BK, Kandall SR, Falciglia H: Sudden unexpected death in infants of narcotic-dependent mothers, *Early Hum Dev* 2:219-225, 1978.
652. Finnegan LP: In utero opiate exposure and sudden infant death syndrome, *Clin Perinatol* 6:163-180, 1979.
653. Chavez CJ, Ostrea EM, Stryker JC, Smialek Z: Sudden infant death syndrome among infants of drug-dependent mothers, *J Pediatr* 95:407-409, 1979.
654. Kandall SR, Gaines J, Habel L, Davidson G, et al: Relationship of maternal substance abuse to subsequent sudden infant death syndrome in offspring, *J Pediatr* 123:120-126, 1993.
655. Wilson GS, McCreary R, Kean J, Baxter JC: The development of preschool children of heroin-addicted mothers: A controlled study, *Pediatrics* 63:135-141, 1979.
656. Kaltenbach KA, Finnegan LP: Prenatal narcotic exposure: Perinatal and developmental effects, *Neurotoxicology* 10:597-604, 1989.
657. van Baar A, de Graaff BMT: Cognitive development at preschool-age of infants of drug-dependent mothers, *Dev Med Child Neurol* 36:1063-1075, 1995.
658. Ornoy A, Segal J, Bar-Hamburger R, Greenbaum C: Developmental outcome of school-age children born to mothers with heroin dependency: Importance of environmental factors, *Dev Med Child Neurol* 43:668-675, 2001.
659. Raye JR, Dubin JW, Blechner JN: Fetal growth retardation following maternal morphine administration: Nutritional or drug effect? *Biol Neonate* 32:222-228, 1977.
660. Zagon IS, McLaughlin PJ: Effect of chronic maternal methadone exposure on perinatal development, *Biol Neonate* 31:271-282, 1977.
661. Zagon IS, McLaughlin PJ: Effects of chronic morphine administration on pregnant rats and their offspring, *Pharmacology* 15:302-310, 1977.
662. Zagon IS, McLaughlin PJ: The effects of different schedules of methadone treatment on rat brain development, *Exp Neurol* 56:538-552, 1977.
663. Zagon IS, McLaughlin PJ: Morphine and brain growth retardation in the rat, *Pharmacology* 15:276-282, 1977.
664. Zagon IS, McLaughlin PJ: Perinatal methadone exposure and brain development: A biochemical study, *J Neurochem* 31:49-54, 1978.
665. McLaughlin PJ, Zagon IS, White WJ: Perinatal methadone exposure in rats: Effects on body and organ development, *Biol Neonate* 34:48-54, 1978.
666. Slotkin TA, Whitmore WL, Salvaggio M, Seidler FJ: Perinatal methadone addiction affects brain synaptic development of biogenic amine systems in the rat, *Life Sci* 24:1223-1229, 1979.
667. Zagon IS, McLaughlin PJ: Neuronal cell deficits following maternal exposure to methadone in rats, *Experientia* 38:1214-1216, 1982.
668. Hammer RP, Ricalde AA, Seatriz JV: Effects of opiates on brain development, *Neurotoxicology* 10:475-484, 1989.
669. Ricalde AA, Hammer RP: Perinatal opiate treatment delays growth of cortical dendrites, *Neurosci Lett* 115:137-143, 1990.
670. Stiene-Martin A, Gurwell JA, Hauser KF: Morphine alters astrocyte growth in primary cultures of mouse glial cells: Evidence for a direct effect of opiates on neural maturation, *Dev Brain Res* 60:1-7, 1991.
671. Hammer RP, Hauser KF: Consequences of early exposure to opioids on cell proliferation and neuronal morphogenesis. In Miller MW, editor: *Development of the Central Nervous System: Effects of Alcohol and Opiates*, New York: 1992, Wiley-Liss.
672. Kuhn CM, Windh RT, Little PJ: Effects of perinatal opiate addiction on neurochemical development of the brain. In Miller MW, editor: *Development of the Central Nervous System: Effects of Alcohol and Opiates*, New York: 1992, Wiley-Liss.
673. Harper RG, Solish GI, Purow HM, Sang E, et al: The effect of a methadone treatment program upon pregnant heroin addicts and their newborn infants, *Pediatrics* 54:300-305, 1974.
674. Kaltenbach K, Graziani LJ, Finnegan LP: Methadone exposure in utero: Developmental status at one and two years of age, *Pharmacol Biochem Behav* 1(Suppl 1):15-17, 1979.

675. Wilson GS, Desmond MM, Wait RB: Follow-up of methadone-treated and untreated narcotic-dependent women and their infants. Health, developmental, and social implications, *J Pediatr* 98:711-716, 1981.

676. Chasnoff IJ, Hatcher R, Burns WJ: Polydrug- and methadone-addicted newborns: A continuum of impairment? *Pediatrics* 70:210-213, 1982.

677. Rosen TS, Johnson HL: Children of methadone-maintained mothers: Follow-up to 18 months of age, *J Pediatr* 101:192-196, 1982.

678. Kaltenbach K, Finnegan LP: Developmental outcome of children born to methadone-maintained women: A review of longitudinal studies, *Neurobehav Toxicol Teratol* 6:271-275, 1984.

679. Lifschitz MH, Wilson GS, Smith EO, Desmond MM: Fetal and postnatal growth of children born to narcotic-dependent women, *J Pediatr* 102:686-691, 1983.

680. Blinick G, Jerez E, Wallach RC: Methadone maintenance, pregnancy, and progeny, *JAMA* 225:477-479, 1973.

681. Strauss ME, Andresko M, Stryker JC, Wardell JN: Methadone maintenance during pregnancy: Pregnancy, birth and neonate characteristics, *Am J Obstet Gynecol* 120:895-900, 1974.

682. Rahbar F: Observations on methadone withdrawal in 16 neonates, *Clin Pediatr* 14:369-371, 1975.

683. Blinick G, Wallach RC, Jerez E, Ackerman BD: Drug addiction in pregnancy and the neonate, *Am J Obstet Gynecol* 125:135-142, 1976.

684. Ostrea EM, Chavez CJ, Strauss ME: A study of factors that influence the severity of neonatal narcotic withdrawal, *J Pediatr* 88:642-645, 1976.

685. Connaughton JF, Reeser D, Schut J, Finnegan LP: Perinatal addiction: Outcome and management, *Am J Obstet Gynecol* 129:679-686, 1977.

686. Madden JD, Chappel JN, Zuspan F, Gumpel J, et al: Observation and treatment of neonatal narcotic withdrawal, *Am J Obstet Gynecol* 127:199-201, 1977.

687. Aylward GP: Methadone outcome studies: Is it more than the methadone? *J Pediatr* 101:214-215, 1982.

688. Doberczak TM, Kandall SR, Friedmann P: Relationships between maternal methadone dosage, maternal-neonatal methadone levels, and neonatal withdrawal, *Obstet Gynecol* 81:936-940, 1993.

689. Shaw NJ, McIvor L: Neonatal abstinence syndrome after maternal methadone treatment, *Arch Dis Child Fetal Neonatal Ed* 71:F203-F205, 1994.

690. Martinez A, Kastner B, Taeusch HW: Hyperphagia in neonates withdrawing from methadone, *Arch Dis Child Fetal Neonatal Ed* 80:F178-F182, 1999.

691. Berghella V, Lim PJ, Hill MK, Cherpes J, et al: Maternal methadone dose and neonatal withdrawal, *Am J Obstet Gynecol* 189:312-317, 2003.

692. Kuschel CA, Austerberry L, Cornwell M, Couch R, et al: Can methadone concentrations predict the severity of withdrawal in infants at risk of neonatal abstinence syndrome? *Arch Dis Child Fetal Neonatal Ed* 89:F390-393, 2004.

693. McCarthy JJ, Leamon MH, Parr MS, Anania B: High-dose methadone maintenance in pregnancy: Maternal and neonatal outcomes, *Am J Obstet Gynecol* 193:606-610, 2005.

694. Rosen TS, Pippenger CE: Pharmacologic observations on the neonatal withdrawal syndrome, *J Pediatr* 88:1044-1048, 1976.

695. Kandall SR, Gartner LM: Late presentation of drug withdrawal symptoms in newborns, *Am J Dis Child* 127:58-61, 1974.

696. Dole VP, Kreek MJ: Methadone plasma level: Sustained by a reservoir of drug in tissue, *Proc Natl Acad Sci U S A* 57:10, 1973.

697. Marcus J, Hans SL, Jeremy RJ: Differential motor and state functioning in newborns of women on methadone, *Neurobehav Toxicol Teratol* 4:459-462, 1982.

698. Wogelius P, Norgaard M, Gislum M, Pedersen L, et al: Maternal use of selective serotonin reuptake inhibitors and risk of congenital malformations, *Epidemiology* 17:701-704, 2006.

698a. Alwan S, Reefhuis J, Rasmussen SA, Olney RS, et al: Use of selective serotonin-reuptake inhibitors in pregnancy and the risk of birth defects, *N Engl J Med* 356:2684-2692, 2007.

698b. Louik C, Lin AE, Werler MM, Hernandez-Diaz S, et al: First-trimester use of selective serotonin-reuptake inhibitors and the risk of birth defects, *N Engl J Med* 356:2675-2683, 2007.

699. Chambers CD, Johnson KA, Dick LM, Felix RJ, et al: Birth outcome in pregnant women taking fluoxetine, *N Engl J Med* 335:1010-1015, 1996.

700. Dahl ML, Olhager E, Ahlner J: Paroxetine withdrawal syndrome in a neonate, *Br J Psychiatry* 17:391-392, 1997.

701. Nijhuis IJM, Rooij GWM, Bosschaart AN: Withdrawal reactions of a premature neonate after maternal use of paroxetine, *Arch Dis Child Fetal Neonatal Ed* 84:F77, 2001.

702. Isbister GK, Dawson A, Whyte IM, Prior FHC, et al: Neonatal paroxetine withdrawal syndrome or actually serotonin syndrome? *Arch Dis Child Fetal Neonatal Ed* 85:F147-F148, 2001.

703. Stiskal JA, Kulin N, Korem G, Ho T, et al: Neonatal paroxetine withdrawal syndrome, *Arch Dis Child Fetal Neonatal Ed* 84:F134-F135, 2001.

704. Nordeng H, Lindemann R, Perminov KV, Reikvam A: Neonatal withdrawal syndrome after in utero exposure to selective serotonin reuptake inhibitors, *Acta Paediatr* 90:288-291, 2001.

705. Jaiswal S, Coombs RC, Isbister GK: Paroxetine withdrawal in a neonate with historical and laboratory confirmation, *Eur J Pediatr* 162:723-724, 2003.

706. Costei AM, Kozer E, Ho T, Ito S, et al: Perinatal outcome following third trimester exposure to paroxetine, *Arch Pediatr Adolesc Med* 156:1129-1132, 2002.

707. Zeskind PS, Stephens LE: Maternal selective serotonin reuptake inhibitor use during pregnancy and newborn neurobehavior, *Pediatrics* 113:368-375, 2004.

708. Kallen B: Neonate characteristics after maternal use of antidepressants in late pregnancy, *Arch Pediatr Adolesc Med* 158:312-316, 2004.

709. Moses-Kolko EL, Bogen D, Perel J, Bregar A, et al: Neonatal signs after late in utero exposure to serotonin reuptake inhibitors: Literature review and implications for clinical applications, *JAMA* 293:2372-2383, 2005.

710. Sanz EJ, DelasCuevas C, Kiuru A, Bate A, et al: Selective serotonin reuptake inhibitors in pregnant women and neonatal withdrawal syndrome: A database analysis, *Lancet* 365:482-487, 2005.

711. Levinson-Castiel R, Merlob P, Linder N, Sirota L, et al: Neonatal abstinence syndrome after in utero exposure to selective serotonin reuptake inhibitors in term infants, *Arch Pediatr Adolesc Med* 160:173-176, 2006.

712. Malm H, Klaukka T, Neuvonen PJ: Risks associated with selective serotonin reuptake inhibitors in pregnancy, *Obstet Gynecol* 106:1289-1296, 2005.

713. Wen SW, Yang Q, Garner P, Fraser W, et al: Selective serotonin reuptake inhibitors and adverse pregnancy outcomes, *Am J Obstet Gynecol* 194:961-966, 2006.

714. Ferreira E, Carceller AM, Agogue C, Martin BZ, et al: Effects of selective serotonin reuptake inhibitors and venlafaxine during pregnancy in term and preterm neonates, *Pediatrics* 119:52-59, 2007.

715. Nulman I, Rovet J, Stewart DE, Wolpin J, et al: Neurodevelopment of children exposed in utero to antidepressant drugs, *N Engl J Med* 336:258-262, 1997.

716. Casper RC, Fleisher BE, Lee-Ancajas JC, Gilles A, et al: Follow-up of children of depressed mothers exposed or not exposed to antidepressant drugs during pregnancy, *J Pediatr* 142:402-408, 2003.

717. Bleyer WA, Marshall RE: Barbiturate withdrawal syndrome in a passively addicted infant, *JAMA* 221:185-186, 1972.

718. Ostrea EM Jr: Neonatal withdrawal from intrauterine exposure to butalbital, *Am J Obstet Gynecol* 143:597-598, 1982.

719. Desmond MM, Schwanecke RP, Wilson GS, Yasunaga S, et al: Maternal barbiturate utilization and neonatal withdrawal symptomatology, *J Pediatr* 80:190-197, 1972.

720. Maurer HM, Wolff JA, Finster M, Poppers PJ, et al: Reduction in concentration of total serum bilirubin in offspring of women treated with phenobarbitone during pregnancy, *Lancet* 2:122-124, 1968.

721. Trolle D: Decrease of total serum-bilirubin concentration in newborn infants after phenobarbitone treatment, *Lancet* 2:705-708, 1968.

722. Ramboer C, Thompson RP, Williams R: Controlled trials of phenobarbitone therapy in neonatal jaundice, *Lancet* 1:966-968, 1969.

723. Victor M: The alcohol withdrawal syndrome: Theory and practice, *Postgrad Med* 47:68-72, 1970.

724. Schaefer O: Alcohol withdrawal syndrome in a newborn infant of a Yukon Indian mother, *Can Med Assoc J* 87:1333-1334, 1962.

725. Nichols MM: Acute alcohol withdrawal syndrome in a newborn, *Am J Dis Child* 113:714-715, 1967.

726. Pierog S, Chandavasu O, Wexler I: Withdrawal symptoms in infants with the fetal alcohol syndrome, *J Pediatr* 90:630-633, 1977.

727. Rosett H, Ouellette EM, Weiner I, Owens F: Therapy of heavy drinking during pregnancy, *Obstet Gynecol* 51:41-46, 1978.

728. Robe LB, Gromisch DS, Iosub S: Symptoms of neonatal ethanol withdrawal, *Curr Alcohol* 8:484-493, 1981.

729. Coles CD, Smith IE, Fernhoff PM, Falek A: Neonatal ethanol withdrawal: Characteristics in clinically normal, nondysmorphic neonates, *J Pediatr* 105:445-451, 1984.

730. Mulder EH, Morssink LP, Van Der Schee T, Visser GH: Acute maternal alcohol consumption disrupts behavioral state organization in the near-term fetus, *Pediatr Res* 44:774-779, 1998.

731. Owen JR, Irani SF, Blair AW: Effect of diazepam administered to mothers during labor on temperature regulation of neonate, *Arch Dis Child* 47:107-110, 1972.

732. Cree JE, Meyer J, Hailey DM: Diazepam in labour: Its metabolism and effect on the clinical condition and thermogenesis of the newborn, *Br Med J* 4:251-255, 1973.

733. Schiff D, Chan G, Stern L: Fixed drug combinations and the displacement of bilirubin from albumin, *Pediatrics* 48:139-141, 1971.

734. McCarthy GT, O'Connell B, Robinson AE: Blood levels of diazepam in infants of two mothers given large doses of diazepam during labor, *Br J Obstet Gynaecol* 80:349-352, 1973.

735. Laegreid L, Olegard R, Waistrom J, Conradi N: Teratogenic effects of benzodiazepine use during pregnancy, *J Pediatr* 114:126-131, 1989.

736. Laegreid L, Hagberg G, Lundberg A: The effect of benzodiazepines on the fetus and the newborn, *Neuropediatrics* 23:18-23, 1992.

737. Mazzi E: Possible neonatal diazepam withdrawal: A case report, *Am J Obstet Gynecol* 129:586-587, 1977.

738. Rementeria JL, Bhatt K: Withdrawal symptoms in neonates from intrauterine exposure to diazepam, *J Pediatr* 90:123-126, 1977.

739. Erkkola R, Kangas L, Pekkarinen A: The transfer of diazepam across the placenta during labor, *Acta Obstet Gynecol Scand* 52:167-170, 1973.

740. Morselli PL, Principi N, Tognoni G, Reali E, et al: Diazepam elimination in premature and full term newborns and children, *J Perinat Med* 1:133-141, 1973.

741. Laegreid L, Olegard R, Conradi N, Hagberg G, et al: Congenital malformations and maternal consumption of benzodiazepines: A case-control study, *Dev Med Child Neurol* 32:432-441, 1990.

742. Laegreid L, Hagberg G, Lundberg A: Neurodevelopment in late infancy after prenatal exposure to benzodiazepines: A prospective study, *Neuropediatrics* 23:60-67, 1992.

743. Bergman U, Rosa FW, Baum C, Wiholm BE, et al: Effects of exposure to benzodiazepine during fetal life, *Lancet* 340:694-696, 1992.

744. Athinarayanan P, Pierog SH, Nigam SK, Glass L: Chlordiazepoxide withdrawal in the neonate, *Am J Obstet Gynecol* 124:212-213, 1976.

745. Musa BA, Smith CS: Neonatal effects of maternal clomipramine therapy, *Arch Dis Child* 54:405-407, 1979.

746. Cowe L, Lloyd DJ, Dawling S: Neonatal convulsions caused by withdrawal from maternal clomipramine, *Br Med J* 284:1837-1838, 1982.

747. Rumack BH, Walravens PA: Neonatal withdrawal following maternal ingestion of ethchlorvynol (Placidyl), *Pediatrics* 52:714-716, 1973.

748. Salguero CH, Villarreal JE, Hug CC Jr, Domino EF: Propoxyphene dependence, *JAMA* 210:135-136, 1969.

749. Wolfe RC, Reidenberg M, Vispo RH: Propoxyphene (Darvon) addiction and withdrawal syndrome, *Ann Intern Med* 70:773-776, 1969.

750. Kane FJ Jr, Norton JL: Addiction to propoxyphene, *JAMA* 211:300, 1970.

751. Tyson HK: Neonatal withdrawal symptoms associated with maternal use of propoxyphene hydrochloride (Darvon), *J Pediatr* 85:684-685, 1974.

752. Klein RB, Blatman S, Little GA: Probable neonatal propoxyphene withdrawal: A case report, *Pediatrics* 55:882-884, 1975.

753. Alarcon RD, Gelfond SD, Alarcon GS: Parental and oral pentazocine abuse, *Johns Hopkins Med J* 129:311-318, 1971.

754. Goetz RL, Bain RV: Neonatal withdrawal symptoms associated with maternal use of pentazocine, *J Pediatr* 84:887-888, 1974.

755. Preis O, Choi SJ, Rudolph N: Pentazocine withdrawal syndrome in the newborn infant, *Am J Obstet Gynecol* 127:205-206, 1977.

756. Scanlon JW: Pentazocine and neonatal withdrawal symptoms [letter], *J Pediatr* 85:735-736, 1974.

757. Kopelman AE: Fetal addiction to pentazocine, *Pediatrics* 55:888-889, 1975.

758. Reeds TO: Withdrawal syndrome in the neonate associated with maternal pentazocine abuse [letter], *J Pediatr* 86:324, 1975.

759. Dunn DW, Reynolds J: Neonatal withdrawal symptoms associated with "T's and blues" (pentazocine and tripelennamine), *Am J Dis Child* 136:644-645, 1982.

760. Chasnoff IJ, Hatcher R, Burns WJ, Schnoll SH: Pentazocine and tripelennamine ("T's and blues"): Effects on the fetus and neonate, *Dev Pharmacol Ther* 6:162-169, 1983.

761. Caplan LR, Thomas C, Banks G: Central nervous system complications of addiction to "T's and blues", *Neurology* 32:623-628, 1982.

762. Van Leeuwen G, Guthrie R, Strange F: Narcotic withdrawal reaction in a newborn infant due to codeine, *Pediatrics* 36:635-636, 1965.

763. Mangurten HH, Benawra R: Neonatal codeine withdrawal in infants of nonaddicted mothers, *Pediatrics* 65:159-160, 1980.

Index

Ventriculomegaly–cont'd
  in Dandy-Walker malformation, 38
  in Joubert syndrome, 39, 39f
  in Walker-Warburg syndrome, 76
  isolated mild, 36
  management of, 35-36
  of fourth ventricle, 38, 39, 39f, 40-41
Ventriculoperitoneal shunts. *See* Shunts.
Ventriculostomy
  in bacterial meningitis, 940
  indications for, 942-943
Vermian agenesis, familial, 40, 40f, 40t
Vermian atrophy/hypoplasia, in hypoxic-
    ischemic encephalopathy, 351, 433
Vermian malformations, 37-40, 37t
Vertebrobasilar aneurysms, rupture of,
    506-507
Vertical gaze palsies, 139
Vestibulospinal tract, 748
Vidarabine, for herpes simplex virus
    infection, 884
Vigilance, evaluation of, 126, 127t
Viral infections. *See also specific infections.*
  adenovirus, 904
  brain stem auditory evoked responses in,
    157-158
  cytomegalovirus, 852-862
  enterovirus, 895-900
  herpes simplex virus, 874-884
  HIV, 889-895
  lymphocytic choriomeningitis in, 903
  TORCH, 851, 852-889, 852t
  varicella, 900-903
  West Nile virus, 904
Viral meningitis
  in enterovirus infections, 895-900, 897t.
    See also Enterovirus infections.
  in varicella, 901-902
Vision assessment, 127-128, 135
Vision impairment, 135-136
  diagnosis of, 127-128, 135
    visual evoked potentials in, 159-160,
      160f
  in hypoxic-ischemic encephalopathy,
    432, 433, 435
  in rubella, 872
  in syphilis, 887
  in toxoplasmosis, 864-867
  optic nerve hypoplasia and, 135-136
Visual cortex
  development of, 85, 87f
  functional MRI of, 191
  photic stimulation of, 191
Visual evoked responses, 158-160,
    159f, 160f
  in bilirubin encephalopathy, 640-641,
    641f
  in hypoxic-ischemic encephalopathy,
    443, 443t
Visual hyperattentiveness, in hearing
    loss, 140
Vitamin(s)
  deficiencies of, neural tube defects and,
    17-19, 18t, 19t
  supplemental, in pregnancy, 17-19,
    18t, 19t
Vitamin A, teratogenicity of, 1023
Vitamin B$_{12}$, 692-695
  for methylmalonic acidemia, 695
Vitamin E, for germinal matrix-
    intraventricular hemorrhage, 555-556,
    556t
Vitamin K
  deficiency of
    anticonvulsant-induced, 1009-1010

Vitamin K–cont'd
  hemorrhage in
    intracranial, 497-498, 506
    systemic, 506
  maternal supplementation of, in
    anticonvulsant therapy, 1010-1011
  neuroprotective effects of, 285, 290
  prenatal, for intraventricular hemorrhage
    prevention, 549
Vocal cord paralysis, 834, 834t
  in birth trauma, 980
  sucking/swallowing problems in, 143
Volume expansion, in germinal matrix-
    intraventricular hemorrhage, 529
Von Gierke disease, 777f
Von Recklinghausen disease,
    macrencephaly in, 60

W

Waardenburg syndrome, 141
Walker-Warburg syndrome, 8, 71t, 75-77,
    810-816, 810t. *See also* Congenital
    muscular dystrophy.
  clinical features of, 810, 810t
  gyral abnormality in, 811, 812f
  imaging studies in, 811
  laboratory studies in, 810-811
  management of, 815
  pathogenesis and etiology of, 814-815
  pathology of, 813
  type II lissencephaly in, 8, 71t, 75-77,
    76f. *See also* Lissencephaly, type II.
Watershed infarct, 356-359, 356f-361f
Weakness. *See also* Neuromuscular
    disorders.
  arthrogryposis multiplex congenita and,
    759
  cerebellar malformations and, 769
  etiology of, 144-145
  facial, 139-140, 140t, 978-980
  in arthrogryposis multiplex congenita,
    775
  in bilirubin encephalopathy, 635
  in chronic motor-sensory
    polyneuropathies, 778-783
  in congenital myotonic dystrophy, 802
  in Dandy-Walker syndrome, 769
  in developmental disorders, 768-769
  in hypermagnesemia, 790
  in hypothyroidism, 768
  in hypoxic-ischemic encephalopathy,
    403, 404, 433, 767
  in metabolic disorders, 767
  in motor disorders
    of neuromuscular junction, 784-793
    of peripheral nerves, 777-784
    with lesions at lower motor neuron,
      769-777
    with lesions below lower motor
      neuron, 767-769
  in myasthenia, 784-790
  in oculocerebrorenal syndrome of
    Lowe, 768
  in parasagittal cerebral injury, 433
  in peripheral nerve disorders, 145,
    777-784
  in poliomyelitis, 777
  in Pompe disease, 776
  in Prader-Willi syndrome, 768
  in spinal cord disorders, 769
  in spinal cord injury, 968, 969
  in Werdnig-Hoffmann disease, 770, 770f
  muscle level and, 801, 802t
  traumatic, 768

Weakness–cont'd
  vs. hypotonia, 144. *See also* Hypotonia.
Weaver syndrome, macrencephaly and, 60
Weight
  birth
    blood pressure and, 453, 453f
    brachial plexus injury and, 972
  brain, glucose metabolism and, 593,
    594f
Werdnig-Hoffmann disease
  anterior horn cells in, 772-773, 772t
  arthrogryposis multiplex congenita in,
    761-762
  course of, 771, 771t
  cranial nerve nuclei in, 773, 773f
  creatine kinase in, 771
  electromyography in, 754, 754f, 771-772
  etiology of, 773-774
  genetic factors in, 773-774, 773f
  hypotonia and weakness in, 145
  laboratory studies in, 771-772
  management of, 774
  muscle biopsy in, 772, 772f
  nerve conduction velocity in, 772
  neurological features of, 769-771
  neuronal-axonal polyneuropathy in, 782
  neuropathology of, 772-773, 772t
  pathogenesis of, 773-774
  sucking/swallowing problems in, 143
  tongue fasciculations in, 144
  topography of, 773
  variants of, 774-775, 775t. *See also* Spinal
    muscular atrophy.
  vs. Pompe disease, 776
  vs. Zellweger syndrome, 732-733
West Nile virus infection, 904
West syndrome, 435
Whistling face, 759
White blood cells, in cerebrospinal fluid,
    154, 155t
  in bacterial meningitis, 930-931, 930t,
    931t
White matter
  abnormalities of
    hypotonia and weakness and, 145
    in Aicardi-Goutieres syndrome, 719t,
      730, 731f
    in Alexander disease, 719t, 725-727,
      726f
    in bacterial meningitis, 924-925
    in Canavan disease, 719t, 724-725,
      725f
    in carbohydrate-deficient glycoprotein
      syndromes, 732t, 736-737, 737f
    in Cockayne syndrome, 729-730
    in congenital muscular dystrophy, 807,
      807t, 808, 810t, 811, 812-813,
      812f
    in germinal matrix-intraventricular
      hemorrhage, 544, 545, 545f, 545t,
      546-547. *See also* Periventricular
      hemorrhagic infarction.
    in HIV infection, 891-892, 891f,
      892f
    in hypoxic-ischemic encephalopathy,
      251, 253, 254t, 280-291, 407-408,
      408t. *See also* Hypoxic-ischemic
      encephalopathy, white matter
      injury in.
    in Krabbe disease, 719t, 727, 728f,
      729f
    in Leigh syndrome, 734-736, 736t
    in maple syrup urine disease, 656,
      658t
    in nonketotic hyperglycinemia, 662